Neurological Rehabilitation

FOURTH EDITION

Neurological Rehabilitation

FOURTH EDITION

DARCY A. UMPHRED, PhD, PT
Professor
Graduate Program in Physical Therapy
University of the Pacific
Stockton, California

International Lecturer, Consultant,
Private Practitioner
Partners in Learning Clinics
Carmichael, California

with illustrations by Jeb Burton,
Steve Schmidt, and Ben Burton

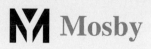 Mosby

A Harcourt Health Sciences Company

St. Louis London Philadelphia Sydney Toronto

Mosby

A Harcourt Health Sciences Company

Acquisitions Editor: Andrew Allen
Developmental Editor: Rachael Zipperlen
Copy Editing Supervisor: Lee Ann Draud
Production Manager: Peter Faber
Illustration Specialist: Rita Martello

FOURTH EDITION
Copyright © 2001, 1995, 1990, 1985 by Mosby, Inc.

NOTICE

Pharmacology is an ever-changing field. Standard safety precautions must be followed, but as new research and clinical experience broaden our knowledge, changes in treatment and drug therapy may become necessary or appropriate. Readers are advised to check the most current product information provided by the manufacturer of each drug to be administered to verify the recommended dose, the method and duration of administration, and contraindications. It is the responsibility of the treating physician, relying on experience and knowledge of the patient, to determine dosages and the best treatment for each individual patient. Neither the publisher nor the editor assumes any liability for any injury and/or damage to persons or property arising from this publication.

THE PUBLISHER

Mosby, Inc.
A Harcourt Health Sciences Company
11830 Westline Industrial Drive
St. Louis, Missouri 63146

Printed in the United States of America.

Library of Congress Cataloging-in-Publication Data

Neurological rehabilitation/[edited by] Darcy A. Umphred; with illustrations by Jeb Burton, Steve Schmidt, and Ben Burton.—4th ed.

p. ; cm.

Includes bibliographical references and index.

ISBN 0–323–00936–0

1. Nervous system—Diseases—physical therapy.   2. Nervous system—Diseases—Patients—Rehabilitation.   I. Umphred, Darcy Ann.

[DNLM: 1. Nervous System Diseases—rehabilitation. WL 140 N49265 2001]

RC350.P48 N487 2001
616.8'0462—dc21   2001030283

International Standard Book Number: 0–323–00936–0

Last digit is the print number: 9   8   7   6   5   4   3   2   1

Dedicated

To
Gordon, Jeb, Benjamin, and my
mother, Janet, whose love, patience,
and understanding constantly give me
strength.

To
All those special people whose
insights, wisdom, guidance, and
patience have helped to give the
authors of these chapters their unique
gifts and talents, as well as their
willingness to share their thoughts
with all of you.

To
A very dear friend, colleague, and
past chapter author—Mary Jane
Bouska. So many master clinicians
and true leaders in the field of
neurological rehabilitation have left
us. Mary Jane certainly fell into the
category of clinical master and
paradigm shifter and will be missed
by all who knew her and were
fortunate to call her a friend.

To
Life, to each person's journey and to
all those who give opportunities for
others' growth along that journey.
Special thanks to my immediate
family and all my friends and
colleagues I hold so close to my heart.
Because of all of you, my journey has
been constantly renewed with love,
warmth, and guidance. No one could
feel wealthier than I.

Contributors

LESLIE ALLISON, MS, PT
Doctoral student, University of
Maryland, College Park, Maryland
Balance and Vestibular Disorders

MYRTICE B. ATRICE, BS, PT
Clinical Supervisor, Spinal Cord Injury
Program, Shepherd Center, Inc., Atlanta,
Georgia
Traumatic Spinal Cord Injury

**WILLIAM G. BOISSONNAULT,
MSc, PT, DPT**
Assistant Professor, Program in Physical
Therapy, University of Wisconsin–
Madison, Madison, Wisconsin; Assistant
Professor, University of St. Augustine
Center of Health Sciences, St.
Augustine, Florida; Instructor, Krannert
School of Physical Therapy, University of
Indianapolis, Indianapolis, Indiana;
Clinical Assistant Professor, College of
Allied Health Sciences, University of
Tennessee–Memphis, Memphis,
Tennessee
*Differential Diagnosis Phase 1:
Medical Screening for the Therapist*

**JENNIFER M. BOTTOMLEY,
PhD, PT**
Core Faculty, Harvard University
Division on Aging, and Adjunct Faculty,
Massachusetts General Hospital Institute
of Health Professions, Boston;
Consultant, Geriatric Rehabilitation
Program, Wayland, Massachusetts
*Alternative and Complementary
Therapies: Beyond Traditional
Approaches to Intervention in
Neurological Diseases, Syndromes,
and Disorders*

DARBI M. BREATH, MS, OTR
Clinical Instructor, Louisiana State
University Health Sciences Center;
Motor Specialist, Medical Center of
Louisiana, New Orleans, Louisiana
Learning Disabilities

**GORDON U. BURTON, PhD,
OTR**
Chair and Professor, Department of
Occupational Therapy, San Jose State
University, San Jose, California
*Psychosocial Aspects of Adaptation
and Adjustment During Various
Phases of Neurological Disability*

NANCY BYL, PhD, PT
Chair, Department of Physical Therapy
and Rehabilitation Science, and
Administrative Director, Peter Ostwald
Health Program for Performing Artists,
Department of Neurology, University of
California, San Francisco, San Francisco,
California
*Interventions for Neurological
Disabilities*

BEATE CARRIÈRE, PT, CIFK
Clinical Specialist, Kaiser Permanente,
Baldwin Park, California
*The Pelvic Floor Treatment of
Incontinence and Other Urinary
Dysfunctions in Men and Women*

**LAURIE E. CHAIKIN, MS, OTR,
OD**
Private practice, Castro Valley, California
*Disorders of Visual and Visual-
Perceptual Dysfunction*

**CORRIE J. CHRISTIANSEN, MS,
PT**
Physical Therapist, Barrow Neurological
Institute, St. Joseph's Hospital and
Medical Center, Phoenix, Arizona
Brain Tumors

CAROL M. DAVIS, EdD, PT
Professor, Division of Physical Therapy,
University of Miami School of Medicine,
Coral Gables, Florida
*Alternative and Complementary
Therapies: Beyond Traditional
Approaches to Intervention in
Neurological Diseases, Syndromes,
and Disorders*

PETER I. EDGELOW, MA, PT
Assistant Clinical Professor, Graduate
Program in Physical Therapy, University
of California, San Francisco, San
Francisco; Senior Physical Therapist,
Physiotherapy Associates, Hayward,
California
*Beyond the Central Nervous System:
Neurovascular Entrapment
Syndromes*

DONNA EL-DIN, PhD, PT
Chair and Distinguished Professor,
Department of Physical Therapy,
Eastern Washington University, Cheney,
Washington
*Introduction: Theoretical Foundations
for Clinical Practice*

DEBRA FRANKEL, MS, OTR
Senior Analyst, Abt Associates, Inc.,
Cambridge, Massachusetts
Multiple Sclerosis

KENDA FULLER, PT, NCS
Affiliate Faculty, Physical Therapy
Program, University of Colorado, and
Department of Physical Therapy, Regis
University, Denver, Colorado; Physical
Therapist, South Valley Physical
Therapy, Englewood, Colorado
Balance and Vestibular Disorders

**MARY LOU GALANTINO, PhD,
PT**
Associate Professor, Program in Physical
Therapy, Richard Stockton College of
New Jersey, Pomona; Clinical Assistant
Professor, Department of Rehabilitation
Medicine, University of Medicine and
Dentistry of New Jersey, New
Brunswick, New Jersey; Consultant,
Department of Physical and
Occupational Therapy, University of
Pennsylvania, Philadelphia, Pennsylvania
*Alternative and Complementary
Therapies: Beyond Traditional
Approaches to Intervention in
Neurological Diseases, Syndromes,
and Disorders; Human
Immunodeficiency Virus (HIV)
Infection: Living with a Chronic
Illness*

JON D. HACKE, MA, PT, ATC
Clinical Assistant Professor, Division of Physical Therapy, University of North Carolina at Chapel Hill, Chapel Hill, North Carolina
Electrodiagnosis and Electrotherapeutic Interventions

ANN HALLUM, PhD, PT
Associate Dean, College of Health and Human Services, San Francisco State University, and Professor, Graduate Program in Physical Therapy, University of California, San Francisco/San Francisco State University, San Francisco, California
Neuromuscular Diseases

OSA JACKSON, PhD, PT
Director of Physical Therapy Center, Feldenkrais Practitioner and Assistant Trainer, Rochester Hill, Michigan
Brain Function, Aging, and Dementia

EVE KARPINSKI, BS
Doctoral Student, Columbia University School of Nursing, New York, New York
Alternative and Complementary Therapies: Beyond Traditional Approaches to Intervention in Neurological Diseases, Syndromes, and Disorders

JEFF KAUFFMAN, MD
Holistic Health Associate, Sacramento, California
Alternative and Complementary Therapies: Beyond Traditional Approaches to Intervention in Neurological Diseases, Syndromes, and Disorders

CAROLYN KELLY, MS, PT
Assistant Professor, Texas Women's University, Houston, Texas
The Postpolio Syndrome

LAURIE KENNY, MS, PT
Clinical Specialist, Occupational Health Department, Kaiser Foundation Hospital, Oakland, California
Beyond the Central Nervous System: Neurovascular Entrapment Syndromes

KRISTIN J. KROSSCHELL, MA, PT
Adjunct Clinical Instructor, Department of Physical Therapy and Human Movement Sciences, Northwestern University Medical School, Chicago; Pediatric Clinical Coordinator, Health South Pediatrics, Wilmette, Illinois
Congenital Spinal Cord Injury

ROLANDO T. LAZARO, MS, PT, GCS
Assistant Professor, Department of Physical Therapy, School of Pharmacy and Health Sciences, University of the Pacific; Director of Rehabilitation Services, Meadowood Health and Rehabilitation Center, Stockton, California
Differential Diagnosis Phase 2: Examination and Evaluation of Disabilities and Impairments; Interventions for Neurological Disabilities

RACHEL O'HARA LOPEZ, MPT
Physical Therapist and Staff Specialist, Barrow Neurological Institute, St. Joseph's Hospital and Medical Center, Phoenix, Arizona
Brain Tumors

DONNA J. MAEBORI, MS, PT
Physical Therapist and Clinical Specialist in Chronic Pain, Providence St. Vincent Hospital, Portland, Oregon
Alternative and Complementary Therapies: Beyond Traditional Approaches to Intervention in Neurological Diseases, Syndromes, and Disorders

KAREN L. MCCULLOCH, MS, PT, NCS
Clinical Assistant Professor, Division of Physical Therapy, University of North Carolina at Chapel Hill, Chapel Hill, North Carolina
Electrodiagnosis and Electrotherapeutic Interventions

SHARI L. MCDOWELL, BS, PT
Education Coordinator, Shepherd Center, Inc., Atlanta, Georgia
Traumatic Spinal Cord Injury

MARSHA E. MELNICK, PhD, PT
Professor, Graduate Program in Physical Therapy, University of California San Francisco/San Francisco State University, San Francisco, California
Basal Ganglia Disorders: Metabolic, Hereditary, and Genetic Disorders in Adults; Movement Dysfunction Associated with Cerebellar Problems

LINDA MIRABELLI-SUSENS, MS, PT
Private Practitioner, St. Petersburg, Florida
Pain Management

SARAH A. MORRISON, BS, PT
Day Program Manager, Shepherd Center, Inc., Atlanta, Georgia
Traumatic Spinal Cord Injury

CHARLENE NELSON, MA, PT
Associate Professor Emerita (retired), Division of Physical Therapy, University of North Carolina at Chapel Hill, Chapel Hill, North Carolina
Electrodiagnosis and Electrotherapeutic Interventions

CHRISTINE A. NELSON, PhD, OTR
NDT Coordinator-Instructor, Neurodevelopment Therapy Association, Clinical Coordinator, Centro de Aprendizaje, The Learning Center, Cuernavaca, Morelos, Mexico
Cerebral Palsy

ROBERTA A. NEWTON, PhD, PT
Professor, Department of Physical Therapy, College of Allied Health Professions, Temple University, Philadelphia, Pennsylvania
Contemporary Issues and Theories of Motor Control: Assessment of Movement and Posture

BARBARA OREMLAND, MEd, PT
Physical Therapy Consultant, Baltimore, Maryland
Movement Dysfunction Associated with Cerebellar Problems

KARLA M. PHILLIPS, BA, BSPT
Staff Physical Therapist, Barrow Neurological Institute, St. Joseph's Hospital and Medical Center, Phoenix, Arizona
Brain Tumors

REBECCA E. PORTER, PhD, PT
Assistant Professor of Physical Therapy, Indiana University, Indianapolis, Indiana; Graduate Program Chair, Neurology Specialty, Rocky Mountain University of Health Professions, Provo, Utah
Inflammatory and Infectious Disorders of the Brain

WALTER RACETTE, BS, CPO
Clinical Instructor in Orthopaedics, University of California, San Francisco, San Francisco, California
Orthotics: Evaluation, Prognosis, and Intervention

CAROL RITBERGER, PhD
Medical Institute, BCR Enterprises, Pollock Pines, California
Alternative and Complementary Therapies: Beyond Traditional Approaches to Intervention in Neurological Diseases, Syndromes, and Disorders

CLINT ROBINSON, 8th DEGREE
Owner, Robinson's Taekwondo, Sacramento, California
Alternative and Complementary Therapies: Beyond Traditional Approaches to Intervention in Neurological Diseases, Syndromes, and Disorders

MARGARET ROLLER, MS, PT
Assistant Professor, Physical Therapy Program, Department of Health Sciences, California State University, Northridge, Northridge; Physical Therapist, UCLA Medical Center, Los Angeles, California
Differential Diagnosis Phase 2: Examination and Evaluation of Disabilities and Impairments; Interventions for Neurological Disabilities

HOWFI L RUNION, PhD, PA-C
Professor of Neurophysiology and Pharmacology, School of Pharmacy and Health Sciences, University of the Pacific, Stockton, California
The Impact of Drug Therapies on Neurological Rehabilitation

SUSAN D. RYERSON, MA, PT
Clinical Consultant and Lecturer; Partner, Making Progress, Alexandria, Virginia
Hemiplegia

WARREN G. SANGER, PhD
Professor of Pediatrics and Pathology, University of Nebraska Medical Center; Director, Human Genetics Laboratories, Munroe Meyer Institute, University of Nebraska Medical Center, Omaha, Nebraska
Genetic Disorders: A Pediatric Perspective

JANE W. SCHNEIDER, PhD, PT
Assistant Professor, Physical Therapy and Human Movement Sciences, Northwestern University Medical School; Senior Physical Therapist, Children's Memorial Hospital, Chicago, Illinois
Congenital Spinal Cord Injury

BETSY SHANDALOV, BS, OTR/L
Clinical Supervisor, Spinal Cord Injury Program, Shepherd Center, Inc., Atlanta, Georgia
Traumatic Spinal Cord Injury

LAURA K. SMITH, PhD, PT
Consultant, Postpolio Clinic, Institute for Rehabilitation and Research, Houston, Texas
The Postpolio Syndrome

TIMOTHY J. SMITH, PhD, RPh
Associate Professor of Pharmacology, Department of Physiology and Pharmacology, University of the Pacific, Stockton, California
The Impact of Drug Therapies on Neurological Rehabilitation

BRADLEY W. STOCKERT, PhD, PT
Associate Professor, Department of Physical Therapy, University of the Pacific, Stockton, California
Beyond the Central Nervous System: Neurovascular Entrapment Syndromes

WAYNE A. STUBERG, PhD, PT, PCS
Associate Professor, Division of Physical Therapy Education, University of Nebraska Medical Center; Director, Physical Therapy, Munroe Meyer Institute, University of Nebraska Medical Center, Omaha, Nebraska
Genetic Disorders: A Pediatric Perspective

MARCIA W. SWANSON, PhD, MPH, PT
Lecturer, Department of Rehabilitation Medicine, University of Washington; Pediatric Physical Therapy Specialist, Center on Human Development and Disability, University of Washington, Seattle, Washington
Low Birth Weight Infants: Neonatal Care and Follow-Up

JANE K. SWEENEY, PhD, PT, PCS
Graduate Program Chair, Doctor of Science Program in Pediatric Physical Therapy, Rocky Mountain University of Health Professions, Provo, Utah; Private Practitioner/Owner, Pediatric Rehab Northwest, Gig Harbor, Washington
Low Birth Weight Infants: Neonatal Care and Follow-Up

STACEY E. SZKLUT, MS, OTR
Guest Lecturer, Boston University, Boston; Clinical Director, Occupational Therapy Associates, Watertown, Massachusetts
Learning Disabilities

DARCY A. UMPHRED, PhD, PT
Professor, Graduate Program in Physical Therapy, University of the Pacific, Stockton; International Lecturer, Consultant, Private Practitioner, Partners in Learning Clinics, Carmichael, California
Alternative and Complementary Therapies: Beyond Traditional Approaches to Intervention in Neurological Diseases, Syndromes, and Disorders; Differential Diagnosis Phase 1: Medical Screening for the Therapist; Differential Diagnosis Phase 2: Examination and Evaluation of Disabilities and Impairments; Interventions for Neurological Disabilities; Introduction: Theoretical Foundations for Clinical Practice; The Limbic System: Influence over Motor Control and Learning

JOHN UPLEDGER, DO
Developer, CranioSacral Therapy, The Upledger Institute, Palm Beach Gardens, Florida
Alternative and Complementary Therapies: Beyond Traditional Approaches to Intervention in Neurological Diseases, Syndromes, and Disorders

RICHARD V. VOSS, DPC, MSW
Assistant Professor, Undergraduate Social Work Department, West Chester University, West Chester, Pennsylvania
Alternative and Complementary Therapies: Beyond Traditional Approaches to Intervention in Neurological Diseases, Syndromes, and Disorders

PATRICIA A. WINKLER, MS, PT
Affiliate Faculty, Regis University, Denver; President, South Valley Physical Therapy, Englewood, Colorado
Traumatic Brain Injury

Preface to the Fourth Edition

Each edition of this book brings new insights, new visions, and new avenues for therapists to advance their respective analytical and clinical skills when assisting individuals with neurological impairments to improve their quality of life. Many individuals within the professions of physical and occupational therapy and related health care disciplines and patients throughout the world have helped to guide the evolution of patient care and outcome evidence to demonstrate the efficacy of interventions. As the complexity of physical systems interactions slowly unravels before the practicing clinician, the possibilities of new variables that affect outcomes will always challenge the mind of the learner. Having a tether to basic neuroscience allows therapists of today and those of the future to stretch to limits and levels of understanding that boggle the rigid linear thinker of today and yesterday. Thus, this edition is dedicated to the visionaries who are willing to stretch our professions to the unknowns of the future while grounding us to the efficacy of today's practice. This book mirrors a family dedicated to the advancement and quality of life of others. It belongs not to the publisher, the editor, or even the chapter authors. It belongs to the learner—those students who are willing to question today's practice and look toward new and innovative ways to provide better patient care, to prevent disabilities, and to enhance the quality of life of all patients who cross their paths.

Twenty-one years and three previous editions have passed since this book was conceived. In the evolution of a person, the attainment of 21 years usually signifies adulthood and maturity. Twenty-one years of evolution of this book has encompassed new visions, greater efficacy within health care delivery, advancements in science and intervention strategies, and certainly many more questions than answers. Maturity can never be obtained, because new visions constantly suggest a new beginning. The journey has led the reader from a book whose initial problem-solving focus was understanding medical diagnosis and science as it related to neurological problems to a book whose focus is impairment/disability diagnosis and the ways in which science, disease/pathology, objective measurements of functional behavior, and intervention strategies interact. During these two decades, the therapeutic management of clients has undergone many stages of evolution. Efficacy of treatment based on research versus philosophy of treatment based on belief has become the choice of intervention procedures. This shift in paradigm from specific treatment approaches to a prob-

lem-solving model that looks at the impairment, functional limitations, and potential disability of the client seems to lead the transformation in approach. As these problem-solving approaches become operational, more effective, reliable, and valid therapeutic examinations and management strategies are being presented in the literature. Yet, our understanding of how humans learn, relearn, or adapt is far from reaching closure. Neuroplasticity, once thought impossible, has become a focus word in the area of neurological rehabilitation. Given the many unknowns and the fact that what is "known" often changes daily, all learners are challenged to keep a mind open to change and to new learning while holding on to a flexible paradigm that allows the comfortable examination, evaluation, and treatment of clients within a dynamic, ever-changing environment.

Cost of services, managed care environments, limitations in visits, and practice patterns all create challenges to today's professional. Young therapists are expected to graduate from school and immediately practice as experienced clinical problem solvers. Young colleagues feel they are expected to know the answers, not to discover them. Yet, within the clinical arena, problem-solving success is always dependent on one variable, and that variable is the patient. As long as the unique qualities of the patient are considered, a therapist will be able to select examination procedures and appropriate interventions once clinical reasoning is employed.

This book is designed to provide the practitioner and advanced therapy student with a variety of problem-solving strategies that can be used to tailor treatment approaches to individual client needs and cognitive style. The treatment of persons with neurological disabilities requires an integrated approach involving therapies and treatment procedures used by physical, occupational, and recreational therapists; nurses; pharmacists; orthotists; physicians; and a variety of other health care providers. Contributors to this book were selected for their expertise and integrated knowledge of various subject areas. The result is, we hope, a blend of state of the art information about the therapeutic management of persons with neurological disabilities.

This book is organized to provide the student with a comprehensive discussion of all aspects of neurological rehabilitation and to facilitate quick reference in a clinical situation. Section I, "Theoretical Foundations for Clinical Practice," constitutes an overview of foundational theories. This includes the entire diagnostic process used by occupational and physical therapists. Section II, "Management of Clinical Problems," offers an in-depth discussion and analysis of the therapeutic management of the most common neurological disabilities encountered by physical and occupational therapists. Section III, "Neurological Disorders and Applications Issues," is devoted to recent advances in general approaches to intervention and rehabilitation that might affect any of the diagnostic categories discussed in Section II.

Special features within all three parts are examinations, evaluations, prognosis, and intervention strategies using sound clinical reasoning. Case studies are presented throughout the book to help the reader with the problem-solving process.

A study guide follows the last chapter to help the new learner identify the key points within each chapter. This study guide is not meant to be all-inclusive; it merely identifies key points the author wishes the learner to grasp on first reading the chapter.

A glossary of specific terminology used by occupational and physical therapists should be of equal value to students and practitioners.

During the conceptualization and preparation of all four editions, many individuals gave time, guidance, and emotional support. To all those people I extend my sincere appreciation. There are many people to thank for help in the preparation of this fourth edition: the authors, the illustrators, each person assisting during the process of publication, and the patients. No person could have accomplished the end product alone. Yet, during the reediting process some specific individuals came to deserve special recognition and thanks:

- Jeb Burton, a creative and brilliant young professional who has taken very complex concepts and transformed them into illustrations that all can comprehend.

- The staff at Harcourt Health Sciences who worked on the publication of this edition: Andrew Allen, Acquisitions Editor; Rachael Zipperlen, Developmental Editor; Lee Ann Draud, Copy Editing Supervisor; and Pete Faber, Production Manager.
- All the teachers and healers who have crossed my path in the last 35 years and helped me to continually realize that before we can find answers, design research projects, and establish efficacy, we must identify and acknowledge unknowns and formulate questions.
- Each family member or significant other who encouraged and supported us from the moment we began the process to the day the book reached the learner.
- My entire family, all of whom helped me make the time to complete this manuscript.
- My two sons, Jeb and Ben, whose support I have had since the beginning of this book. As small children during its conception, their tolerance far exceeded their age. As young adults, their support and guidance always gives me strength.
- Last, my husband, Gordon, who is the only one who truly knows what demands this book has made on me and everyone around me. His support has never dwindled, nor his acceptance of my choices.

This book was conceived 21 years ago. It was visibly presented to the world 16 years ago. Both those dates have great significance in the life of humans, yet for this book represent mere milestones in evolution. We are all interconnected in a tapestry that has allowed this book to evolve into what it is today. For that, I give thanks as an author and as the editor but most importantly as a learner. Let us all hope that this book only reflects the evolution of our respective professions and will help colleagues continue to grow for many years to come.

Darcy A. Umphred

Contents

Theoretical Foundations for Clinical Practice

CHAPTER 1

Introduction: Theoretical Foundations for Clinical Practice

DARCY A. UMPHRED, PhD, PT • DONNA EL-DIN, PhD, PT

Key Words

- clinical problem solving

- diagnostic model: examination, evaluation, diagnosis, prognosis, intervention

- disablement model

- empowerment

- learning environment

- systems model

- visual-analytical problem solving (VAPS)

- wholistic model for health care delivery

Objectives

After reading this chapter the student/therapist will:

1. Understand the concepts of an interlocking systems model.

2. Analyze the diagnostic process using a disablement model of impairment/disabilities, including evaluation, diagnosis, prognosis, intervention, and documentation.

3. Analyze each component of a systems model, including cognitive, affective, and motor subsections and how it relates to function and dysfunction of the central nervous system.

4. Synthesize the importance of the clinical triad and how each aspect of the triad affects the way the therapist interacts with the client and the environment.

5. Identify the components of the clinical learning environment and how it affects clinical practice.

6. Analyze the difference between verbal and visual-analytical problem solving.

Although a physical therapist (PT), occupational therapist (OT), or other health care professional may focus on a specific area of central nervous system (CNS) processing, a thorough understanding of the client as a total human being is critical for high-level professional performance. With the use of a problem-solving clinical diagnosis, prognosis approach, this book orients the student and clinician to the understanding and treatment of impairments and disabilities caused by a variety of common neurological problems. A secondary objective is the development of a theoretical framework that uses techniques for enhancing functional movement, enlarging the client's repertoire for movement alternatives, and creating an environment for improvement in functional activities and quality of life.

Evaluation, prognosis, and intervention methodology incorporates all aspects of the client's CNS- and non–CNS-related clinical problems. The role of specific disciplines has not been defined. In the area of neurological disabilities, the overlap of basic knowledge and practical application of intervention techniques is so great that delineation of professional roles is often an administrative decision. Selection of intervention strategies that have been demonstrated as efficacious is the focus, yet complementary or traditional approaches that remain or are becoming a common standard of intervention are included.

A clinical problem-solving approach is used because it is logical and adaptable, and it has been recommended by many professional studies during the past 25 years.[2, 5, 24, 44] The concept of clinical decision making based in problem-solving theory has been stressed throughout the literature over the past two decades and clearly identifies the therapist's responsibility to examine, evaluate, analyze, draw conclusions, and make decisions regarding prognosis and treatment alternatives.[11, 14, 16, 17, 23, 32, 39, 41, 46] Section I lays the foundation of knowledge necessary to understand and implement a problem-oriented approach to clinical care. The basic knowledge of the human body is constantly expanding and often changing in content, theory, and clinical focus. Section I reflects that change in both philosophy and scientific research. The roles therapists are playing and will be asked to play in the future are changing.[3, 29] In many states, clients are now able to use direct access, which required therapists to screen systems for disease and pathology to make appropriate referrals (see Chapter 2) as well as make a differential diagnosis within that therapist's respective scope of practice (see Chapter 3). Section I has been designed to identify and delineate large conceptual areas that the reader needs to understand to synthesize all aspects of the problem-solving process from the moment a history is taken to the selection of intervention strategies (see Chapter 4). Section II deals with specific clinical problems, beginning with pediatrics and ending with senescence. In Section II each author follows the same problem-solving format to enable the reader either to focus more easily on one specific neurological problem or to address the problem from a large perspective. Authors vary in their use of specific cognitive strategies or methods of addressing a specific neurological deficit. A variety of strategies for examining clinical problems are presented to enable the reader to see variations on the same theme and thus allow better adaptation to individual cases. Because clinicians tend to adapt learning devices to solve specific problems, many of the strategies used by one author apply to situations addressed by other authors. Readers are encouraged to use flexibility in selecting treatment with which they feel comfortable and to be creative when implementing any scheme.

Changes in examination and evaluation methodology are reflected in many clinical problem chapters. Identification of objective measurement tools as well as a shift from a medical to an impairment/function/disability diagnostic process is reflected in all clinical problem chapters. Change is inevitable and a problem-solving philosophy must reflect those changes.

Section III of the text focuses on clinical topics that might be appropriate for any one of the clinical problems discussed in Section II. Chapters have been added to reflect changes in the focus of therapy as it evolves as an emerging flexible paradigm. These changes incorporate not only the interactions of professional disciplines within the Western medical allopathic model of health care delivery but also additional delivery approaches as well as the influence of cultural and ethnic belief systems, family structure, and quality of life issues.

Evaluation tools presented throughout the text should help the reader identify many objective measurement scales. The reader is reminded that although a tool may be discussed in one chapter, its use may have application

to many other clinical problems. The same is true of treatment suggestions and problem-solving strategies used to analyze motor control problems.

The Study Guide of questions and where the answers may be found has been included to assist the new learner as well as the instructors in determining major areas of focus as identified by the authors. This book has been designed both to help the new learner begin the problem-solving, clinical reasoning path of neurological rehabilitation as well as aid the practicing clinician. For that reason, the Study Guide should help focus early learning. As the reader develops more clinical understanding, returning to the book for a more in-depth analysis of specific clinical problems will allow the learner to use this text for many years as a reference for all aspects of clinical problem solving.

CHANGING WORLD OF HEALTH CARE

To understand why impairment/disability models have become the accepted models used by PTs and OTs when evaluating, diagnosing, deciding a prognosis, and treating clients with disabilities resulting from neurological problems, the reader must first analyze the evolution of health care within our culture. This understanding must begin first with the allopathic medical model because this model has been the dominant model of health care in Western society.[26] It forms the conceptual basis for health care in industrialized countries in the Western hemisphere. The model assumes that illness has an organic base that can be traced to discrete molecular elements. The origin of disease is found at the molecular level of the individual's tissue. The first step toward alleviating the disease is to identify the pathogen that has invaded the tissue and, after proper identification, to apply appropriate treatment techniques.

It is implicit in the model that specialists who are professionally competent have the sole responsibility for the identification of the cause of the illness and for the judgment as to what constitutes appropriate treatment. The medical knowledge required for these judgments is thought to be the domain of the professional medical specialists and therefore inaccessible to the public. Yet, PTs and OTs have never been responsible for the treatment of diseases or pathology with which a specific neurological client presents. Instead, we have always focused on the impairments and disabilities caused by the specific disease or pathology. Simultaneously, we have also had to understand the interactions of all other systems and how they compensated for or were affected by the original medical problem. As our roles within Western health care delivery have become clearer, so has the role of the consumer.

Levin[22] points out that there is a lot that consumers can do for themselves. Most people can assume responsibility to care for minor health problems. Use of nonpharmaceutical methods to control pain (e.g., hypnosis, biofeedback, meditation, and acupuncture) is becoming common. The recognition of the value of approaching illnesses with a wholistic approach is receiving increasing attention in society. Treatment of emotional needs as well as physical needs during illness has been advocated as a way to help individuals regain some control over their lives.

A wholistic model of health care seeks to involve the patient in the process and take the mystery out of health care for the consumer. Successful outcome measures are shifting from the traditional measure of whether the person lives or dies as the outcome indicator of success in health care to the quality of a person's life. The use of the phrase "quality of life" or living implies more than physical health. It implies that the individual is mentally and emotionally healthy as well. It is a holistic (holos, from the Greek, meaning "whole") model of health care that takes the other dimensions of a person's being into consideration regarding health. Hippocrates emphasized treatment of the person as a whole. He also emphasized the influence of society and of the environment on health.

A wholistic approach to health care acknowledges that multiple factors are operating in disease, trauma, and aging and that there are many interactions among the factors. Social, emotional, environmental, political, economic, psychological, and cultural factors are all acknowledged to influence health and one's potential to maintain health, to regain health after insult, or to maintain a quality of health in spite of existing disease or illness. An approach that takes this perspective centers its philosophy on the individual. The individual with this orientation is less likely to have the physician look only for the chemical basis of his or her difficulty and ignore the psychological factors that may be present. Similarly, the importance of focusing on an individual's strengths while helping to eliminate impairments and disabilities in spite of existing disease or pathology plays a critical role in this wholistic model. Thus the roles the PT and OT will play in the future of health care delivery can be large.

The health care delivery system in Western society has to serve all of the citizens. Given the variety of economic, political, cultural, and religious forces at work in American society, education of the people in regard to their health care is probably the only method that can work in the long run. With the limitations placed on delivery, the client's responsibility to health and healing is continuing to increase. The future task of PTs and OTs will be to "cultivate people's sense of responsibility toward their own health and that of the community." Education is an effective approach with perhaps the most potential to move us toward a concept of preventive care.

In-depth Analysis of the Wholistic Model

Carlson[9] thinks that pressure to change to wholistic thinking in medicine continues as a result of a societal change in its perspective of the rights of individuals. A concern to keep the individual central in the care process will continue to grow in response to continued technological growth that threatens to dehumanize care even more. The wholistic model takes into account each person's unique psychosocial, political, economic, environmental, and religious needs as they affect the individual's health.

The nation faces significant social change in the area of health care. The coming years will change the access to health care for our citizens, the benefits, the reimbursement process for providers, and the delivery system. Health care providers have a major role in the success of the final product. The Pew Health Professions Commission[34] identified issues that must be addressed as any new system is developed, implemented, and addressed. Most, if not all, of the issues involve close interactions of the provider and client. These issues include (1) the need of the provider to stay in step with client needs; (2) the need for flexible educational structures to address a system that reassigns certain responsibilities to other personnel; (3) the need to redirect national funding priorities away from narrow, pure research access to include broader concepts of health care; (4) the licensing of health care providers; (5) the need to address the issues of minority groups; (6) the need to emphasize general care with less concentration on educating specialists; (7) the issue of promoting teamwork; and (8) the need to emphasize the community as the focus of health care. There are other important issues, but the last to be included here is mentioned in more detail because it is relevant to the consumer.

The Pew Commission[34] concludes that the public has not been educated about the health care workforce and the consumer's role in it. Without the consumer's understanding during development of a new system, the system could omit several opportunities for enrichment of design. Without the understanding of the consumer during implementation of a new system, the consumer might block delivery systems because of lack of knowledge.

All of the information about health care reform conveys with certainty the role of the client as the center of the focus of care. The client will assume greater involvement, greater responsibility, and greater control of the personal care process.

Providers will be more willing to include the client, will design care for the client, and will be better able to educate the client, address the issues of minority clients, and become proactive team caregivers. The influence of such methods will extend to the community and lead to greater patient/client satisfaction. Similarly, this direction will open to the consumer new direct access to providers within many health care delivery professions. The potential for occupational and physical therapy to become a primary provider of health care in the twenty-first century is becoming a reality within the military system as well as in one large health maintenance organization in California. The role a therapist in the future will play as that primary provider will depend on that clinician's ability to screen for disease and pathology, examine and evaluate clinical signs that will lead to diagnoses and prognosis, as well as select appropriate interventions that will lead to the most efficacious, cost-effective treatment.

Neurological rehabilitation will take place in a conceivably changed environment and with a changed delivery system in the year 2000. The balance between visionary and pragmatist must be maintained.

Client-centered care is a reality. As visionaries we will find new ways of sharing information with our client; computers will aid in this effort. The provider will set functional outcomes and work to accomplish performance goals. More people will be involved in the care process, and the process will extend on a continuum from acute care through to the home setting. As a pragmatist, the provider must continue to enhance health care on a daily basis for each client. The case can be made that the most powerful tool for successful outcome is education.

THERAPEUTIC MODEL OF HEALTH CARE DELIVERY

Traditional Therapeutic Models

Keen observers of human movement and how movement distortions or limitations altered functional control developed models of therapeutic interventions from the past such as the Bobath, Brunnstrom, Feldenkrais, Ayers, Rood, Klein-Vogelback, Knott, and Voss approaches. These were the first behavioral-based models introduced within the health care delivery system and have been used by practitioners within the professions of physical and occupational therapy. These individuals, as master clinicians, tried to explain what they were doing and why their respective approaches worked. From their teachings, various philosophical models evolved. These models were isolated models of therapeutic intervention and were based on successful treatment procedures as identified through observation and described and demonstrated by the teachers of those approaches. The model of health care under which these approaches were used was an allopathic model of Western medicine.

During the past decades, both short-term and full-semester courses, as well as literature related to treatment of clients with CNS dysfunction, have been divided into units labeled according to these techniques. Often, inter-relation and integration among techniques were not explored. Clinicians bound to one specific treatment approach without the theoretical understanding of its step-by-step process may have lacked the base for a change of direction of intervention when a treatment was ineffective. It was difficult therefore to adapt alternative treatment techniques to meet the individual needs of clients. As a result, clinical problem solving was impeded, if not stopped, when one approach failed, because little integration of theories and methods of other approaches was ever stressed in the learning process. Similarly, because of specific treatment having a potential effect on multiple systems and that treatment's specific interaction with the unique characteristics of the client's clinical problem, establishing efficacy using a Western research reductionistic model became extremely difficult. This does not negate the potential usefulness of any treatment intervention, but it does create a dilemma regarding efficacy of practice. Similarly, the rationale used to explain these therapeutic models was based on an understanding of the nervous system as described in the 1950s. That understanding has dramatically changed. With the basic neurophysiological rationale for explaining these approaches under fire for validity and the inability to demonstrate efficacy of these approaches using traditional research methods, many of these treatment approaches are no longer introduced to the student during academic training. Yet, if these master clinicians were much more effective than their clinical counterparts, then the contrived therapeutic nature of their interventions may still be valid in certain clinical situation, but the neurophysiological explanation for the intervention may be very different. Similarly, to make statements today saying that these masters did not use theories of motor learning or motor control yet motor learning occurred in their clients seems contradictory. What can be said is that these masters did not verbally know current theories because they did not exist but they may have allowed the client to direct the treatment and the successful intervention reflected in current theories today.

Today's Health Care Models

As clinicians, *especially PTs and OTs*, moved toward establishment of models based on functional needs of the client and outcomes of the care process, more generic conceptualizations were created that were based on the interactions of multiple systems within the human body.

This systems model easily integrates into behavioral models for evaluation, diagnosis, prognosis, and intervention of physical disabilities. Today, the models are considered *Disablement models* as presented by Nagi[30, 31] and the World Health Organization.[47] As therapeutic emphasis has shifted away from a medical model to a disablement model,[30] the primary focus of evaluation, prognosis, and intervention is on the impairment (systems interaction) and how those system interactions affect functional outcomes (Fig. 1–1). Whether the functional limitations and strengths lead to a disability or to adaptation and adjustment will determine the eventual quality of life and empowerment an individual will have over his or her life. Within each component of the disablement paradigm, risk factors occur that can be environmental, psychosocial, or CNS related. These risk factors can positively or negatively affect the process and eventual outcome. Although therapists today are familiar with disablement models, other practitioners or providers of health services may not have the same depth of understanding. For that reason, PTs and OTs need to know how to communicate their models of practice to others who use different frameworks when drawing conclusions regarding patient needs.

Within the present health care delivery system, three conceptual frameworks for client/provider interactions are commonly used. Each framework serves a different purpose and is used accordingly to the goals of the desired outcome and the group interpreting the results (Fig. 1–2). The three primary models include (1) the statistical model, (2) the medical diagnostic model, and (3) the behavioral/disablement model. A fourth possibility may still be found using a philosophical or belief model such as those described by master clinicians from the past such as the Rood, Knott, or Bobath. These philosophical models when applied to functional outcomes would be included with today's disablement model and incorporate a systems approach.

In today's health care arena, the PT and OT must make certain critical decisions before beginning service. With the limitations of visits and the extent of the clinical problems often contradictory, a therapist must determine

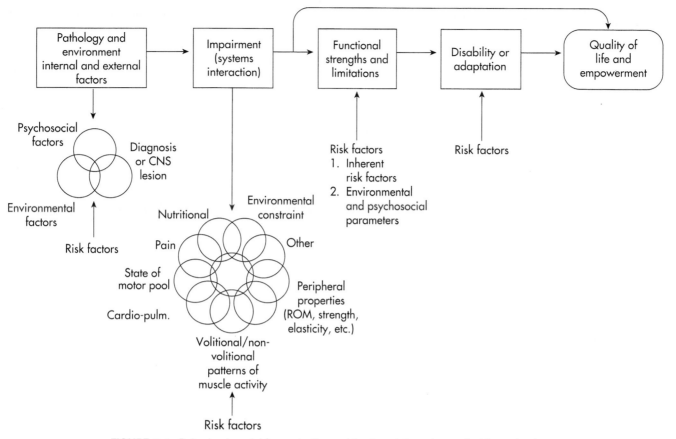

FIGURE 1–1. Behavioral model for evaluation and treatment: based on a disablement schema.

how best to meet the needs of the patient given the environment of service. Similarly, efficacy of any intervention may be questioned by anyone, including the client, the family, the doctor, the third-party payer, or the lawyer. Thus, outcome tools that clearly measure the prognosis made need to be carefully considered. Before selection

of an appropriate evaluation tool, the specific purpose for the request for evaluation and the model by which to interpret the meaning of the data must be identified. Regardless of the tool selected, third-party payers are concerned with the statistics obtained through the assessment. If the therapist scores a number 12 one week and

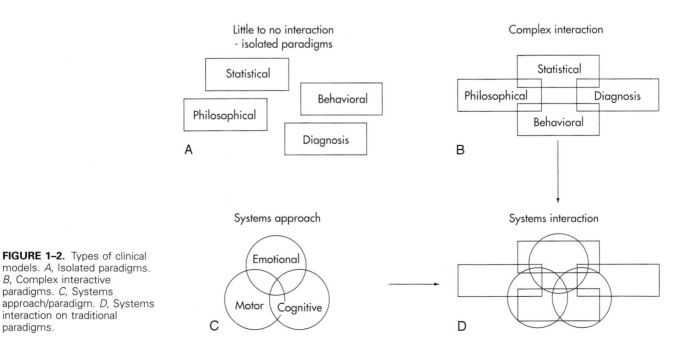

FIGURE 1–2. Types of clinical models. *A,* Isolated paradigms. *B,* Complex interactive paradigms. *C,* Systems approach/paradigm. *D,* Systems interaction on traditional paradigms.

a number 14 the next, and the payer knows a score of 16 means the individual's chance of falling is near normal, then the payer often permits additional visits. Those payers have little interest in the reasons why the client moved from a score of 12 to 14, only that the person is improving. This model is based on number crunching or gross quantitative measurements and relates closely to a statistical model. If today's clinicians do not provide these types of quantitative measurements, payment for services often is denied.

Physicians are educated to use a medical disease/pathology diagnostic model for setting expectations of improvement or lack thereof. In patients with neurological dysfunction, physicians generally formulate their medical diagnosis based on complex, highly technical examinations such as magnetic resonance imaging (MRI), computed tomography (CT), positive emitting transaxial tomography (PETT), evoked potentials, and laboratory studies. When abnormal results are correlated with gross clinical signs and patient history such as high blood pressure, diabetes, or head trauma, a medical diagnosis is made along with an anticipated course of recovery or disease progression. This medical diagnostic model is based on an anatomical and physiological belief of how the brain functions and may or may not correlate with the behavioral/disablement model used by therapists.

A behavioral/disablement model evaluates motor performance based on two types of measurement scales. One type of scale measures functional activities, which range from simple movement patterns such as rolling to complex patterns such as dressing, playing tennis, or using a word processor. These tools would be considered disability measurements. The second type of measurement tools look at specific component of various systems and measures impairments within those respective areas. For example, if the system to be assessed was biomechanical, a simple tool such as a goniometer that measures joint range of motion might be used, whereas a complex mo-

tion analysis tool might be used to look at interactions of all joints during a specific movement. This second type of measurement specifically looks at impairments. Chapter 3 has been designed to help the reader clearly differentiate these measurement tools and how they might be used in the diagnosis, prognosis, and selection of intervention strategies.

All previously presented models can stand alone as acceptable models for health care delivery (see Fig. 1–2A) or can interact or interconnect (see Fig. 1–2B). These interconnections should validate the accuracy of the data derived from each model. The concept of an integrated problem-solving model, or CNS systems model, does not depend on any one of the previously mentioned models and does identify the components within the CNS that make up the client's internal world and how life and internal mechanisms affect the systems (see Fig. 1–2C).

A last model, which identifies the three general neurological systems found within the human nervous system, can be incorporated into each of the other models separately or when they are interconnected (see Fig. 1–2D). A systems/behavioral model that focuses on the neurological systems is much more than just motor and its motor components, or cognition with its multiple cortical facets, or the affective/emotion limbic system with all its aspects. The complexity of a neurological systems model (Fig. 1–3), whether used for statistics, for medical diagnosis, or for behavioral analysis, cannot be oversimplified. As the knowledge bank of central and peripheral system function increases, as well as their interactions with other functions within and outside the body, the complexity of a systems model also enlarges. The reader must remember that each component within the nervous system has many interlocking subcomponents and that each of those components can be evaluated separately. Each component has many parts, and each of those parts could be assessed quantitatively. Those quantitative and qualitative measurements related to specific areas of function are the

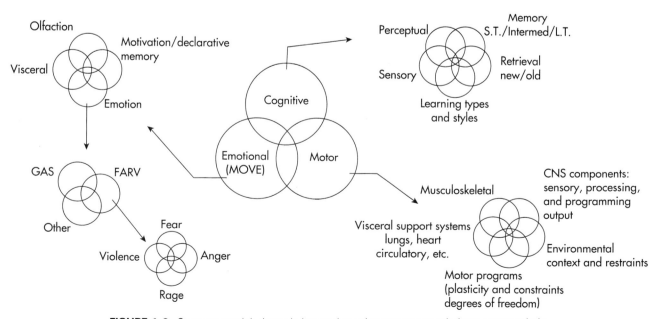

FIGURE 1–3. Systems model: dynamic interactive subcomponents: whole to part to whole.

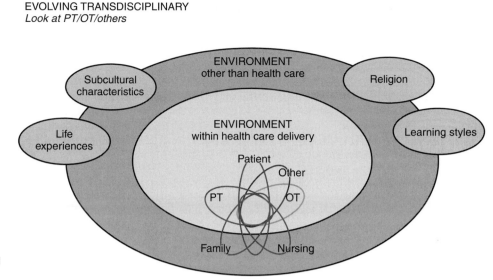

EVOLVING TRANSDISCIPLINARY
Look at PT/OT/others

FIGURE 1–4. Transdisciplinary model for delivery paradigms.

guidelines therapists use to establish problem lists and intervention sequences. Those small yet critical components, *considered impairments*, are of little concern within a general statistics model and may have little bearing on the medical diagnosis made by the doctor.

In addition to the Western health care delivery paradigms would be the interlocking roles identified within an evolving transdisciplinary model (Fig. 1–4). Within this model, the environments experienced by the client both within the Western health care delivery system and those environments external to that system are interlocking; they influence each other and affect the ultimate outcome demonstrated by the client. Because all of these once-separate worlds encroach on or overlay each other and ultimately affect the client, practitioners are now operating in a wholistic environment and must become open to alternative ways of practice. Some of those alternatives will fit neatly and comfortably with Western medical philosophy and be seen as complementary. Others may be seen in sharp contrast, with conflicts seen as insurmountable. Until approaches have gone beyond belief of their effects, therapists will always need to expend additional focus measuring quantitative outcomes and analyzing accurately functional responses. Because the research is not available does not mean the approach has no efficacy. It may be that the complexity of the tools needed to measure the therapeutic interactions are not yet available. Thus, the clinician needs to learn to be totally honest with outcomes, and the importance of quality of care and quality of life remains the primary objective for patient management.

EFFICACY

When considering any model of health care delivery, the question the therapist must ask is which model will provide the most efficacious care. Due to the nature of their education, therapists will never diagnose disease or pathology but must be able to screen systems for the purpose of referral. Similarly, choosing a test to meet a third-party payer's statistical requirements may not be the most valid instrument for use with that client but will get reimbursed. Choosing interventions only because they are acceptable within a critical pathway of recovery after an identified neurological insult will not be questioned but may not match the needs of the particular client.

Health care today demands the therapeutic health care model be efficient, be cost effective, and result in measurable outcomes. The message being given today might be considered to reflect that the "end justifies the means." This hypothesis has come to fruition through the linear thought process of established scientific research. Yet, when a wholistic model is accepted, it becomes apparent that the tools are not yet available to simultaneously measure the interactions of all systems and all models. Thus, we must guard against the reductionistic research of today that has the potential to restrain our evolution and choice of therapeutic interventions. Therapeutic discovery usually precedes validation through scientific research and leads the way to efficacious care. If research and efficacious care always have to come before the application of therapeutic procedures, nothing new will evolve. The range of therapeutic applications will become severely limited and the evolution of neurological care stopped.

Clinicians need to identify which of their therapeutic interventions have demonstrated positive outcomes and which have not. Those that remain in question may still be judged as useful. The bases for that judgment may be a client satisfaction variable that is not measurable with today's research tools. For example, in a course taught by one of us, a neurosurgeon asked the question: "Do you know how to prove the theories of intervention you are teaching?" The answer was YES. "All I need is two dynamic positive emitting transaxial tomography units that can be worn on both the client's and the therapist's heads while performing therapeutic interventions. I also need a computer that will correlate simultaneously all synaptic interactions between the therapist and the client in order to prove the therapeutic effect." The doctor said: "We don't have that tool!" The response was: "you did not ask me if the research tools were available, only if I know how to obtain an efficacious result." Thus, the creativity of the therapist will always bring the professions to new visions of reality. That reality when proven to be efficacious assists in validating the accepted interventions used by the professional. The therapist has a responsibility to the scientific community . . . but also, to the client.

DIAGNOSIS: A PROCESS USED BY ALL PROFESSIONALS WHEN DRAWING CONCLUSIONS

Diagnosis when made by a physician is considered a medical diagnosis and is a conclusion drawn regarding specific diseases and pathological processes within the human body. Diagnosis when made by a PT or OT is a conclusion drawn regarding specific disabilities and the bodily system impairments that have interacted to cause the disability. The disability itself may or may not reflect specific disease or pathology but does reflect specific impairments. PTs and OTs using disablement models are becoming comfortable with the term *diagnosis* and the conceptual understanding that the diagnosis made by a therapist is very different from that made by a physician. For the past 30 years, therapists have been receiving referrals from other health care practitioners that state: **"evaluate and treat."** In the domain of neurological rehabilitation, similar referral patterns have been identified and physicians have made the majority of those referrals.[8] The process of evaluation would include both selection and administration of examination procedures, including impairment and disability measurements, as well as interpreting those results. Once the interpretation has been made, a therapist must draw conclusions regarding those results and their interactions. That interpretation leads to the **diagnosis.** The interpretation of the evaluation results and their interaction with therapist's and client's desired outcomes, available resources, and client's potential lead to the **prognosis.** Selection of the best and most efficient resources or "road map" to the desired outcome will lead to **treatment intervention.**

The process used by therapists is complex and clearly is divided into two specific phases of differential diagnosis (Fig. 1–5).

Phase 1: Differential Diagnosis: System Screening for Disease/Pathology

With the increasing use of direct access and the length of time therapists spend with clients, clinicians have become acutely aware of the need to screen systems for disease and pathology. Accreditation standards for both PTs and OTs require the new learner to develop these skills before graduation. This screening process is used to determine whether the client should be referred to another practitioner such as a physician or can progress to diagnosis, prognosis, and intervention within the specific discipline. Thus, phase 1 of differential diagnosis separates a client's clinical problems into those that fall within a therapist's

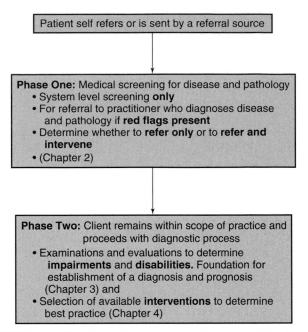

FIGURE 1–5. The diagnostic process used for best practice by physical and occupational therapists.

scope of practice and those that do not. If the phase 1 differential diagnosis shows signs and symptoms totally outside a therapist's scope of practice, then a referral to an appropriate practitioner must be made. If the signs and symptoms fall both within the clinician's scope of practice as well as overlap with other disciplines, the therapist must refer with adequate information and decide (1) to treat to prevent problems until the other practitioner's treatment can be performed, (2) to treat to eliminate disabilities in spite of the pathological process, or (3) to treat to eliminate disabilities and impairments and therefore correct the pathological process. In some cases, the overlapping with other disciplines may not necessitate an immediate referral but interactions must be made when needed to ensure the best outcome from intervention. Chapter 2 has been designed to help the reader grasp a better understanding of phase 1 of differential diagnosis. This form of system screening is part of history taking and may be redone if the therapist has questions regarding changes in body systems. Once a clinician determines that the client's need for service falls within his or her respective scope of practice, then phase 2 differential diagnosis begins.

Phase 2: Differential Diagnosis Within a Therapist's Scope of Practice

The client's signs and symptoms now fall clearly within a disablement model (see Fig. 1–1), and the therapist needs to identify functional difficulties and disabilities. Depending on the client's specific needs and expectations, these functional expectations may be activities of daily living, job requirements, or leisure activities. An in-depth conceptual framework for selection of appropriate examination procedures needed to evaluate and draw appropriate diagnostic conclusion can be found in Chapter 3.

Two important clinical components affect the accuracy of the diagnostic conclusion drawn. First, the clinician must establish an "honesty of results." This fact seems obvious, but with the pressures of third-party payers, family members, other providers of care, and the desire to have the client improve, it is not difficult to draw a conclusion regarding what is desired as outcomes versus what is truly present. The second factor deals with the honesty of the interaction between the therapist and the client. This "bonding" is critical for accuracy of examination results. Safety, trust, and acceptance of the client as a human being plays a key role in outcome and thus in efficacy of practice. The reader is referred to Chapter 6 to get a greater understanding of the impact this bonding has on clinical outcomes.

The specific cognitive process used by therapists before formulation of a diagnosis might be conceptualized as a nine-step process. As the therapist enters into the clinical environment of the client, he or she would collect data that might be relevant to analysis of the clinical problem (step 1). The therapist must take that array of divergent information and converge his or her thought process onto relevant data while disregarding what may be nonrelevant information (step 2). This body of knowledge is then differentiated into various body systems that might be affected by identified problems. If a specific system does not seem to be affected, then it can be eliminated, at least temporarily, from the diagnostic process (step 3). Generally, a clinician will perform functional activity testing at this time to obtain a general understanding of the functional strengths and limitations of the individual (step 4). After observing the patterns of movement and specific responses of the client to the evaluation procedures, the therapist will once again diverge his or her thought process back to separate large body systems to identify the system as having problems (step 5). The therapist will further subdivide these systems into their components to assess specific subsystem deficits as well as strengths (step 6). This will give the therapist objective measurements of impairments that are recognized as deficits within any subsystem. This aspect of the problem-solving process will give clusters of specific signs and symptoms that will help direct the therapist to a clinical diagnosis. Once the therapist has obtained these clusters of symptoms within specific subsystems, two additional convergent steps need to be completed. First, subsystem identification of impairments as well as lack of impairments will help the clinician determine what aspect of each body system is affected by the impairments (step 7). Second, how those impairments affect the interaction of the major system with other major body systems is determined (step 8). The eight steps tell the therapist exactly why the client has difficulty with specific functional activities. The problem list that incorporates the severity of impairments that have interacted to cause loss of function gives the clinician a clinical diagnosis. The number and extent of impairments along with an understanding of the cause of loss of function will lead the therapist to establishment of various prognoses and identification of optimal intervention strategies. The last step (step 9) requires the therapist to diverge his or her thought processes back to the client's total environment to determine the accuracy of the diagnosis, prognosis, and selected treatment interventions as they interact with the client as a whole. Although some completion of this diagnostic process may occur within minutes after a client and therapist begin their interactions, the process is ongoing, and at any time a therapist may need to go back to previous steps to obtain and analyze new and relevant information.

PROGNOSIS: HOW LONG WILL IT TAKE TO GET FROM POINT A TO POINT B?

If a client has a variety of disabilities and impairments within a major system, then a variety of prognoses may be formulated. These prognoses identify the time or number of treatments it will take to get from the existing functional limitations and identified disabilities (point A) to the desired outcomes (point B). The outcomes will state whether the intervention will eliminate functional limitations through (1) changes and learning within the client as an organism or (2) modification of the external environment. Once a diagnosis has been established, there are many factors that a therapist must consider when making a prognosis. Some factors are related to the internal environment of the client, such as number and extent of impairments, condition or decondition of the client, the ability and motivation to learn, and the disease or pathology that lead to the existing neurological condition. The client's support systems dramatically impact on prognosis. Cultural and ethnic pressures, financial support to promote independence, availability of appropriate skilled professional services, prescribed medications, and the interaction of all of these factors need to be considered. Specific environmental factors such as belief in health care and agreement about who has the responsibility for healing can create tremendous conflict between current health care delivery systems, the client, the family, and You, the clinician. All of these variables affect prognosis. The last aspect of determining prognosis relates to empowerment of the client. Who sets the goals? Who determines function? Who identifies when a therapeutic intervention should be used versus a life activity? If consensus to these questions cannot be found by the therapist and the client, then conflict between anticipated and actual outcome will result and an identified prognosis is not achieved.

Once prognoses have been established, the therapist's next step is to identify the intervention strategies that will guide the client to the desired outcome within the time frame identified.

DOCUMENTATION

Documentation of the therapeutic intervention is integral to the process. Although the responsibility of documenting care has always been assumed by providers, there is added emphasis in today's health care environment, as well as a renewed respect for the importance of the issue. A documentation approach designed to reflect the care

PROBLEM	CAUSE(S)	INTERVENTION(S)
Walk 100 yards	a. hip pain	1. electrotherapy 2. relaxation exercise 3. mobilization
	b. retracted pelvis	1. P.N.F. 2. Positional release 3. mobilization 4. strengthening exercise

FIGURE 1–6. An example worksheet.

of the client in today's system has been designed by El-Din and Smith.[12] The system is termed DEP. It consists of three sections named Data, Evaluation, and Performance Goals.

The system is characterized by centering its focus on the client and the client's functional abilities. The goals of the client are expressed in functional outcome terms that are measurable. The goals are developed in the form of hypotheses.

The therapist begins the process by taking a client history in the usual manner. The first section of DEP, **Data**, consists of both subjective and objective categories of information. The section is a listing of the assessments performed. These categories are not different from those named in the most usual documentation approach, except that information is prioritized according to the information needed for the therapeutic intervention. Thus, there may be a subjective statement followed by an objective bank of assessment, followed by a subjective measure of how it felt to do the objective activity. It is the responsibility of the provider to prioritize the information. All of the assessments are of value, and measuring subjective improvement may take precedence over objective assessment.

The second section of DEP, **Evaluation**, consists of the evaluation of the assessments conducted in the first section (Data). The therapist begins by writing a sentence, "The client is able to . . ." The therapist lists the major functional activities the client is able to perform. The statements are selected according to the assessments already performed and based on agreement with the client that they are of importance. The statement forms a baseline for the process. An example would be, "The client is able to walk 10 yards."

The second statement follows the functional baseline and states "The client is unable to . . ." These statements are (1) written in functional terms (2) developed in agreement with the client, and (3) selected according to the perceived need for therapy and usually parallel to the baseline statements. A statement in this category might be, "The client is unable to walk 100 yards." The statement provides a literal contrast between the level of performance relative to the client at this point in time and the desired outcome performances that are amenable to therapeutic intervention.

At this point, for each of the statements of "The client is unable to . . . ," there is a worksheet to be used that will help the therapist link the problem (client is unable to) with the reason for the problem, as well as that therapist's selection of approach to the problem. The worksheet (Fig. 1–6) is developed with the following three headings: problem, cause(s), and intervention(s). "The client is unable . . ." statement is the problem, and the therapist lists probable causes for the problem and then, for each cause, lists the interventions possible. The function to be addressed is stated (problem), the causes are listed, and interventions are listed for each of the causes. The therapist is now ready to move to Performance Goals.

The third section, **Performance Goals**, permits the therapist to state functional outcome goals in the form of measurable hypotheses. The therapist will state each of the problems and, for each, will then link a cause with an intervention, using measurable terms, to form a hypothesis.

The statements in this section will begin, "The client will be able to . . ." An example would be, "The client will be able to walk 25 yards in 2 weeks because of reduced pain, given an intervention of mobilization exercises to the hip."

The time taken to set up this hypothesis requires only measures to be inserted in a daily log (Fig. 1–7). Yet the

PROGRESS NOTES:

The client will be able to walk 25 yards, owing to reduced hip pain:		
Date _____ Pain level _____	Date _____ Pain level _____	Date _____ Pain level _____

FIGURE 1–7. Progress notes.

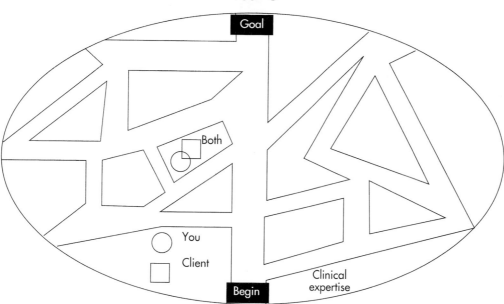

FIGURE 1–8. Concept of clinical mapping.

information remains understandable to the client, the therapist, peers, and third-party payers. These progress notes are uncluttered and contain only measurable terms with room for comment if desired.

The DEP model of documentation produces a clear framework from which to record and follow client progress. The goals are stated in measurable functional terms throughout and are developed in order of importance to the client. The number of goals developed by the therapist takes into account the realistic probability of effectiveness of intervention, environment in which the intervention will likely take place, and support systems available to the client. As the process goes forward, the therapist may add, delete, or change the functional goal, and so states that on the client's record. Further information about this process may be obtained by contacting the authors.[12]

INTERVENTION

The therapist/client chooses nonrestrictive and restrictive treatment environments to best achieve the identified prognosis. It is the therapist's responsibility to select appropriate intervention strategies that will best guide the learner to the desired outcome. Depending on the level of function of the client, some interventions will be contrived and require the therapist to guide or limit the client's selection of CNS choices whereas others will be directed toward the client's practicing functional control without clinician interference. The available choices will depend on the therapist's skill and available intervention strategies as well as on the client's ability to direct and control his or her CNS function. Yet, freedom within that established existing environment must exist if learning by the client is to occur. Another way to consider interven-

tion is to refer to it as a clinical map (Fig. 1–8). Within the map, a therapist, through professional education, efficacy of preexisting clinical pathways, and clinical experience, can generally identify the most expedient way to guide a client toward the prognosed outcome. When the specific client enters into this interaction, slight variations off the existing pathway may lead to quicker outcomes. If the client diverges away from the desired end product, it is the therapist's responsibility to guide that individual back into the clinical map. For example, if a therapist and client are working on coming to standing patterns and the client begins to fall, the therapist would need to guide the client back into the desired movement patterns and not allow the fall. In that way the client is working on the identified outcome. Falling as a functional activity should be taught as a different intervention and would be considered part of a different clinical map. The degree to which the therapist needs to control the response of the client will determine the extent to which the intervention would be considered contrived. Contrived interventions can lead in time to functional independence of the client; but as long as the therapist needs to control the environment, functional independence has not been achieved. There are many ways to get to a desired outcome. Having the client buy into the intervention will lead to the best result but does require trust of the therapist as a guide or teacher. For a more thorough discussion of intervention strategies the reader is referred to Chapter 4.

The majority of interventions used as treatment for clients with CNS damage incorporate principles of CNS function, neuroplasticity, and evaluation and treatment based on control over functional behaviors and adaptation to various environmental contexts. Thus, the basic science of central and peripheral nervous system function and behavioral analysis of movement must be included within any conceptual model used as a foundation for the entire diagnostic process.

Of considerable significance also is the client/therapist interaction, which is labeled the *learning environment*. This may be the critical factor in clinical success or failure of therapeutic intervention. The interrelationships between understanding of neural function, variability in functional movement within the context of the environment, and the therapist/client learning environment could be considered a conceptual triad. All aspects occur simultaneously; yet each component has unique characteristics and influences the clinical performance of the therapist. Although each component is explored separately in the following pages, the reader should retain the image of the entire model. This approach should help develop a gestalt, that is, a picture of the client as a total human being even though a specific aspect of therapy may be the focus. When the client is not viewed as a whole being, the therapist often misses critical response patterns, such as movement in another body part, a grimace, or an autonomic response. These responses may be the key to successful goal attainment or client/therapist rapport.

Concept of Human Movement: a Range of Observable Behaviors

As researchers continue to unravel the mysteries of brain function and learning, understanding of how children and adults learn initially or relearn after insult is often explained with new and possibly conflicting theories. Yet behavioral responses observed as functional patterns of movement, whether performed by a child, adolescent, young adult, or older person, are still visually identified by a therapist, family member, or innocent observer as either normal or abnormal.

Human beings exhibit certain movement patterns that may vary in tonal characteristics, aspects of the specific movement sequences, and even the sequential nature of development. Yet the range of acceptable behavior does have limitations, and variations beyond those boundaries are recognizable by most people. A 5-year-old child may ask why a little girl walks on her toes with her legs stuck together. If questioned, that same 5-year old may be able to break down the specific aspects of the movement that seem unacceptable. From birth a sighted individual has observed normal human movement. Because the range of behaviors identified as normal has been established, the concept behind normal human movement can be considered a constant. This concept does provide flexibility in analysis of normal movement and its development. Some children choose creeping as a primary mode of horizontal movement, whereas others may scoot. Both forms of movement are normal for a young child. In both cases each child would have had to develop normal postural function in the head and trunk to carry out the activity in a normal fashion. Thus, for the child to develop the specific functional motor behavior, the various components or systems involved in the integrated execution of the act would require modulation in a plan of action. Because the action must be carried out in a variety of environment contexts, the child would need the opportunity to practice those contexts, self-correct to regulate existing plans, identify error, and refine for skill development. Thus, each movement has a variety of complex

systems interactions, which when summated are expressed by means of the motor pool to striated muscle function. The specifics of that function, whether fine or gross motor or total body or limb specific, still reflect the totality of the interaction of those systems. No matter the age of the individual, the motor response still reflects that interaction; and the behavior can be identified as normal and functional, functional but limited in adaptability, or dysfunctional and abnormal. Because of the simplicity or complexity of various movements and the components necessary for modulatory control over various movement, therapists can (1) look at any movement pattern, (2) evaluate its components, (3) identify what is missing, and (4) incorporate treatment strategies that help the client achieve the desired function outcome.

One can feel confident that no infant will be born, jump out of the womb, walk over to the doctor and shake hands, or say "hi" to mom and dad. Instead, the infant must integrate the motor plans leading to normal rolling and head control. These plans will be modified and reintegrated along with other plans to develop normal motor control in more complex movement patterns. Each pattern and movement from one pattren to another requires time and repetition for mastery and CNS maturity.

Two very important aspects of the clinical problem-solving process emerge. First, the evaluation of motor function is based on the interaction of all the components of the motor system and the cognitive and affective influences over this motor system as stated previously. Second, rehabilitation treatment strategies become clear when the therapist observes a client trying to perform specific functional behaviors and recognizes what aspects of the movement are deficient, absent, distorted, or inappropriate when cross-referenced with the desired outcome (the diagnostic/prognosis process). These behaviors, although dependent on many factors, are consistent regardless of age. Certain aged clients may not have had the opportunity to maturate to the desired skill, whereas others may have lost the skill due to changes within his or her CNS or disuse. In either case, the normal accepted patterns and range of behaviors remain the same. If an individual wishes to walk to the bathroom, falling will not lead to the desired outcome.

Concept of CNS Control: a Multicomplex Control System

The concept of CNS control is based on a therapist's understanding of the CNS and how it regulates response patterns. This understanding, which requires in-depth background in neuroanatomy and neurophysiology, gives the therapist the basis for clinical application and treatment. Understanding the intricacies of neuromechanisms provides therapists with direction as to when, why, and in what order to use clinical treatment techniques. Behaviors are based on maturation, potential, and degeneration of the CNS. Each behavior observed, sequenced, and integrated as a treatment protocol should be interpreted according to neurophysiological and anatomical principles. Unfortunately, our knowledge of behavior is ahead of our understanding of the intricate mechanism of the

CNS. Thus, the correlation of vital links between observed behavior and CNS processing is not always known.

Because information about the functioning of the CNS is constantly increasing, the rationale for the use of certain treatment techniques may also change. This change can create frustration among therapists who desire solutions and treatment rationales that are reliable, valid, and constant. Because it is unrealistic to expect to know all the answers, therapists should keep abreast of the literature and be open to new ideas. Chapters 4, 5, and 6 have additional information and references on CNS function.

Concept of the Learning Environment

Critical to the clinical triad of our conceptual model is the concept of the learning environment. Clinicians spend a lifetime learning and teaching yet probably never intensively reflect on how they learn or how others learn from them. Understanding personal learning styles and how that leads to perceptions and response helps the clinician understand why he or she behaves in certain ways. It also helps in becoming tolerant of clients and their variance with the motor, affective, and cognitive systems. By assessing the client for intact subcomponents of all three systems, the therapist/client will have a better understanding of (1) how the client best learned, (2) whether those processes are still available, and (3) the potential for alternative learning mechanisms to access the motor systems. The master clinician seems to know how to manipulate the environment by both increasing and decreasing all variables, similar to the way in which a conductor modulates a large orchestra. It is beautiful to watch but difficult to grasp its complexity.

Awareness of and sensitivity to this learning process is vital. Gifted clinicians can be found in each field of the health care system. When these individuals are observed treating clients, it often seems as if the clients demonstrate marked improvement, show a high potential for future achievement, and experience carryover in learning. A phenomenon can be seen even in a short time spent observing the clinician with the client. The observing therapist may write down step by step what the master therapist does with the client and may formulate it into an optimal treatment plan. Yet the therapist may attempt the plan with a client and find that it does not work, that the client is unable to function at the high level expected and may indeed be successful only with those skills already acquired. This leaves the clinician frustrated and the client unable to achieve the desired level of function.

The question arises as to why the sequence worked effectively with one therapist on one day and not on the next with the other therapist. Many answers can be hypothesized. First, the gifted clinician has some "magic healing power." Second, the gifted clinician did not tell the observing group what was truly going on. Third, the second clinician's skills are inadequate for effective therapy. Fourth, the client did not practice; thus there was little carryover. Fifth, the initial clinician used extrinsic feedback to correct the movement problems and there was little intrinsic carryover. For most clients, tremendous carryover occurred, but difficulty arose in making transitions to new functions not addressed by the master clinician and taught by the regular therapist. This carryover suggests that the initial clinician did use treatment concepts (either consciously or intuitively) that reflect motor control and learning theory. Although any one of the five explanations comes quickly to mind, a more accurate explanation may be found by analyzing the learning environment.

Each clinician, as well as each client, processes millions of bits of sensory data each second. How that information is processed and how appropriate response patterns are implemented constitute a unique characteristic of each individual. When two people are interacting, as in a client/therapist relationship, each person is responding to the moment-to-moment changes occurring within the environment. At no time is that environment the same. Thus, the therapist has the responsibility of interacting dynamically with the client to create an optimal situation. An analogy might be made between the therapist and a multimillion-channel biofeedback system. The more skillful the therapist, the more channels he or she is able to modulate. The therapist is responsible not only for processing information within his or her CNS, but also for directing the way the client processes within his or her CNS. This interaction is not just a sensorimotor exchange but incorporates the entire client/therapist interaction. Thus, perceptual, cognitive, and affective channels must be established, and a method of processing the data flowing through those channels must be found. Master therapists seem to grasp this totality and create a treatment sequence that guides the client toward optimal independence. It does not seem to be the sequential steps themselves that are the clues to successful treatment but rather the dynamic interaction of the therapist and client taking those steps. Thus, a different therapist using the same sequential steps with the same client might be unsuccessful. The difference in interaction may account for the failure or success of that treatment plan, carryover, and long-term retention.

If indeed the learning environment must be client/therapist dependent, then regimented, preestablished treatment plans would not promote optimal learning for each client because they could not take into consideration individual differences. Clients often need acute care, rehabilitation, or home health services, whether they have sustained a CNS insult or a severe orthopedic injury. During their recovery process they may need to learn or relearn motor strategies to perform activities of daily living (ADL). The individual who is relearning to walk after a stroke, a total hip replacement, or an amputation faces an environment that is different in place and time from the one in which that individual took his or her first steps. Additional problems of distorted and diminished sensory input, processing of cognitive, perceptual, and affective data, and motor output may confound the relearning process. Seldom in a rehabilitation setting can a client be a passive participant while a clinician acts on that person. For this reason, no matter what the therapist's background, knowledge, or clinical skill, both the client and the therapist are actively involved in what can be referred to as the clinical learning environment. Success within this area depends on the therapist's problem-solving abilities, flexibility in creating environments conducive to client learning, sensitivity to client needs, and various opportunities for the client to gain personal control over his or her life, both internally and externally.

The concept of the learning environment is the most abstract and complex of the three concepts in the clinical triad model. For that reason it is by far the hardest to present in concrete terms. Both simultaneous and successive components formulate and maintain this environment. At any one moment multitudinous input events occur simultaneously and continuously. Thus, a temporal ordering of successive events plays a role in the CNS response to the environment. To comprehend the dynamics of this interaction and be able to function with optimal success, the clinician must:

- Understand the learning process to provide an environment that promotes learning.
- Investigate the input, processing, feedforward, feedback, and output system as a vital servomechanism for higher-order learning.
- Understand higher-order processing, procedural learning, practice scheduling, reinforcement concepts, and other motor control principles if carryover of treatment into other environments, such as the home, is to be expected.
- Differentiate how he or she learns from how the client learns. If these learning styles conflict, then the clinician needs to teach through the client's preferential systems or learning styles.
- Be aware simultaneously of the motoric, affective, and cognitive aspects of an individual, no matter what the clinical emphasis might be at any one time.

To fully understand the learning environment, four distinct components of the learning environment can be identified: the internal and external environments of the client and the internal and external environment of the clinician (Fig. 1–9).

The client's internal environment is an obvious focus of all health care professionals. A lesion has occurred within the system and is affecting how the entire mechanism functions. If the lesion occurred before initial learning, then habilitation must take place. Although a learning style has not yet been established, the individual probably has a genetic predisposition. The therapist should test the (inexperienced) CNS by creating experiences in various contexts that require a variety of types of higher-order processing to discover optimal methods of learning that best suit the CNS of the client. Then the therapist can focus treatment on the most effective strategies. If previous learning has occurred and preferential systems have been established, then the therapist needs to know what they are and whether they have been affected by the insult so that proper rehabilitation can be instituted. The use of preferential modes such as visual versus verbal or kinesthetic versus verbal does not mean that other modes are ineffective, nor do all modes function optimally in any given situation.

One way to determine general preestablished preferential styles is by taking a thorough history. Leisure activities and job choice often give clues to learning styles. For example, a client who loved to take car engines apart or build model ships demonstrates preference to visual-spatial learning style, whereas another client, whose preference for pure enjoyment was sitting in a chair with a novel, demonstrates a probable preference toward verbal learning. Again, this does not mean both clients could not selectively use both methods, but it does illustrate preference. Both the position of the lesion and preferential learning styles can play a key role in matching the leaner with a particular environment and in identifying potential. If a client has suffered massive insult to the left temporal lobe and before the trauma showed poor ability in using the right parietooccipital lobe, then spatial or verbal strategies may be ineffective in the relearning process. However, a client with the same lesion who had high-level right parietooccipital function before the insult will probably learn at a much faster rate if visual-kinesthetic strategies are used to promote learning.

The client's external environment is the second critical component. All external stimuli, including noise, lighting, temperature, touch, humidity, and smell, modulate the client's internal responses. This external input can invoke negative and positive influences on the internal mechanism and alter the client's ability to manipulate his or her world. Because a therapist should make every effort to be aware of what is happening to the client externally, knowing generally what is happening within and outside the hospital is important. Any behavioral change displayed by the client, such as mood, attitude, or muscle tone change, should serve as an indicator to the therapist that a change may have occurred. Following up that observation by determining what happened can help the therapist not only in understanding but also in assisting the client to deal with environmental change or in obtaining additional professional assistance.

The clinician should also be aware of personal internal

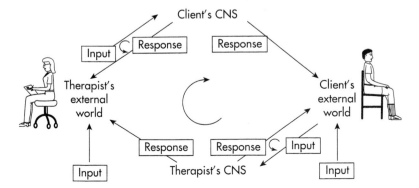

FIGURE 1–9. Clinical learning environment.

and external factors that influence patient responses. Everyone has preferential styles of teaching and learning; yet many may be unaware of what they are and how they affect outlook on life and interaction with other people. A common example of a mismatch of styles is what happens when two people are arguing opposing sides of a political issue. Although both individuals may process the same data, they may also have different learning strategies and come up with very different conclusions.

The interplay of learning styles occurs continually in an academic setting. A student who is asked the question, "what do you want out of this course?" would probably say, "A good grade." Getting a good grade requires doing well on course requirements, including tests. High test performance usually requires not only demonstrating knowledge of materials presented but also integration of the concepts when the student addresses teacher-formulated questions. When the clinician relates the same concepts to a client, it is important that the clinician be aware of the client's behaviors and responses and adapt to the client rather than having the client adapt to the therapist.

This external/internal interaction concept brings up another important clinical consideration. As students, most of us probably "clashed" with one or two teachers with whose learning styles we could never identify. That is, we as learners probably cannot or will not adapt to all learning styles. For that reason there may be some clients whom we cannot teach and some also who cannot learn through our approach. When that seems evident, a shift of therapists is most appropriate for the rehabilitation process to succeed.

The fourth component of the learning environment is the clinician's external environment. It is generally expected that personal life should never affect professional work. To accept this assumption, however, may be to deny that emotions affect behavioral patterns (see Chapter 6). When an individual is feeling poorly, emotionally upset, or under stress, response patterns vary without cognitive awareness. For example, suppose that Mr. Smith, who has a hypertonic condition because of a cerebrovascular accident, comes down early for therapy each morning, has a cup of coffee, and chats while you write notes. If one day you are under extreme stress and do not feel like interacting as Mr. Smith rolls his wheelchair into your office, you might say, "Mr. Smith, I'll be with you in a few minutes. Go over to the mat, lock your brakes, pick up the pedals, and we'll transfer when I get there." Mr. Smith will quickly identify a change in your behavior. He believes you are a professional and that your personal life will not affect your job. Thus he may draw a logical conclusion—that he must have done something to change your behavior. When you go to transfer him, you notice he is more hypertonic than usual and ask, "Is something bothering you? You are tighter than usual," and so goes the interaction. Your external environment altered your internal state and, thus, normal response patterns. In turn, you altered Mr. Smith's external environment, changing his internal balance, and created a change of emotional tone that resulted in increased hypertonicity.[27, 28] If, instead of interacting with Mr. Smith as if nothing were wrong, you informed him you were upset over something unrelated to him, you might avoid creating a negative environment. First, you let Mr. Smith know that there are days that you are upset and have mood changes. As he accepts your changes as normal, you help him realize he can have similar "off" days. Second, you give him an opportunity to offer his assistance to comfort or help you if he so desires. Such behavior encourages interdependence and social interaction, long-term goals for all rehabilitation clients.

Although each client is unique and thus analysis of specifics related to the learning environment is difficult, certain basic learning principles can be formulated. Six clinically significant learning concepts have been selected from many that have been established.[10, 18, 19] Basic learning principles relevant to clinical performance may be summarized as follows:

1. Individuals need to be able to solve problems and practice those solutions as motor programs if independence in daily living is desired. They need to use intrinsic feedback systems to modulate feedforward plans as well as correct existing plans.
2. Although assigned functional tasks must be challenging, there must be a possibility of success.
3. When tasks are difficult or unfamiliar (new problem), an individual will revert to safer or more familiar motor program or ways to solve the problem to succeed at the functional task.
4. When working on learning within one area of the CNS, learning also occurs simultaneously in many areas.
5. Motivation is necessary to drive the individual to try to experience what would be considered unknown. Simultaneously, success of the activity is critical to keep the individual motivated to continue to practice.
6. Clinicians need to be able to analyze an activity as a whole, determine its components, and use problem-solving strategies to design good individual programs. At the same time, if independence in living skills is an objective, the therapist needs to teach the client those same problem-solving strategies rather than teaching the solution.

Although all six learning concepts seem simple, their application within the clinical setting is not always as obvious. Principles 1 and 2 are intricately linked with the appropriateness and difficulty of tasks presented to clients. If a client is asked to perform a task such as standing, rolling, relaxing, dressing, or maneuvering a wheelchair, a problem has been presented that requires a sequence of acts leading to a solution. To succeed, the client must be able to plan the entire task and modulate all motor control during the sequence of the entire activity. If steps are unmastered, if sequencing is inappropriate or absent, or if motor control systems are not modulated accurately, dependence on the clinician to solve the problem is reinforced. If the clinician can differentiate missing components (impairments) from functioning systems creating an environment that encourages and allows the CNS to adapt and learn ways to regain that control will lead to optimal self-empowerment of the client and help eliminate disabilities. Error in practice to intrinsically self-correct is critical for motor learning. Error that always leads to failure does not help the client learn avenues of adaptation. Linked intricately with success is the challenge of the task. The greater its difficulty or complexity, the greater the challenge and, consequently, the greater the satisfaction of success.

There is a subtle interplay in degree of difficulty, challenge, and success. Selecting tasks that are age appropriate, clinically relevant, and goal related is a challenge to the therapist. For the patient to be successful the therapist must be a creative problem solver and knowledgeable about the client's needs, abilities, and goals. If the tasks are too simple or if the client considers them unimportant, boredom will ensue and progress may diminish. If the tasks are too difficult, the client may feel defeated and turn away from them. In such cases a child tends to withdraw physically, whereas an adult usually avoids the problem. Being late to therapy, having to leave early, needing to go to the bathroom, and scheduling conflicting sessions are all avoidance behaviors that may be linked to inappropriate tasks.

The third learning principle describes a behavior inherent in all people: reversal. When confronted by a problem, individuals revert to patterns that produce feelings of comfort and competence when solving the problem. In Figure 1–10, a 2-year-old child is confronted with just such a conflict. The bridge he wants to cross is unstable. The task goal is to cross the bridge; how that is accomplished is not as relevant as the task specificity. Therefore, the child chooses a 6-month-old behavior and thus scoots. On gaining confidence, the child sequences from scooting to four-point bunny hopping, then crawling, on to cruising, and finally to reciprocal walking. The child's reversal lasted approximately 2 minutes. Although reverting to more familiar or comfortable ways of solving problems is normal, it creates constant frustration in the clinic if it is prolonged. For example, if a hemiplegic client has spent a week modifying and controlling a hypertonic upper-extremity pattern during a simple task and is now confronted with a more difficult problem, the hypertonia will most likely return. If another client has successfully worked to obtain the standing position and then is asked to walk, the strong synergistic patterns that had been controlled may return. The pattern or plan for standing is different than that of walking, and the emotional implications of walking are very high. Returning to a more stereotypical pattern should be anticipated and the client prepared. Anticipating that less efficient patterns will usually return as the tasks demanded increase in complexity, the clinician can attempt to modify the unwanted responses. The key to comprehension of this concept is not the behavior itself; instead, it is the attitude of a therapist toward a new task presented to the client. If the clinician expects the client to be successful, the client will also expect success. If failure occurs, both parties will be disappointed and a potentially negative clinical situation will be created; however, if the client succeeds, both will have expected the result and their attitude will be neither excited nor depressed. On the other hand, a clinician that expects the client to revert to an old behavior can prepare the client. If the client reverts, neither party will be disappointed; but if no reversion occurs, both will be excited, pleased, and encouraged by the higher functional

skill. By understanding the concept, the clinician can maintain a very positive clinical environment without the constant negative interference of perceived failure when a client does revert.

The fourth learning principle deals with the totality of the client. Whether the area of emphasis is motor performance, emotional balance, or perceptual integration, all areas are affected. Therefore, understanding and respect for all areas are important if optimal client function is a primary objective. This does not suggest that therapists should address each aspect of personality; however, integration of the client's physical, mental, and spiritual areas should be a responsibility of the staff. Awareness of possible adverse effects of one learned behavior on other CNS functions can help avoid potential problems. For example, if working on lower-extremity patterns creates extreme upper-extremity hypertonicity through associated patterns, the clinician is not dealing with the client as a whole.

The unknown creates fear as well as curiosity for most individuals, and the fifth concept points out that for most clients the unknown is all-encompassing whatever the degree of prior learning. For a client whose only difficulty is a flaccid upper extremity, functional activities such as toileting, dressing, or eating will be troublesome and unfamiliar. Motivation is a critical factor for success. Maintaining motivation to try while ensuring a high degree of success is an important teaching strategy that tends to encourage present and future learning.

An additional comment regarding clients who lack motivation should be made. If a client wants to be totally dependent and has no need to become independent, then a therapist will probably fail at whatever task is presented. For example, Mr. Brown, a 63-year-old bank president with a wife, four children, and ten grandchildren, survives an operable brain tumor with residual right hemiparesis and minimal cognitive-affective deficits. The client's work history indicates that he was highly success oriented. Unknown to most persons is that for 63 years Mr. Brown desired to be a passive-dependent person but circumstances never allowed him to manifest those behaviors. With the neurological insult he is in a position to actualize his needs. Until the client desires to improve, therapy will probably be ineffective. Thus, motivating the client becomes critical and might be accomplished in a variety of ways. Knowing that Mr. Brown values privacy, especially with respect to hygiene, that he thoroughly enjoys dancing and bird watching in the forest, and that he ascribes importance to being accepted in social situations, such as cocktail parties, helps the therapist create a learning environment that motivates this client toward independence. Being independent in hygiene requires certain combinations of motor actions, including sitting, balance, and transfer skills. Being able to bird watch deep in an unpopulated forest requires ambulation skills, tolerance to the upright position for extended periods of time, and endurance. Being socially accepted depends to a large extent not only on grooming but on normal movement patterns, especially in the upper extremity and trunk. Creating a therapeutic environment that stresses independence in the three goals identified by the client will simultaneously create further independence in other ar-

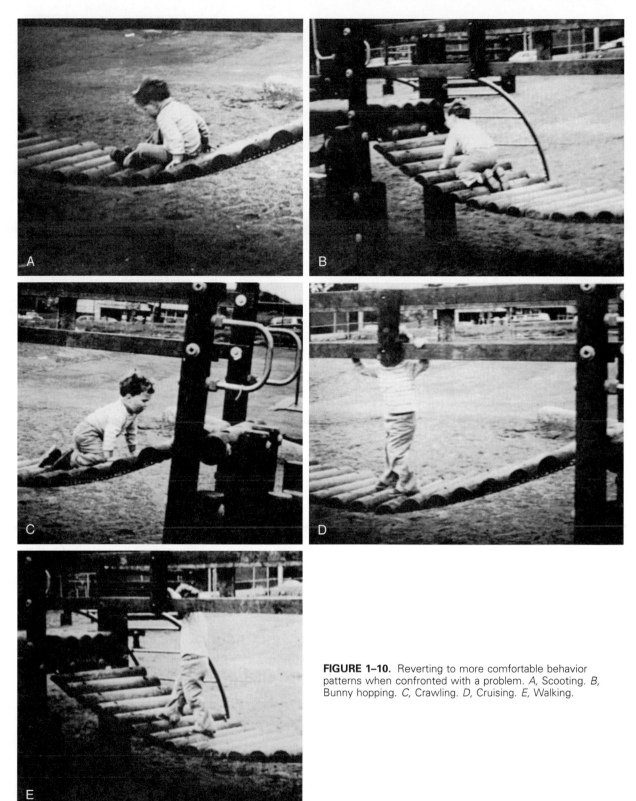

FIGURE 1–10. Reverting to more comfortable behavior patterns when confronted with a problem. *A,* Scooting. *B,* Bunny hopping. *C,* Crawling. *D,* Cruising. *E,* Walking.

eas. Whether the client decides to return to banking and other activities in conflict with his personality will need to be addressed later. Another way to motivate Mr. Brown is to place him in an environment in which he is not satisfied, such as a nursing home or his own home with an assistant rather than his wife to help him with his needs. Dissatisfaction with the current environment will generally motivate an individual to change. Obviously, creating a positive environment for change versus a negative one would be the method of choice.

Many additional learning principles from the fields of education, development, and psychology can be used to explain behavioral responses seen in our clients. It is not expected that all therapists will intuitively or automatically know how to create an environment conducive to help the patient achieve optimal potential. Yet all can become better at creating a maximal learning environment by understanding how people learn.

The principles presented in Chapter 1 deliver a strong message: individuals need to solve problems and must want to solve the problem given a chance that the solutions will be successful. Unless the task fits the individual's current capability, adaptation using whatever is available will become the consensus that drives the motor performance. Learning is taking place in all aspects of life, and the client must ultimately take responsibility for the means to solve the problem.

Health Care Through the Medical Model and Strengthening of Professional Organizations

Active participation in life and in relationships promotes learning. Rogers[36] defines significant learning as learning that makes a difference, which affects all parts of a person. We have spoken of a relationship—educational or learning in nature and centered on an individual's health. Additionally, one of the individuals involved in the relationship (the therapist) has knowledge that is to be imparted to or skills to be practiced by the other. The relationship "works" if the learning environment facilitates exchange. The concept of equal partners is crucial. The issue and practice of informed consent is not just political or ethical; it is central to client care. Voluntarism has to be practiced by both practitioner and client alike. Each has a moral obligation to facilitate the process of health care within the moment. Although the Western world of medicine has steadily climbed a path toward excellence in medical technology, it has not as easily recognized the client's need to assume an equal role in the decision making or for the practitioner to seek the client's help? Although the medical model continues to be perpetuated, consumers are now seeking to play a more active role in their health care.

Clients, or consumers of health care, are becoming aware of the impact of medicine's control over their lives. This awareness has been fueled by the price they are paying for that health care. A recent Surgeon General's report confirms that expenditures for health are increasing. In addition, preventive care assumes major importance in view of the fact that 75% of all deaths today are the result of degenerative diseases, such as heart disease, cerebrovascular accidents, and cancer. Like other major causes of death, accidents (cited as the most frequent cause of death in persons younger than age 49) are increasingly linked to lifestyles.

Individuals in the health care professions internalize values during their training that reinforce the traditional professional attitude alluded to earlier. Many of these values do not support a partnership relationship with the client. Although society is beginning to question the traditional role of the health care professional as the expert, the professional training and organizations resist the pressure to change the image. The professions still hold the image of great authority given to them by the public and fostered through increased political activity.

The major purpose of the patient's relationship with the health care professional is to exchange information useful to both in the health care of the client. McNerney[26] calls health education of the client the missing link in health care delivery. As the gap grows between technology and the users of that technology, client health education becomes more important than ever. McNerney[26] notes that although health care providers are now making efforts to educate their clients, they are doing so with little consistency, enthusiasm, theoretical base, or imagination and often with little coordination with other services. The health care professional continues to receive training and embrace professional organizational membership that places a premium on control of information and control of the decision making. There should be a special effort to introduce health education concepts into the basic educational programs of health care professionals.

When patients are given more information about their illnesses, and retain the information, they express more satisfaction with their caregivers. A study by Bertakis[7] tested the hypothesis that patients with greater understanding and retention of the information given by the physician would be more satisfied with the doctor/patient relationship. The experimental group received feedback and retained 83.5% of the information given them by the doctor. The control group received no feedback and retained 60.5% of the information. Not surprisingly, the experimental group was more satisfied with the doctor/patient relationship.

If the client is to be informed and included in the treatment process, client health education will have to go beyond the present styles of information giving. If the client is to assume some of the responsibility for his or her therapy, the therapist will have to facilitate that involvement. The attitude of the therapist toward educating clients about their health could affect his or her ability to facilitate client involvement in the care process.

The more the professional sees himself or herself as the expert, the less likely he or she will be to see the client as capable of responsibility or expertise in the care process. If communication skills and health education were a part of medical school and the other health care professional school curricula, perhaps the health care professionals would temper their assumption of the "expert" professional role. Payton[33] points out that it is the client alone who can ultimately decide whether a goal is worth working for. Careful planning can be influential in helping all providers include the client in the process.

The health care delivery system in the United States has to serve all of the citizens. That is no easy task. The United States is a society of great pluralism. It is a free society. It is a society that is used to being governed by persuasion, not coercion. Given the variety of economic, political, cultural, and religious forces at work in American society, education of the people in regard to their health care is probably the only method that can work in the long run. The future task of health education will be to "cultivate people's sense of responsibility toward their own health and that of the community." Health education is an effective approach with perhaps the most potential to move us toward a concept of preventive care.

Becker and Maiman[6] discussed Rosenstock's Health Belief model as a framework to account for the individual's decision to use preventive services or engage in preventive health behavior. They cite noncompliance with a physician's recommendation in about one third of all patients. Action taken by the individual, according to the model, depends on the individual's perceived susceptibility to the illness, his or her perception of the severity of the illness, the benefits to be gained from taking action, and a "cue" of some sort that triggers action. The cue could be advice from a friend, reading an article about the illness, a television commercial, and so on. In some way, the person is motivated to do something.

Split-brain research, research in the functions of the left and right halves of the brain, seems to be a pertinent area of mind/body research. The left hemisphere of the brain processes experiences in a factual, logical, and analytical way, whereas the right half appears to process the same experiences in the form of images and impressions. The recognition that one half of the brain may be designed to record the impressionistic part of an experience gives further credibility to including the individual's accounts of his or her feelings and emotions as a part of the input for diagnosis of illness.

Freymann[15] ponders the strange logic of traditional medicine, which rewards the specialist who confines his or her practice to a very few and shows little concern for a public health physician whose field is broad and who treats so many. Dramatic traditional medicine does not result in many health benefits for large numbers of people.

McKay[25] asks to what extent health care providers are willing to commit themselves to explore and implement alternative forms of health care. The provider/client relationship becomes very important to a successful therapeutic outcome, as does health education and promotion of positive health behaviors. Health care providers seem to forget that well-being calls for wellness of the mind, body, and environment. Although they may talk about supporting a focus on health they continue to focus on disease. The training that health care providers receive makes disease more interesting than wellness.

Saward and Sorenson[38] observe that the mass media has promoted the technology of health care. The consumer thus has a heightened expectation of the quality of care he or she will receive. However, we should avoid excesses in the other extreme. If society adheres to inappropriate lifestyles, the health care professional cannot turn around and blame the victim for bringing on the illness and absolve himself or herself from responsibility. Wholistic health care carried to an extreme might result in "blaming the victim." Saward and Sorenson see that, in the extremes, the medical model and the wholistic model of health care have different objectives; evolve from different historical, philosophical, and economic perspectives, and use practitioners with essentially different training and outlook on health care. Perhaps, they suggest, two health care systems should be available to people instead of one.

Szasz and Hollender[43] described five basic relationships between providers and clients on a continuum from a provider-dominated relationship, consistent with the medical model, through a mutual participation relationship, to a relationship where the client accepts the larger share of responsibility, which is consistent with the wholistic model. Whether the client takes some responsibility for his or her care depends a great deal on whether the health care provider gives some to him or her.

Fink[13] also recognized the importance of the provider/patient relationship and made three points about it. The first is that a relationship between them is implicit. The second is that what the relationship becomes is mutually agreed on, consciously or not. Third, whatever the form of the relationship, it should meet the needs and health care requirements of the particular patient.

The relationship of the therapist and client has also been called "the emotional bridge over which the more mechanical forms of treatment are conducted."[21] The psychological makeups of the therapist and of the client have an impact on the relationship that is established. The psychological development of both of them during their growth stages of dependency, aggressiveness, and ability to subordinate personal gratification must be acknowledged as having an effect on the relationship.

The illness or trauma of the client that represents a disintegrating force in his or her life may represent an opportunity for the therapist to grow professionally. The client and the therapist may have different psychological backgrounds; and although the client is usually there because of the medical crisis, the therapist may be there for purposes of personal growth, financial gain, prestige, and unconscious gratification in influencing the lives of others through professional skill.

A large amount of time is spent by therapists in face-to-face patient contact.[35] In this respect, the therapist has an advantage over most other health care practitioners who see the patient at infrequent intervals and who seldom touch the patient as a PT or OT does. The physical contact itself may provide psychological support and promote a close relationship between the therapist and the patient. It is important then that the therapist be aware of the importance of the relationship itself. The therapist's attitudes and values can affect the expectations of patients regarding the outcome of treatment. The patient's expectations can be made realistic if he or she is an active participant in care from the start. Any process that involves personal commitment and purports to effect change should focus on the person seeking help. An attitude of acceptance of the patient as an equal in the process may be of healing value by itself and referred to as empowerment.

As the consumer becomes more involved, so should the family. The family is seldom brought into the practice. Sasano and colleagues[37] described a patient program that includes the family. They made some comments relative to therapy's inclusion of the family in the care process. Patients were happier with the family involved; the family members felt less anxious and could be more supportive. All of these factors facilitate the work of the therapist. The therapist, however, must be willing to facilitate the involvement of the family members and help them learn to take responsibility for some of the care and decision making. Most health care professionals are not conditioned to the patient's assuming greater authority. Family members cannot take responsibility for the care unless the therapist allows the family members to assume that role.

The therapist is caught up in the same problems of the health care system as other health care professionals. Inflation has caused profit to become a more important motive for setting priorities in our clinics than human considerations. Research is heavily focused on technical procedures, yet the relationship with patients in the care process is vital. Singleton[42] labeled this phenomenon a paradox in therapy. Despite the commitment to humanistic service on which the profession was founded, the service rendered is mechanistic.

Is the patient approached like a machine? Has scientific technology captured the therapist's attention to the extent that he or she ignores patient care procedures that cannot or have not been scientifically analyzed? Alexander[1] sees the necessity of reorganizing the education and work of the therapist to encourage a humanistic approach to care. To what degree, Alexander[1] asks, are we "masters or servants to our patients?" The educational programs could emphasize whole-patient treatment, increase communication skills and interdisciplinary awareness and videotape students as they interact with others, and encourage role-playing. Finally, he proposes that although restructuring educational experiences is useful, selection procedures also have to be considered.

If medicine succeeds in bringing humanistic medicine into focus and shifting some emphasis from a scientific technology approach, it is conceivable that some people currently suited to practicing therapy would find it intolerable to do so in the future.

Neurological clients interact with the medical community for short or long periods of time. They present neurological problems of all types that are sudden or insidious. All aspects of human function are represented in the variety of problems. If individual beliefs and values energize and motivate physical behavior, think of the possibilities for stimulating wellness.

The change in roles described previously require a professional who demonstrates a characteristic flexibility. There is a potential for the selection of many roles, responsibilities, and choices along the care pathway. The therapist working with the client with neurological problems must always be ready to respond to triggers anywhere along the pathway from early intervention, midway during a crisis, or later during chronic or long-term care, because they signal a need for change. Of equal importance, the path must be well documented to empower the therapist to reflect on current and prognosticated treatment intervention.

CLINICAL PROBLEM SOLVING

The last concept to be presented within this chapter focuses on the development of problem-solving strategies. The health care professions are stressing the importance of problem-solving skills, development of a problem list for each patient to identify the clinical diagnosis and prognosis, constant reassessment of the problem list, and documentation of client progress during therapy. Schools are basing entire curriculum designs on problem-solving principles. Developing good problem-solving skills is paramount for high-level clinical reasoning and performance. The clinician examines/evaluates the client, establishes relevant goals with the client, and then teaches the client the best solution to a specific problem. Unfortunately, teaching a solution to a problem can often be synonymous with teaching a splinter skill, that is, a skill that has no application to similar functional activities. For example, a therapist might identify that Janet needs to learn to perform a standing pivot transfer. They repeatedly practice the skill of transferring from a wheelchair to the toilet in the clinic. The independence that Janet achieves in this activity may not carry over to other transfer activities or even other toilets. Therefore, teaching the client to solve problems in a variety of environmental contexts while self-correcting errors within the motor plan must accompany skill acquisition if that individual is to reach optimal independence (see Chapters 4 and 5 for additional information on motor control and learning).

A theoretical model that integrates the traditionally separate cognitive subject areas of behavioral analysis, applied neuroanatomy and neurophysiology, and learning theory has already been presented. This section deals with a specific problem-solving format that can be applied to this model. This format serves as the basis for the clinical problem chapters within Section II of this book (see Chapters 8 through 26). Chapter 33 introduces complementary clinical treatment models or paradigms that present additional options. Today's clinician needs to keep his or her mind open to options while grounding treatment choices to identifiable outcomes. The second topic discussed here consists of additional suggestions regarding problem-solving strategies, such as formulation of a client profile and visual-analytical problem solving.

Problem-Solving Format

Although cognitive strategies vary when a clinician approaches a specific clinical problem, an identifiable format is generally followed and will be consistent within all chapters in Section II. The format has at least five areas: (1) existence of the problem (anticipated medical and impairment/disability aspects), (2) evaluation procedures (outcome measures typically used for this clinical problem), (3) goal selection (prognosis accepted as typical standard of practice), (4) treatment planning (choosing the best interventions to obtain desired goals), and (5) specific psychological aspects and adjustment (modifying the solution to individual needs).

Before evaluating a clinical problem and formulating a diagnosis, an understanding of the general characteristics of the dysfunction is important. The neuroanatomical and physiological aspects of a problem and how they affect the client's general performance provide scientific understanding of the problem. Comprehension of typical clinical signs, as well as stages of recovery from acute to long-term rehabilitation, also provides vital background knowledge. Pharmacological considerations and medical management during various phases of recovery or progress can change the response to and direction of a treatment program. All of this background information, in addition to the client's individual characteristics, helps the therapist conceptualize the nature of the problem and formulate a problem list. Although the clinician needs to remain flexible and to accept clinical signs as they occur, grasp of a total concept of the problem provides direction for evaluation, diagnosis, prognosis, and treatment planning. Conceptualizing the clinical problem or observing the client's behavior leads the clinician to formulate questions that focus attention on both selection of intervention procedures and direction of treatment.

Once a clinical problem has been identified and a problem list has been formulated, evaluation procedures are selected. The selection of testing procedures may vary according to clinical preference, clinically established procedures, and client deficits, but it should be thorough, objective, and inclusive of all areas. Specific areas of evaluation have already been presented. Again, the choice of a specific evaluation form is not a critical issue. How the therapist extracts information from an evaluation is critical to the problem-solving/diagnostic process. Through experience clinicians learn to identify additional data not considered part of the test item. For example, a therapist who is evaluating rolling and observes a strong shift in muscle tone as the head turns to the side that prevents rolling may decide that the client is incapable of rolling or cannot roll because of a strong tonal shift with head turning. The more observant and knowledgeable therapist, however, might conclude that the client has persistence of a central pattern generator that is triggered by head rotation. The interaction of the central pattern generator and the stimulus would be considered a reflexive response called an asymmetrical tonic neck reaction (ATNR). This reaction not only prevents rolling but may also affect many other ADL tasks. The therapist who identifies that the client cannot roll has answered the test questions appropriately. The therapist who can pinpoint the observed behavior and recognize its manifest pattern and that it has the potential of affecting other functional activities can extract a large amount of pertinent, additional data that can be used when progressing to other functional tasks. These data provide direction for further examination/evaluation procedures, diagnosis, prognosis, and possible selection of a variety of intervention protocols. Specific suggestions regarding development of these strategies for extracting additional information are discussed later in the section dealing with visual-analytical problem solving.

Caution must be observed regarding conceptualization of a clinical problem and the examination procedures selected to measure outcomes. Biasing findings of an evaluation to fit what is perceived as the problem is an issue all clinicians need to address. The clinician must allow the specific clinical signs of the patient to direct evaluation findings, goal setting, and treatment planning. Preconceptions based on familiarity with the medical diagnosis and general impairment/disabilities associated with that clinical problem can negate both the client's individuality and his or her specific needs.

The ability to reexamine, alter existing diagnoses and expected prognosis, and change intervention strategies needs to be part of an ongoing problem-solving process. Clinical signs often vary quickly. Observation of finite as well as gross changes in impairments and disabilities plays a key roll in establishing and reestablishing goals. Goals that seem appropriate for one phase of recovery or disease may need to change quickly as the phase changes. The clinician who uses high-level clinical problem-solving strategies identifies finite clinical signs that indicate a phase change and therefore reestablishes new goals without losing precious time. For example, if a hemiplegic client has severe hypertonicity in the biceps and no palpable tone in the triceps, one goal might be to reduce tone in the biceps and facilitate triceps activity. A clinician would never isolate those two muscles without considering the rest of the client's arm, shoulder, and trunk; but for minimizing complexity, the following treatment focuses on the two identified muscle groups. Placing the biceps in extreme stretch will inhibit that muscle's action by means of its tendon organs (see Chapter 4). Simultaneously, the tendon organs will facilitate the triceps. Tapping and vibration of the triceps during a weight-bearing pattern while the other arm is reaching for a cup or performing some functional activity should further facilitate this action. The assumption has been made that the biceps, as well as higher centers in the CNS, are inhibiting the triceps. Thus, by inhibiting the biceps' function and using facilitative techniques, the therapist hopes that triceps activity will develop. Instead of low or normal tone development in the triceps, however, hypertonicity may ensue. If that is the case, the specific goal needs to be modified as soon as excessive tone is palpated. If not, triceps tone may become severe, causing additional problems. Once these contrived therapeutic interventions are no longer needed, the client needs to practice uses of all the muscle groups in various functional activities to reach functional outcomes as identified in the prognosis and objectively measured using appropriate evaluation tools.

Intervention procedures are established in terms of treatment objectives. Although the problem-solving protocol seems to follow a temporal, step-by-step sequence, in reality many aspects are occurring simultaneously as a system analysis. The focus may be on evaluation, but treatment is also intricately intertwined; and during treatment a reevaluation is ongoing. Understanding the neurophysiological processes being modulated during a intervention should give the clinician flexibility to alter treatment strategies including type, duration, and amplitude to meet the dynamic needs of the client. Similarly, that knowledge also helps the clinician establish environments that encourage clients to self-correct, thus eliminating the need for extrinsic feedback from the therapist, and promotes greater carryover in learning.

The last area generally affecting the problem environment, and thus the strategies used by the therapist, is specific psychosocial aspects and adjustment during various stages of recovery. An in-depth discussion of this area is presented in Chapters 6 and 7. Although many therapists working with clients with physical disabilities focus their treatment on physical health and not on the social and adjustment aspects, the psychological state of the client affects the outcome of all other areas, including control over functional movement.

Problem solving is continually implemented by therapists from the moment they learn they will be treating specific clients to the moment those clients leave the clinical environment. Gifted therapists are often thought to have intuition. Yet intuitive behavior is based on experience, a thorough knowledge of the area, sensitivity to the total environment, and ability to integrate the three and respond optimally. Intuitive abilities may be equated with high-level problem-solving skills (see Chapter 6 for additional information on intuitive behavior). In that respect each clinician should, with learning and practice, become more skillful and thus a better problem solver. One very important aspect of clinical problem solving is the ability of clinicians to ask pertinent questions as they evaluate, conceptualize about, and treat their clients. How these questions are formulated and the answers documented vary among therapists, but the result is the formulation of a profile for each client.

The Client Profile

A therapist reads charts to gain background information on a client before or at the initial meeting. In the past, emphasis was to get a "feeling for" the client. Instead, time might be better spent gathering useful information about specific areas: cognition, affect, and motor. Because these three areas are interwoven, the therapist needs to focus not only on each of them but also on their interaction. To optimize treatment effectiveness, clinicians should ask questions whose answers will give them valuable information regarding the client's past, present, and potential status as well as provide indicators of the most effective learning environment.

Cognitive Area. Perception and cognition cannot be separated. Perception lays the foundation for higher-level cognition, but there is also spiral overlapping that cannot be overlooked. It would appear that as perception develops, it lays the foundation for cognitive development, which, along with perception, matures and sequences to higher and higher levels. Within the cognitive domain four general areas are identified: (1) sensory input, (2) perceptual awareness and development, (3) preferential higher-order cognitive systems, and (4) level of cognition. All play important roles in the optimal function of the client within the cognitive domain. The following box summarizes pertinent questions a clinician must answer with regard to the cognitive area of the client's profile. Somatosensory retraining has become an important component of intervention strategies and is discussed in Chapter 4.

Affective Area. The affective or emotional area directly influences the client's level of cognition. Simultaneously, all other cognitive domains can be affected by or affect the emotional factor and responses of the client. When considering the affective domain, at least four general areas should be explored: (1) level of adjustment to disability, (2) level of emotional control, (3) attitude, and (4) social adjustment. Questions arise within each category that indicate the client's emotional status and how it will affect a therapeutic environment. See the box on

---

COGNITIVE AREA QUESTIONS FOR CLIENT PROFILE

A. Sensory input: awareness level
   1. What sensory systems are intact?
   2. Are any sensory systems in conflict with others?
   3. If conflict between systems is present, to which system does the client pay attention?
B. Perceptual awareness and development
   1. What specific perceptual processing deficits does the client have, and how would that affect motor performance?
   2. Do the perceptual problems relate to input distortion, processing deficits, or both? If input distortion is alleviated, is information processed appropriately?
C. Preferential higher-order cognitive system
   1. Was or is the individual's primary preferential system verbal or spatial?
   2. Is the client's preferential system different from yours? If so, can you work through the client's system?
   3. Is the client's preferential system affected by the clinical problems?
   4. Can the client adequately use nonpreferred systems?
D. Level of cognition
   1. Is the client functioning on a concrete, abstract, or fragmented level?
   2. Does the client's level of cognition change? If so, when and why?
   3. Is the client realistic? Does the client exercise judgment? If so, when? If not, when and why?
   4. Which systems or individuals are interfering with or distorting potential? (Systems within the individual and the environment around the client, such as the staff, the family, and the other patients, must be considered.)

---

page 25, and for additional information refer to Chapter 6 and 7.

Somatomotor Area. The motor system as a system is extremely complex. As knowledge of the central pattern generator, motor control function, plasticity of the nervous system, and ways to develop motor learning has become part of clinical practice, specific questions need to be formulated to obtain information that will help guide the therapist into appropriate functional training activities with the client. Most therapists are more comfortable addressing both the sensory and the motor control areas than either the affective or cognitive systems. Four identifiable categories (see the box on page 25) have been presented, although many additional focal areas could have been presented.

Summary. Linking the cognitive, affective, somatosensory, and somatomotor domains is the key to providing a productive and satisfying clinical learning environment for both the therapist and the client. Identification of overlapping problems is important. The client's affective

AFFECTIVE AREA QUESTIONS FOR CLIENT PROFILE

A. Level of adjustment or stage of adjustment to the disability
1. At what level or stage of adjustment is the client with respect to the disability?
2. At what level of adjustment is the family?
3. Will the level of adjustment of the client or family affect treatment?
4. If emotions are affecting treatment, what can be done to eliminate this problem?
B. Level of emotional control
1. Can the client exercise impulse control?
2. When does degree of emotional or impulse control vary?
3. How did and does the client respond to stress?
4. How did and does the client respond to perceived success and failure?
5. What types of stresses outside of the specific physical disability are being placed on the client?
C. Attitude (attitude toward the disability is covered to some degree under level of acceptance, although additional information needs to be gathered)
1. Before the onset of disability what was the client's attitude toward disabilities, and specifically, those related to his or her primary deficit?
2. What is the client's attitude toward your professional domain?
3. What is the family's attitude toward disabilities, especially those related to its family member?
4. What is the family's attitude toward your professional domain?
D. Social adjustment
1. At what social-developmental stage is the client's performance?
2. Is the social interaction in alignment with cognitive and sensorimotor stages of development?
3. Are the family's social interactions and expectations at the level of the client's performance?
4. Is the client's level of social adjustment the same as the rehabilitation team's level of expectation?
5. Is the client aware of his, her, or others' socially appropriate behavior?

A clinical example is used here to help the reader through the various questions posed in the client profile. Mary H. is a 22-year-old client with closed-head injuries who has been admitted to Jones Rehabilitation Hospital after a 2-month stay in an acute care facility following an automobile accident. At the time of the insult Mary was a senior at X University. Her major was architectural engineering, and her primary interests were sports such as tennis, skiing, and track. She was to be married after graduation. The accident, which killed her fiancé, occurred on the way home from a beer party. The doctor reported that on admission to the rehabilitation hospital, Mary was awake and verbally responded to questions, but articulation and monotone difficulties made her responses

SENSORIMOTOR AREA QUESTIONS FOR CLIENT PROFILE

A. Level of motor performance with respect to performance
1. Is the client's level of motor performance or sensory and motor integration congruous with the staff's expected performance level?
2. Is the client's level of motor control integration congruous with the family's expected performance level?
3. Is the client's level of motor function congruous with his or her expected level of performance?
B. Functional skills
1. What functional skills does the client perform in a normal fashion?
2. What functional skills does the client perform in an abnormal manner?
3. What functional skills has the client learned to perform that are reinforcing stereotypical patterns or hindering normal movement?
4. What functional skills does the client and family consider of primary importance? Will splintering these skills hinder normal learning?
C. Abnormal patterns
1. What patterns are present?
2. When are these normal and abnormal patterns observed? Do they vary according to spatial positions?
3. Is there ever a shifting or altering in degree of these abnormal patterns? If so, under what circumstances does this variance occur?
D. Degree of cortical override
1. Does the client need to inhibit abnormal output by intentional thought, or does he or she use procedural adjustment through normal feedforward mechanisms?
2. What amount of energy is being used to override abnormal output?
3. Can the client use cognitive systems to control motor output?
4. What amount of energy are you demanding the client to use when attending to the task? Are you asking the client to attend totally to the specific motoric task, or are you overloading the system to take away some cortical attending?

response at any one time will influence both cognitive processing and motor performance. This effect may be extreme or mild, either positive or negative, and in many situations will need to be clearly identified for optimal performance outcomes. Cognitive-perceptual processing by the client will often determine the learning environment to be used, the sequences for treatment, and estimated time needed for therapeutic intervention. The motor output area is a main system the client uses to express thoughts, feelings, and demonstrate independence to family, therapists, and community. This motor area cannot be evaluated effectively by itself while negating the cognitive-perceptual and the affective-emotional areas. If that rigidity becomes a standard of care, accurate prognosing and selection of appropriate interventions will continue to be inconsistent and lack efficacy.

almost incomprehensible. Her volitional motor skills were limited because of extreme hypertonicity. Mary seemed depressed and exhibited bursts of anger at seemingly insignificant problems.

Many of the questions on the client profile cannot be answered on initial evaluation. Answers to specific questions will also change as Mary's neurological condition changes. The Functional Independence Measure (FIM),[20] presented in the conceptual model section, is the evaluation form used at Jones Rehabilitation Center along with range of motion and sensory test forms and the Southern California sensory integration battery.[4]

When the therapist addresses the cognitive profile, certain directional indicators can be identified. Mary's visual system has deficits that cause distortion in the perception of her spatial world. Her proprioceptive-vestibular system is intact, but her visual deficits override former sensory systems. Thus, when sitting, Mary leans 30 degrees to the left with both head and trunk and perceives that she is in a vertical position. With her eyes closed, she still remains off vertical but can reposition herself to vertical when proprioceptive-vestibular cues are given. Knowing that one system is intact but overridden, a therapist can increase both temporal and spatial input through that modality to increase awareness. That increased awareness may help correct the deficit system. One way this might be accomplished would be asking the client to assume different positions while supine. The therapist instructs Mary to close her eyes and feel her position in space, adding approximation down through head and shoulders and quick stretch to appropriate muscle groups. Then the clinician takes Mary out of the position and asks her to reassume it. The goal would be accurate assumption of a totally symmetrical position. This first step toward reorientation to verticality is accomplished in a nonstressful position, thus eliminating anxiety, undue emotional tone, and conflicting input stimuli. Knowing that the client's preferential systems, based on her career choice and leisure activities, were visual-spatial and kinesthetic and that certain sensory systems critical to higher perceptual-cognitive performance in these areas are still intact reveals (1) which modality to use to introduce input if external augmented input is necessary and (2) which teaching strategies should be most beneficial to this client. That is, the client should be treated and taught using spatial and kinesthetic patterns of movement rather than through verbal commands or visual demonstration of desired behavior, at least initially. Thus Mary's intact systems and her preferential modes of thought are tapped. Once an accurate form of communication has been established, other forms such as visual demonstration or verbal instruction can be presented. Then additional questions posed in the profile can be addressed.

As the clinician focuses on the cognitive-perceptual area, the affective area can also be explored. Most of the questions listed under level of emotional control in the affective area outline can be answered while evaluating cognitive-perceptual performance. Many other questions can be answered by spending a few minutes with Mary's family members. Getting at least two other individuals' opinions of Mary's level of adjustment, emotional control, and attitude helps eliminate individual bias. Thus, it might be assumed that Mary highly valued her physical status, that she was always uncomfortable around anyone with a physical disability, and that she had a quick temper and was intolerant toward failure. The therapist can assume that these values and behavior patterns have not changed drastically. In fact, the clinician might expect that these attitudes might at times be exaggerated until Mary has adjusted to her disability, or they may even be retained forever. Her temper and intolerance toward failure need to be considered when establishing a treatment protocol. Success will be critical to motivate Mary in a rehabilitation setting, and her temper should help the therapist regulate the success/failure ratio and thus the task variation used during treatment.

Just as the affective domain influences and is influenced by the cognitive-perceptual systems, the somatomotor area affects and is affected by the first two systems. The entire evaluation process may begin by using a functional ADL form. Answers can also be found to questions in the other areas of the profile. In actuality, all areas should be addressed simultaneously while focus is placed on a specific impairment, such as state of the motor pool, postural integrity, muscle strength, synergy dominance, and so on. If during a functional task Mary can remember a three-step sequence in the arms or the legs but not a six-step sequence of arms and legs together might suggest a temporal sequencing problem and that further evaluation is indicated to determine the degree of difficulty. Although this problem is perceptual-cognitive, it would severely hamper motor performance. If Mary were unable to perform a relatively simple perceptual-motor sequence as identified in the task of rolling over from a supine position, the frustration she would feel when asked to do a standing pivot transfer might be enormous. Although rolling in horizontal is a very different motor program than the vertical stand-pivot transfer, the complexity of the transfer requires many more components of the motor system to interlock and function together. Rolling does not require the same degree of motor control, even though in some patients it may be a more difficult plan. If Mary simultaneously was obligated or limited to certain patterns of movement, she may have difficulty performing successfully either functional task. The interaction of a reflex pattern such as the ATNR and Mary's poor temporal sequencing might limit the number of ADL tasks she would be asked to perform. Her intolerance to failure should alert the therapist to avoid test items in which there is a great likelihood for failure.

Answers to questions in the motor area of the profile should direct the clinician to areas in which Mary can succeed, areas in which she will definitely fail, and areas that are still doubtful. That is, Mary may be able to perform any three- or four-step sequence in prone and supine positions but will have difficulty changing positions due to a central pattern generator's response to external stimuli such as turning of the head. Sitting activities are limited as a result of the visual-perceptual distortions of verticality and their influence over muscle tone in the vertical position. Standing, ambulation, and complex ADL tasks, such as dressing, should be considered extremely difficult because of the multitudinous impairments within the motor system, the complex sequencing of the tasks, and the complex interaction of muscle function in all parts of the body during these complex activities. Selection of these tasks as treatment procedures to make the client feel more normal may in reality clearly identify her disability, may cause extreme frustration and anger, and may dissolve the client/therapist rapport. Identifying motor activities or functional activities that Mary can run independently without contrived therapeutic intervention should help motivate her to continue to learn as well as regain functional control over her motor system.

Once the therapist has a clear understanding of the client's strengths and weaknesses, specific clinical problems can be identified and treatment procedures selected that allow flexibility in treatment sessions. Many treatment suggestions for various problems can be found in Chapters 8 through 33.

Visual-Analytical Problem Solving

The last section of this chapter deals with a specific type of problem-solving strategy that has definite clinical significance: the area of visual-analytical problem solving (VAPS).

Problem solving has become a major issue in professional development, and the question arises as to whether all problem-solving strategies are the same. Some strategies may be more appropriate for clinical performance and others more relevant to academic achievement. The answer is still hypothetical, because no empirical research has been found that addresses all these specific questions. However, at least one research study was undertaken to identify a particular problem-solving strategy that seems to have important clinical application.[45] VAPS is defined as the ability to look at a complex array of visual stimuli, identify the critical attributes, and then use appropriate strategies to solve simple to complex problems. The solution to those problems stems from the original visual information. The following is an example of the use of VAPS:

Mrs. J. sustained a closed-head injury 4 months ago and has just been referred to your rehabilitation center. She was brought down in a wheelchair and placed against the wall in between two other clients (complex array of simultaneous visual stimuli). She first turns to the right to look at another client, then turns to the left (successive and simultaneous visual stimuli). You note as you are treating another client that, as Mrs. J. turns her head (critical attributes of the visual array), she has strong changes in muscle tone and that she has an obligatory bilateral ATNR. From that information you could determine many difficulties and failures that would occur if you gave an ADL test to this individual.

One problem encountered when making the transition from an academic to a clinical environment is having intellectual knowledge but being unable to associate that knowledge with the simultaneous and ongoing observation and palpation conducted in the clinic. Therefore, many therapists believe that information learned in the classroom is irrelevant to the clinical environment. Another problem some students face is the frustration of working with a highly gifted therapist who cannot verbalize what is being done or why it works but can demonstrate the behavior or technique extremely well. A plausible explanation for problems of transference is that part of the high-level problem solving needed in the clinic is based on a nonverbal strategy. To communicate this nonverbal, visual-analytical model, one must translate it into verbal language; and this is very difficult because visual-analytical thought is both simultaneous and sequential. For example, a therapist who pictures a client progressing through a transfer from the wheelchair to the bathtub might visualize the activity as if observing the client from the front, the side, the back, or even from above. In fact, visualizing the movement from all directions gives additional information regarding the behavioral aspect of the client's transfer abilities. There is no rule to tell the therapist from which direction to order such visualization. The combined visualizations make up the total picture, and it is the total picture that is important. Language, on the other hand, is dominated by rules. Those rules are specific and have very clearly defined temporal sequencing. Thus, translating a simultaneous process occurring internally into a temporal sequence to discuss all components changes the consistency of the thought process. Reflecting back on the original problem, a student would need to translate theoretical knowledge that has definite temporal rules into a simultaneous process observed in the clinic. The student must recognize that many gifted therapists cannot explain verbally what they know spatially. Therefore, when asked to explain the treatment procedure, they translate only fragments of the whole, which is often of little help to the student.

A similar example would be taking a picture of a beautiful sunrise over a huge mountain range while the photographer sits at the mouth of a large lake that is absorbed into the mountain landscape. The photographer is engrossed with the whole experience. The totality of the multisensory, three-dimensional emotional interaction needs to be caught forever in the picture. When the picture is developed, the photographer discovers that the camera was unable to capture the whole. In fact, it recorded only a small portion of the original scene. The disappointed photographer may try to explain to friends who are looking at the picture what was really occurring, which would probably lead to frustration and a comment such as, "well, you just had to be there."

To perceive the clinical implications of visual-analytical problem solving, understanding of its sequential steps is paramount. Although this concept tends to use a nonverbal mode of thought, it is not suggested that language be omitted from this strategy. Indeed, language may be critical in storage and retrieval of these images from memory. Development of the sequence seems to be hierarchical, consisting of three general categories: (1) visual recognition, (2) spatial orientation, and (3) spatial transformation.

The first step, visual recognition, implies the ability to recognize key attributes of the visual array and pull out those pieces of information necessary to begin to solve problems. Obviously, this means clinicians need to have mastery of visual information relevant to their professional responsibilities. Students often have difficulty generalizing information obtained at this level of visual recognition. An example would be a student who learns to evaluate the strength of the quadriceps muscle in a sitting position and thus assumes that this is the only position in which the strength of the muscle can be tested. Or, if students study a reflex such as the ATNR and visually learn the motor pattern, they often hold the visual image of a child in the ATNR pattern. That is, they are unable to recognize the ATNR pattern in adults who demonstrate the same programmed response. The student stores the visual recognition with tremendous restrictions and thus limits clinical application of that information.

If visual content in one spatial position has been mastered, the second phase of the sequence, spatial orientation, can be addressed. This strategy requires identification of the key visual elements in various spatial planes. For example, if the clinical problem required the therapist to recognize an ATNR in sitting, four-point, and standing positions, a spatial orientation strategy would be used, which can easily be applied in the clinic. For instance, a therapist may be giving an ADL evaluation and may ask Mrs. J. to transfer in and out of the tub to the right. She fails because she is unable to bend her hip and knee to clear the tub while she is looking at her knee or its placement in the activity. One therapist might identify only that Mrs. J. failed to transfer to the right, thus deciding that the best strategy would be to teach her to transfer to the left: a compensatory skill. A second therapist might realize that Mrs. J. failed because she has a dominant ATNR to the right. The second clinician not only identified that Mrs. J. failed but also why she failed. Knowing the reason gives the therapist freedom to select alternative treatment programs, such as teaching the client to modify the influence of the ATNR in tub transfer to the right, thereby eliminating the need for teaching a compensatory strategy. This would also be true in all ADL activities that require head turning, such as dressing, eating, and climbing into a car. Recognition of the ATNR in sitting position is a spatial orientation strategy because the therapist has gone beyond recognizing this reflex in the supine position. This second stage requires that the clinician visually recognize behavioral patterns in the three-dimensional external world. An important key to successful use of this strategy is allowing oneself the visual freedom to see what is actually present instead of preconceiving and then cognitively altering what one is seeing. Having predetermined questions relevant to specific clinical problems is an important aspect of problem solving. Having preconceived answers limits the flexibility of the clinician, decreases alternatives to treatment planning, and often limits the potential of the client.

The third stage, spatial transformation, requires a higher degree of spatial analysis. Up to this point, internalizing complex spatial or visual images was not necessary, although some imagery may have been used. That is, many people use compensatory verbal strategies to try to interpret what is being seen in the external world. Spatial visualization implies first that complex visual images are being manufactured within the mind of the observer. Then the individual must transpose one image on top of another or, while looking at one image, transform it (through the CNS), enabling the observer to view it simultaneously from a different position. For example, a woman may be looking at a picture of a lake in the mountains. If within her CNS she could form an image of that picture as if she were on the other side of the lake looking across the lake and at herself, then that would be visualization transformation.

A clinical example of spatial transformation is knowing a client has an ATNR to the right from observing that individual's behavior in a sitting position and being able to transpose that behavior into a visual image of a transfer activity and determine at what point in the transfer the client would have difficulty or would fail. This could be accomplished before confronting the client with that task. If a therapist knows a client is going to fail, there is little reason to attempt the task. Thus, an evaluation could be used to maintain an environment that provides positive reinforcement.

This type of spatial thought process involves visually breaking down the observed environment into its component parts and then progressing visually through each component. The clinician is also confronted with less complex clinical problems. If, simultaneously, a total picture of the client can be maintained, then a high-level clinical problem-solving strategy has been achieved. This manipulation of total-to-part to total-to-part is considered a highly integrated cortical function requiring both hemispheres.[40] An example is a clinician who recognizes that as Janie walks across the floor she is using a combination of the ATNR, symmetrical tonic neck reflex (STNR), positive supporting reactions, static postural tone, and moderate equilibrium reactions. The combination of tonal patterns creates a bizarre movement sequence that cannot be explained as a single act. Yet, when the act is broken into components, the summative tonal response resulting from the combined influence of the various patterns and reactions and their respective external stimuli clearly explains the abnormal movement sequence. Treating each component problem separately and recombining the newly learned normal strategies lead to a more normalized gait pattern. That is, the whole is observed, the parts are detected and treated, and then the whole is reassembled in a new order to allow better functions. From a motor learning perspective this might be considered a whole-to-part-to-whole learning sequence.

The development of visual-spatial strategies for use in visual-analytical problem solving is not specifically taught in schools. Yet these skills may provide an explanation of what is often called a therapist's intuitive gift. Academicians are beyond the point of accepting the premise that all problem-solving strategies are the same. Identifying in the next decade which problem-solving strategies lead to high-level clinical performance is a major objective for health care professionals. Learning such skills before entry into a clinical setting should ease the transition between the highly verbal environment of the classroom and the highly visual and kinesthetic environment in the clinic. How to develop this skill depends on the student's preferential learning styles and ability to change learning styles when necessary.

Some general suggestions can help all learners. The first step is to master visual content of normal movement and postural patterns. Pictures or slides, where the visual stimuli can be held for extended periods of time, help the learner identify specific patterns without the demand of recognizing the pattern in a movement sequence. Next, the visual strategy should be mastered during a movement pattern. This requires recognition of key visual elements while additional simultaneous and successive visual input is present. When this is accomplished in one spatial position, the same problems should be practiced in all spatial positions. Viewing videotapes or movies of individuals in a clinical setting can practice this second strategy.

The third strategy, visual transformation, requires the ability to internalize those images recognized in the first two stages. This can be practiced externally before the learner is asked to internalize two sequential images, place them on top of each other, and visualize the summative effect. Slide frames of a normal movement pattern can be taken and placed in front of the learner. A second visual input—such as the presence of a stimulus for the ATNR, as well as the response pattern—can be drawn, pictured on film, or discussed to help the learner visualize it internally. The end product of the second pattern can then be overlaid on the first sequence. At some time the motor response may coincide with the desired effect; at another time the stimulus for the second response may not be present in the first movement pattern. Finally, with the stimulus present, the desired response of the first pattern may conflict with that of the second, and thus the summative effect would cause deviation from normal movement. This strategy of summating externally two or more response patterns can then be practiced with internal visualization. The use of language to clarify visual images should help the learner make the transition from verbal to visual-spatial thought. Feeling and observing tonal changes in the client while visualizing what these total patterns look like should also help the learner begin to develop some of these higher-level visual-spatial strategies.

CONCLUSION

The fourth edition of this textbook hopes to project the reader into the clinical practice of the twenty-first century. As the professions continue to evolve in depth and breathe, the future will encapsulate the knowledge, skill, and lessons of the past and the needs and problems of present and immediate health delivery systems while maintaining unique scopes and parameter of practice in an ever-changing environment. The professions must adapt and embrace change without losing the integrity and philosophical reasons why they came into existence. The only concept that is guaranteed in the future is change. Both physical and occupational therapy are dynamic professions with the ability to adapt and evolve to provide the health care service expected and deserved by the consumer. The future is up to every practitioner. The consumer of our services is dependent on our willingness to learn, adapt and provide the best service, for the least cost with the best outcomes. We have done that in the past and are doing it in the present, and there is little reason to anticipate a change in that direction in the future.

REFERENCES

1. Alexander DA: Yes, but what about the patient? Physiotherapy 59:391–394, 1973.
2. American Occupational Therapy Association: Standards of practice for occupational therapy in schools. Am J Occup Ther 34:900–903, 1980.
3. American Physical Therapy Association: Guide to physical therapy practice. Phys Ther 77:1163–1650, 1997.
4. Ayers AJ: Sensory Integration and Learning Disabilities. Los Angeles, Western Psychological Services, 1972.
5. Barr J (coordinator): Curriculum Planning Workshop, Midwinter Combined American Physical Therapy Association Sections Meeting, Washington, DC, 1976.
6. Becker M, Maiman L: Sociobehavioral determinants of compliance with health and medical care recommendation. Med Care 13:10–24, 1975.
7. Bertakis K: The communication of information from physician to patient: A method for increasing patient practice. J Fam Pract 5:217–222, 1977.
8. Byl NN, Duncan MS, Lewton DA, et al: Characteristics of physician referrals to physical therapists. JSOPTA, in review.
9. Carlson RJ: Holism and reductionism as perspectives in medicine and patient care. West J Med 131:466–470, 1979.
10. Cronback LJ, Snow RE: Aptitudes and Instructional Methods. New York, Irvington Publishers, 1977.
11. Des Marchais JE, Dumais B, Pigeon G: From traditional to problem-based learning: A case report of complete curriculum reform. Med Educ 26:190–199, 1992.
12. El-Din DJ, Smith GJ: The DEP Model of Documentation 1998. (Available from WA Cheney, Department of Physical Therapy, Eastern Washington University, 99004.)
13. Fink D: Holistic health: The evolution of western medicine. In Flynn P (ed): The Healing Continuum. Bowie, MD, Robert J. Brady Co, 1980.
14. Foster MA: Family systems theory as a framework for problem solving in pediatric physical therapy. Pediatr Phys Ther 3(2):70–73, 1992.
15. Freymann JG: Medicine's great schism, prevention vs. cure: An historical interpretation. Med Care 13:525–536, 1975.
16. Hayes KW: The effect of awareness of measurement error on physical therapists' confidence in their decisions. Phys Ther 72:515–525, 1992.
17. Hayes KW, Sullivan JE, Huber G: Computer-based patient management problems in an entry level physical therapy program. J Phys Ther Educ 1(5):65–71, 1991.
18. Hunt DE: Matching models in education, Ontario Institute for Students in Education Monograph Series No. 10, Toronto, Ontario, 1974.
19. Joyce B, Weil M: Models of Teaching. Englewood Cliffs, NJ, Prentice-Hall, 1972.
20. Keith RA, Hamilton BB, Sherwin FS: The Functional Independence Measure: A New Tool for Rehabilitation. New York, Springer, 1987.
21. Leopold RL: Patient-therapist relationship: Psychological considerations. Phys Ther 34:8–13, 1954.
22. Levin L: Forces and issues in the revival of interest in self-care impetus for redirection in health. Health Educ Monogr 5:115, (summer) 1977.
23. Magistro C et al: Diagnosis in physical therapy: A roundtable discussion. PT Magazine 1(6):58–65, 1993.
24. May BJ: An integrated problem-solving curriculum design for physical therapy education. Phys Ther 57:807–815, 1977.
25. McKay S: Holistic health care: Challenge to providers, J Allied Health 9:194–201, 1980.
26. McNerney WJ: The missing link in health services. J Med Educ 50:11–23, 1975.
27. Moore JC: The limbic system. Workshop presented in San Francisco, February 1980.
28. Moore JC: Neuroanatomical structures subserving learning and memory. In Fifteenth Annual Sensorimotor Integration Symposium, San Diego, July 1987.
29. Moyers PA: The guide to occupational therapy practice. Am J Occup Ther 53(3), 1999.
30. Nagi S: Some Conceptual Issues in Disability and Rehabilitation. Washington, DC, American Sociological Association, 1965.
31. Nagi S: Disability Concepts Revisited: Implication for Prevention, Washington, DC, National Academy Press, 1991.
32. Norton BJ: Report on colloquium on teaching clinical decision making. J Phys Ther Educ 6(2):58–66, 1992.
33. Payton OD: Patient participation in program planning: A manual for therapists. Philadelphia, FA Davis, 1990.

34. Pew Health Professions Commission: Healthy America: Practitioners for 2005. San Francisco, University of California, 1991.

35. Pratt JW: A psychological view of the physiotherapist's role. Physiotherapy 64:241–242, 1978.

36. Rogers C: A humanistic concept of man. In Farsom R (ed): Science and Human Affairs. Palo Alto, CA, Science and Behavior Books, 1965.

37. Sasano E et al: The family in physical therapy. JAPTA 57:153–159, 1977.

38. Saward E, Sorenson A: The current emphasis on preventive medicine. Science 200:889–894, 1978.

39. Schmidt HG: The psychological basis of problem-based learning: A review of the evidence. Acad Med 67:557–565, 1992.

40. Schmidt RA: Motor Control and Learning: A Behavior Emphasis, 2nd ed. Champaign, IL, Human Kinetics, 1988.

41. Shipp KM: Clinical decision making: Osteoporosis to manage fragility. PT Magazine 1(10):70–77, 1993.

42. Singleton M: Profession—a paradox? JAPTA 60:439, 1980.

43. Szasz TS, Hollender MH: A contribution to the philosophy of medicine. Arch Intern Med 97:585–592, 1956.

44. Umphred D: Teaching, Thinking and Treatment Planning. Unpublished master's thesis. Boston, Boston University, July 1971.

45. Umphred D: Visual Analytical Problem Solving. Unpublished doctoral dissertation. Syracuse, NY, Syracuse University, 1978.

46. Weinstein CJ: Movement science: Its relevance to physical therapy. Phys Ther 70:759–762, 1990.

47. Wood P: International Classification of Impairments, Disabilities & Handicaps (ICIDH). Geneva, Switzerland, World Health Organization, 1980.

Differential Diagnosis Phase 1: Medical Screening for the Therapist

WILLIAM G. BOISSONNAULT, MSc, PT, DPT • DARCY A. UMPHRED, PhD, PT

Key Words

– Differential Diagnosis Phase 1

– Differential Diagnosis Phase 2

– medical screening

– referral

– systems screening

Objectives

After reading this chapter the student/therapist will:

1. Identify the difference between Differential Diagnosis Phase 1, medical screening, and Phase 2, diagnosis of impairments and disabilities.

2. Analyze the concept for system and subsystem screening.

3. Develop a mechanism for system screening to be used with clients with preexisting neurological dysfunction.

4. Comprehend the significance and importance of medically screening all clients interacting in a therapeutic environment with an occupational or physical therapist.

Traditionally, the term *differential diagnosis* has referred to a process used by physicians to diagnose disease. This process typically involves three distinct steps. Step 1 is taking a thorough history, including an investigation of the patient's medical history, presenting complaints, and a review of systems. Step 2 is the performance of the physical examination. This history and the findings of the physical examination will lead to a diagnosis or to step 3: the identification of necessary tests, including laboratory tests, diagnostic imaging modalities, and so on. The goal of the three steps is the formulation of a specific diagnosis that will lead to the implementation of the appropriate medical treatment.

Although physical therapists (PTs) and occupational therapists (OTs) have long relied on examination findings to determine if a patient should be referred to a physician or to develop an appropriate treatment plan, the use of the term *differential diagnosis* is relatively new for both professions. For PTs, the differential diagnostic process fits within the Patient/Client Management Model described in *The Guide to Physical Therapist Practice*[1] (Fig. 2–1). The therapist attempts to organize the history and physical examination (including tests and measures) findings into clusters, syndromes, or categories. There are certain clusters of findings that suggest the presence of

disease and warrant communication with a physician. There are other symptoms and signs that are consistent with conditions that fit the disablement framework. These conditions are inherent in the interrelationships between impairments, functional limitations, and disability and are appropriate for physical or occupational therapy interventions.[1, 8, 9, 11] The process of differentiating the cluster of findings that warrant communication with a physician regarding concerns about a patient's health status versus those that do not will be called Differential Diagnosis Phase 1.[12] If the decision is reached that the symptoms and signs do fall within the scope of practice of PTs and OTs, a second level of differential diagnosis occurs. Now the therapist attempts to categorize the examination findings into the specific diagnostic categories that will specifically guide the choice of treatment interventions and the development of a prognosis. This second level of diagnosis is called Differential Diagnosis Phase 2[12] and is the focus of Chapters 3 and 4. Figure 2–2 illustrates where Differential Diagnosis Phase 1 and Phase 2 fit into the Patient/Client Management Model.

The purpose of this chapter is to discuss the medical screening components associated with Differential Diagnosis Phase 1, including identification of health risk factors, recognizing atypical symptoms and signs, and review

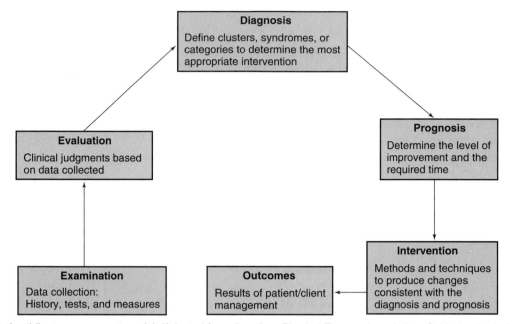

FIGURE 2–1. Patient/client management model. (Adapted from American Physical Therapy Association: Guide to physical therapist practice. Phys Ther 77:1180, 1997, with permission of the American Physical Therapy Association.)

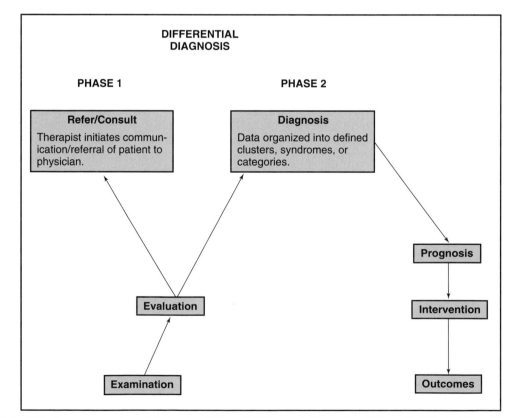

FIGURE 2–2. Patient/client management model showing Differential Diagnosis Phase 1 and Phase 2. (Adapted from Umphred DA: Chair, Diagnostic Task Force, State of California, 1996–2000. California Chapter of American Physical Therapy Association.)

of systems. Methods to collect this information during a patient examination are also presented. Patient cases are used to illustrate the important medical screening principles.

DIFFERENTIAL DIAGNOSIS PHASE 1: MEDICAL SCREENING

As opposed to Phase 2, the goal of Differential Diagnosis Phase 1 is NOT to formulate a specific diagnosis. In fact, labeling a cluster of examination findings when referring a patient to a physician because of health status concerns (e.g., peptic ulcer disease, endometriosis) could place the therapist outside the scope of his or her practice. Formulating such a diagnosis is not necessary to meet the responsibility of identifying when the patient's needs appear to fall beyond the scope of the therapist's practice or expertise. Recognizing symptoms and signs more suggestive of disease and communicating these findings to the patient's physician is necessary to meet our profes-

sional responsibilities. It is then up to the physician to rule out the presence of specific disease entities.

The purpose of the therapist's medical screening is to (1) identify existing medical conditions, (2) identify symptoms and signs suggesting that an existing medical condition is worsening, (3) identify neurological manifestations that suggest an acute or life-threatening crisis, and (4) identify symptoms and signs suggestive of the presence of an occult disease. This medical screening takes place within the framework of an established PT's or OT's examination. Figure 2–3 is an example of an examination scheme leading to the decision of treating the patient, treating AND referring the patient, or referring the patient. The following material focuses on the components of this scheme most directly related to the medical screening process.

Identifying Patients at Risk

An important aspect of the medical screening process is identifying existing health risk factors. There are numer-

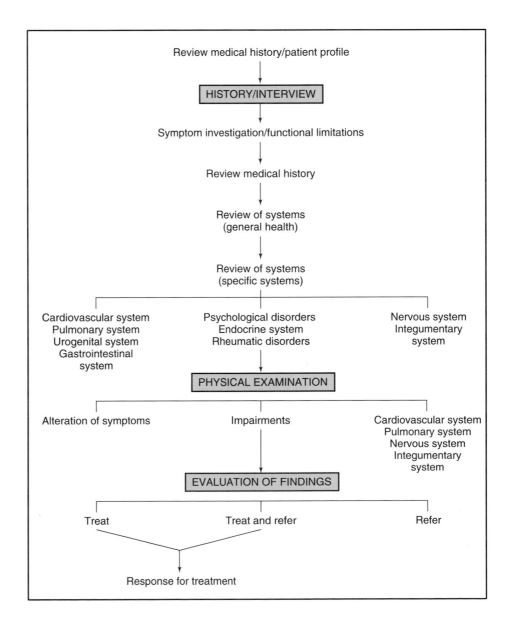

FIGURE 2–3. Patient examination scheme. (Taken from notes from course by WG Boissonnault, 1998.)

Medical History Questionnaire

Name:_____ Age _____

SS#: _____ Occupation: _____

Leisure activities: _____

I. Are you currently being seen by any of the following professionals:

A. General medical doctor (MD)	Yes	No
B. Medical specialist (MD)	Yes	No
If yes: please specify _____		
C. Osteopathic doctor	Yes	No
D. Physical/occupational therapist	Yes	No
E. Chiropractor	Yes	No
F. Psychiatrist/psychologist	Yes	No
G. Alternative medical practitioner	Yes	No
If yes: please specify _____		

If you have been seen by any of the above practitioners within the last year, please discuss the reasons:

_____
_____
_____

II. Have you EVER been diagnosed as having the following condition(s)?

A. Stroke	Yes	No
B. Seizure disorders	Yes	No
C. Migraines	Yes	No
D. Other neurologic problems:	Yes	No
Specify _____		
E. Depression	Yes	No
F. Cancer: Specify _____	Yes	No
G. High blood pressure	Yes	No
H. Heart condition	Yes	No
I. Emphysema	Yes	No
J. Asthma	Yes	No
K. Tuberculosis	Yes	No
L. Diabetes	Yes	No
M. Rheumatoid arthritis	Yes	No
N. Other arthritic disease	Yes	No
O. Kidney disease	Yes	No
P. Anemia	Yes	No
Q. Hepatitis	Yes	No
R. Circulatory problems	Yes	No
S. Thyroid problems	Yes	No
T. Skin problems	Yes	No
U. Digestive problems	Yes	No
V. Bowel or bladder problems	Yes	No
W. Chemical dependency (e.g., alcoholism)	Yes	No
X. Unexplained falls	Yes	No
Y. Cognitive dysfunction	Yes	No
Z. Genetic disorders	Yes	No
AA. Other _____	Yes	No

Please list all surgeries/hospitalizations including dates and reasons.

Date   Surgery/hospitalization/reason

_____ _____
_____ _____

Are you being or have you been treated for musculoskeletal injuries (fracture, dislocations, repetitive strains, joint instability)? If so, please state:

Date   Injury

_____ _____
_____ _____

Are you being or have you been treated for neuromuscular problems (weakness, pain, spasticity, incoordination, dizziness, tremor)? If so, please state:

Date   Injury

_____ _____
_____ _____

Has anyone in your immediate family (parents, sisters, brothers) ever been treated for any of the following:

A. Stroke	Yes	No
B. Seizure disorders	Yes	No
C. Parkinson's disease	Yes	No
D. Multiple sclerosis	Yes	No
E. Other neurologic problems _____	Yes	No
F. Mental illness	Yes	No
G. Cancer	Yes	No
H. High blood pressure	Yes	No
I. Heart condition	Yes	No
J. Breathing problems	Yes	No
K. Diabetes	Yes	No
L. Arthritic disease	Yes	No
M. Kidney disease	Yes	No
N. Anemia	Yes	No
O. Vascular problems	Yes	No
P. Thyroid problems	Yes	No
Q. Skin problems	Yes	No
R. Chemical dependency (e.g., alcoholism)	Yes	No
S. Learning disabilities	Yes	No
T. Cognitive dysfunction	Yes	No
U. Genetic disorders	Yes	No

Please list any PRESCRIPTION medications you are currently taking (include pills, injections, patches, etc.)

_____
_____
_____
_____

Please list any OVER-THE-COUNTER MEDICATIONS you are taking:

_____
_____
_____
_____

Please list any *prescriptions* or *over-the-counter* medications you were taking prior to your current problems

_____
_____
_____

How much caffeinated coffee or other caffeinated beverages do you drink per day? (number of cups/cans/bottles) _____

Do you smoke?   Yes   No
  If yes: How many packs per day?   _____

Do you drink alcohol?
  If yes: How many days per week
     do you drink?   _____   days/week
  If yes: How many drinks per sitting? _____ drinks/sitting
     (Note: one beer or one glass of wine equals 1 drink)

If you use marijuana or other
  substances, how often?   _____   days/week

FIGURE 2–4. Self-administered questionnaire to collect medical history information. (Adapted from Boissonnault WG, Koopmeiners MB: Medical history profile: Orthopaedic physical therapy outpatients. J Orthop Sports Phys Ther 20 [2]:2–10, 1994. with permission of the Orthopaedic and Sports Sections of the American Physical Therapy Association.)

ous factors that increase the risk of developing disease, including age, sex, race, occupation, leisure activities, pre-existing medical conditions, medication usage (over-the-counter and prescription drugs), family medical history, tobacco use, and substance abuse.

Of these, a personal history of an existing medical condition and a positive family history (e.g., mother and aunt with a history of breast cancer, father diagnosed with prostate cancer at the age of 58 years) are the most relevant risk factors for the potential presence of an occult condition. In addition, often the history of a previous episode of depression, for example, significantly increases the risk of having a second episode compared with the risk of someone who has never had an episode of depression having an initial episode.[2] The greater the number of existing risk factors, the more vigilant the therapist should be for the presence of clinical manifestations suggestive of disease and the more extensive the other medical screening components will need to be.

There are different methods to collect this medical history/patient profile information, including a review of the medical record and use of a self-administered questionnaire. Figure 2–4 is an example of a self-administered questionnaire that could be completed by the patient, a family member, and/or a caregiver. As noted in Figure 2–3, a review of this information before beginning the examination should occur if possible. The therapist will have a head start in terms of organizing the history and physical examination, knowing what to prioritize and at least initially what parts of the examination can be deemphasized.

Affirmative answers to previous/current illnesses should direct the therapist to consider what the potential impact may be on the patient's complaints, choice of examination and treatment techniques, rehabilitation potential, and risk for additional illness. For example, the presence of existing chronic kidney disease should alert the therapist to numerous potential complications. Chronic renal failure could result in fatigue, weakness, and impaired concentration, all of which could interfere with rehabilitation efforts. Chronic renal failure could also result in paresthesia and muscle weakness, which could mistakenly be associated with other neurological conditions. Osteoporosis can also be associated with chronic renal failure. This potential association should direct the therapist to use techniques that carry reduced risk of skeletal injury. A series of follow-up questions for the affirmative answers will assist the therapist in determining the relevance (if any) of each item (Fig. 2–5 for examples of follow-up questions for some of the information categories).

Having the self-administered questionnaire completed before the scheduled time of the initial visit will improve the therapist's efficiency. Mailing the questionnaire to the patient before the visit or having the patient arrive 10 to 15 minutes before the appointment would allow for the form being completed without taking time away from the actual examination itself. Once completed, taking 1 to 2 minutes to scan the questionnaire should be all that is necessary for the therapist to begin formulating questions and organizing the physical examination.

Symptom Investigation

A significant aspect of the medical screening process involves the interpretation of a patient's description of symptoms, functional limitations, and the physical examination findings. Descriptions of symptoms associated with neuromusculoskeletal impairments (loss or abnormality of

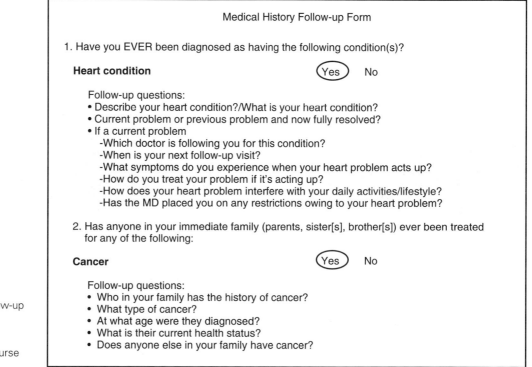

FIGURE 2–5. Potential follow-up questions for affirmative answers on the self-administered questionnaire. (From WG Boissonnault, course notes, 1998.)

physiological, psychological, or anatomical structure or function) generally reveal a fairly consistent and predictable pattern of onset and change over a 24-hour period. In addition, the neurological and musculoskeletal impairments noted during the physical examination should match up with the functional limitations described by the patient or the caregiver. If these expectations are not met, it does not necessarily mean the patient has cancer or infection, but doubt should be raised on the therapist's part whether therapy is indicated.

Patients who are not aware of how a condition appropriate for therapy should present may seek therapy experiencing symptoms that are better addressed by a physician as opposed to a PT or OT. For example, Mr. S. suffered a cardiovascular accident 6 months ago with resultant mild residual left hemiplegia. At the time of discharge from rehabilitation services he was independent in all activities of daily living, but residual left upper extremity weakness remained. When visiting his internist for a routine checkup, he complained that over the past 3 weeks, he had lost some functional skills, including having difficulty with self-care. The physician then referred Mr. S. to your clinic for evaluation and treatment. Mr. S. states he has been less active and just needs some help regaining his motor function. During the history he states he is experiencing a deep, dull, aching sensation in the lower lumbar spine and right buttock. He assumes it has developed due to his inactivity and thus saw no reason to bother the physician with this problem. As Mr. S.

continues to describe his difficulties, he also notes a constant deep ache in the right shoulder that he relates to increased use of his right arm to compensate for the left arm weakness. The physical examination of the low back, pelvis, and right shoulder reveals that the existing symptoms do not vary with active/passive range of motion, resisted testing, or postural holding. In addition, quantity of motion is normal for these regions and motor programming appears intact. At this point you cannot explain the symptoms from an impairment standpoint; therefore, depending on other examination findings, including the patient profile and medical history, communication with the internist may be warranted. The following information describes some of the subcategories associated with symptom investigation.

Location of Symptoms

A body diagram can be a valuable tool to document location of symptoms expressed verbally or nonverbally by patients with identified neurological deficits. Besides pain and altered sensation, patterns of abnormal tone, asymmetrical posturing, and areas of weakness can also be noted on the body diagram (Fig. 2–6). Numerous body structures are potential pain generators, including visceral structures. Figure 2–7 and Table 2–1 illustrate local and referred pain patterns from various visceral organs. The fact there is so much overlap between pain location associated with visceral disease and neuromusculoskeletal

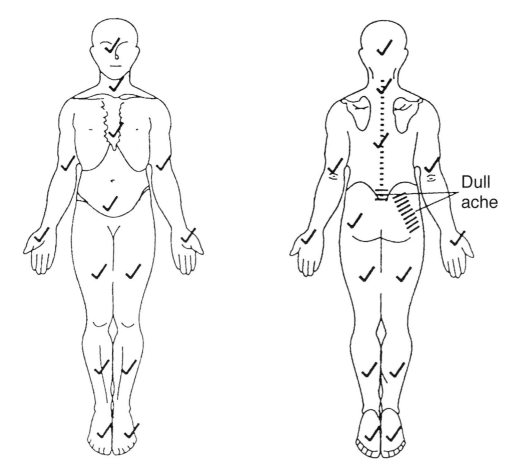

Dull ache

FIGURE 2–6. Body diagram illustrating symptom location. Body areas with no known symptoms or abnormalities are marked with a "check" mark. (From Boissonnault WG [ed]: Examination in Physical Therapy Practice—Screening for Medical Disease, 2nd ed. New York, Churchill Livingstone, 1995.)

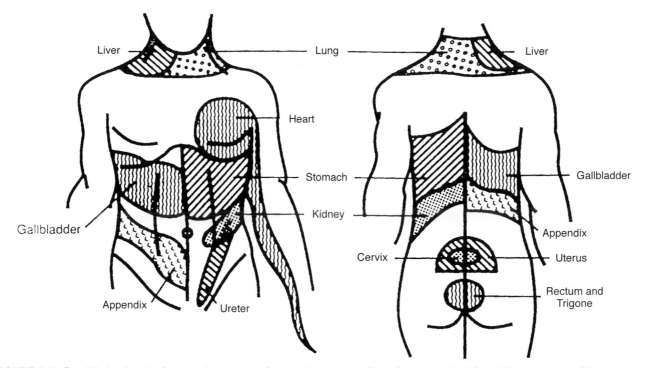

FIGURE 2–7. Possible local and referred pain patterns of visceral structures. (From Boissonnault WG [ed]: Examination in Physical Therapy Practice—Screening for Medical Disease, 2nd ed. New York, Churchill Livingstone, 1995.)

conditions results in this information alone being of minimal use in differentiating musculoskeletal from nonmusculoskeletal conditions. Being familiar with the visceral pain patterns will be extremely important, however, when deciding which body systems to screen during the review of systems.

24-Hour Report

Aspects of the patient's presenting complaint other than symptom location are very relevant to the differential diagnostic process, in particular the 24-hour report and the onset of symptoms. Pain, paresthesia, and numbness associated with neuromusculoskeletal impairments typically change in a consistent manner over a 24-hour period. The patient will report that the symptom intensity increases with the assumption of specific postures such as left side lying or sitting or with specific activities such as walking, driving, or 2 hours of computer work. Conversely, patients typically can relate paresthesia or pain relief with avoiding certain postures or activities, the assumption of certain postures, wearing an arm sling, and so on. If the pattern of symptom aggravation and alleviation is that there is no consistent pattern such as pain that comes and goes independent of the patient's posture, activities, or time of day or paresthesia or pain that moves from one body region to another inconsistent with common pain referral patterns or identified medical conditions, the therapist should start thinking whether physical or occupational therapy is what the patient truly needs.

History of Symptoms

The therapist must also scrutinize the patient's report of the onset of the symptoms. Pain and paresthesia/numb-ness associated with neuromusculoskeletal impairments typically can be related to trauma, either on a macro or a micro level or a medical event such as a cerebrovascular accident. More often than not it is repetitive overuse or cumulative trauma that leads to tissue breakdown and inflammation (see Chapter 12) Patients with neurological impairments resulting in postural abnormalities and abnormal movement patterns are at risk for such conditions. If a patient's symptoms are truly insidious, meaning not related to macro or micro trauma, or there has not been a significant change in activity level that reasonably accounts for the complaints, the therapist should again be concerned about the source of the symptoms. A worsening of symptoms (e.g., numbness, weakness, spasticity) associated with an existing medical condition should be investigated by the therapist with the same scrutiny; is there a reasonable explanation for the worsening? An increase in the intensity of the complaints or the involvement of additional body regions could signal a progression of the disease.

The physical examination including tests and measures also holds important clues related to the source of the symptoms and whether therapy is appropriate. The therapist should have expectations of physical examination findings based on the existing medical diagnosis and data from the history. There should be a correlation between the described functional limitations and the noted impairments. The right shoulder pain Mr. S. was experiencing is an example. One would have expected to be able to increase or decrease the intensity of the ache with palpation, movement assessment, or special tests. Not only was the therapist unable to alter the ache, but the shoulder motion and motor programming also appeared intact. Essentially there is nothing for the therapist to treat. The

TABLE 2-1. Visceral Pain Patterns

Structure	Segmental Innervation	Possible Areas of Pain Referral
Pelvic Organs		
Uterus including uterine ligaments	T10–L1, S2–4	Lumbosacral junction
		Sacral
		Thoracolumbar
Ovaries	T10–11	Lower abdominal
		Sacral
Testes	T10–11	Lower abdominal
		Sacral
Retroperitoneal Region		
Kidney	T10–L1	Lumbar spine (ipsilateral)
		Lower abdominal
		Upper abdominal
Ureter	T11–L2, S2–4	Groin
		Upper abdominal
		Suprapubic
		Medial, proximal thigh
		Thoracolumbar
Urinary bladder	T11–L2, S2–4	Sacral apex
		Suprapubic
		Thoracolumbar
Prostate gland	T11–L1, S2–4	Sacral
		Testes
		Thoracolumbar
Digestive System Organs		
Esophagus	T6–10	Substernal and upper abdominal
Stomach	T6–10	Upper abdominal
		Middle and lower thoracic spine
Small intestine	T7–10	Middle thoracic spine
Pancreas	T6–10	Upper abdominal
		Lower thoracic spine
		Upper lumbar spine
Gallbladder	T7–9	Right upper abdominal
		Right middle and lower thoracic spine, including caudal aspect scapula
Liver	T7–9	Right middle and lower thoracic spine
Common bile duct	T6–10	Upper abdominal
		Middle thoracic spine
Large intestine	T11–12	Lower abdominal
		Middle lumbar spine
Sigmoid colon	T11–12	Upper sacral
		Suprapubic
		Left lower quadrant of abdomen
Cardiopulmonary System		
Heart	T1–5	Cervical anterior
		Upper thorax
		Left upper extremity
Lungs and bronchi	T5–6	Ipsilateral thoracic spine
		Cervical (diaphragm involved)
Diaphragm (central portion)	C3–5	Cervical spine

Adapted from Boissonnault WG, Bass C: Pathological origins of trunk and neck pain: I. Pelvic and abdominal visceral disorders. J Orthop Sports Phys Ther 12:192–207, 1990, with permission of the Orthopaedic and Sports Sections of the American Physical Therapy Association.

inability to alter a patient's complaints and the lack of neuromusculoskeletal impairments one would expect with the medical diagnosis and the reported functional limitations should again raise concern about the source of the symptoms.

Review of Body Systems

The review of systems allows for a general screening of body systems for symptoms suggesting the presence of an adverse drug reaction, occult disease, or worsening of an existing medical condition. Suspicions of any of these scenarios would warrant communication with a physician. Checklists of symptoms and signs for each body system can be used by the physical and occupational therapist during the patient interview (see the box on page 40). To keep the checklists relatively short, the therapist should investigate presenting complaints/symptoms and the patient's medical history before the review of systems as noted in Figure 2–3. For example, on review of the cardiovascular system checklist in the following box, important items appear to be omitted, such as chest pain, claudication and a history of heart problems, hypertension, high cholesterol, and circulatory problems. If symptoms have already been investigated using a body diagram, one would already know if the patient has chest pain. If symptom change (aggravation or alleviation) over a 24-hour period has already been investigated, one would

TABLE 2-2. Linking Pain Patterns and Visceral Systems

Pain Location	Visceral Systems
Right shoulder (including shoulder girdle)	Pulmonary Cardiovascular Gastrointestinal
Left shoulder (including shoulder girdle)	Cardiovascular Pulmonary
Upper/midthoracic spine	Cardiovascular Pulmonary Gastrointestinal
Lower thoracic and upper/midlumbar spine	Peripheral vascular Pulmonary Gastrointestinal Urogenital
Lumbopelvic region	Gastrointestinal Urogenital Peripheral vascular

know if claudication was an issue. Finally, if the patient's medical history has already been discussed, one would know if heart problems, hypertension, or circulatory problems existed.

All of the checklists on page 40 need not be used for each and every patient. The location of symptoms will direct the therapist in deciding which checklists should be included in the initial examination. Figures 2–7 and Table 2–1 can be used to link pain location with visceral systems that could be the source of the complaints, and Table 2–2 provides a summary of potential pain locations and disease of the pulmonary, cardiovascular, gastrointestinal, and urogenital systems. Other symptom characteristics can also alert the therapist for the possible involvement of the endocrine, nervous, and psychological systems. Symptoms, including pain and paresthesias that come and go irrespective of posture, activity, or time of day and that appear to move among the various body regions can be associated with these systems as well as the visceral systems. Besides the location and characteristics of symptoms a patient's medical history will help the therapist decide which systems to screen. A positive medical history, such as a heart problem, would direct the therapist to investigate the patient's condition, including possible use of the cardiovascular checklist as well as the questions listed in Figure 2–5.

Use of a general health checklist (see box on page 41) can assist the therapist in prioritizing the inclusion of the checklists in the review of systems checklists box during the initial visit. The symptoms noted in this checklist can be associated with disease of most of the body's systems.

If the patient or caregiver (on the patient's behalf) replies yes to any of these items (as well as for the items in the review of systems checklists box the therapist must determine whether there is a reasonable explanation for the complaint and if the physician is aware of the complaint and, if so, has the complaint(s) worsened since the patient last saw the physician? When the explanation for the affirmative answer is not satisfactory, the physician is unaware of the complaint, or the symptom is worsening, communication with the physician is warranted. All of the checklists do not need to be covered during the initial

visit. If the patient says "no" for each of the general health items, the presenting complaints vary consistently over a 24-hour period, and the onset of the presenting complaints is explainable, the therapist can proceed with the evaluation of specific impairments and functional limitations with some confidence that therapy is appropriate and Differential Diagnosis Phase 2 is recommended. The review of systems takes on a lower priority. The result is that the therapist could decide to delay the use of the appropriate review of systems checklists until the patient's second or third visit. If the patient answers yes to general health items and presents with an inconsistent pain pattern, the appropriate review of systems takes on a higher priority and should be covered during the initial visit.

Integumentary System

Screening the integumentary system is not typically based on the presence or absence of pain, paresthesia, or numbness. As with the nervous system, some degree of screening of the integumentary system occurs with every patient regardless of the presenting diagnosis. Skin cancer has the highest incidence of all the cancers, and therapists generally see a number of exposed body areas during the postural assessment and regional examination that make up the physical examination. In fact, as noted in Figure 2–3, screening the skin begins during the history. During the interview the therapist can be looking at areas of exposed skin such as the face, neck, arms, and feet. As with screening the other body systems, the therapist's goal is not to identify a melanoma or differentiate squamous cell versus basal cell carcinoma but simply to identify skin lesions with atypical presentations. Once the patient is referred to the physician, disease will be ruled out or diagnosed. The box labeled "Skin Lesion Screening" on page 41 can be used to assess any mole or other skin marking. The items noted are atypical for a benign lesion.[10]

If the therapist notes any of these findings, and the patient reports a recent change in the size, color, or shape of the lesion and that a physician has not looked at the lesion, a referral would be warranted.

Besides skin lesions, abnormal general skin color can be a manifestation of a number of conditions. Table 2–3 summarizes abnormal skin color changes. Occasionally, some of the most obvious abnormalities are the most difficult to note when one is so focused on items more directly related to therapeutic intervention.

Nervous System

As with the integumentary system, the nervous system is screened for all patients. The review of systems checklists box includes items that provide a very general screening of the nervous system. The therapist should be vigilant for the presence of any of these items in all patients during the initial and subsequent visits. For patients with preexisting findings from this checklist, the therapist must be vigilant for a worsening of the symptoms. Covering the items in the nervous system checklist should add little time to the therapist's initial examination. Assessing for facial asymmetries and tremors can take place during the

REVIEW OF SYSTEMS CHECKLISTS

Cardiovascular

- dyspnea
- orthopnea
- palpitations
- pain with sweats
- syncope
- peripheral edema
- cough

Gastrointestinal

- difficulty with swallowing
- heartburn, indigestion
- specific food intolerance
- bowel dysfunction
  - color
  - frequency
  - shape/caliber
  - constipation/diarrhea
  - incontinence

Urogenital

- urinary
  - frequency
  - urgency
  - incontinence
  - reduced force of stream
  - difficulty initiating
  - dysuria
  - color
- reproductive: male
  - urethral discharge
  - impotence
  - dyspareunia
- reproductive: female
  - vaginal discharge
  - dyspareunia
  - change in menstruation
    - frequency and length of cycle
    - dysmenorrhea
    - blood flow
  - date of last period
  - number of pregnancies
  - number of deliveries
  - menopause

Psychological (Depression)

- depressed/irritable mood
- psychomotor agitation/retardation
- apathy
- sleep disturbance
- weight gain/loss
- fatigue
- feelings of worthlessness
- impaired concentration
- suicide ideation (recurrent)

Pulmonary

- dyspnea
- onset of cough
- change in cough
- sputum
- hemoptysis
- stridor
- wheezing

Nervous

- impaired balance
- impaired gross movement patterns
- impaired mentation
- tremors
- muscle atrophy
- asymmetrical facial features
  - facial contour
  - ptosis
  - pupil abnormalities
  - strabismus

Endocrine

- arthralgias
- myalgias
- neuropathies
- cold/heat intolerance
- skin/hair changes
- fatigue
- weight gain/loss
- polyuria
- polydipsia

---

interview. Observing balance, movement patterns, and muscle atrophy can occur while watching the patient ambulate into the examination area, during the interview, and as the patient changes positions during the physical examination. Lastly, impaired mentation may become apparent during the interview or the physical examination as the patient struggles to appropriately answer questions or follow directions.

The following patient case illustrates the importance of this general screening:

A 55-year-old elementary school teacher was referred with a diagnosis of cervical degenerative disk disease at C5–6 and C6–7. Her chief presenting complaint was posterior cervical aching and a sense of neck weakness. Functionally, the patient's primary concern was her increasingly difficult time making it through her work day. She taught first-grade students, so much of her work day was spent with her neck and trunk in a forward flexed position. The patient stated this persistent flexion posturing is a significant factor for the worsening of her symptoms as her work day progresses. As the interview continued, a tremor of the patient's right hand and forearm was

---

GENERAL HEALTH CHECKLIST

Fatigue
Malaise
Fever/chills/sweats
Nausea
Unexplained weight change
Unexplained paresthesia/numbness
Unexplained weakness
Unexplained cognitive and emotional changes

SKIN LESION SCREENING

Multi-variant color
Black or blue-black color
Friable tissue
Ulcerations
Irregular borders
Nondistinct ("fuzzy") borders
Six millimeters or larger in diameter
Asymmetrical shape

---

observed as the arm rested on her thigh. When questioned about the observed tremor she stated it started 4 or 5 months ago. She admitted the tremor appeared to be getting worse and that she did not mention it to the physician. There were no other positive neurological findings noted. After completing the initial examination the concern about the tremor was discussed and the patient consented to allow her primary care physician (the referring physician) to be called to discuss the finding. The physician facilitated a referral of the patient to a neurologist. Approximately 1 month later, after the neurology consultation and tests, the patient was diagnosed with Parkinson's disease. During that month the patient continued to receive physical therapy care for her cervical complaints.

DEPRESSION

Depression is a commonly encountered psychological disorder and is associated with significant morbidity and mortality.[2, 3, 5, 7] The review of systems checklists box (page 40) contains the checklist of items the therapist can use to help make the decision to refer a patient for consultation. If the patient presents with suicide ideation, the physician should be contacted before the patient leaves the clinic. For the first eight items on the depression checklist, concern should be raised when the therapist detects four to five of the items being present daily for a minimum of 2 weeks *and* the patient is having difficulty functioning at home, work, or school, socially, or in reha-

bilitation. Of the four to five items, one of them should be the depressed/irritable affect or apathy. An exception to the 2-week time frame is during periods of bereavement. When faced with a significant loss it will not be uncommon for people to experience a number of the checklist items as they go through the grieving process.[2] It is reasonable for these people to experience these symptoms for up to 2 months. A neurological event such as a cerebrovascular accident could easily trigger a major clinical depressive disorder, and the depression could significantly impede rehabilitation progress. The therapist may be in the position to facilitate a psychological consultation.

RESPONSE TO TREATMENT

Frequently during Differential Diagnosis Phase 1 the therapist will decide referral of the patient to a physician is not warranted and will proceed to Differential Diagnosis Phase 2. As treatment is initiated and progressed the therapist must remain vigilant for the appearance of symptoms and signs discussed throughout this chapter. In addition, correlating subjective and objective changes as treatment progresses will help the therapist decide if further intervention is warranted or referral back to the

---

● TABLE 2-3. Abnormal Color Changes of the Skin

Color Change	Physiological Change	Common Causes
White, pale (pallor)	Absence of pigment or pigment changes	Albinism (albinos), lack of sunlight
	Blood abnormality	Anemia, lead poisoning
	Temporary interruption or diversion of blood flow	Vasospasm, syncope, stress, internal bleeding
	Internal disease	Chronic gastrointestinal disease, cancer, parasitic disease, tuberculosis
Blue (cyanosis)	Decreased oxygen in blood (deoxyhemoglobin)	Methemoglobinemia (oxidation of hemoglobin), high blood iron level, cold exposure, vasomotor instability, cerebrospinal disease
Yellow	Jaundice, excess bilirubin in blood, excess bile pigment	Liver disease, gallstone blockage of bile duct, hepatitis (conjunctivae are also yellow)
	High levels of carotene in blood (carotenemia)	Ingestion of food high in carotene and vitamin A
Gray	High level of metals in body	Increased iron, bronze/gray; increased silver, blue/gray
Brown (hyperpigmentation)	Disturbances of adrenocortical hormones	Adrenal pituitary Addison disease

From Shapiro C, Skopit S: Screening for skin disorders. In Boissonnault WG (ed): Examination in Physical Therapy Practice—Screening for Medical Disease, 2nd ed. New York, Churchill Livingstone, 1995.

physician is appropriate. For example, if a patient reports a significant improvement or worsening, one would expect the therapist to note a corresponding change in posture, movement ability, palpatory findings, or neurological status. If the appropriate correlation between patient report and physical examination findings is not found, the therapist should begin considering that therapy may not be warranted. A careful review of systems and symptom investigation would again be necessary as part of the return to Differential Diagnosis Phase 1.

CONCLUSION

If all diseases presented as a high fever, hemoptysis, and blood in the urine, the medical screening process would be a simple one. Unfortunately, many diseases are initially manifested by subtle complaints, intermittent symptoms or mild pain, stiffness, and paresthesias. If these complaints are brought to a physician's attention by the patient, they often are not severe enough to warrant extensive diagnostic testing. Many patients simply ignore symptoms or physiological changes, rationalizing that everything is okay or it may be they simply do not like to see doctors or are too busy. All of the scenarios can account for patients with occult disease seeing therapists. The fact that PTs and OTs tend to spend a moderate amount of time with patients over a period of weeks can facilitate the detection of subtle manifestations. In addition, as therapists develop rapport with patients, the patients may be willing to share information they were uncomfortable disclosing initially.

The responsibilities of the PT and OT related to screening for symptoms and signs that indicate the involvement of another health care practitioner are clearly stated in the *Guide to Physical Therapist Practice*[1] and *The Guide to Occupational Therapy Practice*.[8] The process associated with Differential Diagnosis Phase 1 allows for the appropriate medical screening yet keeps therapists within their scope of practice. The therapist simply communicates to the physician the list of clinical findings. The physician will determine if medical tests (step 3) are needed to rule out or diagnose specific diseases. Facilitat-ing the timely referral of patients to physicians is an important role for therapists working within a collaborative medical model. It is this model that best serves the needs of our patients. For additional information related to the medical screening process the readers are directed to two other textbooks.[4, 6]

With changes in health care delivery and physicians also being asked to see more patients in less time, the importance of all health care practitioners including an adequate medical screening component to their examination is critical. If quality of life issues are truly an important component of health care delivery, then Differential Diagnosis Phase 1, medical screening, has and will continue to be a professional expectation and responsibility placed on each PT and OT. As consumers are accessing therapeutic services through more direct means, that responsibility will remain and grow in importance as part of our education and practice.

REFERENCES

1. American Physical Therapy Association: Guide to physical therapist practice. Phys Ther 77:1163–1650, 1997.
2. American Psychiatric Association: Diagnostic and Statistical Manual of Mental Disorders [DSM-IV]. Washington, DC, American Psychiatric Association, 1994.
3. Boissonnault WG: Prevalence of comorbid conditions, surgeries and medication use in physical therapy outpatient population: A multicentered study. J Orthop Sports Phys Ther 29:506–519, 1999.
4. Boissonnault WG (ed): Examination in Physical Therapy Practice—Screening for Medical Disease, 2nd ed. New York, Churchill Livingstone, 1995.
5. Boissonnault WG, Koopmeiners MB: Medical history profile: Orthopaedic physical therapy outpatient. J Orthop Sports Phys Ther 20:2–10, 1994.
6. Goodman CC, Snyder TE: Differential Diagnosis for the Physical Therapist, 3rd ed. Philadelphia, WB Saunders, 1999.
7. Jette DU, Jette AM: Physical therapy and health outcomes in patients with spinal impairments. Phys Ther 76:930–941, 1996.
8. Moyers PA: The Guide to Occupational Therapy Practice. Am J Occup Ther 53:247–322, 1999.
9. Physical Disability. Special Issue. Phys Ther 74:375–506, 1994.
10. Sauer GC: Manual of Skin Diseases, 6th ed. Philadelphia, JB Lippincott, 1991.
11. Verbrugge L, Jette A: The disablement process. Soc Sci Med 38:1–14, 1994.
12. Umphred DA (Chair): Diagnostic Task Force and Special Project. California Chapter American Physical Therapy Association, 1996–2000.

Differential Diagnosis Phase 2: Examination and Evaluation of Disabilities and Impairments

ROLANDO T. LAZARO, MS, PT, GCS • MARGARET ROLLER, MS, PT • DARCY A. UMPHRED, PhD, PT

Chapter Outline

Key Words

- Differential Diagnosis Phase 2
- disabilities
- evaluation
- examination
- impairments

Objectives

After reading this chapter the student/therapist will:

1. Clearly differentiate diagnosis of impairments and disabilities from medical diagnosis performed by the physician.

2. Identify the difference between a disability and an impairment.

3. Comprehend the scope of disability and impairment examinations and how the results of those tests interact and present themselves as movement disorders.

4. Apply the concepts of objective measurements to demonstrate efficacy of outcome of interventions.

5. Identify which tests are available and how to find them in the literature.

From the beginning of the evolution of practice, clinicians have been expected to examine a client's performance and draw conclusions from the examination. The synthesis of information gathered has led to the establishment of short- and long-term goals as well as the selection of appropriate intervention strategies. Today, clients are typically referred for physical and occupational therapy, with "Evaluate and treat" orders as the standard referral pattern used by physicians. Once a client enters into a therapeutic environment, whether through self-referral or referral from another medical practitioner, clinicians must first determine whether the individual is medically stable at a body system level (see Chapter 2) and an appropriate candidate for therapeutic intervention. Once medical screening has been completed and the therapist determines that there are no red flags to suggest that the client needs to be referred back for additional disease/pathology examination, then the client enters into Phase 2 of the evaluation process (Fig. 3–1). Critical to this phase is a solid understanding of the disablement model because this is the foundation of a strong diagnostic process (see Chapter 1).

Numerous tools are used to examine clients who present with physical complaints. Many of these tools directly measure the impairments of a client as they examine specific strengths and weaknesses within the body systems. Each impairment tool is intended for a specific purpose and is designed to supply the user with a given outcome measure in a predetermined set of values.

Other tools measure a client's functional abilities or disabilities. These tools are designed to examine the performance of a client during various functional skills and activities of daily living. Functional tools also supply the user with a predetermined set of values. These tools, however, do not directly supply information about the cause of the client's disability. The user must extrapolate information from the results of each functional test and then choose the appropriate impairment measurement tools to determine the combination of impairments that may be contributing to the found disability.

To be able to provide information that is meaningful in determining the best possible intervention for a particular patient, the examination tools selected by the clinician must be objective and reliable. These tools should also

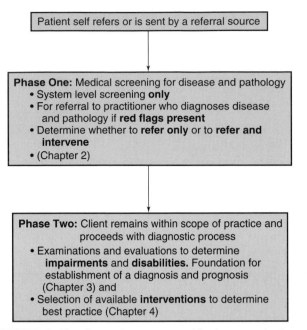

FIGURE 3–1. The diagnostic process used for best practice by physical and occupational therapists.

communicate necessary information in a language that is understandable to all health care professionals, as well as the payer responsible for funding the services.

This chapter has been developed to help the reader through the problem-solving and decision-making process for selecting appropriate tests. It is not within the scope of this chapter or text to explain each examination tool in detail. However, the reader is presented with an extensive list of impairment and disability tests with related references as a guide in determining the appropriate examination tools for a particular client (see Appendix 3–A at the end of this Chapter).

THE DIAGNOSTIC PROCESS

As mentioned previously, it is important for the clinician to have a comprehensive understanding of the disablement model. As the clinician begins to sift through information obtained from the various examination procedures, it is appropriate to identify the impairments that cause the particular disability or functional limitation. The clinician must consider all aspects of the client's multiple body and environmental systems during this process. The clinician should also be sensitive to the individual's perception of the effect that these impairments have on the person and how they relate to society, how they impose social limitations, and/or how the particular impairments or disabilities lead to a handicap or a decreased quality of life.

In the clinical environment the clinician first identifies the client's presenting disabilities or functional limitations through disability testing and then examines the subsystem impairments that directly cause or may have contributed to these disabilities or functional limitations. Therefore, instead of approaching the examination process as

"impairment leading to disability," the clinician actually performs a "disability and then impairment causing the disability" analysis. This process not only streamlines the examination but also assists the clinician in focusing on the problems and the interaction of the systems causing the various disabilities and thus helps to delineate how the disability will be impacted by the resulting therapeutic intervention. Some impairments may be the result of the disease or pathology, reflecting a medical referral, and others may be reflective of life experiences and previous traumas.

Disabilities

Disability or functional limitation is defined as the restriction of the ability to perform—at the level of the whole person—a physical action, activity, or task in an efficient, typically expected and competent manner.[3] It is important to observe the client during the performance of functional tasks and motor patterns to determine the functions that the client is unable to execute or has difficulty performing (disabilities) to determine the cause of the dysfunctional movement patterns. It is not uncommon for a client to present with multiple disability interactions. In this case, the examiner must attempt to determine the primary disability or primary complaint. This will guide the process of choosing the appropriate functional tool(s) to use during the examination.

Functional tools are designed to measure and score a client during the performance of various functional tasks. Each functional tool is designed to measure a specific type of functional ability. Most tools test a range of skills from walking ability to balance ability during the performance of functional tasks or a combination of the two. Some tests are quick and easy to set up and perform (e.g., Functional Reach Test, Tinetti Performance Oriented Mobility Assessment [POMA]), whereas others are lengthy and take longer to administer (e.g., Berg Balance Test, Functional Independence Measure [FIM]). There are advantages and disadvantages to both of these types of tests. Those that are the quickest to administer generally measure fewer functional skills and do not give information on the total functioning of a client. However, if the user properly identifies the client's problem and is able to focus on the most efficient way of measuring it, a quick functional test can be the most beneficial to use. Those tests that take a bit longer to administer and assess multiple skills supply the user with a more comprehensive picture of the client's functional abilities, generally in various domains such as gross mobility, self-care, cognitive ability, communication ability, and others.

Outcome scales for functional tests are generally in ordinal numerical format (e.g., FIM, Barthel Index, Katz Index of Activities of Daily Living). Each has its own unique point value and range, varying from a two- to three-point scale (e.g., Tinetti POMA) to a seven-point scale (e.g., FIM). A few tools supply ratio scale data (e.g., the Timed Up and Go Test [TUG] and modified TUG [mTUG], Functional Reach Test, and other measures of gait speed). Ratio scale data are easier to compare and to measure incremental changes in function.

Impairments

Impairment is defined as the loss or abnormality of physiological, psychological, or anatomical structure or function.[3] An efficient examination process first includes the use of disability measures and functional tools to identify the client's primary functional problems. From this information the clinician extrapolates the primary impairments that are suspected to be creating or contributing to the client's functional limitations. The clinician may then choose to proceed to examine these impaired systems directly by using tests and measures designed to supply objective information regarding the status of each involved body system. This entire process helps the clinician identify the most important problems affecting the client in the least amount of time. Knowledge of the status of involved body systems helps guide choices for therapeutic intervention and goal setting. It also assists in predicting how the client's disabilities may be impacted by the resulting intervention.

Objective examination results are gained from both functional testing and impairment testing. These results supply the information base on which to set goals, determine intervention strategies, and measure progress. The clinician must also consider the nature of the neurological, neuromuscular, or musculoskeletal condition or medical diagnosis in the planning of treatment and goal setting. The potential impact of the intervention to the impairments, disabilities, and handicaps for chronic, degenerative conditions is generally quite different from that of acute, nonprogressive, or acquired conditions. The projected length of time to treat and functional outcomes at the end of treatment episodes will also differ greatly depending on the nature of the disease or disorder.

After the identification of the disabilities or functional limitations, and the impairments that may be causing them, the clinician may decide between three possible intervention scenarios: (1) the correction of impairments that may lead to the correction of disabilities, (2) the correction of the disability itself through enhancement of existing strengths, or (3) compensation for noncorrectable limitations through alterations in the external environment.

The clinician needs to make the distinction between primary impairments, which are a direct consequence of the client's specific disease or pathology, and secondary impairments, which occur as sequelae to the disease or rehabilitation process or due to aging, disuse, repetitive strain, lifestyle, and so on. Moreover, the clinician must remember that although disabilities are usually caused by a combination of specific impairments, it is possible that impairments may not result in specific disabilities for a particular client. If this is the case, the clinician should make a determination regarding whether these impairments, if left uncorrected, will result in the development of disabilities at a later time.

The ultimate goal of any therapeutic intervention program is to attain the highest level of health and wellness possible. Measurement tools that the clinician chooses to use also need to reflect this end result. For example, "traditional" impairment measurements may indicate that a client demonstrated increased shoulder range of motion by 25 degrees. The more important question should be how this increase in range of motion affects the client's ability to perform a functional task such as dressing. The clinician is therefore encouraged to consider the functional implications of these measurements to obtain results that are more meaningful for the client.

The clinician is always faced with the challenge of identifying and administering examination tools that will not only reflect the client's level of health and wellness but also reflect the client's functional improvement as a result of the intervention provided. Disability tests and functional measurement tools can be used as a baseline measure for those functional skills. However, these tools typically require a large improvement in a client's functional performance for a corresponding change in the disability grade to be seen. Results obtained from impairment tests can fill in the large gaps between numerical scores on disability scales with objective measurements and trends in the direction toward improvement before any change is demonstrated on disability scales.

Table 3–1 illustrates impairments that are considered to be central neurological versus peripheral or environmental in origin. The column on the left illustrates the components of motor control within the systems that are traditionally considered central. These components are further discussed in detail in various sections of this book. Some qualitative and quantitative measures commonly used to assess these systems are referenced in Appendix 3–A.

The column on the right identifies impairments in systems traditionally considered peripheral and environmental. Range of motion (ROM) is one example of a common musculoskeletal system examination procedure. Clinicians depend heavily on ROM measurements as an

●
T A B L E   3 – 1 .   Identification and Classification of Impairments

Impairments Within the Central Nervous System	Impairments Within the Peripheral Nervous System and Interaction with the Environment
1. State of the motor pool	1. Range of motion
2. Synergies (volitional or reflexive)	2. Muscle strength or power
3. Postural integration	3. Cardiac function
4. Balance	4. Respiratory function
5. Speed of movement	5. Circulatory function
6. Timing	6. Other organ and system interaction
7. Reciprocal movements	7. Environmental task
8. Trajectory or pattern of movement	8. Endurance
9. Accuracy	9. Psychosocial factors
10. Task content	
11. Emotional influences	
12. Sensory organization: somatosensory mapping	
13. Perception/cognition	
14. Hormonal/nutritional	
15. Levels of consciousness	

essential component of their examination and consequent evaluation process. It is imperative that the data obtained from this procedure be reliable. It has been suggested that the main source of variation in the performance of this procedure is methodology and that by standardizing the procedure improved reliability can be realized.[64]

An impairment of lack of ROM can be the result of other impairments. ROM measurements may be used to determine the effect of tone, balance, movement synergies, and so on on the neuromuscular system and, ultimately, on behavior. Most importantly, the clinician needs to remember that the ROM needed to perform a functional activity is more critical than the "normal," anatomical, biomechanical ROM values and must be considered when labeling and measuring impairments. For example, full ROM in the shoulder is seldom needed unless activities of daily living require it, such as a tennis serve or placing objects overhead at work. When needed for specific tasks, goniometric measurements are appropriate, but at other times a functional range measurement may be just as reliable.

Muscle strength testing is another commonly used examination procedure. Clinicians employ various methods of quantifying this measurement, including "traditional" manual muscle testing and the use of a dynamometer.

As with ROM, strength should be correlated with the patient's functional performance. Again, the clinician may find a client to have 3/5 strength in the shoulder flexor muscle groups, or find grip strength to be 50 kg, but the more important question should be "What does this mean in terms of the client's ability to perform activities of daily living?" The clinician is also advised to make the distinction among strength, power production, and muscular endurance as it relates to function. A client may have sufficient lower-extremity strength and power to get up from the seated position; however, this does not necessarily mean that the client has muscular endurance to perform the task repeatedly during the day as part of normal everyday activities.

The functioning of the cardiac, respiratory, and circulatory systems significantly affects a client's performance. Blood pressure, heart rate, and respiration give the clinician signs of the patient's medical stability as well as the ability to tolerate exercise. The clinician may also obtain pulmonary function tests for ventilation, pulmonary mechanics, lung diffusion capacity, or blood gas analysis after determining that the client's pulmonary system is a major factor affecting medical stability and functional progress. Various exercise tolerance tests also attempt to quantify functional work capacity and serve as a guide for the clinician when performing cardiac and pulmonary rehabilitation.

A client who presents with difficulty performing activities of daily living and who has neurological impairments in the central motor, sensory, perceptual, and/or integrative systems needs to undergo examination procedures to establish the level of impairment of each involved system and to determine if and how that system is contributing to the deficit motor behaviors. Functional evaluation tools employed may include the FIM, the Barthel Index, the Tinetti POMA, and/or the mTUG Test. The results of these tests will help to steer the clinician toward the most useful impairment tools to use to evaluate limitations in the various body systems. Impairment tools may include the modified Ashworth Scale for spasticity, the Upright Motor Control Test for lower-extremity motor control, the Clinical Test of Sensory Integration on Balance (CTSIB) or the Sensory Organization Test (SOT) for balance and sensory integrative problems, and/or computerized tests of limits of stability on the NeuroCom Balance Master, among others (see Appendix 3–A).

The clinician is also advised to investigate the interaction of other organs and systems as they relate to the patient's disabilities. For example, electrolyte imbalance, hormonal disorders, or adverse drug reactions (see Chapter 32) may explain impairments and disabilities noted in the other interacting systems.

CHOOSING THE APPROPRIATE EXAMINATION TOOL

The ability to choose the appropriate examination tool(s) for a particular client will depend on several factors:

1. The client's current functional status (ambulatory vs. nonambulatory)
2. The client's current cognitive status (intact vs. confused/disoriented)
3. The clinical setting in which the person is being evaluated for treatment (acute hospital vs. rehabilitation vs. outpatient vs. skilled care vs. home care)
4. The client's primary complaints (pain vs. weakness vs. impaired balance)
5. The client's goals and realistic expectation of recovery (acute injury vs. chronic problem vs. progressive disease process)

The evaluator should select examination tools that will measure the client's primary problems (impairments and disabilities) and supply outcome measures that are needed to set realistic treatment goals and plan efficient and effective intervention strategies. To choose a functional tool the clinician is advised to select one that contains component skills that the particular client is having difficulty with. Those component skills of the tool in which the client's performance is poor will disclose the client's disabilities. Those skills in which the client performs well determine the client's strengths. The evaluator must then focus on the client's disability measurements as determined by the results of functional test(s) to determine the impairment tests that will next be performed. For example, if the client demonstrates difficulty in rising from a chair during a functional test (e.g., FIM, Tinetti POMA) and scores low on this skill on the outcome measure, the clinician must then closely examine the skill of coming to stand to determine the cause of the disability. The problem may be that the client cannot generate adequate muscle power to push up from the chair or perhaps that the client does not have adequate ROM in the hip or the ankle joints to rise from the chair. It may be a problem with dynamic balance during the transitional movement or once standing. Any impairment that is identified during performance of the functional skill needs to be measured more specifically. It is up to the examiner to determine the next best steps to take to target the client's problems as efficiently as possible, to measure and record the needed outcomes, and to then set treatment goals and design the best intervention to remediate the problems.

Many of the examination tools that measure a client's ability to perform functional activities have been accepted as valid, reliable, and useful for the justification of payment for services rendered. The number of functional limitations and the extent of the client's disabilities is often a reason why an individual either accessed therapy services directly or was referred by a medical practitioner. For this reason, the third-party payer expects to receive reports concerning positive changes in the client's functional status for therapeutic services to be justifiable. The initial list of functional limitations or disabilities helps the therapist determine the extent, expectations, and direction of intervention, but it does not determine why those limitations exist. This is the question that is critical to answer as part of the evaluation process. Examination tests and procedures that identify specific system and subsystem impairments help the therapist determine causes for existing disabilities and functional limitations. These tools need to be objective, reliable, and sensitive enough to provide needed communication to third-party payers to explain the subsystem's baseline progress during and after the intervention. These tools should also supply explanations for residual difficulties in the event that the disabilities themselves do not demonstrate significant objective change or show progress within the time frame estimated.

USING THE EVALUATION PROCESS TO LINK IMPAIRMENTS AND DISABILITIES TO INTERVENTION

After obtaining objective measures for functional limitations/disabilities and systems and subsystems impair-

ments, clinicians must determine whether the impairments and/or the disabilities are changeable given the limitations in the number of treatment interventions. In certain situations a disability may be remediated and become more functional, although the component impairments contributing to it may remain unchanged. In other situations, impairment measures may significantly improve but the disability may remain unaltered. This is especially true when one impairment is significantly improved; however, functional progress is masked by the contribution of other impairments.

To be able to structure and summarize the relationship of disabilities and impairments and assess the effect of the intervention on a particular patient, a clinical decision-making matrix may be used (Fig. 3–2).

The interactions and interrelationships of both the identified disabilities and impairments provide the clinician with an initial status or problem list specific to that individual. That list, or the interactions of the impairments and disabilities, helps to formulate a diagnosis for the movement dysfunction. Similarly, owing to the objective nature of the components within that diagnosis, a target status to be reached at the conclusion of therapeutic intervention can be estimated. That target status is both impairment and function driven and traditionally would be considered a list of outcome goals. The interactions between impairments and their related disabilities make up the unique problem map of that individual and direct the clinician toward selecting optimal interventions.

The difference between the initial and the target status as well as the time frame and estimated number of visits needed to reach the target outcome is the prognosis by the clinician. Once the clinician has measured and identified specific functional limitations and their respective impairments, he or she then has an excellent opportunity to conceptually understand how various impairments affect multiple disabilities and which impairments are disability specific.

INITIAL STATUS	TARGET STATUS	PROGNOSIS
Disability 1 status _____	Disability 1 status _____	Disability 1 # of visits _____
Impairment 1 status _____	Impairment 1 status _____	Impairment 1 # of visits _____
Impairment 2 status _____	Impairment 2 status _____	Impairment 2 # of visits _____
Impairment 3 status _____	Impairment 3 status _____	Impairment 3 # of visits _____
Disability 2 status _____	Disability 2 status _____	Disability 2 # of visits _____
Impairment 4 status _____	Impairment 4 status _____	Impairment 4 # of visits _____
Impairment 5 status _____	Impairment 5 status _____	Impairment 5 # of visits _____
Impairment 6 status _____	Impairment 6 status _____	Impairment 6 # of visits _____
Disability 3 status _____	Disability 3 status _____	Disability 3 # of visits _____
Impairment 7 status _____	Impairment 7 status _____	Impairment 7 # of visits _____
Impairment 8 status _____	Impairment 8 status _____	Impairment 8 # of visits _____
Impairment 9 status _____	Impairment 9 status _____	Impairment 9 # of visits _____

FIGURE 3–2. Clinical decision-making matrix.

To effectively use this matrix, the clinician identifies and records the patient's disabilities and the impairments that are potentially causing each particular disability. As the clinician gathers the information, it is important to remember that a particular impairment may cause multiple disabilities. If such is the case, this particular impairment must therefore be documented under each particular disability on the matrix. During the patient's initial examination session, the clinician determines the treatment goals by projecting the changes to the disabilities and their corresponding impairments (target status). The clinician also makes the determination of the number of visits necessary to achieve the target status for each impairment or disability (prognosis). The clinician will periodically assess the achievement of the target status after intervention sessions and will modify the target status and prognosis as necessary. (See Chapter 1 for further recommendations regarding documentation.)

The following case scenario clearly synthesizes the clinical examination and evaluation process employed by physical and occupational therapists.

Assume that a clinician had been called in to examine a client who has suffered an anoxic event after heart surgery. The client's cognitive skill is within normal limits and he is highly motivated to get back to his normal activities. He is retired, loves to walk in the park with his wife and go on bird watching experiences in the mountains with their group of friends. The clinician must select which functional tests to use to obtain an objective initial status and target the client's disabilities. Currently, the client requires assistance with all gross mobility skills and is demonstrating difficulty balancing in various postures and activities of daily living. After functional testing, the client demonstrates significant limitations in the activities of coming to sit, sitting, coming to stand, standing, walking, dressing, and grooming. If the client is moderately dependent in all seven activities and requires assistance to perform those functions, then, depending on the functional tests used, he will most likely be scored between "unable" and "independent" on a given scale. Assume that the client also displays impairment limitations in flexor range of motion at the hip joints because of both muscle/fascia tightness and hypertonicity within the extensor muscle groups, although he has compensated to some degree and is able to perform bed mobility independently. Upper-extremity control is within normal limits, and thus the client is capable of performing many activities of daily living as long as his lower trunk and hips are placed in a supportive position and hip flexion is not required. The client has general weakness from inactivity as well as power production problems in his abdominals and hip flexor muscles owing to the dominance of extensor tonicity. Once he is brought to stand, the extensor patterns of hip and knee extension, internal rotation, slight adduction, and plantarflexion are present. He can actively extend both legs after being placed in flexion, but he is limited in the production of specific fine and gross motor patterns. Thus, a resulting balance impairment is present owing to the inability to adequately access appropriate balance synergies caused by the presence of tone, limb synergy production, and weakness in the antagonists to the trunk and hip extensors. With the use of augmented intervention (see Chapter 4), the client is noted to possess intact postural and procedural balance programming; however, both functions are being masked by existing impairments. The decision is made to perform impairment measures, including range of motion at the hip, knee, and ankle joints; power production within both the abdominal and hip flexor muscle groups; volitional and nonvolitional synergic programming; balance; posture; and volitional control over muscle tone. The amount of range and power production needed as well as the specific synergic programming required will vary according to the requirements of the functional activities performed.

Using the clinical decision-making matrix, the clinician will conclude that the target impairment measurements will vary from one disability to the next. Looking at Figure 3–2, assume Disability 1 is sitting and Disability 2 is coming to stand. Assume Impairment 1 is biomechanical range of motion. Because Impairment 1 is a contributing cause of Disability 1 and Disability 2, the clinician must document Impairment 1 under both Disability 1 and Disability 2. The initial measurement obtained by the clinician for Impairment 1 within Disability 1 and Disability 2 will therefore be the same value. However, as the clinician makes the determination of the target status of Impairment 1, the target value of this impairment may be different for Disability 1 as opposed to Disability 2. Going back to the example presented earlier, the target measure for Impairment 1 (biomechanical range of motion) may be different for Disability 1 (sitting) and Disability 2 (coming to stand) because different amounts of range of motion are needed to achieve the desired functional tasks.

These objective measurements help the clinician explain which outcomes would be expected to be achieved first and why. These measurements are recorded as part of intervention charting and help to objectively demonstrate that the client is improving toward functional independence. They also give an indication of what the client still needs to reach the desired outcome, the rate of learning that is taking place, and an estimation of recovery time that is still required. These objective measurements give to the clinician and the client a better avenue to discuss expectations with family members, other medical practitioners, and third–party payers. In the previous example, assume that, after intervention, biomechanical range of motion in the hip was achieved. However, this improvement did not result in an improvement in the disability because synergic programming prevented adequate hip flexion during one or more functional activities. Understanding and measuring the difference between lack of range due to muscle/fascia tightness versus lack of range due to synergic patterning helps clinicians communicate why a client is successful in one activity and still needing assistance in another.

Impairment and disability scores supply statistically important measurements that can then be used to discuss the limitations placed on the therapeutic environment by fiscal intermediaries. Therapists must be very clear when documenting the initial status and the target status for clients so that the recommended intervention and length of stay may be justified (see Fig. 3–2).

When making a determination of the potential impact of the intervention on improving the client's problems,

CASE 3–1

C.B. is a 27-year-old white woman who was admitted to the hospital 3 days ago with acute onset and rapidly progressing distal to proximal weakness and sensory loss, greater in the lower extremities than in the upper extremities. The client reports right great toe numbness and weakness and tripping on the carpet at home the night before admission. She went to bed with increased weakness and numbness in both legs and with difficulty walking. At admission through the emergency department she also reported numbness in both hands.

Medical diagnosis was Guillain-Barré syndrome. Prior level of function indicates that the client was an active, independent woman who worked full-time performing computer data entry. She lived at home with her husband and two children. There are four steps with a rail to enter the house and a flight of stairs to access bedrooms.

The client was transferred to the neurology unit of the acute hospital. She was started on intravenous immunoglobulin (IV Ig) treatment and pain medication every 4 hours. A Foley catheter was inserted for bladder control, and the client was supplied with thromboembolic disease (TED) hose and intermittent compression pumps on both legs for deep venous thrombosis prophylaxis.

Phase 1 screening indicates that the client's past medical history is noncontributory. There are no acute or active diseases or pathologies that may contraindicate physical or occupational therapy intervention. There is a precaution against overfatiguing the client; otherwise, the physician assessed the client's medical condition to be stable. At this point PT/OT examination and evaluation may be indicated to provide further insight into the necessity of therapeutic intervention. An order was received for "PT/OT evaluation and treatment as indicated." The patient's goal is to be able to walk, return home to the family, and be able to return to work full time.

Phase 2 examination proceeded to identify impairments, disabilities, and handicaps, as well as to gain an understanding of the potential systems interactions that may influence progress. In this particular case, a decision was made to perform disability testing first to identify the specific functional limitations of the patient and then to selectively identify possible systems impairments that may be causing the disability. Functional assessment indicated that the patient requires moderate assistance to roll to the left/right side and to scoot.

She also required moderate assistance to move from supine to sit and to transfer from sit to stand. Her blood pressure, heart rate, respiration, and oxygen saturation remained within safe limits throughout these changes in body position. She demonstrated fair sitting balance and poor standing balance. She was able to ambulate using a front-wheeled walker approximately 10 feet with moderate assistance of one person.

As mentioned earlier, the identification of potential impairments was done after disability testing to streamline the examination process. After performing the functional examination the therapist postulated that the client might have motor weakness, sensory deficits, pain, and a decrease in endurance that may be causing the functional limitations. Manual muscle testing revealed lower-extremity strength of 1/5 both ankle motions, 2/5 both knees, and 3−/5 both hips. Upper extremities tested as 1/5 finger flexors (incomplete grip), 2/5 wrist motions, and 3+/5 both elbow motions. Shoulders and trunk were within functional limits for all motions. Sensory testing indicated absent touch and proprioceptive sensations from the foot to the knee of both lower extremities, with impaired sensation from the thigh to the hips. Both hands and wrists tested absent to touch and proprioception, with the elbows and shoulders testing intact. The client's endurance was limited to short bouts of activity (3 to 5 minutes), with rapid muscular and cardiovascular fatigue. All of these impairments help to explain the resulting disabilities tested earlier.

The multidisciplinary Functional Independence Measure (FIM) could give insight into this patient's ability to function in multiple systems and categories. As the client regains strength and peripheral sensory ability, she may be able to perform the Tinetti Performance Oriented Mobility Assessment (POMA), the Berg Balance Test, the modified Timed Up and Go (mTUG) Test, and the Functional Reach Test. These functional assessments paint a better picture of what the client can and cannot do, as well as provide a way to measure functional progress in various activities throughout rehabilitation.

In choosing the appropriate functional tool, the clinician must also consider the "ceiling and floor effect" of many of the functional tools. In this particular case, the patient is probably unable to perform the Functional Reach Test but may be appropriate for beginning the balance portion of the POMA.

---

clinicians must remember that a key factor in this process of examination and evaluation is the acceptance of the disability and/or impairment by the client. A disability or impairment may be clearly identified by a functional test or impairment test; however, the client may deny that a problem even exists. Acceptance of the disability by the client and a willingness to change are critical to the client's compliance with the intervention strategy.

REFERENCES

1. Alexander NB, et al: Rising from a chair: Effects of age and functional ability on performance biomechanics. J Gerontol 46:M91, 1991.
2. Allison SC, et al: Reliability of the Modified Ashworth Scale in the assessment of plantarflexor muscle spasticity in patients with traumatic brain injury. Int J Rehabil Res 19:67, 1996.
3. American Physical Therapy Association: Guide to Physical Therapy Practice, Virginia, APTA, 1997.
4. Amundsen LR: Isometric muscle strength testing with fixed-load cells. In Amundsen LR (ed): Muscle Strength Testing: Instrumented and Non-instrumented Systems. New York, Churchill Livingstone, 1990.
5. Andrews AW: Hand held dynamometry for measuring muscle strength. J Hum Muscle Perform 1:35, 1991.
6. Andrews AW, et al: Normative values for isometric muscle force measurements obtained with hand-held dynamometers. Phys Ther 76:248, 1996.
7. Arthur A, Jagger C, Lindesay J, et al: Using an annual over-75 health check screen for depression: Validation of the short Geriatric Depression Scale (GDS15) within general practice. Int J Geriatr Psychiatry 14:431–439, 1999.
8. Bass H, et al: Value and appropriate use of rating scales and apparative measurements in quantification of disability in Parkinson's disease. J Neural Transm Park Dis Dement Sect 5:45, 1993.
9. Beaton D, Richards RR: Assessing the reliability and responsiveness of 5 shoulder questionnaires. J Shoulder Elbow Surg 7:565, 1998.
10. Bechtol CO: Grip test use of dynamometer with adjustable hand spacing. JAMA 36:820, 1954.
11. Beck AT, Steer RA: Depression Inventory. Psychological Corporation, 555 Academic Court, San Antonio, TX 78204.
12. Berg K: Measuring Balance in the Elderly: Validation of an Instrument [dissertation]. Montreal, Canada, McGill University, 1993.
13. Berg K, et al: Measuring balance in the elderly: Preliminary development of an instrument. Physiother Canada 41:304, 1989.
14. Berg K, et al: The Balance Scale: Reliability assessment with elderly residents and patients with an acute stroke. Scand J Rehabil Med 27:27, 1995.
15. Berg KO, et al: Measuring balance in the elderly: Validation of an instrument. Can J Public Health 83(suppl 2):S7, 1992.
16. Bergner M, et al: The sickness impact profile: Conceptual formulation and methodology for the development of a health status measure. Int J Health Serv 6:393, 1976.
17. Bergner M, et al: The Sickness Impact Profile: Development and final revision of a health status measure. Med Care 19:787, 1981.
18. Bernhardt J, et al: Changes in balance and locomotion measures during rehabilitation following stroke. Physiother Res Int 3:109, 1998.
19. Beurskens AJ, et al: Measuring the functional status of patients with low back pain: Assessment of the quality of four disease-specific questionnaires. Spine 20:1017, 1995.
20. Black FO, et al: Normal subjects' postural sway during the Romberg test. Am J Otolaryngol 3:309, 1982.
21. Boake C: Supervision rating scale: A measure of functional outcome from brain injury. Arch Phys Med Rehabil 77:765, 1996.
22. Bohannon RW: Muscle strength testing with hand-held dynamometers. In Amundsen LR (ed): Muscle Strength Testing: Instrumented and Non-instrumented Systems. New York, Churchill Livingstone, 1990.
23. Bohannon RW: Reference values for extremity muscle strength obtained by hand-held dynamometry from adults aged 20 to 79 years. Arch Phys Med Rehabil 78:26, 1997.
24. Bohannon RW, et al: Decrease in timed balance test scores with aging. Phys Ther 64:1067, 1984.
25. Bohannon RW, Smith MB: Interrater reliability of a modified Ashworth scale of muscle spasticity. Phys Ther 67:206, 1987.
26. Boss BJ, et al: A self-care assessment tool (SCAT) for persons with spinal cord injury: An expanded abstract. Axone 17:66, 1996.
27. Brandstater M, et al: Hemiplegic gait: Analysis of temporal variable. Arch Phys Med Rehabil 65:583, 1983.
28. Brazier JE, et al: Validating the SF-36 health survey questionnaire: New outcome measure for primary care. BMJ 305:160, 1992.
29. Bucks RS, et al: Assessment of activities of daily living in dementia:

30. Burckhardt CS, et al: The fibromyalgia impact questionnaire: Development and validation. J Rheumatol 18:728, 1991.
31. Byl NN, Sinnott PL: Variations in balance and body sway in middle-aged adults. Spine 16:325, 1991.
32. Carr JH, et al: Investigation of a new motor assessment scale for stroke patients. Phys Ther 65:175, 1985.
33. Cella DF, et al: Validation of the functional assessment of multiple sclerosis quality of life instrument. Neurology 47:129, 1996.
34. Chandler JM, et al: Balance performance on the postural stress test: Comparison of young adults, healthy elderly and fallers. Phys Ther 70:410, 1990.
35. CIR Systems, Inc. P.O. Box 4402, Clifton, NJ 07012.
36. Cohen H, et al: A study of the clinical test of sensory interaction and balance. Phys Ther 73:346, 1993.
37. Cohen RA, et al: The Extended Disability Status Scale (EDSS) as a predictor of impairments of functional activities of daily living in multiple sclerosis. J Neurol Sci 115:132, 1993.
38. Cress ME, et al: Continuous-scale physical functional performance in healthy older adults: A validation study. Arch Phys Med Rehabil 77:1243, 1996.
39. Crum RM, et al: Population-based norms for the Mini-Mental State Examination by age and educational level. JAMA 269:2386, 1993.
40. Csuka M, McCarty DJ: Simple method for measurement of lower extremity muscle strength. Am J Med 78:77–81, 1985.
41. Daley K, et al: Reliability of scores on the stroke rehabilitation assessment of movement (STREAM) measure. Phys Ther 79:8, 1999.
42. Davidoff G, et al: Galveston Orientation and Amnesia Test: Its utility in the determination of closed head injury in acute spinal cord injury patients. Arch Phys Med Rehabil 69:432, 1988.
43. de Bruin AF, et al: The sickness impact profile: SIP68, a short generic version: First evaluation of the reliability and reproducibility. J Clin Epidemiol 47:863, 1994.
44. de Haan R, et al: The clinical meaning of Rankin "handicap" grades after stroke. Stroke 26:2027, 1995.
45. Di Fabio RP: Sensitivity and specificity of platform posturography for identifying patients with vestibular dysfunction. Phys Ther 75:290, 1995.
46. Di Fabio R, Seay R: Use of the "fast evaluation of mobility, balance, and fear" in elderly community dwellers: Validity and reliability. Phys Ther 77:904, 1997.
47. Ditunno JF Jr: Functional assessment measures in CNS trauma. J Neurotrauma 9(suppl 1):S310, 1992.
48. Dix MR, Hallpike CS: Pathology, symptomatology and diagnosis of certain disorders of the vestibular system. Proc R Soc Med 45:341, 1952.
49. Donaghy S, Wass PJ: Interrater reliability of the Functional Assessment Measure in a brain injury rehabilitation program. Arch Phys Med Rehabil 79:1231, 1998.
50. Duncan PW, et al: Functional reach: A new clinical measure of balance. J Gerontol 45:M192, 1990.
51. Duncan PW, et al: Functional reach: Predictive validity in a sample of elderly male veterans. J Gerontol 47:M93, 1992.
52. Duncan PW, et al: Reliability of Fugl-Meyer assessment of sensorimotor recovery after CVA. Phys Ther 63:1606, 1983.
53. Ekdahl C, et al: Standing balance in healthy subjects. Scand J Rehabil Med 21:187, 1989.
54. Fike ML, Rousseau E: Measurement of adult hand strength: A comparison of two instruments. Occup Ther J Res 2:43, 1982.
55. Flannery J: Cognitive assessment in the acute care setting: Reliability and validity of the Levels of Cognitive Functioning Assessment Scale (LOCFAS). J Nurs Meas 3:43, 1995.
56. Flannery J: Using the levels of cognition functioning assessment scale with patients with traumatic brain injury in an acute care setting. Rehabil Nurs 23:88, 1998.
57. Folstein MF, et al: Mini-Mental State—a practical method for grading the cognitive state of patients for the clinician. J Psychiatr Res 12:189, 1975.
58. Franchignoni FP, et al: Trunk control test as an early predictor of stroke rehabilitation outcome. Stroke 28:1382, 1997.
59. Fugl-Meyer AR, et al: The post-stroke hemiplegic patient: A method for evaluation of physical performance. Scand J Rehabil Med 7:13, 1975.

Development of the Bristol Activities of Daily Living Scale. Age Ageing 25:113, 1996.

60. Functional Independence Measure. Guide for the Uniform Data Set for Medical Rehabilitation (Adult FIM) Version 5.0. Buffalo, NY 14214, State University of New York at Buffalo, 1996.

61. Gajdosik RL, Bohannon RW: Clinical measurement of range of motion: Review of goniometry emphasizing reliability and validity. Phys Ther 67:1867, 1987.

62. Gerety MB, et al: Development and validation of a physical performance instrument for the functionally impaired elderly: The Physical Disability Index (PDI). J Gerontol 48:M33, 1993.

63. Giacino JT, et al: Monitoring rate of recovery to predict outcome in minimally responsive patients. Arch Phys Med Rehabil 72:897, 1991.

64. Gillian J, Barstow M: Range of Motion. In Van Deusen, Brunt (eds): Assessment Techniques in Occupational Therapy and Physical Therapy. Philadelphia, WB Saunders, 1997, pp 50–51.

65. Gill-Thwaites H: The Sensory Modality Assessment Rehabilitation Technique—a tool for assessment and treatment of patients with severe brain injury in a vegetative state. Brain Inj 11:723, 1997.

66. Giorgetti MM, et al: Reliability of clinical balance outcome measures in the elderly. Physiother Res Int 3:274, 1998.

67. Gloth FM III, et al: Reliability and validity of the frail elderly functional assessment questionnaire. Am J Phys Med Rehabil 74:45, 1995.

68. Gloth FM III, et al: The frail elderly functional assessment questionnaire: its responsiveness and validity in alternative settings. Arch Phys Med Rehabil 80:1572, 1999.

69. Goetz CG, et al: Teaching tape for the motor section of the unified Parkinson's disease rating scale. Mov Disord 10:263, 1995.

70. Goetz CG, et al: Utility of an objective dyskinesia rating scale for Parkinson's disease: Inter- and intrarater reliability assessment. Mov Disord 9:390, 1994.

71. Goodkin DE, et al: Inter- and intrarater scoring agreement using grades 1.0 to 3.5 of the Kurtzke Expanded Disability Status Scale (EDSS). Multiple Sclerosis collaborative research group. Neurology 42:859, 1992.

72. Gowland C, et al: Measuring physical impairment and disability with the Chedoke-McMaster Stroke Assessment. Stroke 24:58, 1993.

73. Granger CV, et al: Outcome of comprehensive medical rehabilitation: Measurement of PULSES profile and the Barthel index. Arch Phys Med Rehabil 60:145, 1979.

74. Granger CV, Hamilton BB: Outcome of comprehensive medical rehabilitation: Measurement by PULSES Profile and the Barthel Index. Arch Phys Med Rehabil 60:145, 1979.

75. Gregson JM, et al: Reliability of the Tone Assessment Scale and the modified Ashworth scale as clinical tools for assessing poststroke spasticity. Arch Phys Med Rehabil 80:1013, 1999.

76. Guyatt GH, Sullivan MJ, Thompson PJ, et al: The six-minute walk: A new measure of exercise capacity in patients with chronic heart failure. Can Med Assoc J 132:919–923, 1985.

77. Hagell P, Widner H: Clinical rating of dyskinesias in Parkinson's disease: Use and reliability of a new rating scale. Mov Disord 14:448, 1999.

78. Hamid MA: Clinical patterns of dynamic posturography. In Arenberg IK (ed): Dizziness and Balance Disorders: An Interdisciplinary Approach to Diagnosis, Treatment, and Rehabilitation. Amsterdam/New York, Kugler Publications, 1993.

79. Hamilton M: Hamilton Rating Scale for Depression. J Neurol Neurosurg Psychiatry 23:56–61, 1960.

80. Helmes E, et al: Standardization and validation of the Multidimensional Observation Scale for Elderly Subjects (MOSES). J Gerontol 42:395, 1987.

81. Herdman S: Assessment and treatment of balance disorders in the vestibular-deficient patient. In Duncan P (ed): Balance: Proceedings of the APTA Forum. Alexandria, VA, APTA, 1989.

82. Herdman SJ: Vestibular Rehabilitation. Philadelphia, FA Davis, 2000.

83. Hislop HJ, Montgomery J: Muscle Testing: Techniques of Manual Examination. Philadelphia, WB Saunders, 1995.

84. Hogue CC, et al: Assessing mobility: The first step in falls prevention. In Funk SG, et al (eds): Key Aspects of Recovery: Improving Nutrition, Rest and Mobility. New York, Springer Publishing, 1990.

85. Holden MK, et al: Clinical gait assessment in the neurologically impaired: Reliability and meaningfulness. Phys Ther 64:35, 1984.

86. Holden MK, et al: Gait assessment for neurologically impaired patients: Standards for outcome assessment. Phys Ther 66:1530, 1986.

87. Holol MJ, et al: Disease steps in multiple sclerosis: A longitudinal study comparing disease steps and EDSS to evaluate disease progression. Mult Scler 5:349, 1999.

88. Hooper J, et al: Rater reliability of Fahn's tremor rating scale in patients with multiple sclerosis. Arch Phys Med Rehabil 79:1076, 1998.

89. Horak F: Clinical measurement of postural control in adults. Phys Ther 67:1881, 1987.

90. Hoyt ML, Alessi CA, Harker JO, et al: Development and testing of a five-item version of the Geriatric Depression Scale. J Am Geriatr Soc 47:873–878, 1999.

91. Huntington Study Group: Unified Huntington's Disease Rating Scale: Reliability and consistency. Mov Disord 11:136, 1996.

92. Hurley AC, et al: Assessment of discomfort in advanced Alzheimer patients. Res Nurs Health 15:369, 1992.

93. Hutchinson J, Hutchinson M: The Functional Limitations Profile may be a valid, reliable and sensitive measure of disability in multiple sclerosis. J Neurol 242:650, 1995.

94. Iversen IA, Silbenberg NE, Stever RC, Shhoening HA: The revised Kenny Self-Care Evaluation: A Numerical Measure of Independence in Activities of Daily Living. Minneapolis, MN, Sister Kenny Institute, 1973.

95. Jacobsen GP, Newman CW: The development of the Dizziness Handicap Inventory. Arch Otolaryngol Head Neck Surg 116:424, 1990.

96. Jenkinson C, et al: The Parkinson's Disease Questionnaire (PDQ-39): Development and validation of a Parkinson's disease summary index score. Age Ageing 26:353, 1997.

97. Jennett B, Bond M: Assessment of outcome after severe brain damage: A practical scale. Lancet 1:480, 1975.

98. Jennett B, Teasdale G: Management of Head Injuries. Philadelphia, FA Davis, 1981.

99. Juarez VJ, Lyons M: Interrater reliability of the Glasgow Coma Scale. J Neurosci Nurs 27:283, 1995.

100. Katz S, Down TD, Cash HR, Grotz RC: Progress in the Development of ADL. Gerontologist 10:20–30, 1970.

101. Katz SFA, et al: Studies of illness in the ages: The index of ADL: Standardized measure of biological and psychosocial function. JAMA 185:914, 1963.

102. Keith RA, et al: The functional independence measure: A new tool for rehabilitation. In Eisentberg MG, Grzesiak RC (eds): Advances in Clinical Rehabilitation, vol 1. New York, Springer Verlag, 1987.

103. Kellor M, et al: Hand strength and dexterity: Norms for clinical usage. Am J Occup Ther 25:77, 1971.

104. Kendall FP, McCreary EK: Muscles Testing and Function. Baltimore, Lippincott, Williams and Wilkins, 1993.

105. Klein RM, Bell B: Self-care skills: Behavioral measurement with the Klein-Bell ADL Scale. Arch Phys Med Rehabil 63:335–338, 1982.

106. Kopp B, et al: The Arm Motor Ability Test: Reliability, validity, and sensitivity to change of an instrument for assessing disabilities in activities of daily living. Arch Phys Med Rehabil 78:615, 1997.

107. Kurtzke JF: A new scale for evaluating disability in multiple sclerosis. Neurology 5:580, 1955.

108. Kurtzke JF: Rating neurologic impairment in multiple sclerosis: An expanded disability status scale (EDSS). Neurology 33:1444, 1983.

109. Lawton MP, Brody EM: Assessment of older people: Self-maintaining in instrumental activities of daily living. Gerontologist 9:179–186, 1969.

110. Leary P: Motor control assessment. In Montgomery P, Connoly B (eds): Motor Control and Physical Therapy: Theoretical Framework and Practical Applications. Chattanooga, TN, Chattanooga Group, 1991.

111. Linacre JM, et al: The structure and stability of the Functional Independence Measure. Arch Phys Med Rehabil 75:127, 1994.

112. Loewen SC, Anderson BA: Reliability of the Modified Motor Assessment Scale and the Barthel Index. Phys Ther 68:1077, 1988.

113. Lundin-Olsson L, et al: Attention, frailty, and falls: The effect of a manual task on basic mobility. J Am Geriatr Soc 46:758, 1998.

114. Lynch SM, et al: Reliability of measurements obtained with a modified functional reach test in subjects with spinal cord injury. Phys Ther 78:128, 1998.

115. MacKenzie DM, et al: Brief cognitive screening of the elderly: A comparison of the Mini-Mental State Examination (MMSE), Abbreviated Mental Test (AMT) and Mental Status Questionnaire (MSQ). Psychol Med 26:427, 1996.
116. Mahoney FI, Barthel DW: Functional evaluation: The Barthel index. MD State Med J 14:61, 1965.
117. Mahurin RK, DeBettignies BH, Pirozzolo FJ: Structured assessment of independent living skills: Preliminary report of performance measure of functional abilities in dementia. J Gerontol 46:58–66, 1991.
118. Marder SR: Psychiatric rating scales. In Kaplan HJ, Saddock BJ (eds): Comprehensive Textbook of Psychiatry, 6th ed, vol 1. Baltimore, Williams and Wilkins, 1995, pp 619–635.
119. Marino RJ, Goin JE: Development of a short-form Quadriplegia Index of Function scale. Spinal Cord 37:289, 1999.
120. Marshall SC, et al: Validity of the PULSES profile compared with the Functional Independence Measure for measuring disability in a stroke rehabilitation setting. Arch Phys Med Rehabil 80:760, 1999.
121. Martin DP, et al: Comparison of the Musculoskeletal Function Assessment questionnaire with the Short Form-36, the Western Ontario and McMaster Universities Osteoarthritis Index, and the Sickness Impact Profile health-status measures. J Bone Joint Surg Am 79:1323, 1997.
122. Mathias S, et al: Balance in elderly patients: The "get-up and go" test. Arch Phys Med Rehabil 67:387, 1986.
123. Mathiowetz V, et al: Grip and pinch strength: Normative data for adults. Arch Phys Med Rehabil 66:69, 1985.
124. McDonald TW, Franzen MD: A validity study of the WAIT in closed head injury, Brain Inj 13:331, 1999.
125. McGavin CR, et al: Twelve minute walk test for assessing disability in chronic bronchitis. BMJ 1:822, 1976.
126. McPherson KM, et al: An inter-rater reliability study of the Functional Assessment Measure (FIM + FAM). Disabil Rehabil 18:341, 1996.
127. McRae PG, et al: Physical activity levels of ambulatory nursing home residents. JAPA 4:264, 1996.
128. Mngoma NF, et al: Resistance to passive shoulder external rotation in persons with hemiplegia: Evaluation of an assessment system. Arch Phys Med Rehabil 80:531, 1999.
129. Moskowitz E, McCann CB: Classification of disability in the chronically ill and aging. J Chron Dis 5:342–346, 1957.
130. Nashner L: Evaluation of postural stability, movement, and control. In Hasson S (ed): Clinical Exercise Physiology. Philadelphia, CV Mosby, 1994.
131. Nashner L: Sensory, neuromuscular, and biomechanical contributions to human balance. In Duncan P (ed): Balance: Proceedings of the APTA forum, Alexandria, VA, American Physical Therapy Association, 1990.
132. Neal LJ: Current functional assessment tools. Home Health Nurse 16:766, 1998.
133. Nelson AJ: Functional ambulation profile. Phys Ther 54:1059–1064, 1974.
134. NeuroCom Balance Master LOS test.
135. Newton R: Review of tests of standing balance abilities. Brain Inj 3:335, 1989.
136. Nyein D, et al: Can a Barthel score be derived from the FIM? Clin Rehabil 13:56, 1999.
137. Oliver R, Blathwayt J, Brackley C, Tamaki T: Development of the Safety Assessment of Function in the Environment for Rehabilitation (SAFER tool). Can J Occup Ther 60:78–82, 1993.
138. O'Sullivan SB, Schmitz TJ: Physical Rehabilitation: Assessment and Treatment. Philadelphia, FA Davis, 1994.
139. Pandyan AD, et al: A review of the properties and limitations of the Ashworth and modified Ashworth Scales as measures of spasticity. Clin Rehabil 13:373, 1999.
140. Podsiadlo D, Richardson S: The timed "Up & Go": A test of basic functional mobility for frail elderly persons. J Am Geriatr Soc 39:142, 1991.
141. Pollard WE, et al: The Sickness Impact Profile: Reliability of a health status measure. Med Care 14:146, 1976.
142. Poole JL, Whitney SL: Motor assessment scale for stroke patients: Concurrent validity and interrater reliability. Arch Phys Med Rehabil 69:195, 1988.
143. Powell LE, Myers AM: The activities-specific balance confidence (ABC) scale. J Gerontol 50A(1):M28, 1995.
144. Price LG, Hewett HJ, Kay DR, Minor MM: Five Minute Walk Test of Aerobic Fitness for People with Arthritis. Arthritis Care Res 1:33–37, 1988.
145. Protas EJ, Cole J: Reliability of the 3-minute walk test in elderly post-op patients. J Cardiopulm Rehabil 3:36.
146. Radosevich DM, et al: Health Status Questionnaire (HSQ) 2.0: Scoring Comparisons and Reference Data. Health Outcomes Institute, 1994.
147. Rancho Los Amigos Hospital: Levels of Cognitive Function in Brain Injury. Downey, CA, Rancho Los Amigos Medical Center, Adult Brain Injury Service.
148. Rancho Los Amigos Hospital: Gait Analysis Form. Downey, CA, Rancho Los Amigos Hospital.
149. Rappaport M, et al: Evaluation of coma and vegetative states. Arch Phys Med Rehabil 73:628, 1992.
150. Ravaud JF, et al: Construct validity of the Functional Independence Measure (FIM): Questioning the unidimensionality of the scale and the "value" of FIM scores. Scand J Rehabil Med 31:31, 1999.
151. Ravnborg M, et al: The MS Impairment Scale: A pragmatic approach to the assessment of impairment in patients with multiple sclerosis. Mult Scler 3:31, 1997.
152. Ren XS, et al: Short-Form Arthritis Impact Measurement Scales 2: Tests of reliability and validity among patients with osteoarthritis. Arthritis Care Res 12:163, 1999.
153. Reuben DB, Siu AL: An objective measure of physical function of elderly outpatients: The physical performance test. J Am Geriatr Soc 38:1105, 1990.
154. Richards M, et al: Interrater reliability of the Unified Parkinson's Disease Rating Scale motor examination. Mov Disord 9:89, 1994.
155. Roth EJ, et al: Impairment and disability: Their relation during stroke rehabilitation. Arch Phys Med Rehabil 79:329, 1998.
156. Sager MA, et al: Hospital admission risk profile (harp): II Identifying older patients at risk for functional decline following acute medical illness and hospitalization. J Am Geriatr Soc 44:251, 1996.
157. Sanford J, et al: Reliability of the Fugl-Meyer assessment for testing motor performance in patients following stroke. Phys Ther 73:447, 1993.
158. Schmidt RT, Toews J: Grip strength as measured by the Jamar dynamometer. Arch Phys Med Rehabil 5:321, 1970.
159. Schoppen T, et al: The timed "up and go" test: Reliability and validity in persons with unilateral lower limb amputation. Arch Phys Med Rehabil 80:825, 1999.
160. Schuling J, et al: The Frenchay Activities Index: Assessment of functional status in stroke patients. Stroke 24:1173, 1993.
161. Sharrack B, et al: The psychometric properties of clinical rating scales used in multiple sclerosis. Brain 122:141, 1999.
162. Shields RK, et al: Reliability, validity, and responsiveness of functional tests in patients with total joint replacement. Phys Ther 75:169, 1995.
163. Shumway-Cook A, Horak F: Assessing the influence of sensory interaction on balance. Phys Ther 66:1548, 1986.
164. Shumway-Cook A, Horak F: Rehabilitation of the patient with vestibular deficits. Neurol Clin 8:441, 1990.
165. Shumway-Cook A, McCollum G: Assessment and treatment of balance disorders in the neurologic patient. In Montgomery T, Connolly B (eds): Motor Control Theory and Practice. Chattanooga, TN, Chattanooga Corp, 1990.
166. Siesling S, et al: A shortened version of the Unified Huntington's Disease Rating Scale. Mov Disord 12:229, 1997.
167. Stebbins GT, Goetz CG: Factor structure of the Unified Parkinson's Disease Rating Scale: Motor examination section. Mov Disord 13:633, 1998.
168. Stebbins GT, et al: Factor analysis of the motor section of the Unified Parkinson's Disease Rating Scale during the off-state. Mov Disord 14:585, 1999.
169. Stineman MG, et al: The Functional Independence Measure: Tests of scaling assumptions, structure, and reliability across 20 diverse impairment categories. Arch Phys Med Rehabil 77:1101, 1996.
170. Studenski S, et al: Predicting falls: The role of mobility and nonphysical factors. J Am Geriatr Soc 42:297, 1994.
171. Sunderland T, et al: Clock drawing in Alzheimer's disease: A novel measure of dementia severity. J Am Geriatr Soc 37:725, 1989.
172. Tangalos EG, et al: The Mini-Mental State Examination in general medical practice: Clinical utility and acceptance. Mayo Clin Proc 71:829, 1996.

173. Tesio L, et al: A short measure of balance in multiple sclerosis: Validation through Rasch analysis. Funct Neurol 12:255, 1997.

174. Thapa PB, et al: Clinical and biomechanical measures of balance as fall predictors in ambulatory nursing home residents. J Gerontol A Biol Sci Med Sci 51:M239, 1996.

175. Tinetti ME: Performance-oriented assessment of mobility problems in elderly patients. J Am Geriatr Soc 34:119, 1986.

176. Tinetti ME, et al: Falls efficacy as a measure of fear of falling. Gerontol Psychol Sci 45:239, 1990.

177. Tinetti ME, Powell L: Fear of falling and low self-efficacy: A cause of dependence in elderly persons. J Gerontol 48:35, 1993.

178. Tran PV, et al: Validation of an automated up-timer for measurement of mobility in older adults. Med J Aust 167:434, 1997.

179. Treves TA, et al: Interrater agreement in evaluation of stroke patients with the unified neurological stroke scale. Stroke 25:1263, 1994.

180. Turner-Stokes L, et al: The UK FIM + FAM: Development and evaluation. Functional Assessment Measure. Clin Rehabil 13:277, 1999.

181. Umphred DA, et al: Reliability of the modified timed up and go test (mTUG). In review, 2000.

182. Umphred DA, et al: Validity of the modified timed up and go test (mTUG). In review, 2000.

183. van der Putten JJ, et al: Measuring change in disability after inpatient rehabilitation comparison of the responsiveness of the Barthel index and the Functional Independence Measure. J Neurol Neurosurg Psychiatry 66:480, 1999.

184. Van Straten A, et al: A stroke-adapted 30-item version of the Sickness Impact Profile to assess quality of life (SA-SIP30). Stroke 28:2155, 1997.

185. VanSwearingen JM, et al: The modified Gait Abnormality Rating Scale for recognizing the risk of recurrent falls in community-dwelling elderly adults. Phys Ther 76:994, 1996.

186. Waters RL, et al: Energy-speed relationship of walking: Standard tables. J Orthop Res 6:215, 1988.

187. Waters RL, et al: Prediction of ambulatory performance based on motor scores derived from standards of the American Spinal Injury Association. Arch Phys Med Rehabil 75:756, 1994.

188. Watson YI, et al: Clock completion: An objective screening test for dementia. J Am Geriatr Soc 41:1235, 1993.

189. Weiner DK, et al: Does functional reach improve with rehabilitation? Arch Phys Med Rehabil 74:796, 1993.

190. Weiner DK, et al: Functional reach: A marker of physical frailty. J Am Geriatr Soc 40:203, 1992.

191. Westaway MD, et al: The patient-specific functional scale: Validation of its use in persons with neck dysfunction. J Orthop Sports Phys Ther 27:331, 1998.

192. Wheeler AH, et al: Development of the Neck Pain and Disability Scale: Item analysis, face, and criterion-related validity. Spine 24:1290, 1999.

193. Whipple R, Wolfson LI: Abnormalities of balance, gait, and sensorimotor function in the elderly population. In Duncan P (ed): Balance: Proceedings of the APTA Forum. Alexandria, VA, American Physical Therapy Association, 1990.

194. Whitney SL, et al: A review of balance instruments for older adults. Am J Occup Ther 52:666, 1998.

195. Whitney SL, et al: The activities-specific balance confidence scale and the dizziness handicap inventory: A comparison. J Vestib Res 9:253, 1999.

196. Wilk K: Dynamic muscle strength testing. In Amundsen LR (ed): Muscle Strength Testing Instrumented and Non-instrumented Systems. New York, Churchill Livingstone, 1990.

197. Willoughby EW, Paty DW: Scales for rating impairment in multiple sclerosis: A critique. Neurology 38:1793, 1988.

198. Winograd CH, et al: Development of a physical performance and mobility examination. J Am Geriatr Soc 42:743, 1994.

199. Wolfson L, et al: Gait assessment in the elderly: A gait abnormality rating scale and its relation to falls. J Gerontol 45:M12, 1990.

200. Wolfson LI, et al: Stressing the postural response: A quantitative method for testing balance. J Am Geriatr Soc 34:845, 1986.

201. Yavuz N, et al: A comparison of two functional tests in quadriplegia: The Quadriplegia Index of Function and the Functional Independence Measure. Spinal Cord 36:832, 1998.

202. Yesavage JA, et al: Development and validation of a geriatric depression screening scale: A preliminary report. J Psychiatr Res 17:37, 1983.

203. Zafonte RD, et al: Relationship between Glasgow Coma Scale and functional outcome. Am J Phys Med Rehabil 75:364, 1996.

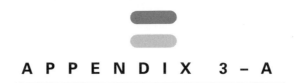

Functional vs. Impairment vs. Health Status/Quality of Life (QOL) Examination Tools

BALANCE IMPAIRMENT TESTS

Clinical Test of Sensory Integration on Balance (CTSIB)[37, 163–165]
Dynamic Posturography[31, 45, 53, 78, 86, 87]
Fukuda Stepping Test[150]
Functional Reach Test (LOS)[50, 51, 150]
Hallpike-Dix Test[48]
LOS Test on Balance Master[134]
Nudge/Push Test[110]
Oculomotor and Vestibuloocular Tests[81, 82]
Postural Stress Test[34, 199, 200]
Postural Sway During Quiet Standing[174]
Romberg Test[20, 135]
Sensory Organization Test (SOT)[130, 131, 134]
Sharpened Romberg Test (EO/EC)[135, 150]
Stand One Leg, Eyes Open/Eyes Closed (SOLEO/EC)[24, 135, 150]
Timed Balance Tests: feet together, etc.[24]

GAIT IMPAIRMENT TESTS

Automated Up-Timer[178]
Clinical Gait Assessments[27, 85, 198]
Functional Ambulation Profile[133]
Gait Abnormality Rating Scale (GARS)[185, 193, 203]
GAITRite System[35]
RLAH Gait Evaluation Form 1[148]

COGNITIVE STATUS TESTS

Abbreviated Mental Test (AMT)[115]
Mental Status Questionnaire (MSQ)[115]
Mini-Mental State Examination (MMSE)[38, 39, 57, 115, 172]

STRENGTH TESTS

Grip Strength Dynamometry[5, 6, 10, 22, 23, 54, 103, 123, 158, 196]
Manual Muscle Testing[4, 40, 83, 104]

SPASTICITY TESTS

Ashworth Scale[139]
Modified Ashworth Scale (MAS)[2, 25, 139]

RANGE OF MOTION TESTS

Objective Measurements of ROM[61]

DEPRESSION SCALES

Beck Depression Inventory[11]
Geriatric Depression Scale (five-item)[90]
Geriatric Depression Scale (GDS15)[7, 202]
Hamilton Rating Scale for Depression[79]
Zung Depression Scale[118]

DISABILITY SCALES (GENERAL PURPOSE)

Barthel Index[116, 183]
DUKE Mobility Skills Protocol (HMS)[84, 170, 189, 190]
Frail Elderly Functional Assessment Questionnaire (FEFA)[67, 68]
Functional Assessment Measure (FIM + FAM)[49, 60, 126, 180]
Functional Independence Measure (FIM)[102, 111, 136, 150, 169, 193]
Katz Index of Activities of Daily Living[100, 101]
OASIS (home health comprehensive)[132]
OPCS Scales of Disability[130]
PULSES Profile[73, 74]

FUNCTIONAL BALANCE ASSESSMENTS

Berg Balance Scale[12–15]
Functional Reach Test (FR)[50, 51, 174, 190]
Modified Functional Reach Test[114]
Repetitive Reach Test (RR)[18]
Step Test[18]
Tandem Gait[66]
Tinetti Performance Oriented Mobility Assessment (and mobility/gait)[175–177]

BALANCE AND MOBILITY ASSESSMENTS

Fast Evaluation of Mobility, Balance, and Fear (FEMBAF)[46]
Get Up and Go Test (GUG)[122]
Modified Timed Up and Go Test (mTUG)[181, 182]
Physical Performance Test (PPT)[153, 194]
Timed Up and Go—Manual Test (TUG manual)[113, 159]
Timed Up and Go Test (TUG)[140, 159]
Tinetti Performance Oriented Mobility Assessment[175]

FUNCTIONAL GAIT ASSESSMENTS

3 minute walk test[145]
5 minute walk test[144]
6 minute walk test[76]
12 minute walk test[125]

TESTS OF PHYSICAL FUNCTION IN THE ELDERLY

Automated Up-Timer[178]
Frail Elderly Functional Assessment Questionnaire (FEFA)[68]
Modified Gait Abnormality Rating Scale (GARS-M)[127, 185]
Physical Disability Index (PDI)[62]
Physical Performance and Mobility Examination (PPME)[198]
The Physical Performance Test (PPT)[195]
Timed Chair Rise[1]
Timed Chair Stands[174]

ACTIVITIES OF DAILY LIVING (ADL) SCALES

Katz Index of Activities of Daily Living[100, 101]
Kenny Self-Care Evaluation[94]

Klein-Bell Activities of Daily Living Scale[105]
Physical Self-Maintenance Scale[109]
PULSES Profile[120, 129]
Structured Assessment of Independent Living Skills (SAILS)[117]
The Safety Assessment of Function and the Environment for Rehabilitation (SAFER)[137]

FALLS EFFICACY SCALES

Activities-specific Balance Confidence (ABC) Scale[143, 195]
Falls Efficacy Scale (FES)[177]

NONEQUILIBRIUM COORDINATION TESTS (RAMs)[138]

(includes Rapid Stepping Tests,
Heel-to-Toe Transition, Heel-to-Shin, and
Rapid Alternating Movement Tests)

DIAGNOSIS-SPECIFIC TOOLS

Stroke Tools

Arm Motor Ability Test (AMAT) (ADL)[106]
Chedoke-McMaster Stroke Assessment[72]
Frenchay Activities Index (disability and handicap)[160]
Fugl-Meyer Test[52, 59, 157]
LIDO Active System: Resistance to Passive Shoulder ER[128]
Modified Motor Assessment Scale (MMAS)[112]
Motor Assessment Scale (MAS)[32, 142]
National Institute of Health Stroke Scale (NIHSS)[155]
PULSES Profile[73, 74]
Rankin Scale (disability and handicap index)[44]
Stroke Rehabilitation Assessment of Movement (STREAM)[41]
Stroke-Adapted 30-item Sickness Impact Profile (SA-SIP 30)[184]
Tone Assessment Scale[75]
Trunk Control Test (TCT)[58]
Unified Neurological Stroke Scale (UFNSS)[179]

Brain Injury Tools

Coma Recovery Scale (CRS)[63]
Coma/Near-Coma (CNC) Scale[149]
Disability Rating Scale[47]
Galveston Orientation and Amnesia Test (GOAT)[42]
Glasgow Coma Scale (GCS)[97–99, 203]
Glasgow Outcome Scale (GOS)[97, 98]
Levels of Cognitive Functioning Assessment Scale (LOFCAS)[55, 56]
Rancho Los Amigos Levels of Cognitive Functioning[147]
Sensory Modality Assessment Rehabilitation Technique (SMART)[65]
Supervision Rating Scale (SRS)[21]
Western Neuro Sensory Stimulation Profile (WNSSP)[65]
Wolinsky Amnesia Information Test (WAIT)[124]

Parkinson's Disease/Huntington's Disease Tools

Obeso Dyskinesia Rating Scale[71, 77]
Parkinson's Disease Questionnaire (PDQ-39)[96]
Schwab-England Activities of Daily Living Score[8]
Unified Huntington Disease Rating Scale (UHDRS)[91, 154]
Unified Parkinson's Disease Rating Scale: Motor Examination[69, 70, 154, 157, 167, 168]

Dizziness/Vestibular Disease

Dizziness Handicap Inventory[95]
Timed Object Transfer Task[37]

Multiple Sclerosis Tools

Cambridge Multiple Sclerosis Basic Score (CAMBS)[161]
Disease Steps[87]
EQUI-SCALE[173]
Fahn's Tremor Rating Scale (FTRS)[88]
Functional Assessment of Multiple Sclerosis (FAMS)[33]
Illness Severity Score (ISS)[93]
Kurtzke Extended Disability Status Scale (EDSS)[71, 89, 107, 108, 199]
Multiple Sclerosis Impairment Scales[151]
Scripps Neurological Rating Scales (SNRS)[161]
The Functional Limitations Profile (FLP)[93]

Spinal Cord Injury Tools

American Spinal Injury Association Functional Classification of Spinal Cord Injury (ASIA Scale)[37, 186, 187]
Capabilities of Upper Extremity (CUE)[119]
Quadriplegia Index of Function Scale (QIF)[201]
Self-Care Assessment Tool (SCAT) (ADLs)[26]
Short-form Quadriplegia Index of Function Scale (QIF)[119]

Dementia, Cognitive Status—Elderly

Bristol Activities of Daily Living Scale[29]
Multidimensional Observation Scale for Elderly Subjects (MOSES)[80]
Structured Assessment of Independent Living Skills (SAILS)[117]

Alzheimer's Tools

Clock Drawing Test for Dementia Severity in Alzheimer's[171, 188]
Discomfort Assessment for Alzheimer's[92]

Orthopedic Tools

Fibromyalgia Impact Questionnaire (FIQ)[30]
Million Visual Analogue Scale[19, 192]
Modified-American Shoulder and Elbow Surgeons Form[9]
Neck Pain and Disability Scale[192]
Oswestry Low Back Pain Disability Questionnaire[19, 192]
Pain Disability Index[192]
Patient-specific Functional Scale[191]
Roland (back pain) Questionnaire[19, 192]
Short-form Arthritis Impact Measurement Scales (AIMS2-SF) (OA)[152]
Shoulder Pain and Disability Index[9]
Shoulder Severity Index[9]
Simple Shoulder Test[9]
Subjective Shoulder Rating Scale[9]
The Iowa Level of Assistance Scale (TJR)[162]

Health Status Tools

Arthritis Impact Scale[152]
Health Status Questionnaire[146]
Hospital Admission Risk Profile[156]
McMaster University Osteoarthritis Index[121]
Musculoskeletal Function Assessment Questionnaire[121]
Short-form 36 Health Survey Questionnaire (SF-36)[28]
Sickness Impact Profile (SIP)[16, 17, 141]
The Parkinson's Disease Questionnaire (PDQ-39)[96]
The Sickness Impact Profile (SIP68)[43]
Western Ontario Osteoarthritis Index[121]

CHAPTER 4

Interventions for Neurological Disabilities

DARCY A. UMPHRED, PhD, PT • NANCY BYL, PhD, PT • ROLANDO T. LAZARO, MS, PT, GCS
• MARGARET ROLLER, MS, PT

Key Words

– contrived therapeutic procedures

– functional training

– motor learning

– neuroplasticity

– somatosensory retraining

Objectives

After reading this chapter the student/therapist will:

1. Develop an appreciation for the complexity of motor responses, the multitudinous ways to influence those behaviors, and the theories that lay the foundation for motor learning.

2. Identify variables that affect neuroplasticity and how to create environments that optimize learning.

3. Differentiate functional training, contrived interventions, and somatosensory retraining and their appropriate selection as intervention strategies.

4. Differentiate feedback/feedforward systems and therapeutic procedures to delineate variables that may affect both positively and negatively complex motor responses.

5. Analyze how to differentiate between extrinsic and intrinsic feedback as a contrived versus a functional therapeutic procedure.

6. Identify procedures and sequences that best meet the client's needs and help regain the highest quality of life.

7. Identify the importance of collaboration with the client, the client's support systems, and the best practice standards available to optimize outcome after interventions.

Before discussing therapeutic intervention procedures, the therapist must identify the learning environment within which the client will perform. As discussed in Chapter 1, that environment is made up of the therapist and the client, all internal body control mechanisms of the client, and the external restraints of the world. Although this text focuses on functional deficits arising from internal peripheral and central nervous system (CNS) mechanism problems, the reader must always consider the client as a totality and include within the analysis how other organ or body systems will be affected by or affect the outcome of therapeutic intervention. An examination/evaluation (see Chapter 3) is performed before intervention to establish objective measurements; to help the clinician diagnose functional limitations and impairments, as well as determine a prognosis of the outcomes based on the patient's potential for functional improvement, motivation, family support, financial support, and cultural biases; and to guide selection of intervention strategies.

Using current motor control/learning theories and systems models, the therapist must also determine the flexibility and/or inherent motor control the client demonstrates while executing functional activities. During the evaluation phase, the therapist must break down the components of movement and determine which, if any, are causing distortions or inefficient execution of the overall plan. The therapist must examine, analyze, and diagnose the strengths and limitations of the client's motor systems including but not limited to range of motion (ROM), muscle strength, state of the motor pool or pattern generators, synergies (volitional and reflexive), postural integrity, balance, rate, timing, and trajectory of movement. In addition, this motor analysis must occur within the larger context of the environment, ethnic and social diversity, sensory status, and learning capacity of the client. Functional goals must be established that lead to the client's control over his or her environment and whenever possible lead to or maintain the quality of life desired by the client.

When selecting treatment interventions the therapist must differentiate between somatosensory retraining, functional motor retraining, and augmented facilitory treatment intervention. All three intervention methodologies include a variety of interventions, each based on different strategies and rationale that contribute to the expected outcome. All three intervention methods can be used simultaneously, but the clinician needs to determine which aspect of the intervention falls into which methodology. If not, even though outcomes can be measured, determination of how and why the outcomes were influ-

enced by the intervention becomes very confusing and very hard to understand. Without the understanding of the interactions of the intervention and the outcome, future clinical decision making remains unpredictable and unique practice patterns and pathways hard to identify with consistency.

The reader must also remember that intervention encompasses multiple interactive environments where intervention decisions are often made moment by moment during any one treatment period. The challenge to the educated professional is to determine what is being done, why it is working, how to continue, and how to determine the progress of the successful intervention. The professional must also determine how to empower the client to take over the intervention with inherent, automatic mechanisms that lead to fluid, flexible, functional outcomes independent of both the therapist and the environment within which the activity is occurring.

OVERVIEW OF NEUROLOGICAL REHABILITATION AND MOTOR LEARNING THEORY

Therapeutic interventions that are focused on restoring functional skills of individuals with various forms of neurological problems have been part of the scope of practice of physical therapists (PTs) and occupational therapists (OTs) since the beginning of both professions. Similarly, nurses, speech pathologists, recreational therapists, orthotists, physical medicine and rehabilitation physicians, special educators, and dance and music therapists also focus on various aspects of regaining functional control. Each profession has a unique education, unique models for intervention, and often the belief that his or her respective professional training is the only and the best to guide the patient toward the best outcome. In reality, no profession has the time or knowledge to develop a practitioner who can evaluate and treat all aspects of each client's mind, body, and spirit. Each professional has a unique skill to offer, and these skills need to be matched to the client and available to the client when needed.

When looking at the educational training of PTs and OTs, these two professions emerge with a complementary background to examine, evaluate, determine a prognosis, and implement interventions that empower clients to regain functional control of activities of daily living (e.g., getting out of bed, bathing, walking, and eating, as well as working, playing, and socially interacting). Both professionals understand how all aspects of the nervous system and the organs that support that system express themselves through motor control and motor output. These two professionals are specialists in the analysis of movement with the scientific background to understand why the movement is occurring, what the strengths and limitations are within the system to support that movement, and how different types of intervention can facilitate functional movement strategies that ultimately carry over into functional life activities. PTs and OTs are also very knowledgeable about neurological and organ system disease and how progression of these pathological states affects motor performance and quality of life as well as about assistance and support needed to help clients maintain functional skills during transitional disease states. Similarly, therapists are currently taught how to minimize impairments within the sensory and motor systems before functional loss. Early intervention before disability can help prevent dysfunction as well as save millions of health care dollars.

History of Development of Interventions for Neurological Disabilities

In the 1950s, the interventions by PTs and OTs were very separate. Generally, PTs worked on gross motor activities with specific emphasis on the lower extremities and the trunk, whereas OTs worked on the upper extremities and fine motor activities. Both professions focused on daily living skills, with those involving the arms falling within the domain of the OT and those involving the legs falling within the domain of the PT. Activities that required gross motor skills such as walking, running, and crutch walking fell within the purview of the PT, whereas brushing the hair and eating were the responsibility of the OT. Today, this approach is considered ridiculous owing to our understanding of motor learning and programming. In the past, it was also accepted that the PT worked on specific problems such as weakness, inflexibility, lack of coordination, and voluntary control, whereas the OT worked on functional activities integrated within the environment as well as the patient's emotional needs and desires. Using the terminology of the twenty-first century, PTs were trained to identify and correct impairments that could lead to physical disability, whereas OTs were trained to identify and minimize the disabilities that resulted from the impairments. Thus, after the onset of a stroke, the PT would strengthen and evaluate range of motion of the leg, whereas the OT would encourage the patient to try to functionally use the arm. The PT would be preparing the patient to transfer out of bed as well as get into and out of a chair and then helping the patient walk, whereas the OT would be preparing the patient to use the arm in functional activities. Both hoped the patient would accept life with new challenges. What both professions discovered was that the patient generally did not regain normal motor control. He or she might be able to walk and may be able to move the shoulder, but the movement strategies were generally stereotypical and abnormal in patterns. There was also minimal recovery of functional hand use. Although functional independent skills were usually achieved, normal movement patterns and normal motor

control were rarely restored and quality of life was clearly impacted for the patient and his or her family.

During the decade or two before the 1960s, some very talented and intelligent clinicians began to question the traditional intervention strategies used by the OT and PT. These pioneers[*] in neurological rehabilitation set the stage for the development of new concepts that infiltrated basic science into the clinical arena. Thus, the intervention strategies of Jean Ayers, Berta Bobath, Signe Brunnstrom, Margaret Knott/Dorothy Voss, Margaret Rood, Susanne Klein-Vogelbach, and others became popular. Colleagues observed these master clinicians and could easily see that the new interventions provided a much better outcome than previous interventions. Each approach focused on multisensory inputs introduced to the client in controlled and identified sequences. These sequences were based on the inherent nature of synergistic patterns[9, 228] and motor patterns observed in humans[9, 34, 228] and lower-order animals[97] or a combination of the two.[176, 288] Each method focused on the individual client, the specific clinical problems, and the availability of alternative treatment approaches within each established framework. Certain methods traditionally emphasized specific neurological disabilities. Cerebral palsy and head injuries in children[22, 34, 236, 288] and hemiplegia in adults[32, 40, 55, 213] were the two most frequently identified diagnostic categories. In the past two decades substantial clinical attention has also been paid to children with learning and language difficulties.[10, 102] Now, these concepts and treatment procedures have been applied across the age spectrum for all types of medically diagnosed neurological problems seen in the clinical setting. This expansion of the use of any of the methods for any pathology seems to be a natural evolution given the structure and function of the CNS and commonalities in impairments and disabilities manifested by insults from disease, injury, or degeneration of the brain.

Unfortunately, dogmatism still persists with respect to territorial boundaries identified by clinicians using some specific intervention methods. On the other hand, intervention approaches such as proprioceptive neuromuscular facilitation (PNF) are now integrated into the care of clients with orthopedic problems as well as patients with neurological impairments. Today, it seems there are more commonalities than differences among the various approaches to rehabilitation.

For example, assume a client with hemiplegia exhibited signs of a hypertonic upper-extremity pattern of shoulder adduction, internal rotation, elbow flexion, and forearm pronation with wrist and finger flexion. Brunnstrom would have identified that pattern as the stronger of her two upper-extremity synergies.[40] Michels, although using an explanation similar to Brunnstrom's to describe the pattern, would have elaborated and described additional upper-extremity synergy patterns.[213] Bobath would have asserted that the client was stuck in a mass-movement pattern resulting from abnormal postural reflex activity.[32] Although the conceptualization of the problem certainly determined treatment protocols, the pattern all three

---

[*]See references 9, 22, 34, 40, 55, 64, 70, 102, 105, 107, 112, 174, 176, 189, 213, 216, 257, 275, 278, 288, and 289.

clinicians would have worked toward was shoulder abduction, external rotation, elbow extension, forearm supination, and wrist and finger extension. The rationale for the use of this pattern within an intervention period would vary according to the philosophical approach. One clinician might describe the pattern as a reflex-inhibiting position. Another would describe the pattern as the weakest component of the various synergies, whereas still another might identify the pattern as producing an extreme stretch and rotatory element that reciprocally inhibited the spastic pattern. How a clinician sequenced treatment from the original hypertonic pattern to the goal pattern correlated with functional movement would vary. Some would facilitate push-pull patterns in supine, side lying, and rolling. Others would look at propping patterns in sitting or at weight-bearing patterns in prone, over a ball or bolster, or in partial kneeling. All have the potential of eliciting the functional pattern and modifying the hypertonic pattern. One method may have been better than the others, but in truth improved performance may have stemmed not from the method itself but rather from the preferential CNS biases of the client and the variability of application skills among the clinicians themselves. That is, when using augmented feedback to modulate the motor system's response to an environmental demand, without the understanding of all the additional augmented feedback applied simultaneously, the individual patient and the variations in outcome from patient to patient would vary, making the efficacy of intervention very questionable.

Because of the overlap of treatment methodologies and the infiltration of therapeutic management into all avenues of neurological dysfunction, various multisensory models were developed during the early 1980s,[56, 67, 102, 116, 130, 140] and these have continued to evolve into acceptable methodologies in today's clinical arena. Although these models attempted to integrate existing techniques, in reality they have created a new set of wholistic treatment approaches. The ultimate goal would be to develop one all-encompassing methodology that allows the clinician the freedom to use any method that is appropriate for the needs and individual learning styles of the client as well as tap the unique individual differences of the clinician. Although that approach does not yet exist, its development will be a challenge to future therapists.

Therapists of today either continue to embrace traditional intervention approaches or have replaced them with applications of new motor control, motor learning theories, or dynamic systems theories. When confronted with a similar upper-extremity pattern described in the past, today's therapist may also work on the same pattern during a functional activity, because control of that combination of movement responses and thus modulation over those central pattern generators will allow the patient opportunities to experience functional movement that is task oriented and environmentally specific while allowing practice to enhance motor learning and carryover.[68] With a better scientific basis for understanding the function of the human nervous system, how the motor system learns and is controlled, and how other systems both internal and external to the CNS modulate response patterns, today's clinicians have many additional options for selection of intervention strategies. Whether a patient would initially benefit best from somatosensory retraining, functional retraining, or a more traditional augmented/contrived treatment environment is up to the clinician and the specific needs identified during the examination and evaluation process.

No matter what treatment methodology is selected by a clinician, all intervention should focus on the active learning process of the client. The client should never be a passive participant, even if the level of consciousness is considered vegetative. With all interventions requiring an active motor response, whether to change an impairment such as increasing or reducing the rate of a motor response or the tonal state of the combined central pattern generators or cause a functional response during an activity, the client's CNS is being asked to process and respond to the external world at multisegmental levels. That response needs to become procedural and run by the patient without any augmentation to be measured as functional independence. In time, the ultimate goal is for the client's internal drive system to self-regulate and orchestrate modulation over this adaptable and dynamic motor system in all functional activities and in all external environments.

A problem-oriented approach to treatment of any impairment and/or the residual disability implies that flexibility and adaptation are key elements in recovery. However, adaptation should not be random, disjointed, or non–goal oriented. It should be based on methods that provide the best combination of available treatment alternatives to meet individual needs. This adaptation achieved through development of a clinical knowledge bank enables the therapist to match treatment alternatives with the patient's impairments, disabilities, handicaps, and objectives for function. A professionally educated therapist no longer bases treatment on identified recipes, although the ingredients for those recipes may be alternative treatment tools if, and only if, the client needs them. Treatment is based on an interaction among basic science, applied science, a therapist's skills, and client objectives.

Motor Learning Concepts as a Basis for Intervention Design

Variables Controlled Outside the Motor System

When considering motor learning, the therapist must first differentiate general factors affecting motor performance. Some factors are under the control of the cognitive and emotional systems, and others are controlled by the motor system itself. These various factors or concepts of motor learning have been presented in Figure 4–1. There are many cognitive factors such as arousal, attention, and cortical pathways related to declarative learning that have specific influences over observable disabilities after neurological insult. Other factors such as motivation, limbic connections to cortical pathways, and emotional stability also dramatically affect motor performance and declarative learning. Some of these factors may also cause functional disabilities. Therapists need to learn how to discriminate between cortical somatosensory and limbic

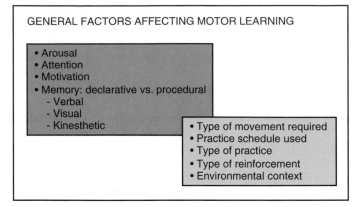

FIGURE 4-1. Concepts affecting motor learning.

emotional problems. Similarly, clinicians need to identify how these two systems affect motor output. With that differentiation, PTs and OTs will be able to separate specific motor system deficits from dysfunction within other areas of the CNS. Similarly, motor learning concepts that relate specifically to the motor system need to be understood and incorporated into all interventions to achieve optimal outcomes in the least amount of time within the least restrictive environment.

Another variable that is outside the motor system itself is consideration of the environmental context within which the client must perform the functional activity. If motor programming and learning is limited, then practicing activities close to if not specific to the functional performance needed by the patient becomes critical. For example, assume a client has limited visits and when returning home will spend the majority of the day on a boat in an armless chair while fishing. Independent sitting is the functional activity listed as the important goal, with the lack of sitting balance as the impairment that limits the functional skill. Because the client will sit either in a lounge chair at home that requires no balance or in a fishing chair on a boat that requires balance on a compliant surface, the environment in which the therapist needs to practice must incorporate either sitting on compliant surfaces or sitting on a hard-surfaced chair that has been placed on a compliant surface. In that way, the therapist is matching the therapeutic environment with the context of the life activity set as a goal by the patient. The closer the therapeutic environment matches the environmental context, the more likely the patient will learn the procedural program needed to gain functional independence within the established activity.

Variables That Are Motor System Specific

If prior procedural learning has occurred, then creating an environment that allows the program to run in the least restrictive environment should lead to the most efficient outcome in the shortest time.[319] If a patient needs to learn a new program, such as walking with an extension synergy, then goal-directed, attended practice with guided feedback is necessary.

Identifying what motor programs are available under what conditions allows the therapist to match existing programs with functional activities, to determine whether

deficits are present, and to anticipate problems. Similarly, knowing available programs and the subcomponent necessary to run those programs aids the therapist in the selection of intervention procedures.

If the client has permanent damage to either the basal ganglia or the cerebellum, then retaining the memory of new motor programs may be difficult and substitution approaches may become necessary. Through evaluation the clinician needs to determine whether anatomical disease or pathology is actually causing procedural learning problems. However, because of the plasticity of the CNS, significant recovery or adaptation may occur after attended goal-directed repetitive behavior.[210]

There are four traditional components of motor learning that must be considered during any intervention.[271] These four components include the type of movement required (Fig. 4–2), the type of practice environment (see Fig. 4–2), the practice schedule itself (Fig. 4–3), and the best reinforcement schedule to bring about the quickest, most efficient and effective motor responses to environmental demands (Fig. 4–4).

Timing of the intervention related to recovery of motor function is also important. There is evidence that aggressive therapy staged too close to the neural injury could increase the extent of damage in the brain and spinal cord. Thus, while goal-directed rehabilitation training has been shown to enhance recovery[231, 321] there is a window of healing that is needed. The time parameters of this window are not yet clearly defined, but they are particularly applicable in the acute inpatient setting.

Stages of Motor Learning

Motor learning is an intricate balance between the feedforward and feedback sensorimotor systems. When observing the sequential activities of the child walking off the park bench, a clear (Fig. 4–5) understanding of this relationship of height and falling is established. In frame A, the child is running a feedforward program for walking. The cerebellum is procedurally responsible for that activity and will correct or modify the walking when necessary to attain the directed goal. Unfortunately, a simple correction of walking is not adequate for the environment presented in frame B. The cerebellum has no prior knowledge of the feedback presented in this second frame and thus is still running a feedforward program for stance on

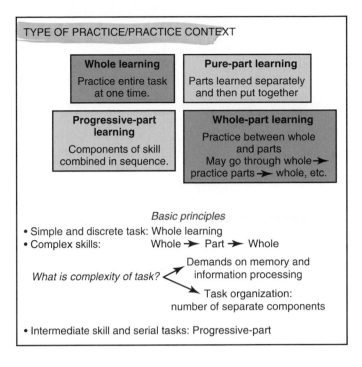

FIGURE 4–2. Type of practice/practice concept.

the left leg and swing on the right leg. The somatosensory cortices are processing a massive amount of mismatched information from the proprioceptive, vestibular, and visual receptors. In addition, the dopamine receptors are activated during the goal-driven behaviors, creating a balance of inhibition and excitation. To prepare for falling, the somatosensory system must generate a sensory plan and then relay that plan to the motor system through the sensorimotor feedback loop. The feedforward system will tell the basal ganglia and the cerebellum to brace and prepare for impact. The basal ganglia initiate the program, and the cerebellum carries out the procedure as observed in Figure 4–5C. The child succeeds at the task. It is possible that this experience created a new procedural program that would be labeled jumping. The entire process of the initial motor learning took 1 to 2 seconds. Because of the child's motivation and interest, the program was mass practiced for the next 30 to 45 minutes. This would be the initial acquisition phase and will help the nervous system store the motor program to be used

for the rest of his life. If this program is to become a procedural skill, practice must continue within similar environments and conditions. Ultimately, the errors will be reduced and the skill will be refined. Finally, with practice, the program will enter the retention phase as a high-level skill. The skill can still be modified in terms of force, timing, sequencing, and speed and be able to be transferred to different settings. This ongoing modification and improvement is the hallmark of true procedural learning.

Systems Interactions: Motor Responses Represent Consensus of CNS Systems

Three Systems Within the CNS

Motor behavior reflects not only motor programming but also the interaction of cognitive, affective, and somatosensory variables. Without a motor system, neither the cogni-

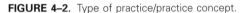

PRACTICE SCHEDULE
Practice vs. rest periods (time between practice)

Mass practice
- Schedule: Daily consecutive session
- Similar to rehabilitation setting

Distributed practice
- Schedule
  - 3 × per week
  - 2 × per week
  - 1 × per week
- Similar to outpatient setting or fixed home program

Random practice
- No fixed schedule
- Empowered client to practice at own pace

General concepts
- Some activities mass practice leads to higher performance—others distributed or random.
- Novel skills probably require more intensive mass practice.
- Even if performance decreases during practice session, learning may increase.

FIGURE 4–3. Practice schedule.

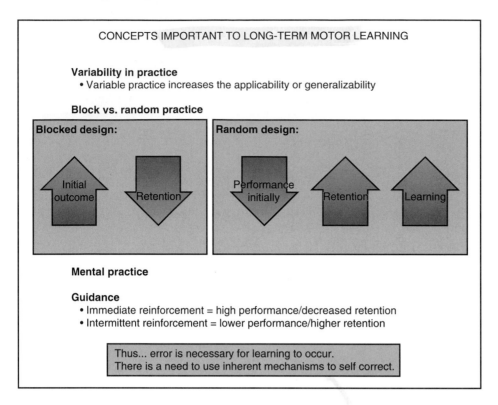

FIGURE 4–4. Concepts important to long-term motor learning.

tive nor the emotion systems have a way to express and communicate inner thoughts to the world. The cognitive and emotional systems can positively or negatively affect motor responses. The significance of the somatosensory or perceptual/cognitive cortical system must also be emphasized. The somatosensory association areas play a critical role in the ideational and constructional aspects of the motor program itself. With deficits within this system, clients will often demonstrate significant distortions in motor control even without a specific motor impairment.

An example of this problem might be an individual who had a stroke and developed a "pusher syndrome." The motor behavior shown by this client would be pushing off vertical generally in a posterolateral direction. Physically correcting the client's posture to vertical will not eliminate the original behavior because it does not stem from a motor problem but rather a visual-perceptual problem within the somatosensory cortices. Although a therapist might want to augment intervention by trying to push the patient to vertical, the patient will resist that movement

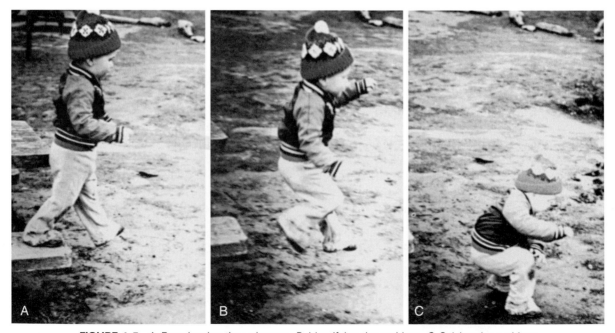

FIGURE 4–5. A, Experiencing the unknown. B, Identifying the problem. C, Solving the problem.

pattern. Functional training becomes frustrating to both the patient and the therapist because the impairment does not fall within the motor system itself. Somatosensory retraining might be the best intervention strategy for this type of problem because of impairment is within the sensory processing centers.

If a patient's insult falls within the limbic/emotional system, then motor behavior could also be affected. The motor dysfunction will be very different from the dysfunction reflecting damage to the sensory cortices. For years it has been common knowledge that individuals who are depressed will demonstrate motor signs of withdrawal (e.g., flexion). If the posture of flexion was created by a chemical response related to depression, then somatosensory retraining would have a limited effect on behavior. Similarly, functional training may initially modify the impairments, but without changes within the limbic system itself no permanent change will be achieved. Instead, augmenting the input to alter the emotional system and then reinforcing self-control could create the best potential outcome.

For many clinical problems functional retraining of the motor system through attended, sequenced, repetitive practice could lead to greater functional gains even though the impairments may never be eliminated. That is, muscle strengthening and programming co-activation to enable joint stability could restore client independence. Given the complexity of impairments and function in a patient with a neurological insult, a therapist may need to use all three types of intervention procedures to affect all areas of the CNS simultaneously. The decision of which intervention is most appropriate or which should be emphasized falls within the professional judgment of the clinician.

In the clinical environment, the most effective and efficient treatment for the neural insult is the one that is matched to the client's expectations and motivation, the neural injury, the healing process, and the physiological potential for recovery. This requires a dynamic interaction between the client, the therapist, the family, science, and technology. The knowledge base of science includes an understanding of the disease process, all body systems interactions both outside and within the nervous system, neuroanatomy/neurophysiology, and the principles of neuroplasticity. Within the following section a more in-depth discussion of neuroplasticity has been presented to introduce or refamiliarize the reader with this rapidly enlarging and evolving component of neuroscience.

PRINCIPLES OF NEUROPLASTICITY: IMPLICATIONS FOR NEUROREHABILITATION

Research, Rehabilitation, and Practice

Rehabilitation is the process of maximizing learning. The integration of basic neuroscience into clinical practice is critical to guiding the questioning of the researcher and maximizing the recovery of the patient. The 1990s were referred to as the "Decade of the Brain." Over a ten-year period, researchers made striking discoveries that

changed the perspective on the adaptability of the CNS. Neuroscientists and clinicians documented that the CNS was adaptable not only during development but also throughout life. The CNS can recover from serious disease and injury through spontaneous adaptation and healing. However, we also know that the extent of the recovery can be enhanced with environmental enrichment and behavioral training. Even the physiological effects of aging can be slowed if neurons remain actively engaged and goal-oriented behavior is rewarded. Unfortunately, despite this revolutionary growth of knowledge regarding the neural mechanisms that facilitate adaptation, implementation of this knowledge into clinical practice has been limited. The lack of integration of basic science and clinical practice can be attributed to the researcher, the clinician, the patient, and the third-party payer.

All too often the researcher is in the laboratory carrying out research experiments without tying together the experimental specific outcomes with the learning environment of the clinical world. Although the researchers actively communicate with others in their fields and attend professional meetings in the areas of special interests, the conferences rarely are of interest to both the scientist and the clinician. Thus, many basic science researchers rarely have contact with clinicians. Some are only interested in pursuing the next basic scientific experiment and they do not care about implications for clinical practice. It would be beneficial if there were more integrative neuroscience conferences that linked the scientist in the laboratory to the practitioner in the clinic.

Sometimes, practicing neurorehabilitation clinicians fail to apply basic science findings to change practice. Familiar treatment approaches dominate practice even when there is little validation that they are successful. Some practitioners are simply unfamiliar with the current basic neuroscience literature, others are familiar with recent research findings but do not know how to translate these findings into practice, and still others are unwilling to accept that the basic research findings provide sufficient evidence to support broad-based changes in practice. Failure to integrate basic science and clinical practice significantly impairs the potential for recovery for patients with disabling neurological problems.

In some situations, the patient could be the obstacle to successful recovery and neural adaptation. To achieve maximum plasticity, the patient must be engaged in attended, goal-directed behaviors. There is no measurable neural adaptation with passive movements or passive stimuli. To achieve a change in neural response, the patient has to attend to the stimulus and make a decision about it. This has to be done repetitively. There are instances when patients are not convinced that their efforts will make a difference. In other cases the patient is not motivated to be compliant. In still other situations, the neural insult itself alters patient motivation and/or cognition, creates emotional instability, or leads to neglect of one or more parts of the body. These latter conditions can interfere with the ability to participate in a meaningful way in goal-directed, even positively rewarded behaviors.

Another failure to bring scientific evidence into practice is the obstacle created by living in a society in which the economics of health care drive the system, rather than the science or the benefit to the patient. When a physician or a therapist recommends a new approach to intervention, the third-party payer may deny payment for service it considers "experimental." Further, third-party payers may disagree that findings from animal studies should be applied to human subjects. For example, studies show that the greatest spontaneous recovery after a cardiovascular accident occurs in the first 30 days. When the physician refers patients for continued therapy after 30 days, the third-party payer denies reimbursement for services despite the evidence that the CNS can be modified under conditions of goal-oriented, repetitive, task-relevant behaviors well after 30 days. It has also been shown that neural adaptation is even greater when environmental conditions and sensory inputs are enriched.[231]

As the science of neuroplasticity continues to develop, it is critical that ways be found to improve the interface between the scientist, the practitioner, the patient, and the third-party payer. This partnership could be reinforced with increased collaborative research between basic scientists and rehabilitation practitioners. In addition, it is critical that third-party payers be regularly informed about current research findings both in the basic sciences and in the clinic.

Integration of Sensory Information and Motor Control

In virtually all higher-order perceptual processes, the brain must correlate sensory input with motor output to assess the body's interaction with the environment accurately. A problem in the somatic motor system impacts the motor output system. Both systems are independently adaptive, but functional neural adaptation involves an interaction of adaptation in both systems. Although these two systems operate differently, they are hopelessly intertwined in the healthy nervous system.

The sensory system provides an internal representation of the outside world that guides the movements that make up our behavioral repertoire. These movements are controlled by the motor systems of the brain and the spinal cord. Our perceptual skills are a reflection of the capabilities of the sensory systems to detect, analyze, and estimate the significance of physical stimuli. (See the Augmented Therapeutic Intervention section within this chapter for a detailed discussion of each sensory system.) Our agility and dexterity represent a reflection of the capabilities of the motor systems to plan, coordinate, and execute movements. The task of the motor systems in controlling movement is the reverse of the task of sensory systems in generating an internal representation. Perception is the end product of sensory processing, whereas an internal representation (an image of the desired movement) is the beginning of motor processing.

Sensory psychophysics looks at the attributes of a stimulus: its quality, intensity, location, and duration. Motor psychophysics considers the organization of action, the intensity of the contraction, the recruitment of distinct populations of motor neurons, the accuracy of the movement, the coordination of the movements, and the speed of movement. In both the sensory and motor systems, the complexity of behaviors depends on the multiplicity of modalities available. In sensation, there are the distinct modalities of pain, temperature, light touch, deep touch, vibration, and stretch, whereas in the motor system can be found the modalities of reflex responses, rhythmic motor patterns, and voluntary movements.[252] Although all motor movements require integration of sensory information, the relationship is particularly complex in voluntary motor movements. Voluntary motor movements require contraction and relaxation of muscles, recruitment of appropriate muscles, appropriate timing and sequencing of muscle contraction and relaxation, the distribution of the body mass, and appropriate postural adjustments required to achieve the movement.

Within each movement, there must be adjustments to compensate for the inertia of the limbs and the mechanical arrangement of the muscles, bones, and joints both before and during movement to ensure and maintain accuracy. The control systems for voluntary movement include (1) the continuous flow of sensory information about the environment, position and orientation of the body and limbs, as well as the degree of contraction of the muscles; (2) the spinal cord; (3) the descending systems of the brain stem; and (4) the pathways of the motor areas of the cerebral cortex, cerebellum, and basal ganglia. Each level of control is based on the sensory information that is relevant for the functions it controls. This information is provided by feedback, feedforward, and adaptive mechanisms. These control systems are organized both hierarchically and in parallel. The hierarchical organization permits lower levels to generate reflexes without involving higher centers, whereas the parallel system allows the brain to process the flow of discrete types of sensory information to produce discrete types of movements.[28, 77]

Ultimately, the control of graded fine-motor movements gets down to the sensory organ of the muscle spindle, which contains the specialized elements that sense muscle length and the velocity on changes in length. In conjunction with the Golgi tendon organ, which senses muscle tension, the muscle spindle provides the CNS with continuous information on the mechanical state of the muscle. Ultimately, the firing of the muscle spindles depends on both muscle length and the level of gamma activation of the intrafusal fibers based on the interpretation by the CNS of the signals from the muscle spindles. This illustrates the close relationship between sensory and motor processing and the integral relationship between the two when discussing neuroplasticity.[149]

Foundation for the Study of Neuroplasticity

The principal models for studying cortical plasticity have been based on the representations of hand skin and hand movements in the New World owl monkey (*Aotus*) and the squirrel monkey (*Saimire*). These primate models have been chosen because their central sulci usually do not extend into the hand representational zone in the anterior parietal (S1) or posterior frontal (M1) cortical fields. In other primates the sulci are deep and interfere with accurate mapping. Albeit there are differences in

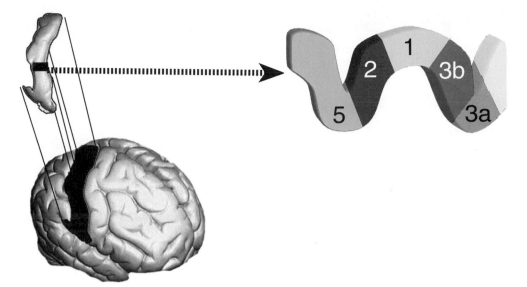

FIGURE 4–6. Classification and anatomical locations of cortical map.

hand use among primates, in all of the primates the hand has the largest topographical representation for the actual size of the extremity, the detail of this representation is distinct, and the hand has the greatest potential for skilled movements and sensory discrimination. However, the findings from studies of this cortical area are applicable across the cortex.[207, 209] Refer to Figure 4–6 to identify specific anatomical locations and their respective classifications.

Neuroplasticity: Principles of Neural Adaptation

In neural adaptation (neuroplasticity), the fundamental questions are: As we learn, how does the brain change its representations of inputs and actions? What is the nature of the processes that control the progressive elaboration of performance abilities? In different individuals, what are the sources of variance for emergent performance abilities? What changes in cortical plasticity facilitate the development of "automatic" motor behaviors? Why are some behaviors not improved indefinitely?

The most informative studies on neuroplasticity are those specifically directed toward defining changes induced by learning. One approach has been to document the patterns of distributed neural response representation of specific inputs before and after learning. In particular, neuronal responses have been measured in the primary auditory, somatosensory, and motor cortices in animals. These animal studies have been paired with behavioral studies in humans. Both the animal and human studies provide strong inference for the ability of the brain to functionally self-organize, not only during development but also in adulthood as well as after injury. Based on some basic studies, one can outline the basic cortical plasticity processes that contribute to learning. These are summarized in the following box and in Table 4–1 and discussed in detail in the ensuing pages.

1. With learning, the distributed cortical representations of inputs and brain actions "specialize" in their representations of behaviorally important inputs and actions in skill learning.

This specialization develops in response to selective cortical neuron responses specialized to demands of perceptual, cognitive, and motor skill learning.[200, 201, 205, 212] This adaptation has been clearly documented in animal studies. For example, if an animal is trained to make progressively finer distinctions about specific sensory stimuli, then cortical neurons come to represent those stimuli in a progressively more specific and progressively "amplified" manner.

2. There are important behavioral conditions that must be met in the learning phase of plasticity.

a. If behaviorally important stimuli repeatedly excite cortical neuron populations, the neurons will progressively grow in number.

b. Repetitive, behaviorally important stimuli processed in skill learning lead to progressively greater specificity in the spectral (spatial) and temporal dimensions.

c. The growing numbers of selectively responding neurons discharge with progressively stronger temporal coordination (distributed synchronicity).

Thus, through the course of progressive skill learning, a more refined basis for processing stimuli and generating the actions critical to the skilled tasks is enabled by the multidimensional changes in cortical responses. Consequently, specific aspects of these changes in distributed neuronal response are highly correlated with learning-based improvements in perception, motor control, and cognition.[231, 261, 262, 321] In these processes, the brain is not simply changing to record and store content. Instead the cerebral cortex is selectively refining its processing capacities to fit each task at hand by adjusting its spectral/spatial and temporal filters. Ultimately, it establishes its own general processing capabilities. This "learning to learn" determines the facility with which specific classes of information can be stored, associated, and manipu-

T A B L E   4 – 1. Summary of Principles of Neuroplasticity as Applied to Rehabilitation

Requisites for Learning: Guidelines for Applying the Principles of Neuroplasticity in Treatment	Evidence of Measurable Neuroplastic Changes* After Intervention
Therapeutic Activities 1. Activities must be attended-goal directed. 2. Behaviors must be motivating/fun. 3. Behaviors must be repeated (and variable). 4. Behaviors should be linked temporally and spatially but not simultaneous in time. 5. Behaviors must be rewarded. 6. Give feedback on performance accuracy. 7. Make stimulus strength adequate for detection. 8. Stimulation and behavioral expectations must be progressed in difficulty. 9. Stimulus-induced behaviors need to be integrated into meaningful function. 10. Behaviors should be age appropriate. 11. Behaviors should be integrated across sensory modalities. 12. Make sensory input relevant to desired outputs. 13. Repeat behaviors over time. 14. Match training behaviors with recovery/developmental periods. 15. Strengthen responses with multisensory modalities. 16. Begin stimulation by using the most mature or capable sensory receptors. 17. Behaviors should be performed in different environmental contexts. 18. Do training in the gravitational positions that facilitate task achievement. 19. Preferred behaviors should be rewarded and negative behaviors punished. 20. Accurate behaviors should be repeated.	*Anatomical/Physiological Principles* 1. Increase in the area of representation 2. Smaller receptive fields 3. Increased density of receptive fields 4. Improved organization 5. Improved order of representation 6. Increased myelination 7. Increased complexity of dendrites 8. Increased strength (amplitude) of evoked responses 9. Decreased latency of response 10. Increased consistency of response (e.g., density of neuronal response) 11. Improved selective excitation 12. Improved autogenic and surround inhibition 13. Improved neurochemical transmission 14. Normalized location/translocation 15. Normalized pattern of response 16. Increased interconnectedness 17. Spread of healthy neurons to take over function in areas where damage occurred 18. Early achievement of developmental milestones 19. Increased specificity of neuronal firing 20. Improved synchrony of neuronal firing 21. Spatial representational mapping consistent with coincident temporal events 22. Increased salience of neuronal responses 23. Increased interrelatedness of temporally related neuronal firing 24. Change in number and complexity of synapses 25. Improved resistance to representational degradation

*Measurements were made with a variety of techniques, including neurophysiological mapping after craniotomies, electroencephalography, magnetic source imaging, functional magnetic resonance imaging, electromyography, cortical response mapping with positron emission tomography, and neurochemical analysis of neurotransmitters, growth hormones, inhibitors, corticosteroids, etc.

lated. These powerful self-shaping processes of the forebrain machinery are operating not only on a large scale during development but also during experience-based management of externally and internally generated information in adults. This self-shaping with experience allows the development of hierarchical organization of perception, cognition, motor, and executive management skills.

3. In learning, selection of behaviorally important inputs is a product of strengthening input-coincidence–based connections (synapses).

The process of coincidence-based input co-selection leads to changes in cortical representation. Coincident, temporally and spatially related events that fire together are strengthened together. In skill learning, this principle of concurrent input co-selection results from repetitive practice that includes:

a. *A progressive amplification of cell numbers engaged by repetitive inputs*[159, 261, 262]
b. *An increase in the temporal coordination of distributed neuronal discharges evoked by successive events that mark features of behaviorally important inputs is a consequence of a progressive increase in positive coupling between nearly simultaneously engaged neurons within cortical networks*[261, 312]
c. *A progressively more specific "selection" of all of*

those input features that collectively represent behaviorally important inputs, expressed moment by moment in time[159, 312]

Thus, skill learning results in mapping temporal neighbors in representational networks at adjacent spatial locations when they regularly occur successive in time.[6, 62, 210]

The basis of the functional creation of the detailed, representational cortical maps converting temporal to spatial representations is related to the hebbian change principle.[139] The hebbian plasticity principle applies to the development of interconnections between excitatory and inhibitory inputs within the cortical pyramidal neurons as well as their connections to extrinsic inputs and outputs. Based on the hebbian principle, the operation of coincidence-based synaptic plasticity in cortical networks results in the formation, strengthening, and continuous recruitment of neurons within neuronal "assemblies" that "cooperatively" represent behaviorally important stimuli.

4. Plasticity is constrained by anatomical sources and convergent-divergent spreads of inputs. Every cortical field has:

a. *Specific extrinsic and intrinsic input sources*
b. *Specific dimensions of anatomical divergence and convergence of its inputs, limiting dynamic combination hebbian input co-selection capacities*[199, 211]

SUMMARY: PRINCIPLES OF NEUROPLASTICITY (NEURAL ADAPTABILITY)

1. With learning, the distributed cortical representations of inputs and brain actions "specialize" in their representations of behaviorally important inputs and actions for skill learning.
2. There are important behavioral conditions that must be met in the learning phase of plasticity that enable growth in the number of neuron populations excited, progressively greater specificity in the neuronal representations, and progressively stronger temporal coordination.
3. In learning, selection of behaviorally important inputs is a product of strengthening input-coincidence–based connections (synapses).
4. The scale of plasticity in progressive skill learning is massive.
5. Enduring cortical plasticity changes appear to be accounted for by local changes in neural anatomy.
6. Cortical plasticity processes in child development represent progressive, multiple-staged skill learning.
7. Cortical field–specific differences in input sources, distributions, and time-structured inputs create different representational structures.
8. Temporal dimensions of behaviorally important inputs influence representational "specialization."
9. The integration time ("processing time") in the cortex is itself subject to powerful learning-based plasticity.
10. Learning is modulated as a function of behavioral state.
11. There are constraints that limit the magnitude of plasticity, such as:
    a. Competition between plasticity processes
    b. Anatomical sources and convergent-divergent spreads of inputs
    c. Time constants governing coincident input co-selection
    d. Achievable coherences of extrinsic and intrinsic cortical input sources
    e. Top-down organizational influences on cortical representational plasticity

Anatomical input sources and limited projection overlap both to enable change by establishing input-selection repertoires and determine the limits for change. There are relatively strict anatomical constraints at the "lower" system levels, where only spatially (spectrally) limited input-coincidence–based combined outcomes are possi-ble. In the "higher" system hierarchies, anatomical projection topographies are more powerful with neurons and neuronal assemblies developing that respond to complex combinations of features of real-world objects, events, and actions.

5. Plasticity is constrained by the time constants governing coincident input co-selection and by the time structures and potentially achievable coherence of extrinsic and intrinsic cortical input sources.

To effectively drive representational changes with coincident input-dependent hebbian mechanisms, temporally coordinated inputs are prerequisite, given the short durations (milliseconds to tens of milliseconds) of the time constants that govern synaptic plasticity in the adaptive cortical machinery (see reference 44 for review). Consistently noncorrelated or low-discharge-rate inputs induce negative changes in synaptic effectiveness. In addition, stimuli occurring repetitively simultaneous in time can also degrade the representation. These negative effects also contribute importantly to the learning-driven "election" of behaviorally important inputs.

6. Cortical field–specific differences in input sources, distributions, and time-structured inputs create different representational structures.

For example, there are significant differences in the activity from afferent inputs from the retina, skin, or cochlea generated in a relatively strictly topographically wired V-1 (area 17), S-1 proper (area 3b), or A-1 (area 43) compared with the inferotemporal visual, insular somatosensory, dorsotemporal auditory, or prefrontal cortical areas that receive highly diffuse inputs (see Fig. 4–6). In the former cases, very heavy schedules of repetitive, temporally coherent inputs are delivered from powerful, redundant projections from relatively strictly topographically organized thalamic nuclei and lower-level, associated cortical areas. Whereas neighboring neurons can share some response properties, neurons or clusters of neurons respond selectively to learned inputs. These neurons are distributed widely across cortical areas and share less information with neighboring neurons. In the "lower" levels, afferent input projections from any given source are greatly dispersed. Highly repetitive inputs are uncommon, inputs from multiple diffuse cortical sources are more common as well as more varied, and complex input combinations are in play. These differences in input schedules, spreads, and combinations presumably largely account for the dramatic differences in the patterns of representation of behaviorally important stimuli at "lower" versus "higher" levels.[211]

Despite these differences in representational organization across the cortex, the cortex does progressively differentiate cortical cells to accomplish specific operational tasks. There is a serial progression of differentiation to allow the development of functional organization that allows an individual to progressively master more and more elaborated and differentiated perceptual, cognitive, monitoring, and executive skills.

The sources of inputs and their field-specific spreads

and boundary limits, the distributions of modulatory inputs differentiated by cortical layer in different cortical regions, the basic elements and their basic interconnections in the cortical processing machine, and crucial aspects of input combination and processing at subcortical levels are inherited (see reference 269 for review). Although these inherited aspects of sensory, motor, and cortical processing circuit development constrain the potential learning-based modification of processing within each cortical area, representation changes can occur as a result of environmental interaction and purposeful behavioral practice.

7. Temporal dimensions of behaviorally important inputs also influence representational "specialization."

In at least four ways, the cortex refines its representations of the temporal aspects of behaviorally important inputs during learning.

First, the cortex generates more synchronous representations of sequenced and coincident associative input perturbations or events, not only recording their identities but also marking their occurrences (for examples, see references 172, 192, 205, 261, 311, 312, and 320). It appears to be primarily achieved through increases in positive coupling strengths between interconnected neurons participating in stimulus- or action-specific neuronal cell assemblies.* The strength of the interconnectedness:

- Increases representational salience as a result of downstream neurons being excited as a direct function of the degree of temporal synchronization of their inputs.
- Increases the power of the outputs of a cortical area to drive downstream plasticity. Hebbian plasticity mechanisms operating within downstream cortical (or other) targets also have relatively short time constants. The greater the synchronicity of inputs, the more powerfully those change mechanisms are engaged.
- Confers immunity to noise. By simple information abstraction/coding, the distributed neuronal representation of the "signal" (a temporally coordinated, distributed neuronal response pattern representing the input or action) is converted at the entry levels in the cortex into a form that is not as easily degraded or altered by "noise."
- Confers robustness of complex signal representation for spatially or spectrally incomplete or degraded inputs.

Second, the cortex can select specific inputs through learning to exaggerate the representation of specific input time structures. Conditioning a monkey or a rat with stimuli that have a consistent, specific temporal modulation rate or interstimulus time, for example, results in a selective exaggeration of the responses of neurons at that rate or time separation. In effect, the cortex "specializes" for expected relatively higher-speed or relatively lower-speed signal event reception.

Both electrophysiological recording studies and theoretical studies suggest that cortical networks richly encode

the temporal interval as a simple consequence of cortical network dynamics.[41, 42] It is hypothesized that the cortex accomplishes time-interval and duration selectivity in learning by positively changing synaptic connection strengths for input circuits that can respond with recovery times and circuit delays that match behaviorally important modulation frequency periods, intervals, or durations. However, studies on including excessive, rapid, repetitive fine-motor movements can sometimes lead to serious degradation in representation if the adjacent digits are driven nearly simultaneous in time. This may be associated with negative learning and a loss of motor control.[52]

Third, the cortex links representations of immediately successive inputs that are presented in a learning context. As a result of hebbian plasticity, it establishes overlapping and neighboring relationships between immediately successive parts of rapidly changing inputs yet retains its individualized, distinct cortical representation.[202, 210]

Fourth, the cortex generates stimulus sequence-specific ("combination-sensitive") responses, with neuronal responses selectively modulated by the prior application of stimuli in the learned sequence of temporally separated events. These "associative" or "combination-sensitive" responses have been correlated with evidence of strengthened interconnections between cortical cell assemblies representing successive event elements separated by hundreds of milliseconds to seconds in time.[225, 270] The mechanisms of origin of these effects have not yet been established.

8. The integration time ("processing time") in the cortex is itself subject to powerful learning-based plasticity.

Cortical networks engage both excitatory and inhibitory neurons by strong input perturbations. Within a given processing "channel," cortical pyramidal cells cannot be effectively reexcited by a following perturbation for tens to hundreds of milliseconds. These integration "times" are primarily dictated by the time for recovery from inhibition, which ordinarily dominates post-stimulus excitability. This "integration time," "processing time," or "recovery time" is commonly measured by deriving a "modulation transfer function," which defines the ability of cortical neurons to respond to identical successive stimuli within cortical "processing channels." For example, these "integration" times normally range from about 15 to about 200 ms in the primary auditory receiving areas.[24, 88, 274] Progressively longer processing times are recorded at higher system levels (e.g., in the auditory cortex, they are approximately a syllable in length, 200 to 500 ms in duration) in the "belt cortex" surrounding the primary auditory cortex.[161]

These time constants govern—and limit—the cortex's ability to "chunk" (i.e., to separately represent by distributed, coordinated discharge) successive events within its processing channels. Both neurophysiological studies in animals and behavioral training studies in human adults and children have shown that the time constants governing event-by-event complex signal representation are highly plastic. With intensive training in the right form, cortical "processing times" reflected by the ability to

---

*See references 13, 20, 27, 79, 87, 96, 117, 136, 137, 183, 184, 187, 208, 212, 214, 224, 245, 285, 293–295, and 311.

accurately and separately process events occurring at different input rates can be dramatically shortened or lengthened.[4, 166, 171, 206]

9. Plasticity processes are competitive.

If two spatially or spectrally different inputs are consistently delivered nonsimultaneously to the cortex, cortical networks generate input-selective cell assemblies for each input and actively segregate them from one another.[122, 123, 171, 284, 312] Boundaries between such inputs grow to be sharp and are substantially intensity independent. Computational models of hebbian network behaviors indicate that this sharp segregation of nonidentical, temporally separated inputs is accomplished as a result of a wider distribution of inhibitory versus excitatory responses in the emerging, competing cortical cell assemblies that represent them.

This hebbian network cell assembly formation and competition appears to account for how the cortex creates sharply sorted representations of the fingers in the primary somatosensory cortex.[6, 203] The hebbian network probably accounts for how the cortex creates sharply sorted representations of native aural language–specific phonemes in lower-level auditory cortical areas in the auditory/speech processing system of humans. If inputs are delivered in a constant and stereotyped way from a limited region of the skin or cochlea in a learning context, that skin surface or cochlear sector is an evident competitive "winner."[258, 261] By hebbian plasticity, the cortical networks will co-select that specific combination of inputs and represent it within a competitively growing hebbian cell assembly. The competitive strength of that cooperative cell assembly will grow progressively because more and more neurons are excited by behaviorally important stimuli with increasingly coordinated discharges. That means that neurons outside of this cooperative group have greater numbers of more coordinated outputs contributing to their later competitive recruitment. Through progressive functional remodeling, the cortex clusters and competitively sorts information across sharp boundaries dictated by the spectrotemporal statistics of its inputs. On the one hand, if it receives information on a very heavy schedule that sets up competition for a limited input set, it will sort competitive inputs into a correspondingly small number of largely discontinuous response regions.[180, 181]

Competitive outcomes are, again, cortical level dependent. The cortex links events that occur in different competitive groups if they are consistently excited synchronously in time. At the same time, competitively formed groups of neurons come to be synchronously linked in their representations of different parts of the complex stimulus and collectively represent successive complex features of the vocalization through the coordinated activities of many groups.

Neurons within the two levels of the cortex surrounding A-1 (see Fig. 4–6) have greater spectral input convergence and longer integration times that enable their facile combination of information representing different spectrotemporal details. Their information extraction is greatly facilitated by the learning-based linkages of cooperative groups that deliver behaviorally important inputs in a highly salient, temporally coordinated form to these fields. With their progressively greater space and time constants, still higher-level areas organize competitive cell assemblies that represent still more complex spectral and serial-event combinations. Note that these organizational changes apply over a large cortical scale. In skill learning over a limited period of training, participating neuronal members of such assemblies can easily be increased by many hundredfold, even within a primary sensory area like S-I area 3b or A-1.[52, 171, 260, 261, 312]

In extensive training in complex signal recognition, more than 10% of neurons within temporal cortical areas can come to respond highly selectively to a specific, normally rare, complex training stimulus. The distributed cell assemblies representing those specific complex inputs involve tens or hundreds of millions of neurons and are achieved by enduring effectiveness changes in many billions of synapses.

10. Learning is modulated as a function of behavioral state.

At "lower" levels of the cortex, changes are generated only in attended behaviors.[3, 159, 259, 260, 262, 313] Trial-by-trial change magnitudes are a function of the importance of the input to the animal as signaled by the level of attention; the cognitive values of behavioral rewards or punishments; and internal judgments of practice trial precision or error, based on the relative success or failure of achieving a target goal or expectation. Little or no enduring change is induced when a well-learned "automatic" behavior is performed from memory without attention. It is also interesting to note that at some levels within the cortex, activity changes can be induced even in nonattending subjects under conditions in which "priming" effects of nonattended reception of information can be demonstrated.

The modulation of progressive learning is also achieved by the activation of powerful reward systems releasing the neurotransmitters noradrenaline, norepinephrine, and dopamine (among others) through widespread projections to the cerebral cortex. Noradrenaline plays a particularly important role in modulating learning-induced change in the cortex.[171, 172, 313]

Note that the cortex is a "learning machine" in the sense that during the learning of a new skill, neurotransmitters are all released trial by trial with application of the behaviorally important stimulus and/or behavioral rewards. If the skill can be mastered and thereafter replayed from memory, its performance can be generated without attention. That results in a profound attenuation of the modulation signals from these neurotransmitter sources; plasticity is no longer positively enabled in cortical networks.

11. Top-down influences constrain cortical representational plasticity.

Attentional control flexibly defines an enabling "window" for change in learning.[4] Progressive learning generates progressively more strongly represented goals and expectations,[59, 167] which feed back both all across representational systems that are undergoing change and to modulatory control systems weighing performance success and error. Strong intermodal behavioral and representational effects have also been recorded in experiments that might be interpreted as shaping expectations in monkeys.[132, 150] These shaping expectations would be similar to those observed in a human subject employing multisensory inputs such as auditory, visual, and somesthetic information to create integrated phonological representations, to create the movement trajectory patterns that underlie precise hand control, or to make a vocal production.

12. The scale of plasticity in progressive skill learning is massive.

Cortical representational plasticity must be viewed as arising from multiple-level systems that are broadly engaged in learning, perceiving, remembering, thinking, and acting. Any behaviorally important input (or consistent internally generated activity) engages many cortical areas and, with repetitive training, drives all of them to change.[201, 204, 211] Different aspects of any acquired skill are contributed from field-specific changes in the multiple cortical areas that are remodeled in its learning.

In this kind of continuously evolving representational machine, perceptual constancy cannot be accounted for by locationally constant brain representations; relational representational principles must be invoked to account for it.[201, 244] Moreover, representational changes must obviously be coordinated level to level. It should also be understood that plastic changes are also induced extracortically. Although it is believed that learning at the cortical level is usually predominant, plasticity induced by learning within many extracortical structures significantly contributes to learning-induced changes that are expressed within the cortex.

13. Enduring cortical plasticity changes appear to be accounted for by local changes in neural anatomy.

Changes in synapse turnover, synapse number, synaptic active zones, dendritic spines, and the elaboration of terminal dendrites have all been demonstrated to occur in a behaviorally engaged cortical zone.[43, 44, 93, 111, 127, 168, 173] Through many changes in local structural detail, the learning brain is continuously physically remodeling its processing machinery across the course of child development. However, this physical remodeling also can occur after behavioral training in an adult who has suffered a neural insult.

14. Cortical plasticity processes in child development represent progressive, multiple-staged skill learning.

There are two remarkable achievements of brain plasticity in child development. The first is the progressive shaping of the processing to handle the accurate, high-speed reception of the rapidly changing streams of information that flow into the brain. In the cerebral cortex, that shaping appears to begin most powerfully within the primary receiving areas of the cortex. With early myelination, the main gateways for information into the cortex are receiving strongly coherent inputs from subcortical nuclei, and they can quickly organize their local networks on the basis of coincident input co-selection (hebbian) plasticity mechanisms. The self-organization of the cortical processing machinery spreads outward from these primary receiving areas over time to ultimately refine the basic processing machinery of all of the cortex. The second great achievement, which is strongly dependent on the first, is the efficient storage of massive content compendia, in richly associated forms.

During development, the brain accomplishes its functional self-organization through a long parallel series of small steps. At each step, the brain masters a series of elementary processing skills and establishes reliable information repertoires that enable the accomplishment of subsequent skills. Second- and higher-order skills can be viewed as both elaborations of more basic mastered skills and the creation of new skills dependent on combined second- and higher-order processing. That hierarchical processing is enabled by greater cortical anatomical spreads, by more complexly convergent anatomical sources of inputs, and by longer integration (processing, recovery) times at progressively higher cortical system levels, which allows for progressively more complex combinations of information integrated over progressively longer time epochs as one ascends across cortical processing hierarchies.

As the cortical machinery functionally evolves and consequently physically "matures" through childhood developmental stages, information repertoires are represented in progressively more salient forms (i.e., with more powerful distributed response coordination). Growing agreement directly controls the power of emerging information repertoires for driving the next level of elaborative and combinatorial changes. It is hypothesized that it also directly enables the maturation of the myelination of projection tracts that deliver outputs from functionally refined cortical areas. More mature myelination of output projections also contributes to the power of this newly organized activity to drive strong, downstream plastic change through the operation of hebbian plasticity processes.

As each elaboration of skill is practiced, in a learning phase, neuromodulatory transmitters enable change in the cortical machinery and the cortex functionally and physically adapts to generate the neurological representations of the skill in progressively more selective, predictable, and statistically reliable forms. Ultimately, the performance of the skill concurs with the brain's own accumulated, learning-derived "expectations." The skill can now be performed from memory, without attention. With this consolidation of the remembered skill and information repertoire, the modulatory nuclei enable no further change in the cortical machinery. The learning machine, the cerebral cortex, moves on to the next elaboration. In this way the cortex constructs highly specialized processing machinery that can progressively produce great towers of automatically performable behaviors and great progressively maturing hierarchies of information-processing machinery that can achieve progressively more powerful complex signal representations, retrievals, and associations. With this machinery in a mature and thereby efficiently operating form, there is a remarkable capacity for reception, storage, and analysis of diverse and complexly associated information.

The flexible, self-adjusting capacity for refinement of the processing capabilities of the nervous system confers the ability of our species to represent complex language structures, to develop high-speed reading abilities, to develop a remarkably wide variety of complex modern-era motor abilities, to develop the abstract logic structures of the mathematician or software engineer or philosopher—to create elaborate, idiosyncratic, experience-based behavioral abilities in all of us.

How Are Learning Sequences Controlled? What Constrains Learning Progressions?

Perhaps the most important basis of control of learning progressions is representational consolidation. Through specialization, the trained cortex creates progressively more specific and more salient distributed representations of behaviorally important inputs. Growing representational salience increases the power of a cortical area to effectively drive change wherever outputs from this evolving cortical processing machinery are distributed (e.g., in "higher system levels distributed and coordinated [synchronized] responses" more powerfully drive downstream hebbian-based plasticity changes).

A second very powerful basis for sequenced learning is progressive myelination. At the time of birth, only the core "primary" extrinsic information entry zones (A-1, S-I, V-1) in the cortex are heavily myelinated.[103, 322] Across childhood, connections to and interconnections between cortical areas are progressively myelinated, proceeding from these core areas out to progressively "higher" system levels. Myelination in the posterior parietal, anterior, and inferior temporal and prefrontal cortical areas is not "mature" in the human forebrain until 8 to 20 years of age. Even in the mature state, it is far less developed at the "highest" processing levels.

Myelination controls the conduction times and therefore the temporal dispersions of input sources to and within cortical areas. Poor myelination at "higher" levels in the young brain is associated with temporally diffuse inputs. They cannot generate reliable representational constructs of an adult quality because they do not as effectively engage input-coincidence–based hebbian plasticity mechanisms. That ensures, in effect, that plasticity is not enabled for complex combinatorial processing until "lower" level input repertoires are consolidated (i.e., become stable, statistically reliable forms).

Although myelination is thought to be genetically programmed, some scientists hypothesize that myelination in the CNS is also controlled by emerging temporal response coherence, and is achieved through temporally coordinated signaling from the multiple branches of oligodendrocytes that terminate on different projection axons in central tracts and networks. It has been argued that central myelination is positively and negatively activity dependent and that distributed synchronization may contribute to positive change.[76] If the hypothesis that coherent activity controls myelination proves to be true, then emerging temporal correlation of distributed representations of behaviorally important stimuli is generated level by level. This is done by changes in coupling in local cortical networks in the developing cortex. It would also directly drive changes in myelination for the outputs of that cortical area. These two events in turn would enable the generation of reliable and salient representational constructs at that higher level. By this kind of progression, skill learning is hypothesized to directly control progressive functional and physical brain development through the course of child development. This is accomplished both by refining ("maturing") local interconnections through response dynamics of information processing machinery at successive cortical levels and by coordinated refinement ("maturing") of the critical information transmission pathways that interconnect different processing levels.

Another constraint in the development of neural adaptation may be the development of mature sleeping patterns, especially within the first year of life.[145] Sleep both enables the strengthening of learning-based plastic changes and resets the learning machinery by "erasing" temporary nonreinforced and nonrewarded, input-generated changes produced over the preceding waking period.[51, 165, 254] The dramatic shift in the percentage of time spent in rapid-eye-movement sleep is consistent with a strong early bias toward noise removal in a very immature and poorly functionally unorganized brain. Sleep patterns change dramatically in the older child, in parallel with a strong increase in its daily schedule of closely attended, rewarded, and goal-oriented behaviors. This research will need to be explored in greater detail when relating this data to patients with CNS damage. This population often has poor breathing habits and capabilities that lead to decreased oxygenation and often broken sleep cycles. How much either impairment breakdown or the interaction of the two diminishes neuroplasticity has yet to be determined.

Top-down modulation controlling attentional windows and learned predictions (expectations and behavioral goals) must all be constructed by learning. Delays in goal development could also create an important constraint for the progression of early learning. In the very young brain, prediction and error-estimation processes would be weakened because stored higher-level information repertoires are ill formed and statistically unreliable. As the brain matures, stored information progressively more strongly and reliably enables top-down attentional and predictive controls, progressively providing a stronger basis for success and error signaling for modulatory control nuclei and progressively enabling top-down syntactic feedback to increase representational reliability.

Attention, reward and punishment, accuracy of achievement of goals, and error feedback gate learning through a modulatory control system are critical for learning. The modulatory control systems that enable learning are also plastic, with their process of maturation providing constraint or facilitation for progressive learning. These subcortical nuclei are signaled by complex information feedback from the cortex itself. The salience and specificity of that feedback information grows over time. The ability to provide accurate error judging or goal-achievement signaling must grow progressively. The nucleus basalis, nucleus accumbens, ventral tegmentum, and locus coeruleus must undergo their own functional self-organization based on hebbian plasticity principles to achieve "mature" modulatory selectivity and power. The progressive maturation of the modulatory control system occurs naturally with development or training. This system can provide another important constraint on skill development progression and regulation of axial/trunk postural and balance control as well as fine-motor coordination.

What Facilitates the Development of Permanent "Automatic" Motor Behaviors?

The creation and maintenance of cortical representations are functions of the animal's or human's level of attention at a task. Cortical representational plasticity in skill acquisition is self-limiting. As the behavior comes to be more "automatic," it is less closely attended and representational changes induced in the cortex fade and ultimately disappear or reverse (unlearning effects).[135, 230] The element of behavioral performance that enables maintenance of the behavior with minimum involvement of the cortical learning machinery is probably stereotypical movement sequence repetition. As a movement behavior is practiced, an effective, highly statistically predictable movement sequence is adopted that enables the storage of the learned behavior in a permanent form that requires only minimal or no behavioral attention. If behavioral performance declines or behavioral or brain conditions change to render a task more difficult, attention to the behavior will again need to increase, producing an invigorated cortical response to the new learning challenge.

By this view the cerebral cortex is clearly a learning machine. William James[158] was the first to point out that the great practical advantage for a self-organizing cortex was the development of what he called "habits." When a skill is overlearned, it will engage pathways that are so reliable that they can be followed without attention.

Why are some habits retained and others lost? Can sensorimotor learning be sustained when the adaptive representations of the learned behavior "fade" in the cerebral cortex? These areas have not been well researched. However, there are several possibilities. Habits could come to be represented in an enduring form extracortically. The cortex could modify processing in the spinal cord, the basal ganglia, red nucleus, and/or the cerebellum. For example, the learning of manual skills requires a motor cortex, but overlearned motor skills may not be very significantly reduced by the induction of a wide area 4 lesion.

Another possibility is that behaviorally induced cortical changes endure in a highly efficient representational form that can sustain the representation of its key features on the cortex itself, engaging only limited distributed populations of cortical neurons to represent the behavior with high fidelity. Thus, recall of past learning may take less time to restructure than to reformat entirely new learning, whether it be a cognitive or motor task. The fact that a monkey improves discriminative abilities or

movement performance after modifying the cortical neuron response with heavily practiced behaviors supports this alternative. However, many behaviors, such as musical performance, require constant attended practice at a highly cognitive level to maintain both the representational changes and the performance.

Summary

Over the years, learning has been tied to critical periods of development. Particularly in terms of language, it was assumed that if a particular skill or behavior was not accomplished during the critical period, the opportunity to acquire that skill had been lost. Although learning progression is heightened during certain periods, learning is not limited to that period alone.

Development actually refers to a process of neural and behavioral self-organization resulting from a physiological and developmental maturation of the nervous system. However, with increasing interaction with the environment, the brain changes its capacity from a simple to an incredibly specialized representational machine that is adapted to meet the specific inputs that engage it. Language is probably one of the most sophisticated examples of a specialized process at multiple levels. First the brain has to learn to put meaning into words. Over time one is exposed to millions of English words even though one may not consciously understand all of them. Yet, as an individual grows, attends school, and continues to interact in more sophisticated interactions, the brain adapts and develops massive, language-specific specialization.

The beauty of the brain is that as it self-organizes, it also stores the contents of its learning, creating a foundation that increases in depth and breadth until it can begin to make predictions on even novel inputs to facilitate acute and efficient operations. The earlier the exposure occurs, the easier it is for the competitive neuronal processes to adapt and to make extensive connections. With growing neuronal specificity and salience, more powerful predictions are continued until there is greater learning and mastery.

Probably the most important thing that has been learned during the twentieth century is that the brain is a learning machine that operates throughout life. The aging process can take a toll on the ability to store information and may reduce both the complexity of the information that is processed and that individual's ability to remember. If an individual is conscious of good hydration and balanced nutrition and regularly engages in goal-directed activities that include intimate interactions with the environment and with people, then CNS pathways of representation and prediction can not only be preserved but also continue to adapt. Continuing to engage neuronal populations also has the potential to slow down the aging process. Thus, whereas the critical period can be viewed as developing more power specialization in the cortex, cortical plasticity does not shut down after the critical period. Instead, at times other than the critical period, therapists may well be driving improvements in individuals who have abnormalities in development or who develop abnormalities due to injury or disease.

It is now known that learning is not necessarily specifically staged. Rather, complex abilities develop more from systems interaction and integration. Therapists must develop the ability to determine what inputs are reliable and salient and which most effectively create functional and physical brain maturation, adaptation, and learning. As an individual continues to gather information, the nervous system adapts. In the face of different types of challenges (structural, emotional, pathological), clinicians must develop more effective strategies that can be used to facilitate neural adaptation, learning, substitution, and representational changes that will allow individuals to maintain meaningful function despite anatomical or physiological variances in structure.

It should be clear that to meet the conditions of neural adaptability, behaviors must be attended, repetitive, goal directed, integrated into functional activities, and carried out over time with an increasing number of coincident events. Although strong behavioral events can be associated with measurable neural adaptability, new neural connections and synapses must be strengthened with repetition and increased complexity. Clients with CNS disorders may have damaged certain areas of the brain, but that does not mean there is no potential for adaptation and learning. Creating the best environment to learn a skill may initially need to be contrived, with limitations controlled externally by the therapist's hands or clinical arena. In time, those limitations must be eliminated and variability within the natural environment reintroduced to obtain true learning and ultimate neuroplasticity.

To provide adequate repetition and learning, rehabilitation programs must include strong, carefully outlined home programs. Therapists need to invest significant time in educating patients and their families about the principles of neuroplasticity to empower them to continue to create progressive learning activities. Patients should come back periodically to see the therapist to also discuss ways to continue to encourage learning. Patients must become their own best therapist. They must be motivated to continue to challenge themselves with progressive, attended behavioral activities that get integrated into functional activities. Individuals must work hard to avoid learning negative patterns of movement and behaviors that degrade the neuronal response as opposed to enriching it.

The maximum attainment of skilled performance cannot necessarily be determined. The original injury can only be used as an estimate of the damage with some indicators for prognosis and recovery. The rest of the success of rehabilitation and restoration of function will reside with the motivation and commitment of the individual. See the following box for a summary of functional outcomes. How that motivation and commitment is initially established and continually reinforced is based on the patient, the therapist's interactive skills and emotional bond (see Chapter 6), and the family and support system surrounding the client (see Chapter 7).

INTERVENTION STRATEGIES

Functional Training

Functional training is a method of retraining the motor system using repetitive practice of functional tasks in an

---

FUNCTIONAL OUTCOMES OF SUCCESSFUL NEURAL ADAPTATION AFTER REHABILITATION

1. Improved fine and gross motor coordination
2. Improved sensory discrimination
3. Improved balance and postural control
4. Faster reaction time
5. Improved accuracy of movements
6. Improved rhythm and timing of movements
7. Improved memory storage, organization, and retrieval
8. Improved alertness and attention
9. Improved sequencing
10. Improved logic, complexity, and sophistication of problem solving
11. Enhanced language skills (verbal and nonverbal)
12. Improved interpersonal communication
13. Increased sense of well-being
14. Increased insight
15. Increased self-confidence
16. Improved self-image
17. Enhanced signal/noise detection; able to make finer distinctions
18. Increased ability to "chunk" information for memory and use
19. Enhanced learning skills including faster learning
20. Early achievement of developmental milestones
21. Decreased hyperactivity and sensory defensiveness
22. Expanded ability to perform a skill from memory
23. Flexible behaviors; variability in task performance
24. Expanded flexibility for experience-based learning

---

attempt to reestablish the client's ability to perform activities of daily living. This method of training is a common and popular intervention strategy employed by clinicians, owing to the fact that it is a relatively simple and straightforward approach to improving deficits in function. Because of its inherent simplicity, functional training is sometimes misused or abused by clinicians, often leading to additional problems for the client. The clinician is therefore advised to use a sound diagnostic process before making the decision to approach a specific clinical problem or condition through the use of functional training.

In Chapter 3 the steps involved in the examination process were explained in detail and the intricate relationship of impairments, disabilities, and handicaps in the rehabilitation process were discussed. Functional training can be implemented once the clinician has identified the client's functional limitations/disabilities. The clinician must first answer the question: "What can the client *Not* do?" Once these functional tasks have been identified, the clinician can proceed to guide the client in performing and practicing these difficult tasks.

Functional Training's Effect on Disabilities

The main focus of functional training is the correction of disabilities (functional limitations). However, through repetitive practice of functional tasks and gross motor patterns, many of the client's impairments will also be affected. For example, if a therapist practices sit-to-stand transfers with a client in a variety of environments and performs multiple repetitions of each type of transfer, not only will learning be reinforced, but the client will also gain strength in the synergistic patterns of the lower extremities that work against gravity to concentrically lift the client off of the support surface and eccentrically lower him or her down. Weight bearing through the feet in a variety of degrees of ankle dorsiflexion during transfer training will effectively place the ankles in functional positions. The act of standing also facilitates the trunk and neck extensors to affect postural control. Varying the speed of the activity during the treatment will stimulate cerebellar adaptation to the movement task. Moving from one position to another and with the head in a variety of positions stimulates the vestibular apparatus and may assist in habituating a hypersensitive vestibular system and allow the client to change body positions, with a higher quality of life. Repetitive practice also affects the vasomotor system and may assist in habituating postural hypotensive responses.

If the presence of a particular disability can be explained as being caused by a specific impairment, then correcting the impairment may correct the disability. For example, if it was determined that a client's inability to stand up from the sitting position was caused by the presence of lower-extremity weakness, then lower-extremity strengthening exercises need to be targeted during therapeutic intervention. It is difficult to predict, however, whether lower-extremity strengthening alone will create improved lower-extremity function. The strengthening intervention selected should reflect the task and the environment within which the impairment was identified. Training within this context should facilitate the correction of the disability. The clinician should attempt to create a training situation so that the client may be able to run the necessary motor programs with all of the necessary subsystems in place. In this example, training the lower extremities using cuff weights is much less likely to automatically result in the improvement of sit-to-stand function than if the strength training was in a functional activity. That is, it may be better to train the sit-to-stand pattern using various surface heights than to perform squat patterns that closely resemble the same motor pattern to train the systems in the appropriate synergies, posture, and environment in which they are required to function.

The decision to treat the impairments causing the disabilities or to correct the disabilities themselves is influenced by myriad factors. It would appear that for certain tasks to be completed, the client must possess a "threshold amount" of basic components to perform the task if movement is to be possible. These components include such factors as cognitive ability and motivation. By having the client control a pattern using a functional motor task within a very narrow biomechanical window at first, then widening this window as motor learning improves would be one way to use functional training and augmented impairment correction simultaneously. The therapist must accept that when the biomechanical window is narrowed, the functional treatment intervention is controlled by the therapist and augmented to allow the client to succeed and correct errors within a limited environment. In this situation the patient is functionally training with environmental limitations. Without correcting these components, it would be impossible for the clinician to achieve any functional improvement. Moreover, if the clinician attempts to have the client run the entire motor program outside of the available "normal" window by providing extrinsic assistance to enable the client to perform the task, the resulting movement is often minimally functional, if not unsafe for the client. Without analyzing impairments and their effect on disabilities and only running functional training in distorted and abnormal patterns, this method of "intervention" may also have the potential of resulting in more impairments or disabilities in the future.

A good example of this is the "nag-and-drag" method of gait training in the parallel bars. This method finds the therapist literally dragging the client through the length of the parallel bars in an attempt to elicit some sort of movement response from the client. The therapist then labels this procedure "gait training." Clearly, this approach will result in the client eventually learning dysfunctional or running inefficient motor programs. Before long, as the client learns to run these dysfunctional programs procedurally, the clinician will realize that he or she has created a bigger problem, which may require a considerable amount of time and resources to undo the damage that was created by limiting the available movement strategies, limiting the variability within practice, and ultimately restricting the plasticity of the nervous system. Similarly, forcing the axial trunk musculature to compensate for lack of motor control within the elbow and wrist will result in dysfunctional upper-extremity movement patterns.

Concept of Critical Pathways

Another intervention approach that evolved as an offshoot of functional training is clinical pathways. These pathways were established by different health care institutions for many medical diagnoses to ensure consistency of practice between medical professionals and that all of a client's needs are met in a timely manner and to facilitate discharge and maximize independence in the shortest amount of time possible. In the rehabilitation setting, these pathways are timelines with corresponding "milestones" in the patient's functional progress. Figure 4–7 is an example of one pathway.

These pathways assist the facility by reducing the amount of paperwork generated per client case. Charting is generally done by exception, rather than narration. If

UCLA MEDICAL CENTER
Name: Ischemic Stroke, Pathway 2, Severe Motor Deficit, Likely d/c to Rehab or Nursing Facility
Physician: _____
Case Manager/CNS: _____
Chief Resident: _____

ADDRESSOGRAPH

Indicators	Admit to: Neurology Service 0 to 12 Hours Post Onset	Day 1 12-72 Hours Post Onset	Day 2	Day 3	Day 4	Day 5	Day 6
MD Responsibilities	Immediately notify Stroke Team for hyperacute therapy evaluation; Notify Primary Care MD; Detailed physical/neurologic exam, history, review labs	Notify Primary Care MD*; Patient exam, review all labs; Discuss probable d/c date and needs with pt/family	Pt exam, review labs; Discuss Rehab/SNF placement with family	Pt exam, review labs; Arrange primary care, neuro f/up; Write d/c prescriptions	Pt exam, review labs; Arrange primary care, neuro f/up if d/c; Write prescriptions if d/c home or dictate d/c summary if d/c rehab/SNF	Patient exam, review all labs; Arrange primary care, neuro f/up if d/c; Write prescriptions if d/c home or dictate d/c summary if d/c rehab/SNF	Pt exam, review labs; Arrange primary care, neuro f/up dictate d/c summary for rehab/SNF
Monitoring	VS/Neuro q 2 hours; Cardiac monitor; Strict I&Os	VS/Neuro q 2 hours; Daily weight; Cardiac monitor; Strict I&Os	VS/Neuro q 4 hours; Cardiac monitor, prn; Strict I&Os	VS/Neuro q 4 hours; Strict I&Os; Daily weight	VS/Neuro q 4 hours; Daily weight; Strict I&Os	VS/Neuro q 4 hours; Strict I&Os	VS/Neuro q 4 hours
Assessment	Nursing assess skin integrity, Assess for fall risk, aspiration risk, assess for usual bowel pattern	Assess for potential discharge needs	Assess for discharge options		Physicians assess need for daily weights	Physicians assess need for Strict I&Os	
Diagnostic/Lab	CXR, ECG, CBC, platelets, PT/PTT, lytes, BUN, creat, gluc, CPK, U/A; Module #1: Additional Labs; Module #6: Neuroimaging	Module #6: Neuroimaging; Module #7: Carotid Duplex; Module #8: Cardiac ECHO; ECG, CXR, CBC, platelets, PT/PTT, lytes, BUN, creat, gluc, U/A; Module #1: Additional Labs	Fasting lipid panel; Module #6: Neuroimaging; Module #7: Carotid Duplex; Module #8: Cardiac ECHO				
Treatment/ Medications/IV	IV NS with 20meq KCl at 100 cc/hr; Thrombolysis protocol if qualifies; Module #2: Antithrombotics; Tylenol, prn, MOM, prn; Module #3: DVT prophylaxis; Pressure ulcer prevention protocol; Straight cath q 8 hr, prn; Seizure/aspiration/fall precautions	IV NS with 20meq KCl at 100 cc/hr, if indicated; Module #2: Antithrombotics; Tylenol, prn, MOM, prn; Module #3: DVT Prophylaxis; Straight cath q 8 hr, prn; Guaiac all stools; ROM q 8 hours	Module #2: Antithrombotics; Tylenol, prn, MOM, prn; Module #3: DVT Prophylaxis; Straight cath q 8 hr, prn; Guaiac all stools; ROM q 8 hours	Module #2: Antithrombotics; Tylenol, prn, MOM, prn; Module #3: DVT Prophylaxis; Straight cath q 8 hr, prn; Guaiac all stools; ROM q 8 hours	Module #2: Antithrombotics; Tylenol, prn, MOM, prn; Module #3: DVT Prophylaxis; Straight cath q 8 hr, prn; Guaiac all stools; ROM q 8 hours	Module #2: Antithrombotics; Tylenol, prn, MOM, prn; Module #3: DVT Prophylaxis; ROM q 8 hours	Module #2: Antithrombotics; Tylenol, prn, MOM, prn; Module #3: DVT Prophylaxis; ROM q 8 hours
Nutrition	NPO	Module #4: Dysphagia Assessment; Module #5: Diet Orders	Assess and advance as tolerated	Assess and advance as tolerated	Assess and advance as tolerated	Assess and advance as tolerated	Assess and advance as tolerated
Activity/Safety	Bedrest with head of bed ↑30°	Bedrest with head of bed ↑30°; Bathroom privileges after 24 hours, if patient safe to ambulate	OOB to chair, advance as tolerated	OOB to chair, advance as tolerated	Advance as tolerated	Advance as tolerated	Advance as tolerated
Education	Orient to 7West routine	Begin discharge teaching if appropriate: activity and meds; Begin stroke education program; Discharge planning	Discharge teaching activity and meds; Discharge options	Advance stroke education program; Discharge teaching	Advance stroke education program; Discharge teaching	Advance stroke education program; Discharge teaching	Advance stroke education program; Discharge teaching; Complete discharge teaching, provide appropriate hand-outs and follow-up appointments
Consults	PT, OT; Speech, prn; CNS Case Manager; Neurology if not neuro primary; Cardiology and Infect. Disease, prn	PT, OT; Speech, prn; CNS Case Manager; Discharge Planner; Social Worker, prn; Neuro Rehab Team; Neurology if not Neuro primary; Cardiology and Infect. Dis., prn	CNS Case Manager; Neurology if not Neuro primary; Cardiology and Infect. Dis., prn	CNS Case Manager; Neurology if not Neuro primary; Cardiology and Infect. Dis., prn; Home Health Liaison, prn	CNS Case Manager; Neurology if not Neuro primary; Cardiology and Infect. Dis., prn	CNS Case Manager; Neurology if not Neuro primary; Cardiology and Infect. Dis., prn	CNS Case Manager; Neurology if not Neuro primary; Cardiology and Infect. Dis., prn
Expected Outcomes	Initial assessment of stroke etiology concluded; Research protocol initiated; Adequate hydration maintained; Pt/family will verbalize usual hospital routine	Initial assessment of stroke etiology concluded; Adequate hydration maintained; Pt/family will verbalize stroke definition, likely cause of own stroke; PTT in target range, of applicable; PT/OT/Speech Therapy evals initiated	Stroke etiology clarified; Adequate hydration maintained; No S&S of decreased bodily function; Pt/family will verbalize risk factors for stroke, s/s TIA and stroke; PTT in target range, if applicable; PT/OT/Speech evals complete, therapy initiated; Pt/family verbalize safe d/c plan	Long term stroke prevention strategy selected; Adequate hydration maintained; No S&S of decreased bodily function; Pt/family demonstrate progress in stroke education program; Pt/family verbalize safe d/c plan; PTT in target range, if applicable	Long term stroke prevention strategy selected; Adequate hydration maintained; No S&S of decreased bodily function; Pt/family demonstrate progress in stroke education program; PTT in target range, if applicable; Bowel and bladder program established; If discharged, all expected outcomes on Day 6 must be met	Pt/family demonstrate progress in stroke education program; Adequate hydration maintained; No S&S of decreased bodily function; PTT in target range, if applicable; If discharged, all expected outcomes on Day 6 must be met	Pt participates in ADLs with assistance; Pt can tolerate OOB and sit in chair 2 consecutive hours; Pt can tolerate 2-3 hours/day of acute rehab, if applicable; Pt/family understand and support rehab/SNF goals; Pt/family know facility to which patient will go, approx LOS, plan for Home Care upon d/c; Pt/family can state S&S of TIA/stroke, risk factors of stroke; Pt/family can state when to notify physician, activity restrictions, f/up appointments
Shift RN Signature	AM Admit D. N.	D. N.	D. N.	D. N.	D. N.	D. N.	D. N.
Initial/ Signature							

FIGURE 4–7. Example of critical pathway. (Copyright February 1996, Regents of the University of California [UCLA Clinical Effectiveness]. Adapted with permission.)

the pathway is followed and the client stays on track with predetermined plans, then the component parts of the pathway are simply checked off. If the patient deviates from the primary pathway or has a complicating event that occurs during the duration of his or her recovery, then the patient "falls off the pathway" and is handled according to a compilation of signs and symptoms that is generally customary for that clinical setting. The concept of clinical pathways works well for predictable diseases, diagnoses, and surgical procedures that follow a generally uncomplicated rehabilitation pathway, such as total joint arthroplasty, coronary angioplasty, and mild stroke. It becomes more difficult to predict the course of recovery and the functional outcomes when the disease or pathology is progressive, degenerative, or chronic, such as an exacerbation of multiple sclerosis; or in the presence of neoplasms; or after a severe insult to the CNS. Clinical pathways should never be used as a justification for denying care to a particular patient. When the patient is unable to follow a normal clinical pathway, the clinician should identify the unique factors in the patient's physical and medical functioning that prevent him or her from following a more "traditional" path of functional progress. As more and more institutions use the concept of clinical pathways as an essential and viable approach to the management of the patient, there is a need to evaluate the outcomes following these pathways to ensure efficacy of the particular intervention strategy.

Selection of Functional Training Strategies

The question exists: what is the "ideal" procedure for effectively and efficiently utilizing functional training as a treatment intervention? First, it is suggested that the clinician identify and select procedures that will use the client's strengths to regain lost function and correct impairments—"what can the client do?" The clinician is also advised to avoid activities that may be too difficult and elicit compensation strategies that may result in the development of abnormal, stereotypical movement and potentially create additional impairments. The therapist's decision regarding what functional patterns or activities to practice, and in what order, will depend on several factors. The therapist must choose functional activities that are necessary for the client to obtain independence before being discharged home or managed with less help. For PTs, safe transfers and ambulation are generally the disabilities that are focused on in this case. For OTs, independent bathing, dressing, and feeding are major focuses. Yet both professionals also need to decide the activities that the patient or the patient's family wants to improve on to enhance the quality of life for everyone involved in the person's case. The ability to get in and out of a car might be the most important activity for the client to learn because he or she needs to take frequent trips to the doctor's office. Lastly, it is suggested that the clinician modify or "shrink" the environment to allow normal motor programs to run. The environment can be progressively "enlarged" to allow the client to perform the activity in a functional context. Although this narrowing of the functional environment would be considered a contrived environment and must not be recorded as func-

tional as defined in a functional/disability examination, it may allow the nervous system the opportunity to control and modify the motor programs within the limitations of its plasticity at the moment. As learning and repetition assist the CNS in widening the response pattern during a functional activity, the client's ability to respond to variance within the environment will enlarge and assist in gaining greater independence. An example of this application might be training a client to squat to pick up an object such as a shoe from the floor (stand-to-sit transfer). The client is first guided down to sitting onto a very large ball or hi-low table that only allows the client to sit one fourth to one half of the way down before returning to stand. As the client develops increased strength and balance and improved control over abnormal limb synergies and tone in this pattern, then a smaller ball or a lower point on the hi-low table can be used. Finally, the client is asked to sit down on a ball that is at a 90-degree angle or onto a chair. Once the client can sit down and regain a vertical position, the next task will be to sit down, relax, and then stand up. Once that activity is done easily, the client will be functional in sit to stand and reversing the movement pattern.

Although many clinicians understand the importance of running motor tasks within an appropriate biomechanical/musculoskeletal/sensorimotor window in which the client has the ability to perform procedures functionally, one may argue that in many cases this particular type of treatment strategy is simply not possible in a real-world situation. For example, given the present health care environment, if the client is given a limited number of visits to achieve the desired outcome, the clinician may conclude that he or she has no choice but to "allow as many degrees of freedom as possible" or, in other words, to "force the window open" no matter the abnormal movement patterns used or the limitations in independent functional control that they may produce.

In summary, the clinician should first identify and emphasize the client's strengths ("What can the client do?") and use those strengths to efficiently and effectively achieve functional change. Next, the clinician must prioritize what systems or activities the client truly needs to change. The choice of what activities to emphasize during therapeutic training always poses a dilemma to therapists. Although it may be ideal for the client to eventually be able to ambulate independently on all surfaces without any assistance or reach for any object in and from any spatial position, it may be more important initially for the client to be able to safely transfer from the bed to the wheelchair, sit independently while someone assists with dressing, or walk and transfer onto and off the commode independently at home. One should keep in mind that, although several skills may be learned by training them simultaneously, it may make more sense to concentrate on the safe performance of one or two necessary functional tasks rather than to end up being able to perform multiple tasks that require considerable outside assistance for safety. The need to work functionally on additional activities may also be an opportunity for the clinician to request additional therapy visits for the client, arguing that there is a reasonable expectation that more intervention would result in an increase in function and a decrease in the risk for potential injury than if the intervention were not continued. The use of valid and reliable functional outcome measures becomes critically important in case management. These tools objectively measure the effect of the intervention, help predict the potential risks if the therapy is not continued, and ultimately aid in the justification to continue therapeutic intervention.

Case Study: Bed Mobility

Teaching the client to roll in bed can be approached in a variety of ways to accomplish the goal. The entire rolling pattern may be practiced with enough assistance for the client to be able to accomplish the goal, but little enough such that the client must use the maximum amount of power and ROM available in key movement patterns.

ROLLING IN BED

The patient is a 73-year-old man, status postischemic infarct in the frontoparietal cortex with resultant left hemiplegia, hemisensory deficit, and left homonymous hemianopia. The patient demonstrates visual-spatial inattention to the left environment. The client must learn to roll independently in bed for comfort and function. An example of a treatment session aimed at reaching the goal of independent rolling to the right and left may include the following sequence of activities: (1) begin in side lying on one side; (2) ask patient to tip back a few degrees and then return to the side-lying position; and (3) progressively increase the degree the patient must roll backward, assisting him as needed. By the end of several repetitions the patient may be rolling from supine to side lying.

Conclusion

Often, clients with neurological trauma or disease cannot begin therapy with functional training because of the degree and extent of both impairments and disabilities within the sensory cortices or the limbic or motor systems. Therapists must then choose augmented therapeutic interventions that externally guide the client's learning through hands-on and environmentally controlled treatment techniques. It is again cautioned that the therapist never consider these interventions as the client demonstrating functional independence because the individual's success is based on external control of the environment and not on internal self-regulation by the client. The clinician must continually strive to transfer that control to the client by widening the window of independence and limiting the hands-on or verbal guidance used during therapy.

Augmented Therapeutic Intervention Classification

As discussed within the previous section, some treatment alternatives require little if any hands-on therapeutic manipulation of the client during the activity. For example, the patient practices transfers on and off many support surfaces with standby guarding only. Thus, the client self-corrects or uses inherent feedback mechanisms to self-correct error to refine the motor skill. This ultimate empowerment of the client allows each individual to adapt and succeed at self-motivated and identified objectives.

Often, allowing the client to try to succeed independently enables the therapist to evaluate what components of the task the client can control and what components are not within the client's adaptable capabilities, especially if normal, fluid, efficient and effortless movement is the desired outcome. In some cases the therapist may use hands-on or adaptive aids, which would augment the environment and allow the client to succeed at the task *but* would be considered contrived or noninherent feedback.

Such contrived techniques make up a large component of the therapist's specific intervention strategies. The difference between contrived and functional or intrinsic might be the need for the therapist to be part of the client's external environment for the client to succeed at the task. The therapist must recognize that as long as the therapist is part of that environment, the client is not functionally independent. Even if the client succeeds at the activity, the augmentation needed to succeed has changed the outcome, and without such intervention the patient would not have been successful. Thus, any contrived therapeutic technique or intervention must at some time be removed from the environment. The client must assume total ownership for the functional responses. Then and only then has independence been achieved. At that time functional retraining can be used with the intent of enlarging the environmental parameters to allow for maximal independence. Figure 4–8 illustrates this concept of functional versus contrived intervention and must be constantly considered throughout any treatment session. At times, selecting functional activities without the use of contrived or augmented procedures may not help the patient achieve the desired outcome. Thus, contrived techniques are often the early choices for treatment. It cannot be emphasized enough that once the client has the ability to perform without augmented methods and does so in functional, efficient ways, those techniques need to be selectively eliminated.

Even though a clinician has chosen to augment the clinical environment, the client needs to learn efficient motor behaviors within the limitations of that environment. The client needs to direct the therapist's decision-making strategies by the plans selected as motor responses to a given task. If the response is effortless, efficient, and noninjurious to any part of the body and meets the client's expectations and goals, then the therapist knows the strategies selected were effective. If the response does not meet the desired goal for any reason, then the therapist must determine why. Many correct solutions may answer the question "why?" Which solution is best may be more client than approach dependent. Yet if flexibility means that the therapist selects any component of any method that helps the client reach an objective, then the therapist is confronted with hundreds—if not thousands—of various treatment procedures. If the treatment procedures used introduce information to the client through sensory systems, then, from a neurological perspective, a limited number of input systems or modalities are available. The myriad treatment procedures are transduced into neurochemical and electrophysiological responses that must travel along a limited number of pathways. Thus, many different treatment procedures

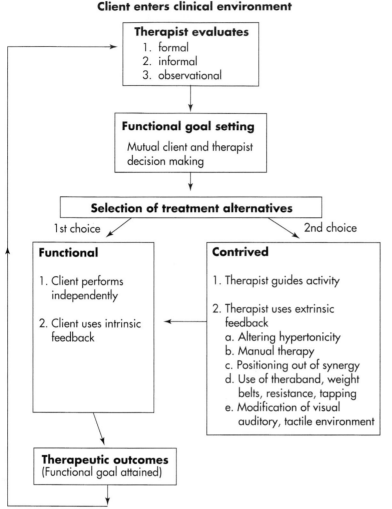

FIGURE 4–8. Contrived versus functional therapeutics.

may produce similar types of neurotransmission. The temporal and spatial sequencing or timing of the input will vary according to the technique and the specific application. The clinician has little basis for decision making without a comprehensive understanding of the neurophysiology of (1) the various techniques introduced to modify input, (2) the potential interactions that information will have with various connections within the CNS, (3) prior learning and ability for new learning, and (4) the client's willingness and motivation to adapt.

The number of available contrived or augmented feedback techniques is almost infinite. In this section an overview is presented of a classification system that can be used to help the reader develop a greater understanding of why certain responses occur and why the selection of certain techniques is appropriate, given the outcome expectations after intervention. This section focuses on intervention strategies accepted and used within the traditional Western health care model, whereas in Chapter 33 alternative approaches to intervention not necessarily classified as traditional within this chapter are introduced.

When considering the selection of a contrived intervention to augment sensory input, appropriate selection of

specific techniques can be made by using a classification schema. The primary goal of this section is to help the reader develop such a classification system—a system based on the primary input modality used when introducing a stimulus or augmented treatment technique. The reader has been provided with an in-depth reference to the specific neurophysiological basis behind each of these systems, and only a brief overview has been included. In-depth discussion of some basic treatment strategies, in addition to an explanation of less familiar techniques, is found within the body of this section. Although only the primary input system is identified, at no time do we suggest it is the only input system affected.

For example, when a proprioceptor is introduced, tactile cutaneous receptors are also simultaneously firing. If there is a "noise" component (such as with vibration), then auditory input has been triggered as well. There is evidence that a given sensory modality may "cross over" or fuse with a completely different modality, helping in the synthesis of motor responses. In addition, there is evidence that the principles of neuroplasticity are applicable across modalities (e.g., auditory, linguistic, visual, vestibular, somatosensory). Sometimes responses occur in a modality that does not appear to be related. For example, olfaction may improve tactile sensitivity of the hand. This concept is called cross-modal training or stimulation.[94, 126] Yet a classification schema based on a primary modality promotes logical problem solving because the therapist can select from available treatment procedures that theoretically provide similar information to the CNS and help in the organization of appropriate motor responses. The motor system and its various motor programmers adapt to the environment to achieve functional motor output toward a goal. Feedback is critical for adaptation and change. Feedback in this chapter is considered a mechanism to help the client's CNS optimally learn and adapt and not to facilitate a hard-wired reflexive response. Therapists must realize that even if the primary goal may be to facilitate or dampen a motor system response through multiple interlooping tracts, diverging pathways may also connect with endocrine, immune, and autonomic systems. At this time it is not known how much input leads to somatosensory remapping, which ultimately affects motor performance versus directly affecting motor programming. According to motor control theory, the clinical picture is a consensus of all systems interacting (see Chapter 5). Research tools are not yet available to measure those systems interacting simultaneously; thus, isolated causation is not known at this time. Efficacy must then be based on outcomes, with an understanding of the best available scientific knowledge as a rationale for why the outcome is present.

Therefore, within this section, the classification system is based on identified input, observed responses, hypothesized neuromechanisms, current research on the function of the CNS, and the various systems involved in the control and modification of responses. An understanding of normal processing of input and its effect on the motor systems helps the clinician evaluate and use the intact systems as part of treatment. When the response to certain stimuli does not help the client select or adapt a desired motor response, then the classification schema provides the clinician with flexibility to select additional options. This can be done by spatially summating input, such as using stretch, vibration, and resistance simultaneously, or temporally summating input, such as increasing the rate of the quick stretch or increasing the time between inputs to give the system ample time to respond.

Many factors can influence motor behavior, such as the methods of instruction, the resting condition of the nervous system before introducing stimulus feedback, synaptic connections, cerebellar/basal ganglia or cortical processing, retrieval from past learning, motor output systems, or internal influences and balance. Figure 4–9 illustrates this total system. Its clinical implications become clearer if the therapist retains a visual image of the client's total nervous system, including afferent input, intersystem processing, efferent response, and the multiple interactions on each other. At any moment in time multiple stimuli are admitted into a client's input system. Before that information reaches a level of primary processing, it will cross over at least one synaptic junction. At that time the information may be inhibited, excited, changed or distorted, or allowed to continue without modification. If the information is inhibited, then no response will be observed, even if it were considered reflexive. If it is changed, then the processing of the input will vary from the one normally anticipated. The end product after multiple system interactions will either be close to or farther away from the desired motor pattern. Furthermore, sensory processing can take place at many segments of the nervous system. Although the CNS is not hierarchical, with one level in total control over another, certain sys-

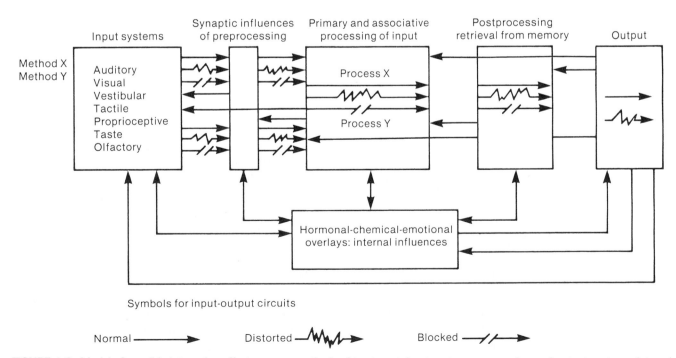

FIGURE 4–9. Model of possible interactive effects among methods of treatment, input systems, processing and output systems, internal influences, and feedback systems.

tems are biased to effect various motor responses. At the spinal level the response may be phasic and synergistic. Brain stem mechanisms may evoke flexor or extensor biases, depending on various motor systems and their modulation. Cerebellar, basal ganglionic, thalamic, and cortical responses may be more adaptive and purposeful. Thus, the therapist must try to discern where the input or the feedback is being short circuited.

The same three alternatives—inhibiting (dampening), distorting, or normal processing—can occur anywhere in the system. Finally, motor output is programmed and a response is observed. If the response is considered normal, the clinician assumes that the system is intact with regard to the use and processing of the input. If the response is distorted or absent, little is known other than there is a lack of the normal processing somewhere in the CNS. Internal influences also need to be considered because they affect each aspect of the system. Once normal processing is identified, understanding of deficit systems and potential problems can be analyzed more easily. To reiterate, this requires awareness of the totality of the individual, that is, the client's personal preference of stimuli and the uniqueness of processing and internal influences. A systems model requires simultaneous processing of multiple areas with interactions relaying in all directions. A client's CNS and peripheral nervous system (PNS) is doing just that, and the therapist must develop a sensitivity toward the client as a whole while interacting with specific components. (See Chapters 5, 6, 7, and 33 for additional information.) The classification system presented in this section will only help the reader organize one component affecting the entire clinical environment.

It is the therapist's responsibility to select methods most efficacious and effective for each client's needs. This viewpoint, based on a variety of questions, leads to a problem-oriented approach to intervention. Because the output or response pattern is based on alpha motor neuron discharge and thus extrafusal muscle contraction, the first question is posed: what can be done to alter the state of the alpha motor neuronal pool or motor generators? Second, what input systems are available, either directly or indirectly, that will alter the state of the motor pool? Third, which techniques use these various input systems as their primary modes of entry into the CNS? Fourth, what internal mechanisms need modification or adaptation to produce a desired behavior response from the client? Fifth, which input systems are available to alter the internal mechanism and what outcomes are expected? Sixth, what combination of input stimuli will provide the best internal homeostatic environment for the client to learn and rehearse a more optimal response pattern? For example, assume that a client with a residual hemiplegia due to a middle cerebral artery problem has a hypertonic lower extremity that produces the pattern of extension, adduction, internal rotation of the hip, extension of the knee, and plantarflexion inversion of the feet. The answers to the first two questions are based on the knowledge that the proprioceptive and exteroceptive systems can drastically affect spinal central pattern generators and that these input systems are intact at a spinal, brain stem,

cerebellar, and thalamic level and may even project to the cortex.

Appropriate selection of specific techniques—such as prolonged stretch using the tendon organ to modulate the hypertonic pattern, quick stretch or light touch to the antagonistic muscle, or any other treatment modality within the classification schema—provides viable treatment alternatives. Awareness that the client's response pattern is an inherent synergistic pattern and that it is further elicited by pressure to the ball of the foot leads to a better understanding of the clinical problem. Knowing that the client is unable to combine the alternative patterns, such as hip flexion and knee extension, needed for the latter aspects of swing through and early aspects of heel strike in gait, the therapist can use the other inherent processes to elicit these and other patterns. Finally, techniques such as combining standing and walking with application of quick stretch, vibration, or rotation or having the client reach for a target or follow a visual stimulus while walking provide a variety of combinations of therapeutic procedures to help the client learn or relearn normal response patterns. Furthermore, this approach gives the clinician a choice of various procedures and promotes a learning environment that is flexible, changing, and interesting. The therapist must make the transition from applying contrived therapeutic procedures during functional tasks to allowing the client to practice the task without the therapist interceding with external feedback. In that way the client uses inherent feedback to self-correct. This self-correction leads to independence and adaptability (see Fig. 4–8).

A variety of sensory classification systems have been accepted by physiologists, neuroanatomists, and therapists. To avoid confusion about which nerve fiber is being discussed, the two primary methods of classification, along with a description of the functional component, have been included in Table 4–2 for easy referral. Each system will be presented separately to help the reader separate out a classification scheme. The primary sensory input systems include proprioception, exteroception, vestibular, vision, auditory, taste, and smell. These inputs integrate pathways among the thalamus, the sensory and motor cortices, the cerebellum, the reticular formation, and the basal ganglia.

Proprioceptive System

Proprioception as an input system has a direct effect on program generators at the spinal level.[163] Due to its importance in motor learning and motor adaptation to new or changing environments, however, proprioception also has significant connections to the cortical and cerebellar neural networks. Its divergent pathways have synapses within both the brain stem and diencephalon, as well as the spinal system. It demonstrates how a systems model functions. Proprioceptive input can potentially influence multiple levels of CNS function, and all of those levels can potentially modulate the intensity or importance of that information through many different mechanisms.[46, 163] Proprioceptors are found in three peripheral anatomical locations: the muscle spindle, the tendon, and

T A B L E   4 – 2. Classifications of Peripheral Nerves According to Size

Gasser-Erlanger	Lloyd	Motor (functional component)	Sensory (functional component)
A Fibers: large myelinated fibers with a high conduction rate			
Aα	Ia	Large, fast fibers of the alpha motor system (large cells of anterior horn to extrafusal motor fibers)	Muscle spindle: primary afferent endings (primary stretch or low threshold stretch: Ia tonic responds to length, Ia phasic responds to rate)
	Ib		Golgi tendon organ for contraction: responds to tendon stretch or tension
Aβ	II		Muscle spindle: secondary afferent endings—tonic receptors responding to length
			Exteroceptive afferent endings from skin and joints: respond to light or low threshold stretch
Aγ 1 and 2	II	Gamma motor system (small cells of anterior horn to intrafusal motor fibers)	Bare nerve endings: joint receptors, mechanoreception of soft tissues—exteroceptors for pain, touch, and cold (low threshold)
AΔ	III		
B Fibers: medium-sized myelinated fibers with a fairly rapid conduction rate			
Bβ		Preganglionic fibers of autonomic system (effective on glands and smooth muscle; motor branch of alpha): unknown function	
C Fibers: small, poorly myelinated or unmyelinated fibers having the slowest conduction rate; augmentation and recruiting occurs within the nervous system after stimulation of these fibers has ceased			
	IV	Postganglionic fibers of sympathetic system	Exteroceptors: pain, temperature, touch

the joint. The afferent receptors responsible for relaying sensory information through those sites are discussed in the following subsections.

MUSCLE SPINDLE

Varied in function, the muscle spindle plays an important role in ongoing modulation of the alpha motor neurons innervating the extrafusal muscle within which it is located. This is accomplished through simultaneous modulation of both the gamma and alpha motor neurons during functional activities. Spindle afferents also polysynaptically facilitate agonistic synergies while dampening antagonists and their synergies. Information is simultaneously sent through ascending pathways to the ipsilateral cerebellum and contralateral parietal lobe. Consequently, the spindle system seems to play an important role as an ongoing peripheral feedback mechanism to various centers within the CNS. These centers in turn regulate the continuous neuroexcitation at the brain stem and spinal cord level. Gamma innervation regulates the degree of internal stretch on the noncontractile portion of the spindle. Internal stretch, along with the external stretch of gravity, positioning, and therapeutic procedures, in turn helps modulate the efferent responses.[275]

Certain spindle afferents are length receptors and respond to length changes placed on the noncontractile portion of the spindle. This length change can result from a mechanical external force, such as positioning or stretch to the muscle, or from an internal mechanism caused by intrafusal muscle contraction. Spinal motor generators and supraspinal influences modulate both the alpha and gamma motor neuron activity to produce flexibility in regulation over patterns of striated muscle contraction. As long as the spindle has enough internal sensitivity, any therapeutic technique that creates a length change to the spindle has the potential of firing these length receptors. Other receptors respond to rate of stretch versus length change. Techniques such as quick stretch, vibration, and tapping cause a rapid rate change within the spindle and thus potentially facilitate their receptors. The importance of muscle spindle afferent input as a treatment technique may lie in its ultimate influence over the cerebellum and basal ganglia to change existing programs permanently. Its direct influence over the spinal system is most likely short lived and has little long-term effect, although neuroplasticity within the spinal cord is possible. Cerebellar and basal ganglia/frontal lobe influence over brain stem motor nuclei and their modulation over interneurons within the spinal pattern generators should lead to change of existing output patterns (Fig. 4–10).

Table 4–3 lists a variety of treatment procedures believed to use the proprioceptive muscle spindle system as a primary mode of sensory stimulation. The varying intensity, amount of tension, or rate of the stimuli, in addition to the original length of the muscle fiber before application of the stimulus, will determine which sensory receptor within the spindle is firing. Remember, afferent information is projecting to many areas above the spinal system, and the result will be regulation or modulation ultimately affecting activity.[163]

Resistance. Resistance is often used to facilitate intrafusal and extrafusal muscle contraction. Resistance can be applied manually, mechanically, and by the use of gravity. Resistance recruits more motor units. Although muscles can contract both in an isometric and isotonic fashion, most contractions are a mixture of the two. Certain muscle groups, such as the flexors, benefit from isometric exercise, as well as isotonic exercise in both eccentric and concentric modes. Under normal circumstances the flexors are used for repetitive or rhythmical activities. The extensors, on the other hand, usually remain contracted in an effort to act against the forces of gravity. Therefore, the extensor groups benefit best from isometric and eccentric resistance.[121]

When resistance is applied to a voluntary muscle, spin-

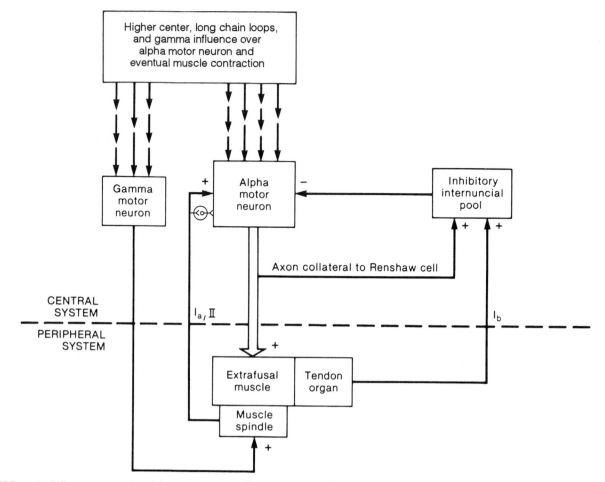

FIGURE 4–10. Influences over the alpha motor neuron. The summation of all facilitory and inhibitory activity on the alpha motor neuron will determine the response of the muscle.

T A B L E   4 – 3. Proprioceptive Muscle Spindle System

Receptor	Stimulus	Nature of Response
Ia tonic	Length	Monosynaptic and polysynaptic facilitation of agonist
Ia phasic	Rate of change in length	Polysynaptic inhibition of antagonist and antagonistic synergy
		Polysynaptic facilitation of agonistic synergy
		Input to cerebellum
		Input to opposite parietal lobe
		Specific responses open for question:
II	Length	Monosynaptic facilitation of agonist
		Polysynaptic facilitation of specific muscle groups, depending on muscle function of tissue where II originates
		Transmittal of information to higher centers

Possible Treatment Alternatives
Resistance
Quick stretch to agonist
Tapping: tendon and muscle belly
Reverse tapping: gravity stretches; tapping agonist into shortened range
Positioning (range)
Electrical stimulation
Pressure or sustained stretch
Stretch pressure
Stretch release
Vibration within a facilitory frequency
Gravity as a prolonged stretch
Active motion

dle afferent fibers and tendon organs fire in proportion to the magnitude of the resistance. Resistance is more facilitative to an isometrically contracted muscle than to an isotonic contraction.[10] As isometric resistance is increased or continued, more motor units are recruited, thereby increasing the strength of extrafusal contraction.[275] Eccentric isotonic contraction refers to the lengthening of muscle fibers to resist force, as in lowering the arms while holding a heavy object. Eccentric contraction uses less metabolic output and promotes strength gains in less time.[275] However, all types of muscle contraction will promote increased strength. Resistance is an important clinical treatment and has been used and will continue to be used by clinicians within multiple treatment philosophies over the next millennium.[40, 176, 268, 289, 302]

Tapping. Three types of tapping techniques are commonly used by therapists. Tapping of the tendon is a fairly nondiscriminatory stimulus. Physicians use this technique to determine the degree of stretch sensitivity of a muscle. A normal response would be a brisk muscle contraction. Because of the magnitude of the stimulus and the direct effect on the alpha motor neuron, this technique is not highly effective in teaching a client to control or grade muscle contraction. Instead, tapping of the muscle belly, a lower-intensity stimulus, is more satisfactory. Reverse tapping is a less frequently described technique but can be used. The extremity is positioned so gravity promotes the stretch, instead of the therapist manually tapping or actively inducing muscle stretch. Once the muscle responds, the therapist taps or passively moves the extremity to help the muscle obtain a shortened range. An example of reverse tapping would be tapping the elbow when the client is bearing weight on the extended elbow and actively trying to achieve full elbow extension. Gravity quickly stretches the triceps. Timing of this technique is important. If the therapist taps the elbow toward extension when the flexors' motor neurons are sensitive, then those flexor muscles may respond to the stretch and contract. If the timing follows the quick stretch to the extensor, then the flexors will be dampened and active extension more likely a motor response.

Positioning (Range). The concept of submaximal and maximal range of muscles is highly significant to clinical application. Bessou and colleagues[23] monitored the neuronal firing of muscle spindles at different ranges of motion. Upper motor neuron lesions can alter the sensitivity of the spindle afferent reflex arc fibers by not using presynaptic inhibition to normally dampen incoming afferent activity.[49] Therefore, ROM should be carefully assessed on an individual basis particularly in a patient with an upper motor neuron lesion to determine what is the maximal or submaximal range for an individual.

Electrical Stimulation. For in-depth discussion of the use of electrical stimulation both as an evaluation and a treatment modality, see Chapter 28. Electrical stimulation has the potential to be an excellent muscle spindle facilitory technique, especially if additional therapeutic tools, such as resistance, are included. Electrical stimulation delivered to create muscle contraction is beneficial, but electrical stimulation as a sensory stimulus is less effective as a learning tool because there are no sensory receptors for electrical currents and thus they are not represented as a unique stimulus on the somatosensory cortex.

Stretch Pressure. The muscle belly is the stimulus focus of stretch pressure. This approach would obviously not be used on a hypertonic muscle because it would increase the tone, but it could be used on the antagonist muscle to inhibit a hypertonic agonist.[94, 110] Generally, this type of stimulus is applied and maintained for a period of time (e.g., 5 to 10 seconds). It is not a quick stimulus.

Stretch Release. This technique is performed by placing the fingertips over the belly of larger muscles and spreading the fingers in an effort to stretch the skin and the underlying muscle. The stretch is done firmly enough to temporarily deform the soft tissue so the cutaneous receptors and Ia afferent fibers may produce facilitation of the target muscle.

Manual Pressure. Manual pressure can be facilitory when applied as a brisk stretch or friction-like massage over muscle bellies. The speed and duration at which the manual pressure is applied determine the extent of recruitment from receptors. Paired with volitional efforts, manual pressure can lead to motor learning.

Vibration. Bishop[25, 26] wrote an excellent series of articles on the neurophysiology and therapeutic application of vibration. High-frequency vibration (100 to 300 hertz [Hz] or cycles per second) applied to the muscle or tendon elicits a reflex response referred to as the tonic vibratory response. Tension within the muscle will increase slowly and progressively for 30 to 60 seconds and then plateau for the duration of the stimulus.[188] Some researchers found that at cessation of the input, the contractibility of the muscle was enhanced for approximately 3 minutes.[188, 309] The discrepancy in the research may reflect the way the individual is using the input, both from a motor generator perspective as well as from supraspinal modulation over the importance of the input, which may affect the overall learning and plasticity of the CNS.

To facilitate hypotonic muscle, the muscle belly is first put on stretch and then vibratory stimuli are applied.[133] To inhibit a hypertonic muscle, the antagonistic muscle could be vibrated.[25, 133] The use of vibration can be enhanced by combining it with additional modalities such as resistance, position, and visually directed movement. Vibration also stimulates cutaneous receptors, specifically the pacinian corpuscles, and thus can also be classified as an exteroceptive modality.[282] Because of its ability to decrease hypersensitive tactile receptors through supraspinal regulation, local vibration is considered an inhibitory technique (it is also discussed later in the section on exteroceptors—maintained stimulus). Therapists have reported that vibration over acupressure points can modulate localized pain syndromes. It seems to trigger A-delta exteroceptive fibers, which in turn dampen the effect of C fibers. (See Chapter 29 for more information on the treatment of pain.)

Farber[94] summarized the use of vibration and clearly identified precautions that must be taken. Frequencies over 200 Hz can be damaging to the skin. We have found frequencies over 150 Hz to cause discomfort and even pain. Thus, it is recommended that vibrators registering 100 to 125 Hz be used. Most battery-operated hand vibrators function at 50 to 90 Hz.[70] Frequencies below 75 Hz are thought to have an inhibitory effect on normal muscle.[188] Cutaneous pressure is also known to cause inhibition, so if it is combined with a vibration technique that is being used to augment a muscle contraction, it can only serve to cancel out the desired effects.

Amplitude or amount of displacement must also be considered when analyzing vibration as a modality. It has been reported that high amplitude causes adverse effects, especially in clients with cerebellar dysfunction.[26] Vibration is not recommended for infants, because their nervous system is not yet fully myelinated and it might cause too much stimulation. The reader is also cautioned about using vibration over areas that have been immobilized because of the underlying vascular tissue potential for clotting. Vibration on or near these blood vessels could dislodge a clot, causing an embolism. Vibration also needs to be used cautiously over skin that has lost its elasticity and is very thin (e.g., that in older persons) because the friction itself from the vibration can cause tearing.

THE TENDON ORGAN

The Golgi tendon organ is a specialized receptor located in both the proximal and the distal musculotendinous insertions. In conjunction with the muscle spindle, the tendon organ plays an important role in the mediation of proprioception.[63, 148, 217]

The principal role of the tendon organ is to monitor muscle tension exerted by the contraction of the extrafusal muscles. Research has demonstrated that the tendon organ is highly sensitive to tension and acts conjointly with the muscle spindle to inform higher centers of ongoing environmental demands to modulate or change existing plans, which, in turn, regulate tonicity and compliance of extrafusal muscles.[68, 163] The tendon organ (Ib) signals not only tension but also rate of change of tension and provides the sensation of force as the muscle is working.[131]

A fundamental difference between the Golgi tendon organ and the muscle spindle is that the muscle spindle detects length, whereas the tendon organ monitors tension and force. Motorically, the muscle spindle and the tendon organ spinal effect are exact opposites.[63, 68, 193] The muscle spindle regulates reciprocal inhibition, whereas the tendon organ modulates autogenic inhibition. In multiarthrodial muscles (superficial flexors and adductors), small-range repeated contractions will reduce hypertonicity in hypertonic muscles.[82, 148] This is thought to occur due to flexor reflex afferent activity along with higher-center adaptation and modulation over those afferents.[69]

Clinically, this autogenic inhibition is seen in clients with upper motor neuron lesions. Usually, the patient has some degree of hypertonicity. As the hypertonic extremity is passively moved through range of motion, resistance is felt and then suddenly "melts away," allowing more freedom of movement. The exact mechanism that dampens the hypertonicity is not known. It appears that other joint and cutaneous receptors could be sending signals to supraspinal centers, as well as the tendon organ, and it most likely is a cumulative effect.[163]

There appears to be a delicate balance between inputs that trigger inhibitory and excitatory loops within the central motor system. These peripheral input systems provide feedback control mechanisms to inform the CNS about the length, speed of movement, and contraction of a given muscle. Therefore, this balance between feedback mechanisms providing information to the CNS and the interpretation of that information is not only basic to the control of fine movements but also to decision making when feedforward plans need changing to adapt to the environmental demands. Table 4–4 lists a variety of known treatment approaches that use the tendon organ to inform higher centers regarding needed change and regulation over spinal generators.

Inhibitory Pressure. Pressure has been used therapeutically to alter motor responses. Mechanical pressure (force), such as cones, pads, or the orthokinetic cuff developed by Blashy and Fuchs,[31] provided continuously is inhibitory. That pressure seems most effective on tendinous insertions. It is hypothesized that this deep, maintained pressure activates pacinian corpuscles, which are rapidly adapting receptors. A variety of researchers have studied these receptors and their relationship to regulating vasomotor reflexes,[301] pain modulation,[242] and dampening other sensory system influence on the CNS.[309]

This inhibitory pressure technique also works when pressure is applied across the longitudinal axis of a tendon. The pressure is applied across the tendon with increasing pressure until the muscle relaxes. Constant pressure applied over the tendons of the wrist flexors may dampen flexor hypertonicity as well as elongate the tight fascia over the tendinous insertion (see Chapter 33 for additional information).

Pressure over bony prominences has modulatory effects. A common example is pressure on the medial aspect of the calcaneus, which dampens plantarflexors and allows contraction of the lateral dorsiflexor muscles. Pressure over the lateral aspect of the calcaneus also dampens calf muscles to allow for contraction of the medial dorsiflexor muscles.[268] Localized finger pressure applied bilaterally to acupuncture points has been shown to relieve pain and reduce muscle tone.[196–198] This technique has also been found to be particularly effective when used in a low-stimuli environment and when combined with deep breathing.

This combination of pressure (manually applied), environmental demands (low), and parasympathetic activity (slow, relaxed breathing) illustrates various systems interacting together to create the best motor response. The real world requires the client to respond to many environmental conditions while relaxed or under stress. Thus, once a client begins to demonstrate normal adaptable motor responses, the therapist needs to change the conditions and the stress level to allow the client to practice variability. That practice should incorporate motor error, especially error or distortions in the plan, yet still achieve the desired goal. As the client self-corrects, greater demand and variability should be introduced.[271]

THE JOINT

From a neurophysiological standpoint, joint movement provides the cerebellum and cortical sensory and motor

T A B L E 4 – 4. Proprioceptive Tendon Organs and Joints

Receptor	Stimulus	Response
Tendon Organ		
Tendon organ 1b	Tension on extrafusal muscle	Polysynaptic inhibition of agonist, facilitation of antagonist spinal level circuitry; supraspinal regulation

Possible Treatment Suggestions
1. Extreme stretch
2. Deep pressure to tendon
3. Passive positioning in extreme lengthened range
4. Extreme resistance: more effective in lengthened and shortened range
5. Deep pressure to muscle belly to put stretch on tendon
6. Small repeated contractions with gravity eliminated

Type of Joint		
I $(6–9 \mu)$	Static and dynamic joint tension: muscle pull	?: Facilitates postural holding: joint awareness
II $(9–12 \mu)$	Dynamic: sudden change in joint tension	?: Facilitates agonist and awareness of joint motion: range
III $(13–17 \mu)$	Dynamic: linked to GTO traction; activates in extreme range	?: Inhibits agonist
IV $(2–5 \mu \leq 2 \mu)$	Pain	?: Inhibits agonist

Possible Treatment Alternatives
1. Manual traction (distraction) to joint surfaces to facilitate joint motion
2. Manual approximation (compression) to joint surfaces to facilitate co-contraction or postural holding
3. Positioning: gravity used to approximate or apply traction
4. Weight belts, shoulder harnesses, and helmets to increase approximation
5. Wrist and ankle cuffs to increase traction
6. Wall pulleys, weights, manual resistance
7. Manual therapy[189]
8. Elastic tubing to provide compression during movement

nuclei with constant information about body position and movement.[71] It appears that the diarthrodial joints contain the greatest number of receptors with the capacity to respond to the slightest change of angle between two bony articulations.

Four major types of joint receptors are described in the literature. Anatomically, these receptors are localized in the joint capsules and ligaments.[46, 163] In general, joint receptors adapt slowly. Joint receptors have different thresholds for the rate of movement and the degree of angulation and thus play a key role in providing information about movement and position and also play a role in sensory mapping in area 3a.[8, 52, 292] These impulses project to many areas within the brain involved in both perception of the body in space and motor control over the body. Feedback to many areas is not crucial unless the existing environment does not match the predetermined feedforward motor plan. If input matches the existing expectation, it is erased. When the input does not match what is expected from the predicted motor behavior, a change or modification in motor output or plan is needed to meet the desired goal. At this time feedback is critical, and without it the client will not have adequate adaptive mechanisms to rapidly change to environmental demands or demonstrate fine-motor control. How the motor programmers adapt, learn, and change is discussed throughout this text both from a basic science as well as an outcome perspective.

Type III Golgi-type endings are slowly adapting joint receptors and seem to provide the brain with information about joint position.[46, 64, 193]

Type II Golgi-Mazzoni corpuscles are rapidly adapting. Higher concentrations of these receptors have been found in the connective tissues of the hands. These corpuscles function principally as detectors of rapid joint movements. They have also been found to discharge under deep pressure and vibration stimulus.[292]

Type I Ruffini's corpuscles respond vigorously with a volley of impulses at the beginning of joint movement and taper off to a steady state of firing at different angular positions. Ruffini's corpuscles monitor both the rate and direction of joint movement.[46, 288]

Free nerve endings are contiguous with unmyelinated group IV or C fibers. It has been speculated that they provide a crude awareness of initial joint movement and the signaling of joint pain.[101, 193, 307] Although laboratory studies have analyzed these receptors in isolation, when functioning together with all other input and regulatory systems it is thought that they operate more like an orchestra, whereby various rates of firing patterns are determined by both internal and external mechanisms. Thus, when treatment is considered, the therapist needs to consider the system as part of a whole, not as an isolated receptor whose rate of firing can be modified.

Studies reveal that an unidentified set of muscle afferent fibers and cutaneous receptors both contribute to the sense of movement and position.[193] Hence it may be safe to say that the somatosensory system works cooperatively as a unit in terms of both sensory processing and motor output.[113]

Because joint receptors are stretched and compressed during joint movement, they are in a good position to transmit signals regarding joint position, direction, and velocity of movement, but not force. Force sensations seem to be mediated by the receptors of the muscles and tendon organs. The joint receptors lend themselves well to treatment techniques. As already stated, the joint receptors are both slow and fast adapting. They exert strong influences on the motor system and ultimately on musculature. Joint receptors are sensitive to movement, position, traction, compression, and palpation. For clinical purposes, a variety of potential treatment approaches focus on the joint receptor (see Table 4–5).

COMBINED PROPRIOCEPTIVE INPUT TECHNIQUES

Many techniques succeed because of the combined effects of multiple input. Some of these combined techniques include jamming; ballistic movements; total positioning; PNF patterns; postexcitatory inhibition with stretch, range, rotation, and shaking; heavy work patterns; Feldenkrais[98, 99, 155]; and manual therapy.[48, 189]

Jamming. Jamming is usually applied to the ankle and knee with the intent of dampening plantarflexion while facilitating postural co-contraction around the ankle. The client can be placed in a side-lying position, can sit on a chair or mat, or can be positioned over a bolster with the hip and knee in some flexion. This flexion dampens the total extension pattern, including the plantarflexor muscles. With release of plantarflexion these muscles are placed on extreme stretch to maintain the modulation. In this position, intermittent joint approximation of considerable force is applied between the heel and knee. If the client is sitting, this approximation can easily be applied by pounding the heel on the floor and controlling a counterforce at the knee. Once co-contraction is minimally palpated, the clinician should initiate a movement pattern such as partial weight bearing to further encourage the CNS to readapt with postural control. This technique can also be used to dampen flexion of the wrist and fingers by focusing on appropriate upper-extremity patterns, modulating flexor reflex afferent activity, and applying a large amount of joint approximation between the heel of the hand and the elbow. To augment functional outcomes, the technique should be incorporated into functional training to get better somatosensory responses, improved representation of the involved body part, and greater functional carryover.

Ballistic Movement. Ballistic movements or pendular exercises are effective because of their combined proprioceptive interaction. The client is asked to initiate a movement, such as shoulder flexion while prone over a table with the arm hanging over the side. As the muscle approaches the shortened range, the amount of ongoing gamma afferent activity decreases. Thus, both the agonist alpha motor neuron bias and the inhibition of Ia and II receptors of the antagonistic alpha motor neurons decrease. Simultaneously, the antagonistic muscle is being placed on more and more stretch. This stretch, as well as the lack of inhibition on the antagonistic alpha motor neurons, will encourage the antagonistic muscle to begin contraction and reverse the movement pattern. The tendon organs also play a key role in ongoing inhibition. As the muscle approaches the shortened range and tension on the tendon becomes intense, the tendon organ increases its firing, thus inhibiting the agonist muscle in the shortened range while facilitating the antagonistic muscle. This technique is highly movement oriented, and the traction applied to the shoulder joint while swinging the arm further facilitates the movement. These ballistic movements are part of the program generators within the

spinal system and are certainly more complex than a reflex response. Supraspinal influence over a preprogrammed activity also plays a role in the effectiveness of this treatment. The specific rationale for why ballistic movements have functional carryover may be explained by recent research about cerebellar function and the importance of mechanical afferent input in regulation over movement (see Chapter 24).

The clinician using this technique must exercise caution. ROM can easily be obtained through pendular movement. Consequently, the clinician must always determine before therapy the reasons for specific clinical signs and whether the total problem will be corrected through an activity such as a ballistic movement. This is the diagnostic responsibility of the professional. If only one component of the problem is alleviated, such as limitation of range, while lack of postural tone or joint stability possibly increases in severity, then additional techniques must be combined with this treatment modality. For example, assume that the rotator cuff muscles are slightly torn and the movers of the shoulder are superficially splinting to prevent further tearing. Instructing the client to hold the humerus in the glenohumeral joint by active contraction of the rotator cuff muscles will facilitate postural holding and strengthen the torn muscles. Having the client simultaneously perform a ballistic movement with the arm will expedite shoulder movement, thus preventing unnecessary splinting and possible limitation of joint range.

Total-Body Positioning. Total-body positioning implies the use of positioning and gravity to dampen afferent activity on the alpha motor neurons and thus cause a decrease in tone, or relaxation.[240] Today, the rationale for why relaxation of striated muscle occurs after this treatment would imply that the effect of the flexor reflex afferents is being dampened by a combination of input and interneuronal activity. These changes in the state of the muscle tone will not be permanent and will revert back to the original posturing unless motor learning and adaptation within the central programmer occur simultaneously. Thus, for this treatment to effect permanent change, a large number of systems need modification. This modification can be augmented by techniques that facilitate autogenic inhibition, reciprocal innervation, labyrinthine and somatosensory influences, and cerebellar regulation over tone.[170] Changing the degree of flexion of the head also alters vestibular input and the state of the motor pool. But, again the CNS of the client needs to be an active participant and will ultimately determine whether permanent learning and change are programmed.

Proprioceptive Neuromuscular Facilitation Patterns. To analyze and learn the patterns and techniques that constitute PNF, a total approach to treatment, refer to the texts by Knott, Voss, Adler,[179] and Sullivan and colleagues.[289] This approach is being used extensively in orthopedic as well as neuromuscular problems, and the research on this method has been studied more in lower motor neuron and musculoskeletal problems than in upper motor neuron lesions.[48]

Postexcitatory Inhibition with Stretch, Range, Rotation, and Shaking. The concept of postexcitatory inhibition (PEI) is based on the action potential or electrical response pattern of a neuron at the time of stimulation, as well as the entire phase response until the neuron returns to normal. At the time of stimulation, the action potential will build and go through an excitatory phase. The neuron then enters an inhibitory phase or refractory period during which further stimulation is not possible. This is referred to as the PEI phase or postsynaptic afferent depolarization (PAD).[94] These phase changes are extremely short and, in normal muscle, asynchronous with respect to multiple neuronal firing. In a hypertonic muscle more simultaneous firing occurs. When the muscle is lengthened, and thus tension is created, more fibers will be discharged. It is hypothesized that if the hypertonic muscle is placed at the end of its spastic range and a quick stretch is applied and held, then total facilitation followed by total inhibition will occur because of postexcitatory inhibition. As the inhibition phase is felt, the therapist can passively lengthen the spastic muscle until the facilitory phase sets in repolarization. At that time the clinician holds the lengthened position. Increased tone will ensue, followed by inhibition and continued lengthening. Holding the range (not allowing concentric contraction during the excitatory phase) is critical. If the muscle is held as the tone increases, the resistance and stretch are then maximal and probably further facilitate the inhibitory phase.

At a certain point in the range, if the muscle is not limited by fascial tightness, the hypertonic muscle will become dampened and tone will disappear. It is thought that at this time either the tendon organ activity takes over and maintains inhibition or flexor reflex afferents are modified, thus creating an inhibitory range where antagonistic muscles can be more easily initiated and controlled by the client. If this technique is performed in a pure plane of motion, the clinician will find it a time-consuming procedure. Range can be achieved quickly by integrating a few additional techniques, that is, incorporating rotatory patterns of movement. For example, if the spastic upper extremity is positioned in the pattern of shoulder adduction, internal rotation, elbow flexion, wrist pronation, and finger flexion, then a pattern in the exact opposite direction can be incorporated to include external rotation of the shoulder and supination of the wrist. Every time the clinician begins to lengthen the spastic extremity, those rotatory patterns should be used. This should be done both on initial stretch and hold and during the inhibitory phase. Rotation seems to lengthen the inhibitory phase and allows additional range. If the clinician adds a quick stretch to the antagonistic muscle during the inhibitory phase of the agonistic muscle, then further facilitation of the antagonistic muscle will occur. Because the agonistic muscle is in an inhibitory phase, movement in and out of its spastic range should not affect it. Yet the quick stretch facilitation of the antagonistic muscle inhibits the spastic agonistic muscle and again lengthens the inhibitory phase. This entire procedure occurs quite quickly. An observer might say that the clinician shakes the hypertonicity out of the arm. The shaking action is thought to be the quick stretch as well as joint oscillations. The degree of success depends on the therapist's sensitivity to the tonal shifts or phase changes occurring in the

client. These tonal shifts are automatic and not under the client's conscious control. The technique does not teach the client anything and should only be used to maintain ROM and to create an optimal environment to encourage the client to initiate normal antagonistic control. This is also a good technique for a family to help with at home to set a better stage for exercises.

Rood's Heavy Work Patterns. Today, the concepts of motor learning more clearly explain why postural holding for periods of time and eccentric lengthening in and out of the shortened range are effective treatment techniques. If repetition within the environmental context leads to motor learning, then the postural systems need to learn co-activation within the shortened range of the postural pattern and need to practice directing the limbs during both closed-chained and open-chained activities.

Feldenkrais. Feldenkrais' concepts[98, 99] of sensory awareness through movement place emphasis on relaxation of muscle on stretch and distracting and compressing joints for sensory awareness. Both techniques reflect combined proprioceptive techniques. Taking muscles off stretch slows down general afferent firing and thus overload to the CNS. Compression and distraction of joints enhance specific input from a body part while simultaneously facilitating input of a lesser intensity from other body segments. This combined proprioceptive approach enhances body schema awareness in a relaxed environment. It also integrates empowerment of the client by using visualization and asking for volitional control. (See Chapter 33 for additional information.)

Manual Therapy: Specifically Maitland's. "The peripheral and central nervous systems need to be considered as one since they form a continuous tissue tract."[98] Manual therapy or mobilization of joint or soft tissue structures is not specific to orthopedic conditions, nor are neurotreatment principles ineffective on orthopedic patients. Irrespective of the diagnostic reason, whether pathology or impairment driven leading to joint immobility, the functional consequences can be synonymous. With the immobility of joints, the peripheral nerve begins to lose its adaptability to change in the length of the nerve bed. This change in neural elasticity then creates additional problems in connective tissue function, which in turn may affect the function of the motor system's control over the musculoskeletal component.[47, 48] For this reason alone, discussion of musculoskeletal mobilization needs to be included in this section as a component of classification.

"Pathological processes may interfere with both of these mechanisms: extraneural pathology will affect the nerve/interface relationship and intraneural pathology will affect the intrinsic elasticity of the nervous system."[47] Patient complaints of pain that limits functional movement constitute the primary reason clients get referred to a therapist for a musculoskeletal evaluation. Besides subjective and observational evaluation, the physical examination must include tension tests that are used to determine the degree of pain and joint limitation, to differentiate between somatic and radicular symptoms, and to identify adverse neurophysiological changes in the

PNS.[47] "The increased muscle tone (in a peripheral injury) is considered to be a protective mechanism for the inflamed tissue."[92] This increase in tone may be due to a dampening of presynaptic activity of the flexor reflex afferent by supraspinal mechanisms. This same mechanism may be triggered by a CNS injury. The difference between the orthopedic and neurological patient may be the trigger to the CNS. In a central lesion the motor generators are often not adequately maintained after injury, which results in hypotonicity. The hypotonicity causes peripheral instability, stretches peripheral tissue, and potentially causes peripheral damage. In both orthopedic and neurological cases, there is peripheral instability, the first due to peripheral damage and the second due to hypotonicity. The CNS response to the instability may be the same: an increase in muscle tone by dampening presynaptic inhibition. A result of a decrease in presynaptic inhibition on incoming afferents would cause an increase in spinal generator activity. With an isolated musculoskeletal problem and an intact CNS, the motor system would have the adaptability and control to modulate the spinal generators and isolate only those components in which an increase in tone might directly affect the problems. The client with CNS may lose some of the flexibility of the motor system's control over the pattern generators, and thus high-tone synergistic patterns may develop.

In either case, the peripheral system needs to be evaluated and intervention provided when necessary. Tension tests look for adverse responses to physical examination of neural tissues. These adverse responses are muscle tone increases as a result of painful provocation of sensitized neural tissue nociceptors attempting to prevent further pain by limiting the movement of the neural tissue.[92] Pain increases tone and leads to limited range of passive movement.[92, 178] Pain-free range suggests CNS sensitivity to the large, highly myelinated alpha fibers and functions in a discriminatory manner. Pain range encompasses the degree of joint motion where neural length as well as nociceptors in the skin, fascia, muscles, and joints play a primary role in CNS attention and protection. Inflammation of neural tissue can also cause the nociceptors to become hypersensitized or more reactive to mechanical or chemical changes. This is particularly true in the joint when the nociceptors react significantly to movement at the end ranges.[47]

Treatment will be based on the degree of immobility, the pain range, the site of the irritability, and the degree of pain. Butler[48] not only looks at joint problems but also considers many joint problems as having adverse neural dynamics (tension on the PNS). Treatment still incorporates Maitland's grades of passive movement listed in Figure 4–11, but with consideration across the length of the neural tissue across multiple joints.

Butler[47] divides treatment of the joint into three categories: limitations, pain, and adverse mechanical tension. When analyzing selective nervous system mobilization as identified by Butler, the therapist needs to mobilize the nervous system and its surrounding fascia rather than stretching it. These techniques may be either gentle (grade 1) or strong (grade IV), through the range (grades II and III), or at end range only (grade IV). Different

Grades of Movement

Grade I A small amplitude movement performed near the beginning of range.

Grade II A large amplitude movement carried well into range. It's a movement that occupies any part of the range that is free of pain or resistance.

Grade III A large amplitude movement that moves up to the limit of range or into resistance.

Grade IV A small amplitude movement performed near the end of range or slightly into resistance.

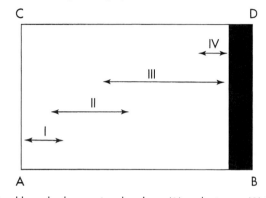

Maitland has also been using the pluses (1) and minuses (2) in his grades of movement for many years now. It enables the therapist to communicate better with other therapists as well as treat the patient with accuracy and skill.

Grade IV－－: just nicking resistance

Grade IV－: touching resistance

Grade IV: into resistance about 25%

Grade IV＋: into resistance about 50%

Grade IV＋＋: into resistance about 75%

FIGURE 4–11. Grades of movement. (Adapted from Maitland's Theory of Joint and Tissue Mobilization by John Sievert, PT, GDMT. From Course Notes, Graduate Diploma in Manipulative Therapy, Curtin University of Technology, Perth, WA, 1990; and from Maitland GD: Peripheral Manipulation, 3rd ed. Boston, Butterworth Heinemann, 1991.)

disorders (irritable versus nonirritable) will require different treatment approaches.

Treatment must interface with related tissues. When joint immobility is interfaced with muscle and fascia tightness, all components must be treated simultaneously. If the focus of treatment is the correction of joint and muscle signs, the constant reassessment of nervous system effect is crucial. This aspect would seem even more crucial in clients with CNS and PNS injuries. The treatment may be direct or indirect. Direct intervention refers to procedures directed to rebalance the neuromusculoskeletal system through strengthening and increasing ROM to improve motor control. Indirect treatment includes the use of movement patterns, especially posture-based patterns. When individuals experience nervous system changes, static and dynamic postural patterns often emerge as compensatory reactions to the problem state. Pain posturing, tension, or stiffness due to prolonged positioning, and forced postures due to synergy patterns, to name a few, all seem to respond well to indirect treatment with or without passive CNS mobilization. The use of posture-based movement patterns during functional activities also provides for variability and repetition and thus should lead to greater carryover in motor learning.

Many manual therapy approaches affect and use the proprioceptive system as a means to change motor responses. The reader is again reminded that the proprioceptive system affects all systems within the CNS and vice versa. The end effect of all systems interactions will be intrinsic reinforcement of existing behavior or will change and adapt behavior to meet intrinsic and extrinsic demands. The behavior observed by the therapist as the client initiates motor strategies in response to functional goals will be a consensus of all these interactions.

Exteroceptive/Cutaneous Sensory System

The somatosensory system is usually subdivided into two distinct systems. One system is phylogenetically older and nonspecific in nature. The other system is phylogenetically newer and specific in function. The concept of the dual quality of the somatosensory system was first suggested by Head.[138] Today, the systems are described in more anatomical terms as the spinothalamic (mediates more protective stimuli) and the lemniscal (mediates discriminative aspects of somatic sensibility) systems, which include both exteroceptive and proprioceptive information.[10, 221]

A fundamental understanding of the anatomy and physiology of the dual sensory systems is important before undertaking therapeutic intervention techniques. The afferent information entering the lemniscal system originates from either a peripheral or cranial nerve. These interneurons are large and well myelinated. Therefore, signals are transmitted rapidly, with a minimum of three synaptic relays. A striking characteristic of this system is its somatotopic organization. There is an orderly spatial topographical representation of the surface of the skin in the fiber bundles of the dorsal columns and the synaptic organization of the thalamus. This highly developed organization of sensory relays allows discrimination among specific proprioceptive and tactile stimuli. This system transmits conscious proprioceptive and kinesthetic information such as touch, pressure, localization, contour, quality, and spatial details of mechanical stimuli.[46, 323]

The spinothalamic system's ascending impulses either terminate in or send collateral connections to the reticular formation. These fibers continue upward to synapse with the nonspecific thalamic nuclei (medial) and then diverge to make connections with practically all regions of the cerebral cortex. Other collaterals of this system project to the regulators of the autonomic nervous system (ANS), limbic system, and brain stem nuclei.[46, 163]

Because the spinothalamic system synapses with the reticular formation and the ANS, it serves more as an energizing or arousal mechanism to potentially harmful stimuli. Therefore, this system is involved in perception of pain, light touch, pleasurable sexual sensations, and aversive stimuli and in the production of primitive orientations and preprogrammed and protective responses.[38, 46, 266]

This subdivision into spinothalamic and lemniscal systems can mislead one into thinking that they can be activated separately. Most sensory stimuli will activate both systems simultaneously—for example, light touch. The lemniscal system can carry both exteroceptive and proprioceptive stimuli. However, it is possible to "load" one system more than the other by using selective stimuli in a fast or slow manner.[10]

Poggio and Mountcastle[246] suggest that the lemniscal system can have an inhibiting influence on the spinothalamic system. Ayers[11] and Wilbarger[316] have proposed that "touch defensiveness" constitutes the predominance of the spinothalamic (protective) system over the lemniscal system. Many of the therapeutic techniques used in sensory integrative therapy are designed to activate the lemniscal system and establish a better balance between the two systems. In addition, the facial region receives its sensory innervation from the trigeminal nerve, which can be regarded as a third somatosensory system because it supplies a body surface that is outside the dermatomal segments supplied by the spinal cord.[221] A soft, low-intensity stimulation to the facial region can elicit a relaxation response, because the soft tissues are also richly innervated by the parasympathetic nervous system.[128, 157] Wilbarger[316] postulates that if the protective system becomes hypersensitive, its generalized effect will lead to sympathetic overactivity, avoidance behaviors of all types, inability to handle or dampen extraneous input, and potential attention deficits. By desensitizing the touch system through maintained deep rubbing with a surgical-type scrub brush or other maintained stimuli, she states the system will dampen its firing, and the discriminatory (lemniscal) system can begin to function. This discriminatory system will further override the older system and help to reestablish better homeostasis.

The exteroceptive system can be considered as a whole system or divided into sensory end organs located in the superficial layers of the skin, the subcutaneous layers, the dermis, and the external mucous membranes.[282] Some authors include the special sense organs and/or cranial nerves, such as gustational, olfactory, visual, and auditory, as part of the exteroceptive system. This section describes only the nonencapsulated and encapsulated end organs found in the skin around hairs and does not include special senses.

The skin, being the organ of touch, is activated by stimuli from outside the body. Therefore, the exteroceptors inform the CNS about changes taking place in the external environment. These receptors tend to be especially sensitive to specific kinds of energy, such as pain, temperature, touch, and pressure. Before an exteroceptor will discharge, it must receive the appropriate amount of energy, which is called the adequate stimulus. Exteroceptors also have different thresholds. When the stimuli are adequate the neuron reaches its action potential and discharges according to the intensity of the stimulus.[124, 282] The duration of discharge depends on the receptor's ability to adapt. Some receptors adapt quickly, and others adapt slowly.

Exteroceptors innervate certain areas of the skin in a distinct fashion. The area of skin innervation is called a receptive field. There is a large variation in the number of receptors and the rate they transmit information from a given field of glabrous, nonhairy skin.[23, 242] For example, the palmar surface of the hand contains a greater number of receptors than the dorsal surface. There is a greater density of small receptor fields because the hands are used for fine motor skill, prehension, and touch and thus need to have greater representation within the cortical area.[154, 163, 325]

DIFFERENTIATION OF RECEPTOR SITE AS AUGMENTED INTERVENTION

Humans have many different types of tactile receptors. Some are superficial, and others are deep. These receptors have been identified within the next subsection in order to discuss their use as augmented intervention strategies.

Free Nerve Endings. Free or bare nerve endings are phylogenetically the oldest unencapsulated receptors (see Table 4–2). Free nerve endings transmit pain, temperature, and light-touch sensations.[124] Sensitivity to cold stimuli is 10 times greater along the midline than in the extremities.[64, 163] Free nerve endings seem to serve as primitive protective receptors because they are centrally located and alert the organism to potential dangers to vital organs.

Hair Receptors. In general, hair receptors cause an excitatory response because the reticular-activating system links to the ANS. Stimulation to hair follicles or skin located on a dermatome at the same segmental level can facilitate the underlying muscle.[91, 139] However this stimulus activates a cutaneous sensorimotor reflex. The reflex sends impulses along the alpha (group II) fibers to the interneurons and alpha motor neurons that terminate at the myoneural junction of the skeletal muscle.[91, 139] This creates a dermatome-myotome relationship.

Merkel's Disks. Slowly adapting touch-pressure receptors, Merkel disks (group II) are highly responsive to slow movements across the skin surface and to light pressures. These receptors have also been associated with the sense of tickly and pleasurable touch.[46, 64]

Meissner's Corpuscles. Meissner's corpuscles as receptors are highly discriminative, providing an instantaneous sense of contact and flutter sensation. These receptors are used in two-point discrimination and stereognosis. There is some evidence that elderly individuals have a reduction of sensation resulting from a combination of skin inelasticity and loss of Meissner's corpuscles.[255, 256]

Pacinian Corpuscles. Pacinian corpuscles are located deep in the dermis of the skin: in viscera, mesenteries, and ligaments, and near blood vessels. Interestingly, they are most plentiful in the soles of the feet, where they seem to exert some influence on posture, position, and ambulation.[255] The pacinian corpuscles adapt very quickly, and they are activated by deep pressure and quick stretch of tissues.[91]

A list of treatment techniques using the tactile or exteroceptive system as their primary mode of entry can be found in Table 4–5.

TREATMENT ALTERNATIVES USING THE EXTEROCEPTIVE SYSTEM

The function of the exteroceptive system is to inform the nervous system about the surrounding world. The CNS will adapt behavior to coexist and survive within this environment. Although many protective responses are patterned within the motor system, these patterned responses can be changed or modulated according to momentary inherent chemistry, attitude, motivation, alertness, and so on. Different from some of the other treatment approaches, the function of the exteroceptive input system is not reflexive but rather informative and adaptable.

Quick Phasic Withdrawal. The human organism reacts to painful or noxious stimuli at both conscious and unconscious levels. If the stimulus is brief and of noxious quality, it will elicit a protective reaction of short duration using the long-chain spinal reflex loops. Simultaneously, afferent impulses ascend to higher centers to evoke prolonged emotional-behavioral responses. Stimuli such as pain, extremes in temperature, rapid movement, light touch, and hair displacement are the most likely to cause this reaction by activating free nerve endings. These stimuli are perceived as potentially dangerous and communicate directly with the reticular-activating system and nonspecific thalamic nuclei. These structures have diffuse interconnections with all regions of the cerebral cortex, ANS, limbic system, cerebellum, and motor centers in the brain stem. Observing clients' behavior in chronic pain problems, these responses seem to become habitual and may lead to somatosensory remapping, making it hard to differentiate protective from discriminatory information.

There are some real therapeutic limitations to using stimuli that "load" the spinothalamic system. A painful stimulus will be excitatory to the nervous system and produce a prolonged reaction after discharge. According to Wall's "gate-control" theory,[101, 185, 310] all sensory afferent neurons converge and synapse in the dorsal horn in an area called the substantia gelatinosa. Curiously, the large, more discriminatory fibers do outnumber the small fibers.[315] Therefore, physical activity, frequent positioning, deep pressure, and proprioceptive and cutaneous stimulation should cause enough impulses to converge on cells within the substantia gelatinosa to close the gate and thus block transmission of pain messages to the brain. Studies have demonstrated that physical activity (types of physical stress) stimulates the production of endorphins, which in turn release opiate receptors and act as the body's own morphine for pain control[36, 189, 190, 197] (see Chapters 29 and 32).

Because light touch has both a protective and discriminatory function, techniques such as brushing or stroking the skin with a soft brush have the potential of informing the CNS about (1) texture, object specificity, and error in fine motor responses or (2) danger (eliciting a protective response). If a protective response is triggered, the specific withdrawal pattern will depend on a variety of cir-

TABLE 4-5. Exteroceptive Input Techniques

Receptors	Stimuli	Response*
Free nerve endings: C + A fibers	Pain, temperature, touch	Seems to protect and alert, perception of temperatures, protective withdrawal
Hair follicles	Mechanical displacement of hair receptors	Increased tone of muscle below stimulus site
Merkel's disk	Touch: pressure receptors	Touch identification
Meissner's corpuscles	Discriminative touch	Postural tone; two-point discrimination
Pacinian corpuscles	Deep pressure and quick stretch to tissue, vibration	Position sense, postural tone and movement
Ruffini's corpuscles	Touch mechanoreceptor	Touch/spatial discrimination

Suggested Treatment Procedures Using Cutaneous Stimuli

Quick phasic withdrawal

1. Stimuli
   a. Pain
   b. Cold: one-sweep with ice cubes—Rood's quick ice
   c. Light touch: brush (quick stroking), finger, feather
2. Response
   a. Stimulus applied to an extensor surface: elicits a flexor withdrawal
   b. Stimulus applied to flexor surface: may elicit flexor withdrawal or withdrawal from stimulus into extension

Repetitive icing should be used with caution because of rebound effect.

Prolonged icing

1. Stimuli
   a. Ice cube
   b. Ice chips and wet towel
   c. Bucket of ice water
   d. Ice pack
   e. Immersion of body part or total body
2. Response: inhibition of muscles below skin areas iced

Neutral warmth

1. Stimulus
   a. Air bag splints
   b. Wrapping entire body or individual body part with towel
   c. Tight clothing such as tights, fitted turtleneck jerseys
   d. Tepid water or shower
2. Response: inhibition of area under which neutral warmth was applied

Light touch/rapid stroking: to facilitate muscle below stimulus area

Maintained pressure or slow, continuous stroking with pressure

*Response: adaptation of many cutaneous receptors to stimulus, thus decreasing exteroceptive input, decreasing reticular activity, and decreasing facilitation of muscles underlying stimulated skin.

cumstances. If the stimulus is applied to an extensor surface, then a flexor withdrawal will be facilitated. If the stimulus is placed on a flexor surface, one of two responses occurs. First, the client might withdraw from the stimulus, thus going into an extensor pattern. Second, the stimulus may elicit a flexor withdrawal and cause the client to go into a flexor pattern. Which pattern occurs depends on preexisting motor programming bias as a result of positioning and the predisposition of the client's CNS. Both responses would be considered normal. The condition or emotional state of the nervous system and whether the stimulus is considered threatening also determine the sensitivity of the response, again reinforcing the systems' interdependence. These responses are protective and do not lead to repetition of movement and not motor learning. For that reason, along with the emotional and autonomic reactions, a phasic withdrawal to facilitate flexion or extension is not recommended as a treatment approach unless all other possibilities have been eliminated.

Short Duration: High-Intensity Icing. Cold is another stimulus that the nervous system perceives as po-

tentially dangerous. The use of ice as a stimulus to elicit desired motor patterns is an early technique developed by Rood. Her technique was referred to as repetitive icing. An ice cube is rubbed with pressure for 3 to 5 seconds or used in a quick-sweep motion over the muscle bellies to be facilitated. This method would activate both exteroceptors and proprioceptors and causes a brief arousal of the cortex. This method can produce unpredictable results. Although initially a phasic withdrawal pattern generator response will be activated immediately after the reflex has taken place, the "rebound" phenomenon deactivates the muscle that has been stimulated and lowers the resting potential of the antagonistic muscle.[276] Therefore, a second stimulus to the same dermatome/myotome neural network may not elicit a second response. But, because of reciprocal innervation, the antagonistic muscle may effect a rebound movement in the opposite direction. Icing may also cause prolonged reaction after discharge because of the connections to the reticular system, limbic system, and ANS. Thus, the ANS would be shifted toward the sympathetic end. Too much sympathetic tone causes a desynchronization of the cortex.[14] Although the resting state of the spinal generator may be altered briefly, if the heightened state persists it is most likely due to fear or sympathetic overflow. This state is destabilizing to the system and most likely will not lead to any motor learning. Because of unpredictable response patterns to Rood's repetitive icing, this technique is seldom used.

The therapist is cautioned not to use short-duration, high-intensity icing to the facial region above the level of the lips, to the forehead, or to the midline of the trunk. These areas have a high concentration of pain fibers and a strong connection to the reticular system.[64, 263]

Ice should not be used behind the ear because it may produce a sudden lowering of blood pressure.[52] The therapist should also avoid using ice in the left shoulder region in patients with a history of heart disease because referred pain secondary to angina pectoris manifests itself in the left shoulder area, indicating the cold stimulus might cause a reflexive constriction of the coronary arteries.[314] In addition, the primary rami located along the midline of the dorsum of the trunk have sympathetic connections to internal organs. The cold stimulus may alter organ activity and perhaps produce vasoconstriction, causing increased blood pressure and less blood supply to the viscera.[11, 229]

Brief administration of ice can have beneficial effects if the nervous system's inhibitory mechanisms are in place. For instance, in children with learning disabilities or adults with sensorimotor delays, the application of ice to the palmar surface of the hands will cause arousal at the cortical level because of the increased activity of the reticular activating system. This arousal response presumably produces increased adrenal medullary secretions, resulting in various metabolic changes. Therefore, icing should be used selectively. If the patient has an unstable ANS, it should be eliminated as a potential sensory modality.[108]

Prolonged Use of Ice. A variety of approaches incorporate prolonged icing techniques. The proprioceptive neuromuscular facilitation approach may be the most common.[176] Inhibition of hypertonicity or pain is the goal for the use of any of these methods. With prolonged cold the neurotransmission of impulses, both afferent and efferent, is reduced. Simultaneously, the metabolic rate within the cooled tissue is reduced (see Chapter 29). Caution must be exercised with regard to the use of this modality. However, for effective treatment results, the client (1) should be receptive to the modality, (2) should be able to monitor the cold stimulus (sensory deficits should not be present), and (3) should have a stable autonomic system to prevent unnecessary adverse effects of hypothermia.

Ice massage is a form of prolonged icing and is often used to treat somatic pain problems. It is also used over high-toned muscles to dampen striated muscle contractions. Caution must be used when eliminating pain without correcting the problem causing pain. For example, if instability causes muscle tone and pain, then icing might decrease pain while causing additional joint instability and potential damage. The end result would be an increase, not decrease, in pain as well as motor dysfunction.

Neutral Warmth. Like icing, this approach alters the state of the motor generators, either directly or indirectly through afferent input. According to Farber,[95] the length of application depends on the client. A 3- to 4-minute tepid bath may create the same results as a 15-minute total body-wrapping procedure. As with any input procedure, the effects should be incorporated into the therapeutic session to maximize the effect and promote client learning. Johnstone uses air splints effectively as a neutral warm treatment intervention in which she has clients work on functional activities.[160] If neutral warmth is applied as an isolated intervention, the client may feel relaxation or a decrease in discomfort, but neuroplastic CNS changes are very unlikely, owing to the lack of repetition, attention, and error correction by the client during activities.

Maintained Stimulus or Pressure. Because of the rapid adaptation of many cutaneous receptors, a maintained stimulus will effectively cause inhibition by preventing further stimuli from entering the system. This technique is applied to hypersensitive areas to normalize skin responses. Vibration, used alternately with maintained pressure, can be highly effective. It should be remembered that these combined inputs use different neurophysiological mechanisms. It is often observed that low-frequency maintained vibration is especially effective with learning-disabled children who have hypersensitive tactile systems that prevent them from comfortable exploration of their environment. By having them use vibration themselves on the extremities, their hypersensitivity systems seem to normalize and they become receptive to exploring objects. If that exploration is accompanied by additional prolonged pressure, such as digging in a sandbox, the technique seems to be more effective due to the adaptive responses of the nervous system.

Maintained pressure approaches using elastic stockings, tight form-fitting clothing (e.g., wet suits, Gore-Tex biking clothing), air splints, and other techniques can be incorporated into a client's daily activity without altering lifestyle. In this way clients can self-regulate their systems, allowing greater variability in adapting to the environment. Owing to the multisensory and multineuronal pathways used when augmenting peripheral input, traditional linear, allopathic research on human subjects is extremely difficult to design or measure with control. But outcome studies demonstrating efficacy is possible. Initially, efficacy was acceptable through observation. Now it is time to repeat studies using objective measures to demonstrate the same outcome.

Vestibular System

The vestibular apparatus is a mechanoreceptor.[46] Peripheral proprioceptive receptors inform the CNS where the body is in space, and the vestibular system relays information about the head position and linear acceleration in space. Because the vestibular system is intimately connected to the auditory, visual, proprioceptive, and motor systems, it works interactively to modulate important functions.[71, 84] The vestibular system has been credited with influencing muscle tone and maintaining visual gaze, spatial directionality, clarity of the image when the head is moving or the object is moving, and head and body orientation. It also influences learning and emotional development.[218, 318]

The vestibular system has two distinct receptor areas. The vestibule (utricle and saccule) is located between the semicircular canals and the cochlea. It is often called the static labyrinth because it elicits tonic reflexes in postural muscles in response to changes in head and body positions and gravitational influences.[163] The anatomical arrangement of the hair cell receptors within the vestibule allows sensory receptors to be highly responsive to changes in head position. As the head is tilted to one side, the force of gravity displaces the otolithic membrane, which causes the cilia of the hair cell to bend. This bending or shearing action causes the hair cell to discharge and transmit afferent impulses to the CNS.[19]

The hair cells are tonic receptors and, even in the neutral position, are constantly discharging. The bending of the cilia in a single hair cell in one direction will cause an increase in firing, and bending in the opposite direction will cause a slowing of the rate of discharge.[46, 163]

The saccule lies between the utricle and cochlear duct. The majority of the cilia (hair cells) in the saccule are arranged in a side-lying fashion when the head is in the normal upright position. Therefore, if the head moves in a vertical plane (e.g., nodding), the cilia will discharge. Any up-and-down motion, including bouncing on a trampoline, is an adequate stimulus to the cilia in the saccule. In contrast, the majority of the cilia in the utricle are arranged vertically and the head is in the upright position. Thus, linear acceleration and deceleration in the horizontal plane are adequate stimuli for the cilia in the utricle. One may think of a child in a prone position propelling down an incline on a scooter board. As the child hits the horizontal plane the head is upright, causing the cilia to deflect and discharge. Quick deceleration, caused by running into a mat on the floor, causes the hair cells to whip forward, deflecting the cilia once again. In most instances, the cilia in both the sacculus and utriculus are sensitive to a variety of stimuli. For example, forward and backward movements will activate cilia in both chambers. In summary, the adequate stimuli for the cilia of the utricle and saccule (vestibule) are the static position of the head in space and linear acceleration and deceleration in horizontal and vertical planes. The greatest tonal changes occur in extensor groups of the postural muscles. In addition, the vestibule (saccule and utricle) contributes to the maintenance of righting reactions, especially head position in space.

Rood[268] suggested that the side-lying position of the head is useful to diminish unwanted extensor tone caused by poorly integrated labyrinthine information. In this position the symmetrical input of the vestibular receptors on the vestibular nuclei is eliminated, modifying the outflow of the vestibulospinal tract and thus its influence over postural extensors.

The semicircular canals are referred to as the kinetic labyrinth, because they respond to movements of the head. The semicircular canals also exert influences on the limbs and the extraocular muscles of the eyes, as well as assist in equilibrium responses and orientation in space.

The semicircular canals are arranged approximately at right angles to one another, one for each axis of rotation. The anterior and posterior canals are sensitive to movement in the sagittal plane. The horizontal canal reacts to rotation around the central body axis.[163, 219] Any angular (rotatory) acceleration or deceleration of the head will displace and causes the semicircular canal receptors to fire.[19, 163, 318]

The semicircular receptors are not responsive to prolonged spinning at constant velocity. Numerous physiological studies[16, 128] have demonstrated that during the beginning of rotation the receptors fire at a greater rate. If the rotation is continued, the receptors gradually reassume their resting position in about 20 seconds. When rotation is stopped, deflection again occurs but in the opposite direction because the endolymph fluid continues to circulate through the canals. After 10 to 30 seconds, the endolymph stops circulating and the receptors return to their resting positions and resume a tonic level of discharge. During this time, a normal nystagmus can be observed.

Based on this information, prolonged spinning is physiologically nonproductive. It should be remembered that the initial acceleration is the force that causes firing at a greater rate. Also, the semicircular canals are most responsive to short rotational movements as opposed to prolonged rotation.[71] A good formula for semicircular canal stimulation is to spin the subject approximately 10 times in 20 seconds, stop abruptly, wait about 20 seconds, and spin again at the same rate in the opposite direction. Spinning that includes alternation of direction (e.g., right then left) maintains adaptive firing. It is also beneficial to consider the position of the head while spinning. For example, if the subject is side lying on a large spinning apparatus, the endolymph fluid in both the anterior and posterior canals will circulate, causing a more powerful response. If functional movement is not incorporated along with attention (e.g., spelling words or counting), learning will not occur as motor programs.

Spinning is not to be used without proper precautions. In infants and disinhibited patients it may induce seizures or depress respiration. It is best to allow patients to control the initial rate of spinning or vestibular stimulation so they can accommodate to the stimulus.

To review, the receptors of the vestibule (macula) seem to be concerned with static orientation of the head in space and "directionality." In this context, directionality refers to the ability to move from a beginning point A to a designated point B without becoming disoriented or veering off in the wrong direction. For example, we rely on the macula for orientation when we are swimming underwater. Because the feet are not in contact with the ground and gravitational forces are altered, the proprioceptors in joints and muscles provide little information about position in space. Thus, the brain is not receiving its normal proprioceptive input from the legs and postural muscles. In addition, vision is of little assistance because to work properly the cornea must have air in front of it. Water causes a refractive error and vision becomes distorted.[125] Consequently, if the vestibular mechanism were not receiving gravitational feedback, the underwater swimmer would become disoriented and unable to determine the direction of the surface.

The semicircular canals detect movements of the head in all planes and are involved in the maintenance of the upright posture. The pathways of the semicircular canals are extremely important for visual gaze, ocular movements, and alignment of head and body. The connections of the semicircular canals and the otoliths work cooperatively with the joint receptors of the neck to accomplish head and neck-righting reactions.[9, 102, 219]

VESTIBULAR TREATMENT ALTERNATIVES

Because the vestibular system is a unique sensory system, critical for multisensory functioning, it is a viable and powerful input modality for therapeutic intervention (see Chapter 21). Because any static position as well as any movement pattern will facilitate the labyrinthine system, vestibular function and dysfunction play a role in all therapeutic activities. To conceptualize vestibular stimulation as spinning or angular acceleration minimizes its therapeutic potential and also negates an entire progression of vestibular treatment techniques.[95, 140, 143, 144] Horizontal, vertical, and forward-backward movements occur very early in development and should be considered one viable treatment modality. These movements seem to precede side-to-side and diagonal movements, which are followed by linear acceleration and end with rotatory movements. All of these movements can be done with assistance or by the client independently in all functional activities. It is important to remember that the rate of vestibular stimulation determines the effects. A constant, slow, repetitive rocking pattern, irrespective of plan or direction, generally causes inhibition of total-body responses, whereas a fast spin or fast linear movement tends to heighten both alertness and the motor responses. Again, the vestibular mechanism is only one of many that influence the motor system. Thus, the system interaction must be constantly reassessed.

General Vestibular Treatment Technique with Sensory Systems Intact. As already indicated, constant, slow, repetitive rocking patterns, irrespective of plane or direction, generally cause inhibition of the total-body responses. Yet any stimulus has the potential of causing undesired responses, such as increased or decreased tone. When this occurs, the procedure should be stopped and reanalyzed to determine the reason for the observed or palpated response. For example, assume that a client, whether a child with cerebral palsy, an adolescent with head trauma, or an adult with anoxia, exhibits signs of severe generalized extensor hypertonicity in the supine position. To dampen the general motor response, the therapist decides to use a slow, gentle rocking procedure in supine position and discovers that the hypertonicity has increased. Obviously, the procedure did not elicit the desired response and alternative treatment is selected, but the reason for increased hypertonicity needs to be addressed.

It is possible that the static positioning of the vestibular system is causing the release of the original tone and that by increasing vestibular input the tone also increases. It may also be that the facilitory input did indeed cause

inhibition, but the movement itself caused fear and anxiety, thus increasing preexisting tone and overriding the inhibitory technique. Instead of selecting an entirely new treatment approach, a therapist could use the same procedure in a different spatial plane, such as side lying, prone, or sitting. Each position affects the static position of the vestibular system differently and may differentially affect the excessive extensor tone observed in the client. The vertical sitting position adds flexion to the system, which has the potential of further dampening extensor tone. This additional inhibition may be necessary to determine whether the slow rocking pattern will be effective with this client. It would seem obvious that if a vestibular procedure were ineffective in modifying the preexisting extensor tone, then using a powerful procedure, such as spinning, is inappropriate. Selection of treatment techniques should be determined according to client needs and disability. Clients with either an acoustic tumor that perforates into the brain stem or with generalized inflammatory disorders may be hypersensitive to vestibular stimulation, whereas other clients, such as a child with a learning disability, may be in need of massive input through this system. Heiniger and Randolph[140] and Farber[94, 95] present an in-depth analysis of various specific vestibular treatment procedures commonly used in the clinic. A general summary of the treatment suggestions is summarized in the box on page 95.

General Body Responses Leading to Relaxation. Any technique performed in a slow, continuous, even pattern will cause a generalized dampening of the motor output.[152] During handling techniques, these procedures can be performed with the client in bed, on a mat while horizontal, sitting at bedside or in a chair, or standing. The movement can be done passively by the therapist or actively by the client. Carryover into motor learning will best be accomplished when the client performs the movement actively, without therapeutic assistance. In a clinical or school setting, a client who is extremely anxious, hyperactive, and hypertonic may initiate slow rocking to decrease tone or feel less anxious or hyperactive. The reduction of clinical signs allows the client to sit with less effort and to be more attentive to the environment, thus promoting the ability to learn and adapt.

It is the type of movement, not the technique, that is critical. The concept of slow, continuous patterns is used in Brunnstrom's rocking patterns[40] in early sitting, in proprioceptive neuromuscular facilitation mat programs, and in gymnastic ball exercise programs; the use of these patterns can be observed in every clinic. Although the therapist may be unaware of why Mr. Smith gets so relaxed when slowly rocked from side to side in sitting, this procedure elicits an appropriate response. The nurse taking Mr. Smith for a slow wheelchair ride around the hospital grounds may do the same thing. Once the relaxation or inhibition has occurred, the groundwork for a therapeutic environment has been created to promote further learning, such as activity of daily living (ADL) skills. The technique in and of itself will relax the individual but not create change or learning.

Pelvic mobilization techniques in sitting use relaxation from slow rocking to release the fixed pelvis. This release

TREATMENT SUGGESTIONS*

General Body Responses Leading to Relaxation

1. Slow rocking
2. Slow anterior-posterior: horizontal or vertical movement (chair, hassock, mesh net, swing, ball bolster, carriage)
3. Rocking bed or chair
4. Slow linear movements, such as in a carriage, stroller, wheelchair, or wagon
5. Therapeutic and/or gymnastic ball

Techniques to Heighten Postural Extensors

1. Rapid anterior-posterior or angular acceleration
   a. Scooter board: pulled or projected down inclines
   b. Prone over ball: rapid acceleration forward
   c. Platform or mesh net: prone
   d. Slides
2. Rapid anterior-posterior motion in prone, weight-bearing patterns such as on elbows or extended elbows while rocking and crawling
3. Weight-shifting in kneeling, ½ kneel, or standing

Facilitory Techniques Influencing Whole-Body Responses

1. Movement patterns in specific sequences
   a. Rolling patterns
   b. On elbows, extended elbows, and crawling: side by side, linear and angular motion
2. Spinning
   a. Mesh net
   b. Sit and spin toy
   c. Office chair on universal joint
3. Any motor program that uses acceleration and deceleration of head
   a. Sitting and reaching
   b. Walking
   c. Running
   d. Moving from sit to stand

Combined Facilitory and Inhibitory Technique: Inverted Tonic Labyrinthine

1. Semi-inverted in-sitting
2. Squatting to stand
3. Total inverted vertical position

*Remember that all of these treatment suggestions involve other input mechanisms and all aspects of the motor system and its components.

allows for joint mobility and thus creates the potential for pelvic movement performed passively by the therapist, with the assistance of the therapist, or actively by the client. This technique often combines vestibular with proprioceptive techniques, such as rotation and elongation of muscle groups, which physiologically modify existing fixed tonal response through motor mechanisms or systems interactions. Simultaneously, slow, rhythmic rocking, especially on diagonals, is used to incorporate all planes of motion and thus all vestibular receptor sites to get maximal dampening effect, whether directly through the vestibulospinal system or indirectly through the cerebellum or another motor system. The same pelvic mobility can be achieved by placing the patient (child or adult) over a large ball. The ball must be large enough for the patient to be semiprone while arms are abducted and externally rotated and legs relaxed (either draped over the ball or in the therapist's arms). Again, this position allows for maintained or prolonged stretch to tight muscles both in the extremities and trunk while doing slow, rhythmical rocking over the ball. The pelvis often releases, and the patient can be rolled off the large ball to stand on a relaxed pelvis preliminary to gait activities.

Techniques to Heighten Postural Extensors. Any technique that uses rapid anteroposterior or angular acceleration of the head and body while the client is prone will facilitate a postural extensor response. Scooter boards down inclines, rapid acceleration forward over a ball or bolster, going down slides prone, or using a platform or mesh net to propel someone will all facilitate a similar vestibular response of righting of the head with postural overflow down into the shoulder girdle, trunk, hips, and lower extremities. Rapid movements while on elbows, on extended elbows, and in a crawling position can also facilitate a similar response. Depending on the intensity of the stimulus, the response will vary. In addition, the client's emotional level during introduction to various types of stimuli may cause differences in tonal patterns. Clinical experience has shown that facilitory vestibular stimulation promotes verbal responses and affects oral motor mechanisms. Children with speech delays will speak out spontaneously and respond verbally.

Because facilitory vestibular stimulation biases the sympathetic branch of the ANS, drooling diminishes and a generalized arousal response occurs at the cortical level. Therefore, the appropriate time to teach adaptive rehabilitative techniques is after vestibular stimulation.[163]

Facilitory Techniques Influencing Whole-Body Responses. Tactile, vestibular, and proprioceptive inputs also assist in the regulation of the body's responses to movement.[10, 94] As stated previously, the vestibular system, when facilitated with fast, irregular, or angular movement, such as spinning, not only induces tonal responses but also causes massive reticular activity and overflow into higher centers. Thus, increased attention and alertness are often the outcome. The tracts going from the spinal cord, brain stem, and higher subcortical structures must be sufficiently intact to permit the desired responses from this type of input. If a lesion in the brain stem blocks higher-center communication with the vestibular apparatus, then massive input may cause a large increase in abnormal tone. The therapist needs to closely monitor any distress or ANS anomalies.

Total-Body Relaxation Followed by Selective Postural Facilitation. The use of the inverted position in therapy has become increasingly more popular in recent years. Early research on the labyrinth's influence on posture and the influence of the inverted position showed that total inversion (angle of 0 degrees) produced maximal postural extensor tone, and the normal upright position elicited maximal flexor tonicity.[240] There seems to be much confusion in the literature about the clinical effects of inversion. The initial research was performed on anesthetized animals and may not be representative of how the human CNS responds to inversion as a system. Kottke[179] reports that the static labyrinthine reflex is maximal when the head is tilted back in the semireclining position at an angle of 60 degrees above the horizontal. Conversely, minimal stimulation occurs when the head is prone and down 60 degrees below the horizontal position. Stejskal[287] studied the effects of the tonic labyrinthine position in hypertonic patients. This study failed to show labyrinthine reflexes in subjects with hypertonia.

The explanation for this incongruity seems to be one of interpretation. Any time a subject is put on a tilt table or even a scooter board, the weight bearing of the body on the surface must cause firing of the underlying exteroceptors while gravity pulls on the proprioceptors. This position also has the potential of creating fear.[83] As the body shifts and presses onto the underlying surface, stretch reflexes associated with posture and movement must contribute some bias to muscle tone.[323] In addition, if the subject is flexing or extending the head, the proprioceptors of the neck could also alter the muscle tone of the limbs.[266]

Another factor that contributes to tonal changes in the extremities is the cervicoocular reflex.[16, 17] Reflex eye movements to center the eyes as the body or neck rotates also exert influences on the muscles of the limbs. Because all the influences brought about by gravity and postural mechanisms in a clinical situation cannot be controlled, the inverted position appears to be an interplay of cutaneous receptors, proprioceptors, and tonal changes in the labyrinthine system.[239]

Several highly recognized therapists have reported using the inverted position as a therapeutic modality.[95, 140, 288] Generally, the inverted position produces three major changes. First, because of the gravitational forces on circulation, the carotid sinus sends messages to the medulla and cardiac centers that ultimately lower heart rate, respiration, and resting blood pressure through peripheral dilation, creating a parasympathetic response pattern. This position may be contraindicated for certain patients with a history of cardiovascular disease, glaucoma, or completed stroke. Clients with unstable intercranial pressure, for example, those with traumatic head injuries, coma, tumor, or postinflammatory disorders, and many children with congenital spinal cord lesions would also be at high risk for further injury if the inverted position were used. However, this position has been used with some success for adult patients with hypertension. In any case, scrupulous recording of blood pressure and other ANS effects should be taken before, during, and after positioning.

Another benefit of the inverted position is generalized relaxation. Farber[95] recommends its use as an inhibitory technique. Because the carotid sinus stimulates the parasympathetic system, the trophotropic system is influenced and muscle tonicity is reduced. This has been found to be beneficial to patients with upper motor neuron lesions and also to children who exhibit hyperkinetic behavior.

Heiniger and Randolph[140] report that severe hypertonicity in the upper extremities is noticeably reduced.

The third benefit of the inverted position is an increased tonicity of certain extensor muscles. This phenomenon is not purely a function of the labyrinth; it is also a result of activation of the exteroceptors being stimulated by the body's contact with the positioning apparatus.[239] Therapists have capitalized on this reaction to activate specific extensor muscles of the neck, trunk, and limb girdles.[179, 266, 287]

Because the inverted position decreases hypertonicity and hyperactivity and facilitates normal postural extensor patterns, the responses to the technique should be incorporated into activities. For example, if the position of total inversion over a ball is used, then postural extension of the head, trunk, and shoulder girdles and hips should be facilitated next. Additional facilitation techniques, such as vibration or tapping, could help summate the response. Resistance to the pattern in a functional or play activity would be the ultimate goal. If the inverted position is used in a squat pattern, then squatting to standing against resistance would probably be a primary goal. This can be accomplished by the therapist positioning his or her body behind and over the child, not only to direct the child initially into the inverted position but also to resist the child coming to stand. If the inverted position is used in sitting, activities of the neck, trunk, and upper extremities would be the major focus after the initial responses.

Because the inverted position elicits both labyrinthine and ANS responses, this technique needs to be cross-referenced within the classification schema. Because of its ANS influence, close monitoring is important for all clients placed in an inverted position. As with all labyrinthine treatment techniques, this approach, considered a normal, inherent human response, is used outside the therapeutic setting. For example, standing on one's head in a yoga exercise causes the same physiological state as that observed in the clinic. In many respects the yoga stance is done for the same reasons: decreasing hypertonicity (generally caused by tension), relaxation, and increasing postural tone and altered states of consciousness. Clients can certainly be taught to control their own ANS activity and hypertonicity by placing their hands between their legs when they need a generalized dampening effect on motor generators. Thus, when accessing and incorporating other approaches, the therapist analyzes each specific technique using a critical neuroscience frame of reference.

This section has described procedures that use the vestibular system as a primary input modality to alter the client's CNS. If the client's vestibular system itself is dysfunctional, it has the potential of altering the functional state of the motor system.

PERIPHERAL AND CENTRAL VESTIBULAR PROCESSING DEFICITS

A variety of clinical symptoms are associated with unilateral and bilateral vestibular dysfunction. Unilateral problems present as vertigo, nausea, dizziness, and postural instability, whereas bilateral problems include those mentioned earlier along with blurred vision, oscillopsia, and gait ataxia.[146, 147] When clinical symptoms persist, vestibular therapy seems to be an effective treatment approach but must be patient specific and based on whether the function of the vestibular system is reduced or absent.[118, 147] In cases of total vestibular loss, treatment approaches will either teach the client a substitution approach using proprioception and vision or a combination approach using both substitution and adaptation in clients with reduced vestibular function. A variety of researchers[143, 144, 146, 147, 281] have shown therapeutic intervention to be the most effective treatment for most clients. (See Chapter 21 for an in-depth discussion of vestibular deficits.)

Shumway-Cook and Horak[280, 281] found that with testing, some children and adults who demonstrated clinical vestibular impairment did not have true vestibular deficits but demonstrated impaired postural reactions under all conditions of sensory conflict among visual, vestibular, and somatosensory systems. They concluded that these patients had an integrative central processing disorder and recommended treatment that dealt with the total sensorimotor system. Approaches such as sensory integrative therapy,[215] Feldenkrais,[324] or neurodevelopmental therapy (NDT)[215] might be possible options. The critical link or recommendation would be to integrate all treatment activities into normal activities that the client is self-motivated to practice under conditions of specific attention in a variety of ways (e.g., walking) on an unstable surface, on support surfaces with eyes closed while head turning, and while counting backward).

Autonomic Nervous System

The ANS has become a focus of clinical interest.[140] Traditionally, the ANS regulates, adjusts, and coordinates visceral activities. Many aspects of emotional behavior and primitive drives are controlled by the ANS.[108, 228, 229] The intricate interconnections between the ANS and CNS have led clinicians to discover viable treatment approaches that depend on both systems.[94, 140] The importance of these interconnections seems obvious. If the external world is threatening the system, then both somatic and visceral systems need to modify responses to optimally protect the organism. For example, if your visual system identifies an angry bear ready to attack you as you walk through the forest, both autonomic and somatic responses are needed. Your somatic system needs to ready your neuromuscular system for immediate action. Your autonomic system needs to ready your heart and respiration for increased rate to provide oxygen and nourishment to muscles for increased metabolism. Your emotional system needs arousal to attend to and deal efficiently with the crisis. All systems must react simultaneously and at appropriate intensities to protect the organism from imminent danger. If any system malfunctions and creates too little or too much output, imbalance and inefficiency result. This decreases your flexibility and ability to solve the problem and remove yourself from the dangerous environment[314] (see Chapter 6).

The input and processing systems, as well as the ANS itself, are often impaired in clients with brain damage. This can create ANS responses that are not always appropriate to the situation as well as limbic responses that affect motor performance (see Chapter 6). Understanding the intricate balance of sympathetic and parasympathetic responses of the ANS and how these behaviors affect functional output is important to conceptualizing the client's total needs. All systems within the CNS will change if the person perceives imminent danger, whether real or imaginary. The clinician will observe these altered responses to the environment, for example, in a gait session or an ADL task. Anxiety level, emotional responses, increased blood pressure, heart rate, and respiration, hypertonicity, and hyperactivity are but a few of the signs a therapist might use to identify an ANS response. These signs should alert and orient the clinician to the causes of the change. Slight alterations in the external environment are often sufficient to produce homeostasis. For example, if when standing a client feels he is falling forward, it is important to check the patient's perception, even if the therapist believes it to be inaccurate. If the perception is wrong, then the clinician needs to help the client relearn perception of vertical. If the perception is correct, the client's response is appropriate and provides important internal feedback. Even more important, the therapist has respected and responded to the opinion and judgment of the client. This helps begin and kindle trust and mutual respect, important clinical tools for modifying the client's ANS responses to new situations.[61, 108]

The ability to differentiate tone created by emotional responses versus tone resulting from CNS damage is a critical aspect of the evaluation process. Emotional tone can be reduced when stress, anxiety, and fear of the unknown have been reduced. This is true for all individuals. The client with brain damage is no exception. Seven treatment modalities that normally produce a parasympathetic or decreased sympathetic (flight/fight) response are listed below[305]:

1. Slow, continuous stroking for 3 to 5 minutes over the paravertebral area of the spine
2. Inversion, eliciting carotid sinus reflex and tonic labyrinthine response (refer to vestibular section)
3. Slow, smooth, passive and active assistive movement within a pain-free range (Maitland's grade II movements)[189]
4. Maintained, deep pressure on the abdomen, palms, soles of the feet, peroneal area, and skin rostral to the top lip
5. Deep breathing exercises (see Chapter 12)
6. Progressive muscle relaxation
7. Cranial sacral manipulation (see Chapter 33)

When pressure is applied to both the anterior and posterior surfaces of the body, measurable reductions may be recorded in pulse rate, metabolic activity, oxygen consumption, and muscle tone.[291, 296]

These pressure techniques are identified as an intricate part of the many intervention approaches such as therapeutic touch,[257, 314] Feldenkrais,[98, 99, 155, 324] Maitland,[189] and myofacial release.[18, 22, 197, 297, 299] Although not verbally identified, other techniques (e.g., NDT,[32, 33] Rood,[94, 140, 288] Brunnstrom,[40] and PNF[289]) also place an important emphasis on the response of the patient to the therapist's touch.

TREATMENT ALTERNATIVES

Slow Stroking. Slow stroking over the paravertebral areas along the spine from the cervical through lumbar components will cause inhibition or a dampening of the sympathetic nervous system. The technique is performed while the client is in the prone position. The therapist begins by stroking the cervical paravertebral region in the direction of the thoracic area, using a slow, continuous motion with one hand. Usually a lubricant is applied to the skin, and the index and middle fingers are used to stroke both sides of the spinal column simultaneously. Once the first hand is approaching the end of the lumbar section, the second hand should begin a downward stroking at the cervical region. This maintains at least one point of contact with the client's skin at all times during the procedure. The technique is applied for 3 to 5 minutes—and no longer—because of the potential for massive inhibition or rebound of the autonomic responses.[10, 152] It is also recommended that at the end of the range of the last stroking pattern, the therapist maintain pressure for a few seconds to alert both the somatic and visceral systems that the procedure has concluded. Eastern medicine recognizes the importance of the ANS in total-body regulation to a greater extent than Western medicine. The concepts of meridians and acupressure/acupuncture points are all intricately intertwined with the ANS (see Chapter 33). For that reason, a technique such as slow stroking would potentially interact with meridians and does extend over the row of acupoints referred to as "shu points" and relates to visceral reflexes connecting smooth muscle and specific organ systems. It is believed that this continuous, slow, downward pressure modulates the sympathetic outflow, causing a shift to a parasympathetic reaction or relaxation. Whether the result of the pressure on the sympathetic chain, some energy pressure over meridian points, a pleasant sensation, or something unknown, slow stroking does elicit relaxation and calming.[94, 140] Clients with large amounts of body hair or hair whorls are poor candidates for this procedure because of the irritating effect of stroking against the growth patterns and the sensitivity of hair follicles.

Slow, Smooth, Passive Movement Within Pain-Free Range. Increasing ROM in painful joints is a dilemma frequently encountered by therapists caring for clients with neurological damage. Having the client communicate the first perception of pain and then moving the limb in a slow, smooth motion toward the pain range elicit a variety of behaviors. First, the client generally gestures or verbalizes that pain is present 10 to 15 degrees before it may, in reality, exist. This behavior may occur because the patient during previous treatment interventions learned that therapists often responded to the client's statement of pain by saying, "Let's just go a little farther." That additional range is usually 10 to 15 degrees. By stopping at the stated point of pain, retreating back into a pain-free area, and approaching again, possibly with a slight variation in the rotatory direction, the client will often relinquish the safety range and a true picture of the pain range is obtained. The second finding is that if the motion toward the pain range is slow, smooth, and continuous, very frequently much of the range that was initially painful becomes pain free. The hypothesis is that slow, continuous motion is critical feedback for the ANS to handle imminent discomfort. The slow pattern provides the ANS time to release endorphins, thus modifying the perception of pain and allowing for increased motion. If the therapist stabilizes the painful joint and prevents the possibility of that joint going into the pain range, rapid, oscillating movements can often be obtained within the pain-free range. This maintains joint mobility and often, as an end result, increases the pain-free range. This technique is not unique to the treatment of clients with neurological problems; it is often used as a manual therapy procedure.[101, 194, 197] Furthermore, one can move slowly into a range that actually shortens muscles. If held for 30 seconds, the muscle that is too short can relax, promoting greater motion in the opposite direction. This can be called strain/counterstrain, inhibiting firing by maintaining a position of active insufficiency, making the muscle too short.

Manual therapy[189, 302] can be used to describe the pain and joint changes occurring at the joint level. As the fields of orthopedics and neurology merge into one system,[48] with the brain acting as an organ controlling the entire system and its components, the question of whether the pain reduction is centrally or peripherally triggered may be an important one. It is probably both. For example, thumb pain can increase the sensation of the nervous system to the point that even cutaneous and proprioceptive receptors act as nociceptors.

Maintained Pressure. Farber[95] discusses a variety of techniques that facilitate a reduction of tone or hyperactivity. Pressure to the palm of the hand or sole of the foot, to the tip of the upper lip, and to the abdomen all seem to produce this effect. The pressure need not be forceful, but it should be firm and maintained.[115] This same technique is defined as inhibitory casting when applied through the use of an orthosis (see Chapter 31).

Progressive Muscle Relaxation. Progressive muscle relaxation is practiced during both meditation and treatment approaches such as Feldenkrais.[115, 126, 324] These methods of relaxation tend to trigger parasympathetic reactions, which in turn slow down heart rate and blood pressure and trigger slow, deep breathing (see Chapters 12 and 33).

Cranial Sacral Manipulation. Summarizing the complexity of cranial sacral theory is not within the scope of this book. The reader is referred to references to gain a global understanding of the treatment interactions and the ANS response to cranial therapy as well as a brief discussion in Chapter 33.[18, 305] This treatment approach needs to be more intensively researched in terms of physiological effects and clinical effectiveness.

Olfactory System: Smell

The sense of smell is the least understood of all the senses. Because of the inaccessibility of the olfactory receptors, to date little research has been conducted. Unfortunately, there are more theories than facts about how odors are sensed.[157]

Although the olfactory epithelium occupies an area only about the size of a dime, it is estimated to contain 100 million receptor cells.[31] These have an equal number of fibers but converge on principal neurons at a ratio of 1,000:1.[63] How the receptor cells transduce odors into meaningful perception of smell is not well understood. One theory suggests that different odors do selectively activate some receptors and not others.[64, 279] Other theories suggest that odorous molecules simply alter the sodium permeability of the receptor membrane and cause an inactivation of enzymes, thus changing its chemical reactions and electrical states.[156]

Findings indicate that humans can distinguish between 2000 and 4000 different odors. What is more confusing is that individual perception of the same odor will vary considerably; what is nauseating to one may be fragrant to another.[95, 235, 326] Receptors for smell adapt rather quickly to a constant stimulus. Physiological studies indicate that olfactory receptors adapt as much as 50% during the first few seconds of stimulation.[53, 250] The strength of the odor has to change by approximately 30% before the receptors are reactivated. There is also some evidence that part of the adaptation takes place in the CNS.

One of the most remarkable characteristics of the olfactory system is that some impulses travel from the receptors through alternative routes and synapses to the temporal and frontal lobes without passing through the thalamus. All other major sensory systems must pass through a relay in the thalamus en route to the cortex.

Smell evokes different responses by means of the limbic system's control over behavior. Pleasant odors, such as vanilla or perfume, can evoke strong moods. Unpleasant odors can facilitate primitive protective reflexes, such as sneezing and choking. Sharp-smelling substances such as ammonia can elicit a reflex interruption of breathing.[218]

As a result of arousal, protective reflexes, and mood changes caused by odors, the use of smell as a treatment modality has been implemented especially during feeding procedures. Odors such as vanilla and banana have been used to facilitate sucking and licking motions.[286] Ammonia and vinegar have been used clinically to elicit withdrawal patterns and increase arousal in semicomatose patients.[153] When using odors as a stimulant, the therapist must be aware of all behavior changes occurring within the client. Arousal, level of consciousness, tonal patterns, reflex behavior, and emotional levels all can be affected by odor. Because of limited research in this area, caution must be exercised to avoid indiscriminate use of the olfactory system. Odors such as body odor, perfumes, hair spray, and urine can affect the client's behavior even though the smell was not intended as a therapeutic procedure. Some clients, especially those with head traumas and inflammatory disorders of the CNS, often seem to be hypersensitive to smell. In these cases the therapist needs to be aware of the external olfactory environment surrounding the client and to make sure those odors that are present facilitate or at least do not hinder desired response patterns.[86]

Many clinical questions arise regarding smell as a therapeutic modality. If the choice of odors is pleasant versus noxious, a pleasant odor will theoretically be perceived in a way that should be enjoyable, relaxing, and thus potentially tone reducing. On the other hand, noxious odors should have a sympathetic reaction and, although causing one to become alert, may also create a fight/flight internal reaction that, if repeated frequently, could cause an adverse response to the client's perception of the world. This has the potential of having a profound effect on his or her feelings toward the therapist and the therapeutic environment. The effect may not be observable until the client reaches a level of consciousness or motor skill in which he or she has some ability to react.

Gustatory Sense: Taste

The sense of taste is a chemical sense, involving not only the receptors of the tongue but also olfaction and tactile receptors. Therefore, the term *taste* encompasses not only gustatory sensations derived from food but also the smell, temperature, and texture of the material to be ingested.[57]

Four primary taste sensations have been identified: salty, sour, bitter, and sweet. These primary tastes are believed to blend together in various combinations to form additional tastes, similar to the way mixing the colors yellow and blue produces green. Histologically, the taste buds appear to be the same, yet they tend to be selective to specific stimuli. Action-potential studies have shown that any one taste bud will respond to all four primary tastes.[129] However, the quantitative responses differ considerably, allowing some buds to respond more vigorously to bitter and some to sour, sweet, or salty stimuli. It is also commonly known that regions of the human tongue vary in sensitivity to the four primary tastes. The base of the tongue best detects bitter, the sides detect sour, and the tip is sensitive to sweet substances. The ability of taste buds to discriminate changes in concentration of a substance is relatively crude; a 30% change in concentration is needed before a difference in taste intensity is detected.[94, 232, 243]

Afferent transmission of impulses from taste receptors may travel to the CNS by three cranial nerves. Taste sensations from the base of the tongue are served by the glossopharyngeal nerve (cranial nerve IX); the sides and the tip are served by the vagus nerve (cranial nerve X) and the facial nerve (cranial nerve VII). The pharyngeal surface of the tongue is innervated by the laryngeal branch of the vagal nerve (cranial nerve X). Taste buds begin to degenerate during the fifth decade of life, contributing to diminished taste sensation in the elderly.[63, 64]

Taste sensation adapts rapidly. Action-potential studies have shown that when first stimulated, taste buds fire a burst of impulses and only partially adapt. As with the olfactory system, the additional adaptation is suspected to come from the CNS.[163, 220] As the neurons terminate on the somatesthetic region of the temporal lobe, adaptation may be occurring there.[46, 163]

Gustatory input is generally used as part of feeding and prefeeding activities. As already mentioned, the oral region is sensitive not only to taste but also to pressure, texture, and temperature. For that reason feeding would be classified as a multisensory technique that uses gustatory input as one of its entry modalities. Specific input modalities are based on the combined taste, texture, temperature, and affective response pattern. That is, a banana and an apple both may be sweet, yet the textures vary greatly. When mashed, both fruits may have a pudding-like texture, yet the client's emotional response may differ. Disliking the taste of banana but enjoying apple may cause startling differences in the client's response to various sensations. Thus, the importance of the clinician's sensitivity to the client's response patterns within each sensory modality cannot be overemphasized.[94]

Auditory System

The auditory system is fundamental to survival and also to human communication. Together with vision, the auditory system enables human beings to perceive events in the external world that take place at a distance from the body as well as to localize in space the exact position of a sound.[46]

The auditory nerve shares a common cranial nerve (VIII) with the vestibular system, thus creating a close anatomical and physiological relationship between these two senses.[216] Thus, individuals with hearing loss may show simultaneous vestibular imbalances. Approximately 10% of adults suffer to some extent from hearing loss, with hearing loss even greater in the elderly. Therapists need to discuss with clients whether they have difficulty hearing specific tones or frequencies. Similarly, clients with auditory figure-ground problems will have difficulty hearing in noisy environments, and compensatory types of communication may need to be used.

The auditory pathway to the CNS is very diffuse and complex. Information about sound is sent ipsilaterally and contralaterally to the auditory cortex at the superior temporal gyrus or area 41. As information ascends toward the cortex, synapsing within a variety of nuclear masses, all information will synapse in the inferior colliculus within the midbrain as well as the medial geniculate nucleus of the thalamus. Other collaterals pass directly to the reticular-activating system. There are also important connections to the cerebellum, particularly in the event of a sudden noise.[46, 163] Once sound reaches the superior temporal a sound is "heard," but more specific recognition requires connections with additional auditory associative centers.[58, 63, 163]

Descending fibers from the cortex as well as efferent pathways within the brain stem auditory complex project ipsilaterally through the cochlear nerve back to both the inner and outer hair cells of the cochlea. The efferents are important to auditory sensitivity and selective tuning of the cochlea. With this efferent control over the auditory afferents, the cortex has a way of focusing in on certain sounds while ignoring others.[46] This may be the mechanism for auditory figure-ground or selective hearing. Similarly, fibers leaving the inferior colliculi project into the tectum of the midbrain and help modify the effects of the tectospinal tract and automatic turning of the head in response to sound.[163]

TREATMENT ALTERNATIVES

Because of the complexity of the auditory system, a potentially large number of input modalities exists. Although some of them might not be considered traditional thera-

peutic tools, they are nonetheless techniques that affect the CNS. Some treatment alternatives focus on:

Quality of voice (pitch and tone)
Quantity of voice (level and intensity)
Affect of voice (emotional overtones)
Extraneous noise (sound)
Auditory biofeedback
Language
Levels, volume, and affect of voice

The therapist's voice can be considered one of the most powerful therapeutic tools. Even constant sound has the ability to cause adaptation of the auditory system and thus inhibition of auditory sensitivity.[49] Similarly, intermittent, changing, or random auditory input can cause an increase in auditory sensitivity.[109] Because of auditory system connections, an increase or decrease in initial input or auditory sensitivity has the potential of drastically affecting many other areas of the CNS.[85] The connections to the cerebellum could affect the regulation of muscle tone. The collaterals projecting into the reticular formation could affect arousal, alertness, and attention, in addition to muscular tone. The importance of voice level has been acknowledged by colleagues for decades with respect to encouraging clients to achieve optimal output or maximal effort. The use of voice levels is a critical aspect of the entire PNF approach.[108, 289] Yet the volume or intensity of a therapist's voice is only one aspect of this important clinical tool. Through clinical observation, it has been observed that clients respond differently to various pitches. The response patterns and specific range of comfortable pitch seem to be client dependent. The concept that each individual may have a range within the musical scale or even a specific note that is optimal for his or her biorhythm function has been posed by one composer-musician.[39] This concept needs research verification but may prove to relate to one of those innate talents some therapists have that distinguish them as gifted therapists.

The emotional inflections used by the clinician certainly have the potential of altering client response. For example, assume the therapist asks Tim, a child with cerebral palsy, to walk. The specific response from the child may vary if the clinician's voice expresses anger, frustration, encouragement, disgust, understanding, or empathy. Knowing which emotional tone best coincides with a client's need at a particular moment may come with experience or sensitivity to others' unique needs.

Extraneous Noise. The varying level of sound or extraneous noise in a clinical setting can at times be overwhelming. Dropping of foot pedals, messages over loudspeakers, conversations, typewriters, printers, telephones, moans, a jackhammer outside the clinic, water filling in a tank, a drip in a faucet, whirlpool agitators, a burn patient screaming, and a child crying all are encountered in the clinical environment, and all could be occurring simultaneously. A therapist whose CNS is intact usually can inhibit or screen out most of the irrelevant sound. A client with CNS damage may not have the ability to filter his or her sensitivity to all these intermittent noise sensations. The protective arousal responses these sounds might produce in a client could certainly elevate tone, block attention to the task, heighten irritability, and generally destroy client progress during a therapy session. Awareness of the noisy environment and the client's response to it not only is important for treatment modalities but also is critical to the problem-solving process.

Decreasing auditory distracters or sudden noises can drastically improve the client's ability to attend to a task and/or succeed at the desired movement.[120] The therapist is reminded that if the environment has been externally adapted for a client to procedurally and successfully practice the goal, then independence in that functional skill has not been achieved. Reintroduction of the noises of the external world must be incorporated into the client's repertoire of responses so that the individual can feel competent in dealing with any auditory environment the world might present.

Music as an adjunct to therapy has been suggested as a viable way to help clients develop timing and rhythm to a movement sequence (see Chapter 22 for a discussion of basal ganglia disorders). Consistent sound waves and tempos, such as soft music, allow the patient to develop a neuronal model or an engram for the stimulus. The use of background music during therapy sessions enables the patient to make an association to the sounds, producing an autonomically induced relaxation response to a particular musical composition.[65]

Music is used for encouraging not only motor function but also memory[251] and socialization.[234, 247] Rhythmic sound perceived as an enjoyable sensation certainly has the effect of creating motor patterns in response to that rhythm. Individuals, young and old, will tap their fingers or feet to a beat. If the beat has words, people will often sing along, recalling from memory the appropriate words. The movement, memory, and willingness to interact are all critical aspects of the therapeutic environment.[1] Having clients dance with a significant other twice a day to music they have enjoyed in the past encourages both the physical function and the social bonding so important for quality of life.[3] Music affects heart rate, blood pressure, and respiration. It has even been suggested that easy listening music may bolster the immune system.[61, 106, 183]

Auditory Biofeedback. Biofeedback as a total therapeutic modality is discussed under the treatment sections in Chapters 28 and 29. Auditory biofeedback is generally thought of as a procedure in which sound is used to inform the client of specific muscle activity. The level or pitch may change in relation to strength of muscle contraction or specific muscle group activity. Yet auditory biofeedback also encompasses feedback as simple as a foot slap that communicates that a client's foot is on the floor or verbal praise after a successful therapeutic session. The importance of the auditory feedback system as a regulatory mechanism between internal and external homeostasis cannot be overlooked. However, the clinician should not assume that this system is intact and can automatically be used as a normal feedback mechanism for clients with CNS damage.[5, 126]

Language. Although most therapists thoroughly appreciate the complexity of the language system as a whole, they have little if any in-depth background to help them

understand the components or the sequences leading to the development of language.[50] Thus, many therapists are extremely frustrated when confronted with clients who show perceptual or cognitive deficits involving the auditory processing system.

Therapists easily identify language comprehension difficulties with adults who have first language differences and with young children because of their age and lack of language experience. Nevertheless, many clients have a language processing dysfunction that leads to communication difficulties, both in reception and appropriate expression. The elderly often can understand a conversation in a quiet room but have difficulty in rooms that are noisy.[85] The environment within which communication occurs can drastically affect both reception and the ability to express back to the world inner feelings and thoughts.[61] Creating an environment conducive to that exchange will dramatically affect the motivation and drive of a patient within the therapeutic setting.[106]

Visual System

Vision is considered the most important and dominant sensory modality. The eye is the most complex of all the sense organs in our body. Its uniqueness is attributed to the biochemical or biophysical mechanism used to transduce a light stimulus to a neurological action potential. The retina, which makes up a major portion of the inside of the eye, is where light energy is transformed into neuronal-electrical impulses. Once transformed, the information must reach one of two sensory photoreceptors: the rods and cones. The rods are reactive to light intensity, that is, shades of gray. Unable to distinguish different colors, rods are said to provide "night vision." The cones (about 6 million) are responsible for color vision and require more light energy to become activated. A central part of the retina, called the fovea, is in direct line with the lens and cornea. Therefore, when we fixate on an object, the image of that object is projected upside down and backward on the fovea.[151, 163] Once information reaches these sensory receptors, a complex interaction among chemical reactions, cell membrane ion transport, action potential generation, and synaptic activity takes place that will terminate with axons of neurons leaving the eye and projecting down the optic nerve.[129, 163, 273]

Each optic nerve consists of about 1 million nerve fibers. The combined 2 million nerve fibers of both optic nerves make up about 38% of all sensory and motor fibers entering and leaving the CNS.[163] The optic nerve contains two types of fibers: large, fast-conducting fibers concerned with visual perception and small, slower-conducting fibers concerned with reflexive activity. Fibers originating in the nasal halves of each retina cross in what is referred to as the optic chiasm. Conversely, the fibers originating in the temporal portion of the retina pass through the chiasm without crossing. The fibers from the temporal side also carry the fibers from the fovea (macula), where visual acuity is sharpest.[151, 163]

Once the optic nerve passes through the optic chiasm, it is referred to as the optic tract. These anatomical relationships of visual fields and distribution of axonal tracking help therapists understand why clients have specific field loss and the functional extent of the impairment. Once the optic tract reaches the thalamus, synapses, and proceeds as the geniculocalcarine tract, it again divides and radiates onto the top and bottom of the calcarine fissure. If lesions occur along either portion of these radiations, variance in field deficits result and thus affect a client's functional sight.[151] Once primary sight has reached the occipital lobe, an individual sees, but for those images to have meaning additional associative aspects of this cortical lobe must be activated. Once that occurs, a individual will display visual perception[151] (see Chapter 27). The visual system is extremely helpful to medical personnel for diagnosing disorders of the CNS. The eye provides a window through which a physician can examine the integrity of blood vessels and neurological tissue. Because the system extends through so much of the subcortical and cortical regions of the brain, many disorders manifest themselves in the visual system. Aside from the more obvious visual field problems, nervous system disorders can interrupt visual reflexes and impede eye movements.

Eye movements are subserved at the cortical and subcortical levels. Areas 18 and 19 of the occipital lobe produce a reflexive visual pursuit in response to visual stimuli. Voluntary eye movements elicited on command derive from neurons in the frontal lobe of the cortex (area 8). Protective reflexes, such as blinking and quick localization of eyes, head, and neck toward a startling stimulus, are mediated by the retinotectal system (superior colliculus). Reflex eye movements activated by rotation of the head are mediated at the brain stem level by the vestibular system. The sizes of the pupil and lens are reflexively controlled by light stimulus. Pretectal areas, such as the Edinger-Westphal nucleus of cranial nerve III, act on the sphincter muscle of the iris and the ciliary muscle. Psychosocial research has demonstrated that pupils dilate and constrict in response to emotional feelings elicited by a visual stimulus.[64] Objects that are pleasing to the eye cause the pupil to dilate, whereas repugnant visual stimuli constrict the pupil. The higher-level cortical association pathways are very complex, and our understanding of them continues to grow.[163]

Child development studies suggest that the efficiency with which an infant uses its eyes is a strong indicator of verbal ability and performance on intelligence tests.[37] The therapist should reinforce eye pursuits by pointing out objects in the environment and by encouraging the hand to follow the eye toward the object. According to Stejskal,[287] the eyes turn toward an object, the head has a natural tendency to turn, and when the neck rotates, a volley of neuromuscular events take place that better enable the upper extremities to perform a task such as reaching. Program generators are much more than a pure reflex action and thus manifest motor response with great adaptability and variability within the environment.

Because of the complexity of the visual system, treatment procedures can vary from simple to extremely complex. Simple treatment alternatives, such as hues or types of lighting, are often overlooked by therapists; yet they have the potential of altering patient response. Complex treatment procedures, such as those discussed in Chapter 27, are also often ignored by therapists because of a lack of understanding of and frustration with the visual system. Although we are not suggesting that all therapists become experts in visual processing and training, clinicians should become more aware of this input system, its potency as a treatment modality, and, when damaged, its devastating effect on normal response patterns.

TREATMENT ALTERNATIVES

Because light is an adequate stimulus for vision, any light, no matter the degree of complexity, has the potential to affect a client's CNS. That input not only reaches the optic cortex for sight recognition and processing but also projects to the cerebellum through the tectocerebellar tract and affects the reticular-activating and limbic systems through the interneuronal pathway. It even has influence over cervical spinal generators through the tectospinal tract.[46, 100] Thus, as long as light is entering a client's CNS, it has the potential of altering response patterns either directly—through the tectospinal system or the corticospinal system through occipitofrontal radiations—or indirectly through the influence of the ANS and limbic system on muscle tone resulting from emotional levels.[72]

The five categories of visual-system treatment alternatives should not be considered fixed, all-inclusive, or without overlap. The first three categories (color, lighting, and visual complexity) are common everyday visual stimuli. Combined, they make up the visual world.

Colors. By varying the colors or by changing hues, tones, or the type of lighting and degree of complexity of the combined visual stimuli, the treatment modality and the way the CNS processes it change.[119, 300, 308] Because the visual system tends to adapt to sustained, repetitive, even patterns, any input falling under those parameters should elicit visual adaptation.[113, 163, 250] This adaptation response will lead to decreased firing of sensory afferent fibers and have an overall effect of decreasing CNS excitation. A clinician would expect to see or palpate a decrease in muscle tone, a calming of the client's affective mood, and a generalized inhibitory response. Cool colors, a darkened room, and monotone color schemes all seem to have an inhibitory effect.

In contrast, intermittent visual stimuli, bright colors, bright lights, and a random color scheme seem to alert the CNS and have a generalized facilitory effect.[66] Research in the 1980s in the area of criminology has produced evidence to suggest that specific shades of colors can produce either a sedating response (such as certain pinks) or general arousal (certain blues).[227] Although a tremendous amount of research is required to substantiate these results if the clinician is to apply them with confidence, research is beginning to show that specific shades of colors and hues may drastically affect a client's general response to the world and specific response to a therapy session.[306] Within the next few years, many facts regarding the reaction of the CNS to specific visual stimuli may be uncovered, and the clinician will be responsible for integrating this new information into the present categorization scheme.[267] In Holland at the Institute de Hartenbuer, playrooms have been designed in different colors.[105] Except for color all rooms are exactly the same and originate from a central hub or core.[105] Children are allowed to select which room they wish to play or be treated in. Children seem to pick the color room that most suits their moods and alertness and creates an environment in which they can learn.[105]

Lighting. Two types of lighting are found in a clinical environment. Fluorescent or luminescent lighting comes by definition from a nonthermal cold source. This type of lighting is generally emitted by a high-frequency pulse. Umphred[303] has found that many individuals within a normal population complain that this high-frequency flutter is irritating and causes distraction. For this reason, it is recommended that each clinician observe clients' responses to various types of lighting to determine whether fluorescent visual stimuli cause undesirable output. This is especially true with clients who already have an irritated CNS, such as those with inflammatory disorders, head trauma, or seizure disorders. The clinician should also remember that clients frequently lie supine and look directly at overhead lighting, whereas the therapist looking at the client is unaware of that particular visual stimulus.

Incandescent lights by definition come from hot sources and emit a constant light without a frequency. The brightness of this type of lighting has the potential of altering CNS response. The visual system quickly responds to bright lights with pupil constriction. After prolonged exposure to a bright environment, the visual system adapts and becomes progressively less sensitive to it.[113, 163] Similarly, when exposed to darkness, the retina becomes more sensitive to small amounts of light. Because of the response of the visual system to incandescent lighting, it is recommended that a therapist monitor the brightness of the lighting, especially preceding any type of visual-perceptual training or visually directed movement.

Although the sun is a natural source of light, it is not generally the primary source in a clinical setting. The sun can effectively be used as indirect lighting, thus eliminating the problems produced by artificial lighting. Sunlight is also more acceptable psychologically. Some clinics have designed the buildings to allow for maximum use of natural light.[102]

Visual Complexity. The visual system is the primary spatial sense for monitoring moving and stationary objects in space.[142] An infant continually refines the ability to discriminate objects in external space until capable of identifying specific objects amid a complex visual array.[250] When brain damage occurs, the ability to identify objects, localize them in space, pick them out from other things, and adapt to their presence may be drastically diminished.[11] Because of the distractibility of many clients, reducing the visual stimuli within their external space can help them cope with the stimuli to which they are trying to pay attention. Using rooms that have been stripped of such stimuli as furniture and pictures can reduce not only distractibility but also hyperactivity and emotional tone. If this method of reduction of stimuli is used, the clinician must remember that this procedure has a sequential component. The client must once again adapt to extraneous visual stimuli. Thus, as the client's coping mechanisms improve, the therapist needs to monitor and change the

visual environment. The therapist can monitor the amount of input according to the response patterns of the client but in time needs to have the client function in everyday environments and practice adaptation.

Cognitive-Perceptual Sequencing with the Visual System. In sighted individuals the visual system is important in integrating many areas of perceptual development, such as body schemes, body image, position in space, and spatial relationships.[11] Vision as a processing system is so highly developed and interrelated with other sensory systems that, when intact, it can be used to help integrate other systems.[141] Conversely, if the visual system is neurologically damaged, it can cause problems in the processing of other systems.

For example, assume that a child is asked to walk a balance beam while fixating on a target. The child is observed falling off the beam. On initial assessment vestibular-proprioceptive involvement would be primarily suspected. On further testing the therapist might discover that the child, while looking at the target, switches the lead eye in conjunction with the ipsilateral leg. As the child switches from right to left eye, the target will seem to move. Knowing the wall is stationary, the child will assume the movement is caused by body sway, will counter the force, and will fall off the beam. The problem is a lack of bilateral integration of the visual system versus other sensory modalities. The visual system deficit is overriding normal proprioceptive-vestibular input to avoid CNS confusion. Unfortunately, the client is attending to a deficit system and negating intact ones. This visual conflict would be overriding the normal processing of intact systems.

This same problem of the visual system overriding other inputs is often seen when clients are trying to relearn the concept of verticality. Clients with hemiplegia who demonstrate a "pusher" syndrome illustrate this conflict. Because the intact visual system can often be used to help reintegrate other sensory systems, the reverse should also occur. Teaching clients to attend to vestibular-proprioceptive cues while vision is occluded or visual stimuli tremendously reduced will help them orient to intact systems. Once the orientation is reestablished, visual input will often be perceived in a more normal fashion.

Familiarity with the visual-perceptual system and its interrelationships with all aspects of the therapeutic environment is crucial if the clinician is to have a thorough concept of the client's problem. (See Chapter 27 for specific information regarding visual deficits and treatment alternatives.)

COMPENSATORY TREATMENT ALTERNATIVES

The visual system can be used effectively as a compensatory input system if the sensory component of the tactile, proprioceptive, or vestibular system has been lost or severely damaged. The procedure of using vision in a compensatory manner should not be attempted until the clinician is convinced the primary systems will not regain needed input for normal processing. Although vision can direct and control many aspects of a movement, it is not extremely efficient and seems to take a tremendous amount of cortical concentration and effort.[303, 304] Vision was meant to lead and direct movement sequences.[142, 287] If used to modify each aspect of a movement, it cannot warn or inform the CNS about what to expect when advancing to the next movement sequence. Thus, using vision to compensate eliminates one problem but also takes the visual system away from its normal function. For example, assume that a hemiplegic man is taught to use vision to tell him the placement of his cane and feet, thus decreasing his need to attend to proprioceptive cues. When advancing to ambulatory skills such as crossing the street, the client may be caught in a dilemma. As he is crossing the street, if he attends to the truck coming rapidly down the road, he will not know where his cane or foot are and thus become anxious and possibly fall. If, on the other hand, he attends to his foot and cane, he will not know if the truck is going to hit him. That may increase emotional tone and make it difficult to move. If normal sensory mechanisms could be reintegrated, this client would have freedom to respond flexibly to the situation. Thus, caution should be exercised to avoid automatic use of this high-level system to compensate for what seem to be depressed or deficit systems.

Visual input should be used to check or correct errors if other systems are not available. Movement should be programmed on a feedforward mode unless change is indicated. Vision often recognizes the need for that change. If a client is taught a motor strategy in which vision is used as feedback to direct each component of the pattern, the pattern itself will generally be inefficient and disorganized and will lack the automatic nature of feedforward procedural motor plans. If the client is too anxious to practice the procedure physically without overusing vision, then visual mental practice can be introduced.

INTERNAL VISUAL PROCESSING: "VISUALIZATION TECHNIQUES" OR "MENTAL IMAGERY"

The use of visualizing some aspect of bodily function has been and continues to be used in many forms of therapy.[38] It has been shown that individuals can modulate their immune responses through visualization.[283] Smith and co-workers[283] showed that individuals could dictate through their thoughts and visualization various control over what was thought to be mindless internal processes. These concepts have been used therapeutically but usually when the client is resting or totally relaxed.[98, 99, 324]

More recently, technology in neuroscience has allowed for the measure of blood flow (positive emitting transaxial tomography) and magnetic resonance imaging while engaging the brain in functional mental tasks. All areas of the brain except the cerebellum appear to be activated during intense goal-directed mental imagery. Given the task is not motorically executed, errors in rhythm and accuracy are not made, and thus the cerebellum is not recruited for correction. This suggests that mental imagery can be used to restore a function that might have been lost due to a stroke or other type of injury. Visual imagination has the benefit of allowing correct task performance when physical limitations may prevent normal

task completion. This could prevent abnormal learning (e.g., like that which develops from abnormal posturing in gait in a stroke patient who lacks the voluntary control to ambulate and integrate a primitive synergy). For additional information, see the section on somatosensory discrimination.

Today, these concepts can be integrated during active treatment in a variety of ways. Before a client begins to initiate a plan of movement, the therapist could ask the client to close his or her eyes and imagine the movement and what it felt like in that functional activity before the CNS injury. In this way, the patient is using prior memory and visualization to access the motor systems and hopefully initiate better motor plans. Similarly, if during a movement plan the state of the motor generators builds to such a level that the client is becoming dysfunctional, the therapist can stop the movement; ask the client to visualize a calm, quiet place; and then continue with the movement pattern when the tone is reduced or extraneous patterns cease. The client can be asked to practice mental imagery of the task until he or she can accomplish it normally and then finally carry it over to the real environment. For example, a client may have practiced transferring during an intervention session in which the therapist, using augmented treatment, kept the patient within a biomechanical window. During the interval between sessions, the patient is asked to visualize at least a couple of times an hour, performing transfers initially from the same surface practiced and later to other surfaces. At the follow-up session, the therapist will often be able to tell if the patient has done the visualization. If the patient did practice, there is often carryover into the skill performance. If the patient forgot to practice, often the skill has reverted back to the initial level of learning, with little carryover from the last intervention.

Another way to use the visual system to access the processing strategies of the client is to observe his or her eye gaze. Neurolinguistic theory postulates that the eyes gaze in the direction of brain processing.[14, 177] Figure 4–12 illustrates the eye gaze direction along with the suggested processing activity. For example, a client who needs to

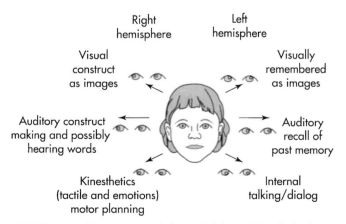

FIGURE 4–12. Eye gaze: correlation with lobe and hemispheric processing based on right-handed individuals. (Adapted from a handout from New Learning Pathways, Denver, 1988. Illustrations by Ben Burton.)

access and process motor plans through the frontal lobe will look down. A client who needs to visually construct an idea of something new will look up and to the right. Various cortical lobes and hemispheres serve specific global processing functions. There are many ways to apply and interpret this theory. By observing the patient's eye gaze, the therapist can determine if processing is conducted in what would be believed to be the appropriate areas. Even more clinically relevant is observing where the eyes are gazing before and during successful functional activities. It may be that the area once used in processing is no longer available to do the function. If gazing to the right and down always leads to motor success, then the therapist can empower the patient to look down and right before dressing or transferring. Similarly, if a patient always looks down at the feet during ambulation, the reason may not be "to look at the feet" but instead may be accessing the motor cortex to gain better motor function. By asking the client to visualize the movement before and during the activity, the head often comes to a posturally correct position as the eyes gaze upward toward the occipital lobe. If the client is asked to walk while visualizing the movement, again the therapist may find a more upright, posturally efficient pattern. Once the program is set and practice scheduling begun, the patient may no longer need to look down and into the frontal lobe. Thus, in this case, the client not only learned the procedure but also avoided practicing and learning a posturally incorrect ambulation strategy.

Combined Multisensory Approaches

Although all techniques have the potential of being multisensory, the specific mode of entry may focus on one sensory system, as already described, or it may target two or more input modalities. Table 4–6 categorizes a variety of treatment techniques that are clearly multisensory. The therapist, analyzing how the summated effect of the combined input influences client performance, gains direction in anticipating treatment outcomes in terms of the problem-solving process. Because the potential combinations of multisensory classification are enormous, only a few examples of combinations are included in the text to illustrate the process a clinician might use when classifying a new technique. When clinicians select augmented treatment interventions to help a client as part of somatosensory retraining or functional retraining or to establish a procedural program, the basic science understanding behind the clinical decision helps develop questions for future research, determine a prognosis regarding outcomes, and rationally explain why or why not an intervention was efficacious. Clinical decisions must ultimately be made regarding which techniques should be eliminated first as the patient progresses. These decisions must be based on neurophysiological understanding and on client need. A simple rule a therapist might follow would be to take away the least natural technique first. That technique would be the most artificial or contrived. For example, a therapist might teach a client to assist with elbow flexion during a feeding pattern by (1) vibrating the biceps, (2) quick tapping the biceps, or (3) quick

stretching the biceps a little beyond midrange using gravity. The first option would be the least natural and obviously the least socially acceptable at a dinner party. The third option is the most natural and closest to the real environment the client will need to function within. Remember, these contrived techniques are used to assist clients who cannot control or perform the motor programs or functional activities without assistance or who need assistance in learning to modulate motor control for greater functional adaptability and independence.

Within the following section are examples of combined multisensory approaches that might be used to augment sensory feedback to obtain a better environment for regaining functional control.

Sweep Tapping. Many isolated techniques, such as sweep tapping[94] or rolling,[40] would be considered primarily proprioceptive-tactile in sensory origin. During sweep tapping the clinician first uses a light-touch sweep pattern over the back of the fingers of one of his or her hands. This stimulus is applied quickly over the dermatome area that relates to muscles the client is to contract. Second, the therapist applies some quick tapping over the muscle belly of the hypotonic muscle. The first technique is tactile and believed to stimulate the reflex mechanism within the cord to heighten motor generators and increase the potential for muscle contraction. The second aspect, tapping, is a proprioceptive stimulus used to facilitate afferent activity within the muscle spindle, thus further enhancing the client's potential for muscle contraction. At the same time the client will be asked to voluntarily activate the motor system, which then automatically augments tactile, proprioceptive, and auditory input with functional control.

Rolling of the Hand. Before Brunnstrom's rolling pattern is implemented, the client's upper extremity is placed above 90 degrees to elicit a Souques sign. This decreases abnormal, excessive tone in the arm, wrist, and hand.[40] This phenomenon may well be a proprioceptive reaction of joints and muscle. The rolling technique consists of two alternating stimulus patterns. The wrist and fingers are placed on extensor stretch. The ulnar side of the volar component of the hand is the stimulus target. A light-touch sweeping pattern is applied to the hypothenar aspect, which has the potential of eliciting an automatic opening of the hand beginning with the fifth digit.[40] Immediately after the light touch, a quick stretch is applied to the wrist and finger extensors. These two techniques are applied quickly and repeatedly, thus giving the visual impression that the therapist is rolling his or her hand over the ulnar aspect of the dorsum of the client's hand. In reality, tactile and proprioceptive stimuli are being effectively combined to facilitate the central pattern generators responsible for the extensor motor neurons controlling the wrist and finger musculature. Because the tone is felt in the client's extensors and thus induces relaxation of the hypertonic flexors, the therapist can more easily open the client's hand. As the client obtains volitional control, some resistance can be added by the therapist to further facilitate wrist and finger extension. A hemiplegic client can also be taught to use this combined

TABLE 4-6. Combined Input Sensory Systems: Treatment Modalities

Technique	Proprioceptive: Joint, Tendon, Spindle	Exteroceptive	Vestibular	Gustatory	Olfactory	Auditory	Visual	ANS	Inherent Response — Labeled	Inherent Response — Not Labeled
Sweep tapping[94]	X	X							Automatic extension of hand	
Brunnstrom's rolling (hand)[40]	X	X								?
Raimiste's sign[40]	X	X								
Stretch pressure[94]	X	X								
Digging in sand, etc.	X	X					?			
Gentle shaking[94]	X		X							
Prone activities over ball[50, 94]	X	X	X				X		Automatic righting of head (tectospinal/vestibulospinal)	
Sitting activities on ball[50]	X	?	X			?	X	X	OLR and balance (all systems)	
Mat activities	X	X	X				?			
Resistive exercises										
1. Resistive rolling	X	X	X			If verbal command	If visual leads			Rotatory integration
2. Resistive patterns: PNF[176, 289]	X	X	Depends on pattern			X	X			
3. Resistive gait	X	?	Depends on pattern			If verbal command	X			
4. Isokinetics	X	Some					X			
5. Wall pulleys	X		X (if done in body rotation)				X (if guided toward target)			
6. Rowing[40]	X	?	X			If verbal command	X			Body rotation
Feeding[50, 94, 223]										
1. Maintained pressure: walking to back of tongue	X	X		?	?					
2. Resistive sucking										
a. Straw	X	X		?	?					
b. Popsicle	X	X		X	X				X	
3. Use of textures										
a. Peanut butter	X	X		X	X				X	
b. Apple sauce	X	X		X	X					
4. Maintained pressure to top lip	X	X						X		Automatic closing of mouth

Technique						Comments
Inverted TLR[94,140]	X	X	?		X	
Touch bombardment[94]	X	X	X		X	Decreased hypersensitive tactile system and thus withdrawal pattern: stereognosis
1. Tactile discrimination in sand, etc.	X				X	
2. Pool therapy	X	X			X	
Joint compression more than body weight[189,288]	X				X	
Throwing and catching						
1. Balloon	?	X			X	
2. Heavy ball	X	?	X	? Result of light touch	X	? (withdrawal to light touch)
Variance in movement						
1. Quick action directed by vision	X		X	X	X	
2. Postural activities in front of mirror	X	?	X	X		
3. Therapist using voice command to assist client with movement	X		X		X	
High-level movement						
1. Walking balance beam	X	X	?	? If visually directed	X	Labyrinthine righting and equilibrium; possible OLR
2. Trampoline activities	X	X		If visually directed	X	OLR and equilibrium
3. Running, jumping, skipping	X					

approach to open the affected hand and give it increased range. This technique is a noninvasive, relaxing approach to opening the hand stuck in wrist and finger flexion hypertonicity. The technique itself also seems to trigger spinal generator patterns that dampen the existing neuron network. It does not teach the patient anything unless that individual begins to assist or take over control of the extensor pattern. This usually occurs first by the therapist feeling the flexors relax when the patient is trying to extend the wrist and fingers even if no active extension is palpated. Encouraging the patient at this time that he or she is thinking correctly is very important motivation for continued practice.

Withdrawal with Resistance. A therapist could combine the technique of eliciting a withdrawal with resistance to the withdrawal pattern. This can be an effective way to release hypertonicity, especially in the lower extremities. The withdrawal can be elicited by a thumbnail, a sharp instrument, a piece of ice, or any adequate light-touch stimulus to the sole of the foot. As soon as the flexor withdrawal is initiated, the therapist must resist the entire pattern. Once the resistance is applied, the input neuron network changes and the flexor pattern is maintained through the proprioceptive input caused by resistance to the movement pattern. The one difficulty with this technique is the application of resistance. The withdrawal pattern directly affects alpha motor neurons innervating those muscles responding in the flexor pattern and simultaneously suppresses alpha motor neurons going to the antagonistic muscles. If the antagonistic muscles are hypertonic, then initially the hypertonicity is dampened within the alpha motor neurons' neuronal pool. Because of the pattern itself, as soon as the flexor response begins, a high-intensity quick stretch is applied to the extensor muscles. If resistance is not applied to the flexors to maintain inhibition over the antagonistic muscles, the extensors will respond to the stretch. The client will very quickly return to the predisposed hypertonic pattern and may even exhibit an increase of abnormal tone. This extensor response is a complex reaction within the spinal generators. The therapist should instruct the patient to assist with the flexor pattern to recruit other components of the motor system to enhance the system's modulation over the spinal generators.

Touch Bombardment. Another example of a proprioceptive-tactile treatment technique is modification of a hypersensitive touch system through a touch-bombardment approach. The goal of this approach is to bombard the tactile system with continuous input to elicit light-touch sensory adaptation or desensitization. Deep pressure is applied simultaneously to facilitate proprioceptive input and conscious awareness. Proprioceptive discrimination and tactile-pressure sensitivity are thought to be critical for high-level tactile discrimination and stereognosis. A hypersensitive light-touch system elicits a protective, altering, withdrawal pattern that prevents development of this discriminatory system and the integrated use of these systems in higher thought. This method of treatment can be implemented by having an individual dig in sand or rice. The continuous pressure forces adaptation of the touch system, and the resistance and deep pressure enhance the proprioceptive-discriminatory touch system by a very complex adaptation process that most likely affects all areas involved in light and discriminatory touch, as well as the complex interaction of all motor system components.

Pool therapy can be used effectively for the same purpose, with the added advantage of neutral warmth. Any client perceiving touch as noxious, dangerous, and even life threatening will not greatly benefit from any therapeutic session in which touch is a component part. Touch includes contacts such as touching the floor with a foot, reaching out and touching the parallel bar railings, and touching the mat. The client may not respond with verbal clues such as "Don't touch me" or "When I touch the floor it hurts" but will often respond with increased tone, emotional or attitude changes, and avoidance responses. Nevertheless, this treatment approach has application in many areas of intervention with clients having neurological deficits. As an adjunct to this method, a clinician should cautiously apply light touch when in contact with the client. Deep pressure or a firm hold should elicit a more desirable response for the client even if the light-touch system is functional.[115, 197] The use of Gore-Tex material for clothing can greatly enhance the client's ability to tolerate the external world, where light-touch encounters cannot be avoided.

The therapist may also consider systematic desensitization as a strategy to integrate the touch system. By allowing patients to apply the stimuli to themselves, they can grade the amount that they can tolerate. In this respect they are empowered to control their own environment. They can practice adaptation in many situations. When the environment seems overwhelming, they have learned techniques to dampen the input both from within their own systems and by controlling the external world. For example, the therapist may place a box containing objects of different textures before the patient and encourage exploration and active participation to learn which textures are acceptable or offensive. A gradual exposure to the offensive stimuli will raise the threshold of the mechanoreceptors in the skin. There are also the benefits to the patient of being in control of the stimulus and having awareness of the treatment objective. In addition, vibratory stimuli through a folded towel provide proprioceptive input to desensitize the touch system.[11, 115, 309] Desensitizing the touch system from a need to protectively withdraw is an important process within the CNS if normal stereognosis is to develop.

Taping. Taping procedures used in peripheral orthopedic muscle imbalances and pain have the same potential for patients with neurological problems. This adaptation would be a modification of both splinting and slings. Although no research has been done to demonstrate efficacy for taping peripheral instability due to CNS dysfunction, the concepts and ideas remain the same. Taping hypotonic muscle groups into a shortened range should effectively reduce the mechanical pull on both the muscle groups and joints and prevent the CNS from developing the need for compensatory stabilization. If hypertonicity is the result of peripheral instability, then taping a hypertonic muscle into its shortened range should stabilize the peripheral system and eliminate the need for the CNS to create the hypertonic pattern. On the other hand, taping can also be used to heighten information about proprioception and joint position, providing feedback to avoid hyperextension or hypermobility of a joint. This is especially true when there is an imbalance of intrinsics and extrinsics in the hand.

Oral-Motor Interventions. The complexity of combined proprioceptive-tactile input becomes enhanced by adding another sensory input, such as taste. Implementations of one of a variety of feeding techniques clearly identify the complexity of the total input system. When taste is used, smell cannot be eliminated as a potential input, nor can vision if the client visually addresses the food. The following explanation of feeding techniques is included to encourage the reader to analyze the sensory input, processing, and motor response patterns necessary to accomplish this ADL task. The complexity of the interaction of all the various systems within the CNS is mind boggling, but if the motor response is functional, effortless, and acceptable to the client and the environment, then the adaptation should be facilitated after attended repetitive behaviors.

Several feeding techniques have been developed by Knickerbocker,[1, 75] Mueller,[223] Farber,[94] Rood,[268] and Huss.[152] These techniques are not easily mastered or understood through reading alone. Competency in feeding techniques is best achieved from empirical experience under the guidance of a skilled instructor.

The facial and oral region plays an important role in survival. Facial stimulation can elicit the rooting reaction. Oral stimulation facilitates reflexive behaviors, such as sucking and swallowing. Deeper stimulation to the midline of the tongue causes a gag reflex. These reactions and reflexes are normal patterns for the neonate. When these reactions/reflexes are depressed or hyperactive, therapeutic intervention is a necessity. Oral facilitation is an important treatment modality for infants and children with CNS dysfunction. Therapeutic intervention during the early stages of myelination can be crucial to the development of more normalized feeding and speech patterns.

Similarly, adults suffering neurological impairment often have difficulty with oral motor integration. Problems with swallowing, tongue control, and hypersensitive and desensitive areas within the oral cavity and also with mouth closure and chewing are frequently observed in adults with CNS damage.

Before implementing basic feeding techniques, clinicians need to understand how the CNS and peripheral nervous system work collaboratively with the musculoskeletal system to control and perform these very complex oral-motor functional movements.[46, 163, 317]

Feeding therapy is preceded by observation and examination. With a pediatric client, the therapist should observe breathing patterns while the client is feeding to determine if the child can breathe through the nose while sucking on a nipple. In addition, the child's lips should form a tight seal around the nipple. Formal assessments should include functional assessments, developmental milestones, and behavioral manifestations. Medical charts and results from neurological examinations should be consulted for baseline data.

Postural mechanisms can influence feeding and speech patterns in clients with neurological dysfunction.[261, 288] A client with a strong extensor pattern may have to be placed in the side-lying, flexed position to inhibit the forces of the extensor pattern. The ideal pattern for feeding is the flexed position, which promotes sucking and oral activity. Basic reflexes such as rooting, sucking, swallowing, and bite and gag reactions should be elicited and graded in children and evaluated in adults. The head needs to be in slight ventroflexion to pull in the postural stabilization of the neck and tongue. This is necessary to effectively facilitate programs that provide functional swallowing and control of foods by the tongue.

The facial region and the mouth have an extraordinary arrangement of sensory innervation. Therefore, oral techniques must be used with utmost care. Anyone who has visited the dentist can attest to the feeling of invasiveness when foreign objects are placed in the mouth. With this in mind, the therapist should begin each treatment session by moving the autonomic continuum toward the parasympathetic end. Activation of the parasympathetic system should lower blood pressure, decrease heart rate, and, more importantly, increase the activity of the gastrointestinal system. Neutral warmth, the inverted position, and slow vestibular stimulation should help to promote parasympathetic "loading." Another approach that is applicable to feeding techniques is the application of sustained and firm pressure to the upper lip. An effective inhibitory device is a pacifier with a plastic shield that applies firm pressure on the lips. Perhaps this is why a pacifier is a "pacifier." Adults can acquire resistive sucking patterns with a straw and plastic shield and achieve the same results.

Sometimes children or adults are not cooperative and will not open their mouths. Rather than pry the mouth open, the jaw is pushed closed and held firmly for a few seconds. On releasing the pressure, the jaw reflexively relaxes. The receptors in the temporomandibular joint and tooth sockets may be involved in the production of this response.

A common problem seen in neurologically impaired infants and adults with head trauma is the "hyperactive tongue," which is often accompanied by a hyperactive gag reflex. To alleviate this problem, the receptors have to be systematically desensitized. The technique called tongue walking has met with clinical success.[95, 140] It entails using an instrument such as a swizzle stick or tongue depressor to apply firm pressure to the midline of the tongue. The pressure is first applied near the tip of the tongue and progressively "walked back" in small steps. As the instrument reaches the back of the tongue, the stimulus sets off an automatic swallow response. The instrument is withdrawn the instant the swallow is triggered. This technique is repeated anywhere from 5 to 30 times a session, depending on individual responses.

Another technique, which might be called deep stroking, is used to either elicit or desensitize the gag reflex. Again, an instrument such as a swizzle stick is used to apply a light stroking stimulus to the posterior arc of the mouth. The instrument should lightly stretch the lateral walls of the palatoglossal arch of the uvula. Normally, the palatoglossal muscle elevates the tongue and narrows the fauces (the opening between the mouth and the oropharynx). Just behind the palatoglossal arch lies another called the palatopharyngeal arch. Normally, this structure elevates the pharynx, closes off the nasopharynx, and aids in swallowing. Touch pressure to either arc incites the gag reflex. This touch pressure should be carefully calibrated. A hyperactive gag reflex may be best diminished by prolonged pressure to the arcs, whereas light, continuous stroking may be more facilitory in activating a hypoactive gag reflex. A child or adult who has been fed by tube for extended periods of time will often have both hypersensitive reactions in various parts of the oral cavity and hyposensitive areas in other locations. This needs to be assessed to formulate a complete picture of the client's difficulties.

The use of vibration over the muscles of mastication appears to be physiologically valid. Muscle spindles have been identified in the temporal and masseter muscles.[67] Selected use of vibration on the muscles of mastication enhances jaw stability and retraction. To facilitate protraction the mandible is manually pushed in.[94, 134]

To promote swallowing, some therapists use manual finger oscillations in downward strokes along the laryngopharyngeal muscles and follow up with stretch pressure. Ice is beneficial as a quick stimulus to the ventral portion of the neck or the sternal notch. In addition, chewing ice chips provides a thermal stimulus to the oral cavity and a proprioceptive stimulus to the jaw and teeth; it also increases salivation for swallowing.

It is recommended that a therapist work closely with a colleague who has experience working with functional feeding before independently beginning to work with clients. The possible complications that might develop with individuals aspirating food cannot be overemphasized.

The therapist can quickly realize that feeding as a proprioceptive, tactile, and gustatory input modality is extremely complex and often incorporates other sensory systems. Breaking down the specific approaches into finite techniques helps the clinician categorize each component and then reassemble them into a whole. The job of dividing and reassembling the parts becomes more and more difficult as the number of input systems enlarges.[314]

Head and Body Movements in Space. Proprioceptive and vestibular input is one of the most frequently combined techniques used by therapists. In fact, client success in almost all therapeutic tasks depends on the coordinated input of these two sensory modalities.

If the head is moving in space and gravity has not been eliminated from the environment, vestibular and proprioceptive receptors will be firing to inform the CNS whether it should continue its feedforward pattern or adapt the plan because the environment no longer matches the programmed movement. Depending on the direction of the head motion and the way gravity is affecting joints, tendons, and muscle, the specific body response will vary according to the degree of flexibility within the motor system. Bed mobility, transfers, mat activities, and gait all incorporate these two modalities.

Although all these functional movements can be performed without these feedback mechanisms, the CNS cannot adapt effectively to changing environments without input from these systems. For that reason alone a thorough examination of the integrity of both systems and the effect of their combined input seems critical if any ADL activity is to be used as a treatment goal.

The use of a large ball or a gymnastic exercise ball can be classified under the category of proprioceptive-vestibular input. Many activities can be initiated over a ball. When a child or adult is prone on a ball, righting of the head can often be elicited by quickly projecting the child forward while the therapist exerts control through the feet, knees, or hips. If the weight of the head is greater than the available power, then a more vertical and less gravitationally demanding position can be used. As the head begins to come up, approximation of the neck can be added. Vibration of the paravertebral muscles might also assist. Rocking forward or bouncing the client who is weight bearing on elbows or extended elbows would facilitate postural weight-bearing patterns through the two identified sensory input systems. Having a client sitting on a gymnastic ball doing almost any exercise will require vestibular and proprioceptive feedback to make appropriate adaptive responses. The combination seems to play a delicate role in the maintenance of normal righting and the equilibrium response so important in functional independence.

A trampoline, balance board, or a similar apparatus has the potential of channeling a large amount of vestibular-proprioceptive input into the client's CNS. In fact, a trampoline is so powerful it can often overstimulate the client and cause excitation or arousal in the CNS.

The trampoline and balance board are generally used to increase balance reactions, orient the client to position in space and to verticality, and increase postural tone. A client with poor balance, poor postural tone, and/or inadequate position in space and verticality perception may be justifiably fearful of these two apparatuses because of the rate, intensity, and skill necessary to accomplish the task. Because fear creates tone and that tone may be in conflict with the motor response from the client, caution must be exercised with either modality. (See Chapter 21 for further discussion of the interactions of sensory systems and balance.)

Gentle Shaking. A specific technique of gentle shaking can be listed under a combined vestibular, muscle spindle, and tendon category. This technique is performed while the client is in a supine position and the head ventroflexed in midline. The head is flexed 35 to 40 degrees to reduce the influence of the otoliths and unnecessary extensor tone through the lateral vestibulospinal tract. This flexed position should be maintained throughout the procedure. The therapist places one hand under the client's occiput and the other on the forehead. Light compression is applied to the cervical vertebrae. This technique activates the deep-joint receptors (C1 to C3) and muscle spindles in the neck along with the vestibular mechanism, which in turn connects with the cerebellum and motor nuclei with the brain stem. If the technique is performed slowly and continuously in a rhythmical motion, total-body inhibition will occur. If the pattern is irregular and fast, facilitation of the spinal motor generators will be observed.

Any one of these techniques can be implemented as a viable treatment approach in considering vestibular-proprioceptive stimuli. The selection of an approach or a method will depend on client preference, client response, the clinician's application skills, and the need for therapeutic assistance.

Summary of Techniques Incorporating Auditory, Visual, Vestibular, Tactile, and Proprioceptive Senses

Most therapeutic activities activate five sensory modalities: auditory, visual, vestibular, tactile, and proprioceptive. Auditory and visual inputs are used as the therapist talks to the client and demonstrates the various movement or response patterns to be accomplished during an activity. As the client moves, vestibular, tactile, and proprioceptive receptors are firing as inherent feedback systems. Thus, the complexity of any activity with respect to analysis of primary input systems is enormous. Even a sedentary activity such as card playing requires a certain amount of proprioception for postural background adaptations, tactile input from supporting body parts and limbs, and visual input for perception and cognition.

Thus, when considering the categorization of techniques—such as a PNF slow reversal,[176] a Brunnstrom marking time,[40] marking time with music,[7, 45] Feldenkrais' sensory awareness through movement,[98, 99] NDTs,[33, 54] Rood's mobility on stability,[268, 288] or any mat or ADL activity—the therapist must observe the sensory systems being bombarded during the activity. At the same time, if the therapist has determined which sensory systems are intact, which are suppressed, and which seem to be registering faulty data, then altering duration and intensity of stimuli through any one system and the combined input through all modalities creates tremendous flexibility in the clinical learning environment. Understanding this diagnostic process leads to more accurate prognosis and selection of appropriate interventions. Highly gifted therapists seem to know instinctively which input systems to use. One skill that seems consistent among master clinicians is a highly developed sensitivity to the client's responses. Simultaneously, they adjust the quantity and duration of combined input to best meet the needs of the client. They release external control and encourage the client to use normal, inherent monitoring systems to adapt to changing environments as soon as the client is able to function independently. That control may begin with a part of the range of a functional skill and not necessarily the entire functional activity itself. The key to carryover will be the client's empowerment over his or her motor control system and the degree of practice, self-monitoring, and adaptation available to the client. By analyzing and categorizing input as well as patients' responses, many therapists may develop skills that were initially considered out of reach.

Innate CNS Programming

The responses of peripheral and central nervous systems (PNS and CNS) to various external stimuli deter-

mine the individuality of an organism and its survival potential in the environment. As organisms become more and more complex, the types of external stimuli as well as the internal mechanisms designed to deal with that input also increase in complexity. As the CNS develops structurally and functionally, inherent control over responses to certain common environmental stimuli seems to be manifested. Different areas of the motor system play different roles in the regulation of motor output. No area is dominant over another. Each area is interdependent on both the input from the environment and the intrinsic mechanisms and function of the nervous system.

As mentioned earlier, the PNS is intricately linked to the CNS and vice versa. Damage to one could potentially alter the neuropathways, their function, and ultimately behavior anywhere along the dynamic loops. Nevertheless, although researchers today emphasize the dynamic interactions of all components, clinicians have observed for decades different motor problems when different areas of the brain are damaged. Thus, when discussing clients with neurological damage, it seems paramount to identify inherent synergy patterns available to humans, especially if those patterns become stereotypical and limit the client's ability to adapt to a changing environment.

The authors do not recommend or discredit the use of any stereotypical or patterned response as a treatment procedure. Acknowledging the presence and stressing the importance of knowing how these motor programs affect clients' functional skills are important. Without this knowledge, therapists working with either children or adults with CNS dysfunction limit their understanding of the normal CNS, normal motor control mechanism and its components, and the interactive effect of all systems on the end product: a motor response to a behavioral goal.

To conceptualize a systems model, the reader must replace the hypothesis of a stimulus-response–based concept of reflexes[68] with a theory of neuronetworks that may be more or less receptive to environmental influences. That sensitivity is modulated by a large number of interconnecting systems throughout the CNS, as well as the internal molecular sensitivity of the neurons themselves. Specific patterns seem to be organized or programmed at various levels or areas within the CNS. These synergies or patterned responses are thought to limit the degrees of freedom available to programming centers such as the basal ganglia and cerebellum[70, 170] and enable more control over the entire body. Having soft-wired, preprogrammed, patterned responses allows organizing systems to activate entire sequences of plans as well as modify any components within the total plan. Modification and adaptation then become the goal or function of the motor system in response to both internal and external goal-directed activities. The specific location of soft-wired programs is open to controversy, as is the complexity of programming at any level within the CNS. Recognizing that these neuronetworks exist with or without external environmental influences would suggest that patterns can and will present themselves without an identified stimulus. In the past, when an external influence was not correlated with an identifiable stereotypical motor pattern, it was referred to as a synergy. When a stimulus was identifiable, the entire loop was called a reflex. Reflexes and preprogrammed, soft-wired neuronetworks such as walking are interactive or superimposed on one another to form the background combinations for more complex program interactions. This superimposed network may encompass spinal and supraspinal co-activity, which makes it very difficult to specify a level of processing. The exact control mechanisms that regulate the specific pattern may again be a shared responsibility throughout the nervous system, thus providing the plasticity observed when disease, trauma, or environmental circumstances force adaptation of existing plans, as discussed in the neuroplasticity section.

One way to conceptualize this complex neuronetwork is to picture a telephone system linking your home to any other home in any city in any country on earth. If the relay between a friend in New York and you in California develops static, the system may self-correct, relay through another area, or even traject through a nonwired mechanism such as a satellite. The options are infinite, but priorities for efficiency and adaptability exist both within the telephone network and the brain. If the wires to your home are cut, the phone will not ring. If your peripheral nerve is cut or the alpha motor neuron damaged, the muscle will not contract. If the relay centers at one end of your block are short-circuiting and not working properly, then your phone and those of your neighbors may still function, but not in a fluid or specific manner. That is, someone may be calling your neighbor but both your phone and your neighbor's phone might ring. Spinal involvement can create a similar problem. The muscles are innervated, the input from the environment accurate, but the neuronetwork faulty. Regulation or modulation may be less efficient or controlled, but the system will use all available resources to try to respond to internal and external environmental requirements. This rule seems consistent throughout the nervous system, and the degree of plasticity is tremendous.[81]

When specific patterned responses are observed, the reader must always hold simultaneously the interaction of all other motor programming options. In this way the therapist can easily conceptualize the variations within one response and the reason why, under different environmental and internal constraints, the motor response pattern may show great variations within the same general plan. Similarly, the expected motor response may not be observable even though it would seem appropriate and anticipated. The clinician must remember that the more complex the action (e.g., rolling vs. dressing vs. playing hockey), the greater the need for integration and coordination over pattern generators. Similarly, the more complex the desired action (especially in new learning), the greater the potential for needed perceptual/cognitive and affective interactions, as well as the greater the potential for gratification and also for failure.

Certain patterned responses or neuronetworks might be considered more simplistic or protective in function. These patterns were once thought to be hard-wired spinal reflexes. It is now known that these reflexes, as well as very complex pattern generators, exist at the spinal level and that their responses affect brain stem, cerebellar, and cortical actions. These centers simultaneously affect the specifics of the spinal neuronetwork responses. With cli-

ents who have low functional control over the spinal or brain stem motor networks, identification of existing patterns, optional patterns as a response to environmental demands, and obligatory patterns not within the control of the client's intentional repertoire of patterns becomes a critical evaluative component before prognosing or identifying the most appropriate interventions.

Recognizing specific patterns and how those patterns and others might affect functional movement or positional patterns has clinical significance. A child with spastic cerebral palsy, for instance, shows extension and "scissoring" when the pads of the feet are stimulated. Sometimes the extension pattern is so strong that the child will arch backward. Sustained positions that oppose pathological patterns are believed to elicit autogenic inhibition. Contraction-relaxation techniques also work on the autogenic inhibition principle.[176]

Just as afferent input can be used to alter tone and elicit movement, it can also become an obstacle when the therapist tries to coordinate complex movement patterns. A persistent grasp pattern is a common occurrence in children and adults with a CNS insult. This dominant grasp is often reinforced by the client's own fingers and frequently prevents functional use of the hand. If a withdrawal pattern is elicited every time a client is touched, the client not only will be unable to explore the environment through the tactile-proprioceptive systems but also will experience arousal by the influence of the cutaneous system over the reticular activating system. Severe agitation could likely be a behavioral outcome from such a persistent reflex.

As with any treatment procedure, a clinician should determine whether the technique will help the client obtain a higher level of function. The clinician must learn to recognize not only specific patterns but also what combinations of responses of pattern generators would look like. If the reader overlaid the map of the pattern generators for any combination of programs, a complex neuronetwork would result. To some it would verify chaos theory, and to others it would verify the end result of multiple systems interacting. The neuronetwork complexity of multiple input can be overwhelming. Thus, a therapist must always be observant of the specific behavioral response and the moment-to-moment changes in behavior during a treatment session, even if the specific neuronetwork is not understood.

The clinician needs to observe whether the specific patterned response is (1) triggered by afferent input, (2) triggered by volitional intent, or (3) activated without environmental input or cortical intent. In the third case, the entire motor system needs to be evaluated to determine which portion might be modulating the observable behavior. Differentiating these motor components will help in prognosing and selecting interventions.

Wholistic Treatment Techniques Based on Multisensory Input

As already mentioned, a variety of accepted treatment methodologies exist. Each approach focuses on multisensory input introduced to the client in controlled and identified sequences. These sequences are based on the inherent nature of synergistic patterns,[9, 228] the patterns observed in humans[9, 34, 278] and lower-order animals,[97] or a combination of the two.[176, 288] Each method focuses on the total client, the specific clinical problems, and alternative treatment approaches available within each established framework. Certain methods have traditionally emphasized specific neurological disabilities. Cerebral palsy in children[24, 34, 236, 288] and hemiplegia in adults[33, 40, 55, 213] are the two most frequently identified. In the past two decades substantial clinical attention has been paid to children with learning difficulties.[10, 102] Yet the concepts and treatment procedures specific to all the techniques have been applied to almost every neurological disability seen in the clinical setting. This expansion of the use of each method seems to be a natural evolution because of the structure and function of the CNS and commonalities in clinical signs manifested by brain insult.

Clinical Example: How to Use a Classification Scheme When Selecting an Augmented Intervention Program

CLINICAL PROBLEM: LACK OF HEAD CONTROL

There is a potential for lack of head control among young, developmentally delayed children or in individuals after a severe injury to the CNS. For that reason it is a common clinical problem. Furthermore, because of the importance of head and neck control, virtually all functional activities are affected by its absence.

Before discussing a classification schema, the clinical problem must be analyzed and identification made of those sensory and inherent input systems to be facilitated. In considering the specific problem of lack of head control, let us assume that Timothy, a 16-year-old with a closed-head injury, suffered a lesion within his CNS 3 months ago. He has the following signs regarding head control:

- Mild extensor hypertonicity is present in the supine position, and Timothy is unable to flex and rotate his head off the mat.
- In prone position, extensor hypertonicity is absent, and hypotonicity prevails. The client is able to briefly bob his head off the mat in a hyperextension pattern. Mild tonal shifts occur to either side when the head is turned and when it is symmetrically flexed or extended.
- Timothy is unable to roll or perform any functional activity in the horizontal plane.
- When placed in long sitting position, he is unable to hold the position or sit with flexed hips and extended knees. His head remains in total flexion with his chin on his chest.
- When sitting over a table mat, he is unable to hold his position. General hypotonicity prevails, although slightly more flexion is palpable. His head remains flexed. When asked to pick up his head, he extends into a hyperextension pattern followed by extensor relaxation into flexion.
- He is unable to hold the head in a postural co-activation pattern in a vertical position.
- Timothy does not mind being touched and responds well to handling techniques.

From the analysis of these clinical signs, the following clinical interpretations are presented.

1. In the horizontal position, Timothy has persistence of a motor program that is enhanced by the spatial position and its influence on the vestibular system. The result might be considered persistence of a tonic labyrinthine reflex. In this client the dominant synergic pattern is extension. While he is supine, extension prevails. While he is prone, extension is inhibited, although flexion tone is not dominant. Because of the persistence of hyperactivity among the extensor motor generators, the ability to initiate rolling using a neck-righting pattern is prevented. The presence of a mild, asymmetrical tonic neck reflex to both sides and a symmetrical tonic neck reflex has been noted. Because of his instability and low tone, Timothy seems to be using these stereotypical patterns volitionally to assist in gaining some control over his motor patterns. In prone position, Timothy has the ability to move into a neck extension or optic and labyrinthine righting (OLR) pattern but is unable to hold it. Thus, movement and range are present but postural holding is missing.

2. As a result of ventroflexion of the head in sitting, the vestibular apparatus is placed in a position similar to that when prone. In a like manner, the total patterns remain fairly consistent. The increase in flexor tone may result from the positioning of hip and knee flexion and kyphosis of the back. The inability to flex the hips with knee extension suggests that total tonal patterns or synergies are dominant. The client is unable to break out of those dominant patterns. Dominant OLR is not present.

3. When asked, Timothy carries out the command to the best of his motor ability. This suggests the presence of some intact verbal processing, which is translated into appropriate motor acts. Similarly, when asked to pick up his head, he does just that, suggesting some perceptual integrity of body image, body schema, and position in space. Knowing where his head is in space and where to reposition it also suggests that some proprioceptive-vestibular input and processing are occurring.

4. Timothy's enjoyment of being moved in space as related to handling techniques suggests proprioceptive-vestibular integrity. Similarly, his tactile systems seem to be functioning in a discriminatory manner and modifying negative responses of withdrawal and arousal. However, specific tactile perception would need a great deal of further testing. Thus, he demonstrates functional strengths in cognition and perception, in limbic motivation, in some areas of sensory integrity, and in control over available but limited motor programming. Yet, performance on any functional test would result in identification of an individual whose functional limitations prevent him from independence in any activity. Prognosis would need to be guarded until the therapist had an opportunity to augment the environment to determine how quickly he regained control and retained the learning. The initial prognosis is assumed to focus on development of head control as a preliminary and necessary motor program for all

functional daily living activity. The estimated time it will take to regain this function would not be identified until after the first intervention session.

Behavioral Diagnosis: The client is unable to functionally control his head in any position in space that limits independence in all functional activities. Lack of postural co-activation and adequate control over the motor generators has led to imbalances in the tonal characteristics of flexor and extensor patterns with the compensatory development of stereotypical patterns of movement.

Goal of Intervention Program: Development of independent head control initially in a narrow vertical window with the intent of enlarging that window to include all space positions.

Now that the clinical problem has been analyzed and the goal of development of head control set, an intervention sequence or protocol must be established. Timothy lacks head control in all planes and in all patterns of movement. Thus, flexors and extensors must be facilitated to develop a dynamic co-activation or postural holding pattern of the neck. The categorization scheme can now be of some assistance. The therapist can ask, "Are there any inherent mechanisms that enhance flexors or extensors in a holding pattern?" OLR should elicit the desired response. Similarly, the clinician can ask, "Are there any inherent motor programs that would prevent righting of the head to face vertical OLR?" The tonic labyrinthine reflex (TLR) would block or modify the facilitation of OLR. Knowing the TLR is most dominant in horizontal and least dominant (if at all affected) in vertical is of clinical significance. It is also important to know that the OLR is most frequently tested in a vertical position and seems most active in that position. Awareness that the client is sensitive to total patterns (e.g., flexion facilitates flexion or extension facilitates extension) gives additional treatment clues.

After all this information is assimilated, the following treatment protocol could be established.

To enhance neck flexors, the client will be placed in a totally flexed position in vertical, with the head positioned in neutral. The client will be rocked backward toward supine, allowing gravity to quick stretch the flexors (Fig. 4–13A). As soon as the neck flexors are stretched, the head should be tapped forward and then back to vertical but not beyond. This avoids hyperextension, extreme stretch to the proprioceptors, and the horizontal supine position of the labyrinths, all of which dampen the flexors and facilitate the extensors. The quick stretch and position should optimally facilitate OLR, which should activate the neck flexors. The total flexion of the body similarly facilitates the neck flexors. Once the neck flexors respond, Timothy can be rocked farther and farther backward while maintaining the head in vertical or ventroflexion (see Fig. 4–13B). Once Timothy can be rocked from vertical to horizontal and back to vertical while maintaining good flexor neck control, his CNS has demonstrated inherent control and modification over the stereotypical patterns, such as the TLR in supine with respect to its influence over the neck musculature. This rocking maneuver can be done on diagonals to practice flexion and rotation (see Fig. 4–13C), the key to eliciting a neckrighting, rolling pattern from supine to prone. The total flexed pattern can also be altered by adding more and more extension of the extremities. This decreases the external facilitation to the flexors and demands that Timothy's CNS take more and more control (internal regulation). Additional treatment procedures can be extracted from a variety of sensory categories. To add additional proprioceptive input, any one of those listed techniques might be used. The rotation and speed of the rocking pattern affect the vestibular mechanism. Auditory and visual stimuli can be used effectively. If the therapist takes a position slightly below the client's horizontal eye level, the client (to look at the therapist) will need to look down and flex his head, thus encouraging the desired pattern. Any type of visual or auditory stimulus that directs the client into the desired pattern would be appropriate. The therapist must remember that neck flexion is one of the identified goals. Rotation was added to incorporate and set the stage for inherent programming that will lead to rolling, coming to sit, and reaching while sitting. Since the postural extensor component still needs integration, total head control has not been attained. To facilitate neck extension, a procedure similar to the one

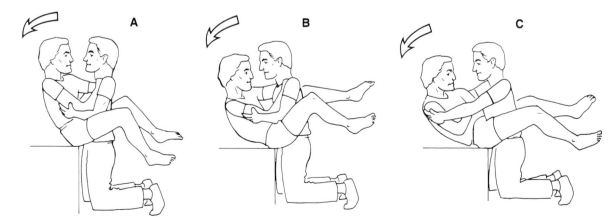

FIGURE 4–13. Development of flexor aspect of head control. *A,* Vertical position: head at midline and midrange (total body flexion) to optimally facilitate neck flexors. *B,* Facilitating symmetrical neck flexion, using position, gravity, and flexor positions. *C,* Facilitating flexion and rotation to develop pattern necessary for neck-righting pattern.

for flexion can be established. A vertical position, thus eliminating the influence of the TLR, would again be the starting position of choice.

With extension facilitating extension, the client should be placed in as much extension as possible without eliciting excessive extensor tone. An inverted labyrinthine position, a kneeling position, or a standing position would be viable spatial patterns to facilitate OLR of the head and co-activation of postural extensors. The vestibular system sensory category can be checked to identify the treatment procedure for use with an inverted labyrinthine position. The kneeling or standing position places the client in a vertical position with hip and trunk extension. Kneeling rather than standing is used first because of the influence of the positive supporting reaction in standing and the massive facilitation of total extension. Kneeling avoids total extension while maintaining a predominant extensor pattern. As a result of the gravitational pull of body weight through the joints, approximation to facilitate postural extension is constantly maintained. The upper extremities can be placed in shoulder abduction and external rotation, which tends to inhibit abnormal upper-extremity flexor tone and facilitate postural tone into the shoulder. This extensor tone has the potential through associated spinal reactions to facilitate neck and trunk extension. The arms can be placed in this position over a bolster or ball or by the therapist handling the client from the rear (Fig 4–14A). The head should begin again in a neutral position. The client is rocked forward (see Fig. 4–14B) to facilitate optic and labyrinthine righting of the head and to elicit a quick stretch to the postural extensors. If the head begins to fall forward, the therapist can tap the client's forehead immediately after the quick stretch. This tapping action is the reverse tap procedure described under the muscle spindle proprioceptive category. The tapping is done to passively move the head back to vertical.

A variety of additional procedures can easily be combined to summate facilitation to the postural extensors. Tapping, vibration, and approximation through the head to the shoulders are only a few of the proprioceptive modalities. All would be facilitory. A variety of auditory and visual stimuli could be used to orient the client to a position in space and thus righting of the head. Techniques listed under the exteroceptive and vestibular sys-

tems could also be part of the treatment protocol. The therapist would want to sequence the client toward prone while the head remained in a vertical postural holding pattern. As the therapist rocks the client toward prone again, a rotatory component should be added (see Fig. 4–14C). The client will extend and rotate to counterbalance the movement, thus incorporating the neck-righting pattern of extension and rotation necessary when rolling from prone to supine. Resistance to neck extension with or without rotation is an important element in regaining normal functional control. The client is alert and has some functional use of the arms and legs. This rocking pattern in kneeling can be done as a functional activity. The therapist asks the client to assist in reaching toward an object with one upper extremity. The therapist can guide the client in the reaching pattern in a forward, sideward, or cross-midline direction. While reaching, the client can be rocked forward to elicit right and equilibrium reactions. By incorporating an activity into the treatment of head control, the client not only is entertained but also attends to the task rather than cognitively trying to keep his head up. In this way automatic head control is facilitated, and often postural patterns follow. In a partial kneeling pattern the client can be sequenced to on-elbow over a bolster or ball or on a chair. These activities should be sequenced from vertical to prone to ensure both total postural programming in prone and optimal integration of OLR, as well as letting the client experience control of various motor strategies in many different environmental contexts.

Once the client can maintain good flexor, extensor, and rotational components of head control, the activity should, if possible, be practiced with the client's eyes closed. If the client can still maintain head control, labyrinthine righting would be adequate for any functional activity. If the client loses head control, then additional labyrinthine facilitation would be indicated. If a client uses only vision to right the head, then any time vision is needed to lead or direct another activity, head control might be lost. Because symmetrical vestibular simulation plays a key role in activating the neck muscles to hold the head in vertical, it also is a key element leading to the perception of vertical and all the directional activities sequencing out of the concept of verticality. The postural extensor programming for head control needs to be practiced in a

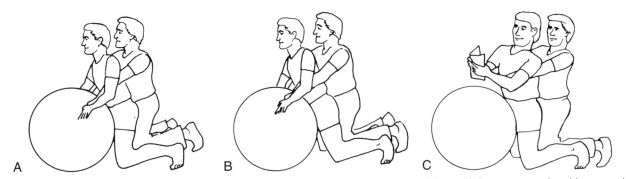

FIGURE 4–14. Development of extensor aspect of head control. *A*, Vertical position: head midline with long extensor in midrange and postural extensors in shortened range; body in postural weight-bearing pattern. *B*, Facilitating symmetrical extension of head, trunk, and hips while inhibiting abnormal upper extremity tone. *C*, Facilitating head and trunk extension and rotation to encourage neck righting pattern; client reaches for an object, which is then placed on the opposite side.

standing position as well as a sitting position. The client needs to be able to stand quietly without excessive extension to run both postural and balance programs. Similarly, he needs to be able to sit with hip flexion while co-activating postural extension in the trunk and neck.

Head control is a complex motor response. A therapist can facilitate inherent mechanisms to assist a client in regaining function. Simultaneously, multitudinous external input techniques classified under the various sensory modalities and combined modalities can be used to give the client additional information. Awareness of one technique and the ability to categorize it appropriately allow easy identification and implementation of many additional approaches. The therapist always needs to remember that the client must practice the behavior (head control) in a variety of spatial positions during various functional activities. This practice must be functional and no longer contrived.

Somatosensory Discrimination and Interventions

When considering intervention options, a third category of treatment must also be considered. Given that there is strong evidence that the nervous system is adaptable, when there are signs of neural dysfunction, planned, attended repetitive behaviors can be designed to restore normal neural function. In this chapter on interventions, we have concentrated primarily on using the sensory input system as a way to facilitate motor outputs. However, there are times when the somatosensory system is dysfunctional as a result of either developmental delay, injury, or high levels of repetitive fine-motor use of the hand, chronic pain, or learned dysfunction. Even though the patient may not be complaining of sensory dysesthesia, numbness, or tingling, the therapist should determine the accuracy of sensory discriminative processing and the accuracy of performance of fine-motor skills such as writing, using a computer keyboard, or playing an instrument to be certain there are no underlying sensory problems, even though the patient may be complaining of pain or problems of motor control.

Brief Review of Somatosensory Neuroanatomy

The somatosensory system is complex.[164] It includes the primary sensory cortex in the parietal lobe and all of the pathways between the somatosensory cortex, the thalamus, the motor cortex, the basal ganglia, the cerebellum, and the spinal cord. The primary sensory cortex is an afferent input system, receiving information from the environment through the receptors in the skin and from the body through the muscle afferents, the Golgi tendon organs, and the joint proprioceptors. Information is carried from the receptors up the spinal cord to the medial lemniscus and the thalamus to the somatosensory cortex.

The somatosensory system includes four major modalities: discriminative touch, proprioception, nociception, and temperature. Discriminative touch helps us recognize the size, shape, and texture of objects as well as their movement across the skin. Proprioception is concerned with the sense of static position and movement of limbs and the body. Nociception is the signaling of tissue damage referred to as pain. Temperature sense includes warmth and coldness. The peripheral anatomy of the somatosensory system includes the sensory receptors, the peripheral nerve (carrying information to the spinal cord), the interneurons (excitatory and inhibitory), the dorsal column pathway in the spinal cord (carrying information to the medial lemniscus), the axons from the medial lemniscus projecting to the thalamus in the ventral posterior medial and ventral poster lateral nuclei, and then finally the projections to the primary somatosensory cortex in the postcentral gyrus of the parietal lobe. Sensations of pain and temperature are carried by the anterolateral system in the spinal cord to the thalamus. A discussion of these same receptors and their importance as feedback during hands-on augmented therapeutic interventions can be found in the section under Intervention: Augmented Treatment Techniques in this chapter. The sensations of pain and temperature are not addressed in this section but can be found in Chapters 11 and 29.

The somatosensory cortex has three major divisions: the primary (S-I) and the secondary (S-II) somatosensory cortices and the posterior parietal. See Figure 4–6 for orientation of cortical structures and their traditional classification. The primary S-I is divided into four areas: Brodmann's areas 1, 2, 3a, and 3b. Most of the thalamic fibers terminate in areas 3a and 3b. The cells in areas 3a and 3b then project to Brodmann's areas 1 and 2. Some of the thalamic neurons project directly to Brodmann's areas 1 and 2 and to the adjacent secondary somatosensory cortex (S-II). S-II is also innervated by neurons from each of the four areas of S-I. The projections from S-I are required for the perceptual function of S-II. If S-I connections are removed, it prevents stimuli applied to the skin of the hand from activating neurons in S-II. This outcome is most apparent when you obliterate area 3a. But removal of S-II has no effect on the response of neurons in S-I. Some thalamic neurons project to the posterior parietal cortex. The projections from the ventral posterolateral thalamus project to 3a and 3b and area 1. These pathways are most sensitive to cutaneous touch. Projections from the ventral posterolateral thalamus and the ventrolateral thalamus project to area 3a. Other neurons from the ventrolateral thalamus project to areas 1 and 2.

The sensory and motor hand regions in S-I and M-1 have been referenced most extensively in the study of neuroplasticity. In S-I, the area 3b has an unusually large topographical representation of the skin compared with the proportional size of the hand relative to the rest of the body. There is less precise representation in area 3a and areas 1 and 2. In area 3b, it is also most precisely and distinctly represented. The orderly representation of the digits makes it particularly sensitive to the measurement of change. However, these studies focusing on defining the characteristics of neuroplasticity are applicable to other somatotopic areas of the CNS. The hand representations in the cortical areas of 3b have a roughly mirror image topographic relationship with duplicative palmar representations between areas 3a, 3b, and 1.[207, 226, 290] These cortical representations have been described in

S-I in humans,[241] macaque monkeys,[226] New World owl monkeys,[207, 209] squirrel monkeys,[21, 209, 290] spider monkeys,[253] cebus monkeys, and marmosets.

Some New World monkeys have exaggerated representations of their fingernails that are used on a heavy behavioral schedule in grasping. The representation of the thumbs of humans and apes is proportionally large. In general, all primates have a similar general layout for the representation of the hand. The radial margin is lateralward and discontinuously related to the face. The digits and palmar pads are represented in order proceeding medialward in the cortex, in a radial to ulnar sequence across the hand. The wrist and forearm are represented medial to the hand representation. However, the representation of 3b is fairly consistent across species, with more variations by species and within species for 3a, 1, 2, and 5.[209]

Sensory information in all primates including humans is serially processed through relay regions. The relay nuclei are composed of projection neurons that send axons to the next relay nucleus in the ascending pathways. Each projection neuron receives synaptic input from many afferent axons. Most commonly, the sensory inputs to relay cells follow a pattern of extensive convergence and divergence. In addition to activating relay cells, afferent fibers also activate interneurons, both excitatory and inhibitory. These interneurons contribute to the processing of incoming sensory information by modulating the firing of the projection neurons. The firing pattern of the projection neurons reflects transformation of the signal by the cells of the nucleus.

There are three types of inhibitory pathways: feedforward, feedback, and distal inhibition. These are local inhibitory mechanisms operating within a relay nucleus. Feedforward (or reciprocal) inhibition allows activity in one group of neurons to inhibit a different group of neurons. Feedforward inhibition permits a singleness of action (winner takes all). This ensures that only one of two or more competing responses is expressed. Feedback (recurrent inhibition) allows the most active neurons to limit the activity of all adjacent elements are less active. This enhances the contrast in firing patterns between the actively firing cells and the surrounding, less active neurons. These types of inhibition create a central zone of active neurons surrounded by a ring of less active neurons. By enhancing or amplifying the contrast between the highly active cells and their neighbors, the cellular interactions contribute to selective perception (attend to one stimulus and not another).

There is no inhibition in the peripheral receptor in the somatosensory system. Inhibitory actions are common in all relay nuclei (e.g., both feedforward and feedback inhibitions are present in the dorsal column nuclei). The afferent fibers inhibit the activity of cells in the dorsal column nuclei that surround the cells they excite (feedforward inhibition). Active cells in a nucleus inhibit the less active cells by recurrent collateral fibers (feedback inhibition), sharpening the contrast between the active cells and their neighbors. Neurons from more distant sites such as the motor cortex and the brain stem can also inhibit and control the flow of information from the relay nuclei (called distal inhibition) operating mostly on presynaptic terminals Thus, higher areas of the brain are able to control the sensory inflow from the peripheral receptors.

Total removal of S-I (areas 3b, 3a, 1, and 2) produces deficits in position sense and the ability to discriminate size, texture, and shape. Thermal and pain sensibilities are altered but not abolished. Lesions in area 3b produce deficits in discrimination of the texture, size, and shape of objects. Lesions in area 2 alter only the ability to differentiate the size and shape of objects. 3b is the principal target for the afferent projections from the ventral posterolateral nucleus of the thalamus. The projections to area 1 are concerned primarily with texture, whereas the projections to area 2 are concerned with size and shape.

S-II receives inputs from all areas of S-I. Thus, a lesion of S-II causes severe impairment in the discrimination of both shape and texture as well as preventing animals from learning new tactile discrimination tasks based on the shape of an object. Thus, damage to the posterior parietal cortex creates complex abnormalities in attending to sensations from the contralateral half of the body.

Sensory information is topographically organized in the primary somatic cortex. The body surface and deep tissues are also represented in a topographical order in the thalamus and the dorsal column nuclei. Each part of the body is represented in the brain in proportion to its relative importance in sensory perception. The face is large compared with the back of the head. The index finger is large compared with the big toe. This distortion reflects differences in innervation density in different areas of the body. Each of the four areas in Brodmann's classification has its own map (3a, 3b, 1, 2). In addition, area S-II has its own map. Each area has its own somatosensory inputs. Each central neuron has its own receptive field on the skin. The cortical neurons in the somatosensory system respond only to stimulation of a specific area of the skin. Any point on the skin is represented in the cortex by a population of cells connected to the afferent fibers that innervate that point on the skin. Stimulation of the skin excites very specific cortical neurons.

The receptive fields have four important features: their size, distribution, modifiability, and fine structure. Where there is unusual sensitivity to touch in the body (e.g., lips and fingers), there are a large number of receptors per unit area and the receptive fields are very small. The fingertips have the highest density of receptors (about 2500/cm^2). Three fifths of these receptors are Meissner corpuscles, one third are Merkel cells, and the remainder are pacinian and Ruffini corpuscles. They are innervated by myelinated axons. Each afferent fiber connects to about 20 Meissner corpuscles, and each corpuscle receives two to five afferent fibers. As you move up the arm, the receptive fields become larger and decreased in density and there is a reduction in fineness of sensory discrimination.

The receptor cell has its greatest discharge at the center of the receptive field and its weakest around the perimeter. There is a gradient of excitatory activity within the receptive field and a gradient of inhibition. The inhibition is also greatest at the center of the field and decreases with distance from the center. Inhibition is delayed. Inhibition occurs after excitation. At each relay station in the somatic afferent system, a stimulus in the excitatory center of the receptive field produces a peak of excitation that is surrounded by a population of inactive (inhibited) cells. This spatial distribution sharpens the peak activity within the brain.

Spatial discrimination is the ability to distinguish two closely placed point stimuli as two rather than one. Two stimuli applied to different positions on the skin set up excitatory gradients of activity in two cell populations at every relay point in the somatosensory system. The activity in each population of cells has its own maximal region of activity or peak, and the perception of two points rather than one occurs because two distinct populations are active. Each neuron population has a central excitatory zone surrounded by a weaker excitatory zone. It is further depressed by the inhibitory surround, which sharpens each peak and further enhances the distinction between the two peaks.

When the two stimuli are brought closer together, the activity of the two populations tends to overlap so that the section between the two peaks can become blurred. As they get closer and closer, the inhibition produced by each summates. This allows the peaks of activity to be sharpened. When two stimuli keep getting closer and occur within a single large receptive field, the separation of the two stimuli becomes encoded as a single population of receptors. When two stimuli are widely separated they elicit separate, distinguishable, high-frequency responses. When these are coincident in time, it allows two different behaviors to be programmed and mapped together. This is a type of learning that facilitates improved skill, even automation of learning. As the separation narrows, the frequency decreases and the duration of neuronal firing decreases.

Somatosensory Discrimination Deficits: Degradation

Although rapidly adapting receptors can distinguish spacing between stimuli as small as 1 mm, ultimately the spacing is further reduced until no difference between stimuli can be distinguished. This can be a form of neuroplasticity that represents negative learning or degradation. Now two sensory stimuli come in to adjacent digits, for example, and no longer are interpreted as separate stimuli but the same stimulus. Thus, the stimulus is interpreted as the same one across the adjacent digits, which may interfere with individualized, coordinated, rapid fine-motor movement. This is hypothesized to be the underlying cause of occupational hand cramps that can develop in people who perform high levels of repetition as part of their job. The representation of the involved hand on the primary sensory cortex may become smaller than normal, with larger than normal receptive fields. In addition, the location of the hand area differs from normal and the order of the digits may not be sequential.[15, 52, 60, 90] This same change in location and area of representation has also been observed in patients with chronic pain.[104, 298]

This type of degradation might be more likely to occur when the stimuli are both cutaneous and deep, particularly when stretch stimuli impact fast twitch, fatigable fibers. The fast twitch fatigable fibers have a large cell body. The slow fatigue resistance cells have a small cell body. The intermediate fibers, which are fast twitch, fatigue-resistant fibers, have an intermediate-sized cell body. With stimulation or activation, the small cell bodies are activitated first. With an increase in strength of contraction, the larger cell bodies are recruited. The slow fatigue-resistant fibers can fire with a consistent amplitude over 60 minutes; the fast twitch, fatigue-resistant fibers can fire consistently up to 50 minutes, whereas the fast twitch fatigable fibers lose their force at 4 minutes.[45, 78]

In a muscle, when the firing rate gets to 80 Hz, there is an unfused tetanus. At 100 Hz, there is a fused tetanus and no muscle twitches are definable. The muscle stays in a fixed contraction. Interestingly, when an individual contracts a muscle voluntarily, even against resistance, the contraction rarely exceeds 25 Hz.[45]

Another possible learned degradation would be having the agonists and the antagonists always contract simultaneously instead of reciprocally. If this was repeated during all voluntary motor contraction, they could become learned. It is then possible that a stretch of the spindle would lead to an exaggerated muscle contraction of both the agonist and the antagonist rather than a reciprocal response. This simultaneous contraction of agonists and antagonists interferes with graded muscle contractions, again interfering with normal, coordinated voluntary muscle movements.[233, 237, 264]

Specific Afferent Sensitivity and Cortical Representation

Each nerve cell is responsive to one modality: touch, pressure, temperature, or pain. Neurons mediating touch are responsive to superficial tactile stimuli but not deep stimuli. Neurons responsive to superficial stimuli are more specialized. Some are responsive to movement of hairs, whereas others respond to a steady indentation of skin. One modality tends to dominate in each of Brodmann's areas. Muscle stretch is dominant in 3a, and information from cutaneous receptors is dominant in 3b. Deep-pressure receptors are dominant in area 2; and in area 1, rapidly adapting cutaneous receptors are dominant. Furthermore, there is a column for rapidly adapting and one for slowly adapting receptors in S-I, area 3b. Each relay nucleus has some level of adaptation similar to the receptors. The signal received by the input to the cortex reproduces the stimulus features encoded by the receptors in the skin.

The somatosensory cortex is arranged in six cellular layers, and there is no correlation between layers and neuron type. In all six layers, neurons within a column or slab of cortex running from the cortical structure to the white matter respond as one class of receptors. Some columns are activated by rapidly adapting cutaneous receptors of the Meissner type, some by slowly adapting cutaneous receptors of the Merkel type, and others by movement of the hair cells or the subcutaneous, rapidly adapting pacinian receptors.

Although each of the four areas of the primary somatosensory cortex (3a, 3b, 1, 2) receives input from all areas of the body surface, one modality tends to dominate in each area: area 3a = muscle stretch; area 3b = cutaneous; area 2 = deep pressure; and area 1 = rapidly adaptive cutaneous. Each layer also has connections with different parts of the brain. Layer 6 projects back to the thalamus, layer 5 projects to the subcortical structures, layer 4 receives information from the thalamus, and layers 1, 2, and 3 project to other cortical regions.

Tactile perception is determined by the response properties of the receptors that are matched with those of the CNS. Rapidly adaptive skin receptors connect to rapidly adapting neurons in the thalamus that connect to neurons in 3b and 3a. S-I slowly adapting receptors connect to neurons in the thalamus, as well as 3b and 3a.

The neural representation of the surface texture of objects in areas 3b and 1 has been studied. Awake monkeys were stimulated with embossed letters. When the letter was moved across the skin, the response of a single neuron to a stimulus moved systematically across the receptive field could be assumed to represent the response of a pulsation of neurons with similar response properties of slowly and rapidly adapting receptors in the skin (e.g., Merkel cells, Meissner cells). In area 3b, the first stage of processing from the projections of the skin receptors gave rise to sharp images. In the later stages in area 1, the responses were more abstract.[29, 30]

To sense the texture, form, and motion of an object, integration of information from many different mechanoreceptors sensitive to superficial tough, deep pressure and position of the finger and hand is required (stereognosis). Four factors are involved: (1) response properties of the neurons at successive levels of sensory processing become more complex; (2) submodalities converge on one common cell; (3) the size of the receptive field gets larger; and (4) profiles of responding populations of neurons change (e.g., cells in the hand region of the somatosensory cortex respond briskly to three-dimensional objects placed within the receptive fields, particularly movement of objects across the skin; the same cells do not respond to point stimuli like cells at earlier relays).

Neurons involved in inputs of 3b and 3a can respond to single and multiple static and dynamic point stimuli. Neurons in areas 1 and 2 also respond to these types of stimuli. These neurons have complex response properties (e.g., responding to movement across the skin). This type of sensory analysis permits stereognosis (the perception of the three-dimensional shape of objects). The convergent projections for 3a and 3b into areas 1 and 2 permit neurons in areas 1 and 2 to respond to complex features such as edge orientation. Neurons in 3b and 1 respond only to touch. Neurons in 3a respond to position senses, and those in area 2 respond to both, particularly when an object is held in the hand.

Three types of neurons respond to movement. Motion-sensitive neurons respond to movement in all directions. Direction-sensitive neurons respond much better to movement in one direction. Orientation-sensitive neurons respond best to movement along a specific axis of the receptive field. Feature-detecting neurons are sensitive to stimulus direction and orientation and are found in area 1 and more extensively in area 2. These areas are more concerned with stereognosis and with discriminating the direction of movement of objects on the skin. These complex stimulus properties arise not from the thalamic input but from cortical projections from area 3a. The convergent projections from areas 3a and 3b into areas 1 and 2 also permit neurons in areas 1 and 2 to respond to other complex features. Neurons in areas 3b and 1 respond only to touch. Neurons in areas 3a respond only to position sense, and certain neurons in area 2 have both inputs.

Receptive fields are small in areas 3a and 3b (sites of initial inputs of S-I). Neurons in areas 1 and 2 receive inputs from 3a and 3b and also have their own neurons projecting on the fingers. Inputs for the finger areas are commonly adjacent to one another, and cells respond most effectively when adjacent fingers are stimulated, as when the hand is used to hold and manipulate an object. These complex cells in areas 1 and 2 become active during movements of the hand around an object. These complex cells also seem to have a role in stereognosis.

Inputs for finger areas are usually adjacent to one another, and cells respond most effectively when adjacent fingers are stimulated, as when the hand is used to hold and manipulate objects. Areas 1 and 2 are activated when the hand is actually moving objects.

Increase in complexity is important in perception and skilled movements. Area 2 sends somatosensory inputs from the entire body surface to the primary motor cortex. There is also some inhibition produced by neurotransmitters (e.g., gamma-aminobutyric acid [GABA]) that inhibit cortical cells. Reversible inhibition of neural activity in area 2 can be produced pharmacologically (GABA agonist). This leads to an inability to assume functional postures of the hand and coordinate the fingers. The somatosensory area protects the motor cortex and Brodmann's areas 5 and 7. Cells detecting complex information receive inputs from several modalities and are often related to movement. Cutaneous information is integrated into visual information and with other system activities in the brain stem, thalamus, and temporal lobe concerned with attention.

Tactile information from the periphery reaches the cortex by several pathways, all carrying redundant as well as unique information. Also, many pathways project to more than one cortical area. This parallel processing is designed to allow different neuronal pathways and brain relays to deal with the same sensory information in slightly different ways. Neurons in areas 2 and 1 are involved in the later stages of somatosensory processing and have more complex feature-detecting properties receiving convergent input from a number of other modalities. More complicated processing is carried out with object manipulation. In addition, the somatosensory cortex sends outputs to the posterior parietal cortex, where further integration takes place and an overall picture of the body is formed.

The convergent projections from 3a and 3b into areas 1 and 2 permit neurons in areas 1 and 2 to respond to complex features such as edge orientation. Neurons in areas 3b and 2 respond only to touch, and neurons in area 3a respond only to position sense. Area 2 neurons have both; thus, neurons respond best when an object is held in the hand and manipulated. Areas 1 and 2 also are activated when the hand is actually moving around objects.

The somatosensory areas also project to the posterior parietal cortex (Brodmann's areas 5 and 7). The cells that have complex projections receive inputs from several modalities that are often related to movement. Thus, information from tactile discrimination and position sense is integrated with visual information and neural information from the brain stem, thalamus, and temporal lobe.[86]

Sensory Receptor Interactions with Sensory Discrimination

Although each sensory receptor is described in detail under the Augmented Therapeutic Intervention section of this chapter, these receptors are discussed within this section to help the reader develop an understanding of how these receptors work to aid somatosensory discrimination. These receptors are classified as proprioceptors (position and location in space) or exterosensory receptors, providing information about the environment primarily through the superficial skin and some of the deep skin receptors. Proprioception is considered position sense, and kinesthesia is movement position.

PROPRIOCEPTION: SENSORY RECEPTORS IN THE MUSCLE AND THE TENDON

The proprioceptors include the muscle spindle, the Golgi tendon organ, and the joint receptors (free nerve endings, Ruffini corpuscles, and pacinian corpuscles). The proprioceptive system modulates the alpha motor neurons. Muscle spindle afferents also facilitate polysynaptically agonistic synergies while dampening antagonists. Information from the muscle spindle is simultaneously sent through ascending pathways to the ipsilateral cerebellum and contralateral parietal lobe.

The muscle spindle plays an important role in ongoing peripheral feedback mechanisms within the CNS, regulating continuous neuroexcitation at the level of the spinal cord and brain stem. These fibers do not contribute to muscle force but rather to length.

The Golgi tendon organ and the muscle spindles together provide complementary information about the mechanical state of muscle, length, and degree of tension. Information on length is used by the brain to determine the position of the limb segment. The length of the muscle varies with the angle of the joint. The information from the Golgi tendon organ is useful for maintaining a steady grip on objects and compensatory for fatigue (e.g., steady neural drive). Muscle stretch fires the spindle afferent, whereas, the Golgi tendon organ only shows light, inconsistent increases. When the muscle contracts after motor nerve stimulation, the firing rate of the Golgi tendon organ increases where the spindle decreases.

EXTEROCEPTOR SYSTEM: SOMATOSENSORY SYSTEM

In the exteroceptor system, there are sensory end organs located primarily in the superficial and subcutaneous layers of the skin. The somatosensory receptors are densest in the fingertips, the lips, and the tip of the tongue and have the greatest capacity for fine discrimination of touch stimuli. The sense of touch is most discriminative in the fingertips. Humans can feel the shape and texture of objects from information transmitted to the brain from mechanoreceptors in the fingers. The somatic modalities are segregated functionally in the CNS, and they are combined for coherent perception. These areas also contain more encapsulated receptors and more afferent neurons, also transmitting along thicker fibers. They also have the greatest representation on the cortical gyri.

There are four types of receptors in the skin. The rapidly adapting Meissner corpuscles are in the superficial skin (providing an instantaneous sense of contact and flutter).[29] The slowly adapting Merkel cells are also in the superficial skin. These group II receptors respond to slow movements across the skin and light pressure, which is associated with pleasure.[30] Meissner's corpuscles are used in two-point discrimination and stereognosis. The deeper subcutaneous tissue contains the rapidly adapting pacinian corpuscles, which respond to vibration (and provide information on posture, position, and ambulation).[222] These adapt very quickly and are activated by deep pressure and quick stretch, which also stimulate the muscle spindle.[86, 141, 191] The slowly adapting Ruffini corpuscles are also deep.[29] They respond to rapid indentation of the skin.

Tactile information from the periphery reaches the cortex by several pathways, carrying unique and redundant information. Also, parallel ascending pathways project to multicortical areas. So there are five representations of the body surface in the parietal cortex: one in S-II and four in S-I. This allows parallel processing to enable neural pathways to send the brain relays to deal with the same information in different ways. Information from S-I (area 2) sends information from the entire body surface to the primary motor cortex.

Assessment of Somatosensory Function

When evaluating the somatosensory system, it is important to provide multiple trials of stimuli to measure localization of light touch, kinesthesia, two-point discrimination, stereognosis, graphesthesia (interpretation of passive stimuli delivered to the skin), proprioception, and perception of sharpness and dullness. Two-point discrimination and detection of sharp and dull are traditionally included in the neurological examination. A discriminator can be used for easy testing of two-point discrimination.[186] Tests of localization, kinesthesia, stereognosis, and graphesthesia can be found in the Jean Ayres Sensory Integration and Praxis Test.[12] However, because this test is normed on children, tests of stereognosis may need to be elaborated, such as with the key test (matching a key by tactile exploration to a Xerox of the key).[195] It is also important to measure the strength of grip,[272] pinch, and strength of intrinsics to make sure there is no weakness associated with the sensory dysfunction.[169] The patient should complete several standardized fine-motor tasks, such as the Purdue Pegboard Test,[182] tapping speed,[238] and motor reaction time.[35] For measuring subtle changes over time, it can be helpful to videotape the patient doing several fine-motor tasks, such as using the computer, playing an instrument, or writing. An ordinal scale can be created to grade the quality of movement, again to standardize the measurement and quantify change. Furthermore, the patient should complete some type of functional independence measure to document how much an upper-extremity problem interferes with the ability to care for oneself and work.

Intervention: Sensory Discriminative Retraining

The intervention strategies for retraining sensory discrimination are based on the principles of neuroplasticity (see Table 4–1). It should be remembered, however, that the sensory and motor systems are intimately linked. Thus, while one is focused on improving the responsiveness and the accuracy of the somatosensory system, the ultimate goal is usually to improve fine-motor voluntary control.

To set the stage for the patient to benefit from sensory retraining of the hands in particular, the patient must become more aware of how he or she uses the involved extremity, particularly the hand. Appendix 4–A describes recommended strategies for how to use the hands in a stress-reduced way. If one works on sensory retraining and the individual continues to overuse unnecessary forces for self-care, then even effective retraining will not have the maximum benefit on restoration of function.

Appendix 4–B summarizes some activities recommended for sensory discriminative retraining. All activities must be attended, and all sensory modalities should be included. For the most part, the eyes must be closed because patients will depend on vision when the eyes are open, especially when somatosensory feedback is decreased. The sensory stimulation tasks must progress in difficulty. The emphasis initially should be on the cutaneous receptors (light touch). The performance accuracy should be close to 80%. All trials should involve feedback to determine if performance was correct. The tasks should be performed in different contexts and with the patient in different positions to maximize information processing from all possible sensory areas. When a sensory stimulus is delivered to the fingers, the most involved digits should be targeted. Stimulation should be on the distal pads and the side of the fingers to help restore the individual nature of the digits. The stimulation should involve active and passive stimulation with static and moving stimuli. It is critical to have someone assist by providing these passive stimulation challenges. Furthermore, it is important to move from meaningful letters and numbers to designs to increase the challenge of the sensory task. The sensory task ultimately needs to be incorporated into functional tasks, particularly those that are difficult for the patient. There must be significant repetition in the performance of these tasks. The patient probably needs to spend at least 1 to 1.5 hours a day doing specific sensory discrimination tasks. Ultimately, computer-based sensory games may help drive faster change in the nervous system.

Some people with somatosensory degradation also have problems with movement control (e.g. focal hand dystonia).[15, 52] There is an intimate close relationship between all higher-order perceptual and movement processes. The brain must correlate sensory inputs with motor outputs to accurately assess the body's interaction with the environment. Thus, dysfunction in sensory processing can lead to serious problems in motor control.[163] To carry out effective sensory discriminative retraining, it is important not to elicit abnormal movements and tension. When abnormal patterns of movement are repeated, they, too, can be learned; however, this would be considered negative learning. Movement problems have also been noticed in patients with chronic pain. Coincidentally, cortical differences have also been reported in the primary sensory cortex for patients with chronic pain, similar to those reported in patients with hand dystonia.[104, 298]

The deep receptors should also be included in retraining. Appendix 4–B summarizes some activities that can be used to facilitate the sensitivity and accuracy of these deep receptors. Even though the deep receptors are in area 3a, they provide information on proprioception and kinesthesia through deep pressure, tapping, weight bearing, and muscle stretch. These receptors also contribute information to the sensorimotor feedback loop that guides graded contractions and coordinated movements. Deep pressure can also contribute toward object recognition (size, shape, and attributes). Static and dynamic joint position and location sense should also be addressed to help improve motor control and control joint movement. These stimulation activities should be distinguished from discriminative touch. By having subjects practice lifting items of the same and different weights with rough surfaces such as Velcro applied, it is possible to begin to enhance gradations of force. Subjects will squeeze objects with a smooth surface harder than the same objects with a rough surface. Practicing controlled grasp and release strategies in functional tasks also contributes toward the development of proprioception and kinesthesia. Giving the extremity some resistance is another method of enhancing proprioception. Each of the behaviors must require a decision and be rewarded with feedback.

Sometimes it is difficult to perform sensory retraining activities without causing abnormal motor movements. This may be an indication to use imagery instead of physical practice. Imagery involves creating an internal representation of an object or a task without physical operation on the object or the task. Thus, in sensory discriminative programs, visual imagery, motor imagery, and/or mental rehearsal of a sequential task such as playing an instrument may assist the patient in restoring a sense of "normality." It has been well established that mental practice is successful in improving performance in sports.[249] It has also been used extensively in trying to control physiological states such as blood pressure[2, 8, 73, 265] and to increase immunity to fight cancer.[76]

Current technology has allowed us to measure the blood flow in the brain while individuals are imaging. The hypothesis is that direct matching predicts the areas that contain the neurons that discharge during action execution regardless of how action is elicited. At least a subset of the neurons should encode the action as carried out as well as imagined. Thus, the cortical areas should have motor properties that become more active when the action to be executed is elicited by observation or imaging of the task. Recent research suggests that visual imagery is associated with increased activity in the somatosensory cortex, whereas motor imagery is associated with increased activity in the motor cortex.[74] In both types of imagery as well as actual motor performance, the same cortical area is recruited.[73] However, during imaged performance, the cortical activity level is approximately 30% of that measured during actual task performance.[248] Abbruzzese and associates [1] note that the excitability of the human cortex increases both during execution and mental imagination of a sequential finger task but not a repetitive finger movement. This suggests that retraining must be goal oriented, attended, and variable, not simple, simultaneous, or repetitious without attention.

Appendix 4–C outlines some of the functions that patients who have somatosensory problems associated with chronic pain or movement dysfunction are encouraged to visually image. Some patients can perform mental imagery more easily than others. Patients have to be able to isolate themselves, focus intensively on the task at hand, and be uninterrupted in this process. During a session, an individual should focus on this aspect of retraining for approximately 45 minutes to an hour. Patients may find it helpful to purchase a book on how to do imagery, take a course on mental imagery, or work with an individual counselor who can help them with this process.

In summary, sensory discriminative retraining as discussed within this section includes a complex process of retraining that adapts the principles of neuroplasticity to restore normal sensory and motor function. The retraining program is comprehensive, addressing first prevention and stress-free use of the arms. This specific sensory retraining includes both concerns about superficial somatosensory receptors and proprioceptive or deep receptors. The specific sensory discriminative activities are supplemented with visual imagery, motor imagery, and mental practice to facilitate maximum restoration of function.

CONCLUSION

There are treatment techniques that are universally applied to the very young and the very old. As discussed under the Neuroplasticity section, the CNS is in a constant state of change throughout life. The brain is unique to each individual. Each brain has idiosyncrasies but also has an enormous number of predictable responses. These factors affect the success or failure of a client/therapist interaction. After thorough evaluation the therapist must decide which treatment is appropriate and the most efficient course of intervention. The options include functional retraining, augmented and contrived intervention using a classification scheme, or somatosensory reintegration. No matter the intervention, the therapist must cognitively organize intervention options while developing a greater clinical repertoire of intervention strategies.

When specific augmented interventions are needed, the therapist must select specific treatments according to the needs of the client, the time available for therapy, the level and extent of the impairment/disability involvement, the motivation of the client and his/her family, the creativity of the therapist, the pathology, and the course of a disease process. A therapist must choose whether somatosensory retraining, functional training, augmented treat-

ment interventions, or any combination of these three will provide the client with the most efficacious, cost-effective, and quickest map to functional independence or maximal quality of life. How each therapist combines the interventions with the client's specific needs will vary according to education, belief, skill, and openness to learning from the total environment itself.

REFERENCES

1. Abbruzzese G, Trompetto C, Schieppati M: The excitability of the human motor cortex increases during execution and mental imagination of sequential but not repetitive finger movements. Exp Brain Res 111:476–472, 1966.
2. Achterberg J: Imagery in Healing: Shamanism and Modern Medicine. Shambhala, Boston, Shambhala, 1985.
3. Ahissar E, Vaadia E, Ahissar M, et al: Dependence of cortical plasticity on corelated activity of single neurons and on behavioral context. Science 257:1412–1415, 1992.
4. Ahissar M, Hochstein S: Attentional control of early perceptual learning. Proc Natl Acad Sci U S A 90:5718–5422, 1993.
5. Aitkin LM: The auditory system. In Bjorklund A, Hokfeld T, Swanson LW (eds): Handbook of Chemical Neuroanatomy, Vol 7, Integrated Systems of the CNS Part II. New York, Elsevier, 1989.
6. Allard TA, Clark SA, Jenkins WM, Merzenich MM: Reorganization of somatosensory area 3b representation in adult owl monkeys following digital syndactyly. J Neurophysiol 66:1048–1058, 1991.
7. Allensworth A: A practical guide to the use of music with geriatrics. Aging Perfections 16(1):9, 1993.
8. Andrew BL, Dodt E: The deployment of sensory nerve endings at the knee joint in a cat. Acta Physiol Scand 28:287–296, 1953.
9. Ayers AJ: Sensory Integration and Learning Disabilities, Los Angeles, Western Psychological Services, 1972.
10. Ayers AJ: The Development of Sensory Integrative Theory and Practice. Dubuque, IA, Kendall/Hunt Publishing Co, 1974.
11. Ayers AJ: Sensory Integration and the Child. Los Angeles, Western Psychological Services, 1979.
12. Ayers A: Sensory Integration and Praxis Test (SIPT) Manual. Los Angeles, CA, Western Psychological Association, 1989.
13. Baddeley A, Wilson BA: A developmental deficit in short-term phonological memory: Implications for language and reading. Memory 1:65–78, 1993.
14. Bandler R, Grindler J: The Structure of Magic. Palo Alto, CA, Science and Behavior Books, 1975.
15. Bara-Jimenez W, Catalan H, Hallett M, Gerloff C: Abnormal somatosensory homunculus in dystonia of the hand. Ann Neurol 44:828–831, 1998.
16. Barnes GR: Head-eye coordination in normals and in patients with vestibular disorders. Proceedings of the Barany Society, Uppsala, Sweden. Adv Otorhinolaryngol 25:15, 1978.
17. Barnes GR, Forbat LN: Cervical and vestibular afferent control of oculomotor response in man. Acta Otolaryngol (Stockh) 88:79–87, 1979.
18. Barnes JF: Myofascial Release, 3rd ed. Paoli, PA, Rehabilitation Service, 1990.
19. Barr ML, Kiernan JA (eds): The Human Nervous System: an Anatomical Viewpoint, 6th ed. Philadelphia, JB Lippincott, 1990.
20. Benasich AA, Tallal P Auditory temporal processing thresholds, habituation, and recognition memory over the first year. Infant Behav Develop 19:339–356, 1996.
21. Benjamen RM, Walker WI: Somatic receiving areas of cerebral cortex in the squirrel monkey (Saimie sciureus). J Neurophysiol 20:286–299, 1957.
22. Bertoti DB: Effect of therapeutic horseback riding on posture in children with cerebral palsy, Phys Ther Forum 68:1505–1512, 1988.
23. Bessou P, Burgess PR, Perl ER, Taylor CB: Dynamic properties of mechanoreceptors with unmyelinated (C) fibers. J Neurophysiol 34:116–131, 1971.
24. Bieser A, Moller-Preuss P Auditory responsive cortex in the squirrel monkey: Neural responses to amplitude-modulated sounds. Exp Brain Res 108:273–284, 1996.
25. Bishop B: Vibration stimulation: I Neurophysiology of motor re-

sponses evoked by vibratory stimulation. Phys Ther 54:1273–1281, 1974.

26. Bishop B: Vibratory stimulation: II. Vibratory stimulation as an evaluation tool. Phys Ther 55:29–33, 1975.

27. Bishop DV: The underlying nature of specific language impairment. J Child Psychol Psychiat Allied Discipl 33:3–66, 1992.

28. Bizzi E, Abend W: Posture control and trajectory formation in single and multi-finger movements. In Desmedt JE (ed): Motor Control Mechanisms in Health and Disease. Advances in Neurology, vol 39, New York, Raven Press, 1983, pp 31–45.

29. Blake DT, Hsiao SS, Johnson K: Neural coding mechanisms in tactile pattern recognition: The relative contributions of slowly and rapidly adapting mechanoreceptors to perceived roughness. J Neurosci 17:7480–7489, 1997.

30. Blake DT, Johnson KO, Hsiao SS: Monkey cutaneous SAI and RA responses to raised and depressed scanned patterns: Effects of width, height, orientation, and a raised surround. J Neurophysiol 78:2503–2517, 1997.

31. Blashy MRM Fuchs R: Orthokinetics: A new receptor facilitation method. Am J Ther 8:5, 1959.

32. Bobath B: Adult Hemiplegia: Evaluation and Treatment 2nd ed. London, William Heinemann Medical Books, 1978.

33. Bobath B: Abnormal Postural Reflex Activity Caused by Brain Lesions, 3rd ed. Frederick, MD, Aspen Publications, 1985.

34. Bobath K, Bobath B: Cerebral palsy. In Pearson PH, Williams CE (eds): Physical Therapy Services in Developmental Disabilities, Springfield, IL, Charles C Thomas, 1972.

35. Bohannon RW: Stopwatch for measuring thumb movement time. Percept Mot Skills 81:122–126, 1995.

36. Booker J: Pain: It's all in your patient's head (or is it)? Nursing 82:47–51, 1982.

37. Borenstein M, Sigman M: Infant Intelligence quotient predictable by gaze. Child Dev 57:251–274, 1987.

38. Brecker LR: Imagery and ROM combine to create. Adv Phys Ther 5(2):18–19, 1994.

39. Brewer S: Personal correspondence with composer, pianist, and theoritician in use of sound in harmony with body rhythms, August 1983.

40. Brunnstrom S: Movement Therapy in Hemiplegia, 2nd ed. Philadelphia, JB Lippincott, 1992.

41. Buonomano DV, Hickmott PW, Merzenich MM: Context-sensitive synaptic plasticity and temporal-to-spatial transformations in hippocampal slices. Proc Natl Acad Sci U S A 94:10403–10408, 1997.

42. Buonomano DV, Merzenich MM: Temporal information transformed into a spatial code by a network with realistic properties. Science 267:1028–1030, 1995.

43. Buonomano DV, Merzenich MM: Net interaction between different forms of short-term synaptic plasticity and slow-IPSPs in the hippocampus and auditory cortex. J Neurophysiol 80:1765–1774, 1998.

44. Buomomano DV, Merzenich MM: Cortical plasticity: From synapses to maps. Ann Rev Neurosci 21:149–186, 1998.

45. Burke RE, Rudomin P, Zajac FE: Catch property in single mammalian motor units. Science 168:122–124, 1974.

46. Burt AM: Textbook of Neuroanatomy. Philadelphia, WB Saunders, 1993.

47. Butler DS: Adverse mechanical tension inthe nervous system: A model for assessment and treatment. Aust J Physiother 35:227–238, 1989.

48. Butler DS: Mobilization of the Nervous System. New York, Churchill Livingstone, 1991.

49. Butler RA: The cumulative effects of differential stimulus repetition rates on the auditory evoked response in man. Electroencephalogr Clin Neurophysiol 35:337–345, 1973.

50. Buttram B, Brown G: Developmental Physical Management for the Multi-disabled Child. Tuscaloosa, University of Alabama Press, 1977.

51. Buzski G: Memory consolidation during sleep: A neurophysiological perspective. J Sleep Res 1:17–23, 1998.

52. Byl H, Merzenich MM, Jenkins WM: A primate genesis model of focal hand dystonia and repetitive strain injury: I. Learning-induced dedifferentiation of the representation of the hand in the primary somatosensory cortex in adult monkeys, Neurology 47:508–520, 1996.

53. Cain WS (ed): Odors, evaluation utilization and control. Ann NY Acad Sci 2371:439, 1974.

54. Campbell S: Clinics in Physical Therapy, 2nd ed, vol 5. New York, Churchill-Livingstone, 1992.

55. Carr JH, Sheperd RB: A motor Relearning for Stroke. Frederick, MD, Aspen Publishers, 1987.

56. Carr JH, Sheperd RB: Movement Science: Foundations for Physical Therapy in Rehabilitation. Frederick, MD, Aspen Publishers, 1987.

57. Case J: Sensory Mechanisms: Current Concepts in Biology. New York, Macmillan, 1966.

58. Cauna N: The effects of aging on the receptor organs of the human dermis. In Montagna W (ed): Advances in Biology of Skin, Vol 6, Aging, New York, Pergamon Press, 1965.

59. Chelazzi L, Duncan J, Miller EK, Desimone R: Responses of neurons in inferior temporal cortex during memory-guided visual search. J Neurophysiol 80:2918–2940, 1998.

60. Chen R, Hallett M: Focal dystonia and repetitive motion disorders. Clin Orthop Rel Res 351:102–106, 1998.

61. Cherney L: Aging and communication. In Lewis C (ed): Aging: The Health Care Challenge. Philadelphia, FA Davis, 1989.

62. Clark SA, Allard T, Jenkins WM, Merzenich MM: Receptive fields in the body-surface map in adult cortex defined by temporally correlated inputs. Nature 332:444–445, 1988.

63. Cohen H (ed): Neuroscience Rehabilitation. Philadelphia, JB Lippincott, 1993.

64. Colavita F: Sensory Changes in the Elderly. Springfield, IL, Charles C Thomas, 1978.

65. Cook J: The therapeutic use of music: A literature review. Nurs Forum 20(3):252–256, 1981.

66. Cooper BA, Letts L, Rigby P: Exploring the use of color cueing on an assistive device in the home: Six case studies. Phys Occup Ther Geriatr 11(4):47, 1993.

67. Cooper S: Muscle spindles in the intrinsic muscles of the human tongue. J Physiol 122:193, 1953.

68. Craik R: Abnormalities of motor behavior. In Lister MJ (ed): Contemporary Management of Motor Control Problems. Norman, OK, Foundation for Physical Therapy, 1991.

69. Craik R: Spasticity revisited. In APTA Combined Section Meetings, New Orleans, Louisiana, 1996.

70. Crutchfield CA, Barnes MR (eds): Motor Control and Motor Learning in Rehabilitation, 2nd ed. Atlanta, Stokesville Publications, 1993.

71. de Groot J: Correlative Neuroanatomy, 21st ed. San Mateo, CA, Lange Medical Publications, 1991.

72. Debenham G: The healing art. Can Med Assoc J 149:1994, 1993.

73. Decety J: Do imagined and executed actions share the same neural substrate? Brain Res Cogn Brain Res 1996 3:87–93, 1996.

74. Decety J, Perani D, Jeannerod M, et al: The neurophysiological basis of motor imagery. Behav Brain Res 77:45–52, 1996.

75. Demerens C, Stankoff B, Logak M, et al: Induction of myelination in the central nervous system by electrical activity. Proc Natl Acad Sci U S A 93:9887–9992, 1996.

76. Derogatis R, Abeloff MD, Melisaratos N: Psychological coping mechanisms and survival time in metastatic breast cancer. JAMA 242:1504–1508, 1979.

77. Desmedt JE: Patterns of motor command during various types of voluntary movement in man. In Evarts EV, Wise SP, Bousfield D (eds): The Motor System in Neurobiology. New York, Elsevier, 1995, pp 133–139.

78. Desmedt JE, Godaux E: Fast motor units are not preferentially activated in rapid voluntary contractions in man. Nature 267:717–719, 1977.

79. DeWierdt J: Spectral processing deficit in dyslexic children. Appl Psychol 9:163–174, 1989.

80. DiGuisto EL, Bond N: Imagery and the autonomic nervous system: Some methodological issues. Percept Motor Skills 48:427–438, 1979.

81. Dobkin B: Neuroplasticity: Key to recovery after CNS injury. West J Med 159:56–60, 1993.

82. Downie RA: Cash's Textbook of Neurology for Physiotherapists. Philadelphia, JB Lippincott, 1986.

83. Duensing F, Schaefer KP: The activity of various neurons of the reticular formation of the unfettered rabbit during head turning and vestibular stimulation. Arch Psychiatr Nervenkr 201:97–122, 1960. (In German).

84. Duncan PW (ed): Balance proceedings of the APTA Forum. Alexandria, VA, APTA, 1989.

85. Dwyer B: Detecting hearing loss and improving communication in elderly persons. Focus Geriatr Care Rehabil 1(16):3–4, 1987.

86. Eckert E: Muscle and movement. In Animal Physiology: Mechanisms and Adaptations, 3rd ed. New York, Freeman, 1988.

87. Eden GG, Stein JF, Wood HM, Wood FB: Temporal and spatial processing in reading disabled and normal children. Cortex 31:451–468, 1995.

88. Eggermont JJ: Temporal modulation transfer functions for AM and FM stimuli in cat auditory cortex: Effects of carrier type, modulating waveform and intensity. Hear Res 74:51–66, 1994.

89. Eklund G, Hagbarth KE: Normal variability of tonic vibration reflexes in man. Exp Neurol 16:80–92, 1966.

90. Elbert T, Candia V, Altenmuller E, et al: Alteration of digital representations in somatosensory cortex in focal hand dystonia. Neuroreport 9:3571–3575, 1998.

91. Eldred E: Peripheral receptors: Their excitation and relation to reflex patterns. Am J Phys Med 46(1):69–72, 1967.

92. Elvey RL: Physical evaluation and treatment of neural tissues in disorders of the neuromusculoskeletal system: Neural and brachial plexus tension. Course handout. San Jose, CA, Northeast Seminars, unpublished.

93. Engert F, Bonhoeffer T: Dendritic spine changes associated with hippocampal long-term synaptic plasticity. Nature 399:66–70, 1999.

94. Farber S: Sensorimotor Evaluation and Treatment Procedures, 2nd ed. Indianapolis, Indiana University—Purdue University at Indianapolis Medical Center, 1974.

95. Farber S: A multisensory approach to neurorehabilitation. In Farber S (ed): Neurorehabilitation: A Multisensory Approach, Philadelphia, WB Saunders, 1982.

96. Farmer ME, Klein R: The evidence for a temporal processing deficit linked to dyslexia: A review. Psychonom Bull Rev 2:460–493, 1995.

97. Fay T: The neurophysical aspects of therapy in cerebral palsy. In Payton OP, Hirt S, Newton RA: Neurophysiologic Approach to Therapeutic Exercise. Philadelphia, FA Davis, 1978.

98. Feldenkrais M: Awareness Through Movement. New York, Harper & Row, 1977.

99. Feldenkrais M: The Elusive Obvious. Cupertino, CA, Meta Publication, 1981.

100. Felton DL, Felton SY: A regional and systemic overview of functional neuroanatomy. In Farber SA (ed): Neurorehabilitation: a Multisensory Approach. Philadelphia, WB Saunders, 1982.

101. Fields HL: Pain. New York, McGraw-Hill, 1987.

102. Fisher AG, Murray EA, Bundy AC: Sensory Integration: Theory & Practice, Philadelphia, FA Davis, 1991.

103. Fleschig P: Anatomie des menschlichen Gehirns und Ruckenmarks auf myelogenetischen Grundlage. Liepzig, Georg Thieme, 1920.

104. Flor H, Braun C, Elbert T, Birbaumer N: Extensive reorganization of primary somatosensory cortex in chronic back pain patients. Neurosci Lett 224:5–8, 1997.

105. Flynn J: Snoezelen. Ede, Holland, Hartenberg, 1986.

106. Frank A, Maurer P, Shepherd J: Light and sound environment: A survey of neonatal intensive care units. Phys Occup Ther Pediatr 11(2):27–45, 1991.

107. Freeman G: Hippotherapy/therapeutic horseback riding. Clin Man Phys Ther 4(3):20–25, 1984.

108. Gandhavadi B, et al: Autonomic pain: Features and methods of assessment. Pain 71:85–90, 1982.

109. Gardner E: Fundamentals of Neurology. Philadelphia, WB Saunders, 1975.

110. Garliner D: Myofunctional Therapy. Philadelphia, WB Saunders, 1976.

111. Geinisman Y, deToledo-Morrell L, Morrell F, et al: Structural synaptic correlate of long-term potentiation: Formation of axospinous synapses with multiple, completely partitioned transmission zones. Hippocampus 3:435–445, 1993.

112. Gelb M: Body Learning—an Introduction to the Alexander Technique. London, Auburn Press, 1981.

113. Geldard FA: The Human Senses, 2nd ed. New York, John Wiley & Sons, 1972.

114. Gelhorn E: Principles of Autonomic-Somatic Integration: Physiological Basis and Psychological and Clinical Implication. Minneapolis, University of Minnesota Press, 1967.

115. Gerhart KD, et al: Inhibitory receptive fields of primitive spinothalamic tract cells. J Neurophysiol 46:1309–1325, 1981.

116. Gilfoyle EM, Grady AP, Moore JC: Children Adapt. Thorofare, NJ, Charies B Slack, 1981.

117. Giliam RB, Cowan N, Day LS: Sequential memory in children with and without language impairment. J Speech Hear Res 38:393–402, 1995.

118. Gill-Body KM, et al: Physical therapy management of peripheral vestibular dysfunction: Two clinical case reports. Phys Ther 74:130–142, 1994.

119. Gimbel T: Healing Through Colour. Suffron Halden, England, CW Daniel, 1980.

120. Gladsone VS: Hearing loss in the elderly. Am J Phys Occup Ther Geriatr 2:5–20, 1992.

121. Gould JA: Orthopedic and Sports Physical Therapy. St. Louis, CV Mosby, 1990.

122. Grajski KA, Merzenich MM: Hebb-type dynamics is sufficient to account for the inverse magnification rule in cortical somatotopy. Neural Computation 2:74–81, 1990.

123. Grajski KS, Merzenich MM: Neuronal network simulation of somatosensory representational plasticity. In Touretzky DL (ed): Neural Information Processing Systems, vol 2. San Mateo, CA, Morgan Kaufman 1990.

124. Granit R: Receptors and Sensory Perception. New Haven, CT, Yale University Press, 1967.

125. Green JH: Basic Clinical Physiology. Oxford, Oxford University Press, 1973.

126. Greenberg JH, et al: Metabolic mapping of functional activity in human subjects with the fluorodeoxyglucose technique. Science 212:678–680, 1981.

127. Greenough WT, Chang FF: In Peters A, Jones EG (eds): Cerebral Cortex, vol 7. New York, Plenum, 1988, pp 335–392.

128. Groen JJ: Vestibular stimulation and its effects from the point of view of theoretical physics. Neurology 21:380, 1961.

129. Groer MW, Shekleton ME: Basic Pathophysiology, 2nd ed. St. Louis, CV Mosby, 1983.

130. Grollman S: The Human Body—its Structure and Physiology, 2nd ed. New York, Macmillan, 1970.

131. Guyton A: Basic Neuroscience: Anatomy and Physiology. Philadelphia, WB Saunders, 1991.

132. Haenny PE, Maunsell JH, Schiller PH: State dependent activity in monkey cortex: II. Retinal and extraretinal factors in V4. Exp Brain Res 69:245–259, 1988.

133. Hagbarth KE, Eklund G: Tonic vibration reflexes in spasticity. Brain Res 2:201–203, 1966.

134. Hagbarth KE, Wohlfart G: The number of muscles in cat in relation to the composition of the muscle nerves. Acta Anat 15:85, 1952.

135. Haier RJ, Siegel BV, MacLachlan E, et al: Regional glucose metabolic changes after learning a complex visuospatial/motor task: A positron emission tomographic study. Brain Res 570:134–143, 1992.

136. Harel S, Nachson I: Dichotic listening to temporal tonal stimuli by good and poor readers. Percept Motor Skills 84:467–473, 1997.

137. Harl R, Kiesila P: Deficit of temporal auditory processing in dyslexic adults. Neurosci Lett 205:138–140, 1990.

138. Head H: Studies in Neurology, vol 2. Oxford, Oxford University Press, 1920.

139. Hebb DO: The Organization of Behavior. New York, Wiley, 1949.

140. Heiniger MC, Randolph SL: Neurophysiological Concepts in Human Behavior. St. Louis, CV Mosby, 1981.

141. Heinsen A: Visual Motor Development. Palo Alto, CA, Learning Opportunities: Stanford Professional Center, 1973.

142. Henderson A: Body schema and the visual guidance of movement. In Henderson A, Coryell J (eds): The Body Senses and Perceptual Deficit. Boston, Boston University Press, 1973.

143. Herdman SJ: Assessment and treatment of balance disorders in the vestibular-deficient patient. In Duncan PW (ed): Balance. Alexandria, VA, APTA, 1990.

144. Herdman SJ: Exercise strategies in vestibular disorders. Ear Nose Throat 68:961–964, 1990.

145. Hopson JA: The Dreaming Brain. New York, Basic Books, 1989.

146. Horak FB, et al: Vestibular function and motor proficiency in children with impaired hearing, or with learning disability and motor impairment. Dev Med Child Neurol 30:64–79, 1988.

147. Horak FB, et al: Effects of vestibular rehabilitation on dizziness and imbalance. Otolaryngol Head Neck Surg 106:175–180, 1992.

148. Houk J, Hennemou E: Responses of Golgi tendon organs. J Neurophysiol 30:466–489, 1967.
149. Houk JD, Rymer WA: Neural control of muscle length and tension. In Brooks VB (ed): Handbook of Physiology, Section 1: The Nervous System, Vol II, Motor Control Part 1. Bethesda, MD, American Physiological Society, 1981, pp 257–323.
150. Hsiao SS, O'Shaugnessy DM, Johnson KO: Effects of selective attention on spatial form processing in monkey primary and secondary somatosensory cortex. J Neurophysiol 70:444–457, 1993.
151. Hubel D, Weisel T: Brain mechanisms of vision. Sci Am 241:130–162, 1979.
152. Huss J: Sensorimotor Treatment Approaches in Occupational Therapy. Philadelphia, JB Lippincott, 1971.
153. Huss J: Workshop, San Jose State University, Neurophysiological approaches to treatment. Unpublished class notes, 1980.
154. Iggo A: A single unit analysis of cutaneous receptor with C afferent fibers. CIBA foundation groups. Springfield, IL, Charles C Thomas, 1967.
155. Jackson O: Clinics in Physical Therapy, vol 14, Therapeutic Considerations for the Elderly. New York, Churchill Livingstone, 1987.
156. Jackson O: The Feldenkrais method: A personalized learning model. In Lister MJ (ed): Contemporary Management of Motor Control Problems. Norman, OK, Foundation for Physical Therapy, 1991.
157. Jacob S, Francone C: Structure and Function in Man, 3rd ed. Philadelphia, WB Saunders, 1974.
158. James W: The Principles of Psychology, vol 1. New York, Dover, 1890.
159. Jenkins WM, Merzenich MM, Ochs M, et al: (1990) Functional reorganization of primary somatosensory cortex in adult owl monkeys after behaviorally controlled tactile stimulation. J Neurophysiol 63:82–104, 1990.
160. Johnstone M: Restoration of Normal Movement after Stroke. New York, Churchill Livingstone, 1995.
161. Kaas JH, Hacket TA, Tamo MJ: Auditory processing in primate cerebral cortex. Current Opin Neurobiol 9:164–170, 1999.
162. Kandel ER, Schwartz JH, Jessell TM: Essentials of Neural Science and Behavior. Norwalk, CT, Appleton Lange, 1995.
163. Kandel ER, Schwartz JH, Jessell TM: Principles of Neural Science, 3rd ed. New York, Elsevier Medical Science, 1991.
164. Kandel ER, Schwartz JH, Jessel TM: Principles of Neural Science, 4th ed. New York, McGraw-Hill, 2000.
165. Karni A: When practice makes perfect. Lancet 345:395, 1995.
166. Karni A, Sagi D: Where practice makes perfect in texture discrimination: Evidence for primary visual cortex plasticity. Proc Natl Acad Sci U S A 88:4966–4970, 1991.
167. Kaster S, Pinsk MA, deWeerd P, et al: Increased activity in human visual cortex during directed attention in the absence of visual stimulation. Neuron 22:751–761, 1999.
168. Keller A, Arissian K, Asanuma H: Synaptic proliferation in the motor cortex of adult cats after long-term thalamic stimulation. J Neurophysiol 68:295–308, 1992.
169. Kellor M, Frost J, Silverberg N, et al: Norms for clinical use, hand strength and dexterity. Am J Occup Ther 25(2):77–83, 1971.
170. Keshner EA: How theoretical framework biases evaluation and treatment. In Lister MJ (ed): Contemporary Management of Motor Problems. Norman, OK, Foundation for Physical Therapy, 1991.
171. Kilgard MP, Mezenich MM: Cortical map reorganization enabled by nucleus basalis activity. Science 279:1714–1718, 1998.
172. Kilgard MP, Merzenich MM: Plasticity of temporal information processing in the primary auditory cortex. Nature Neurosci 1:727–731, 1999.
173. Kleim JA, Swain RA, Czerlanis CM, et al: Learning-dependent dendritic hypertrophy of cerebellar stellate cells: Plasticity of local circuit neurons. Neurobiol Learn Memory 67:29–33, 1997.
174. Klein-Vogelbach S: Functional Kinetics. New York, Springer-Verlag, 1995.
175. Knickerbocker H: A Holistic Approach to the Treatment of Learning Disorders. Therefore, NJ, Charles B Slack, 1980.
176. Knott M, Voss DE: Proprioceptive Neuromuscular Facilitation. New York, Harper & Row, 1968.
177. Knowles R: Through neurolinguistic programming. Am J Nurs 83:1010, 1983.
178. Kornberg C, McCarthy T: The effect of neural stretching techniques on sympathetic outflow to the lower limbs. J Orthop Sports Phys Ther 16:269–274, 1992.
179. Kottke F: The neurophysiology of motor function. In Kottke F, Stillwell K, Lehmann J (eds): Handbook of Physical Medicine and Rehabilitation, 3rd ed. Philadelphia, WB Saunders, 1982.
180. Kuhl PK: Human adults and human infants show a "perceptual magnet effect" for the prototypes of speech categories, monkeys do not. Percept Psycho 50:93–107, 1991.
181. Kuhl PK: Learning and representation in speech and language. Curr Opin Neurobiol 4:812–822, 1994.
182. Lafayette Instrument Company, PO Box 5729, Lafayette IN 47903. (317) 423–1505. Purdue Pegboard, Model 32020, Instructions and Normative Data
183. Leonard LB Children with Language Impairment. Cambridge, MA, MIT Press, 1998.
184. Leonard LB, Bortoline U: Grammatical morphology and the role of weak syllables in the speech of Italian-speaking children with specific language impairment. J Speech Hear Res 41:1363–1374, 1998.
185. Lim RK: Pain. Annu Rev Physiol 32:269, 1970.
186. Louis S, Greene TL, Jacobson KE, et al: Evaluation of normal values for stationary and moving two point discrimination in the hand. Hand Ther 9A:552–555, 1984.
187. Lundberg I: Why is learning to read a hard task for some children. Scand J Psychol 39:155–167, 1998.
188. Maisden DC, Meadows JC, Hodgson HJ: Observations on the reflex response to muscle vibration in man and its voluntary control. Brain 42:829–846, 1969.
189. Maitland GD: Peripheral Manipulation, 3rd ed. Boston, Butterworths, 1992.
190. Marx J: Analgesia: How the body inhibits pain perception. Science 195:471–473, 1977.
191. Mathews PBC: Proprioceptors and their contribution to somatosensory mapping: Complex messages required complex processing. Can J Physiol Pharmacol 66:430–438, 1988.
192. McAnally KE, Stein JF: Auditory temporal coding in dyslexia. Proc R Soc Lond 263:961–965.
193. McCloskey DI: Kinesthetic sensibility. Physiol Rev 58:763–813, 1978.
194. McCormack GL: Pain management: A role for occupational therapists. Am J Occup Ther 43:4, 1988.
195. McKenzie A: A new test to measure stereognosis: Key Test Abstract. Presented before the annual meeting of the California Chapter of the APTA, Sacramento, October 1997.
196. Melzack R: Myofascial trigger points: Relations to acupuncture and mechanisms of pain. Arch Phys Med Rehabil 62:47–50, 1981.
197. Melzack R, Konard KW, Dubrobsky B: Prolonged changes in the nervous system activity produced by somatic and reticular stimulation. Exp Neurol 25:416–428, 1969.
198. Melzack R, Still well DM, Fox EJ: Trigger points and acupuncture points for pain: Correlations and implication. Pain 1:3–23, 1977.
199. Merzenich MM: Development and maintenance of cortical somatosensory representations: functional "maps" and neuroanatomical repertoires. In Barnard KE, Brazelton TB (eds): Touch: The Foundation of Experience. Madison, WI, International Universities Press, 1990, pp 47–71.
200. Merzenich MM, Allard T, Jenkins WM: Neural ontogeny of higher brain function: Implications of some recent neurophysiological findings. In FranzÈn O, Westman P (eds): Information Processing in the Somatosensory System. London, Macmillan, 1991, pp 293–211.
201. Merzenich MM, deCharms RC: Neural representations, experience and change. In Llinas R, Churchland P (eds): The Mind-Brain Continuum. Boston, MIT Press, 1996, pp 61–81.
202. Merzenich MM, Grajski KA, Jenkins WM, et al: Functional cortical plasticity: Cortical network origins of representational changes. Cold Spring Harbor Symp Quant Biol 55:873–887, 1991.
203. Merzenich MM, Jenkins WM: Cortical representation of learned behaviors. In Anderson P (ed): Memory Concepts. Amsterdam, Elsevier, 1993, pp 437–453.
204. Merzenich MM, Jenkins WM: Reorganization of cortical representations of the hand following alterations of skin inputs induced by nerve injury, skin island transfers, and experience. J Hand Ther 6:89–104, 1993.
205. Merzenich MM, Jenkins WM: Cortical plasticity, learning and

learning dysfunction. In Julesz B, Kovacs I (eds): Maturational Windows and Adult Cortical Plasticity. New York, Addison-Wesley, 1995, pp 247–272.

206. Merzenich MM, Jenkins WM, Johnson P, et al: Temporal processing deficits of language-learning impaired children ameliorated by training. Science 271:77–81, 1996.

207. Merzenich MM, Kaas JH, Sur M, Lin CS: Double representation of the body surface within cytoarchitectonic areas 3b and 1 in "S1" in the owl monkey (Aotus trivirgatus). J Comp Neurol 181:41–73, 1978.

208. Merzenich MM, Miller S, Jenkins WM, et al: Amelioration of the acoustic reception and speech reception deficits underlying language-based learning impairments. In Euler C v (ed): Basic Neural Mechanisms in Cognition and Language. Amsterdam, Elsevier, 1998 pp 143–172.

209. Merzenich MM, Nelson RJ, Kaas JH, et al: Variability in hand surface representations in areas 3b and 1 in adult owl and squirrel monkeys. J Comp Neurol 258:281–296, 1987.

210. Merzenich MM, Recanzone GH, Jenkins WM: How the brain functionally rewires itself. In Arbib M, Robinson JA (eds): Natural and Artificial Parallel Computations. New York, MIT Press, 1991.

211. Merzenich MM, Sameshima K: Cortical plasticity and memory. Curr Opin Neurobiol 3:187–196, 1993.

212. Merzenich MM, Tallal P, Peterson B, et al: Some neurological principles relevant to the origins of—and the cortical plasticity based remediation of—language learning impairments. In Grafman J, Cristen Y (eds): Neuroplasticity: Building a Bridge from the Laboratory to the Clinic. New York, Springer-Verlag, 1998, pp. 169–187.

213. Michels E: Motor behavior in hemiplegia. Phys Ther 45:759–767, 1965.

214. Mills M, Cohen BB: Developmental Movement Therapy. Amherst, MA, The School for Body/Mind Centering, 1979.

215. Montgomery PC: Neurodevelopmental treatment and sensory integrative theory. In Lister MJ (ed): Contemporary Management of Motor Control Problems. Norman, OK, Foundation for Physical Therapy, 1991.

216. Moore JC: Cranial nerves and their importance in current rehabilitation techniques. In Henderson A, Coryell J (eds): The Body Senses and Perceptual Deficit. Boston, Boston University Press, 1973.

217. Moore JC: The Golgi tendon organ and the muscle spindle. Am J Occup Ther 28:415–420, 1974.

218. Moore JC: The Limbic System. Class notes from Bay Area Sensory Symposium, San Francisco, CA, February 1980.

219. Moore JC, Umphred DA: The Vestibular-Visual-Cervical Triad: Foundations for Balance, Posture, Position Sense and Movement and Treatment Implications. San Francisco, 1993.

220. Moulton DG, Turk A, Johnston JW (eds): Methods in Olfactory Research. London, Academic Press, 1975.

221. Mountcastle VB (ed): Sensory receptor and neural encoding: Introduction to sensory processes. In Medical Physiology, 14th ed, vol 2. St. Louis, CV Mosby, 1979.

222. Mriganka S, Wall JT, Kaas JH: Modular distribution of neurons with slowly adapting and rapidly adapting responses in area 3b of somatosensory cortex in monkeys. J Neurophysiol 52:724–742.

223. Mueller HA: Facilitating feeding and prespeech. In Pearson PH, Williams CE (eds): Physical Therapy Services in the Developmental Disabilities. Springfield, IL, Charles C Thomas, 1972.

224. Nagarajan S, Mahncke H, Salz T, et al: Cortical auditory signal processing in poor readers. Proc Natl Acad Sci U S A 96:6483–6488, 1999.

225. Naya Y, Sakai K, Miyashita Y: Activity of primate inferotemporal neurons related to a sought target in pair-association task. Proc Natl Acad Sci U S A 93:2664–2669, 1996.

226. Nelson RJ, Smith BN, Douglas VD: Relationship between sensory responsiveness and premovement activity of quickly adapting neurons in area 3b and 1 of monkey primary somatosensory cortex. Exp Brain Res 84:75–90, 1991.

227. Ninth National Conference on Juvenile Justice: Open forum discussion. Atlanta, GA, March 1982.

228. Noback CR, Strominger NL, Demarest RJ: The Human Nervous System: Introduction and Review, 4th ed. Philadelphia, Lea & Febiger, 1991.

229. Normell LA: The cutaneous thermoregulatory vasomotor response in healthy subjects and paraplegic men. Scand J Clin Invest 4(33):133–138, 1974.

230. Nudo R, Jenkins W, Merzenich M, unpublished observations, 1998.

231. Nudo RJ, Milliken GW, Jenkins WM, Merzenich MM: Use-dependent alterations of movement representations in primary motor cortex of adult squirrel monkeys. J Neurosci 16:785–807, 1995.

232. Oakley B, Benjamin RM: Neurological mechanisms of taste. Physiol Rev 46:173, 1966.

233. Odergren T, Iwassaki N, Borg J, Foressberg H: Impaired sensory-motor integration during grasping in writer's cramp. Brain 119 (pt. 2):569–583, 1996.

234. Olderog Millard KA, Smith JM: The influence of group singing on the behavior of Alzheimer's disease patients. J Music Ther 26:58–70, 1989.

235. Ottoson D: Experiments and concepts in olfactory physiology. Progr Brain Res 23:83–138, 1967.

236. Page D: Neuromuscular reflex therapy as an approach to patient care. Am J Phys Med 46:816–837, 1967.

237. Panizza M, Hallett M, Nilsson J: Reciprocal inhibition in patients with hand cramps. Neurology 39:85–89, 1989.

238. PAR Finger Tapper User's Guide, Psychological Assessment Resources, Inc., 1992. PO Box 998/Odessa, Florida 33556 1–800 331TEST.

239. Parker DE: The vestibular apparatus. Sci Am 243(11):118–130, 1980.

240. Payton OP, Hirt S, Newton RA: Scientific Bases for Neurophysiologic Approaches to Therapeutic Exercise: An Anthology. Philadelphia, FA Davis, 1978.

241. Penfield W, Boldrey E: Somatic motor and sensory representations in the cerebral cortex of man as studied by electrical stimulation. Brain 60:389–443, 1937.

242. Pertovaara A: Modification of human pain threshold by specific tactile receptors. Acta Physiol Scand 107:339–341, 1979.

243. Pfaffman C: Taste, its sensory and motivating properties. Am Sci 52:187–206, 1964.

244. Phillips WA, Singer W: In search of common foundation for cortical computation. Behav Brain Sci 20:657–722, 1997.

245. Plaut DC, McClelland JL, Seidenberg MS, Patterson K: Understanding normal and impaired word reading: Computational principles in quasi-regular domains. Psychol Rev 103:56–115, 1996.

246. Poggio GF, Mountcastle VB: A study of the functional contributions of the lemniscal and spinothalamic systems to somatic sensibility. Bull Johns Hopkins Hosp 106:266–316, 1960.

247. Pollack NJ, Namazi KH: The effect of music participation on the social behavior of Alzheimer's disease patients. J Music Ther 29(1):54–67, 1992.

248. Porro Ca, Francescato MP, Cettolo V, et al: Primary motor and sensory cortex activation during motor performance and motor imagery: A functional magnetic resonance imaging study. J Neurosci 16:7688–7698, 1996.

249. Porter K, Foster J: The Mental Athlete. New York, Ballantine Books, 1986.

250. Pribram KH: Languages of the Brain: Experimental Paradoxes and Principles in Neuropsychology. Englewood Cliffs, NJ, Prentice-Hall, 1971.

251. Prickett CA, Moore RS: The use of music to aid in the memory of Alzheimer's patients. J Music Ther 28(2):101–110, 1991.

252. Prochazka A, Hulliger: Muscle afferent function and its significance for motor control mechanisms during voluntary movements in cat, monkey and man. In Desmedt JE (ed): Advances in Neurology, Vol 39: Motor Control Mechanisms in Health and Disease. New York, Raven Press, 1983, pp 93–132.

253. Pubois BH, Pubols LM: Somatotopic organization of spider monkey somatic sensory cerebral cortex. J Comp Neurol 141:63–76, 1971.

254. Qin YL, McNaughton BL, Skaggs WE, Barnes CA: Phil Trans R Soc Lond 352:1525–1533, 1997.

255. Quillian TA: Neuro-cutaneous relationships in fingerprint skin. In Kornhuber H (ed): The Somatosensory System. Sachs, Germany, Thieme, 1975.

256. Quillian TA, Ridley A: The receptors community in the fingertip. J Physiol 216:15–17, 1971.

257. Quinn JF: Building a body of knowledge-research on therapeutic touch, 1974–1986. J Holistic Nurs 6(1):37–45, 1988.

258. Recanzone GH, Merzenich MM, Dinse HR: Expansion of the cortical representation of a specific skin field in primary somatosensory cortex by intracortical microstimulation. Cerebral Cortex 2:181–196, 1992.

259. Recanzone GH, Merzenich MM, Jenkins WM: Frequency discrimination training engaging a restricted skin surface results in an emergence of a cutaneous response zone in cortical area 3a. J Neurophysiol 67:1057–1070, 1992.

260. Recanzone GH, Merzenich M, Jenkins WM, et al: Topographic reorganization of the hand representational zone in cortical area 3b paralleling improvements in frequency discrimination performance. J Neurophysiol 67:1031–1056, 1992.

261. Recanzone GH, Merzenich MM, Schreiner CS: Changes in the distributed temporal response properties of SI cortical neurons reflect improvements in performance on a temporally-based tactile discrimination task. J Neurophysiol 67:1071–1091, 1992.

262. Recanzone GH, Schreiner CE, Merzenich MM: Plasticity in the frequency representation of primary auditory cortex following discrimination training in adult owl monkeys. J Neurosci 13:87–103, 1993.

263. Reith E, Breidenbach B: Textbook of Anatomy and Physiology, 2nd ed. New York, McGraw-Hill, 1978.

264. Ridding MC, Sheehan G, Rothwell JC, et al: Changes in the balance between motor cortical excitation and inhibition in focal, task-specific dystonia. J Neurol Neurosurg Psychiatry 59:493–498, 1995.

265. Rizzolatti G, Fadiga L, Gallese V, Fogassi L: Brain Res Cong Brain Res 3:131, 1996.

266. Roberts TDM: Neurophysiology of Postural Mechanisms. New York, Plenum, 1967.

267. Roitman DM: Age-associated perceptual changes and the physical environment: Perspectives on environmental adaptation. Isr J Occup Ther 2:14–27, 1993.

268. Rood M: The use of sensory receptors to activate, facilitate and inhibit motor response, autonomic and somatic in developmental sequence. In Scattely C (ed): Approaches to Treatment of Patients with Neuromuscular Dysfunction, Third International Congress, World Federation of Occupational Therapists. Dubuque, IA, William Brown Group, 1962.

269. Rubenstein JLR, Rakic P: Special issue: Genetic control of cortical development. Cerebral Cortex 9:521–654, 1999.

270. Sakai K, Miyashita Y: Neural organization for the long-term memory of paired associates. Nature 354:152–155, 1991.

271. Schmidt RA: Motor learning principles for physical therapy. In Lister MJ (ed): Contemporary Management of Motor Control Problems. Norman, OK, Foundation for Physical Therapy, 1990.

272. Schmidt RT, Towws JV: Grip strength as measured by the Jamar dynamometer Arch Phys Med Rehabil 52:321–327, 1970.

273. Schraidt R: Fundamentals of Sensory Physiology. Berlin, Springer-Verlag, 1978.

274. Schreiner CE, Urbas JV: Representation of amplitude modulation in the auditory cortex of the cat: II. Comparison between cortical fields. Hear Res 32:49–63, 1988.

275. Seivert J: Manual Therapy: Maitland's Concepts, 1993.

276. Selbach H: The principle of relaxation occillation as a special instance of the law of initial value in cybernetic functions. Ann NY Acad Sci 98:1221–1228, 1962.

277. Serizawa K: Tsubol—vital points for oriental therapy. Tokyo, Japan Publishing, 1976.

278. Seufert-Jeffer U, Jeffer EK: An introduction to the VOJTA Method. Clin Man Phys Ther 2(4):26–29, 1982.

279. Shepard GM: Synaptic organization of the mammalian olfactory bulb. Physiol Rev 52:864–917, 1972.

280. Shumway-Cook A: Equilibrium deficits in children. In Woolcott MH, Shumway-Cook A (eds): Development of Posture and Gait Across the Lifespan. Columbia, SC, University of South Carolina, 1989.

281. Shumway-Cook A, Horak FB: Rehabilitation strategies for patients with vestibular deficits. Neurol Clin 8:441–457, 1990.

282. Sinclair D: Cutaneous Sensation. London, Oxford University Press, 1967.

283. Smith GR, et al: Psychological modulation of the human immune response to varicela zoster. Arch Intern Med 145:2110–2112, 1985.

284. Somers DC, Todorov EV, Siapas AG, et al: A local circuit approach to understanding integration of long-range inputs in primary visual cortex. Cerebral Cortex 8:204–217, 1998.

285. Spitz RV, Tallal P, Flax J, Benasich AA: Look who's talking: A prospective study of familial transmission of language impairments. J Speech Lang Hear Res 40:990–1001, 1997.

286. Steiner JE: Innate discriminative human facial expressions to taste and smell stimulations. Ann NY Acad Sci 237:229–233, 1974.

287. Stejskal L: Postural reflexes in man. Am J Phys Med 58:1–24, 1979.

288. Stockmeyer SA: An interpretation of the approach of Rood to the treatment of neuromuscular dysfunction. Am J Phys Med 46:900–961, 1967.

289. Sullivan PE, Markos PD, Minor MA: An Integrated Approach to Therapeutic Exercise. Reston, VA, Reston Publishing, 1982.

290. Sur M, Nelson RHJ, Kaas JH: The representation of the body surface in somatic koniocortex in the Prosimian (Galago senegalensis). J Comp Neurol 180:381–402, 1980.

291. Takagi K, Kobagasi S: Skin pressure reflex. Acta Med Biol 4:31–37, 1956.

292. Talbot WH, et al: The sense of flutter-vibration: companion of the human capacity with response patterns of mechanoreceptive afferents. J Neurophysiol 31:301–334, 1968.

293. Tallal P, Miller SL, Bedi G, et al: Acoustically modified speech improves language comprehension in language-learning impaired children. Science 271:81–84, 1996.

294. Tallal P, Piercy M: Defects of non-verbal auditory perception in children with developmental aphasia. Nature 241:468–469, 1973.

295. Tallal P, Piercy M: Developmental aphasia: Rate of auditory processing and selective impairment of consonant perception. Neuropsychologia 13:69–74, 1974.

296. Tappan FM: Healing Massage Techniques: Holistic, Classic and Emerging methods 2nd, ed. Norwalk CT, Appelton & Lange, 1988.

297. Taylor TC: Myofascial release techniques. Phys Ther Forum 5(23):2–4, 1986.

298. Tinazzi M, Zanette G, Volpato D, et al: Neurophysiological evidence of neuroplasticity at multiple levels of the somatosensory system in patients with carpal tunnel syndrome. Brain 121:1785–1794, 1998.

299. Travell J: Myofascial Pain and Dysfunction. Baltimore, Williams & Wilkins, 1983.

300. Treisman A, Gormican S: Feature analysis in early vision: Evidence from search asymmetries. Psychol Rev 95:15–48, 1988.

301. Tuttle R, McClearly J: Mesenteric baroreceptors. Am J Physiol 229:1514–1519, 1975.

302. Twomey LT, Taylor JR: Physical Therapy of the Low Back, 2nd ed. New York, Churchill Livingstone, 1994.

303. Umphred DA: Clinical observations, 1967 to 1994.

304. Umphred DA: Integrated approach to treatment of the pediatric neurologic patient. In Campbell SK: Clinics in Physical Therapy: Pediatric Neurologic Disorders. New York, Churchill Livingstone, 1984.

305. Upledger J: Craniosacral Therapy, 5th ed. Seattle, Eastman Press, 1986.

306. Valdez P: Emotion responses to color. Doctoral dissertation, University of California at Los Angeles, 1993.

307. Vallbo AB, et al: Somatosensory, proprioceptive, and sympathetic activity in human peripheral nerves. Physiol Rev 59:919–951, 1979.

308. Van Houten R, Rolider A: The use of color mediation techniques to teach number identification and single digit multiplication problems to children with learning disability. Educ Treat Child 13:216, 1990.

309. Verrillo R: Change in vibrotactile thresholds as a function of age. Sens Processes 3:49–59, 1979.

310. Wall P: The gate control theory of pain mechanisms. Brain 101 (March):1, 1978.

311. Wang X, Merzenich MM, Beitel R, Schreiner C: Representation of species-specific vocalizations in the primary auditory cortex of the marmoset monkey: Spectral and temporal features. J Neurophysiol 74:1685–1706, 1995.

312. Wang X, Merzenich MM, Sameshima K, Jenkins WM: Remodelling of hand representation in adult cortex determined by timing of tactile stimulation. Nature 378:71–75, 1995.

313. Weinberger NM: Learning-induced changes of auditory receptive fields. Current Opin Neurobiol 3:570–577, 1993.

314. Weiss SJ: Psychophysiologic effects of caregiver touch on incidence of cardiac dysrhythmia. Heart Lung 15:495–502, 1986.

315. West A: Understanding endorphins: Our natural pain relief system. Nursing 2:50–53, 1981.
316. Wilbarger P: Advanced course for treatment of sensory defensiveness. In Symposium on Intervention for Persons with Mild to Severe Dysfunction. Minneapolis, 1994, unpublished.
317. Willis WD, Grossman RG: Medical Neurobiology, 3rd ed. St. Louis, CV Mosby, 1981.
318. Wilson V, Peterson B: The role of the vestibular system in posture and movement. In Mountcastle VB (ed): Medical Physiology, 14th ed, vol 2. St. Louis, CV Mosby, 1989.
319. Winstein CJ: Designing practice for motor learning: Clinical implications. In Lister MJ (ed): Contemporary Management of Motor Control Problem. Norman, OK, APTA, 1991.
320. Wright B, Lombardino LJ, King WM, et al: Deficits in auditory temporal and spectral resolution in language-impaired children. Nature 387:176–177, 1997.
321. Xerri C, Stern J, Merzenich MM: Alterations of the cortical representation of the rat ventrum induced by nursing behavior. J Neurosci 14:1710–1721, 1994.
322. Yakolev PI, Lecours AR: The myelogenetic cycles of regional maturation of the brain. In Minkowski A (ed): Regional Development of the Brain in Early Life. Oxford, Blackwell Scientific, 1967, pp. 3–70.
323. Young RR: The clinical significance of exteroceptive reflexes. In Desurdet JE (ed): New Developments in Electromyography and Clinical Neurophysiology, vol 3. Basel, Karger, 1973.
324. Zemack-Bersin D, Zemach-Bersin K, Resse M: Relaxercise: The Easy New Way to Health and Fitness. New York, Harper & Row, 1990.
325. Zotterman Y: Sensory Functions of the Skin in Primates. Oxford, Pergamon Press, 1976.
326. Zwaardemaker H: Physiology of Smell. London, Collier Macmillan, 1895.

APPENDIX 4 – A

Biomechanical Stress-Free Hand Techniques

A. General Comments Regarding Stress-Free Use of the Hand
1. Strengthen the small muscles inside the hand (intrinsics) to facilitate stability.
   a. Give resistance to spreading fingers apart (try not to use muscles that straighten the fingers).
   b. Try to hold the fingers together while you use your other hand to try and spread them apart.
   c. Bend the fingers at the large knuckle to 90 degrees (metacarpophalangeal joint) by placing the back of the hand against the edge of a table. Now, one finger at a time, try to keep the fingers straight as you use the other hand to try and bend the finger, giving resistance at the distal segment of the finger.
2. Use the small muscles of the hands in functional activities.
   a. Initiate bending the fingers from the base (the large metacarpophalangeal joint); try to do this without bending the fingers at the other joints and without using the muscles that bend the distal finger joints.
   b. Avoid heavy gripping; squeeze only when necessary. For example, do not (1) squeeze the steering wheel, (2) exercise while holding on to free weights, or (3) squeeze a ball or strengthen the grip in other ways.
   c. When reaching for something, keep the hand relaxed. When you contact the object, let the surface of the object open the hand. For example, when you reach for your cup, let the cup open the hand. Do not use the handle. When you drop your hand onto the keyboard, let the keyboard open the hand; do not actively spread the fingers.
3. Stop precise, rapid, forceful finger flexion and extension movements of the hand.
   a. Transfer the work from the fingers to the forearm. For example,
      1) Lift the fingers by rotating the forearm into supination (palm up); let the shoulder externally rotate if necessary.
      2) When the hand is pronated (palm down), let the elbow swing away from the side a little if necessary to keep the hand relaxed (some internal rotation of the shoulder can take the stress off the forearm).
   b. Use the hand in a natural functional position (rounded palm from the base of the thumb to the base of the fifth finger and rounded from the tips of the fingers to the wrist). Thus, all of the finger joints are slightly bent, the palm is round, and the wrist is extended about 15 degrees. When your arms are at your side, this will usually be the position of the hand.
   c. Do not let the fingers collapse or hyperextend on the surface when they are down on a surface.
      1) Practice dropping the hand onto a surface and maintaining the roundness of the hand (a small soft ball under the palm may be used for assistance).
      2) Lean lightly onto the hand while it is on a flat surface and keep the round shape of the hand.
      3) Thread the fingers of one hand through the fingers of the other hand to help stabilize the hand when placing weight onto the hand, as in 2.
      4) Put a soft, flexible ball about 2 inches in diameter on the table; roll the palm of the hand over the ball and let the finger pads drop onto the surface.

B. Using the Keyboard Safely
1. Sit with feet flat on the floor. Sit tall with hips about 90 degrees (vary this posture throughout the day).
   a. Place the computer screen at or slightly below eye level.
   b. Keyboard height should be adjusted to maintain elbow flexion at about 80 degrees (positioned in approximately 110 degrees of extension). Forearms should be angled toward the floor and not resting on the table. If it is difficult to let your hands rest lightly on the keyboard with the wrist floating, it may be helpful to have a pillow on your lap, where the forearms receive positive sensory information to help them relax.
   c. Place the screen about 2 feet away from the eyes for the majority of work; pull the screen closer as necessary for close work.
   d. Consider getting special antiglare glasses for computer terminal display work or use a screen glare protector.
2. Look at the contour of the hand when it is at your side; maintain that position as the hand is dropped on the keyboard.
3. Keep the wrist in neutral (0–10 degrees' extension) on the keyboard (floating). Do not rest your wrist on a "wrist rest." Resting the wrist and forearm on the work surface will increase the pressure in the carpal tunnel and force all of the work to be done with the fingers. If you have a wrist pad, think of the pad as a sensory *tickle* to let you know that your wrists should be floating above the rest.
4. Have all of the fingers resting down on the keyboard. Do not let any of the fingers fly up. Also note that all fingers should be resting down. Continue this resting down even when one finger is engaged in depressing a key. Do not allow the adjacent fingers to extend to get them away from the active finger.
5. It is not necessary to actively lift the fingers after pressing down. Sometimes it is enough simply to release the pressure down.
6. Change the fulcrum of movement from the fingers of the hand to the elbow and shoulder.
   a. Allow the elbow to move freely.
   b. Use the shoulder and the trunk to move up and down the keyboard of a piano.
7. Do not curl the fingers when striking the keys. Avoid using the tips, but rather use the pads of the fingers. Initiate the movement at the base joint of the fingers. Imagine that you are using muscles inside your hand and not the long muscles that bend the fingers.
8. Avoid reaching one finger out in isolation from the others.
9. Do not squeeze the mouse; drape your hand on the mouse.

a. Keep your wrist in neutral.

b. Do not activate the mouse button by lifting and bending the index finger.

c. Use rotation of the forearm to activate the button on the mouse.

d. Make sure the mouse is close to you and that the arm is not extended out to the side. Place a cover for the mouse over the number keys, if necessary, to keep the arm closer to your trunk.

10. Take regular breaks.

a. Do diaphragmatic breathing and gentle range of motion exercises. Place the arms on the desk and bend the trunk over the arms.

b. Consider obtaining the software that forces a computer break through a screen reminder.

C. Writing

1. The fulcrum for the movement for writing should be the shoulder and elbow, not the fingers.

2. The hand should be round and relaxed.

3. Hold the pen between the second and third fingers rather than the thumb and index finger. Practice this way of holding the pen. The hand should be open, thumb resting down.

a. Move the pen from the elbow and shoulder; keep wrist and fingers still.

b. Hold the pen lightly.

c. If you must write in the traditional way, hold the pen lightly and try a larger pen, but still do not squeeze the pen.

d. Practice making circles, loops, large numbers, and letters. Consider practicing by writing in shaving cream, finger paints, or water.

e. Practice picking up the pen and putting it down without feeling any tension.

f. Let the arm rest lightly on the table and comfortably on the ulnar side. Avoid resting the elbow on the surface. If there is inadequate pronation, allow the shoulder to move out a little into abduction and internal rotation.

g. Mentally review relaxed writing before beginning to write with a new technique.

h. Let all fingers rest down. Do not hold any fingers up off of the pen.

4. Place a mirror up in front of your hand as you write and notice if it appears relaxed.

5. Put the pen down if any signs of stress develop.

D. Daily Activities in the Kitchen

1. Use two hands to hold a pot or a frying pan.

2. Use an electronic can opener and jar opener.

3. Use an electronic blender rather than hand stirring.

4. Use a chopper so you avoid heavy cutting.

5. Stand close to the sink and the work surface so you do not have to have your arms out too far in front of you.

6. Get close to the table for setting the table; avoid having to lean over; bend at the knees.

7. If you are short, stand on a stool to work at the sink.

8. If you are tall, consider raising the refrigerator up taller so you do not have to lean over.

9. When eating, hold the utensils lightly.

10. When cutting, use the weight of the trunk to assist.

E. Driving

1. Use a lumbar roll in your seat to support your lower back.

2. Pull the seat close to the steering wheel so you do not have to reach out so far for the gas pedal.

3. Sit tall and try to drive without stress.

4. Turn your trunk in the opposite direction that you want to look, and this will allow you to use your whole body for turning, avoiding excessive pressure at the neck.

5. Mentally rehearse and review calm, alert driving.

6. Do not squeeze the wheel in a death grip. Hold the steering wheel by gently pushing your arms together. You only need to hold the wheel with a palmar squeeze when turning.

7. Keep your arms comfortably at your sides.

8. Do not grip the shift bar; press the palm of your hand down on the shift bar to shift. You may even want to allow your trunk to move with your arm while shifting.

F. Other Household Activities

1. Do not grip objects too firmly; keep hands open and adduct the arms (pull them toward midline).

2. Always bend your knees to pick up objects.

3. Be careful to avoid leaning over and grabbing the bedding (e.g., when making the bed, ask someone to do it with you; otherwise, make one side of the bed at a time).

4. Put items at eye level; avoid putting things over your head for which you have to reach out and up.

5. Walk close to the vacuum cleaner; try to hold it where you do not have to reach your arms out.

6. Do not lean over from the waist for dusting; if necessary, dust while kneeling or wipe the floor while you are on your knees; hold the dustcloth lightly.

Specific Sensory Discrimination Activities
Instructions for Patients

The purpose of these activities is to place demands on the receptors of the skin, the receptors in the muscle, and the receptors in the joints to restore normal sensitivity and accuracy of sensory information processing. By improving the accuracy of sensory discrimination under conditions of high levels of attention, it should be possible to restore the normal somatosensory representation of the hand in the primary sensory cortex. It is essential to begin this process of retraining to restore the distinct differentiation of the somatosensory representation of the hand before emphasizing activities for restoring normal fine-motor control.

A. Emphasis on Superficial Sensory Receptors (Light Touch)
1. In all regular activities, increase the opportunity to feel objects in your environment and decide what the objects are without looking at them.
2. Develop a variety of sensory tasks you can do by yourself.
   a. Put small objects in bowls of rice or beans and reach in and try to find and match the objects.
   b. Hang objects from a door jam; start the objects swinging and allow them to stimulate across your hand. See if you can differentiate the different objects as they move across your hand.
3. Modify the intensity of the sensory stimuli; increase the challenge and complexity of the stimuli you are trying to identify and change the environment in which you are exploring a sensory stimulus.
   a. Draw shapes and letters in shaving soap; draw big letters and then small letters.
   b. Palpate objects in water or other media for identification; have the water be still and then agitate the water so it is harder.
4. Put pairs of coins and objects in your pocket and try to match them or discriminate between them.
   a. Purchase clay that can be molded and shaped and then heated until firm.
   b. Place or draw different shapes on the clay; always draw a pair that can be matched.
5. Have a friend help you. Ask this friend to write things on your hands and fingers while you are not looking at your fingers.
   a. Identify the letters/numbers/words/shapes verbally.
   b. When it is easy to get the letters correct, have your friend draw designs that must be redrawn on a piece of paper. Ask your friend to give you feedback about the drawing to make sure the drawing matches the stimulus.
      1) Check the angles where the lines meet.
      2) Note accuracy of detection of curves.
      3) Note if all parts of the design are placed in the right relationship and orientation (spatial accuracy).
      4) Note if the design is the correct size.
      5) Check whether the drawing has some elaborate components that were not actually drawn on the surface of the skin.
   c. Ask your friend to provide a sensory stimulus and define a task you are supposed to do when you feel the stimulus (e.g., when I tap with this sharp object, I want you to tap once, but when I touch you with this dull object, I want you to tap twice).
   d. Have a friend draw designs on your finger, and then you copy the designs you felt on the area of the skin where drawn (pay close attention to orientation, angles, curves).
   e. Make the drawings smaller and smaller to increase the challenge of detection.
   f. Stimulate with hot, cold, sharp, and dull stimuli and ask patient to identify the stimulus.
6. Play games that require heavy discrimination of sensory information through the skin of the fingers.
   a. Play dominoes with the eyes closed.
   b. Play pick-up sticks.
   c. Play shape games (e.g., match a shape to an opening when eyes are closed, such as Perfection)
   d. Put together puzzles that have a raised surface (eyes closed).
   e. Play Scrabble with raised or indented letters.
7. Get "stickers" with different shapes; place them on plastic and then feel them and match them.
8. Sew different buttons on cloth and try to match them.
9. Glue alphabet soup onto cards and palpate the letters.
10. Play games that require orientation in place without the benefit of vision.
    a. Play pin the tail on the donkey.
    b. Walk through the house with your eyes closed and hands out to catch yourself if needed.
11. Take construction paper and create pairs of letters, shapes, or other designs by pressing heavily with the pen; this will create a raised surface on the other side.
    a. With eyes closed, palpate and try to find matching pairs.
    b. Turn the paper in different directions to make the exploration different.
12. Make a grab bag of items and have patient reach into the bag and identify by gentle touch.
13. Create other sensory games that require planning and control and can be done without vision.
14. Obtain Braille workbooks and learn to read Braille.
    a. If you have trouble with your affected side, try with the unaffected side.
    b. Do not tense your hand as you feel the letters and do not extend the adjacent digits away.
    c. Work your hands smoothly over the dots. You can improve your skill, getting other workbooks for the blind.
    d. Get a Braille deck of cards and play cards.
    e. Obtain "object cards" where the object is described in Braille.
15. Place raised numbers and designs on the computer keyboard and try to determine what the number/shape is before striking the key; make some labeled letter match or mismatch the key itself.

16. Ask your friend to stroke affected areas of your hand and arm with different surfaces (rough, smooth, cold, hot); then have your friend stroke an adjacent uninvolved area with the same stimulus. You should try to make the sensations in the different areas feel the same.

17. Paste matched pairs of items on a card and try to find the matched pairs (eyes closed).
    a. Paste matched pairs of buttons on a card.
    b. Paste alphabet soup letters on a card.
    c. Paste magnetic letters and other shapes on a card.

B. Emphasis on Proprioception/Kinesthesia
1. Create games in which a part of an object or a piece of a picture has to be placed on the right place on a picture or on an object.
    a. Create games in which objects have to be moved to certain distances that are variable.
    b. Create objects of the same weight and place different types of surfaces on the object (e.g., Velcro, sandpaper, slipper) and practice picking up and moving the object with minimal effort.
    c. Assemble puzzles by feeling with your eyes closed.
    d. Work with a friend and practice copying movements together.
    e. Tap one finger while others are resting down.
    f. Bring arms up over head and tap one finger at a time.
    g. Bend wrist with one hand and bend elbow with other arm.
    h. Circle wrist to the right (right hand) and circle to the left with left hand.
    i. Have a friend give you a little resistance as you move one finger up and down.
    j. Draw different angles of the fingers and wrist on a piece of paper. Then you try to copy the angles without looking at your finger or wrist. Check to see how accurate you are.
    k. See if you can rent a continuous passive motion machine. Set the machine at different speeds, and try to follow the movements of the machine, carefully timing the movements.

2. Practice grasping objects of different sizes with minimum graded force.

3. Practice throwing objects of different size; practice throwing them to a particular spot.

4. Have someone make a video performing the target task that you are having trouble with. Then try to copy the movements. Watch the movements carefully and imagine that the movements are your hands moving.

Imagery, Mental Rehearsal, and Mental Practice to Restore Normal Hand Representation

A. General Comments About Imagery

It is critical to restore a total sense of wellness and control of your hand/arm. Initially, this may be difficult because of pain, difficulty with the control of movement, or the fact that you cannot imagine that the hand/arm could be normal again. One way to begin to restore the normal information processing system so you can use your hand normally is to begin by changing how the hand and the task you are trying to perform are represented in your brain (the internal representation of that injured part). It is important to be able to restore the normal image of the part; that it is how it used to be and how it will be again. In the process of restoring normal control, it is also important to begin to use the hand normally and not increase the pain or repeat the abnormal movements. Thus, visually imagine your hand and how it looks. Making your hand look like the other hand is a good beginning. Then begin to create a motor image of the hand in which you begin to imagine using it normally to perform all of the usual and normal tasks. You can start by imaging small parts of a larger task and then finally the whole task and then related skills and activities that would go along with the task.

The evidence is clear that you can activate both the motor and sensory representations of your hand as well as the function you are completing with your hand. For example, you have several maps on your brain that represent the motor and sensory aspects of your body. Also, well-learned functions are mapped in a different part of your brain. When you visually image a body part, you will activate the somatosensory cortex. When you imagine doing the task (motor imagery), you will also activate the motor cortex. When you both visually and motorically imagine completing the task in your mind, you will activate the cortical areas representing the part of your body that is moving as well as the part of the brain that is devoted to completing that task (e.g., walking, writing, playing an instrument). The intensity with which the neurons fire when you are imaging is less than the intensity of firing when you are actually performing the task. Try to imagine without mistakes. This will reinforce the positive aspects of the sensorimotor feedback. You must imagine without interruption and you must repeat the imaging process with a high level of concentration to help the nervous system learn. If you are imaging and you run into difficulty completing a task normally, try to focus on the source of the difficulty, including asking your inner self what barriers are getting in the way. Once you can get insight into these barriers, you should be able to break them down.

B. Suggestions for Goal-Directed Imaging

1. Set goals for yourself to specifically improve the function of your hand. First start with imagining that your hand and arm feel normal. Then focus on improving performance on one aspect of the task that is bothering you.

Then, as you begin to perform different parts of the task normally, finally imagine completing the entire task.
   a. First focus on healing the tissues.
      1) Focus on bringing the blood to the tissues.
      2) Imagine the blood carrying important elements to the area of injury (e.g., the growth factors and oxygen that are requisites for healing tissues).
      3) Imagine that an injury causes inflammation that triggers the healing response (e.g., laying down collagen [scar]). Also imagine that the body modifies the scar tissue and tries to keep it mobile.
   b. Mentally visualize the anatomy, physiology, and kinesiology of the hand.
      1) Imagine the bones gliding smoothly on each other.
      2) Imagine the muscles being strong.
      3) Imagine normal movement patterns.
      4) Imagine normal sensation in the hand.
      5) Imagine pain-free movement.
      6) Imagine the hand being quiet and relaxed.
      7) Imagine smooth control of the hand and no extraneous movements.
   c. Imagine the hand is working just like the other hand.
   d. Imagine using the hand as you used to use it. Go back in time to when your hand felt good and you did not have any problems.
   e. When mentally practicing and imaging, there should be no distractions. Spend at least 60 minutes a day normalizing the hand and imagining how good it feels.
   f. Mentally practice and perform the target task without any signs of strain or pain.
   g. Concentrate and mentally review each of the components of the hand working normally.
   h. Concentrate on the free flow of rhythmic movements of the hand/arm as you walk.
2. Recapture the excitement of using your hand without effort and without pain while playing your instrument or working at your job.
3. Reinforce the image of a normal hand by using a mirror.
   a. Put both hands on the table.
   b. Block the affected hand from view by putting it behind the mirror.
   c. Place the mirror in such a position that you can see the unaffected side in the mirror; in the mirror, the hand looks like your affected arm.
   d. Do common movements with the unaffected side (e.g., writing, making circles, tapping a finger) and have the affected hand copy the mirror image.
4. Take time to review your upper extremity and your body as a whole. Imagine your body is healthy. Imagine the healthy flow of blood into all of your tissues. Feel an increase in the heat of the arm/hand.

Contemporary Issues and Theories of Motor Control: Assessment of Movement and Posture

ROBERTA A. NEWTON, PhD, PT

Key Words

– motor and postural control theories
– neurological assessment

Objectives

After reading this chapter the student/therapist will:

1. Identify the difference between motor control–based theory and reflex/hierarchical-based theory.

2. Identify and analyze the parameters of motor and balance control.

3. Compare the various elements of motor control and identify how each factor might affect balance and movement.

4. Recognize how motor and postural control theory can be applied to the assessment and treatment of clients with neurological dysfunction.

Foundation sciences fundamental to physical therapy and occupational therapy assessment and treatment are motor control, motor learning, and motor development. Therapists need an understanding of neural regulation of movements, how movement patterns or motor behavior is learned, and how motor behavior changes across the life span in healthy people. A framework for typical motor behavior is necessary to understand how motor behavior is altered in persons with neurological dysfunction. As new information about motor control, learning, and life span development becomes available, principles that form the bases for assessment and treatment are reassessed, modified, or replaced with newer principles of motor control.

This chapter has two purposes: (1) to provide the reader with a review of current models used to represent neural regulation of motor control leading to posture and movement in all aspects of life activities and (2) to describe some deficits of motor control using these models and the ways in which therapists can use this schema to evaluate patients with neurological dysfunction.

A model is a schematic representation of a theory and, in this context, how the nervous system regulates motor behavior. Many motor and postural control models exist because researchers use different approaches to develop and test theories. All models have limitations and are constantly changing as researchers gain new information and as technological advances are made. A theory that is constantly tested and undergoing change is better than outdated theory or no theoretical framework. Early researchers used visual observation and palpation to develop models of motor control. Today, researchers use a variety of techniques and tools reflective of their level of interest. These include, for example, electromyography, film analysis, force plates, electron microscopy, transcranial magnetic stimulation, and functional magnetic resonance. Finally, models may portray only a small part of the nervous system; for example, a model of spinal cord control mechanisms examining regeneration of the lesioned spinal cord would not include higher-center control processes. Other models may be more wholistic. For example, systems modeling may be used to investigate the interrelationships among various brain centers and spinal pattern generators to examine recovery of hand function in clients with hemiplegia resulting from a cerebrovascular accident.

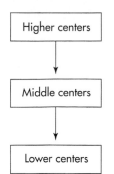

FIGURE 5–1. Model of a hierarchy of motor control.

Motor control theories serving as a basis for predicting motor responses during patient assessment and treatment as well as functional outcome should have a broad scope. A therapist using a spinal level reflex model, for example, may inaccurately predict motor behavior because this model does not consider regulation of motor behavior by higher brain centers. This model assumes the patient is a passive recipient rather than an active participant. Selecting and using a proper model is important for the analysis and treatment of individuals with posture and movement dysfunction.

A CLASSICAL MODEL OF MOTOR CONTROL

The hierarchy model is the base for traditional neurological therapy. A description of the hierarchy, its application to pathophysiology and motor control, and its limitations is presented. The hierarchy model proposes that a higher-center commander select and delegate the motor program to subordinate centers for execution (Fig. 5–1). The midbrain, brain stem, and spinal cord are considered subordinate centers. Motor programs are assumed stored at the highest level and are not influenced by feedforward or feedback mechanisms during execution of the movement. Feedback loops are included in contemporary hierarchical models of motor control. Although information about the internal and external environment is available before and after the execution of the movement, the commander does not necessarily incorporate the information during subsequent movements.

When disease or injury damages the highest center, dissolution of the whole nervous system occurs.[23] The more stable lower and evolutionarily older nervous centers located in the midbrain and brain stem control movement. Movements represented at the lower levels of the nervous system are reflexive, that is, stereotypical and not capable of modification when the external or internal environmental conditions necessitate a change. Damage to the highest centers also results in a poverty of motor responses (negative deficit) or an overreadiness of the nervous system to remain active (positive deficit).

The hierarchy model for motor control represents the state of science from the middle of the nineteenth century to the early twentieth century. Although this model has limitations, it was the basis for development of the disciplines of neurology and neurological physical therapy. Since the incorporation of the hierarchy model into physical therapy theory, researchers have developed other theories for the regulation of posture and movement. The hierarchical model is useful to examine motor activity that occurs without feedback; however, this model is of limited use when trying to understand the interrelationships of brain centers for planning, initiating, or learning motor activities.

CONTEMPORARY MODELS OF MOTOR CONTROL

Researchers adopted the term *systems* from engineering to describe the relationship of various brain and spinal centers working together with the use of feedback (Fig. 5–2). Sensation is the process whereby receptors receive information relative to the internal and external environment. The receptors encode the information for transmission to various regions of the nervous system. The central nervous system (CNS) receives and interprets the sensations based on present experiences, the present state of the internal and external environment, and memory of

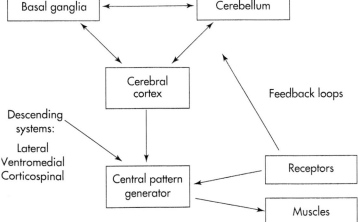

FIGURE 5–2. Systems model of motor control.

similar situations. This process is termed *perception*. Processing this information in the context of a goal (motor activity to be achieved) leads to the development of a movement (and postural) strategy. This operation is termed *response selection*, that is, choosing the most contextually appropriate movement strategy to meet the needs of the individual and the constraints of the environment. The strategy is executed (response execution) by the muscles and joints. The observable motor behavior is the result of perception and then the selection and execution of the appropriate motor and postural responses using both feedforward and feedback mechanisms.

Researchers have garnered principles and concepts from different disciplines to develop the systems approach to motor control, for example, neuroscience theory, principles of nonlinear phenomena in physics, and Bernstein's[3] degrees of freedom. Some of the principles and concepts included in systems theory are described later. The concepts presented in this section are representative of systems theory and dynamic action theory and by no means are inclusive of all the concepts contained in these multifaceted and complex theories. Comprehensive discussions of these theories are found elsewhere.[3, 18, 29, 38, 42]

Principles and Concepts Related to Contemporary Motor Control Theories

As mentioned earlier, contemporary motor control models have a similar set of assumptions and concepts; yet each model contains additional assumptions and concepts. Described in this section are elements from the various contemporary theories that are useful for the description of motor and postural control in clients with neurological dysfunction, as well as in healthy individuals. These elements can be components of a theory, or a single element can represent a theory. They do not stand alone to explain motor control in the healthy individual or the individual with neurological dysfunction. Rather, they are interrelated. The interaction of these various elements produces the emergent motor and postural behavior in response to the environmental and task demands of the situation.

Multiple Descending Pathways to Regulate Posture and Movement. A traditional hierarchical model assumes only one descending, voluntary pathway. Regulation of posture and movement is more complex, as demonstrated by a descending model proposed by Laurence and Kuypers.[25, 26] The descending pathways are categorized into the medial descending system, the lateral descending system, and the cortical corticospinal system. The medial descending system, primarily represented by the vestibulospinal pathways, projects bilaterally to spinal level neuronal pools to provide antigravity regulation, that is, to control proximal limb girdle and trunk musculature to maintain the upright position so that the face is vertical and the mouth is horizontal. The lateral descending systems, primarily represented by the reticulospinal pathways, provide regulatory control over the limb musculature. The third system, the corticospinal tract, provides regulation and control of fine finger fractionation. Thus, the corticospinal system is not considered the "volitional" control system as suggested in the hierarchical model.

Lesioning the corticospinal system in monkeys did not result in loss of volitional control. To expand their model, the cortical system, including the corticobulbar system, provides regulation and control over all synergies, both movement and balance movement patterns. The rubrospinal tract is small in humans, and its function in the regulation of upper-extremity flexor activity is assumed a function of the lateral corticospinal tract.

Central Pattern Generator or Reflex. Traditionally, in the hierarchical model, the basic spinal level unit is the reflex. If a particular stimulus activates receptors, a single stereotypical motor response results. In systems theory developed from a neuroscience perspective, the basic spinal level unit is the central pattern generator (CPG).[6, 7] Evidence for CPGs has been found in many vertebrates, including humans. CPGs are diagramed as oscillators to denote their rhythmical activity. One model postulates that one half of the oscillator controls flexor synergies and the other half is responsible for extensor synergies, thereby controlling the muscles of an entire limb.[13] More discrete oscillators are postulated to regulate individual pairs of antagonistic muscles.[15] Coupling oscillators within a single limb permits multijoint intralimb coordination, and coupling oscillators between limbs produces interlimb coordination and allows for a variety of movement patterns. For example, a loose coupling of interlimb oscillators permits homolateral, homonymous, and cross-diagonal locomotor patterns.

If a single stimulus activates a CPG, a series of motor responses occurs. The rhythmical pattern (emergent property) produced by an oscillator can remain activated without additional sensory input. Rhythmical activity in a spinal level reflex occurs only by additional sensory stimuli (Fig. 5–3).

Perturbations or disturbances during the rhythmical activity can affect the timing or amplitude of the response of the synergy. For example, a perturbation can occur

A. A single response per stimulus

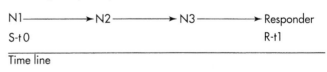

B. Emergent property: more than one response

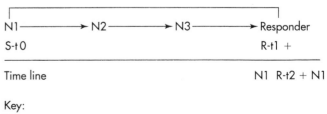

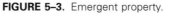

Key:
N = neuron
S-t0 = start time
R-t = response 1; response 2, etc.

FIGURE 5–3. Emergent property.

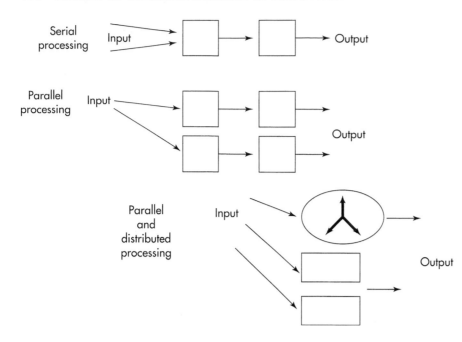

FIGURE 5–4. Methods of information processing.

during locomotion by placing an obstacle in the path. Portions of the CPGs can alter the timing or amplitude of the response without altering the rhythm. Spinal level neurons such as Renshaw cells or IA inhibitory interneurons have been identified as potential contributors to this modulation.[14]

Information Processing. The configuration of the systems model lends itself to many modes to process information. Serial processing denotes a specific order of processing (Fig. 5–4) of information by various centers. Information proceeds lockstep through each center. Parallel processing denotes processing of information by more than one center simultaneously or nearly simultaneously, and that information can be used for more than one activity. A third and more flexible type of processing of information is parallel-distributed processing.[35] This type of processing combines the best attributes of serial and parallel processing. That is, when the situation demands serial processing, this type of activity occurs. At other times, parallel processing is the mode of choice. For optimum processing of information from internal and external sensory information with various regions of the brain, a combination of both parallel and serial processing is the most efficient mode. The type of processing depends on constraints of the situation. For example, maintaining balance after an unexpected external perturbation requires rapid processing, whereas learning to voluntarily shift the center of gravity to the limits of stability requires a different combination of processing modes.

In summary, processing reinforces and refines the motor patterns that are used. Processing permits the organism to initiate compensatory strategies if the wrong motor pattern is selected or if an unexpected perturbation occurs. Lastly, processing permits learning.

Movement Patterns Arising from Self-Organizing Subsystems. Coordinated movement patterns are developed from the dynamic interaction of subsystems in relation to internal and external constraints. Therefore, movement patterns used to accomplish a goal are contextually appropriate and arise as an emergent property of subsystem interaction. Several principles relate to self-organizing systems: reciprocity, distributed function, consensus, and emergent properties.[9]

Reciprocity implies information flow between two or more neural networks. These networks can represent specific brain centers, for example, the cerebellum and basal ganglia (see Fig. 5–2). Alternatively, the neural networks can be interacting neuronal clusters located within a single center, for example, the basal ganglia. One model to demonstrate reciprocity is the basal ganglia regulation of motor behavior through direct and indirect pathways to cortical areas. One pathway, the more direct pathway from the putamen to the globus pallidus internal segment, provides net inhibitory effects. The more indirect pathway from the putamen through the globus pallidus external segment and subthalamic nucleus provides a net excitatory effect on the globus pallidus internal segment. Alteration of the balance between these pathways is postulated to produce motor dysfunction.[1, 10] An abnormally decreased outflow from the basal ganglia is postulated to produce involuntary motor patterns such as chorea, hemiballism, or tremor. Alternatively, an abnormally increased outflow from the basal ganglia is postulated to produce rigidity, as observed in individuals with Parkinson's disease.

Distributed function presupposes that a single center or neural network has more than one function. The concept also implies that several centers share the same function. For example, a center may serve as the coordinating unit in one task and may serve as a pattern generator or oscillator to maintain the activity in another task. An advantage of distributing function among groups of neurons or centers is to provide centers with overlapping or redundant functions. Neuroscientists believe such redundancy is a safety feature. If a neuronal lesion occurs, other centers can assume critical functional roles, thereby producing recovery from CNS dysfunction.

Consensus implies that motor behavior occurs when a majority of brain centers or regions reach a critical threshold to produce activation. Consensus also functions to filter extraneous information or information that does require immediate attention. If, however, a novel stimulus enters the system, it carries more weight and receives immediate attention. A novel stimulus may be new to the system or may reflect a potentially harmful situation.

Emergent properties may be understood in the adage, "the whole is greater than the sum of its parts." The concept implies that brain centers and not a single brain center work together to produce movement. An example of the emergent properties concept is continuous repetitive activity (oscillation). In Figure 5–3A, a hierarchy is represented by three neurons arranged in tandem. The last neuron ends on a responder. If a single stimulus activates this network, a single response occurs. What is the response if the neurons are arranged so that the third neuron sends a collateral branch to the first neuron in addition to the ending on the responder? In this case (see Fig. 5–3B), a single stimulus activates neuron No. 1, which in turn activates neurons No. 2 and No. 3, causing a response as well as reactivating neuron No. 1. This neuronal arrangement produces a series of responses rather than a single response. This process is also termed *endogenous activity*.

Another example of an emergent property is the production of motor behavior. Rather than having every motor program stored in the brain, an abstract representation of the intended goal is stored. At the time of motor performance, various brain centers use present sensory information, with past memory of the task to develop the appropriate motor strategy. This concept negates a hard-wired motor program concept. If motor programs were hard-wired and if a motor program existed for every movement ever performed, the brain would need a huge storage capacity.

Controlling the Degrees of Freedom. Combinations of muscle and joint action permit a large number of degrees of freedom that contribute to movement. A system with a large number of degrees of freedom is called a *high-dimensional system*. For a contextually appropriate movement to occur, degrees of freedom need to be constrained. Bernstein[3] suggested that the number of degrees of freedom could be reduced by muscles working in synergies, that is, coupling muscles and joints of a limb to produce functional patterns of movement. Therefore, the functional unit of motor behavior is a *synergy*, also called coordinative structure. By reducing the degrees of freedom, a high-dimensional system becomes a low-dimensional system, that is, a system with fewer degrees of freedom. For example, a functional synergy pattern for the lower extremity can be a step. Locomotion occurs by linking together the functional synergies of other limbs (interlimb coordination).

Functional synergy implies that muscles are activated in an appropriate sequence and with appropriate force, timing, and directional components. These components can be represented as fixed or "relative" ratios. The relative parameters are also termed *control parameters*. Scaling control parameters leads to a change in motor behav-

ior to accomplish the task. For example, writing your name on the blackboard exemplifies scaling force and timing. Scaling is the proportional increase or decrease of the parameter to produce the intended motor activity.

Coordinated movement is defined as an orderly sequence of muscle activity in single functional synergy or the orderly sequence of functional synergies with appropriate scaling of activation parameters necessary to produce the intended motor behavior. Uncoordinated movement can occur at the level of the scaling of control parameters in one functional synergy or inappropriate coupling of functional synergies. The control parameter of duration will be used to illustrate scaling. If muscle A is active for 10% of the duration of the motor activity and muscle B is active 50% of the time, the fixed ratio of A/B is 1:5. If the movement is performed very slowly, the relative time for the entire movement increases. Fixed ratios also increase proportionally. Writing your name on a blackboard very small or very large yields the same results—your name.

When performing a repetitive movement such as elbow flexion and extension, the biceps and triceps muscles need to be active at certain times to maintain the repetitive motion. If the biceps demonstrates a delayed onset and longer duration of activity that continued into the time of activation of the triceps muscle, the movement would appear uncoordinated. If muscle A had a delayed onset and the same duration, the movement would not appear to be smooth. Patients with neurological dysfunction demonstrate alterations in the timing of muscle activity in a functional synergy or in coupling of functional activities to produce movement.[32, 39]

Fixed ratios such as amplitude and timing are incorporated into a synergy to decrease the degrees of freedom. The relative parameters of the synergy provide the flexibility or adaptability of the system for task accomplishment; however, the movement pattern may be self-limiting or limited by constraints imposed by the environment or the body. The amplitude of writing on a blackboard is limited by the height of the blackboard, the length of the arm, and the overall height of the person stretching to make the letter larger.

These functional synergies are not hard-wired but represent emergent properties. They are flexible and adaptable to meet the needs of the task and the environmental constraints. They can be described in terms of timing, for example, timing of the flexion and extension phases, and in terms of phasing, that is, when the flexion and extension phases occur in relation to one another. The movement can also be described in terms of the positional relationship between joints. These descriptors of motor behavior have been termed *order parameters*. In summary, the nervous system is organized to limit the degrees of freedom to accomplish the task. Limiting the degrees of freedom implies that a finite number of strategies are available to accomplish the goal.

Finite Number of Movement Strategies. The concept of emergent properties could conceivably imply an unlimited number of movement strategies available to perform a particular task. As stated earlier, limiting the degrees of freedom decreases the number of strategies available for selection. In addition, constraints imposed by the internal environment (e.g., musculoskeletal system, cardiovascular system, metabolic activity, cognition) and external environment (e.g., support surface, obstacles, lighting) limit the number of movement strategies. Horak and Nashner observed that a finite number of balance strategies was used by individuals in response to externally applied linear perturbations on a force plate system.[20] Using a life span approach, VanSant identified a limited number of movement patterns for the upper limb, head-trunk, and lower limb for the task of rising from supine to standing.[43]

The combination of these strategies produces variability in motor behavior. Although an individual has a preferred or modal profile, the person can combine the strategies in the various body regions to produce a different movement pattern to accomplish the task.

Variability of Movements Implies Normalcy. Age, activity level, the environment, constraints of the task, and neuropathology affect the selection of patterns. When change occurs in one or more of the neural subsystems, a new movement pattern emerges. The element that causes change is called a control parameter. For example, an increase in the speed of walking occurs until a critical speed and degree of hip extension is reached, thereby switching the movement pattern to a run. When the speed of the run is decreased, there is a shift back to the preferred movement pattern, that is, walking. A control parameter then shifts the individual into a different pattern of motor behavior.

This concept underlies theories of development and learning. Development and learning can be viewed as moving the system from a stable state to a more unstable state. When the control variable is removed, the system moves back to the early, more stable state. As the control variable continues to push the system, the individual spends more time in the new state and less time in the earlier states until the individual spends most of the time in the new state. When this occurs, the new state becomes the preferred state. Moving or shifting to the new preferred state does not obviate the ability of the individual to use the earlier state of motor behavior. Therefore, new movement patterns take place when critical changes occur in the system due to a control parameter.

Functional limitations and neuropathology also shift the individual to different patterns of motor behavior. The musculoskeletal system, by nature of the architecture of the joints and muscle attachments, can be a constraint on the movement pattern. An individual with a functional contracture may be able to bend a joint only so far into the range, thereby decreasing the movement repertoire available to the individual. Such a constraint produces adaptive motor behavior. Dorsiflexion of the foot needs to meet a critical degree of toe clearance during gait. If there is functional limitation in dorsiflexion, then biomechanical constraints imposed on the nervous system will produce adaptive motor behaviors (e.g., toe clearance during gait). Changes in motor patterns during the task of rising from supine to standing are observed when healthy individuals wear an orthosis to limit dorsiflexion.[23]

An individual uses preferred movement patterns that are stable yet flexible enough to meet the ever-changing environmental conditions. These preferred, not obligatory, movement patterns are considered *attractor* states. That is, the individual can choose to use another movement pattern to accomplish the task. Older adults may choose movement patterns that decrease the risk of falling. The choice may be in response to age-related declines in the sensory systems or a fear of falling. For example, when performing the Multi-directional Reach Test (MDRT),[31] the older adult may choose to reach forward, backward (lean), or laterally without shifting the center of gravity toward the limits of stability. The older adult can perform a different reach if asked but prefers a more stable pattern.

An obligatory or stereotypical movement pattern suggests that the individual does not have the capability to adapt to a new situation or cannot use a different movement pattern to accomplish the task. This inability may be due to internal constraints that are functional or pathophysiological. The patient who had a cerebrovascular accident has CNS constraints that limit the number of different movement patterns that can emerge from the self-organizing system. With recovery, the patient is able to select and use additional movement strategies. Cognition and the capability to learn may also limit the number of movement patterns available to the individual and the ability of the person to select and use new or different movement patterns.

Obligatory or stereotypical movement patterns also arise from external constraints imposed on the organism. Consider the external constraints placed on the concert violin player. These external constraints include, for example, the length of the bow and the position of the violin. Repetitive movement patterns leading to cumulative trauma disorder in healthy individuals can lead to muscular and neurological changes.[2, 4, 16] Over time, changes in dystonic posturing and changes in the somatosensory cortex have been observed. Although one hypothesis considers that the focal dystonia results from sensory integrative problems, an observable result is a stereotypical motor problem.

A key to the assessment and treatment of individuals with neurological dysfunction lies in variability of movement and in the notion that variability is a sign of normalcy and stereotypy is a sign of dysfunction.

To review, the nervous system responds to a variety of internal and external constraints to develop and execute motor behavior that is age appropriate and efficient to accomplish the task. Efficiency can be examined in terms of metabolic cost to the individual, type of movement pattern used, the preferred or habitual movement (habit) used by the individual, and time to complete the task. The term *attractor state* is used in dynamic systems theory to describe the preferred pattern or habitual movement.

The concepts of motor efficiency and preferred movement patterns are important for neurological rehabilitation. The patient with a neurological deficit may have a limited repertoire of movement strategies due to the neurological insult. The patient experiments with different motor patterns to learn the most efficient and energy-conserving motor strategy to accomplish the task. Therapists can refine the task based on safety issues and the patient's capability to accomplish the task using a variety of movement strategies rather than using one, stereotypical strategy.

Role of Sensory Information. The CNS uses sensory information in a variety of ways to regulate posture and movement. Before movement is initiated, information about the position of the body in space, body parts to one another, and environmental conditions is obtained from sensory receptors. This information is used in the selection and execution of the movement synergy. During movement, various neural centers (e.g., cerebellum) use feedback to compare the actual motor behavior with the intended motor behavior. If the actual and intended motor behaviors do not match, an error signal is produced and alterations in the motor behavior occur. In some instances, the control system anticipates and makes corrective change before the detection of the error signal. This anticipatory correction is termed *feedforward* control.

Ballistic movements do not rely on sensory feedback loops to modify the program as it is being executed because the execution phase occurs very quickly. In this instance, feedback is received in the form of knowledge of results after the execution of movement. Most naturally occurring movements are classified as nonballistic and therefore operate on feedforward and feedback mechanisms.

Another role of sensory information is to revise the reference of correctness (central representation) before executing the motor program again. For example, a young child standing on a balance beam with the feet close together falls off the balance beam. An error signal occurs because of the mismatch between the intended motor behavior and the actual motor behavior. If the child knows that the feet were too close together when the fall occurred, then the child will space the feet farther apart on the next trial. The information about what happened, falling or not falling, is called knowledge of results. The CNS can store knowledge of results and use it when planning movement strategies for balancing on any narrow object (e.g., balance beam, log, or wall).

Several researchers investigated whether peripheral feedback is necessary during the execution phase of movement.[28, 37, 41] Rothwell and colleagues[28, 37] studied a patient with a unilateral deafferented upper extremity due to peripheral sensory neuropathy. The man could write sentences with his eyes closed and drive a car with a manual transmission without watching the gearshift, but he had difficulty with fine motor tasks, such as buttoning a shirt and using a knife and fork. He was unable to sustain a muscle contraction using a pincer grasp when asked to perform the task with eyes closed and could not learn to drive a new car with a manual transmission. Based on these observations, continued peripheral feedback may not be necessary when executing a learned motor behavior. However, peripheral feedback is necessary during the acquisition or learning of new motor behaviors that are not inherent.

Errors in Motor Control. When the actual motor behavior does not match the intended motor behavior, one or several errors may be postulated to produce this mismatch. This section describes several types of errors. The following scenario can be used to illustrate various types of errors. A person is standing at a curb waiting for the light to change. The individual is unexpectedly pushed from behind and attempts to make a balance response, for example, sway at the ankle to maintain the upright position. A loss of balance is indicative that one or several errors occurred. First, the individual selected the wrong movement strategy. Although sway about the ankle is a proper strategy to maintain balance, it was inappropriate for this situation because the person fell. Second, the individual selected the appropriate motor program but used inappropriate scaling of relative parameters (in this instance an inappropriate scaling of amplitude of the response in relation to the perturbing force). Third, the individual may not have accurately accessed and perceived the initial sensory conditions, (e.g., unable to ignore sensory conflicts). If a car were passing in front of the individual, the individual might perceive that he or she was moving sideways, thereby relying on altered or inaccurate information for selection of the motor program.

Errors also occur when unexpected factors disrupt the execution of the program. For example, an individual walks on a moving sidewalk. When the individual steps off the sidewalk, a disruption in walking occurs. The first few steps are not smooth because the person needs to switch movement strategies from one incorporating a moving support surface to one incorporating a stationary support surface.

Errors occur in the perception of sensory information, in selection of the appropriate motor program, in selection of the appropriate variable parameters, or in the response execution. Patients with a neurological deficit may demonstrate a combination of these errors. Therefore, an assessment of motor deficits in clients includes analysis of these types of errors.

All individuals, both healthy individuals and those with CNS dysfunction, make errors in motor programming. These errors are assessed by the CNS and are stored in past memory of the experience. Errors in motor programming are extremely useful in learning. Learning can be viewed as decreasing the mismatch between the intended and actual motor behavior. This mismatch is a measure of the error; therefore, a decrease in the degree of the error is indicative of learning. Errors, then, are a very important part of the rehabilitation process. The ability of the patient to detect an error and correct it to produce appropriate motor behavior is one key to recovery.

Summary. The previous components of contemporary motor control theories are interrelated. Movement is an emergent property that arises from the cooperative working of neural centers that assess information from the internal and external environments, process the information with past memories, and produce a movement strategy that is appropriate to the situation and accomplishes the task. The movement pattern has appropriate amplitude, duration, and sequencing of synergies. It is efficiently executed, both in terms of metabolic efficiency and movement efficiency. Movement efficiency in terms of energy expenditure relates to the appropriate controlling of the multiple of degrees of freedom at the various joints to accomplish the movement. The movement is accomplished with the flexibility and adaptability to be modified if new constraints are imposed during the execution of the movement. The movement pattern used by the individual is the preferred movement pattern selected by that individual to accomplish the task and not an obligatory pattern. Once the task is accomplished, elements of the task are stored in motor memory. The representation of the movement pattern that is stored may be modified as a result of learning and development.

Regulation of Posture and Equilibrium

Postural and equilibrium reactions are those automatic responses to maintain the organism in the erect position and to maintain the head in space (face vertical and mouth horizontal). These responses are accomplished through the integration of sensory input from the vestibular, visual, and somatosensory systems. Stabilization of the head in space for gaze control will be described first, followed by a brief description of balance responses (see also Chapter 21).

Head Stabilization in Space

The phrase "stabilization of the head in space" refers to a dynamic equilibrium incorporating the alignment of the head on the trunk during movement to maintain gaze stability.[8] Vestibulocollic, vestibulospinal, and tonic neck reflexes and righting reactions assist with head stabilization in space by coordinating the neck, trunk, and limb musculature to maintain or regain a stable platform for the eyes. When the head or trunk is tilted or rotated in space or body parts are rotated in relation to one another (e.g., body on body righting reaction), automatic reactions are evoked. They oppose the motion resulting from the perturbing force to maintain or regain equilibrium of the head and body in space.

Another function of the vestibular reflexes, particularly the vestibulocollic reflex, is to dampen the tendency for oscillatory motion of the head. Based on the biomechanics of the head/neck system, a resonant frequency of 2 to 3 Hz is likely to produce oscillation of the head. To maintain a stable gaze, this oscillation is regulated by a negative reflex loop associated with the vestibulocollic reflex system. The cervicocollic reflex also assists to stabilize the head.[33] Proprioceptors, primarily muscle spindles from muscles of the neck, provide sensory feedback for this reflex. Although this reflex has been demonstrated in decerebrate animals, it has been difficult to elicit in alert animals. The vestibular reflexes and this stretch reflex may be operating over the same circuitry, thereby making it more difficult to isolate and study. An investigation of these systems in a gravity environment and in a gravity-eliminated environment is ongoing.[17, 34]

The roles of the tonic neck reflexes and of righting reactions are also important in the coordination of postural reactions. The tonic neck reflex can be considered to assist in the regulation of the neck-trunk-limb–coordinated linkage operated through proprioceptors. Depending on the direction of the tilt, the tonic reflexes

may oppose vestibular reflexes. For example, forward tilting of the head in a quadruped results in upper limb flexion by means of the tonic neck reflexes and upper limb extension by means of the vestibulospinal reflexes. When the reflexes are combined, tilting of the head maintains the neutral limb-trunk posture to support the animal.

Gaze stabilization is regulated by the vestibuloocular reflex and the optokinetic systems. The function of these systems is to maintain a stable retinal image during head motion. Oscillopsia indicates that the retinal image is not stable during movement, that is, the stable world appears to move. The vestibuloocular system tends to operate during higher speeds of rotation whereby the semicircular canals can monitor the precise velocity of head rotation. The optokinetic system tends to be most efficient at low speeds of rotation whereby the photoreceptors detect both the speed and direction of the image passing across the retinal field. Both systems activate extraocular muscles to produce a counterrotation of the eyes.

The vestibuloocular reflex functions to produce counterrotation in the eyes in response to head rotation, thereby maintaining a stable gaze in the line of sight. Eye rotation is limited by the excursion in the eye socket; therefore, compensatory movements are necessary. Compensatory movement during maintained head rotation is termed *nystagmus*, and consists of two phases, a slow phase that compensates for head rotation and a quick phase that returns the eye back to the center of the orbit. If the counterrotation of the eyes matches the rotation of the head, then the strength of this linkage, or gain, is 1. If the gain is 0.5, it signifies a mismatch between the rotation of the head and counterrotation of the eyes such that the eye movement undercompensates head movement by one half. That is, the eyes rotate half as far as head rotation. Alternately, a gain of 2 indicates that the eyes are overcompensating and rotating twice as far as head rotation. The cerebellum assists in maintaining the gain of the vestibuloocular reflex.[27]

Other eye movements controlled by a complex neural system are saccades and smooth pursuit. Saccades are small gaze-shifting movements that operate quickly to keep the eyes in position. Input from vision, the somatosensory system, and the auditory system is used by the saccadic system to regulate eye movement to maintain the line of gaze.[14] Saccadic movements are necessary to scan the visual world, and smooth pursuit movements are used to maintain the eyes on target. The cerebellum is involved in the regulation of both of these tasks. Eye movements are extremely important for aligning (righting) and maintaining (equilibrium) the body in space.

Regulation of Balance

Balance reactions occur to maintain or regain the center of gravity (center of mass) over the base of support (see Chapter 21). Base of support is defined as the boundary whereby shifts of the center of gravity can occur using one movement strategy without losing balance or necessitating a change in the movement strategy. Alternately, posture defined from a biomechanical point of view is body segment orientation to one another and in space. These automatic reactions occur during static positions such as sitting and quiet standing, and they occur during transition phases, that is, from one position to another position (e.g., sit to stand, walk, and turn). Balance reactions operative over long ascending and descending pathways are sometimes termed *long-loop reflexes*.

Balance responses may be classified as *anticipatory* or *compensatory*. Anticipatory balance responses are those postural changes that occur before the perturbing force, whereas compensatory balance responses occur as a result of the perturbing force. A perturbing force may be voluntary, for example, reaching for an object moves the center of gravity close to the limits of the base of support. In anticipation of reaching, electromyographic activity occurs in lower-extremity musculature before the initiation of electromyographic activity in the upper extremity to counter the destabilizing effect that the reach will produce. Alternately, a compensatory balance response is activated by an external perturbing force. The balance responses to maintain or regain the center of gravity over the base of support occur within 90 ms of the external perturbing force.

As discussed earlier, a finite number of movement strategies are available for response selection. These strategies were observed during externally applied linear perturbations in the laboratory setting. The *ankle strategy* is a synergy whereby muscle activation occurs at the ankle and temporally spreads to more proximal musculature. A greater linear perturbation or unexpected rotation about the ankle results in the selection of a different movement strategy, *hip strategy*. If the perturbation is such that the hip and ankle strategies are not successful, then the individual takes a step to prevent falling, *step strategy*. The time the individual has to react to maintain balance and prevent falling is extremely short, occurring approximately 90 ms after the disturbance. Coupling muscles together into functional synergies and limiting the number of movement strategies available decrease the time for response.

Balance reactions occurring during routine activities of daily living incorporate a combination of these lower-extremity movement patterns with trunk and upper limb patterns. Response selection is based on the conditions of the perturbation, the initial position of the individual, environmental conditions, past experiences, and the goal. These are the same conditions as those described earlier that pertain to the regulation of movement. Conditions of the perturbation include the amplitude, velocity, and direction of the perturbing force. The initial position of the individual incorporates the position of the individual in space and the relationship of the person's body parts to each other. Also included is the biomechanical, neurological, and general physiological status of the individual. Environmental conditions include the stability of the support surface, objects in the environment, and the condition of the lighting. The goal to be achieved in this particular scenario is to maintain or regain the center of mass over the base of support so the individual does not fall.

Errors in the selection and execution of balance responses occur both in healthy individuals and those with neurological disorders. Both groups of individuals may be unable to resolve conflicts that arise from the sensory processing of information from the visual, somatosensory, and vestibular systems. The result may be the selection and execution of an inappropriate balance response. The appropriate balance response may be selected, but there may be an inappropriate scaling of control parameters. For example, an individual with cerebellar dysfunction may demonstrate increased amplitude of the balance response in relation to an externally applied linear perturbation.[11] An individual with traumatic brain injury may select the appropriate movement strategy but with a delayed onset.[30] An individual with Parkinson's disease may have difficulty selecting a single movement strategy.[21] Selecting two movement strategies in response to externally applied linear perturbation results in decreasing all the degrees of freedom imposed by the selection of the two strategies. A more rigid posture ensues that potentially destabilizes the individual.

ASSESSMENTS BASED ON CONTEMPORARY MOTOR AND BALANCE CONTROL THEORIES

Many evaluative methods are used to assess motor and postural control in clients with neurological dysfunction. How the therapist uses and interprets the data is based on contemporary theories of motor and balance control and on considering the client as an active participant and not a passive recipient in the evaluation procedure. Evaluation procedures are designed to determine how the individual's physical, mental, and cognitive status affects motor abilities. Furthermore, evaluation procedures are valid and reliable tools to determine functional outcome. A custom-designed evaluation approach is used because the mechanism of injury or disease, secondary brain damage, recovery rate, and functional outcome differ in every individual. One strategy to assess the client with neurological dysfunction is to assess the individual's previous and present activity levels.

Activity Level

Unobtrusive evaluation at bedside or in the clinic provides an excellent opportunity to examine functional activity level and observe compensatory or preferred movement strategies used by the individual. Another unobtrusive observation period can be "staged"; for example, the client is asked to assist the clinician to move objects off a low mat table, or the client is asked to remove his shoes and socks. During these observation times, the patient is not "performing" a motor task and a more natural pattern of motor behavior may be observed. A patient may sit on the floor to remove shoes and socks because the floor is more stable than sitting on a low mat table. In this instance, the therapist has the opportunity to observe the movements used by the patient to reach the floor, the mobility and stability patterns used while the shoes and socks are being removed, and the movement strategy used to get up from the floor. Stability, transition phases, and movements occurring with the various tasks are observed and documented.

Items incorporated in an assessment of activity level vary depending on the age of the patient, severity of complaints, observational analysis before the evaluation, and the physical, cognitive, and behavioral status of the individual. For example, an elderly patient with CNS dysfunction may have preexisting movement and balance dysfunction owing to the aging process. Activity level, however, should not be based solely on the assumption that elderly persons are more inactive than younger adults. Inactive elderly and inactive college-aged individuals have lower functional patterns for righting reactions when coming to standing from supine than their active cohorts.[43] Assessment of activity level involves employment status, including type of work (sedentary or active); participation in leisure activities, both organized and solo (sports, choir, bridge, walking, gardening); and the effect of the preexisting and existing dysfunction on current activity levels in terms of assistance with activities of daily living, work, and leisure activities.

Another important facet is to identify activities the individual believes he or she can no longer perform because of the motor control problem or loss of confidence. Tasks used in the evaluation should be similar to those activities the patient can perform and those activities that are familiar to the individual. The inability to perform a new task may be due to CNS damage or the inability of the individual to understand and carry out an unfamiliar task. Tasks can incorporate transitional movements moving from supine to sit, sit to stand, bending down and reaching for something on the floor, walking and turning the head, and reaching in various directions. Functional activity permits analysis of motor and postural control, interplay between the individual and the environment, and the ability of the individual to function safely in the everyday home and work environment.

Physical deconditioning decreases general flexibility, endurance, and strength and predisposes the individual to movement instability. Biomechanical factors such as the degree of motion between the head and neck, intersegmental rotation of the trunk, and degree of movement in the lower extremities are examined as the individual performs a functional activity. A decrease in range of motion may be due to a functional biomechanical loss or to a motor control problem that alters the timing of the movement. For example, a patient with a cerebrovascular accident may exhibit footdrop. Initially, the footdrop is due to alteration in the movement pattern due to the loss of CNS control for the timing and sequencing of interlimb muscle activity. If the footdrop persists, biomechanical changes contribute to the deficit in the lower-extremity movement pattern.

Another element to consider is metabolic change or a reduced exercise capacity. Inactivity deconditions the cardiovascular and pulmonary systems, which results in a decreased ability to perform routine activities of daily living. The resulting decline increases stress on these physiological systems when the patient is asked to perform a task. A task as simple as walking up several steps can cause the individual to exceed his or her exercise capacity. When the decreased aerobic capacity is coupled with alterations in the CNS or biomechanical system, a cycle occurs in which a reduced exercise capacity leads to an increase in inactivity, which further reduces exercise capacity. This cycle can also cause a loss of self-confidence. Lastly, the motor and postural control systems are assessed according to the ability of the individual to perform the activity smoothly and efficiently. A more detailed discussion follows.

USE OF MOTOR CONTROL PARAMETERS TO ASSESS POSTURE AND MOVEMENT DEFICITS IN CLIENTS WITH NEUROLOGICAL DISEASE OR TRAUMA

Patients with neurological disease are unable to generate "normal" motor behavior because the CNS deficit has altered the integrative capability of the brain. Biomechanical and metabolic factors are also altered. The movement pattern executed by the patient is considered a functional movement pattern used to accomplish the goal. Depending on the pathophysiology of the trauma and secondary complications, the pattern may not be efficient in terms of neurological, biomechanical, or metabolic costs to the system. Nevertheless, the pattern is the preferred pattern (emergent property) arising from a self-organizing system that permits the individual to function. This preferred pattern is a result of the constraints imposed on the individual by the neurological condition as well as of the constraints imposed by the environment and the task. The use of assistive devices may further increase the costs to the system.[19] For example, a person using a walker will have an altered gait pattern, resulting in increased metabolic costs. Prolonged use of the walker alters the biomechanical and neurological relationship for postural alignment and the location of the center of mass.

Evaluation and treatment should focus on those movement parameters that have been altered and the way in which the individual can optimally function in a particular task. To guide the evaluation of posture and movement, several general questions can be addressed. For example, what is the activity level of the person? Is the person able to safely function in the everyday environmental home and work setting? Does the person have the capability to generate movement strategies, and is the person capable of learning new motor strategies?

Another guiding factor is the life span developmental status of the person. A young child with cerebral palsy has a reference of correctness about movement that is based on the constraints imposed from the condition. An adult with an acute CNS deficit may have either a preinjury reference of correctness or a postinjury reference of correctness that may or may not be compatible with the new constraints imposed by the acute neurological condition. For example, a client with a cardiovascular accident may exhibit a list to the involved side while sitting but perceives that he or she is sitting upright.

Specific questions relative to motor control also guide the assessment. For example, is the individual appropri-

CASE 5–1   PERSON WITH PARKINSON'S DISEASE

When evaluating motor control deficits in the client with Parkinson's disease, the severity of the disease, the activity level of the person, and the medication schedule are important considerations. Described below are several motor control deficits that are evident in this disease. Figure 5–4 can be used to guide the evaluation.

The Get Up and Go Test can be used to assess both gait and transition phases of a stand up, walk, and turn task. Alterations in stride length, speed, and frequency produce changes in the gait pattern in the person with Parkinson's disease. The person may demonstrate a gait pattern with decreases in amplitude of leg movement, duration of the gait cycle, trunk rotation, and arm swing. Small, shuffling steps and a festinating gait are also observed. The festinating gait occurs in an attempt to maintain the center of gravity over the base of support in the individual with a flexed posture. A decrease in righting and equilibrium reactions also contributes to instability in gait. Whenever the preferred speed and frequency parameters are altered in any movement, they can increase metabolic costs and alter the ability of the individual to safely complete the functional movement with appropriate coordination of postural and motor control. In fact, any gait deficit increases metabolic costs.

The difficulty in initiating gait, or "freezing," is another observable motor control problem.[5] Freezing refers to a failure in gait initiation and can be assessed at different times in the Get Up and Go Test. Freezing can occur when the person rises from the chair, turns at the end of 3 meters, and turns and then sits down in the chair. Freezing also occurs when the target is approached (i.e., destination freezing), when an obstacle is encountered, or spontaneously. This deficit is attributed to the imbalance of the direct and indirect pathways from the basal ganglia.[40]

Overshoot of the 10-meter line before turning may be demonstrated. Although clients with Parkinson's disease are able to prepare the motor strategy and use advance information, the primary problem is the slow onset of execution of movement.

To illustrate the multiple motor control deficits, imagine a patient performing the Get Up and Go Test. The person is asked to stand up from a chair, walk a specified distance, turn around, walk back to the chair, and sit down. The person may have difficulty accelerating and decelerating to turn around and may have difficulty decelerating when approaching the chair and sitting down. These motor control deficits exhibited in the patient with Parkinson's disease are numerous and intertwined. The severity of these motor control deficits is influenced by the progression of the disease. As mentioned earlier, the client cannot appropriately control the increase and decrease in the rate of force production, which is evident in the acceleration and deceleration phases of the movement. If the rate of force production is altered, amplitude of force production may also be affected.

The person may have decreased ability to predict and prepare the motor pattern for turning before the actual turn. There appears to be a slow initiation of the turning task. This phenomenon could be due to the inability to sequence the motor behavior as a whole. Several researchers have observed that the person completes one movement before starting the next movement in the sequence rather than executing a smooth, ongoing movement pattern.[39] Another reason for the decrease in the ability to perform this task smoothly is the patient's dependence on visual feedback. Relying more heavily on visual feedback to accomplish a task slows the movement.

The movement deficits observed may also be due to the inability to effectively coordinate movements such as those observed between postural and motile components of the task. Postural strategies may be classified on a continuum that includes postural preparations, postural accompaniments, and postural reactions.[12] The person with Parkinson's disease may not predict and make appropriate postural adjustments before the movement and may have deficits in postural reactions (i.e., righting and equilibrium reactions). When patients are externally perturbed, some researchers[18, 21] noted that simultaneous activation of two balance strategies occurs, whereas others[24, 36] noted a decrease in functional activation of muscles, particularly around the ankle.

In the case of the Get Up and Go Test, movement and balance strategies are assessed when the client stands up and sits down. If the client does not use a controlled descent into the chair but rather flops, what are the possible causes for the sudden descent? The individual's preferred pattern may be to flop into the chair; the individual may not be able to predict the time and force needed to activate the muscles for a smooth descent; the individual may be deconditioned and does not have the strength or endurance to perform a smooth descent; or the individual may not have the balance strategies required to perform this maneuver.

In summary, to assess the patient with Parkinson's disease or any other neurological deficit, all aspects of motor control need to be examined as the individual executes a variety of functional tasks. The patient may have multiple motor and postural control deficits; only a few were examined in the example. It is not within the scope of this section to present all the motor and postural control deficits but to highlight the complexity of patients with neurological pathophysiology. Accurate identification of motor control problems in clients assists in the development of effective treatment goals and plans (see Section II).

ately processing sensory information? Is the person generating an appropriate motor response? Can the individual modify the motor response to accomplish the task, or does the person use limited or obligatory motor patterns? Is the person selecting the appropriate motor strategy, but parameters such as amplitude, timing, and phasing are not appropriate? The clinician identifies inappropriate parameters of motor control. The therapist then develops a hypothesis(es) pertaining to alterations in the motor control system, in the physiological system, or in the biomechanical systems and uses this hypothesis(es) as a basis for treatment. Treating the patient and assessing the outcome are the means to test the hypothesis.

These examples are only a few of the guiding questions that can be asked relative to motor and postural control. Once the therapist observes the patient, the therapist can formulate hypotheses on what factors are contributing to the deficits in motor behavior. Observational analysis can be used to focus the remainder of the evaluation in a more contextually appropriate manner. The more focused questions can be used to test the hypotheses. Often, a single factor does not produce the motor deficit but rather an interaction of present and past constraints. The satisfying part of an evaluation is to be able to test and rule out hypotheses. Theoretically, by ruling out hypotheses, the treatment program can become more focused and effective. A list of a large variety of assessment tools can be found in Chapter 3 and those located within this chapter identified in the appendix at the back of this book.

REFERENCES

1. Alexander GE, DeLong MR, Crutcher MD: Do cortical and basal ganglionic motor areas use "motor programs" to control movement? In Cordo P, Harnad S (eds): Movement Control. New York, Cambridge University Press, 1994, pp 54–63.
2. Barr AF, Barbe MF, Vincent KK: Behavioral and histological changes in a rat model of an upper extremity cumulative trauma disorder. Phys Ther 79(5):S54, 1999.
3. Bernstein N: Coordination and Regulation of Movement. New York, Pergamon Press, 1967.
4. Byl N, Merzenich MM, Cheung S, et al: A primate model for studying focal dystonia and repetitive strain injury: Effects on the primary somatosensory cortex. Phys Ther 77:269–284, 1997.
5. Brown P, Steiger MJ: Basal ganglia gait disorders. In Bronstein AM, Brandt T, Woollacott M (eds): Clinical Disorders of Balance, Posture and Gait. London, Arnold, 1996, pp 156–167.
6. Bussel B, Roby-Brami A, Yakovleff A, Bennis N: Late flexion reflex in paraplegic patients: Evidence for a spinal stepping generator. Brain Res Bull 22:53–56, 1989.
7. Calancie B, Needham-Shropshire B, Jacobs P, et al: Involuntary stepping after chronic spinal cord injury: Evidence for a central rhythm generator for locomotion in man. Brain 117:1143–1159, 1994.
8. Cromwell RL, Newton RA, Carlton LG: Horizontal plane head stabilization during locomotor tasks. J Motor Behav (in press, 2000).
9. Davis WJ: Organizational concepts in the central motor networks of invertebrates. In Herman RM, Grillner S, Stein PSG, Stuart DG (eds): Neural Control of Locomotion. New York, Plenum Press, 1976, pp 265–291.
10. DeLong MR: Primate models of movement disorders of basal ganglia origin. Trends Neurosci 13:281–285, 1990.
11. Diener H-C, Dichgans J: Cerebellar and spinocerebellar gait disorders. In Bronstein AM, Brandt T, Woollacott M (eds): Clinical Disorders of Balance, Posture and Gait. London, Arnold, 1996, pp 147–155.
12. Frank JS, Earl M: Coordination of posture and movement. Phys Ther 70:855–863, 1990.
13. Gelfand IM, Orlovsky GN, Shik ML: Locomotion and scratching in tetrapods. In Cohen AH, Rossignol S, Grillner S (eds): Neural Control of Rhythmic Movements in Vertebrates. New York, Wiley Publishers, 1988.
14. Glimcher PW: Eye movements. In Zigmond MJ, Bloom FE, Landis SC, et al (eds): Fundamental Neuroscience. San Diego, Academic Press, 1999, pp 993–1010.
15. Grillner S: Neurobiological bases of rhythmic motor acts in vertebrates. Science 228:143–149, 1989.
16. Hallett M: Is dystonia a sensory disorder? Ann Neurol 38:139–140, 1995.
17. Herdman SJ: Vestibular Rehabilitation. Philadelphia, FA Davis, 1994.
18. Heriza C: Motor development: Traditional and contemporary theories. In Contemporary Management of Motor Control Problems. Proceedings of the II STEP Conference, Fredericksburg, VA, Foundation for Physical Therapy, 1991.
19. Holt KG: Toward general principles for research and rehabilitation of disabled populations, Phys Ther Practice 2(2):1–18, 1993.
20. Horak FB, Nashner LM: Central programming of postural movements: Adaptation to altered support surface configurations. J Neurophysiol 55:1369–1381, 1986.
21. Horak FB, Nutt JG, Nashner LM: Postural inflexibility in parkinsonian patients. J Neurol Sci 111:46–58, 1992.
22. Jackson H: The Croonian Lectures on evolution and dissolution of the nervous system: Lecture 2. BMJ 660–663, 1884.
23. King LA, VanSant AF: The effect of solid ankle foot orthoses on movement patterns used to rise from supine to stand. Phys Ther 75:952–964, 1995.
24. Lauk M, Chow CC, Lipsitz LA, et al: Assessing muscle stiffness from quiet stance in Parkinson's disease. Muscle Nerve 22:635–639, 1999.
25. Lawrence DG, Kuypers HGJM: The functional organization of the motor system in the monkey: I. The effects of bilateral pyramidal lesions. Brain 91:1–14, 1968.
26. Lawrence DG, Kuypers HGJM: The functional organization of the motor system in the monkey: II. The effects of lesions of the descending brainstem pathways. Brain 91:15–36, 1968.
27. Lisberger SG: Properties of pathways subserving long-term adaptive plasticity in the vestibulo-ocular reflexes in monkeys. In Ruben RW, et al (eds): The Biology of Change in Otolaryngology. Amsterdam, Elsevier, 1986, pp 171–183.
28. Marsden CD, Rothwell JC, Day BL: The use of peripheral feedback in the control of movement. In Evarts EV, Wise SP, Bousfield D (eds): The Motor System in Neurobiology. Amsterdam, Elsevier Biomedical Press, 1985.
29. Newell KM, Corcos DM (eds): Variability and Motor Control. Champaign, IL, Human Kinetics Publishers, 1993.
30. Newton RA: Balance abilities in individuals with moderate and severe traumatic brain injured patients. Brain Injury 9:445–451, 1995.
31. Newton RA: Balance screening of an inner city older adult population. Arch Phys Med Rehabil 78:587–591, 1997.
32. Nutt J, Marsden C, Thompson P: Human walking and higher-level gait disorders, particularly in the elderly. Neurology 43:268–279, 993.
33. Peterson B, Goldberg J, Bilotto G, Fuller J: Cervicocollic reflex: Its dynamic properties and interaction with vestibular reflexes. J Neurophysiol 54:90–109, 1985.
34. Peterson B, Richmond F (eds): Control of Head Movement. New York, Oxford University Press, 1988.
35. Prihram KH: Holonomic Brain Theory: Cooperation and Reciprocity in Processing the Configural and Cognitive Aspects of Perception. Hillsdale, NJ, Erlbaum, 1988.
36. Rogers MW: Motor control problems in Parkinson's disease. In Contemporary Management of Motor Control Problems. Proceedings of the II STEP Conference, Fredericksburg, VA, Foundation for Physical Therapy, 1991.
37. Rothwell JC, Traub MM, Day BL, et al: Manual motor performance in a deafferented man. Brain 105:515–542, 1982.
38. Schoner G, Kelso JAS: Dynamic pattern generation in behavioral and neural systems. Science 239:1513–1520, 1988.
39. Sharmann S, Norton BJ: The relationship of voluntary movement to spasticity in the upper motor neuron syndrome. Ann Neurol 2:460–465, 1977.

40. Stelmach GE, Phillips IG: Movement disorders: Limb movement and the basal ganglia. Phys Ther 71:60–67, 1991.

41. Taub E: Movements in nonhuman primates deprived of somatosensory feedback. Exerc Sport Sci Rev 4:335–374, 1976.

42. Tuller B, Turvey MT, Fitch HL: The Bernstein perspective: II. The concept of muscle linkage or coordinative structure. *In* Kelso JAS (ed): Human Motor Behavior: An Introduction. Hillsdale, NJ, Erlbaum, 1982.

43. VanSant AF: A lifespan perspective of age differences in righting movements. Motor Dev Res Rev 1:46–63, 1997.

CHAPTER 6

The Limbic System: Influence over Motor Control and Learning

DARCY A. UMPHRED, PhD, PT

Key Words

- amygdala
- declarative memory
- emotional behavior
- F²ARV (Fear/Frustration, Anger, Rage, Violence) continuum
- general adaptation syndrome (GAS)
- hippocampus
- intuition
- limbic system
- MOVE
- reverberating loops or circuits

Objectives

After reading this chapter the student/therapist will:

1. Identify the complexity of the limbic complex and its influence over behavioral responses.

2. Differentiate between limbic motor control responses and cerebellar/basal ganglia motor regulation.

3. Identify different emotional or limbic responses and their influence on the spinal and brain stem motor generators.

4. Differentiate between declarative and procedural learning.

5. Analyze client's functional responses to environmental demands and determine if the limbic complex has negatively or positively influenced the observable behavior.

6. Analyze the influence intuition and spirituality may have on therapist and client behavior.

The understanding of the nervous system becomes more and more complex as scientists answer research questions and unravel new unknowns. Many grounded neuroscience questions about the limbic system still puzzle basic researchers. As our understanding enters into areas of alternative medicine, new questions will develop. Still the complexity of the human organism is a totality made up of many interlocking parts. The totality is like a completed puzzle. The learner should hold the visualization of the entire puzzle and then take a few pieces apart. The puzzle may initially consist of 5 to 10 pieces that fit together but when rejoined give the learner a feeling of accomplishment and intellectual mastery. The process of unlocking and reassembling the puzzle while either subdividing each original puzzle piece or adding new pieces is the journey a learner begins in school and can, if so chosen, continue

throughout life. The emotions felt by the learner and the ability to have the intellectual memory of the learning are limbic functions and thus play an important role in all of our lives.

In many curriculums the limbic system is only discussed in a basic science course of neuroanatomy/neurophysiology. In others, the limbic role in declarative memory and or/emotional responses is presented as part of a discussion on memory or cognitive function within a psychology course. Few faculty believe they have opportunity or time to present the limbic system's role in observable motor behavior whether that behavior is being expressed by the client or the therapist. This chapter has been written to provide the reader with the realization that without an understanding of limbic interactions and modulations over motor expression, the reliability and validity of measurements of motor performance will always be in question. Similarly, owing to the limitations of visits in today's health care delivery service models and the dependency on home programs, without a keen awareness of limbic responses to therapeutic interventions, a therapist will have little guarantee of compliance by the patient or caregivers. The limbic system drives behavior not through motor programming or comprehension of the task but rather through willingness to participate in the activity and/or engage in the learning. Therapists today often say: "I have no time to talk to the patient." Given the limited time available, the response I give is: "I do not have enough time not to talk to the patient!" Bonding is even more important today because empowering the patient to self-learning through less supervised or hands-on repetitive practice requires a patient who is willing and motivated to continue to learn and practice. That desire to improve can be self-motivated, but very often it is instilled by the clinician that the patient trusts and feels clearly has his or her best interests as primary goals. Through interactions, the patients know that their desires, interests, and needs as unique and valued members of society are considered and that they are not just other patients who have specific diagnoses, are placed on critical pathways, are administered drugs, will be on to the next facility in a couple of days, and have lost all individuality. That feeling of security and safety is what bonds a patient to a therapist along the journey of learning.

Before understanding and becoming compassionate to the needs of other people such as patients with signs and symptoms of neurological problems, therapists need to understand their own limbic system and how that affects others that might interact with them. Because both occupational and physical therapy professions have evolved to using enablement models and systems interactions to explain movement responses of their respective client population, the importance of separating limbic from true motor or cognitive impairments will help guide the clinician toward intervention strategies that will lead to the quickest and most efficacious outcomes. The complexity of the anatomy, physiology, and neurochemistry of the limbic complex baffles the minds of basic science doctoral students. Yet a therapist deals on a moment-to-moment functional level with the limbic system of clients throughout the day. Figure 6–1 illustrates the interlocking/codependency of all major central nervous system (CNS) components with the environment. At no time does any system stand in isolation. Thus, from a clinical perspective the therapist should always maintain focus on the whole environment and all major interactive components within it, while directing attention to any specific component.

The primary purpose of this chapter is to discuss the influence of the limbic system on motor learning, motor performance, and functional independence in life activities. If a person is scared, fearful, or apprehensive, motor performance and ability to learn either motor skill or intellectual information will be very different[30, 37, 44, 47, 71, 73, 82] from that of an individual who feels safe and functions inherently with control.[63, 71]

After injury to any part of the body, but especially the CNS, an individual will naturally have reservations or

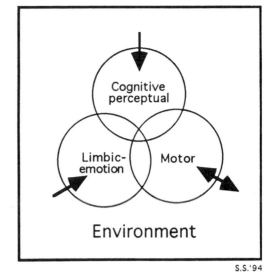

FIGURE 6–1. Interlocking/co-dependency of all major central nervous system components.

fears about the unknown future. Yet, that individual needs to be willing to experience the unknown to learn and adapt. The willingness, drive, and adaptability of that individual will affect the optimal plasticity of the CNS. The limbic system is a key player that drives and motivates that individual. The lack of awareness of that variable or its effect on a patient will ultimately eliminate efficacy of interventions. Similarly, if this system is overwhelmed either internally or externally, it will dramatically affect motor learning as well as cognitive, syntactical learning. At the conclusion of this chapter it is hoped that therapists will comprehend why there is a need to learn to modulate this system into chemical balance so that patients can functionally control movement and experience cognitive learning. Then therapists need to reintroduce emotions into the activity and allow the patient to once again experience success.

For the new learner, the first section of the chapter is a discussion of limbic behavior and how to begin to differentiate true motor responses from those entangled in limbic interactions. For colleagues desiring more in-depth discussion of the basic neuroscience, the second section delves into the anatomy and physiology, the biology of learning and memory, and neurochemistry. The last section opens up paradigms of possibilities for future research and presents questions that have not begun to be answered.

THE FUNCTIONAL RELATIONSHIP OF THE LIMBIC SYSTEM TO CLINICAL PERFORMANCE

The Limbic System's Role in Motor Control, Memory, and Learning

It is not easy to find a generally accepted definition of the "limbic system or complex," its boundaries, and the components that should be included. Mesulam[86] likens this to a fifth century BC philosopher's quotation: "the nature of God is like a circle of which the center is everywhere and the circumference is nowhere." Brodal[14] suggests that functional separation of brain regions becomes less clear as we discover the interrelatedness through ongoing research. He sees the limbic system reaching out and encompassing the entire brain and all of its functional components and sees no purpose in defining such subdivision. Although the anatomical descriptions of the limbic system may vary from author to author, the functional significance of this system is widely acknowledged in defining human behavior and behavioral neurology. To go one step farther, the link between emotions, electrochemical energy, and healing has been researched for decades by a therapist who once practiced as a neuroscience therapist and worked with patients with CNS problems.[60] This system may be the link to establishing efficacy in alternative medical practices.[101]

Brooks[15] divides the brain into the limbic brain and the nonlimbic sensorimotor brain. The sensorimotor portion is involved in perception of nonlimbic sensations and motor performance. He defines a component of the limbic brain as primitive, essential for survival, sensing the "need" to act, and thereby initiating need-directed motor activity for survival. The limbic brain also has the capability for memory and can select what to learn from experience. Brooks also defines the two limbic and nonlimbic systems functionally and not anatomically, because their anatomical separation according to function is almost impossible and changes with the task specificity (Fig. 6–2).

Kandel and others[63] state that behavior requires three major systems: the sensory, the motor, and the motivational or limbic. When analyzing a seemingly simple action, such as swinging a golf club, we recruit our sensory system for visual, tactile, and proprioceptive input to guide the motor systems for precise, coordinated muscle recruitment and postural control. The motivational (limbic) system does the following: (1) provides intentional drive for the initiation, (2) integrates the total input, and (3) plays a role in motor expression. The motivational system plays a role in control of both the autonomic and the somatic sensorimotor system. It thereby plays a role in controlling the skeletal muscles through input to the frontal lobe and brain stem and the smooth muscles and glands through the hypothalamus, which lies at the "heart" of the limbic system (Fig. 6–3). Noback and others[94] state that "the limbic system is involved with many of the expressions that make us human, namely, emotions, behaviors, and feeling states." That humanness also has individuality. Our unique memory storage, our variable responses to different environmental contexts, and our control or lack thereof over our emotional sensitivity to environmental stimuli all play roles in molding each one of us. Because of this uniqueness, each therapist and each client need to be accepted for their own individuality.

Broca[13] first conceptualized the anatomical regions of the limbic lobe as forming a ring around the brain stem. Today, neuroanatomists do not differentiate an anatomical lobe as limbic but rather refer to a complex system that encompasses cortical, diencephalon, and brain stem structures.[63] This description is less precise and encompasses, but is not limited to, the orbitofrontal cortex, hippocampus, parahippocampal gyrus, cingulate gyrus, dentate gyrus, amygdaloid body, septal area, hypothalamus, and some nuclei of the thalamus.[9, 63] Anatomists stress the importance of looking at interrelated segments or loops within the limbic region and include fiber bundles such as the fornix, mamillothalamic fasciculus, stria terminalis, medial forebrain bundle, and the stria medullaris as part of the system.[9, 18, 21] These multiple nuclei and interlinking

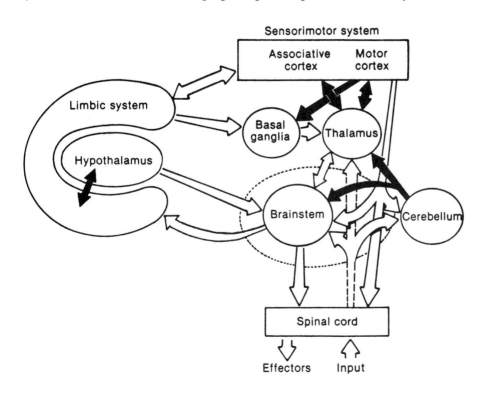

FIGURE 6–2. Divisions and interconnections between the limbic and nonlimbic cortices (sensory and motor areas).

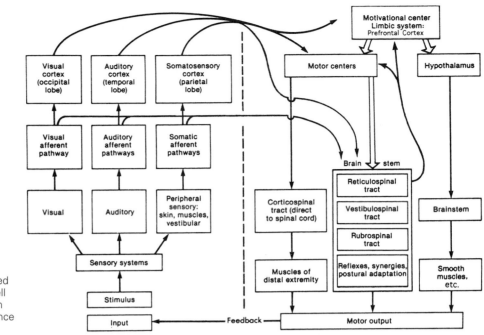

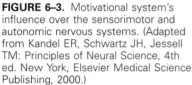

FIGURE 6-3. Motivational system's influence over the sensorimotor and autonomic nervous systems. (Adapted from Kandel ER, Schwartz JH, Jessell TM: Principles of Neural Science, 4th ed. New York, Elsevier Medical Science Publishing, 2000.)

circuits play crucial roles in behavioral and emotional changes,[17, 31, 34] declarative memory,[3, 132] and motor expression.[58] The loss of any link can affect the outcome activity of the whole circuit. Thus, damage to any area of the brain can potentially cause malfunctions in any or all other areas, and the entire circuit may need reorganization to restore function.

Researchers do not ascribe a specific single function to CNS formations but see each as part of a system, participating to various degrees, in the multitude of behavioral responses (see Chapters 4 and 5 for additional information). Therefore, the loss of any part of higher centers or the limbic system may not be clearly definable functionally, and the return of function is not always easy to predict.

Recovery of function after injury may involve mechanisms that allow reorganizing of the structure and function of cortical, subcortical, and spinal circuits. In very young infants, areas within opposite hemispheres may "take over" function, whereas in more mature brains reorganization of existing systems seems to be the current accepted hypothesis within the expanding knowledge of neuroplasticity.[36] For complex behavior, such as in motor functioning requiring many steps, the limbic system, cortex, hypothalamus, basal ganglia, and brain stem work as an integrated unit, with any damaged area causing the whole system to malfunction. A loss of function or a change in behavior cannot necessarily be localized as to the underlying cause. A lesion in one area may cause secondary dysfunction of a different area that is not actually damaged.

The complexity of the limbic system and its associative influence over both the motor control system and cortical structures are enormous. A therapist dealing with a client with motor control or learning problems needs to understand how the limbic system affects behavioral responses. The knowledge base focuses not only on the client's

deficits but also on the integrative function of the therapist. This understanding should lead to a greater awareness of the clinical environment and the factors within the environment that cause change. Without this knowledge of how to differentiate systems, objective measurements of motor performance or cognitive abilities may be inconsistent without any explanation. Similarly, with excessive limbic activity, clients' ability to store and retrieve either declarative or procedural learning may be negatively affected, thus limiting the patients' ability to benefit from traditional interventions and potentially regaining their respective highest quality of life.

The Limbic System's Influence on Behavior: Its Relevance to the Therapeutic Environment

Levels of Behavioral Hierarchies: Where Does the Limbic System Belong?

Strub and Black[124] view behavior as occurring on distinct interrelated levels, which represent behavioral hierarchies. Starting at level one, a state of alertness to the internal and external environment must be maintained for motor or mental activity to occur. The brain stem reticular activating system brings about this state of general arousal by relaying in an ascending pathway to the thalamus, the limbic system, and the cerebral cortex. To proceed from a state of general arousal to one of "selective attention" requires the communication of information to and from the cortex, thalamus, and the limbic system and its modulation over the brain stem and spinal pattern generators.[58, 63]

Level two of this hierarchy lies in the domain of the hypothalamus and its closely associated limbic structures. This level deals with subconscious drives and innate instincts. The survival-oriented drives of hunger, thirst, temperature regulation, and survival of the species (sex) and the steps necessary for drive reduction are processed here, as well as learning and memory. Most of these activities relate to limbic functioning.

On level three, only cerebral cortical areas are activated. This level deals with abstract conceptualization of verbal or quantitative entities.

Level four behavior is concerned with the expression of social aspects of behavior, personality, and lifestyle. Again, the limbic system and its relationship to the frontal lobe are vital here.

The interaction of all four levels leads to the integrative and adaptable behavior seen in humans. Our ability to become alert and protectively react is balanced by our previous learning, whether it is cognitive-perceptive, social, or affective. Adaptability to rapid changes in the physical environment, in lifestyles, and in personal relationships results from the interrelationships or complex neurocircuitry of the human brain. When insult occurs at any one level within these behavioral hierarchies, all levels may be affected.

As Western medicine is unraveling the mysteries behind the neurochemistry of the limbic system° and alternative medicine is establishing efficacy for various interventions philosophies (see Chapter 33), a fifth level of limbic function may become the link between the hard science of today and the unexplained mysteries. Those medical mysteries would be defined as unexplained, yet identified events that have either been forgotten or hidden from the world by those scientists. Mysteries such as why some people heal from terminal illnesses spontaneously, various others heal in ways not accepted by traditional medicine yet heal nonetheless, and still others just die without any known disease or pathology.[60, 101, 114] One critical component everyone identifies as part of that unexplained healing is a belief by the client that he or she will heal. That belief has a strong emotional component[101] and that may be the fifth level of limbic function. How conscious intent drives hypothalamic autoimmune function is yet to be unraveled scientifically, yet clinicians often observe these patient changes. Through observation it becomes apparent that clients who believe they will get better often do and those who believe they will not, often don't. Whether belief comes from a religious, spiritual, or hard science paradigm, that belief drives behavior and that drive has a large limbic component.

The Limbic System MOVEs Us

Moore[90] eloquently describes the limbic system as the area of the brain that moves us. The word "MOVE" can be used as a mnemonic for the functions of the limbic system.

LIMBIC SYSTEM FUNCTION

Memory/motivation: drive
   Memory: attention and retrieval
   Motivation: desire to learn, try, or benefit from the
      environment

Olfaction (especially in infants)
   Only sensory system that does not go through the
      thalamus as its second-order synapse in the sensory pathway before it gets to the cerebral cortex
Visceral (drives: thirst, hunger, and temperature regulation; endocrine functions)
   Sympathetic and parasympathetic reactions
   Peripheral autonomic nervous system (ANS) responses
      that reflect limbic function
Emotion: feelings and attitude
   Self-concept and worth
   Emotional body image
   Tonal responses of motor system
   Attitude, social skills, opinions

As seen in this outline, the "M" depicts the drive component of the limbic system. Before learning, an individual must be motivated to learn, to try to succeed at the task, to solve the problem, or to benefit from the environment. Without motivation the brain will not orient itself to the problem and learn. Motivation drives both our cortical structures to develop higher cognitive associations as well as the motor system to develop procedures or motor programs that will enable us to perform movement with the least energy expenditure and most efficient patterns available. Once motivated, the individual must be able to pay attention and process the sequential and simultaneous nature of the component parts to be learned, as well as the whole. Thus, there is an interlocking dependency between somatosensory mapping of the functional skills[105] (cognitive), attention (limbic) necessary for any type of learning, and the sequential, multi- and simultaneous programming of functional movement (motor). The limbic amygdala and hippocampal structures and their intricate circuitries play a key role in the declarative aspect of memory. Once this syntactical, intellectual memory is learned, taken out of short-term memory by passing through limbic nuclei, the information is stored in cortical areas and can be retrieved at a later time without limbic involvement.

The "O" refers to olfaction or the incoming sense of smell, which exerts a strong influence on alertness and drive. This is clearly illustrated by the billions of dollars spent annually on perfumes, deodorants, mouthwashes, and soap as well as scents used in stores to increase customers' desires to purchase. This input tract can be used effectively by therapists who have clients with CNS lesions such as internal capsule and thalamic involvement. The olfactory system synapses within the olfactory bulb and then with the limbic system structures and then may go directly to the cerebral cortex without synapsing in the thalamus. Although collaterals do project to the thalamus, unlike all other sensory information, olfaction does not need to use the thalamus as a necessary relay center to access the cortical structures, although many collaterals also project there.[63] Other senses may not be reaching the cortical levels, and the client may have a sensory-deprived environment. Olfactory sensations, which enter the limbic system, may be used to calm or arouse the client. The specific olfactory input may determine whether the person remains calm or emotionally aroused[10] Pleasant odors would be preferable to most people. With the limbic systems influence on tone production through brain stem modulation, this is one reason why aromatherapy causes relaxation and is used by many massage therapists.

A comatose and seemingly nonresponsive client may respond to odor or be highly sensitive to it. The therapist needs to be acutely aware of the responses of these patients, because these responses may be autonomic instead of somatomotor.

The "V" represents visceral or autonomic drives. As noted earlier, the hypothalamus is nestled within the limbic system. Thus, regulation of sympathetic and parasympathetic reactions, both of the internal organ systems and the periphery, reflect ongoing limbic activity. Obviously, drives such as thirst, hunger, temperature regulation, and sexuality are controlled by this system. Clients demonstrating total lack of inhibitory control over eating or drinking or manifesting very unstable body temperature regulation may be exhibiting signs of hypothalamic/pituitary involvement and/or direct pathways from hypothalamus to midbrain structures.[33, 63]

Less obvious autonomic responses that may reflect limbic imbalances often go unnoticed by therapists. When the stress of an activity is becoming overwhelming to a client, he or she may react with severe sweating of the palms or an increase in dysreflexic activity in the mouth area rather than heightened motor activity. A therapist must continually monitor this aspect of the client's response behaviors to ascertain that the behaviors observed reflect motor control and not limbic influences over that motor system.

If the sensory input to the client is excessive whether through internal or external feedback, the limbic system may go into an alert, protective mode and will not function at the optimal level, and learning will diminish. The client may withdraw physically or mentally, lose focus or attention, decrease motivation, and become frustrated or even angry. The overload on the reticular system may be the reason for the shutdown of the limbic system and not the limbic system itself. Both are part of the same neuro-loop circuitry. All of these behaviors may be expressed within the hypothalamic/autonomic system as output, no matter where in the loop the dysfunction occurs. The evaluation of this system seems even more critical when a client's motor control system is locked, with no volitional movement present. Therapists often try to increase motor activity through sensory input; however, they must cautiously avoid indiscriminately bombarding the sensory systems. The limbic system may demonstrate overload, whereas the spinal motor generators reflect inadequate activation. Although the two systems are different, they are intricately connected, and the concept of massively bombarding one while ignoring the other does not make sense from any learning paradigm, but especially from a systems model where consensus creates the observed behavior. To illustrate this concept, think of an orchestra leader conducting a symphony. It would make no sense if one half of the brass section got sick to have the violin section play louder. Instead, the conductor would need to quiet the violin section to allow the brass component to be heard.

"E" relates to emotions, the feelings, attitudes, and beliefs that are unique to that individual. These beliefs include psychosocial attitudes and prejudices, ethnic upbringing, cultural experiences, religious convictions, and concepts of spirituality.[101] All these aspects of emotions link especially to the amygdaloid complex of the limbic system and orbitofrontal activity within the frontal lobe.[129] This is a primary emotional center, and it regulates not only our self-concept but our attitudes and opinions toward our environment and the people within it.

Self-concept is the emotional aspect of body image. For example, assume that one morning I looked in the mirror and said, "The poor world, I will not subject it to me today." I then go back to bed and eat nothing for the rest of the day. The next day I get up and look in the same mirror and say, "What a change, I look trim and beautiful. Look out world, here I come!" In reality, my physical body has not been altered drastically, if at all, but my attitude toward that body has changed. That is, the emotional component of my body image has perceptually changed.

A second self-concept deals with my attitude about my worth or value to society and the world and my role within it. Again, this attitude can change with mood, but more often it seems to change with experience. This aspect of client/therapist interaction can be critical to the success of a therapeutic environment. Two examples will be given to illustrate this point, with the focus of bringing perceived roles into the therapeutic setting:

Your client is Mrs. S., a 72-year-old woman with a left cerebrovascular accident (CVA). She comes from a low socioeconomic background and was a housekeeper for 40 years for a wealthy family of high social standing. When addressing you (the therapist) she always says "yes, ma'am" or "no, ma'am," and does just what was asked, no more and no less. It may be very hard to empower this client to assume responsibility for self-direction in the therapeutic setting. Her perceived role in life may not be to take responsibility or authority within a setting that may, from her perception, have high social status, such as a medical facility. She also may feel that she does not have the right or the power to assume such responsibilities. Success in the therapeutic setting may be based more on changing her attitudes than on her potential to relearn motor control. That is, the concept of empowerment may play a crucial role in regaining independent functional skill and control over her environment.

Your client is a 24-year-old lumberjack who suffered a closed-head injury during a fall at work. It is now 1 month since his accident, and he is totally alert, verbal, and angry and has moderate to severe motor control problems. During your initial treatment you note that he responds very well to handling. He seems to flow with your movement and with your assistance is able to practice much higher level motor control within a narrower biomechanical window; although at times he needs your assistance, you release that control whenever possible to empower him to control his body. At the end of therapy he sits back in his chair with much better residual motor function. Then he turns to you (the female therapist) and instead of saying, "That was great," he says, "You witch, I hate you." The inconsistency between how his body responded to your handling and his attitude toward you as a person may seem baffling, until you realize that he has always perceived himself as a dominant male. Similarly, he perceives women as weak, to be protected, and in need of control. If his attitude toward you cannot be changed to see you in a generic professional role, he will most likely not benefit as much from your clinical skills and guidance as a teacher.

Preconceived attitudes, social behaviors, and opinions have been learned by filtering the input through the limbic system. If new attitudes and behaviors need to be learned after a neurological insult, the intactness, especially of the amygdaloid pathways, seems crucial. Damage to these limbic structures may prevent learning; and thus socially maladaptive behavior may persist, making the individual less likely to adapt to the social environment.

As our feelings, attitudes, values, and beliefs drive our behaviors both through attention and motor responses, the emotional aspect of the limbic system has great impact on our learning and motor control. If a patient is not motivated and places little value on a motor output, then complacency results and little learning will occur. On the other hand, placing an extremely high value on a motor output as a pure expression of motor control without interlocking that control with limbic influence may lead to inconsistent responses, lack of compliance, and thus lack of learning and carryover.

MOTIVATION AND REWARD

Moore[91] considers motivation and memory as part of the MOVE system. Stellar and Stellar[123] link motivation with reward and help, illustrating how the limbic system learns through repetition and reward. They state that the concept of motivation includes drive and satiation, goal-directed behavior, and incentive. They recognize that these behaviors maintain homeostasis and ensure the survival of the individual and the species. Although the frontal lobe region appears to play an important role in self-control and execution activities, these functions seem to require a close interlocking neuronetwork between cognitive representation within the frontal regions and motivational control provided by limbic and subcortical structures.[129]

Motivated behavior is geared to reinforcement and reward, which is based on both internal and external feedback systems. Repeated experience of reinforcement and reward lead to learning, changed expectancy, changed behavior, and maintained performance.[69] Repetition with the feeling of success (reinforcement) is a critical element in the therapeutic setting, and consistently making the task more difficult just when the client feels ready to succeed will tend to decrease reinforcement/reward and thus lessen the client's motivation to try. With the pressure placed on therapists to produce changes quickly, repetition and thus long-term learning are often jeopardized, and this may have a dramatic effect on the quality of the client's life and the long-term treatment effects once he or she leaves the medical facility. Motor control theory (see Chapter 5) coincides with limbic research regarding reinforcement. Inherent feedback within a variety of environmental contexts and allowing for error leads to greater retention. Repetition or the opportunity to

practice a task (motor or cognitive) in which the individual desires to succeed will lead to long-term learning. Without practice or motivation the chance of successful learning is minimal to nonexistent.

Integration of the Limbic System as Part of a Whole Functioning Brain

Motivation, alertness, and concentration are critical in motor learning because they determine how well we pay attention to the learning and execution of any motor task. These processes of learning and doing are inevitably intertwined: "we learn as we do, and we do only as well as we have learned."[15]

Both motivation ("feeling the need to act") and concentration are contributed by the limbic system. The amygdaloid complex with its multitude of afferent and efferent interlinkages is especially adapted for recognizing the significance of a stimulus, and it assigns the emotional aspect of feeling the need to act. These neuroanatomical loops have tremendous connections with the reticular system. Hence, some authors call it the reticulolimbic system.[63, 91] The interaction of the limbic system and the motor generators of the brain stem and ultimate modulation over the spinal system lead to need-directed and, therefore, goal-directed motor activity. It also filters out the significant from the nonsignificant information by selective processing and storing the significant for memory, learning, and recall.

Goal-directed or need-directed motor actions are the result of the nervous system structures acting as an interactive system. Within this system (Fig. 6–4), all components share responsibilities. The limbic system and its cortical and subcortical components represent the most important level. In response to stimuli from the internal or external environment, the limbic system initiates motor activity out of the emotional aspect of feeling the need to act. This message is relayed to the sensory areas of the cerebral cortex, which could entail any one or all association areas for visual, auditory, tactile, olfactory, gustatory, or proprioceptive input. These areas are located in the prefrontal, occipital, parietal, and temporal lobes, where they analyze and integrate sensory input into an overall strategy of action or a general plan that meets the requirements of the task. Therefore, these cortices recognize, select, and prepare to act as a response to relevant sensory cues when a state of arousal is provided by reticular input. The limbic cortex (uncus, parahippocampal gyrus/isthmus, cingulate gyrus, and septal nucleus) has even greater influence over the sensorimotor cortices through cingulate gyrus, both directly and indirectly through association areas. The thalamus, cerebellum, and basal ganglia contribute to the production of the specific motor plans. These messages of the general plan are relayed to the projection system. The limbic structures through the cingulate gyrus also have direct connections with the primary motor cortex. This certainly has the potential to assist in driving fine motor activities through corticobulbar and corticospinal tracts. The thalamus, cerebellum, basal ganglia, and motor cortices (premotor, supplementary motor, and primary motor) contribute to the production of the specific motor plans.[63] Messages regarding the sensory

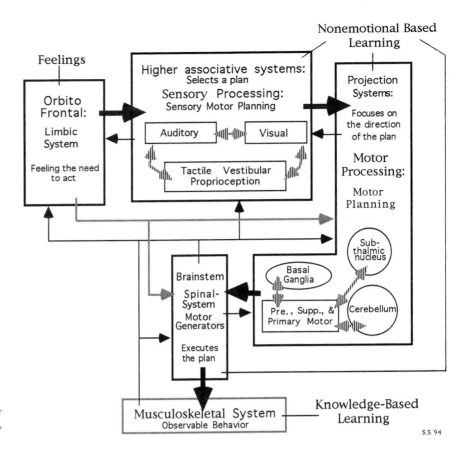

FIGURE 6–4. Functional and dynamic hierarchy of systems based on both limbic and motor control interactions. (Adapted from Brooks VB: The Neural Basis of Motor Control. New York, Oxford University Press, 1986.)

component of the general plan are relayed to the projection system where they are transformed into refined motor plans. These plans are then projected throughout the motor system to modulate motor generators throughout the brain stem and spinal system.[63] Limbic connections with (1) cerebellum, basal ganglia, and frontal lobe[63] and (2) the motor generator within the brain stem[58] enable further control of limbic instructions over motor control or expression. If the limbic and the cognitive systems decide not to act, goal-driven motor behavior will cease. An individual's belief (emotional and spiritual) can inhibit even the most basic survival skills, as has been clearly shown throughout history when individuals' religious beliefs were pitted against vicious predators and those people chose not to defend themselves.

Within the projection system and motor planning complexes, the specifics are programmed and the tactics are given a strategy. In general, the "what" is turned into "how" and "when." The necessary parameters for coordinated movement are programmed here as to intensity, sequencing, and timing to carry out the motor task. These programs that incorporate upper motor neurons and interneurons are then sent to the brain stem and spinal motor generators, which in turn through lower motor neurons send orders regarding the specific motor tasks to the musculoskeletal system. (See Chapters 4 and 5 for more specific in-depth discussion.) The actions performed by each subsystem within the entire limbic/motor control complex constantly loop back and communicate to all subsystems to allow for adjustments of intensity and duration and to determine whether the plan remains the best

choice of responses to an ever-changing three-dimensional world.

The limbic system has one more opportunity to modify and control the central pattern generators and control the body and limbs through direct connections to the spinal neuronetwork.[51, 58, 59, 93] That is, the limbic system can alter existing motor plans by modulating those generators up and down or altering specific nuclear clusters and varying the patterns themselves. Therapists as well as the general public see this in activities where emotions are high, no matter the emotion itself. Thus, for a therapist to get a true picture of a patient's motor system's function, the limbic system should be flowing in neutral or balance without strong emotions of any kind. Generally, that balance seems to reflect itself in a state of safety, trust, and compliance.

In summary, the limbic complex generates need-directed motor activity and communicates that intent throughout the motor system.[58, 59] This step is vital to normal motor function and thus client care. Clients need the opportunity to analyze correctly both their internal environment (their present and feedforward plans and their emotional state) and the external world around them requiring action on a task. The integration of all this information should produce an appropriate strategy for the present activity. These instructions must be correct and the system capable of carrying out the motor activity. If the motor system is deficit, lack of adaptability will be observed in the client. If the limbic complex is faulty, the same motor deficits might present themselves. The therapist must differentiate what is truly a motor system problem verses a limbic influence over the motor system problem.

Schmidt[112] stresses the significance of "knowledge of results feedback" as being the information from the environment that provides the individual with insights into task requirements. This insight helps the motor system correctly select strategies that will successfully initiate and support the appropriate movement for accomplishing the task. This knowledge of results feedback is required for effective motor learning and to form the correct motor programs for storage. The following example is presented to help the reader understand the limbic role in this motor programming.

You are sitting in your new car. The dealer has filled the tank with necessary fuel. The engine mechanism is totally functional with all its wires and interlocking components. The engine will not perform without a mechanism to initiate its strategies or turn on the system. The basal ganglia/frontal lobe motor mechanism plays this role in the brain. In a car you have a starter motor. Yet, the starter motor will not activate the motor system without your intent and motivation to turn the key and turn on the engine. The limbic complex serves this function in the brain. Once you have turned the key, the car is running and ready for your guidance. Whether you choose reverse or first gear usually depends on prior learning unless this is a totally new experience. Once the gear is selected, the motor system will program the car to run according to your desires. It can run fast or slow, but to change the plan both a purpose and a recognition that change is necessary are required. The car has the ability to adapt and self-regulate to many environmental variables, such as ruts or slick pavement, to continue running the feedforward program, just as many motor systems within your CNS play that function. The limbic system may emotionally choose to drive fast, whereas your cognitive judgment may choose otherwise. The end result will drive your pedal and brake pressure and ultimately regulate the car. The components discussed play a critical role in the total function of the car just as all the systems within your CNS play a vital role in regulating your behavioral responses to the environment.

Brooks[15] distinguishes insightful learning, which is programmed and leads to skills when the performer has gained insight into the requirements, from discontinuous movements, which need to be replaced by continuous ones. This process is hastened when clients understand and can demonstrate their understanding of what "they were expected to do." Improvement of motor skills is possible by using programmed movement in goal-directed behavior. The reader must be cautioned to make sure the client's attention is on the goal of the task and not on the components of the movement itself. The motor plan needs programming and practice without constant cognitive overriding. The limbic/frontal system helps drive the motor toward the identified task or abstract representation of a match between the motor planning sequence and the desired outcome.

Without the knowledge of results, feedback, and insight into the requirements for goal-directed activity, the learning is performing by "rote," which merely utilizes repetition without analysis, and little meaningful learning or building of effective motor memory in the form of motor holograms will be minimal. Children with cognitive and limbic deficits can learn basic motor skills through repetition of practice, but the insights and ability to transfer that motor learning into other contexts will not be high (see Chapters 10 and 11).

Schmidt[112] suggests that, to elicit the highest level of function within the motor system and to enable insightful learning, therapy programs should be developed around goal-directed activities, which means a strong emotional context. These activities direct the client to analyze the environmental requirements (both internal and external) by placing the client in a situation that forces development of "appropriate strategies." Goal-directed activities should be functional behavior and thus involve motivation, meaningfulness, and selective attention. Functional and somatosensory retraining uses these concepts as part of the intervention (see Chapter 4). Specific techniques such as proprioceptive neuromuscular facilitation (PNF), neurodevelopmental therapy (NDT), Rood, and Feldenkrais can be incorporated into goal-directed activities in the therapy programs, as can any treatment approach as long as it identifies those aspects of motor control and learning that lead to retention and future performance and allow the patient to self-correct.[112] With insights into the learned skills, clients will be better able to adjust these to meet the specific requirements of different environments and needs, using knowledge of response feedback to guide them. The message then is to design exercises or programs that are meaningful and need-directed, to motivate clients into insightful goal-directed learning. Thus, understanding the specific goals of the client is critical and will only be obtained by interaction with that client as a person with needs, desires, and anticipated outcomes. A therapist cannot assume that "someone wants to do something." The goal of running a bank may seem very different from that of bird-watching in the mountains, yet both may require ambulatory skills. If a client does not wish to return to work, then a friendly smile and stating, "Hi, I'm your therapist and I'm going to get you up and walking so you can get back to work," may lead to resistance and decreased motivation. In contrast, by knowing the goal of the client, a person highly motivated to ambulate may be present in the clinic every day to meet the goal of bird-watching in the mountains although never wishing to walk back into the office at work.

Clinical Perspectives

THE CLIENT'S INTERNAL SYSTEM INFLUENCES OBSERVABLE BEHAVIOR

At least once a year almost any local newspaper will carry a story that generally reads as follows:

Seventy-nine-year-old, 109-pound arthritic grandmother picks up car by bumper to free trapped 3-year-old grandson.

All of us read these articles and at first doubt their validity and then question the sensationalism used by the reporter. I would also question such news reporting if, at age 13, I had not seen three teenage boys pick up a 1956 Chevrolet and put it back in the garage in its correctly parked position. The boys had moved the car because they feared that if they did not put the car back into its original parked position, their parents would find out that they had driven the car without a license or permission. That elderly lady picked up the car out of fear of severe injury to her grandchild. Emotions can create tremendous high tonal responses, either in a postural pattern such as in a temper tantrum or during a movement strategy such as picking up a car. Similarly, fear can immobilize a person and make it impossible to create enough tone to run a motor program or actually move. Separating power or tone production due to strong emotions versus motor system control is an aspect of therapeutic evaluation often overlooked.

LIMBIC CONTINUUMS

All clinicians need to understand and recognize two powerful limbic motor response programs: the F²ARV and the general adaptation syndrome (GAS). These continuums need to be monitored frequently with all patients with CNS injury and evaluated and recorded if response patterns exceed normal expectations.

F²ARV (Fear/Frustration, Anger, Rage, Violence) Continuum. One sequence of behaviors used to describe the emotional circuitry of the amygdala is called the F²ARV (Fear/Frustration, Anger, Rage, Violence) continuum[91] (Fig. 6–5). This continuum begins with fear, often exhibited as frustration by children, teens, and young adults. If the event inducing the fear/frustration continues to heighten, anger will often develop. Anger is a neurochemical response perceived and defined by the cognitive aspect of our cortex as anger. If the neurochemical response continues to build, the anger of the person may go into rage (internal chaos) and, finally, violence (motor response). How quickly any individual will progress from fear to violence depends on many factors. First, the initial wiring or genetic neurochemical predisposition will influence behavioral responses. Second, soft-wired or conditioned responses resulting from environmental influences and reinforcement patterns will determine output. For example, it is commonly known that abusive parents were usually abused children; they learned that anger quickly leads to violence, and that the behavior of violence was acceptable. Third, the stimulus initiating the continuum and its intensity will determine the level of response.

The neurochemistry within the individual's CNS, whether inherently active or released into the system through drugs or injury, will have great influence on the plasticity of the existing wiring.[43] When the chemistry or wiring becomes imbalanced owing to damage, environmental stress, learning, or other potentially altering situations, then the control over this continuum may also change.[36, 63]

Therapists need to be acutely aware of this continuum in clients who have diffuse axonal shearing within the limbic complex. Diffuse axonal shearing most commonly is seen and reported in research on head trauma. As a result, lesions within the limbic structures may result in an individual who progresses down this continuum at a rapid speed.[17] This point cannot be overemphasized. Patients who have difficulty in this area may physically strike out at a therapist out of frustration. The result may be a broken nose or blackened eye of the therapist. Now fear has been instilled in the therapist. Two continuums are interacting. By understanding "why the patient acted out," the therapist retains cognitive distance and potentially chemical control over his or her own limbic reactions. Knowing the social history of the client and the causation of the injury often can help the therapist gain insight into how an individual patient might progress down this continuum. Not all head-injured patients had prior difficulty with the F²ARV continuum, but, similarly, many individuals received their head injuries in violent confrontational situations.

General Adaptation Syndrome. The autonomic responses to stress have been identified as following a specific course of behavioral changes and are referred to as the general adaptation syndrome.[9, 78, 115] The sequential stages of this syndrome directly relate to limbic imbalance and can play a dramatic role in determining client progress. This stress can be caused by pain, the illness itself, ramification of the illness, confusion, sensory overload, and a large variety of other potential sources. Initial reaction to stress or neurochemical imbalance creates a state of alarm and triggers a strong sympathetic nervous system reaction. Heart rate, blood pressure, respiration, metabolism, and muscle tonus will increase. At this stage, the grandmother lifts the car off the child. If the overstimulation or stress does not diminish, the body will protect itself from self-destruction and trigger a parasympathetic response. At this time, all the symptoms reverse and the client exhibits a decrease in heart rate, blood pressure, and muscle tonus. The bronchi become constricted, and the patient may hyperventilate and become dizzy, confused, and less alert. As the blood flow returns to the periphery, the face may flush and the skin may become hot. The patient will have no energy to move, will withdraw, and again will exhibit signs of flexion, adduction, internal rotation, and lack of postural tone.

This stress or overstimulation syndrome is characterized by common symptoms.[129] If the acute symptoms are not eliminated, they will become chronic and the behavior patterns much more resistant to change.

General adaptation syndrome is often seen in the elderly, with various precipitating health crises,[78] and also in infants (see Chapter 8), head trauma victims, and other clients with neurological conditions. What causes the initial alarm can range from internal instability and minimal to mild external stress, to minimal internal instability, and to severe external sensory bombardment. Head traumas, inflammatory problems, and tumors often create hypersensitivity to external input such as noise, touch, or light. Normal clinical environments may create a sensory overload and trigger this general adaptation syndrome.

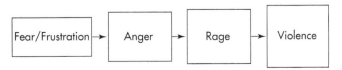

FIGURE 6–5. Fear/Frustration (F²), Anger, Rage, Violence: F²ARV continuum.

In the elderly, stresses such as change of environment, loss of loved ones, failing health, and fears of financial problems can each cause the client's system to react as if overloaded. Our elderly clients usually have two or more of these issues to deal with while trying to benefit from a therapeutic setting that demands their full attention for effective functioning. No wonder so many older clients shut down, withdraw from the therapeutic environment, and eventually withdraw from the entire world and become resistant and confused.

It is logical to assume that because of the autonomic responses that this syndrome evokes, strong interactions exist with the hypothalamus and limbic system. Stress, no matter what the specific precipitating incident (confusion, fear, anxiety, grief, and pain), has the potential of triggering the first steps in the sequence of this syndrome. The clinician's sensitivity to the client's emotional system will be the therapeutic technique that best controls and reverses the acute condition. Decreasing stimulation versus increasing facilitation may lead to attention, calmness, and receptiveness to therapy. When the client feels control over his or her life has been returned or at least the individual is consulted regarding decisions, resistance to therapy or movement often is released and stress is reduced. Even semicomatose clients can participate to some extent. As a clinician begins to move a client, resistance may be encountered. If slight changes are made in rotation or trajectory of the movement pattern, the resistance is often lessened. If the clinician initially feels the resistance and overpowers it, total control has been taken from the client. Instead, if the clinician moves the patient in ways his or her body is willing to be moved, respect has been shown and overstimulation potentially avoided.

No single input causes these reactions, nor does one treatment counteract its progression. Being aware of clinical signs is critical. Another important therapeutic skill is not prejudging withdrawn clients by assuming that they need more stimulation to regain function. The specific techniques appropriate for treating this syndrome are tools all therapists possess. How each clinician uses those tools is a critical link to success or failure in clinical interaction.

EMOTIONS EXPRESSED THROUGH MOTOR PROGRAMMING

Emotions throughout the existence of humankind have been identified in all cultures. A child knows when a parent is angry without the patient saying anything. A stranger can recognize someone who is sad or depressed. People walk to the other side of the road to avoid having to be close to someone who seems enraged. What is it that is recognized? Are emotions recognizable? Emotions are expressed through motor output and thus have the potential of impacting functional motor control. The extent and intensity are up to the therapist to evaluate.

Anger. Anger itself creates tone through the amygdaloid's influence over the basal ganglia and the sensory and motor cortices and their influence over the motor control system. This is clearly exhibited in a child throwing a temper tantrum (Fig. 6–6) or an adult putting his fist through a wall. How far a client or a friend will progress through the F^2ARV continuum (discussed in the previous

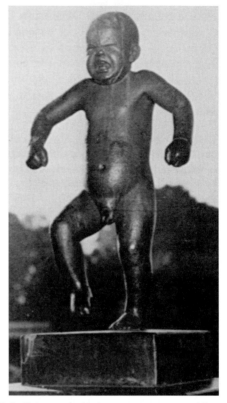

FIGURE 6–6. Extensor behavior responses caused by anger. ("Angry Boy," Vigelund Sculpture Grounds in the Frogner Park, Oslo, Norway. Adapted from photo by Normann.)

section) depends on a large number of variables. From observation, it is clear that clients do not want to lose control and progress to rage or violence, which often causes embarrassment. This fear, in and of itself, may be frustrating and trigger the continuum. When a client loses that control the therapist must first determine whether the therapist forced the client beyond his or her ability to control. If so, changes within the therapeutic environment need to be made to allow the client opportunities to develop control and modulation over that continuum. Creating opportunities to confront frustration/fear or even anger in real situations while the client practices modulation that will lead to independence or self-empowerment. The client simultaneously needs to practice self-directed motor programming without these emotional overlays. Thus, true motor learning can result. In time, practicing the same motor control over functional programs while confronted with a large variety of emotional situations should lead to independence in life activities and thus be a therapeutic goal.

Similarly, being unaware of a client's anger may lead the therapist to the false assumption that that individual has adequate inherent postural tone to perform activities such as independent transfers. If the client is angry with the therapist and performs the transfer only to "get the therapist off his or her case," when the client is sent home he or she may be unable to create enough postural extension to perform the transfer. Thus, this transfer skill was never functionally independent because the test measurements were based on limbic/frontal influence over the extensor component of the motor system. The client needs to learn how to do the activity without the emotional overlay. When a therapist is unwilling, unaware, or unable to attend to these variables, the reliability or accuracy of functional test results becomes questionable if not inaccurate.

Grief, Depression, or Pain. Emotions such as grief or depression can be expressed by the motor system.[63, 131] The behavioral responses are usually withdrawal, decreased postural adaptation, and often a feeling of tiredness and exhaustion (Fig. 6–7). Sensory overload, especially in the elderly, can create the same pattern of response of flexion, internal rotation, and adduction. Again, due to the strong emotion factor these motor responses are considered the result of the limbic system's influence over motor control.[58] Learned helplessness is another problem that therapists need to avoid. When patients are encouraged to become dependent, their chances of benefiting from services and regaining motor function are drastically reduced.[70, 79] The concept of pain and pain management is discussed in detail in both Chapters 12 and 29. Whether the pain is peripherally induced or centrally induced because of trauma or emotional overload, often the same motor responses will exist. That withdrawn flexor pattern makes postural activities exhausting because of the work it takes to override the existing central pattern generators. Thus, daily living activities, which constantly require postural extension against gravity, may be perceived as overwhelming and just not worth the effort. The therapist needs to learn to differentiate peripheral physical pain from central and/or emotional pain. To the patient, "pain is pain!"[74]

Bonding Projects Relaxation, Whereas Lack of Bonding Reflects Isolation. Because of the potency of the limbic system's connections into the motor system, a therapist's sensitivity to the client's emotional state would obviously be a key factor in understanding the motor responses observed during therapy. In Figure 6–8 an entire spectrum of motor responses can be observed in the four statues. A client who feels safe can relax and participate in the learning without strong emotional reactions. The woman being held in Figure 6–8 is safe and relaxed. The man and woman are interacting through touch with warmth and compassion that is often observed when colleagues watch a "master clinician" treating a client. The client and clinician seem to flow together during the treatment as one motor system. When looking at the man and woman, it becomes obvious that the two figures could not be separated, for they are one piece of art. In today's health care environment and with the stress on the client running and self-correcting motor programming, many therapists assume that they need not or should not touch the patient. This conclusion may be accurate when considering the motor system in isolation

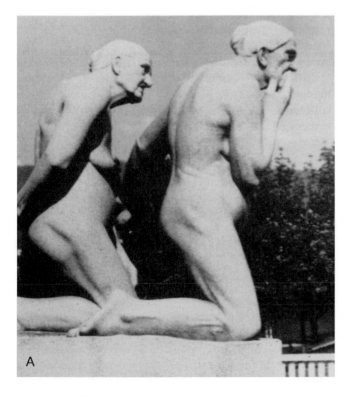

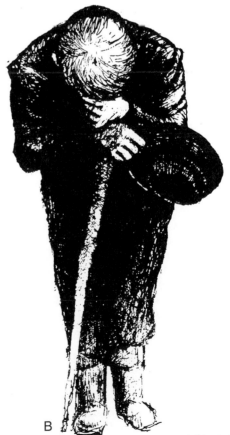

FIGURE 6–7. *A,* Behavior responses elicited by concern, pain, and grief. *B,* Pain or grief elicits flexion and can modify postural extension. (*A,* Vigelund Sculpture Grounds in the Frogner Park, Oslo, Norway. Adapted from photo by Normann.)

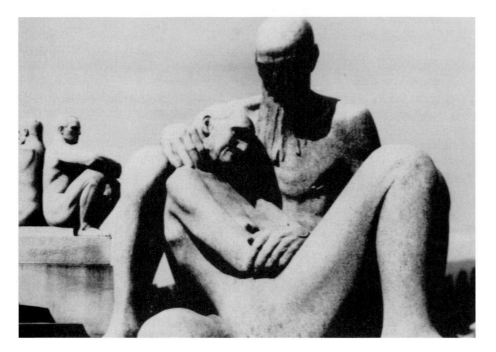

FIGURE 6–8. Grief, depression, and compassion responses are seen in the center figures, and rigid, stoic, distancing behaviors are observed in the two left statues. (Vigelund Sculpture Grounds in the Frogner Park, Oslo, Norway. Adapted from photo by Normann.)

and having concluded that the patient can self-correct error in motor programs. When correction by the therapist is through words rather than touch, it is external feedback where the auditory system has replaced the somatosensory system. The voice, as well as touch, can be soothing and instill confidence. Yet, language in and of itself will not replace the trust and safety felt both physically and emotionally through the deep pressure of touch. Bonding and trust occur much more often through touch than through verbal conversational.

Referring again to Figure 6–8, the statue on the left of the two men could represent two unique pieces of art. Those two men have no bonding. In fact, if the artist could have brought them closer together, they would just have rejected or repelled each other with greater intensity. One can see that if one of the men were the therapist and one the patient, little learning would be occurring. The therapist could not do anything to the other person (and vice versa) without that person perceiving the act as invasive. The therapist's responsibility is to open the patient's receptiveness to learning, not to close it.

These pictures clearly illustrate two types of therapist/client interactions. If an artist can clearly depict the tonal characteristics of emotion, certainly the therapist should be able to recognize those behaviors in the client. If a client is frustrated or angry and simultaneously has rigidity, spasticity, or general high tone, then a therapist might spend the entire session trying to decrease the motor response. If the client could be helped to deal with the anger or frustration during the therapy session and thus release the emotion, then the specific problems could be treated effectively. Differentiating the limbic system component from the motor control system and establishing treatment protocols for each may not be within the spectrum of a therapist's skills. Thus, working simultaneously with another professional such as a psychologist, social worker, or neuropsychologist may be an acceptable alternative approach. This co-treatment will allow all as-

pects of the client to be addressed simultaneously. Carryover of procedural learning (motor learning; see discussion of neurobiology of learning and memory for details) into adaptive motor responses needs to be practiced with consistency.[63] The influence of the limbic system in a client with large mood swings may drastically alter the consistent responses of the motor systems and thus dampen the procedural learning and limit the success of the therapeutic setting.

LIMBIC CONCEPTS THAT INFLUENCE THERAPIST/CLIENT INTERACTIONS: OBSERVATIONS OF MASTER CLINICIANS AT WORK

Although some colleagues might see this section as irrelevant to patient care, it has been presented for those who strive to understand and become the clinical masters of the future. As the professions of Occupational and Physical Therapy are considered both "arts" and "sciences," then linking the art to the science may allow new learners to obtain clinical skill and sensitivity earlier than "masters of the past."

How a clinician reacts at any given moment during a therapeutic session depends on both the client's and the clinician's declarative problem-solving skills, their procedural motor skills (see discussion of neurobiology of learning and memory), and their emotional drive to be part of the learning environment. Therefore, the sensitivity and specific level of attention of the therapist toward all responses of the client depend, to a large extent, on the clinician's limbic system and his or her interest and commitment to the patient and their mutual learning environment.

In an analysis of what differentiates a truly gifted or master clinician from a group of highly skilled and talented colleagues, the following philosophical verbal concepts are often expressed:

- That person has a rare gift.
- That person seems to intuitively know what to do or what the client needs.
- When that clinician treats a client, the two seem to flow together in their movements.
- The client seems to totally trust that clinician; I have never seen that before.
- I cannot believe that the client accurately did that with that clinician; before, the client was too afraid.

Many factors in an interactive setting, such as therapy, cannot be identified, but certain limbic/emotional factors may play a role in that gifted clinician's skill. Some of those factors are discussed next. This discussion in no way encapsulates all limbic variables within an interaction, only those that I believe safe to share and have had opportunity to repetitively observe as behaviors and interactions.

Trust/Responsibility. Trust is a critical component of a successful therapeutic session. The therapist gains the client's trust by his or her actions. Honesty and truth lead to trust.[60, 75] Telling someone you will not hurt them and then continually ranging a joint beyond a pain-free range is neither honest nor truthful and will not lead to trust. That trust can be earned by stopping as soon as the client verbalizes pain or shows pain with a body response such as a grimace or you as a therapist feel the presence of pain. This concept of not producing pain whenever possible cannot be overemphasized. The phrase "No pain, no gain!" is often used both by athletes trying to improve performance or by therapists and doctors trying to motivate their patients. Why does something have to hurt to get better? Pain is present because of danger and potential harm, not for pleasure. Why can't the phrase "Gain without pain!" be just as appropriate? People often ask me: "How do I deal with pain?" I respond with "I am not the colleague to ask because I first feel the pain, next I get rid of the pain, and then I treat the CNS problems!"

What does "feel the patient's pain" refer to? First, a therapist needs to assess the biomechanics of the joint(s) where pain is expressed. Second, the muscle fascial tightness needs to be examined. Third, the motor programming available to the patient during movement of the joint(s) during functional activities needs to be assessed. All three of these actions and their interactions do not necessarily explain the causation of the pain, but they do help a therapist draw conclusions about the pain. A fourth variable exists that is much harder to explain or validate scientifically. It seems as if "I feel the pain in my body." Maybe I include all types of information from the examination and project that information onto my somatosensory cortex and into my body image, but "I feel the pain" and thus have limbic associations to that feeling.

Second, I get rid of the pain, if possible. Using all the therapeutic techniques such as manual therapy for biomechanical alinement and joint mobility, fascial and muscle mobilization to get filament gliding, and rotation with elongation or compression to get changes in the motor programs helps, but in addition "I feel the pain, bond with it, and then, through visualization and touch, draw it away from the patient. While in Germany in 1996, I asked Suzanna Klein Vogelbach about this phenomenon.

She was a true master clinician. All the other master clinicians in the area of neurorehabilitation whom I had known were deceased at that point in time. Her responses to my questions were preceded with long pauses because of the sensitivity and lack of scientific scrutiny of her responses. Yet, she acknowledged she also felt the physical and emotional pain of her patients and that she too drew it out with her hands. She paused one moment, smiled, and then stated, "but sometimes they pull it back in!"

Pain is a complex phenomenon, and the more it is understood, the more complex it becomes. Being sensitive to a patient's pain, no matter the cause, and working with the patient to eliminate that pain often lead to very strong bonding and trust that will lead to compliance and learning. Ignoring the pain may be perceived as insensitivity and lack of caring, which can lead to distrust and often resistance to learning or performance.

A personal limbic experience helped teach me the previous lesson. It occurred while giving birth to our second son. The doctor finally said, "Push" and as I did our son's head compressed my sciatic nerve and I stopped pushing. I said, "Please reposition my left leg (which was strapped into a stirrup) because the head of the baby is pushing on my sciatic nerve." Everyone ignored me, and as my pelvic muscles started to contract the doctor again said "Push." I refused and again stated the problem. The doctor then said: "Honey, you are having a baby and it is going to hurt!" I again stated my dilemma. The nurse finally said, "What did you say?" I repeated and she said "Oh!" and adjusted my leg, and in one push my son was born. Compliance to participate is limbic, and limbic has tremendous control over intentional movement, no matter the context of the environment.[60]

Once a client gives his or her trust, a clinician can freely move or move with a client and little resistance because of fear, reservations, or need to protect self will be felt or observed. Trust does not mean lack of awareness of potential danger; it means acceptance that although the danger is present, the potential of harm, pain, or disaster is very slight and the expected gain is worth the risk. In Figure 6–9, the student's trust that the instructor will not hurt her can be seen by her lack of protective responses and by her calm, relaxed body posture. The student is aware of the potential of the kick but trusts her life to the skills, control, and personal integrity of the teacher. Those same qualities are easily observed when watching a gifted clinician treat clients. The motor activities in a therapeutic setting are less complex than in Figure 6–9, but in no way are they less stressful, less potentially harmful, or less frightening from the client's point of view.

Therapists must trust themselves enough to know that they can effect changes in their clients. Understanding their own motor system, how it responds, and how to use their hands, arms, or entire body to move someone else is based partly on procedural skills, partly on declarative learning, and partly on self-confidence or self-trust. Trusting that they have the skill to implement that motor response has a limbic component. If a therapist has self-doubts about therapeutic skills, it will change performance, which will alter input to the client. This altered

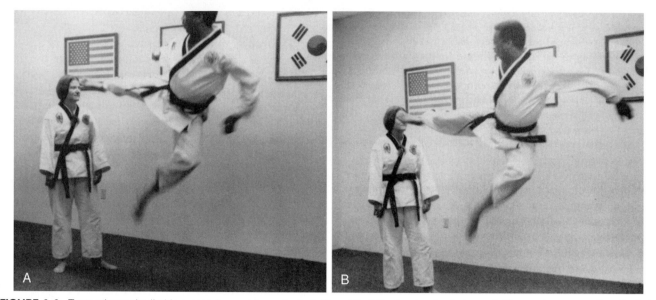

FIGURE 6–9. Trust relaxes the limbic system's need to protect. *A,* The skill of the teacher is obvious. *B,* The student trusts that she is in no danger.

input can potentially alter the client's output and vary the desired responses.

Very close to the concept of trust is the idea of responsibility. Accepting responsibility for our own behavior seems obvious and is totally accepted as part of a professional role. Accepting and allowing the client the right to accept responsibility for his or her own environment are also key elements in creating a successful clinical environment and an independent person. Figure 6–10 illustrates the concept through the following example:

The teacher (or therapist) asked the student (or client) to perform a motor act. In the figure, the act was to perform a kick to the teacher's head. The kick was to be very strong or forceful and completed. The student was

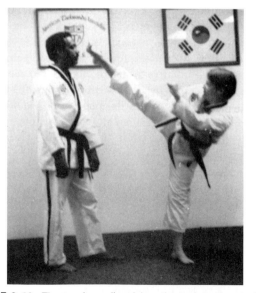

FIGURE 6–10. The teacher relinquishes the task to the student, and the student trusts the teacher is right even if self-doubt exists.

told not to hold back or stop the kick in any way, yet the kick was to come within a few inches of the teacher's head. This placed tremendous responsibility on the student. One inch too far might dangerously hurt the instructor, yet one inch too short was not acceptable. The teacher knew the student had the skill, power, and control to perform the task and then passed the responsibility to the student. She was hesitant to assume the responsibility, for the consequence of failure could have been very traumatic, but the student trusted that the teacher would not ask for the behavior unless success was fairly guaranteed. That trust reduced anxiety and the neurochemical effects on the motor system, thus giving her more motor control over the act. Once the task was completed successfully, the student gained confidence and could repeat the task with less fear or emotional influence while gaining refinement over the motor skill.

Although the motor activities described in this example are more complex than those required by therapists and clients, the dynamics of the environment relate consistently with client/therapist roles and expectations. A gifted clinician knows that the client has the potential to succeed. When asked to perform, the client trusts the therapist and assumes the responsibility for the act. The therapist can facilitate the movement or postural pattern, thereby ensuring that the client succeeds. This feeling of success stimulates motivation for task repetition, which ultimately leads to learning. The incentive to repeat and learn becomes self-motivating and then becomes the responsibility of the client. The limbic complex and its interwoven network throughout the nervous system play a key role in this behavioral drive. The task itself can be simple, such as a weight shift or postural co-activating in a sitting pattern, or as complex as getting dressed or climbing onto and off of a bus. No matter what the activity, the client needs to accept responsibility for his or her own behavior before independence in motor functioning can be achieved. Although the motor function itself is not limbic, many variables that lead to success, self-motivation, and feelings of independence are directly related to limbic and prefrontal lobe circuitry.

Dedication to Reality. Another component of a successful clinical environment deals with learning on the part of the therapist. A master clinician sees and feels what is happening within the motor control output system of the client. That therapist does not get stuck with what he or she has been taught but uses that as a foundation for additional learning. Learning is constantly correlated to memories and new experiences. Each client is a new map, sketchy at the beginning, that needs to be constantly revised as the terrain (client) changes. Similarly, the therapist will be able to transfer one motor activity into another spatial position. That is, the therapist can let go of an outdated map or treatment technique and create a new one as the environment and motor control system of the client changes. This transference or letting go of old maps or ideas is true for both the client and therapist. If a position, pattern, or technique is not working, then the clinician needs to change the map or directions of treatment and let the client teach the therapist what will work. The ability to change and select new or alternative treatment techniques is based on the attitude of the therapist toward selecting alternative approaches. Willingness to be flexible is based on confidence in oneself, a truly emotional strategy or limbic behavior. Master clinicians have learned that the answers to the patient's puzzle are within the patient, not the textbooks.

Figure 6–11 depicts two maps with a beginning point and a terminal outcome or goal in each. The parameters

Outside Clinical Expertise of Two Disciplines

MAPPING

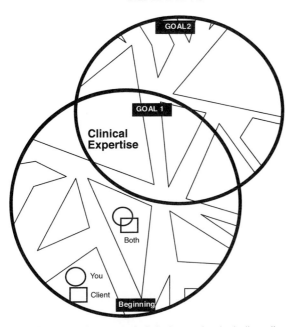

FIGURE 6–11. Concept of clinical mapping including client and therapist and the interactions and importance of overlapping professional goals and staying within the professional expertise.

of the first map illustrate the boundaries of that therapist's experience and education. The clinician, through training, can identify what would seem to be the most direct and efficient way or path toward the mutually identified goal of the therapist and client. When the client becomes a participant within the environment or map, what would seem like a direct path toward a goal might not be the easiest or most direct for the client. If empowerment of the client leads to independence, then allowing and encouraging the client to direct therapy may provide greater variability, force the client to problem solve, and lead to greater learning. The therapist needs to recognize when the client is not going in the direction of the goal. For example, the client is trying to perform a stand-pivot transfer and instead is falling. If it is important to practice transfers, then practicing falling is inappropriate and the environment (either internal or external) needs modification. Falling can be learned and practiced at another time. Once both strategies are learned, the therapist must empower the patient to the ownership of the map. In the examples of transferring, if the therapist asks the client to practice transfers and if the client starts to fall, a change in required motor behavior must be made and the opportunity given to the client to self-correct. In that way the client is gaining independent control over a variety of environmental contexts and outcomes. Within the same figure (see Fig. 6–11) is a second map. That second map might represent another professional's interaction and goal with the same client. It is during these overlapping interactions that both professionals can empower the patient to practice and that practice will help lead to those functional goals established by both practitioners. In some situations one profession may guide a client toward obtaining the functional skill necessary for the second profession to begin guiding the client toward the expected outcomes of the second profession. These interlocking dependencies of the client and the professions are illustrated in Figure 6–11. If the client begins therapy striving for the first goal and ends at the functional outcome of the second goal, then additional functional outcomes have been achieved and both professions interacted in the ultimate prognosis of the patient. That interaction requires respect and openness of both professionals toward each other as well as the client. Those attitudes and ultimate behaviors are limbic driven.

Vulnerability. To receive input from a client that is multivariable and simultaneous, a therapist has to be open to that information. If a clinician believes that he or she knows what each client needs and how to get those behaviors before meeting the client, then the client falls into a category of a recipe for treating the problem. Using the recipe does not mean the client cannot learn or gain better perceptual/cognitive, affective, or motor control, but it does mean that the individuality of the person may be lost. A more individualized approach would allow the clinician to identify through behavioral responses the best way for the client to learn how to sequence the learning, when to make demands of the client, when to nurture, when to stop, when to continue, when to assist, when to have fun, when to laugh, or when to cry. An analogy might be going to a fast food restaurant versus a restaurant where each aspect of the meal is tailored to one's taste. It does not mean that both restaurants are not selling digestible foods. It does mean that at one eating place the food is mass produced with some choices, but individuality, with respect to the consumer, is not an aspect of the service. Unfortunately, managed care, limited visits, reduced time for treatment, and therapists' level of frustrations all are pushing therapeutic interventions toward a "one size fits all" philosophy that may increase the time needed for learning not reduce it.

To be open totally to processing the individual differences of the client, the clinician must be relaxed and nonthreatened and feel no need to protect himself or herself from the external environment. The clinician is highly vulnerable because he or she is open to new and as yet unanalyzed or unprocessed input. Being open must incorporate being sensitive to not only the variability of motor responses but also to the variability of emotional responses on the part of the client. This vulnerability leads to compassion, understanding, and acceptance of the client as a unique human being. It can also be exhausting. Therapists need to learn ways to allow openness without taking on the emotional responsibility of each patient.

Limbic Lesions and Their Influence on the Therapeutic Environment

Many lesions or neurochemical imbalances within the limbic system drastically affect the success or failure of physical, occupational, and other therapy programs. This chapter does not discuss in detail specific problems and their treatment, but instead it is hoped that identification of the limbic involvement may help the reader develop a better understanding of specific neurological conditions and carry that knowledge into Section II where the specific clinical problems are discussed.

SUBSTANCE ABUSE (see Chapter 22)

The anterior temporal lobe (especially the hippocampus and amygdala) has a lower threshold for epileptic seizures than other cortical structures.[33, 63] This type of epilepsy is produced by use of systemic drugs such as cocaine and alcohol. This type of seizure is often accompanied by sensory auras and alterations in behavior, with specific

focus on mood shifts and cognitive dysfunction.[119] Obviously, the precise association between behavior and emotions or temporolimbic and frontolimbic activity is not understood, yet the associations and thus their impact on a therapeutic setting cannot be ignored.[1, 9]

Whether street bought, medically administered, or ingested for private or social reasons (such as in alcohol consumption), drugs and alcohol can have dramatic effects on the CNS. Korsakoff's syndrome, caused by chronic alcoholism and its related nutritional deficiency, is identified by the structural involvement of the diencephalon with specific focus on the mamillary bodies, and the dorsal medial and anterior nucleus of the thalamus[63] usually shows involvement (see the anatomy section and Fig. 6–12). This syndrome is not a dementia, but rather a discrete localized pathological state with specific clinical signs. The most dramatic sign observed in a client with Korsakoff's syndrome is severe memory deficits. These deficits involve declarative memory and learning losses, but the most predominant problem is short-term memory loss. As the disease progresses, clients generally become totally unaware of their memory loss and are unconcerned. Initially, confabulation may be observed, but in time most clients with a chronic condition become apathetic and somewhat withdrawn and are in a profound amnesic state. They are trapped in time, unable to learn from new experiences because they cannot retain memories for more than a few minutes and are unable to maintain their independence[33, 79]; many may become street people.

The use of alcohol affects not only adults but also children and adolescents. Still another population of children suffering from alcohol abuse has surfaced as a specific clinical problem. These children are infants who suffer from the effects of fetal alcohol syndrome. A variety of researchers have investigated the effects of alcohol and other toxic drugs on neuromotor and cognitive development.[27, 55, 98, 106, 113]

ALZHEIMER'S DISEASE (see Chapter 26)

In Alzheimer's disease, the hippocampus and nucleus basalis are the most severely involved structures, followed by neurofibrillar degeneration of anterotemporal, parietal, and frontal lobes.[9, 33, 79]

Initially, the symptoms fall into several categories: emo-

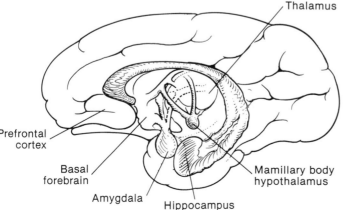

FIGURE 6–12. Anatomy of the limbic system: schematic illustration.

tional, social, and cognitive. Usually the symptoms have a gradual onset. Depression and anxiety often are seen during the early phases because of the neuronal degeneration within the prefrontal lobes and limbic system.[104] During the second stage, the emotional, social, and intellectual changes become more marked. Clients have difficulty with demands, business affairs, and personal management. Their memory and cognitive processing continue to deteriorate, whereas their awareness of the problem is often still insightful, causing additional anxiety and depression. During this phase clients may be unable to recognize familiar objects and become scared because they are losing control of the environment both internally and externally. Thus, the client may become combative out of a defensive (fight/flight) autonomic response. For that reason, therapists need to make sure the client feels safe during therapy to optimize the learning and compliance. The third phase manifests itself with moderate to severe aphasic, apraxic, and agnostic problems. Object agnosia, the failure to recognize objects, is a typical sign of advancing Alzheimer's disease. Distractibility and nonattentiveness are also common signs of this third stage. The final stage is marked by an individual who is noncommunicative, with little meaningful social interaction, and who often takes on the features of the Kluver-Bucy syndrome. Thus, they exhibit emotional outbursts, inappropriate sexual behaviors, severe memory loss, constant mouth movements, and often a flexor-type postural pattern. In this latter phase, the client is virtually decorticate and clinically indistinguishable from persons suffering from other dementias.

The continual degeneration of the limbic system is a key distinguishing factor in Alzheimer's disease.[81, 124] Many clients are misdiagnosed as having other problems such as intracranial tumors, normal-pressure hydrocephalus, multiinfarct dementia, or alcoholic/chronic drug intoxication.[6] Similarly, many clients with tumors, multifaceted dementias, alcoholism, or heart attacks resulting in hippocampal damage may be diagnosed with Alzheimer's disease. When the disease is correctly evaluated and diagnosed, however, it becomes obvious that the limbic-cortical area involved from phase one through the last phase is interacting with other areas of the brain and constantly affecting the behavioral patterns of the patient. Owing to the neurochemical sensitivity and production within the limbic system, drugs are often used to try to prevent or slow down the progression of Alzheimer's disease (see Chapter 32). Similarly, with some patients with Alzheimer's disease, a genetic predisposition has been found[38, 63, 77, 99]; thus, gene therapy may prove in the future to have great therapeutic value.

HEAD INJURY (see Chapter 14)

Traumatic Injury. One potentially severe limbic problem that can be present after traumatic closed head injury is diffuse axonal injury.[2, 8] The long associative bundles or fibers that transverse the cortex on a curved route can be sheared by an impact or a blow to the head. One of these long associative bundles is the cingulate fasciculus, which coordinates the amygdala and hippocampal projections to and from the prefrontal cortex. Many basic perceptual strategies, such as body schema, hearing, vision, and smell, are linked into the emotional and learning centers of the limbic system through the cingulate fasciculus. Thus, declarative learning through sensory/cognitive processing can become impossible. If the pathways to and from the hippocampus and amygdala are sheared bilaterally, total and permanent global anterograde amnesia will be present.[53, 124] If destruction of both tracts on one side occurs, but the contralateral side is left intact, the individual can compensate, but learning will be slower or the rate of processing delayed.[91] If only one tract on one side is damaged, such as the tract to and from the hippocampus, the amygdaloid system on the same side will compensate but be slower than without the lesion.[91] Thus, the specific degree of involvement will vary and depend on the extent of shearing. Those people with total shearing on both sides will usually be in a deep coma and will not survive the injury.[5] Those individuals with less severe insult will show signs ranging from total amnesia to minor delays in declarative learning.[8]

Cerebral contusions (bruises) have long been a primary sign of traumatic head injury.[97] Regardless of impact, the contusions are generally found in the frontal and temporal regions. The regions most frequently involved are orbitofrontal, frontopolar, anterotemporal, and lateral temporal surfaces.[8] The limbic system's connection to these areas would suggest the potential for direct and indirect limbic involvement. The greater the contusion, the greater the likelihood that the limbic structures might simultaneously be involved. Impulsiveness, lack of inhibition, and hyperactivity are a few of the clinical signs associated with orbitofrontal/limbic involvement. The dorsomedial frontal region, involved in the hippocampal-fornix circuit (once referred to as Papez circuit), when damaged, seems to induce a pseudodepressed state, including slowness, lack of initiation, and perseveration.

Nontraumatic Head Injuries: Anoxic/Hypoxic Brain Injury. Lack of oxygen to the brain, regardless of the cause, seems not only to have a dramatic effect throughout the cortex but also selectively damages the hippocampal regions.[8] The loss of hippocampal declarative memory systems bilaterally would certainly provide one reason for the slowness in processing so commonly observed in head injury. A hypothesis could also be made regarding the limbic system's interrelation with other cortical and brain stem structures. In cases of hypoxia, many structures feeding into the limbic system are potentially affected, so information sent to the limbic system may be distorted. These distortions could cause tremendous imbalances within the limbic processing system, with not only attention and learning problems but also hypothalamic irregularity often seen in head trauma.

A therapist always needs to understand the environment within which the injury occurred. If the injury was due to a violent confrontation, such as a fight or a frightful experience such as a near-drowning, the emotional system had to be at a high level of metabolic activity at the time of the insult. If the event was anoxic, then those areas with the highest oxygen need or at the highest metabolic state might be the most affected or damaged after the event. Knowing that information, a therapist's analytical problem-solving strategies should guide them toward limbic assessment.

Summary of Limbic Problems with Head-Injured Clients. The behavioral sequelae following any head injury reflect many signs of limbic involvement. In both pediatric and adult studies, behaviors of impulsiveness, restlessness, overactivity, destructiveness, aggression, increased tantrums, and socially uninhibited behaviors (lack of social skills) are frequently reported. These behaviors all reflect a strong emotional or limbic component. After discussion of Moore's concept of a limbic system that MOVEs us and the F²ARV continuum regarding emotional control over noxious or negative input, it is no wonder so many clients have difficulty with personal and emotional control over their reactions to the therapeutic world. If the imbalance were within the client, then the external environment would be one possible way to help center the client emotionally. This centering requires that the therapist be sensitive to the emotional level of the client. As the client begins to regain control, an increase in external environmental demands would challenge the limbic system. If the demand is excessive, the client's emotional reaction as expressed by motor behavior should alert the therapist to downgrade the activity level.

Head injuries affect many areas of the CNS. A client with spasticity, rigidity, or ataxia may exhibit an increase in those motor responses when the limbic system becomes stressed. Learning to differentiate a motor control problem from a limbic problem that influences the motor control systems requires that the therapist be willing to address the cause of the problems and their treatment. Each client is so different and in each moment has the potential of affecting the limbic system with great variance. Thus, the therapist needs to give undivided attention to the client at all times and be willing to make moment-to-moment adjustments within the external environment to help the client maintain focus on the desired learning.

CEREBROVASCULAR ACCIDENTS
(see Chapter 25)

The most common insult results in occlusions within tributaries of the middle cerebral artery.[63] When this occlusion is in the right hemisphere, studies have shown that clients are often confused and exhibit metabolic imbalance.[111] The primary problem of this confused state is inattention. After brain scans, it has been shown that focal lesions existed within both the reticulocortical and limbic cortical tracts, suggesting direct limbic involvement in many middle cerebral artery problems.[86]

Many clients with a cerebrovascular accident do not have direct limbic involvement, yet the stresses placed on the client, whether external or internal, are often reflected in the limbic system's influence over the motor control systems. Everyday existence as well as performance of the motor task required during therapy is usually valued highly in the client's life. This value or stress placed on the limbic system overflows into the motor system and never allows it to relax, as observed by noting the increase of tonus in the nonaffected leg. The client is usually unaware of this buildup of tonus but can release it once attention is drawn to it. If attention is never directed toward these tension buildups, a therapist trying to decrease tonus in the affected arm or leg will always be interacting with the associated patterns from the less-involved extremities.

TUMOR (see Chapter 23)

Any brain tumor, whether or not directly affecting the limbic structures, will certainly arouse the limbic system because of the stress, anxiety, and emotional overlays of the diagnosis. The degree of emotional involvement will obviously affect the declarative learning of the client as well as the limbic system's influence over motor response.

Tumors specifically arising within limbic structures can cause dramatic changes in the client's emotional behavior and level of alertness, especially with hypothalamic tumors. The behaviors reported include aggressiveness, hyperphagia, paranoia, sloppiness, manic symptoms, and eventual confusion.[63] Tumors within the hypothalamus cause not only behavioral abnormalities but also autonomic endocrine imbalances, including body temperature changes, menstrual abnormalities, and diabetes insipidus.[124]

When the tumor is located within the frontal and temporal lobes associated with limbic structures, psychiatric problems may manifest, ranging from depression to schizoid psychosis.[124] Amnesia has been reported in tumor patients with dorsomedial thalamus, fornix, midbrain lesions, and reticulolimbic pathway lesions. This again reinforces the importance of the limbic system's role in storage.[124]

VENTRICULAR SWELLING AFTER SPINAL DEFECTS IN UTERO, CNS TRAUMA, AND INFLAMMATION (see Chapters 14, 15, and 17)

Although the effects of ventricular swelling after trauma, inflammation, and in utero cerebrospinal malformations are not discussed in great detail in the literature with respect to limbic involvement, the proximity of the lateral and third ventricle to limbic structures cannot be ignored. It is common knowledge that most people when exposed to hot, humid weather begin to swell; become more irritable, less tolerant, and moody; and may complain of headaches. Some people become aggressive, others lethargic. All these behaviors are linked to some extent with limbic function. Thus, ventricular swelling causing hydrocephalus, whether caused by trauma, inflammation, or obstruction, would potentially affect the limbic structures. Reported behavioral changes such as seizures, memory and learning problems, personality alternations, alertness, dementia, and amnesia can be tied to direct or indirect limbic activity.[63]

SUMMARY OF CLINICAL PROBLEMS AFFECTED BY LIMBIC INVOLVEMENT

It is easy to identify limbic problems when the behaviors deviate drastically from normal responses. It is much more difficult to determine subtle behavior shifts in clients. The therapist should be sensitive to these minor mood shifts, because they may represent early signs of future problems. Similarly, noting that a particular client is always irritable and has difficulty learning on hot days should help direct the therapist toward establishing a treatment session that regulates humidity and temperature to optimize the learning environment. The limbic system is not just a neurochemical bundle of nuclei and axons found within the brain. It is a pulsating center that links perception of the world and the way an individual responds to that perception. Quality of life is a value and that value has a strong limbic component. If functional outcomes leading to maintaining or improving quality of life of our clients is the goal of both physical and occupational therapy, then the limbic system is no less important during examination, evaluation, prognosis, and intervention than the motor system itself.

THE NEUROSCIENCE OF THE LIMBIC SYSTEM

Basic Anatomy and Physiology

A very brief overview of the anatomy and physiology of the limbic system is presented in the following sections. The reader is referred to a variety of textbooks for a more in-depth understanding of this system.[60, 63, 101]

Basic Structure and Function

The limbic system can best be visualized as consisting of cortical and subcortical structures with the hypothalamus in the central position (Figs. 6–12 and 6–13). The hypothalamus is surrounded by the circular alignment of the subcortical limbic structures vitally linked with each other and the hypothalamus. These structures are the amygdaloid complex, the hippocampal formation, the nucleus accumbens, the anterior nuclei of the thalamus, and the septal nuclei (see Fig. 6–12). These structures are again surrounded by a ring of cortical structures collectively called the "limbic lobe," which includes the orbitofrontal cortex, the cingulate gyrus, the parahippocampal gyrus, and the uncus. Other neuroanatomists also include the

olfactory system and the basal forebrain area (see Fig. 6–13). Vitally linked and often included in the limbic system as the "mesolimbic" part is the excitatory component of the reticular activating system and other brain stem nuclei of the midbrain. Some consider components of the midbrain a very important region for emotional expression.[34] Derryberry and Tucker[34] found that attack behavior aroused by hypothalamic stimulation is blocked when the midbrain is damaged and that midbrain stimulation can be made to elicit "attack behavior" even when the hypothalamus has been surgically disconnected from other brain regions. Recent research has clearly identified the neurochemical precursors to this aggressive behavior.[31, 63, 73, 92] This "septo-hypothalamic-mesencephalic" continuum, connected by the medial forebrain bundle, seems to be vital to the integration and expression of emotional behavior.[72] The linking of other brain structures to emotions came initially from the work of Papez,[100] who first identified the hippocampal-fornix circuit. He saw this as a way of combining the "subjective" cortical experiences with the emotional hypothalamic contribution. Earlier, Broca[13] labeled the cingulate gyrus and hippocampus "circle" as "the great limbic lobe." These concepts were combined by Maclean[83] into the construct of the limbic system.

Kluver and Bucy[66] linked the anterior half of the temporal lobes and the amygdaloid complex to the limbic system. They showed changes in behavior, with specific loss of the amygdaloid complex and anterior hippocampus input resulting in (1) restless overresponsiveness, (2) hyperorality of examining objects by placing them in their mouths, (3) psychic blindness of seeing and not recognizing objects and the possible harm they may entail, (4) sexual hyperactivity, and (5) emotional changes characterized by loss of aggressiveness. These changes have been named the Kluver-Bucy syndrome.[9, 18, 33] A myriad of connections link the amygdala to the olfactory pathways,

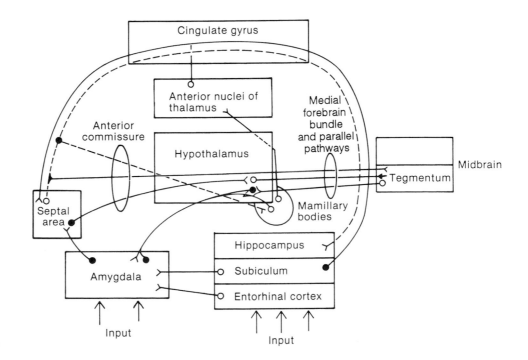

FIGURE 6–13. Limbic system circuitry with parallel and reverberating connections as well as medial forebrain bundle.

the frontal lobe and cingulate gyrus, the thalamus, the hypothalamus, the septum, and the midbrain structures of the substantial nigra, locus coeruleus, periaqueductal gray matter, and the reticular formation. The amygdala receives feedback from many of these structures it projects to by reciprocal pathways.

At the heart of the limbic system is the hypothalamus. The hypothalamus, in close reciprocal interaction with most centers of the cerebral cortex, the amygdala, hippocampus, pituitary gland, brain stem, and spinal cord, is a primary regulator of autonomic and endocrine functions and controls and balances homeostatic mechanisms. Autonomic and somatomotor responses controlled by the hypothalamus are closely aligned with the expression of emotions.[93, 131]

In the temporal lobe, anteromedially, are the amygdaloid complex of nuclei, with the hippocampal formation situated posterior to it. Located medial to the amygdala is the basal forebrain nuclei, which receive afferent neurons from the reticular formation, the hypothalamus, and the limbic cortex. From this basal forebrain efferents project to all areas of the cerebral cortex, the hippocampus, and amygdaloid body, providing an important connection between the neocortex and the limbic system. These nuclei represent the center of the cholinergic system, which supplies acetylcholine to limbic and cortical structures involved in memory formation. Depletion of acetylcholine in clients with Alzheimer's disease relates to their memory loss.[9, 93]

Interlinking the Components of the System

The limbic system has many reciprocating interlinking circuits between its component structures, which provide for much functional interaction and also allow for ongoing adjustments with continuous feedback (Fig. 6–14).[63, 93] The largest pathway is the fornix.

Another limbic pathway is the stria terminalis, which originates in the amygdaloid complex and follows a course close to the fornix to end in the hypothalamus and septal regions. The amygdala and the septal region are also connected by a short direct pathway called the diagonal band of Broca. A third pathway, the uncinate fasciculus, runs between the amygdala and the orbitofrontal cortex.[63]

The medial forebrain bundle and other parallel circuits (see Fig. 6–13) are vital connections of the limbic system. These pathways course through the lateral hypothalamus and terminate in the cingulate gyrus in its ascending limb and in the reticular formation of the midbrain in its descending part and have strong interconnections and control over the periaqueductal gray area.[93] These links enable the limbic system itself and the non–limbic-associated structures to act as one neural task system. No portion of the brain, whether limbic or nonlimbic, has only one function.[63] Each area acts as an input-output station. At no time is it totally the center of a particular effect, and each site depends on the cooperation and interaction with other regions.

During the past decade anatomical pathways have been identified that are descending motor tracts that terminate in the caudal brain stem and spinal cord.[58] These pathways help modulate the activity level of somatic and autonomic motor neurons. Some of these tracts receive direct and indirect afferent information from the periphery and are part of the interneuronal projection system to motor neurons. They are found in the caudal brain stem, spinal cord, and between the two, and play a role in the generation of fixed action patterns such as biting and swallowing, which have a strong emotion context linked to the motor program. Some of the pathways are linked with the ventromedial and lateral systems, identified for many years as part of both the proximal/axial and distal motor control system modulated by a variety of structures.[93] The last tracts are the most recently discov-

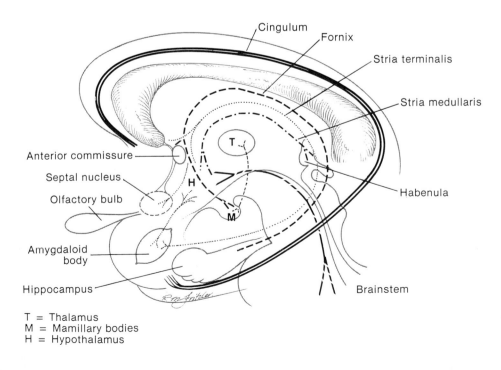

FIGURE 6–14. Interlinking neuron network within the limbic system. (Adapted from Kandel ER, Schwartz JH, Jessell TM: Principles of Neural Science, 5th ed. New York, Elsevier Medical Science Publishing, 2000.)

T = Thalamus
M = Mamillary bodies
H = Hypothalamus

ered. They connect the limbic system to the brain stem and spinal neuronal pools. These tracts do not seem to synapse on what would be considered true motor nuclei of the brain stem (e.g., red nucleus, vestibular nuclei, lateral reticular nuclei, interstitial nuclei of Cajal, or inferior olive). However, these new pathways do connect with raphe nuclei, periaqueductal gray matter, and locus coeruleus. The medial components of these tracts originate within the medial portion of the hypothalamus, and the lateral portion originates in the limbic system (lateral hypothalamus, amygdala, and bed nucleus of the stria terminalis). The prefrontal area may be the master controller over this regulatory system, but that is yet to be determined.

The functional motor implication of these tracts is determined by whether the fibers project as part of a medial or lateral descending system. The medial system, through the locus coeruleus, periaqueductal gray matter, and raphe spinal pathways, plays a role in the general level of activity of both somatosensory and motor neurons. Thus, the emotional brain or limbic system has an effect on both somatosensory input and motor output. These fibers can alter the level of excitation to the first synapse of somatosensory information, thus altering the processing or importance of that information as it enters the nervous system. Similarly, it can alter the level of motor generators involved in motor expression, which may account for the extension with anger and flexion with depression. The lateral system seems to be involved in more specific motor output related to emotional behavior and may explain some of the loss of fine motor skill when placed in an emotional situation such as competition.[58] To differentiate whether the tonal conditions of a client are due to limbic imbalance or problems within the traditionally accepted motor system, the clinician would need to observe the emotional state and how it changes within the client. If the abnormal state consistently alters with mood shifts, then limbic involvement causing motor control disturbances would be identified.

Neurobiology of Learning and Memory

Functional Applications for an Intact System

"Ultimately, to be sure, memory is a series of molecular events. What we chart is the territory within which those events take place."[90]

The brain stores sensory and motor experiences as memory. In processing incoming information, most sensory pathways from receptors to cortical areas send vital information to the components of the limbic system. For example, extensions can be found from the visual pathways into the inferior temporal lobe (limbic system).[63, 87] Visual information is "processed sequentially" at each synapse along its entire pathway, in response to size, shape, color, and texture of objects. In the inferior temporal cortex, the total image of the item viewed is projected. In this way the sensory inputs are converted to become "perceptual experiences." This also applies to other sensory stimuli, such as tactile, proprioceptive, and vestibular. The process of translating the integrated perceptions into memory oc-

curs bilaterally in the limbic system structures of the amygdala and the hippocampus.[4, 12, 16, 26, 39, 40, 57, 63, 93, 127]

Before delving into the limbic system's impact on learning and memory, a clear understanding of what is meant by these functions is needed.

Current theories support a "dual memory system" using different pathways in the nervous system. Terms such as *verbal* and *nonverbal*, *habit* versus *recognition*, *extrinsic* and *intrinsic*, and *procedural* and *declarative* have been given to these two memory systems. These systems do not operate autonomously, and many therapeutic activities seem to combine these memory systems to achieve functional behavior.[63]

For this discussion, two specific categories of learning—declarative and procedural—will be used, although in today's neuroscience environment implicit and explicit memory is used as frequently. Declarative (explicit) memory entails the capability to recall and verbally report experiences. This recall requires deliberate conscious effort, whereas the procedural counterpart is the recall of "rules, skills, and procedures (implicit)"[63] and can be recalled unconsciously.

Procedural learning is vital to the development of motor control. A child first receives sensory input from the various modalities through the thalamus, terminating at the appropriate sensory cortex. That information is processed, a functional somatosensory map is formulated,[11, 105] and the information is programmed and relayed to the motor cortex. From there, it is sent to both the basal ganglia and the cerebellum to establish plans for postural adaptations, refinement of motor programs, and coordination of direction, extent, timing, force, and tone necessary throughout the entire sequence of the motor act. Storage and thus retrieval of memory of these semiautomatic motor plans are thought to occur throughout the motor control system.[63]

The frontal lobe, basal ganglia, and cerebellum are critical nuclei for changing and modulating existing programs.[63] Many interlocking neuronetworks establish pathways allowing for the conceptualization of research on motor theory concepts of reciprocity, distributed function, consensus, and so on (see Chapters 4 and 5). Procedural learning and memory do not *necessitate* limbic system involvement as long as an emotional value is not placed on the task. This memory deals with skills, habits, and stereotyped behaviors. This motor system is involved in developing procedural plans used in moving us from place to place or holding us in a position when we need to stop.[63]

Unlike procedural learning and memory, declarative (explicit) learning and memory require the wiring of the limbic system. This type of thought deals with factual, material, semantic, and categorical aspects of higher cognitive and affective processing. A strong emotional and judgmental component is linked with declarative thought. Thus, as soon as a motor behavior has value placed on the act, it becomes declarative as well as procedural, and the limbic system may become a key element in the success or failure of that movement.[48] Most functional tasks or activities practiced in a clinical setting have value attached to them. That value can be clearly seen by

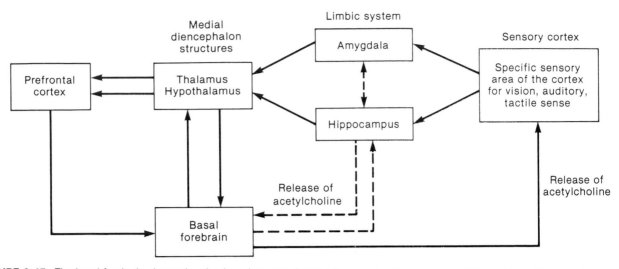

FIGURE 6–15. The basal forebrain closes the circuit and causes changes in sensory area neurons, which could lead to correct perception and stored memory. This is totally neurochemical dependent.

observing the emotional intent placed on the activity by the client.

The two reverberating or reciprocal pathways, or circuits, within the limbic system most intimately involved in declarative learning are (1) the amygdaloid, dorsomedial thalamic nucleus, and cortical pathways and (2) the hippocampal, fornix, anterior thalamic nucleus, and cortical pathways.

The hippocampus may be more concerned with sensory and motor signals relating to the external environment, whereas the amygdala is concerned with those of the internal environment. They both contribute in relation to the significance of external or internal environmental influences.[40, 102, 103, 120–122]

The amygdaloid circuits seem to deal with strongly emotional and judgmental thoughts, whereas the hippocampal circuits are less emotional and more factual. The amygdala may be more involved in emotional arousal and attention, as well as motor regulation, whereas the hippocampus may deal with less emotionally charged learning. These limbic circuits seem crucial in the initial processing of material that leads to learning and memory. Once the thought has been laid down within the cortical structures, retrieval of that specific intermediate and long-term memory does not seem to require the limbic system, although new associations will need to be run through the system.[12, 26, 32, 40, 63]

A third component in the memory pathway involves the medial diencephalon, a structure that contains the thalamic nucleus. When this region is destroyed by neurotrauma such as strokes, neoplasms, infections, or chronic alcoholism, global amnesias result, owing to the destruction of the amygdala and hippocampus. The amygdala and hippocampus send fibers to specific target nuclei in the thalamus, and the destruction of these tracts also causes the same amnesic effect. It appears that the limbic system and the diencephalon cooperate in the memory circuits. The medial diencephalon seems to be another relay station along the pathway that leads from the specific sensory cortical region to the limbic structures in the temporal lobe to the medial diencephalic structures and ending in the ventromedial part of the prefrontal cortex (Fig. 6–15).[50, 63]

According to Figure 6–15, memories may be stored in the sensory cortex area where the original sensory input was interpreted into "sensory impressions." Today, concepts regarding memory storage suggest that declarative memory is stored in categories similar to a filing system. Those categories or files seem to be stored in several cortical areas bilaterally depending on the context.[46, 84] This system allows for easy retrieval from multiple areas. Memory has stages and is continually changing. Thus, to go from short-term to long-term memory, the brain must physically change its chemical structure (a plastic phenomenon). Memory first begins with a representation of information that has been transformed through processing of perceptual systems. The transferring of this new memory into a long-lasting chemical bond requires the neuronetwork of the limbic complex. Owing to the multiple tracts or parallel circuits in and out of the limbic system and throughout neocortical systems, clients, even with extensive lesions, can often learn and store new information.[63] This may also explain why damage to the limbic system structures does not destroy existing memory nor make it unavailable, because it is actually stored in many places throughout the neocortex. The circular memory circuit illustrated in Figure 6–14 shows only one system. The reader must remember that many parallel circuits function simultaneously. The circular memory circuit shown reverts back to the original sensory area after activation of the limbic structures to cause the necessary neuronal changes that would inscribe the event into retrievable stored memory. This information can be recognized and retrieved by activation of storage sites anywhere along the pathway.[63]

The last station or system to be added to the circuit is the "basal forebrain cholinergic system," which delivers the neurochemical acetylcholine to the cortical centers and to the limbic system with which it is richly linked. The loss of this neurotransmitter is linked to memory malfunctioning in Alzheimer's disease. Performance of visual recognition memory can be augmented or impaired by administration of drugs that enhance or block the action of acetylcholine.[67]

It has also been shown that the amygdala and hippocampus are both interchangeably involved in recognition memory. The hippocampus is vital for memory of location of objects in space, whereas the amygdala is necessary for the association of memories derived through the various senses with a specific recognition recall. For example, a whiff of ether might bring to mind a painful surgical experience or the sight of some food may cause a recall of its pleasant smell. Removal of the amygdala brings out the behavior shown in Kluver-Bucy syndrome. For clients with this neurological problem, familiar objects do not bring forth the correct associations of memories experienced by sight, smell, taste, and touch and relate them to objects presented. Association of previously presented stimuli and their responses appear to be lost. Animals without amygdaloid input had different response patterns that ignored previous fears and aversions. Thus the amygdala adds the "emotional weight" to sensory experience.[88] Loss of the amygdala also loses the positive associations and reward and thereby alters the shaping of perceptions that lead to memory storage.

When stimuli are endowed with emotional value or significance, attention is drawn to those possessing emotional significance, selecting these for attention and learning. This would give the amygdala a "gatekeeping" function of selective filtering. The amygdala may enable emotions to influence what is perceived and learned by reciprocal connection with the cortex. Emotionally charged events will leave a more significant impression and subsequent recall. The amygdala alters perception of afferent sensory input and thereby affects subsequent actions.

In humans, memory functioning has been associated with the phenomenon of long-term potentiation observed in hippocampal pathways.[50] This potentiation of synaptic transmission, lasting for hours, days, and weeks, occurs after brief trains of high-frequency stimulation of hippocampal excitatory pathways.[9] Whether this phenomenon is caused by alteration at the presynaptic or postsynaptic terminals has not been established. The question remains whether there is an increased amount of neurotransmitter released presynaptically (glutamate)[50] or whether the expected amount is producing a heightened postsynaptic response. Or, are both sites involved?[63] Even a third hypothesis regarding nonsynaptic neurotransmission or exocytoses with receptor sites on the surface of neuron beyond postsynaptic cites may in the future help guide our understanding of memory and memory storage.[63, 93]

Learning and memory evoke alterations in behavior that reflect neuroanatomical and neurophysiological changes.[61, 63] These include the phenomenon of long-term potentiation as an example of such changes. The hippocampus demonstrates the importance of input of long-term potentiation in associative learning. In this type of learning, two or more stimuli are combined. Tetanizing of more than one pathway needs to occur simultaneously. When only one pathway is tetanized, the effect is decreased synaptic transmission. Long-term potentiation, requiring the cooperative action of numbers of co-active fibers, is engendered and formed by the "associative" interaction of afferent inputs. Thus, long-term potentiation serves as one model for understanding the neural mechanism for associative learning.

Learning/Memory Problems After Limbic Involvement

For initial declarative learning and memory, the combination of hippocampus and amygdala of the limbic system is required.[63] For memory formation to occur, there must be a storing of the "neural representation" of the stimuli in the association and the processing areas of the cortex. This storage occurs when sensory stimuli activate a "cortico-limbo-thalamo-cortical" circuit.[63] Although there is not one single all-purpose memory storage system, this circuit serves as the "imprinting mechanism," reinforcing the pathway that activated it. On subsequent stimulation, a stimulus recognition or recall would be elicited. In associative recall, stored representations of any interconnected imprints could be evoked simultaneously.[63]

A vital processing area for all sensory modalities is located in the region of the anterior temporal lobe. This area is directly linked with the amygdala and indirectly with the hippocampus. The hippocampus and amygdala are also linked both structurally and functionally to each other and to specific thalamic nuclei. Clients with temporal epileptic seizures and whose temporal lobes have been surgically removed developed global anterograde amnesia; that is, amnesia developed for all senses and no new memories could be formed. Experimental removal of only the hippocampus does not bring about these changes, although processing is slowed down. When both the hippocampus and the amygdala are removed bilaterally, the amnesia is both retrograde and global. It is postulated that the amygdala is the area of the brain that adds a "positive association," the reward part to stimuli received and passed through processing. In this way, stimulus and reward are associated by the amygdala, and an emotional value is placed on it.[53]

It appears that limbic involvement in the declarative memory creates a chemical bond that allows cortical storage of "stimulus representation" necessary for subsequent recognition and recall of the information.[12, 26, 39, 63, 102]

When analyzing declarative and procedural learning from a clinical reference, a separation of functional mediation can be observed. Clients with brain lesions localized in the limbic system components of the amygdala and hippocampus have the ability to acquire and function with "rule-based" games and skills but have lost the capacity to recall how, when, or where they gained this knowledge or to give a description of the games and skills learned. Relating this to clinical performance, clients may develop the skill in a functional activity but not the problem-solving strategies necessary to associate danger or other potentially harmful aspects of a situation that may develop once out of the purely clinical setting.[8, 17, 25, 45, 69] Similarly, if a client needs to learn a procedural task such as walking, transfers, eating, and so on, it may be extremely important to direct the attention off the task while the task is being practiced procedurally.

Neurochemistry

Discussion of the limbic system's intricate regulation of many neurochemical substances is not within the scope of this chapter. Yet therapists need to appreciate how potent this system can be with respect to neurochemical reactions. The amount of research reflecting new understanding of the neurochemistry role on brain function is inundating the pharmacological research literature on a monthly basis.[28, 96, 128]

The hypothalamus, the physiological center of the limbic system (see Figs. 6–2 and 6–13), is involved in neurochemical production and is geared for passage of information along specific neurochemical pathways. Guyton[52] considers it the major motor output pathway of the limbic system, which also communicates with every part of this system. Certain nuclei of the hypothalamus produce and release neuroactive peptides that have a long-acting effectiveness as neuromodulators. As such, they control the levels of neuronal excitation and effective functioning at the synapses. By their long-lasting effects, they regulate motivational levels, mood states, and learning. These peptide-producing neurons extend from the hypothalamic nuclei to the ANS components and to the nuclei of the limbic system, where they modulate neuroendocrine and autonomic activities.[52] The importance of these neuropeptides are being recognized as research begin to unravel the mysteries of the limbic systems role in regulation of affective and motivated behaviors.[63, 89, 93]

Lesions in the medial hypothalamus affect hormone production and thus alter regulation of many hormonal control systems.[63] For example, clients with medial hypothalamic lesions may have huge weight gains because of the increase of insulin in the blood, which increases feeding and converts nutrients into fat. Similarly, this weight gain may be caused by hyperphagic responses resulting from the loss of satiety. General hyperactivity and signs of hostility after minimal provocation can also be observed. These problems are often encountered in patients with head trauma.

Lesions in the lateral hypothalamus lead to damage of dopamine-carrying fibers that begin in the substantia nigra and filter through the hypothalamus to the striatum. Lesions, either along this tract or within the lateral hypothalamus, lead to aphagia and hypoarousal. Decreased sensory awareness contributing to sensory neglect is also present in lateral hypothalamic lesions. The decreased awareness may be caused by a decrease of orientation to the stimuli versus awareness of the stimuli once they are brought to conscious attention. These lesions cause the client to exhibit marked passivity with decreased functioning.

As noted earlier, depression is clearly identified as a limbic function. A functional deficiency in monoamines, especially serotonin, is hypothesized to be a primary cause of depression.[108] The serotonin systems originate in the rostral and caudal raphe nuclei in the midbrain. Ascending serotonergic tracts start in the midbrain and ascend to the limbic forebrain and hypothalamus; they are concerned with mood and behavior regulation. Damage with direct or indirect limbic involvement results in the client exhibiting depression. Descending pathways to the substantia gelatinosa are involved in pain mechanisms and have also been linked through a complex sequence of biochemical steps to the increased sensitization of the presynaptic terminals of the cutaneous sensory neurons, leading to a hyperactive withdrawal reflex or hypersensitivity to cutaneous input.[63] This would account for the behavior patterns seen in clients with head trauma, when the therapist sees a flexed posture with a withdrawn or depressed affect yet with an extremely sensitive tactile system.

It is hypothesized that the underlying pathophysiology of one form of schizophrenia involves an excessive transmission of dopamine within the mesolimbic tract system.[63] The dopaminergic cell bodies are located in the ventral tegmental area and the substantia nigra. Some of these neurons project to the limbic system. These projections go to the nucleus accumbens, the stria terminalis nuclei, parts of the amygdala, and the frontal entorhinal and anterior cingulate cortex. It is the projection to the nucleus accumbens that seems critical, because of its influence over the hippocampus, frontal lobe, and hypothalamus. This nucleus may act as a filtering system with respect to affect and certain types of memory, and the dopaminergic projections may modulate the flow of neural activity.[63] The flat affect seen in clients with Parkinson's disease and the paranoid/schizophrenic behaviors observed in some clients with CNS damage may directly reflect back to these mesolimbic dopaminergic systems.

The specific roles of the noradrenergic pathway are numerous and affect almost all parts of the CNS. The center for the noradrenergic pathways is located within the caudal midbrain and upper pons. Its nucleus is referred to as locus coeruleus. This nucleus sends at least five tracts rostrally to the diencephalon and telencephalon.[63] Of specific interest for this discussion are the projections to the hippocampus and amygdala. The axons of these neurons modulate an excitatory effect on the regions where they terminate.[20] Thus, the activation of this system will heighten the excitation of the two nuclei within the limbic system intricately involved in declarative learning and memory. Hyperactivation may cause overload or the lack of focus of attention. Decreased activity may prevent the desired responses. Attention to task may depend on ongoing noradrenergic stimulation. These tracts from the midbrain rostrally play a key role in alertness. The correlation of alertness and attention to performance of motor tasks as well as to learning can be demonstrated.[63] Again, these research findings reiterate previous statements regarding a therapist's role in balancing the neurochemistry within the client's limbic system. From a clinical perspective, a therapist will observe a relaxed, motivated, alert participant in the learning environment and will observe better carryover because the chemical interactions will only enhance the learning.

More than 200 neurotransmitters have been identified within the nervous system.[63] How each transmitter and the interaction of multiple transmitters on one synapse affect any portion of the CNS is still unclear. Certainly, some relationships have been identified. Novelty-seeking behavior of the limbic system seems to be dopamine dependent,[55] whereas melatonin receptors seem to coordinate circadian body rhythm.[80] Adrenal corticosteroids modulate hippocampal long-term potentiation.[45] The specifics of the total complexity are still beyond the grasp of human understanding.

In conclusion, the neurochemistry of the limbic system is intricately linked to the neurochemistry of the brain. All systems within the limbic circuitry seem to be interdependent, with the summation of all the neurochemistry being the determinants of the specific processing of information. Similarly, the interdependence of the limbic system to almost all other areas of the brain and the activities of those areas at any time reflect the complexity of this system.

THE LIMBIC CONNECTIONS TO THE "MIND, BODY, SPIRIT" PARADIGM

As a neuroscientist, safe and deep within a Western allopathic model of linear research, establishing efficacy and evidence-based practice for what is taught to new learners is critically important. Yet, there are too many unexplainable behavioral unknowns occurring daily in the clinical environment that cannot be researched using standard Western research tools common to physical and occupational therapists. Thus, establishing efficacy for intervention when variables are not identifiable is often not possible at this time. After 30 years of clinical practice and hearing Western doctors saying "PT and/or OT just make the patients FEEL BETTER," it is obvious that many doctors first do not understand the depth and breadth of our professions or what is provided to the clients. Second, those doctors do not understand the limbic interconnections to "feel better" and how that might drive the neuroplasticity of the CNS and the autoimmune system's response to disease or pathology.

The success or failure of many forms of alternative medical practice and for that matter Western allopathic medicine and therapeutic practices may very well be due to the limbic system. If a patient "believes" an intervention will work, even if it is a placebo, the chances of success far exceed those when the patient does not think it will work. If it is a placebo and the body heals, then logic dictates that the body and the mind did the healing. How that occurs is yet to be totally determined, but enough research substantiates that neurochemical changes as well as neuroelectrical changes occur within an individual's physical body when the individual believes that change is possible.[60, 101] When I was a novice therapist, a nurse once told me: "I am very glad you are not a nurse because you are so idealistic. You believe these comatose patients are going to wake up and walk out of here. And what is even worse is that most of them do!" That moment should have told me that I was going to clash with allopathic doctrine throughout my professional career, but instead I was confused with her term *idealistic*. For, if the patients awoke and walked back into life, then was that not a realistic expectation? In that same job situation, my boss asked me to treat all the vegetative patients and once they were awake, my colleagues would treat them from there. My response was: "Emotionally for both the patient and myself, I could not do that. Once I bonded with a person, gained his/her trust, and the

patient was willing and capable of regaining consciousness, I could not just drop them and go onto another person." The significance of that statement took many years to understand, and it was not until I began my study of the limbic system that I truly comprehended the accuracy of my perception.

After 30 years of practice and often in front of colleagues in workshop situations, I have observed during treatment many patients move from a level 2, 3, or 4 on the Rancho Consciousness Scale to a level of 6, 7, or 8. For that reason alone, I cannot deny that something more than just "feeling good" occurs during physical or occupational therapy interventions. When working with clients, I find myself feeling very open and bond with something that is neither "physical" or "mental" and thus my only option left as a definition is "spiritual." If, when treating a vegetative patient, that bond tells me he or she wants to regain consciousness and the respective physical body seems capable, then the treatment is goal directed and the decision of the outcome is selected by the patient. The map has been established, and together the patient and I proceed. Like all therapists the intervention will be guided by the motor control of the patient and the window within which the patient can run those programs. At times, when treating vegetative clients, I am unable to locate the "spirit"; at other times it feels as if that person has not decided whether to venture to an awake state, but more often I sense a frightened, confused individual who just wants to find his or her way back to what we call "life." Those patients often gain consciousness during therapy. It is not a miracle nor can I even say, "I healed anything." The term *healing* referred to a concept of "whole." The only person who can regain the structure of the whole is the patient. As a therapist I am a teacher or a guide, helping others relearn and regain control over their lives. If after a 30-minute treatment session, a person regains feeling and control of an extremity after 18 years post stroke, or regains functional use of a hand 6 years post incomplete spinal injury, there is more to the intervention than following a critical pathway or a treatment regimen geared to all individuals at a specific stage of a disease process. One variable that always seems to be present when clients regain what seems like dramatic recovery is strong motivation to retain the control and an appreciation for the instruction. A strong bond or compassionate appreciation for each other always seems to be present as another interlocking variable. Thus, the question arose over 20 years ago: "What is spirituality?" It is a variable very difficult to define. That variable when researched has been shown to affect health and healing in individuals with health problems. The concept of "spirituality" and "healing" are both words that each individual defines according to his or her own beliefs, cultural experiences, and use of verbal language. The literature is available for those who wish to pursue this topic.* Within this chapter a system that affects all areas of the CNS and peripheral function has been discussed. How this system is affected by or affects one's spirituality is open for years of future study. Yet, if spirituality affects healing and an individual's belief that this potential is available,

---

*See references 5, 25, 42, 49, 54, 56, 64, 65, 68, 76, and 125.

then this variable may play a critical role in compliance and potentially has a very strong limbic interaction. Ignoring this variable is not different from ignoring perception when dealing with motor behavior.

Until we can measure simultaneous synaptic activity of all interactions within the therapist's and the client's CNS, we will not, from a grounded neuroscience efficacy base, be able to demonstrate exactly what occupational or physical therapists do. Until then outcomes need to be measured objectively. Even if interactions seem unmeasurable and subjective, clinicians still need to record the event and not bury it deep somewhere in a subconscious level. The mind, the body, and the spirit are connected as a whole. If therapists treat only one part, it may help the whole, but if the whole is treated simultaneously, the outcome is more likely to change the whole.

After years of clinical experience and thousands of patients responding positively to various interventions, the question arises regarding clinical decision making and choice of interventions. There is not "a variable" that has been identified that guides that decision. It has been shown that humans bring to consciousness about 10% of all incoming information. Yet, the human brain is making decision using 100% of the input information. Given that relationship, quite a bit of human decision making may be based on unconscious information regarding the external world.[63] Thus the word all neuroscientists shutter over, *intuition*, may, to a large extent, be the unraveling of that unconscious data. I have effectively taught colleagues how to feel blood pressure and heartbeats of clinical partners by just barely touching the top of the hand, which might be explained by the high level of sensitivity of receptors in our skin.[95] If a clinician can sense an autonomic response when touching a patient's skin, then knowing how the limbic system is interacting with the motor system can also be deduced. This would allow the clinician to determine how fast to move the patient during an activity without ever needing to increase the state of the motor generators due to heightened fear. In this case, it would look intuitive because one clinician seems to know how fast to move the patient and another clinician has no idea how to make that decision. This is a case of one clinician being open to receiving information and processing it. The other therapist, for some reason, is either not receiving or not processing the available information. This is not an example of "intuition."

Intuition has been a source of fascination over centuries. Recently, with consumer dissatisfaction with health care and insurgence of alternative medical practices, intuition has again sparked the interest of scholars and the public. To many it reflects mystery, magic, and even voodoo. Those individuals with a strong ethnic, cultural, and even religious bias may find it hard to scientifically analyze this strategy. For over 25 years my husband has answered questions I have posed in my mind. It took half of that time for my left brain to actually accept that I was not subvocalizing the thought or that he could not have extrapolated the thought from the environmental stimuli. Yet, he constantly tells me he hears me. Obviously, my thoughts have traveled to his primary and associative receiving areas of his left temporal lobe and he hears the thought. The dilemma that confronted me is: "If the information did not input through his eighth cranial nerve, how did it enter into his system?" That is intuition—knowing without entering the data through traditional input systems. The next question is: "What is intuition?" Unfortunately, after 20 years of study I cannot answer that question, but I can say it is something, it can be learned, and master clinicians use it as a part of their clinical decision making even if they choose not to verbalize it to their colleagues or even acknowledge it within their conscious mind. There is a lot of research and literature available regarding intuition.[24, 29, 41, 60, 62, 117, 126] Yet, the answer to that simple question "what is intuition?" is unavailable. No answer exists that has shown to be efficacious and reliable. It may be that intuition is more than one variable and can be accessed through more than one way. In fact, after studying various alternative medical practices, all using very different interventions based on different philosophies and belief systems, it seems as if everyone may be tapping into the same system just opening to that system through different doors. In the 1960s I was presenting an integrated approach to neurological disabilities and integrating various treatment philosophies using the behavioral responses of patients to guide intervention. I was told, at that time, that it could not be done and that I would potentially injure patients by using approaches from different philosophical techniques. Today, of course, with our understanding of motor control and motor learning, that approach from the 1960s is what we do. I now present the same model when looking at complementary approaches to intervention and the concept of intuition. Bonding, dedication to the patient, openness to listening to the patient, not only a willingness to learn but an insatiable appetite to continue learning, and the ability to let go of one's importance and just be another person within the environment all seem to be the variables that open one's intuition and thus may be the best place for a learner to begin studying how to develop this skill. It would seem as if intuition is like an aptitude. Some come in already with a high level of potential, others are nurtured to develop that potential, and still others never have an opportunity or are within an environment to develop those strategies. Some individuals have had strong intuitive senses from childhood but share those experiences with few, if any, others. Until 19 years ago, I hid that aspect of my person because I was a neuroscientist and wanted to be grounded in scientific efficacy like all my other colleagues. Unfortunately, my clinical experiences did not allow me to hide that intuitive aspect of my clinical decision making. After treating a head-injured woman who presented herself at a Rancho level 3 and left 30 minutes later volitionally moving both independently and with command without cognitive confusion, I shared with my colleagues this woman's medical and social history. That information was critical to their understanding the course of progression of this women throughout rehabilitation. I discussed her social background, her education, her family, her children, and her husband, who had shot her in the head. This all makes perfect sense, until the head of the department asked me: "how I knew that information." I said: "I read it in the chart." She informed me that I did not see the chart.

I said, "You told me." She responded with: "We did not discuss the case!" I asked her if I was wrong and she said "no." In fact, she was amazed at how accurate I was and just wondered how I knew that. At that moment, my life was changed. I could no longer hide whatever this "intuition" was, nor could I truthfully tell colleagues I am sharing what I do during interventions without bringing up this topic and saying I can only tell you ways to develop it. I cannot tell you exactly what it is because I do not know. The future will unravel those answers. What I have found is that "masters," whether they are doctors, therapists, or teachers, often use this additional source of information gathering to help them in their clinical reasoning. I do not make this statement lightly nor without tremendous professional risk. Thus, I will leave you with an interaction that solidified my belief. A few years ago, I was a keynote speaker at a "Neurosurgical Conference on Brain Tumors." I was the token "other," nonneurosurgeon. I presented the topic of the "Limbic System's Influence on Motor Output." With this audience, I, of course, used charts and pictures and based every sentence on research. At dinner that night the master neurosurgeon asked if he could sit next to me. I was aghast, a little nervous but honored nonetheless. He opened by saying: "I think many PTs and OTs are intuitive." With that, I knew him, his life, his experiences, and so on. I responded with: "Yes, it is like walking into a room, looking at a patient, knowing where and what type of tumor he has, and using instruments to validate what you already know!" He responded with: "Yes, it is exactly like that!" I do not need to continue to discuss our interaction that night but let me leave you with the thought that even the master neurosurgeon used intuition as a variable in clinical decision making. No one uses intuition as the only variable; it just gives additional information that helps in the final process of clinical reasoning. It would seem as though intuition has a strong limbic interaction. Intuition is knowing something and as a result may bring on great emotion, such as "I know, thus I fear." If the sequence of events begins with an emotion and leads to what is perceived as knowledge I would question that intuition was a driving force. "I fear, thus I think I know" may not be intuitively driven. Intuition is knowing with emotional balance, not without emotion. To become truly intuitive one needs to become emotionally centered. In our everyday world this emotional balance is extremely difficult. It is even harder to find that balance in a clinical arena where patients are coming in faster, often in multiple numbers, and staying for shorter periods of time. That does not mean it is not our responsibility to find those avenues to provide better care within the existing environment, it just says the challenges and questions are there. Intuition seems to be a variable that gives some colleagues additional information that is then used as part of the clinical reasoning process. Intuition as a variable needs to be identified, studied, researched, and taught once clearly understood. It is up to all of us to find the answers to these questions and the solutions to today's clinical problems and develop evidence-based practice in order to progress into the twenty-first century.[107]

SUMMARY

The complexity and interwoven neurological network of the limbic system may seem overwhelming. A reader who tries to grasp all parts on first study will feel lost and defeated—a true limbic emotion. Thus this chapter was presented in three parts. The first part introduces the system and its potential clinical application. This section, in and of itself, has many interwoven components, for nothing in the limbic system functions in isolation. Yet the mysteries of this complex neurological network when solved may hold the answers to many clinical questions regarding the art and gift of a master clinician. The second part introduces in more detail the basic anatomy and physiology of the limbic system. It is hoped that once the student/clinician has been drawn to the conclusion that this system may be a key to clinical success, he or she might be willing to delve into the science of the system. This path of exploration is challenging, difficult, and frustrating at times but certainly worth the effort once understanding is achieved. The last section opens up the mind of the readers when and if they so choose to address these unknown variables. The limbic system is very complex, is very interactive with all parts of the human body, and may hold many answers about patients' responses. The reader's journey has just begun, and the future will open up many more avenues of research and clinical study as well as many more questions.

REFERENCES

1. Adamec R: Kindling, anxiety, and limbic perspectives. In Wada JA (ed): Advances in Behavioral Biology. New York, Plenum Press, 1990.
2. Adams JH, et al: Diffuse axonal injury due to nonmissile head injury in humans: An analysis of 45 cases. Ann Neurol 12:557–563, 1982.
3. Aggleton JP, et al. Removal of the hippocampus and transection of the fornix produce comparable deficits on delayed non-matching to position by rats. Behav Brain Res 52:61–71, 1992.
4. Alkire MT, Haier RJ, Fallon JH, Cahill L: Hippocampal, but not amygdala, activity at encoding correlates with long-term, free recall of nonemotional information. Proc Natl Acad Sci U S A 95:14506–14510, 1998.
5. Anadaraijah G: Spirituality and medicine. J Fam Pract 48:389, 1999.
6. Appel SH (ed): Current Neurology, vol 6. Chicago, CV Mosby, 1986.
7. Arnsten AFT: The biology of being frazzled. Science 280:1711–1712, 1998.
8. Auerbach SH: Neuroanatomical correlates of attention and memory disorders in traumatic brain injury: An application of neurobehavioral subtypes, J Head Trauma Rehabil 1(3):1–12, 1986.
9. Barr ML, Kiernan JA (eds): The Human Nervous System: An Anatomical Viewpoint, 6th ed. Philadelphia, JB Lippincott, 1993.
10. Bell IR, Miller C, Schwartz GE: An olfactory-limbic model of multiple chemical sensitivity syndrome: Possible relationships to kindling and affective spectrum disorders. Biol Psychiatry 32:218–242, 1992.
11. Blais C: Concept mapping of movement: Related knowledge. Percept Mot Skills 76:767–774, 1993.
12. Bluck MA, Myers CE: Psychobiological models of hippocampal function in learning and memory. Ann Rev Psychol 48:481–512, 1997.
13. Broca P: Anatomie comparée des circonvolutions cérébrales: Le grand lobe limbique et la scissure limbique dans la séries des mammifères. Rhone Antropol 1:385, 1878.
14. Brodal A: Neurological Anatomy in Relation to Clinical Medicine, 5th ed. New York, Oxford University Press, 1992.
15. Brooks VB: The Neural Basis of Motor Control. New York, Oxford University Press, 1986.
16. Bunsey M, Eichenbaum H: Conservation of hippocampal memory function in rats and humans. Nature 378:255–257, 1996.
17. Burns LH, Robbins TW, Everitt BJ: Differential effects of excitotoxic lesions of the basolateral amygdala, ventral subiculum and

medial prefrontal cortex on responding with conditioned reinforcement and locomotor activity potentiated by intro-accumbens infusion of D-amphetamine. Behav Brain Res 55:167–183, 1993.

18. Burt AM: Textbook of Neuroanatomy. Philadelphia, WB Saunders, 1993.

19. Cahill L: Interactions between catecholamines and amygdala in emotional memory: Subclinical and clinical evidence. Adv Pharmacol 42:964–967, 1998.

20. Cai Z: The neural mechanism of declarative memory consolidation and retrieval: A hypothesis. Neurosci Biobehav Rev 14:295–304, 1990.

21. Carpenter MB: Core Text of Neuroanatomy, 4th ed. Baltimore, Williams & Wilkins, 1991.

22. Carr DB, Sesack SR: Hippocampal afferents to the rat prefrontal cortex: Synaptic targets and reaction to dopamine terminals. J Comp Neurol 369:1–15, 1996.

23. Cohen J: Gut reaction is your best guide. New Scientist, March 8, 1997.

24. Cohen J, Steward I: That's amazing, isn't it? New Science, January 17, 1998.

25. Colon K: The healing power of spirituality. Minn Med 79:12–18, 1996.

26. Cohen NJ, Poldrack RA: Memory for items and memory for relations in the procedural/declarative memory framework. Memory 5:131–178, 1997.

27. Conry J: Neuropsychological deficits in fetal alcohol syndrome and fetal alcohol effects. Alcohol Clin Exp Res 14:650–655, 1990.

28. Coull JT, Buchel C, Friston KJ, Frith CD: Noradrenergically mediated plasticity in a human attentional neuronal network. Neuroimage 10:705–715, 1999.

29. Courchesme E: Neuroanatomic imaging in autism. Pediatrics 87:781–790, 1991.

30. Davis M: The role of the amygdala in fear and anxiety. Annu Rev 15:333–375, 1992.

31. Davis M: Are different parts of the extended amygdala involved in fear versus anxiety. Soc Biol Pathways 44:1239–1247, 1998.

32. Decker MW, Curzon P, Brioni JD: Influence of separate and combined septal and amygdala lesions on memory, acoustic startle, anxiety, and locomotor activity in rats. Neurobiol Learn Mem 64:156–168, 1995.

33. deGroot J: Correlative Neuroanatomy. Norwalk, CT, Appleton & Lange, 1991.

34. Derryberry D, Tucker DM: Neural mechanism of emotion. J Consult Clin Psychol 60:329–338, 1992.

35. Diano S, Naftolin F, Horvath TL: Gonadal steroids target AMPA glutamate receptor–containing neurons in the rat hypothalamus, septum and amygdala: A morphological and biochemical study. Endocrinology 138:778–789, 1997.

36. Dobkin BH: Neuroplasticity: Key to recovery after central nervous system injury, West J Med 159:56–60, 1993.

37. Dougherty DD, Shin LM, Alpert NM, et al: Anger in healthy men: A PET study using script-driven imagery. Biol Psychiatry 46:466–472, 1999.

38. Ehrenkrantz D, Silverman JM, Smith CJ, et al: Genetic epidemiological study of maternal and paternal transmission of Alzheimer's disease. Am J Med Genet 88:378–382, 1999.

39. Eichenbaum H: Declarative memory: Insights from cognitive neurobiology. Annu Rev Psychol 48:547–572, 1997.

40. Eichenbaum H: How does the brain organize memories? Science 277:330–335, 1998.

41. Epstein S, Donovan S, Denes-Raj V: The missing link in the paradox of the Linda problem: Beyond knowing and thinking of the conjunction rule, the intrinsic appeal of heuristic processing. Personality Soc Psychol 25:204–214, 1999.

42. Fallot RD: Recommendations for integrating spirituality in mental health services. New Dir Ment Health Serv 80:97–100, 1998.

43. Falls WA, Miserendino MJ, Davis M: Extinction of fear-potentiated startle: Blockage by infusion on an NMDA antagonist into the amygdala. J Neurosci 12:854–863, 1992.

44. Fendt M, Fanselow MS: The neuroanatomical and neurochemical basis of conditioned fear. Neurosci Biobehav Rev 23:743–760, 1999.

45. Filipine D, et al: Modulation by adrenal steroids in limbic function. J Steroid Biochem 39:245–252, 1991.

46. Gabrieli JD: Disorders of memory in humans. Curr Opin Neurol Neurosurg 6(1):93–97, 1993.

47. Gisquet-Verrier P, Dutrieux G, Richer P, et al: Effects of lesions to the hippocampus on contextual fear: Evidence for a disruption of freezing and avoidance behavior but not context conditioning. Behav Neurosci 113:507–522, 1999.

48. Glisky EL: Acquisition and transfer of declarative and procedural knowledge by memory-impaired patients: A computer data-entry task. Neuropsychologia 30:899–910, 1992.

49. Goddard NC: Spirituality as integrative energy: A philosophical analysis as requisite precursor to holistic nursing practice. J Adv Nurs 22:805–815, 1995.

50. Greenberg DA, Aminoff MJ, Simon RP (eds): Clinical Neurology. Norwalk, CT, Appleton & Lange, 1993.

51. Groenewegen HJ, Wright CI, Beijer AVJ: The nucleus accumbens: Gateway for limbic structures to reach the motor system? Prog Brain Res 107:485–511, 1996.

52. Guyton A: Basic Neuroscience: Anatomy & Physiology. Philadelphia, WB Saunders, 1991.

53. Haist F, Shimamura AP, Squire LR: On the relationship between recall and recognition memory. J Exp Psychol Learn Mem Cogn 18:691–702, 1992.

54. Hamilton J: Yes, religion and spirituality do matter in health. Altern Ther Health Med 5(4):18, 1999.

55. Harris SR, et al: Effects of prenatal alcohol exposure on neuromotor and cognitive development during early childhood: A series of case reports. Phys Ther 73:608–617, 1993.

56. Hawks SR, Huyll ML, Thalman RL, Richins PM: Review of spiritual health: Definition, role, and intervention strategies in health promotion. Am J Health Promot 9:371–378, 1995.

57. Helmstaedter C, Grunwalk T, Lehnertz K, et al: Differential involvement of left temporolateral and temporomesial structures in verbal declarative learning and memeory: Evidence from temporal lobe epilepsy. Brain Cogn 35:110–131, 1997.

58. Holstege G (ed): Descending Motor Pathways and the Spinal Motor System: Limbic and Non-limbic Components. New York, Elsevier Science Publications, 1991.

59. Holstege G, Bandler R, Saper CB: The emotional motor system. Prog Brain Res 107:3–6, 1996.

60. Hunt VV: Infinite Mind: Science of the Human Vibrations of Consciousness. Malibu, CA, Malibu Publishing Co, 1996.

61. Izquierdo I, Medina JH: Memory formation: The sequence of biochemical events in the hippocampus and its connection to activity in other brain structures. Neurobiol Learn Mem 68:285–316, 1997.

62. Johnson KE, Mervis CB: Impact of intuitive theories on feature recruitment throughout the continuum of expertise. Memory Cogn 26:382–401, 1998.

63. Kandel ER, Schwartz JH, Jessell TM: Principles of Neural Science, 5th ed. New York, Elsevier Medical Science Publishing, 2000.

64. Karasu TB: Spiritual psychotherapy. Am J Psychother 53:143–162, 1999.

65. Kligman E: Alternative medicine. Iowa Med 87:232–234, 1997.

66. Kluver H, Bucy PC: Preliminary analysis of functions of the temporal lobes in monkeys. Arch Neural Psychiatry 42:979, 1939.

67. Knopman D: Long-term retention of implicitly acquired learning in patients with Alzheimer's disease. J Clin Exp Neuropsychol 13:880, 1991.

68. Koenig HG, et al: Religion, spirituality, and medicine: A rebuttal to skeptics. Int J Psychiatr Med 29:123–131, 1999.

69. Kostandov EA: Organization of human higher cortical functions with different forms of reinforcement, Neurosci Behav Physiol 19:93–102, 1989.

70. Lachman HM: Alterations in glucocorticoid inducible RNAs in the limbic system of learned helpless rats. Brain Res 609:110–116, 1993.

71. Lachman ME, Howland J, Hennstedt S, et al: Fear of falling and activity restriction: The survey of activities and fear of falling in the elderly (SAFE). J Gerontol B Psychol Sci Soc Sci 53:43–50, 1998.

72. LeDoux J: Emotional networks and motor control: A fearful view. In Holstege G, Bandler R, Saper (eds): Progress in Brain Research, vol 107. Elsevier Science Amsterdam, 1996.

73. LeDoux J: Fear and the brain: Where have we been, and where are we going? Soc Biol Psychiatry 44:1229–1238, 1998.

74. Lenz FA, Bracely RH, Zirh AT, et al: The sensory-limbic model of pain memory. Pain Forum 6(1):22–31, 1997.

75. Leonard G: The Silent Pulse. New York. Bantam Books, 1981.

76. Levey AL, Heilman CJ, Lah JJ, et al: Presenilin-1 protein expression in familial and sporadic Alzheimer's disease. Ann Neurol, 41:742–753, 1997.

77. Levin JS, Larson DB, Puchalski CM: Religion and spirituality in medicine: Research and education. JAMA 278:792–793, 1997.

78. Lewis CB: Aging: The Health Care Challenge. Philadelphia, FA Davis, 1990.

79. Lewis CB, Bottomley JM: Geriatric Physical Therapy: A Clinical Approach. Norwalk, CT Appleton & Lange, 1994.

80. Lindross OF, Leinonen LM, Laakso ML: Melatonin binding to the anteroventral and anterodorsal thalamic nuclei in the rat. Neurosci Lett 143:219–222, 1992.

81. Libon DJ, Boganoff B, Cloud BS et al: Declarative and procedural learning, quantitative measures of the hippocampus, and subcortical white alterations in Alzheimer's disease and ischaemic vascular dementia. J Clin Exp Neuropsychol 20:30–41, 1998.

82. Liu CY, Wang SJ, Fun JL, et al: The correlation of depression with functional activity in Parkinson's disease. J Neurol 244:493–498, 1997.

83. Maclean PD: Role of transhypothalamic pathways in social communication. In Morgane PJ, Panksapp J (eds): Handbook of the Hypothalamus, vol 3. New York, Marcel Dekker, 1981.

84. McKee RD, Squire LR: On the development of declarative memory. J Exp Psychol Learn Mem Cogn 19:397–404, 1993.

85. Menza MA, et al: Dopamine-related personality traits in Parkinson's disease. Neurology 43:505–508, 1993.

86. Mesulam MM: Principles of Behavioral Neurology. Philadelphia, FA Davis, 1985.

87. Mishkin MA, Appenzeller T: The anatomy of memory. Sci Am 256:680, 1987.

88. Mishkin M, et al: An animal model of global amnesia. In Cashin S (ed): Alzheimer Disease: A Report of Progress. New York, Raven Press, 1982.

89. Mitrovic I, Napier TC: Substance P attenuates and DAMGO potentiates amygdala glutamatergic neurotransmission within the ventral pallidum. Brain Res 792:193–206, 1998.

90. Moore JC: Review of neurophysiology as it relates to treatment: personal notes. San Francisco, 1980.

91. Moore JC: Neuroanatomical structures subserving learning and memory. In Fifteenth Annual Sensorimotor Integration Symposium, unpublished manual, San Diego, July 1987.

92. Morris JS, Ohman A, Dolan RJ: Conscious and unconscious emotional learning in the human amygdala. Nature 393:467–474, 1998.

93. Nieuwenhuys R: The greater limbic system, the emotional motor system and the brain. Prog Brain Res 107:510–580, 1996.

94. Noback CR, Strominger NL, Demarest RJ: The Human Nervous System: Introduction and Review, 4th ed. Philadelphia, Lea & Febiger, 1991.

95. Ogawa H: The Merkel cell as a possible mechanoreceptor cell. Prog Neurobiol 49:317–334, 1996.

96. Ogren SO, Schott PA, Kehr J, et al: Modulation of acetylcholine and serotonin transmission by galanin: Relationship to spatial and aversive learning. Ann NE Acad Sci 863:342–363, 1999.

97. Ommaya AIC, Gennarelli TA: Cerebral concussion and traumatic unconsciousnes. Brain 24:1181, 1974.

98. Osborn JA, Harris SR, Weinberg J: Fetal alcohol syndrome: Review of the literature with implication for physical therapists. Phys Ther 73:599–607, 1993.

99. Osterlund MK, Keler E, Hurd YL: The human forebrain has discrete estrogen receptors alpha messager RNA express high levels in the amygdaloid complex. Neuroscience 95:333–342, 2000.

100. Papez JW: A proposed mechanism of emotions. Arch Neurol Psychiatry 38:725, 1937.

101. Pert CB: Molecules of Emotion: The Science behind Mind-Body Medicine. New York, Touchstone, 1997.

102. Poldrck RA, Gabrieli JDE: Functional anatomy of long-term memory. J Clin Neurophysiol 14:294–310, 1997.

103. Reber PJ, Knowlton BJ, Squire LR: Dissociable properties of memory systems: Differences in the flexibility of declarative and nondeclarative knowledge. Behav Neurosci 110:861–871, 1996.

104. Reding M, et al: Depression in patients referred to a dementia clinic: A three-year prospective study. Arch Neurol 42:894, 1985.

105. Rijntjes M, Dettmers C, Buchel C, et al: A blueprint for movement: Functional and anatomical representations in the human motor system. J Neurosci 19:8043–8048, 1999.

106. Rosenthal M, et al (eds): Rehabilitation of the Adult and Child with Traumatic Brain Injury. Philadelphia, FA Davis, 1990.

107. Rosswurm MA, Larrabee JH: A model for change to evidence-based practice. Image J Nurs Sch 31:317–322, 1999.

108. Ruat M, et al: Molecular cloning characterization and localization of a high-affinity serotonin receptor activating cAMP formation. Proc Natl Acad Sci U S A 90:8547–8551, 1993.

109. Saito H, Matsumoto M, Tagashi H, Yoshioka M: Functional interaction between serotonin and other neuronal systems: Focus on in vivo microdialysis studies. Jpn J Pharmacol 70:203–225, 1996.

110. Sapolsky RM: Why stress is bad for your brain. Science 273:749–751, 1996.

111. Schmidley JW, Messing RO: Agitated confusional states in patients with right hemisphere infarctions. Stroke 15:883, 1984.

112. Schmidt RA: Motor learning principles for physical therapy. In Lister MJ (ed): Contemporary Management of Motor Control Problems. Norman, OK, Foundation for Physical Therapy, 1991.

113. Schneider JW, Chasnoff IJ: Motor assessment of cocanin/polydrug-exposed infants at age 4 months. Neurotoxicol Teratol 14:97–101, 1992.

114. Segal B: Love, Medicine, & Miracles: Lessons Learned About Self-Healing from a Surgeon's Experience with Exceptional Patients. New York, Harper Collins, 1986.

115. Selye H: The Stress of Life. New York, McGraw Hill, 1959.

116. Servan-Schreiber D, Perlstein WM, Cohen JD, Mintun M: Selective pharmacological activation of limbic structures in human volunteers: A positron emission tomography study. J Neuropsychiatry Clin Neurosci 10:148–159, 1998.

117. Shirley DA, Langan-Fox J: Intuition: A review of the literature. Psychol Rep 79:563–584, 1996.

118. Smith BR, Dudek FE: Amino acid-mediated regulation of spontaneous synaptic activity patterns in the rat basolateral amygdala. J Neurophysiol 76:1958–1967, 1996.

119. Spiers PA: Temporal limbic epilepsy and behavior. In Mesulam MM (ed): Principles of Behavioral Neurology. Philadelphia, FA Davis, 1985.

120. Squire LR: The medial temporal lobe memory system. Science 253:1380–1386, 1991.

121. Squire LR: Memory and the hippocampus: A synthesis from findings with rats, monkeys, and humans. Psychol Rev 99:195–231, 1992.

122. Squire LR, Zola SM: Structure and function of declarative and nondeclarative memory systems. Proc Natl Acad Sci U S A 93:13515–13522, 1996.

123. Stellar JR, Stellar E: The Neurobiology of Motivation and Rewards. New York, Springer-Verlag, 1985.

124. Strub RL, Black FW: Neurobehavioral Disorders: A Clinical Approach. Philadelphia, FA Davis, 1988.

125. Sulmasy DP: Is medicine a spiritual practice? Acad Med 74:1002–1005, 1999.

126. Taggart WM, Valenzi E, Zalka L: Rational and intuitive styles: Commensurability across respondents' characteristics. Psychol Rep 8:23–33, 1997.

127. Thompson RF: Are memory traces localized or distributed? Neuropsychologia 29:571–582, 1991.

128. Toni N, Buchs PA, Nikonenko I, et al: LTP promotes formation of multiple spine synapses between axon terminal and a dendrite. Nature 402:421–425, 1999.

129. Tucker DM, Derryberry D: Motivated attention: Anxiety and the frontal executive functions. Neuropsychiatry Neuropsychol Behav Neurol 5:233–252, 1992.

130. Vizi ES, Kiss JP: Neurochemistry and pharmacology of the major hippocampal transmitter systems: Synaptic and nonsynaptic interaction. Hippocampus 8:566–607, 1998.

131. Waxman SG: Clinical observations on the emotional motor system. Prog Brain Res 107:595–604, 1996.

132. Zola MS, et al: Damage to the perirhinal cortex exacerbates memory impairment following lesions to the hippocampal formation. J Neurosci 13:251–265, 1993.

Psychosocial Aspects of Adaptation and Adjustment During Various Phases of Neurological Disability

GORDON U. BURTON, PhD, OTR

Key Words

- adaptation
- adjustment
- bonding
- cognitive age
- coping
- family network
- loss and grief
- problem solving
- sensuality
- sexuality
- support systems

Objectives

After reading this chapter the student/therapist will:

1. Describe adaptation and adjustment as a flexible and flowing process, not as static stages.

2. Describe elements of the grief process that deal with age, cognition, and developmental level.

3. Respect aspects of sensuality and sexuality in treatment and consider them when treating the client.

4. Integrate the family of the client and the client's styles of coping into therapeutic treatment strategies to be used in the clinic.

5. Integrate the elements of problem solving, loss, cognitive functioning, coping, sensuality, as well as significant others' coping and learning styles into the treatment process to encourage adaptation.

IMPAIRMENT AND DISABILITY

Every individual must adapt and adjust to changes in life on a daily basis. We hope we adjust to the everyday stresses but there are situations that may overwhelm us. Work stress can create a situation that may stimulate a person who may not have "snapped" to break down and react in what appears to be inappropriate ways.[58] These are all examples of impairments that result in disability due to stress. The advent of a physical disability may provide the stress that will result in the failure of a person to adjust or adapt due to impairments.

Why worry about adjustment or adaptation? If you have had a major stress in your life, such as the loss of a loved one or a divorce, you may have experienced a lack of concentration or an inability to function effectively. This is a natural experience and a part of life that all people have at some time, but it gives the therapist some minor insight into what a client goes through when confronted with the multiple major stresses that accompany a physical disability.

The adjustment process is a dynamic state that is always in process.[94] We have some good days and some bad ones (feel good about ourselves or not). When we feel "in balance" we are more productive and are able to incorporate new strategies and concepts into our life. When we are out of balance we find it hard to accept new concepts or incorporate new activities into our lives. Thus, the therapist must encourage growth and adaptation into the treatment of the client.[82, 97] If this area is not recognized or encouraged, the client may engage in maladaptive strategies.[180] Sometimes it is hard to distinguish between adaptive and maladaptive behaviors. The client may be angry, but this may be good and stimulate positive strategies for change, or the anger can be used for negative self-defeating behaviors and strategies. Superficial observation may not be enough to distinguish between one or another. The therapeutic session and the environment should be designed to stimulate positive adaptation for the client and help the client incorporate these strategies into everyday life for the growth of the client and the family.[30, 82] If this is done, the chances for compliance and the incorporation of positive changes in the client's life will improve and the quality of life will be greatly enhanced.[82, 94, 175, 177]

Impairments in relation to psychosocial adjustment relate to how the person is able to cope and adapt to the radical changes and demands of the situation.[126] The impairment may be new, such as in the case of brain damage or chemical imbalances, or it may have been premorbid in the case of a person who was just barely functioning before the stress and extra demands of a disability. The underlying problem will result in functional problems and resulting disability. The psychosocial impairment or impairments are very often hard to tease out from the other impairments and disabilities in a traumatic event or even from a chronic problem. This coupled with the fact that the person may have had several impairments or presently has several new impairments or a combination of these complicates the problem for the therapist, the client, and the family. Think of yourself becoming disabled by a spinal cord injury at the C2–3 level. Might you have underlying psychological impairments that may never have been displayed or expressed if you had never had been exposed to this stressful experience?

The resulting functional disability limits the person's ability to enjoy and be productive in life activities.[131] At times it may be hard or impossible to ascertain why specific behaviors are being displayed by the client.[116] Is anger the impairment that results in the disability, or is it the disability that results from another impairment? In some cases the physical disability may have been caused by the impairment, impulsiveness, or anger.

Just looking at a person's behavior will not necessarily tell you the motivation behind it. Some people use anger or religious activities to grow and adapt, and others use it to hide from adaptation. Compliance with therapy can also be a sign of future adaptation or of just going through the paces and not adapting. Unfortunately, if people go through therapy just doing what they have to do ("doing

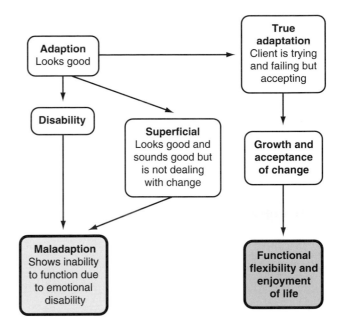

FIGURE 7–1. Possible directions of the adaptive process.

time"), when they get home or stop therapy they may not be able to adapt to the changes in the rest of their life. Whenever possible in therapy the functional activity should be presented and structured to promote empowerment, problem solving, and adjustment. Adjustment and adaptation to life is a dynamic process that allows for the person to interact with life in a meaningful and productive way that encourages the person to enjoy life (Fig. 7–1).[82, 116, 135, 176] We see the client at a very stressful time, and we need to make this time as productive for the client and the family as possible.

OVERVIEW

Psychological Adjustment

Theoretical foundations for adjustment to disability in practice appear to be elusive because it is a fluid process: all people are constantly changing. This is especially true for people who have recently become physically disabled. They do not reach a certain state of adjustment and stay there but progress through a series of adaptations. Therapists commonly see clients in a crisis state[48] and therefore identify their adjustment pattern from this frame of reference. How well the client adjusts to crisis, however, does not necessarily indicate how well the individual will adjust to all aspects of the disability or the rate of progress from one adaptation to another.[3, 14, 56, 66, 119, 169, 173] Disabilities are a massive insult to a person's self-perception.[6, 12, 16, 132] A month, or even a year, after the injury may not be long enough to put the disability into perspective.[6, 14, 49, 56, 99–102]

For most people, progressing from the shock of injury to the acceptance of, and later adaptation to, disability is a process fraught with psychologic ups and downs. Several authors have discussed the possible stages of adjustment and grieving.[56, 134, 144, 173] The research of Kubler-Ross[106] into death and dying also has application to this topic of adjustment to disability. She discusses the concept of loss and grief in relation to life; loss of function may result in just as profound a reaction. Peretz[136] discusses the grieving process in relationship to loss of role function as well as loss of body function. These losses must be grieved for before the client can benefit from therapy or adjust to a changed lifestyle and body. Therapists must be aware that the client can and must deal with the death of certain functional abilities.

The concept of stages of adjustment has been questioned,[48] and a call for more empirical research into adaptation and adjustment has been made.[21, 60, 100] Several studies have given some attention to this concept, but much more work is needed.

The components of successful psychological adjustment to a physical disability are varied. To bring a client to a level of function that is of the highest quality possible for that individual, therapists must look wholistically at the psychosocial aspects and at the adjustment processes involved, evaluate each component, and integrate the processes into the therapeutic milieu to promote growth in all areas. There is more to evaluation and treatment than just the physical component; the mind and body have interrelated influences, and both must be understood, evaluated, and treated individually and as a whole.

This chapter explores the processes of adjustment and adaptation, as well as the influences of culture and societal values as they affect the physically disabled person. The importance of loss as a psychological component will be examined as it relates to the body, sexuality, the personality, and the family. Age will also be discussed as a factor in adjustment to disability. The importance of focusing on the strengths of the client, the family, and the support system, rather than on the weaknesses of the disability, will also be explored.

This overview is designed to help therapists think of the client as a whole person, not as a diagnosis to be handled in some prescribed way. As fellow human beings, therapist and client are in the rehabilitation process together.

Adjustment Using the Stage Concept

Each person has his or her own coping style, and each should be allowed to be unique. Kerr[89] describes five stages of adjustment:

Shock: "This really isn't happening to me."
Expectancy for recovery: "I will be well soon."
Mourning: "There is no hope."
Defense: "I will live with this obstacle and beat it." (healthy attitude) "I am adjusted, but you fail to see it." (neurotic attitude)
Adjustment: "It is part of me now, but it is not necessarily a bad thing."

In light of current research, it is important for the therapist to realize that these are not lockstep stages and are to be thought of as concepts to help with the understanding of common reactions of all individuals.[114]

Shock. The client in shock does not recognize that anything is actually wrong. He or she may totally refuse to accept the diagnosis. The client may even laugh at the concern expressed by others. This stage is altered when the person has an opportunity to test reality and finds that the physical condition is actually limiting performance. If this stage continues, it may signify either a lack of mental health or an inability to cognitively realize the situation.

Expectancy for Recovery. The client in this stage is aware that he or she is "ill" but also believes that recovery will be quick and complete. The person may look for a "miracle cure" and may make future plans that require total return of function. Total recovery is the only goal, even if it takes a great deal of time and effort to achieve. Key signs of this stage are resentment of loss of function and the feeling that the whole body is necessary to do anything worthwhile. The staff can stimulate a change from this stage by giving clear statements to the client that the damage is permanent, by transferring the person home or to the rehabilitation unit, or by discontinuing therapy. Any one of these occurrences can help make the client realize the permanence of the disability.

Mourning. During the stage of mourning the individual feels all is lost, that he or she will never achieve anything in life. Suicide is often considered. The person may feel that characteristics of the personality (such as courage or fight) have also been lost and must be mourned as well. Thus, motivation to continue therapy, to work on improving, may be absent. The prospect of total recovery can no longer be held, but, at the same time, there appears to be no other acceptable alternative. This feeling of despair may be expressed as hostility, and, as a result, therapists may view the individual as a "problem patient." It is possible for a client to remain at this stage with feelings of inadequacy, dependency, and hostility. However, it is also possible for therapeutic intervention to facilitate movement to the next stage by creating situations in which the client may feel that "normal" aspirations and goals can be achieved. In this circumstance, "normal" would not include such low-level activities as dressing or walking—activities that were taken for granted before the injury—but would include doing the work he or she was trained to do. These activities would also include playing with or caring for a child or family. This would be seen as self-actualization by Maslow.[115]

Defense. The defense stage has two components. The first represents a healthy attitude in which the client actually starts coping with the disability. The client can take pride in his or her accomplishments, work to improve independence, and become as normal as possible. The person is still very much aware that barriers to normal functioning exist and is bothered by this fact but also realizes that some of the barriers can be circumvented. This healthy defensive stage can be undermined and possibly destroyed by well-meaning family, friends, and therapists who encourage the individual to see only the positive aspects and who do not allow the client to examine feelings about the restrictions and barriers of the condition. Conditions that lead to the final stage of adjustment may either be the client realizing that the whole body is not needed to actualize his or her life goals or that needs behind the goals can be actualized in other ways. A therapist should watch for opportunities to facilitate this transition.

The negative alternative during the defensive stage is the neurotic defensive reaction. This is typified by the client refusing to recognize that even a partial barrier exists to meeting normal goals. The client may try to convince everyone that he or she has adjusted.

Adjustment. In the final stage, adjustment, the person sees the disability as neither an asset nor a liability but as an aspect of the person, much like a large nose or big feet. The disability is not something to be overcome, apologized for, or defended. Kerr[59] refers to two aspects or goals of this stage. The first goal is for the person to feel at peace with his or her god: the client does not feel that he or she is being punished or tested. The second goal is for the client to feel that he or she is an adequate person, not a second-class citizen. Kerr[90] believes that "It is essential that the paths to those more 'abstract goals' be structured if the person is to make a genuine adjustment." She also believes that it is the health care professional's job to offer that structure.

Acceptance or adjustment is at least as hard to achieve and maintain in life for the disabled person as happiness and harmony are for all people. Adjustment connotes putting the disability into perspective, seeing it as one of the many characteristics of that person. It does not mean negating the existence of or focusing on the condition. Successful adjustment may be defined as an ongoing process in which the person adapts to the environment in a satisfying and efficient manner. This is true for all human beings, able-bodied or disabled. There are always obstacles to overcome in attempting the goal of a happy and successful life.[12, 21, 84]

People and circumstances change. Maintaining a balanced state of adjustment is not easy, especially for the disabled person. I recall a woman who had achieved a stable state of acceptance of her quadriplegic condition. She called in a panic because, as she saw it, she "wasn't adjusted anymore." She had moved into a college dormitory and wanted to go out for a friendly game of football with her new friends but suddenly saw how disabled she was. She had grown up in a hospital and had never had to face this situation. After discussing this, she was able to put things into perspective and was able to talk over her feelings of isolation with her friends, who, without hesitation, altered the game to include her. Keeping a balanced perspective is hard in a world that changes constantly.

White[183] states that without some performance, there can be no affecting the environment and, thus, no sense of self-satisfaction. Fine[43] and King[95] point out that without satisfaction from affecting the environment, reinforcement is insufficient to carry on the behavior and the behavior will be extinguished. Thus, satisfaction and performance must be linked. If the patient has not adjusted to his or her new body, however, little satisfaction can be gained from such everyday activities as walking, eating, or rolling over in bed.[144] To define adjustment on a purely performance basis is to run the risk of creating a "me-chanical person" who might be physically rehabilitated, but, once discharged, may find that he lacks satisfaction, incentive, and purpose. The psychological state of adjustment is what makes self-satisfaction possible.

King's Model of the Adaptive Process

The therapist can use the concept of the adaptive process to organize therapy sessions that promote the adjustment process as well as attain physical goals. In so doing, the therapist will be promoting and teaching performance and working toward the eventual achievement, client satisfaction.

King[95] describes four characteristics of the adaptive process. They can be worked on singly or simultaneously, and they can be thought of as the means to reach the goal of Kerr's[90] final stage of adjustment. These characteristics are active response, incorporation of the environment, response organized unconsciously, and self-reinforcing adaptation.

Active Response. In general, therapy encourages an active response by the client against the environment.[30] The client is expected to produce action to improve. Interaction with environmental factors can be seen even if there is little functional ability, as in the case of a high-level quadriplegic client whose main avenue of interaction is verbal but whose influence can change the environment.

Incorporation of the Environment. Another characteristic of the adaptive process is use of the environment to stimulate adaptive responses.[30, 176] An example of this would be setting up a graded walking program that takes the client from a smooth surface, to a rug, and eventually to grassy and rocky terrain. The adaptive process would be enhanced if at the time of discharge the client was not only able but also confident of his or her ability to walk over the lawn to reach the house from the surrounding perimeter.

Response Organized Unconsciously. King[95] believes that an unconsciously organized response is achieved most effectively by directing the client's conscious attention to a task or an object while allowing the subconscious centers to integrate the response. The example in the previous paragraph can be used to illustrate this characteristic. The client's objective (conscious mind) may be set on getting across a lawn to get into her or his house, but the therapist's goal would be to stimulate automatic equilibrium reactions at a subconscious level. Unconscious adaptive responses generalize to other situations more easily than cognitively taught "splinter skill" reactions. As soon as the client cortically attends to equilibrium, the automatic postural changes are, by definition, lost. That is, if the task is procedural, attention needs to be placed on something else while the client practices the activity.

Self-Reinforcing Adaptation. Each successful adaptation stimulates the next more complex step. It is essential for the client to succeed because this success stimulates progression to the next more complex "task." It should be remembered that the "task" is adjustment and that the activity only facilitates adaptation or adjustment. Thus, the therapist does not need to feel disheartened if the client learns to get into and out of his or her house but does not want to start mountain climbing: the goal of the adaptive process is adjustment in as near a normal pattern as possible for that client.

SUMMARY

Combining knowledge of Kerr's stages of adjustment, as outlined previously, with the adaptive process gives the therapist a reality-based, evaluative treatment framework. The stage of adjustment can be assessed, and the adaptive process characteristics can be drawn on in treatment to facilitate progression toward psychological acceptance of the disability as well as to promote physical improvement.

For example, if a person is in the mourning stage of adjustment, the therapist, knowing that the defense stage usually follows, can encourage and support the client's entrance into this next stage by adapting a situation that meets the goal of the defense stage—beating the obstacles of disability. The adaptive process may also be used to structure the therapeutic activities that facilitate an active response to overcome the disability, using the environment to organize the response subcortically in such a way that it is self-reinforcing. For example, the client might want to call his or her spouse, and the therapist may be working cortically on increasing upper-extremity strength and wheelchair mobility. The client could be told that the only accessible phone is up a steep ramp and that the client must push himself or herself up there to use the phone in privacy. The therapist might also add that it always seems that obstacles are in the way of the disabled and that the client must explore methods to deal with these problems. As the client accomplishes the task, not only will the objectives of strength and wheelchair mobility be realized but the client may start thinking that he or she may be able to beat the effects of the disability, thus moving the client from the mourning stage to the defense stage. No single experience will cause this to happen, but if therapy is designed to encourage adjustment and adaption, the client will tend to progress faster and with less trauma.

AWARENESS OF PSYCHOLOGICAL ADJUSTMENT IN THE CLINIC, SOCIETY, AND CULTURE

The problem for the therapist in treating a person with a disability is to see the disability in perspective: to see the whole person in the client's own world and in the context of society and a given time. After this difficult task is achieved, the therapist must develop a program that will appropriately stimulate the client and all significant others around the client to pursue the highest-quality life possible. The successful and skilled therapist evaluates the client's physical capabilities but does not stop there. At some level, assessment of the more subtle psychological aspects of the client's ability to function is needed. This includes the client's family network (support system) and its ability to adjust to the imminent change in lifestyle.

The rest of this section introduces the reader to some of the psychological change components that may be assessed. The last section will attempt to demonstrate possible ways that these components can be taken into account as an aspect of therapy.

Societal and Cultural Influences

From an early age, people in our society are exposed to misconceptions regarding the disabled person.[6, 12, 72] Some of these misguided perceptions are that the physically disabled person is also retarded, not employable, dependent, helpless, asexual, unlovable, and miserable. If a first- or second-grade child is asked how a retarded person walks, the common response is the demonstration of a hemiplegic gait and posture with one arm going into a flexion synergy. This child has already learned not only the "role" of the physically disabled but will have also incorporated other misconceptions about how a disabled person acts. If these misconceptions were held before injury, then it is only reasonable for the newly disabled person to be inclined to fulfill these perceived role expectations.[12, 72] Thus, the client may undergo a radical change in the perceived self (how the person sees himself or herself) as a result of the "new" role expectations. Even worse, the family members and medical personnel may hold the same expectations of the disabled person and thus reinforce the helpless, dependent role.[1, 60, 61, 70, 80]

If in the therapeutic environment, however, the client and family have their misconceptions challenged constantly, they may start reformulating their concept of the role of the disabled person. As this process progresses, therapists and other staff can help make the expectations of the disabled person more realistic. Therapists can schedule their clients at times when they will be exposed to people making realistic adjustments to their disabilities. Use of successfully rehabilitated individuals as staff members (role models) can help to dispel the misconception that disabled people are not employable.[1, 113]

This process of adaptation to a new disability can be considered as a cultural change from a majority status (able bodied) to a minority status (disabled). Part of the adaptation process can be considered as an acculturation process, and the therapist can help facilitate this process.[12, 15] The cultural background of the individual also contributes to the perception of disability and to the acceptance of the disabled person. Trombly[172] states that perception and expression of pain, physical attractiveness, valuing of body parts, as well as acceptability of types of disabilities can be culturally influenced. One's ethnic background can also affect intensity of feelings toward specific handicaps, trust of staff,[172] and acceptance of therapeutic modalities.[7, 116, 171]

The successful therapist will be sensitive to the cultural values of the client and will attempt to present therapy to the client in the most acceptable way. For example, in the Mexican culture it is not polite to just start to work with a client; rapport must first be established. Sharing of food may provide the vehicle to accomplish rapport. Thus, the therapist might schedule the first visit with a Mexican client during a coffee break. The therapist must remember that the dysfunctional client may be the one who can least be expected to adjust to the therapist and that the therapist may need to adjust to the client, especially in the early stages of therapy.

Gaining trust is one of the crucial links in any meaningful therapeutic situation.[105] Trust will create an environment that facilitates communication, productive learning, and exchange of information.[123] Trust is important in all cultures and will be fostered by the therapist who is sensitive to the needs of the client. This sensitivity is necessary with every client but will be manifested in many different ways, depending on the background and needs of the individual in therapy. A client of one culture may feel that looking another person in the eyes is offensive, whereas in another culture refusal to look into someone's eyes is a sign of weakness or lack of honesty (shifty-eyed).[69] Thus, although it is impossible to know every culture or subculture with which the therapist may come into contact, the therapist must attempt to be sensitive to the background of the client. Even if the therapist knows the cultural norms, not every person follows the cultural patterns, and thus every client needs to be treated as an individual in the therapeutic relationship. It should be the therapist's job to be sensitive to the subtle nonverbal and verbal cues that indicate the level of trust in the relationship.

Trust is often established in the therapeutic relationship through physical activities. The act of asking a client to transfer from the chair to the bed can either build trust or destroy the potential relationship. If the client trusts the therapist just enough to follow instructions to transfer but then falls in the process, it may take quite some time to reestablish the same level of trust, assuming that it can ever be reestablished. This trusting relationship is so complex and involves such a variety of levels that the therapist should be as aware of attending to the client's security in the relationship as to the physical safety of the client in the clinic.[105] If the client believes that the therapist is not trustworthy in the relationship, then it may follow that the therapist is not to be trusted when it comes to physical manipulation of a disabled body. If the client does not know how to use the damaged body and thus cannot trust the body, then lacking trust in the therapist will only compound the stress of the situation.[105] (See Chapter 6 for more information on some of the neurological components of this interaction.)

The client's culture may be alien to the therapist, even though they may be from the same geographical region. A client's problems of poverty, unemployment, and a lack of educational opportunities[1, 71] can all result in the therapist and client feeling that therapy will be unsuccessful, even before the first session has begun. Such preconceived concepts held by both parties may not be warranted and must be examined.

Cultural and religious values may also result in the client feeling that he or she must pay for past sins by being disabled and that the disability will be overcome after atonement for these sins. Such a client may not be inclined to participate in or enjoy therapy. The successful therapist does not assault the client's basic cultural or religious values but may recognize them in the therapy sessions. If the therapist feels that the culturally defined problems are impeding the therapeutic process, the therapist may offer the client opportunities to reexamine these cultural "truths" and may help the client redefine the way the disability and therapy is seen. Religious counseling could be recommended by the therapist, and follow-up support in the clinic may be given to the client to view therapy not as undoing what "God has done" but as a way of proving religious strength. Reworking a person's cultural/religious (cognitive) structure is a very sensitive area, and it should be handled with care and respect and with the use of other professionals (social workers and religious and psychological counselors) if needed.

The hospital staff can be encouraged to establish groups in which commonly held values of clients can be examined and possibly challenged.[12, 34–37, 41, 84] Such groups can lead the client to a better understanding of priorities and may help the person see the relevance of therapy and the need to continue the adjustment process. This can also prepare the client to better accept the need for support groups after discharge. The therapist may be able to use information from such group sessions to adjust the way therapy sessions are presented and structured to make therapy more relevant to the client's values and needs. Value groups or exercises[150, 161] can be another means used by the therapist for evaluation and understanding of the client.

Values, roles, and body parts may all be grieved for by the client. This is especially true during the mourning stage of adjustment. The following section will look at ways of grieving and will explore some possible losses the therapist may not be alert to.[31, 51, 62, 70, 84, 127]

Examination of Loss

Reaction to loss has been examined by Peretz.[136] Nine types of bereavement states are described:

1. Normal grief
2. Anticipatory grief
3. Absent, delayed, and inhibited grief
4. Chronic grief
5. Depression
6. Hypochondriasis
7. Development of psychophysiological reactions
8. Acting out
9. Neurotic and psychotic states

The individual with normal grief alternates from shock and incomprehension to bewilderment and weeping, which may give way to guilt feelings, irrational anger, and even depressive symptoms. Progress can be judged by a gradual return to the client's level of functioning before the loss. The person with anticipatory grief is grieving for a loss that has not yet taken place. This may be grieving for loss of function or role even before the loss is documented. The client with absent, delayed, and inhibited grief may postpone grief until the crisis is past; or he or she may hide grief, not expressing it and not getting the necessary support. These individuals have been noted to experience "anniversary reactions" (reexperiencing loss at some later date such as the "anniversary" of the accident or diagnosis of the disability). With chronic grief the patient is in a state of persistent mourning, and no change in lifestyle or environment will be tolerated. Sadness, tension, and gloom characterize the individual in the emotional state of depression. The client may feel sorry for himself or herself and may be rendered nonfunctional. Psychotherapy or chemotherapy may be necessary. The patient with hypochondriasis may express anxiety regarding a physical concern (other than the disability) to avoid dealing with the disability. Usually there is no physical cause for the anxiety expressed, but the symptoms may exist. With development of psychophysiological reactions, depression or loss may be expressed through somatic symptom formation, such as a decreased immune defense system, colitis, hypertension, duodenal ulcers, and other illnesses. These illnesses may become so severe as to cause the person's death. One of the complicating aspects of disability can be the development of depression and the resulting decrease in quality of life.[24, 58, 66, 74, 85, 87, 128, 139]

This is true for both the client and the family as well.[154, 156, 179] The quality of life for all involved can be impacted by this often undetected complication. Quality of life can be impacted by many aspects of life: mastery,[98] access,[142] marital status and physical independence,[103] and meaningful occupation.[176] Further research and documentation are needed in this area. Acting out is an attempt to avoid the pain of loss by turning attention to something else. This can be done through involvement in acceptable activities, such as work, or unacceptable activities, such as drug use (abuse). Neurotic and psychotic states may take numerous forms depending on the psychological predisposition of the person.

Knowledge of the types of bereavement as described by Peretz[136] can be used by the therapist to better understand the client's reactions to loss and will allow the therapist the possibility of adjusting the treatment approach to the client's type of bereavement.[106] This knowledge of the grief process can be applied to clients who have terminal illnesses in an attempt to increase the client's quality of life.

Cognitive Age and Loss

The cognitive age of the person experiencing the loss is another aspect that therapists sometimes fail to consider. Harper and Bhattarai[72] and Krause and Crewe[101] have pointed out that the age of the person dealing with loss affects his or her reaction. It seems likely that this concept may be generalized to further understand loss of function.[3, 52, 72, 153]

The child who is younger than 5 years of age views loss as a temporary, reversible phenomenon. From age 5 to 9 years, the average child views death or loss as final but remote. The child thinks of the dead person as someone who went away on a long trip or as someone who will not be around anymore. It is not until the person is older than the age of 9 that the child perceives loss as permanent. Dunton[42] cites the following case history:

A typical family with three children ages 11, 9, and 4 years suffered the sudden loss of a beloved pet dog. When informed of the sad event the 11-year-old responded at first by saying

nothing. Slowly the tears welled up in his eyes and he began to cry softly. When he regained his composure he said, "It's such a horrible thing—it's all over." The 9-year-old listened quietly to the news and said, "He has gone a long way. We'll have to get another one." The 4-year-old looked puzzled and said repeatedly, "What happened? Why are you crying? Let's go get him!"

As a result of brain damage or shock, cognitive levels in the adult may regress after injury, much as reflex development may regress. The client may be functioning at a low cognitive level and may not be capable of understanding the permanence of the loss suffered. Disabled parents and spouses will have to deal with their children's reactions to the parent's loss in a manner appropriate to the cognitive level of each child.[43, 44, 52, 72, 73, 84, 187] Values clarification groups can be used to help the family deal with adjustment to loss.[150, 161] The very act of being aware of cognitive levels of dealing with loss may help family members and therapists accept how the others are dealing (or not dealing) with the loss.[16, 21, 43, 44, 177]

Preschool-aged children often believe that the disability is a punishment and that they must have done something very wrong to deserve such a punishment.[151] It is thus important to stress that a disability is not a punishment and that accidents and disabilities happen to good people. In this way the therapist dispels the next logical concept—that therapy is further punishment and that the client needs to be punished.

Loss and the Family

In this chapter, the client's support system is referred to as the family. The family may be composed of spouses, parents, children, lovers (especially in gay and lesbian relationships), friends, employers, or interested others—church groups, civic organizations, or individuals. The people in the support system may go through the same stages of reaction and adjustment to loss that the client does.[14, 43, 48, 54, 72, 154, 155]

Family Needs

The family will, at least temporarily, experience the loss of a loved member from the normal routine. During the acute stage the family may not have concrete answers to basic questions regarding the extent of injury, the length of time before the injured person will be back in the family unit, or possibly whether the person will live.

During this phase, the family network will be in a state of crisis.[14, 73, 79, 154] New roles will have to be assumed by the family members, and the "experts" will not even tell them for how long these roles must be endured. If children are involved, they will probably demand more attention to reassure themselves that they will remain loved. Depending on the child's age, the child will have differing capabilities in understanding the loss (see the section on examination of loss). Each member of the family may react differently to bereavement, and each may be at a different stage of adjustment to the disability (see the section on adjustment). One member may be in shock and deny the disability, whereas another member is in mourning and verbalizes a lack of hope. The family crisis that is caused by a severe injury cannot be overstated.[14, 43, 72, 120, 128, 149, 154, 155]

Role changes in the family may be dramatic.[44, 62, 70, 84, 120, 128, 174] Members who have never driven may need to learn how; one who has never balanced a checkbook may now be responsible for managing the family budget; and those who have never been assertive may have to deal forcefully with insurance companies and the medical establishment.[14, 24, 44, 148, 177]

The family may feel resentment toward the injured member. This attitude may seem justified to them as they see the person lying in bed all day while the family members must take over new responsibilities in addition to their old ones. The medical staff may not always understand the stress that family members are under and may react to the resentment expressed either verbally or nonverbally with a protective stance toward the client. Siding with the "hurt" client may alienate the family from the medical staff and may also drive a permanent wedge between family members.

Parental Bonding and the Disabled Child

The parent bonding process is complicated and is still being studied.[25, 96] This process (attachment) may start well before the child is even conceived.[96] The parents often think about having a child and plan and fantasize about future interactions with the child. After conception the planning and fantasizing increase. During the pregnancy the fetus is accepted as an individual by the mother[96] and father, and after the birth of the child the attachment process is greatly intensified. The "sensitive period" is the first few minutes to hours after the birth. During this time the parents should have close physical contact with the child to strongly establish the attachment that will later grow deeper.[96, 184] There is an almost symbiotic relationship between mother and child at this time: infant and mother behaviors complement each other (e.g., nursing stimulates uterine contraction). It is important at this point for the child to respond to the parents in some way so that there is an interaction. In the early stages of bonding, seeing, touching, caring for, and interacting with the child allow for the bonding process. When this process is disturbed for any reason, such as congenital malformations or hospital procedures for high-risk infants, problems may occur later. The occurrence of battered child syndrome and failure to thrive has been noted to be higher than the norm when the child is born prematurely or when there is poor (or lack of) bonding at an early age.[96] Klaus and Kennell[96] have recommended elements that increase the chances of parental bonding: (1) special needs during pregnancy and birth dealt with to support the parents; (2) parent preparation, education, and support; (3) need for a companion at labor and especially at birth; and (4) enhancing attachment—privacy and contact with the child and each other.

When the parents are told that their child is going to be malformed or disabled, it is a massive shock. The parents must start a process of grieving. The dream of a "normal" child must be given up, and the parents must go through the loss or "death" of the child they expected before they can accept the new child. Parents often feel guilty. Shellabarger and Thompson[159] state that parents feel the deformed child was their failure.[48] Fathers are the most distressed about the child initially. The disabled child will always have a strong impact on the family, sometimes a catastrophic one.[3, 14, 48, 159]

Parents must be encouraged to express their emotions, and they must be taught how to deal with the issues at hand. Techniques for accomplishing these goals are discussed in later sections.[159, 170, 184]

The Child Dealing with Loss

If a parent is injured, the young child may experience an overwhelming sense of loss. Child care may be a problem, especially if the primary caregiver is injured. The child will probably feel deserted by the injured parent and may demand the attention of the remaining parent. This will increase the strain on all family members.[44, 166]

If the child is the client, his or her life will have undergone a radical change: every aspect of the child's world will have altered. Loved objects and people will help to restore the child's feeling of security. It is of major importance to explain to the child in very simple terms what is going on and to allow the child the opportunity to express feelings both verbally and nonverbally (perhaps using play as the medium of communication).

The hospital setting is threatening to all people, but children are especially susceptible to loss of autonomy, feelings of isolation, and loss of independence. Bentovim and Nelson (see Chapter 9) have stated that the severity of the disability is not as important a variable in the emotional development of the child as are the attitudes of parents and family.[3, 14, 72] Parents must attempt to be aware of the child's inability to understand the permanence (or transience) of the loss of function.[3, 52] They will also need to help the child feel secure by bringing in familiar and cherished objects. A schedule should be established and kept to promote consistency. Play should be encouraged, especially that which allows the child to vent feelings and deal with the new environment. Any procedures or therapies should be presented in a relaxed way (fun, if possible), so that the child has time to think and to feel as comfortable as possible about the change.[16] The parents may often need to be reminded to pay attention to the nondisabled children in the family during this acute stage.

The Adolescent Dealing with Loss

The adolescent is subject to all of the feelings and fears that other clients express. Adolescents are in a struggle to obtain autonomy and independence, and they often are ambivalent about these feelings. When an adolescent is suddenly injured and has to cope with being disabled, it can be a massive assault on the individual's development.[21, 55]

The adolescent appears to react differently from other age groups to the knowledge of his or her own terminal illness. The adolescent often feels that he or she has gone through a very painful process (initiation) that will soon lead to the "joys and rights" of adulthood. Unlike persons in older age groups who might feel that they can look back and gain solace from the past,[166] the adolescent feels that he or she will have what Solnit and Green[166] term "death before fulfillment" and thus may react by feeling cheated by life. This same pattern may occur with the disabled adolescent. The therapist must be acutely aware of these feelings so that therapy may be presented in the most effective manner for the client to find challenge and fulfillment in life.

Family Maturation

The family also has a maturational aspect. If the injured person is a child and if the family is young with dependent children at home, the adjustment may not be the problem that it would be for a family whose children are older. In the latter case, parents have begun to experience freedom and independence, and they may find adjusting to a return to a restricted lifestyle difficult, or even intolerable. They may have the feeling that they have already "put in their time" and should now be free. If the disability interrupts the child's developmental process, future conflict may arise because the parents will eventually want retirement, relaxation, and freedom. Parents may feel guilty about and try to repress this normal response.

The reverse may also be true. The parents may be feeling that the children have left them ("empty nest syndrome"), and they may be too willing to welcome a "dependent" family member back into the home. This may lead to excessive dependence or anger toward the parents on the part of the client. All of these factors must be taken into consideration by the therapist when therapy is presented to the client and family.

The therapist can develop a greater understanding of the client and family by being aware of the normal human developmental patterns as discussed by Sheehy[158] and Lewis.[110] These patterns identify some of the major hurdles that must be overcome in the client's life.

Coping with Transition

In the acute stage of a family member's injury, the family must be helped to deal with the crisis at hand. During this phase, the family must first be allowed to cope with the emotional impact of what is happening with a loved one. Second, the family should be helped to see the situation as a challenge that, if overcome, will facilitate growth. Third, adaptation within the family unit must occur to overcome the situation. Brammer and Abrego[13] have developed a list of basic coping skills that they have broken into five levels. In the first level the person becomes aware of and mobilizes skills in perceiving and responding to transition and attempts to handle the situation. In the second level the person mobilizes the skills for assessing, developing, and using external support systems. In level three the person can possess, develop, and use internal support systems (develop positive self-regard and use the situation to grow). The person in level four must find ways to reduce emotional and physiological distress (relaxation, control stimulation, and verbal expression of feelings). In level five the person must plan and implement change (analyze discrepancies, plan new options, and successfully implement the plan). Using this model, the therapist and family can evaluate the coping skill level of the family. The therapist and staff can then help promote movement toward the next level of coping with the transition. These levels are also broken into specific skills and subskills so that the therapist can grade them further.

One of the more damaging aspects of hospitalization to all involved is that the hospital staff focuses on the disability rather than on the individual's strengths.[1, 54, 92] Centering on the disability can lead to a situation where client, family, and staff see only the disability and not the potential ability of the client.

Decentering from the disability will be examined further in this chapter. If the family relationship was positive before the insult and if the client is cognitively intact, then the focus should be directed toward the relationship's strengths as well as toward the client's and family's individual strengths.[147] In the initial acute stage of adjustment, crisis intervention may help the family use its strengths and at the same time deal with the situation at hand.

To adequately deal with the crisis, the family should:

- Be helped to focus on the crisis caused by the disability, identify the situation to stimulate problem solving; identify and deal with doubts of adequacy, guilt, and self-blame; identify and deal with grief work; identify and deal with anticipatory worry; and be offered basic information and education regarding the crisis situation.
- Be helped to create a bridge to resources in the hospital and in the community for support, as well as to see their own family resources.
- Be helped to remember how they have dealt successfully with crises in the past and to implement some of the same strategies in the present situation.

Working with the family as a unit during crisis will help strengthen the family and facilitate more positive attitudes toward the client, thus improving the client's attitudes or feelings toward the injury and hospitalization.[23, 70, 84, 99, 122] Encouraging family-unit functioning in this situation will decrease the amount of regression displayed by the client. If the family is encouraged to function without the client, however, more damage than good may be done.[21, 48]

Awareness of Sexual Issues

Sexuality is usually one of the last areas to be assessed by clinical staff, but it is one area mentioned as having great importance to family members and the client.[109] Sexuality involves more than just the sex act; it incorporates characteristics such as sexual attraction, sexual identification, sexual confidence, and sexual validation.[32] It is a predictor of adjustment to disability, of success in vocational training, and of marital satisfaction when the woman is disabled.[160] Sexuality (sensuality) is representative of how the person is dealing with her or his world. If the person feels inadequate as a sexual, sensual, and lovable human being, there is little chance that he or she will also feel motivated to pursue other avenues of life.[146, 160, 163] This area of function must be assessed with great sensitivity to the individual's feelings.[27, 108, 145, 146]

The framework for assessing sexuality differs with the

therapist. Some therapists see sexuality as an activity of daily living and incorporate it into this evaluation. Others feel the client needs information about body mechanics to perform the sex act; thus, positioning and reflex inhibiting patterns are assessed. Still others have found it a motivating force when range of motion and muscle control are worked on. A further discussion of these concerns follows in the section on adult sexuality.

Development of Sensuality (Sexuality)

Even before birth, the sense of touch[93, 124] and the ability to distinguish pleasurable and unpleasurable tactile sensations begin to develop. Pleasurable feelings are comforting, and attempts are made to prolong them; for example, a baby cries when nursing is stopped. If satisfaction is not derived from this interaction on a regular basis, a feeling of anxiety may develop and the child may withdraw from interaction with others and distrust may develop.[124] If pleasure in interaction with others is obtained in the first 3 years, the ability to maintain the warmth of being close and being nourished is translated into trust (that all needs will be satisfied by the caretaker) and lovability (bonding). It is here that a sense of intimacy is initiated.[28, 104, 124, 165] Ego and sensuality are refined as the child develops the ability to stimulate and satisfy itself. By the age of 5, the ability to explore the world by using the hands and mouth, as well as other parts of the body, allows the person to develop communication, self-gratification, and a feeling of competence.[165, 183]

This feeling of competence is derived from the effective use of the body to make itself feel good and to accomplish tasks. By the age of 8, body parts and body processes are usually named and the child perceives the body as good. At this time intimacy between the self and another person is further refined, as are roles. During puberty, body changes and sexual tension are heightened.[63, 124] Self-acceptance is based on the person's perception of how effectively he or she has accomplished the previous tasks.[185]

The preceding is an oversimplification of the first 20 years of life, but the role of sensuality and sensation cannot be overemphasized. This is especially true for those professionals who constantly interact with clients in a physical manner. The intervention the therapist provides when the client is, or feels he or she is, in a dependent state can have direct impact on how the client may perceive himself or herself in the future.

Pediatric Sensuality

The child needs to learn to enjoy his or her body. The therapist should help the client to distinguish between therapeutic touch and "fun" sensual touch, such as tickling or cuddling. It is important for clients to distinguish between the two so that they do not "turn their bodies off" to touch. For example, a woman with cerebral palsy stated during an interview that therapy was either painful or so clinical that she disassociated herself from sensations in her body during therapy. Later in life this became a problem when she was married. She stated that it took 7 years of marriage before she could enjoy the sensations

of being touched by her husband. She also stated that it was a revolutionary concept for her that a vibrator could be used to give pleasure.

The therapy session should also help the client develop a sense of personal ownership of the body.[2, 29, 105, 124] This aspect is often neglected when working with children.[2, 63, 165] The therapist often does not ask permission to touch a client, thus suggesting that the client lacks the right to control being touched by others. The last thing the therapist would desire to communicate, especially to a child, is that any person has the right to handle and touch the client's body. Child molestation is just beginning to be recognized as a problem in this country, with possibly one third of the female and male population being victimized.[2] It is hard to think of a more likely victim than a person who has (unintentionally) been taught that he or she does not have the right to say "No" to being touched, and who cannot physically resist unwanted advances and in some cases cannot even communicate that abuse has taken place. The effects of this can be seen in adults. When one client was asked why tone increased in her lower extremities when she was touched, her response was "I was sexually abused by my father in the name of therapy, and therapy and sexual abuse are synonymous at this point." No wonder she had been resistant to reentering therapy!

One way of helping clients "own" their bodies (besides asking permission to touch) is by naming body parts and body processes using correct terminology (as opposed to baby talk), thus making it possible for the client to communicate and relate appropriately.[2, 18, 47, 124, 162, 165] This can be accomplished as the need arises, or it can be encouraged through the use of anatomically correct puzzles or dolls during therapy sessions.

One goal of therapy may be to develop the concept that the body (in the case of persons with the congenital disabilities) or the "new body" (in the case of those with acquired disabilities) is acceptable and good,[63, 105] thus giving the client a more positive attitude toward his or her body and toward therapy. This attitude can be encouraged by pointing out a particularly positive aspect of the client's body and mentioning this regularly. The feature could be the hair, eyes, or a smile, but it should be an aspect of the client that can be seen and commented on by others as well. Commenting on how well the body feels when it is relaxed or how good the sun feels on the body helps the client recognize that the body can be a positive source of pleasure.

Another message that can affect the client in later life is the concept that the disabled are asexual and will never have sexual needs or partners.[104, 148] Although it may not be appropriate to deal directly with the concept in therapy with a child, the therapist might mention that he or she knows of a person with disabilities, such as the client's disability, who is married or who has children. In this way the therapist communicates that there is a possibility that the "normal" sex roles of the child may be fulfilled in the future. Without this possibility being presented, the child may think that there is no chance that all the movies, books, and television programs that deal with normal adult interactions apply to the disabled, a belief that leads to poor socialization and further alienation.[19, 28, 104, 138, 148]

Adult Sexuality

Adaptive devices can be a detriment to one's perceived sexuality. It can be hard to see oneself as sexy with an indwelling catheter or braces, but by discussing this topic the client can get some ideas as how to handle difficult situations when they arise.[18, 28, 75, 104, 129, 148] Discussing positioning to reduce pain and spasticity or to enable the client to more comfortably engage in sexual relations will help the client deal with problems before they reveal themselves. Because sexual hygiene may be considered as an activity of daily living, it may fall within the domain of therapy.

The client may feel that his or her sexual identity is threatened by a newly acquired disability and may try to assert his or her sexuality through jokes, flirting, or even passes toward the therapist. In these cases it is important for the therapist to realize that what is often being looked for is the confirmation that the client is still a sexual and sensual human being; thus, the therapist's response is very important.[11, 18, 65, 118, 148, 168] If the therapist rejects or even ridicules the client, it may be a very long time before the client can even think of attempting such a confirmation of personal attractiveness. The client may feel that because the therapist rejects the client and the therapist is familiar with the disabled, there is little chance anyone who is not familiar with the disabled could accept the client as lovable.[67] The therapist should not be surprised by such advances and should deal with the situation in a professional manner. The therapist should also realize that approximately 10% of the population is homosexual and be prepared for advances from clients of the same sex. The therapist may need to remember that the therapist should not attempt to change the client's sexual orientation nor be offended but instead be as professional in dealing with this client as with any other. All of the therapist's interactions should be directed toward creating an environment that will promote a stronger and more well-adjusted client.[18, 148]

The therapist's response to sexual advances must be tempered with an understanding of the possible cause for the behavior. The client may be cognitively impaired and may not even be aware of the inappropriateness of some forms of sexual behavior, or the client may be trying to control others through acting-out behaviors. The client may have been sexually aggressive even before the injury. At no time should the therapist allow himself or herself to be sexually harassed. If the therapist feels harassed, the therapist must take control of the situation and find a way to stop the client's behavior. This is usually achieved by confronting the issue. Not dealing with inappropriate behavior will allow it to continue and may be detrimental to the client and the medical staff.[18, 118, 168]

Nowinski and Ayers[130] found that sexuality was of great concern to most people with physical disabilities. As Bogle and Shaul[9] state, it is difficult to see oneself as lovable and huggable when surrounded by hard, cold, and usually unsightly braces.[28, 75, 128, 148] The therapist can assist the client in moving through the stages of self-awareness to the reinstatement of self-appreciation that precede positive feelings that he or she is still sensual, sexual, and huggable. This process can be done through everyday interaction; it may entail encouraging the family to embrace the client and may even call for the therapist to role model these behaviors at times.[38] The therapist may provide reading materials to the client and family directly by reviewing and answering questions or indirectly by having such books as *Enabling Romance*,[104] *Reproductive Issues for Persons with Physical Disabilities*,[75] *Sexuality and the Person with Traumatic Brain Injury: A Guide for Families*,[67] *Who Cares?*,[33] *Sexuality and Physical Disability*,[17] *Sexual Options for Paraplegics and Quadriplegics*,[125] *Sexual Function in People with Disability and Chronic Illness*,[164] or the *Hite Report* on female[77] and male sexuality[78] available. In this way, the individual and significant others are made aware of possible options for the expression of intimacy and of the fact that this part of life is not over.

Because the therapist is in a situation of one-to-one treatment involving touching, moving, and handling the client's body, he or she may frequently be a natural person from whom the individual may seek information. If this natural curiosity does not appear to be forthcoming, however, the therapist can give the client an opening. For example, during an evaluation of motor skills, the person may be asked if there are any problems in such areas as sexual positioning. The topic need not be pursued any further by the therapist, but when the client is ready to deal with the subject area, he or she will probably remember that the therapist brought it up and may be a person to approach when dealing with these issues.[59, 107, 163]

Other ways of presenting sexual information are to have literature available on the client's ward so that those who are interested may pursue the topic in private, to have a group discussion (interested clients, clients and significant others, or whatever group the client and therapist might choose to assemble), or to have literature in the department waiting room.

It is important for the therapist to be aware of some of the aspects of sexuality that may or may not be affected by a disability. Fertility is seldom affected in women.[175, 181, 182] Men, on the other hand, may experience dysfunction of the penis and testicles and/or fertility.[40, 112, 143] Devices may be used and adapted to allow for sexual gratification of the client (masturbation) or significant others. Stimulant drugs such as Viagra or other aids may be used to enhance a person's sex life. Safe sex is even more of a problem for clients who may be inclined to get infections,[67, 104] especially in or around the genitals, because this may provide an avenue for transmission of disease. Sensation should be checked and sexual activities modified (or the client should be alerted to the problem) to avoid breakdowns or medical complications. Positioning modifications may be needed to allow for better energy conservation, joint protection, motor control, maintenance of muscle and skin integrity, and pleasure. Clients may have questions regarding modifications that may be needed for the use of birth control devices or contraindications regarding the use of such devices. Complications may arise due to pregnancy that may affect function and mobility of the client. Delivery may present some unique situations that may also need to be dealt with. After delivery the disabled parent may require modifications to the wheelchair or consultations may be needed to achieve an optimal level of function in the parenting role. All of these possibilities point to the fact that sexual issues must be dealt with throughout the treatment of all individuals with disabilities.[75, 104, 140, 175] The therapist may approach these needs or aspects of function while taking a client's sexual history. Clients have repeatedly called for more attention to be paid to sexual concerns. This is not sex counseling or therapy, and the therapist should not try to deal with deep psychosexual issues. The therapist should be informed and should provide information that relates to the therapist's areas of expertise, especially as other medical personnel may not have the knowledge to correctly analyze the components of some of these activities.[68, 75, 81, 104, 186]

All of the clinical problem areas that need assessment and evaluation and that have been mentioned previously are examined in relation to treatment planning in the clinical setting in the following sections.

TREATMENT VARIABLES IN RELATION TO THERAPY

This section examines issues the therapist and staff should know to create a therapeutic environment that will facilitate psychological adjustment and independence of the disabled client. The physical and the attitudinal environment of the treatment facility plays a major role in the way the client views the services that are rendered.

Recall a time before you became a member of the medical community. Think about how awe-inspiring the people in white coats were, how strange the smells of the hospitals were, how busy it all seemed, and how puzzling the secret medical language was. It all seemed overwhelming then, and it still is to newcomers, especially newly admitted patients and their families. The hospital usually appears impersonal,[76] sterile, monotonous, and confusing; and all status accumulated outside the hospital means little inside.

The therapist needs to take the setting into account when dealing with the client. The environment can be altered in a variety of ways. Therapy staff could wear street clothes, decorate the department or hospital with posters and lively colors, and allow clients to bring some personal items into the hospital.

The nature of the therapy process can often lead the therapist to see only the disability and not the person, as occurs for example when a client is referred to by his or her disability, rather than by name. This stereotyping of disability can lead the therapist to concentrate on the lack of ability rather than on the strengths of the client. The real danger is that the client and family will also start to focus on the disability of the client and feel that their family relationship is now permanently altered. The accuracy of this perception may have to be evaluated as part of the adjustment process. The wife of a man with paraplegia said with a sudden burst of insight, "I didn't marry him for his legs—this doesn't change that much." Very often so much attention is directed toward the disability that tunnel vision develops. One way to try to get a better perspective is to look at the bigger picture. A variety of questions can be asked that may help the therapist gain a greater insight into the client as a person:

- Who will marry this person and why?
- What are his or her good points?
- What will this person do for a living?
- What will this person do for enjoyment?
- How will this person bring others enjoyment?
- What would this person be doing if there was no disability?
- How is the disability stopping the person from actualizing their goals? (these are the goals that need to be worked on)

Similar questions can be asked of the client to explore ways of helping the client have a meaningful life:

- What do you look like and function like now?
- What will you look like after therapy?
- What important things would you be doing now if you were not in need of treatment?
- What activities or forms of productivity were you involved in before and which were important to you?
- Which of these things do you still do?
- What if anything is preventing you from doing these things now?
- How does this condition affect your being a lover of life, family, significant other, and so on?
- How will this condition affect your important life goals, activities, and your ability to do meaningful activities?
- How much different would your life look if it were not for this condition?
- Will any of the above be stopped by your condition and if so how?

After the therapist is aware of the strengths of the client, these strengths may be capitalized on in therapy to help the client realize them and build confidence. Clients often reported that they were not complimented in therapy and especially that they never received feedback that their bodies were desirable[9] or that they were doing things correctly.[1, 22, 66, 67, 75, 146] A logical thought by the client is "if the therapist cannot see anything desirable about me, and the therapist deals with the disabled all the time, then there must not be anything good about me." Positive, sincere comments to client and family can add a motivational factor to treatment that may have been missing.[1, 22, 99]

The last and possibly the most important aspect in creating an environment that will foster growth and adjustment in the client is a staff that is well adjusted and aware of their own personal needs. Just as coping skills are necessary for the client, the staff, too, must be capable of coping with the stresses of the emotional and physical pain of the client and the client's family. The therapist must also deal with his or her own personal reactions to the sometimes devastating situations others are in.[1, 46, 99] Exposure to such situations often elicits introspection on the part of the staff that can result in emotional turmoil for staff members and affect their own personal relationships. This emotional energy needs to be directed in a productive way so that the energy does not turn into chaos within the staff interaction and/or become a destructive force on the client.

To decrease the possibly distractive nature of this emotional energy, the staff should be made aware of their own coping styles, and they should be allowed to vent their reactions to particularly distressing client case loads in a positive, supportive group. Group meetings can be used to handle some of the inevitable tension, especially if there is a respected member who is skilled in group work. This is not a psychotherapy session but rather an opportunity to test reality and remove tension before it is incorrectly directed toward fellow staff members. These sessions can make use of the four elements of crisis intervention mentioned in the previous section, as well as information from Combs and others.[31, 99, 121] Other times that this stress reduction can be achieved are in supervision or during coffee breaks, as long as the sessions are productive.

The staff can use these sessions to better understand their reactions to stress and to explore their coping styles.[26, 46, 62, 99, 121] Ideally, this knowledge of coping styles and stress reduction will decrease staff burnout as well as aid the staff to help clients and their families deal with stress more successfully.[21, 26, 46, 121]

The need to have a staff that is supportive is of paramount importance, because the attitude of rehabilitation personnel has emerged as one of the chief motivating factors in rehabilitation.[48, 84, 91] Rogers and Figone[145] developed several suggestions that the therapist could benefit from when trying to create a supportive environment:

1. It is helpful to use the same staff member to develop the relationship and to provide continuity of care.
2. Concerned silence is most appreciated, although pushing is sometimes necessary.
3. Staff members should anticipate the need to repeat information graciously.
4. Cumbersome and hard to repair adaptive equipment should not be used after discharge.
5. Give clients responsibility so that they feel they have some control over therapy.
   a. The client should be allowed to pick his or her own advocate from the team.
   b. The client should be given a choice of activities (e.g., which exercise comes first).
   c. Professionals should avoid placing the client in an inferior status. In time the client starts thinking this way (feeling like a "second-class citizen").
6. Psychological support was attributed to noncounseling personnel. Personal matters were better discussed with staff members with whom the client had developed a relationship.[14, 99, 148]
7. Willingness to allow the client to try and fail is more helpful than controlling the client.

CONCEPTUALIZATION OF ASSESSMENT AND TREATMENT

Assessment

The one component that weaves through all of Rogers and Figone's[145] seven points is the need for the therapist to be involved with the client in a therapeutic relationship, that is, to know where the client is "coming from."

To know where the client is coming from is to be aware of and sensitive to the person's total psychosocial frame of reference.[14, 99]

The therapist who knows his or her own beliefs, reference points, and prejudices can evaluate whether an assessment result or treatment sequence reflects the client's needs and values or those of the therapist. In the first half of this chapter, several assessments were discussed that could be summarized into the following three major components:

1. Preinjury
   a. Values and prejudices (value systems, culture, and prejudgments) of the client and family members before the injury
   b. Developmental stage of the client and family members
   c. Cognitive level of the client and family members
   d. Ability of the client and family members to handle crisis
2. Components to be evaluated leading to adjustment
   a. Loss and grief process for the client and family members
   b. Adjustment process for the client and family members
   c. Transitional stages for the client and family members
   d. Role changes for the client and family members
   e. Age or cognitive level of client and family members[5, 14, 21, 99]
   f. Sexual adjustment for the client and spouse
3. Techniques used to elicit adjustment and independence
   a. Crisis intervention strategies
   b. Letting the client and family take control
   c. Expression of emotion—both verbally and nonverbally
   d. Problem solving
   e. Role playing
   f. Praise
   g. Education
   h. Support groups

Once an assessment has been made of the client and family member's stages of psychological adjustment, of the client's occupational history and roles, as well as of their preinjury attitudes and beliefs, a treatment protocol can be established. This protocol will need to incorporate steps toward stage change and possibly attitudinal change. Because these changes require learning on the part of the client and family, an environment that optimally facilitates these changes must be established.[51, 70, 141]

Therapy can be seen as a form of education in which the client and the client's family are taught how the client should use his or her body. The education process is not limited to the physical aspects of therapy, however. The client is also taught how to look at and think about the body and the disability. If the staff is nonverbally telling the client and the family that the client is not capable of making decisions and of being independent, it follows that the client may indeed feel dependent and incapable of making decisions. Giles[62] and others[4, 7, 127, 155, 157, 160] stated that there was an inverse relationship between independence and distress. Distress causes further anxiety and decreases the learning potential of the client. There are ways, however, for the therapist to encourage independence on the part of the client and his family.

Specific Therapeutic Interventions

Problem-Solving Process

The family unit, including the client, should be encouraged to take active control over as much of the client's care and decision making as possible. This can be done in every phase of the rehabilitation process. A family conference with the rehabilitation staff should actively involve the client and family in all stages of planning and treatment up to and including discharge. The family (including the client) should be briefed ahead of time to prepare questions that they want answered or problems that need to be addressed. Rogers and Figone[145] report that conferences with family members that excluded the client engendered suspicion[14, 62, 127]; therefore, if the client is capable, the client may educate the family in regard to what is happening in the hospital and in rehabilitation. Conversely, family involvement facilitates and shortens the rehabilitation process and reintegration into the community.[3, 7, 127, 155, 157, 160] The family can also be educated regarding the side effects and interactions of medication with publications such as the *Physicians' Desk Reference*.[137] Later in the rehabilitation process the client and family can be encouraged to arrange transportation services, find and evaluate housing, and supervise attendant care. All of these activities allow the client and the family to be more in control of the environment and, thus, to feel independent.

In the context of one-to-one therapy, client responsibility and independence can be fostered by giving choices. Making a decision about the order of treatment activities (such as in which direction to roll one's wheelchair first) can give the individual a sense of self-worth that can continue to grow. This should lead the client and family toward believing that they are strong, with rights that need to be met. Moving out of the role of the victim, the client begins to exercise responsibility and to take action, such as applying for extended health benefits or getting a second consultation when an important medical decision needs to be made. If the client and family start to realize that they do not have to be a casualty of the medical establishment and if they find ways to control the medical establishment,[5, 14, 50, 127, 174] they are better able to discard the role of victim.

In some centers, such as the occupational therapy clinic at San Jose State University, the client is even taught the art of self-defense to make sure that the client never has to fall into the victim (dependent) role. It should be noted, however, that this knowledge on the part of the client and family can be used in ways that the therapist may not always agree with. At such times it may help to adopt a philosophical attitude toward the situation and to view it as a positive direction for the client in terms of moving from victim to advocate in the rehabilitation process.

The steps of crisis intervention, which were mentioned in the previous section, can be used to help the family understand and analyze their needs in the crisis situation. Once the family has discovered that they are in crisis, they will then be able to create strategies that they can use to overcome present and future problems.

Problem solving is another element the therapist may use to help the client and family gain independence and control.[4, 5, 9, 14, 84, 127] Rather than having the client routinely learn how to accomplish a specific task, the client or family should be encouraged to think through the process, from the problem to the solution, and to accomplishment of the task. To achieve this activity analysis, the client would have to know the basic principles behind the activity[145] and may then be responsible for educating the family. An example of this would be a transfer from the wheelchair to the toilet. If the therapist simply has the client memorize the steps in the task, the client or family members will not necessarily be able to generalize this procedure to a transfer to the car. If the client learns the principles of proper body mechanics, work simplification, and movement, the client or family member may be able to generalize this information to almost any situation and to solve problems later when the therapist is unavailable.[4] Rogers and Figone[145] have noted that even though the client and family may fail at times during these trials, the therapist should let them be as independent and responsible as possible: let them try it their way, even if they are not successful the first time.

Pictures or slides of a restaurant, movie theater, or public building can be used to facilitate discussion and problem solving by the family unit when analyzing potential architectural barriers in the environment. Thus, in the future, when the family is presented with a problem or a barrier, they will have the resources to overcome it rather than be devastated by it.

Role playing in combination with support groups can also be used to defuse potentially painful situations and operate independently. While still in the safe environment of the rehabilitation setting, simulations of incidents can be created for the family and client to practice problem solving with supervision. They can be asked what they would do when a stranger (possibly a child) approaches the client and asks why he or she is in a wheelchair or is disabled or what they would do when a waiter asks the family member to order for the disabled client. All of these situations are potentially devastating for all involved; however, if role playing and support groups are used in advance to help all members of the family (client included) to satisfactorily handle and feel in control of the situation, the family will not be as likely to be traumatized by a similar occurrence. The result is that the family will not be as inclined to be overwhelmed by social situations and will be able to socialize in a much freer, more gratifying way.[86, 172] Cognitive-behavioral therapy has been used for clients and spouses with success.[34-36] Psychosocial support groups have been called for throughout the literature.[86, 87, 131, 138, 152, 176, 177]

Throughout the therapeutic process the client and the family need to be praised frequently, and credit needs to be given for the gains made by the client and family members. Granted, the therapist may have engineered the gains, but the family and client are the ones who need the reinforcement. Through gratifying experiences the family will unite to overcome the disability. They need to know that they can survive in the world without having the medical staff constantly there to solve the family's problems. In short, they need the strategies and resources that will allow them to be independent outside the medical model.

Yet another way to encourage independence can be applied to working with parents of disabled children.[45, 169] The parents should be educated about normal and abnormal growth and development, including physical, cognitive, and emotional growth, so that the family can maintain some perspective and objectivity about their child's various levels.[3, 6, 72, 84, 176, 165] The parents can then better understand the needs of the disabled and nondisabled children in the family. Armed with this knowledge, the parents and children will not be frustrated with unreal expectations or unreal demands. Educations of the parents could take place at local colleges, the hospital, or even in a parent's group.

Support Systems

Groups are often used to increase motivation, provide support, increase social skills, instill hope, and help the client and family realize that they are not the only ones who have a disabled family member. This will help the client and family establish a more accurate set of perceptions about the disabled individual and allow for greater independence of the client and family.[14, 84, 100] Problem solving can be encouraged and value systems can be clarified. Client and/or family support groups can be used to relieve pressure that might otherwise be vented in therapy. Livneh and Antonak[114] found that in a chronic-care ward family involvement helped the client and the family improve their status. Schwartzberg[157] and Schulz[155] and others[5, 48, 50, 51] have reported great success in the use of support groups with individuals who had brain damage. Support groups can also be used to educate the client about the client's disability to increase independence.[5, 48, 123, 127, 155, 157, 160] Kreuter,[103] Taamla and colleagues,[169] and Wade[178] found that independent physical functioning and knowledge about one's condition were exceedingly important in moving through the phases of the rehabilitation process.[82, 98, 131, 142] A guide to facilitating support groups has been published by Boreing and Adler,[10] and it has been found to be useful, especially by lay people establishing such groups.[84, 123, 155, 157, 178]

Establishment of Self-Worth and Accurate Body Image

Self-worth is composed of many aspects, such as body image, sexuality, and the ability to help others and to affect the environment. The body image of a client is a composite of past and present experiences and of the individual's perception of those experiences. Because body image is based on experience, it is a constantly changing concept. An adult's body image is substantially different from that which he or she held as a child and will no doubt change again as the aging process continues. A newly disabled person is suddenly exposed to a radically

new body, and it is that individual's job to assess the body's sensations and capabilities and develop a new body image. Because the therapist is at least partially responsible for creating the environmental experiences from which the client learns about this new body, he or she should be aware of the concept. In the case of an acute injury, the client has a new body from which to learn. The therapist can promote positive feelings as he or she instructs the client how to use this new body and to accept its changes.[12, 48, 92, 101, 104, 146, 148]

Because in "normal" life we slowly observe changes in our bodies, such as finding one gray hair today and watching it take years for our hair to turn totally white, we have the luxury of slowly adapting to the "new me." This usually does not happen quite so slowly and "naturally" with a disability. This sudden loss of function creates a void that only new experiences and new role models can fill.

The loss of use of body parts can cause a person to perceive the body as an "enemy" that needs to be forced to work or to compensate for its disability. In all cases the body is the reason for the disability and the cause of all problems. The need for appliances can create a sense of alienation and lack of perceived "lovability" resulting from the "hardness of the hardware." People tend to avoid hugging someone who is in a wheelchair or who has braces around the body, because of the physical barrier and because of the person's perceived fragility[124]; the disabled person is certainly not perceived as soft and cuddly.[12, 17, 104, 124] Both the perception that they are not lovable and their labored movements can sap the energy of the disabled for social interaction. To accept the appliances and the dysfunctional body in a way that also allows the disabled person to feel sexy and sensual is surely a major challenge.

In the case of a chronically disabled person, the therapist is attempting to teach the client how to change the previously accepted body image to one that would allow and encourage more normal function. In short, the therapist has two roles. One role is to take away the disabled body image of the chronically disabled person, such as the person with cerebral palsy or Parkinson's disease. The second is the opposite sequence, that is, to teach a functional disabled body image to a newly disabled person. The techniques may be the same, but in both cases the client will have to undergo a great amount of change. The chronically ill person has based his or her life on the concept that the reason for not accomplishing many things was the disability. If the therapist can change the client's ability level, the individual must now change self-expectations. The newly disabled person must now also change expectations; however, he or she has little concept of what is realistic to expect of this new body. At this point, role models can be used to help shape the client's expectations. If the client does not adjust to this new body and change his or her body image and self-expectations, life will be impoverished for that individual. Pedretti[133] states that the client with low self-esteem often devalues his or her whole life in all respects, not just in the area of dysfunction.[7, 66, 74, 75, 104, 129, 141]

One way the client can start exploring this new body is by exploring it for sensation and performance. The male client with a spinal cord injury may touch the whole body to see how it reacts.[28] For example, is there a way to get the legs to move using reflexes? What, if anything, stimulates an erection? Can positioning the legs in a certain way aid in rolling the wheelchair or make spasms decrease? Such exploration will start the client on the road to an informed evaluation of his abilities.

The therapist's role is to promote expansion of the client's realistic perceptions of body functioning. Exercises can be developed that encourage exploration of the body by the individual and, if appropriate, the significant other. Functioning and building an appropriate body image will be more difficult if intimate knowledge of the new body is not as complete as before injury.[14] Books on body massage or exercises, similar to those found in *Your*

Child's Sensory World,[111] can be used to establish such programs. The successes the client experiences in the clinical setting coupled with the client's familiarity with his or her new body will result in a more accurate body image and will contribute to the client's feelings of self-worth.

As mentioned earlier in this chapter, sexuality and sensuality have an enormous impact on how the person feels about his or her adequacy and self-worth.[28, 129, 167] Societal members often evaluate each other on appearance and sensuality (or sexual attractiveness) and may avoid those who are perceived to have deficits.[9, 104] Sensuality and sexuality are some of the major ways that humans express their intimate beings, and in Western society the expression of the physical intimacy is closely associated with

---

CASE 7–1   PUTTING EVALUATIONS AND TECHNIQUES INTO PRACTICE

Joan, a married 30-year-old woman, has suffered a T2 spinal cord injury. She has worked as a computer programmer for the past 8 years, except for a short maternity leave when she gave birth to her daughter, who is now 6 years old. Joan was always very active physically and often stated that she felt sorry for her physically disabled neighbor because the neighbor could not hike, be active, or enjoy the outdoors. Joan's husband, age 33, is attempting to visit Joan regularly and care for their daughter, a role that is new for him.

The therapist has assessed several things regarding Joan's developmental stage, adjustment stage, social/cultural influences, and family adjustment reactions. The two adult family members are probably in Sheehy's[158] "catch-30" stage, in which the person reevaluates his or her life and relationships. Joan already "knows" that the physically disabled cannot enjoy a physically active life and is also feeling that everything she has worked for in her career is lost. She appears to be in the mourning stage of adjustment. Her daughter and husband are having to adjust to radical role changes. Cognitively, Joan's young daughter is not going to understand the permanence of the disability and may be inclined to act out as the result of the turmoil. The husband will have to be assessed to determine his stage of adjustment to her disability.

The therapist has determined that Joan's transfers need further work but would like to use the adaptive process to stimulate adjustment. The therapist has devised a treatment session to meet the goals of promoting the defense stage of adjustment, decreasing her prejudice against the disabled, encouraging problem solving, increasing her feelings of self-worth, proving to her that she can take care of her daughter through interacting with children, as well as having her decenter her focus from her disability to her ability. The therapist has contacted the recreational therapist (who is a para-

plegic) to plan a collaborative session at the park across the street from the hospital. Because the recreational therapist works in the pediatrics ward, it is determined that the children with spina bifida should come and play tag transferring from log to log in the playground.

The stage is now set. Joan will be asked to help supervise the children. The adaptive process will be used to teach Joan how to transfer using the environment. The transfer will be organized subcortically because she will be attending cortically to the children's needs and to the game itself. Joan will be actively affecting her personal environment, and if everything goes well, the act of helping the children will increase her self-worth and will also be self-reinforcing. Within this treatment session, the therapist has used the recreational therapist as a role model to change Joan's prejudice against the disabled being active in the outdoors as well as to show Joan that she can still be a parent even though she is disabled. The therapist may also increase Joan's knowledge of how to interact with children from a wheelchair by giving a few hints and then having Joan transfer up a set of stairs to reach one of the children.

If we want to carry this scenario further, the therapist could introduce Joan to a child who is interested in computers and who needs help with a programming problem (Joan's computer background will be used, which will increase Joan's feelings of self-worth and help her focus on her abilities rather than on her disabilities). On the way back to the ward, the therapist and Joan may discuss how the family is dealing with the crisis they are in and help her realize how the family has made it through other crises in the past and how those previously successful strategies could be used in this situation. Support groups may be mentioned as resources. The session may end with Joan planning the next therapy session and thus starting to take control of her life.

love. Thus, a client who feels incapable of expressing sensuality or sexuality may see himself or herself as incapable of loving and being loved. Because love and acceptance are primary driving forces in a human's life,[117] the inability to perceive the self as capable of loving would be devastating.[66]

The last aspect of self-worth to be mentioned here is often overlooked in the health fields: it is the need that people have to help others.[57] People often discover that they are valuable through the act of giving. Self-worth is increased by seeing others enjoy and benefit from the individual's presence or offering. Situations in which the client's worth can be appreciated by others may be needed. Unless the client can contribute to others, the client is in a relatively dependent role, with everyone else giving to him or her without the opportunity of giving back. Achieving independence and then reaching out to others, with therapeutic assistance if necessary, facilitates the individual's more rapid reintegration into society. The therapist should take every opportunity to allow the client to express self-worth to others through helping.

The Adult Client with Brain Damage

The adult client with brain damage and the needs of the family will be specifically, yet briefly, examined here because brain damage affects the cognitive and emotional system of the client. When a person receives brain injury and is hospitalized, emotional support for the family (client included) is the primary need to be met initially. Pearson[133] feels that it is not the function of the support but the emotional tone of the support that is most important. The therapist should attempt to convey warmth and a caring attitude, especially during the family's initial contacts. Typical complaints about the acute period involve impersonal hospital routines and lack of definite information about the patient's status.[75, 84, 129, 169] Unfortunately, definite information is usually not available at the earliest stages.

Later, the family must deal with the physical changes in the client's body; what may be even more injurious to the family is the psychological, cognitive, and social changes in the client.[3, 8, 12, 14, 48, 49] People with cerebrovascular accidents have been found to be more clinically depressed than orthopedic patients. The libido[8, 83] and emotional systems are also affected.[67, 75, 129, 164] It has further been shown that persons who survive a cerebrovascular accident or other impairment and who have a full return of function do not return to normal life because of a lack of social and emotional skills.[7, 49, 88, 110, 176] Families of cerebrovascular accident victims have also reported that social reintegration is the most difficult phase of rehabilitation. Lack of socially appropriate behaviors has been one of the most troublesome complaints of people who deal with the person with chronic brain injury.[67] Therapists may be able to help alter this syndrome by encouraging appropriate behavior and by structuring therapy situations to reteach the client interaction skills. A technique called structured learning therapy[39, 64, 67] has been used with schizophrenics, and although this approach has not been used by enough clinics to judge its

effectiveness completely, it appears to be a promising approach.

Better follow-up care needs to be implemented when dealing with the adult with brain damage.[14, 20, 48, 84, 86, 87, 131] It may not be possible for the client and family to constantly come to the clinic for support and follow-up, but telephone conversations can be scheduled on a periodic basis, or the exchange of letters or audiotapes can also be used. With the increased availability of video recorders, the day may come when a follow-up may be performed on videotapes sent by clients living in rural areas. Support groups are being used increasingly to facilitate client and family adjustment and accommodation to disability, as well as reentry into the community.°

REFERENCES

1. Abresch RT, Seyden NK, Wineinger MA: Quality of life: Issues for persons with neuromuscular diseases. Phys Med Rehabil Clin North Am 9:233–248, 1998.
2. Andrews AB, Veronen LJ: Sexual assault and people with disabilities. J Soc Work Hum Sexuality 8:137–159, 1993.
3. Asarnow RF, Satz P, Light R: Behavior problems and adaptive functioning in children with mild and severe closed head injury. J Pediatr Psychol 16:543–555, 1991.
4. Baker LL: Problem solving techniques in adjustment services. Vocation Eval Work Adjust Bull 25(3):75–76, 1992.
5. Balcazar FE, et al: Empowering people with physical disabilities through advocacy skills training. Am J Community Psychol 18:281–296, 1990.
6. Baxter C: Investigating stigma as stress in social interactions of parents. J Ment Defic Res 33:446–455, 1989.
7. Belgrave FZ: Psychosocial prediction of adjustment to disability in African Americans. J Rehabil 57:37–40, 1991.
8. Berrol S: Issues of sexuality in head injured adults in sexuality and physical disability. In Bullard DG, Knight DE (eds): Sexuality and Physical Disability. St. Louis, CV Mosby, 1981.
9. Bogle JE, Shaul SL: Body image and the woman with a disability. In Bullard DG, Knight DE, (eds): Sexuality and Physical Disability. St. Louis, CV Mosby, 1981.
10. Boreing ML, Adler LM: Facilitating support groups: An instructional guide. Educational Monograph No. 3. San Francisco, Department of Psychiatry, Pacific Medical Center, 1982.
11. Boyle PS: Training in sexuality and disability: Preparing social workers to provide services to individuals with disabilities. J Soc Work Hum Sexuality 8(2):45–62, 1993.
12. Braithwaite DO: From majority to minority: An analysis of cultural change from ablebodied to disabled. Int J Intercultural Relations 14:465–483, 1990.
13. Brammer LM, Abrego PJ: Intervention strategies for coping with transitions. Counsel Psychol 9(2):19, 1981.
14. Brooks DN: The head-injured family. J Clin Exp Neuropsychol 13:155–188, 1991.
15. Brown SE: Creating a disability mythology. Int J Rehabil Res 15:227–233, 1991.
16. Bukowski WM, Hoza B: Popularity and friendship: Issues in theory, measurement, and outcomes. In Berndt T, Ladd G, (eds): Contributions of Peer Relationships of Children's Development. New York, Wiley, 1989.
17. Bullard DG, Knight DE: Sexuality and Physical Disability. St. Louis, CV Mosby, 1981.
18. Burton GU: Sexuality and physical disability. In Pedretti LW (ed): Occupational Therapy: Practice Skills for Physical Dysfunction, 5th ed. St. Louis, CV Mosby, 2000.
19. Burton GU: Sexuality: An activity of daily living. In Early MB (ed): Physical Dysfunction Practice Skills for the Occupational Therapy Assistant. St. Louis, CV Mosby, 1998.
20. Burton L, Volpe B: Sex differences in the emotional status of traumatically brain-injured patients. J Neurol Rehabil 2:151–157, 1993.

°See references. 5, 7, 12, 20, 48, 51, 84, 99, 123, 127, 155, and 157.

21. Cairns D, Baker J: Adjustment to spinal cord injury: A review of coping styles contributing to the process. J Rehabil 59(4):30–33, 1993.
22. Capell B, Capell J: Being parents of children who are disabled. *In* Bullard DG, Knight DE (eds): Sexuality and Physical Disability. St. Louis, CV Mosby, 1981.
23. Charlifue SW, et al: Sexual issues of women with spinal cord injuries. Paraplegia 30(3):192–199, 1992.
24. Clarke PJ, Black SE, Badley EM, et al: Handicap in stroke survivors. Disabil Rehabil 21:116–123, 1999.
25. Coffman S: Parent and infant attachment: Review of nursing research 1981–1990. Pediatr Nurse 18:421–425, 1992.
26. Cohen MZ, Sarter B: Love and work: Oncology nurses' view of the meaning of their work. Oncol Nurs Form 19:1481–1486, 1992.
27. Cole TM: Gathering a sex history from a physically disabled adult. Sex Disabil 9(1):29–37, 1991.
28. Cole SS, Cole TM: Sexuality, disability, and reproductive issues for persons with disabilities. *In* Haseltine FP, Cole SS, Gray DB (eds): Reproductive Issues for Persons with Physical Disabilities. Baltimore, Paul H. Brookes, 1993.
29. Cole SS, Cole TM: Sexuality, disability, and reproductive issues through the life span. Sexuality Disabil 11:189–205, 1993.
30. Collins LF: Easing client transition from facility to community. OT Practice 1(4):36–39, 1996.
31. Combs AW, et al: Helping Relationship. Boston, Allyn & Bacon, 1971.
32. Corbett KS, Klein S, Bregante JL: The role of sexuality and sex equity in the education of disabled women. Peabody J Educ 64(4):198–211, 1987.
33. Cornelius DA, et al: Who Cares? Baltimore, University Park Press, 1982.
34. Craig AR, Hancock K, Chang E, Dickson H: Immunizing against depression and anxiety after spinal cord injury. Arch Phys Med Rehabil 79:375–377, 1998.
35. Craig AR, Hancock K, Dickson H, Chang E: Long-term psychological outcomes in spinal cord injured persons: Results of a controlled trial using cognitive behavior therapy. Arch Phys Med Rehabil 78:33–38, 1997.
36. Craig A, Hancock K, Chang E, Dickson H: The effectiveness of group psychological intervention in enhancing perceptions of control following spinal cord injury. Aust N Z J Psychiatry 32:112–118, 1998.
37. Craig A, Hancock K, Dickson H: Improving the long-term adjustment of spinal cord–injured persons. Spinal Cord 37:345–350, 1999.
38. Daniels SM: Critical issues in sexuality and disability. *In* Bullard DG, Knight SE (eds): Sexuality and Physical Disability. St. Louis, CV Mosby, 1981.
39. Davis RE: Family of physically disabled children: Family reactions and deductive reasoning. N Y State J Med 75:1039, 1975.
40. Ducharme SH, Gill KM: Management of other male sexual dysfunction. *In* Sipski ML, Alexander CJ (eds): Sexual Function in People with Disability and Chronic Illness. Rockville, MD, Aspen, 1997.
41. Dunn, KL: Sexuality education and the team approach. *In* Sipski ML, Alexander CJ (eds): Sexual Function in People with Disability and Chronic Illness. Rockville, MD, Aspen, 1997.
42. Dunton HD: The child's concept of death. *In* Schoenberg B, et al: Loss and Grief: Psychological Management in Medical Practice. New York, Columbia University Press, 1970.
43. Fine SB: Resilience and human adaptability: Who rise above adversity? 1990 Eleanor Clark Slagle Lecture. Am J Occup Ther 45:493–503, 1991.
44. Fine S: Interaction between psychosocial variables and cognitive function. *In* Royeen CB (ed): American Occupational Therapy Association Self-Study Series on Cognitive Rehabilitation. Rockville, MD, American Occupational Therapy Association, 1993.
45. Finnie NR: Handling the Young Cerebral Palsied Child at Home, 2nd ed. New York, EP Dutton, 1974.
46. Fisher M: Can grief be turned into growth? Staff grief in palliative care. Prof Nurse 7(3):178–182, 1991.
47. Fitz-Gerald M, Fitz-Gerald DR: Involvement in sex education. Volta-Review 89(5):96–110, 1987.
48. Flagg-Williams JB: Perspectives on working with parents of handicapped children. Psychol Schools 28:238–246, 1991.
49. Fleming JM, Mass F: Prognosis of rehabilitation outcome in head injury using the disability rating scale. Arch Phys Med Rehabil 75:159–162, 1994.
50. French S: Researching disability: The way forward. Disabil Rehabil 14(4):183–186, 1992.
51. Fuhrer MJ, et al: Depressive symptomatology in persons with spinal cord injury who reside in the community. Arch Phys Med 74:255–260, 1993.
52. Furman RA: The child's reaction to death in the family. *In* Schoenberg B, et al: Loss and Grief, New York, Columbia University Press, 1970.
53. Gage M: The appraisal model of coping: An assessment and intervention model for occupational therapy. Am J Occup Ther 46:353–362, 1992.
54. GAP, Group for the Advancement of Psychiatry: Caring for People with Physical Improvements: The Journey Back. Washington, DC, American Psychiatric Press, 1993.
55. Gardner B: Ways of Coping: Adolescents with Spinal Cord Injury Compared with Able-Bodied Adolescents. San Jose, CA, San Jose State University, 1993.
56. Garske GG, Turpin JO: Understanding psychosocial adjustment to disability: An American perspective. Int J Rehabil Health 4(1):29–37, 1998.
57. Geis HJ: The problem of personal worth in the physically disabled patient. Rehabil Lit 33(2):34, 1972.
58. Gelenberg A: Depression is still unrecognized and undertreated. Arch Intern Med. 159(15), 1999.
59. Gender AR: An overview of the nurse's role in dealing with sexuality. Sex Disabil 10(2):71–70, 1992.
60. Gerhart KA, Weitzenkamp DA, Kennedy P, et al: Correlates of stress in long-term spinal cord injury. Spinal Cord 37(3):183–190, 1999.
61. Gething L: Judgements by health professionals of personal characteristics of people with visible physical disability. Soc Sci Med 34:809–815, 1992.
62. Giles GM: Illness behavior after severe brain injury: Two case studies. Am J Occup Ther 48:247–255, 1994.
63. Goldberg RT: Toward an understanding of the rehabilitation of the disabled adolescent. Rehabil Lit 42(3–4):66, 1981.
64. Goldstein AP, et al: Skill Training for Community Living. New York, Pergamon Press, 1976.
65. Goldstein H, Runyon C: An occupational therapy education module to increase sensitivity about geriatric sexuality. Phys Occup Ther Geriatr 11(2):57, 1993.
66. Gorman C, Kennedy P, Hamilton LR: Alterations in self-perceptions following childhood onset of spinal cord injury. Spinal Cord 36:181–185, 1998.
67. Griffith ER, Lemberg S: Sexuality and the Person with Traumatic Brain Injury: A Guide for Families. Philadelphia, FA Davis, 1993.
68. Grossenbacher NL: The trauma of spinal cord injury on the adolescent. Occup Ther Health Care 2(3):79–90, 1985.
69. Hall ET: The Hidden Dimension. Garden City, NJ, Doubleday Anchor Books, 1966.
70. Hallett JD, et al: Role change after traumatic brain injury in adults. Am J Occup Ther 48:241–246, 1994.
71. Hammond DC: Cross-cultural rehabilitation. *In* Stubbins J (ed): Social and Psychological Aspects of Disability. Baltimore, University Park Press, 1977.
72. Harper DC, Bhattarai PK: Children's attitudes toward disabilities in Nepal. Dev Med Child Neurol. 31(35):1989.
73. Harvey RM: The relationship of values to adjustment in illness: A model for nursing practice. J Adv Nurs 17:467–472, 1992.
74. Hartkopp A, Bronnum-Hansen H, Seidenschnur AM, Biering-Sorensen F: Suicide in a spinal cord injured population: Its relation to functional status. Arch Phys Med Rehabil 79:1356–1361, 1998.
75. Haseltine FP, Cole SS, Gray DB: Reproductive Issues for Persons with Physical Disabilities. Baltimore, Paul H. Brookes, 1993.
76. Heiskill LE, Pasnau RD: Psychological reaction to hospitalization and illness in the emergency dept. Emerg Med Clin North Am 9:207–218, 1991.
77. Hite S: The Hite Report on Female Sexuality. New York, Dell Publishing, 1976.
78. Hite S: The Hite Report on Male Sexuality. New York, Random House, 1981.
79. Humphry R, Gonzalez S, Taylor E: Family involvement in practice: Issues and attitudes. Am J Occup Ther 47:587–593, 1993.

80. Hwang K: Living with a disability: A woman's perspective. *In* Sipski ML, Alexander CJ: Sexual Function in People with Disability and Chronic Illness. Rockville, MD, Aspen, 1997.

81. Jackson AB, Wadley V: A multicenter study of women's self-reported reproductive health after spinal cord injury. Arch Phys Med Rehabil 80:1420–1428, 1999.

82. Jonsson AL, Moller A, Grimby G: Managing occupations in everyday life to achieve adaptations. Am J Occup Ther 53:353–362, 1999.

83. Kaitz S: Strategies to prevent caregiver fatigue. Headlines, May/June:18–19, 1993.

84. Kasowski JC: Family recovery: An insider's view. Am J Occup Ther 48:257–258, 1994.

85. Kauhanen M, Korpelainen JT, Hiltunen P, et al: Poststroke depression correlates with cognitive impairment and neurological deficits. Stroke 30:1875–1880, 1999.

86. Keefe FJ, Caldwell DS, Baucom D, et al: Spouse-assisted coping skills training in the management of knee pain in osteoarthritis: Long-term followup results. Arthritis Care Res 12:101–111, 1999.

87. Kemp BJ, Krause JS: Depression and life satisfaction among people aging with post-polio and spinal cord injury. Disabil Rehabil 21(5–6):241–249, 1999.

88. Kemp BJ, Adams BM, Campbell ML: Depression and life satisfaction in aging polio survivors versus age-matched controls: Relation to postpolio syndrome, family functioning, and attitude toward disability. Arch Phys Med Rehabil 78:187–192, 1997.

89. Kerr N: Understanding the process of adjustment to disability. J Rehabil 27(6):16, 1961.

90. Kerr N: Understanding the process of adjustment to disability. *In* Stubbins J (ed): Social and Psychological Aspects of Disability. Baltimore, University Park Press, 1977.

91. Kerr N: Staff expectations for disabled persons. *In* Stubbins J (ed): Social and Psychological Aspects of Disability. Baltimore, University Park Press, 1977.

92. Kettl P, et al: Female sexuality after spinal cord injury. Sex Disabil 9:287–295, 1991.

93. Kewman D, Warschausky LE, Warzak W: Sexual development of children and adolescents. *In* Sipski ML, Alexander CJ: Sexual Function in People with Disability and Chronic Illness. Rockville, MD, Aspen, 1997.

94. Kibele A, Padilla R, Burton GU: The psychosocial issues of physical illness and disability. *In* Cara E, MacRae A: Psychosocial Occupational Therapy in Clinical Practice. Albany, Delmar, 1998.

95. King LJ: Toward a science of adaptive responses. Am J Occup Ther 32:429, 1978.

96. Klaus MH, Kennell JH: Maternal-Infant Bonding, 2nd ed. St. Louis, CV, Mosby, 1982.

97. Klausner EJ, Alexopoulos GS: The future of psychosocial treatments for elderly patients. Psychiatr Serv 50:1198–1204, 1999.

98. Koplas PA, Gans HB, Wisely MP, et al: Quality of life and Parkinson's disease. J Gerontol A Biol Sci Med Sci 54(4):M197–M202, 1999.

99. Koscuilek JF, McCublin MA, McCublin HI: A theoretical framework for family adaptation to head injury. J Rehabil 59(3):40–45, 1993.

100. Krause JS, Crewe NM: Long-term prediction of self-reported problems following spinal cord injury. Paraplegia 28:186–202, 1990.

101. Krause JS, Crewe NM: Chronological age, time since injury, and time of measurement: Effect on adjustment after spinal cord injury. Arch Phys Med Rehabil 72:91–100, 1991.

102. Krause JS: Ageing and life adjustment after spinal cord injury. Crawford Research Institute, Shepherd Center, Atlanta, Georgia, USA. Spinal Cord 36:320–328, 1998.

103. Kreuter M, Sullivan M, Dahllof AG, Siosteen A: Partner relationships, functioning, mood and global quality of life in persons with spinal cord injury and traumatic brain injury. Spinal Cord 36:252–261, 1998.

104. Kroll K, Klein EL: Enabling Romance. New York, Harmony Books, 1992.

105. Krueger DW: Rehabilitation Psychology. Rockville, MD, Aspen Systems Corporation, 1984.

106. Kubler-Ross E: On Death and Dying. New York, Macmillan, 1969.

107. Lefebvre KA: Sexual assessment planning. J Head Trauma Rehabil 5(2):25–30, 1991.

108. Lefebvre KA: Performing a sexual evaluation on the person with disability or illness. *In* Sipski ML, Alexander CJ: Sexual Function in People with Disability and Chronic Illness. Rockville, MD, Aspen, 1997.

109. Lemon MA: Sexual counseling and spinal cord injury. Sex Disabil 11(1):73–97, 1993.

110. Lewis SC: The Mature Years. Thorofare, NJ, Charles B. Slack, 1979.

111. Liepmann L: Your Child's Sensory World. New York, Dial Press, 1973.

112. Linsenmeyer TA: Management of male infertility. *In* Sipski ML, Alexander CJ (eds): Sexual Function in People with Disability and Chronic Illness. Rockville, MD, Aspen, 1997.

113. Livneh H: A unified approach to existing models of adaption to disability. J Appl Rehabil Counsel 17(2):6, 1986.

114. Livneh H, Antonak RF: Reactions to disability: An empirical investigation of their nature and structure. J Appl Rehabil Couns 21(4):13–20, 1990.

115. Maslow A: Motivation and Personality, 2nd ed. New York, Harper & Row, 1970.

116. Mauras-Neslen, Neslen SE: The therapeutic alliance: Enhancing client-practitioner relationships. OT Practice 1(4):20–27, 1996.

117. Maze JR: The complementarity of object-relations and instinct theory. Int J Psychoanalysis 74:459–470, 1993.

118. McComas J, et al: Experiences of students and practicing physical therapists with inappropriate patient sexual behavior. Phys Ther 73:762–769, 1993.

119. McCubbin MA, McCubbin HI: Family stress theory and assessment: The resiliency model of family stress, adjustment, and adaptation. *In* McCubbin HI, Thompson AI, (eds): Family Assessment Inventories for Research and Practice. Madison, WI, University of Wisconsin–Madison, 1991.

120. McKinley W, Brooks D, Bond M: Post-concussional symptoms, financial compensation, and outcome of severe blunt head injury. J Neurol Neurosurg Psychiatry 46:1084–1091, 1983.

121. McLaughlin AM, Erdman J: Rehabilitation staff stress as it relates to patient acuity and diagnosis. Brain Inj 6(1):59–64, 1992.

122. McNeff EA: Issues for the partner of the person with a disability. *In* Sipski ML, Alexander CJ: Sexual Function in People with Disability and Chronic Illness. Rockville, MD, Aspen, 1997.

123. Miller L: When the best help is self-help, or everything you always wanted to know about brain injury support groups. Cogn Rehabil 10(6):14–17, 1992.

124. Mims FH, Swenson M: Sexuality: A Nursing Perspective. New York, McGraw-Hill, 1980.

125. Mooney TO, et al: Sexual Options for Paraplegics and Quadriplegics. Boston, Little, Brown, 1975.

126. Moyers PA: The guide to occupational therapy practice. J Occup Ther 53(3), 1999.

127. Nadig PW: Vacuum constriction devices in patients with neurogenic impotence. Sex Disabil 12(1):99–106, 1994.

128. Neau JP, Ingrand P, Mouille-Brachet C, et al: Functional recovery and social outcome after cerebral infarction in young adults. Cerebrovasc Dis 8:296–302, 1998.

129. Neistadt ME, Freda M: Choices: A Guide to Sex Counseling with Physically Disabled Adults. Malabar, FL, Krieger, 1987.

130. Nowinski JK, Ayers T: Sexuality and major medical conditions. *In* Bullard DG, Knight SE (eds): Sexuality and Physical Disability. St. Louis, CV Mosby, 1981.

131. Pain H: Coping with a child with disabilities from the parents' perspective: The function of information. Child Care Health Dev 25:299–312, 1999.

132. Parker JG, Asher SR: Peer relations and later personal adjustment: Are low accepted children at risk? Psychol Bull 102:357–389, 1987.

133. Pearson R: Support: Exploration of a basic dimension of informal help and counseling. Personnel Guidance J 61(2):83, 1982.

134. Pedretti LW: Occupational Therapy: Practice Skills for Physical Dysfunction, 5th ed. St. Louis, CV Mosby, 2000.

135. Pentland W, Harvey AS, Walker J: The relationships between time use and health and well-being in men with spinal cord injury. J Occup Sci 5(1):14–25, 1998.

136. Peretz D: Reaction to loss. *In* Schoenberg B, et al (eds): Loss and Grief. New York, Columbia University Press, 1970.

137. Physicians' Desk Reference, 56th ed. Montvale NJ, Medical Economics Books, 1999.

138. Post MW, de Witte LP, van Asbeck FW, et al: Predictors of health status and life satisfaction in spinal cord injury. Arch Phys Med Rehabil 79:395–401, 1998.

139. Prince MJ, Harwood RH, Thomas A, Mann AH: A prospective population-based cohort study of the effects of disablement and social milieu on the onset and maintenance of late-life depression. The Gospel Oak Project VII. Psychol Med 28:337–350, 1998.

140. Resources FRI: Resources for people with disabilities and chronic conditions, 2nd ed. Lexington, KY, Resources for Rehabilitation, 1993.

141. Revenson TA, Felton BJ: Disability and coping as predictors of psychological adjustment to rheumatoid arthritis. J Consult Clin Psychol 57:344–348, 1989.

142. Richards JS, Bombardier CH, Tate D, et al: Access to the environment and life satisfaction after spinal cord injury. Arch Phys Med Rehabil 80:1501–1506, 1999.

143. Rivas DA, Cancellor MB: Management of erectile dysfunction. In Sipski ML, Alexander CJ (eds): Sexual Function in People with Disability and Chronic Illness. Rockville, MD, Aspen, 1997.

144. Rodrigue RR: Psychological crises of the ill and handicapped. Emotional First Aid 2(1):44, 1985.

145. Rogers JD, Figone JJ: Psychosocial parameters in treating the person with quadriplegia. Am J Occup Ther 33:432, 1979.

146. Romeo AJ, Wanlass R, Arenas S: A profile of psychosexual functioning in males following spinal cord injury. Sex Disabil 11:269–276, 1993.

147. Rose MH: The concepts of coping and vulnerability as applied to children with chronic conditions. Issues Compr Pediatr Nurs 7(4–5):177, 1984.

148. Sandowski C: Responding to the sexual concerns of persons with disabilities. J Soc Work Hum Sexual 8(2):29–43, 1993.

149. Santoro J, Spiers M: Social cognitive factors in brain injury–associated personality change. Brain Inj 8:256–276, 1994.

150. Satir V: Peoplemaking. Palo Alto, CA, Science & Behavior Books, 1972.

151. Schalen W, et al: Psychosocial outcome 5–8 years after severe traumatic brain lesions and the impact of rehabilitation services. Brain Inj 8:49–64, 1994.

152. Schanke AK: Psychological distress, social support and coping behaviour among polio survivors: A 5-year perspective on 63 polio patients. Disabil Rehabil 19(3):108–116, 1997.

153. Schoenberg B, et al: Loss and Grief. New York, Columbia University Press, 1970.

154. Scholte OP, Reimer WJ, de Haan RJ, et al: The burden of caregiving in partners of long-term stroke survivors. Stroke 29:1605–1611, 1998.

155. Schulz CH: Helping factors in a peer-developed support group for persons with a head injury: II. Survivor interview perspective. Am J Occup Ther 48:305–309, 1994.

156. Schulz R, Beach SR: Caregiving as a risk factor for mortality: The caregiver health effects study. JAMA 282:2215–2219, 1999.

157. Schwartzberg SL: Helping factors in a peer-developed support group for persons with a head injury: I. Participant observer perspective. Am J Occup Ther 48:297–304, 1994.

158. Sheehy G: Passages. New York, EP Dutton, 1976.

159. Shellabarger SG, Thompson TL: The clinical times: Meeting parental communication needs throughout the NICU experience. Neonatal Network, 12(2):39–45, 1993.

160. Sigler G, Mackelprang RW: Cognitive impairments: Psychosocial and sexual implications and strategies for social work intervention. J Soc Work Hum Sexual 8(2):89–106, 1993.

161. Simon SB, et al: Values Clarification. New York, Hart Publishing Co, 1972.

162. Sipski ML: Performing the medical sexual history and physical. In Sipski ML, Alexander CJ: Sexual Function in People with Disability and Chronic Illness. Rockville, MD, Aspen, 1997.

163. Sipski ML, Alexander CJ: Impact of disability or chronic illness on sexual function. In Sipski ML, Alexander CJ (eds): Sexual Function in People with Disability and Chronic Illness. Rockville, MD, Aspen, 1997.

164. Sipski ML, Alexander CJ: Sexual Function in People with Disability and Chronic Illness. Rockville, MD, Aspen, 1997.

165. Smith M: Pediatric sexuality: Promoting normal sexual development in children. Nurse Practitioner 18(8):37–44, 1993.

166. Solnit AJ, Green M: The pediatric management of the dying child. In Solnit A, Provence S (eds): Modern Perspectives in Child Development. New York, International Universities Press, 1963.

167. Spanbock P: Children and siblings of head injury survivors: A need to be understood. J Cogn Rehabil 10(4):8–9, 1992.

168. Stockard S: Caring for the sexually aggressive patient: You don't have to blush and bear it. Nursing. 21(11): 72–73, 1991.

169. Taanila A, Jarvelin MR, Kokkonen J: Parental guidance and counselling by doctors and nursing staff: Parents' views of initial information and advice for families with disabled children. J Clin Nurs 7:505–511, 1998.

170. Tedder TL: Using the Brazelton Neonatal Assessment Scale to facilitate the parent-infant relationship in a primary care setting. Nurse Practitioner 16(3):26–36, 1991.

171. Tharp RG: Cultural diversity and treatment of children. J Consult Clin Psychol 59:799–812, 1991.

172. Trombly CA: Occupational Therapy for Physical Dysfunction, 2nd ed. Baltimore, Williams & Wilkins, 1989.

173. Vander Kolk CJ: Client credibility and coping styles. Rehabil Psychol 36(1):51–62, 1991.

174. Vickery DM, Fries JF: Take care of yourself: A consumer's guide to medical care. Reading, MA, Addison-Wesley, 1976.

175. Verduyn WH: Spinal cord injured women, pregnancy, and delivery. Sex Disabil 11:29–43, 1993.

176. Viemero V, Krause C: Quality of life in individuals with physical disabilities. Psychother Psychosom 67:317–322, 1998.

177. Vogel LC, Klaas SJ, Lubicky JP, Anderson CJ: Long-term outcomes and life satisfaction of adults who had pediatric spinal cord injuries. Arch Phys Med Rehabil 79:1496–1503, 1998.

178. Wade OT: Is stroke rehabilitation worthwhile? Curr Opin Neurol Neurosurg 6(1):78–82, 1993.

179. Weitzenkamp DA, Gerhart KA, Charlifue SW, et al: Spouses of spinal cord injury survivors: The added impact of caregiving. Arch Phys Med Rehabil 78:822–827, 1997.

180. Weitzner MA, McMillan SC: Quality of life in cancer patients: Use of a revised hospice index. Cancer Pract 6(5):282–288, 1998.

181. Welner SL: Management of female infertility. In Sipski ML, Alexander CJ: Sexual Function in People with Disability and Chronic Illness. Rockville, MD, Aspen, 1997.

182. Whipple B, McGreer KB: Management of female sexual dysfunction. In Sipski ML, Alexander CJ: Sexual Function in People with Disability and Chronic Illness. Rockville, MD, Aspen, 1997.

183. White W: The urge towards competence. Am J Occup Ther 26(6):271, 1971.

184. Yellott G: Promoting parent-infant bonding. Prof Nurs 6:519–520, 1991.

185. Zani B: Male and female patterns in the discovery of sexuality during adolescence. J Adolesc 14:163–178, 1991.

186. Zorzon M, Zivadinov R, Bosco A, et al: Sexual dysfunction in multiple sclerosis: A case-control study: I. Frequency and comparison of groups. Mult Scler 5:418–427, 1999.

187. Zurmohle UM, Homann T, Schroeter C, et al: Psychosocial adjustment of children with spina bifida. J Child Neurol 13:64–70, 1998.

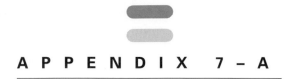

Support Groups That May Assist the Therapist and Client

Administration on Developmental Disabilities
U.S. Department of Health and Human Services
330 C Street, SW
Washington, DC 20201
(202) 245–2890

American Coalition for Citizens with Disabilities
1346 Connecticut Avenue, NW
Washington, DC 20036

American Genetic Association
P.O. Box 39
Buckeystown, MD 21717
(301) 695–9292

American Heart Association
7320 Greenville Avenue
Dallas, TX 75231

Arthritis Foundation
3400 Peachtree Road, NE, Suite 1106
Atlanta, GA 30326

Association for Persons with Severe Handicaps
7010 Roosevelt Way, NE
Seattle, WA 98115
(206) 523–8446

Beach Center on Families and Disability
c/o Life Span Institute, University of Kansas
3111 Haworth Hall
Lawrence, KS 66045
(913) 864–7600; FAX (913) 864–7605

Center for Independent Living
2539 Telegraph Avenue
Berkeley, CA 96704
(415) 841–4776

Closer Look
National Information Center for the Handicapped
Box 1492
Washington, DC 20013

Coalition on Sexuality and Disability
132 East Twenty-Third Street
New York, NY 10010
(212) 242–3900

Council for Exceptional Children
1920 Association Drive
Reston, VA 22091–1589
(703) 620–3660

Disabled American Veterans
National Headquarters
P.O. Box 14301
Cincinnati, OH 45250–0301
(606) 441–7300

Epilepsy Foundation of America
1828 L Street NW, Suite 406
Washington, DC 20036

Federation for Children with Special Needs
95 Berkeley Street, Suite 104
Boston, MA 02116
(617) 482–2915

Information Center for Individuals with Disabilities
20 Park Plaza, Room 330
Boston, MA 02116

Interdisciplinary Special Interest Group on Head Injury
American Congress of Rehabilitation Medicine
5700 Old Orchard Road
Skokie, IL 60077
(708) 966–0095

National Association for Retarded Citizens
2709 Avenue E East
Arlington, TX 76011

National Association of the Physically Handicapped, Inc.
76 Elm Street
London, OH 43140

National Center for Youth with Disabilities
Adolescent Health Program
University of Minnesota
P.O. Box 721–UMHO
Harvard Street at East River Road
Minneapolis, MN 55455
(800) 333–NCYD or (612) 626–2825

National Committee to Prevent Child Abuse (NCPCA)
332 S. Michigan Avenue, Suite 1600
Chicago, IL 60604
(312) 663–3520; TDD (312) 663–3540; (800) 835–2671

National Council on Disability
800 Independence Avenue, SW, Suite 814
Washington, DC 20591
(202) 267–3846; (202) 267–3232 (TT); FAX (202) 453–4240

National Council on Independent Living (NCIL)
Troy Atrium
4th Street and Broadway
Troy, NY 12180
(518) 274–1979; (518) 274–0701 (TT); FAX (518) 274–7944

National Head Injury Foundation, Inc.
1140 Connecticut Avenue, NW, Suite 812
Washington, DC 20036
(202) 296–6443

National Rehabilitation Information Center
8455 Colesville Road, Suite 935
Silver Spring, MD
20910–3319 (800) 346–2742

Office for Handicapped Individuals
U.S. Department of Health and Human Services
200 Independence Avenue, SW
Washington, DC 20201
(202) 245–6568

President's Committee on Employment of People with
   Disabilities
P.O. Box 17413
Washington, DC 20041
(703) 471–5761

Sex Information and Education Council of the United States
84 Fifth Avenue, Suite 407
New York, NY 10011

Sexuality and Disability Training Center
University of Michigan Medical Center
Department of Physical Medicine and Rehabilitation
1500 E. Medical Center Drive
Ann Arbor, MI 48109
(313) 936–7067

Stroke Clubs of America
805 Twelfth Street
Galveston, TX 77550
(409) 762–1022

Task Force on Sexuality and Disability of the American
   Congress of Rehabilitation Medicine
5700 Old Orchard Road
Skokie, IL 60077
(708) 966–0095

Well Spouse Foundation
P.O. Box 28876
San Diego, CA 92198–0876
(619) 673–9043; in New York (914) 357–8513; FAX (914)
   368–4336

WEB SITES

Abledata Assistive Technology
http://www.abledata.com/

Alliance for Technology Access
http://www.ataccess.org/

American Foundation for the Blind
http://www.afb.org/

Associated Blind, Inc.
http://www.tabinc.org/

Disability Social History Project
http://www.disabilityhistory.org/

Don Johnston Incorporated
http://www.donjohnston.com

Dragon Systems
http://www.dragonsys.com

Educational Services/Support Groups of the Rehabilitation
   Institute of Chicago
http://www.rehabchicago.org/community/support.htm

Empowerment Zone
http://www.empowermentzone.com/

General Disability Resources
http://www.nccn.net/~freed/gendisrc.htm

GW Micro
http://www.gwmicro.com

Henter-Joyce, Inc.
http://www.hj.com

IBM Via Voice
http://www-4.ibm.com/software/speech/

National Federation of the Blind
http://www.nfb.org/

National Women's Health Information Center
http://www.4women.gov/wwd/

Prentke Romich Company
http://www.prentrom.com

Rehabilitation Engineering and Assistive Technology Society of
   North America
http://www.resna.org/

Sexual Health Network Home Page
http://www.sexualhealth.com

Snap Alternative Medicine
*http://pacbell.snap.com/LMOID/resource/
   0.566.–156.00.html?st.sn.fdts.0.sp-156*

U.S. Department of Labor: ETA Disability Online
http://www.wdsc.org/disability/

Wheelchairnet (Virtual Wheelchair Community)
http://www.wheelchairnet.org/

Management of Clinical Problems

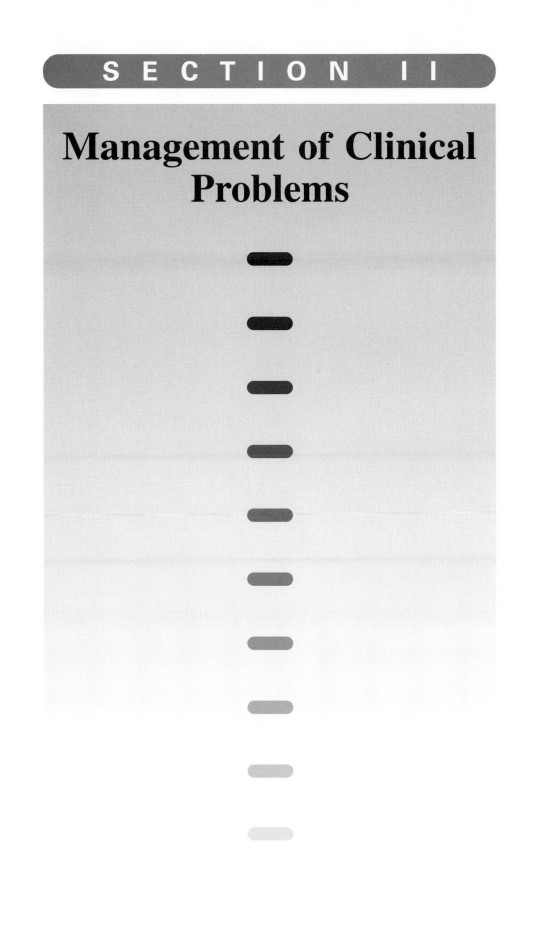

Low Birth Weight Infants: Neonatal Care and Follow-Up

JANE K. SWEENEY, PhD, PT, PCS • MARCIA W. SWANSON, PhD, MPH, PT

Chapter Outline

Key Words

- high-risk clinical signs

- neonatal neuropathology

- neuromotor assessment

- neuromotor intervention

- NICU environment

- parent instruction

- physiological and musculoskeletal risks

- subspecialty training

Objectives

After reading this chapter the student/therapist will:

1. Discuss three theoretical frameworks guiding neonatal therapy services in the NICU.

2. Identify the physiological and structural vulnerabilities of preterm infants that predispose them to stress during neonatal therapy procedures.

3. Outline supervised clinical practicum components and pediatric clinical experiences to prepare for entry into NICU practice.

4. Describe how the grief process may affect behavior and caregiving performance of parents of LBW neonates.

5. Differentiate the developmental course and neuromotor risk signs in infants with emerging neuromotor impairment from the clinical characteristics of infants with transient movement dysfunction.

6. Identify instruments for neuromotor examination of high-risk infants in NICUs and in follow-up clinics and compare psychometric features of the tests.

7. Describe program plans for LBW infants in NICU and home settings.

In the past four decades, specialized neonatal intensive care units (NICUs) and technological advances have contributed to a dramatic decline in neonatal mortality, particularly among low birth weight (LBW; defined as less than 2500 g) infants. Between 1960 and 1983 the rate of survival for infants of birth weights between 500 and 1000 g increased from 1% to 45%, and from 42% to 85% for neonates weighing between 1000 and 1500 g.[28, 39, 91] Within the past 10 years, further gains have been achieved for the smallest group, extremely low birth weight infants (ELBW; <1000 g). For neonates weighing between 500 and 800 g at birth, the survival rate increased from 40% in the 1980s to 60% in the 1990s.[91, 159] Because premature birth is associated with an increased risk of neurological injury, the improved survival of very small infants is associated with an increased prevalence of major and minor neurodevelopmental disabilities. Over the past 20 years, the prevalence of children with cerebral palsy has increased an estimated 20%, with the rise occurring primarily among very low birth weight (VLBW, <1500 g) infants, in whom there has been a threefold increase in cerebral palsy.[28, 39, 93, 159, 169, 206]

Although new diagnostic techniques, such as cranial ultrasonography, can document brain injury during the neonatal period, prediction of subsequent neurodevelopmental outcome is still unreliable and imprecise. Careful developmental assessment continues to be required during the outpatient phase of care for NICU graduates. Pediatric therapists serve the increasing numbers of surviving neonates at developmental risk by (1) providing valuable diagnostic data through neurological and developmental examination, (2) facilitating and coordinating interdisciplinary case management for infants and parents, and (3) reinforcing the preventive aspects of health care through early intervention and long-term developmental monitoring.

This chapter focuses on LBW infants and their parents during the clinical management phases of inpatient neonatal intensive care and outpatient follow-up. A theoretical framework for neonatal practice and an overview of neonatal neuropathology related to movement disorders are presented. In-depth discussion in the neonatal section includes indications for referral based on risk, neurological examination instruments, high-risk profiles in the neonatal period, treatment planning, and therapy strategies in the NICU. The section on outpatient follow-up focuses on a service delivery model for a high-risk infant clinic and includes neuromotor examination and evaluation, clinical decision making, and selected intervention strategies.

THEORETICAL FRAMEWORK

Concepts of dynamic systems, neonatal behavioral organization, and parental hope and empowerment provide a theoretical framework for neonatal therapy practice. In this section are three models that provide a theoretical structure for practitioners designing and implementing neuromotor and neurobehavioral programs for LBW infants and their parents.

Dynamic Systems

Dynamic systems theory applied to infants in NICUs refers, first, to the presence of multiple interacting structural and physiological systems within the infant to produce functional behaviors and, second, to the dynamic interactions between the infant and the environment(s). In Figure 8–1, neonatal movement and postural control are targeted as a core focus in neonatal therapy with overlapping and interacting influences by cardiopulmonary, behavioral, neuromuscular, musculoskeletal, and integumentary systems. A change or intervention affecting one system may diminish or enhance stability in the other dynamic systems within the infant. Similarly, a change in the infant's environment may impair or improve the infant's functional performance.

This theory guides the neonatal practitioner to consider the many potential physiological and anatomical influences (dynamic systems within the infant) that make preterm infants vulnerable to stress during caregiving procedures, including neonatal therapy. Dynamic systems theory also emphasizes the contributions of the interacting environments of the NICU, home, and community in constraining or facilitating the functional performance of LBW infants.[219]

Synactive Model of Infant Behavior

The synactive model of infant behavioral organization is a specific neonatal dynamic systems model for establishing physiological stability as the foundation for organization of motor, behavioral state, and attention/interactive behaviors in infants. Als[6, 7] and co-workers[8] described a "synactive" process of four subsystems interacting as the neonate responds to the stresses of the extrauterine envi-

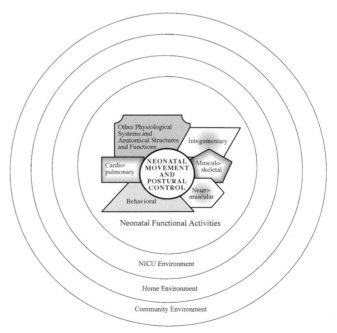

FIGURE 8–1. Dynamic systems within neonates and interacting external environments influencing functional performance. (From Sweeney JK, et al: Practice guidelines for the physical therapist in the NICU. Pediatr Phys Ther 11:119, 1999.)

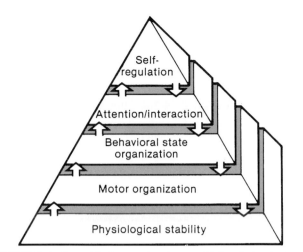

FIGURE 8–2. Pyramid of synactive theory of infant behavioral organization with physiological stability at the foundation.

ronment. They theorized that the basic subsystem of physiological organization must first be stabilized for the other subsystems to emerge and allow the infant to maintain behavioral state control and then interact positively with the environment (Fig. 8–2).

To evaluate infant behavior within the subsystems of function addressed in the synactive model, Als[7] and coworkers[8] developed the Assessment of Preterm Infant Behavior. With the development of this assessment instrument, a fifth subsystem of behavioral organization, self-regulation, was added to the synactive model. The self-regulation subsystem consists of physiological, motor, and behavioral state strategies used by the neonate to maintain balance within and between the subsystems.[127] For example, many preterm infants appear to regulate overstimulating environmental conditions with a behavioral state strategy of withdrawing into a drowsy or light sleep state, thereby shutting out sensory input. The withdrawal strategy is used more frequently than crying because it requires less energy and less physiological drain to immature, inefficient organ systems.

Fetters[78] placed the synactive model within a dynamic systems framework to demonstrate the effect of a therapeutic intervention on an infant's multiple subsystems (Fig. 8–3). She explained that although a neonatal therapy

intervention is offered to the infant at the level of the person, outcome is measured at the systems level, where many subsystems may be affected. For example, the motor outcome from neonatal therapy procedures is frequently influenced by "synaction," or simultaneous effects, of an infant's physiological stability and behavioral state. Physiological state and behavioral state are therefore potential confounding variables during research on motor behavior in neonatal subjects. Neonatal therapists may find this combined dynamic systems and synactive framework helpful in conceptualizing and assessing changes in infants' multiple subsystems during and after therapy procedures.

Hope-Empowerment Model

A major component of the intervention process in neonatal therapy is the interpersonal helping relationship with the family. A hope-empowerment framework (Fig. 8–4) may guide neonatal practitioners in building the therapeutic partnership with parents, facilitating adaptive coping, and empowering them to participate in caregiving, problem solving, and advocacy. The birth of an infant at risk for a disability, or the diagnosis of such a disability, may create both developmental and situational crises for the parents and the family system. The developmental crisis involves adapting to changing roles in the transition to parenthood and in expanding the family system. Although not occurring unexpectedly, this developmental transition for the parents brings lifestyle changes that may be stressful and cause conflict.[1]

A situational crisis occurs from unexpected external events presenting a sudden, overwhelming threat or loss for which previous coping strategies either are not applicable or are immobilized.[43, 114] The unfamiliar, high-technology, often chaotic NICU environment creates many situational stresses that challenge parenting efforts and destabilize the family system. The language of the nursery is unfamiliar and intimidating. The sights of fragile, sick infants surrounded by medical equipment and the sounds of monitor alarms are frightening. The high frequency of seemingly uncomfortable but required medical procedures for the infant are of financial and humanistic concern to parents. No previous experiences in everyday life

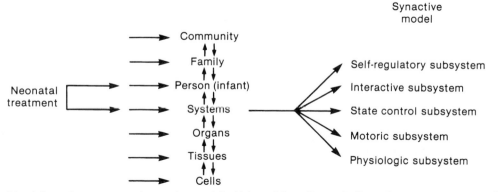

FIGURE 8–3. Combined dynamic systems and synactive models. (Adapted from Fetters L: Sensorimotor management of the high-risk neonate. Phys Occup Ther Pediatr 6:217, 1986.)

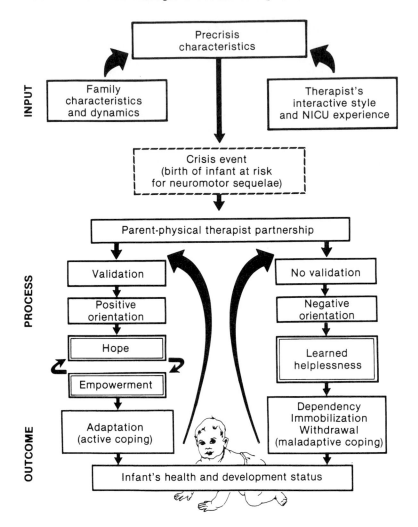

FIGURE 8–4. Hope-empowerment *(left)* versus learned helplessness *(right)* processes of the therapeutic partnership between parents and neonatal therapist.

have prepared parents for this unnatural, emergency-oriented environment.

The quality and orientation of the helping relationship in neonatal therapy affect the coping style of parents as they try to adapt to developmental and situational crises (see Fig. 8–4). Although parents and neonatal therapists come into the partnership with established interactive styles and varying life and professional experiences, the initial contacts during assessment and program planning set the stage for either a positive or a negative orientation to the relationship.

Despite many uncertainties about the clinical course, prognosis, and quality of social support, a positive orientation is activated by validation or acknowledgment of parents' feelings and experiences. Validation then becomes a catalyst to a hope-empowerment process in which many crisis events, negative feelings, and insecurities are acknowledged in a positive, supportive, nonjudgmental context where decision-making power is shared.[158] In contrast, a negative orientation may be facilitated inadvertently by information overloading without exploration and validation of parents' feelings, experiences, and learning styles. This may lead to magnified uncertainty, fear, and powerlessness with the perception of excessive complexity in the proposed neuromotor intervention.

In a hope-empowerment framework, parent participa-

tion in neuromotor intervention allows sharing of power and responsibility and promotes continuous, mutual setting and revision of goals with reality grounding. Adaptive power can be generated by helping parents stabilize and focus energy and plans and by encouraging active participation in intervention and advocacy activities.[158] Exploring external power sources (e.g., Parents of Prematures or Parent-to-Parent support groups) early in the therapeutic relationship may help parents with focusing and mobilizing.[147]

Hope and empowerment are interactive processes. They are influenced by existential philosophy: the hope to adapt to what is and the hope to later find peace of mind and meaning for the situation, regardless of the infant's outcome. In describing the effect of a prematurely born infant on the parenting process, Mercer[146] related that "hope seems to be a motivational, emotional component that gives parents energy to cope, to continue to work, and to strive for the best outcome for a child." She viewed the destruction of hope as contributing to the physical and emotional withdrawal observed frequently in parents who attempt to protect themselves from additional pain and disappointment and then have difficulty reattaching to the infant.

In a hope-empowerment context, parent teaching activities are carefully selected to contribute to pleasurable interaction between infant and parent. Gradual participation in infant care activities and therapeutic handling in the NICU provides experience and builds confidence for carryover to the home environment.

Conversely, if the parents' learning styles, goals, priorities, values, time constraints, energy levels, and emotional availability are not considered in the design of the developmental program, the parents may experience failure, loss of self-esteem, powerlessness, immobilization, or dependency. The neonatal therapist may recognize signs of learned helplessness in parents when they show nonattendance, noncompliance, negative interactions with infant and staff, or hopeless outlook during bedside teaching sessions.

New events in the infant's health or developmental status may create new crises and destabilize the coping processes.[1] In long-term follow-up many opportunities occur within the partnership to validate new fears and chronic uncertainties within a hopeful, positively oriented helping relationship. The alleviation of hopelessness is a critical helping task in health care. This model provides a conceptual framework for sharing with parents and caregivers the gifts of hope and power.

NEUROPATHOLOGY OF MOVEMENT DISORDERS

The neurodevelopmental outcome for infants born prematurely, or for term infants with prenatal or birth complications, depends on the *timing* of a brain injury, as well as on the *nature* of an insult to the developing brain. Different components of the fetal central nervous system are more vulnerable to noxious events or exposures at specific times in the maturational process. For example, insults occurring early in pregnancy typically result in neural tube defects, dysmorphic features, and congenital malformations. The subcortical periventricular region of the fetal brain is more vulnerable to injury during the gestational period spanning the late second trimester and early third trimester, whereas the basal ganglia and cerebral cortex are more susceptible as the fetus approaches term. This selective vulnerability is related to the temporal sequence of maturation of specific structures and systems within the fetal brain, including vascular networks, metabolic processes, and myelination of the neural axons.

During the past decade, improved technology and higher-resolution imaging equipment have provided more detailed insight into neurological structures and physiology, and previously held views regarding the development and pathology of the fetal brain are being revised. It is now generally recognized that the neuropathology most directly related to movement disorders in preterm infants involves areas of the brain that are composed primarily of "white matter," as opposed to the "gray matter" areas, such as the cerebral cortex, striatum, and cerebellum.[126] As stated by Paneth and co-authors, "The cardinal feature of brain damage in the preterm infant is injury to the hemispheric white matter."[163]

The white matter is composed of axons and axon tracts that transmit nervous system impulses from one area of the brain to other areas of the central and peripheral

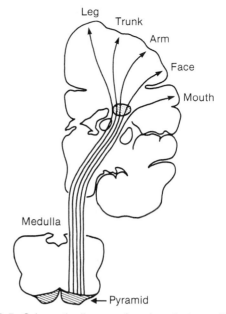

FIGURE 8–5. Schematic diagram of corticospinal tract fibers that extend from the motor cortex through the periventricular region into the pyramid of the medulla.

nervous systems. The characteristic white color of white matter is derived from the myelin sheath of fatty acid that surrounds the axons. Because white matter regions include a predominance of motor projection fiber bundles, impairment of motor function is a logical consequence of injury in this location. Figure 8–5 illustrates the vulnerability of the medial corticospinal tract fibers that extend from the motor cortex through the periventricular region. The two primary lesions of white matter, *periventricular leukomalacia* (PVL) and *periventricular hemorrhagic infarction* (PHI), are described, as well as other lesions that commonly occur in the preterm infant, *germinal matrix and intraventricular hemorrhage* (GM/IVH), and the neuropathology that is more typically seen in the term infant.

Germinal Matrix/Intraventricular Hemorrhage

The most common type of brain lesion occurring in the premature infant is hemorrhage, which typically originates in the subependymal layer of the germinal matrix (GM) and extends into the intraventricular space of the lateral ventricles (IVH). GM/IVH occurs in 20% to 30% of LBW infants, which represents a decline from a level of 40% to 50% over a decade ago.[141, 164, 168, 232, 233] The reduction in the incidence of IVH is due to improved neonatal management, including administration of indomethacin to high-risk neonates.

The GM is the source of the neuroblasts, or germinal cells of the cerebrum, and the glioblasts, which subsequently differentiate into astrocytes and oligodendrocytes. Toward the end of the second trimester of gestation, the GM is a region of high metabolic activity, and the endothelial walls of the vasculature in this area are immature and fragile. This anatomical vulnerability, coupled with the immaturity of vascular autoregulation at this time, contributes to the susceptibility to GM hemorrhage in response to fluctuations in cardiovascular pressure. In the majority of cases of GM hemorrhage, blood extends into the lateral ventricles and GM/IVH may or may not be accompanied by distention or dilatation of the ventricles.

Severity of GM/IVH is typically graded according to the location of the blood and the presence of ventricular dilatation. The criteria for grades I through III IVH are presented in Table 8–1. Earlier descriptions of IVH often included another category, "grade IV IVH," described as an extension of the IVH into the brain parenchyma. However, this lesion is no longer recognized as a progression of IVH and is presently referred to as *periventricular hemorrhagic infarction* (PHI).[164, 232] Hydrocephalus, or progressive dilatation of the ventricles, is a major complication of GM/IVH. A distinction is made by some neuropathologists between *hydrocephalus*, which is ventricular enlargement resulting from disruption of cerebrospinal fluid absorption by a blood clot or other condition, and *posthemorrhagic ventriculomegaly*, which occurs subsequent to PVL or PHI.[232] In the posthemorrhagic type, ventricular enlargement is believed to result from passive expansion of the ventricles into adjoining periventricular areas of damaged white matter tissue, not because of increased intracranial pressure.[126, 164]

The relationship between GM/IVH and neurodevelopmental outcome has been investigated extensively since cranial ultrasononography became a routine NICU procedure for VLBW infants in the 1980s. However, reliable and consistent prediction is complicated by variations in the grading criteria used to describe the severity of IVH and in the outcome measures used in follow-up. Longitudinal studies that relate neonatal brain abnormalities to long-term outcome are often based on cranial ultrasound examinations performed with less sophisticated technology, as well as on less knowledge about neonatal pathology, than currently available. Consequently, earlier studies are more likely to associate adverse neurodevelopmental outcomes with GM/IVH, whereas more recent investigations evaluate outcome in relation to concurrent abnormalities, such as PHI and PVL, in addition to GM/IVH.[238] Because specific neonatal brain lesions usually do not occur in isolation but exist with other pathological features, attribution of a neurodevelopmental disability to a specific type of lesion can be misleading.

The neurodevelopmental outcome of infants with grade I or II hemorrhage is generally recognized to be favorable, with the majority of infants showing no adverse sequelae[16, 77, 171] (Table 8–2). Paneth and colleagues sup-

TABLE 8–1. Grades of Germinal Matrix/Intraventricular Hemorrhage

Grade	Description of Hemorrhage
I	Germinal matrix hemorrhage (no intraventricular hemorrhage)
II	Intraventricular hemorrhage into lateral ventricle(s) (no ventricular distention)
III	Intraventricular hemorrhage with distention of lateral ventricle(s)

TABLE 8–2. Neurodevelopmental Outcome of LBW/VLBW Infants Relative to Presence of GM/IVH

Grade of Hemorrhage	Outcome	
	Major Disability	Cerebral Palsy
I	5%	0
II	15%	0–5%
III	25–60%	25–50%

Data from references 16, 77, 119, 163, 172, and 232.

port this finding: "Since the germinal matrix is destined to involute, . . . and bleeding into the ventricles likewise in itself does not interfere with the function of any part of the brain: it is reassuring to discover that GM/IVH—the most common neurologic lesion in preterm infants, . . . is not associated with a substantial risk of later disability."[163] On the other hand, grade III IVH (i.e., IVH with ventriculomegaly) is associated with an increased risk of major neurological impairment.[16, 77, 119, 172] Cerebral palsy has been reported to occur in 30% to 70% of neonates with persistent ventricular enlargement, and even transient ventriculomegaly appears to be associated with a greater incidence of neurodevelopmental disability (Fig. 8–6).[2, 16, 119, 126]

Periventricular Hemorrhagic Infarction

Periventricular hemorrhagic infarction refers to a relatively large region of hemorrhagic necrosis in the periven-

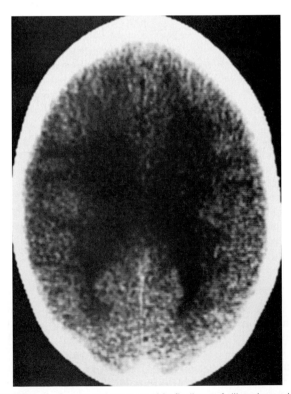

FIGURE 8–6. Computed tomographic findings of dilated ventricles from a child with the spastic diplegia category of cerebral palsy.

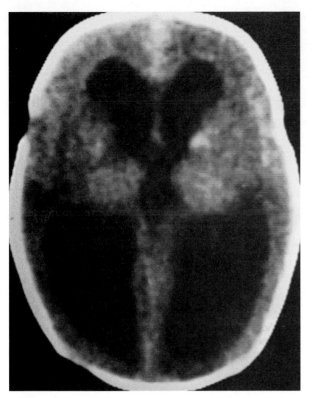

FIGURE 8–7. Computed tomographic findings of ventriculomegaly and hydrocephalus in an infant with periventricular hemorrhagic infarction.

tricular white matter. PHI occurs in approximately 15% of infants with GM/IVH, primarily those with grade III IVH.[232] The majority of PHI lesions occur in conjunction with a GM hemorrhage or IVH on the same side of the brain (Fig. 8–7). PHI has a characteristic fan-shaped distribution that corresponds to the distribution of the medullary veins in the periventricular white matter.[163, 232] These observations, as well as other characteristics of this lesion, contribute to the current hypothesis that PHI is caused by venous infarction resulting from compression or obstruction of the medullary veins by a GM/IVH blood clot.[168] The concept of "grade IV IVH" that was described in earlier literature has generally been replaced by the current view of PHI as a lesion that is independent from IVH but may result as a complication of GM/IVH.[163] PHI in the LBW infant is associated with significantly increased risk for adverse neurological sequelae. Cerebral palsy, predominantly of the spastic quadriplegic or hemiplegic type, reportedly occurs in 60% to 80% of infants with this type of lesion[2, 16, 53, 232, 238] (Table 8–3).

Periventricular Leukomalacia

Periventricular leukomalacia refers to areas of cellular necrosis of the white matter in a specific location in the fetal brain, adjacent to the external angles of the lateral ventricles. The terminology of PVL, which was derived from neuropathological studies that were done before the time of routine ultrasonography, does not accurately describe the appearance of this lesion on cranial ultrasonograms of surviving preterm infants. However, whereas some researchers recommend alternate designations, such as *white matter damage*, PVL remains the most widely used term. PVL occurs primarily in preterm infants, particularly those born between 28 and 32 weeks' gestation. Ultrasound studies with serial scans of VLBW infants indicate that 15% to 30% of surviving neonates demonstrate areas of periventricular echogenicity. For the majority of infants, PVL is apparently transient; cystic PVL reportedly occurs in 5% to 11% of VLBW infants.[67, 163, 188, 238]

The primary pathological manifestation of PVL consists of focal, or localized, areas of cellular necrosis believed to represent axonal degeneration. These areas are seen as echodensities on cranial ultrasonograms. Sequential cranial ultrasonograms of surviving neonates reveal a typical evolutionary course beginning with areas of increased echogenicity in the periventricular region. Over a period of days, cavitation occurs in these echodense areas, which then evolve into either small localized cysts, usually in the frontoparietal area, or extensive cystic lesions in the occipital and frontoparietal white matter.[77, 163] This process of cyst formation occurs over a course of weeks so identification and classification of PVL will depend on the timing, as well as on the number, of ultrasound studies performed in an infant. Further investigation of these lesions with magnetic resonance imaging (MRI) has revealed that the areas of localized brain injury are usually accompanied by broader, more diffuse regions of white matter damage, extending beyond the periventricular area and often not detectable by routine cranial ultrasonography.[67, 116] In contrast to the process of cyst formation, some echodense areas in the periventricular region resolve without evidence of residual abnormality and are referred to as transient periventricular echodensities (TPE), or "flares."[49, 59, 188]

The pathogenesis of PVL is believed to involve ischemia coupled with unique aspects of the fetal brain. The characteristic location of PVL in the periventricular region appears to be related to the vascular distribution in this area. Earlier theories were based on the concept of "watershed" areas, described as boundary zones between arterial sources that might be inadequately perfused and therefore susceptible to ischemic injury.[232] Whereas this "watershed" view has not been upheld by recent neuropathological and ultrasonographic investigation, researchers continue to suspect that the localized distribution of PVL is related to a susceptibility to ischemia that is related to critical stages of vascular development in this region.[163]

T A B L E 8 – 3. Neurodevelopmental Outcome of LBW/VLBW Infants Relative to Periventricular Hemorrhagic Infarction (PHI)

| Severity of PHI | Outcome | |
	Cerebral Palsy	Cognitive Disability
Localized	60–80%	30–50%
Extensive	80–100%	40–50%

Data from references 16, 67, 163, 232, and 237.

A second key feature in the pathogenesis of PVL is the vulnerability of the cellular tissue at the time of injury. During the period between 28 and 34 weeks' gestation, myelin, which facilitates the transmission of nerve impulses, is deposited around the axons projecting through the periventricular region. Myelin is produced by glial cells, the oligodendrocytes, in a predictable sequence of time and location within the fetal brain during the latter half of gestation and the first year of life. Myelination appears to occur earlier in the deep white matter areas of the frontal, occipital, and parietal regions and progresses to the temporal lobe and cortical areas later.[2, 19, 163] Histological studies of areas of PVL reveal specific damage to the myelin-producing glial cells and infiltration by hypertrophic astrocytes, the progenitors of glial cells. The process of myelination, in which oligodendrocytes differentiate to produce the myelin sheaths, requires high levels of energy and glucose to synthesize the lipids and cholesterol necessary for myelin composition. It is hypothesized that during critical periods of gestation when the oligodendrocytes are differentiating within the fetal brain, these cells are more susceptible to toxic influences, such as increased concentrations of glutamate and nitrous oxide.[126]

The relationship between PVL observed on neonatal cranial ultrasonography and neurovelopmental outcome depends primarily on the location, the extent, and the duration of periventricular echodensity and on the degree of cavitation or cyst formation (Table 8–4). Transient echodensities that resolve within 2 to 4 weeks appear to be of little prognostic significance relative to major disability. In contrast, infants with large cystic lesions, usually seen in the frontoparietal or frontparietooccipital areas of the brain, are at high risk for major neurodevelopmental disability.[2, 67, 149, 163, 192] Bilateral cystic PVL is associated with spastic quadriparesis, whereas asymmetrical cysts are typically associated with spastic diplegia or hemiplegia.[150] Smaller areas of localized cystic PVL have been associated with less severe cerebral palsy in 50% to 60% of the cases.[67] Echodense areas that persist but without apparent cyst formation, observed in 10% to 20% of VLBW infants, are associated with more variable outcome.

The relationship between neonatal PVL and subsequent motor disability is further supported by MRI studies of older children. MR images of children with spastic cerebral palsy have consistently revealed atrophy of white matter and high-intensity areas adjacent to the lateral ventricles.[49, 67, 116, 157] In one study of *nondisabled* VLBW children at 6 years of age, periventricular gliosis that was observed in the white matter was associated with fine and gross motor deficits and inferior performance on tests of visual-perceptual function.[229]

Selective Neuronal Necrosis

Selective neuronal necrosis (SNN) refers to a type of brain injury that usually results from a neonatal hypoxic-ischemic event.[232] As the name indicates, it is characterized by necrosis of neurons with a characteristic distribution in multiple areas of the brain. The primary regions of injury are the cerebral cortex, hippocampus, and cerebellum in the term infant; components of the brain stem (pons and inferior nuclei) in the LBW infant; and the basal ganglia and thalamus for both term and preterm infants. Severe oxygen deprivation appears to be a major factor in the pathogenesis of SNN, and SNN is frequently associated with intrapartum asphyxia in the full-term infant.[232] Although the hypoxic-ischemic event, such as total or near-total asphyxia, may be a global insult to the central nervous system, the selective vulnerability of specific areas of the brain is believed to reflect varying levels of metabolic activity in different regions at the time of injury. The neurological sequelae associated with SNN are related to the specific sites of necrosis. Injury in the cerebral cortex is associated with mental retardation and a high incidence of seizures; neuromotor consequences, including hypotonia, spastic quadriplegia, and ataxia, result from damage in the cerebellum, basal ganglia, and regions of the motor cortex.

Parasagittal Cerebral Injury/Focal (Multifocal) Ischemic Brain Necrosis

Two lesions that are primarily seen in full-term infants are parasagittal cerebral injury and focal/multifocal ischemic brain necrosis. Parasagittal cerebral injury, characterized by diffuse cortical atrophy and cystic lesions in the subadjacent white matter, occurs predominantly in the parietooccipital region. This type of injury, which is associated with perinatal asphyxia in term infants, is usually bilateral with fairly symmetrical distribution between the two hemispheres.[232] The most frequent long-term neurodevelopmental consequence of parasagittal cerebral injury is spastic quadriparesis. Focal ischemic brain necrosis refers to injury due to infarction that leads to necrotic areas within a particular vascular distribution. The middle cerebral artery is the most common vascular site of injury in the term infant, occurring more frequently on the left side of the brain.[120] The neurodevelopmental consequences of this type of injury are determined by the location and extent of the lesion. Spastic hemiparesis, especially right hemiplegia, is the most common outcome, as well as spastic quadriparesis and seizures.

CLINICAL MANAGEMENT: NEONATAL PERIOD

Pediatric therapists with precepted subspecialty training in neonatology and infant therapy can expand neonatal

---

T A B L E 8 – 4. Neurodevelopmental Outcome of LBW/VLBW Infants Relative to Periventricular Leukomalacia (PVL)

	Outcome	
Severity of PVL	Mild Motor Deficits	Cerebral Palsy
Transient echodensities ("flares")	0–30%	4–10%
Persistent echodensities without cyst formation	0–30%	7–15%
Periventricular leukomalacia		
Localized cysts		25–67%°
Extensive cysts		70–100%°

°Bilateral cysts are associated with increased likelihood of poor outcome.
Data from references 16, 67, 110, 163, and 188.

medicine efforts by creating clinical protocols and pathways designed to optimize the development and interaction of neonates and parents. The therapeutic partnership between parents and neonatal therapists during developmental intervention in the NICU sets the stage for competency in caregiving and compliance with follow-up in the outpatient period. General aims of NICU clinical management of infants at risk for neurological dysfunction, developmental delay, or musculoskeletal complications are to (1) promote posture and movement appropriate to gestational age and medical stability, (2) support symmetry and biomechanical alignment of extremities and trunk while multiple lines and equipment are required, (3) decrease potential musculoskeletal deformity and acquired joint-muscle contractures, (4) foster infant-parent attachment and interaction, (5) modify sensory stimulation in the infant's NICU environment to promote behavioral organization and physiological stability, (6) provide consultation or direct intervention for neonatal feeding dysfunction and oral-motor deficits, (7) enhance parents' caregiving skills (feeding, dressing, bathing, positioning of infant for sleep, interaction/play, and transportation), and (8) prepare for hospital discharge and integration to home and community environments.

Educational Requirements for Therapists

Examination and treatment of neonates are advanced-level, not entry-level, clinical competencies. Neonatology is a subspecialty within the specialty areas of pediatric physical therapy and pediatric occupational therapy. No amount of literature review, self-study, or experience with other pediatric populations can substitute for clinical training with a preceptor in an NICU. The potential for causing harm to medically fragile infants during well-intentioned intervention is enormous.[167] The ongoing clinical decisions made by neonatal therapists in evaluating and managing physiological and musculoskeletal risks while handling small (2 or 3 lb), potentially unstable infants in the NICU should not be a trial-and-error experience at the infants' expense. Therapists with adult-oriented training and even those with general pediatric clinical training (excluding neonatal) are not qualified for neonatal practice without a supervised clinical practicum (usually 2 to 3 months). The NICU is not an appropriate practice area for physical therapy assistants, occupational therapy assistants, or student therapists on affiliations, for the following reasons, outlined by Sweeney and colleagues: "handling of vulnerable infants in the NICU requires ongoing examination, interpretation, and multiple adjustments of procedures, interventions, and sequences to minimize risk for infants who are physiologically, behaviorally, and motorically unstable or potentially unstable."[219] The physical or occupational therapy assistant and student therapist are not prepared, even with supervision, to "provide moment-to-moment examination and evaluation of the infant and have the ability or modify or stop preplanned interventions when the infant's behavior, motor, or physiological organization begins to move outside the limits of stability with handling or feeding."[219]

Delineation of advanced-level roles, competencies, and knowledge for the physical therapist[219] and the occupational therapist[10] in the NICU setting have been described separately by national task forces from the American Physical Therapy Association and the American Occupational Therapy Association. These practice guidelines provide a structure for assessing competence of individual therapists working in NICU settings and offer a framework for designing clinical paths for specific neonatal therapy services.

A gradual, sequential entry to neonatal practice is advised by building clinical experience with infants of term gestation as well as with physiologically fragile older infants and children and their parents. The experience may include managing caseloads of hospitalized children on physiological monitoring equipment, external feeding lines, and supplemental oxygen or ventilators. Participating in discharge planning and in outpatient follow-up of high-risk neonates are other options for providing exposure to examination, intervention, and family issues when the infants and parents are more stable. This clinical experience and a precepted practicum in the special care nursery offer the best preparation for appropriate, accountable, and ethical practice in neonatal therapy.[219, 220]

Indications for Referral

Research efforts in recent years have been directed toward determining which neonates will have adverse neurodevelopmental outcomes. Specific prenatal, perinatal, and neonatal conditions that are associated with an increased likelihood of long-term neuromotor disability have been identified as risk factors.[30, 111] However, the predictive value of these risk factors is compromised by the absence of uniform or consistent definitions, differences in the study samples and follow-up procedures, and lack of standard measures of neurodevelopmental outcome. Moreover, ongoing changes in obstetrical and neonatal procedures limit the applicability of findings from longitudinal studies of infants born in earlier eras of NICU care.

Tjossem's categories[224] of biological, established, and social risk provide a framework for categorizing indicators for neonatal therapy referral. An overview of developmental risk categories and risk factors for neonatal therapy referral is listed in the box on page 212 to assist clinicians in developing a referral mechanism for a clinical protocol based on risk categories.

Biological Risk. Biological risk refers to neurodevelopmental risk due to medical or physiological conditions in the prenatal, perinatal, or neonatal period.[30, 224] Biological risks include placental abnormalities, labor/delivery complications, prenatal infection, and teratogenic factors. Examples of biological risk factors include asphyxia, neonatal seizures, prenatal exposure to cocaine or alcohol, and the cranial ultrasound abnormalities described earlier. Birth weight is a strong predictor of outcome; in general, lower birth weight is associated with greater risk for adverse developmental outcome.[28, 91, 153]

Respiratory disease is generally considered to be an important risk factor for motor and cognitive disability in LBW infants. Although the presence of respiratory dis-

DEVELOPMENTAL RISK INDICATORS FOR NEONATAL THERAPY REFERRAL

Biological Risk

Birth weight of 1500 g or less

Gestational age of 32 weeks or less

Small for gestational age (less than 10th percentile for weight)

Prenatal exposure to drugs or alcohol

Ventilator requirement for 36 hours or more

Intracranial hemorrhage: grade III

Periventricular leukomalacia

Muscle tone abnormalities (hypotonia, hypertonia, asymmetry of tone/movement)

Recurrent neonatal seizures (3 or more)

Feeding dysfunction

Symptomatic TORCH infections (toxoplasmosis, rubella, cytomegalovirus infection, herpesvirus type 2 infection)

Meningitis

Asphyxia with Apgar score less than 4 at 5 minutes

Multiple birth

Established Risk

Hydrocephalus

Microcephaly

Chromosomal abnormalities

Musculoskeletal abnormalities (congenitally dislocated hips, limb deficiencies, arthrogryposis, joint contractures, congenital torticollis)

Brachial plexus injuries (Erb's palsy, Klumpke's paralysis)

Myelodysplasia

Congenital myopathies and myotonic dystrophy

Inborn errors of metabolism

Human immunodeficiency virus infection

Down syndrome

Environmental/Social Risk

High social risk (single parent, parental age younger than 17 years, poor-quality infant-parent attachment)

Maternal drug or alcohol abuse

Behavioral state abnormalities (lethargy, excessive irritability, behavioral state lability)

---

ease alone does not appear to be predictive of neurodevelopmental outcome,[27] severity of disease does appear to be related to long-term outcome. Infants with chronic lung disease or bronchopulmonary disease have been found to be at increased risk for cerebral palsy and other neurodevelopmental abnormalities compared with preterm infants without bronchopulmonary disease.[2, 40, 231] Prolonged mechanical ventilation and duration of supplemental oxygen were associated with increased risk of neurodevelopmental disability in some studies.[40, 204] Administration of surfactant in the neonatal period has reduced the incidence and severity of respiratory disease in VLBW infants but has not been associated with a decline in neurodevelopmental disability in these children.[2]

Established Risk. Established risk is the risk for neurodevelopmental deficits associated with a diagnosis that is clearly established in the neonatal period. Included in this category are congenital malformations, chromosomal abnormalities, central nervous system disorders, and metabolic diseases with known developmental sequelae.

Environmental/Social Risk. Environmental/social risk involves developmental risk related to competency in parenting roles and factors in family dynamics.[124, 203] Such risk may be heightened by prolonged hospitalization of infants with suboptimal levels of stimulation and interaction (overstimulation or deprivation) in the intensive care nursery environment, inadequate infant-parent attach-

ment, insufficient educational preparation of parents for caregiving roles, meager financial resources, and limited or absent family support to assist in taking care of and nurturing the infant in the home environment.

It is common for LBW neonates to have a combination of risk factors from more than one major category. For example, an infant born prematurely to a single mother who is in a drug treatment program because of her use of heroin during pregnancy is considered to be at both biological and environmental risk. In-depth study of perinatal and neonatal medicine and related obstetrical, neonatal nursing, and neonatal therapy literature is recommended before beginning to develop a neonatal therapy protocol or clinical pathway and participate on the special care nursery team.

Neonatal Neurological Assessment

Multiple neonatal neurological and neurobehavioral examinations have been developed to assess the integrity of the nervous system, to calculate gestational age, and to describe newborn behavior.[11, 41, 82, 129, 189] Six frequently used instruments are the Clinical Assessment of Gestational Age,[72] the Newborn Maturity Rating,[17] the Neurological Examination of the Full-term Infant,[179] the Brazelton Neonatal Behavioral Assessment Scale,[36] the Neurological Assessment of the Preterm and Full-term Newborn Infant,[74] and the Assessment of Preterm Infant

Behavior.[6] These instruments were selected to familiarize the reader with a range of neurological and behavioral tools used in current practice for management of both preterm and term infants. Most of these instruments offer quality data on motor performance and interactional behavior that are essential for developing individualized treatment plans.

Clinical Assessment of Gestational Age in the Newborn Infant. The Clinical Assessment of Gestational Age in the Newborn Infant[72] was developed by Dubowitz and associates from data for a total of 167 preterm and full-term infants (28 to 42 weeks' gestation) tested within 5 days of birth. It focuses on criteria for calculation of gestational age from a composite of 10 neurological and 11 external features.

This test rates criteria on a four-point scale; it is commonly administered by nurses or physicians in the newborn nursery. The accuracy (95% confidence limit) of the gestational age score is determined within a variation of ±2 weeks on any single assessment. This measurement error can be decreased to approximately ±1.4 weeks when two separate assessments are performed. From the analyses of multiple assessments on 70 of the 167 infants, the age score was equally reliable in the first 24 hours of age as during the next 4 days of life. The behavioral state(s) of the infant during the assessment is not considered a significant variable in the examination.

Calculation of gestational age is an important adjunct to all other neonatal assessment tools: it guides practitioners in interpreting neurological and behavioral findings relative to the expected performance of neonates at various gestational ages. Additional guidelines on gestational differences in neurological, physical, and neuromuscular maturation can be found in the work of Lubchenco[129] and Amiel-Tison.[11–13]

Newborn Maturity Rating. Ballard and colleagues designed a simplified modification of the Dubowitz gestational age tool. It has been widely adopted because of the time efficiency (3 to 4 minutes versus 10 to 15 minutes) and the elimination of active tone items, which are difficult to evaluate reliably in physiologically unstable newborns. The Ballard instrument involves only six physical and six neurological criteria with a 0 to 5 scale and a maturity rating beginning at 20 weeks. It is designed to be used for neonates from birth through 5 days of age and has demonstrated concurrent validity with the Dubowitz gestational age calculation tool.[17, 18]

The Neurological Examination of the Full-Term Infant. The Neurological Examination of the Full-Term Infant[179] was designed by Prechtl to identify abnormal neurological signs in the newborn period. The examination was developed from an investigation of more than 1350 newborns and was standardized on infants born at the gestational age of 38 to 42 weeks. If the test is used in premature infants who have reached an age of 38 to 42 weeks of gestation, lower resistance to passive movements (lower tone) may be expected. Delay of testing until a minimum of 3 days of age is advised to maximize the stability of behavioral states and neuromotor responses for improved reliability and validity of results.

The pattern of examination includes an observation period and an examination period. A 10-minute screening examination is offered to determine if the full 30-minute assessment of posture, tone, reflexes, and spontaneous movement is required. Although specific requirements for examiner training are not addressed, Prechtl offers a flow diagram (Fig. 8–8) to assist clinicians with organizing the neurological examination process. Significant findings from the examination are summarized in the following categories: (1) quality of posture, spontaneous movement, and muscle tone (consistency and resistance to passive movement), (2) presence of involuntary or pathological movements (clonus, tremor, athetoid postures or movements), (3) behavioral state changes and quality of cry, and (4) threshold/intensity of responses to stimulation. Because of the transient pattern of neurological signs and rapid changes in the developing nervous system, Prechtl advises repeated examinations to monitor neurological status.

Neonatal Behavioral Assessment Scale (NBAS). To document individual behavioral and motoric differences in term infants, Brazelton and colleagues developed a neonatal behavior scale to assess neuromotor responses within a behavioral state context.[36] The 30- to 45-minute examination consists of observing, eliciting, and scoring 28 biobehavioral items on a 9-point scale and 18 reflex items on a 4-point scale. The reflex items are derived from the neurological examination protocol of Prechtl and Beintema.[180]

The scale was designed to assess newborn behavior in healthy 3-day-old term (40-week gestation) white infants whose mothers had minimal sedative medication during an uncomplicated labor and delivery. Use of this examination with preterm infants requires modification of the examination procedure to the environmental constraints of an intensive care nursery and interpretation of findings relative to the gestational age and medical condition of the infant. For preterm infants approaching term (minimum of 36 weeks of gestation), nine supplementary behavioral items are offered. Many of these items were developed by Als[6] for use with preterm and physiologically stressed infants.

Although the mean scores are related to the expected behavior of 3-day-old term infants, the NBAS is considered an appropriate assessment tool from 37 weeks of gestation until 44 weeks of gestation. Extended use of this scale for older infants was reported by Provost,[181, 182] who described the methods for and results from administering the scale with the Kansas Supplements (five additional items on a 9-point scale) to 11 normal, full-term infants during the first 4 months of life.

The NBAS outlines six behavioral state categories: deep sleep, light sleep, drowsiness/semidozing, quiet alert, active alert, and crying. Behavioral state prerequisites are provided for each biobehavioral and reflex item to reduce the state-related variables in testing. During the assessment the examiner systematically maneuvers the infant from the sleep states to crying and back to the alert states to evaluate physiological, organizational, motoric, and interactive capabilities during stimulation and physical handling. The scoring is based on the infant's best perfor-

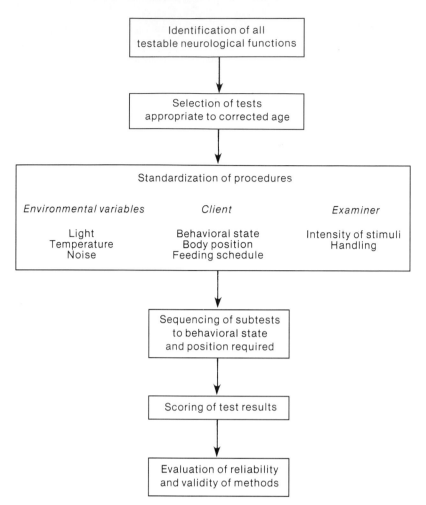

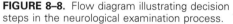

FIGURE 8–8. Flow diagram illustrating decision steps in the neurological examination process.

mance, with flexibility allowed in the order of testing, repetition of items encouraged, and scheduling of the assessment midway between feedings to give the infant every advantage to demonstrate the best possible responses.

Four dimensions of newborn behavior are analyzed in the Brazelton Scale: interactive ability, motor behavior, behavioral state organization, and physiological organization. Interactive ability describes the infant's response to visual and auditory stimuli (Fig. 8–9), consolability from the crying state with intervention by the examiner, and ability to maintain alertness and respond to social/environmental stimuli.

Motor behavior refers to the ability to modulate muscle tone and motor control for the performance of integrated motor skills, such as the hand-to-mouth maneuver, pull-to-sit maneuver, and defensive reaction (e.g., removal of cloth from face). In the assessment of behavioral state organization, the infant's ability to organize behavioral states when stimulated and the ability to shut out irritating environmental stimuli when sleeping are analyzed. Physiological organization is analyzed by observing the infant's ability to manage physiological stress (changes of skin color, frequency of tremulous movement in the chin and extremities, number of startle reactions during the assessment).

Performance profiles of worrisome or deficient interactive-motoric and organizational behavior are identified by clusters of behavior associated with potential developmental risk.[8, 124, 208] The cluster systems are highly useful for clinical interpretation and for data analysis aspects of clinical research.[243]

Definite strengths of the NBAS are the well-defined indicators of autonomic stress, the analysis of the coping ability of high-risk infants to external stimuli and handling, and the quality of infant-examiner interaction. These features generate specific findings to assist therapists in grading the intensity of assessment and treatment within each infant's physiological and behavioral tolerance and in guiding the development of parent teaching strategies to address the individual behavioral styles of infants. The Brazelton Scale has proved to be more sensitive to the detection of mild neurological dysfunction in the newborn period than have classic neurological examinations that omit the behavioral dimensions.

Participation of the parent in the newborn assessment may yield long-term positive effects on infant-parent interaction and later on cognitive and fine motor development. Widmayer and Field[241] reported significantly better face-to-face interaction and fine motor/adaptive skills at 4 months of age and higher mental development scores at 12 months of age when teenage mothers of preterm

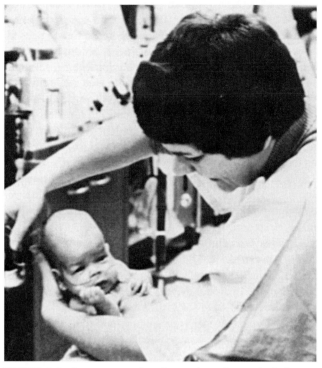

FIGURE 8–9. Assessment of auditory orientation to the bell during neonatal assessment using the Brazelton Neonatal Behavioral Assessment Scale.

streamlined neurological and neurobehavioral assessment designed by Dubowitz and Dubowitz to provide a systematic, quickly administered (10 to 15 minutes) examination applicable to both premature and full-term infants. A distinct advantage of this tool is the minimal training or experience required by the examiner.

The test includes multiple neurobehavioral components of the Brazelton NBAS: The six behavioral state categories and nine neurobehavioral items are scored on a condensed five-point grading scale and sequenced according to the intensity of response. These neurobehavioral items, selected to reflect higher neurological functioning than the brain stem level reflex responses, consist of the following: (1) habituation to light and sound while sleeping, (2) auditory and visual orientation responses (Fig. 8–10), (3) quality and duration of alertness, (4) defensive reaction to a cloth over the face, (5) peak of excitement—the infant's overall responsiveness and variability of behavioral states during the examination, (6) irritability—the frequency of crying to aversive stimuli during reflex testing and handling throughout the examination, and (7) consolability—the ability after crying to reach a calm state independently or with intervention by the examiner. The appearance of the eyes (sunset sign, strabismus, nystagmus) and the quality of the cry are included in the neurobehavioral category because they also require the awake state for testing.

(mean gestational age at birth: 35.1 weeks) infants were given Brazelton Scale demonstrations. These demonstrations were scheduled when the premature infants had reached an age equivalence of 37 weeks' gestation.

Nugent[155, 156] developed parent teaching guidelines for using the Brazelton Scale as an intervention for infants and their families. Published by the March of Dimes Birth Defects Foundation, the guidelines offer strategies for interpreting each item according to its adaptive and developmental significance, descriptions of the expected developmental course of the behavior (item) over several months, and recommendations for caregiving according to the infant's response to the item.

Four films are available for examiner training.[38] In addition, administration and scoring of the NBAS in 15 to 25 infants are recommended to establish reliable testing and interpretation skills. Certification for use of the Brazelton Scales in research is coordinated through The Brazelton Center for Infants and Parents, Children's Hospital, Boston, Massachusetts.[37] Wilhelm[243] recommends NBAS training for clinicians beginning to develop competence in examining at-risk infants. She explains that it provides a system for developing basic handling skills with full-term, healthy infants without concerns of stressing medically fragile preterm infants during the training period. Learning the Brazelton Scale before the Assessment of Preterm Infant Behavior provides familiarity with similar testing and scoring procedures for preterm infants.[243]

Neurological Assessment of the Preterm and Full-Term Newborn Infant. The Neurological Assessment of the Preterm and Full-Term Newborn Infant[74] is a

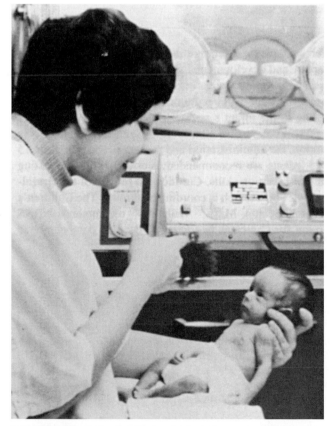

FIGURE 8–10. Evaluation of visual orientation responses (i.e., visual fixation and horizontal tracking) during the Dubowitz Neurological Assessment.

The 15 items that assess movement and tone and the 6 reflex items evolved from clinical trials on 50 full-term infants using the Clinical Assessment of Gestational Age by Dubowitz and colleagues,[72] the Neurological Examination of the Newborn by Parmelee and co-workers,[165] and the Neurological Examination of the Full-Term Newborn Infant by Prechtl.[179] The examination format was then used during a 2-year period on over 500 infants of varying gestational ages. The authors did not present reliability data in the manual but described modification of the protocol during their clinical trial phase that promoted objectivity in scoring and a high interrater reliability among examiners, regardless of experience level.

The examination protocol is outlined and illustrated on a two-page form with space allowed for comments. The illustrated form is constructed to accommodate both baseline and repeat assessments, and it can be effectively combined with an additional narrative impression and treatment goals/plan for neonatal therapy programs. Because a total or summary score is avoided in this examination and because emphasis is given instead to patterns of responses, selected parts of the protocol are appropriate for the assessment of premature or acutely ill infants on ventilators, incubators, or attached to monitoring or infusion equipment. It is recommended that the scheduling of examinations occur two thirds of the way between feedings.

Dubowitz and Dubowitz[74] do not have long-term follow-up data beyond 1 year with this examination. Instead they present and discuss seven case histories, describe experiences using the tool in the evaluation of infants with intraventricular hemorrhage, and report outcome data at 12 months of age. The abnormal neonatal clinical signs that correlated with long-term neurological sequelae were persistent asymmetry, decreased lower extremity movement, and increased tone. Infants with IVH had significantly higher incidence of abnormally tight popliteal angles, reduced mobility, decreased visual fixing and following, and roving eye movements.

Dubowitz and associates[73] reassessed 116 infants (27 to 34 weeks of gestation) at 1 year of age. Of 62 infants assessed as neurologically normal in the newborn period, 91% were also normal at 1 year of age. Of 39 infants assessed as neurologically abnormal in the newborn period, 35% were found to be normal at 1 year of age. According to Wilhelm,[243] the predictive value of a negative test with this instrument was 92%, but the predictive value of a positive test was only 64%.

Clinicians interested in using the Neurological Assessment for Preterm and Full-Term Infants in clinical studies may assign numerical values to the range of descriptive criteria within the items under each major examination category. This technique was used by Morgan and colleagues[147] in efforts to quantitate neonatal neurological status for data analysis.

Interpretations of evaluative findings from the Neurological Assessment for Preterm and Full-Term Newborn Infants for neonatal therapy practice are described comprehensively in a case study format by Heriza[104] and Campbell.[42] Dubowitz[71] discussed the clinical significance of neurological variations in infants and offered decision guidelines to clinicians on when to worry, reassure, and intervene with developmental referrals.

Assessment of Preterm Infant Behavior. Als[6] designed the Assessment of Preterm Infant Behavior (APIB) to structure a comprehensive observation of a preterm infant's autonomic, adaptive, and interactive responses to graded handling and environmental stimuli. As described previously in the theoretical framework section, this assessment is derived from synactive theory and is focused on assessing the organization and balance of the infant's physiological, motor, behavioral state, attention/interaction, and self-regulation subsystems. The APIB follows similar testing sequences and scoring as for the NBAS, with increased complexity and expansion for premature infants.

Administration and scoring of the APIB require 2 to 3 hours per infant, depending on examiner experience. Although the APIB may be an instrument of choice for the clinical researcher, it is not practical (time efficient) for many neonatal clinicians with heavy caseloads in managed care environments.

Extensive training and reliability certification are required to safely administer and accurately score and interpret the test for clinical practice or research. The training is available in Boston and Tucson.[8]

Neonatal Individualized Developmental Care and Assessment Program. Als[7] and colleagues[8, 9] developed the Neonatal Individualized Developmental Care and Assessment Program (NIDCAP) to document the effects of the caregiving environment on the neurobehavioral stability of neonates. This naturalistic observation protocol includes continuous observation and documentation at 2-minute intervals of an infant's behavioral state and autonomic, motor, and attention signals with simultaneous recording of vital signs and oxygen saturation. This documentation occurs before, during, and after routine caregiving procedures. A narrative description of the infant's responses to the stress of handling by the primary nurse and to auditory and visual stimuli in the NICU environment is provided for developing care plans. Options are described in the care plans for reducing aversive environmental stimuli and adapting physical handling procedures. This clinical tool allows neonatal therapists to determine the infant's readiness for assessment and intervention by observing the baseline tolerance of the infant to routine nursing care before superimposing neonatal therapy procedures.[218] Examiner training in the NIDCAP may be coordinated through the National Training Center at the Children's Hospital, Boston, Massachusetts.[218]

Summary. It is essential that practitioners be aware of the normative and validation data and of the predictive characteristics of the test(s) administered to allow appropriate interpretation of the results. Specific clinical training with a preceptor is essential to accurately administer, score, and interpret neonatal assessment instruments; to establish interrater reliability; and to plan treatment based on the evaluative findings. Even low-risk, healthy preterm infants are vulnerable to becoming physiologically and behaviorally destabilized during neurological assessment procedures.[216, 217, 226, 242] This risk is reduced with precepted clinical training in the NICU.

Testing Variables

Neuromuscular and behavioral findings in the newborn period may be influenced by several variables. Increased reliability in examination results and in clinical impressions may occur when these variables are recognized.[14, 52] Medication may produce side effects of low muscle tone, drowsiness, and lethargy. Such medications include anticonvulsants, sedatives for diagnostic procedures (CT scan, electroencephalography, electromyography), and medication for postsurgical pain management. Intermittent subtle seizures may produce changes in muscle tension and in the level of responsiveness. These may be mild, ongoing seizures that present in the neonate as lip smacking or sucking, staring or horizontal gaze, apnea, bradycardia, or stiffening of the extremities more frequently than as clonic movement. Fatigue from medical/nursing procedures can result in decreased tolerance to handling, decreased interaction, and magnified muscle tone abnormalities. Fatigue may also result when neurodevelopmental assessment is scheduled immediately after laboratory (hematologic) procedures, suctioning, ultrasonography, or respiratory (chest percussion) therapy. Metabolic/physiological signs such as tremulous movement in the extremities may be linked to conditions of metabolic imbalance (hypomagnesemia, hypocalcemia, hypoglycemia); low muscle tone may be associated with hyperbilirubinemia, hypoglycemia, hypoxemia, and hypothermia.[14, 31]

Treatment Planning

Level of Stimulation. The issue of safe and therapeutic levels of sensory and neuromotor intervention is a high priority in the design of developmental intervention programs for infants who have been unstable medically. The concept of "infant stimulation," which was introduced by early childhood educators to describe general developmental stimulation programs for healthy infants, is highly inappropriate in an approach based on concepts of dynamic systems, infant behavioral organization, and individualized developmental care.

For intervention to be therapeutic in a special care nursery setting, the amount and type of touch and kinesthetic stimulation must be customized to each infant's physiological tolerance, movement patterns, unique temperament, and level of responsiveness. Rather than needing more stimulation, many infants, especially those with hypertonus or those with tremulous, disorganized movement, have difficulty adapting to the routine levels of noise, light, position changes, and handling in the nursery environment. General, nonindividualized stimulation can quickly magnify abnormal postural tone and movement, increase behavioral state lability and irritability, and stress fragile physiological homeostasis in preterm or chronically ill infants. Implementation of careful physiological monitoring and graded handling techniques are essential to prevent compromise in patient safety and to facilitate development. Infant modulation, rather than stimulation,

is the aim of intervention. Techniques of sensory and neuromotor facilitation and inhibition developed for caseloads of healthy infants and children are usually inappropriate for the developmental needs and expectations of an infant with physiological fragility and with gestational age younger than term.

Physiological and Musculoskeletal Risk Management. Many maturation-related anatomical and physiological factors predispose preterm infants to respiratory dysfunction (Table 8–5). For this reason many LBW neonates will require the use of a wide range of respiratory equipment and physiological monitors (Table 8–6). Pediatric therapists preparing to work in the NICU and those involved with designing risk management plans are referred to Crane's overview[55–57] of neonatal cardiopulmonary management for therapists and Peter's[169] analysis of physiological stress in preterm neonates during routine nursing procedures.

In this subspecialty of pediatric practice, neonatal therapists are responsible for the prevention of physiological jeopardy in LBW infants during developmental intervention in special care units. Before examination, discussion with the supervising neonatologist is advised regarding specific precautions and the safe range of vital signs for each infant. Medical update and identification of new precautions by the nursing staff before each intervention session are recommended because new events in the last few hours may not be recorded or fully analyzed at the time therapy is scheduled. It is essential that the nurse be invited to maintain ongoing surveillance of the infant's medical stability during neonatal therapy activities in case physiological complications occur. If medical complications develop during or after therapy, immediate, compre-

---

TABLE 8–5. Factors Contributing to Pulmonary Dysfunction in Preterm Neonates

Anatomical	Physiological
Capillary beds not well developed before 26 weeks of gestation	Increased pulmonary vascular resistance leading to right-to-left shunting
Type II alveolar cells and surfactant production not mature until 35 weeks of gestation	Decreased lung compliance Diaphragmatic fatigue; respiratory failure
Elastic properties of lung not well developed	Decreased or absent cough and gag reflexes; apnea
Lung "space" decreased by relative size of the heart and abdominal distention	Hypothermia and increased oxygen consumption
Type I, high-oxidative fibers compose only 10% to 20% of diaphragm muscle	
Highly vascular subependymal germinal matrix not resorbed until 35 weeks of gestation, increasing infant's vulnerability for hemorrhage	
Lack of fatty insulation and high surface area/body weight ratio	

From Crane L: Physical therapy for the neonate with respiratory disease. In Irwin S, Tecklin JS (eds): Cardiopulmonary Physical Therapy, St. Louis, CV Mosby, 1985.

TABLE 8-6. Equipment Commonly Encountered in the NICU

Equipment	Description
Radiant warmer	Unit composed of mattress on an adjustable table top covered by a radiant heat source controlled manually and by servocontrol mode. Unit has adjustable side panels. *Advantage:* provides open space for tubes and equipment and easier access to the infant. *Disadvantage:* open bed may lead to convective heat loss and insensible fluid loss.
Self-contained incubator (Isolette)	Enclosed unit of transparent material providing a heated and humidified environment with a servo system of temperature monitoring. Access to infant through side portholes or opening side of unit. *Advantage:* less convective heat and insensible water loss. *Disadvantage:* infection control; more difficult to get to infant; not practical for a very acutely ill neonate.
Thermal shield	Plexiglas dome placed over the trunk and legs of an infant in an Isolette to reduce radiant heat loss.
Oxygen hood	Plexiglas hood that fits over the infant's head; provides environment for controlled oxygen and humidification delivery.
Mechanical ventilator	
Pressure ventilator	Delivers positive-pressure ventilation; pressure-limited, with volume delivered dependent on the stiffness of the lung.
Volume ventilator	Delivers positive-pressure ventilation; volume-limited, delivering same tidal volume with each breath.
Jet ventilator	Ventilator that delivers short bursts of air at high rates of flow; provides high-frequency jet ventilation.
Nasal and nasopharyngeal prongs	Simple system for providing continuous positive airway pressure consisting of nasal prongs of varying lengths and adaptor to pressure-source tubing.
Resuscitation bag	Usually a self-inflating bag with a reservoir (so high concentrations of oxygen may be delivered at a rapid rate) attached to an oxygen flowmeter and a pressure manometer.
Electrocardiogram; heart rate, respiratory rate, and blood pressure monitor (cardiorespirograph)	Usually one unit will display one or more vital signs on oscilloscope and digital display. High and low limits may be set, and alarm sounds when limits exceeded.
Transcutaneous oxygen ($TcPo_2$) monitor	Noninvasive method of monitoring partial pressure of oxygen from arterialized capillaries through the skin. The electrode is heated, placed on an area of thin epidermis (usually abdomen or thorax). The monitor has capability of providing both a digital display and a continuous recording of $TcPo_2$ values.
Intravenous infusion pump	Used to pump intravenous fluids, intralipids, and transpyloric feedings at a specific rate. Pump has alarm system and capacity to monitor volume delivered, obstruction of flow, and other parameters.
Neonatal vital signs monitor	Measures mean blood pressure and mean heart rate from plastic blood pressure cuff; values are digitally displayed on monitor.
Pulse oximeter	Measures peripheral oxygen saturation and pulse from a light sensor secured to the infant's skin; values are digitally displayed on the monitor; some models have continuous recording of values on strip charts.

Modified from Crane L: Physical therapy for the neonate with respiratory disease. *In* Irwin S, Tecklin JS (eds): Cardiopulmonary Physical Therapy, St. Louis, CV Mosby, 1985.

hensive co-documentation of the incident with the supervising nurse and discussion with the neonatology staff are essential to analyze the events, outline related clinical teaching issues, and minimize legal jeopardy.

Areas of particular concern during neonatal therapy activities include the following: potential incidence of fracture, dislocation, or joint effusion during the management of limited joint motion; skin breakdown or vascular compromise during splinting or taping to reduce deformity; apnea or bradycardia during therapeutic neuromotor handling with potential deterioration to respiratory arrest; oxygen desaturation or regurgitation and aspiration during feeding assessment or oral-motor therapy; hypothermia from prolonged handling of the infant away from the neutral thermal environment of the incubator or overhead radiant warmer; and propagation of infection from inadequate compliance with infection control procedures in the nursery. Signs of overstimulation may include labored breathing with chest retractions, grunting, nostril flaring, color changes (skin mottling to red or cyanotic appearance), frequent startles, irritability or drowsiness, sneezing, gaze aversion, bowel movement, and hiccups.[8, 127] Signals of overstimulation expressed through infants' motor systems are finger splay (extension and abduction posturing), arm salute (shoulder flexion with elbow extension), and trunk arching away from stimulation.[8]

Even a baseline neurological examination, usually presumed to be a benign clinical procedure, may be destabilizing to the newborn's cardiovascular and behavioral organization systems. The physiological and behavioral tolerance of low-risk preterm and full-term neonates to evaluative handling by a neonatal physical therapist was studied in 72 newborn subjects.[217] During and after administration of the Neurological Assessment of the Preterm and Full-Term Newborn Infant, preterm subjects (30 to 35 weeks of gestation) had significantly higher heart rate; greater increase in blood pressure; decreased peripheral oxygenation inferred from mottled skin color; and higher frequencies of finger splay, arm salute, hiccups, and yawns than in full-term subjects. Neonatal practitioners must examine the safety of even a neurological examination and weigh the risks and anticipated benefit of the procedure given the expected physiological and behavioral changes in low-risk, medically stable neonates.[216, 242]

High-Risk Profiles. Three general high-risk profiles are observed from a dynamic systems perspective. These profiles identify movement abnormalities, related temperament/behavioral characteristics, and interactional styles associated with motor status.

The first high-risk profile involves the irritable hypertonic infant. These infants classically have a low tolerance level to handling and may frequently reach a state of overstimulation from routine nursing care, laboratory procedures, and the presence of respiratory and infusion equipment. They express discomfort when given quick changes in body position by caregivers and when placed in any position for a prolonged time. Predominant extension patterns of posture and movement are associated with this category of infants. Quality of movement may appear tremulous or disorganized with poor midline orientation and limited antigravity movement into flexion as a result of the imbalance of increased proximal extensor tone. Visual tracking and feeding may be difficult because of extension posturing or the presence of distracting, disorganized upper-extremity movement. In addition, increased tone with related decreased mobility in oral musculature may complicate feeding behavior. Hypertonic infants frequently demonstrate poor self-quieting abilities and may require consistent intervention by caregivers to tolerate movement and position changes. These temperament characteristics and the signs of neurological impairment discussed earlier may place infants at considerable risk for child abuse or neglect as the stress and fatigue levels of parents rise and as coping strategies wear thin during the demanding care required by irritable, hypertonic infants.[114, 144]

Conversely, the lethargic hypotonic infant excessively accommodates to the stimulation of the nursery environment and can be difficult to arouse to the awake states even for feeding. The crying state is reached infrequently, even with vigorous stimulation. The cry is characteristically weak, with low volume and short duration, related to hypotonic trunk, intercostal, and neck accessory musculature and decreased respiratory capacity. These infants are exceedingly comfortable in any position, and when held they easily mold themselves to the arms of the caregiver. Depression of normal neonatal movement patterns is common. To compensate for low muscle tone when in the supine position, some preterm infants appear to push into extension against the surface of the mattress in search of stability. Although potentially successful in generating a temporary increase in neck and trunk tone, the extension posturing from stabilizing against a surface in supine lying interferes with midline and antigravity movement of the extremities. Such infants respond dramatically to containment positioning in side-lying and

prone. Drowsy behavior limits these infants' spontaneous approach to the environment and decreases their accessibility to selected interaction by caregivers. Feeding behavior is commonly marked by fatigue, difficulty remaining awake, weak sucking, and incoordination/inadequate rhythm in the suck-swallow process, with the need for supplementation of caloric intake by gavage (oral or nasogastric tube) feeding. The risk for sensory deprivation and failure to thrive is high for hypotonic infants because they infrequently seek interaction, place few if any demands on caregivers, and remain somnolent.

The third high-risk profile is the disorganized infant with fluctuating tone and movement, who is easily overstimulated with routine handling but remains relatively passive when left alone. Disorganized infants usually respond well to swaddling or to containment when handled. When calm, these infants frequently demonstrate high-quality social interaction and efficient feeding with coordinated suck-swallow sequence. When distracted and overstimulated, however, these infants appear hypertonic and irritable. Caregiving for intermittently hypertonic, disorganized, irritable infants can be frustrating for parents unskilled in reading the infant's cues, in implementing consolability and containment strategies, and in pacing during feeding.

While these profiles address the extremes in motor and behavioral interaction, they suggest a need for identifying different tolerance levels of handling neonates with abnormal tone and movement, even though long-term developmental goals may be similar. Few neonates will demonstrate all behaviors described in the high-risk profile, but outpatient surveillance of neonates with worrisome or mildly abnormal motor and interactive behavior is advised to monitor the course of those behaviors and the developing styles of parenting.

Timing. The timing of neurodevelopmental examination and treatment for infants with high-risk histories or diagnoses is based on the medical stability of the infant and, in some centers, gestational age. All therapy activities need to be synchronized with the intensive care nursery schedule so that nursing care and medical procedures are not interrupted.

Neonatal therapists should not interrupt infants in a quiet, deep sleep state but instead wait about 15 minutes until the infant cycles into a light, active sleep or semi-awake state. Higher peripheral oxygen saturation has been correlated with quiet rather than with active sleep in neonates. Preterm infants reportedly have a higher percentage of active sleep periods, in contrast to the higher percentage of quiet sleep observed in full-term infants.[95] Allowing the preterm infant to maintain, rather than interrupting, a deep, quiet sleep is a therapeutic strategy for enhancing physiological stability.

Timing of parent teaching sessions is most effective when readiness to participate in the care of the infant is expressed. Some parents need time and support to work through the acute grief process related to the birth of an imperfect child before participation in developmental activities is accepted. Other parents find the neonatal therapy program to be a way of contributing to the care of their infant that also helps them cope with overwhelming fears, stresses, and grief.

Treatment Strategies

This section addresses components of treatment designed to enhance movement, minimize contractures and deformity, promote feeding behaviors appropriate to corrected age, develop social interaction behaviors, and foster attachment to primary caregivers. The areas of developmental intervention presented are management approaches to body positioning, extremity taping, graded sensory and neuromotor intervention, neonatal hydrotherapy, and oral-motor/feeding therapy; parent teaching is discussed here and on page 231. In managing an intensive care nursery caseload, the constant physiological monitoring, modifying of techniques to adapt to the constraints of varying amounts of medical equipment, scheduling of intervention to coincide with visits of the parents and peak responsiveness of the infants, and ongoing coordination and reevaluation of goals, plans, and follow-up recommendations with the nursery staff create many interesting challenges and demand a high degree of adaptability and creativity from the clinician. Willingness to change a preestablished assessment plan, treatment strategy, or therapy schedule to meet the immediate needs of the infant, parents, or nursery staff is paramount. For some infants with prolonged periods of only borderline stability with handling, a discharge examination with recommendations for follow-up care may be the best practice. Productivity standards of billable hours used for other caseloads of stable pediatric or adult clients in the hospital are not appropriate for the NICU setting and require negotiation and reinterpretation with rehabilitation department managers to protect both the infant and the neonatal therapist.

Positioning. A diligently administered positioning program can greatly assist infants on mechanical ventilators, under hood oxygen, or in incubators to simulate the flexed, midline postures of the normal full-term newborn swaddled in a bassinet. Preterm infants characteristically demonstrate low postural tone, with the amount of hypotonia varying with gestational age. Infants born prematurely do not have the neurological maturity or the prolonged positional advantage of the intrauterine environment to assist in the development of flexion. They are instead placed unexpectedly against gravity and presented with a dual challenge of compensating for maturation-related hypotonia and adapting to ventilatory and infusion equipment that frequently reinforces extension of the neck, trunk, and extremities.

The imbalance of excessive extension can occur quickly in preterm infants from repeated efforts to gain postural stability in the nonfluid extrauterine environment by leaning into or stabilizing against a firm mattress while in the supine position. De Groot[65] explained the postural behavior of preterm infants as an imbalance between low passive muscle tone and active muscle power. She theorized that because preterm neonates have prolonged periods of immobility (often in the supine position), exaggerated active muscle power may be observed in the extensor musculature, particularly in the trunk and hips. This imbalance of extension is viewed as non-optimal muscle power regulation that may negatively influence postural stability, coordinated movement, and later hand and perceptual skills.[65]

The neonate may attempt to posturally stabilize by hyperextending the neck in supine or side-lying positions to compensate for maturation-related hypotonia. According to Bly[33] and Quinton,[183] neck hyperextension posturing may herald the development of a host of related abnormal postural and mobility patterns to compensate for inadequate proximal stability. Both authors suggested that in some high-risk infants, excessive postural stabilizing into neck hyperextension may contribute to sequential blocking of mobility in the shoulder, pelvis, and hip regions. The potential components of this high-risk postural profile follow:

Hyperextended neck
Elevated shoulders with adducted scapulae
Decreased midline arm movement (hand-to-mouth)
Excessively extended trunk
Immobile pelvis (anterior tilt)
Infrequent antigravity movement of legs
Weight bearing on toes (supported standing)

The use of blanket or cloth diaper rolls or customized foam inserts in a neonatal positioning program can modify the increasing imbalance of extension in preterm or chronically ill infants and promote movement and postural stability from positions of flexion. Postural principles to incorporate into a positioning program include neutral head alignment on trunk, scapular abduction to encourage engagement of hands at midline, posterior pelvic tilt, and symmetrical flexion of the legs. After the infant is facilitated into a flexed position in the side-lying position, posterior rolls behind the head, trunk, and thighs provide a surface against which the infant can posturally stabilize while a flexed midline position is maintained (Fig. 8–11). An additional anterior roll between the extremities and the use of a pacifier may promote further midline stabilization in flexion (Fig. 8–12). Small neonates can be maintained in a flexed, symmetrical position in a circular nest formed from a long blanket roll. Larger neonates may need additional stabilization from a folded blanket or stockinette band tucked over the nest of blanket rolls (Fig. 8–13). Cloth buntings with circumferential body-straps and a foot roll (Fig. 8–14) provide positioning support and containment of extremity movement.

Endotracheal tube placement frequently contributes to the neck hyperextension posture in infants who require mechanical ventilation (Fig. 8–15). This iatrogenic component can be avoided by repositioning the ventilator hoses to allow enough mobility for slightly tucked chin and partially flexed trunk posture. For neurologically impaired infants with severe pulmonary disease necessitating prolonged ventilatory support, inattention to the alignment of the neck and shoulders may lead to the development of a contracture in the neck extensor muscles (Fig. 8–16).

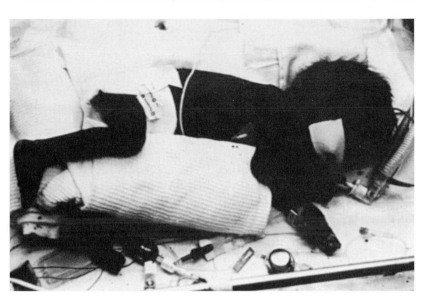

FIGURE 8–11. Positioning with diaper rolls to reduce extension posturing.

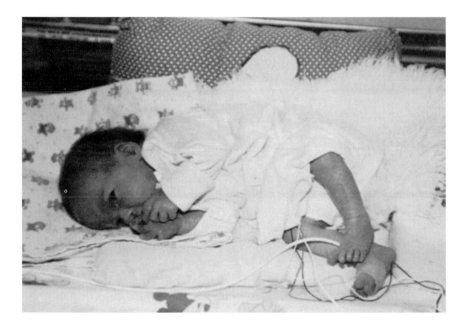

FIGURE 8–12. Pacifier promotes flexion and long roll allows anterior and posterior containment of flexed side-lying position.

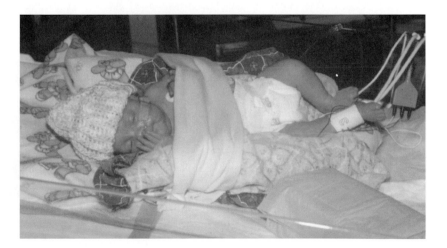

FIGURE 8–13. A 6-inch-wide cotton stockinette is used to stabilize anterior and posterior rolls around the infant's body.

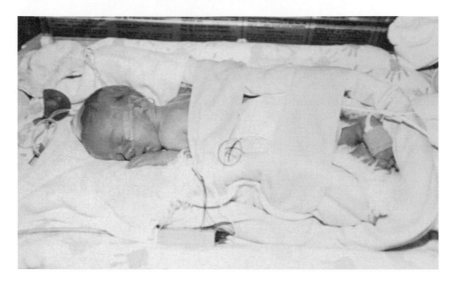

FIGURE 8–14. Use of cloth bunting with circumferential straps, interior foot roll, lateral rolls, and sheepskin to promote body containment in prone flexion.

Owing to enhanced extremity and trunk flexion in the prone position, improved oxygenation[136, 234] and less crying, even infants on ventilators (Fig. 8–17) are now routinely positioned in prone. Placing infants on a sheepskin surface (see Fig. 8–14) offers increased tactile input and has been correlated with increased weight gain in LBW infants compared with a matched group of infants on standard cotton sheets.[200] Thin, gel-filled, disc-shaped plastic head pillows of varying depths are options for distributing pressure on the side of the infant's head to reduce lateral head flattening in infants with extremely low birth weight.

Water- or gel-filled mattresses may contribute to a nursery positioning program by providing a soft surface that is not conducive to postural fixing. Other recognized advantages of waterbeds include increased vestibular and proprioceptive stimulation, decreased apnea, reduced head flattening, and improved skin condition.[50, 117, 135] After the infant is moved from intensive care to intermediate care, transition from a waterbed to a standard mattress is recommended to allow time for adaptation to the type of mattress likely to be used at home.

The neonatal therapist provides consultation on body alignment of infants in car seats when the LBW infant has failed the peripheral oxygen saturation test in the car seat, usually conducted by the neonatal nurse before discharge. Some infants require the use of a car bed with

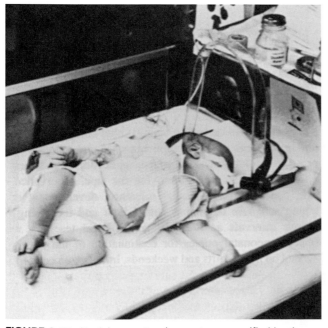

FIGURE 8–15. Neck hyperextension posture magnified by the position of the endotracheal tube.

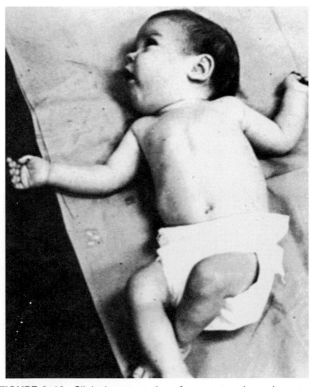

FIGURE 8–16. Clinical presentation of contracture in neck extensor muscles related to hyperextension posture during prolonged mechanical ventilation.

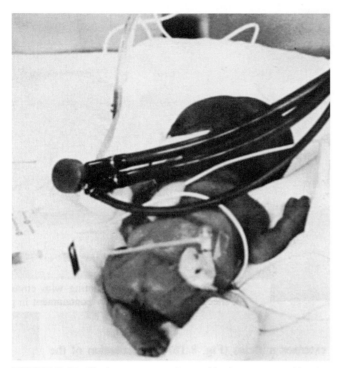

FIGURE 8–17. Flexion posture enhanced in the prone position by the influence of the tonic labyrinthine reflex.

body harness when they are unable to tolerate the semi-upright position of a car seat without oxygen desaturation.

Multiple studies of the effects of body positioning of neonates in NICU settings were reviewed and analyzed by Long and Soderstrom.[128] Continued research efforts are needed to measure effects of positioning and also the risk-benefit effects of other neonatal therapy interventions to guide future directions of neonatal practice.

Extremity Taping. The presence of perinatal elasticity encourages early management of congenital musculoskeletal deformities in the neonatal period (birth to 28 days of age). A temporary ligamentous laxity is presumed to be present in the neonate because of transplacental transfer of relaxin and estrogen from the mother. In addition to the influence of maternal hormones, the rapid growth of the neonate can foster correction of malalignment if the deforming forces are managed expediently. This peak period of hyperelasticity offers pediatric therapists with advanced orthopedic expertise many opportunities to manage congenital joint deformities.[103]

Intermittent taping of foot deformities (Fig. 8–18) has been more adaptable to the nursery setting than either casts or splints and is more effective in gaining mobility than range of motion exercises. Access to the heel for drawing blood, inspection of skin and determination of vascular status, and placement of intravenous lines can be accomplished with the tape in place or by temporary removal of the tape as needed. Therapists without a sound knowledge of arthrokinematic principles and techniques should not attempt the taping procedure, because it involves articulation of the joint(s) into a corrected position before taping. Other components of the taping process include application of an external skin protection solution under the tape, application of an adhesive removal solution when removing the tape, observance of skin condition and vascular tolerance, development of a taping schedule beginning with 1 hour and increasing by 1-hour intervals as tolerated, and clinical teaching with selected neonatal nurses for continuation of the taping if needed on night shifts and weekends. Infants with congenital foot deformities required shorter periods of casting in the outpatient period after taping of the extremity (Fig. 8–19) was implemented during the inpatient phase. In 18 years of my experience using silk tape to reduce deformity in neonates, neither skin nor vascular complications have occurred, even in infants with absent lower-extremity sensation resulting from meningomyelocele. Taping is not appropriate for medically fragile infants on minimal handling protocols or for infants younger than 30 to 32 weeks of gestation because of potential epidermal stripping from tape removal or vascular compromise from inadvertent, excessive compression by either the tape or the underwrap layer.

The availability of thin self-adherent foam material now allows taping on an underwrap (bandage) layer, rather than on the infant's skin (Fig. 8–20). Although this method creates a definite advantage in skin protection, it may cover the calcaneal region for blood drawing. Compromise in alignment may occur if the underwrap layer is applied loosely; conversely, restriction in circulation may be observed by edema or purple-blue color changes in the toes if the underwrap is excessively tight around the foot or ankle.

Infants with wristdrop from radial nerve compression related to intravenous line infiltration also benefit from the use of taping (Fig. 8–21). The wrist is supported in a functional position of slight extension. As muscle function returns, the taping is used intermittently to reduce fatigue and overstretching of the emerging, but still weak, wrist extensor musculature.

Therapeutic Handling. Use of tactile, vestibular, proprioceptive, visual, and auditory stimuli to facilitate infant development has been reported and reviewed by many authors.[81, 112, 118, 125, 186, 196, 203, 239] Selection and application of the sensory or neuromotor treatment options in neonatal therapy must occur with judicious attention to preven-

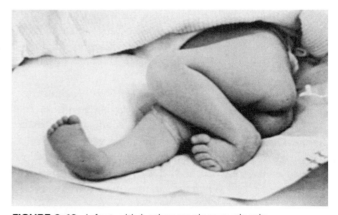

FIGURE 8–18. Infant with lumbar meningomyelocele demonstrating marked varus foot deformities before taping.

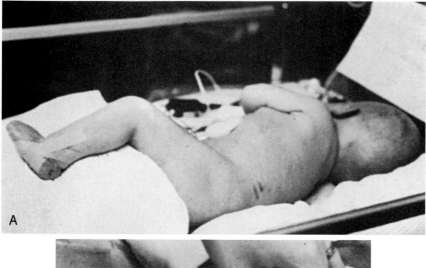

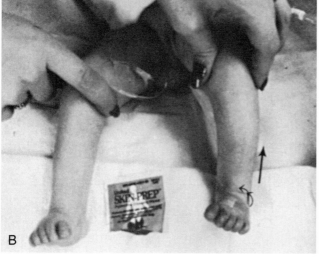

FIGURE 8–19. Significant correction in alignment of varus foot deformities in neonate with a lumbar meningomyelocele. *A*, Lateral stirrup with open heel taping procedure. *B*, Moderate correction.

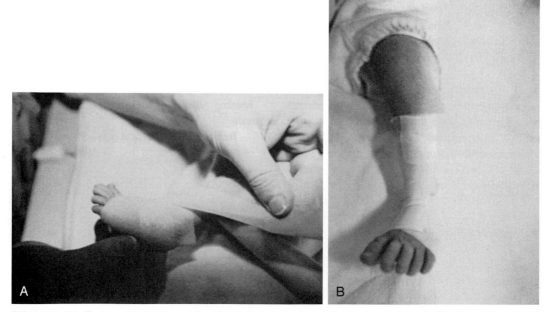

FIGURE 8–20. Taping of varus foot deformity. *A*, Thin foam layer. *B*, Silk tape in lateral stirrup over foam layer.

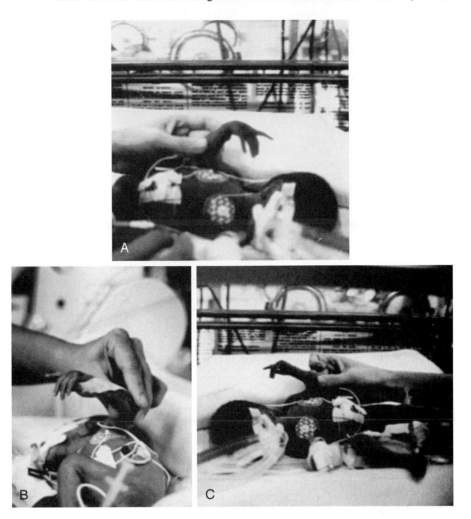

FIGURE 8–21. Management of wristdrop in medically fragile neonate. *A,* Wristdrop before taping. *B,* Taping procedure. *C,* One week after taping.

tion of sensory overload and related physiological consequences. Decision making on the type, intensity, duration, frequency, and sequencing of intervention within the context of infant physiological and behavioral stability can be learned only in a mentored clinical practicum in the NICU setting. The current general guidance on intervention is more observation, less handling, protection from bright lights and loud conversation, and readiness for handling based on behavioral and physiological cues of the infant.[9, 31, 112]

Primary aims of therapeutic handling include assisting the newborn to achieve maximum interaction with parents and caregivers and facilitating the experience of postural and movement patterns appropriate to the infant's adjusted gestational age. Helping infants to reach and maintain the quiet, alert behavioral state and age-appropriate postural tone appears to enhance opportunities for visual and auditory interaction and for antigravity movement experiences. The typical early movement experiences include hand-to-mouth movement, scapular abduction/adduction, anterior/posterior pelvic tilt, free movement of the extremities against gravity, and momentary holding of the head in midline.[33, 42]

Behavioral state and some movement abnormalities can be modified by creative swaddling and gentle weight shifts and nesting in the caregiver's lap. Swaddling the infant in a blanket with flexed, midline extremity position appears to promote flexor tone, increase hand-to-mouth awareness, inhibit jittery or disorganized movement, and elicit quiet, alert behavior. These effects can also be accomplished in skin-to-skin holding of infants against the parent's chest, a procedure now commonly adopted in NICUs in North America.[31] Application of neonatal therapy techniques must be contingent on both the infant's readiness for interaction and the need for a recovery break in interaction because of sensory overload. Teaching parents and caregivers to read and respond to the infant's motor cues for interaction, feeding, change of body position, and rest breaks is a critical quality-of-life component in the infant's NICU therapy program.

Incorporation of selected sensory and neuromotor activities into routine nursing care in the NICU increases developmental opportunities for the neonate during prolonged hospitalization.[31, 235] While feeding the infant in an incubator, the nurse may facilitate head lifting and momentary maintenance of the head in midline during the "burping" process in supported sitting (Fig. 8–22). Techniques for inhibiting trunk and lower extremity hypertonus may be added during diaper changes. Modulated visual and auditory interaction may be integrated into nearly all parts of infant care (Fig. 8–23), or they may be specifically reinforced as appropriate (e.g., visual

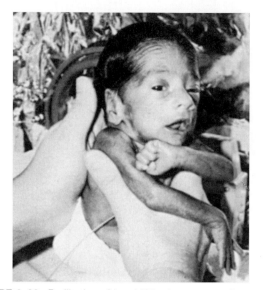

FIGURE 8–22. Facilitation of head lifting by a neonatal nurse while "burping" the infant after feeding.

orientation to human face, color photograph of family members' faces, or brightly colored animal toy; auditory orientation to human voice, taped soft conversation by parent reading a story, or taped sounds of nature).

A semi-inverted supine flexion position (Fig. 8–24) with preterm neonates should be used with caution to facilitate elongation of neck extensor muscles and decrease the neck hyperextension posture. This position may compromise breathing from positional compression of the chest and from potential airway occlusion associated with maximal flexion of the neck. The use of cardiorespiratory and oxygen saturation monitors during therapeutic handling activities is recommended for objective measurement of physiological tolerance. Although the peripheral oxygen saturation values from monitors may be intermittently unreliable because of motion artifacts from either the

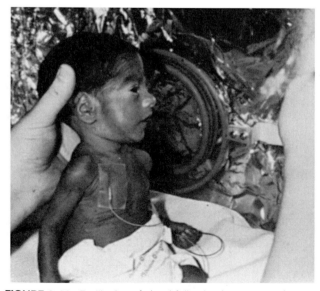

FIGURE 8–23. Facilitation of visual following by a neonatal nurse during a change of the infant's position in the isolette.

infant's spontaneous movement or the therapist's handling of the infant, reliable readings of oxygen saturation may be taken approximately 1 minute after the infant's body is not moved.

Easily overstimulated preterm infants may not tolerate multimodal sensory stimulation but may instead respond to a single sensory stimulus.[29, 31, 239] Implementation of a positioning program, oral-motor therapy, environmental modifications, and reinforcement of developmental activities with parents can be instituted only in collaboration with the shifts of bedside nurses who are in charge of the infant's 24-hour day in the NICU. Collaboration with nurses is a major component of precepted neonatal therapy training and requires integration into and valuing of the unique culture of the NICU.[218] Part of NICU culture is the unique ecology of environmental light and sound modifications, medical procedures, equipment, and caregiving patterns. Observing and analyzing the effects of the environment on an infant's behavior, physiological stability, postural control, and feeding function are critical elements to establish a prehandling baseline status before each neonatal therapy contact.[218]

Neonatal Hydrotherapy. Modified for use in an intensive care nursery setting, the traditional physical therapy modality of hydrotherapy has been adapted and implemented into neonatal therapy programs. Neonatal hydrotherapy was conceptualized in 1980 at Madigan Army Medical Center in Tacoma, Washington, and results of a pilot study of physiological effects were reported in 1983.[215]

Indications for referral of medically stable infants to the hydrotherapy component of the neonatal therapy program include the following: (1) muscle tone abnormalities (hypertonus or hypotonus) affecting the quality and quantity of spontaneous movement and contributing to the imbalance of extension in posture and movement (Fig. 8–25); (2) limitation of motion in the extremities related to muscular or connective tissue factors; and (3) behavioral state abnormalities of marked irritability during graded neuromotor handling or, conversely, excessive drowsiness during "handling" that limits social interaction with caregivers and lethargy that contributes to feeding dysfunction.

Infants are considered medically stable for aquatic intervention when ventilatory equipment and intravenous lines are discontinued and when temperature instability and apnea or bradycardia are resolved. A standard plastic bassinet serves as the hydrotherapy tub, and the water temperature is prepared at 37.8°C to 38.3°C (100°F to 101°F). An overhead radiant heater is used to decrease temperature loss and enhance thermoregulation in the undressed infant. Agitation of the water is not included in the hydrotherapy protocol in the NICU.

After receiving medical clearance and individualized criteria for the maximum acceptable limits of heart rate, blood pressure, and color changes during hydrotherapy from the neonatal staff, the baseline heart rate and blood pressure values are recorded and pretreatment posture and behavioral states are observed. The undressed infant is swaddled and moved into a semiflexed, supine position. The blood pressure cuff is placed around the distal tibial

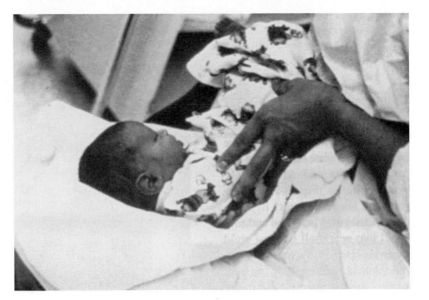

FIGURE 8–24. Potential respiratory compromise to the infant from neck extensor muscle elongation in excessively flexed position while in supine position.

region to continuously measure heart rate and blood pressure at 2-minute intervals during the 10-minute water immersion period. After being lifted into the water, the infant is given a short period of "quiet holding in the water" without body movement or auditory stimulation to allow behavioral adaptation to the fluid environment (Fig. 8–26). A second caregiver (e.g., nurse or parent) is recruited to stabilize the infant's head and shoulder girdle region while the neonatal therapist provides support at the pelvis (Fig. 8–27).

The movement techniques involve midline positioning of the head and slow, graded movement incorporating slight flexion and rotation of the trunk, followed (if tolerated) by progression distally to the pelvic girdle region and, finally, to the shoulder girdle and neck regions. After guided trunk extensor flexion with partially dissociated movement at the shoulder or pelvic girdle, most infants will demonstrate active extremity movement in the water. The improved range and smoothness of spontaneous extremity movement is facilitated by the buoyancy and surface tension of the water. Movement experiences in the supine, side-lying, and prone positions are offered as tolerated. If the movement therapy becomes stressful, with agitation or crying by the infant, body movement is stopped immediately and the infant is either consoled or removed from the water and held with warmed towels. Compromise in hemodynamic stability (increased heart rate, increased blood pressure, decreased respiratory rate) and a decrease in arterial oxygen tension during crying have been well documented in neonates recovering from respiratory distress syndrome.[68] Careful monitoring of behavioral tolerance to hydrotherapy (with avoidance of crying) is considered critical for reducing physiological risk with hydrotherapy.

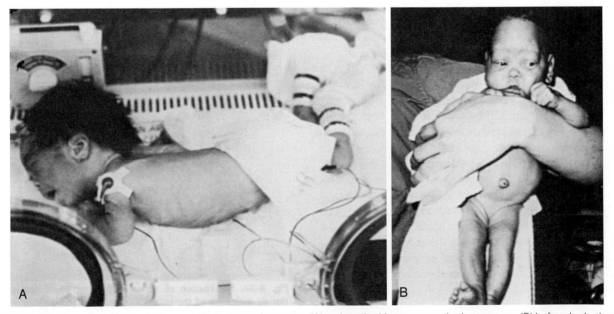

FIGURE 8–25. Neonates demonstrating opisthotonic trunk posture *(A)* and marked lower-extremity hypertonus *(B)* before hydrotherapy.

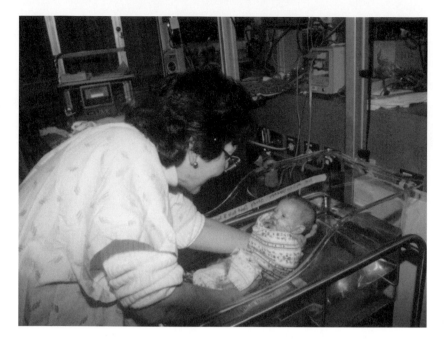

FIGURE 8–26. Adjustment to water immersion before introducing guided movement during neonatal hydrotherapy.

Multiple therapeutic benefits have been observed from selective use of 10-minute aquatic intervention sessions. Improved postural tone with semiflexed posture is obtained with less time and effort by the therapist and with higher behavioral tolerance by the infant than when a similar therapeutic handling approach is used without the medium of water. Postural tone changes are frequently maintained for 2 to 3 hours when aquatic intervention is followed by flexed, midline body positioning in the sidelying or prone position on a water mattress or supported against rolls. Enhancement of visual and auditory orienta-

tion responses (i.e., visual fixing and tracking, auditory alerting, and localization to human voices), prolonged high-quality alertness, and longer periods of social interaction with caregivers are demonstrated during and after hydrotherapy sessions. Significant improvement in feeding performance may occur when hydrotherapy is scheduled 30 minutes before feeding to prepare the infant for arousal to the quiet, alert state and for flexed, midline postural changes for optimal feeding. As with all neonatal therapy interventions, possible adverse effects of fatigue and temperature loss during hydrotherapy must be care-

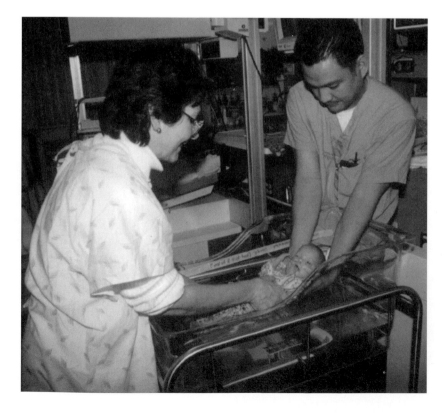

FIGURE 8–27. Swaddled infant is supported in neonatal hydrotherapy tub by neonatal physical therapist and neonatal nurse. The blanket is gradually loosened to encourage spontaneous, mid-range movement of the extremities.

fully monitored, so that exhaustion of the infant with a deterioration in feeding abilities does not establish a need for gavage feeding. Mild flexion contractures of knees and elbows and dynamic hip adduction contractures can be safely and quickly reduced by gentle muscle elongation techniques in warm water.

Therapeutic bathing techniques are incorporated into the parent teaching program to foster early parent participation in child care and in specific neonatal therapy activities during the inpatient period to prepare for carryover into the home environment. This early pleasurable involvement of parent and child in hydrotherapy and therapeutic bathing may provide a strong base for future participation in aquatics as a family leisure sports activity and, if needed, as an adjunct to an outpatient therapy program.

When oriented to treatment goals and trained in specific hydrotherapy techniques for individual infants, the nursing staff can effectively carry on the hydrotherapy program established by the neonatal therapist. This release of the neonatal therapist's role to nurses allows additional use of hydrotherapy on evening and night shifts and continued teaching and supervision of parents during evening and weekend visits (Fig. 8–28).

An additional advantage of neonatal hydrotherapy is cost effectiveness with the use of equipment readily available in the newborn nursery and the short time period (10 minutes) required for therapeutic bathing. It becomes labor efficient for the neonatal therapist when hydrotherapy is incorporated into nursing care plans and conducted by nurses and parents, with the therapist assuming a supervisory role.

Although many clinical benefits may be obtained by judicious use of hydrotherapy in the newborn nursery, pilot study data obtained on physiological changes in high-risk infants during hydrotherapy clearly indicate a physiological risk.[215] This risk (7% increase in blood pressure and heart rate in the pilot sample) must be carefully evaluated relative to each infant's general medical stability and baseline heart rate and blood pressure status before

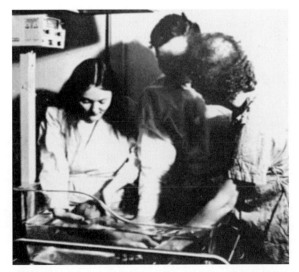

FIGURE 8–28. Parents being trained in hydrotherapy techniques for later therapeutic bathing at home.

hydrotherapy can be included safely in a neonatal therapy program. In collaboration with the neonatology and nursing staff, the therapist must use preestablished criteria for general medical stability and the maximal limits during hydrotherapy for blood pressure, heart rate, and acceptable color changes; this step is essential for risk management. Physiological monitoring of mean blood pressure and heart rate by a neonatal vital signs monitor during aquatic intervention is recommended. The blood pressure cuff is a pneumatically driven device that is not electronically connected to the infant and can be safely immersed in water. Because hypothermia is a recognized risk with hydrotherapy, body temperature should be measured routinely before and after the hydrotherapy session using a thermometer with a digital display. A risk-benefit analysis of the potential physiological risk to each infant and the expected therapeutic benefits is strongly advised before incorporating hydrotherapy techniques into a neonatal therapy program.

Oral-Motor Therapy. Feeding difficulties are common among LBW infants, owing in part to neurological immaturity, depressed oral reflexes, prolonged use of an endotracheal tube for mechanical ventilation, or insufficient postural tone. Because the behavioral state affects the quality of feeding behavior, feeding performance may be improved significantly by specific arousal or calming procedures before feeding. Other variables influencing feeding may include decreased tongue mobility, presence of tongue thrusting, decreased lip seal on nipple, nasal regurgitation, tactile hypersensitivity in the mouth, inefficient and uncoordinated respiratory patterns, insufficient proximal stability from hypotonic neck and trunk musculature, and hypertonic posturing of the neck and trunk in extension.[35, 244]

Two instruments for assessing oral-motor and feeding behaviors in the nursery are the Neonatal Oral-Motor Assessment Scale (NOMAS)[35] and the Nursing Child Assessment Feeding (NCAF) Scale.[21] The NOMAS is used to evaluate the following oral-motor components during sucking: rate, rhythmicity, jaw excursion, tongue configuration, and tongue movement (timing, direction, and range). Tongue and jaw components are analyzed during nutritive and nonnutritive sucking activity. Cut-off scores were derived from a pilot study[35] with the instrument: a combined score of 43 to 47 indicated "some oral-motor disorganization"; a score of 42 or less indicated oral-motor dysfunction. The absence of a category to evaluate breathing pattern, work of breathing/respiratory exertion, and physiological variables during feeding limits the use of this instrument to low-risk, healthy neonates.

The NCAF Scale is used to analyze parent-infant feeding interaction. It provides a method for evaluating the responsiveness of parents to infant cues, signs of distress, and social interaction opportunities during the feeding process. In concurrent validity studies, NCAF Scale scores were positively correlated with the Home Observation for Measurement of the Environment Inventory at 8 months (r = .72) and at 12 months (r = .79).[21]

Management strategies during feeding may include semiflexed, upright positioning with light support under the chin (Fig. 8–29). Techniques such as tactile facilitation

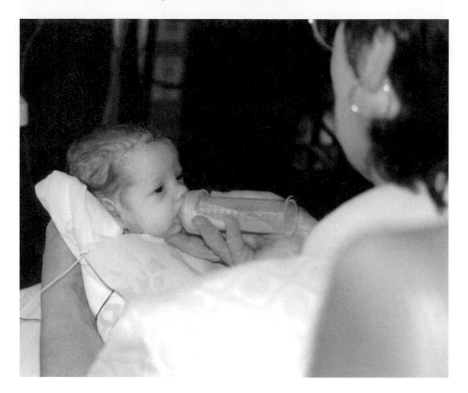

FIGURE 8–29. Swaddled preterm infant fed in semi-upright position with light support under chin.

of the facial muscles, judicious tactile stimulation of specific intraoral structures, use of a pacifier during gavage feedings, light manual support to the jaw or lip, and thickening of formula are frequent components of oral-motor therapy programs.[97, 244]

For some infants, oral intake by bottle may be improved by selecting a nipple with a flatter shape, larger hole, and softer, lower resistance to compression than those for standard newborn nipples. Wolf and Glass[86, 244] advise evaluating the flow rate of liquid from various types of nipples and analyzing the effect of nipple size, shape, and consistency on an infant's sucking proficiency. Feeding infants in the side-lying position may improve tongue position, particularly if marked tongue retraction is present (Fig. 8–30). The timing of movement therapy or neonatal hydrotherapy 30 minutes before feeding may

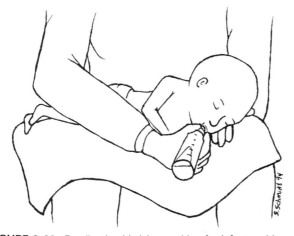

FIGURE 8–30. Feeding in side-lying position for infants with marked tongue retraction.

significantly improve performance by preparation of postural tone, facilitation of oral musculature, and enhancement of alertness.

Infants with oral facial anomalies (e.g., cleft lip and palate, hypoplastic mandible) often respond to bottle feeding with a Haberman feeder (Medela Inc., McHenry, IL), which allows control of the flow rate through a valve. The Haberman feeder is an ideal option for infants with large bilateral cleft lip and palate because formula can be released from nipple compression alone, rather than by generating negative pressure for suction. The feeding performance of infants with severe cleft palate deformities may be improved by a dental obturator. This custom-fabricated prosthesis is inserted before feeding to cover the defect in the palate. The increasing popularity of breast-feeding has encouraged the development of breast-feeding aids (e.g., Lact-Aid, Division of J.J. Avery, Inc., Denver). These devices allow supplementation of oral intake during breast feeding through a small tube that goes to the mouth from a presterilized bag containing infant formula.

Expected outcomes of oral-motor treatment supported by clinical research include (1) increased number of nutritive sucks after perioral stimulation,[123] (2) increased volume of fluid ingested during nipple feedings,[226] (3) decreased number of gavage feedings and earlier bottle feeding,[140] (4) accelerated weight gain,[140] and (5) earlier hospital discharge.[140] Measel[140] found that use of a pacifier during tube feedings allowed hospital discharge 4 days earlier for experimental subjects (n = 29) than for controls (n = 30). With the cost of NICU care at approximately $2000 per day, a discharge 4 days earlier for infants with alterations in feeding may represent a saving of $8000 per infant.

Monitoring the infant's physiological tolerance, breathing pattern, and work of breathing is critical during oral-motor examination, intervention, and feeding trials.[244] Heart rate values may be monitored from either the cardiorespirograph or with peripheral oxygen saturation from a pulse oximeter. Color changes, diminished tone in facial muscles, and behavioral stress cues (e.g., restlessness, trunk arching) must be carefully monitored to allow appropriate response to early signs of fatigue, overexertion, and potential airway management difficulty. Regurgitation with aspiration of milk or formula into the lungs may occur during feeding trials with complications of pneumonia, cardiopulmonary arrest, and associated asphyxia. Because of these risks, feeding trials should not be attempted by neonatal therapists untrained in managing the respiratory and general physiological monitoring components of neonatal feeding.[86]

Success during feeding activities enhances parent-infant interaction and perceived competency in parenting. Parents of infants with feeding dysfunction describe higher stress than that reported by parents of infants who are gaining weight and feeding satisfactorily. Because oral-motor dysfunction has been reported as an early functional deficit in infants at high risk for later neuromotor sequelae,[199] early support to parents coping with a challenging feeding situation builds competence in caregiving and also commitment to continuity in outpatient developmental monitoring.

Parent Support

Grief Process. Strong, continuous support is essential to help parents through perhaps the most frightening crisis in their adult lives—the potential death or disability of their infant.[121, 145] It is not uncommon for parents to initially establish emotional and physical distance from the infant as they cope with the knowledge that the infant may die. During this time of anticipatory grief, peer-group support by other parents of prematurely born children can be of immeasurable value. Actively listening to the parents' feelings and concerns and providing support, without judgment, through their episodes of detachment and anger are critical. Although long-range plans include parent participation in all aspects of the developmental program, the timing and amount of initial teaching must be individualized to the levels of stress and acute grief present.

When an infant dies, the neonatal therapist begins the important work of closure. This work includes attending memorial or funeral services to support the family and initiating a personal closure process. Neonatal therapists are advised to find a senior nurse mentor to guide them through the closure process of identifying and dealing with frustrations and other feelings regarding the infant and family. Finding meaning and value in the process of caregiving rather than solely in functional outcomes is an important task in the work of closure and in preventing professional burnout.

Parent Teaching. Components of the parent teaching process may include (1) discussion of the program goals and services in the NICU; (2) orientation to the interdisciplinary follow-up plan after discharge; (3) guidelines for recognizing and understanding the infant's temperament, stress cues, and ability to interact with the environment; and (4) specific instructions on selected developmental activities and therapeutic handling techniques. When used in conjunction with verbal instructions and demonstrations, a packet of written guidelines and pictures that are individualized to the infant's needs may improve parents' overall skills and understanding of the program.

Occasionally, when geographical distance prevents participation by parents in the neonatal therapy program, the infant's individualized developmental plan may be mailed and later reviewed at discharge or during outpatient follow-up. During times of separation, telephone contact with parents helps to foster attachment to the infant and to explain the purpose and content of the home developmental intervention program and provides opportunity to discuss the critical need for follow-up. Parents need this ongoing dialogue to make the infant seem real to them and to allow ventilation of their fears and concerns during the separation.

Teaching strategies are most effective when they are adapted to the learning style of the parents. This may involve more demonstrations and an increased opportunity for supervised practice for some parents, particularly those with reading or language difficulties that limit use of a written instructional packet. Cultural caregiving practices of the family may require elimination of common procedures such as use of pacifiers for nonnutritive sucking or hand-to-mouth engagement.

In the neonatal period, the quality of infant-parent attachment and the comfort level and proficiency in routine caregiving and therapeutic handling set the stage for later parenting styles. Helping parents find and appreciate a positive aspect of the neonate's motor or other developmental behaviors gives them a spark of hope from which emotional energy can be generated to help them through the marathon of the NICU experience. Empowering parents early in their parenting experience with the infant is crucial. In the life of the child, the effects of parent empowerment will last far longer than neonatal movement therapy and positioning strategies.

CLINICAL MANAGEMENT: OUTPATIENT FOLLOW-UP PERIOD

Purpose of Outpatient Follow-Up for the At-Risk Infant

Systematic follow-up of the at-risk infant after discharge from the NICU is an essential component of the clinical management of high-risk infants. The purpose of this follow-up is threefold:

1. To monitor and manage ongoing medical issues, such as respiratory problems and feeding difficulties.
2. To provide support and guidance to parents and caregivers in care and nurturing of at-risk infants.
3. To assess the developmental progress of infants to ensure that neuromotor impairments and delays in motor development can be identified and intervention initiated as early as possible.

Issues of assessment, intervention, and developmental profiles of the high-risk infant after discharge from the NICU are discussed in this section.

Medical Management. The routine medical care of LBW infants after discharge may be provided by a pediatrician, family practitioner, or health professional. The LBW infant is frequently followed by a number of additional professionals, including neurologists, ophthalmologists, cardiac or pulmonary specialists, nutritionists, public health nurses, physical and occupational therapists, and infant educators. Communication among these specialists is often minimal, especially when they are located at different facilities, and access to providers may be restricted by policies of managed care systems. The parent or caregiver is often confronted with conflicting opinions, demands, and expectations of the family and infant. The follow-up clinic can play a valuable role in this situation by providing case management to assist the caregivers in coordinating necessary services, to verify that all needs of the infant are being met, and to help the parents set realistic goals and priorities for themselves and their child.

Family Support. The stress that a vulnerable, premature, or at-risk infant brings to a family is well documented. Grief, anger, and depression are common reactions to the trauma and anxiety of an unanticipated premature birth.[121] The caregivers of high-risk infants are required to become knowledgeable about complex medical terminology and equipment. At discharge, they often become responsible for the administration of multiple medications of varying dosages, cardiopulmonary resuscitation procedures and equipment, and complicated feeding schedules requiring daily measurement and recording of nutritional intake and output. In addition, families often must cope with a tremendous financial obligation and deal with different billing agencies and funding sources.

These stresses and demands are even more overwhelming for parents who are young, single, or non–English-speaking. In contrast to the case in the 1980s, a greater proportion of at-risk infants seen in follow-up clinics are living with caregivers other than their biological mothers. These caregivers may include other relatives, such as single fathers, grandparents, aunts, and uncles; foster care providers; or preadoptive parents. At the same time, the changing demographics of American society are reflected in the increasing ethnic diversity of LBW infants. Whether they are recent immigrants to the United States, seasonal workers, or residents of an ethnic neighborhood, parents from minority ethnic groups are frequently overwhelmed by the complexities and procedures of a large medical institution. To adequately serve this population, a follow-up clinic team should have access to interpreters and should include social workers who are knowledgeable about community resources outside of the predominant culture. Cultural competence, defined as performing "one's professional work in a way that is congruent with the behavior and expectations that members of a distinctive culture recognize as appropriate among themselves," is an essential prerequisite for professionals working in a high-risk infant follow-up clinic.[132] For the physical thera-

pist conducting an evaluation, cultural competence includes familiarity with differing cultural norms regarding personal interaction, child-rearing practices, and family dynamics.

The LBW or at-risk infant may be irritable, hypersensitive to stimulation, less responsive to the affective interactions of adults, and more irregular in sleeping and feeding schedules compared with the term infant.[63] The demands that such an infant places on the caregivers can be extremely stressful, especially when there are other siblings in the home, financial concerns, and sleep deprivation. While these stresses may resolve as the infant's schedule and temperament become more stable, some studies raise concerns about their long-term impact on the parent-infant relationship and the infant's social and affective development.[20, 58]

The pediatric therapist in the follow-up clinic must be sensitive to these issues and concerns. Because social work and/or nursing services may not be routinely available, the therapist, within the context of the examination, needs to be alert to cues in the behavior of the infant or caregiver that may be indicative of problems in the home. Thoughtful questions regarding daily routines, feeding patterns, the sleep schedule of the caregiver as well as the infant, the caregiver's impression of the infant's temperament, and the availability of supportive resources can prompt a discussion of concerns that may not be readily communicated to a pediatrician or other professionals involved in the child's care.

Examination of Neurodevelopmental Status. LBW infants are at increased risk for neurodevelopmental disabilities so close follow-up is necessary during the first 6 to 8 years of life. Compared with that in term infants, the incidence of cerebral palsy is greater for LBW infants and the rate of cerebral palsy increases with decreasing birth weight levels (Table 8–7).[28, 76, 93, 170, 207] Cerebral palsy is one of several major neurological conditions that are sequelae of prematurity; others include mental retardation, hydrocephalus, sensorineural hearing loss, visual impairment, and seizure disorder. When examined as a group, these major disabling conditions occur more frequently in LBW infants, and the incidence increases as the birth weight and gestational age of the infant decreases (Table 8–8).[32, 76, 90, 240]

LBW infants are also at increased risk for more subtle neurodevelopmental disabilities, including visual-motor dysfunction, speech and language deficits, reading and math problems, balance and coordination impairment, and behavioral disorders, such as attention deficit and hyperactivity.[91, 195, 206, 222, 240] Longitudinal studies indicate

TABLE 8–7. Incidence of Cerebral Palsy Relative to Birth Weight

Birth Weight (g)	Incidence
>2500	<1%
1500–2500	5–8%
1000–1500	10–17%
<1000	20–30%

Data from references 16, 28, 90, 110, 172, and 237.

TABLE 8 – 8. Incidence of Major Neurodevelopmental Disability Among Preterm Infants Relative to Birth Weight

Birth Weight (g)	Disability*
>2500	4–5%
1500–2500	5–20%
1000–1500	15–25%
<1000	20–40%

*Cerebral palsy, mental retardation, blindness, seizures, sensorineural hearing loss, hydrocephalus.
Data from references 16, 77, 90, 148, and 240.

that by school age approximately one half of all LBW infants will have educational and learning deficits, compared with a reported rate of 24% in the general population.[90, 240] Overall, it is estimated that 10% to 30% of LBW infants will have "major" disabilities and another 40% have "minor" disabilities.

A primary objective of developmental follow-up in at-risk infants is the early identification of neurodevelopmental disabilities so that therapeutic intervention can be initiated. LBW infants who participate in a follow-up clinic program have been shown to have advanced performance on cognitive measures and to receive more intervention services compared with nonmonitored infants.[130, 205] Motoric benefits of early intervention for high-risk infants have not been clearly demonstrated by research findings.[87, 113, 138, 185, 193, 201, 227, 236] The lack of substantiating evidence is due, in part, to the methodological challenges presented by research in this area. The variability of LBW infants and the difficulty of early diagnosis, the heterogeneity of neurodevelopmental outcomes such as cerebral palsy, and the limitations of existing assessment instruments are just some of the obstacles to the efforts to conduct efficacy studies of early intervention for this population.

Early identification of a developmental disability remains an important goal. A confirmed or tentative diagnosis can direct the family toward intervention services, financial resources, and social supports. Systematic follow-up and recognition of developmental problems in a high-risk infant provides a major role in supporting the relationship between an infant and the caregiver. An infant with a developmental disability often does not interact in the same ways as those seen in typically developing infants and may evoke negative maternal responses of anxiety, frustration, or withdrawal.[146, 246] Diagnosis of a neurodevelopmental disability often facilitates dialogue about parental concerns and questions and can assist caregivers in their process of acceptance of a disability and of adjustment of their expectations.

High-Risk Infant Follow-Up Clinic: A Model

The developmental progress of an at-risk infant requires careful monitoring, with regular evaluation at designated intervals in the first years of life. An organizational model of a high-risk infant follow-up clinic is shown in Figure 8 31. It is based on the protocol of the High Risk Infant Follow-up Clinic (HRIF Clinic) of the Center on Human Development and Disability (CHDD) at the University of Washington in Seattle, Washington.

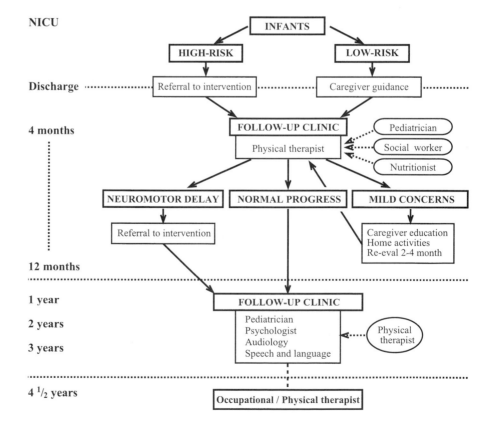

FIGURE 8–31. Organizational model of a follow-up clinic for infants at risk for neurodevelopmental disabilities. Infants are evaluated through the interdisciplinary clinic from the time of discharge from the neonatal intensive care unit. When problems are identified, referrals are made to appropriate specialists.

Before discharge from the NICU, infants who are considered to be at very high risk (infants with seizures, cystic PVL, chronic lung disease, feeding problems, or obvious neurological abnormalities) are identified. The high-risk infant receives therapeutic intervention as described in the section of this chapter on management in the neonatal period. Infants who do not exhibit specific signs of abnormality are closely monitored but do not receive individual intervention. For the LBW infant who is growing appropriately, the role of the physical therapist is primarily to instruct nurses and caregivers in positioning and handling techniques that will support and promote normal development.

At discharge, infants who demonstrate atypical development or signs of abnormal neuromotor function are referred directly to therapy programs within the local community. It is recommended that intervention be provided in the home, if possible, to minimize the stress for the infant and family and to reduce exposure to infection. Infants who do not require therapy services at the time of discharge from the NICU are scheduled for an evaluation in the follow-up clinic and referred to a community pediatrician for medical management.

Age Correction. Premature infants are scheduled for evaluations in the follow-up clinic according to their corrected age (age adjusted for weeks of prematurity). The issue of whether to adjust for prematurity when assessing cognitive or motor development is an ongoing question.[2, 137, 161, 177] Several studies have demonstrated that if chronological or unadjusted age is used for standardized testing, the premature infant who is developing appropriately will have a low developmental quotient and test scores indicative of motor delay.[2, 3, 66, 161, 177, 228] If age is adjusted for prematurity, the performance of the premature infants is comparable to that of full-term infants at 1 year. Although some investigators caution that adjustment for prematurity tends to result in overcorrection, particularly for infants born at less than 33 weeks' gestation,[122] the general consensus is that premature infants should be evaluated according to their corrected age.[15]

The decision regarding correction for gestational age in a follow-up clinic should be based on the objectives and testing protocol for that clinic. Consideration should be given to the following factors: (1) the testing instruments used, with attention to the competencies evaluated by the tool and the number of preterm infants in the normative sample, and (2) the overall purpose of the evaluation and whether the emphasis is on screening or diagnosis. In the High-Risk Infant Clinic at the University of Washington, premature infants born when younger than 37 weeks' gestational age are assessed according to their corrected age level through 8 years of age. However, developmental quotients in the normal range do not preclude concerns or referral to intervention services when neuromotor or behavioral abnormalities are observed.

Follow-Up Clinic Evaluation Schedule. The basic schedule of evaluations for infants and children in the follow-up clinic is shown in Table 8–9. Although the first routine appointment is at 4 months (corrected age), infants may be seen earlier at the recommendation of the hospital discharge team, physical therapist, community

TABLE 8–9. High-Risk Infant Clinic: Scheduled Evaluations

Corrected Age of Child	Examiner(s)*	Standard Tests Administered
4 months	Physical therapist	Movement Assessment of Infants (MAI) Bayley Scales of Infant Development (BSID)
	Pediatrician°	
1 year	Pediatrician	Denver Developmental Screening Test (DDST) Neurological examination
	Psychologist Audiologist Physical therapist°	BSID
2 years	Pediatrician	Neurological examination DDST
	Psychologist Physical therapist°	BSID
3 years	Pediatrician	DDST Neurological examination
	Psychologist	Stanford-Binet Peabody Picture Vocabulary Test
	Phsyical therapist° Speech/audiologist°	
4½ years	Pediatrician	DDST Neurological examination
	Psychologist	Wechsler Preschool and Primary Scale of Intelligence (WPPSI)
	Occupational therapist	Peabody Developmental Motor Scales (PDMS) Miller Assessment of Pre-Schoolers
	Phsyical therapist° Speech/audiologist°	
6 years	Pediatrician	DDST Neurological examination
8 years	Psychologist	Wechsler Intelligence Scale for Children—Revised (WISC-R) or WPPSI Peabody Individual Achievement Test (PIAT)
	Physical therapist° Speech/audiologist°	

°Consultant examiner.

pediatrician, public health nurse, or caregiver. The examinations and test instruments typically administered by each specialist are listed in Table 8–9.

Four-Month Evaluation. Four months of age is an optimal time for the initial follow-up evaluation for the following reasons:

1. Infant examinations are better predictors than neonatal examinations. The neonatal period and the first 2 to 3 months of life are characterized by variability in infant behavior and motor skills, as well as instability of muscle tone and reflex activity.[7, 8] Longitudinal studies

with sequential examinations indicate that neonatal examinations are less accurate in long-term prediction of neurodevelopmental outcome than examinations administered to older infants.[75, 160, 175, 185]

2. Four months is a critical time in the developmental maturation of infants. In the typically developing infant, muscle tone tends to be stable,[92, 185] the influence of primitive reflexes is minimal,[22] balance reactions are emerging, and functional skills are present with orientation around the midline (Fig. 8–32). For most LBW infants, medical concerns have resolved at this age and caregivers are raising questions about developmental expectations. Although it is not possible to make definitive predictions about long-term prognosis for a preterm infant at this age, the predictive accuracy of evaluation at 4 months has been shown to be comparable to that of evaluations at later ages.[212] A comprehensive developmental assessment at 4 months' adjusted age can document an infant's current level of performance and provide a baseline for subsequent evaluations.

In the High-Risk Infant Clinic at the University of Washington, the physical therapist assumes the role of case manager for the 4-month evaluation and for other scheduled evaluations up to 12 months of age. During the first year of life, infants express their capabilities and neurological integrity primarily through movement, so the physical therapist, as a specialist in movement, is the most appropriate professional to observe and coordinate the evaluation. By using the Movement Assessment of Infants (MAI)[46] and the Bayley Scales of Infant Assessment (BSID-II),[24] the therapist examines both the neuromotor and developmental status of the infant. (The infant evaluation and the clinical decision-making process of the physical therapist are described in greater detail later in this chapter.)

At the 4-month evaluation, the developmental pediatrician provides medical consultation at the request of the therapist when health, neurological, or medical concerns are observed during the evaluation. A nutritionist is available to address feeding issues, growth concerns, and nutritional problems, which are not uncommon among preterm infants. Because of the increasing number of infants born to single women, mothers of minority ethnic groups, and women using illicit substances during pregnancy, a social worker is an important member of the follow-up clinic team. The social worker evaluates the family's home and living situation, identifies indicators of environmental risk, and assists the caregiver in accessing necessary financial and personal resources.

One-Year (Two/Three-Year) Evaluation. Beginning at 1 year of age, the High-Risk Infant Clinic evaluations become increasingly multidisciplinary as the infant becomes a more complex individual. The clinic schedule is designed to allow for assessment of maximal areas of competency without exhausting the infant and family. Because the infant was evaluated by the physical therapist during the first year of life, a neuromotor evaluation is not routinely scheduled. Motor skills are assessed by the psychologist and by the pediatrician using the BSID and the Denver Developmental Screening Test (DDST). The physical therapist is available for consultation if motor delay or neuromotor concerns are noted.

Four-and-a-Half–Year Evaluation. A routine evaluation scheduled at 4½ years of age enables the follow-up team to inform and assist families as they are making decisions regarding school entry. In addition to assessment by the psychologist, speech pathologist, and pediatrician, the occupational or physical therapist evaluates the child's motor development. Particular attention is given to balance and coordination and to fine motor and perceptual-motor skills. Depending on the needs of the individual child, the concerns of the caregivers, and the time available for the evaluation, the therapist may use the Peabody Developmental Motor Scales (PDMS), the Beery Test of Visual-Motor Integration (VMI), the Miller Assessment of Pre-School, or other standard assessments. At this age, a major goal of the follow-up evaluation is to identify

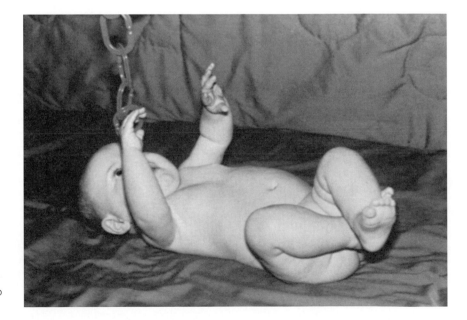

FIGURE 8–32. Normal full-term infant at 4 months of age demonstrating symmetrical alignment of trunk and extremities, functional movement against gravity, and no influence of the tonic labyrinthine reflex.

problems that might compromise learning and to assist the family in obtaining appropriate services to minimize the effect of any deficits on the child's school performance.

Neuromotor Assessment of the At-Risk Infant

Neuromotor Assessment Tools: Purpose and Clinical Use. Evaluation of the at-risk infant using a quantitative, standard assessment tool serves two major purposes in a follow-up clinic:

1. *Documentation of the infant's motor status relative to developmental norms or relative to the infant's performance on previous examinations.* The information is used to determine the child's developmental progress, rate of change, or extent of motor delay. Achievement of this objective is determined by the scope and focus of the assessment tools used in the evaluation.
2. *Identification of a neuromotor impairment to initiate appropriate intervention services.* Early identification is not simply a task of detecting signs of neuromotor deviation. The challenge is to identify those infants who are most likely to have an abnormal neurodevelopmental outcome. Achievement of this objective is determined by the *predictive validity* of the assessment tools that are used.

Evaluation of Predictive Validity of Infant Assessment Tools. A primary goal of the neuromotor evaluation is prediction of the long-term developmental outcome of the child based on a clinical examination of the infant. The ability to accurately achieve this goal depends not only on the clinical experience and expertise of the therapist but also on the predictive accuracy or validity of the assessment tool being used. The predictive validity of a test is defined in terms of **sensitivity** and **specificity** and **positive** and **negative predictive values**[194] (Table 8–10).

The **sensitivity** of a test evaluates how *sensitive* the test is in its ability to identify a defined developmental problem, such as cerebral palsy. In the testing situation described here, sensitivity is calculated as the proportion of children with abnormal neurodevelopmental outcome who were correctly identified as "abnormal" when examined as infants. **Specificity** refers to how *specific* the test is in identifying *only* the defined developmental problem and not overdiagnosing by identifying children who do not have the problem. Specificity is calculated as the proportion of children with normal developmental outcome who were correctly identified as "normal" when examined as infants. The children with normal developmental outcome who were inaccurately classified as "abnormal" by the infant test are referred to as *false positives;* that is, they were falsely determined by the test to be positive for the developmental problem. On the other hand, children who were classified as "normal" when tested as infants but subsequently are diagnosed with cerebral palsy are described as *false negatives* because the test falsely indicated that they were negative for the developmental problem.

The **positive predictive value** of a test refers to the accuracy of the infant test in its classification of infants as "abnormal." For example, of the infants who were identified as "abnormal" or "suspect" by the infant test the proportion of infants who are actually diagnosed with cerebral palsy represents the *positive predictive value.* The *negative predictive value* refers to the accuracy of the infant test in its classification of infants as "normal." It is calculated as the proportion of infants categorized as "normal" who actually have normal developmental outcome. To the therapist in a follow-up clinic, it may appear that the positive and negative predictive values of a given test would be most useful, because they indicate the probability of a given outcome for an infant being tested. However, predictive value is not a stable measure of the predictive validity of a test, because the predictive values vary according to the prevalence of the developmental problem within a group or population of infants. When a condition occurs commonly, the positive predictive value will be relatively high. When the outcome of interest is rare, the positive predictive value will be relatively low. Further discussion about test evaluation and measurement can be found in a number of excellent resources that are available to the therapist.[178, 194]

Examples of Infant Assessment Tools. In addition

T A B L E 8 – 10. Predictive Validity of an Infant Assessment Tool

Infant Test	Outcome (at Specified Age in Childhood)		
	Normal	Abnormal	
No risk	a Correct nonreferrals	b Incorrect nonreferrals (false negatives)	a + b = Total nonreferrals
Risk	c Incorrect referrals (false positives)	d Correct referrals	c + d = Total referrals
	a + c = Total normal at outcome	b + d = Total abnormal at outcome	

Sensitivity = d/b + d × 100 = percentage of abnormal children who were correctly identified as "no-risk" by the infant test
Specificity = a/a + c × 100 = percentage of normal children who were correctly identified as "risk" by the infant test
Positive predictive value° = d/c + d × 100 = percentage of infants identified as "risk" by the infant test who had abnormal outcome
Negative predictive value° = a/a + b × 100 = percentage of infants identified as "no risk" by the infant test who had normal outcome

°Positive and negative predictive values will vary according to the prevalence of the abnormal outcome within the study population.

to the tools described previously for the assessment of the neonate, a number of testing instruments have been designed for evaluation of the infant. Based on their content, infant assessment instruments can be viewed within two broad categories: comprehensive/developmental and neuromotor/motor. The BSID-II[24] and the DDST are comprehensive tests that assess the developmental status of infants across several domains of function. On the other hand, neuromotor assessments such as the Movement Assessment of Infants (MAI)[46] and the Neurological Evaluation of the Infant and Newborn[13] or the Alberta Infant Motor Scale (AIMS),[176] which assesses gross motor skills, primarily focus on one functional area.

The choice of instrument for a particular clinical situation will depend on the emphasis and purpose of the clinic, as well as on the professional disciplines that are represented in the follow-up team. Neurological findings may be the most useful indicator of impairment in the neonate or young infant, because this is a time when behavioral responses are influenced by the infant's affective state and motor skills are rudimentary. As the infant matures, neuromotor integrity is manifested by the acquisition of motor skills. For infants older than the age of 3 months, longitudinal research indicates that observed neuromotor abnormalities are predictive of later cerebral palsy only when accompanied by delay in one or more developmental milestones.[75, 212] A brief review of the infant assessment tools commonly used in follow-up clinics is presented next.

Bayley Scales of Infant Development. The BSID-II[24] is a standardized assessment of the cognitive and motor abilities of infants and children between the ages of 2 months and 3 years. The test is divided into two primary areas. The Mental Scale is composed of items rating performance in the areas of problem solving, memory, visual perception, learning, and verbal communication; the Motor Scale evaluates gross and fine motor skills. For infants younger than 12 months of age, successful performance on the Mental Scale requires competency in visual following and fine motor manipulation; the scale becomes more heavily weighted toward language items at the older age levels. The Motor Scale is predominantly an assessment of gross and fine motor milestones, with visual-perceptual skills included in the recent edition. The BSID-II also provides a Behavior Rating Scale that evaluates the child's behavior during the testing session.

The BSID was first published in 1969 in a format that has been used extensively in clinical and research settings throughout the United States. The BSID-II, a revised version of the BSID, was published in 1993. The goals of the revision process included updating the normative data, extending the upper age level of the test from 30 to 42 months, and adding more relevant test items and materials. The revised test was standardized on 1700 young children representing a distribution of race, gender, geographical regions, and level of parent education as an indicator of socioeconomic status. In addition, approximately 370 children with various clinical diagnoses, including autism, Down syndrome, developmental delay, preterm birth, and prenatal exposure to drugs, were tested with the BSID-II. Test scores from these children were not included in the normative data and are intended to provide a "baseline of performance" for children with these diagnostic conditions.[24]

Administration procedures and grading criteria are clearly described in the manual. Items are scored on the basis of presence or absence of response. The raw scores are converted to standard scores, the Mental Developmental Index (MDI) and the Psychomotor Developmental Index (PDI), both of which have a mean of 100 and a standard deviation variation of ± 15. The authors note that scores on the BSID-II are lower than the scores derived from the original BSID, with the Mental Scale 12 points lower on average and the Motor Scale 10 points lower.[24] A "moderate" level of correlation was demonstrated between the original BSID and the BSID-II: $r = 0.62$ for the Mental Scale and $r = 0.63$ for the Motor Scale.

Test-retest reliability was evaluated for the BSID-II using a sample of 175 children aged 1, 12, 24, and 36 months.[24] The "stability coefficients" for ages 1 and 12 months were $r = 0.83$ for the Mental Scale and $r = 0.77$ for the Motor Scale. Interrater reliability, determined with a sample of 51 children, was 0.96 for the Mental Scale and 0.75 for the Motor Scale.[17] Concurrent validity of the BSID-II was evaluated by comparing the BSID-II scores with those obtained for a variety of assessment tools, including tests of language, cognitive, and intellectual function. The correlations between the Mental Scale and subscales of language and cognitive tests ranged from 0.57 to 0.99, indicating positive correlations that were considered to be in the moderate to high range. The strongest correlation for the BSID Motor Scale was obtained with the Motor subscale of the McCarthy Scales of Children's Abilities ($r = 0.59$).[24] The predictive validity of 4-month scores on the Motor Scale of the original BSID relative to subsequent cerebral palsy was poor, but it was more accurate for the older infant.[160, 191] No predictive validity was provided for the BSID-II in the manual for the revised version of the test.

The expanded age range and updated normative data offered by the BSID-II enhance its overall utility as an assessment tool. However, several areas of weakness have been identified in the BSID-II, particularly in its use with preterm infants.[83, 152, 191] The problems result primarily from the item set format of the revised version of the test. Unlike in the testing protocol of the original test, the administration of items and the scoring procedures for the BSID-II are based on item sets. The appropriate item set for an individual child is usually determined according to the "child's chronological age," but the examiner is told to "select the item set that you feel is closest to the child's current level of functioning based on other information you might have."[24] The option to begin testing at different item sets, which can yield different raw scores for the same infant, introduces a level of variability in administration procedures and test results that is inconsistent with the purpose of a standardized test.[83] This problem is magnified for preterm infants because it places even greater importance on the decision of whether to test the infant according to chronological or corrected age.[191]

In spite of these limitations the BSID-II is widely used throughout the United States. Until the administration and scoring issues are addressed by the test developers, and the testing procedures are clarified and universally followed, therapists using this tool should define and clearly state the protocol adopted by their clinical or research setting. Interpretation of test results, especially those for high-risk or premature infants, should be done with caution and the potential for variation in test results should be acknowledged.

Movement Assessment of Infants. The MAI[46] was originally developed by physical therapists specifically for use in a high-risk infant follow-up clinic. The MAI provides a systematic examination of muscle tone, primitive reflexes, automatic reactions of balance and equilibrium, and volitional gross and fine motor skills.

In the MAI manual, the authors outlined the following clinical uses: (1) to identify motor dysfunction in infants up to 12 months of age, (2) to establish the basis for an early intervention program, (3) to monitor the effects of physical therapy on infants or children whose motor behavior is at or below the level for 1 year of age, (4) to assist in data collection and clinical research on motor development through the use of a standard system of movement assessment, and (5) to teach skilled observation of movement and motor development through evaluation of normal and handicapped children.[46] The MAI has been used in clinical, research, and intervention settings with infants with a broad range of conditions and diagnoses, including Down syndrome,[94, 98, 184] prenatal exposure to alcohol and drugs,[79, 198, 213] and human immunodeficiency virus (HIV)–positive status,[101] and it has been used extensively with LBW and preterm infants.[61, 98, 173–175, 210, 212]

The MAI can be administered in 20 to 30 minutes, with additional time required for scoring, parent counseling, and rest/feeding breaks for the infant. A flexible order of testing is allowed, but grouping of items by the position of the infant (supine, prone, sitting, vertical suspension, standing, prone suspension) is advised to minimize fatigue and stress. The items in the categories of Primitive Reflexes, Automatic Reactions, and Volitional Movement are graded on a four-point ordinal scale; Muscle Tone items are scored on a six-point scale. The MAI manual includes a full description of the examination and administration procedures with detailed scoring criteria for each item.

The MAI provides a scoring profile based on the neuromotor performance expected for 4- and 8-month-old infants. A comprehensive full-scale score, the "total risk score," is derived, with higher scores indicating greater deviation from the norm. For a sample of typically developing full-term 4-month-olds, reported MAI total risk scores ranged from 0 to 13, with a mean of 5.9 and standard deviation of ±3.2; at 8 months the mean total risk score was 5.9, range 0 to 10, and standard deviation of ±2.4.[210] The MAI provides subscale scores for each of the four categories of the test as well as individual item scores.

Early studies of interrater reliability examining the percent of agreement between the MAI scores given to full-term infants by different examiners reported 90% reliability,[46] whereas a later study reported 72% interrater reliability and 76% test-retest reliability.[100] A more recent investigation with high-risk infants reported interrater and

test-retest reliability, measured by intraclass correlation coefficients, of 0.91 and 0.79, respectively.[34] Concurrent validity between the MAI and the BSID Motor Scale was reported as −0.63.[99]

Preliminary findings originally reported in the MAI manual suggested that total risk scores greater than 7 were indicative of neuromotor delay or abnormality.[46] However, later studies with full-term and premature infants indicated that a score of 10 is a more useful cutpoint for prediction of neuromotor disability.[63, 96, 197, 210, 212] The predictive validity of the MAI has been examined in relation to developmental outcome as measured by performance on the BSID and by pediatricians' assessments of childhood neurological status. The correlations between MAI scores at 4 and 8 months and MDI and PDI scores at 1 and 2 years of age have been shown to be highly significant.[99, 212] In a follow-up study of LBW infants weighing 1750 g or less, MAI total risk scores at 4 and 8 months of greater than or equal to 10 were highly predictive of cerebral palsy at 18 months (Table 8–11).[212] The predictive validity of the MAI has also been demonstrated for infants with bronchopulmonary disease.[131]

Chandler Movement Assessment of Infants Screening Test (CMAI-ST). The CMAI-ST is a 10- to 15-minute screening tool for health care professionals in primary care (pediatricians, family practice physicians, and nurse practitioners), designed to identify infants needing referral for definitive neurological and developmental assessment.[45] The test retains the basic categories of the MAI, but it is limited to selected items that are considered to be most predictive of movement disorders. All items on the CMAI-ST are scored on a three-point scale. Reported interrater and test-retest reliability ranges from 87% to 97% and from 81% to 92%, respectively.[45] Normative data have been collected on full-term infants from 1.5 to 12.5 months of age. Publication of the CMAI-ST will occur after the collection of normative data has been completed.

Alberta Infant Motor Scale. The AIMS[176] was designed to evaluate gross motor function in infants from birth to independent walking, or birth to 18 months. The stated purposes of the AIMS are (1) to identify infants who are delayed or deviant in their motor development and (2) to

---

● **T A B L E   8 – 11. Predictive Validity of Infant Assessment Tools**

Assessment	Sensitivity (%)	Specificity (%)	Positive PV (%)	Negative PV (%)
4-Month Examination				
BSID, Motor Scale	17	97	57	70
MAI	83	78	59	85
MAI	73	93	58	96
AIMS	77	82	39	96
8-Month Examination				
BSID, Motor Scale	77	88	63	82
MAI	96	65	52	91
MAI	96	80	43	99
AIMS	91	86	50	98

AIMS, Alberta Infant Motor Scale; BSID, Bayley Scales of Infant Development; MAI, Movement Assessment of Infants; PV, predictive value.
Data from references 61, 62, and 212.

evaluate motor maturation over time. The AIMS is described as an "observational assessment" that requires minimal handling of the infant by the examiner. The test includes 58 items, organized by the infant's position, designed to evaluate three aspects of motor performance: weight-bearing, posture, and antigravity movements. The normative sample consisted of 2200 infants born in Alberta, Canada.

Raw scores obtained on the AIMS can be converted to percentile ranks for comparison with the motor performance of the normative sample. Test-retest and interrater reliabilities, established on normally developing infants, ranged from 0.95 to 0.98 depending on the age of the child. The AIMS reportedly had high agreement with the Motor Scale of the BSID and the Gross Motor Scale of the Peabody Developmental Motor Scales (PDGMS) (r = 0.93 and r = 0.98, respectively).[176] An evaluation of concurrent validity between the AIMS and the MAI at 4 and 8 months demonstrated "good" agreement (r = 0.70 and r = 0.84, respectively)[60] The predictive validity of the AIMS is presently being evaluated to determine appropriate cutoff points to distinguish deviant or abnormal performance and to assess its predictive accuracy.[61]

Predictive Validity of Infant Assessment Tools. Table 8–11 shows the sensitivity and specificity of several infant assessment tools. It can be seen that more thorough instruments, such as the Neurological Examination of the Newborn and Infant[13] and the MAI,[46] have a high sensitivity but a relatively low specificity. Instruments that are less detailed, such as the AIMS, tend to have higher specificity but lower sensitivity. High sensitivity indicates that infants with a neuromotor impairment are unlikely to be "missed," or falsely identified as "normal," in a follow-up assessment; but low specificity suggests that infants who do not have a neuromotor impairment are more likely to be inappropriately identified as "abnormal." The balance between specificity and sensitivity can be altered by changing the cutoff score: a higher score will reduce the sensitivity of the test but increase the specificity.

A recent study of 164 high-risk infants compared the predictive ability of the AIMS, the MAI, and the PDGMS administered at 4 and 8 months of age relative to motor outcome at 18 months.[62] At 4 months, the MAI with a cut-point of 10 or higher provided the best combination of specificity and sensitivity values, as well as the highest positive predictive value, compared with the other assessments. For the AIMS, the 10th centile rank was determined to provide the optimal predictive accuracy at this age. At 8 months, the MAI and the AIMS were comparable in their combined sensitivity and specificity, with a 5th or 10th centile cut-point recommended for the AIMS. The positive predictive value of the AIMS was higher than that of the MAI at this age.

The positive predictive values for the MAI at 4 and 8 months were 58.3% and 42.9%, respectively, and for the AIMS, 39.5% and 50.0%, respectively (based on a cut-point of 10%).[62] These figures indicate that for this sample, approximately one half of the infants who were identified as "at risk" by the MAI or the AIMS had an abnormal outcome. On the other hand, negative pre-

dictive values for both the AIMS and the MAI were consistently above 90% at both the 4- and 8-month examinations. These results demonstrate that a negative, or "normal," rating for an infant is a more stable prediction of outcome than a positive, or "abnormal," rating.

The choice of assessment instrument and cutoff score should be determined according to the purpose and objectives of the follow-up clinic and the population of infants that will be evaluated. If the primary goal is to detect possible signs of early neuromotor abnormality so that infants at increased risk for disability can be monitored more closely, a test with a high sensitivity is most desirable. This may be an important consideration for a regional clinic, or a clinic in a high-risk social environment where regular follow-up visits or ongoing medical supervision is not routine. When it is likely that a high-risk infant will not be seen again for 8 to 12 months, or the family may be lost to regular medical follow-up, even *potential* problems need to be identified and addressed. On the other hand, in a clinical situation where a high-risk infant is monitored regularly or where a test result of "abnormal" dictates referral to intervention services, high specificity would be of greater priority to prevent unnecessary stress to the family or inappropriate utilization of limited therapy resources.

High-Risk Clinical Signs. Longitudinal studies of LBW infants have been used to identify specific clinical signs or conditions that are most predictive of abnormal neurodevelopmental outcome, such as cerebral palsy. The conclusions among studies are inconsistent owing to the lack of standard criteria for the risk variables, demographic and clinical variation in the study samples, and the use of different outcome measures. Results from these studies are summarized in Table 8–12.

Neonatal Period. During the neonatal period and first 1 to 2 months' post-term age, clinical signs considered to be indicative of neuromotor abnormality include stiff, jerky movements or a paucity of movement. Heinz Prechtl and his colleagues have developed an assessment technique that is based on the recognition of "General Movements" that occur at specific times during matura-

---

TABLE 8–12. Clinical Characteristics of Transient Dystonia

Neonatal Period
Neck extensor hypertonia
Hypotonia
Irritability; lethargy

4 Months of Age
Increased muscle tone in extremities
Truncal hypotonia
Scapular adduction/shoulder retraction
Persistent reflexes: asymmetrical tonic neck reflex; positive support reflex
Asymmetry

6–8 Months of Age
Increased muscle tone in lower extremities
Truncal hypotonia; minimal trunk rotation
Immature postural reactions
Immaturity of fine motor skills

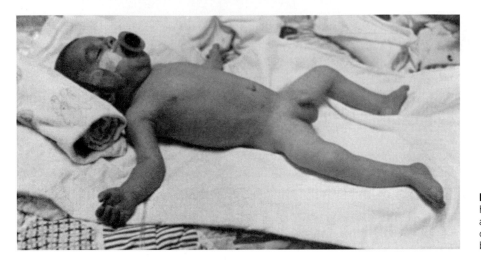

FIGURE 8–33. Posture characteristic of hypotonia with minimal movement against gravity in unswaddled 4-month-old preterm infant with bronchopulmonary dysplasia.

tion. Abnormal general movements are characterized as movements with "reduced complexity and a reduced variation. They lack fluency and frequently have an abrupt onset with all parts of the body moving synchronously ....."[92] Persistence of these movements is considered to be predictive of cerebral palsy and/or cognitive impairment.[92]

Infancy. At 4 months of age, hypertonicity of the trunk or extremities is recognized as a high-risk clinical sign.[12, 13, 84, 98, 212] Neck extensor hypertonicity has been reported to be highly predictive of cerebral palsy.[75] This finding correlates with neck hyperextension and shoulder retraction associated with the tonic labyrinthine reflex in supine, which has been identified as a high-risk sign by other studies.[98] However, although neck hypertonicity was the single item that was most predictive of cerebral palsy in one study, the majority of infants (60%) who exhibited this clinical sign did not subsequently develop cerebral palsy.[75] Hypotonicity of the trunk at 3 months of age has also been associated with abnormal developmental outcome[84] (Fig. 8–33).

The predictive value of primitive reflexes has been debated extensively. Reflexes and neurological signs, such as the asymmetrical tonic neck reflex (ATNR) and tremulousness, have been correlated with cerebral palsy in some studies[75, 190, 249] but not in others.[98] Of the four sections of the MAI, Primitive Reflexes has been found to be the least predictive of later outcome.[99, 212] The positive support reflex, as manifested as stiff extension of the lower extremities when the infant is held in supported standing, is frequently cited as a high-risk sign, but this posture is seen in both term and LBW infants and has not been consistently associated with adverse sequelae.[98, 212, 228] Persistent reflex activity and asymmetry have been identified as early signs of athetoid cerebral palsy, which is more common among term infants.[248] In Figure 8–34 a dominant ATNR posture is demonstrated by a 4-month-old infant with athetoid cerebral palsy. Immaturity of automatic reactions of balance and equilibrium at 4 months, including head righting and the Landau reaction, has been found to be a significant predictor of abnormal neurological outcome.[98]

Recent research has also emphasized the importance of an infant's spontaneous, active movements compared with reflex or passive responses in determining risk for neurodevelopmental disability. Systematic observation of the kicking activity of LBW infants indicates that infants with neurological impairment demonstrate less alternate kicking movement compared with that in normally developing LBW infants.[70] Abnormal patterns of kicking, including simultaneous flexion and extension of the hips and knees, were associated with subsequent cerebral palsy.[247] Abnormalities of kicking described by Prechtl as "cramped-synchronized"—that is, limited in variety and characterized by "rigid movement with all limbs and the trunk contracting and relaxing almost simultaneously"—were observed in 3-month-old infants who were subsequently diagnosed with cerebral palsy.[230]

In addition to qualitative differences in motor function, delayed acquisition of motor milestones is an important

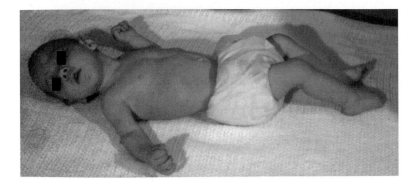

FIGURE 8–34. Dominant asymmetrical tonic neck reflex in 4-month-old infant with athetoid cerebral palsy.

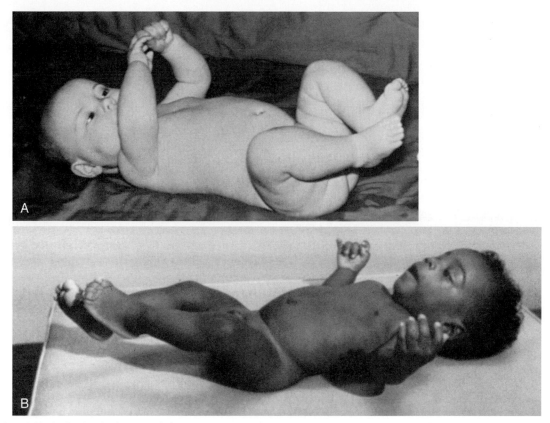

FIGURE 8–35. *A*, Typically developing term infant at 4 months of age demonstrating ability to bring hands to midline and elevate legs with flexion and abduction of hips and dorsiflexion of ankles. *B*, Infant diagnosed with cerebral palsy at 5 months of age; note inability to bring hands to midline because of shoulder retraction, extension and adduction of hips with limited movement into flexion, and plantarflexion of ankles.

indicator of neuromotor impairment. Several investigations of the predictive validity of the MAI found Volitional Movement to be the most predictive MAI category at 4 and 8 months.[99, 212] This finding is supported by other studies in which delayed developmental milestones were significant predictors of later cerebral palsy[4, 75] (Fig. 8–35). In particular, delay in achievement of later milestones, such as sitting without support, creeping on hands to knees, and pulling to stand, was found to be useful in identifying infants with neuromotor impairment.[4]

Challenges to Prediction of Neurodevelopmental Outcome

Accurate prediction of neurodevelopmental outcome of LBW infants on the basis of standard neuromotor tests is particularly challenging because of several complicating factors.

Impact of Medical Status on Test Performance. LBW infants often exhibit motor delay or neuromotor deviations because of their health or medical status, not because of neurological impairment. Two primary examples are (1) residual influences from habitual positioning in the NICU and (2) chronic medical conditions.

Variations in Posture and Movement Due to Residual Influences from the Period of Hospitalization in the NICU. Although current NICU positioning and handling procedures are sensitive to the developmental needs of

the neonate, provision of life-sustaining interventions is often the priority concern. Infants who have spent prolonged periods of time in the supine position, with minimal support to their shoulders or hips, are likely to maintain a posture of shoulder retraction and diminished flexion activity (see Fig. 8–33). On follow-up evaluation, these infants are typically delayed in reaching skills and in their ability to achieve antigravity postures.

LBW infants frequently exhibit asymmetry that may be related to position in utero or to prolonged positioning in the NICU necessitated by surgical or medical intervention. On a follow-up examination, this asymmetry may appear as visual orientation to one side of the body, more mature upper extremity skill on the same side, and asymmetry of primitive reflex activity. Physical deviations, such as tightness of neck musculature on the preferred side and relative weakness of the opposing muscles, or cranioplagia, may be present.[66, 210] Asymmetrical motor function resulting from in utero or NICU positioning can usually be distinguished from early spastic hemiplegia or other hemisyndromes by clinical examination and by review of the infant's medical history.[66, 212] Positional asymmetry is generally not associated with differences in muscle tone between the two sides of the body or with neuromotor abnormalities, such as fisting of the hand on the less active side. Caregivers are advised to promote symmetrical posture through their physical handling of the infant, placement of the infant in relation to toys, social activity in the room, and use of cushions or rolls to maintain midline positioning for the infant's head and proximal musculature.

Prolonged Retardation of Motor Development Because of Chronic Medical Conditions, Such as Bronchopulmonary Dysplasia. Infants with chronic lung disease typically exhibit low muscle tone, delayed gross motor function, and immature balance reactions. Motor skills are often delayed as long as the infant's pulmonary capacity is compromised, but the rate of developmental progress typically accelerates when the respiratory condition resolves.[130, 131] Intervention for infants with persistent respiratory disease includes providing reassurance and support to the caregivers who are dealing with the demands and stresses of parenting a medically fragile child. Caregivers are advised to avoid aggressive physical activity and excessive sensory stimulation that could cause fatigue or tax the infant's limited respiratory capacity. At the same time, it is important that the child be given opportunities to develop skills in nonmotor arenas. Adaptive positioning techniques enable the infant to be supported in age-appropriate postures, such as prone-lying or upright sitting, that are necessary for the development of hand function, vestibular responses, and social skills, without major expenditure of energy.

Transient Dystonia. During the first year of life, up to 60% of all LBW infants, as well as a number of full-term infants, exhibit abnormal neurological signs that subsequently resolve without evidence of major neurodevelopmental sequelae.[54, 64, 69, 88, 143, 174] This phenomenon is referred to as "transient dystonia." The abnormalities are initially observed in the first 4 months of life, are most prominent between 4 and 8 months, and usually resolve by 1 year of age (Fig. 8–36). The clinical characteristics of transient dystonia described most frequently are summarized in Table 8–12.

The presence of these findings on clinical examination poses a challenge to the physical therapist because they are often undistinguishable from clinical signs considered to be indicative of early cerebral palsy (Table 8–13). Longitudinal studies suggest that infants with transient neuromotor abnormalities may be at increased risk for long-term neurodevelopmental problems. Infants who demonstrated abnormal neurological findings during the first 12 months, although considered to be developmentally normal at 1 year of age, reportedly had a higher incidence of mental, motor, and behavioral deficits in

TABLE 8–13. Clinical Signs Indicative of Possible Neuromotor Impairment in LBW/VLBW Infants

Neonatal Period
Abnormal muscle tone
Jerky, stiff movements
Tremulousness
Abnormal or absent cry; abnormal eye movements

4 Months of Age
Hypertonicity: limited passive mobility in hips, ankles, or shoulders; neck extensor hypertonicity
Truncal hypotonicity
Abnormal kicking with simultaneous bilateral leg movements of flexion and extension
Persistent, dominant reflexes: asymmetrical tonic neck reflex; tonic labyrinthine in supine
Motor delay in: head control, hands to midline, support in prone position
Fisted hands

6–8 Months of Age
Hypertonicity of extremities
Persistent, dominant reflexes: asymmetrical tonic neck reflex, tonic labyrinthine in supine, positive support
Delayed postural reactions: head righting, equilibrium reactions
Delayed motor skills: rolling, sitting, support in prone position, reach and grasp
Persistent asymmetry with differences in muscle tone and functional skill

preschool and at school age.[13, 69, 88] However, a definite relationship between transient abnormalities in infancy and long-term developmental outcome has not been confirmed by other studies.[64, 143, 209]

Abnormal neuromotor signs, even if they appear to be transient, should not be considered as clinically insignificant. They may indicate a child who is at risk for subtle neuromotor problems that will not be functionally evident until school age. Furthermore, neuromotor deviations, although transient, may interfere with the infant's ability to form attachments with caregivers. The infant who arches back into extension instead of cuddling, has poor head control and difficulty establishing eye contact, or stiffens when held may contribute to feelings of frustration, inadequacy, or resentment in caregivers. Instruction in handling techniques to minimize these postures, as well as informing caregivers that these behaviors reflect neurological instability commonly seen in LBW infants, is often valuable intervention during this "transient" period.

Differences Between Preterm and Term Infant Neuromotor Function. The motor development of LBW infants differs from that of typical full-term infants even when not compromised by chronic illness or neurological impairment. When compared with full-term infants, healthy premature infants demonstrate variations in their passive and active muscle tone. They initially tend to have greater joint mobility, such as an increased popliteal angle and low muscle tone in the trunk.[133, 210] In the older infant, increased extremity tone is often present, particularly in the hips and ankles.[177, 210] Comparison studies have frequently noted that preterm infants tend to exhibit more neck hyperextension and scapular adduction

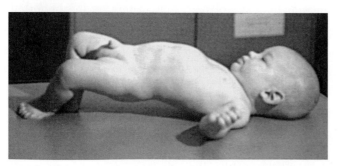

FIGURE 8–36. Preterm infant at 4 months of corrected age demonstrating excessive trunk arching and shoulder retraction, but developmental outcome was normal at 1 year.

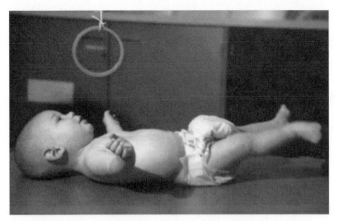

FIGURE 8–37. Healthy preterm infant at 4 months of corrected age demonstrating neck hyperextension, scapular adduction/shoulder retraction, and limited antigravity movement into flexion.

and fewer antigravity movements in supine[84, 85, 88, 89, 210, 228] (Fig. 8–37).

Primitive reflexes, such as the ATNR, the Moro reflex, and the positive support reflex, persist longer in LBW infants, even when assessed at corrected age.[65, 134, 228] Balance responses, such as protective extension reactions of the arms, are generally less mature in the healthy premature infant when compared with full-term infants of comparable age (Fig. 8–38). Gross and fine motor skills, especially activities requiring active flexion, such as bringing hands to midline and feet to hands; truncal stability, required for head control and upright sitting; and, trunk rotation, seen in rolling and transitional movements, are frequently delayed relative to standard norms.[89, 210]

LBW infants exhibit more asymmetry in their active movements compared with full-term infants, but asymmetry is usually not observed in their passive tone or reflex activity.[66, 210] One group of investigators concluded that "these findings convey an important clinical message: if motor asymmetries are only restricted to the facet of active muscle power, then they are unlikely to be of central origin and as such should not be seen as a sign of neurological impairment. In short, they constitute a typical feature of the post-term development of relatively healthy preterm infants."[66] For most premature infants, these early variations in movement and posture eventually resolve. However, in the first months of life, neuromotor deviations may influence the infant's performance on a standard assessment of motor function or neurological status.

In Utero Exposure to Drugs and Other Substances. Infants with a history of in utero exposure to illicit drugs, such as marijuana, cocaine, or methadone, may exhibit deviations in their neuromotor behavior. Neonatal abstinence syndrome, predominantly observed in infants exposed to heroin or methadone, is characterized by irritability, tremulousness, and inconsolability. Treatment of neonatal abstinence syndrome with morphine or other medications during the neonatal period usually leads to resolution of the symptoms within 2 to 4 weeks.

Since 1985, when "crack" cocaine became widely available to women of child-bearing age, many term gestation and LBW infants have been exposed prenatally to cocaine. Reliable documentation of the effects of in utero cocaine exposure on the neurobehavioral outcome of the neonate and infant is limited. Results vary, and reported findings are frequently compromised by methodological limitations of the research.[211] Studies suggest that prenatal cocaine exposure is associated with tremulousness, irritability, hypertonia, abnormal reflexes, and motor impairment in the neonatal period.[25, 47, 151, 154] These findings are not consistently observed and, when present, often do not persist beyond 2 to 4 months of age.

Longitudinal research specifically addressing motor outcomes in infants beyond the neonatal period has yielded inconsistent results. Follow-up studies using the BSID have generally observed no statistically significant differences in the PDI scores of exposed and nonexposed infants when examined at 6, 12, 24, or 30 months of age.[5, 47, 106, 107] Cocaine exposure also was not associated with significant differences in scores on the Peabody Developmental Motor Scales (PDMS) at 6 or 15 months.[79] How-

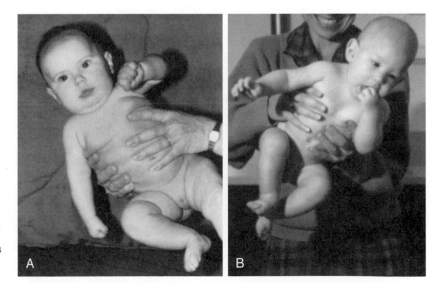

FIGURE 8–38. *A,* Normal full-term infant at 4 months of age demonstrating lateral head righting. When tipped to the side she is able to maintain her head in midline. *B,* Healthy preterm infant at 4 months of age demonstrating immature lateral head righting. When the body is tipped to one side, the head also leans toward that side.

ever, a preliminary report from one study indicated inferior fine motor performance on the PDMS at 24 months of age in a group of infants exposed prenatally to cocaine.[80]

Studies using the MAI as an outcome measure have detected subtle but statistically significant differences in the neuromotor function of cocaine-exposed infants.[79, 198, 213] Prenatal cocaine exposure was associated with higher total risk scores at 4 and 8 months, with significant differences in muscle tone, primitive reflexes, and volitional movement. Individual clinical findings included tremulousness, extension posturing with shoulder retraction, fisted hands, inability to bring hands to midline, and less mature head balance in the infants prenatally exposed to cocaine.[198, 213] Further evidence suggests that infants exposed through the third trimester of pregnancy may be at increased risk for adverse neuromotor outcomes.[213]

The long-term implications of cocaine-related neuromotor or behavioral deviations observed in exposed infants are not known. Follow-up studies have generally found no significant differences on standardized test performance between children with prenatal cocaine exposure and a comparable control group. However, in some recent longitudinal studies evaluating children at school age, prenatal cocaine exposure was associated with increased risk for deficits in visual-motor skills, language, and attentional behavior.[26, 102, 187] Further research is required to determine if neuromotor abnormalities detected in infancy are related to adverse long-term developmental outcome.

Clinical Decision Making in the High-Risk Infant Follow-Up Clinic

During the past 10 to 20 years, advances in multiple areas have dramatically increased the amount of information and knowledge available to the therapist working in a high-risk infant follow-up clinic. Evidence-based medical practice requires the therapist to access objective, scientifically based evidence and to incorporate this knowledge into the formation of diagnostic and therapeutic decisions. More sophisticated imaging techniques, assessment tools with improved predictive accuracy, and high-risk factors identified by longitudinal research provide the substance for evidence-based decisions. Yet, as is indicated by the material presented earlier, no single source of information currently offers a means of establishing a definitive and reliable prognosis for the neurodevelopmental outcome of the preterm infant.

During the follow-up clinic evaluation, the therapist administers the standardized assessment procedures, obtains information from the caregivers, and observes the movements and behavioral responses of the infant. The information and impressions gained are evaluated within the context of the infant's medical, social, and environmental history to form a hypothesis regarding the infant's neuromotor status and prognosis. Although this process is very individualized, because it is influenced by the therapist's own clinical experience and by the characteristics of the infant, an informed clinical judgment should be reached in an organized, systematic way. Clinical decisions should be based on the integration of knowledge derived from valid research with the therapist's clinical experience and expertise and with the values and priorities of the family.

General Guidelines. The clinical decision-making process for at-risk infants occurs within a framework of general guidelines regarding the neurodevelopmental outcome of LBW infants. These guidelines are based on the clinical and research evidence presented earlier.

1. Risk for adverse neurodevelopmental outcome is increased by the presence of specific abnormal neurological signs, but the majority of infants with any abnormal sign develop normally.
2. A normal neonatal or infant assessment is more predictive than an abnormal examination.
3. Multiple factors are more predictive of neurodevelopmental outcome than single factors, emphasizing the need for a comprehensive evaluation.
4. Periodic, sequential examinations over time are the most useful method of determining the developmental outcome of an individual infant.

A conceptual model provided by Aylward is used to understand and categorize the variations that are observed in an infant's neuromotor function.[15] In this model, three types of developmental abnormality are described: (1) *delay*, which occurs when a child does not achieve an expected developmental milestone; (2) *dissociation*, a difference in the developmental rate of two different aspects of development (e.g., cognitive and motor); and (3) *deviation*, "an atypical developmental indicator."[15]

Clinical Decision-Making Pathway. A model of the clinical decision-making process for the pediatric therapist in a follow-up clinic is shown in Figure 8–39. It is based on a model of clinical decision making that was developed for pediatric physical therapists working within an interdisciplinary assessment team.[221] The model is composed of a series of alternating "action steps," of data collection and assessment procedures, and "decision steps" of analysis, interpretation, and planning. The sequential order of the steps is intended to reflect the thought process and is not necessarily a linear progression of events.

Action Step 1: Obtain Relevant History. The therapist reviews the infant's medical history with particular attention to events or conditions that are known to be associated with neurological risk or adverse outcomes. For the infant born prematurely, key risk factors including extremely low birth weight (<1000 g), abnormal findings on cranial ultrasonography, neonatal seizures, or infectious conditions should be noted. For the full-term infant, indicators of birth asphyxia or trauma, infection, and genetic or metabolic disorders are highlighted. Evidence of prenatal exposure to illicit drugs or alcohol, and the timing and extent of exposures during pregnancy, should also be noted. Attention is given to the source and reason for the referral: is this a routinely scheduled examination for a graduate of the NICU, or is this an infant who has raised specific concerns for caregivers or medical professionals? Specific concerns of caregivers are an important consideration, although parents' overall perceptions of the developmental status of their high-risk infant do not correlate well with clinical assessment.[115] Background information

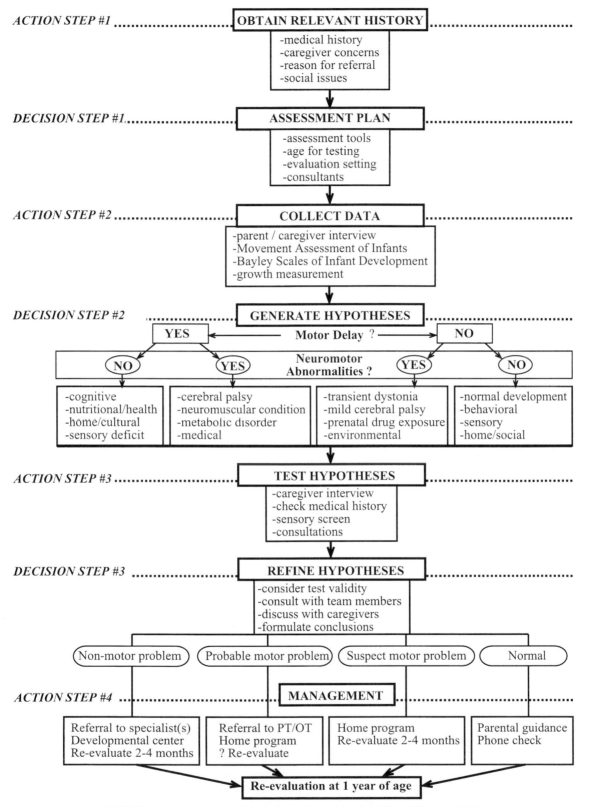

FIGURE 8–39. Decision-making pathway in the high-risk infant follow-up clinic.

about the social environment is also reviewed to identify risk factors, as well as to ascertain available resources and level of support for the caregivers.

Decision Step #1: Assessment Plan. On the basis of the information gained, the therapist anticipates the central questions and issues that need to be addressed in the evaluation and decides on an appropriate assessment plan. This includes consideration of the testing instruments to be used, the evaluation setting and format, and the interdisciplinary team members to be included. For standardized tests to be administered, the therapist must determine the appropriate age level for initiation of testing. The age level will be determined by the choice of chronological or corrected age, as well as preliminary evidence suggesting that the child may be functioning below expected age level.

Consideration is also given to medical conditions or sensory impairments that would require alterations of the standardized testing procedures. For example, an infant who is medically fragile and still receiving oxygen support might be unable to tolerate the amount of physical handling and stimulation in a typical evaluation period. The needs and concerns of the caregivers should also be anticipated. Parents from a high-risk social background may benefit from consultation with a social worker and a confidential testing situation; non–English-speaking parents will require an interpreter.

Action Step #2: Collect Data. The initial interview enables the therapist to establish a relationship with the parents or caregivers, to elicit their perception of the infant's developmental status and their specific concerns and questions, and to explain the evaluation process. If the infant is awake and alert at the outset of the examination period, lengthy detailed discussion should be avoided to ensure that the assessment will be completed before the infant becomes tired or fatigued. The organization of the evaluation session allows for a logical sequence of testing and an efficient use of time, while maintaining the flexibility to respond to the infant's cues and needs. Test items that require the infant's compliance and cooperation, such as items of the Mental Scale of the BSID, are ideally administered first; activities that may be stressful, such as balance reactions and growth measurements, are done later in the evaluation.

Decision Step #2: Generate Hypotheses. Beginning with the initial review of the medical history and throughout the evaluation, the therapist formulates hypotheses regarding the infant's neurodevelopmental status. Two questions underlie the overall assessment process.

Is motor development delayed? Determination of the level of motor function is based on the infant's performance on the standardized tests, observations of the child's movement activities, and the therapist's knowledge of normal development in the first year of life. For the preterm infant, this question involves a decision regarding the use of chronological or corrected age; if corrected age is used, the accuracy of the gestational age estimate must be considered.

Is neuromotor function abnormal or deviant? Identification of neuromotor abnormalities is based on test results, clinical observations of the infant's movements and behavior throughout the assessment period, and the therapist's own experience and knowledge of atypical or abnormal neuromotor function.

By considering these questions within a matrix configuration, four potential hypothetical situations can be derived. Whereas such a matrix is a simplistic representation, it accurately presents the major issues to be addressed in the evaluation of a high-risk infant.

1. ***If motor development is delayed relative to the infant's age (corrected or adjusted age for the preterm infant) and the quality of movement is abnormal,** the possibility of cerebral palsy or other neuromuscular condition must be seriously considered.*

A number of longitudinal studies conclude that the early signs of neurodevelopmental disabilities, such as cerebral palsy, include both motor delay and neuromotor deviations. Neuromotor abnormalities that are not associated with delayed motor skills appear to be of minimal clinical significance. When accompanied by delayed motor function, neuromotor deviations have greater prognostic value. The age of the infant and testing conditions are critical factors because, at a given age, absent skills may be just emerging and deviant responses may be exaggerated by stress, fatigue, or illness.

2. ***If motor development is delayed or immature, but the quality of movement appears to be normal with no evidence of neuromotor abnormalities,** nonmotor problems should be considered as potential causes of the motor delay.*

Possible reasons for a motor delay include medical conditions, such as bronchopulmonary dysplasia; health or nutritional problems, such as failure to thrive; a cognitive deficit that diminishes the child's lack of motivation to move or explore; and a sensory defect, such as a vision or hearing impairment. Environmental conditions within the home can also contribute to delayed motor function as measured by a standardized test. For example, since the introduction of the "Back to Sleep" campaign designed to reduce the risk of sudden infant death syndrome, infants typically spend less time in the prone position and healthy full-term infants are delayed in their acquisition of rolling on the Denver Developmental Screening Test.[108] Extended time spent in a baby walker has been associated with delayed achievement of sitting, creeping on hands and knees, and independent ambulation.[113, 207, 223]

Ethnic or racial variations may account for an apparent delay in motor development if an infant is evaluated by a test that has been normed on infants of different ethnic group or groups. Compared with white infants, black infants exhibit higher muscle tone and achieve gross motor milestone at an earlier age.[3, 44, 48, 51] Full-term Asian, Asian-American, and Native American infants reportedly achieve gross and fine motor milestones at a slower pace.[48] Asian-American infants demonstrated longer persistence of primitive reflexes, delayed maturation of automatic reactions, and more asymmetries when evaluated with the MAI.[225] In addition to biological differences between infants of different racial backgrounds, cultural variations in child-rearing techniques can influence the rate of motor development. In some African and Asian cultures, the floor or ground is considered to be unclean and mothers are warned about negative spiritual consequences if an infant is placed on the floor before 6 months of age.

3. If neuromotor abnormalities are observed but motor development is not delayed, *early signs of mild cerebral palsy should be considered as one of several possible conditions.*

Mild diplegia or hemiplegia may first appear between 4 and 8 months of age as subtle asymmetries or muscle tone variations that are not likely to compromise motor function until the infant begins to crawl on hands and knees, pull to stand, or perform skilled bimanual activities. However, in the preterm infant, neuromotor variations without motor delay are more likely to be manifestations of transient dystonia. If the infant has a history of prenatal exposure to cocaine or other substances such as methamphetamines or heroin, characteristic neuromotor deviations may be observed but are usually not associated with definite delay of motor skills. Environmental influences may also account for deviations in the quality of movement. For example, infants who spend extended time in baby walkers, jumpers, or nonmobile standing devices may exhibit excessive toe-standing and limited mobility in ankle dorsiflexion.

4. If the examination reveals no delay in motor function and no abnormalities in the quality of the infant's movement, *the therapist may assume normal neurodevelopmental status but needs to explore alternative conditions.*

Consideration should be given to other possible reasons for the caregiver's or referring professional's concerns. A problem that is perceived as a neuromuscular impairment, such as paucity of active movement, minimal exploration of the environment, or failure to manipulate toys, may in fact be the consequence of a cognitive or sensory impairment. parents may be concerned by differences they observe between the motor development of their child and that of other infants of comparable age, or between siblings, particularly among nonidentical multiple birth siblings. For the parents or caregivers of an LBW infant, the therapist should emphasize the importance of using the infant's corrected age to determine developmental expectations, especially during the first 1 to 2 years of life. Furthermore, an infant's individual personality or body type can be a major factor in rate and style of development. Active infants with firm, strong neuromuscular structures typically achieve gross motor milestones earlier than infants with calm, placid personalities and large, chubby infants. It is essential that a therapist in a follow-up clinic be aware of the broad range of variability in the pace and age of acquisition of gross motor milestones in the normally developing infant.[61]

Action Step #3: Test Hypotheses. Initial hypotheses and assumptions can be verified or substantiated by additional testing and probing into the infant's medical or environmental history. Further discussion with the infant's care-givers may reveal health or nutritional conditions that could compromise physical growth or indicate other developmental influences within the infant's home. In general, open-ended questions elicit more relevant and informative responses and may be less threatening and intrusive than inquiries directed toward a specific answer. For example, a request to "Tell me what your baby's typical day is like" or "Where does your baby like to spend her time?" will provide a more complete view of the home environment and appear less challenging than "Do you put your baby in a baby walker?"

A review of the infant's birth and neonatal history may validate examination findings or cast doubts on a hypothesis being considered. For example, cranial ultrasound documentation of periventricular leukomalacia on the right side of the brain would provide support for suspicion of a neuromotor impairment on the left side of the body. On the other hand, a benign birth history for a term infant with a tendency to stand on her toes and immature of motor development would argue against an hypothesis of early cerebral palsy.

Consultation with or examination by other specialists may be warranted. For an infant with motor delay who exhibits no neuromotor abnormalities but shows inadequate physical growth, examination by the pediatrician or nutritionist may reveal health conditions that account for the motor delay. Immaturity in fine motor skills or asymmetrical development with persistent orientation to one side may be evidence of a visual impairment.

Decision Step #3: Refine Hypothesis. In formulating a final hypothesis, the validity of the test results must be considered. Performance on a standardized test may be compromised if the infant is fatigued, ill, exhibiting stranger anxiety, or unable to cope with the demands and stimulation of a testing situation. If this is a concern, the therapist can verify with the caregiver whether the observed responses and behaviors are representative of the infant's abilities and temperament typically observed at home.

Discussion with other members of the interdisciplinary follow-up clinic team is often helpful, especially when ambiguities or inconsistencies are present in the overall clinical picture. Although other team members may not have examined or observed the infant, they may be able to offer insights based on their own clinical experience when presented with a given constellation of factors. For example, a psychologist may recognize early signs of autistic behavior or a pediatrician may suspect a particular genetic disorder in an infant whose developmental profile is inconsistent with the therapist's expectations.

Finally, but most importantly in the clinical decision-making process, the therapist reviews the test results, clinical observations, and tentative conclusions with the infant's caregivers. A diagnosis is based on the expertise of the interdisciplinary professionals and the clinical, medical, and technological resources available to the follow-up clinic. However, it is important to acknowledge the individuality of the developmental course and outcome of each high-risk infant, the broad range of factors that influence an infant's development, and the limitations of a single assessment in an unfamiliar environment. A summary discussion with the parents or caregivers allows the therapist to present the clinical impressions of the follow-up team as well as the limitations of long-term prognosis for LBW infants and to assess the compatibility between the diagnostic hypotheses and the caregivers' perception of their infant.

Action Step #4: Management. In accordance with the protocol of the High Risk Infant Follow-up Clinic at the University of Washington, the infant who demonstrates normal neuromotor and developmental progress at the 4-month evaluation is scheduled for a follow-up evaluation at 1 year of age (corrected age). The parents or caregivers are informed of their infant's performance on the standard tests as well as the therapist's overall impressions and conclusions. In addition to reviewing the infant's abilities in various domains of competency (e.g., gross motor, fine motor, language), the child's personal strengths, such as sociability, alertness, inquisitiveness, or persistence, are emphasized. Recommendations for developmental activities and handling skills are given when appropriate, and caregivers are advised regarding expectations for their child's developmental activities in the next months. They are encouraged to call the therapist if they have questions about their child's developmental progress. If the therapist has noted a minor concern, such as a subtle asymmetry, an interim telephone call can verify that motor development is proceeding appropriately.

If the infant demonstrates definite neuromotor abnormality with motor delay (Fig. 8–40) or shows strong evidence of a neurodevelopmental disability, the child is referred to an appropriate intervention program. An infant who has only motor disability, without evidence of deficits in other areas, is usually referred to a pediatric therapist in the local community. The infant with delays in multiple areas of development may be referred to a developmental program with comprehensive, interdisciplinary services.

At 4 months of age, many LBW infants demonstrate immaturity or mild neuromotor abnormality. In this situation, the therapist gives parents or caregivers recommendations for methods of handling and positioning, as well as activities to facilitate normal developmental progress. Reevaluation is scheduled at an interval of 2 to 4 months based on the therapist's level of concern, the caregivers' preferences and concerns, and geographical, financial, and transportation considerations. At follow-up examination, the infant's neurodevelopmental status is reassessed.

If neuromotor abnormalities are still present, or if the infant's progress in acquisition of motor skills is below the expected rate, the infant is referred for intervention. If previous neuromotor concerns have resolved and motor development is progressing appropriately, the infant is scheduled to return for the 1-year evaluation.

At all follow-up visits, caregivers are advised about appropriate expectations for development in the subsequent months as well as hazards and risks. Particular emphasis is given to issues of safety, which often include injuries associated with infant walkers and the need for a "safe place" where an infant who has learned to crawl or walk can be confined. Caregivers are advised to introduce their infants to a playpen or other restrictive area before the time of independent mobility and to place the infant in this "safe place" whenever they are unable to provide constant supervision for their child.

NEUROMOTOR INTERVENTION

Levels of Intervention for the High-Risk Infant

Therapeutic intervention for the high-risk infant in the outpatient phase after discharge from the NICU occurs at multiple levels. Type and intensity of intervention depend on (1) the needs of the infant and family, (2) the structure and organization of the follow-up clinic, and (3) the availability of resources in a particular clinical and geographical setting.

Assessment as Intervention. The clinical assessment of an infant is a unique opportunity for intervention on behalf of the infant and his family. For the full potential of this interaction to be realized, parents or caregivers must be informed and involved participants in the assessment process, not passive observers. The focus of intervention in this context is on parent or caregiver support with two primary components: (1) *education* and (2) *positive reinforcement for parenting skills*.

Education. The educational component of intervention includes enabling the parents of an at-risk infant to recognize their child's unique capabilities and strengths as well as his or her ability to respond to and influence the surrounding environment. Caregivers learn about their infant's individual responses to stimuli: for example, what causes their child to attend and what elicits stress reac-

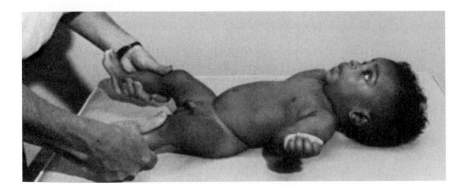

FIGURE 8–40. Infant diagnosed with cerebral palsy at 5 months of corrected age; limited hip abduction is demonstrated with passive mobility.

tions. Parent education includes describing typical characteristics and common developmental patterns of the LBW or medically fragile infant that may differ from expectations that are based on observations or published descriptions of healthy full-term infants. Parents of at-risk infants are informed about the appropriate sequence and pace of development for their child so they will be realistic in their expectations and interpretation of the child's progress. This anticipatory guidance enables parents to prepare for and maximize learning opportunities.

Reinforcement for Parenting Skills. During the follow-up examination, opportunities to provide positive reinforcement to caregivers need to be emphasized. It is especially important that parents of a high-risk infant who responds inconsistently to affective cues be given positive feedback and affirmation for their investment of emotion and energy.[245] They should be reassured that they are providing appropriate and beneficial parenting and reminded that the infant's behavioral responses reflect neurobehavioral immaturity or instability, rather than an unpleasant "personality" or negative affective feelings toward the caregiver.

Intervention as Instruction in Home Management. A critical component of intervention is instruction in specific activities and handling techniques for home management. The recommendations are based on the therapist's knowledge of the infant's medical and neurological history, current health status, and findings from the neurodevelopmental assessment. The overall purpose may be to maximize a healthy child's growth potential or to promote developmental progress in an infant who demonstrates delay or neuromotor abnormality. In either case, it is essential that the parent or caregiver have a clear understanding of the purpose of the activity, what motor behavior it is intended to facilitate or counteract, the underlying neurodevelopmental process that the activity will support, and the desired response on the part of the infant. This enables the parent to participate more creatively in the process of intervention by adapting and modifying the recommendations according to the infant's responses and progress of the infant at home.

Although handling recommendations are specific to the individual child, some intervention activities are applicable to many preterm infants. These include the following:

Activities to Counteract Shoulder Retraction. Up to 50% of LBW infants reportedly demonstrate shoulder retraction.[85] This posture inhibits the infant's ability to bring hands to midline and often results in delayed achievement of upper-extremity skills and rolling. To overcome shoulder retraction, play activities and carrying techniques that bring shoulders forward and hands to midline are encouraged.

Reaching. Most premature infants are immature in their reaching skills, reducing their ability to interact with their environment. Activities to counteract shoulder retraction will promote reaching, but it is also essential that LBW infants be provided with opportunities to practice this skill. Often infants who are ready to initiate reaching at 3 to 4 months of age have only a visually stimulating mobile suspended beyond their reach in the

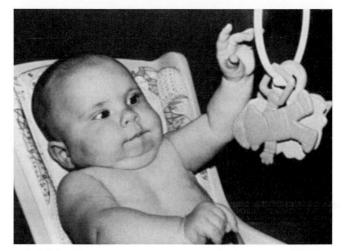

FIGURE 8–41. Toys suspended directly in front of infant to encourage symmetrical reaching and midline orientation of head.

crib. Caregivers are advised to hang toys *within the child's reach* in the crib, playpen, or other suitable place. Objects that are suspended, rather than handed to or placed in front of the infant, are preferred to promote the development of directed reach and grasp as well as shoulder stability (Fig. 8–41). Activity gyms that stand upright on the floor, which are commercially available and relatively inexpensive, are highly recommended for LBW infants.

Centering and Symmetrical Orientation. Midline positioning of head with symmetrical alignment of the trunk and extremities is encouraged to counteract the residual effects of asymmetrical positioning in utero or during hospitalization. Midline orientation will reduce the influence of the ATNR and promote symmetrical function of the right and left sides of the body. Asymmetry that is not caused by neurological dysfunction tends to resolve when positioning and environmental influences are modified.

Prone Positioning. Active play time in the prone position is beneficial for the development of postural control of the neck and back and of shoulder stability in weight-bearing. Prone lying also counteracts extension posturing because influence of the tonic labyrinthine reflex in prone contributes to extremity flexion. However, parents of vulnerable premature infants are often hesitant to place their infants in the prone position. LBW infants, particularly infants who have relatively large heads and are visually attentive, often demonstrate a low tolerance for prone positioning. Caregivers are advised to gradually increase duration of the prone lying according to the infant's tolerance. Visually stimulating toys and objects, including mirrors and the faces of siblings or caregivers, can be placed on the floor in front of the infant to encourage acceptance of the prone position. A roll or wedge positioned under the infant's axillae will facilitate the ability to push up in prone, particularly for the infant with low muscle tone. An infant who is apprehensive or stressed when placed on the stomach may tolerate prone lying on the caregiver's chest, where reassuring eye contact can be maintained.

Head Balance. Balance activities to develop active head

control are frequently recommended for LBW infants. Tilting responses are usually achieved most effectively with the infant in the parent's lap. Instruction to the caregivers often includes demonstration and practice using a doll, as well as the infant. Emphasis is placed on the importance of (1) adequate trunk support; (2) movement through small ranges; (3) slow, graded motion; (4) the desired head-righting response; and (5) sensitivity to indications of stress or fatigue.

Limited Use of Infant Jumper or Baby Walker. For infants with increased lower-extremity tone or a tendency for toe-standing, the use of baby walkers and jumpers is discouraged because they may increase stiffness and extension posturing of the legs.[105] Moreover, mobile baby walkers are associated with a high risk of injury, including serious trauma such as burns, drowning, and severe head injuries resulting from falls down stairs.[109, 166, 214, 223] However, baby walkers are usually very enjoyable for infants and may provide caregivers with some needed moments of respite within a stressed household. Hence, when recommending that time in a baby walker or jumper be restricted, it is important for the therapist to assist the caregivers in finding alternative methods of positioning and amusement for the infant. Parents are often reluctant to discard a baby walker, believing that it promotes early ambulation and is beneficial for infants. Informing caregivers of the hazards of infant walkers and of research findings that indicate walker use may delay the acquisition of gross and fine motor skills enhances the likelihood of their cooperation.[109, 113, 202, 223]

Intervention as Ongoing Therapy. Referral to a regular program of therapeutic intervention is usually made after at least two assessments in the follow-up clinic and a trial period of interim home activities. Criteria for referral include the following:

1. Persistent or progressive indications of abnormal tone
2. Developmental delay in motor skills or postural reactions
3. Increasing asymmetry or disparity between right and left sides of the body, especially if accompanied by tone differences
4. Loss of joint mobility
5. Feeding difficulties

As described in the clinical decision-making pathway presented earlier, a referral for intervention is determined after consideration of several key factors including the following:

1. Infant's medical status
2. Concerns and priorities of parents or caregivers
3. Home environment
4. Availability of therapy services relative to geographical, financial, and personnel factors

Effectiveness of Early Therapy for Infants

Critical Analysis of Evidence. The effectiveness of therapy for high-risk or neurologically abnormal infants has been addressed by numerous studies and reviews with inconclusive and, at times, conflicting results.[23, 87, 138,] [162, 173, 193, 201, 203, 227, 236] The therapist whose clinical responsibilities include referring high-risk infants to intervention programs or providing intervention to high-risk infants must critically analyze these studies with respect to the validity of the research methodology and to clinical relevance. Specific questions to be addressed include the following:

1. Is the sample of infants or subjects receiving intervention "at risk" or neurologically abnormal? Are these infants similar to the infants seen in the therapist's own clinic situation?
2. Are the comparison groups of subjects similar in all relevant factors other than the intervention being studied?
3. Are the intervention techniques used clearly described and are they consistent with conventional therapy practice?
4. Is the frequency of therapy an accurate and realistic representation of the standard of practice?
5. Is the duration and timing of intervention appropriate and relevant to what is known about change in motor function and critical periods of development?
6. Is the quality and amount of parent or caregiver participation documented, evaluated, and realistic?
7. Are the outcome measures of the study appropriate relative to the subjects included in the study sample and to the methods and objectives of the intervention?

Characteristics of Positive Intervention for the At-Risk Infant. A review of early intervention programs that demonstrated measurable positive change highlights several characteristics of effective intervention.[138, 139, 162, 185, 201, 227]

High Degree of Parent Involvement. The parents or caregivers must be active participants in the therapy session as well as the therapy program at home. This requires that activities and techniques to be carried out by the parents are comprehensible and manageable by them. Infants often spend much of their time in the care of other adults besides their parents, such as relatives or day-care providers. Instructions or recommendations that are given in the therapy session must be easily communicated to all of the infant's caregivers.

Comprehensive Program of Developmental Intervention. Motor skills cannot be addressed in isolation from other aspects of an infant's development. To improve quality of life, not just quality of movement, the therapist must include the broad perspective of infant learning and development.

Well-Defined Curriculum of Sequential Activities. Physical therapy for infants has traditionally been implemented through a flexible and variable selection of therapy activities rather than a structured curriculum. However, a defined program of learning objectives and activities enables the therapist and caregivers (as well as day-care providers and others participating in the infant's care) to have a clear and consistent understanding of the current therapeutic activities, the goals of the program, and the steps involved in achieving those goals.

Intervention for a LBW Infant. The therapy program for an infant ideally incorporates the preceding recommendations into a treatment plan that is individualized for the infant and the home environment. Progress is monitored by systematic, quantified evaluation performed at regular intervals. Effectiveness of therapy is determined relative to the rate of progress and the specified goals for each infant.

The long-range goals of an intervention program for an infant with a neurodevelopmental disability must be realistic and stated in terms of clear, measurable objectives. When defining goals, it is important for therapists to make distinctions among (1) objectives that are generally accepted as achievable by therapy, (2) objectives that are presumed to be achievable through therapy but objective evidence is not available; and (3) changes that are not within the domain or capability of physical therapy. Examples of objectives in these categories are provided in Table 8–14.

For example, physical therapy cannot "cure" cerebral palsy (i.e., it cannot heal areas of damaged brain tissue). LBW infants who demonstrate neurological abnormalities and who receive therapy and subsequently show no residual signs of abnormality demonstrate a clinical course typical of transient dystonia, in which the neuromotor abnormalities resolve without intervention. To imply that the therapy "cured" the cerebral palsy is a misrepresentation and a disservice to families, funding agencies, and the profession. Nevertheless, the benefit of the support and guidance provided by the therapist to the family during this critical time of intervention should not be underestimated.

Therapists and other professionals are mandated to conduct research to evaluate the effectiveness of interventions that purport to modify movement and posture, or to improve motor function, in infants with neurological impairments. Other benefits of intervention, including prevention of contractures or deformities, design and modification of adaptive equipment, functional training, assistance in home management, and parent satisfaction, also need to be assessed and documented. Further research on the efficacy of physical therapy is required, especially by therapists working with this population who can address the clinical questions that are most important

to the quality of life for the LBW infant and the infant's family.

SUMMARY

This chapter on the NICU management and follow-up of at-risk neonates and infants presented three theoretical models for NICU practice, reviewed neonatal neuropathology related to movement disorders, and described expanded professional services for at-risk neonates and infants in a relatively new subspecialty within pediatric practice. Pediatric therapists participating in intensive care nursery and follow-up teams in the care of high-risk neonates and their parents are involved in an advanced-level practice area that requires heightened responsibility for accountability and for precepted clinical training (beyond general pediatric specialization) in neonatology and infant therapy techniques. Practice guidelines for the NICU from national task forces representing the American Physical Therapy Association and American Occupational Therapy Association indicate roles, proficiencies, and knowledge for neonatal therapy and designate the NICU as a restricted area of practice to therapy assistants, aides, and entry-level students on affiliation.

Inherent in this subspecialty practice is the challenge to design comprehensive neonatal therapy protocols and clinical paths that include standardized examination instruments, comprehensive risk-management plans, long-term follow-up strategies, and systematic documentation of outcome. Ongoing analyses of the physiological risk/therapeutic benefit relationship of neuromotor and neurobehavioral treatment for chronically ill and LBW infants must guide the NICU intervention process. The quality of collaboration between therapists and neonatal nurses largely determines the success of neonatal therapy implementation during the 24-hour care environment of the nursery.

Pediatric therapists working in neonatal units are encouraged to participate in follow-up clinics for NICU graduates to identify and analyze the development of movement dysfunction and behavioral sequelae that may, in the future, be minimized or prevented with creative neonatal treatment approaches. The important preventive aspect of neonatal treatment must be guided by careful analyses of neurodevelopmental and functional outcomes in the first year of life.

The LBW or medically fragile infant is at increased risk for major and minor neurodevelopmental problems that may be manifested in infancy or not became evident until childhood. Prenatal and perinatal risk factors serve to identify infants who have a greater likelihood of neurological complications, but the relationship between single factors and outcome is neither direct nor consistent. Abnormal neurological signs in the first year are also not reliably predictive of abnormal outcome. Attempts to identify factors that definitively indicate significant brain injury are complicated by changing NICU technology, management procedures, environmental variables, and the variability among and within individual infants.

In deciding whether and when an infant requires regular intervention, consideration must be given both to the

---

TABLE 8 – 14. Efficacy and Feasibility of Physical Therapy Intervention for At-Risk Infants

Realistic Goals of Physical Therapy	Potential Goals of Physical Therapy Not Yet Documented	Goals Not in Domain of Physical Therapy
Home management of disability (feeding, handling)	Change abnormal motor patterns	Cure cerebral palsy
Equipment design for position and function	Prevent physical deformities	Release contractures
Parent support and guidance	Minimize long-term neurodevelopmental abnormalities by early therapy	
Documentation of motor development in at-risk infants		

potential for abnormalities to resolve during the first year and to the time span that may elapse before definitive evidence of cerebral palsy. The pediatric therapist's long-term clinical management of the at-risk infant is guided by the developmental course of the individual infant over time, including behavioral and cognitive growth as well as neuromotor progress, considered within the context of the priorities and values of the family.

CASE STUDIES

CASE 8–1   HIGH-RISK INFANT 1

The infant was born prematurely at 29 weeks of gestation with a birth weight of 940 g. Her neonatal course was complicated by idiopathic respiratory distress syndrome, which was treated with surfactant.

She was first evaluated in the high-risk infant follow-up clinic at 4 months' corrected age (6 months' chronological age). Her mother stated that the infant had had several respiratory illnesses since she was discharged from the NICU. She also reported that this infant felt "tense" compared with her older child, who had been born at term, and seemed to be "a little behind" in her development. On the Bayley Seales of Infant Development II (BSID-II) her scores were Mental Scale score (MDI) of 94 and Motor Scale score (PDI) of 82. On the Movement Assessment of Infants (MAI), this infant had a total risk score of 7. She had mildly increased muscle tone in her lower extremities, which was evident in mild resistance to passive range of motion of her hips and ankles. She demonstrated persistent primitive reflexes, including an asymmetrical tonic neck reflex, a Moro reflex, and influence of the tonic labyrinthine reflex in supine. Head balance was immature, but emerging righting reactions were noted. When the infant was observed in supine her posture was extended, but she was beginning to bring her hands to midline. In prone, she had started to push up on elbows but posture was immature. Her parents were given recommendations for handling to include carrying position with shoulders forward to inhibit retraction, frequent play in the prone position, and increased opportunities for reaching in supine.

The infant returned at 8 months' corrected age. Her mother reported that she had made progress in some areas because she could now roll and was talking more but she had just started sitting up by herself and was not yet stable in sitting. She said that the "stiffness" was less evident, but the infant did not like to play when on her "tummy" and preferred to be in the baby walker. BSID-II scores at this time were MDI of 101 and PDI of 81. The MAI total risk score was 9. Increased muscle tone observed previously was less evident and she had full mobility in her hips but some resistance to passive movement of her ankles. Muscle tone of the trunk was mildly hypotonic but she demonstrated age-appropriate antigravity movements in all positions. Primitive reflexes were no longer evident except for the positive support reflex, which was seen in a tendency to stand on her toes when weight bearing on her feet. Balance reactions were present but immature in some areas, including head righting into flexion and protective extension reactions. In volitional skills, the infant was now sitting independently for up to 30 seconds, could roll from supine to prone, and could pivot on her stomach. She could pick up a block with either hand and transfer objects. Immaturity was seen in her sitting balance, her inability to move out of sitting, and her failure to progress forward on the floor. She attempted to pick up a pellet but was unable to do so. Her parents were advised to discontinue using the baby walker and to maximize play time on the floor. Because the infant reportedly enjoyed watching her 4-year-old sibling it was recommended that he play on the floor beside her. Her mother was also advised to provide the infant with tiny edible bits of food to practice fine dexterity.

When seen at 12 months' corrected age, the infant had an MDI of 108 and a PDI of 88. Although not yet not walking independently, she was cruising with good weight shift and balance. She was able to creep reciprocally on hands and knees and pulled to stand. She picked up a pellet with an inferior pincer grasp. No deviations of muscle tone or reflex development were observed during examination by the developmental pediatrician. The infant was developing normally and will return for follow-up at 2 years of age. Her parents were advised to call if she was not walking within 2 months or if they had any concerns regarding her pattern of independent walking.

In the management of this child who demonstrated abnormal signs, the primary responsibilities of the pediatric therapist were ongoing assessment and parental guidance and teaching. Although there were initial concerns about this infant because of muscle tone and reflex deviations, it would have been inappropriate to diagnose her with a particular condition. When followed over time, the abnormalities resolved and proved to be transient. This child should continue to be followed in the high-risk infant clinic because she remains at risk for neurodevelopmental problems, which may not become evident until school age.

CASE 8–2   HIGH-RISK INFANT 2

The infant was born prematurely at 29 weeks of gestation with a birth weight of 1200 g. The neonatal course was complicated by idiopathic respiratory distress syndrome and persistent apnea and bradycardia. Cranial ultrasonography revealed a left subependymal hemorrhage with ventriculomegaly and left-sided periventricular leukomalacia.

She was first seen in the high-risk infant follow-up clinic at 4 months' corrected age (6 months and 17 days' chronological age). The parents stated that they had no specific concerns regarding their daughter's development. On the Bayley Scales of Infant Development II (BSID-II) the infant received a Mental Scale score (MDI) of 96 and a Motor Scale score (PDI) of 87. On the Movement Assessment of Infants (MAI) the infant received a total risk score of 14. Muscle tone was normal at rest but increased when she was active or agitated. Tone in the lower extremities was mildly increased with restricted passive mobility in the hip abductors and gastrocsoleus muscles bilaterally. In supine, she frequently was in an extended posture and brought her hands to midline only once during the examination. In prone, she was able to push up and elevate her head while kicking actively. In the prone suspended position, she showed good postural elevation but movements were stiff. Persistent primitive reflexes included the tonic labyrinthine reflex in supine, asymmetrical tonic neck reflex, neonatal positive support reflex, and bilateral ankle clonus. Plantar grasp with toe curling was observed on the right. Righting and equilibrium reactions were emerging. She showed a mature Landau with full extension in prone suspension, which is atypical for her age. In volitional movement, mild asymmetry was evident, because she had difficulty bringing her right arm forward in prone and brought her left arm to midline more frequently. Her kicking pattern in supine was low and she did not elevate her hips. On the right side, hip extension was accompanied by knee extension and plantarflexion of the ankle. She was not yet reaching out for objects, and her hands were frequently fisted, particularly on the right. Her parents were helped with handling skills to reduce shoulder retraction and extension posturing and to facilitate more symmetry in movements and posture. They were advised to return in 6 months.

When the family returned for a follow-up visit at 6 months they reported that their daughter was making good progress but she continued to prefer use of her left hand in spite of their efforts to encourage use of the right hand. At this evaluation her MDI was 94, her PDI was 83, and the MAI total risk score was 13. The infant had made the following developmental progress: (1) rolling from supine to prone (over the right side only), (2) beginning sitting balance, and (3) reaching out and grasping objects. She showed a preference for greater skill and dexterity with her left hand. Occasional fisting was still observed on the right hand. She transferred objects only from right to left. Muscle tone continued to be increased in the lower extremities with restricted passive mobility of the gastrocsoleus muscles bilaterally. Toe clawing was observed on the right with minimal spontaneous dorsiflexion observed on this side. Primitive reflexes were integrated except for persistent neonatal positive support and asymmetrical tonic neck reflex to the right. Automatic reactions were improved, but balance responses were asymmetrical with equilibrium reactions and protective extension reactions delayed on the right. Although the developmental progress was encouraging, the persistent asymmetry remained a major concern. The infant was referred to a developmental intervention program with the recommendation that she receive regular therapy in her home at least once a week.

The infant was seen in the follow-up clinic at 12 months' corrected age (14 months' chronological age). On the BSID, the MDI was 95 and the PDI was 82. She now was creeping reciprocally on hands and knees. When she pulled to stand she consistently brought the left foot up first. She cruised at furniture with a tendency to stand on her toes on the right. She picked up cubes with either hand but showed partial palmar grasp on the right. She picked up a pellet with an inferior pincer grasp on the left but scooped it into the palm of the right hand. Muscle tone continued to be mildly increased in the lower extremities with tight heelcords, particularly on the right. She sat independently, but her back was not straight. When moving into and out of sitting, she lacked full trunk rotation and weight was generally over her left hip. Language development was considered appropriate for her age. The infant was diagnosed with mild right hemiplegic cerebral palsy. It was recommended that she continue in the intervention therapy program and return for reevaluation at 2 years of age.

In the management of this child, the role of the pediatric therapist was assessment of neurodevelopmental status and referral to therapy when it became evident that the abnormalities of muscle tone were persisting and interfering with her developmental progress. It should be noted that this child's MDI scores were in the normal range at both the 4- and 8-month examinations. Because the BSID-II does not require infants to perform tasks with both hands, a normal score can be obtained using just one side of the body. This child should continue to be followed in the high-risk infant clinic after 2 years of age to provide periodic reassessment and guidance to the family as they confront questions of school placement and program planning for their child.

REFERENCES

1. Affleck G, et al: Mothers, fathers, and the crises of newborn intensive care. Inf Mental Health J 11:12, 1990.
2. Allan WC, et al: Antecedents of cerebral palsy in a multicenter trial of indomethacin for intraventricular hemorrhage. Arch Pediatr Adolesc Med 151: 580, 1997.
3. Allen MC, Alexander GR: Gross motor milestones in preterm infants: Correction for degree of prematurity. J Pediatr 116:955, 1990.
4. Allen MC, Alexander GR: Using gross motor milestones to identify very preterm infants at risk for cerebral palsy. Dev Med Child Neurol 34:226, 1992.
5. Allesandri SM, Bendersky M, Lewis M: Cognitive functioning in 8- to 18-month-old drug-exposed infants. Dev Psych 34:565, 1998.
6. Als H: Toward a synactive theory of development: Promise for the assessment and support of infant individuality. Inf Mental Health J 3:229, 1982.
7. Als H: A synactive model of neonatal behavioral organization: Framework for the assessment of neurobehavioral development in the premature infant and for support of infants and parents in the neonatal intensive care environment. Phys Occup Ther Pediatr 6(3/4):3, 1986.
8. Als H, et al: Individualized behavioral and environmental care for the VLBW preterm infant at high risk for bronchopulmonary dysplasia: NICU and developmental outcome. Pediatrics 78:1123, 1986.
9. Als H, et al: Individualized developmental care for the very low-birth-weight preterm infant: Medical and neurofunctional effects. JAMA 272: 853, 1994.
10. American Occupational Therapy Association, Neonatal Intensive Care Unit Task Force: Knowledge and skills for occupational therapy practice in the neonatal intensive care unit. Am J Occup Ther 47: 1100, 1993.
11. Amiel-Tison C: Neurological evaluation of the maturity of newborn infants. Arch Dis Child 43:89, 1968.
12. Amiel-Tison C: Does neurological assessment still have a place in the NICU? Acta Paediatr Suppl 416:31, 1996.
13. Amiel-Tison C, Grenier A: Neurological Assessment During the First Year of Life. New York, Oxford University Press, 1986.
14. Avery GB, Fletcher M, MacDonald MG.: Neonatology: Pathophysiology and Management of the Newborn. Philadelphia, Lippincott, Williams & Wilkins, 1999.
15. Aylward GP: Conceptual issues in developmental screening and assessment. J Dev Behav Pediatr 18:340, 1997.
16. Aziz K, et al: Province-based study of neurologic disability of children weighing 500 through 1249 grams at birth in relation to neonatal cerebral ultrasound findings. Pediatrics 95:837, 1995.
17. Ballard JL, et al: A simplified score for assessment of fetal maturation of newly born infants. J Pediatr 95:769, 1979.
18. Ballard JL, et al: New Ballard Score, expanded to include extremely premature infants. J Pediatr 119:417, 1991.
19. Barkovich AJ, Truit CL: Brain damage from perinatal asphyxia: Correlation of MR findings with gestational age. AJNR 11:1087, 1990.
20. Barnard KE, et al: Developmental changes in maternal interactions with term and preterm infants. Infant Behav Dev 7:101, 1984.
21. Barnard KE, Eyres SJ: Feeding scale. In Child Health Assessment (DHEW publication No. HRA 79–25). Hyattsville, MD, U.S. Department of Health, Education, and Welfare, Health Resources Administration, Bureau of Health Manpower, Division of Nursing.
22. Bartlett D: Primitive reflexes and early motor development. J Dev Behav Pediatr 18: 151, 1997.
23. Barrera ME, et al: Early home intervention with low-birth-weight infants and their parents. Child Dev 57:20, 1986.
24. Bayley N: Manual for the Bayley Scales of Infant Development, 2nd ed. New York, The Psychological Corp, 1993.
25. Beltran RS, Coker SB: Transient dystonia of infancy: A result of intrauterine cocaine exposure? Pediatr Neurol 12:354, 1995.
26. Bender SL, et al: The developmental implications of prenatal and/or postnatal crack cocaine exposure in preschool children: A preliminary report. J Dev Behav Pediatr 16:418, 1995.
27. Bennett FC, et al: Hyaline membrane disease, birth weight, and gestational age. Am J Dis Child. 136:888, 1982.
28. Bhushan V, Paneth N, Keily JL: Impact of improved survival of very low birth weight infants on recent secular trends in the prevalence of cerebral palsy. Pediatrics 91:1094, 1993.
29. Blackburn ST: Fostering behavioral development of high-risk infants. JOGN Nurs 12:76, 1983.
30. Blackburn ST: Assessment of risk: Perinatal, family, and environmental perspectives. Phys Occup Ther Pediatr 6(3/4):105–120, 1986.
31. Blackburn ST, VandenBerg KA: Assessment and management of neonatal neurobehavioral development. In Kenner C, et al (eds): Comprehensive Neonatal Nursing. Philadelphia, WB Saunders, 1993.
32. Blitz RK, et al: Neurodevelopmental outcome of extremely low birth weight infants in Maryland. Maryland Med J 46:18, 1997.
33. Bly L: The components of normal movement during the first year of life. In Slayton DS (ed): Development of Movement in Infancy. Chapel Hill, University of North Carolina Press, 1981.
34. Brander R, et al: Inter-rater and test-retest reliabilities of the movement assessment of infants. Pediatr Phys Ther 5:9, 1993.
35. Braun MA, Palmer MM: A pilot study of oral-motor dysfunction in "at-risk" infants. Phys Occup Ther Pediatr 5:13, 1985.
36. Brazelton TB, Nugent JK: Neonatal behavioral assessment scale, 3rd ed. In Clinics in Developmental Medicine, No. 137. London, Mac Keith Press, 1995.
37. Brazelton neonatal behavioral assessment scale certification program: Brazelton Center for Infants and Parents, Children's Hospital Medical Center, 300 Longwood Avenue, Boston, Massachusetts.
38. Brazelton neonatal behavioral assessment scale training films: Cambridge, MA, Educational Development Corporation.
39. Brothwood M, et al: Mortality, morbidity, growth and development of babies weighing 501–1000 grams and 1001–1500 grams at birth. Acta Paediatr Scand 77:10, 1988.
40. Bull MJ, Bryson CQ, Schreiner RL: Perinatal status and neonatal treatment as predictors of the neurologic integrity and development of very low birth weight infants. J Perinatol 5:16, 1988.
41. Burns WJ, et al: Developmental assessment of premature infants. J Dev Behav Pediatr 3:12, 1982.
42. Campbell SK: The infant at risk for developmental disability. In Campbell SK (ed): Decision Making in Pediatric Neurologic Physical Therapy. Philadelphia, Churchill Livingstone, 1999.
43. Caplan G: Patterns of parental response to the crises of premature birth. Psychiatry 23:365, 1970.
44. Capute AJ, et al: Normal gross motor development: The influence of race, sex, and socioeconomic status. Dev Med Child Neurol 27:635, 1985.
45. Chandler LC: Neuromotor assessment. In Gibbs ED, Teti DM, (eds): Interdisciplinary Assessment of Infants: A Guide for Early Intervention Professional. Baltimore, Paul H. Brookes, 1990.
46. Chandler LS, Andrews MS, Swanson MW: Movement Assessment of Infants: A Manual. Rolling Bay, WA, Authors, 1980.
47. Chiriboga CA, et al: Neurological correlates of fetal cocaine exposure: Transient hypertonia of infancy and early childhood. Pediatrics 96:1070, 1996.
48. Cintas HM: Cross-cultural variation in infant motor development. Phys Occup Ther Pediatr 8:1, 1988.
49. Cioni G, et al: MRI findings and sensorimotor development in infants with bilateral spastic cerebral palsy. Brain Dev 19:245, 1997.
50. Clark JE: Waterbeds: Therapeutic devices for handicapped children. Phys Ther 61:1175, 1981.
51. Cohen E, et al: Evaluation of the Peabody Developmental Gross Motor Scales for your children of African American and Hispanic ethnic backgrounds. Pediatr Phys Ther 11:191, 1999.
52. Coleman M: Congenital brain syndromes. In Coleman M (ed): Neonatal Neurology. Baltimore, University Park Press, 1981.
53. Cooke RWI: Cerebral palsy in low birthweight infants. Arch Dis Child 65:201, 1990.
54. Coolman RB, et al: Neuromotor development of graduates of the neonatal intensive care unit: Patterns encountered in the first two years of life. J Dev Behav Pediatr 6:327, 1985.
55. Crane L: Physical therapy for the neonate with respiratory disease. In Irwin S, Tecklin JS (eds): Cardiopulmonary Physical Therapy. St. Louis, CV Mosby, 1985.
56. Crane L: Cardiorespiratory management of the high-risk neonate: Implications for developmental therapists. Phys Occup Ther Pediatr 6(3/4):255, 1986.

57. Crane L: The neonate and child. *In* Frownfelter DL (ed): Chest Physical Therapy and Pulmonary Rehabilitation: An Interdisciplinary Approach, 3rd ed. Chicago, Year Book Medical Publishers, 1983.

58. Crnic KA, et al: Social interaction and developmental competence of preterm and full-term infants during the first year of life. Child Dev 54:1199, 1983.

59. Dammann O, Leviton A: Duration of transient hyperechoic images of white matter in very-low-birthweight infants: A proposed classification. Dev Med Child Neurol 39:2, 1997.

60. Dancsak M, et al: Concurrent validity of two infant motor scales: The Alberta Infant Motor Scale (AIMS) and the Movement Assessment of Infants (MAI). Dev Med Child Neurol 35(Suppl 69):4, 1993.

61. Darrah J, et al: Intra-individual stability of rate of gross motor development in full-term infants. Early Hum Dev 52:169, 1998.

62. Darrah J, Piper M, Watt MJ: Assessment of gross motor skills of at-risk infants: Predictive validity of the Alberta Infant Motor Scale. Dev Med Child Neurol 40:485, 1998.

63. Davis DH, Thoman EB: Behavioral states of premature infants: Implications for neural and behavioral development. Dev Psychobiol 20:25, 1987.

64. D'Eugenio DB, et al: Developmental outcome of preterm infants with transient neuromotor abnormalities. Am J Dis Child 147:570, 1993.

65. de Groot L: Posture and motility in preterm infants. Annotation. Dev Med Child Neurol 42:65, 2000.

66. de Groot L, Hopkins B, Touwen B: Motor asymmetries in preterm infants at 18 weeks corrected age and outcomes at 1 year. Early Hum Dev 48:35, 1997.

67. DeVries LS, et al: Correlation between the degree of periventricular leukomalacia diagnosed using cranial ultrasound and MRI later in infancy in children with cerebral palsy. Neuropediatrics 24:263, 1993.

68. Dinwiddle R, et al: Cardiopulmonary changes in the crying neonate. Pediatr Res 13:900, 1979.

69. Drillien CM: Abnormal neurologic signs in the first year of life in low-birthweight infants: Possible prognostic significance. Dev Med Child Neurol 14:575, 1972.

70. Droit S, Boldrini A, Cioni G: Rhythmical leg movements in low-risk and brain-damaged preterm infants. Early Hum Dev 44:201, 1996.

71. Dubowitz L: Neurologic assessment. *In* Ballard R (ed): Pediatric Care of the ICN Graduate. Philadelphia, WB Saunders, 1988.

72. Dubowitz L, et al: Clinical assessment of gestational age in the newborn infant. J Pediatr 77:1, 1970.

73. Dubowitz L, et al: Correlation of neurologic assessment in the preterm newborn infant with outcome at 1 year. J Pediatr 105:452, 1984.

74. Dubowitz L, Dubowitz V: The neurological assessment of the preterm and full-term newborn infant. Clinics in Developmental Medicine, No. 79. Philadelphia, JB Lippincott, 1981.

75. Ellenberg JH, Nelson KB: Early recognition of infants at high risk for cerebral palsy: Examination at age four months. Dev Med Child Neurol 23:705, 1981.

76. Escobar GJ, Littenberg B, Petitti DB: Outcome among surviving very low birthweight infants: A meta-analysis. Arch Dis Child 66:204, 1991.

77. Fawer CL, Dievold P, Calame A: Periventricular leucomalacia and neurodevelopmental outcome in preterm infants. Arch Dis Child 62:30, 1987.

78. Fetters L: Sensorimotor management of the high-risk neonate. Phys Occup Ther Pediatr 6(3/4):217, 1986.

79. Fetters L, Tronick EZ: Neuromotor development of cocaine-exposed and control infants from birth through 15 months: Poor and poorer performance. Pediatrics 98:938, 1996.

80. Fewell R, et al: Motor ability of children prenatally exposed to cocaine: The effect of age on motor test results (abstract). Pediatr Phys Ther 9:194, 1997.

81. Field T: Supplemental stimulation of preterm neonates. Early Hum Dev 4:301, 1980.

82. Forslund M, Bjerre I: Growth and development in preterm infants during the first 18 months. Early Hum Dev 10:201, 1985.

83. Gauthier SM, et al: The Bayley Scales of Infant Development II: Where to start? J Dev Behav Pediatr 20:75, 1999.

84. Georgieff MK, et al: Abnormal truncal muscle tone as a useful early marker for developmental delay in low birth weight infants. Pediatrics 77:659, 1986.

85. Georgieff MK, Bernbaum JC: Abnormal shoulder girdle muscle tone in premature infants during their first 18 months of life. Pediatrics 77:664, 1986.

86. Glass RP, Wolf LS: Feeding and oral-motor skills. *In* Case-Smith J (ed): Pediatric Occupational Therapy in Early Intervention, 2nd ed. Boston, Butterworth-Heinemann, 1998.

87. Goodman M, et al: Effect of early neurodevelopmental therapy in normal and at-risk survivors of neonatal intensive care. Lancet 2:1327, 1985.

88. Gorga D, et al: The neuromotor behavior of preterm and full-term children by three years of age: Quality of movement and variability. J Dev Behav Pediatr 12:102, 1991.

89. Gorga D, Stern FM, Ross G: Trends in neuromotor behavior of preterm and full-term infants in the first year of life: A preliminary report. Dev Med Child Neurol 27:756, 1985.

90. Hack M, Klein NK, Taylor HG: Long-term developmental outcome of low birth weight infants. The Future of Children 5:176, 1995.

91. Hack M, Friedman H, Fanaroff AA: Outcomes of extremely low birth weight infants. Pediatrics 98:931, 1996.

92. Hadders-Algra M: The assessment of general movements is a valuable technique for the detection of brain dysfunction in young infants. Acta Paediatr Suppl 416:39, 1996.

93. Hagberg B, Hagberg G: The changing panorama of cerebral palsy—bilateral spastic forms in particular. Acta Paediatr Suppl 416:48, 1996.

94. Haley SM: Sequence of development of postural reactions by infants with Down syndrome. Dev Med Child Neurol 29:674, 1987.

95. Hansen N, Okken A: Transcutaneous oxygen tension of newborn infants in different behavioral states. Pediatr Res 14:911, 1980.

96. Hardy S: Personal communication. Toronto, Ontario, January 1988.

97. Harris M: Oral-motor management of the high-risk neonate. Phys Occup Ther Pediatr 6(3/4):231, 1986.

98. Harris SR: Early neuromotor predictors of cerebral palsy in low-birthweight infants. Dev Med Child Neurol 29:587, 1987.

99. Harris SR, et al: Predictive validity of the Movement Assessment of Infants. Dev Behav Pediatr 5:335, 1984.

100. Harris SR, et al: Reliability of observational measures of the Movement Assessment of Infants. Phys Ther 64:471, 1984.

101. Harris-Copp M: The HIV-infected child: A critical need for physical therapy. Clin Management 8:16, 1988.

102. Hefflefinger A, Craft S, Shyken J: Visual attention in children with prenatal cocaine exposure. J Int Neuropsychol Soc 3:237, 1997.

103. Hensinger RN, Jones ET: Neonatal Orthopedics. New York, Grune & Stratton, 1981.

104. Heriza C: The neonate with cerebral palsy. *In* Scully R, Barnes ML (eds): Physical Therapy. Philadelphia, JB Lippincott, 1989.

105. Holm VA, et al: Infant walkers and cerebral palsy. Am J Dis Child 137:1189, 1983.

106. Hurt H, et al: Cocaine-exposed children: Follow-up through 30 months. Dev Med Child Neurol 16:29, 1995.

107. Jacobson SW, et al: New evidence for neurobehavioral effects of in utero cocaine exposure. J Pediatr 129:581, 1996.

108. Jantz JW, Blosser CD, Fruechting LA: A motor milestone change noted with a change in sleep position. Arch Pediatr Adolesc Med 151:565, 1997.

109. Johnson CF, et al: Walker-related burns in infants and toddlers. Pediatr Emerg Care 6:58, 1991.

110. Jongmans M, et al: Minor neurological signs and perceptual-motor difficulties in prematurely born children. Arch Dis Child Fetal Neonatal Ed 76:F9, 1997.

111. Kaback MM (ed): Prenatal diagnosis. Pediatr Ann 10:13, 1981.

112. Kahn-D'Angelo L: The special care nursery. *In* Campbell SK (ed): Physical Therapy for Children. Philadelphia, WB Saunders, 1994.

113. Kauffman IB, Ridenour M: Influence of an infant walker on onset and quality of walking pattern of locomotion: An electromyographic investigation. Percept Mot Skills 45:1323, 1977.

114. Kenner C: Caring for the NICU parent. J Perinat Neonatal Nurs 4(3):78, 1990.

115. Kim MM, et al: Do parents and professionals agree on the developmental status of high-risk infants? Pediatrics 97:676, 1996.

116. Kokeda T, et al: MR imaging of spastic diplegia: Comparative study between preterm and term infants. Neuroradiology 32:187, 1990.

117. Korner AF, et al: Effects of waterbed flotation on premature infants: A pilot study. Pediatrics 56:361, 1975.

118. Korner AF, Thoman EB: The relative efficacy of contact and vestibular-proprioceptive stimulation in soothing neonates. Child Dev 43:443, 1972.

119. Krishnamoorthy KS, et al: Periventricular-intraventricular hemorrhage, sonographic localization, phenobarbital, and motor abnormalities in low birth weight infants. Pediatrics 85:1027, 1990.

120. Kuban KCK, Leviton A: Cerebral palsy. N Engl J Med 330:188, 1994.

121. Leander D, Pettett G: Parental response to the birth of a high-risk neonate: Dynamics and management. Phys Occup Ther Pediatr 6(3/4):205, 1986.

122. Lems W, Hopkins B, Samson JF: Mental and motor development in preterm infants: The issue of corrected age. Early Hum Dev 34:113, 1993.

123. Leonard E, et al: Nutritive sucking in high risk neonates after perioral stimulation. Phys Ther 60:299, 1980.

124. Lester BB: Data analysis and prediction. In Brazelton TB (ed): Neonatal Behavioral Assessment Scale, 2nd ed. Philadelphia, JB Lippincott, 1984.

125. Levine MS, Kliebhan L: Communication between physician and physical and occupational therapists: A neurodevelopmental based prescription. Pediatrics 68:208, 1981.

126. Leviton A, Gilles F: Ventriculomegaly, delayed myelination, white matter hypoplasia, and "periventricular" leukomalacia: How are they related? Pediatr Neurol 15:127, 1996.

127. Linton PT: Behavioral development of the premature infant. Pediatrics 29:175, 1986.

128. Long T, Soderstrom E: A critical appraisal of positioning infants in the neonatal intensive care unit. Phys Occup Ther Pediatr 15(3):17, 1995.

129. Lubchenco LO: The High Risk Infant. Philadelphia, WB Saunders, 1976.

130. Luchi JM, Bennett FC, Jackson JC: Predictors of neurodevelopmental outcome following bronchopulmonary dysplasia. Am J Dis Child 145:813, 1991.

131. Luther M, Ornstein M, Asztalos E: Predictive value of the Movement Assessment of Infants (MAI) and bronchopulmonary dysplasia as a confounding variable. Pediatr Res 31:254A, 1992.

132. Lynch EW, Hanson MJ (eds): Developing Cross-Cultural Competence: A Guide for Working with Young Children and Their Families. Baltimore, Paul H. Brookes, 1992.

133. Majemer A, et al: A comparison of neurobehavioral performance of healthy term and low-risk preterm infants at term. Dev Med Child Neurol 34:417, 1992.

134. Marquis PJ, et al: Retention of primitive reflexes and delayed motor development in very low birth weight infants. J Dev Behav Pediatr 5:124, 1984.

135. Marsden DJ: Reduction of head flattening in preterm infants. Dev Med Child Neurol 22:507, 1980.

136. Martin RJ, et al: Effect of supine and prone positions on arterial oxygen tension in the preterm infant. Pediatrics 63:528, 1979.

137. Matilainen R: The value of correction for age in the assessment of prematurely born children. Early Hum Dev 15:257, 1987.

138. Mayo NE: The effect of physical therapy for children with motor delay and cerebral palsy. Am J Phys Med Rehabil 70:258, 1991.

139. McCormick MC, et al: The Infant Health and Development Program: Interim summary. J Dev Behav Pediatr 19:359, 1998.

140. Measel CP: Non-nutritive sucking during tube feedings: Effect on clinical course in premature infants. Obstet Gynecol Neonat Nurs 8:265, 1979.

141. Ment LR, et al: Neurodevelopmental outcome at 36 months' corrected age of preterm infants in the multicenter indomethacin intraventricular hemorrhage prevention trial. Pediatrics 98:714–718, 1996.

142. Mercer RT: Nursing Care for Parents at Risk. Thorofare, NJ, Slack, 1977.

143. Michaelis R, et al: Transitory neurological findings in a population of at risk infants. Early Hum Dev 34:143, 1993.

144. Miles MS: Parents of critically ill premature infants: Sources of stress. Crit Care Nurs Q 12(3):69, 1989.

145. Minde K, et al: Impact of delayed development in premature infants on mother-infant interaction: A prospective investigation. J Pediatr 112:136, 1988.

146. Mitchell JS: Taking on the World: Empowering Strategies for Parents of Children with Disabilities. New York, Harcourt Brace Jovanovich, 1982.

147. Morgan AM, et al: Neonatal neurobehavioral examination. Phys Ther 68:1352, 1988.

148. Msall ME, et al: Multivariate risks among extremely premature infants. J Perinatol 14:41, 1994.

149. Murphy DJ, Hope PL, Johnson A: Ultrasound findings and clinical antecedents of cerebral palsy in very preterm infants. Arch Dis Child 74:F105, 1996.

150. Murphy DJ, Hope PL, Johnson A: Neonatal risk factors for cerebral palsy in very preterm infants: Case-control study. BMJ 314:404, 1997.

151. Napiorkowski B, et al: Effects of in utero substance exposure on infant neurobehavior. Pediatrics 98:71, 1995.

152. Nellis L, Gridley BE: Review of the Bayley Scales of Infant Development, 2nd ed. J Sch Psychol 32:201, 1994.

153. Nelson KB, Ellenberg JH: Antecedents of cerebral palsy. N Engl J Med 315:81, 1986.

154. Neuspiel DR, et al: Maternal cocaine use and infant behavior. Neurotoxicol Teratol 13:229, 1991.

155. Nugent JK: The Brazelton Neonatal Behavioral Assessment Scale: Implications for intervention. Pediatr Nurs 42:18, 1981.

156. Nugent JK: Using the NBAS with Infants and Their Families: Guidelines for Intervention. White Plains, NY, March of Dimes Birth Defects Foundation, 1985.

157. Olsen P, et al: Magnetic resonance imaging of periventricular leukomalacia and its clinical correlation in children. Ann Neurol 41:754, 1997.

158. O'Neil S: Personal communication. School of Nursing, University of Washington, Seattle, May 1986.

159. O'Shea TM, et al: Survival and developmental disability in infants with birth weights of 501 to 800 grams, born between 1979 and 1994. Pediatrics 100:982, 1997.

160. Paban M, Piper MC: Early predictors of one year neurodevelopmental outcome for "at risk" infants. Phys Occup Ther Pediatr 7:17, 1987.

161. Palisano RJ: Use of chronological and adjusted ages to compare motor development of healthy preterm and fullterm infants. Dev Med Child Neurol 28:180, 1986.

162. Palmer FB, et al: The effects of physical therapy on cerebral palsy. N Engl J Med 318:803, 1988.

163. Paneth N, et al: Brain Damage in the Preterm Infant. London, MacKeith Press, 1994.

164. Parer JT: Evaluation of the fetus during labor. Curr Probl Pediatr 12:1, 1982.

165. Parmelee AH, Michaelis MD: Neurological examination of the newborn. In Hellmuth J (ed): Exceptional Infant, vol 2. New York, Brunner/Mazel, 1971.

166. Partington MD, et al: Head injury and the use of baby walkers: A continuing problem. Ann Emerg Med 20:652, 1991.

167. Peabody JL, Lewis K: Consequences of newborn intensive care. In Gottfried AW, Goither JL (eds): Infant Stress under Intensive Care. Baltimore, University Park Press, 1985.

168. Perlman JM, et al: Relationship between periventricular intraparenchymal echodensities and germinal matrix–intraventricular hemorrhage in the very low birth weight neonate. Pediatrics 91:474, 1993.

169. Peters K: Does routine nursing care complicate the physiologic status of the premature neonate with respiratory distress syndrome? J Perinat Neonatal Nurs 6(2):67, 1992.

170. Pharaoh POD, Platt MJ, Cooke T: The changing epidemiology of cerebral palsy. Arch Dis Child 75:F169, 1996.

171. Piecuch RE, et al: Outcome of extremely low birth weight infants (500 to 999 grams) over a 12-year period. Pediatrics 100:633, 1997.

172. Pinto-Martin JA, et al: Cranial ultrasound prediction of disabling and nondisabling cerebral palsy at age two in a low birth weight population. Pediatrics 95:249, 1995.

173. Piper MC, et al: Early physical therapy effects on the high-risk infant: A randomized controlled trial. Pediatrics 78:216, 1986.

174. Piper MC, et al: Resolution of neurological symptoms in high-risk infants during the first two years of life. Dev Med Child Neurol 30:26, 1988.

175. Piper MC, et al: The consistency of sequential examinations in the early detection of neurological dysfunction. Phys Occup Ther Pediatr 11:27, 1991.

176. Piper MC, Darrah J: Motor Assessment of the Developing Infant. Philadelphia, WB Saunders, 1994.

177. Piper MC, Darrah J, Byrne P: Impact of gestational age on preterm motor development at 4 months chronological and adjusted ages. Child Care Health Dev 15:105, 1989.

178. Portnoy LG, Watkins MP: Foundations of Clinical Research: Applications to Practice. Norwalk, CT, Appleton & Lange, 1993.

179. Prechtl H: The neurological examination of the full-term newborn infant, 2nd ed. Clinics in Developmental Medicine, No. 63. Philadelphia, JB Lippincott, 1977.

180. Prechtl H, Beintema D: The neurological examination of the newborn infant. Clinics in Developmental Medicine, No. 12. London, Heinemann Educational Books, 1964.

181. Provost B: Normal development from birth to 4 months: Extended use of the NBAS-K: Part I. Phys Occup Ther Pediatr 2:39, 1980.

182. Provost B: Normal development from birth to 4 months: Extended use of the NBAS-K: Part II. Phys Occup Ther Pediatr 1:19, 1981.

183. Quinton M: Personal communication. Neurodevelopmental treatment baby course, Puyallup, Washington, July 1982.

184. Rast M: Motor control in infants with Down syndrome. Dev Med Child Neurol 27:675, 1985.

185. Resnick MB, et al: Developmental intervention for low birth weight infants: Improved early developmental outcome. Pediatrics 80:68, 1987.

186. Rice RD: Neurophysiological development in premature infants following stimulation. Dev Psychol 13:69, 1977.

187. Richardson GA, Conroy ML, Day NL: Prenatal cocaine exposure: Effects on the development of school-age children. Neurotoxicol Teratol 18:627, 1996.

188. Ringelberg J, van de Bor M: Outcome of transient periventricular echodensities in preterm infants. Neuropediatrics 24:269, 1993.

189. Rosenblith JF, Anderson-Huntington R: Behavioral examination of the neonate. In Wilson J (ed): Infants at Risk: Medical and Therapeutic Management, 2nd ed. Chapel Hill, University of North Carolina Press, 1982.

190. Ross G, et al: Perinatal and neurobehavioral predictors of one-year outcomes in infants ≤ 1500 grams. Semin Perinatol 6:317, 1982.

191. Ross G, Lawson K: Using the Bayley II: Unresolved issues in assessing the development of prematurely born children. J Dev Behav Pediatr 18:109, 1997.

192. Roth SC, et al: Relationship between ultrasound appearance of the brain of very preterm infants and neurodevelopmental impairment at eight years. Dev Med Child Neurol 35:755, 1993.

193. Rothberg AD: Six-year follow-up of early physiotherapy intervention in very low birth weight infants. Pediatrics 88:547, 1991.

194. Rothstein JM, Echternach JL: Primer on Measurement: An Introductory Guide to Measurement Issues. Alexandria, VA, American Physical Therapy Association, 1993.

195. Saigal S, et al: Cognitive abilities and school performance of extremely low birth weight children and matched term control children at 8 years: A regional study. J Pediatr 118:751, 1991.

196. Scafidi FA, et al: Effects of tactile/kinesthetic stimulation on the clinical course and sleep/wake behavior of preterm neonates. Infant Behav Dev 9:91, 1986.

197. Schneider JW, Lee W, Chasnoff IJ: Field testing of the Movement Assessment of Infants. Phys Ther 68:321, 1988.

198. Schneider JW, Chasnoff IJ: Motor assessment of cocaine/polydrug exposed infants at age 4 months. Neurotoxicol Teratol 14:97, 1992.

199. Schertzer AL, Tscharnuter I: Early Diagnosis and Therapy in Cerebral Palsy. New York, Marcel Dekker, 1982.

200. Scott S, et al: Weight gain and movement patterns of very low birthweight babies nursed on lambs wool. Lancet 2:1014, 1983.

201. Shonkoff JP, Hauser-Cram P: Early intervention for disabled infants and their families: A quantitative analysis. Pediatrics 80:650, 1987.

202. Siegel AC, Burton RV: Effects of baby walkers on motor and mental development in human infants. J Dev Behav Pediatr 20:355, 1999.

203. Simeonsson RJ, Cooper DH, Scheiner AP: A review and analysis of the effectiveness of early intervention programs. Pediatrics 69:635, 1982.

204. Skidmore MD, Rivers A, Hack M: Increased risk of cerebral palsy among very low-birthweight infants with chronic lung disease. Dev Med Child Neurol 32:325, 1990.

205. Slater MA, et al: Neurodevelopment of monitored versus nonmonitored very low birth weight infants: The importance of family influences. J Dev Behav Pediatr 8:278, 1987.

206. Sommerfelt K, Markestad T, Ellertson B: Neuropsychological performance in low birth weight preschoolers: A population-based, controlled study. Eur J Pediatr 157:53, 1998.

207. Stanley FJ: Survival and cerebral palsy in low birthweight infants: Implications for perinatal care. Paediatr Perinat Epidemiol 6:298, 1992.

208. Stengel TJ: The neonatal behavioral assessment scale: Description, clinical uses, and research implications. Phys Occup Ther Pediatr 1:39, 1980.

209. Stewart KB, et al: Transient neurologic signs in infancy and motor outcomes at 4 1/2 years in children born biologically at risk. TECSE 7:71, 1988.

210. Swanson MW: Neuromotor assessment of low-birthweight infants with normal developmental outcome. Dev Med Child Neurol 31 (Suppl 59):27, 1989.

211. Swanson MW: Neuromotor outcomes of infants exposed prenatally to cocaine: Issues of assessment and interpretation. Phys Occup Ther Pediatr 16:35, 1996.

212. Swanson MW, et al: Identification of neurodevelopmental abnormality at four and eight months by the Movement Assessment of Infants. Dev Med Child Neurol 34:321, 1992.

213. Swanson MW, et al: Prenatal cocaine and neuromotor outcome at four months: Effect of duration of exposure. J Dev Behav Pediatr 20:325, 1999.

214. Swanson MW, Rivara FP, Gomness JM: Baby walkers: Hazardous vehicles for infants. WA Pub Health, Summer, 1994.

215. Sweeney JK: Neonatal hydrotherapy: An adjunct to developmental intervention in an intensive care nursery setting. Phys Occup Ther Pediatr 3:20, 1983.

216. Sweeney JK: Physiological adaptation of neonates to neurological assessment. Phys Occup Ther Pediatr 6:155, 1986.

217. Sweeney JK: Physiological and behavioral effects of neurological assessment in preterm and full-term neonates, abstracted. Physical Occup Ther Pediatr 9(3):144, 1989.

218. Sweeney JK: Assessment of the special care nursery environment: Effects on the high risk infant. In Wilhelm IJ (ed): Physical Therapy Assessment in Early Infancy. New York, Churchill Livingstone, 1993.

219. Sweeney JK, et al: Practice guidelines for the physical therapist in the neonatal intensive care unit (NICU). Pediatr Phys Ther 11:119, 1999.

220. Sweeney JK, Chandler LS: Neonatal physical therapy: Medical risks and professional education. Inf Young Child 2(3):59, 1990.

221. Tatarka ME, et al: The role of pediatric physical therapy in the interdisciplinary assessment process. In Guralnick MJ (ed): Interdisciplinary Clinical Assessment for Young Children with Developmental Disabilities. Baltimore, Paul H. Brookes, 2000.

222. Teplin SW, et al: Neurodevelopmental, health, and growth status at age 6 years of children with birth weights less than 1001 grams. J Pediatr 118:768, 1991.

223. Thein MM, et al: Infant walker use, injuries, and motor development. Inj Prev 3:63, 1997.

224. Tjossem TD: Early intervention: Issues and approaches. In Tjossem TD (ed): Intervention Strategies for High Risk Infants and Young Children. Baltimore, University Park Press, 1976.

225. Toy CC: Performance of 6-month-old Asian American infants on the Movement Assessment of Infants: A descriptive study. Masters' thesis, University of Washington, Seattle, WA, 1997.

226. Trykowski L, et al: Enhancement of nutritive sucking in premature infants. Phys Occup Ther Pediatr 1:27, 1982.

227. Turnbull JD: Early intervention for children with or at risk of cerebral palsy. Am J Dis Child 147:12, 1993.

228. Valvano J, DeGangi GA: Atypical posture and movement findings in high risk pre-term infants. Phys Occup Ther Pediatr 6:71, 1986.

229. van der Bor M, den Ouden L, Guit GL: Value of cranial ultrasound and magnetic resonance imaging in predicting neurodevelopmental outcome in preterm infants. Pediatrics 90:196, 1992.

230. van der Heide J, et al: Kinematic and qualitative analysis of lower-extremity movements in preterm infants with brain lesions. Phys Ther 79:546, 1999.

231. Vohr BR, et al: Neurodevelopmental and medical status of low-birthweight survivors of bronchopulmonary dysplasia at 10 to 12 years of age. Dev Med Child Neurol 33:690, 1991.
232. Volpe JJ: Neurology of the Newborn, 3rd ed. Philadelphia, WB Saunders, 1995.
233. Volpe JJ, Koenigsberger R: Neurologic disorders. *In* Avery GB (ed): Neonatology, 2nd ed. Philadelphia, JB Lippincott, 1981.
234. Wagaman MJ, et al: Improved oxygenation and lung compliance with prone positioning of neonates. J Pediatr 94:787, 1979.
235. Webb ZW: Developmental care in the neonatal intensive care unit. Dimens Crit Care Nurs 1:221, 1983.
236. Weidling AM, et al: A randomized controlled trial of early physiotherapy for high-risk infants. Acta Paediatr 85:1107, 1996.
237. Weisglas-Kuperus N, et al: Minor neurological dysfunction and quality of movement in relation to neonatal cerebral damage and subsequent development. Dev Med Child Neurol 36:727, 1994.
238. Whitaker AH, et al: Neonatal cranial ultrasound abnormalities in low birth weight infants: Relation to cognitive outcomes at six years of age. Pediatrics 98:719, 1996.
239. White-Traut R, et al: Responses of preterm infants to unimodal and multimodal sensory intervention. Pediatr Nurs 23:169, 1997.
240. Whitfield MF, Eckstein RV, Holsti L: Extremely premature (<800 g) schoolchildren: Multiple areas of disability. Arch Dis Child 77:F85, 1997.
241. Widmayer SM, Field TM: Effects of Brazelton demonstrations for mothers on the development of preterm infants. Pediatrics 67:711, 1981.
242. Wilhelm IJ: The neurologically suspect neonate. *In* Campbell SK (ed): Pediatric Neurologic Physical Therapy. New York, Churchill Livingstone, 1985.
243. Wilhelm IJ: The neurobehavioral assessment of the high-risk neonate. *In* Wilhelm IJ (ed): Physical Therapy Assessment in Early Infancy. New York, Churchill Livingstone, 1993.
244. Wolf LS, Glass RP: Feeding and Swallowing Disorders in Infancy: Assessment and Management. Tucson, Therapy Skill Builders, 1992.
245. Yoder PJ: Relationship between degree of infant handicap and clarity of infant cues. Am J Mental Defic 91:639, 1987.
246. Yoder PJ, Farran DC: Mother-infant engagements in dyads with handicapped and nonhandicapped infants: A pilot study. Appl Res Ment Retard 7:51, 1986.
247. Yokochi K, et al: Leg movements in the supine position of infants with spastic diplegia. Dev Med Child Neurol 33:903, 1991.
248. Yokochi K, et al: Motor function of infants with athetoid cerebral palsy. Dev Med Child Neurol 35:909, 1993.
249. Zaferiou DI, Tsikoulas IG, Kremenopoulos GM: Prospective follow-up of primitive reflex profiles in high-risk infants: Clues to an early diagnosis of cerebral palsy. Pediatr Neurol 13:148, 1995.

Cerebral Palsy

CHRISTINE A. NELSON, PhD, OTR

Key Words

– athetosis

– cerebral palsy

– direct versus indirect

– handling

– hypotonia

– intervention

– rhizotomy

– spastic diplegia

– spastic quadriplegia

Objectives

After reading this chapter the student/therapist will:

1. Appreciate the clinical advantages of starting treatment in infancy before abnormal movement patterns are fully established.

2. Identify the parameters of the diagnosis of cerebral palsy, including sensorimotor, family, and psychosocial components.

3. Analyze the multifaceted aspects of the clinical problem and appreciate a multifaceted approach to evaluation and treatment.

4. Identify the appropriate sequence of treatment and its correlation with the clinical problems presented.

5. Recognize the role of the therapist in helping the child reach his or her optimal level of functional independence within the social, familial, and financial challenges of the child's environment.

OVERVIEW

Definitions, Parameters, Anticipated Changes

Cerebral palsy is a sensorimotor disorder that affects the control of posture and movement. It is said to present a "conglomerate of complexities."[2] The diagnosis has historically referred to a lack of oxygen or some related insult to the brain shortly before, during, or shortly after the birth process. There is presently some debate regarding the multiple causations of the condition, some of which are related to problematic development in utero.[52] The repercussions of the insult to the brain fall into patterns that are not always neatly organized. Earlier categorizations of the types of cerebral palsy have proved inconsis-

tent because a single child may move from one diagnostic category to another during the maturational and treatment process and some of the effects on motor development differ related to changes in medication used and birthing practices. The child often has associated perceptual and learning problems, as well as developmental deprivation of movement experience and functional vision difficulties. Record keeping is often inaccurate because of the various definitions and diagnoses applied. In one center a child may be identified as having cerebral palsy, whereas in another the same child may be labeled as having psychomotor dysfunction or developmental delay. Much depends on the level of physician training in the identification of normal and abnormal movement patterns in the young infant.

It has now been established by Dr. Heinz Prechtl

and his associates[58] that reliable identification of affected children is possible within the first 2 to 3 months of life. At times the diagnosis of cerebral palsy is applied to infants who have sustained gross damage to the entire brain or who have conditions such as primary microcephaly or other congenital malformations that alter the prognosis for positive change. As we are confronted by new concepts of brain functioning,[21, 62, 70, 72] we may have to revise our hypotheses of causation of the physical problems as well as our expectations for the evolution of individual children. As a consequence, our therapy focus must evolve to a more functionally specific level.

The Little Club, named for the British physician Dr. John Little, who first defined cerebral palsy, described the condition as "a persistent disorder of movement and posture appearing early in life and due to a developmental nonprogressive disorder of the brain."[64] Dr. Karel Bobath elaborates that "the lesion affects the immature brain and interferes with the maturation of the central nervous system, which has specific consequences in terms of the type of cerebral palsy which develops, its diagnosis, assessment, and treatment."[12]

Another controversy has been the span of time over which the diagnosis may be applied. Vining and colleagues[70] report that their center uses a limit of 3 years of age for applying the diagnosis, whereas the American Academy for Cerebral Palsy and Developmental Medicine (AACPDM) recognizes damage occurring to the central nervous system (CNS) before age 5 years. The age limit that is set is somewhat arbitrary and subject to change, but it tends to recognize the early plasticity of the immature brain. This creates some confusion in specific diagnosis, because there is immediately an overlap with traumatic head injuries, brain infections, near-drownings, and episodes that can directly affect brain function early in life. The therapist, however, will find more similarities than differences in the clinical treatment of the sensorimotor consequences of these events. More complete coverage of related conditions may be found in Chapters 14 and 17.

Prechtl[58, 61] and Milani-Comparetti[50] have presented for our consideration a new classification of cerebral palsy based on characteristic fetal movement patterns. Prechtl[26, 59] and his associates have researched the relationships between pre-birth and post-birth movement over a 20-year period. They have developed an impressive body of knowledge regarding the precise assessment of the quality of spontaneous infant movement patterns, with an interrater reliability of 95% and the use of video recordings. Ultrasonography permits professionals to appreciate the wide variability of movements in utero, as well as the movement responses to specific changes in the external environment. This work helps us to appreciate the continuity of movement patterns from fetal to postnatal life.

Clinically, therapists deal with the observable signs in a child's behavioral responses and quality of movement. Such differences can be evaluated early in development.[14] Early treatment intervention should start between 3 and 5 months of age to be effective. Therapists evaluate the interference of pathological signs and symptoms in comparison with normal or nearly normal responses made by the infant. The lack or distortion of righting reactions against gravity is a strong clue to the presence of a neuromotor disorder.[9, 43] As these righting reactions begin early to integrate movement responses in normal development, they provide one means of early identification of the infant who is in trouble (Fig. 9–1). Early treatment as outlined by Quinton in her lectures uses active facilitation of the righting reactions to normalize the movement patterns of the infant at risk for cerebral palsy. Quinton was the first therapist to dedicate her efforts to early treatment, working in partnership with the Swiss pediatrician Köng.[43] They have shown that informed, individualized home handling can change the outlook for infants who otherwise continue to develop nonfunctional movement patterns and inadequate postural control. Older children also change significantly with intensive physical treatment that takes into account the visual, proprioceptive, and vestibular aspects of the condition. It is essential for therapists to realize that they are dealing with a developing human being with emotional needs—an emerging personality within a personal environment. Physical limitations as well as perceptual distortions need to be assessed. Nothing less than a wholistic view of the problem will change the life pattern of the child and the family who require assistance to make change.[49]

The abnormal signs observed in the infant with neuromotor difficulties can be related to the infant's need to make postural adjustments against gravity with uncoordinated movement of poorly dissociated body parts. Early spontaneous movement patterns presented a poor repertoire, and the "fidgety" peripheral movement patterns described by Prechtl[61] have not developed. The interference with function therefore becomes greater as normal developmental tasks demand more specific control of the body in an upright alignment. To the naive observer the

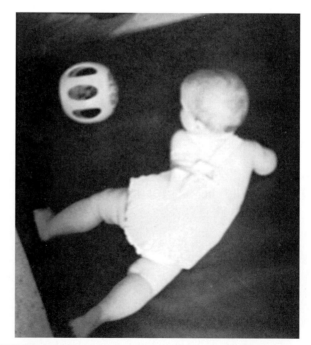

FIGURE 9–1. Normal infants accumulate a multitude of experiences as they move smoothly in their environments.

increased difficulty may give the erroneous impression that the basic condition is worsening. There is no evidence to suggest that the condition itself worsens, but the will of children directs them to use whatever movement potential they possess to explore their environment and to become acquainted with their own bodies. As time goes by the infant establishes habits of postural control that are identified as more indicative of certain types of cerebral palsy. Vining and colleagues[70] state unequivocally that cerebral palsy "is not a specific disease state with an accepted cause, pathogenesis, pathological picture, clinical presentation, treatment, or prognosis." Bobath[11] has documented the course of development in the presence of various forms of cerebral palsy when intervention is not available, but she also stresses the uniqueness of each child and that child's particular constellation of pathological and normal responses. It is true that active use of the abnormal patterns of movement tends to reinforce the pathology and consequently block the expression of the more differentiated normal developmental progression[12] (Fig. 9–2).

The osteopathic profession calls our attention to its correlation of combinations of physical characteristics in infants and young children with cranial findings that offer the possibility of relieving specific pressures that impede proper craniosacral rhythms as well as venous and cerebrospinal fluid circulation.[68] Documentation of cranial abnormalities in the newborn has been in the literature for the past 40 years.[1] The infant or young child treated directly by the cranially oriented osteopathic physician tends to move the head more appropriately, and postural tone is modified.[30] General alertness often changes in a positive way. This primary intervention is accomplished by the osteopathic physician in a limited number of sessions, and the child generally is better able to retain the changes obtained by the therapists in direct therapeutic handling.

Because early development depends so heavily on motor responses, all areas of development are potentially affected by cerebral palsy.[47, 54, 57] There can also be primary physiological limitations due to limited developmental experience. The most common of these is the limited movement of the eyes when adequate head control in all positions fails to develop. There is a paucity of eye movement and frequently limitations in the use of the two eyes together, so the eyes are unable to lead the head movement as they should. Malnourishment, which often compounds the intrauterine conditions, can develop

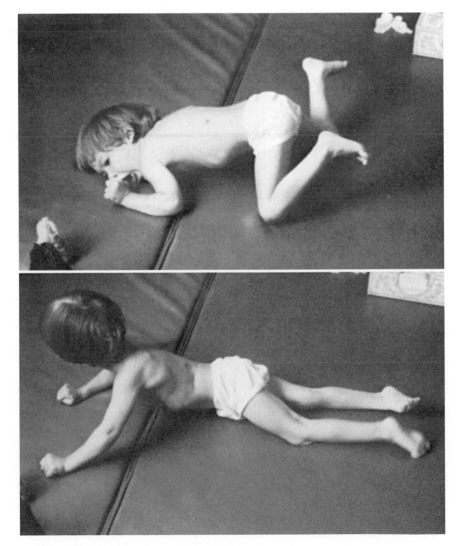

FIGURE 9–2. Attempted movement activates abnormal patterns and restrictions.

because of poor sucking patterns and inadequate processing of ingested food. Low birth weight for age is a significant feature of infants who become identified as having cerebral palsy.[40] Poor circulation relates directly to inadequate respiratory patterns and lack of movement. The sensory system is deprived from the beginning and consequently fails to mature appropriately with the expected matching of incoming information from the sensory receptors.[36] There is no question that cerebral palsy must be considered a sensorimotor developmental dysfunction, and early intervention is important (see Fig. 9–2).

The parents' concern and their feelings of inadequacy in dealing with this atypical infant further compound the developmental frustrations and thus affect personality development of the child. Early therapeutic and educational programming can play a strong role in fostering emotional health for the child and the family.[33] It is essential to support positive developmental responses and to avoid overidentification of inabilities. Parents are caught in the therapist's professional dilemma of symptomatic diagnosis. The very characteristics that constitute the basis for the labeling process are those features that may change with the application of effective treatment strategies.[22] This makes documentation of change and avoidance of premature labeling vital for the continued learning of family and professional alike. Slides, film, or videotape sequences can provide a sample of a child's function on a particular date. The therapist gains much from the review of such visual aids and has a base from which change may be evaluated more objectively.

The outcome for infants with cerebral palsy can be positively influenced by informed and specific therapeutic intervention. Köng[43] has published population statistics that reflect significant reduction in the number of children with all levels of cerebral palsy when therapy was begun between 3 and 5 months of age. Individual cases can also be used as their own control, because the presence of pathology makes certain outcomes predictable with no intervention. Intelligence and motivation also have their roles in anticipating potential direction of change, particularly as the child grows older and initiates more complex functional activity.

Family Reactions

No one ever plans or expects to give birth to a child with a disability. Parents are looking for normal, healthy responses from their infants and consequently allow a wide latitude in their identification of adequate development.[2] In spite of this tendency most parents identify a problem long before it is acknowledged by professionals.[42] Well-intentioned pediatricians are more fully prepared to cope with the medical needs of the normal child and many tend to believe that this child will follow the majority of high-risk infants and outgrow the problematic delay. At our present level of knowledge, only the more severely damaged child is identified at birth, unless the Prechtl evaluation of spontaneous movements is applied. Dealing with preterm infants and their high-risk factors is addressed in detail in Chapter 8.

As the early months pass, parental suspicions accumulate to the point that they can no longer be ignored.

Even when a developmental difficulty is acknowledged, a formal diagnosis may not be applied. Humanistically, this is an advantage to the infant who has some local dysfunction and responds within the normal range of expectation after a relatively brief period of intensive treatment. An infant may be identified as having neuromotor or developmental delay to qualify for treatment services. A series of visits to specialists may be the next experience of the family. It may be assumed that the parents in most instances make clear observations of developmental difficulties during this period, but in general they do not have the background to relate one finding to another nor the cause to the effect. Because there tends to be a reluctance on the part of professionals to begin intervention without a diagnosis, this period of searching by the family may require extended expenditure of time, energy, and financial investment. This investment without immediate return results in varying levels of frustration. Siblings may be somewhat neglected during this critical search for help, and some commercial-style programs increase the abandonment of the family. It is no wonder that parents appear suspicious and less than totally cooperative when they first arrive in the new therapeutic environment.

Diagnosis and the Time of Intervention

When there is an early diagnosis, parents have the opportunity to understand the problem more completely and to participate in helping the infant's development. An early diagnosis, however, may be accompanied by dire predictions as to the limited future of the child. Because these forecasts are presented to the parents in a moment of extreme emotional stress, they tend to make a strong impression. This colors the interaction between parent and infant and may severely restrict the expectations of the parents. The therapist needs to be aware of these early experiences and the parents' view of their child when discussing treatment goals. Even early communicative attempts on the part of the child may be rejected as "not possible" and thus not reinforced. Inexperienced therapists should learn from this situation and avoid giving a specific prognosis until they have sufficient clinical experience to be certain of the observations made.

It is important to encourage the parents to be alert to responses of the infant and young child and to offer consistent psychosocial stimulation. If the infant has merely spent developmental time resting in bed or sitting passively in the same chair at home, the therapist may find deprivation compounding the physical and sensory limitations (Fig. 9–3). Parents often need help in seeing the positive responses and specific changes of their child. They need to acknowledge the child as a unique human being while becoming accurate observers of minor changes in the components of movement control.

Although there is reason to supplement the young child's learning environment when definite limitations exist, clinicians must also maintain a strong sense of respect for the child's capacity to compensate. There are numerous examples of persons developing better than normal intelligence in spite of their inability to move or even speak.[72] Therapists cannot be expected to have all the answers for how this is accomplished, and an honest

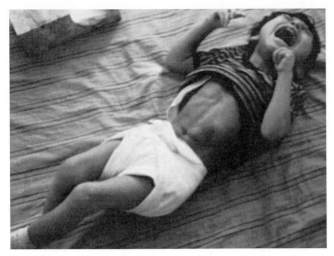

FIGURE 9–3. Emotional reactions are also translated into stronger spastic reactions (see Chapter 6 on the limbic system).

relationship with the family is essential. By keeping a balanced perspective regarding the child's development, therapists can offer meaningful help at the moment when parents are ready to receive it. The child does not exist in a vacuum, nor is treatment the only activity in the life of the family. Parents have individual personalities and life experiences that determine their way of dealing with this life trauma.

The most important contribution of therapists may be their ability to provide practical information based on clinical experience with similar children.[23] It is vital that the guidance offered be appropriate to the family's view of the situation. Once the parents begin to see results from the new positioning and home handling (Fig. 9–4), they find their tension sufficiently reduced and begin to ask questions and regain some confidence in their parenting skills. A problem that is unknown is always more threatening and lacking solutions than one that is understood.

Parents sometimes need specific reminders to avoid focusing all their energy on the disabled child.[40] Siblings often feel as helpless and guilty as the adults in this situation. Their life experience has been altered dramatically. Older children may profit from talking with the therapist directly to understand the movement problems of their sister or brother. It is important to enlist their cooperation in avoiding overstimulation of the affected child and play activities that strengthen abnormal reactions. Some children born into the family after the child with a disability may accept the situation without question. However, others may have vague fears that something like that could happen to them. At times children may find it appealing to have the attention received by the disabled child. Normal siblings may even wish to have cerebral palsy themselves to receive more attention from parents or to experience the relationship that the sibling has with therapists or special teachers. Letting the sibling experience some therapy handling during the last few minutes of the treatment session may help the family situation.

Cultural and familial value systems bear directly on the interaction of the family with the professional help they seek and receive. Socioeconomic factors and the existence of insurance or other third-party payers may determine what assistance the family is able to offer the child. It is always helpful to determine how the family is currently viewing the problem and what they consider to be the major difficulty of the moment. The more that therapists take these psychosocial factors into account, the more effective their influence will be to help the child. (See Chapter 7 on psychosocial adjustment.)

Diagnostic Categorization of the Characteristics of Cerebral Palsy

In general, diagnosis of cerebral palsy suggests that the individual has a lesion within the motor control system with residual disorder of posture and movement control. In addition, the labeling process often identifies the parts of the body that are primarily involved. Diplegia, hemiplegia, and quadriplegia, respectively, indicate that the lower extremities, one side of the body, or all four extremities are affected. This can be misleading to the therapist who is working with infants because these children often change their clinical signs and symptoms and their respective disabilities.

The clinician must be aware that the categorization of cerebral palsy is based on descriptions of observable

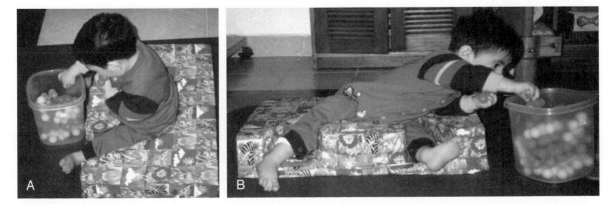

FIGURE 9–4. Use of a simple cut-out space in 3-inch foam gives this 1-year-old child security while requiring more active trunk adaptation.

characteristics; thus it is a symptomatic description. Both Dr. Little, who first identified the condition, and Dr. Winthrop Phelps, who differentiated the characteristic types of cerebral palsy, described the spontaneous movement attempts away from the resting posture. These characteristic movement patterns refer to older children and were identified as spasticity, athetosis, hypotonicity, and ataxia (Fig. 9–5).

The hypertonus of spasticity prevents a smooth exchange between mobility and stability of the body. Constriction of respiratory adaptability occurs with poor trunk control. Incrementation of postural tone occurs with an increase in the speed of even passive movement, and clonus may occur in response to sudden passive movement. Although diagnostic terms reflect the distribution of excessive postural tone, the entire body must be considered to be involved. Spasticity, by nature, involves reduced quantity of movement, which makes its distribution easier to identify. There is also a risk of reduction in the range of limb movements over time when therapy does not include active adaptation in end ranges and organization of postural transitions.[17]

The term *athetosis* refers to a lack of posture and axial/trunk co-activation. The excessive peripheral movement of the limbs occurs without central co-activation. Athetosis may occur with greater involvement in particular extremities, although it most often interferes with postural stability as a whole. Athetoid distribution of postural tone is changeable in force and velocity, particularly during attempted movement by the individual. For this reason these children have a reduced risk of contractures over time. It has been reported that adolescents with athetosis from birth tend to have neck instability, but this may

relate to original findings or to compensatory movement patterns used to function.[34]

Hypotonicity is another category of cerebral palsy, but it may also mask undiagnosed degenerative conditions (see Chapter 10). Hypotonia in a young infant may also be a precursor of athetosis. Often the athetoid movements are not noticed until the infant is attempting antigravity postures, although there may be some disorganization apparent to the careful observer. Tone changes with attempted movement may be present even without the peripheral signs of athetosis. Generalized hypotonia often masks some specific areas of deep muscle tension with accompanying local immobility.

True ataxia is a cerebellar disorder that is seen more frequently as a sequela of tumor removal (see Chapters 23 and 24) than as a problem occurring from birth. Probably because of changes in delivery practices, it seems to occur with less frequency now than it did when Phelps categorized the types of cerebral palsy. Ataxic reactions are often noted in the gait of an athetoid individual. However, more specific analysis may reveal compensatory responses to the athetoid tone changes while the body is in motion through space. (See Chapters 3 and 5 on impairment and disability evaluations and motor control theory.) Clinical experience suggests that a high proportion of these individuals can be assisted more effectively by working with the visual-motor system and functional training than with the postural system alone. Padula[53] is a leader in the specialized field of neurooptometric rehabilitation and has shown impressive change in these clients with prescribed prism additions to acuity-corrected lenses.

There are also children with cerebral palsy who demonstrate athetoid tone changes within a range of hypertonicity or hypertonic distributions of tone superimposed on athetoid disorganization. The developing child may move from one predominant postural pattern to another. Tonus in the proximal joints may be so high that attempted movement results in some athetoid-like movement in the hands or feet. These characteristics change as the proximal movement issues are addressed by the therapist. Attempted speech may be accompanied by limb tension until respiration adequate for speech is facilitated. Treatment intervention will reveal finer nuances of difference in the distribution of postural tone as total patterns are inhibited[51] and reflexive reactions are integrated into functional movement patterns.

These classifications, even when accurately applied, give the therapist only a general idea of the treatment problem and must be supplemented by a specific analysis of posture and movement control during task performance, an interview for home care information, and assessment of treatment responses (see Chapter 3). The therapist is then ready to establish treatment priorities for the individual child.

The visual-motor component of performance must be added to the physical measures for the child with cerebral palsy, because the spatial judgments needed for movement in an upright alignment are visual in nature.[53] Strabismus dysfunctions commonly coexist with cerebral palsy and may cause the child to receive a double image of environmental objects. After an opthalmological examina-

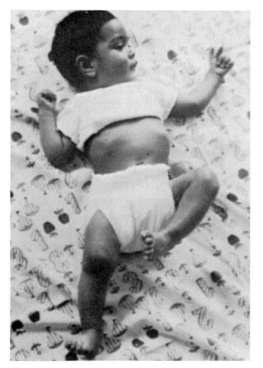

FIGURE 9–5. Asymmetry in this immobile 8 month old is a clue to right hemiparesis caused by porencephaly.

tion to determine the health of the eye structures, a functional vision examination by a behavioral or developmental optometrist will reveal the level of efficiency that the two eyes have achieved in working together, and whether the ability to focus far as well as near ranges is smoothly established. It is important that head control be minimally established before surgical intervention for the eye muscles is considered, although conservative management can make significant positive change in visual function.[56] Padula, a behavioral optometrist specializing in neurooptometric rehabilitation, has described a visual midline shift syndrome in adults with acquired central dysfunction and has applied this information to ambulatory children with cerebral palsy with positive results.[53] A distortion in the perceived visual midline is corrected with the use of prisms, which then permits the child to step into the perceived space with more confidence. By including visual system function as part of the initial evaluation the therapist gains another avenue through which active intervention can be successful.

Many of the characteristics described in the preceding paragraphs also apply to children who have suffered closed head traumas or brain infections. Further information can be obtained in Chapters 14 and 17. Some of the treatment suggestions that follow may also be applied in such cases. As with cerebral palsy, early positioning and handling after trauma may deter later problems.

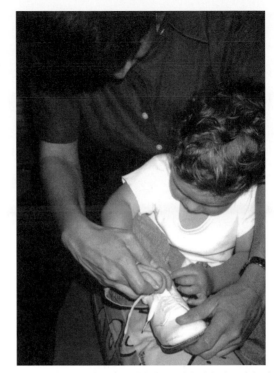

FIGURE 9–6. With assistance, this boy with right hemiplegia is helped to improve his self-esteem by exploring dressing.

EVALUATIVE ANALYSIS OF THE INDIVIDUAL CHILD

Initial Observations

Examination of the individual child begins with careful observation of the interaction between parents and the child, including parental handling of the child that occurs spontaneously (Fig. 9–6). Some additional insight can be gained about the relationship between parent and child by observing how the child is handled both physically and emotionally. Does the child receive and respond to verbal reassurance from the parent in the therapy situation? Are immediate bribes offered to the child? Does parent eye contact increase the child's confidence in responding? Does family communication convey the idea of negativity in the therapy situation or a difficult experience that will soon come to an end? The family orientation will affect the response of the child while working with the therapist.

The therapist working as part of a team may have the advantage of a social worker or psychologist who will relate to the problems and motivations of the parents. Parental responses toward the disabled child arise from their uncertainty, fear, concern for the future, disappointment, distress, and other normal reactions to this unforeseeable life experience. The therapist will observe positive changes in parent orientation to the child as the parents are educated as to what can be done to help their child move forward. They may be further assisted by opportunities to interact with well-adjusted parents of older children.

While observing the child the experienced therapist will want to periodically elicit from the parents their view of the problem. By listening carefully the therapist will also be able to discern the emotional impressions that have surrounded previous experiences with professionals. Sometimes what is not said is more important than what is offered immediately. Listening carefully and clarifying facts are more important than overwhelming the parents with excessive information and suppositions during early contacts. Observation of the family response to information will keep the therapist on track in developing a positive relationship with parents that deepens over time.

The next general step is to observe, in as much detail as possible, the spontaneous movement of the child when separated from the parent. Is the child very passive? Does he or she react to the supporting surface? Are there abnormal patterns of movement to reach a toy (Fig. 9–7)? Are clearly normal responses occurring with specific interference by reflexive synergies or total patterns of movement? Does the child rely heavily on visual communication? Do the eyes focus on a presented object? Do they lead or follow hand activity? Does an effort to move result only in an increase of postural tone with abnormal distribution? Does respiration adapt to new postural adaptations? Is the child able to speak as well while standing as while sitting?

This type of observation is valuable because movement patterns directly reflect the state of the CNS and can generally be seen while the parent is still handling the child.[13] Once the child is on the mat outer clothing can be removed to observe interactions of limbs and trunk. Movement responses of the child can gradually be influenced directly by the therapist. Many disabled children associate immediate undressing in a new environment with a doctor's office, and the chance to establish rapport

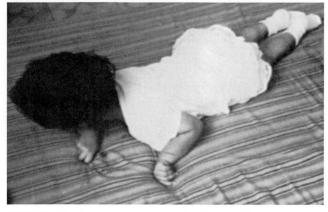

FIGURE 9–7. Play experience or exploration for this child is limited to abnormal patterns of movement.

is lost. In some instances it is preferable to have the parent gently remove the child's clothing or even to leave the child dressed during the first therapy session.

Examination of the child's status is more likely to be adequate if the therapist follows the child's lead when possible. Notes can be organized later to conform to a specific format. It is often possible to jot down essential information while observing the child moving spontaneously or while the parent is holding the child. Reactions to the supporting surface will differ in these circumstances. After the session one can dictate the salient information into a tape recorder, or a videotape can be made to capture the interactions and movement patterns. Attention should be given to the normal movements of the child as well as to those postures that the child spontaneously attempts to control. It is important to notice the interaction between the two sides of the body. In noting abnormal reactions and compensatory movement patterns, one must also indicate the position of the body with respect to the supporting surface. One tends to compile more pertinent data by learning to cluster observations and relating one to the other. Children are vibrant beings. Their choices of position tell us something about their habits and how comfortable they are in this situation. To be the slave of a preformulated sequence destroys the decision-making initiative appropriate to the situation at hand. This is true for the therapist as well as the child.

Each child will differ in ability to separate from his or her parents. Spontaneity of movement, interest in toys, general activity level, and communication skills will also vary from child to child.[32] Responding to the specific needs of the child enables the therapist to set priorities more effectively. If fatigue is likely to be a factor, it is important to evaluate first those reactions that present themselves spontaneously, followed by direct handling to determine near-normal potential for movement. Those movements or abilities for which there is a major interference by spasticity, reflexive responses, or poor balance may be better checked at the termination of the assessment. Information regarding favorite sleeping positions, self-care independence, and chair supports used at home can be requested as the session comes to a close.

Reactions to Placement in a Position

If the child totally avoids certain postures during spontaneous activity, these are likely to be the more important positions for the therapist to evaluate. Placement of the child in the previously avoided position will permit the therapist to feel the resistance that prevents successful control by the child.[51] The parent should play an active role in the assessment whenever possible (Fig. 9–6). Continued dialogue with the parents reveals factors such as the frequency of a poor sitting alignment at home or a habitual aversion to the prone position. Sitting close to the television set or tilting the head when looking at books should also be noted so that functional vision skills can be related to other therapy interventions.[4] These contributions by the parents establish the importance of good observation and the need for parents and therapist to work cooperatively. Therapists of different specialties need to initiate ongoing communication to coordinate therapy objectives.

Following the guide of normal development,[9, 43] infants should be able to maintain a posture in which they are placed before they acquire the ability to move into that position alone.[39] The problems presented by cerebral palsy occur to some extent as a reaction to the field of gravity in which the child moves.[9] Visual perceptions of spatial relationships motivate and determine movement patterns while the child must react at a somatic level to the support surface. It is helpful, therefore, to attempt placement of the infant or child into developmentally or functionally appropriate postures that are not assumed spontaneously (Fig. 9–8). Resistance to placement indicates an increase in tone, a structural problem, or an inability to adapt to the constellation of sensory inputs for that alignment. *A movement that resists control by the therapist will be even less possible for the child.* What appears to be a passive posture may hide rapid increases in hypertonicity when movement is initiated or instability of a proximal joint when weight bearing is initiated. A child may have learned to avoid excitation of the unwanted reactions and may fix the body position to avoid the alignment that cannot be controlled. Another child may enjoy the sensory experience of accelerated changes in postural tone and deliberately set them off.

Abnormal Interferences

Abnormal responses that interfere with postural adjustments by the infant or child with cerebral palsy have not been truly normal at any point in development. Reflexive reactions that are retained beyond the point at which they should have been integrated block the normal differentiation of movement and reflect the inability of the child to dissociate movement responses. Postural transitions or movement sequences become distorted and poorly timed if they are initiated at all. In normal development the integration of reflexive reactions follows a sequence that correlates with the acquisition of motor skills.[9] Fiorentino[29] and others[13, 37] view these early reflexive reactions as the establishment of efficient patterns of movement that are used even in adult life. These synergistic combinations of movement patterns help to limit

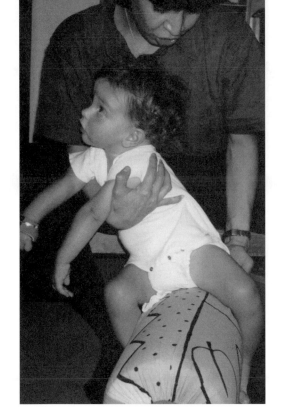

FIGURE 9–8. Crossing of midline and rotational patterns can be exaggerated during undressing and dressing.

degrees of freedom (see Chapter 5) and allow success for a particular movement strategy. They may also be viewed as systematic, organized cues that guide the motor responses.

Hellebrandt and others[37] predictably elicited the asymmetrical tonic neck reflex (ATNR) in normal college students by placing them in a prone position across a hammock-type support. With the subjects blindfolded and the arms unsupported, voluntary turning of the head to the side was resisted by the examiner. The response obtained in the arm position was the typical ATNR with the face arm extended and the skull arm flexed. Children with cerebral palsy will vary greatly as to the amount of effort required to activate a stereotypical synergy. The most severely involved individuals almost never move out of the stereotypical patterns, whereas the mildly involved child who runs or reacts with strong emotion becomes only transiently bound by reflexive reactions. The level at which the reflexive responses interfere with function is significant. The therapist must also be aware of the reflexive synergies most active in each position assumed by the child (Fig. 9–9).

Patterns of movement used by the child to accomplish functional skills of daily living may be limited in degrees of freedom and thus would be considered abnormal. Further development of movement skill can be blocked by continued use of a limited variety of movement patterns. Therapy will then serve to vary and increase the movement repertoire of the child in order to increase functional control over necessary daily tasks. Differentiated levels of motor control are assisted so that the child tends less to plateau in motor development. Parents of the older child may seek help to elaborate the necessary sensorimotor base for more sophisticated and age-appropriate function. These needs may be recognized in new school challenges and social needs. It is more effective to avoid the child's early use of abnormal patterns than to attempt to change established habits superimposed on the use of abnormal synergies.

Children with cerebral palsy can experience successful motor learning when the soft tissue preparation is adequate and tasks are broken down to appropriate motor components. Motor learning depends on many factors,

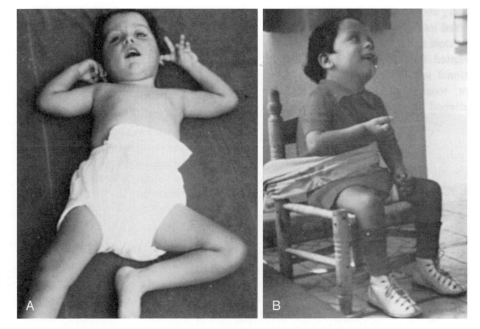

FIGURE 9–9. *A,* Strong asymmetry and abnormal tone in supine. *B,* Simple seating can inhibit strong asymmetry and make function a possibility.

and there is not yet agreement on the motor development process.[20] It is essential to realize that even a dysfunctioning system continues to learn, which offers a new chance for the child with cerebral palsy. By understanding more clearly why abnormal responses become dominant and learning to guide the control of specific components of movement, therapists will become more effective in guiding new motor control.[16] See Chapters 3–5 for additional information.

Primary and Compensatory Patterns

Compensatory patterns must be taken into account when assessing function. They commonly are mistaken for primary postural reactions, possibly resulting from the distribution of spasticity. One of the most common misunderstandings occurs with the presence of the toe-walking response. This position may represent a distribution of postural tone that is stronger in flexor patterns, and the child uses strong extension of the legs to stay upright and counteract hip flexion. In the standing alignment, the body weight is displaced forward, which is often related to a visual misperception of space combined with undifferentiated responses of the legs and lack of lateral weight shift.[5] Then the spastic child counteracts the pull of flexion with a total pattern of extension. The plantarflexion of the foot is only one small component of the total postural picture. This same postural response will be observed in an adult with a shift forward of the visual midlines[4, 53] after head trauma, and the entire postural pattern may change when prism lenses change the individual's visual perception of space.

Careful analysis of the postural adjustments and movement patterns of the child with cerebral palsy is crucial to initiating effective therapeutic intervention. The interaction of many factors creates the final picture of posture and movement control (Fig. 9–10). Normal reactions to abnormal distribution of tone may distort gait as easily as a lack of adequate trunk extension or marked pelvic immobility. Some children have begun to walk without being helped to experience sustained weight-bearing and controlled lateral shifting that reflects good pelvic participation. In addition to the physical factors, the sensory aspects of the condition often interfere with the quality of movement. Tactile sensitivity may interfere with foot placement or prevent sustained grasp of a toy or an eating utensil. Weight-bearing and other firm pressure experiences will change this response. Learning experiences associated with firm pressure input to the hands and feet are missing for the child with cerebral palsy, and the consequent normal evolution of the sensory system is limited.

It is important for the therapist to intervene at the proximal articulation first to determine whether tissue immobility is the interfering factor, and this is especially likely in the case of retraction of the upper limbs, when the shoulders and arms attempt to assist upright head control. The therapist may want to simulate normal weight-bearing by the application of firm pressure against the palms of the hands and the soles of the feet. Postural transitions over the hands and feet need to be experienced with trunk flexion as well as extension. Slight move-

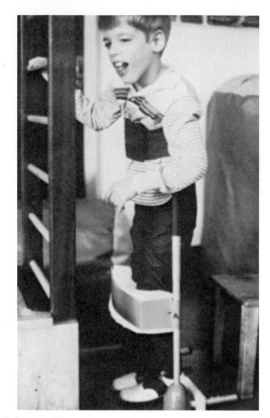

FIGURE 9–10. Through sensorimotor experience, the child in the upright position can help to integrate more normal postural patterns.

ment of the extremity while keeping the limb stable will facilitate the adaptation while weight-bearing. This experience of firm pressure with movement of the body over that point of contact tends to inhibit the tendency for withdrawal and prepare for weight-bearing over the limb.

Consideration of foot support is crucial to influence a more normal distribution of postural tone and a better alignment in weight-bearing.[66] Heavy orthotic controls that completely limit ankle mobility are to be avoided because joint proprioception at the ankle is essential for balance in the upright position. Use of a simple foot orthosis that respects the multiple arches of the foot will guide adequate physical development of the foot and aid the confidence of the child. Careful attention to the dynamic balance of the foot itself gives a stable base that permits mobility in gait. In children with low tone a semisoft foot orthosis that is fitted early often stimulates an increase in spontaneous movement of the extremity.

The orthosis that seems the most efficient and applicable in the clinical setting was developed by Buethorn[18] working in close coordination with physical therapists Hylton and Uhri. Various trim lines address the need for functional ankle stability, but the base gives full support to the foot. A detailed tracing is made of the individual foot, and a plaster cast is made to support the foot medially and laterally. The metatarsal heads and the heel are lowered into carved recesses while the toes are supported only to the extent that relaxation is achieved. Most often the leg is permitted forward-back mobility over the foot. With the additional security of anatomically correct support for the foot, tone is reduced in the legs, and weight bearing is aligned to protect foot development. (For additional information on orthotic devices, see Chapter 31.)

Compensation processes have their positive aspects. The independence finally achieved by the older child reflects his or her intelligence and motivation, as well as the family's attitude toward the child and the disability. The most debilitating handicap of cerebral palsy may be social or psychological, when the child is not accepted by the family and therefore cannot accept himself or herself.[73] This inadequate self-image creates problems in school interaction. Early treatment not only prevents physical limitations but also assists the parents in understanding their child and the influence of a disability on development. The therapist is in a position to encourage development of abilities that emerge so that the child's valuable developmental time is not spent only on remediation.

The Visual System in Cerebral Palsy

The visual system in its development has many parallels with the postural system.[5] Binocular control and freedom of movement are necessary for the system to function properly. Too often a simple screening examination tests acuity at 20 feet on the eye chart or simply checks the health of the eye structure. These tests do not relate to complete function of the visual system as it relates to total development, and particularly as it interacts with deficient motor control.

In the case of a child with cerebral palsy there has often been, by definition, a lack of adequate control of the head position, which would allow the eyes to develop sustained binocular focus and orientation to the environment.[53] Without stable control of the head and neck, it is difficult for the eyes to develop adequate movement. With inadequate alignment of the head in relation to the base of support, the visual system accumulates distortions and inconsistent input, which leads to the formation of an inadequate perceptual base for later learning. Even after improvement in the control of posture and movement, the visual system continues to adapt to the previous faulty learning, resulting in perceptual confusion and inefficient organization of body movement in space. The therapist who is working for improved motor control may notice that such a child reacts very adequately when facing the therapist or a support and that the movement quality seems to disintegrate when the child faces an open space. Adequate visual skills develop from the establishment of a sound experiential base formed by the organized input to and integration of the central and ambient systems.

Working with children with cerebral palsy and with head trauma clients, Padula,[53] a behavioral optometrist, has defined a visual midline shift syndrome that can be easily tested. He has demonstrated impressive change in gait patterns by correcting the visual midline orientation to match the body orientation in space. Athetoid children who have plateaued in physical handling are able to reduce their base of support and their extraneous movement while walking after a few weeks of specific vision

work. Children who walk on their forefoot or their toes, without having true Achilles contractures, also demonstrate a reduction of the forward shift in their visual orientation. In many instances, gait improves immediately by placing the proper lenses on the individual and is further established by using the lenses during facilitated movement provided in the therapy session. The eyes permit the individual to anticipate movement into space and provide constant feedforward to the CNS. This applies to timing of steps in gait as well as to hand coordination activities that require timing of reach and grasp based on visual feedforward.

In some instances there will be an observable movement of the eyes, separating them farther apart or bringing them closer together, as the body has the opposite reaction while the child walks.[4, 5] This suggests that the visual system may try to compensate for inadequacies of the postural system, just as the postural system will adjust the head to accommodate the eyes. Understanding the nature of the ongoing dynamic interaction between these two functional subsystems of the CNS and attending to the needs of a visual-postural orientation will increase the successful evolution of clients with cerebral palsy.

DIRECT INTERVENTION OR CASE MANAGEMENT

Simple documentation of observed changes in a child over a series of regular clinic visits is still too common for many children with cerebral palsy. Regular appointments, with periodic assignment of a new piece of apparatus, do not constitute active treatment. Although physical intervention in the form of direct handling of the child is considered a conservative treatment by most physicians,[54] there are relatively few children who receive sufficient physical treatment at an early age.[35] Therapists need to demonstrate their unique preparation and describe their interventions in ordinary language so that families as well as other health care professionals understand the importance of specific treatment versus general programs of early stimulation that are designed for neurologically normal infants.

The prognosis for change in cerebral palsy is too often based on records of case management rather than on the effect of direct and dynamic treatment by a well-prepared therapist. Bobath[10] documented accurately the developmental sequence expected in the presence of spasticity or athetosis. Her book consolidates some observations of older clients that help professionals understand the uninterrupted effects of the cerebral palsy condition. In any institution one can observe the tightly adducted and internally rotated legs, the shoulder retraction with flexion of the arms, and the chronic shortening of the neck so common as the long-term effects of cerebral palsy. The long-term influence of athetosis results in compensatory stiffness or limited movement patterns to create a semblance of the missing postural stability while a limited number of movement patterns with limited degrees of freedom are used to function.

Responsible surgeons now recognize the improved outcome of their intervention if physical treatment, or a conservative noninvasive therapy, is applied before and after the surgical procedure.[6, 57] Tendon lengthenings for older children with average intelligence may be preceded by muscle energy work or specific stimulation, in which the therapist assists the child in activating the desired muscle group. The therapist may then follow the controlled surgical release with isometric activity inside the cast.[65] Early standing in casts is highly recommended, as are specific footplates, to reduce potential sensory deprivation and to promote more rapid healing with improved circulation.[7, 57, 64]

Within the clinical community there is increasing evidence that soft tissue restrictions further limit spontaneous movement in children with cerebral palsy. That these local myofascial restrictions are often found in infants and very young children suggests that they originate early rather than as a gradual result of faulty movement patterns. Because of the tendency of fascial tissue to change in response to any physical trauma or strong biochemical change, some of these responses might be originating with traumatic birth experiences, and they would be continued by daily use of limited patterns of movement. Tissue restrictions can also occur with immobilization or general infectious processes. Applying specific soft tissue treatment techniques to any person with a neuromotor disorder creates the need for immediate follow-up with appropriate new motor learning activities. Creating excessive tissue mobility in a given area of the body can destroy the delicate patterns of coordination that permit synergic function in the person with cerebral palsy, so functional activation of the body after specific mobilization is strongly recommended. Careful analysis of the movement pattern of the individual child will determine the best location and the sequence for the combined intervention.

Because myofascial changes are closely related to biochemical changes, much research is needed in nutritional supplementation for young children with cerebral palsy. Therapists introducing feeding programs must be very conscious of supporting the establishment of healthy eating habits. In many cases the child has had poor intrauterine development, possibly complicated by an early birth and consequent immaturity. The specialized practice of ecological medicine may provide some specific assistance in this area over time. It is important to have a correct balance of nutrients, both vitamins and minerals, to support optimal growth and development.

There is clear documentation[35, 38] of epidemiological or population changes as a result of early intervention while the CNS is in a period of rapid growth and change. It is also important to offer the flexibility that permits short periods of intensive treatment for an individual child at any age. Informed evaluation by developmentally knowledgeable physicians permits optimal use of effective treatment resources. We have long had evidence that neurological change occurs in small mammals as a result of physical handling and specific environmental experiences.[40] Now evidence for change in the human CNS as a result of therapeutic intervention is accumulating rapidly.[41, 51]

Moore has highlighted some important points for therapists in her concept of increasing functional demands on the system and her observations of the significance of the

neck structures in developmental sequences.[3] The righting reactions used by both Rood and Bobath are completely dependent on neck functions and are possible because of neck mobility. Spastic children often have a lack of developmental elongation of the neck, whereas athetoid children lack neck stability as well as postural co-activation. Moore suggests that our concept of cephalocaudal development should be amended to consider development as beginning at the neck and moving in both a cephalic and caudal direction. This is useful to the therapist who realizes that tone change most often originates with changes in the delicate postural interrelationship between head and body. Tone itself is developing in a caudocephalic direction, whereas antigravity control follows the cervicocephalic cervicocaudal pattern. This is clearly demonstrated when analyzing the electromyographic activity seen in balance synergies and their responses to perturbations (Chapter 21).

In applying Moore's notion of forcing the system, professionals must first gain an understanding of the function of various subsystems as well as the integrative action of the CNS as a whole. Appreciation of the abundance of polysynaptic neurons[3] and parallel processing will provide a much more optimistic view of the therapist's role as a facilitator and feedback organizer for the system. At the same time, therapists have a responsibility to interpret and apply the feedback that they receive from the entire organism. Any stimulus that is of sufficient strength to make a positive change is also capable, under the right circumstances, of making a negative change to influence the quality of output at that moment. For example, excessive treatment to obtain extensor responses in the prone position can result in failure of the neck to elongate and inadequate balance of flexor tone to permit normal standing or postural co-activation in other functional positions, such as sitting.

Therapy intervention is far from innocuous when responsibly applied. A truly eclectic treatment approach comes only after years of experience and a comprehensive understanding of various approaches. The therapist who makes functional changes in the child with cerebral palsy will gradually formulate a personal philosophy of treatment that includes space for new ideas that arise from treatment feedback or from new knowledge about the CNS. One can never learn too much about the intricacies of normal development and its implications. With high-quality treatment intervention there will be no uncertainty about the need for therapy services as a crucial aspect of case management for these children. These interventions need to be reported in the literature as case study outcomes to enrich the depth and breadth of clinical research.

ROLES OF THE THERAPIST

Role of the Therapist in Direct Intervention

The primary role of the therapist is in direct treatment or physical handling of the child that offers opportunities for new motor learning. This should precede and accom-

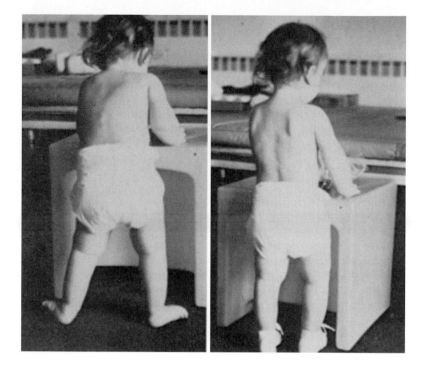

FIGURE 9–11. Supportive shoes for the low-tone child unquestionably facilitate more normal trunk reactions and permit use of the hands for play.

pany the making of recommendations to parents, teachers, and others handling the child. Positioning for home and home handling recommendations should always be tried first by the therapist during a treatment session. As was noted with the initial assessment, many interventions will cause a reaction unique to the particular youngster.[24, 51] It is the role of the therapist to analyze the nature of the response that is accompanied by adaptation inadequacies, to analyze the movement problems, and to choose the most effective intervention (Fig. 9–11). It will then be possible for other persons to manage play activities and supervise independent functioning that reinforce treatment goals.[32]

The therapist working with these children becomes an important and trusted resource to the family. At times the therapist who has had the more consistent contact with the child becomes the facilitator of better communication between the parents and medical or health care professionals. The child who starts early and continues with the same therapist may make of this person a confidant and share concerns that are difficult or uncomfortable for the child to explain to parents.

Nature of Direct Treatment for Specific Problems

The child who is bound within the limitations of hypertonicity suffers first of all from a paucity of movement. Although the hypertonicity may have developed from lack of axial and trunk stabilization due to hypotonicity, disuse of those initially weak or hypotonic muscles will lead to additional weakness over time. As early attempts to move have resulted in the expression of limited synergistic postural patterns, the child often experiences the body as heavy or awkward and loses incentive to attempt movement. The observed tightness in the limbs is not the major problem of these children. The therapist will want

to focus on the abilities to sustain postural control in the trunk. Stability that should be present in the shoulder structure to support good arm movement or in the pelvis to free the leg has not developed. The limb has taken on the role of stabilizer, with an abnormal distribution of excessive tone as a compensatory reaction due to lack of central security. As the trunk tone is normalized through facilitating a variety of postural transitions with the child, the abnormally high tone in the limbs will be reduced. The compensatory reaction is no longer necessary. As the initiation of the central pattern generator that runs postural programs changes within the child, it will be marked by improved limb movement in many children with cerebral palsy and opens the possibility for new learning of more coordinated tasks. Specific work on hand preparation for reach and grasp follows use of the arm for directed movement and often results in improved balance in standing. This is related to freeing the upper body to participate in active balance adaptations.

Postures that are associated with an abnormal distribution of postural tone or that express abnormal patterns of movement should be avoided initially in the treatment process. The therapist will want to return to these positions later to reduce tone in the active posture and gradually demand that the child's nervous system take over control of appropriate sensorimotor programs. Inhibition of one part of a movement range or even one limb must be done in a way that permits the child to activate the body in a functional way. The child who lies in the supine position with extreme pushing back against the surface is rarely seen when treatment has started early. There is a need for the therapist to understand these total patterns to recognize remnants of the total pattern that still interfere with intended movement. The therapist initially eliminates the supine position entirely but would incorporate into the treatment plan the activation of normal flexor tone in sitting with variations of pelvic tilt. Gradually the child is reintroduced to a supine position with postural transitions so that balanced control of the body emerges.

A primary consideration for the child with spasticity is adequate respiratory support for movement. Mobility of the chest wall and abdominal area must be combined with trunk rotation during basic postural transitions. Consideration of age-appropriate speed of movement will guide the therapist to include activities that challenge better respiration and prepare for speech breathing to support vocalization. The therapist will find it helpful to hum or sing or even make silly sounds that encourage sound production by the child during therapy.

In some children, respiratory patterns remain immature and superficial, which may be related to the original insult and the inadequate establishment of functional breathing patterns. A lack of sitting or antigravity postural control limits even the physiological shaping of the rib cage itself, because the ribs do not have an opportunity to change their angle at the spine (see Fig. 9–2). Initial treatment sessions with an older child must take into account the physiological stress induced by respiratory adaptation, and the child's ability to adjust to functional activities must be increased according to respiratory tolerance. The child may literally stop breathing when moving into a new postural alignment. The therapist must give careful support to sustain the transitional posture until breathing resumes. The therapist requires an active respiratory adaptation that will then reinforce postural tone changes in the trunk itself while increasing the variability of postural adaptation. Normal respiratory adaptation will help to maintain normal trunk tone, just as dynamic trunk alignment facilitates good respiration.

When the therapist needs to inhibit unwanted posturing in total patterns, placing the body in a completely opposite alignment should be used with caution. Care must be taken to avoid a complete reversal of the original position, because this will lead to an adaptation to the new extreme alignment. It is more helpful to study the interaction between the central body and the extremities. The therapist can move the body weight over a limb to normalize the postural tone while facilitating functional postural adaptations. The trunk can be helped to experience weight-bearing in a variety of alignments by using inflated balls or rolls that offer a contoured surface. The threshold of the original response is gradually altered so that the child begins to learn a new way of controlling movement. By orienting more to the disordered learning process in movement control[60] the therapist can elicit new improved responses by controlling the body position for the new learning.

When there are distinct differences between the two sides of the body, attention must be given to lateral weight shifts in sitting and standing. Frequently, changes near midline represent the more difficult stimuli for the disorganized system to accept, so the initial therapy sessions may introduce sustained weight-bearing on each side of the body while assisting the sensory adaptation of the more affected side (see Chapter 4). The shoulders may be assisted to align over the hip of the same side, and it may be necessary for the therapist to repeat the experience with a marked pause to allow integration of the new alignment at the sensory or proprioceptive level.

Preparation of lateral shifts in sitting helps to prepare the adaptation of the pelvis that will be needed in standing and later in walking. Young children need special help with rotation of the trunk, which keeps the weight-bearing side relatively forward with dynamic balance of flexion and extension influences.

While working with children and young people with cerebral palsy, the therapist may need to use an intensity of stimulation somewhat beyond the average or typical range. Weight-bearing often must be sustained for a prolonged time, and a full physiological range of limb movement must be prepared, rather than just the part of a range used for a specific function. Therapists are addressing a system that is deficient in its ability to receive, perceive, and utilize the available input. This makes careful analysis and functional orientation of the sensory input essential. If the microcosm of experience given the child during a treatment session is no more intense than an equal amount of time in his or her everyday living environment, the therapist has failed to utilize this unique opportunity to deliver a meaningful message that developmentally integrates the system and encourages the learning of new sensorimotor control.

Reassessment of Direct Treatment

The therapist who is handling a child functions as a sensorimotor extension of the child's CNS, organizing input as to intensity, frequency, and distribution to anticipate a desired response.[63] The child may react positively, negatively, or inadequately to the sensory experience. The therapist is then confronted with the need to evaluate the quality of the motor response, much as an intact system monitors its own output and seeks further experience. The therapist observes whether the needed adaptation has been achieved. Is the body tolerating a variety of positions? Does the child adapt to the supporting surface? Is the movement of a limb graded and without unwanted associated reactions in other parts of the body? Is the child now ready to take over more independent control? By analyzing the answers to such questions the therapist is guided to an appropriate sequence of the session and is enabled to set functional treatment goals and realistically change prognoses.

The therapist acts on these judgments that are made regarding the nature of the response obtained from the child. The next feedback provided for processing by the child's CNS needs to challenge the system while ensuring success and moving toward more normal control.[22] Depending on the technique found to be most effective, the therapist is interrupting the child's customary abnormal feedback to allow new somatosensory and motor learning to occur. At times the input of the therapist may be a slight modification of the child's own response, such as an elongation of a limb as it is being moved. At other times the therapist introduces a sensory substitute for missed developmental experiences. For example, firm pressure on the sole of the foot can be combined with active pushing to simulate weight-bearing in standing. The infant's feet can be placed firmly against a ball surface or against the wall while an adult securely controls the posture. This can provide a component of the sensory experience of normal development (Fig. 9–12). Visual experiences can be altered with prism lenses to cause new postural responses that are guided by the therapist.[53]

Too often professionals consider sensory input to be on a simple graded continuum. The real situation is not so elementary.[24] It must be considered as at least a three-dimensional and possibly a four-dimensional phenomenon that occurs with extreme rapidity in the CNS. Multiple sensory systems are simultaneously activated by most therapeutic input, whereas a variety of sights and sounds may be available in the immediate environment. Memory, previous learning, and cognition are often activated by the therapist-child interaction. The therapist must be accustomed to continuous reassessment of the child's experiential needs compared with the current input provided. The reticular activating system is awakened by the treatment experience and helps to spread the influence to other parts of the CNS. Input modification is determined by the therapist and graded according to the child's response.

To philosophically explore the developmental meaning attached to the sensory experience of normal movement, therapists must take into account the ability to process contrasting stimuli. While several parts of the body are stable, another is moving. Stability of the proximal body permits a limb to extend forcefully or to be maintained in space. Each new level of developmental differentiation or dissociation of movement increases the complexity of processing by the CNS (Fig. 9–13). Stimuli from within the body and from the environment impinge simultaneously on the CNS. This is easily illustrated with a review of self-feeding. Initially the process of guiding a full spoon into the mouth engages the child's full attention. The arm

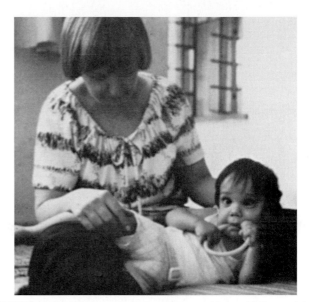

FIGURE 9–13. Treatment sessions can consider a child's need for a teething experience while facilitating good postural patterns and tone distribution.

is lifted at the shoulder to bring the spoon to the level of the mouth before elbow flexion takes the spoon to the face. Between the ages of 2 years and 6 years the self-feeding pattern modifies and the elbow moves down beside the body. Now the motor aspect of the task has become procedural and more efficient, permitting the child to participate in social exchanges with the family at the same time that he or she manages independent self-feeding.

A solid understanding of normal developmental sequences is essential for the clinician providing direct treatment.[8, 13] Early responses of the normal infant change from a self orientation to an environmental orientation as new developmental competence emerges. More sophisticated balance in independent sitting occurs as the ability to pull to standing at a support begins to develop. Such knowledge of developmental details may be applied by the therapist to introduce postural activities at a higher developmental level than the child's present function permits. The assisted self-dressing process is an effective way to introduce and integrate new movement and sensorimotor learning while using established movement skills. To sit well, the child must practice moving over the seat surface, coming in and out of sitting, and control of coming to stand (Fig. 9–14). To walk well, the child may need to run with control by the therapist to allow practice in changing rate, direction, range, and balance. Sitting may be made more dynamic by using a gymnastic ball as a seat. A part of the treatment session is often spent filling in gaps that represent missed developmental experiences, such as squatting to play or coming to stand from kneeling or even attending to specific shifts over midline in prone or supine to move more easily in bed. Activation of the entire body, in different postures, with the most normal alignment and postural tone is vital to maximize the sensory experience of postural control. Specific techniques can be reviewed thoroughly in Chapter 4.

With the athetoid child, the therapist's role relates

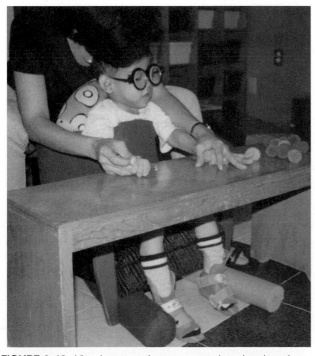

FIGURE 9–12. Visual contact that corresponds to hand motion can be learned with prism lenses that displace the child's perception of spatial relationships.

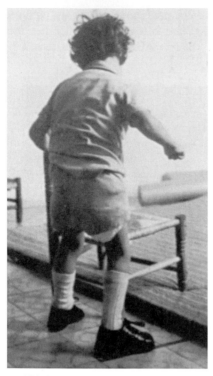

FIGURE 9–14. This boy with hemiplegia tries to move a chair by orienting only his more active side to the task and bearing weight only briefly on the more affected side.

primarily to organization and grading of seemingly erratic movement. Initially, therapists provide the postural control that the child has not been able to achieve independently. Through their handling of the child they give stability from which movement can emerge. At a more sophisticated level the therapist grades the movement of limbs by structuring the postural control of the proximal body, with special attention to head-trunk relationships. It is essential to work closely with a behavioral optometrist with these children in order to include visual feedback and feed forward information. In some instances the therapist may assist a limb to keep a position that elicits active proximal adjustments that are the basis of true postural control. The astute therapist will find that careful analysis of tone changes reveals, in many cases, a predictable pattern. One particular movement will initiate the interfering spasm or series of spasms that interrupt stability. This may be part of a reflexive or synergistic pattern, or it may be an isolated reaction.

It is often useful to check for soft tissue restriction in the localized area. In the ambulatory athetoid child it is often the spontaneous depression or elevation of a scapula or the protraction of a shoulder that initiates tone change throughout the body. If this particular initiating action can be effectively inhibited, while righting reactions of the head and trunk are stimulated, the body begins to build a repertoire of responses that does not include the customary interference. With functional use of the upper extremity for support, reach, and grasp, the client shares with the therapist inhibition of the abnormal response. Gradually, the more normal use of the whole upper trunk integrates the interfering response, resulting in improved

control for a variety of independently controlled postures. The therapist continues to introduce graded stress during treatment sessions to normalize even further the threshold for the unwanted reaction.

Environmental stimuli such as sights, sounds, and social interaction should be considered as stimuli along with positional stress. Visual disorganization is a particularly difficult problem for the athetoid child, and it improves most when balanced activity of the visual and the postural systems has been achieved. Movement control must become procedural if independence is to be accomplished. Thus, distracting the child's cognitive attention off the motor act and onto the activity will allow for better procedural learning. This concept of graded stress is considered more thoroughly in Chapters 6 and 7.

Direct intervention for the hemiplegic child takes into account the obvious difference in postural tone between one side of the body and the other. However, treatment for children that addresses itself only to the more affected side of the body will not prove to be effective. The critical therapeutic experience seems to be that of integration of the two sides of the body. This begins early for the normal infant, with lateral weight shifts in a variety of developmental patterns. This leads to postural organization that permits later reaching for a toy while the body weight is supported with the opposite side of the body. The child with a contrast in the sensorimotor function of the two sides of the body needs to experience developmental patterns that include rotation within the longitudinal body axis and lateral flexion of the trunk, with special emphasis on bringing the more affected side forward. The more affected side needs the experience of supporting the body as well as the experience of initiating movement.

Development of hand use first focuses on bilateral arm activity while keeping the affected hand well within the functional visual field. The infant or young child is helped by working primarily in sitting until dynamic trunk flexion begins to activate. The therapist may find that true flexion of the more affected side of the body is fully as difficult for some children as the initial active elongation of that side. There tends to be a high incidence of soft tissue restrictions in the shoulder and neck of the affected side. Children with hemiplegia have difficulty in sustaining a balanced posture against the influence of gravity, and some begin to struggle to do everything with the less affected side. This characteristic contrast in function may contribute to the development of seemingly hyperactive behavior that is related to the inability of the CNS to resolve contrasting information. Hyperkinetic responses in one side of the body may compensate for relative inactivity in the opposite side. One goal of treatment is to bring these divergent response levels closer together so that the child can experience more comfortable postural change and adapt to later school demands.

The limbs of the hemiplegic child will change in postural tone as the trunk reactions are brought under active control. Specific attention must be given to sensory normalization. The two hands need the experience of sustaining the body weight simultaneously, as do the two feet. Although the more affected hand may not develop sensation adequate for skilled activity, an important treatment goal is sufficient shoulder mobility to move the arm across the body midline and to assume a relaxed alignment during ambulation. Early treatment will increase the possibility that the more affected hand will be used as an assisting or helping hand. There are some children who have such severe sensory loss that active use is minimal, even though considerable relaxation can be achieved.

A strong discrepancy between the sensorimotor experiences of the two sides of the body seems to lead the system to reject one of the messages. This can lead to distortions in verticality and is a major interference in bilateral integration. Functional vision evaluation is important to avoid the midline shift problem that will distort postural control. As body weight is shifted to the more normal side, flexor withdrawal patterns of the limbs increase in frequency and strength in some children. The presence of a lateral visual midline shift may increase the avoidance of weight on the more affected side.[48] One important therapy goal is the achievement of graded weight shift through the pelvis during ambulation (Fig. 9–15).

Treatment preparation must incorporate a wide variety of more basic developmental alignments in which pelvic weight shift is a factor. The choice of prone, moving from sitting to four-point support, or a simple weight shift while sitting on a bench will depend on the movement characteristics observed by the therapist during the session. Diagonal adaptations are useful in normalizing the distribution of tone for upright function. Careful attention must be given to pelvic alignment and mobility because the pelvis has a tendency to be rotated posteriorly on the more affected side in children who have not had good

early therapy. This can cause increased hip flexion later if the child begins to walk with the more affected side held posteriorly, a characteristic that may be observed during analysis of leg position in gait. Dynamic foot supports will facilitate this functional weight shift when the child is not in treatment. The goal of functional movement is best reached through a wide variety of weight-bearing postures, from the obvious developmental alignments to horizontal protective responses or reaching above the shoulders in sitting and standing (Fig. 9–16).

The child with low muscle tone is perhaps the greatest challenge for both therapist and parent. Adequate developmental stimulation is difficult unless positioning can be varied. Placing the child in a more upright alignment, even though it is achieved with complete support initially, seems to aid the incrementation of postural tone. To prepare the low-tone body for function, it is helpful to review the articulations for possible soft tissue restrictions. The neck and shoulder girdle are particularly vulnerable. Strong proprioceptive input while ensuring accurate postural alignment is an important part of the treatment session. Direct push-pull motion of the limbs, which is gentle traction approximation as described by the Bobaths,[11] also assists in maintaining antigravity positions. Positioning at home may include a high table that supports the arms, allows for good trunk alignment, and permits voluntary horizontal arm motion. The therapist must be cautious of high-tone responses to peripheral and trunk instability and initial hypotonicity. This hypertonic response, which can be distributed in the deeper musculature, contributes to fixation rather than differentiated postural control. Even though the child's motor output

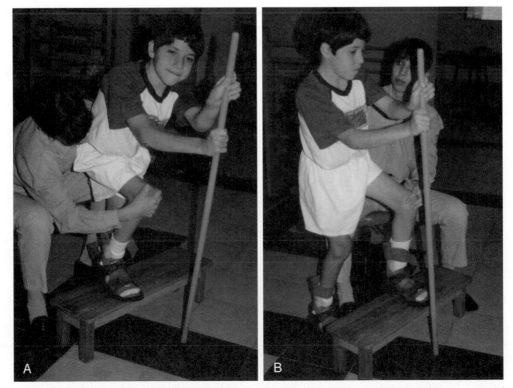

FIGURE 9–15. The two sides of the body (A and B) often respond very differently to the same task, and therapy must be adapted accordingly.

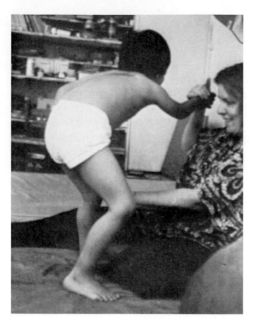

FIGURE 9–16. The experience of coming to stand over the more affected side activates diagonal patterns of postural adjustment.

may remain low, changes in positioning and opportunities to have visual and other sensory experiences will aid learning. Home handling needs to include a variety of positions during each day for seating and play.

The process of undressing and dressing can be a dynamic part of the treatment program for any child. Diagonal patterns of movement that are incorporated into the removal of socks and shoes assist in the organization of midline orientation. Weight shifts and changes in stability-mobility distribution occur throughout the dressing process. Concepts of direction and spatial orientation are applied to the relation of body parts and clothing. Directional vocabulary terms and names of clothing and body parts are learned with this experience. A bench is useful because it permits the adult to sit behind the child who is just beginning to participate actively. The older child with difficult balance reactions can use the bench in a straddle-sit alignment. Aside from the physical and perceptual benefits, this achievement of dressing independently is one that offers the child a feeling of pride and independence. It is also a very practical preparation for the future when it is introduced in keeping with individual developmental and emotional needs.

Developing a Personal Philosophy of Treatment

The practicing therapist continues to learn much about the nuances of normal human development.[24, 28] The dynamic interaction of developmental movement components becomes more significant as the therapist acquires greater clinical experience and recognizes developmental change as a reflection of CNS maturation. Increasing knowledge of the functional nature of sensory systems and CNS processing will influence the choice of treatment techniques (Fig. 9–17). Direct intervention will have

more depth and specificity that improve the child's control of posture and movement while the therapist appreciates the complex interaction of developmental factors in cerebral palsy. Based on individual experience, each therapist develops a personal philosophy of treatment that incorporates new research findings and evolving perceptions of the problem of CNS dysfunction. Without a philosophical orientation for decision making the therapist may succumb to following each promising treatment idea that is learned without having a clear image of the potential benefits for the specific client. Without an internalized treatment goal toward which independent techniques are applied, the result remains ineffective and unconvincing. The therapist in a direct treatment situation must be secure with a concise, personalized visualization of what is to be achieved in each session with the individual child. Repetition that is critical for learning must often be carried out at home, and the therapist becomes responsible for family instruction.

Specialized therapy, like normal development, is potentially a preparation for functional performance. Training in specific coordination skills may be necessary for the older child or adolescent and must begin with a thorough analysis of the whole person who happens to demonstrate the effects of cerebral palsy. Some children have learned self-care along with brothers and sisters. Others have needed therapy guidance for each achievement. Intelligent children with strong motivation may only need some assistance in avoiding use of abnormal reactions, whereas others have poor spatial orientation and minimal motivation to achieve independence. The therapist most often

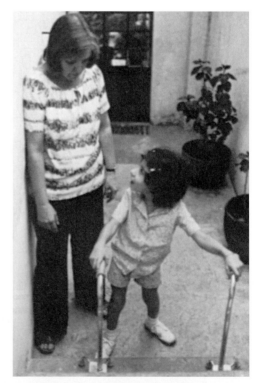

FIGURE 9–17. True ability to "walk" must include problem solving for architectural barriers in the child's own environment.

must appeal to the individual with the problem, because parents are often fatigued and without energy to solve the issue of adolescent life skills.

Adaptations of position and special equipment may be necessary to initiate independent activity for the more severely affected child (Fig. 9–18). Finnie[28] has given many practical suggestions for new therapists and parents. Brereton and associates[15] have done an excellent job of grading perceptual-motor tasks and suggest alternate presentations that may better suit the individual child. Furth and Wachs[31] have presented, in a useful reference that is organized for the busy therapist, precognitive skill development in a visual-motor context that develops a child's thinking strategies.

Active Involvement of the Family

To be successful, active treatment of the child with cerebral palsy includes daily home follow-up in both physical and psychological handling of the child. This allows for variability of practice in different environments, which tends to promote more effective motor learning. Parents who learn to help their child early begin to understand the importance of their participation as well as the nature of their child's disability. This is not easy because parents have suffered damage to their own self-image when they learned of their child's disability. Although they should not be expected to become therapists per se, close observation of treatment sessions offers insight into the child's current strengths and weaknesses.

Parents can consequently adapt their expectations in keeping with the child's ongoing change. Parenting a child with cerebral palsy is no easy task, and the therapist will do well to develop respect for this demanding role. No one provides more for the child with cerebral palsy than the nurturing parent who guides the child to self-acceptance of limitations without destroying personal initiative.

This is the child who most often becomes an independent working adult (Fig. 9–19).

The therapist must give serious thought to priorities in home recommendations. To be considered are the size of the family, outside employment of mother and/or father, physical capabilities of the child, general health status of the child, and psychological acceptance of the problem within the family (Fig. 9–20). The emotional needs of some parents demand a period of less, rather than more, direct involvement with the child. Other parents must be cautioned that repetition of an activity more times than recommended will not result in faster improvement. This impression is sometimes gained from wide advertising of commercial programs that offer the same activity sequence for every child and demand a large number of daily repetitions. Both parent and therapist must appreciate the need for the CNS to have some time to integrate new sensorimotor experiences and to perfect emerging control of postural adjustments. Excessive control of movement patterns by an adult tends to reduce initiation of postural change and decrease active sensorimotor learning. Health needs for good nutrition and adequate rest must also be considered by parents and professionals.

Criteria for Equipment Recommendations

Equipment recommendations must take into account the physical space in the home and the amount of direct treatment available to the child (see Fig. 9–17). Young children in particular can often use normal seating with slight adaptations. This is not only more socially acceptable but also permits changes as required by the child's developmental progress. Portability of supportive seats or standers encourages the family to take the apparatus along for weekend outings or visits to relatives. Chair designs should place children at an age-appropriate level in their environments. This permits a better quality of

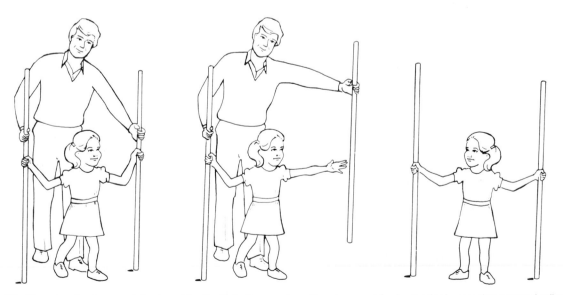

FIGURE 9–18. The use of poles was introduced by the Bobaths as a transitional support for increasingly complex postural adjustments in standing and walking.

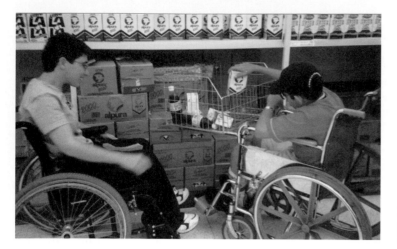

FIGURE 9–19. Therapy goals must incorporate functional activities that lead to personal independence if they are to be pertinent for the older child and adolescent.

visual exploration and facilitates social exchange with siblings and visiting peers.

When planning the amount of physical support needed by the child, the therapist considers varying the structural control in relation to activity (see Fig. 9–18). The child who is merely watching the play of others or a television presentation may successfully control trunk and head balance independently with minimal support. However, concentration on hand skills or self-feeding may necessitate trunk control assistance by a chair insert to avoid the child's use of abnormal reactions. As postural reactions become more integrated and hence more automatic, support should be diminished.

For the more severely disabled child, equipment

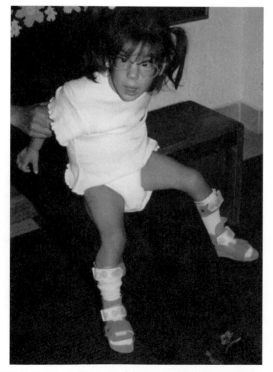

FIGURE 9–20. The ability to adapt to changes in the center of gravity can be practiced at home with the help of an adult.

should be easily and completely washable. Mothers should be able to place special seating inserts into wheelchairs or travel chairs using one hand while holding the child. Wheelchairs should be ordered with consideration for family needs and the child's environment. The most costly does not always offer the best solution. Control straps and seating should be adaptable and allow for future change based on growth and improved function. The severely limited child needs seating changes at least once every hour during the day. Pleasing color, good quality upholstery, and professional finishing are important not only for the child but also for family members, who are accepting the equipment as part of a personal living environment.

As prices rise and the applicability of insurance changes, cost effectiveness must be considered more carefully by the therapist. Parents are often desperate to do everything possible for their child and tend to be very susceptible to high-powered advertising and reassuring sales personnel. By providing a list of essential equipment features, the therapist will aid the parents in becoming informed consumers. Perusal of several catalogs permits some comparison of quality and prices. Periodic review of equipment used by the child will encourage the family to pass along to someone else equipment items that are no longer needed. Investment in expensive equipment also has the hidden effect of influencing both parent and therapist to continue its use when its effectiveness as a dynamic supplement to treatment has passed. For this reason more than any other, large investments must be thoroughly researched as to their long-term applicability for the child.

Special Needs of Infants

The direct treatment of infants deserves special mention, because there are significant differences between the infant and the older child. Aside from the delicate situation of the new parents, the infant is less likely to have a diagnosis and presents a mixture of normal and abnormal characteristics. It is essential that the clinician have a strong foundation in the nuances of normal developmental movement[48, 59] and early postural control. Direct

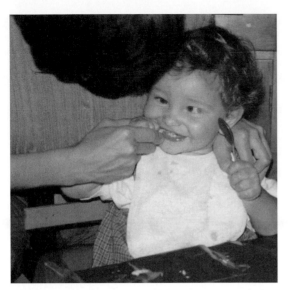

FIGURE 9–21. Therapy gains should be a happy experience whenever possible.

intervention can be offered as a means of enhancing development and overcoming the effects of a difficult or an early birth (Fig. 9–21). It will be important, however, to secure a diagnosis for the infant who reaches 8 or 9 months of age and continues to need therapy.

Infants with early alterations in motor control should be followed until they are walking independently, even if they no longer need weekly therapy. Infant responses can change very rapidly as the therapist organizes the components of movement control. Soft tissue restrictions should be treated initially to have more success with facilitated movement responses. Careful observation is essential, because all but the severely involved infant will change considerably between visits. The therapist should invest some time in training the parents to become skilled observers while appreciating the small gains made by their infant.

Referral to other health care professionals is essential in the presence of possible allergies, new neurological signs, visual or auditory alterations, and persistent reflux. There is always the possibility of convulsions, which can occur for a variety of reasons in infants with neuromotor dysfunction.

Role of the Therapist in Indirect Intervention

For many children with cerebral palsy, active treatment is not available. Geographical isolation, socioeconomic factors, and lack of qualified therapists may interfere with the delivery of direct service. The therapist must then assume the role of teacher, counselor, or consultant. More often the new role emerges as one in which the therapist tries to meet a combination of needs and is frequently frustrated by lack of time, energy, and community resources. The therapist may be a member of a community team that includes a psychologist, a social worker, and a public health nurse. This sometimes creates more of a

behavioral than a traditional medical orientation. Therapists can also be primarily responsible to the public school systems, introducing therapeutic positioning to classroom teachers. For these types of situations the clinician will find videotape a valuable adjunct to direct instruction. The individual child may be filmed with equipment, adequate positions, or therapeutic procedures. Useful topic-oriented videotapes are also available for professionals and families.

Physical Positioning for the Child Who Lacks Direct Treatment

When the therapist receives children who have no access to direct treatment, positioning is of paramount importance. The selected support is used to avoid contractures, scoliosis, and permanent limitations in range of movement. Even the most severely limited child should have a minimum of three positions that can be alternated during the day. In addition, the position selected should be as functional as possible for the individual child. In some cases this may mean encouraging eye contact. For another child, hand use becomes a possibility with proper trunk support.

All supports, whether they be chairs, prone boards, standers, or floor seats, should be checked carefully for their effect on the child's posture. A child may appear to be properly positioned for the first few minutes and then be pulled into excessive flexion or collapse to one side. Positions that appear simple to the therapist may be viewed quite differently by a person who does not have experience with reflexive reactions and postural alignments. It is helpful to have a photo of the client in the chair, with important points of control noted. If the therapist has not seen this particular client over a period of time, careful interview of the family is advisable to understand typical behaviors of the child and to plan some options that respond to problems that might arise.

Communication for the nonverbal client with cerebral palsy must be an integral part of the treatment program.[45] A simple start may be made with pictures to permit choices in food, clothing, and therapy activities. The parents need encouragement to begin the process of letting the child make some simple choices in food, clothing, or preferred activities. Although computers have their place, the child should have the communication device with him or her at all times. Language development in the young child is enhanced by having this type of alternative while articulation is still difficult. Affordable electronic systems, with voice recording, portability, and growth features, are available. Communication can make the difference between passivity and active participation in the environment and can be achieved by coordinating efforts with the speech pathologist.[45]

Consultation for the Family and Other Helpers

If at all possible, some opportunity for in-service exchange should be provided when persons with a variety of professional backgrounds are brought together to accomplish a task. The therapist, along with other specialists, must forfeit some professional jargon in the interest of true communication that benefits the child. One may practice with familiar persons who lack training in therapy to develop the skill of clear instruction. The therapist can try talking this volunteer through the task of positioning a child or feeding the child according to written directions. The therapist should then note the areas of miscommunication and adapt the instructions accordingly.

Therapists should encourage parents, teachers, and others to understand why certain positions are being recommended. This will make them more conscious of both positive and negative changes that may call for further adaptations. Excessive explanation is preferable to a partial understanding or outright confusion as to why positioning may have an effect on the child's development. When feasible, it is helpful to let caregivers assume some abnormal postures to personally feel some of the difficulties that the child experiences. This will offer a guide to helping the child.

Communication systems for the more severely disabled child should be evaluated by the primary therapist to determine which near-normal movement patterns may be used. Repeated activation of total patterns of flexion or extension will eventually interfere with trunk control in sitting and may cause a child to regress physically. Use of head movement is a powerful influence on tone changes that may cause negative regression in postural or visual control. Use of a simple, more proximal response will help toward the goal of better function. A solution that was successful with one athetoid girl of 9 years was moving the elbow back to a switch mounted on the vertical bar of the wheelchair backrest. Any activity that is repeated on a daily basis should be examined in light of possible interference by abnormal patterns. Secure seating for toileting is fundamental for success in the required physiological control. Self-feeding assistance can be most effectively introduced with abduction at the shoulder and the overhand grasp of the normal toddler. This normal alignment fosters the development of proximal control for the child with cerebral palsy and facilitates active grasp of the spoon.

The Therapist in the Schools

Children with mild dysfunction as a result of cerebral palsy may be successfully incorporated into physical education classes if the teacher is prepared to make some small adaptations. Teachers generally appreciate the opportunity to discuss with the therapist specific limitations of the child and those movements that should be encouraged. For better success the disabled child can be incorporated into a class that follows the British form of movement education, which places much less emphasis on intragroup competition and encourages each child to progress at his or her own rate.

Classroom teachers who lack experience with special needs are understandably reluctant to incorporate a disabled child into their classroom until they know the child. A meeting with the therapist might be used to help the child demonstrate his or her strengths and physical

independence. The child may often play an active role in the problem-solving process necessary for a successful classroom experience. Children often have developed their own ways of managing the water fountain, the locker door, or personal care needs. Demonstrating these abilities reinforces strengths rather than limitations and arms the child with some positive responses for curious peers.

NEW DIRECTIONS IN THE COMMUNITY

As programs that hire therapists move into prevention and early intervention, the therapist is dealing directly with a population that is not familiar with therapy per se nor aware of the need for this intervention. The therapist may discover a need to reorient previously accepted concepts of general rehabilitation. Clarification of one's own ideas is essential to establish effective communication with others. In some instances, active intervention to help the child will precede the labeling or diagnostic process and referral to other specialists becomes part of the therapist's responsibility. Philosophically, early therapy becomes an enhancement of normal development rather than a remedial process. This implies introducing new concepts of quality in early child development to the public.

It is important to keep direct, active treatment available for older children, adolescents, and adults who are motivated to change. Now that more effective procedures are available for changing some of the basic neurophysiological characteristics of cerebral palsy, it is possible to obtain change with direct treatment of the older client. Motor learning concepts are better understood (see Chapters 4 and 5) and can be applied after normalizing the tissues that have been unused for so many years. With present program directions many older clients will not have had the opportunity for direct treatment over time by a qualified therapist.

The movement toward a health orientation as opposed to crisis intervention for illness will also affect services for children and adults with cerebral palsy. This population does not have an illness or active disease process and strives to lead as normal a life as possible. Many adults with neuromotor disabilities express their preference to participate in the decisions that are made for them regarding their ultimate lifestyle in the community. Optimal health for the person with residuals of cerebral palsy has yet to be described, and much more data must be collected.

PSYCHOSOCIAL FACTORS IN CEREBRAL PALSY

We have defined cerebral palsy as a condition existing from the time of birth or infancy. The developing child has no memory of life in a different body. Movement limitations circumscribe the horizon of the child's world unless the family is able to provide compensatory experiences. The development of both intelligence and personality relies heavily on developmental experiences and self-expression.

The child with spastic diplegia or spastic quadriplegia may be hesitant in making decisions or reaching out for a new opportunity because the world may seem overwhelming and somewhat threatening. The child may find it easier to withdraw toward social isolation. Parents and professionals can help to avoid these reactions by encouraging independence in thought and in physical tasks. Early choices can be made by the child regarding which clothes to wear or which task to do first. Understanding the child's limitations helps build successes rather than failures. To function in spite of the constraints of spasticity or other movement problems demands considerable effort on the part of the child.

Athetoid children, in contrast, have adapted to failures as a transient part of life. However disorganized their movements, they repeatedly attempt tasks and eventually succeed. Their social interactions reflect this life experience. Most people will sooner or later succumb to the positive smiling approach without analyzing the deeper communication offered by the child. These children are difficult for parents to discipline and structure during their early years. Early treatment with concomitant guidance for young parents does ameliorate some of the problems by making more appropriate the developmental expectations for the child.

Intelligent children with low tone demand that the world be brought to them. Mentally limited children may fail to receive sufficient stimulation for optimal development at their functional level. Many of these children need visual or auditory evaluations and intervention, and some of them need a special educational approach. Whatever the learning potential of the child with cerebral palsy, it is not always evident early. Parents find it difficult to know how to guide a child when they are not certain that an assigned task or patient explanation is understood.

Parental guidance of the disabled child is also influenced by the adults' adaptation to their offspring's problem. They need to have resolved in their own way the emotional impact of the child's disability. Most parents feel inadequate, ignorant, and relatively helpless at being unable to remedy the situation for their child. They need help in feeling good about themselves before they can effectively guide the child toward self-acceptance as an adequate human being. Parents need guidance to provide themselves with opportunities to rest and renew their energies.

The therapist plays an important role in the psychosocial development of children who receive regular treatment. The child may perceive the therapist as a confidant, disciplinarian, counselor, or friend at various stages of development. Some children accept the therapist as a member of their extended family. This is natural considering the extent to which therapists influence clients' own self-awareness through changes in their physical bodies. However, it also places a personal responsibility on the therapist to be cognizant of the ongoing interaction and its effect on the maturational process of the child.

Any evaluation of personality characteristics in a disabled child must take into account the unnatural lifestyle that is superimposed by the need for therapy, medical appointments, and hospitalization. The child is expected to separate from parents earlier than the average child and usually confronts many more novel situations. There is little time or physical opportunity for free play. Continuous demands are placed on children to prove their intellectual potential in evaluations of various types. Their social interaction is most often monitored by adults, while they assume a dependent role. Nonetheless, these children's social acceptance frequently rests on their skill in interacting with persons in their environments. It is not easy to evaluate the evolution of personality without considering these experiential factors.

MEDICAL INFLUENCES ON TREATMENT

Because the problems of cerebral palsy are so varied, the condition lends itself to diverse interventions, some of which have a longer life than others. The cerebellar implant so popular in the late 1970s offered the possibility of regulating tone by supplementing cerebellar inhibition.[23, 24, 64] As time passed, the procedure was used less often and patients had difficulty getting repairs or replacement parts for the implant. The procedure that largely replaced the cerebellar implant was the placement of four electrodes in the cervical area to offer more control over postural tone.[39] These had the advantage of being adjustable so that the individual or a family member could make daily choices as to the optimal tone distribution. In some cases early success gave way to disappointment as the system adapted to the inputs. In some cases the child or adolescent had to make a decision whether movement or speech was more important on a given day. Therapy was always recommended after the procedure, although the nature of the specific program was left to the family to decide.

In 1968 a posterior rhizotomy surgical intervention was developed by Foerster and some success was reported in reducing spasticity.[27, 44] It remained for Peacock to apply the procedure more selectively and functionally and to bring it to the United States from South Africa.[55] Based on his experience, he insisted on daily neurodevelopmental (Bobath) treatment for at least 1 year after the surgical intervention. Electromyographic testing before and during the surgery is used to determine which posterior nerve rootlets are creating the spasticity in the lower extremities.

Typically, the child cooperates actively in treatment as more normal movement patterns are learned. There is a need for the surgical candidate to have some trunk function and fairly normal underlying tone for the selective posterior rhizotomy.[46, 55] The child must also adapt psychologically to the temporary loss of physical control, as the previous ability to walk or move about may be impaired for some months as new patterns of movement are learned. The long-term gains can be impressive, although some therapists state the need for 1 to 3 years of treatment after surgery because of the child's completely new tone distribution. The foundation for success is accurate selection of the child, an experienced surgeon, and careful analysis of therapy goals.[19]

The more recent improvement in the rhizotomy procedure has been developed by Lazareff,[46] who enters two rather than five levels of the spinal column and prefers to work close to the cauda equina, following the technique of Fasano.[27] The children operated on using this limited selective posterior rhizotomy technique tend to recuperate more rapidly, and diplegic children of 6 to 9 years resume walking within weeks. Older clients have a slower process of learning new motor patterns, but the reduction of spasticity frees them for better postural control. More severely involved children can benefit from this intervention as early as 4 years of age. Lazareff prefers to have recommendations from the child's therapist and considers 2 years for CNS maturation plus 2 years of quality therapy as a minimum consideration for the limited selective posterior rhizotomy as an intervention to reduce spasticity. Lazareff has also operated on more severely involved older youngsters, with improvements noted in respiration, postural adaptation, and ease of daily care. Excessive hypotonia is avoided with the limited procedure. Lazareff's most recent publication[47] clearly demonstrates that a more conservative surgical intervention gives the same results as more extensive separation of rootlets. Tone in lower extremities as well as upper body was measured before and after the limited selective posterior rhizotomy to demonstrate clear reduction of tone in both areas.

Orthopedic intervention continues to be effective in cerebral palsy when there are tendon contractures or specific structural limitations that are not accompanied by excessive levels of spasticity.[7, 57] In any surgery the outcome is much improved by close coordination between therapist and surgeon, with a functional orientation toward goal setting for the child. Using early standing postsurgery, dynamic footplates inside the casts, and orthotics to follow cast removal will generally improve functional outcomes. Bone surgeries that offer better joint stability are usually planned for the termination of growth. The orthopedist is also able to guide conservative positioning measures to prevent hip problems due to spasticity while direct treatment intervention continues.

Both orthopedists and neurologists have taken an interest in the use of botulism toxin to block selected muscle responses for a temporary period of time. This permits the therapist to work toward a previously agreed upon goal. New motor learning can occur while the overpowering nonfunctional responses are blocked. In some clients spontaneous movement responses occur that were impossible before the injections. These conservative interventions serve to delay surgery until the child is more capable of responding to postsurgical therapy programs. Children with cerebral palsy differ in the ability to relax completely during sleep, and a small number of them can benefit from inhibitive casting[6] or splints to be used at night. More often this type of positioning is used during therapy sessions and independent ambulation to combine the control with weight-bearing.[71] The orthopedist should participate in any plan for prolonged immobilization or temporary casting that will be used on a 24-hour schedule.

RECORD KEEPING AND CLINICAL RESEARCH

Data collection is an important task in the treatment of cerebral palsy. Change occurs at variable rates, but it is important to document the cause and effect of change whenever possible. Slides or videotapes are useful in recording functional comparisons over time. Film lends itself to a formal frame-by-frame analysis, and digital video now allows a specific analysis of movement sequences. A motor drive unit or automatic advance on a 35-mm single lens reflex camera also records a sample of movement five or more times per second. Placing the subject against a spaced grid in a specific alignment to perform a movement task allows for measurement of efficiency of movement. These ideas may be applied to documentation of treatment effectiveness or analyzed for an understanding of similar movement problems in other clients.

Matching of groups is an approach doomed to failure, or at least to considerable inaccuracy in cerebral palsy because of a wide range of individual differences. It is analogous to making a statement regarding the mean in a widely variable population. This does not mean that methods of intervention or treatment are not measurable or that research is not applicable to the functional problems presented by a diagnosis of cerebral palsy. Once a specific research question has been formulated, systematic recordings of appropriate data can be gathered over time to accumulate the number needed for a viable study. There is value in longitudinal reporting of a single case or a small group of individuals who have some characteristics in common because this aids our understanding of what we need to prevent in the young child to permit optimal function later. (See Chapters 3 and 11 regarding suggestions of impairment and disability measurements to be used as objective measures for functional outcome studies and record keeping.)

The way in which therapists are taught to view a problem determines, to a large extent, the potential range of solutions available to them. Cerebral palsy is a complex of inabilities that cluster about the inadequacy of CNS control and the amazing ability of the human body to compensate. For the purpose of productive study, therapists may look critically at qualities of movement, postural adjustments, timing of movements, or changes in range of functional movement. New areas of motor learning, systems, and chaos theories offer the researcher novel approaches to the challenge of cerebral palsy and the resultant disorder of posture control and movement learning. Environmental factors may have as much influence as specific CNS limitations, and this awareness emphasizes proprioceptive information in early developmental handling. Therapists are improving a disorder of posture and movement through their direct treatment. Analysis of the postural components and movement characteristics will lead to meaningful research more quickly than reliance on the traditional definitions of the medical condition.

CASE STUDIES

To understand the problems of children with cerebral palsy, it is essential to follow some children over time

CASE 9–1 L.P.

A young mother was pregnant with her first child. She was middle class, well nourished, and had no identified risk factors. In her seventh month of pregnancy, her older sister died, causing considerable emotional upheaval. The much anticipated infant was born, small for gestational age, at her correct date. It was theorized that there had been inadequate intrauterine nourishment during the first 6 to 7 months. L.P. weighed 3.5 pounds (1587 g) and was fed initially by nasogastric tube. Her movements were quick and eye movement was very active for a new infant. She was received for therapy at 17 days of age, immediately after hospital discharge.

Initial therapy focus was on the practical task of adequate nutritional intake so that the nasogastric tube could be removed before scarring occurred from repeatedly passing the tube. Swaddling was suggested to calm the infant and assist her organization of body movement. Simple handling was oriented to moving the trunk over midline to let the head follow and assisting the infant to assume age-appropriate antigravity postures.

At 3 years of age L.P. continued to have difficulty with control of her head position in space and was unable to initiate postural change with her head. Her clinical picture was one of low tone with athetoid movement. She could not speak, communicated with looks and a few word approximations, and hitched along the floor in a seated position with one hand supporting.

By 5 years of age L.P. was still receiving therapy three times per week and could walk in a hesitating way with her hands held. At this stage she was evaluated by a behavioral optometrist and started vision therapy to prepare her to participate in preschool activities. As a secondary benefit her balance in walking improved markedly. L.P. began walking up and down 27 steps daily in her new home.

Now at 7 years of age L.P. can walk independently on level surfaces. She has physical therapy once a week and vision therapy once a week to maintain her control of posture and movement. Her school performance is adequate to keep her with her age peers and she attends a regular school.

CASE 9–2 D.D. AND E.D.

D.D. and E.D. were born within 6 months of each other at 6 months and 1 week of gestation. Both were first-born infants for their respective mothers. D.D.'s mother was discovered to have a double uterus when she had a miscarriage early in the pregnancy. E.D. suffered malnutrition during his intrauterine development. D.D. started therapy just before he was 5 months old. E.D. began therapy at almost 7 months old.

At 6 years of age D.D. walks alone with very mild athetotic "overflow." He wears corrective lenses that were fit at 2 years of age and returns for follow-up examinations with the behavioral optometrist once a year. Vision therapy was an important adjunct to physical handling because it introduced changes in spatial perception based on specific sessions with prism lenses. At 4 years of age D.D. was discovered to have a mild to moderate hearing loss and still uses a hearing aid in one ear. He speaks English and Spanish, as do his parents, and he understands the French spoken to him by his grandparents. He functions in a regular school with his age peers and is a well-adapted, active child.

At 6 years of age E.D. presents as a moderately severe diplegic, with some immaturity of hand use and trunk control. He speaks English and Spanish well, although he demonstrates some emotional instability and difficulty in dealing with his disability. He is creative in storytelling and offers to tell original stories for other children in therapy. He is just beginning to walk with a walker within interior environments and with low resistance.

to capture the evolution of family problems. Functional treatment must change according to the developmental level, chronological age, and neuromotor responses of the child. Intervention must be specific to the presenting problem of the moment while considering the missing aspects of complete motor development. The case study comparison of two boys illustrates the typical lack of clinical correlation between history and manifest characteristics of cerebral palsy.

REFERENCES

1. Arbuckle BE: The Selected Writings of Beryl E. Arbuckle. Newark, OH, American Academy of Osteopathy, 1947.
2. Arnold GG: Problems of the cerebral palsy child and his family. Va Med Monthly 103:225–227, 1976.
3. Bach-y-Rita P (ed): Recovery of Function: Theoretical Considerations for Brain Injury Rehabilitation. Berne, Switzerland, Hans Huber, 1980.
4. Benabib RM: Vision Training for Neurologically Impaired Children. Albuquerque, NM, Clinician's View Video, 1993.

5. Benabib RM, Nelson CA: Efficiency in visual skills and postural control: A dynamic interaction. J Occup Ther Pract 3(1), 1991.
6. Bertoti DB: Effect of short leg casting on ambulation in children with cerebral palsy. Phys Ther 66:1522–1529, 1986.
7. Bleck E: Orthopedic Management in Cerebral Palsy. Philadelphia, JB Lippincott, 1987.
8. Bly L: Motor Skills Acquisition in the First Year: An Illustrated Guide to Normal Development. San Antonio, Therapy Skill Builders, 1994.
9. Bobath B: The very early treatment of cerebral palsy. Dev Med Child Neurol 9:373–390, 1967.
10. Bobath B: Abnormal Postural Reflex Activity Caused by Brain Lesions. London, William Heinemann Medical Books, 1975.
11. Bobath B: Motor Development in the Different Types of Cerebral Palsy. New York, William Heinemann Medical Books, 1975.
12. Bobath K: A Neurophysiological Basis for the Treatment of Cerebral Palsy, 2nd ed. Clinics in Developmental Medicine, No. 75, London, William Heinemann Medical Books, 1980.
13. Brazelton TB: Infants and Mothers: Differences in Development. New York, Dell, 1969.
14. Brazelton TB: Neonatal Behavioral Assessment Scale. In Clinics in Developmental Medicine, No. 50, London, William Heinemann Medical Books, 1973.
15. Brereton B, et al: Cerebral Palsy: Basic Abilities. Mosman, NSW, Australia, The Spastic Centre of New South Wales, 1975.
16. Brooks VB: The Neural Basis of Motor Control. New York, Oxford University Press, 1986.
17. Bryce J: The management of spasticity in children. Physiotherapy 62:11, 1976.
18. Buethorn D: Dynamic Ankle Foot Orthotics (manual and video). Albuquerque, Clinician's View, 1992.
19. Cahan LD, et al: Electrophysiologic studies in selective dorsal rhizotomy for spasticity in children with cerebral palsy. Appl Neurophysiol 50:459–462, 1987.
20. Conner F, et al: Program Guide for Infants and Toddlers with Neuromotor and Other Developmental Disabilities. New York, Teacher's College Press, 1978.
21. Cooper IS, et al: Correlation of clinical and physiological effects of cerebellar stimulation. Acta Neurochir (Suppl) 30:339–344, 1980.
22. Crutchfield CA, Barnes MR: Motor Control and Motor Learning in Rehabilitation. Atlanta, Stokesville Publishing Co, 1993.
23. Davis R, et al: Cerebellar stimulation for cerebral palsy. J Fla Med Assoc 63:910–912, 1976.
24. Davis R, et al: Cerebellar stimulation for spastic cerebral palsy: Double-blind quantitative study. Appl Neurophysiol 50:451–452, 1987.
25. Denhoff E, et al: Treatment of spastic cerebral palsied children with sodium dantrolene. Dev Med Child Neurol 17:736–742, 1975.
26. Einspieler C, Prechtl HFR, et al: The qualitative assessment of general movements in preterm, term and young infants: Review of the methodology. Early Hum Dev 50:47–60, 1997.
27. Fasano VA, et al: Long-term results of posterior functional rhizotomy. Acta Neurochir 30(suppl):435–439, 1980.
28. Finnie NR: Handling the Young Cerebral-Palsied Child at Home. New York, EP Dutton, 1975.
29. Fiorentino MR: A Basis for Sensorimotor Development: Normal and Abnormal. Springfield, IL, Charles C Thomas, 1981.
30. Frymann V: Relation of disturbances of craniosacral mechanisms to symptomatology of the newborn: Study of 1,250 infants. J Am Osteopath Assoc 65:1059–1075, 1966.
31. Furth H, Wachs H: Learning Goes to School. New York, Oxford University Press, 1974.
32. Gilfoyle EM, et al: Children Adapt. Thorofare, NJ, Slack, 1981.
33. Goleman D: Emotional Intelligence. New York, Bantam Books, 1995.
34. Haberfellner H, Muller G: Sequelae of head and neck positions on auditory performance. Neuropadiatrie 7:373–378, 1976.
35. Hagberg BA: Epidemiology of cerebral palsy: Aspects on perinatal prevention in Sweden. Neonatal Neurological Assessment and Outcome Report of the 77th Ross Conference on Pediatric Research, 1980.
36. Held R: Plasticity in Sensory-Motor Systems. Sci Am 71–80, 1965.
37. Hellebrandt FA, et al: Methods of evoking the tonic neck reflexes in normal human subjects. Am J Phys Med 41:263–269, 1962.
38. Hochleitner M: Control study of children with cerebral palsy with and without early neurophysiological treatment. Aust Med J 32: 1091–1097, 1977.
39. Hugenholtz H, et al: Cervical spinal cord stimulation for spasticity in cerebral palsy. Neurosurgery 22:707–714, 1988.
40. Illingworth RS: The Development of the Infant and Young Child: Abnormal and Normal, 7th ed. Edinburgh, Churchill Livingstone, 1980.
41. Keshner EA: Re-evaluating the theoretical model underlying the neurodevelopmental theory. Phys Ther 61:1035–1040, 1981.
42. Knoblock H, Pasamanick B (eds): Developmental Diagnosis. Hagerstown, MD, Harper & Row, 1974.
43. Köng E: Very early treatment of cerebral palsy. Dev Med Child Neurol 8:68–75, 1966.
44. Laitinen LV, et al: Selective posterior rhizotomy for treatment of spasticity. J Neurosurg 58:895–899, 1983.
45. Langley MB, Lombardino LJ: Neurodevelopmental Strategies for Managing Communication Disorders in Children with Severe Motor Dysfunction. Austin, TX, Pro-Ed, 1991.
46. Lazareff J, et al: Limited selective posterior rhizotomy for the treatment of spasticity secondary to infantile cerebral palsy: A preliminary report. Neurosurgery 27:535–538, 1990.
47. Lazareff JA, Garcia-Mendez MA, et al: Limited (L4–S1, L5–S1) selective dorsal rhizotomy for reducing spasticity in cerebral palsy. Acta Neurochir 141:743–752, 1999.
48. Leach P: Babyhood. New York, Alfred A Knopf, 1977.
49. MacKeith RC, et al: The Little Club memorandum on terminology and classification of cerebral palsy. Cereb Palsy Bull 1:34–37, 1959.
50. Milani-Comparetti A: Neurophysiologic and clinical implications of studies on fetal motor behavior. Semin Perinatol 5:183–189, 1981.
51. Montgomery PC, Connolly BH: Motor Control and Physical Therapy: Theoretical Framework, Practical Application. Hixson, TN, Chattanooga Group, 1991.
52. Niswander KR: The obstetrician, fetal asphyxia, and cerebral palsy. Am J Obstet Gynecol 133:358–361, 1979.
53. Padula WV: A behavioral vision approach for persons with physical disabilities. Santa Ana, CA, Optometric Extension Program Foundation, 1988.
54. Palmer FB, et al: The effects of physical therapy on cerebral palsy: A controlled trial in infants with spastic diplegia. N Engl J Med 318:803–808, 1988.
55. Peacock WJ, Arens LJ: Selective posterior rhizotomy for the relief of spasticity in cerebral palsy. S Afr Med J 62:119–125, 1982.
56. Pearlstone A, Benjamin R: Ocular defects in cerebral palsy. Eye Ear Nose Throat Mon 48:87–89, 1969.
57. Pettitt B: Surgery of the lower extremity in cerebral palsy: Considerations and approaches. Arch Phys Med Rehabil 57:443–447, 1976.
58. Prechtl HFR: The Neurological Examination of the Full-Term Newborn Infant. Philadelphia, JB Lippincott, 1977.
59. Prechtl HFR: Development of postural control in infancy. In vonEuler C, Forssberg H (eds): Neurobiology of Early Infant Behaviour, Vol 55. Wenner-Gren International Symposium Series. London, Macmillan, 1989.
60. Prechtl HFR: The organisation of behavioural states and their dysfunction. Semin Perinatol 16:258–263, 1992.
61. Prechtl HFR: State of the art of a new functional assessment of the young nervous system: An early predictor of cerebral palsy. Early Hum Dev 50:1–11, 1997.
62. Rosenthal R, et al: Levodopa therapy in athetoid cerebral palsy. Neurology 22:21–24, 1972.
63. Rosenzweig M, et al: Brain changes in response to experience. Sci Am, February 1972.
64. Soboloff HR: Trends in cerebral palsy treatment. Tex Med 66:82–91, 1970.
65. Sussman M, Cusick B: Preliminary report: The role of short-leg tone-reducing casts as an adjunct to physical therapy of patients with cerebral palsy. Johns Hopkins Med J 145:112–114, 1979.
66. Tardieu G, Tardieu C: Cerebral palsy: Mechanical evaluation and conservative correction of limb joint contractures. Clin Orthop 219:63–69, 1987.
67. Trew M, Everett T: Human Movement. Edinburgh, Churchill Livingstone, 1997.
68. Upledger JE, Vredevoogd JD: Craniosacral Therapy. Seattle, Eastland Press, 1983.
69. Van der Knaap MS, et al: Myelination as an expression of the functional maturity of the brain. Dev Med Child Neurol 33:849–857, 1991.

70. Vining E, et al: Cerebral palsy: A pediatric developmentalist's overview. Am J Dis Child 130:643–649, 1976.
71. Watt J, et al: A prospective study of inhibitive casting as an adjunct to physiotherapy for cerebral-palsied children. Dev Med Child Neurol 28:480–488, 1986.
72. Whittaker CK: Cerebellar stimulation for cerebral palsy. J Neurosurg 52:648–653, 1980.
73. Wright BA: Physical Disability—A Psychological Approach. New York, Harper & Row, 1960.

ADDITIONAL READINGS

Alexander R, Boehme R, Cupps B: Normal Development of Functional Motor Skills: The First Year of Life. Tucson, Therapy Skill Builders, 1993.

Ames LB, et al: The Gesell Institute's Child from One to Six: Evaluating the Behavior of the Preschool Child. New York, Harper & Row, 1979.

Aptekar R, et al: Light patterns as means of assessing and recording gait: II. Results in children with cerebral palsy. Dev Med Child Neurol 18:37–40, 1976.

Ashmead D, McCarty M, et al: Visual guidance in infants reaching toward suddenly displaced targets. Child Dev 64:1111–1121, 1993.

Bach-y-Rita P: Brain Mechanisms in Sensory Substitution. New York, Academic Press, 1972.

Barolat G: Dorsal selective rhizotomy through a limited exposure of the cauda equina at L–1. J Neurosurg 75:804–807, 1991.

Beintema DJ: A neurological study of newborn infants. In Clinics in Developmental Medicine, No. 28, London, William Heinemann Medical Books, 1968.

Black R: Visual disorders associated with cerebral palsy. Br J Ophthalmol 66:46–52, 1982.

Bly L, Whiteside A: Facilitation Techniques. San Antonio, Therapy Skill Builders, 1997.

Bock A: Motor control prior to movement onset: Preparatory mechanisms for pointing at visual targets. Expl Brain Res 90:209–216, 1992.

Boehme R: Improving upper body control: An Approach to Assessment and Treatment of Tonal Dysfunction. Tucson, Therapy Skill Builders, 1988.

Bower TGR: The visual world of infants. Sci Am 251:349–357, 1966.

Bower TGR: A Primer of Infant Development. San Francisco, WH Freeman, 1977.

Briggs DC: Your Child's Self-Esteem, 2nd ed. Garden City, NJ, Dolphin Books, 1975.

Buscaglia L: The Disabled and Their Parents: A Counseling Challenge. Thorofare, NJ, Slack, 1975.

Bushnell EW, Boudreau PR: The development of haptic perception during infancy. In Heller MA, Schiff W (eds): The Psychology of Touch. Hillsdale, NJ, Lawrence Erlbaum, 1991, pp 139–161.

Case-Smith J: Comparison of in-hand manipulation skills in children with and without fine motor delays. Occup Ther J Res 13:87–100, 1993.

Case-Smith J, Pehoski C: Development of Hand Skills in the Child. Rockville, American Occupational Therapy Association, 1992.

Chakerian D, Larson N: Effects of upper extremity weight bearing on hand opening and prehension patterns in children with cerebral palsy. Dev Med Child Neurol 35:216–229, 1993.

Clifton R, Rochat P, et al: Multimodel perception in the control of infant reaching. J Exp Psychol 20:876–886, 1994.

Cioni G, Ferrari F, Einspieler C, et al: Neurological assessment of preterm infants: Comparison between observation of spontaneous movements and neurological examination. J Pediatr 130:704–711, 1997.

Connolly KJ (ed): The psychobiology of the hand. In Clinics in Developmental Medicine, No. 147. London, MacKeith Press, 1998.

Corbetta D, Thelan E: The developmental origins of bimanual coordination: A dynamic perspective. J Exp Psychol Hum Percept Perform 22:502–522, 1996.

Cosgrove A, Corry I, Graham J: Botulinum toxin in the management of the lower limb in cerebral palsy. Dev Med Child Neurol 36:386–396, 1994.

Duckman R: Accommodation in cerebral palsy: Function and remediation. J Am Optom Assoc 55:281–283, 1984.

Eccles JC: The Understanding of the Brain, 2nd ed. New York, McGraw-Hill, 1977.

Eliasson G, Forssberg H: Tactile control of isometric fingertip forces during grasping in children with cerebral palsy. Dev Med Child Neurol 37:72–84, 1995.

Erikson E: Toys and Reasons: Stages in the Ritualization of Experience. Philadelphia, WW Norton & Co, 1977.

Featherstone H: A Difference in the Family: Life with a Disabled Child. New York, Basic Books, 1980.

Feldenkrais M: Awareness Through Movement. New York, Harper & Row, 1977.

Ferrari F, Cioni G, Prechtl HFR: Qualitative changes of general movements in preterm infants with brain lesions. Early Hum Dev 23:193–233, 1990.

Fikes T, Klatzky R, Lederman S: Effects of object texture on precontact movement time in human prehension. J Motor Behav 26:325–332, 1994.

Ford E, Englund S: For the Love of Children. Garden City, NY, Anchor Press, 1977.

Forssberg H: The neurophysiology of manual skill development. In Connolly KJ (ed): The Psychobiology of the Hand. In Clinics in Developmental Medicine, No. 147. London, MacKeith Press, 1998.

Friedli W, Hallett M, Simon S: Postural adjustments associated with rapid voluntary arm movement: I. Electromyographic data. J Neurol Neurosurg Psychiatry 47:611–622, 1984.

Gahm NH, et al: Chronic cerebellar stimulation for cerebral palsy: A double-blind study. Neurology 31:87–90, 1981.

Galjaard H, Prechtl HFR, Veličkovič M: Early Detection and Management of Cerebral Palsy. Boston, Martinus Nijhoff, 1987.

Gentile M (ed): Functional Visual Behavior: A Therapist Guide to Evaluation and Treatment Options. Baltimore, American Occupational Therapy Association, 1997.

Girolami G, Campbell S: Efficacy of a neurodevelopmental treatment program to improve motor control in infants born prematurely. Pediatr Phys Ther 6:175–184, 1994.

Gleick J: Chaos: Making a New Science. New York, Viking Press, 1987.

Goffman E: Stigma: Notes on the Management of Spoiled Identity. Englewood Cliffs, NJ, Prentice-Hall, 1963.

Goleman D: Emotional Intelligence. New York, Bantam Books, 1995.

Gordon J, Ghez C: Roles of proprioceptive input in control of reaching movements. In Movement Disorders in Children, vol 36. Basel, Karger, 1991, pp 124–129.

Gormley ME: The treatment of cerebral origin spasticity in children. Neurorehabilitation 12:93–103, 1999.

Graham M, et al: Prediction of cerebral palsy in very low birthweight infants: Prospective ultrasound study. Lancet 2:593–595, 1987.

Harrell R, et al: Can nutritional supplements help mentally retarded children? An exploratory study. Proc Natl Acad Sci U S A 78:574–578, 1981.

Hulme JB, et al: Effects of adaptive seating devices on the eating and drinking of children with multiple handicaps. Am J Occup Ther 41:81–89, 1987.

Jones FP: Body Awareness in Action: The Alexander Technique. New York, Schocken Books, 1976.

Katayama M, Tamas LB: Saccadic eye-movements of children with cerebral palsy. Dev Med Child Neurol 29:36–39, 1987.

Katz K, et al: Seat insert for cerebral-palsied children with total body involvement. Dev Med Child Neurol 30:222–226, 1988.

Kelso J (ed): Human Motor Behavior: An Introduction. Hillsdale, NJ, Lawrence Erlbaum Associates, 1982.

Laborde AT, Weibel ME, et al: Intrathecal baclofen for spasticity of cerebral origin. Neurorehabilitation 12:81–91, 1999.

Leboyer F: Loving Hands: The Traditional Indian Art of Baby Massage. New York, Alfred A Knopf, 1976.

Loria C: Relationship of proximal and distal function in motor development. Phys Ther 60:165–167, 1980.

Menken C, et al: Evaluating the visual-perceptual skills of children with cerebral palsy. Am J Occup Ther 41:646–651, 1987.

Montagu A: Touching, the Human Significance of the Skin, 2nd ed. New York, Harper & Row, 1978.

Nelson KB, et al: Children who "outgrew" cerebral palsy. Pediatrics 69:529–536, 1982.

Nwaobi OM: Seating orientations and upper extremity function in children with cerebral palsy. Phys Ther 67:1209–1212, 1987.

Oetter P, Richter E, Frick S: Integrating the Mouth with Sensory and Postural Functions. Hugo, MN, PDP, 1995.

Ornstein R, Sobel D: The Healing Brain. New York, Simon and Schuster, 1987.

Penn RD: Chronic cerebellar stimulation—a review. Neurosurgery 10:116–121, 1982.

Prechtl FR: Continuity of Neural Functions from Prenatal to Postnatal Life. Philadelphia, JB Lippincott, 1984.

Prechtl HFR: Principles of early motor development in the human. *In* Kalverboer AF, Hopkins B, Geuze RH (eds): A Longitudinal Approach to the Study of Motor Development in Early and Later Childhood. Cambridge, England, Cambridge University Press, 1993, pp 35–50.

Prechtl HFR: State of the art of a new functional assessment of the young nervous system: An early predictor of cerebral palsy. Early Hum Dev 50:1–11, 1997.

Prechtl HFR, Einspieler C: Early abnormal spontaneous movements as a predictor of cerebral palsy. In Veličkovič, M, Neville B (eds): Textbook on Cerebral Palsy. Amsterdam, Elsevier, 1999.

Rast M: The use of play activities in therapy. Developmental Disabilities Special Interest Newsletter, American Occupational Therapy Association, 7:3, 1984.

Reilly M (ed): Play as Exploratory Learning. Beverly Hills, CA, Sage Publication, 1994.

Restak R: The Brain. New York, Bantam Books, 1984.

Rochat P: Self-sitting and reaching in 5 to 8 month old infants: The impact of posture and its development on early eye-hand coordination. J Motor Behav 24:210–220, 1992.

Rolf IP: Rolfing: The Integration of Human Structures. New York, Harper & Row, 1978.

Rose S: The Conscious Brain, updated ed. New York, Vintage Books, 1976.

Ruff HA: The infant's use of visual and haptic information in the perception and recognition of objects. Can J Psychol 43:302–319, 1989.

Russman B, Tilton A, Gormley M: Cerebral palsy: A rational approach to a treatment protocol and the role of botulinum toxin in treatment. Muscle Nerve 6:S181–S193, 1997.

Samples B: Open Mind Whole Mind: Parenting and Teaching Tomorrow's Children Today. Rolling Hills Estates, CA, Jalmar Press, 1987.

Scherzer A, Tscharnuter I: Early Diagnosis and Therapy in Cerebral Palsy. New York, Marcel Dekker, 1982.

Scherzer A, et al: Physical therapy as a determinant of change in the cerebral palsied infant. Pediatrics 58:47–52, 1976.

Sparling J, Walker D, Singdahlsen J: Play techniques with neurologically impaired preschoolers. Am J Occup Ther 38:603–612, 1984.

Stockmeyer SA: An interpretation of the approach of Rood to the treatment of neuromuscular dysfunction. Am J Phys Med 46:900–961, 1967.

Stone LJ, et al: The Competent Infant, Research and Commentary. New York, Basic Books, 1973.

Sweeney JK: The High-Risk Neonate: Developmental Therapy Perspectives. New York, The Haworth Press, 1986.

Szasz S: The Body Language of Children. New York, WW Norton, 1978.

Thelen E: Developmental origins of motor coordination: Leg movements in human infants. Dev Psychobiol 18:1–18, 1985.

Thelen E, et al: Self-organizing systems and infant motor development. Dev Rev 7:39–65, 1987.

Tjossen TD (ed): Intervention Strategies for High-Risk Infants and Children. Baltimore, University Park Press, 1976.

Touwen B: Neurological development in infancy. *In* Clinics in Developmental Medicine, No. 58. London, William Heinemann Medical Books, 1976.

Verny T, Kelly J: Secret Life of the Unborn Child. New York, Delta Books, 1981.

Wann J: The integrity of visual-proprioceptive mapping in cerebral palsy. Neuropsychologia 11:1095–1106, 1991.

Willemson E: Understanding Infancy. San Francisco, WH Freeman, 1979.

Witkin K: To Move, to Learn. New York, Schocken Books, 1977.

Wolf S, Glass R: Feeding and Swallowing Disorders in Infancy: Assessment and Management. Tucson, Therapy Skill Builders, 1992.

Yokochi K, et al: Leg movements in the supine position of infants with spastic diplegia. Dev Med Child Neurol 33:903–907, 1991.

Genetic Disorders: A Pediatric Perspective

WAYNE A. STUBERG, PhD, PT, PCS • WARREN G. SANGER, PhD

Key Words

– evaluation
– functional skills
– genetic disorders
– natural environments
– physical therapist
– occupational therapist

Objectives

After reading this chapter the student/therapist will:

1. Describe the main types of genetic disorders and give examples of each type.

2. Describe the diagnostic approach for genetic disorders.

3. Describe three modes of inheritance for single-gene disorders.

4. Describe the use of and be able to utilize the National Center for Biotechnology web site to look up the pathophysiology, impairments, functional limitations, and disability information on common genetic disorders frequently observed in therapy settings.

5. Explain why it is important to include family members in the planning and development of therapy programs for children with genetic disorders.

6. Describe and give examples of three types of assessment tools and state the intended purpose of each.

7. Describe the importance of developing therapy programs for children that are outcome-focused on functional skills in natural environments.

8. Identify three medical treatments that may be used for children with genetic disorders to ameliorate the effects of the disorder.

9. Explain why it is important for physical and occupational therapists to have knowledge of the services available through genetic counseling.

Genetic disorders in children can result in severe neuro-musculoskeletal impairments and disability. In this chapter we discuss disorders of known genetic origin that physical and occupational therapists are most likely to encounter in therapy programs for children. A nomenclature for genetic disorders and a description of the clinical and laboratory diagnostic processes are presented in the first section. Specific examples of each type are given along with a brief description. A summary of typical clinical signs observed in genetic disorders is presented in the second section.

In the third section the focus is on the physical or

occupational therapist's role in the clinical management of children with genetic disorders. Evaluation procedures, treatment goals and objectives, and general treatment principles and strategies are discussed from a family-centered perspective. The final section includes a discussion of the medical management of genetic disorders and genetic counseling.

AN OVERVIEW: CLINICAL DIAGNOSIS AND TYPES OF GENETIC DISORDERS WITH REPRESENTATIVE CLINICAL EXAMPLES

An accurate diagnosis for a specific genetic disorder (syndrome or disease) is necessary to provide a prognosis and a plan of management for the affected individual. It is also important for the provision of genetic counseling and discussion with other family members about risks for a similar or the same condition. Because of the nearly 4,000 genetic conditions described to this point, evaluation by a clinical geneticist to determine appropriate testing is often needed for accurate diagnosis. The construction of a family history and other medical histories for the child and family is imperative. The medical diagnosis is sometimes made solely on clinical grounds, if laboratory diagnostic procedures do not exist for that condition.

Genetic disorders are typically divided into four categories: chromosomal, single-gene, multifactorial, and mitochondrial.[60] Chromosomal disorders include deletion of a chromosome segment or of an entire chromosome, duplication, and other alterations. When there is a suspicion of a chromosomal syndrome such as a structural chromosome abnormality, chromosome (cytogenetic) studies are typically performed on peripheral blood obtained from the patient. If the clinical suspicion is that of a clinical spectrum associated with some of the known microdeletions, fluorescence in situ hybridization (FISH) procedures, utilizing specific sequence DNA probes, can confirm a specific suspected diagnosis.

Single-gene disorders may be transmitted through three different modes of inheritance: autosomal dominant, autosomal recessive, and sex-linked. In the event of a suspected gene abnormality, specific molecular genetic procedures utilizing unique DNA sequence probes, mutation analysis, or linkage analysis can be performed to confirm single-gene disorders.

Multifactorial disorders are due to a combination of multiple genetic and environmental causes. Mitochondrial disorders are very rare and therefore not specifically addressed in this chapter. They are caused by alterations in the cytoplasmic mitochondrial chromosome.

Table 10–1 shows the categories of genetic disorders and clinical examples of each. The chromosomal and single-gene abnormalities are discussed in this chapter. An in-depth discussion of spina bifida can be found in Chapter 15. Management information on clubfoot can be found in pediatric textbooks that include orthopedic information.[14, 94, 106]

With the completion of the Human Genome Project

TABLE 10–1. Partial Listing of Typical Genetic Syndromes or Diseases

Syndrome or Disease	Approximate Incidence
Chromosomal Abnormalities	
Autosomal Trisomy	
Trisomy 21 (Down syndrome)	1/700 to 1/10,000
Trisomy 18	1/6,000
Trisomy 13	1/15,000 to 2/20,000
Sex Chromosome Abnormality	
Turner syndrome	1/2,500–10,000 females
Klinefelter syndrome	1/1,000 males
Partial Deletion	
Prader-Willi syndrome	1/10,000
Cri-du-chat syndrome	1/20,000
Single-Gene Abnormalities	
Autosomal Dominant	
Osteogenesis imperfecta	1/20,000–30,000
Tuberous sclerosis	1/10,000
Neurofibromatosis	1/3,500
Autosomal Recessive	
Cystic fibrosis	1/2,500–4,000 whites
Hurler syndrome	1/100,000
Phenylketonuria	1/10,000–15,000
Werdig-Hoffmann disease	1/20,000
Sex-Linked	
Fragile X syndrome	1/1,500 males; 1/2,500 females
Hemophilia A	1/10,000 males
Duchenne muscular dystrophy	1/3,500
Multifactorial	
Cleft lip with/without cleft palate	1/500–1,000
Clubfoot (talipes equinovarus)	1/1,000
Spina bifida	1/200–1,000
Mitochondrial	
Mitochondrial myopathy	Rare
Kearns-Sayre disease	Rare
Other	
Rett syndrome	1/15,000

the total human DNA sequence is known, potentially allowing specific DNA testing to be available for nearly all human genetic disorders. This not only allows for accurate and more complete diagnosis but should pave the way for the development of mechanisms for treatment, cure, and prevention of certain genetic conditions.

Chromosome Disorders

Most chromosomal abnormalities appear as an extra chromosome or as a missing chromosome. Others may involve a missing or "extra portion" of a chromosome. The incidence of chromosomal abnormalities among spontaneously aborted fetuses may be as high as 60%. About 1 in 150 live-born infants have a detectable chromosomal abnormality; and in about half of these cases, the chromosomal abnormality is accompanied by congenital anomalies, mental retardation, or phenotypic changes that are manifested later in life.[60] Of the fetuses with abnormal chromosomes that survive to term, about half have sex chromosome abnormalities and the other half have autosomal trisomies.[102]

The following section provides a brief overview on

PART 1—USE OF THE WORLD WIDE WEB (WWW) TO ACCESS INFORMATION ON PATHOPHYSIOLOGY AND IMPAIRMENTS

Maile is a 3-year-old girl with Down syndrome (trisomy 21) who was referred to you for development of a therapy program. You have not worked with children with Down syndrome, but having access to the WWW you decide to look up the syndrome on the electronic database maintained by the National Center for Biotechnology called Online Mendelian Inheritance in Man (OMIM).[82] You activate your WWW browser (a program that runs on an Internet-connected computer and provides access to the WWW) and type in http//www.ncbi.nlm.nih.gov/omim, which is the Internet home page address for OMIM.* At the OMIM home page you select "Search the OMIM Database," which takes you to the area of OMIM where you can search using key words. By typing in "Down syndrome" you are taken to information on trisomy 21, and additional information on Down syndrome can be found on the OMIM web site or the suggested link sites on the WWW. The link sites from the OMIM site include direct access to PubMed, which is the National Library of Medicine search service for Medline and other related databases.[93] These reference tools are highly recommended to the clinician, as the information on and number of new syndromes or diseases with genetic etiology are increasing each year. A concise synopsis of genetic syndromes can also be found in *Smith's Recognizable Patterns of Human Malformation* by Jones if WWW access is not available.[59]

---

*More detailed information on accessing the WWW for genetic information can be found in a review article by Phillips.[87] The article also includes an annotated bibliography of WWW sites related to genetics.

---

common genetic disorders seen by physical and occupational therapists working with children. The section also introduces the reader to use of the world wide web (WWW) to obtain more in-depth and the most current information.

Autosomal Trisomies

Trisomy 21 (47,XY,+21).* The pathophysiology of Down syndrome includes the presence of an extra twenty-first chromosome (trisomy 21), found in 95% of individu-

---

*47,XY,+21 is an example of the typical notation used to denote chromosomal syndromes. The number refers to the number of chromosomes with 47 indicating an extra chromosome being present (46 is the normal number), XY refers to a genetic male, and +21 refers to the extra chromosome being number 21.[59]

als with the diagnosis. The remaining 5% have the mosaic and translocation forms. The incidence of Down syndrome increases with advanced maternal, and possibly paternal, age.[50]

The impairments associated with Down syndrome are numerous. Down syndrome is the most common chromosomal cause of moderate to severe mental retardation.[27, 95] Down syndrome occurs in 1 of every 650 to 1,000 live births and is equally distributed between the sexes.[82]

A list of 10 features characterizing newborns with Down syndrome was published by Hall in 1966.[44] These features included hypotonicity, a poor Moro reflex, joint hyperextensibility, excess skin on the back of the neck, a flat facial profile, slanted palpebral fissures, anomalous auricles, dysplasia of the pelvis, dysplasia of the midphalanx of the fifth finger, and simian creases. In his study of 48 newborns with Down syndrome, Hall[44] reported the frequency of these characteristics to vary from 45% to 90% (Fig. 10–1).

In a longitudinal study of 79 infants with Down syndrome from birth to 10 months of age, Cowie[24] reported the universal finding of marked hypotonicity (which appeared to gradually diminish with age) and the persistence of several primitive reflexes, including the palmar and plantar grasp reflexes, the stepping reflex, and the Moro reflex. She also observed a delay in the development of normal postural tone, as indicated by the severe head lag evident during elicitation of the traction response and the lack of full antigravity extension noted when the Landau response was tested.

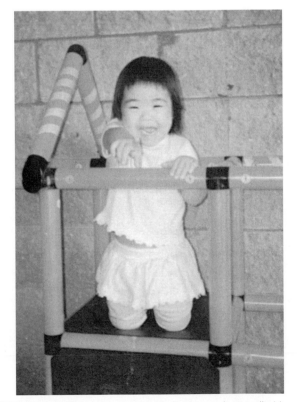

FIGURE 10–1. Two-year-old girl with Down syndrome climbing up playground equipment.

Additional impairments observed in individuals with Down syndrome include congenital heart disease (occurring in 40% of children) and musculoskeletal anomalies such as metatarsus primus varus, pes planus, thoracolumbar scoliosis, patellar instability, and an increased risk for atlantoaxial dislocation.[50] It is particularly important for persons working with infants and children with Down syndrome to be aware of this propensity for atlantoaxial dislocation, which has been observed through radiography in up to 20% of a sample studied.[116] If atlantoaxial instability persists undetected, spinal cord compression with myelopathy may result, leading to leg weakness, decreased walking ability,[84] and increased spasticity or incontinence.[75] Although dislocation is relatively rare, there have been reported cases of quadriplegia.[116]

Craniofacial impairments such as a shortened palate and midface hypoplasia have been noted. These craniofacial differences together with oral hypotonia, tongue thrusting, and poor lip closure frequently result in feeding difficulties at birth.[75]

Impairments of visual and sensory systems are also common in individuals with Down syndrome. As many as 77% of children with Down syndrome have a refractive error (myopia, hyperopia) or astigmatism. Convergent strabismus and nystagmus are also reported.[35] Hearing losses that interfere with language development are reportedly present in 80% of children with Down syndrome. In most cases the hearing loss is conductive; in up to 20% the loss is sensorineural or mixed.[75]

Several researchers have explored the neuropathology associated with Down syndrome. The relatively small size of the cerebellum and brain stem has been widely reported.[27, 86, 96] Marin-Padilla[71] studied the neuronal organization of the motor cortex of a 19-month-old child with Down syndrome and found various structural abnormalities in the dendritic spines of the pyramidal neurons of the motor cortex. He suggested that these structural differences may underlie the motor incoordination and mental retardation characteristic of individuals with Down syndrome. Loesch-Mdzewska[68] also found neurological abnormalities of the corticospinal system (in addition to reduced brain weight) in his neuropathological study of 123 individuals with Down syndrome aged 3 to 62. Crome[26] reported lesser brain weight in comparison with normal persons. Finally, Benda[6] noted a lack of myelinization of the nerve fibers in the precentral area, frontal lobe, and cerebellum of infants with Down syndrome. As McGraw[72] has pointed out, the amount of myelin in the brain reflects the stage of developmental maturation. The delayed myelinization characteristic of newborns and infants with Down syndrome is thought to be a contributing factor to the generalized hypotonicity and persistence of primitive reflexes characteristic of this syndrome.[23]

Trisomy 18 (47,XY, + 18). Trisomy 18 is the second most common of the trisomic syndromes to occur in term deliveries, although far less prevalent than Down syndrome (Fig. 10–2). The incidence has been reported as 1 in 8,000 live births, with females affected more often than males (3:1).[100] As with Down syndrome, advanced maternal age is positively correlated with trisomy 18.[35] Only 10% of infants born with trisomy 18 survive past the first year of life. The survival of girls averages 7 months; the survival of boys averages 2 months.

Individuals with trisomy 18, also known as Edwards syndrome, generally have far more serious organic malformations than seen in those with Down syndrome.[59] Typical malformations affect the cardiovascular, gastrointestinal, urogenital, and skeletal systems. At birth, infants with trisomy 18 are of low birth weight and small stature, with a long narrow skull, low-set ears, flexion deformities of the fingers, and rocker-bottom feet. Muscle tone is initially hypotonic, but it becomes hypertonic.[59] The period of hypertonicity in the early years may change to low tone and joint hyperextensibility by preschool and school age. Microcephaly, abnormal gyri, cerebellar anomalies, mye-

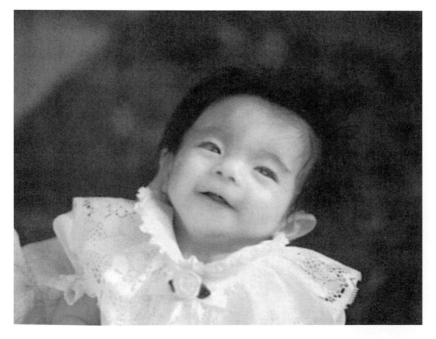

FIGURE 10–2. One-year-old girl with trisomy 18.

lomeningocele, hydrocephaly, and corpus callosum defects have been reported in individuals with trisomy 18.

Common skeletal malformations that may warrant attention from the developmental physical or occupational therapist include scoliosis,[34] limited hip abduction, flexion contractures of the fingers, rocker-bottom feet, and talipes equinovarus.[59] Infants with trisomy 18 may also experience feeding difficulties as a result of a poor suck.[84] Profound mental retardation is another clinical factor that will affect the developmental therapy programs for children with trisomy 18.

Trisomy 13 (47,XY,+13). Trisomy 13 is the least common of the three major autosomal trisomies, with an incidence of 1 in 15,000 to 20,000 live births.[105] As in the other trisomic syndromes, advanced maternal age is correlated with the incidence of trisomy 13.[19] Less than 10% of individuals with trisomy 13 survive past the first year of life.[101]

Trisomy 13 is characterized by microcephaly, deafness, anophthalmia or microphthalmia, and cleft lip and palate.[86] As in trisomy 18, infants with trisomy 13 frequently have serious cardiovascular and urogenital malformations and typically have severe to profound mental retardation. Skeletal deformities and anomalies include flexion contractures of the fingers and polydactyly of hands and feet.[82] Rocker-bottom feet also have been reported, although less frequently than in individuals with trisomy 18. Reported central nervous system (CNS) malformations include arhinencephalia, cerebellar anomalies, defects of the corpus callosum, and hydrocephaly.[113]

Sex Chromosome Disorders

Two of the most prevalent sex chromosome anomalies are Turner syndrome and Klinefelter syndrome.

Turner Syndrome (45,X). Turner syndrome is the most common chromosomal anomaly among spontaneous abortions.[15] Known also as gonadal dysgenesis or 45,X syndrome, Turner syndrome occurs in 1 in 2,500 births.[45] Unlike in the autosomal trisomy syndromes, the incidence of Turner syndrome does not increase with advancing maternal age.

Three characteristic impairments of the syndrome are sexual infantilism, a congenital webbed neck, and cubitus valgus.[111] Other clinical characteristics noted at birth include dorsal edema of hands and feet, hypertelorism, epicanthal folds, ptosis of the upper eyelids, elongated ears, and shortening of all the hand bones.[45] Growth retardation is particularly noticeable after the age of 5 or 6 years, and sexual infantilism, characterized by primary amenorrhea, lack of breast development, and scanty pubic and axillary hair, is apparent during the pubertal years. Ovarian development is severely deficient, as is estrogen production.[82]

Congenital heart disease is present in 20% of individuals with Turner syndrome[21]; 33% to 60% of individuals with Turner syndrome have kidney malformations.[45] There are numerous incidences of skeletal anomalies, some of which may be significant enough to require the attention of a pediatric therapist. Included among these are hip dislocation, pes planus and pes equinovarus, dislo-

cated patella,[45] deformity of the medial tibial condyles, and deformities due to osteoporosis.[54, 82] Decreased lumbar lordosis[43] and idiopathic scoliosis are also common.[34]

Sensory impairments include decrease in gustatory and olfactory sensitivity, deficits in spatial perception and orientation,[74] and moderate hearing loss. (Up to 80% of individuals with Noonan syndrome experience chronic otitis media.[45]) Although the average intellect of individuals with Turner syndrome is within normal limits, the incidence of mental retardation is higher than in the general population.[59]

Klinefelter Syndrome (47,XXY). The most common type of Klinefelter syndrome, XXY, is usually not clinically apparent until puberty when the testes fail to enlarge and gynecomastia occurs.[35] Eighty percent of males with Klinefelter syndrome possess a karyotype of XXY, and the other 10% of cases are variants.[35] The incidence of Klinefelter syndrome (XXY) is about 1 in 1,000 males.[84]

Most individuals with karyotype XXY have normal intelligence, a somewhat passive personality, and a reduced libido. Nearly all individuals with a nonmosaic karyotype are sterile. Individuals with the karyotypes XXXY and XXXXY tend to display a more severe clinical picture. Individuals with XXXY usually have severe mental retardation, with multiple congenital anomalies, including microcephaly, hypertelorism, strabismus, and cleft palate.[82] Skeletal anomalies include radioulnar synostosis, genu valgum, malformed cervical vertebrae, and pes planus. Parental age does not appear to be a factor in the incidence of the more severe types of Klinefelter syndrome.[35]

Partial Deletion Disorders

Cri-du-Chat Syndrome (46,XY,del[5p]). Cri-du-chat syndrome, also referred to as cat-cry syndrome, results from a partial deletion of the short arm of chromosome 5. The incidence of the syndrome is estimated to be 1 case per 20,000 to 50,000 live births.[82] Although approximately 70% of individuals with cri-du-chat syndrome are female, there is an unexplained higher prevalence of older males with this disorder.[11] Advanced parental age is not a factor in the etiology of this syndrome.

Primary identifying characteristics at birth include a definitive high-pitched catlike cry, microcephaly, and evidence of intrauterine growth retardation.[82] The characteristic cry results from abnormal laryngeal development and disappears in the first few years of life.[84] It is not present in all individuals.

Other features of individuals with this syndrome include hypertelorism, strabismus, "moon face," and low-set ears.[82] Associated musculoskeletal deformities include scoliosis, hip dislocations, clubfeet, and hyperextensibility of fingers and toes. Severe mental retardation and muscular hypotonicity are associated with this syndrome, although cases with hypertonicity have also been noted.[98] Severe respiratory and feeding problems have also been reported[84] (Fig. 10–3).

Prader-Willi Syndrome (46,XY,del[15]). The incidence of Prader-Willi syndrome (PWS) is estimated to be 1 in 25,000 births.[82] Characteristics include obesity, hypogonadism, short stature, hypotonia, dysmorphic facial

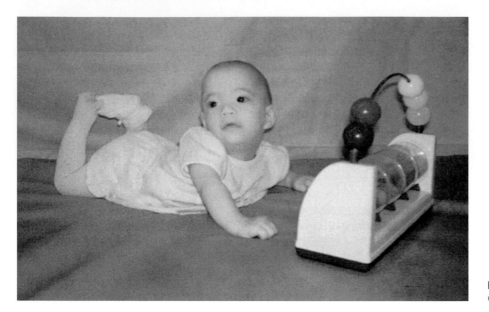

FIGURE 10–3. Nine-month-old girl with cri-du-chat syndrome.

features, dysfunctional CNS performance,[55] and a compulsive preoccupation with food.

PWS is characterized by a distinct combination of physical and behavioral features. Diagnosis is confirmed by chromosome studies and molecular studies. In approximately 70% of cases a microdeletion is noted. The deletion occurs on the paternally derived chromosome.[13]

At least 30 cases of chromosome 15 translocations have been reported in PWS.[66] Parental studies are important in translocation cases because 20% of cases cited in the literature involved familial rearrangements, which may significantly increase the recurrence risk.[95a]

Generalized hypotonia is present at birth and is severe in the majority of cases.[17] Most infants have an expressionless face, flaccid muscles, a weak cry, and little spontaneous movement. Muscle tone generally improves after the first few months of life; however, poor coordination and motor delays persist. Hypotonia often results in a poor suck, with early feeding difficulties and slow initial weight gain.[17] At an average age of 2 years, children develop a persistent appetite and the focus shifts from initial concerns about weight gain to preventing obesity.[69]

The majority of individuals with PWS have mild to moderate mental retardation, although some individuals have IQ scores within normal limits.[69] Maladaptive behaviors such as temper tantrums, aggression, self-abuse, and emotional lability have been reported.[108] As a result of extreme obesity, many individuals with PWS experience impaired breathing that can produce sleepiness, cyanosis, cor pulmonale, and heart failure.[69] Scoliosis is common but does not appear to be related to obesity.[112]

Single-Gene Disorders

Other genetic disorders commonly seen among children in a therapy setting include those that result from specific gene defects. There are three types of specific gene defects: autosomal dominant, autosomal recessive, and sex-linked. Each of these types of inheritance is discussed separately. Several examples of syndromes or disorders associated with each type are presented. They include those most commonly seen in children attending pediatric therapy programs and those of specific neurological importance to physical or occupational therapists.

Autosomal Dominant Disorders

Autosomal dominant disorders occur when one parent is affected with the disorder, although spontaneous cases with no family history also have been reported. Each child of a parent with an autosomal dominant trait has a 50:50 chance of inheriting that trait. Many of these are specific isolated anomalies that may occur in otherwise normal individuals, such as extra digits or short fingers. Other autosomal dominant disorders include syndromes characterized by profound neurological disabilities. Three examples of autosomal dominant disorders that can result in serious neurological disabilities are osteogenesis imperfecta, tuberous sclerosis, and neurofibromatosis. Individuals with these disorders may require intervention from a physical or occupational therapist because of the associated musculoskeletal and neuromuscular impairments that lead to disability.

Osteogenesis Imperfecta. Osteogenesis imperfecta (OI) is a spectrum of diseases that results from deficits in collagen synthesis.[84] The four types of OI are characterized by brittle bones, hyperextensible ligaments, blue sclerae, cardiopulmonary abnormalities, discolored and fragile teeth,[70] and hypotonia.[1] Deafness, secondary to otosclerosis, appears in adulthood and is found in 35% of individuals by the third decade of life.[59]

Type I, the mildest form of OI, is characterized by mild-to-moderate bone fragility and joint hyperextensibility. There are no significant deformities, and individuals with this type are usually ambulatory. Type II, the most severe form, is lethal before or shortly after birth.[90] Children with type III OI present with severe bone fragility and osteoporosis, often experiencing fractures in utero. An autosomal recessive form of OI, type III is characterized by progressive skeletal deformity, scoliosis, triangular facies, large skull, normal cognitive ability, short stature, and limited ambulatory ability.[70, 90] Type IV OI is characterized by more severe bone fragility and joint hyperextensibility than type I. Bowing of long bones, scoliosis, and short stature are common.[70] Children with type IV OI are often ambulatory but may require splinting or crutches. The overall incidence of OI is 1 in 20,000 to 30,000, with types I and IV being the most common. Types II and III have an incidence of 1 in 62,000 and 1 in 68,000, respectively.[70]

The long bones of the lower extremities are most susceptible to fractures, particularly between the ages of 2 to 3 years and 10 to 15 years,[59] with the frequency of fractures diminishing with age.[84] Intramedullary rods inserted in the tibia or femur may minimize recurrent fractures.[96] *Prevention of fractures through careful handling and positioning is the most important goal in working with individuals with OI.* Mobility aids and splinting also can be helpful in preventing fractures.[84] We have found the use of pool therapy to be a valuable treatment strategy for children with OI.

Tuberous Sclerosis. Tuberous sclerosis is characterized by a triad of impairments: seizures, mental retardation, and sebaceous adenomas[96]; however, there is wide variability in expression, with some individuals displaying skin lesions only.[59] Although tuberous sclerosis is inherited as an autosomal dominant trait, 86% of cases occur as spontaneous mutations, with older paternal age a contributing factor. Tuberous sclerosis is a relatively rare condition, with a frequency of 1 in 10,000 births[114]; both sexes are affected equally. Infants are frequently normal in appearance at birth, but 70% of those who go on to show the complete triad of symptoms display seizures during the first year of life.

Hypopigmented macules are often the initial finding. These lesions vary in number and are small and ovoid. Larger lesions, known as leaf spots, may have jagged edges.[84] Sebaceous adenomas first appear between the ages of 4 and 5 years, with early individual brown, yellow, or red lesions of firm consistency in the areas of the nose and upper lips. These isolated lesions may later coalesce to form a characteristic butterfly pattern on the cheeks. Known also as hamartomas (tumor-like nodules of superfluous tissue), the skin lesions are present in 83% of individuals with tuberous sclerosis.[59]

Delayed development is another characteristic during infancy,[25] particularly, in the achievement of motor and speech milestones. Mental retardation occurs in 62% of individuals with tuberous sclerosis.[59] Because of the retardation in motor development, as well as associated rigidity or hemiplegia seen in some cases, children with this disorder may be referred to a developmental physical or occupational therapist.

Ultimately, 93% of individuals who are severely affected develop seizures, usually of the myoclonic type in early life, progressing in later life to grand mal seizures. Seizure development is secondary to the formation of nodular lesions in the cerebral cortex and white matter.[59] Tumors are also found in the walls of the ventricles. Neurocytological examination reveals a decreased number of neurons and an increased number of glial cells as well as enlarged nerve cells with abnormally shaped cell bodies.[82] Surgical excision of seizure-producing tumors has been successful in some cases.[96]

Other associated impairments include retinal tumors and hemorrhages, glaucoma, and corneal opacities.[96] Cyst formation in the long bones and in the bones of the fingers and toes contributes to osteoporosis. Cardiac and kidney involvement[84] and catatonic schizophrenia have also been reported.[96]

Neurofibromatosis. Neurofibromatosis is characterized by flat, light brown skin patches, known as café-au-lait spots, and neurofibromas, or connective tissue tumors of the nerve fiber fasciculus.[8] It is a slowly progressive disease, characterized by an increase in the number of tumors with increasing age. The prevalence of neurofibromatosis is 1 in 3,500.[82] Fifty percent of cases are due to new mutations (usually paternal in origin).[21]

Infants usually appear normal at birth, with the initial symptoms of café-au-lait spots first appearing in early childhood.[59] Neurofibromas may be found in either the peripheral nervous system or the CNS[102] and can lead to secondary impairments such as optic and acoustic nerve damage, paraplegia, quadriplegia,[96] or hemiparesis.[58] Muscle weakness or incoordination, rather than complete paralysis, may be evident.[84] Neurofibromas may also develop in the kidneys, stomach, or heart.[59] Puberty and pregnancy may exacerbate symptoms of this disorder.[8] Three percent of affected individuals have moderate to severe mental retardation, approximately 30% have learning difficulties, and 3% have seizure disorders.[21] Ultimately, 47% of individuals with neurofibromatosis develop some type of neurological impairment.[59]

Cervical paraspinal neurofibromas may develop in late childhood or early adulthood and are a major cause of chronic disability.[29] Scoliosis occurs in up to 5% of individuals with neurofibromatosis.[21] Severe kyphoscoliotic deformities may lead to spinal cord compression or impaired cardiopulmonary function. Kyphosis usually becomes apparent between ages 6 and 10. Other skeletal deformities include pseudoarthrosis of the tibia and fibula, tibial bowing, craniofacial and vertebral dysplasia,[84] rib fusion, and dislocation of the radius and ulna. Differences in leg length also have been noted and may contribute to scoliosis.

Autosomal Recessive Disorders

When both parents are unaffected carriers of the trait, they are heterozygous for the abnormal gene and each of their offspring faces a 25% risk of exhibiting the disorder. When two homozygous affected parents mate, there is a great risk that all children will be similarly affected with the disorder. Consanguinity involving close relatives increases the chance of passing on autosomal recessive traits. Certain types of limb defects, familial microcephaly, and a variety of syndromes such as Hurler syndrome are passed on through autosomal recessive genes. Four examples of autosomal recessive disorders that may be of interest to physical or occupational therapists are presented in this section: cystic fibrosis, Hurler syndrome, phenylketonuria, and Werdnig-Hoffmann disease.

Cystic Fibrosis. Cystic fibrosis (CF) is one of the most common autosomal recessive disorders affecting whites, with an incidence of 1 in 2,000 to 1 in 4,000.[82] The incidence in nonwhites is much less and has been reported at 1 in 17,000 among African Americans. The CF gene has been mapped to chromosome 7, and the protein CF transmembrane regulator (CFTR), which is the product of the gene, has been cloned.[60] CFTR is involved in the regulation of chloride channels of the bowel and lung, which is dysfunctional in CF patients.

The primary impairments include fibrotic lesions of the pancreas, and up to 85% of CF patients have been reported to have pancreatic insufficiency. The inability of the pancreas to secrete digestive enzymes can result in chronic malnutrition. Ten to 20% of newborns with CF also have intestinal tract involvement with a meconium ileus. The sweat glands are commonly affected, with high levels of chloride found in the sweat, which is the basis for the sweat chloride test used in diagnosis. The most serious impairment in CF is the obstruction of the lungs by thick mucus, which leads to chronic pulmonary obstruction, infection that destroys lung tissue, and eventual death from pulmonary disease in 90% of individuals.[60]

Although CF has markedly variable expression, the overall median survival has improved from about 6 years of age in the 1940s to 30 years of age in the 1990s.[60] This improved survival rate is a result of improved antibiotic management, aggressive chest physical therapy, and pancreatic replacement therapy. Postural drainage, percussion, vibration, and breathing exercises are key components of the management program provided by the therapist. Attention to diet is important, and every attempt should be made to maintain a routine exercise program with a goal of helping the children be more active to improve their respiratory status. Overexertion and fatigue are to be avoided in prescribing an exercise program.

Hurler Syndrome (Gargoylism, Mucopolysaccharidosis I). Hurler syndrome is an inborn error of metabolism that results in abnormal storage of mucopolysaccharides in many different tissues of the body.[1] The incidence of Hurler syndrome is estimated to be 1 in 100,000 live births.[82]

Infants born with Hurler syndrome are usually normal in appearance at birth[96] and may be larger in birth weight than their siblings. Symptoms of this progressively deteriorating disease usually appear during the latter half of the first year of life,[101] with the full disease picture apparent by 2 to 3 years of age.[82]

Characteristic physical features include a large skull with frontal bossing, heavy eyebrows, edematous eyelids, corneal clouding, a small upturned nose with flat nasal bridge, thick lips, low-set ears, hirsutism, and gargoyle-like facial features. Growth retardation results in characteristic dwarfism.[1] Some individuals with the physical characteristics of Hurler syndrome have normal intelligence, but the vast majority have mental retardation.[82]

Spastic paraparesis or paraplegia and ataxia[82] also have been observed in individuals with Hurler syndrome. Commonly reported orthopedic deformities include flexion contractures of the extremities, thoracolumbar ky-phosis, genu valgum, pes cavus,[1] hip dislocation, and claw hands secondary to joint deformities.[59] Restriction of neck flexion and extension also may result from hypoplasia of the odontoid process.[84]

Deafness is another frequently reported anomaly.[1] Progressive mental and physical deterioration leads to early death, usually before adulthood.[1] Death is usually secondary to deposits of mucopolysaccharides in the cardiac valves, myocardium, or coronary arteries.[1]

Delayed motor milestones have been noted in later infancy and early childhood, with severe disabilities occurring with increasing age.[84] Adaptive equipment often is needed, and most children with Hurler syndrome become wheelchair users in their later years.[84]

Phenylketonuria. Phenylketonuria (PKU) is the result of one of the more common inborn errors of metabolism. Absence of phenylalanine hydroxylase prevents the conversion of phenylalanine to tyrosine, resulting in an abnormally excessive accumulation of phenylalanine in the blood and other body fluids. If untreated, this metabolic error results in mental and growth retardation, seizures, and pigment deficiency of hair and skin.[99] PKU is most prevalent among individuals of northern European ancestry, with a frequency of 1:10,000 to 1:15,000 births.[102] It is estimated that 1 of every 50 individuals is heterozygous for PKU.

Children born with PKU are usually normal in appearance, with delayed development becoming apparent toward the end of the first year. Parents usually become concerned with their child's slow development during the preschool years.[99] If PKU is untreated, the affected child may go on to develop hypertonicity (75%), hyperactive reflexes (66%), hyperkinesis (50%), or tremors (30%),[64] in addition to mental retardation. IQ levels generally fall between 10 and 50, although there have been reported rare cases of untreated individuals with normal intelligence.[99]

A simple blood plasma analysis, which is mandatory for newborns in many states in the United States, can detect the presence of elevated phenylalanine levels. This test is ideally performed when the infant is at least 72 hours old. If elevated phenylalanine levels are found, the test is repeated, along with further diagnostic procedures. Placing the infant on a low phenylalanine diet can prevent the mental retardation and other neurological sequelae characteristic of this disorder.[99] Follow-up management by an interdisciplinary team consisting of a nutritionist, psychologist, and appropriate medical personnel is advised in addition to the special diet.

Spinal Muscle Atrophy. Spinal muscle atrophy includes a continuum of disorders, with acute infantile spinal muscular atrophy (Werdnig-Hoffmann disease) demonstrating early onset. Intermediate-onset (juvenile) spinal muscle atrophy (Kugelberg-Welander disease) is seen in later childhood.

Werdnig-Hoffmann disease is a progressive, degenerative disorder of the anterior horn cells. It is characterized clinically by severe hypotonicity, generalized symmetrical muscle weakness, absent deep tendon reflexes, and markedly delayed motor development. Intellect, sensation, and sphincter functioning, however, are normal.[51] In one third of individuals with this disorder, onset occurs in utero with a prenatal history of decreased fetal movements during the third trimester. Other neurological signs are observed during early infancy, usually by 6 months of age.[84] Incidence is estimated to be 1 in 20,000 live births.[83]

Diagnosis may be accomplished through electromyography (EMG) and muscle biopsy, which reveal neurogenic atrophy.[49] DNA testing is also now available. Poor head control, froglike positioning of lower extremities,[56] better use of distal than of proximal musculature, and fasciculation and atrophy of the tongue secondary to hypoglossal nucleus involvement[49] are other clinical symptoms. Progressive swallowing problems also have been noted in some cases.[84]

Intercostal muscle weakness leads to diaphragmatic breathing and contributes to the greatly increased susceptibility to pulmonary infection, which usually results in death before the age of 2 years.[82] A few individuals with Werdnig-Hoffmann disease have survived to adolescence but are unable to stand without support.

The intermediate-onset form of spinal muscle atrophy is called Kugelberg-Welander disease, with an age at onset between 3 months and 15 years. Incidence is estimated at 1:24,000 live births.[83] Like the infantile-onset form of spinal muscle atrophy, Kugelberg-Welander disease is characterized by proximal weakness, decreased deep tendon reflexes, and normal intelligence. There is an increased incidence of scoliosis and joint contractures. Chewing and swallowing difficulties are rare. Individuals with this disorder may experience long periods in which the disease appears static, and many survive into adulthood.[84]

Sex-Linked Disorders

The third mechanism for transmission of specific gene defects is through sex-linked inheritance. Two well-known sex-linked diseases are Duchenne muscular dystrophy (see Chapter 13) and hemophilia. In sex-linked disorders, the abnormal gene is carried on the X chromosome. Female individuals carrying one abnormal gene usually do not display the trait because of the dominant normal gene on the other X chromosome. Each son born to a carrier mother, however, has a 50:50 chance of inheriting the abnormal gene and thus exhibiting the disorder. Each daughter of a carrier mother has a 50:50 chance of becoming a carrier of the trait. Three syndromes that result in disability are discussed in this section: hemophilia A, fragile X syndrome, and Lesch-Nyhan syndrome.

Hemophilia A. The term *hemophilia* refers to hemophilia A (factor VIII deficiency), hemophilia B or Christmas disease (factor IX deficiency), and von Willebrand's disease. Hemophilia A is an X-linked recessive bleeding disorder caused by mutations in the factor VIII gene. Hemophilia A is reported to affect 1 in 5,000 to 10,000 males worldwide.[60]

Affected individuals experience hemorrhage into joints and muscles, easy bruising, and prolonged bleeding from wounds. The severity and frequency of bleeding in hemophilia A are inversely related to the amount of residual factor VIII (<1%, severe; 2–5%, moderate; and 5–30%, mild). The proportions of cases that are severe, moderate, and mild are about 50%, 10%, and 40%, respectively.[3] The joints (ankles, knees, hips, and elbows) are frequently affected, causing swelling, pain, decreased function, and degenerative arthritis. Similarly, muscle hemorrhage can cause necrosis, contractures, and neuropathy by entrapment. Hematuria and intracranial hemorrhage, while uncommon, can occur after even mild trauma. Bleeding from tongue or lip lacerations is often persistent.

Treatment includes guarding against trauma and replacement of factor VIII derived from human plasma or recombinant techniques. In the late 1970s to mid 1980s it was estimated that half of the hemophiliacs in the United States contracted hepatitis B or C or human immunodeficiency virus (HIV) infection when treated by donor-derived factor VIII. The initiation of donor blood screening and use of heat treatment of donor-derived factor VIII has almost completely eliminated the threat of infection. Although replacement therapy is effective in most cases, 10% to 15% of treated individuals develop neutralizing antibodies that decrease its effectiveness.[60]

Fragile X Syndrome. Fragile X syndrome is the most common sex-linked inherited cause of mental retardation, with a frequency of 1:1,250 in males and of 1:2,500 in females.[82] A fragile site on the long arm of an X chromosome is present, with breaks or gaps shown on chromosome analysis. Life span is normal.

Eighty percent of males are reported to have mental retardation, with IQs of 30 to 50 being common but ranging up to the mildly retarded to borderline range. Penetrance in the female is reported at only 30%.[60] Other impairments include delayed acquisition of motor milestones, emotional lability, and autistic-like behaviors such as hand biting that have been reported to improve at puberty.

Lesch-Nyhan Syndrome. A sex-linked disorder that leads to profound neurological deterioration is Lesch-Nyhan syndrome, or hereditary choreoathetosis. The primary metabolic defect that characterizes this disorder is a marked overproduction of uric acid (hyperuricemia),[56] which results in a deficiency of hypoxanthine guanine phosphoribosyltransferase (HGPRT) in the brain, liver,[61] and amniotic cells.[10] First described in 1964 by Lesch and Nyhan,[67] the syndrome has an incidence of 1 in 10,000 males.[21] This disorder is detectable through amniocentesis, and genetic counseling is advisable for parents who have already given birth to an affected son.[10]

Infants appear normal at birth but begin to self-mutilate at 1 to 2 years of age by biting their lips. The disorder progresses to more severe forms of self-mutilation in which individuals have been known to bite off their fingertips.[56] In spite of the extreme self-mutilation that characterizes this disorder, pain perception appears to be normal.

Motor development is often normal during the first 6 to 8 months of life. Progressive spastic paresis and athetosis, however, become evident during the latter half of the first year of life. Other neuromotor symptoms include chorea, ballismus, tremor, hyperactive deep tendon reflexes, severe dysarthria, and dysphagia. Bilateral dislocation of hips may occur secondary to the spasticity.[56] An increased incidence of clubfoot deformity has been noted.[29] Growth retardation is also apparent, as well as moderate to severe mental retardation.[82]

Blood and urine levels of uric acid have been decreased successfully through the administration of allopurinol, with resultant decrease in kidney damage.[29] Death usually occurs before adolescence and is often secondary to uremia from gouty nephropathy or to generalized debilitation.[56]

Rett Syndrome. Although Rett syndrome has been reported as an X-linked dominant condition affecting only females and being lethal in males, the inheritance pattern has yet to be fully delineated. More recently, Rett syndrome has been reported in males with a specific mutation of the X chromosome.[19a, 72a] The estimated incidence is 1 in 15,000 births.[39]

The syndrome is characterized by apparently normal development during the first 6 months of life, with deterioration occurring between 6 to 18 months of age.[41] Virtually all language ability is lost, although some children may produce echolalic sounds and learn simple manual signing. Evidence of minimal receptive language skills may be observed. Previously acquired purposeful hand skills are also lost and replaced by stereotypical hand movements. These nonspecific hand movements have been described as hand wringing, clapping, waving, or mouthing. Almost all individuals with Rett syndrome function in the range of severe to profound mental retardation. Although head circumference is normal at birth, deceleration of rate of head growth occurs between 5 months and 4 years of age.[109]

Onset of walking is usually delayed until about 19 months of age; almost one fourth of girls with Rett syndrome never develop independent ambulation skills.[109] Initially, hypotonia may be evident, but with advancing age, spasticity of the extremities develops.[40] Increased muscle tone is usually observed first in the lower extremities, with continued greater involvement than in the upper extremities. Peripheral vasomotor disturbances and muscle wasting have been noted as associated characteristics.[109]

In a report of 16 patients with Rett syndrome, Hennessey and Haas[52] described musculoskeletal deformities in nearly all patients. Fifteen showed clinical evidence of scoliosis, nine showed heelcord tightening, and hip instability was identified as an area of potential concern. Trevathan and Naidu[109] reported scoliosis in 50% of girls with Rett syndrome after the age of 10 years, many of whom required surgical correction.

Seventy percent to 80% of individuals with Rett syndrome develop seizures in the first five years of life. Early electroencephalography can be normal before 2 years of age. Cranial computed tomography results are normal or shows mild generalized atrophy. Breathing dysfunction, including wake apnea and intermittent hyperventilation,[109] is also associated with Rett syndrome. Interventions reported in the literature have focused on splinting,[77] behavioral modification techniques to teach self-feeding skills,[88] music therapy, physical therapy, and occupational therapy.[105]

TYPICAL CLINICAL SYMPTOMS AND COMMON MOTOR PROBLEMS

Specific examples of genetic disorders in children and their accompanying symptomatology were presented in the foregoing section. Table 10–2 summarizes the clinical signs common to many of the disorders. This section describes those common impairments that are most relevant for physical or occupational therapists.

Hypertonicity

Children with hypertonus generally display stiff or jerky movements that are limited in variety, speed, and coordination. Movements tend to be limited to the middle ranges. Total patterns of flexion or extension may dominate, with limited ability for selective joint movements. Motor development of children with hypertonicity may be further complicated by the retention of primitive reflexes, which can result in stereotyped movements that are dependent on sensory input.

Children will learn to use stereotypical patterns of movement to achieve functional goals and are able to activate the muscle synergies of a reflex without sensory feedback.[9] If a goal of therapy is to facilitate functional movement that is not dominated by persistent reflexes, it is critical to practice new motor patterns to accomplish the functional activity for which that reflex is being used. When an older child has used a stereotypical movement and the pattern appears to be the only way the child can perform a task, then therapy to establish a new movement pattern will have a poor prognosis for change. The focus of therapy activities needs to be on active movement of the child and not passive inhibition techniques for the sake of "normalization" of tone and movement because the therapy would not be cost effective and may be detrimental to functional independence.[46]

Differences and similarities observed in children with hypertonicity and hypotonicity are listed in Table 10–2. Although hypertonicity is often used interchangeably with the term *spasticity* (defined as increased resistance to passive stretch), there is growing recognition that muscles may be stiff but not spastic. One explanation for muscles that are stiff but not spastic is that such hypertonicity results from an attempt to control excessive movement at a joint.[9] This may be observed during the learning of a new skill in which there is a need to eliminate some of the excessive movement. Such "fixing" keeps the involved joints fairly rigid, thereby "freezing" nonessential movements and resulting in increased muscle tone or stiffness around that joint. As skill increases, a child learns to control the forces of movement and no longer needs to "fix," thereby allowing a greater variety of movements to occur. If skill does not increase, however, a child may "fix" to compensate for his or her lack of active control, resulting in hypertonus. Another reason for stiffness without the evidence of spasticity may be an increase in connective tissue in the muscle. This has been shown to be a factor in children with cerebral palsy.[107]

TABLE 10–2. Typical Impairments in Selected Genetic Disorders

Genetic Disorder	Hypotonicity	Hypertonicity	Hip Dislocation	Spinal Deformity	Upper Extremity Deformity	Other Deformity	Motor Delays	Cognitive Delays	Cerebellar Dysfunction
Trisomy 21	X			X		X	X	X	X
Trisomy 18	X	X		X	X	X	X	X	
Trisomy 13	X	X			X	X	X	X	
Turner syndrome			X	X		X			
Klinefelter syndrome					X	X			
Cri-du-chat syndrome	X	X	X	X		X	X	X	
Prader-Willi syndrome	X			X		X	X	X	
Osteogenesis imperfecta				X	X	X	X		
Tuberous sclerosis		X		X				X	
Neurofibromatosis		X		X		X			
Untreated phenylketonuria									
Hurler syndrome		X	X	X	X	X	X	X	
Werdig-Hoffmann syndrome	X			X	X	X	X	X	X
Kugelberg-Welander syndrome	X			X		X	X		X
Fragile X syndrome	X			X			X	X	
Lesch-Nyhan syndrome		X	X		X	X	X	X	
Hemophilia A					X	X		X	X
Rett syndrome					X	X	X	X	

297

Hypotonicity

Whereas movements of the child with high muscle tone are generally limited to the mid ranges, children with low muscle tone typically display movements in the extremes of the range. Children with hypotonicity tend to lock weight-bearing joints or assume positions that provide a broad base of support to maximize their stability. Although retention of primitive reflexes is less likely to interfere with the development of functional movement patterns, delays in the development of postural reactions are a major concern (Fig. 10–4). As a result of delays in postural development, children with hypotonicity often learn to rely on sources of external support to maintain upright positions. Limited strength and lack of endurance are often concerns with children who have hypotonicity. Additional concerns may arise from joint laxity.

Hyperextensible Joints

Hyperextensible joints are commonly observed in children with hypotonicity and are noted in many children with genetic disorders. Activities should be modified to avoid undue stress to these joints and the surrounding ligaments, tendons, and fascia. For example, positions that allow knee or elbow joints to lock into extension should be modified so that weight bearing occurs through more neutral alignment. Varying the placement of toys and support surfaces, providing physical assistance, and using adaptive equipment can help modify weight-bearing forces to achieve more neutral alignment. For example, if hyperextensibility of ligaments leads to excessive pronation in stance, the use of ankle-foot orthoses may provide enough support to the structures to allow functional activities in standing (see Chapter 31). For a child who stands

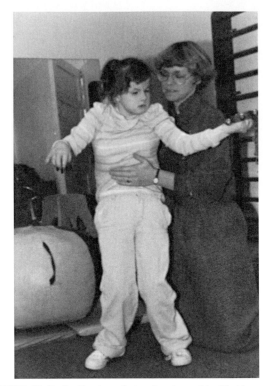

FIGURE 10–5. Facilitation of standing in a girl with trisomy 18.

with knee hyperextension, a vertical stander may allow that child to stand and play at a water table with his or her classmates for extended periods with the knees in a more neutral position. Rather than restricting a child's repertoire of upright positions, it is preferable to modify an activity or provide external support to enable a child to participate fully (Fig. 10–5).

Contractures and Deformities

Skeletal anomalies and deformities are associated with many genetic disorders. The physical or occupational therapist may work with orthopedists, prosthetists, and orthotists to detect and prevent the progression of a variety of conditions. The therapist should be aware of factors that can contribute to the development of deformities in order to prevent or minimize such problems.

Although joint contractures are less likely to occur in a child with hypotonicity, habitual positioning may lead to soft tissue restrictions. For example, children with spinal muscle atrophy often adopt a constant position of wide abduction, external rotation, and flexion at the hips ("frog" or "reverse W" position)[106]; in these children, soft tissue contractures can develop at the hips and knees. Children whose hips are maintained in a position of adduction, flexion, and internal rotation are at risk for hip subluxation or dislocation.[106] Spinal deformities, such as lumbar lordosis and thoracic kyphosis and scoliosis, are also common concerns in children with abnormal muscle tone. An imbalance of muscle tone or strength or immobility may increase the risk of spinal deformity. In general, contractures and deformities are of most concern for children who display a limited variety of postures and movements.

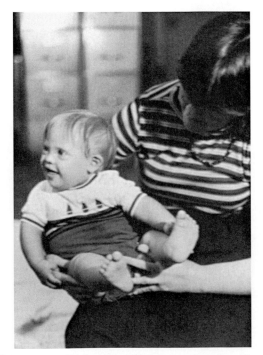

FIGURE 10–4. Facilitation of equilibrium reactions in a 10-month-old child with Down syndrome.

Respiratory Problems

Respiratory problems are often observed in children with hypotonicity or hypertonicity, as well as in children whose respiratory functioning is compromised by chest and skeletal deformities. These children may require mobilization techniques, deep breathing, chest expansion exercises, and postural drainage. Some children may find it difficult to tolerate one position for an extended time owing to respiratory difficulties. For these children, frequent changes of position and use of adapted positioning devices may be necessary. In the case of children with cystic fibrosis a comprehensive program of respiratory care is the primary therapy goal.

FAMILY-CENTERED INTERVENTION FOR CHILDREN WITH GENETIC DISORDERS

This section examines the role of the physical or occupational therapist in providing therapy services for children with genetic disorders. After a discussion of ways in which therapists can support families of children with genetic disorders, evaluation strategies, goals and objectives, and general treatment principles are presented. Throughout this section, emphasis is placed on supporting and including family members in all aspects of therapy and ensuring that therapy programs meet the priorities and needs of family members.[28]

Supporting Families

Therapists working with children with genetic disorders need to recognize and acknowledge the multitude of tasks that all families work to accomplish. In addition to tasks specifically related to caring for their child with a disability, families must perform functions to address the economic, daily care, recreational, social, and educational/vocational needs of both individual members and the family as a whole. As Turnbull and Turnbull[110] have cautioned, each time professionals intervene with families and children, they can potentially enhance or hinder the family's ability to meet important family functions. For example, intervention that promotes a child's social skills can be an important support to positive family functioning. On the other hand, intervention that focuses on a child's deficits can have a negative impact on how the family perceives that child and the place of the child in the family. For therapists to be supportive of families, they must (1) acknowledge the importance of family priorities, (2) respect the family's cultural values, (3) include families as integral team members, and (4) promote and deliver services that build on family and community resources.

Assisting the family in identification of a support group is often helpful for adjustment and ongoing encouragement in coping with issues. A comprehensive web site provided by the Alliance of Genetic Support Groups to locate support groups can be found at http://www.geneticalliance.org.

Assessment Strategies

Knowledge of a child's diagnosis can aid in the selection of appropriate assessment tools and alert the therapist to any potential medical problems or contraindications associated with the specific syndrome that might affect the assessment procedures (tests and measures). Therapists must be careful, however, not to develop preconceived opinions about a child's capabilities based on how other children with similar diagnoses have performed. It is critical to remember that there is wide behavioral and performance variability among children within each genetic disorder. For example, wide variability in the achievement of developmental milestones has been reported among children with Down syndrome.[73]

The assessment process includes many components that in certain areas are specific to the either physical or occupational therapy. For the physical therapist, use of the *Guide to Physical Therapist Practice* is recommended as a framework to identify appropriate tests and measures for impairments or disablities that are identified.[2] For the occupational therapist a very useful reference is the assessment section of the textbook *Occupational Therapy for Children*.[16]

Typically, therapists include in their assessment clinical observations noted during evaluation of the neuromuscular status of the child, such as primitive reflexes, automatic reactions, and muscle tone. For children with orthopedic involvement, assessment of muscle strength, joint range of motion, joint play, and soft tissue mobility is also important. In addition to these types of evaluations, an assessment of the child's developmental level and functional ability should be completed. Such assessments can be used to discriminate between typical and delayed development, to identify the constraints interfering with the achievement of functional skills, and to guide the development of treatment goals and strategies. Most developmental assessment tools fall into one of the following categories: (1) discriminative, (2) predictive, and (3) evaluative measures.[62] Each of these three types of developmental assessment tools yields a different type of information. It is important to understand these differences and the intended purpose for each type of assessment to ensure that evaluation tools are used appropriately.

Discriminative Assessments. A discriminative assessment is used to compare the ability of an individual with the ability of members of a peer group or with a criterion selected by the test author.[62] Such instruments provide information necessary to document children's eligibility for special services but rarely provide information useful for planning or evaluating therapy programs.[49] Norm-referenced tests such as the Bayley Scales of Infant Development (motor and mental scales),[5] the Motor Assessment of the Developing Infant (AIM),[89] the Peabody Developmental Motor Scales,[31] and the Revised Gesell & Amatruda Developmental & Neurological Examination (adaptive, gross and fine motor, language, and personal/social development)[63] are examples of tests used with infants and young children to verify developmental delay or to assign age levels (Fig. 10–6). An example of a norm-referenced assessment tool for older children is the Bruininks-Oseretsky Test of Motor Proficiency.[12]

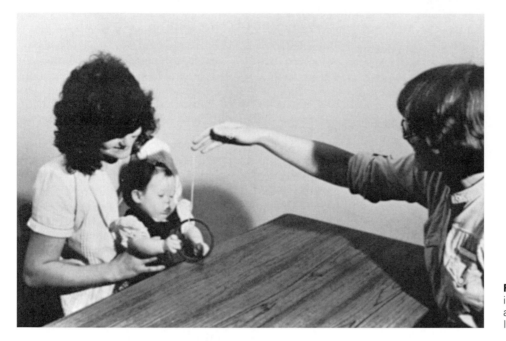

FIGURE 10–6. Four-month-old infant with Down syndrome being assessed on the Bayley Scales of Infant Development.

It may be possible to detect improved motor performance by administering a developmental test used to identify children who have motor delays. Such tests, however, usually cannot detect small increments of improvement, because there are relatively few test items at each age level and developmental gaps between items are often large. In assessing whether intervention has been effective, the use of most discriminative tools does not examine a child's performance of functional activities in natural environments.[49]

Predictive Assessments. Predictive measures are used to classify individuals according to a set of established categories and to verify whether an individual has been classified correctly.[62] Measures designed to predict future performance are often used to detect early signs of motor impairment in infants who are at risk for neuromotor dysfunction.[49] The Movement Assessment of Infants (MAI) was designed to assess muscle tone, reflex development, automatic reactions, and volitional movement of infants in the first year of life.[18] The ability of the MAI to predict later cerebral palsy has been examined.[47]

Evaluative Assessments. An evaluative measure is used to document change within an individual over time or change occurring as the result of intervention.[62] Helping Babies Learn[32] is a curriculum-referenced test that provides information about a child's developmental progress relative to a prespecified curriculum sequence.

To determine whether a child's ability to perform meaningful skills in everyday environments has improved, a functional assessment should be used. Functional assessments focus on the accomplishment of specific daily activities, rather than on the achievement of developmental milestones. Emphasis is placed on the end result in terms of the achievement of a functional task, rather than on the form or quality of the movement. Assistance in the form of people or devices is incorporated into the assessment of progress, with the measurement of progress focusing on the achievement of independence.[43] Qualitative aspects of movement that have important functional implications, such as accuracy, speed, endurance, adaptability, and generalizability, are also considered.

Functional assessments can be used to screen, diagnose, or describe functional deficits and to determine the resources needed to allow the child to function optimally in specific environments (e.g., school, home). Another use of functional assessments is to evaluate the nature of the problem and the specific task requirements limiting function in order to develop educational plans and teaching strategies.[43] A final use of functional assessments is to examine and monitor for changes in functional status. Such assessments can be used for program evaluation and for determining the cost-effectiveness of services or programs. (See Chapter 3 for additional information regarding evaluation tools.)

The Functional Independence Measure (FIM) is an example of a functional assessment. The FIM assesses the effectiveness of therapy on functional dependence in the areas of self-care, sphincter control, mobility, locomotion, communication, and social cognition.[36] Seven levels of functional dependence ranging from total assistance to complete independence are used to determine an individual's status. An adaptation of the FIM places greater emphasis on functional gains as opposed to the level of care. The Wee FIM[37] has been developed for use with children through the age of 6 years.

Another example of a functional assessment is the Tufts Assessment of Motor Performance (TAMP). The TAMP is a standardized, criterion-referenced tool that has been designed to assess functional motor performance in the areas of mobility, dressing, feeding, and communication.[33] Separate pediatric and adult versions are available.

The Pediatric Evaluation of Disability Inventory (PEDI) is a functional assessment that focuses on the domains of self-care, mobility, and social cognition. The PEDI incorporates three measurement scales: (1) the capability to perform selected functional skills, (2) the level of caregiver assistance that is required, and (3) identification of environmental modifications or equipment needed to perform a particular activity.[42] The PEDI has been standardized and normed and is intended for use with children whose abilities are in the range of a typical 6-month-old to 7-year-old child.

The final example of a functional assessment is the School Function Assessment (SFA).[22] The SFA is designed to measure a student's performance in accomplishing functional tasks in the school environment. It is composed of three sections that focus on (1) the student's participation in major school activities, (2) the task supports needed by the student for participation, and (3) the student's activity performance. The SFA is standardized and was conceptually developed to be reflective of the functional requirements of a student in elementary school.

Family-Driven Goals and Objectives

After a child's strengths and needs are evaluated, therapy goals and objectives can be developed. In the past, this has been the responsibility primarily of professionals. More recently, however, professionals have recognized the value of having families guide the process of establishing intervention goals and objectives.[104] This shift toward collaborative goal setting has occurred largely as a result of the belief that families should determine their vision of the future for their children, and professionals should act as consultants and resources to assist families in achieving that vision. When parents and therapists jointly determine goals and the means by which to attain them,[4] parents are more likely to commit time and energy to work toward the goals. For children, these goals are developed within the context of individualized service plans.

Individualized Service Plans. With the enactment of Public Law 94–142 in 1975,[92] physical and occupational therapists working in public school settings were required to establish long-term annual goals and short-term therapy objectives within the framework of each child's individualized education program (IEP). The components of an IEP are as follows[30]:

1. A statement of the child's present levels of educational performance
2. A statement of annual goals, including short-term instructional objectives
3. A statement of the specific special education and related services to be provided to the child
4. The projected dates for initiation of services and the anticipated duration of the service
5. Appropriate objective criteria and evaluation procedures and schedules for determining, at least annually, whether short-term instructional objectives are being achieved

Similar requirements are now in effect for infants receiving early intervention services as a result of the enactment of Public Law 99–457 in 1986 and its revision of Public Law 102–119 (Individuals with Disabilities Education Act) in 1991, which was reauthorized in 1997. An individualized family service plan (IFSP) must be written after a multidisciplinary assessment of the strengths and needs of the child is completed. This assessment must include a family-directed assessment of the supports and services necessary to enhance the family's capacity to meet the needs of their child with a disability.[30] The IFSP must contain the following:

1. A statement of the child's present levels of development (cognitive, speech/language, psychosocial, motor, and self-help)
2. A statement of the family's resources, priorities, and concerns related to enhancing the child's development
3. A statement of major outcomes expected to be achieved for the child and family
4. The criteria, procedures, and timelines for determining progress
5. The specific early-intervention services necessary to meet the unique needs of the child and family including the method, frequency, and intensity of service
6. The natural environments in which services shall be provided
7. The projected dates for the initiation of services and expected duration
8. The name of the service coordinator
9. The procedures for transition from early intervention to the preschool program

Functional Objectives. The development of behaviorally written, measurable therapy objectives is crucial for monitoring the effects of intervention in a child with a genetic disorder. Many of the clinical symptoms listed in the descriptions of genetic disorders described earlier in the chapter may be monitored through systematic, periodic, data-keeping procedures. One example is the monitoring of functional hand skills in girls with Rett syndrome. Periodic vital capacity measures for a child with osteogenesis imperfecta or a child with Werdnig-Hoffmann disease can reflect progress toward a goal of maintaining respiratory function.

Typically, therapy objectives focus on a child's deficits. For example, delays in achieving motor milestones are often used to identify gaps in development, and therapy objectives are written and programs established to address these deficits. When the child meets an objective, new deficits are identified and new objectives are developed. A different approach is to begin with the desired outcome and consider what needs to occur to achieve that outcome.

Goal attainment scaling is a variation of behavioral objectives that detects small, clinically important changes over time.[85] Similar to behavioral objectives, goal attainment scaling requires (1) identification of observable goals, (2) reproducibility of conditions under which performance is measured, (3) measurable criteria for success, and (4) a time frame for goal achievement. In contrast to behavioral objectives, however, goal attainment scaling identifies five possible outcomes with accompanying score values: two outcomes that surpass the expected level, the expected-level outcome, and two outcomes that fall below the expected level. Using five possible levels of attainment, one can determine whether a child has made prog-

CASE 10–1

PART 2—PROGRAM PLANNING

Maile on developmental testing displays deficits in single-leg stance stability. A typical developmental therapy objective might be, "Maile will balance on one foot for at least 3 seconds, two out of three trials." In Maile's IFSP meeting, however, her parents expressed the hope that Maile would be able to play safely with her peers at a neighborhood playground—a more functionally relevant goal. The following therapy objectives were developed to address her need to develop single-limb stance stability within the context of the family-identified goal:

1. With standby assistance, Maile will climb up the rungs of a 4-foot-high slide and seat herself at the top with feet pointed down the decline of the slide by 6/94.
2. Maile will be able to walk independently across a 25-foot stretch of uneven ground (sand or lawn) without falling by 6/94.

ress despite not achieving the expected outcome, or whether progress has exceeded the expected outcome.

Following is an example of the use of goal attainment scaling to assess Maile's first functional objective:

-2 = With physical assistance, Maile will climb up the rungs of a 4-foot-high slide by 6/94.

-1 = With physical assistance, Maile will climb up the rungs of a 4-foot-high slide and seat herself at the top with feet pointed down the decline of the slide by 6/94.

0 = With standby assistance, Maile will climb up the rungs of a 4-foot-high slide and seat herself at the top with feet pointed down the decline of the slide by 6/94.

$+1$ = Maile will climb up and seat herself at the top of a 4-foot-high slide independently, slide down, and stop at the bottom with physical assistance to prevent losing her balance by 6/94.

$+2$ = Maile will climb up and seat herself at the top of a 4-foot-high slide, slide down, and stop at the bottom independently by 6/94.

Rather than focusing on a child's deficits, such "outcome-focused" objectives provide a more positive and supportive context for therapy and at the same time address the family's needs and priorities. This approach to developing therapy goals and objectives in ways that support positive family functioning is also an important aspect of delivering therapy services to children and their families.

General Treatment Principles

Several general treatment principles guide the delivery of therapy services to children with genetic disorders. A description of each of these principles is followed by examples illustrating their applicability to particular children.

Focus on Functional Skills. Many of the classic therapeutic exercise approaches for individuals with neurological disorders are oriented toward making qualitative changes in motor tasks, such as normalizing muscle tone or improving gait symmetry. Often, there is little regard for the functional significance of those changes.[48] More recent therapeutic approaches place less emphasis on such qualitative changes and instead focus on the motor behaviors necessary to acquire functional skills. In this approach, environmental adaptations and assistive technology are used to attain functional outcomes such as independence in self-help skills, communication, and mobility[48] (Fig. 10–7).

This shift to a focus on functional skills is consistent with recent task-oriented approaches to neurological rehabilitation. The task-oriented model assumes that control of movement is organized around goal-directed, functional behaviors rather than on muscle or movement patterns.[57] Intervention, therefore, is aimed at teaching motor problem solving (adaptability to varied contexts), developing effective compensations that are maximally efficient, and providing practice of new motor skills in functional situations. Rather than teaching individuals to perform movement patterns in a controlled therapy setting, this approach focuses on the learning that must take

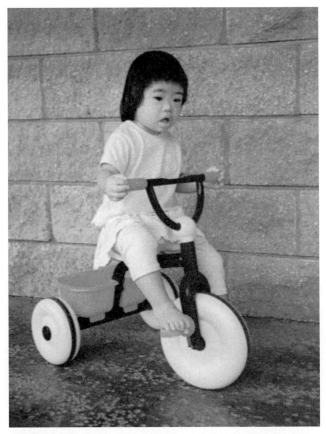

FIGURE 10–7. Child with Down syndrome during practice of functional motor skills.

place for an individual to function independently of a therapist's guidance.[53]

Delivery of Services in Natural Environments. Functional skills are most meaningfully taught and practiced within the context in which they will be used.[79] The movement toward integrating therapy into classroom settings is one example of providing services in a natural environment.[20, 103] In an integrated model of service delivery, therapists work in the classroom with teachers, rather than removing students to an isolated therapy room to provide services. Therapists work closely with the teacher to establish common goals for the student and to devise programs that will allow therapeutic activities to be interwoven into a variety of activities throughout the day in a natural manner.

Another example of providing therapy in a natural environment is providing home-based services for infants and young children. Home-based programs are "normal" options for very young children because the natural environment for most infants and toddlers is the home— either their own or that of a day-care provider.[79] For children who are medically fragile, it is the preferred option for therapy.[97] For other families, transportation to a center-based program may be difficult because of the expense or length of travel required.

Incorporating Therapy Activities into Daily Routines. Therapists need to work collaboratively with families to develop activities that incorporate therapeutic activities into the family's daily routine (e.g., during play, dressing, bathing, meals). Rather than practicing narrowly defined tasks in a controlled clinic environment, therapy activities should be interwoven into a variety of activities throughout the day in a natural manner. Practicing skills in the context of daily routines allows the child to learn to adapt to the real-life contingencies that arise during a functional task.[53] In addition, activities become more meaningful to both the child and the family (Fig. 10–8).

Use of Assistive Technology Devices. As noted previously, an important aspect of providing developmental therapy services is the use of assistive technology devices to maximize a child's functional abilities, level of independence, and inclusion in school and community activities with peers. Examples of assistive technology include mobility devices, augmentative communication devices, and adapted computer keyboards. Assistive technology also includes adaptive devices such as splints, bath chairs, prone standers, and other positioning equipment that can be used to provide optimal body alignment and minimize the risk for contractures/deformities, while encouraging a greater variety of movement patterns. Such devices can be constructed from readily available materials or obtained commercially. The developmental physical or occupational therapist works with the family and other team members to select, construct, and/or order assistive devices, as well as to assist caregivers in the use of the devices.

The case example demonstrates how these general treatment principles are applied to a particular child receiving therapy services. The case example also shows how the family's priorities and needs are considered and

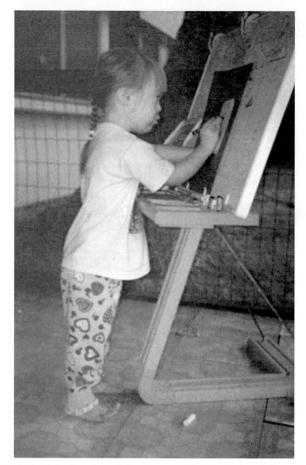

FIGURE 10–8. Practice of developmental skills during daily routine at home.

supported in the planning and delivery of services (see Case 10–1: Part 3, page 304).

MEDICAL MANAGEMENT AND GENETIC COUNSELING

The physical or occupational therapist should have general knowledge of both medical management of children with genetic disorders and genetic counseling for family members. This information allows the therapist to answer the family's general questions and to refer family members to the appropriate persons for more specific information.

Medical Management

Few medical therapies have been successful in treating genetic disorders in children, although a number of strategies for ameliorating isolated symptoms have been reported. Of the genetic disorders discussed in this chapter, the only one for which dramatic results have been achieved through early medical management is PKU. With early diagnosis and immediate implementation of a low-phenylalanine diet, the infant with PKU can be spared the severe mental retardation and other progres-

CASE 10–1

PART 3—INTERVENTION

The primary concerns of the parents were regarding Maile's motor skills involving her playground abilities. Therefore, the therapist scheduled Maile's weekly therapy session during the classroom playground time. In this way, the therapist would be able to help Maile improve her strength, endurance, and coordination in the context in which these skills need to be used. Therapy occurring on the playground will provide opportunities for Maile to learn how to assess the demands of the environment and to match them with her abilities. In this natural setting, she will also learn a variety of strategies to adapt to changing conditions. For example, when faced with the task of negotiating the playground slide, Maile will have to learn how to compensate for her low muscle tone and joint laxity so that she can climb up the ladder to sit on the top of the slide. Working on postural stability, single-leg stance, and shoulder girdle stabilization in this context will be more motivating than practicing these same skills in an isolated therapy room, and will likely be facilitated by Maile's classmates, who can serve as models.

sive neurological impairments that have resulted without treatment.[99]

Medical treatment for the other disorders is not curative but rather palliative or directed at specific associated anomalies. The congenital heart defects present in an estimated 40% to 60% of individuals with Down syndrome can, in most instances, be corrected by cardiac surgery.[75] Orthopedic surgery in the form of insertion of intramedullary rods in the tibia or femur may minimize the recurrence of repeated fractures associated with osteogenesis imperfecta.[106] Surgical correction of scoliosis may be warranted in individuals with neurofibromatosis, Rett syndrome,[109] or Werdnig-Hoffmann disease[65] if the deformity is severe and bracing[78] is not successful. Radiographic screening for atlantoaxial instability in children with Down syndrome can be initiated beginning at age 2 years.[75] If atlantoaxial instability is excessive or results in a neurological deficit, a posterior fusion of the cervical vertebrae is recommended.[84] Surgical removal of obstructive or malignant tumors is advisable in certain cases of neurofibromatosis, as is removal of cerebral nodular growths in individuals with tuberous sclerosis for the control of seizures.

The use of appetite-regulating drugs for individuals with Prader-Willi syndrome has had equivocal results. Surgical interventions such as gastric bypass, small intestinal bypass, and jaw wiring have been attempted for weight control with these individuals but have met with limited success.[69]

Respiratory therapy is an important adjunctive treatment strategy for children with cystic fibrosis or Werdnig-Hoffmann disease[65] and should be implemented as part of the overall therapy program. Specific medical therapies include estrogen therapy to promote feminization in individuals with Turner syndrome and testosterone therapy to enhance secondary sex characteristics in boys with Klinefelter syndrome.[76] The use of anticonvulsants is an important part of seizure management for individuals with Rett syndrome[109] and tuberous sclerosis.[7] To assist in the management of metabolic acidosis and rickets, which are often present in persons with Lowe syndrome, alkali supplements and vitamin D therapy have been used.[56] Allopurinol has been used for individuals with Lesch-Nyhan syndrome to prevent urological complications, although it has no effect on the progressive neurological symptomatology.[29]

The use of large, potentially toxic amounts of vitamins and minerals (the orthomolecular hypothesis) has been proposed for children with many different types of developmental disabilities. This approach has been rejected for children with Down syndrome based on results of several investigations. In addition, supplementation of individual metabolites such as 5-hydroxytryptophan or pyridoxine for children with Down syndrome is ineffective.[38] Proponents of cell therapy, which involves intramuscular injection of fetal lamb brain tissue, claim that many of the morphological and developmental characteristics of Down syndrome can be altered. These claims have not been supported by clinical investigations, and opponents of cell therapy warn of the potential risk for serious allergic reactions.[91]

As of early 2000, more than 400 gene therapy protocols have been approved.[60] Gene therapy can take on many different forms from altering human somatic cells to techniques that involve the replacement of a missing gene product by inserting a normal gene into a somatic cell. Because viruses have the ability to insert their genes into somatic cells attention is being focused on using viruses that have been modified to include the desired genetic information. To date, a gene therapy protocol is under way for Duchenne muscular dystrophy but, otherwise, not for any of the disorders described in this chapter. The interested reader can obtain an up-to-date listing of current gene therapy protocols from the National Institutes of Health's Office of Biotechnology on the WWW at http://www.nih.gov/od/oba/.

In light of the limited medical treatment strategies available for children with genetic disorders, the physical or occupational therapist must be concerned with maximizing the child's developmental or functional potential within the limitations imposed by the lack of possible cures and the prospect of the shortened life span that characterizes many of these disorders. When deterioration of skills is expected, therapy must be directed at maintaining current functioning levels, minimizing decline, and minimizing caregiver support as possible.

Genetic Counseling

Of crucial importance in working with children with genetic disorders and their families is a knowledge of genetic counseling. Developmental physical or occupational therapists must have an understanding of the modes of inheritance of the various genetic disorders, as well as information about the services that can be offered through genetic counseling. Although the physician has primary responsibility for informing the parents of a child with a genetic disorder about the availability of genetic counseling, the close professional and personal relationships that therapists often develop with families may prompt family members to seek this type of information from the therapist.

Although we are certainly not advocating that the therapist serve in the role of genetic counselor, it is important that therapists be aware of the availability and location of genetic counseling services so that they may be assured that parents of a child with a genetic disorder have this information. Most major university–affiliated medical centers provide genetic counseling.

Six steps or procedures in genetic counseling have been discussed by Novitski.[81] The first is to make an accurate medical diagnosis of the child's disorder. In the case of a suspected chromosome abnormality, this usually involves determining the karyotype of the child and possibly karyotypes of parents. Other diagnostic procedures may include a medical examination, FISH, DNA studies, biochemical studies, muscle biopsy, and other laboratory tests.

The next step in genetic counseling is to construct a pedigree or family tree of all known relatives and ancestors of both parents.[81] Pedigree information includes the age at death and cause of death in ancestors, a history of stillbirths and spontaneous abortions, and a history of appearance of any other genetic defects or unknown causes of mental retardation. The country of origin of ancestors is also important, because certain genetic defects, such as PKU, are far more prevalent in families of a particular ethnic origin. Once the defect has been identified and a pedigree constructed, Novitski[81] advises that further information be obtained from one of the comprehensive resource texts on genetic disorders. Informing family members about the characteristics of the disorder and its natural history may diminish fears of the unknown.[17]

The third procedure in genetic counseling is to estimate the risk of recurrence of the disorder.[81] In specific gene defects, the probability of recurrence is fairly straightforward, with a risk of 25% for autosomal recessive disorders and a 50% risk for each male child in sex-linked disorders. These percentages, however, do not hold true in cases of spontaneous mutations. In cases of chromosomal abnormalities, such as Down syndrome, karyotyping is mandated to determine whether the child has the translocation type of Down syndrome. In that case the risk of recurrence is much greater than with a history of standard trisomy 21 Down syndrome.

Informing parents of the probability of recurrence is the next procedure.[81] Novitski points out the common misunderstanding that if a risk is 1:4 for a child to be affected, as in an autosomal recessive disorder, many parents assume that if they have just given birth to a child with the disorder, the next three children should be normal. It is important to explain that each subsequent child faces a 1:4 risk of inheriting the disorder regardless of how many siblings with the disorder have already been born.

The fifth step in genetic counseling is for the parents to decide on the course of action they will take for future pregnancies once the counselor has presented all available facts to them.[81] Some parents may choose not to have any more children; others may elect to undergo prenatal diagnostic procedures for subsequent pregnancies. These decisions rest entirely with the parents and may be influenced by their individual religious or ethical preferences.

Follow-up counseling and review of the most recent advances in medical genetics are the final steps in the genetic counseling procedure.[81] Genetic counseling can play an important role in opening channels of communication between parents, other family members, and their friends; connecting parents and siblings to support groups; and helping families to address their grief, sadness, or anger.[17] The effect of a child's disability on the family may modify the parents' earlier decision to have or not to have more children. Recent medical advances may allow a more certain prenatal diagnosis of specific genetic disorders.

The most common prenatal diagnostic procedure is amniocentesis, which is used to detect early genetic disorders in the fetus at 14 to 16 weeks' gestation. This method involves inserting a long, slender needle through the mother's abdominal wall and into the placenta to extract a small amount of amniotic fluid.[115] Laboratory tests of amniotic fluid reveal all types of chromosome abnormalities, as well as a number of specific gene defects, including Lesch-Nyhan syndrome, and some disorders of multifactorial inheritance, such as neural tube defects.

SUMMARY

In this chapter we have addressed several chromosomal abnormalities and specific gene defects that are most likely to be seen in children in a typical developmental therapy setting. The inclusion of family members in all aspects of therapy has been stressed along with the need to consider family goals, priorities, and resources in the development and implementation of therapy services. The importance of developing functional goals and delivering services in natural environments has also been emphasized. Readers are encouraged to consult the following reference list for further information about genetic disorders not described in this chapter (see especially the work of Connor and Ferguson-Smith,[21] Nora and Fraser,[80] Weatherall,[114] Jorde and associates,[60] and Jones[59]).

ACKNOWLEDGMENTS

The authors wish to acknowledge the contributions of Gay M. Naganuma, Susan R. Harris, and Wendy L. Tada to the writing of the previous edition's version of this chapter.

REFERENCES

1. Aita JA: Congenital Facial Anomalies with Neurologic Defects. Springfield, IL, Charles C Thomas, 1969.
2. American Physical Therapy Association: Guide to physical therapist practice. Phys Ther 77:1163–1674, 1997.

3. Antonarakis SE, Waber PG, Kittur SD, et al: Hemophilia A: Detection of molecular defects and carriers by DNA analysis. N Engl J Med 313: 842–848, 1985.

4. Bailey D: Collaborative goal setting with families: Resolving differences in values and priorities for services. Top Early Childhood Special Educ 7:59, 1987.

5. Bayley N: Bayley Scales of Infant Development, 2nd ed. San Antonio, TX, Psychological Corporation, 1993.

6. Benda CE: The Child with Mongolism (Congenital Acromicria). New York, Grune & Stratton, 1960.

7. Berg BO: Convulsive disorders. In Bleck EE, Nagel DA (eds): Physically Handicapped Children: A Medical Atlas for Teachers. New York, Grune & Stratton, 1975.

8. Berg BO: Current concepts of neurocutaneous disorders. Brain Dev 13:9–20, 1991.

9. Bly L: A historical and current view of the basis of NDT. Pediatr Phys Ther 3:131, 1991.

10. Boyle JA, et al: Lesch-Nyhan syndrome: Preventive control by prenatal diagnosis. Science 169: 688, 1970.

11. Breg WR, et al: The cri du chat syndrome in adolescents and adults: Clinical findings in 13 older patients with partial deletion of the short arms of chromosome no. 5 (5p−). J Pediatr 77: 782, 1970.

12. Bruininks RH: Bruininks-Oseretsky Test of Motor Proficiency: Examiner's Manual. Circle Pines, MN, American Guidance Service, 1978.

13. Butler MG, et al: Clinical and cytogenetic survey of 39 individuals with Prader-Labhart-Willi syndrome. Am J Med Genet 23:793, 1986.

14. Campbell SZ: Pediatric Physical Therapy. Philadelphia, WB Saunders, 1999.

15. Carr DH: Chromosome anomalies as a cause of spontaneous abortion. Am J Obstet Gynecol 97:283, 1967.

16. Cass-Smith J, Allen AS, Pratt PN: Occupational Therapy for Children, 3rd ed. St. Louis, CV Mosby, 1996.

17. Cassidy SB: Management of the problems in infancy: Hypotonia, developmental delay, and feeding problems. In Caldwell ME, Taylor RL (eds): Prader-Willi Syndrome: Selected Research and Management Issues. New York, Springer-Verlag, 1988.

18. Chandler LS, et al: Movement Assessment of Infants: A Manual. Rolling Bay, WA, Chandler, Andrews & Swanson, 1980.

19. Christensen CM: Multicultural competencies in early intervention: Training professionals for a pluralistic society. Infants Young Children 4:49, 1992.

19a. Clayton-Smith J, et al: Somatic mutation in MECP2 as a non-fatal neurodevelopmental disorder in males. Lancet 356 (9232):830–832, 2000.

20. Cole K, et al: Comparison of two service delivery models: In class vs. out of class therapy approaches. Pediatr Phys Ther 1:49, 1989.

21. Connor JM, Ferguson-Smith MA: Essential Medical Genetics, 4th ed. Boston, Blackwell Scientific Publications, 1993.

22. Coster W, Deeney T, Haltiwanger, Haley S: School Function Assessment. San Antonio, TX, Therapy Skill Builders, 1998.

23. Cowie VA: Neurological aspects of the early development of mongols. Clin Proc Child Hosp DC 23:64, 1967.

24. Cowie VA: A Study of the Early Development of Mongols. Oxford, Pergamon Press, 1970.

25. Critchley M, Earl CJC: Tuberose sclerosis and allied conditions. Brain 55:311, 1932.

26. Crome L: The pathology of Down's disease. In Hilliard LT, Kirman BH (eds): Mental Deficiency, 2nd ed. Boston, Little, Brown & Co, 1965.

27. Crome L, Stern J: Pathology of Mental Retardation, 2nd ed. Edinburgh, Churchill Livingstone, 1972.

28. Dunst C, et al: A family systems assessment and intervention model. In Hanft BE (ed): Family Centered Care. Rockville, MD, American Occupational Therapy Association, 1989.

29. Emery AEH, Rimoin DL: Principles and Practice of Medical Genetics, 2nd ed. New York, Churchill Livingstone, 1990.

30. Federal Register, Part II, Department of Education, 34 CFR Parts 300 and 303, Vol 64, No 48, March 12, 1999.

31. Folio MR, Fewell RR: Peabody Developmental Motor Scales, 2nd ed. Austin, TX, PRO-ED, 1983.

32. Furuno S, et al: Helping Babies Learn. Developmental Profiles and Activities for Infants and Toddlers. San Antonio, TX, Communication Therapy Skill Builders, 2000.

33. Gans BM, et al: Description and interobserver reliability of the Tufts Assessment of Motor Performance. Am J Phys Med Rehab 67: 202, 1988.

34. Goldberg MJ: The Dysmorphic Child: An Orthopedic Perspective. New York, Raven Press, 1987.

35. Gorlin RJ: Classical chromosome disorders. In Yunis J (ed): New Chromosomal Syndromes, New York, Academic Press, 1977.

36. Granger CV, et al: Guide for the Use of the Uniform Data Set for Medical Rehabilitation. Buffalo, NY, Research Foundation, State University of New York, 1986.

37. Granger CR, et al: Guide for the Use of the Functional Independence Measure (Wee FIM) of the Uniform Data Set for Medical Rehabilitation. Buffalo, NY, Research Foundation, State University of New York, 1988.

38. Guralnick MJ, Bennett FC: Early intervention for at-risk and handicapped children: Current and future perspectives. In Guralnick MJ, Bennett FC (eds): Effectiveness of early intervention for at-risk and handicapped children. Orlando, FL, Academic Press, 1987.

39. Hagberg B: Rett syndrome: Swedish approach to analysis of prevalence and cause. Brain Dev 7:277, 1985.

40. Hagberg B, et al: A progressive syndrome of autism, dementia, ataxia and loss of purposeful hand use in girls: Rett syndrome: Report of 35 cases. Ann Neurol 14:471, 1983.

41. Hagberg B, et al: Rett syndrome, criteria for inclusion and exclusion. Brain Dev 7:372, 1985.

42. Haley SM, Coster WJ, Ludlow LH, et al: Pediatric Evaluation of Disability Inventory (PEDI), Version 1, Development, Standardization and Administration Manual, 1992, PEDI Research Group, Department of Rehabilitation Medicine, New England Medical Center #75K/R, 750 Washington Street, Boston, MA 02111–1901.

43. Haley SM, et al: Functional assessment in young children with neurological impairments. Top Early Childhood Special Educ 9:106, 1989.

44. Hall D: Mongolism in newborn infants. Clin Pediatr 5:90, 1978.

45. Hall JG, Gilchrist DM: Turner syndrome and its variants. Pediatr Clin North Am 37:1421, 1990.

46. Harris SR: Early intervention: Does developmental therapy make a difference? Top Early Childhood Special Educ 7:20, 1988.

47. Harris SR: Early diagnosis of spastic diplegia, spastic hemiplegia, and quadriplegia. Am J Dis Child 143:1356, 1989.

48. Harris SR: Functional abilities in context. In Lister MJ (ed): Contemporary Management of Motor Control Problems: Proceedings of the II-Step Conference. Alexandria, VA, Foundation for Physical Therapy, 1991.

49. Harris SR, McEwen I: Assessing motor skills. In McLean M, Bailey D, Wolery M (eds): Assessing Infants and Preschoolers with Special Needs, 2nd ed. Englewood Cliffs, NJ, Prentice Hall, 1996.

50. Harris SR, Shea AM: Down syndrome. In Campbell SK (ed): Pediatric Neurologic Physical Therapy, 2nd ed. New York, Churchill Livingstone, 1991.

51. Haslam RHA: Neurological disorders. In Smith DW (ed): Introduction to Clinical Pediatrics, 2nd ed. Philadelphia, WB Saunders, 1977.

52. Hennessey MJ, Haas RH: Orthopedic management of Rett syndrome. J Child Neurol Suppl 3:48–50, 1988.

53. Higgins S: Motor skill acquisition. Phys Ther 71:123, 1991.

54. Hoffenberg R, Jackson WPU: Gonadal dysgenesis: Modern concepts. BMJ 2:1457, 1957.

55. Holm VA: The diagnosis of Prader-Willi syndrome. In Holm VA, Sulzbacher S, Pipes PL (eds): Prader-Willi Syndrome. Baltimore, University Park Press, 1981.

56. Holmes LB, et al: Mental Retardation: An Atlas of Diseases with Associated Physical Abnormalities. New York, Macmillan, 1972.

57. Horak FB: Assumptions underlying motor control for neurologic rehabilitation. In Lister MJ (ed): Contemporary Management of Motor Control Problems: Proceedings of the II-Step Conference. Alexandria, VA, Foundation for Physical Therapy, 1991.

58. Hornstein L, Borcher D: Stroke in an infant prior to the development of manifestations of neurofibromatosis. Neurofibromatosis 2(2):116–120, 1989.

59. Jones KL: Smith's Recognizable Patterns of Human Malformation, 5th ed. Philadelphia, WB Saunders, 1997.

60. Jorde LB, et al: Medical Genetics, 2nd ed. St. Louis, CV Mosby, 2000.

61. Kelley WN: Hypoxanthine-guanine phosphoribosyltransferase deficiency in the Lesch-Nyhan syndrome and gout. Fed Proc 27:1047, 1968.
62. Kirshner B, Guyatt GH: A methodological framework for assessing health indices. J Chron Dis 38:27, 1985.
63. Knobloch H, et al: Manual of Developmental Diagnosis: The Administration and Interpretation of the Revised Gesell & Amatruda Developmental and Neurological Examination. Houston, Gesell Developmental Materials, 1987.
64. Know WE: Phenylketonuria. In Stanbury JB, et al (eds): The Metabolic Basis of Inherited Disease, 3rd ed. New York, McGraw-Hill, 1972.
65. Koehler J: Spinal muscular atrophy of childhood. In Bleck EE, Nagel DA (eds): Physically Handicapped Children: A Medical Atlas for Teachers. New York, Grune & Stratton, 1975.
66. Ledbetter DH, Cassidy SB: The etiology of Prader-Willi syndrome: Clinical implications of the chromosome 15 abnormalities. In Caldwell ME, Taylor RL (eds): Prader-Willi Syndrome: Selected Research and Management Issues. New York, Springer-Verlag, 1988.
67. Lesch M, Nyhan WL: A familial disorder of uric acid metabolism and central nervous system function. Am J Med 36:561, 1964.
68. Loesch-Mdzewska D: Some aspects of neurology of Down's syndrome. J Ment Defic Res 12:237, 1968.
69. Luiselli JK, et al: Issues in Prader-Willi syndrome: Diagnosis, characteristics and management. In Caldwell ME, Taylor RL (eds): Prader-Willi Syndrome: Selected Research and Management Issues. New York, Springer-Verlag, 1988.
70. Marini JC: Osteogenesis imperfecta: Comprehensive management. Adv Pediatr 35:391, 1988.
71. Marin-Padilla M: Pyramidal cell abnormalities in the motor cortex of a child with Down's syndrome: A Golgi study. J Comp Neurol 167:63, 1976.
72. McGraw MB: The Neuromuscular Maturation of the Human Infant. New York, Hafer, 1966.
72a. Meloni I, et al: A mutation in the Rett syndrome gene, MECP2, causes X-linked mental retardation and progressive spasticity in males. Am J Hum Genet 67(4):982–985, 2000.
73. Melyn MA, White DT: Mental and developmental milestones of noninstitutionalized Down's syndrome children. Pediatrics 52:542, 1973.
74. Milunsky A (ed): Genetic Disorders and the Fetus, 3rd ed. Baltimore, Johns Hopkins University Press, 1992.
75. Msall ME, et al: Health, developmental and psychosocial aspects of Down syndrome. Infants Young Children 4:35, 1991.
76. Myhre SA, et al: The effects of testosterone treatment in Klinefelter's syndrome. J Pediatr 76:267, 1970.
77. Naganuma GM, Billingsley FF: Effects of handsplints on stereotypic behavior of three girls with Rett syndrome. Phys Ther 68:664, 1988.
78. Nagel DA: Temporary orthopedic disabilities in children. In Bleck EE, Nagel DA (eds): Physically Handicapped Children: A Medical Atlas for Teachers. New York, Grune & Stratton, 1975.
79. Noonan MJ, McCormick L: Early intervention in natural environments. Pacific Grove, CA, Brooks/Cole Publishing Co, 1993.
80. Nora JJ, Fraser FL: Medical Genetics: Principles and Practice. Philadelphia, Lea & Febiger, 1989.
81. Novitski E: Human Genetics. New York, Macmillan, 1977.
82. Online Mendelian Inheritance in Man (OMIM): Center for Medical Genetics, Johns Hopkins University (Baltimore, MD) and National Center for Biotechnology Information. US National Library of Medicine (Bethesda, MD), 1998. World Wide Web: http//www.ncbi.nlm.nih.gov/omim.
83. Osawa M, Shishikura K: Werdnig-Hoffmann disease and variants. Handbook Clin Neurol 15:51, 1991.
84. Oski FA, et al: Principles and Practice of Pediatrics. Philadelphia, JB Lippincott, 1990.
85. Palisano RJ: Validity of goal attainment scaling in infants with motor delays. Phys Ther 73:651, 1993.
86. Patau K, et al: Multiple congenital anomaly caused by an extra chromosome. Lancet 1:790, 1960.
87. Phillips JA: Surfing the Net for information on genetic and hormone disorders. Growth Genet Horm 15:17–22, 1999.
88. Piazza CC, et al: Teaching self-feeding skills to patients with Rett syndrome. Dev Med Child Neurol 35:991, 1993.
89. Piper MC, Darrah J: Motor Assessment of the Developing Infant. Philadelphia, WB Saunders, 1993.
90. Plumridge D, et al (eds): The Student with a Genetic Disorder. Springfield, IL, Charles C Thomas, 1993.
91. Pruess JB, Fewell RR: Cell therapy and the treatment of Down syndrome: A review of research. Trisomy 21 1:3, 1985.
92. Public Law 94–142. Education for all handicapped children act of 1975 (5.6), 94th Congress, 1st Session, 1975.
93. PubMed. US National Library of Medicine, 8600 Rockville Pike, Bethesda, MD 20894, 1999. World Wide Web: http://www.ncbi.nlm.nih.gov/PubMed.
94. Ratliffe KT: Clinical Pediatric Physical Therapy. St. Louis, CV Mosby, 1998.
95. Robinson NM, Robinson HB (eds): The Mentally Retarded Child: A Psychological Approach. New York, McGraw-Hill, 1976.
95a. Robinson WP, Bottani A, Xie YG, et al: Molecular, cytogenetic, and clinical investigations of Prader-Willi syndrome patients. Am J Hum Genet 49(6):1219–1234, 1991.
96. Rubinstein TH: Cranial abnormalities. In Carter CH (ed): Medical Aspects of Mental Retardation, 2nd ed. Springfield, IL, Charles C Thomas, 1978.
97. Sandall SR: Developmental interventions for biologically at-risk infants at home. Top Early Childhood Special Educ 10:1, 1990.
98. Schneegans E, et al: Un cas de maladie du cri du chat. Délétion partielle du bras court du chromosome 5. Pediatrie 21:823, 1966.
99. Scott CR: Inborn enzymatic errors. In Smith DW (ed): Introduction to Clinical Pediatrics, 2nd ed. Philadelphia, WB Saunders, 1977.
100. Simpson JL, Golbus MS: Genetics in Obstetrics and Gynecology. Philadelphia, WB Saunders, 1992.
101. Smith DW: Clinical diagnosis and nature of chromosomal abnormalities. In Yunis J (ed): New Chromosomal Syndromes. New York, Academic Press, 1977.
102. Solnit A, Stark M: Mourning and the birth of a defective child. In Menolascino FJ (ed): Psychiatric Aspects of the Diagnosis and Treatment of Mental Retardation. Seattle, Special Child Publications, 1971.
103. Sternat J, et al: Occupational and physical therapy services for severely handicapped students: Toward a naturalized public school service delivery model. In Sontag E: Educational Programming for the Severely and Profoundly Handicapped. Reston, VA, Council for Exceptional Children, 1977.
104. Stewart K: Collaborating with families: Reflections on empowerment. In Hanft BE (ed): Family Centered Care. Rockville, MD, American Occupational Therapy Association, 1989.
105. Stewart KB, et al: Rett syndrome: A literature review and survey of parents and therapists. Phys Occup Ther Pediatr 9:35, 1989.
106. Tachdjian MO: Pediatric Orthopedics, 2nd ed. Philadelphia, WB Saunders, 1990.
107. Tardieu G, Tardieu C: Cerebral palsy: Mechanical evaluation and conservative correction of limb joint contractures. Clin Orthop Rel Res 219:63–69, 1987.
108. Taylor RL: Cognitive and behavioral characteristics. In Caldwell ME, Taylor RL (eds): Prader-Willi syndrome: Selected Research and Management Issues. New York, Springer-Verlag, 1988.
109. Trevathan E, Naidu S: The clinical recognition and differential diagnosis of Rett syndrome. J Child Neurol Suppl 3:S6, 1988.
110. Turnbull AP, Turnbull HR: Families, Professionals and Exceptionality: A Special Partnership, 2nd ed. Columbus, OH, Merrill, 1990.
111. Turner HH: A syndrome of infantilism, congenital webbed neck, and cubitus valgus. Endocrinology 23:566, 1938.
112. Wagner CW: Surgical considerations in Prader-Willi syndrome. In Caldwell ML, Taylor RL (eds): Prader-Willi Syndrome: Selected Research and Management Issues. New York, Springer-Verlag, 1988.
113. Warkany J, et al: Congenital malformations in autosomal trisomy syndromes. Am J Dis Child 112:502, 1966.
114. Weatherall DJ: The New Genetics and Clinical Practice, 3rd ed. New York, Oxford University Press, 1991.
115. Werch A: Amniocentesis: Indications, techniques, and complications. South Med J 69:894, 1976.
116. Whaley WI, Gray WD: Atlanto-axial dislocation and Down's syndrome. Can Med Assoc J 123:35, 1980.

Learning Disabilities

STACEY E. SZKLUT, MS, OTR • DARBI M. BREATH, MS, OTR

Key Words

– developmental coordination disorder
   (DCD)

– learning disabilities

– life span disability

– model of disablement

– motor control

– motor learning

– neurodevelopmental treatment
   (NDT)

– nonverbal learning disabilities

– praxis

– sensory integration

– verbal learning impairments

Objectives

After reading this chapter the student/therapist will:

1. Be aware of characteristics that typically identify a child with learning
   disabilities.

2. Become familiar with accepted definitions and terminology used in
   the field of learning disabilities.

3. Develop an historical perspective of brain dysfunction theories in the
   field of learning disabilities.

4. Understand the clinical presentation of subgroups within the learning-
   disabled population.

5. Become familiar with members of the specialist team and service
   provision types for children with learning disabilities.

6. Recognize the characteristics of the child with developmental
   coordination disorder.

7. Identify areas of evaluation to effectively assess motor deficits in the
   child with a learning disability.

8. Become familiar with theoretical development and intervention
   techniques applicable to children with learning disabilities and motor
   deficits.

9. Understand the lifelong ramifications for the individual with learning
   disabilities.

AN OVERVIEW OF LEARNING DISABILITIES

Characteristics

Difficulties in learning may manifest themselves in various combinations of impairments in language, memory, visual-spatial organization, motor functions, and the control of attention and impulses.[58, 90] The characteristics of a child with a learning disability are often diverse and complex. Each child presents with a different composite of impairments, disabilities, functional deficits, and societal limitations. The most commonly recognized performance difficulties in learning are associated with academic success. In most instances, the focus has been on deficits in verbal learning, including difficulties with reading, the acquisition of spoken and written language, and arithmetic. Impairments in nonverbal learning are equally important and more recently recognized. The three primary areas impacted by nonverbal learning disorders include visual-spatial organization, social-emotional development, and sensorimotor performance.[271] In addition to verbal and nonverbal disabilities, specific motor impairments also can be present and impact academic achievement or daily life tasks.[222] Accompanying behavioral disorders may include hyperactivity, lack of attention, and poor impulse control.[3, 160, 271] These learning and behavioral difficulties may be isolated (e.g., academic, motor, or behavioral), combined (e.g., academic and motor), or global (academic, motor, and behavioral).[92]

Definition

The heterogeneity of persons with learning disabilities has made consensus on a single definition difficult. Many disciplines describe learning disabilities according to their own frames of reference. Medical professionals tend to relate the deficit to its etiology, particularly to cerebral dysfunction. Terms historically used include *brain-injured*,[265] *minimal brain dysfunction*,[58] and *psychoneurological disorder*,[202] all implying a neurological cause for the deviation in development. Educational professionals, however, describe the child's difficulties in behavioral or functional terms. Educators view children with learning disabilities as "children who fail to learn despite an apparently normal capacity for learning."[209] Preferred terminology within the academic environment includes *reading disorder, mathematics disorder*, and *disorder of written expression*.[119] Associated behaviors observed include poor impulse control, restlessness, and frustration. Functional difficulties result in unsuccessful participation in classroom activities, playground games, and peer interactions.

These differences in frame of reference have resulted in numerous definitions, labels, and inconsistencies in terminology for children having difficulties in learning.[3, 34, 35, 90, 179, 229] Regardless of the inconsistencies, the salient features of learning disabilities are average to high intelligence and adequate hearing and vision, coupled with a deficiency in learning.[145] Despite these common features and a variety of proposed guidelines, the issue of creating a single, standard definition has not been resolved.[151] The delineation of one accepted definition is essential to consistency in diagnosis, research, and intervention of persons with learning disabilities.

After multiple revisions, the National Joint Committee on Learning Disabilities (NJCLD), which represents six professional organizations, proposed the following definition:

Learning disability is a generic term that refers to a heterogeneous group of disorders manifested by significant difficulties in the acquisition and use of listening, speaking, reading, writing, reasoning, or mathematical abilities. These disorders are intrinsic to the individual and are presumed to be due to central nervous system dysfunction. Even though a learning disability may occur concomitantly with other disabling conditions (e.g., sensory impairment, mental retardation, social and emotional disturbance) or environmental influences (e.g., cultural differences or insufficient/inappropriate instruction), it is not the direct result of those conditions or influences.[115 (pp 77–78)]

This definition describes learning disabilities in terms of function and cause,[284] despite a preference for educationally relevant behavioral terminology and less concern for etiology expressed by a multidisciplinary seminar of experts in special education.[113, 173] The Interagency Committee on Learning Disabilities[143] later recommended expanding this definition by including deficiencies in social skills and the relationship of attention deficits to learning disabilities. For legal and financial reasons, however, this proposal was not accepted by the U.S. Department of Education.[257]

The definition used in educational settings was initially passed in Public Law 94–142 and later incorporated into the Individuals with Disabilities Education Act (Section 602.26). These federal educational regulations specified seven potential areas of specific academic difficulties children with learning disabilities may exhibit: oral expression, listening comprehension, written expression, basic reading, reading comprehension, mathematics calculation, and mathematics reasoning.[209] The development of a uniform educational definition provided guidelines for creating academic programs and delineating appropriate services for children with learning disabilities. Children with learning disabilities are defined by the Individuals with Disabilities Education Act (IDEA) as[141, 230]:

Those children who have a disorder in one or more of the basic psychological processes involved in understanding or in using language, spoken or written, which may manifest itself in imperfect ability to listen, think, speak, read, write, spell, or do mathematical calculations. The term includes conditions such as perceptual disabilities, brain injury, minimal brain dysfunction, dyslexia, and developmental aphasia. This term does not include a learning problem that is primarily the result of visual, hearing, or motor disabilities, of mental retardation, of emotional disturbance, or of environmental, cultural, or economic disadvantage.

The 1997 Amendments of the IDEA redirected the focus of special education services by adding provisions that would enable children with disabilities to make greater progress and achieve higher levels of functional performance by promoting the early identification and provision of services. The rationale for this was based on research and experience demonstrating that the practice of waiting to refer children with significant reading or behavior problems for special education services increased their problems.[225] The new regulations also permit states and local education agencies to service children ages 3 to 9 who have learning problems using "developmental delay" eligibility criteria instead of specific disability categories, which are limited in scope.

Classifications

Binet and Simon's[33] test of intelligence, which enabled an intelligence quotient (IQ) to be calculated, was a landmark in the history of learning disorders.[284] This test was accepted to provide an objective, scientific, and accurate measurement of a child's intellectual potential. An IQ score of 70 or less (i.e., lower than two standard deviations below the mean) was used as the primary diagnostic criterion for mental retardation. Those children with IQ scores greater than 70 who were failing in school sparked off intensive research in child development and child psychology. Debate among practitioners regarding this mathematical criterion continues to this day. The primary concerns are whether the IQ test is an accurate measurement of ability and how skill competency is measured.[284]

Historically, a two-year discrepancy between the child's age and school achievement was the criterion used for the classification of a learning disability. This approach overestimates the possibility of a learning disability for children with low IQ scores and underestimates such disabilities in children with higher IQ scores. A poignant example provided by Gallico and Lewis[92] demonstrates the disadvantages and possible misinterpretation of this classification system. A child who is 9 years old with an IQ of 80 is functioning at a 7-year-old level in school. The two-year discrepancy in age and achievement might deem him as learning disabled. Another child who is 9 years old with an IQ of 130 functioning at an 8-year-old level would not be classified as learning disabled despite the IQ score indicating he should be functioning at a higher age level. This child's functioning level is significantly below his achievement level, indicating that he could have a learning disability. The current qualification for classification of a learning disability varies from state to state.[92]

The two most widely used classification systems are those of the American Psychiatric Association (*Diagnostic and Statistical Manual of Mental Disorders* [*DSM*]) and the World Health Organization (WHO) (*International Classification of Diseases* [*ICD*]). Educational professionals prefer the *DSM* classification for its academic relevance. Neuropsychological test batteries identify cognitive impairments leading to the identification of a specific learning disorder.[119] A variety of specific academically related disorders are outlined in the *DSM*. The latest edition, *DSM-IV*,[6] now classifies learning disabilities under developmental disorders as:

"Disorders usually first diagnosed in infancy, childhood, or adolescence"
  Learning disorders:
  • Reading disorder
  • Mathematics disorder
  • Disorder of written expression
Motor skills:
  • Developmental coordination disorder
Communication disorders:
  • Expressive language disorder
  • Mixed receptive-expressive disorder
  • Phonological disorder
  • Stuttering

The classification system commonly used by therapists is the *ICD*. The *ICD* codes are state mandated and recognized diagnostic codes used for billing and information purposes. In the recent revision, *ICD-10*,[290] "specific delays in development," which included "other specific learning difficulties" was changed to "disorders of psychological development." The term "learning" is no longer part of this classification. This updated classification is as follows:

"Disorders of psychological development"
  • Including specific developmental disorders (SDD) of speech and language (including acquired aphasia with epilepsy)
  • SDD of scholastic skills
  • SDD of motor function
  • Pervasive developmental disorder

Model of Disablement

Beyond classifying learning disabilities as a diagnosis, the National Center for Medical Rehabilitation Research (NCMRR),[205] and the WHO have integrated related approaches to classify functional performance. The conceptual approach, The Model of Disablement, describes the multiple dimensions of disability and identifies various internal and external factors that impact the way a disability manifests.[114] The purpose of this model is to shift classification of a disability to include assessment of functional performance and societal participation, as opposed to solely identifying component deficit areas.

Five dimensions are outlined in the model of disablement. They include pathophysiology, impairments, functional limitations, disabilities, and societal limitations. *Pathophysiology* refers to the underlying disease or injury processes at the tissue or cellular level. Proposed etiological factors related to learning disabilities at this level include brain damage, biochemical abnormalities, genetics, or metabolic disorders. The challenge for interventionists is to recognize the signs and symptoms that verify the diagnosis.[216]

The second dimension of *impairment* includes the organ and system dysfunction that potentially impairs functional performance. Children with learning disabilities may demonstrate impaired balance, endurance, and coordination of movements. Impairments that occur in one or more systems may lead to functional limitations, the third dimension. The challenge for the clinician is to treat impairments within the context of daily functional performance, because impairments do not always result in functional limitation.

Functional limitations involve whole-body functions that are typically assessed, but may or may not receive remediation.[216] For a child with learning disabilities this may include poor hand function in the performance of manipulation activities involved in dressing and handwriting. When functional limitations persist, which are not remediable and cannot be adequately compensated for with assistive technology or other supports, *disabilities* in daily life occur. The child then fails to be an active participant in normal life roles, such as activities of daily living and school tasks. Emotional difficulties, such as depression and decreased self esteem, which may result from learning difficulties, can ultimately impair social interactions.

Community and environmental barriers, called *societal limitations*, also can lead to restriction in social participation. An example of structural or attitudinal barriers that prevent optimal participation in society is a child who cannot use playground equipment because of lack of accessibility. The ultimate goal for the clinician is to facilitate functional abilities and performance, as well as provide necessary supports, so the child can become an active participant in society.

The Model of Disablement proposes that the environment, purpose, and level of participation all should be considered when evaluating performance. Determination of the presence, severity, or kind of disability should be based on a combination of these factors. Within this framework a clinician does not assume a handicap exists due to an impairment but rather considers levels of functional and societal abilities. This allows the therapist to determine intervention needs based on functional performance in relevant environments rather than being driven purely by diagnosis. A 9-year-old child with learning disabilities, for example, might have impairments in motor components of muscle strength and balance. Although these impairments can be identified on assessment, the Model of Disablement suggests that a disability does not exist unless these deficits impact functional performance (e.g., ascending/descending stairs) that limit societal participation (e.g., child cannot leave house independently to go to school or play). If assessment occurs within an academic setting the identified impairments would have to affect successful participation within the educational environment to warrant intervention.

Incidence and Prevalence

According to a 1997 report by the U.S. Department of Special Education, the total number of children, aged 6 to 21, with all types of learning disabilities was approximately 2,507,000.[280] Inconsistencies in the definition of learning disabilities affect the ability to determine accurate numbers of incidence and prevalence, although both have increased greatly. Incidence refers to the number of new cases identified within a given time period; prevalence is the total number of cases in a population at a given time.[153] The estimated prevalence of children with learning disabilities ranges from 1% to 30% of the school population, depending on the criterion used to determine the disability.[3, 119, 171, 243, 291] Incidence of identified cases has grown tremendously, with a 135% gain between 1976 and 1986, whereas the incidence of other disabilities increased by only 16%.[149]

Students diagnosed with learning disabilities are currently the largest percentage of children enrolled in special education programs, ranging from 25% to 65% of the total students with special needs.[3, 149] Shaywitz and Shaywitz[252] reported an estimated 11% of first-grade children have learning disabilities (including those with attention deficit hyperactivity disorders). This figure increased to 12.6% a year later for the same group of children. Learning disabilities occur from two to five times more frequently in boys than in girls, although some authors have estimated the ratio at as high as 10:1.[145, 269] Certain epidemiological samples[31, 252] have found only small differences in the prevalence of boys with learning disabilities over girls.

Perspectives on the Causes of Learning Disabilities

Diverse causes have been proposed for children with learning disabilities and have received varying degrees of empirical support. No one cause exists.[127, 259, 283] Single theories are inadequate to explain the multifaceted nature of this disorder. Frequently studied etiological factors include (1) brain damage or dysfunction due to birth injury, perinatal anoxia, head injury, fetal malnutrition, encephalitis, and lead poisoning; (2) allergies; (3) biochemical abnormalities or metabolic disorders; (4) genetics; (5) maturational lag; and (6) environmental factors, such as neglect and abuse, a disorganized home, and inadequate stimulation.[83, 274, 275] Theories on the cause of learning disabilities were often based on experimental studies of animals, studies of adults with gunshot wounds or other forms of cerebral trauma, or studies of people with epilepsy who have had brain surgery.

Although most researchers emphasize neurological causes of learning disabilities, emotional and environmental causes have been considered. In 1972, Peck and Stackhouse[218] hypothesized that children with reading disabilities were experiencing difficulties due to familial conflict. Bannatyne[28] stated there was a type of dyslexia, termed *primary emotional communicative dyslexia*, that resulted from a poor communicative (language) relationship between the mother and infant. Other researchers hypothesized that learning disabilities resulted from an interaction of organic and nonorganic factors,[185] suggesting that situational influences played an important role in eliciting maladaptive behaviors in children with learning disabilities.

Children with learning disabilities frequently display a composite of neuropsychological symptoms. These symptoms include disorders of speech, spatial orientation, perception, motor coordination, and activity level. Researchers have attempted to identify areas of the brain that may be responsible for these functional limitations. Recent research includes empirical measures of physiological function such as electroencephalogram (EEG), event-related potentials (ERP), brain electrical activity mapping (BEAM), regional cerebral blood flow (rCBF), and positron emission tomography (PET). These measures expand our understanding of brain functioning. Research on the behavioral, physiological, and anatomical levels continues to strengthen the conceptual basis in the field of learning disabilities.[200]

Early attempts at classifying the causes of functional deficits of learning disabilities generated many theories.

The three most accepted theories were delayed development of cerebral dominance, visual-perceptual deficits, and auditory-perceptual deficits with associated language inefficiencies.[285] Although each of these theories has been criticized for being too simplistic to cover the broad spectrum of learning disabilities, all of them have contributed greatly to research and subgrouping within the field of learning disabilities.

Orton's theory of delayed cerebral dominance, for example, was based on his clinical observation of higher incidence of reading problems in children with mixed handedness. He asserted that the left hemisphere did not develop dominance for preferred hand and language processes, which, therefore, led to deficiencies in organizing language information necessary for reading.[210, 285] Although this theory of a dominant side of the brain was refuted by empirical data, several research models evolved, including left hemisphere maturational lag or damage, lack of hemispheric specialization, and inefficient interhemispheric integration.[285]

Left Hemisphere Maturational Lag or Damage

In the early 1970s, researchers proposed that reading problems resulted from a lag in the development of left hemisphere lateralization.[245, 262, 263] These authors suggested a left hemisphere *maturational lag* impacting motor, somatosensory, and language functions in children with dyslexia. This resembled behavioral patterns of chronologically younger children, as opposed to a unique syndrome of disturbance. Geschwind and Galaburda[97] proposed an elaborate model attributing the underdevelopment of the left hemisphere to testosterone, which selectively inhibits maturation of the left hemisphere. Other studies[61, 200] have suggested hemispheric lateralization is present at birth, questioning the tenability of the left hemisphere maturational lag theory. Patterns of behavioral deficits in children with dyslexia also were found to be similar to those of adults who sustained damage to the left hemisphere.[96] Theories of left hemisphere deficiencies continue to be debated and researched.

Lack of Hemispheric Specialization

Research findings on brain function document that certain functions are specialized within each hemisphere.[43, 249] Semmes[249] first hypothesized that the left hemisphere has a more focal, precise organization, with functional units located near each other, facilitating the accurate coding needed for speech. The left hemisphere processes information in a sequential, linear fashion, and is more proficient in analyzing details. Academically, this hemisphere is responsible for recognizing words and comprehending material read, performing mathematical calculations, and processing and producing language.

The right hemisphere is organized diffusely, allowing dissimilar information to be processed simultaneously. This type of organization is advantageous for spatial processing and visual perception. The right hemisphere processes input in a more wholistic manner, grasping the overall organization or the "gestalt" of a pattern.[200, 270]

Functionally, the right hemisphere synthesizes nonverbal stimuli, such as environmental sounds and voice intonation, recognizes and interprets facial expressions, and contributes to mathematical reasoning and judgment. Although the hemispheres vary in the method of organization of input, they both participate in specific academic outcomes such as reading and mathematical concepts.

Specialization of cerebral hemisphere functioning is generally considered an optimal neural basis for learning.[16] Ayres[13] suggested that in some children with learning disabilities, the two hemispheres do not specialize in their functions, implying that neither hemisphere is as effective for specified tasks. Levy and others[174] reviewed a number of studies that support the hypothesis that development of language function in both hemispheres is achieved at the expense of the development of visual-spatial skills. Witelson[288] hypothesized that children with learning disabilities have bilateral representation for spatial function, leading to poor performance on linguistic tasks such as reading, which demands sequential analysis.

Measures of hemispheric specialization are largely inferential, and definitive statements of function are compounded by the complex organization of the brain and the heterogeneity of learning disabilities. Research suggests that children with learning disabilities show different patterns of cerebral organization than normal children.[200, 285] A strict left-right dichotomy is oversimplified, because it does not take into account many aspects of functional brain organization.[200, 285] Luria's[178] neuropsychological theory of brain organization, for example, proposes three basic functional units within the brain: subcortical, anterior, and posterior. According to this theory, communication between these functional units occurs at many levels, with each of the three units involved with the performance of any behavior. This system suggests the nervous system is highly specialized for function. Recently, as physiological measures improve, the emphasis of research has shifted to looking at differential patterns of cortical activation, emphasizing the highly complex nature of information processing within the brain.

Inadequate Interhemispheric Communication

Adequate communication between the cerebral hemispheres is important for many academic tasks. Reading, for example, is a process that requires the participation of both hemispheres and the transfer of information between them. Gazzaniga[95] suggests that aspects of learning difficulties may reflect problems in the "shuttling of information between various specialized processing centers in the brain." Myklebust[203] also believes the primary deficit of some children with learning disabilities is due to one hemisphere not communicating with the other. This lack of hemispheric communication is reflected cognitively by the child's inability to convert verbal learning (left hemisphere) into nonverbal meanings (right hemisphere) and to convert nonverbal learning into verbal expression. Hardy and associates[117] report that this auditory-to-visual processing is critical to academic achievement.

Adequacy of interhemispheric communication also has

been assessed using motor tasks. Badian and Wolff[26] examined motor sequencing abilities in boys 8 to 15 years old with reading disabilities using both single-hand tapping and alternating-hand tapping. Although no differences were found in single hand tapping, boys with reading disabilities showed marked deterioration when performing alternating-hand tapping. The authors suggested that the motor sequencing deficit of children with reading disabilities was the result of inadequate interhemispheric communication. This communication is necessary to coordinate control over the motor actions in the left hand (right hemisphere), motor actions of the right hand (left hemisphere), and hemispheric specialization for temporal sequencing (left hemisphere). The complex bilateral nature of many motor skills lends further support to the theory on the necessity of communication between the two sides of the brain.

Subgroups

As debate continues regarding definition and causes of learning disabilities, discrete subgroups identifying specific learning difficulties also are inconsistent. Although similarities can be found in grouping individuals with learning disabilities by patterns of academic achievement, the categorization appears to vary with the orientation of the researcher, the types of assessments and observations used, and the age and heterogeneity of the sample.[181, 233, 256, 259, 270] This ongoing dilemma affects not only how a diagnosis is determined but also who receives services and how research studies are interpreted.[142, 151, 259]

In early attempts to classify learning disabilities, Denckla and Rudel[74] determined that approximately 30% of the 190 children they assessed by neurological examination could be classified into three recognizable subgroups. The other 70% exhibited an unclassifiable mixture of signs. Of the 30%, the first subgroup was classified as children having a *specific language disability*. These children, who were failing reading and spelling, showed a pattern of inadequacy on repetition, sequencing, memory, language, motor, and other tasks, all of which require rote functioning. The second group had a specific *visual-spatial disability*. These children had average performance in reading and spelling with delayed arithmetic, writing, and copying skills. This subgroup all had social and/or emotional difficulties. The third group manifested as a *dyscontrol* syndrome. These children had decreased motor and impulse control, were behaviorally immature, and were average in language and perceptual functioning.

Rourke identified discrete patterns of academic performance and neuropsychological functioning with his ongoing research.[233] Initially, he drew from research on adults with brain damage that used the Weschler Adult Intelligence Scale (WAIS) to yield a "verbal IQ" (based primarily on language tasks) and a "performance IQ" (based primarily on visual-perceptual and perceptual-motor tasks). Research on adults with brain damage found that patients with left hemisphere dysfunction showed a low-verbal, high-performance WAIS profile with language deficits. Adults with right hemisphere dysfunction presented the opposite profile of high verbal, low performance on the WAIS and exhibited predominantly visual-

constructive deficits. Based on patterns of scores on the Weschler Intelligence Scale for Children (WISC), children aged 9 to 14 were placed into similar subgroups.[232, 235, 236, 255] The performance of the high-verbal, low-performance group was superior for tasks that primarily involved verbal skills, language, and auditory-perceptual skills. In contrast, the high-performance, low-verbal subgroup was superior on tasks that primarily involved visual-spatial skills.

In additional studies of children with learning disabilities, similar subgroups of children were identified.[118] The first group exhibited age-appropriate visual-spatial-organizational, tactile-perceptual, motor, and nonverbal problem-solving skills coupled with poor language skills, including reading and spelling. The second group exhibited strengths in language skills, spelling, and rote verbal memory with difficulties in visual-spatial-organizational, mathematics, balance and equilibrium, discerning social cues, and nonverbal problem solving. This group often had difficulties understanding nonverbal cues, with greater frequencies of emotional problems reported by their parents.[234]

These studies substantiate the need for subgroups of children with learning disabilities and have significant implications for future research and intervention.[11, 12, 20, 25, 124, 233, 255] Trends based on previous studies led to the following subgroups: verbal learning impairments, nonverbal learning disorders, specific motor impairments, and behavior disorders. The characteristics of these subgroups are described next.

Verbal Learning Impairments

Verbal learning impairments typically include dyslexia, dyscalculia, and dysgraphia. Harris[119] classifies these deficits in functional terms with dyslexia including disorders of reading and spelling, dyscalculia labeling a mathematics disorder, and dysgraphia describing a disorder of written expression. These learning disorders may occur individually or concurrently. Although children with reading delays typically exhibit poor spelling skills the reverse is not always observed.[92] Each of these verbal learning impairments will significantly affect academic performance.

DYSLEXIA

Children with dyslexia demonstrate a specific reading problem and language disorder,[92] often proposed to be neurologically based.[106] Neuroanatomical malformations, atypical brain symmetry in the temporal lobe, and anomalies in cerebral blood flow have been observed in children with reading disorders.[83, 119, 259] Recent investigation using ERPs is providing preliminary information on the sequence, timing, and location of neural activity during the reading process. This research suggests that a timing problem in the visual system may be involved in reading disorders.[119]

According to a subcommittee of The World Federation of Neurology (1968), "specific developmental dyslexia" is defined as "a disorder manifested by difficulty in learning to read despite conventional instruction, adequate intelligence, and socio-cultural opportunity."[60] Three to 10% of school-aged children are diagnosed with dyslexia. The ratio of males to females ranges from 2:1 to 4:1.[60, 239]

Classifications of dyslexia are based on types of reading errors and include *visual-spatial, audiophonic,* and *mixed.*[40] Reading skills consist of a combination of visually perceiving words and phonetically decoding letters, morphemes, and words.[105, 119] Children with visual-spatial difficulties often reverse letters, read words backward, and misread similar words (e.g., "when" and "which"). These children must sound out every word and lack the ability to rely on visual word recognition. They tend to read slowly but are good phonetic spellers. Children with audiophonic difficulties are unable to relate letter symbols to sounds. They can often achieve age-appropriate reading skills but have difficulty spelling words.[92] Children with mixed problems show a variety of both types of reading errors.

DYSCALCULIA

Children with dyscalculia have specific difficulties in performing arithmetic functions. This heterogeneous disorder may involve both intrinsic and extrinsic factors.[119] Intrinsic factors are hypothesized to include deficits in visual-spatial skill, quantitative reasoning, memory, or intelligence. Extrinsic factors can be a combination of poor instruction in the mastery of prerequisite skills, sociocultural and economic background, as well as attitude and interest in the subject. The neurological etiology of dyscalculia was initially hypothesized to be right hemisphere dysfunction due to the strong relationship of visual-spatial skills to numerical computation.[119] Further research supports the involvement of both hemispheres because mathematics computation involves a complex relationship of spatial problem solving, sequential analysis, and memory.

The *DSM-IV*[6] defines a "mathematics disorder" as "mathematical ability, as measured by individually administered standardized tests ... substantially below that expected given the person's chronological age, measured intelligence, and age appropriate education." An additional criterion includes "the interference with academic achievement or activities of daily living requiring mathematical ability." Dyscalculia occurs in approximately 6% of school-aged children. Math disorders are represented equally in both sexes but are more prevalent in lower socioeconomic groups.[208]

Various classifications of subtypes within dyscalculia have been proposed based on the development and functional structure of mathematical skills. Specific skills that may be impaired in this disorder include linguistic skills for mathematical terms and concepts and decoding written problems; perceptual skills for recognition of number symbols; attentional ability to copy figures correctly and follow sequenced procedures; and development and memory of basic math facts.[6] Children with mathematics disorder demonstrate a variety of these mathematical difficulties, including recognizing numbers and symbols, performing and applying basic mathematical functions (e.g., addition and subtraction), and maintaining proper order of numbers when performing mathematical calculations.[92, 105] Some children have difficulty with written math problems but can learn practical concepts in functional applications (e.g., using money or measurement concepts in cooking).[248]

DYSGRAPHIA

Children with dysgraphia have specific difficulties in written language production. This heterogeneous disorder is frequently found in combination with other academic and attention disorders.[119] Difficulties in written expression are often underidentified and can be masked by reading disorders or considered to be due to poor motivation. The complex nature of written expression makes finding the etiology difficult. Writing involves integration of spatial and linguistic functions, planning, memory, and motor output. This suggests involvement of both the left and right hemispheres for skill in decoding, spelling, formulating and sequencing ideas, and producing work in correct spatial orientation, all coupled with rules of punctuation and capitalization.

Diagnosis of "disorder of written expression" is dependent on recognition of "writing skills ... substantially below those expected given the person's chronological age, measured intelligence, and age appropriate education," which "significantly interferes with academic achievement or activities of daily living that require composition of written texts."[6] Limited data are available on the prevalence of dysgraphia, which is thought to be as common as reading disorders.[119] Three to 4% of the population has a disorder of written expression.[208]

Classifications of dysgraphia can include penmanship-related aspects of writing (e.g., motor control and execution), linguistic aspects of writing (e.g., spelling and composing), or a combination.[208] The common difficulty is in the expression of thoughts through written language.[119] Sandler and colleagues[244] proposed four subtypes within dysgraphia based on assessment of 190 children aged 9 to 15 with average intelligence. These subgroups include writing disorder coupled with *fine motor and linguistic deficits, visual-spatial deficits, attention and memory deficits,* and *sequencing deficits.* The subgroup that exhibited fine motor and linguistic difficulties also demonstrated delays in decoding and comprehension during reading. Written output was slow, with spelling, punctuation, and capitalization errors. Soft neurological indicators of finger agnosia and mirror movements were present influencing motor output. Children who exhibited visual-spatial deficits as the primary component of writing disorder had normal reading skills. Their difficulties were in written production with inconsistent letter formations and poor spatial organization, including sloping lines, inconsistent spacing, and undefined margins. Decoding difficulties were observed with attention and memory deficits. Spelling was poor and inconsistent. For these children written production and speed were within expected ranges.

When sequencing deficits were present the children exhibited strong reading skills but delayed math computation. A variety of deficits were noted in written production including spelling, letter formation, and legibility. Finger agnosia and difficulties with a task of finger sequencing were commonly reported.

Nonverbal Learning Disabilities

Nonverbal learning disorders affect children in both academic performance and social interactions. Three primary areas affected by nonverbal learning disabilities include visual-spatial organization, sensorimotor integration, and social-emotional development. These functions are all mediated by the right hemisphere. These deficit areas impede the child's performance in constructional tasks, handwriting, and fine and gross motor skills. The social and emotional difficulties for individuals with nonverbal learning disorders are paramount, leading some researchers to label this a *social-emotional learning disability*.[71, 119] Deficits include the inability to read facial expressions and change performance in response to interactional cues. These children cannot appropriately interpret emotional responses made by others or make correct inferences regarding emotional behavior.[119] They are often intrusive and disruptive. Cues received through body language, facial expressions, and voice intonation are unnoticed or misinterpreted. Jokes, metaphors, and implied meanings are not understood, and figures of speech are interpreted on a concrete level.

Children with nonverbal learning disabilities are frequently labeled behavior problems or emotionally disturbed.[271] Accurate diagnosis involves identification of depressed performance IQ in comparison to verbal IQ on the WISC. Sensorimotor deficits in tactile discrimination, body awareness, and balance, coupled with social ineptitude, are the other salient features.[119] Differential diagnosis is essential because nonverbal learning disabilities can occur in conjunction with dyscalculia, attention deficit, adjustment disorder, anxiety and depression, and obsessive-compulsive tendencies.

Nonverbal learning disabilities are frequently overlooked in the educational arena because children with this disorder are highly verbal and develop an extensive vocabulary at a young age. Well-developed memory for rote verbal information positively influences early academic learning of reading and spelling. Yet, these students will have difficulty performing in situations where adaptability and speed are necessary and their written output will be slow and laborious.[270] Nonverbal learning disorders, therefore, are challenging to identify at younger ages but become progressively more apparent and debilitating by adolescence and adulthood.

Nonverbal learning disorders are less prevalent than language-based disorders. Although approximately 10% of the general population is suspected to have an identifiable learning disability, only 1% to 10% of that population would have a nonverbal learning disability (i.e., 0.1% to 1% of the general population). This type of learning disability affects females and males equally, with an uncommon incidence of left-handedness.[271]

Classification of nonverbal learning disorders are based on the domains for processing social signals[119] and include *expressive*, *receptive*, and *mixed*. Expressive deficits are observable in limited facial expression, flat affect, unchanging voice intonation, and robotic speech. Receptive difficulties result in impairments in social understanding with intact affective expression. Mixed disorders couple both expressive and receptive features. Children often lack social reciprocity and awareness of social space.

Specific Motor Impairments

Children with learning disabilities may or may not present with motor coordination problems. Conversely, some children have motor and coordination problems but do not experience learning difficulties. Children with motor impairments typically have difficulty acquiring age-appropriate motor skills and move in an awkward and clumsy manner. Difficulties in daily functional tasks and performance areas (e.g., school and leisure skills) are common. Motor deficits can result from a wide variety of neurological, physiological, developmental, and environmental factors. These impairments can manifest in diverse ways, depending on the severity of the disorder and the areas of motor and social performance affected.

An International Consensus Meeting on Children and Clumsiness was held in 1994 with experts including educators, kinesiologists, occupational therapists, physical therapists, psychologists, and parents. These experts discussed a common name to identify "clumsy" children experiencing movement, coordination, and motor planning difficulties. The term *developmental coordination disorder* (DCD) was identified to distinguish these children from those with severe motor impairments (such as those with cerebral palsy or paraplegia) and children with normal motor movements.

As described in the *DSM-IV* as one of the motor skill disorders, DCD is a "marked impairment in the development of motor coordination that significantly interferes with academic achievement or activities of daily living that is not due to a general medical condition."[6] This condition is not considered benign and is distinct from normal developmental variance, maturational delays, and other medical conditions.[222] An estimated 6% of school-aged children have DCD.[6]

An initial attempt at classifying subtypes within DCD supports the heterogeneity of this group of children.[128] In a sample of 80 children identified as having DCD five patterns of dysfunction were observed.[128] The two largest subgroups had average to above-average visual-perceptual and visual-motor performance, with mild to moderate delays in two of the three gross motor measures (i.e., kinesthetic acuity, static balance, and running). Difficulty with visual-perceptual and visual-motor tasks, as well as kinesthetic acuity and balance, delineated the third largest subgroup. The smallest two clusters had average kinesthetic acuity but experienced difficulty in either visual-perceptual or balance and running.

Behavior Disorders

Behavior disorders associated with learning disabilities include attention deficits, conduct problems, depression, and global behavior problems. Ames[7] stressed that there is no single behavior pattern prevalent in children with learning disabilities. Issues in learning and related behaviors impact each other in a complex manner.

Attention problems can affect behavior, often relating to difficulties with impulse control, restlessness, and irritability, with the inability to sustain attention for learning and peer interactions. These issues frequently coincide with frustration, anger, and resentment, which may manifest as a conduct problem (e.g., verbal and nonverbal aggression, destructiveness, and significant difficulties interacting with peers). Children with learning disabilities often become discouraged and fearful, lose motivation, and develop negative and defensive attitudes. These patterns of behavior frequently worsen with age, contributing to juvenile deliquency.[90] Low self-esteem and depression are common during school years and escalate around age ten.[226]

Children with learning disabilities may initially be an integral part of the social and educational milieu. Poor academic progress, additional prompting needed from teachers, and negative attention for disruptive behaviors can cause children with learning disabilities to perceive themselves as being "different."[107] A self-defeating cycle may be established: the child experiences learning problems, school and home environments become increasingly tense, and disruptive behaviors become more pronounced. These responses, in turn, further affect the child's ability to learn. Lack of success generates more failure until the child anticipates defeat in almost every situation.[291]

Assessment of and Intervention for the Child with Learning Disabilities

Specialists

Evaluation of and intervention for children with learning disabilities must involve interdisciplinary procedures due to the differing constellations of problems in learning disabilities. Remediation of foundational and skill-related deficits is beyond the competency of any one professional group. Most children with learning disabilities are seen by a group of professionals, the make-up of which depends on the purpose, location, philosophical orientation, or availability of resources of a particular program. The box below lists the different professionals and specialists who might participate in assessment or remediation of children with learning disabilities. The types of professionals are grouped into the four categories of education, medicine and nursing, psychology, and special services; and they have been listed only once, although some professions could be categorized in more than one way.

Therapists should be familiar with the roles of the various medical specialists and of primary care physicians. School nursing is mentioned, however, because it is a specialty within nursing. The school nurse is usually the key health care professional in a school system and is responsible for maintaining information about the child's health history, current health status, medication, home environment, family cooperation, and family problems. The school nurse is the primary liaison between the child and the doctor or health clinic and relays information from the school to medical professionals.

Psychologists have two distinct and often separate roles in the care of children with learning disorders. The first role is in psychodiagnosis. Psychological testing is essential in the identification of specific learning problems and may be done by clinical psychologists, school psycholo-

---

TYPES OF SPECIALISTS WORKING WITH CHILDREN WITH LEARNING DISABILITIES

Education
Classroom teacher
Special educator
Learning disability specialist
Psychoeducational diagnostician
Reading specialist
Early childhood education teacher
Physical educator
Adaptive physical educator

Medicine and Nursing
Family physician
Pediatrician
Pediatric neurologist
Psychiatrist
School nurse
Biochemist
Geneticist
Endocrinologist
Nutritionist
Ophthalmologist

Otologist

Psychology
Clinical psychologist
Neuropsychologist
School psychologist
Child psychologist
Counseling psychologist
Guidance counselor

Special Services
Occupational therapist
Physical therapist
Speech and language pathologist
Psycholinguist
Audiologist
Optometrist
Social worker
Recreational therapist
Motor therapist
Perceptual-motor trainer
Vocational education specialist

gists, or clinical neuropsychologists, who specialize in diagnosis of learning disorders with an organic base. The second role of psychologists is to provide mental health services. Children with learning disabilities often have problems with self-esteem and peer relationships, resulting from either primary behavior problems or reactions to failure.

A child with learning disabilities with a primary behavior problem, such as impulsiveness, disinhibited behavior, or hyperkinetic activity, may receive special treatment for the behavior disorder. A behavior modification specialist may be working with parents and teachers to help the child control his or her behavior. The child may receive psychotherapy from a psychologist or psychiatrist, or family therapy may be provided by a social worker, psychologist, or psychiatrist. These latter interventions are usually provided by public or private mental health clinics. Children with learning disabilities with general adjustment problems in peer relationships are often treated within the school setting. School adjustment or guidance counselors offer support and advice on specific academic difficulties, social conflicts, and affective issues. The school psychologist, in addition to the diagnostic role, may offer psychological counseling to students and may help plan strategies for classroom management.

Physical educators, adaptive physical educators, physical therapists, occupational therapists, and developmental optometrists also may be involved in the evaluation. Overlap in the areas assessed may occur. The unique training of each professional influences both the selection of tests and the qualitative aspects of assessment based on observations of a child's performance. Although the evaluations may appear similar, there are differences between professions in orientation and rationale when interpreting dysfunction.

Differences in professional orientation and emphasis in assessment contribute to a comprehensive overview of the child's abilities and relative concerns related to the impairments resulting from the learning disability. Physical educators and adaptive physical educators typically assess skilled tasks necessary for sports-related activities. These include abilities in ball throwing, kicking, catching, jumping, running, and climbing skills. The primary concern of these professionals is the child's physical fitness. Physical therapists' assessment of the child's gross motor development and physical fitness integrate neuromuscular and neurodevelopmental factors. The physical therapy assessment includes observations of muscle strength and tone, postural refinement, reflex integration including automatic reactions, and sensorimotor functions. Occupational therapists consider developmental motor skills and sensory integrative functions that underlie skill development. Fine motor and visual-perceptual motor skills are emphasized with consideration of the impact of motor deficits on functional abilities. The developmental optometrist assesses bilateral eye movements as they relate to visual-perceptual motor skills, recognizing the relationship between vision and movement in development and eye-hand coordination.

Planning an assessment protocol can prevent unnecessary duplication of testing and provide comprehensive information related to the referral concerns. The areas assessed and particular evaluations chosen are dependent on the make up of the professional team, the setting, and the service delivery model. The assessment is driven by the referral concerns and the functional difficulties the child is experiencing. Communication of information between professionals will generate a comprehensive picture of the child's areas of strength and weakness necessary for effective intervention planning.

Coordinating Multiple Interventions

As the number of therapeutic disciplines involved in the assessment and therapeutic management of children with learning disabilities has steadily increased, communication for effective programming has become more challenging. Despite the benefits of specific skills brought to the case by each professional, the huge variety of well-meaning recommendations can result in service delivery overkill. According to Kenny and Burka,[152] our society values highly trained specialists and therefore it is in danger of expanding itself to the "point of logistic chaos." Case Study 11–1 provides an example of the negative impacts of overabundant specialized intervention on the child and family.

Effective coordination of intervention services presents a dilemma because no single discipline has trained its students to handle that role.[152] Rather, the assumption is made that all professionals acquire the ability to coordinate services by virtue of learning their own special skills. Kenny and Burka[152] stress the need for a person to act as coordinator for the management and integration of the multiple interventions received by the child with learning disabilities. They propose that leadership be delegated on a functional rather than on a hierarchical basis. By this, they suggest that the coordinator be the team member who could best service the needs of the child.

Service Delivery Models

Cruickshank and others[62] indicated that one of the major problems confronting the child with learning disabilities was the lack of a true interdisciplinary approach. Each discipline has traditionally been concerned with its own viewpoint in the field of learning disabilities, resulting in research and remediation approaches that are limited in scope. Kenny and Burka[152] emphasize the need for each discipline to accept fully the skills and competence of other disciplines. Gaddes[90] reiterates that territoriality is not necessary because none of the procedures by themselves is complete and adequate for dealing with all children with learning disabilities or with all the deficits of one child. He continues that the superiority of any one method over another has generally not been demonstrated for all children with learning disabilities. Johnson[144] supports this belief, stating that there is no simple response or intervention program for the child with learning disabilities. In creating a plan that truly encompasses and addresses the issues hindering the child's learning within the academic setting, the team must work together to fabricate relevant and inclusive goals and objectives. Goals should be functionally based, with team members collaborating to determine appropriate program outcomes for that child.[79]

The IDEA currently requires that all children in special

CASE STUDY 11–1　　　MATT

Matt is an 8-year-old boy referred for clinic-based physical therapy intervention 1 hour per week for remediation of severe motor coordination and planning problems that accompanied his learning disability. In addition to Matt's weekly treatment sessions, suggestions were made to his mother for a home program to be accomplished three times a week for 15 to 30 minutes each time. Meanwhile, Matt also received other services. Although he was mainstreamed into a regular classroom in accordance with the special education law, he was seen by the resource room teacher on a daily basis and by the adaptive physical education teacher twice a week to meet his specialized needs. The classroom teacher told Matt's mother that it was imperative for Matt to read at least one book a night because he needed additional reading practice. A reading tutor came to Matt's house Saturday morning. Ocular motor problems were identified so he was evaluated by an optometrist, who recommended weekly visits plus ocular exercises for 30 minutes a day. Matt developed secondary emotional problems, partly because he was very bright yet aware of his learning disability and frustrated by it. Thus, Matt also saw a psychotherapist on a weekly basis. The psychotherapist recommended participation in weekly group sessions, in addition to Matt's individual sessions, to help improve peer relationships. Thus, in all, Matt's "therapists" had developed a 12-hour-a-day program for him and his family. It is no wonder that Matt had difficulty in developing peer relationships—he never had time. Matt's schedule also affected interaction in his own family. His mother believed that being a "therapist" to Matt interfered with her role as his mother. She felt unable to carry out the home program and felt guilty for not doing it.

What became apparent with Matt's case is that while each professional involved with him made an important contribution to evaluation and intervention, the massive input, to some extent, had a detrimental effect on Matt and his family. Coordinating interventions and providing additional support at home can create a drain on the family and limit time for family activities and extracurricular participation.

education be educated in the Least Restrictive Environment (LRE). This environment is often mistakenly interpreted as meaning a regular or general special education environment. The LRE should be determined after assessing the individual needs of the child. If services in a regular classroom with supplemental aids and services are not meeting the needs of the child, an alternate environment should be considered.

In some educational settings, children with learning disabilities are given full-time instruction in a special classroom with a small group of other children with learning disabilities. A special education teacher or a learning disability teacher is in charge of the classroom. More commonly, the child is placed in a regular classroom and leaves class for special instruction for some part of the day. The child may go to a resource room, where a special education teacher provides regularly scheduled remedial education for children with a variety of educational handicaps, or the child may receive tutoring from a reading specialist or a private tutor.

Although there is much support for the model of inclusion, this requires members of the team to work closely together with the regular education teacher. This collaborative effort ensures an understanding of the child's special learning needs and incorporation of therapeutic procedures into the regular classroom to facilitate the best learning environment. Within the model of inclusion, therapy services can be provided through a variety of approaches, including direct service, monitoring, and consultation. The child's services should not be provided in isolation from the child's natural environment.[79] This means that regardless of the choice of service provision, the therapist must, at the very least, observe the child within the classroom and other appropriate environments, ensuring that intervention addresses the functional issues of the child within the educational setting.

Summary

A great deal of attention has been focused on the definition of learning disabilities. Various models of classification have evolved with continued revisions. Research has attempted to identify causes and the associated functional deficits of learning disabilities. The heterogeneity of the group suggests a spectrum of factors from neurologically based to environmental. As physiological measures of brain function improve, our theoretical understanding increases. Based on research, subgrouping within learning disabilities has assisted in delineating functional areas of dysfunction and distinguishing associated deficits. The challenge for the clinician is to recognize the multitude of components that interact to impede functional abilities and social participation for the child with learning disabilities.

THE CHILD WITH LEARNING DISABILITIES AND MOTOR DEFICITS

The Occurrence of Developmental Coordination Disorder

Motor deficits are often the most overt sign of difficulty for the child with learning disabilities. Yet they are only one of the multifaceted problems facing these children.

Denckla[72] reported that across the entire spectrum of developmental disabilities the most frequent signs leading to medical referral are those related to motor output. Occupational and physical therapists are frequently asked to provide intervention to enhance functional performance for children with a variety of motor coordination difficulties. The emphasis of this chapter, therefore, relates to children with DCDs.

Specific focus on motor performance does not imply that the motor deficits are the paramount problems of children with learning disabilities or that motor deficits should receive priority over other symptoms. The therapist providing intervention must be aware of the child's strengths and weaknesses and of the characteristics of the child's educational program to effectively plan and implement optimal intervention strategies.

Historical Terminology of Developmental Coordination Disorders

Terms used to describe motor deficits have varied greatly in the literature, research, and clinical practice. Developmental clumsiness was documented as early as the 1900s, when Collier used the term *congenital maladroitness*.[89] Orton[210] first adopted the term *clumsy* or *developmentally clumsy* to refer to children with motor coordination difficulties. He recognized that disorders in praxis and gnosis resulted in clumsiness in physical performance, which he described as similar to a right-handed person trying to use the left hand and said that the child seemed to have two left feet. The child with learning disabilities and motor incoordination has been described in the literature most frequently as "clumsy."[108-111, 125, 140, 282] Clinicians have suggested that this term is pejorative and has unfavorable connotations.[146, 222] Other terminology used to describe children with motor deficits includes motor delayed, physically awkward, perceptual motor deficient,[246] developmentally dyspraxic/apraxic,[11, 16, 21, 282] or having sensory integration dysfunction or developmental output failure.[222]

The revised *DSM-III* introduced the diagnostic label of developmental coordination disorder.[5] This descriptive term was adopted in 1994 at the International Consensus Meeting on Children and Clumsiness to identify and describe the heterogeneous group of children with motor deficits and facilitate communication within the field.[222] In this chapter, the term *DCD* will be used to describe a subgroup of children with learning disabilities who demonstrate motor coordination deficits that interfere with academic achievement, activities of daily living, and social skills. *Motor coordination deficit*, *disorder*, or *disturbance* will be used as general terms to identify disorders that have a motor component.

Motor coordination refers to functions that are more clearly and traditionally defined as motoric and includes gross motor, fine motor, and motor planning (praxis). Gross motor coordination includes motor behaviors concerned with posture and locomotion, ranging from early developmental milestones to finely tuned balance.[133] Fine motor coordination involves motor behavior such as discrete finger movements, manipulation, and eye-hand coordination. Motor planning is used specifically to denote the ability to plan and execute skilled, nonhabitual motor tasks.[14] Visual-motor function can be considered an aspect of motor coordination and is predominantly used in the literature as a synonym for visual constructional abilities. Visual-motor tasks involve the ability to reproduce shapes, figures, or other visual stimuli in written form. This subject is described and discussed in Chapter 27.

Prevalence

Motor difficulties manifest in multiple variations, which skews the ability to accurately document the prevalence of motor deficits within learning disabilities. The child's motor disturbances may be predominantly in gross or fine motor skills, but not necessarily both.[112] Other factors influencing prevalence rates include the criteria used to determine motor dysfunction, differences in types and methods of testing, reliability of the tests used, and heterogeneity of the test sample.[78, 146]

Within the general population the prevalence rates of motor dysfunction for school-aged children range from 5% to 15%.[59, 108, 146] Johnston and colleagues[146] screened 717 five-year olds and 757 seven-year olds and found the prevalence of children with poor coordination to be 6.5% and 7.2%, respectively. In this study boys outnumbered girls by 2:1. In a sample of 19-year-old boys Keogh[154] found 19% to be physically awkward and clumsy.

Various researchers have attempted to identify the prevalence of motor problems in children with learning disabilities. Tarnopol and Tarnopol[268] reported that about 90% of the children with learning disabilities have motor coordination and visual-motor defects. Sugden and Wann[267] found that 29% to 33% of children with learning disabilities also have coordination problems. In other studies, the estimates of motor deficits range from 35% to 60%.[78, 169] A meta-analysis of 1,077 studies concluded that 70% of children with learning disabilities have perceptual-motor difficulties.[150]

Causes of Developmental Coordination Disorders

Debate among researchers and clinicians exists regarding the causes of DCD. Developmental delays, variance from normal development,[222] and physiological factors are the major theories proposed to explain the basis of DCD.[286] The American Academy of Pediatrics issued a statement in 1985 that children with clumsiness are demonstrating a maturational lag that will correct itself over time.[4] Other professionals have attributed motor coordination deficits to a normal variance of development. These proposals suggest that children demonstrating motor coordination disorders will eventually outgrow their motor problems.

Possible physiological origins of motor coordination deficits have addressed unisensory and multisensory processing. The visual system, kinesthetic system, and vestibular system have been explored, individually and in combination. Depth perception and figure-ground perception are hypothesized to provide a foundation for motor movements.[136] Kinesthetic awareness (i.e., awareness of body position in space) can be an important factor in coordination problems and motor skill learning for children with developmental coordination difficulties. The vestibular system mediates movement in space and postural control and stabilizes the eyes during head movements.[15, 84] Fisher suggests the visual and kinesthetic systems work in conjunction for accurate motor performance, hence the support of the multisensory processing theories.[84] Ayres[14, 21] developed the sensory integration theory that suggests that the integration between sensory systems is imperative for motor performance in children. She suggested that normal development depends on intrasensory integration, particularly from the somatosensory and vestibular system.[21] When examining vestibular functioning in children with learning disabilities and coordination problems, difficulty with the integration of vestibular, visual, and somatosensory inputs was exhibited, thereby impacting postural stability.[132]

The perspective on the cause of DCD impacts intervention. When a maturational lag theory is endorsed, the child typically does not receive therapeutic intervention. This "wait and see" attitude can have long-lasting effects on the child's motor development and self-esteem. Attributing the child's problems to normal deviations of development can have similar ramifications. Considering that difficulties simply fall along the normal developmental curve endorses the idea that age-appropriate skills will never be achieved. Physiological theories support intervention that is specific to identified sensory deficits, encouraging unisensory and multisensory interventions to be applied to the child at different developmental stages.[286]

Descriptions of Children with Coordination Deficits

The motor deficits of children with learning disabilities are variable, without a single characteristic pattern.[48] One of the commonly documented findings is the extreme discrepancy in competence over the range of motor skills, with strengths in some motor areas and significant weaknesses in others.[72, 197] Patterns of movement in children are influenced by age, individual variability, and the environment.[177] Presentation of difficulties may change over time depending on developmental maturation and environmental demands. The salient features are coordination difficulties in gross and/or fine motor skills that include decreased speed, anticipation, and grading of movement.[197]

Two approaches are proposed to describe the characteristic motor deficits of the child with DCD. The first approach is based on observations and is descriptive, highlighting the general characteristics of the motor problems. These characteristics are frequently reported by parents and teachers. The second method, termed the *neurological approach*, is based on direct assessment of soft neurological signs. Evaluation of soft neurological signs is typically part of an examination by a pediatric neurologist, although therapists can assess these areas in conjunction with standardized testing. Soft signs may include minor neurological indicators, coordination difficulties, postural/motor impairments, and tactile discrimination deficits.[91]

Descriptive/Observational Approach

Children with DCD are generally described as awkward, with clumsy movements and poor coordination. They often fall, trip, and bump into things, acquiring more than the usual number of bruises. Motor movements are performed at a slower rate despite practice and repetition.[197] These motor problems can affect gross and fine motor skills with related functional limitations, such as running, ball skills, manipulating fasteners, tying shoelaces, and handling objects. Although motor milestones of rolling, sitting, standing, and walking may develop within normal or slow normal limits, there is often a history of relative slowness in self-care skills. Self-care tasks such as dressing, feeding, and use of tools (e.g., a toothbrush) also may be problematic and delayed.

In school, children with DCD may have lowered academic achievement, with any or all areas of learning affected (reading, spelling, writing).[222] When playing, these children are often sedentary, engage in solitary play, and have difficulty mastering puzzles and games.[64] Other play skills, such as riding a tricycle and bicycle, skipping rope, and catching a ball, are often achieved at a later age and seem to take extra effort for the child to perform. Children with DCD often experience secondary low self-esteem,[286] and emotional and behavioral problems because of their motor difficulties. Feelings of incompetence, depression, or frustration are common and experienced as lifelong problems.[55, 176, 222]

Fine motor coordination problems specifically related to academic and play skills also are evident. They may be manifested by reluctance to engage in, or incompetence in, small motor tasks such as coloring and cutting with scissors, or constructive manipulatory play such as block building, tinker toys, Legos, and assembling puzzles. Inefficiencies of fine motor performance may manifest educationally in difficulties with drawing and writing. Impaired drawing ability is characterized by poor motor control, with wobbly lines, inaccurate junctures, and difficulty coloring within the lines. Handwriting is often labored, with spacing and sizing problems evident. Letters may be irregular, illegible, and poorly organized on the page. To compensate for inadequate pencil manipulation, the child may develop a maladaptive grasp and use excess pressure when writing, further contributing to making writing prolonged and laborious. Associated articulatory deficits are often present, possibly because of the fine motor nature demanded for articulation.[14, 21, 54, 172]

Poor motor coordination may present as total-body balance difficulties. Ineptness is most apparent when complex motor activities are attempted. Physical education class often presents major problems. A 9-year-old boy described his motor problems as follows: "When the gym teacher tells us to do something, I understand exactly what he means. I even know how to do it, I think. But my body never seems to do the job."[173] Case Study 11–2 describes the motor difficulties frequently encountered in children with DCD.

Neurological Approach

Children with DCD do not exhibit obvious evidence of neuropathology (i.e., "hard" neurological signs such as a

The following is a mother's description of her child, Paul, who had motor coordination problems and learning disabilities: "I think when Paul was first born I tried to ignore the problem. Paul is a child who never climbed or ran or drew pictures the way other kids did. But until he went to nursery school, I didn't pay much attention to it. Maybe I didn't want to pay attention to it. Maybe I knew it was there and I didn't want to know about it. I'm not sure. But Paul was always a very verbal child and a very creative and imaginative child. He and I had something special because I used to enjoy that kind of creative imaginative play. We used to have our own world of various fantasies, heroes, and places.

"Paul sat up at about 7 months; he crawled and crept on time. He didn't learn to walk until he was about 15 months old. He walked very cautiously holding on and wouldn't let go of anything. He walked late, but he talked early. He said his first clear word, "cat," at 6 months. He knew what a cat was and could relate to it. My husband and I were so enthusiastic about his sounds. In those days they said that if you stimulated your child and talked to him and got him ready to talk, that this was the important thing, and he could read early. I was very concerned that Paul would be able to talk and have a marvelous vocabulary and read because I had a reading disability and a spelling disability.

"When Paul was 4 years old and in nursery school, at my first conference the teacher said, 'Look out the window, Mrs. B. See Paul sitting at the bottom. All the other kids are climbing on top of the jungle gym.' And then she showed me some art work. Paul couldn't cut, he couldn't paste, he couldn't do any of it. We could definitely, at the age of 3 or 4, see his problems. He was very bright, but he couldn't cut, paste, or draw, he couldn't climb, and he really didn't know how to run. That was where his handicaps were first being noticed, more by other teachers and professionals than by my husband and myself.

"When we had to make the decision as to whether to put Paul into kindergarten or hold him back, we were very frustrated by it because Paul was very very bright and very alert. He has always known everything that was going on in the world.

"Now, the kids Paul knows and the kids who know Paul know that he can't do motor tasks and they'll come over and play rocket ships with him.

But there will come a time, as the kids are getting older, that they won't want to do this."

Paul's mother, who also had learning and motor difficulties, described her own disability as follows:

"The hardest course for me was gym. I was unfortunate enough to have the same gym teacher throughout high school. The teacher always used to think I was a lazy kid, that I just never wanted to try to do the exercises. Although I tried, I couldn't do the stunts and tumbling for anything. The other girls would do a somersault and I would still do it like a 4 year old. I'd just about get over.

"I took dance a couple of times. I never could figure out as a kid why I couldn't point my toes. The teacher would say, 'Point your toes' and it never made any sense to me. I always curled my toes up. Only when somebody sat down with me and actually showed me did I know that that was how you were supposed to point your toes. With other kids, they just did what the teacher did. Nobody had to stop and tell them. I was the klutzy kid. I never could do the nice leaps across the floor. But I would try. After two or three sessions my mother stopped giving me lessons. She was probably embarrassed.

"As a girl, it wasn't as traumatic not being athletic. As I got older, the need for a woman to be athletic tended to decrease, whereas for a boy, the need to be athletic and competitive tends to increase. I foresee this as one of the major problems for Paul.

"Most of my life my friendships with people have always relied on other people. I met most of my friends through other friends because I've gone along to things. I think it goes back to being teased as a child, about the things I couldn't do or the way I looked. If you looked at me, I probably looked like a lot of the learning-disabled kids that you see—clothes were not put together properly, shoelaces were untied, my hair was never quite combed properly.

"It was very difficult for me learning how to put on make-up, to use a hairblower. It would take many hours of trying to learn. For a long time, my fingernails were cut very short because I didn't know how to file them. It is still very hard for me to put on eye make-up . . . to look in the mirror and try to figure it out. I still don't feel as though I am completely put together. And I put a lot of effort and energy into looking good."

cerebral lesion). They therefore are often not referred for evaluation until they reach school age. Parents, however, report long-standing coordination problems and associated difficulties.[48] Classic neurological examinations may not identify motor deficits[107, 222] and neurological involve-

ment is not a necessary concomitant of learning disabilities.[3, 289] Subtle abnormalities of the central nervous system are frequently noted by the presence of "soft" neurological signs.[215, 222, 250, 274] Deficits indicative of soft neurological signs include abnormal movements and reflexes, delayed motor milestones, and poor coordination.[59, 266] The following box lists soft neurological signs frequently used to assess this population. The reader is referred to Tupper,[279] Touwen and Prechtl,[273] and Levine and others[173] for more information on the evaluation of soft neurological signs.

Researchers suggest that a high percentage of children

COMMON SOFT NEUROLOGICAL SIGNS USED IN ASSESSMENT OF CHILDREN WITH LEARNING DISABILITIES AND MOTOR DEFICITS

Minor Neurological Indicators

Left-right discrimination

Finger agnosia

Visual tracking

Extinction of simultaneous stimuli

Choreiform movement

Tremor

Exaggerated associated movements

Reflex asymmetries

Coordination

Finger-to-nose touching

Sequential thumb-finger touching

Diadochokinesia

Heel to shin

Slow controlled motions

Postural/motor measures

Muscle tone

Schilder's arm extension posture

Standing with eyes closed (Romberg test)

Walking a line

Tandem walking (forward and backward)

Hopping/jumping/skipping

Ball throw and catch

Imitation of tongue movements

Pencil/paper tasks

Fine motor tasks (bead stringing, block towering)

Sensory

Graphesthesia

Stereognosis

Localization of touch input

Note: There is considerable variation in assessment measures of soft neurological signs for children with learning disabilities, both in what signs are included in assessment and how they are grouped. This chart represents a compilation of possible soft neurological signs.

---

with learning disabilities exhibit certain soft neurological signs. In a study of preschoolers,[164] children who exhibited a greater number of minor neurological indicators had a high likelihood of demonstrating difficulty with tasks of visual perception and gross and fine motor tasks on developmental scales. A National Collaborative Perinatal Project reported that 75% of the more than 2,300 children with positive total "neurological soft sign" ratings had the symptom of poor coordination.[72] Other frequently noted signs seen in these children were abnormal reflexes, abnormal gait, mirror movements, and impaired position sense.

In general, a composite of signs is more predictive of dysfunction than single signs. Children without notable motor difficulties can frequently exhibit one or more soft signs; and, therefore, identification of a single sign must be interpreted cautiously. In a study of 80 children with learning disabilities, the total number of soft signs exhibited was not predictive of learning disabilities.[228] Neurological signs requiring complex processes were found to be the most predictive. Peters and others[220] compared boys with learning disabilities with a normative sample for the presence of 80 signs and found that 44 of the signs significantly discriminated between the groups. Research has suggested that soft neurological signs could be more predictive if they were subgrouped, but no one sign or discrete group of signs currently presents a consistent relationship to learning disabilities.[146]

Kinsbourne[158, 159] stressed the need to view soft signs from a developmental perspective and stated that "soft signs differed from hard signs in that the child's age is the factor that determines whether the sign represents an abnormality." Denckla[70] divided soft signs into two groups—developmental and neurological. Developmental signs imply a state of immature neurological function that is considered to be normal in a younger normal child. These signs include functional articulatory substitution or distortion, motor overflow, right-left confusion, and mild oculomotor difficulties. Neurological soft signs, such as reflex asymmetries, are subtle abnormalities that do not occur at any time during normal development and are possible evidence of brain damage. Tupper[278] has added a third category of signs that results from causes other than neurological damage.

Social and Emotional Consequences of Motor Impairments

Poor motor coordination often results in significant social and emotional consequences. Play, which in the early years of life is in large part motoric, is essential to psychosocial aspects of development, including self-concept and ego development.[10] As early as 1912, Montessori[198] believed that movement was the basis for personality. In addition, the stimulation stemming from socialization and play was essential to the development of motor behavior.[10] The child with poor play skills and coordination is impacted in both aspects.

Development of gross and fine motor skills, coupled with the child's ability to master body movements, enhances feelings of self-esteem and confidence. The extent to which the child's perceptual or motor difficulties impede success will directly affect self-concept.[80, 152, 231] Clumsy children tend to be more introverted and anxious, frequently judging themselves to be both physically and socially less competent.[247] Children with motor deficits may be ostracized by their peers. In one recent study it was found that boys with learning and motor coordination problems demonstrated significantly less effective coping strategies in all domains of functioning than the normative sample.[186] Boys with learning disabilities and poor motor coordination also were found to have lower ratings on measures of self-esteem, happiness, and establishing same-sex social relationships than a matched group of boys with learning disabilities and adequate motor coordination.[251] Shaw and others[251] called this phenomenon "double developmental jeopardy," which refers to the double risk factors of poor self-esteem coupled with learning disabilities and motor deficits.

Being unsuccessful in peer competition, having difficulty with the changing demands of cooperative play, or feeling self-conscious because of their lack of coordination, children with learning disabilities often shy away from participation in games. Adolescents with motor deficits were found to have fewer social pastimes and hobbies than peers their age.[47] Failure at play and social interactions, coupled with the inability to succeed at school serve to compound the child's feelings of worthlessness, increasing inappropriate responses to the demands of society.[10] The impact of motor coordination difficulties on social behavior is exemplified by this statement from a child with learning disabilities and motor deficits.

They always pick me last. This morning they were all fighting over which team had to have me. One guy was shouting about it. He said it wasn't fair because his team had me twice last week. Another kid said they would only take me if his team could be spotted four runs. Later, on the bus, they were all making fun of me, calling me a "fag" and a "spaz." There are a few good kids, I mean kids who aren't mean, but they don't want to play with me. I guess it could hurt their reputation.[173 (p 83)]

Assessment of Motor Impairments

The use of standardized tests can help identify the overall developmental status of a child and examine patterns of impairments, thereby providing clues to underlying deficits and functional limitations.[168] Appendix 11–A provides an overview of standardized tests available for the assessment of motor dysfunction in children with learning disabilities. Uses and limitations of the individual tests and test batteries are listed. Knowledge and understanding of the rules for use and interpretation of standardized tests is a prerequisite. The use of any evaluation tool requires specific training or practice. A therapist should become familiar with all aspects of test administration and scoring procedures of an evaluation and should comply with the training requirements described in the test manual. Administration and interpretation of some tests such as the Sensory Integration and Praxis Tests require special course work and training.

The test descriptions in Appendix 11–A include data on test construction and reliability but not validity. Crite-

ria for a satisfactory standardized test should include validation against external criteria. The fragmented knowledge regarding patterns of motor impairments and functional implications of coordination disorders make it difficult to select appropriate external criteria. Few of the tests for children with learning disabilities reach a desirable level of external validity.[103] The judicious use of the evaluations described in Appendix 11–A must rest on the content validity of the test items. Clinical judgment of the therapist is important in the selection of tests for an assessment protocol. The evaluations must be logical and accurate in assessing the concerns from the parents, teachers, and referral source.

Within the school system the child is assessed for deficits that are educationally relevant. The frame of reference is to evaluate functional skills needed for success in the school environment. Evaluation procedures noted in IDEA (Section 300.532) state that each child's evaluation must be comprehensive to identify all the child's special education and related service needs. When conducting the evaluation, the use of a variety of assessment tools and strategies to gather relevant functional and developmental information is mandated by the IDEA (Section 614). Additional information should be collected from parents, existing data, classroom-based assessments, and observations and assessments made by the teacher and other related personnel. Eligibility for special education or related services is determined by a team of qualified personnel with a copy of the evaluation and eligibility report given to the parent or guardian of the child.[141]

Evaluation also may occur outside the context of the academic environment. Hospital- and clinic-based assessments focus on both medical (physical and psychological health) and educational issues. The frame of reference is diagnostic to determine the type and extent of difficulties in foundational development and skill performance. A variety of standardized and nonstandardized evaluation tools should be employed to assess these areas extensively. Information is gathered from direct observations, as well as reports from parents and input from other professionals interacting with the child. Performance should be assessed in a variety of environments and should include components of skill, functional performance areas, and social and societal participation. Recommendations may be made for further diagnostic assessment, direct remediation, and consultation. Specific recommendations should include activities to enhance performance in the environments and contexts the child functions in on a daily basis.

Qualitative Assessment of Motor Deficits

Identification of subtle motor difficulties is critical and challenging. These subtle motor difficulties initially can be undetected, leading to unrealistic expectations of age-level motor performance. The child's difficulty with skilled, purposeful manipulative tasks or with finely tuned balance activities may not be readily apparent in the classroom or may be perceived as lack of effort. Children with DCD may be able to perform certain motor tasks with a level of strength, flexibility, and coordination that is qualitatively average but must use increased effort and cognitive control for sustained success. Levels of performance in gross and fine motor composites may encompass borderline function. Careful observations are of paramount importance, because the child's deficits are often qualitative rather than quantitative. A child might have age-appropriate balance on testing but lack ability in weight shifting and making quick directional changes, which impacts his or her ability to participate in extracurricular activities such as soccer or baseball. When assessing children with subtle motor deficits, realizing that evaluation tools, for the most part, have been developed for children with moderate-to-severe neurological impairments is important.

Compiling a complete picture of motor deficits in children with learning disabilities involves assessing the following complex skills: (1) postural control and gross motor performance; (2) fine motor and visual motor performance; (3) motor planning; (4) sensory integration; and (5) physical fitness. Each of these interrelated functions is described here as an area of clinical assessment. Greater reliance on tests with normative data may be necessary because children with learning disabilities often exhibit subtle motor dysfunction. Information on age-appropriate performance is not always available, but sources for provisional information are included when possible. Formal tests and test batteries are described in Appendix 11–A to provide sources of normative data that can be used as guides for clinical assessment.

POSTURAL CONTROL AND GROSS MOTOR PERFORMANCE

Muscle Tone and Strength. Low muscle tone and poor joint stability have been identified as characteristic of some children with learning disabilities.[2, 14] Increased tone is not common in children with learning disabilities and may be indicative of mild cerebral palsy. Children with low tone may develop patterns of compensation called *fixing patterns*. These patterns often include elevated and internally rotated shoulders, internally rotated hips, and pronated feet. The child compensates for low tone by using the stable joint positions and holding himself or herself stiffly for increased stability. These patterns may resemble those of children with slightly increased tone. Judgments of inadequate tone are primarily made through clinical observations and felt through a hands-on assessment.

On observation, the child with low tone may look "floppy," have an open mouth posture, lordotic back, sagging belly, and knees positioned closely together. Muscles may be poorly defined and feel "mushy" or soft on palpation, and joints may be hyperextensible. A common method for assessing muscle tone and proximal joint stability involves placing the child in a quadruped position and observing the ability to maintain the position without locking elbows, winging of the scapula, or sagging (lordosis) of the trunk. The therapist can determine joint stability by asking the child to "freeze like a statue." The therapist then provides intermittent pushes to the trunk assessing the child's ability to remain in a static position.

Manual muscle testing can provide detailed information about an impairment in strength of individual muscles but is not regularly used in assessing children with learning disabilities, unless there are concerns of a possible degenerative disease. More appropriately, strength should be assessed by the child's functional ability to move against gravity during activities. Within developmental assessments, the therapist is observing range of motion against gravity in skills such as reaching, climbing, throwing, and kicking. The therapist also can have the child hold positions against gravity to assess strength and endurance (e.g., prone extension and supine flexion).

Early Postural Reflexes. Early reflexes are essential for the development of normal patterns of motor development. These reflexes facilitate movement patterns that are later integrated into purposeful motions.[36] Stereotyped or obligatory responses only occur in pathology and are not expected in the child with a learning disability and motor dysfunction. The residual reactions (e.g., asymmetrical tonic neck [ATNR] and symmetrical tonic neck reflex [STNR]) that might be noted in this population are subtle and most often are seen in stressful nonautomatic tasks. Full integration of these postural reflexes of children who are typically developing is not anticipated until they are 8 or 9 years old,[258, 279] or even later.[116, 240] Assessment for persistence of primitive reflex patterns in children with learning disabilities should emphasize impact on functional aspects of performance.

The effect of lack of integration can be observed during tasks such as writing at a table or gross motor activities such as ball skills and rope jumping. Persistence of these primitive reflexes may be seen in the child's inability to sit straight forward at the table for fine motor or writing tasks. The ATNR influence might be observed by a sideways position at the table with the arm on the face side used in extension. During ball games the child may have diminished ability to throw with directional control because head movements will influence extension of the face-side arm. Another observation of residual ATNR can be seen when the child is asked to pull a rope at midline to propel a swing or scooter board. If the reflex is affecting function, the child may lose the bilateral hold on the rope with changes in head position. Although residual reflex involvement may impact performance on these tasks, many other components are involved that will need consideration.

Righting, Equilibrium, and Balance. Righting and equilibrium are dynamic reactions essential for the development of upright posture and smooth transitional movements. Righting reactions help maintain our head in an upright alignment and are the background for movement between positions.[36, 162] Equilibrium reactions occur in response to a change in body position or surface support to maintain body alignment.[162] In simpler terms, righting reactions get us into a position and equilibrium reactions keep us in that position. Together these reactions provide continuous automatic adjustments that maintain the center of gravity over the base of support and keep the head in an upright position.

Righting and equilibrium (balance) reactions are assessed on an unsteady surface such as a tilt board or large therapy ball. These reactions occur in all developmental and/or functional positions, and complete assessment will consider a range of positions during functional performance in gross and fine motor activities. When testing equilibrium, the child's center of gravity is quickly tipped off balance. The equilibrium response is one of phasic extension and abduction of the downhill limbs for protection and of flexion of the uphill body side for realignment. In daily actions, most of the balance reactions are subtle and occur continuously to relatively small changes in the center of gravity.[162] Subtle shifts of the support surface can be made to assess the child's ability to maintain the head and trunk in a continuous upright position.

The vestibular system plays a role in the mediation and facilitation of reactions for the development of balance.[87, 253] Automatic righting and equilibrium reactions occur as a response to changes in the center of gravity that stimulate the utricles and semicircular canals of the vestibular system. This stimulation "acts on antigravity extensor muscles so as to elicit compensatory head, trunk, and limb movements, which serve to oppose head perturbations, postural sway, or tilt."[85 (p 240)] Sensory input of proprioception and vision plays an even more integral role in balance control than the vestibular system.[253] On assessment of balance, considering these combined sensory inputs is important. The therapist should test balance with the child's eyes open and closed. Assessment can include items that involve visual, proprioceptive, and vestibular dissociation, such as balancing on an unsteady surface (e.g., dense foam or a tilt board), with and without visual orientation.[253] DeQuiros and Schrager,[77] for example, changed consistency of the board to demonstrate vestibular proprioceptive dissociation. The board is a wide walking beam with irregular lengths of polyurethane foam alternating with wood for an inconsistent walking surface. Traditional tests of balance include: (1) the Romberg position—standing with feet together and eyes closed, (2) Mann's position—standing with feet in tandem with eyes closed, and (3) standing on one leg with eyes open and eyes closed. The Sensory Integration and Praxis tests[24] include a 16-item test of standing and walking balance. (See Chapter 21 for additional information on balance.)

Posture. The quality of posture is affected by decreased strength and endurance of the trunk musculature and diminished automatic postural reactions required to maintain a dynamic upright position. The relationship between posture and muscle tone is important to consider. A child has adequate trunk stability when control of the trunk is sufficient "to maintain an erect posture, shift weight in all directions, and use rotation within the body axis."[85 (p 92)] These areas are often deficient in children with learning disabilities and motor dysfunction, impacting both gross and fine motor performance.

The child may fatigue quickly and fall often during gross motor play. Other body parts may be used for additional support because of weak postural musculature, such as placing the head on the ground when crawling up an incline or sticking out the tongue when climbing or pumping a swing. In sitting, a child with diminished postural control will fatigue quickly, either leaning on his or her hands for additional support or moving frequently in and out of the chair. These compensations impact the child's ability to perform fine motor tasks or maintain attention for cognitive learning, because so much effort is exerted on sitting up. Observing the effects of fatigue

is important because both sitting and standing postures may deteriorate over the course of a day. Generally, the problem stems from motor programming problems versus muscle power.

Gross Motor Skills. Children with learning disabilities and DCD may attain reasonably high degrees of motor skill in specific activities. Motor accomplishments frequently remain highly specific to particular motor sequences or tasks and do not necessarily generalize to other activities, regardless of their similarities. When variation in the motor response is required, the response often becomes inaccurate and disorganized. Smyth[260] found that movement time for complex responses was longer for these children. Although children with DCD can sit, stand, and walk with apparent ease, they may be awkward or slow in rolling, coming to standing, running, hopping, and climbing. Skilled tasks such as skipping may be accomplished with increased effort, decreased sequencing and endurance, and associated movements. Gilfoyle and others[98, 99] have described qualitative differences in gross motor skills when observing twins, one demonstrating motor dysfunction and the other demonstrating age-appropriate skills.

Evaluation of motor skills, therefore, should include novel motor sequences[192] and age-appropriate skills. The child, for example, can be asked to imitate a hopping sequence or maneuver around a variety of obstacles. Skills that have been accomplished can be varied slightly (e.g., hopping over a small box). Age-appropriate social participation tasks, such as tag and dodge ball, can be observed for qualitative difficulties in timing and spatial body awareness. Developmentally earlier skills also should be observed to assess the quality of performance. The Bruininks-Oseretsky Test of Motor Proficiency[44] and the Peabody Developmental Motor Scales[88] are examples of standardized assessment of motor skills (see Appendix 11–A). Hughes and Riley[135] have described several other gross motor tasks useful in evaluating minor motor dysfunction.

FINE MOTOR PERFORMANCE

Fine Motor Skill. A child with learning disabilities often demonstrates multiple fine motor concerns. Areas of difficulty typically include the grasp and manipulation of small objects and tools such as a pencil, spoon, or knife. Delays in activities of daily living requiring dexterous hand use such as buttoning, zippering, and shoe tying may be observed. Assessment should include both standardized assessments and structured observations.

Fine motor evaluation should include assessment of proximal trunk control and distal finger movements. Upper-extremity reach and manipulation patterns are thought to be controlled by dual systems.[219] Proximal movements of the trunk and shoulders directly impact distal function.[63] Trunk control and shoulder stability affect the accuracy and control of reaching patterns and create a stable base from which both hands can be used to perform bilateral skills.

The assessment of distal control considers wrist stability, development of hand arches, and separation of the two sides of the hand, all providing a structural basis for the control of distal movement.[29] Qualitative observations of distal fingertip control are separated into manipulative motions labeled translation, shift, and rotation.[80] Translation involves finger motions to move objects into and out of the palm of the hand. Shift is an alternation pattern of the thumb and first finger generally used for the final adjustment of an object. Rotation involves turning an object within the hand. The reader is referred to Exner's[80] works for further explorations of these concepts and the work of Pehoski[219] for more information on developmental trends.

Although standardized assessments such as The Test of Motor Proficiency by Bruininks[44] and the Peabody Developmental Motor Scales[88] have fine motor sections, they do not adequately measure manipulative elements described earlier. Careful observations of movement components during a variety of fine motor tasks are necessary for qualitative analysis. The clinician must have a strong reference base in normal development for accurate assessment. Soft neurological signs, including diadochokinesia (rapid alternation of forearm supination and pronation), sequential thumb-to-finger touching, and stereognosis (identifying objects/shapes without visual input) can provide further qualitative information. Several excellent sources provide provisional information on age-appropriate performance.[69, 173, 273, 274, 278]

Eye-Hand Coordination and Handwriting. The evaluation of eye-hand coordination is best achieved by using standardized test measures. Examples include the Bruininks-Oseretsky Test of Motor Proficiency,[44] Movement-ABC,[126] Gubbay's Tests of Motor Proficiency,[108] the Motor Accuracy Test of the Sensory Integration and Praxis Tests,[24] and the Purdue Pegboard Test.[272] Supplemental clinical observations include the assessment of ball catching and throwing, fine motor tasks such as bead stringing and block towering, and written accuracy tasks of drawing or coloring within a boundary.

Handwriting requires complex integration of fine motor control, motor planning, sensory feedback, and visual-motor integration.[277] Refinements of accuracy and control have been documented up to the age of 14.[292, 293] Despite developmental trends in the child's finger and hand position during writing, the actual type of grasp on the pencil has not been proven to significantly affect the speed and legibility of written work.[293] More important to accuracy is grasp pressure (observationally measured by the angle of flexion in the index finger and the breaking of the pencil during writing) and forearm position.[292] Children who experience difficulties with handwriting commonly produce sloppy work with incorrect letter formations or reversals, inconsistent size and height of letters, variable slant, and irregular spacing between words and letters.[276]

Visual motor integration can be assessed through standardized measures such as The Developmental Test of Visual Motor Integration[32] and the Test of Visual Motor Skills.[105] The production of handwritten work can be assessed utilizing the Evaluation Tool of Children's Handwriting (ETCH).[8] Handwriting samples provide important information regarding functional abilities in written production.

PRAXIS AND MOTOR PLANNING

Praxis involves the ability to plan and carry out a new or unusual action when adequate cognitive and motor skills are present. Derived from the Greek work for acting or doing, praxis means "action based on will."[49] The components of praxis include *ideation* or generating an idea of how one might act in the environment, *planning* or organizing a program of action, and *execution* of the action sequence.[23] Motor planning involves the same components relative to a motor task. Sensory information is considered essential for initiation, execution, and adaptation of motor actions.

Children with praxis difficulties, or dyspraxia, may exhibit a paucity of ideas. The child may enter a room filled with toys or equipment and have limited capacity to experiment and play. Other children with dyspraxia may move from one activity to the next without generating effective plans for participating in, or completing, tasks. Lack of variation and adaptation in play can be another indication of planning problems. At times, children with dyspraxia also may exhibit poor anticipation of their actions. They can quickly engage in play with the equipment, but demonstrate little regard for safety (e.g., kicking a large ball across the room where other children are playing). Observations of typically developing children show continuous modifications in play, with spontaneous adaptations to motor sequences, making explorations varied and increasingly successful.

Kephart[155] describes trouble adapting to changes in external conditions as being a reflection of a child's inability to plan his or her movements. Children with dyspraxia often have difficulties in situations characterized by changing demands, such as unstructured group play. Transitions also may be difficult as they involve the creation or adaptation of a plan. Frustration and difficulties with peer interactions frequently are part of the composite. Often the child with planning problems can clearly see the differences between his or her performance and that of other children the same age, significantly impacting self-esteem.

The child with motor planning deficits has difficulty performing in, and acting on, the environment.[23] Observations of motor planning deficits may include difficulties figuring out new motor activities, disorganized approaches, resistance or inability to vary performance when a task is not successful, and awkward motor execution. Movements are performed with an excessive expenditure of energy and with inaccurate judgment of the required force, tempo, and amplitude.[281] There is an inability to relate the sequence of motions to each other.

Manifestations of poor motor planning ability are apparent in many daily tasks. Dressing is often difficult. The child is not able to plan where or how to move his or her limbs to put on clothes. Problems are often demonstrated in constructive manipulatory play, such as tinker toys, cutting, and pasting. Similarly, learning how to use utensils, such as a knife, fork, pencil, or scissors, is difficult. The child with dyspraxia often has problems with handwriting.

Standardized assessments of praxis include the tests of Postural Praxis, Sequencing Praxis, Praxis on Verbal Command, Oral Praxis, Constructional Praxis, and Design Copy of the Sensory Integration and Praxis Tests.[24] The FirstSTEP[193] is a preschool screening tool with a section assessing motor planning abilities. Clinical observations can add valuable information regarding the child's ability to see the potential for action, organize and sequence motor actions for success, and anticipate the outcome of an action.

SENSORY INTEGRATION

Ayres[14] originally defined sensory integration as "the ability to organize sensory information for use." Information is received through the senses and simultaneously processed and organized throughout the nervous system to learn about and act on the environment. Integration of sensory input impacts regulatory cycles, arousal state, planning, and skilled motor execution.

Information is registered by the sensory receptors, organized, and used in social, motor, and academic learning. The process of scanning incoming information for relevance is called *sensory modulation*. Sensory modulation is important in determining the appropriate action for a situation and regulating arousal. *Discrimination* of sensory input involves discerning subtle differences in sensation to learn about the qualities of objects and refine body movements within space. Both sensory modulation and discrimination are thought to play integral roles in organized motor behavior.[87]

Impairments in processing sensory input can result in motor dysfunction, including immature postural reactions, delayed eye-hand coordination, deficient safety awareness, and motor planning problems.[14, 20, 21] Deficits in registering and discriminating sensory input may be responsible for qualitative motor difficulties in children with developmental coordination disorder. Observations may include awkward timing and movement, poor grading of force, and difficulty performing in situations involving integration of multiple inputs (e.g., gym class).

Types of Sensory Integration Dysfunction. Ayres[11, 13, 15, 19, 24] has described certain characteristics that often co-occur in the child with learning disabilities and relate to deficits in the processing of specific sensory input. These types of sensory integration dysfunction often are associated with deficits in tactile or vestibular-proprioceptive processing. The patterns that have emerged most consistently through factor and cluster analyses impacting motor performance include: (1) disorders in vestibular-proprioceptive discrimination influencing postural-ocular movements, bilateral integration, and sequencing, and (2) deficits in somatosensory discrimination resulting in somatodyspraxia.

Certain indicators of inadequate vestibular functions have been noted in children with learning disabilities. One of the most frequently used measures is the postrotatory nystagmus response (i.e., the back and forth movements of the eyes following rotation of the head). This response is a manifestation of the vestibulo-ocular reflex and is a normal adaptive response designed to reestablish the original fixation on a visual field.[17] DeQuiros and Schrager[77] and Ayres[17, 20] found that more than 50% of the children with learning disabilities they each studied had shortened duration of nystagmus.

Nystagmus is only one manifestation of vestibular functioning. Other indicators, such as *postural and ocular problems*, have been associated with vestibular system dysfunction.[199] The vestibular system serves a primary role in the maintenance of tone, development of postural control, and equilibrium reactions. Inadequate muscle tone and proximal joint stability may be noted on assessment.[14, 66, 199, 211] The child also may show an inability to assume and maintain the prone extension position (head, trunk, and leg extension against gravity). Many children with learning disabilities have immature or poorly developed equilibrium and delayed automatic postural reactions. Standing balance is often deficient,[100] and standing with eyes closed is even more impaired because the child cannot use vision and must rely on vestibular and proprioceptive input.[17, 18] The ability to use the eyes efficiently in space may be hindered because the vestibular system stabilizes the eyes during head and neck movements so that a fixed visual image may be perceived.[14]

Bilateral integration and sequencing deficits are represented by difficulties in coordination of the two body sides, avoidance of crossing the body midline, failure to develop a preferred hand for skill, and possible right-left confusion. Tasks demonstrating these difficulties include problems in jumping with both feet together, reciprocal stair climbing, or skipping. The child who tends to avoid crossing the midline may shift the entire body to avoid crossing the midline or tend to use the right hand on the right body side and the left hand on the left body side. This may interfere with the development of a preferred skilled hand. Difficulties sequencing and projecting body movements in space can be observed through deficits in timing, sequencing and terminating a series of jumps, and running to kick a moving ball.[84]

Somatodyspraxia refers to the subgroup of children with motor planning delays that are hypothesized to result from deficits in tactile and proprioceptive discrimination.[49] Somatosensory input is important for developing awareness of where the body is in space and body scheme. "If the information that the body receives is not precise, the brain has a poor basis on which to build its body scheme."[22 (p 170)] During early development the child experiences much of the environment through the tactile system to gain awareness of his or her own body and discover the nature of objects. Proprioceptive input from the muscles, tendons, joints, and vestibular input from the inner ear work in conjunction with the tactile system to establish body scheme. According to Ayres,[14] motor planning depends strongly on an adequate body scheme to understand one's relationship to the environment.

Ayres has repeatedly linked poor tactile, proprioceptive, and kinesthetic perception with problems in motor planning.[11, 13, 18, 19] Kinesthesia, the conscious perception of the position of body parts and movement, is suggested to have a close association with motor performance and learning.[242] Laszlo and Bairstow[168] have developed a Kinesthetic Sensitivity Test (KST) that measures acuity, perception, and memory. Initial results of a study of 40 children with motor impairments indicated that 73% had deficits in processing kinesthetic input.[167] Hoare and Larkin[129] tested 80 children with motor difficulties using the KST and found that three of the seven kinesthetic measures were deficient in these children. Johnston and associates[146] found that 40% of a sample of 95 children had abnormal proprioception. Slower processing of proprioceptive information was identified in children with motor deficits.[261] Other researchers have emphasized the visual and kinesthetic contributions to movement.[125, 136, 168, 207]

Clinical observation of a child's responses to a variety of sensory inputs and the ability to organize multiple inputs provides essential information regarding the integration of sensory input. Gross and fine motor tasks that involve postural and ocular responses, bilateral motor coordination, planning, and sequencing are end products that reflect sensory integration. The Sensory Integration and Praxis Tests[24] and The Miller Assessment for Preschoolers[191] are used most commonly to assess various aspects of sensory integration function.

PHYSICAL FITNESS

Children with developmental coordination disorder often have performance difficulties in games and athletic activities. As a result, the level of physical fitness, strength, muscular endurance, flexibility, and cardiorespiratory endurance may be poorly developed. Fitness testing of a group of "clumsy" children in a movement program in Australia indicated that the group performed well below average on a number of fitness tests of aerobic/anaerobic capacity, flexibility, strength, and muscular endurance, even when the tasks selected required minimal motor coordination.[165] Tests of flexibility indicated that children who were "clumsy" performed at both ends of the range. Seventy-two percent of the sample scored either below the 25th or above the 75th percentile. One task of the physical therapist is to differentiate between poor physical fitness secondary to low motor activity and problems of low muscle tone, joint limitations, decreased strength, and reduced endurance that reflect a developmental lag or deviation in motor function. Collaboration among the physical educator, the adaptive physical educator, and the physical therapist is critical in these areas. Arnheim and Sinclair[10] and Larkin and Hoare[166] further discuss a physical fitness developmental program for children with problems in motor coordination.

Linking Evaluation to Intervention

After evaluation the therapist must synthesize areas of strength and weakness to address the functional implications of identified deficits. If impairment areas are clearly impacting the child's functional performance within his or her environment, intervention may be warranted. The intervention process begins with identification of the child's specific concerns coupled with corresponding statements of the type and quality of behavior desired as a result of remediation. In other words, the therapist must set treatment goals to be achieved through intervention.

Interpreting test data, integrating findings, identifying functional limitations, and creating goals is a complex process. Initial impressions of the child's areas of difficulty may result in the recommendation for further examination before outlining refined goals relevant to functional performance. Collecting additional assessment information may involve observations in other environments or during functional daily tasks, and/or additional formal testing.

Setting goals for the child with learning disabilities with motor deficits must be based on consideration of a variety of factors:

1. Referral information and age of the child
2. Medical, developmental, and sensory processing history
3. Parents' and teachers' perception of child's strengths and concerns and functional impairments
4. Educational information
   a. Major difficulties experienced in school
   b. How motor problems are interfering with the child's school performance
   c. Current services being received
5. Child's peer relationships, play and leisure activities, and self-esteem
6. Therapists' observations/assessment of the child through informal and formal evaluation, both standardized and nonstandardized
7. Functional expectations and abilities at home and school

Goals for the child with learning disabilities can be stated in terms of long-term or short-term objectives. According to Arnheim and Sinclair,[10] the major long-term objective in remediation of motor impairments for the child with DCD should be:

effective total body management in a wide variety of activities requiring dynamic balance and agility; object management including manipulation, propulsion and reception, emotional control, ability to socialize effectively, a positive self-concept and a sense of enjoyment in movement.

Short-term objectives should be written to reflect a specific behavior or set of behaviors that are attainable within a predetermined time frame of intervention, usually 6 months to 1 year. Bundy[45] indicates that "well written objectives are predictions about how a client will be different, in some meaningful way, as a result of intervention." Behavioral short-term objectives are composed of three parts: (1) the *behavioral statement* is what will be accomplished by the child; (2) the *condition statement* provides details regarding how the skill or behavior will be accomplished; and (3) the *performance statement* denotes how the skill or behavior will be measured for success. The most important consideration is assuring that the goals and objectives chosen are relevant to the child's functional daily performance and are meaningful to the team, including the family, working with the child. Case Study 11–3 provides an example of functional objectives.

Intervention for the Child with Learning Disabilities and Motor Deficits

Roles of the Therapist

Traditionally, occupational and physical therapy was provided in special schools or classes for multiply handicapped children, or in clinics that were completely separated from the educational environment. Integration of services into the public school arena occurred with the establishment of the Education for All Handicapped Act (PL 94–142) and the IDEA. The provision of related

CASE STUDY 11–3　　JONATHAN

Jonathan was a 6 year old referred for an occupational therapy evaluation by his parents and teacher owing to concerns regarding motor skill development. Assessment results revealed several areas of impairment including poor discrimination of his body position and movement in space, diminished postural control and balance reactions, motor planning deficits, delayed eye-hand coordination, qualitative fine motor deficits, and delayed visual-motor integration affecting his handwriting. Jonathan's mother reported that he was clumsy and seemed to bump into things constantly. Of greater concern was that Jonathan seemed fearful of activities that his peers found pleasurable, such as climbing the jungle gym and coming down the slide at the neighborhood playground. Jonathan tended to play on the outskirts of groups. When he did attempt to interact he became angry because the children would not play the game by his rules. At home, Jonathan often was frustrated by tasks of daily living such as putting on his coat, snapping his pants, and tying his shoes. His mother reported that Jonathan frequently called himself "stupid" when he could not independently complete self-care skills.

When determining appropriate behavioral objectives for Jonathan, looking at the areas of functional relevance such as pleasure and safety in gross motor play, peer interactions, and independence in age-appropriate activities of daily living is critical. These areas of concern for Jonathan were consistent with those of his parents. His parents wanted him to feel more competent and less frustrated in play, at home, and at school. Jonathan's goal was to "not be so stupid that kids won't play with me." The occupational therapist believed that through remediation of sensory discrimination and motor deficits Jonathan could develop improved motor competence and planning abilities. This would lead to greater success in peer interactions and improved feelings of self-confidence. Based on these common desires the following goals and objectives were made. Among the many excellent references on writing goals and objectives and functional outcome measures are Arnheim and Sinclair,[10] Dunn and Campbell,[79] Fisher and co-workers,[87] and LaVesser and Bloomer.[169]

One of the general/long-term goals became to *improve Jonathan's gross motor skill development.* Jonathan was interested in learning to ride a bicycle without training wheels and his parents were hopeful that he could become more confident at the neighborhood playground. These behavioral objectives would measure the development of improved proficiency in discrimination of his body in space, postural control balance reac-

tions, and motor planning. The following objectives were written:

1. Jonathan will independently climb the ladder and come down the slide without exhibiting fear, bumping into other children, or falling.
2. Jonathan will develop the ability to ride his bicycle without training wheels in straight lines and will learn to turn corners. (*Note:* Successfully riding the bicycle becomes the performance measure of behavior in this objective.)

To address *improvement in independence for self-care:*

1. Jonathan will put on his coat independently in correct orientation and successfully zipper it four out of five times.
2. Jonathan will successfully tie his shoes without assistance in a timely manner.

To address *greater success in peer interactions:*

1. Jonathan will participate in a structured game, following the rules, for 10 minutes.
2. Jonathan will play outside with the children in the neighborhood without conflict for at least 1 hour.

Although impairment level objectives could have been written to address the same areas, they would have been of limited relevance to Jonathan and the team working with him. Balance and postural control also could be addressed by an objective stating that Jonathan would stand on one foot for 10 seconds. The functional implications of this objective would not have been clear, and Jonathan and his parents would be without an outcome measure that was measurable and meaningful to them. Thus, it would have negated the effects of working as a cohesive team toward a common goal.

When working as a member of a team within the school, behavioral objectives will have implications for the child's performance in the school environment. Within the school system, statements of goals and specific objectives are included in the Individualized Educational Plan (IEP). In Jonathan's case, specific objectives that were meaningful to the classroom situation included the ability to sit in the chair to complete written assignments for 15 minutes and increase accuracy of letter formation, size, and spacing on written assignments. Other areas related to gross and fine motor skills and peer interactions also were influential to Jonathan's success at school. Specific objectives written pertaining to school would have functional outcome measures chosen from tasks within the school environment such as gym class, playground interactions, and classroom expectations.

services, including occupational and physical therapy, as well as special education, is now a mandated part of the educational process. During the past 20 years, occupational and physical therapy services for children with learning disabilities have become increasingly common.

Kalish and Presseller[147] have identified five areas of function for the physical or occupational therapist in the educational environment:

1. Screening and evaluating children with a wide variety of functional deficits
2. Program planning based on evaluating results and related to a child's ability to receive maximum benefit from his educational experiences
3. Treatment activities designed to meet program goals
4. Consultation to teachers, other school personnel, and parents around carryover of services into the classroom and home programming
5. In-service training for individuals and/or groups relative to the needs of handicapped children

Because each of these functions is usually required of the public school therapist, the time available for providing direct services to children may be limited. Intervention services must be done, in part, through consultation to parents, classroom teachers, and physical educators. The child's motor development needs can sometimes be met, wholly or in part, through the physical education program. Through assessment and observation the therapist can identify deficit areas and suggest therapeutic activities that could be incorporated into an adaptive physical education program.

Kalish and Presseller[147] point out the necessity of integrating therapy into the educational process, first by adapting intervention to reinforce educational goals and then by incorporating therapy into routine classroom activities. The therapist must be flexible and discover alternate methods of reaching goals, such as positioning and using unobtrusive adaptive equipment. The teacher's responsibility for all of the children in his or her classroom must always be kept in mind. Before proposing the incorporation of a therapeutic activity into a classroom, feasibility of the activities must be ensured. In some classrooms a teacher's aide might be available for individual attention, but in all instances both the child's time and the teacher's time must be considered in relation to the total program requirements.

Intervention Techniques

Models of intervention used in treating children with motor deficits include direct and indirect therapeutic techniques. Both approaches are necessary when addressing the variety of motor impairments in the child with learning disabilities. Indirect methods provide the foundations for the development of components for functional performance and the generalization of skills. Direct methods enhance a child's motor performance and social participation through skill training. Indirect methods involve "training the brain"[90] and direct methods teach the child what you want him or her to learn by practice and repetition. Ottenbacher[213] proposed that the medical model of intervention resembles the indirect therapeutic

approach and the educational model resembles the direct therapeutic approach. Intervention should be provided in an atmosphere in which these models are synergistic rather than antagonistic.[213] Proportions of direct and indirect therapy utilized are relevant to the child's age, developmental status, and the severity of his or her disability.[89]

Many of the treatment approaches later discussed integrate indirect and direct concepts of intervention. Sensory integration, for example, attempts to modify the neurological dysfunction interfering with motor performance, while emphasizing functional adaptive performance and motor skill development. The neurodevelopmental treatment approach uses handling techniques to inhibit abnormal movement by facilitating normal movement patterns to encourage the acquisition of functional movement skills needed for learning and daily living skills.[65] Motor learning theories aim to adapt the neural structures required to control movement using task-related intervention. Successful intervention for children with learning disabilities should derive from all existing procedures for the management of impairments.

No delineated formulas exist for determining the best intervention approach for an individual child. Each child is unique and presents a new challenge to the therapist when fabricating a functional outcome plan. A chosen intervention approach typically reflects the setting the child is referred to, the therapist's experience and expertise, and the parents' beliefs and goals. Selection of intervention methods is integrally tied to the child's presenting problems and the goals and objectives established as part of the intervention plan.

The intervention methods presented for remediation of motor deficits in the child with learning disabilities are classified as sensory integration; neurodevelopmental; motor control, learning, and development; sensorimotor; motor skill training; and physical fitness.[10, 194] None is mutually exclusive, and each requires a level of training and practice for competence, as well as experience in normal development. Most therapists synthesize information from different intervention techniques and use an eclectic approach, pulling relevant pieces from a variety of intervention modalities to best meet the needs of each child.

SENSORY INTEGRATION

The sensory integration theory was developed and articulated by A. Jean Ayres,[11, 22, 24, 25] with concepts drawn from neurophysiology, neuropsychology, and development. Her purpose in theoretical development was to explain the observed relationship between difficulties organizing sensory input and deficits in academic and neuromotor "learning" observed in some children with learning disabilities and motor deficits.[86] The theory postulates that ". . . learning is dependent on the ability of normal individuals to take in sensory information derived from the environment and from movement of their bodies, to process and integrate these sensory inputs within the central nervous system, and to use this sensory information to plan and organize behavior."[86 (p 4)] Ayres[24] used "learning" in a broad sense to include the development of concepts, adaptive motor responses, and behavioral change. The goal of sensory integration intervention is to elicit responses that result in better organization of sensory input and facilitate the generalization of functional skills.

Ayres[14] proposed that the integration of sensory inputs could be facilitated by providing opportunities for enhanced sensory intake in the context of meaningful activities, resulting in adaptive responses. During intervention, sensory input is provided in a planned and organized manner, while eliciting progressively harder adaptive motor responses. The therapist strives to find activities that are motivating and tap the child's inner drive to encourage adaptation. "Evincing an adaptive behavior promotes sensory integration, and, in turn, the ability to produce an adaptive behavior reflects sensory integration."[14 (p 17)] Effective intervention requires melding the science of a neurophysiological theory with the art of "playing" with the child.

An example of sensory integration intervention for a child with postural difficulties might involve having the child riding a swing pretending to be a fisherman while keeping a lookout for whales that might bump his boat. This "pretend play" scenario taps the child's motivation and inner drive to be productive (fishing), while challenging himself in a dangerous situation (whales). The therapist will adapt this activity in a variety of ways to maintain an appropriate level of challenge and adaptation (adaptive response). The required type and amount of sensory input, postural demands, bilateral control, timing, and planning are all considered and can be adapted to an easier or harder level to maintain adaptation and learning. Sensory input can be controlled through the speed and direction the boat moves and the amount of work the child must do with his arms to propel the boat and catch fish. Additional sensory input can be provided through "rocky seas" and "whales crashing the side of the boat." The boat can facilitate more or less postural adaptation by the amount of support it provides and the speed of its movement. The child can pull a rope to propel the swing, or the therapist can provide the movement to decrease the bilateral coordination and postural demands. A more demanding bilateral response could include pulling a rope and catching a fish simultaneously. Unexpected movements of the boat, fish, and whales will require greater timing and planning for success.

For this intervention technique to be appropriate, the motor and planning difficulties observed in a child with learning disabilities need to be a result of deficits in processing sensory information. Each child's intervention plan should be individualized based on the results of a comprehensive evaluation and responses to sensory input within therapy. Aspects of modulation and discrimination of sensation will be considered for their impact on functional motor performance. Sensory modulation difficulties can result in heightened responsiveness to sensation, thereby increasing the child's arousal level, which can impact successful peer interactions and safety on the playground. Sensitivity to movement input can cause the child to avoid playground equipment or become nauseated during car rides. Discrimination difficulties can significantly impact the quality of motor performance and the acquisition of prepositional concepts (i.e., up, down, left, right, in front of, behind, next to). The child who has difficulty discriminating information from his or her body can exhibit deficits in body awareness, force grading, balance, timing movements in space, bilateral and eye-hand coordination, fine motor control, and handwriting.

Vestibular, proprioceptive, and tactile sensory inputs used in therapy are powerful and must be applied with caution. The autonomic and behavioral responses of the child must be monitored carefully. The therapist should be knowledgeable about sensory integration theory and intervention before using these procedures. Monitoring behavioral responses after the therapy session also is suggested through parent or teacher consultation. Intervention precautions are elaborated by Ayres[14] and Koomar and Bundy.[162]

Research on the Effects of Sensory Integration Procedures. Within the field of occupational therapy, sensory integration is the most well-documented intervention procedure. According to Gaddes,[90] sensory integration is one of the most articulated and best-developed programs of sensorimotor training for children with learning disabilities. Despite this, disagreement persists on the value of this therapeutic modality.

When considering the multiple reviews of sensory intervention *effectiveness*, a lack of consistency and agreement exist.[°] In relation to children with learning disabilities, Hoehn and Baumeister[130] concluded that sensory integration therapy was both unproven and ineffective.

Henderson,[124] however, concluded that "the studies . . . [of sensory integration] provide preliminary evidence of the value of sensory integrative therapy for children with learning disabilities."[124 (p 45)] Clinicians using sensory integration procedures also are convinced of the effectiveness of this treatment approach in making important functional changes. Testimonials from parents of children who have received occupational therapy using sensory integration procedures are frequently heard. Perhaps the inconsistencies noted in research on sensory integration effectiveness are due to the complex characteristics of children receiving intervention and to the challenge of creating a structured research model for an intervention that adapts frequently to the child's changing needs.

The empirical data continue to raise questions about *who, how,* and *what* sensory integration procedures affect.[214] Studies have not adequately controlled for the heterogeneity of children with sensory integration dysfunction. Ottenbacher[212] performed a meta-analysis, based on eight studies of children with a wide range of diagnoses including learning disabilities, mental retardation, aphasia, and children at risk. A study by Densem and co-workers[75] included subjects who "exhibited a wide array of handicapping conditions, including mild mental retardation, behavioral disturbance, mild cerebral palsy, and epilepsy."[75 (p 223)] The variation of this population confused the study results and encouraged the authors to consider not "How effective was the program?" but, rather, "How does it work and for whom?"[75 (p 228)]

Sensory integration effectiveness research also is confounded by variable treatment designs and outcome

---

°See references 9, 50, 51, 56, 130, 137–139, 195, 215, 223, and 224.

measures. Clark and Pierce[57] found 26 effectiveness studies that included four different independent variables including sensory integration procedures, systematically applied vestibular stimulation, multisensory input, and perceptual-motor training. In reviewing effectiveness studies, Cermak and Henderson[50, 51] identified at least six different outcome measures, including academic measures, language outcomes, motor skills, postrotatory nystagmus, self-stimulatory behaviors, and behavioral outcomes. When considering the incredible variation in the approaches within research studies it is understandable that consensus on intervention effectiveness is lacking.

Several studies have demonstrated some improvements in sensory integrative measures.[137–139] In a three-year follow-up study, Wilson and Kaplan[287] found that sensory integration intervention had a more sustained impact on gross motor performance. Humphries and colleagues[139] found that subjects treated with a sensory integration approach showed an advantage in motor planning. Depauw[76] reported sensory integration procedures to be more effective than remedial physical education in improving scores on perceptual-motor and fine motor tests. A recent study of intensive short-term sensory integration intervention with children with special needs demonstrated a reduction in soft neurological signs, extremes of activity level, and increased predictability and adaptability compared with a matched group.[157] Self-esteem was shown to significantly increase in a sample of 67 children with learning disabilities randomized into two groups after sensory integration intervention.[224] The results of these studies suggest that motor and behavior measures may be more effective outcome measures for sensory integration intervention.

Several studies[139, 148, 224] have suggested that sensory integration intervention is not more effective in motor skill development than more traditional skill-based therapies. One recognized confounding variable is the heterogeneity of the study subjects.[170] Another difficulty is in determining the best outcome measures of improved sensory integration. Traditional motor tests may not best reflect the changes in organization, adaptability, and planning that children with sensory integration therapy consistently appear to make. Cermak and Henderson[50, 51] suggest that "organization, learning rate, attention, affect, exploratory behavior, biological rhythm (sleep-wake cycle), sensory responsivity, play skills, self-esteem, peer interactions and family adjustment" are domains that may change with sensory integration treatment.

In her review of sensory integration research with children with learning disabilities, Henderson concluded that the studies "certainly . . . provide sufficient evidence to warrant further investigation of the effects of sensory integrative therapy."[124 (p 45)] In their recent review of sensory integration effectiveness, Miller and Kinnealey[195] suggest that future studies need better controls for homogeneous samples, treatment approach, and more clearly defined hypotheses. The complexity of sensory integration theory, the individualized approaches that treatment warrants, and the difficulty finding sensitive outcome measures create many challenges in designing appropriate and valid research studies.

NEURODEVELOPMENTAL THEORY

Neurodevelopmental treatment (NDT) is a technique formulated by Karel and Bertha Bobath[38, 39] to enhance the development of gross motor skills, balance, quality of movement, and hand skills in individuals with movement disorders.[238] The original framework was based on the hierarchical levels of reflex integration in the nervous system.[39] Abnormal and normal postural reflexes were thought to be the basis of automatic changes in muscle activity[36, 37] Abnormal postural responses were lower level hierarchical reactions that did not integrate into a typical time frame (e.g., ATNR, STNR), thereby inhibiting the development of automatic postural mechanisms. The normal postural reflex action used higher-level righting and equilibrium responses as a foundation for automatic postural reactions, balance, and transitional movement patterns. In this framework the nervous system was viewed as a passive system controlled by sensory feedback.[37] The NDT approach emphasized specific ways to inhibit abnormal reactions and facilitate more normal movement patterns.[227] Treatment techniques were originally designed for individuals with cerebral palsy.

In recent years the hierarchical model of reflex integration has been replaced by the distributed control model of the nervous system. In this model the nervous system is viewed as a dynamic system capable of initiating, anticipating, and controlling movements with ongoing sensory feedforward and feedback.[37] Many factors are recognized as contributing to abnormal movement patterns, including abnormal muscle tone, influence of primitive reflex patterns, delayed development of righting and equilibrium reactions, weakness of specific muscles, inability to counteract the forces of gravity, and deficits in sensory input. The current framework of NDT is to facilitate normal movement patterns so that the individual does not develop abnormal or compensatory patterns, which lends its use to children with more minimal motor involvement. Of particular relevance to the child with learning disabilities with motor deficits is facilitation of improved righting and equilibrium responses, automatic postural adjustments, and balance reactions.

Neurodevelopmental treatment uses physical handling techniques directed toward developing the components of movement that underlie functional motor performance. Movement components of neuromotor maturation, postural alignment and stability, mobility skills, weight bearing, weight shifting, and balance are all foundations for smoothly executed movements in space.[238] This is accomplished through a combination of facilitation and inhibition techniques that use sensory input, particularly tactile-proprioceptive cues. Abnormal movement patterns are prevented whereas normal postural adjustments are guided through key points of control on the body.[65] The ultimate goals of NDT are the normalization of abnormal tonus, facilitation of active adaptive posture and movement, and integration of postural reactions to encourage the acquisition of functional movement patterns needed for learning and daily living skills.[65]

As theory and intervention practices have evolved, the need to promote better movement within the context of functional task performance has been greatly emphasized. Activities incorporate targeted reactions into the specific functional skills the child is working on. The therapist's hands guide the reactions, with the child actively participating in problem solving and adapting performance. Practice of more effective postural reactions and reduction of abnormal movement patterns are embedded into meaningful activities. A skilled therapist balances the quality of movement patterns with the importance of active problem solving and participation in learning new motor tasks.[37] At times, participation and independent task completion are more important than qualitatively normal movement patterns.[227] Knowledge of normal movement patterns, postural control, base of support, and weight shifting are important aspects of this intervention approach.[227]

Research on the Effects of Neurodevelopmental Therapy. NDT is based on principles derived from research in motor development and neurophysiology. The techniques, however, arise from careful and extensive clinical observations. There are few studies that have quantitatively assessed the effectiveness of this intervention technique. One difficulty with designing effectiveness studies to assess NDT is defining appropriate and measurable outcomes. Two studies[120, 221] that used standardized developmental motor tests as a dependent variable did not find significant differences between children treated with NDT techniques and children who were not treated. In her study of infants and toddlers with Down syndrome, Harris[120, 121] utilized individualized specific objective measures as a dependent variable. According to her findings, 80% of the treatment group reached individualized objectives, compared with only 57% of the control group. Harris, however, did not find any significant differences on the standardized motor measures. The appropriateness of these standardized tests in assessing the qualitative motor changes associated with the use of NDT are therefore questioned.

In 1986 Ottenbacher and associates[215] performed a meta-analysis on the use of NDT procedures in the pediatric population and found that the effect was small due to the small number of samples, difficulty in measuring the changes in the quality of movement and posture, and lack of rigorous control. The findings did suggest that individuals receiving NDT or some combination of NDT and other related therapy performed better than 62.2% of the subjects not receiving therapeutic service.

Of the 41 studies initially identified by Royeen and DeGangi[238] for a review of NDT effectiveness, only one quantitative study was performed.[215] Royeen and DeGangi concluded that the effectiveness studies had methodological problems due to the lack of objective outcome measures, overreliance on subjective clinical observations, and small sample size. Of the 19 studies they reviewed, sample populations varied greatly, including adults and children with cerebral palsy and Down syndrome as well as high-risk infants.

No studies were found on the use of this technique for children with learning disabilities and motor deficits. Royeen and DeGangi[238] suggested that more studies are needed. They proposed that the benefits of NDT intervention over time should be investigated before comparison of NDT and other therapeutic approaches.

MOTOR CONTROL, MOTOR LEARNING, AND MOTOR DEVELOPMENT THEORIES

Motor control is the study of the nature and cause of movement, encompassing the control of both posture and movement.[254] The organization and control of processes underlying motor behavior are considered.[281] The mechanism responsible for the control of motor behavior is the primary focus.

The motor control model is developed on the assumption that the neural structures controlling movement must adapt to the constraints of the musculoskeletal system and the physical laws governing motion.[104] Bernstein[30] proposed that the brain has difficulty controlling the many different joints and muscles of the body. The body's biomechanical system has a large number of *degrees of freedom*. Degrees of freedom in the upper extremity, for example, occur within each joint that flexes, extends, or rotates. This creates an incredible complexity and variation of movement patterns that control for functional activities such as handwriting.[30] Bernstein believed that synergies play an important role in decreasing degrees of freedom. Synergies are achieved when muscles work together as a unit.

Another mechanism that decreases the "degrees of freedom" problem is *motor programs*. Motor programs are "command sets," characterized by specific motor patterns which activate in invariant order.[279] When throwing a baseball, for example, the motor program used (the order the muscles fire, the duration of the muscular contraction, and the force levels used) is fixed. A theory incorporating motor programs is the "open-loop theory," or feedforward system. With the feedforward system of control, the nervous system does not rely on peripheral feedback but uses previous motor learning to detect errors in a movement plan before it has been executed, so that the individual can avoid errors in motor performance. The work of Nashner and McCollum[204] indicates that postural control works on a feedforward system. A person makes preparatory postural adjustments before he or she ever initiates a movement.

A feedback, or closed-loop system, depends on the recognition and correction of errors from peripheral feedback for performance. Feedback can be intrinsic or extrinsic. Intrinsic feedback is provided by sensory receptors (e.g., muscle spindles) before, during, and after movement. Extrinsic feedback is provided externally by visual or verbal information or cues.[27] If all movement depended on this type of error correction, human behavior would be extremely slow and inefficient.[241]

Feedforward and feedback work collaboratively during movement. Feedforward is used when initiating movement, and feedback assists in regulating and adapting movements. Both are learned experientially, by practice, and cannot be taught.[37]

Functional motor behaviors are critical regardless of the specific motor control theories adopted. These functional behaviors should occur in the context of a meaningful environment. The influences of environmental factors make task-related interventions essential to the development of motor control. For interventionists, the environments in which children are required to function is of paramount importance. The environment can be considered stable or variable.[279] Home and classrooms can be stable, in that many elements within these settings are fixed and do not change. The heights of the tables, sizes of chairs, and so forth are considered "variable features" within these stable environments. These variable features require a greater amount of motor control as the child must adjust movements and actions to the changing demands. Therapists generally practice in stable environments and therefore must ensure that the children are able to function under varied circumstances encountered in daily life situations. All environments must be assessed critically to determine the actions and adaptations needed to perform functional tasks relative to the child's abilities and demands.[281]

Motor learning refers to the process of acquiring the ability to produce skilled movements[102] or the modifications of movements.[254] The acquisition of motor skills through practice and experience is emphasized.[281] The acquisition of skilled movements not only depends on integration within the nervous system but also is influenced by environmental factors and human biomechanics. The acquisition of the motor behavior, whether through practice or experience, is the focus.

Motor learning occurs when the skill becomes a permanent response, regardless of the environment.[27] Motor learning cannot be directly observed, only noted through the performance of a motor skill.[281] Variables of motor learning applicable to intervention include feedback, practice, and motivation.[27]

During the process of learning, often called the skill acquisition phase, extrinsic feedback (often called knowledge of results) usually is given to the learner. "Feedback is essential for learning, but may not be necessary for the performance of a well learned task."[281 (p 21)] Therapists tend to provide excessive feedback, especially when the performance is below what is expected. Low frequency and fading feedback, progressively decreasing the rate at which feedback is provided, appears to be most effective in facilitating learning.[281] One proposed reason is that the individual does not depend on the feedback when less is provided and can engage in processes that enable learning. During intervention, therapists should allow children the opportunity to self-evaluate and correct their own performance, with only accurate and necessary feedback given. Children should be provided with motor problems that require similar processing but varying outcomes.[27]

Regardless of the intervention approach used, repetition occurs. Practice, in general, is believed to increase learning of a skill or movement. Variations in practice can occur in the order tasks are performed and in the environment where the tasks are practiced and by changing the aspects of the task. Opportunity and variety in practice appear to improve motor learning, particularly when skills are practiced in a random manner. Practice, therefore, should be varied and occur in multiple environments (e.g., home and school) to maximize motor learning. (For additional information on motor control and motor learning see Chapters 4 and 5.)

Motor development is the evolution of motor changes across the life span. This age-related process has been examined in specific age groups and the life span. Changes in motor behavior over time is the primary focus.

A life span approach to motor development has sparked research in the variety of movement patterns used to perform motor tasks from infancy throughout life. Variability in performance has been found to differ with age and activity levels. Two systems theories have explained the variety of motor development. The perceptual-action theory views motor development as functions of the perceptual system and motor system. The dynamic action theory promotes increasing the dimensions of variables until a new action is formed. A child's growth, for example, changes motor behavior. A child's motor behavior when grasping a baseball changes as the size of the hand increases. The emphasis in intervention should therefore be on age-appropriate skills and motor patterns during functional activities, regardless of the impairment.

Components of these theories of motor control appear particularly relevant to the treatment of children with learning disabilities with motor deficits. Progress is seen more rapidly when there is investment in a task-related behavior that is meaningful to the child. Eye-hand coordination tasks, for example, become more meaningful within the context of a game of hot potato or baseball.

Motor learning and control problems typically seen in children with learning disabilities and motor difficulties include clumsiness, difficulty with judging force, timing and amplitude of motions, and deficits in anticipating the results of a motor action. These children often take longer to initiate a motor action and many move in a slow, plodding fashion. Using the concepts of the motor control theories presented here, we can hypothesize that these children are experiencing difficulties with feedforward and feedback systems. Feedforward would be essential to the development of timing body movements in space in relationship to another object. Smyth[260] compared children with motor difficulties with a normal control group on a series of simple and complex movements and found that the group with motor difficulties had a longer reaction time and movement time for complex motions. He hypothesized that these children have a deficit in programming the movements; they need to rely more heavily on feedback for movement control.

Intervention using theories of motor control and learning considers how the child solves movement problems in the environment.[211] For completion of a successful task-oriented movement, the child must conform to the spatial and temporal demands of the environment. Visual and verbal cognitive strategies are used to assist the individual in performing the movement more appropriately. At times specific movement components of a task might be practiced, but they are combined in the context of the entire motor task, concentrating on the specific goal or end product of the task. The clinician should communicate the goal of the task to the child but encourage independent problem solving.

Critique of Motor Control Theories. Current motor control research involves a multidisciplinary effort, including neurophysiology, anatomy, muscle physiology, biomechanics, and behavioral sciences.[42, 104] The great number and variation of theories presented on motor control, learning, and development limit consensus on terminology and definitions. These variations impede the ability to adequately test and compare these theories using samples of children with mild motor difficulties. The variety of theories and terms used to describe motor functioning impedes researchers from understanding and interpreting related research and limits the ability to search for underlying neural mechanisms of dysfunction.[131]

SENSORIMOTOR INTERVENTION

The premise that sensorimotor performance requires organizing sensory information from the environment for use in executing motor actions[175] is the basis of sensorimotor intervention. Evolution of sensorimotor intervention has not revolved around a single, unified theory[101] but has incorporated a variety of theoretical foundations. Techniques developed for children with learning disabilities are a combination of perceptual-motor, neurodevelopmental, motor control, and sensory integration procedures.[82, 99, 175, 194]

The goal of sensorimotor intervention is outcome based, with emphasis on the development of age-appropriate perceptual-motor and gross motor skills. The therapist chooses activities to meet the child's developmental levels, promote sensory and motor foundations, and encourage practice of appropriate motor skills. Gross motor outcomes of improved muscle strength, postural control, balance, equilibrium, and planning are promoted. For the child having difficulty keeping up with the skilled activities in gym class such as rope jumping, components of these activities will be encouraged, with emphasis on sequencing and timing. The therapist may use a heavier jump rope or wrist and ankle weights to provide more sensory information for improved task performance.

In sensorimotor intervention, tasks are chosen for their innate sensory and motor components. The child is directed to activities that encourage the use of his or her body in space to complete a structured motor sequence. Activities incorporate sensory components such as movement (vestibular), touch (tactile), and heavy work for the muscles and joints (proprioception). Environmental concepts such as spatial and temporal sequencing are included in the structure of a motor activity. Play interactions are considered important to encourage sensorimotor integration within the context of meaningful interactions with persons and objects.[175] A child may propel himself or herself prone on a scooter board through an "obstacle maze" while looking for matching shapes, for example. This activity provides tactile and proprioceptive and vestibular sensory input and encourages the development of postural strength and endurance at the same time as it addresses perceptual skill development.

For further discussion of sensorimotor therapy, the reader is referred to the works of Gilfoyle and Grady,[98, 99] Heiniger and Randolph,[122] Knickerbocker,[161] Ayres,[14] and DeQuiros and Schrager.[77] These sources also describe many therapeutic activities for the development of postural functions in children with learning disabilities.

Research on Sensorimotor Intervention. DeGangi and associates[67] identified a gap between theoretical reasoning and current research in sensorimotor intervention. Studies in this intervention technique are limited. In a comparison study, DeGangi and associates[67] found that children provided with structured sensorimotor therapy made greater gains in sensory integrative foundations, gross motor skills, and performance areas such as self-care than children who engaged in child-centered activity.

MOTOR SKILL TRAINING

Motor skill training involves learning skills and subskills functionally relevant to the child's daily performance. Tasks are taught in a sequenced manner by developmental ages or by steps from simple to complex. Evaluation identifies the point at which a child fails, and intervention involves a hierarchy of tasks from gross to fine.[109, 110] Thus, a graded system that includes ongoing evaluation of performance and task acquisition is developed.

Abbie[1] described the motor skills training approach: "One can . . . break down the skills into their simplest forms and give the child opportunities to practice each in as many varied ways as possible so that he does not learn one isolated splinter skill."[1 (p 200)] As an example, Abbie suggested that a child with poor balance in standing practice balance in all positions—kneeling, all fours, sitting, and prone—and on both stable and mobile surfaces. Abbie used multiple approaches, including neurodevelopmental theory, modern dance, and gymnastics.

In general, the recommended approach for motor skill training includes indirect remediation, coupled with direct facilitation of motor skill development.[122] Much of the treatment is directed toward the acquisition of basic skills as described by Abbie.[1, 2] The goal is to provide a great variety of motor activities at the child's developmental motor level to promote motor generalizations. The activities recommended include balance, locomotion, body awareness, and hand-eye coordination. The functional relevance of these skill areas includes being able to sit at the desk within the classroom and complete written work, as well as greater success in recess games such as basketball. Specific skills such as dribbling and foul shooting also may be taught and practiced to facilitate improved social participation.

A final area of skill that should be addressed is activities of daily living. Children with DCD are frequently delayed in the basic self-care skills of tying shoelaces, using a knife and fork, and blowing their nose, as well as generally inefficient in dressing for school.[108, 110] Inadequacy in self-care is a sensitive area for children whose peers have no such difficulty, and teachers and therapists should be aware of a child's need to learn these basic skills.

MONITORING PHYSICAL FITNESS

In addition to the primary deficits in sensory integrative functions and motor skill development, a child with learning disabilities and motor deficits is at risk for poor posture, body mechanics, and physical fitness. Physical fitness, as defined here, includes strength, endurance, speed, agility, flexibility, and cardiorespiratory endurance. Arnheim and Sinclair[10] pointed out that there is a vicious cycle in the relationship between motor ability and physical fitness. The child with poor motor ability avoids physical activity, and the poor fitness that develops through lack of exercise lessens motor ability. A study of 24 7- to 9-year-old boys with DCD[206] found significantly decreased anaerobic performance and peak power and speed, with increased fatigue.

The physiologically based poor posture and inefficient body use can be exaggerated by a secondary disability. The child's poor self-concept may be reflected in a hunched, withdrawn posture and the avoidance of any physical activity beyond that needed in everyday activities. This latter pattern also can be found in children with learning disabilities without a primary motor disability.

The physical therapist should monitor and prevent or correct loss of movement in the joints of the neck and spine and work with the physical educator to ensure that a child receives sufficient exercise to maintain his or her physical fitness. Arnheim and Sinclair[10] presented graded levels of activities for fitness in the four areas of strength and muscular endurance, flexibility, agility and large muscle coordination, and cardiorespiratory endurance. The reader is referred to Arnheim and Sinclair[10] and Larkin and Hoare[165] for further discussion of physical fitness and a developmental program for children with problems in motor coordination.

Summary

Children with learning disabilities frequently have motor coordination problems. The presenting motor deficits may be subtle and difficult to pick up using neurological evaluation or standardized testing. When undetected, motor difficulties may have significant impact on the qualitative development of age-appropriate motor skills, limiting functional performance at home and school. The child's inability to master basic motor skills such as dressing and bicycle riding further affects self-esteem, peer relations, and societal participation.

Motor performance and movement are important aspects of a child's total development, including academic growth. Automatic postural control provides stability needed to sit upright in a chair for participation in academic tasks and freedom of movement for exploration within his or her environment. Movement through space and body awareness precedes prepositional concept development. A child first understands the words up, down, left, and right on his or her own body. A multitude of factors have to be considered in the development of each individual's learning capacities. Lerner stated that:

We cannot conclude that motor development is unimportant or that this aspect of learning should be discarded. Rather, these studies suggest that plans are needed for building the bridge between motor training and academic learning. Efficient motor movement may be a prerequisite but alone it is insufficient.[171 (p 155)]

Many theoretical models have been developed in an attempt to explain the qualitative motor deficits observed in children with learning disabilities as well as to provide constructs to develop intervention programs. All have certain relevance to this population and perhaps to each individual child. Many of the approaches share common assumptions, although rationales and intervention strategies may vary markedly. Several theories and intervention approaches have been presented to give a spectrum of alternatives in working with children with DCD.

Each child presents a unique composite of clinical signs

and functional deficits, and the therapist is challenged to assess the child appropriately, to identify strengths and weaknesses, and to formulate an intervention program that best addresses the underlying deficits in foundation skills and the functional weaknesses in daily life tasks. The experienced interventionist will combine knowledge from many areas of theoretical development and remediation to facilitate the best performance in each child.

LEARNING DISABILITIES ACROSS THE LIFE SPAN

Research with adolescents and adults with learning disabilities has indicated that, for the most part, children do not outgrow learning disabilities. They are a life span disability. Problems tend to persist in some or all of the following areas: attention and activity, cognitive and academic performance, motor skills, emotional adjustment, and social interactions.

Follow-up studies of children with high activity levels indicate that although hyperactivity itself becomes less of a problem as children get older, many other problems exist. Routh and Mesibov[237] found that, of 83 teenagers who had been hyperactive as children, 58% had failed one or more grades in school, many had low self-esteem, and several had been involved in delinquent behavior. Weiss[283] did a 5-year follow-up study of children with hyperactivity and found that 70% had repeated at least one grade as compared with 15% of matched control subjects. In a second 5-year follow-up study, Hoy and colleagues[134] found that although activity declined at adolescence, attentional and stimulus-processing difficulties persisted that affected both academic and social functioning. Overall, results indicated that childhood hyperactivity was often predictive of continued academic failure, poor concentration, impulsivity, behavioral difficulties, and low self-esteem.

Helper[123] reviewed follow-up studies of children with learning disabilities and found that, both emotionally and behaviorally, boys continued to have a much higher frequency of problems than controls. In addition, persistent deficits in learning skills (e.g., reading achievement), along with deficits in attention and information processing were noted. Research also has indicated that there are long-term academic effects of learning disabilities during the school years. To ascertain whether children outgrow learning disabilities, Book[41] tested 472 Utah kindergarten children on standardized tests and assigned each student to one of three categories of presumed risk. Students were retested on academic achievement tests in first through fourth grades. Less than 11% of the students assigned to the high-risk group ever performed above the fiftieth percentile. Only 4% in the lowest-risk group ever performed below the twenty-fifth percentile. Parham's[217] recent four-year longitudinal study of elementary school children supported the belief that children with learning disabilities do not outgrow perceptual-motor problems related to academic achievement.

Within the motor domain, there is increasing evidence that children do not outgrow their deficits despite some arguments to the contrary.[4] Denckla[72, 73] pointed out that although many children with motor difficulties do eventually master specific motor skills, they fail new age-appropriate ones. Longitudinal studies have found an association between childhood motor deficits and later learning difficulties and psychological problems.[53, 176] Cantell and colleagues[47] provided additional evidence in a longitudinal study that adolescents with DCD have lower academic achievement, fewer spare time activities, poor opinion of their competence, and lower aspirations.

Learning disabilities and motor impairments appear to have a persistent effect on self-concept.[222] Of the adolescent populations with learning disabilities or hyperactivity studied, 40% to 60% have low self-esteem.[264] Depression, thoughts of suicide, and low expectations for the future also seemed to be more prevalent in the adolescent with a learning disability.[183]

In recent years, the relationship between learning disabilities and juvenile delinquency has been explored.[165, 291] A high rate of antisocial behavior in adolescence, "trouble

A LETTER FROM AN ADULT WITH A LEARNING DISABILITY

I am 26 years old, a professional bassoonist with a master's degree in Music Performance. My name is Wendy. Through Jane, an occupational therapist, I discovered when I was 24 years old that I had learning problems and sensory integration problems.

I invert letters and especially numbers. When people speak English to me, I feel it's a foreign language. There's translation lag time. When learning new things, I either understand intuitively or never. I can't seem to go through step-by-step learning processes.

Physically, I'm extremely sensitive to motion. When I was little, we moved every year. I spent the first 5 years of my life feeling sick. It seems that I feel everything more strongly than most people. I have an extremely low threshold of pain and even pleasure tends to overload me. If I am touched unexpectedly it hurts; it's so jarring. This causes a lot of problems with interpersonal relationships. I can't stand to have people close to me; it produces an adrenalin reaction.

Motor activities are also a problem; my muscles don't seem to remember past motions. Despite the many times I've walked down steps and through doors, I still have to think about how high to lift my foot and about planning my movements. When eating, I have to think about chewing or I bite my tongue or mouth. I don't think other people think about these things. I'm physically inept; I can bump into the same table 10 times running. I'm always bruised, and as a child people constantly labeled me as clumsy. Physical education courses were hell as a child, especially gymnastics, where you are forced to leave the ground and swing or walk on balance beams or uneven bars. I cannot begin to explain the terror or disorientation.

Academically, I was labeled stupid or, more frequently, lazy. I was told that I was not trying. Actually, my IQ is very high and my coping mechanisms are very complex. If they only knew how hard I was trying. I was lucky because I taught myself to read at an early age. I would never have learned to read otherwise. Even so, my first grade teacher wouldn't believe that I could read so far past my age. She called me a liar when I said that I had finished each stupid "Dick-Jane" book. I was forced to read each one 50 times before she would give me a new one.

Not all teachers were so insensitive. My fourth grade teacher made every effort to let me go at my own pace, letting me read on a college level and do 2 years of math on my own. Left to my own devices, I can learn and love to do so. My fifth grade teacher forced me to do math the long way with steps. I just know the answer by looking at multiplication or division problems, even algebra problems, but to this day I cannot understand how one does it in steps. If a teacher didn't accept this, I was in for a year of hell. I cried a lot in school, from frustration mostly, and I pretended to be sick a lot.

I never had friends until college. I guess I was too different to be acceptable. I grew up in a very rigid, repressive, religious community which made it especially difficult to be accepted. My differences were labeled evil or, at best, I was ignored. I left high school at age 16 for college, where at least I could structure what I wanted to learn. It's never been easy for me to make friends, although it's better now. Music circles tend to be a bit crazy so I fit in more easily.

My learning disabilities still are problems. My motor and learning problems get in the way of my music, but my coping mechanisms are strong. I deal better with my clumsiness now. Just being diagnosed by Jane has made a big difference. To have things labeled, to be told and realize that it's not my fault, has given me a sense of peace. It's also allowed me to turn from inward depression to outward anger at those who labeled me stupid and clumsy. Just being able to admit anger allows one to let it go.

Other than my testing and subsequent conversations with Jane, I have not received treatment for my problems. I believe that adults with my problems can be helped. I wish programs were available in all areas of the country. At age 26, I feel much better about myself than I did even at age 24. It's a matter of growth and coping with major differences.

The greatest advice I would give to educators and therapists working with problem children is: accept. Accept what they can do well; don't make an issue of what they can't do. We all have our strengths and weaknesses. If a child can't do math, so what! Buy the child a calculator and the child will do a lot better with it than with a label of stupidity following her through life.

with the law," or "police contact" are found frequently in follow-up studies of children with learning disabilities.[46, 176] Several studies of delinquent adolescent boys have shown that 25% to 30% have learning disabilities,[81] and Mauser[182] reported that 50% to 70% of juvenile delinquents in his sample exhibited evidence of learning disabilities. Some clinicians believe that the educational and psychological trauma within the classroom may be expressed later as aberrant social functioning in the community.[291]

Less information is available on adults with learning disabilities, in part because "learning disabilities" were not diagnostic entities until the 1960s. Many of the reports on learning disabilities in adulthood are from persons who were diagnosed in their teenage or adult years. Thus, they did not receive the early intervention services that children with learning disabilities are currently receiving. Therefore, we are unable to evaluate the effectiveness of treatment or its impact on long-term disabilities.

Much of our knowledge about the adult with a learning disability today is anecdotal and in the form of case histories. Few research studies have systematically explored the continued effects of a learning disability in adulthood. Review of the literature regarding adults with learning disabilities indicates that difficulties can be expressed throughout the total personality—cognitively, perceptually, and emotionally.[7] Functional difficulties also persist and are seen in vocational adjustment, work management, and social and family interactions.[52]

The same cycles of ineptitude, frustration, and anxiety experienced by the child with learning disabilities may be repeated as an adult. Mrs. B., Paul's mother in Case Study 11–2, articulates this. She was not diagnosed with learning disabilities until age 20. Nevertheless, she completed both college and a master's degree in counseling. Although the academic frustrations were no longer an issue, the learning disability interferes with her work and home performance. Mrs. B. describes her organizational difficulties and identifies a continuous need to make lists to function in her job. She concentrates on not looking "clumsy" and is fearful she will trip over things and look foolish. Learning and accomplishing things continues to require increased effort as compared with her peers. Thus, it is apparent that as an adult, the learning disability continues to present difficulty in functional performance.

A letter from a woman with learning disabilities, motor coordination impairments, and sensory integration problems is included in the box on page 337. She describes how her learning disability affects her current functioning and how it affected her when she was a child.

SUMMARY

Meeting the needs of the child with learning disabilities offers new challenges in occupational and physical therapy. As a result of the passage of PL 94–142 and IDEA, intervention with children is moving from the clinical to academic arena. Providing comprehensive service requires variety in patterns of service delivery, with an increase in consultation and inservice education. When presented with the subtle motor deficits that are frequently part of DCD the therapist must develop and refine skills in assessment and intervention.

Occupational and physical therapists assume an important role in educating the team of professionals and parents to the importance of motor deficits to functional performance and societal participation. Within the school system motor deficits must have educational relevance to warrant remediation. Service provision within the LRE might begin with education of the teacher and accommodations to the classroom. If this approach does not facilitate adequate functional abilities, intervention in or out of the classroom may be warranted.

The child's motor needs must be assessed in the context of overall educational and emotional development. The question is not whether the child *would* benefit from therapy but *which types* of remediation are the most essential for the child at a given time in his or her development. Some children with coordination difficulties cope quite well as long as their problem is recognized. Gubbay says, "Bringing the child into focus by the recognition of his problem immediately reduces the pressures to conform."[110 (p 157)] In an environment where parents, teachers, peers, and the child recognize the nature of the deficit and set reasonable expectations, some children accept their motor disability, and academic skills and alternative forms of recreation assume greater importance.

As this review has indicated, evidence supporting the effectiveness of intervention of motor deficits in children with learning disabilities is as yet fragmentary. Children with learning disabilities present highly variable patterns of disability that make it difficult to predict or measure response to therapy. Continued formal research and careful documentation of clinical outcomes are needed to explore and define the dimensions of motor disorders in children with learning disabilities that are relevant to therapy. Only then can we better categorize children, improve the precision of treatment, and validate theory.

REFERENCES

1. Abbie MH: Physical treatment for clumsy children—not enough? Physiotherapy 64:198, 1978.
2. Abbie MH, et al: The clumsy child: Observations in cases referred to the gymnasium of the Adelaide Children's Hospital over a three-year period. Med J Aust 1:65, 1978.
3. Adelman HS, Taylor L: An Introduction to Learning Disabilities. Glenview, IL, Scott Foresman & Co, 1986.
4. American Academy of Pediatrics: Committee on children with disabilities: School-age children with motor disabilities. Pediatrics 76:648–649, 1985.
5. American Psychiatric Association: Diagnostic and Statistical Manual of Mental Disorders, 3rd ed, revised (DSM-III-R). Washington, DC, American Psychiatric Association, 1987.
6. American Psychiatric Association: Diagnostic and Statistical Manual of Mental Disorders, 4th ed (DSM-IV). Washington, American Psychiatric Association, 1994.
7. Ames TH: Post secondary problems: An optimistic approach. *In* Weber RE (ed): Handbook on Learning Disabilities: A Prognosis for the Child, the Adolescent, the Adult. Englewood Cliffs, NJ, Prentice-Hall, 1974.
8. Amundson SJ: Evaluation of Children's Handwriting (ETCH). Homer, AK, OT Kids, 1995.
9. Arendt RE, MacLean WE, Baumeister A: Critique of sensory integration theory and its application in mental retardation. Am J Ment Defic 92:401, 1988.

10. Arnheim DD, Sinclair WA: The Clumsy Child: A Program of Motor Therapy. St. Louis, CV Mosby, 1979.

11. Ayres AJ: Patterns of perceptual motor dysfunction in children: A factor analytic study. Percept Mot Skills 20:335, 1965.

12. Ayres AJ: Deficits in sensory integration in educationally handicapped children. J Learning Dis 2:160, 1969.

13. Ayres AJ: Characteristics of types of sensory integrative dysfunction. Am J Occup Ther 25:329, 1971.

14. Ayres AJ: Sensory integration and learning disorders. Los Angeles, Western Psychological Services, 1972.

15. Ayres AJ: Types of sensory integrative dysfunction among disabled learners. Am J Occup Ther 26:13, 1972.

16. Ayres AJ: Sensorimotor foundations of academic ability. In Cruickshank WM, Hallahan DP (eds): Perceptual and Learning Disabilities in Children, Vol 2, Research and Theory. New York, Syracuse University Press, 1975.

17. Ayres AJ: Southern California Postrotary Nystagmus Test. Los Angeles, Western Psychological Services, 1975.

18. Ayres AJ: Interpreting the Southern California Sensory Integration Tests. Los Angeles, Western Psychological Services, 1976.

19. Ayres AJ: Cluster analyses of measures of sensory integration. Am J Occup Ther 31:362, 1997.

20. Ayres AJ: Learning disabilities and the vestibular system. J Learning Dis 11:18, 1978.

21. Ayres AJ: Sensory Integration and the Child. Los Angeles, Western Psychological Services, 1980.

22. Ayres AJ: Southern California Sensory Integration Tests Manual, Revised. Los Angeles, Western Psychological Services, 1980.

23. Ayres AJ: Developmental Dyspraxia and Adult Onset Apraxia. Torrance, CA, Sensory Integration International, 1985.

24. Ayres AJ: The Sensory Integration and Praxis Tests. Los Angeles, Western Psychological Services, 1988.

25. Ayres AJ, Mailloux Z, Wendler C: Developmental dyspraxia: Is it a unitary function? Occup Ther J Res 7(2):93, 1987.

26. Badian NA, Wolff PH: Manual asymmetries of motor sequencing in boys with reading disabilities. Cortex 13:343, 1977.

27. Baker B: Principles of motor learning for school-based occupational therapy practitioners. School System Special Interest Section Q 6(2):1–4, 1999.

28. Bannatyne A: Language, Reading and Learning Disabilities. Springfield, IL, Charles C Thomas, 1971.

29. Benbow M: A neurodevelopmental approach to teaching handwriting. Lecture notes from a workshop presented March 1990.

30. Bernstein N: The Coordination and Regulation of Movements. Elmsford, NY, Pergamon Press, 1967.

31. Berry CA, Shaywitz SE, Shaywitz BA: Girls with attention deficit disorder: A silent minority? A report on behavioral and cognitive characteristics. Pediatrics 76:133–136, 1985.

32. Berry KE: Developmental Test of Visual-Motor Integration (VMI), 4th ed. Cleveland, Modern Curriculum Press, 1997.

33. Binet A, Simon T: Le dévelopment de l'intelligence chez l'enfant. Année Psychol 14:1, 1908.

34. Black PE: Brain Dysfunction in Children: Etiology, Diagnosis and Management. New York, Raven Press, 1981.

35. Black PE: Introduction: Changing concepts of "brain damage" and "brain dysfunction." In Black PE (ed): Brain Dysfunction in Children: Etiology, Diagnosis and Management. New York, Raven Press, 1981.

36. Bly L: The Components of Normal Movement During the First Year of Life and Abnormal Motor Development. Oak Park, IL, NDT, 1983.

37. Bly L: A historical and current view of the basis of NDT. Pediatr Phys Ther 3:131–135, 1991.

38. Bobath K: The motor deficits in patients with cerebral palsy. In Clinics in Developmental Medicine, No. 23. London, The National Spastics Society Medical Education and Information Unit in association with William Heinemann Medical Books, 1966.

39. Bobath KA, Bobath B: Neuro-developmental treatment. In Scrutton D (ed): Management of the Motor Disorders in Children with Cerebral Palsy, 2nd ed. Philadelphia, JB Lippincott, 1984.

40. Boder E: Developmental dyslexia: A diagnostic approach based on three typical reading-spelling patterns. Dev Med Child Neurol 15:663–687, 1973.

41. Book RM: Identification of educationally at-risk children during the kindergarten year: A four-year follow-up study of group test performance. Psychol Schools 17:153, 1980.

42. Bradley NS: Motor control: Developmental aspects of motor control in skill acquisition. In Campbell SK (ed): Physical Therapy for Children. Philadelphia, WB Saunders, 1995.

43. Brown JK, Minns RA: The neurological basis of learning disorders in children. In Whitmore K, Hart H, Willems G: A Neurodevelopmental Approach to Specific Learning Disorders. High Holborn, London, MacKeith Press, 1999.

44. Bruininks RH: Bruininks-Oseretsky Test of Motor Proficiency. Minnesota, American Guidance Service, 1978.

45. Bundy A: A conceptual model of school system practice for occupational and physical therapists. Lecture notes from a conference presented in November 1991.

46. Cannon IP, Compton CL: School dysfunction in the adolescent. Pediatr Clin North Am 27:79, 1980.

47. Cantell MH, Marjo H, Smith MM, Ahonen TP: Clumsiness in adolescence: Educational, motor, and social outcomes of motor delay detected at 5 years. Adapted Phys Activity Q 11(2):115–129, 1994.

48. Cermak S: Developmental dyspraxia. In Roy E (ed): Neuropsychological Studies of Apraxia and Related Disorders. New York, Elsevier Science, 1985.

49. Cermak SA: Somatodyspraxia. In Fisher AG, Murray EA, Bundy AC (eds): Sensory Integration: Theory and Practice, Philadelphia, FA Davis, 1991.

50. Cermak SA, Henderson A: The effectiveness of sensory integration procedures: I. Sensory Integration Q 17(4):1–5, 1989.

51. Cermak SA, Henderson A: The effectiveness of sensory integration procedures: II. Sensory Integration Q 18(1):1–17, 1990.

52. Cermak SA, Murray E: The adult with learning disabilities: Where do all the children go? Work 2(2):41–47, 1991.

53. Cermak SA, Trimball H, Coryell J, Drake C: Bilateral motor coordination in adolescents with and without learning disabilities. Phys Occup Ther Pediatr 10:5–18, 1990.

54. Cermak S, Ward E, Ward L: The relationship between articulation disorders and motor coordination in children, Am J Occup Ther 40:546, 1986.

55. Cermak SA, et al: The persistence of motor deficits in older students with learning disabilities, Jpn J Sensory Integration 2:17–31, 1991.

56. Clark FA, Pierce D: Synopsis of pediatric occupational therapy effectiveness: Studies on sensory integrative procedures, controlled vestibular stimulation, other sensory stimulation approaches, and perceptual-motor training. Paper presented at the Occupational Therapy for Maternal and Child Health Conference, Santa Monica, CA, 1986.

57. Clark F, Pierce D: Synopsis of pediatric occupational therapy effectiveness. Sensory Integration 16(2), 1988.

58. Clements SD: Minimal brain dysfunction in children: Terminology and identification. NINDB Monograph No. 3. Washington, DC, U.S. Department of Health, Education, and Welfare, 1966.

59. Cratty BJ: Perceptual and Motor Development in Infants and Children. Englewood Cliffs, NJ, Prentice-Hall, 1986.

60. Critchley M: The Dyslexic Child. London, William Heinemann, 1970.

61. Crowell DH, et al: Unilateral cortical activity in newborn infants: An early index of cerebral dominance? Science 180:205–208, 1973.

62. Cruickshank WM, et al: Learning Disabilities, the Struggle from Adolescence Toward Adulthood. Syracuse, NY, Syracuse University Press, 1980.

63. Danella E, Vogtle L: Neurodevelopmental treatment for the young child with cerebral palsy. In Case-Smith J, Pehoski C (eds): Development of Hand Skills in the Child. Rockville, MD, American Occupational Therapy Association, 1992.

64. Dare MT, Gordon N: Clumsy children: A disorder of perception and motor organization. Dev Med Child Neurol 12:178–185, 1970.

65. DeGangi GA: Perspectives on the integration of neurodevelopmental treatment and sensory integrative therapy. NDTA Newsletter 1(4), January 1990.

66. DeGangi GA, et al: The measurement of vestibular based dysfunction in pre-school children. Am J Occup Ther 34:452, 1980.

67. DeGangi GA, et al: A comparison of structured sensorimotor therapy and child-centered activity in the treatment of preschool children with sensorimotor problems. Am J Occup Ther 47:778–785, 1993.

68. Deloria DJ: Review of Miller Assessment for Preschoolers. In

Mitchell JV Jr (ed): The Ninth Mental Measurements Yearbook. Lincoln, NB, University of Nebraska Press, 1985.

69. Denckla MB: Development of motor coordination in normal children. Dev Med Child Neurol 16:729, 1974.

70. Denckla MB: MBD and dyslexia: Beyond diagnosis by exclusion. Top Child Neurol 19:253, 1977.

71. Denckla MB: The neuropsychology of social-emotional learning disability, Arch Neurol 40:461–462, 1983.

72. Denckla MB: Developmental dyspraxia: The clumsy child. In Levine MD, Satz P (eds): Middle Childhood Development and Dysfunction. Baltimore, University Park Press, 1984.

73. Denckla MB, et al: Motor proficiency in dyslexic children with and without attentional disorders. Arch Neurol 42:228, 1985.

74. Denckla MB, Rudel R: Rapid automatized naming (RAN): Dyslexia different from the other learning disabilities. Neuropsychologia, 14:976, 1976.

75. Densem JF, et al: Effectiveness of a sensory integrative therapy program for children with perceptual-motor deficits. J Learning Dis 22(4):221–229, 1989.

76. Depauw KP: Enhancing the sensory integration of aphasic students. J Learning Dis 11:142, 1978.

77. DeQuiros J, Schrager O: Neuropsychological Fundamentals in Learning Disabilities. San Rafael, CA, Academic Therapy Publications, 1979.

78. Deuel RK, Robinson DJ: Developmental motor signs. In Tupper DE (ed): Soft Neurological Signs. New York, Grune & Stratton, 1987.

79. Dunn W, Campbell PH: Designing pediatric service provision. In Dunn W (ed): Pediatric Occupational Therapy: Facilitating Effective Service Provision. Thorofare, NJ, Charles B Slack, 1991.

80. Exner CE: In-hand manipulation skills. In Case-Smith J, Pehoski C: Development of Hand Skills in the Child. Rockville, MD, American Occupational Therapy Association, 1992.

81. Faigel HC: The learning disabled adolescent. In Gottlieb MI, et al (eds): Current Issues in Developmental Pediatrics: The Learning Disabled Child. New York, Grune & Stratton, 1979.

82. Farber SD: Neurorehabilitation: A Multisensory Approach. Philadelphia, WB Saunders, 1982.

83. Finucci MM: Genetic considerations in dyslexia. In Myklebust HR (ed): Progress in Learning Disabilities, Vol 4. New York, Grune & Stratton, 1978.

84. Fisher AG: Vestibular-proprioceptive processing. In Fisher AG, Murray EA, Bundy AC (eds): Sensory Integration: Theory and Practice. Philadelphia, FA Davis, 1991.

85. Fisher AG, Bundy AC: Vestibular stimulation in the treatment of postural and related disorders. In Payton OD, et al (eds): Manual of Physical Therapy Techniques. New York, Churchill Livingstone, 1989.

86. Fisher AG, Murray EA: Introduction to sensory integration theory. In Fisher AG, Murray EA, Bundy AC (eds): Sensory Integration: Theory and Practice. Philadelphia, FA Davis, 1991.

87. Fisher AG, Murray EA, Bundy AC: Sensory Integration: Theory and Practice. Philadelphia, FA Davis, 1991.

88. Folio MR, Fewell R: Peabody Developmental Motor Scales (PDMS), revised experimental edition. Allen, TX, DLM Teaching Resources, 1983.

89. Ford FR: Diseases of the Nervous System in Infancy, Childhood and Adolescence, 5th ed. Springfield, IL, Charles C Thomas, 1966.

90. Gaddes WH: Learning Disabilities and Brain Function: A Neuropsychological Approach, 2nd ed. New York, Springer-Verlag, 1985.

91. Galaburda AM: Neurology of developmental dyslexia. Curr Opin Neurobiol 3:237–242, 1993.

92. Gallico R, Lewis MEB: Learning disabilities. In Batshaw ML, Perret YM (eds): Children with Disabilities: A Medical Primer, 3rd ed. Baltimore, Paul H Brookes, 1992.

93. Gardner MF: Test of Visual-Motor Skills (TVMS). San Francisco, Psychological and Educational Publications, 1995.

94. Gardner RA, Broman M: The Purdue Pegboard: Normative data on 1334 school children. J Clin Child Psychol 1:156, 1979.

95. Gazzaniga MS: Brain theory and minimal brain dysfunction. Acad Sci 205:89, 1973.

96. Geschwind N: Language and the brain. Sci Am 226:76, 1972.

97. Geschwind N, Galaburda A: Cerebral lateralization: Biological mechanisms, associations, and pathology: I, II, III. Arch Neurol 42:428–459, 521–552, 634–654, 1985.

98. Gilfoyle EM, Grady A: A developmental theory of somatosensory perception. In Henderson A, Coryell J (eds): The Body Senses and Perceptual Deficit. Proceedings of the Occupational Therapy Symposium on Somatosensory Aspects of Perceptual Deficit. Boston, Boston University, 1972.

99. Gilfoyle EM, et al: Children Adapt. Thorofare, NJ, Charles B. Slack, 1981.

100. Gillberg IC: Children with minor neurodevelopmental disorders: III. Neurological and neurodevelopmental problems at age 10. Dev Med Child Neurol 27:3, 1985.

101. Goldman L: Sensory motor activity not necessarily SI. OT Week 2(10):8, 1988.

102. Goodgold-Edwards SA: Clinical application of motor control and motor learning theory. Massachusetts Chapter Physical Therapy Lecture Series, January 1993.

103. Goodwin WL, Driscoll LA: Handbook for Measurement and Evaluation in Early Childhood Education. San Francisco, Jossey-Bass, 1980.

104. Gordon J: Assumptions underlying physical therapy intervention: Theoretical and historical perspectives. In Carr JH, Shepard RB: Movement Science: Foundations for Physical Therapy in Rehabilitation. Rockville, MD, Aspen Publications, 1987.

105. Gordon N: Children with developmental dyscalculia [annotation]. Dev Med Child Neurol 34:459–463, 1992.

106. Gordon N: Dyslexia—why can't I learn to read? In Whitmore K, Hart H, Willems G (eds): A Neurodevelopmental Approach to Specific Learning Disorders. High Holborn, London, MacKeith Press, 1999.

107. Gottlieb MI: The learning-disabled child: Controversial issues revisited. In Gottlieb MI, et al (eds): Current Issues in Developmental Pediatrics: The Learning Disabled Child. New York, Grune & Stratton, 1979.

108. Gubbay SS: The Clumsy Child. New York, WB Saunders, 1975.

109. Gubbay SS: The management of developmental apraxia. Dev Med Child Neurol 20:643, 1978.

110. Gubbay SS: The clumsy child. In Rose FC (ed): Pediatric Neurology. London, Blackwell Scientific Publications, 1979.

111. Gubbay SS, et al: Clumsy children: A study of apraxic and agnosic deficits in 21 children. Brain 85:295, 1963.

112. Haley S, Coster W, Binda-Sundberg K: Measuring physical disablement: The contextual challenge. Phys Ther 74:74–82, 1994.

113. Hall DM: Clumsy children. BMJ 296:375–376, 1988.

114. Hallahan D, Cruickshank W: Psychoeducational Foundations of Learning Disabilities. Englewood Cliffs, NJ, Prentice-Hall, 1973.

115. Hammill DD: On defining learning disabilities: An emerging consensus. J Learning Dis 23(2):74–84, 1990.

116. Hanson C: A study of the presence of the asymmetrical tonic neck reflex in fifth and seventh grade children, master's thesis, 1976, Sargent College, Boston University.

117. Hardy M, et al: Developmental patterns in elemental reading skills: Phoneme-grapheme and grapheme-phoneme correspondences. J Educ Psychol 63:433, 1972.

118. Harnadek MCS, Rourke BP: Principal identifying features of the syndrome of nonverbal learning disabilities in children. J Learning Dis 27(3):144–154, 1994.

119. Harris JC: Developmental Neuropsychiatry: Assessment, Diagnosis, and Treatment of Developmental Disorders, vol II. New York, Oxford University Press, 1998.

120. Harris SR: Effects of neurodevelopmental therapy on motor performance of infants with Down's syndrome. Dev Med Child Neurol 23:477–483, 1981.

121. Harris SR: Physical therapy and infants with Down's syndrome: The effects of early intervention. Rehab Literature 42:339, 1981.

122. Heiniger MC, Randolph SL: Neurophysiological Concepts in Human Behavior. St. Louis, Mosby, 1981.

123. Helper MJ: Follow-up of children with minimal brain dysfunctions: Outcomes and predictors. In Rie HE, Rie ED (eds): Handbook of Minimal Brain Dysfunctions: A Critical View. New York, John Wiley & Sons, 1980.

124. Henderson A: Research in occupational therapy and physical therapy with children. In Camp BW (ed): Advances in Behavioral Pediatrics. Greenwich, CT, Jai Press, 1981.

125. Henderson SE, Hall D: Concomitants of clumsiness in young school children. Dev Med Child Neurol 24:448, 1982.

126. Henderson SE, Sugden D: Movement Assessment Battery for Children (ABC). Kent, England, Psychological Corporation, 1992.

127. Hiscock M, Kinsbourne M: Specialization of the cerebral hemispheres: Implications for learning. J Learning Dis 20(3):130, 1987.
128. Hoare D: Subtypes of developmental coordination disorder. Adapted Phys Activity Q 11:158–169, 1994.
129. Hoare D, Larkin D: Kinaesthetic abilities of clumsy children. Dev Med Child Neurol 33:671–678, 1991.
130. Hoehn TP, Baumeister AA: A critique of the application of sensory integration therapy to children with learning disabilities. J Learning Dis 27:6, 1994.
131. Horak FB: Assumptions underlying motor control for neurologic rehabilitation. In Lister MJ (ed): Contemporary Management of Motor Problems. Alexandria, VA, Foundation for Physical Therapy, 1991.
132. Horak F, Shumway-Cook A, Crowe TK, Black FO: Vestibular function and motor proficiency of children with impaired hearing, or with a learning disability and motor impairments. Dev Med Child Neurol 30:64–79, 1988.
133. Hoskins T, Squires J: Developmental assessment: A test for gross motor and reflex development. Phys Ther 53:117, 1973.
134. Hoy E, et al: The hyperactive child at adolescence: Cognitive, emotional and social functioning. J Abnorm Child Psychol 6:311, 1978.
135. Hughes JE, Riley A: Basic gross motor assessment. Phys Ther 61:503, 1981.
136. Hulme C, et al: Visual, kinaesthetic and cross-modal judgements of length by normal and clumsy children. Dev Med Child Neurol 24:461, 1982.
137. Humphries TW, Snider L, McDougall B: Clinical evaluation of the effectiveness of sensory integrative and perceptual motor therapy in improving sensory integrative function in children with learning disabilities. Occup Ther J Res 13:3, 1993.
138. Humphries T, Wright M, McDougall B, Vertes J: The efficacy of sensory integration therapy for children with learning disabilities. Phys Occup Ther Pediatr 10:3, 1990.
139. Humphries T, et al: A comparison of the effectiveness of sensory integrative therapy and perceptual-motor training in treating children with learning disabilities. Dev Behav Pediatr 13(1):31–40, 1992.
140. Illingsworth RS: The clumsy child. In Bax M, MacKeith RM (eds): Minimal Cerebral Dysfunction: Clinics in Developmental Medicine, No. 10. London, The National Spastics Society Medical Education and Information Unit in association with William Heinemann Medical Books, 1963.
141. Individuals with Disabilities Education Act (IDEA): 1990 Public Law 101–476.
142. Ingersoll BD, Goldstein S: Attention Deficit Disorder and Learning Disabilities, Realities, Myths and Controversial Treatments. New York, Doubleday, 1993.
143. Interagency Committee on Learning Disabilities. Report to Congress Health Resource Extension. (Public Law 99–158.) Washington, DC, October 1985.
144. Johnson D: Paper presented at the 85th Convention of the American Psychological Association, Washington, DC, September 1976.
145. Johnson DJ, Myklebust HR: Learning Disabilities: Educational Practices and Principles. New York, Grune & Stratton, 1967.
146. Johnston O, Short H, Crawford J: Poorly coordinated children: A survey of 95 cases. Child Care Health Dev 13:361–376, 1987.
147. Kalish R, Presseller S: Physical and occupational therapy. J Sch Health 50:264, 1980.
148. Kaplan BJ, et al: Reexamination of sensory integration treatment: A combination of two efficacy studies. J Learning Dis 26:342–347, 1993.
149. Kavale KA, Forness SR: History, definition and diagnosis. In Singh NN, Beale IL: Learning Disabilities: Nature, Theory, and Treatment. New York, Springer-Verlag, 1992.
150. Kavale KA, Nye C: Parameters of learning disabilities in the achievement, linguistic, neuropsychological, and social/behavioral domains. J Spec Educ 19:443–458, 1985–1986.
151. Kavanagh JF, Truss TJ (eds): Learning Disabilities, Proceedings of the National Conference. New York, York Press, 1988.
152. Kenny TJ, Burka A: Coordinating multiple interventions. In Rie HE, Rie ED (eds): Handbook of Minimal Brain Dysfunctions: a Critical View. New York, John Wiley & Sons, 1980.
153. Keogh BK: Learning disabilities: Diversity in search of order. In Wang MC, Reynolds MC, Walberg HJ (eds): The Handbook of Special Education: Research and Practice, vol 2. Oxford, Pergamon Press, 1988.
154. Keogh JF: Incidence and severity of awkwardness among regular school boys and educationally subnormal boys. Res Q 39:806–808, 1968.
155. Kephart NC: Teaching the child with a perceptual-motor handicap. In Bortner M (ed): Evaluation and Education of Children with Brain Damage. Springfield, IL, Charles C Thomas, 1968.
156. King-Thomas L, Hacker B: A Therapist's Guide to Pediatric Assessment. Boston, Little, Brown, 1987.
157. Kinnealey M, Koenig K, Eichelberger-Huecker G: Changes in special needs children following intensive short term intervention. J Dev Learning Dis 3(1):85–103, 1999.
158. Kinsbourne M: Minimal brain dysfunction as a neurodevelopmental lag. Ann NY Acad Sci 205:268, 1973.
159. Kinsbourne M: Editorials: MBD—a fuzzy concept misdirects therapeutic efforts. Postgrad Med 58:211, 1975.
160. Kirk S: National Advisory Committee on Handicapped Children: Special Education for Handicapped Children, First Annual Report. Washington, DC, U.S. Department of Health, Education, and Welfare, 1968.
161. Knickerbocker BM: A Holistic Approach to the Treatment of Learning Disorders. Thorofare, NJ, Charles B. Slack, 1980.
162. Koomar JA, Bundy AC: The art and science of creating direct intervention for theory. In Fisher AG, Murray EA, Bundy AC (eds): Sensory Integration: Theory and Practice. Philadelphia, FA Davis, 1991.
163. Koppitz EM: The Bender Gestalt Test for Young Children. New York, Grune & Stratton, 1963.
164. Landman GB, et al: Minor neurological indicators and developmental function in preschool children. Dev Behav Pediatr 7(2):97–101, 1986.
165. Lane BA: The relationship of learning disabilities to juvenile delinquency: Current status. J Learning Dis 13:20, 1980.
166. Larkin D, Hoare D: Out of Step. Nederlands, West Australia, The Active Life Foundation, 1991.
167. Laszlo JI: Child perceptuo-motor development: Normal and abnormal development of skilled behavior. In Hauert CA (ed): Developmental Psychology: Cognitive, perceptuo-motor, and Neuropsychological Perspectives. North Holland, Amsterdam, Elsevier Science Publishers, 1990.
168. Laszlo JI, Bairstow PJ: Kinaesthesis: Its measurement, training, and relationship to motor control. Q J Exp Psychol 35A:411, 1983.
169. LaVesser P, Bloomer MA: Using functional performance outcomes in a school setting. OT Week 4(38):7, 1990.
170. Law M, Polatajko HJ, Schaffer R, et al: The impact of heterogeneity in a clinical trial: Motor outcomes after sensory integration therapy. Occup Ther J Res 11:3, 1991.
171. Lerner J: Children with Learning Disorders. Boston, Houghton-Mifflin, 1976.
172. Levine M: Pediatric Examination of Educational Readiness at Middle Childhood. Cambridge, MA, Educators Publishing Service, 1985.
173. Levine MD, Brooks R, Shonkoff MD: A Pediatric Approach to Learning Disorders. New York, John Wiley & Sons, 1980.
174. Levy J, et al: Perception of bilateral chimeric figures following hemispheric deconnexion. Brain 95:61, 1972.
175. Linquist JE, Mack W, Parham LD: A synthesis of occupational behavior and sensory integration concepts in theory and practice: I. Theoretical foundations. Am J Occup Ther 36:365–374, 1982.
176. Losse A, et al: Clumsiness in children: Do they grow out of it? A 10-year follow-up study. Dev Med Child Neurol 33:55–68, 1991.
177. Lucas AR: Muscular control and coordination in minimal brain dysfunctions. In Rie HE, Rie ED (eds): Handbook of Minimal Brain Dysfunctions: A Critical View. New York, John Wiley & Sons, 1980.
178. Luria AR: Higher Cortical Functions in Man, 2nd ed. New York, Basic Books, 1980.
179. MacKeith RM: Defining the concept of minimal brain damage. In Bax M, MacKeith RM (eds): Minimal Cerebral Dysfunction. London, The National Spastics Society Medical Education and Information Unit in association with William Heinemann Medical Books, 1963.
180. Mathiowetz V, et al: The Purdue Pegboard: Norms for 14- to 19-year olds. Am J Occup Ther 40:174, 1986.

181. Mattis S, et al: Dyslexia in children and young adults: Three independent neuropsychological syndromes. Dev Med Child Neurol 17:150, 1975.

182. Mauser AJ: Learning disabilities and delinquent youth. Acad Ther 9:389, 1974.

183. Mendelson W, et al: Hyperactive children as teenagers: A follow-up study. J Nerv Ment Dis 153:273, 1971.

184. Michaels WB: Review of Miller Assessment for Preschoolers. In Mitchell JV Jr (ed): The Ninth Mental Measurements Yearbook. Lincoln, University of Nebraska Press, 1985.

185. Michael-Smith H: Reciprocal factors in the behavior syndrome of the neurologically impaired child. In Hellmuth J (ed): The Special Child in Century 21. Seattle, Special Child Publications, 1964.

186. Miller AE: Differences in Coping Strategies Between Boys with Motor Incoordination and Learning Disabilities and Normally Developing Peers. Masters thesis, Boston University, 1994.

187. Miller LJ: Miller Assessment for Preschoolers (MAP). Littleton, CO, The Foundation for Knowledge in Development, 1982.

188. Miller LJ: Longitudinal validity of the Miller Assessment for Preschoolers: Study I. Percept Mot Skills 65:211, 1987.

189. Miller LJ: Differentiating children with school-related problems after four years using the Miller Assessment for Preschoolers. Psychol Schools 25:10, 1988.

190. Miller LJ: Longitudinal validity of the Miller Assessment for Preschoolers: Study II. Percept Mot Skills 66:811, 1988.

191. Miller LJ: Miller Assessment for Preschoolers, manual 1988 revision. San Antonio, TX, The Psychological Corporation, 1988.

192. Miller LJ: The Toddler and Infant Motor Evaluation (TIME). Littleton, CO, The KID Foundation, 1992.

193. Miller LJ: FirstSTEP (Screening Test for Evaluating Preschoolers). San Antonio, TX, The Psychological Corporation, 1993.

194. Miller TG, Goldberg MA: Sensorimotor integration. Phys Ther 55:501, 1975.

195. Miller LJ, Kinnealey M: Researching the effectiveness of sensory integration. Sensory Integration Q 21(2), 1993.

196. Miller LJ, Schouten PGW: Age-related effects on the predictive validity of the Miller Assessment for Preschoolers. J Psycheduc Assess 6(2):99, 1988.

197. Missiuna C: Motor skill acquisition in children with developmental coordination disorder. Adapted Phys Activity Q 11:214–235, 1994.

198. Montessori M: The Montessori Method: Scientific Pedagogy as Applied to Child Education in the Children's Houses. E. George (trans.). New York, FA Stokes, 1912.

199. Montgomery P: Assessment of vestibular function in children. Phys Occup Ther Pediatr 5:33, 1985.

200. Murray EA: Hemispheric specialization. In Fisher AG, Murray EA, Bundy AC: Sensory Integration: Theory and Practice. Philadelphia, FA Davis, 1991.

201. Mutti M, et al: Quick Neurological Screening Test (QNST), revised edition. Novato, CA, Academic Therapy Publications, 1978.

202. Myklebust HR: Learning disabilities: Definition and overview. In Myklebust HR (ed): Progress in Learning Disabilities, Vol 1. New York, Grune & Stratton, 1968.

203. Myklebust HR: Learning disabilities and minimal brain dysfunction in children. In Tower DB (ed): The Nervous System, Vol 3, Human Communication and Its Disorders, New York, Raven Press, 1975.

204. Nashner LM, McCollum G: The organization of human postural movements: A formal basis and experimental synthesis. Behav Brain Sci 8:135–172, 1985.

205. National Institute of Health. Research Plan for the National Center for Medical Rehabilitative Research. NIH Publication No. 93–3509. Bethesda, MD, National Institute of Health, 1993.

206. O'Beirne C, Larkin D, Cable T: Coordination problems and anaerobic performance in children. Adapted Phys Activity Q 2(2):141–149, 1994.

207. O'Brien V, Cermak S, Murray E: The relationship between visual-perceptual motor abilities and clumsiness in children with and without learning disabilities. Am J Occup Ther 42:359, 1988.

208. O'Hare A: Dysgraphia and dyscalculia. In Whitmore K, Hart H, Willems G: A Neurodevelopmental Approach to Specific Learning Disorders. London, MacKeith Press, 1999.

209. Office of Education: Education of Individuals with Disabilities (IDEA), 1990, 20 U.S.C., §1401(1) (15) p. 4.

210. Orton ST: Reading, Writing, and Speech Problems in Children. New York, WW Norton, 1937.

211. Ostronsky KM: Facilitation vs motor control: Clinical management. Am PT Assoc 10(3):34–40, 1990.

212. Ottenbacher K: Identifying vestibular processing dysfunction in learning disabled children. Am J Occup Ther 33:317, 1979.

213. Ottenbacher K: Occupational therapy and special education: Some issues and concerns related to public law 94–142. Am J Occup Ther 36:81, 1982.

214. Ottenbacher K: Sensory integration therapy: Affect or effect. Am J Occup Ther 36:9, 1982.

215. Ottenbacher K, et al: Qualitative analysis of the effectiveness of pediatric therapy. Phys Ther 66:462–468, 1986.

216. Palisano KJ, Campbell SK, Harris SR: Clinical decision-making in pediatric physical therapy. In Campbell SK (ed): Physical Therapy for Children. Philadelphia, WB Saunders, 1995.

217. Parham D: Is sensory integration related to achievement? A longitudinal study of elementary school children. Sensory Integration Q 18(1):9, 16, 17, 1990.

218. Peck BB, Stackhouse T: Reading problems and family dynamics. J Learning Dis 6:506, 1973.

219. Pehoski C: Central nervous system control of precision movements of the hand. In Case-Smith J, Pehoski C (eds): Development of Hand Skills in the Child. Rockville, MD, American Occupational Therapy Association, 1992.

220. Peters JE, Romine RA, Dykman RA: A special neurological examination of children with learning disabilities. Dev Med Child Neurol 17:63–78, 1975.

221. Piper MC, et al: Early physical therapy effects on the high risk infant: A randomized control trial. Pediatrics 78:216–224, 1986.

222. Polatajko HJ: Developmental coordination disorder (DCD): Alias the clumsy child syndrome. In Whitmore K, Hart H, Willems G (eds): A Neurodevelopmental Approach to Specific Learning Disorders. London, MacKeith Press, 1999.

223. Polatajko HJ, Kaplan BJ, Wilson BN: Sensory integration for children with learning disabilities: Its status 20 years later. Occup Ther J Res 12:6, 1992.

224. Polatajko HJ, Law M, Miller J, et al: The effect of a sensory integration program on academic achievement, motor performance, and self-esteem in children identified as learning disabled: Results of a clinical trial. Occup Ther J Res 11:3, 1991.

225. Partnership for Implementing IDEA (PMP): IDEA 1997 and Final Part B Regulations. Benefits to children with disabilities. March 1999. www.ideapolicy.org

226. Rasmussen P, Gillberg C: AD(H)D, hyperkinetic disorders, DAMP, and related behaviour disorders. In Whitmore K, Hart H, Willems G (eds): A Neurodevelopmental Approach to Specific Learning Disorders. London, MacKeith Press, 1999.

227. Rast M: NDT in continuum: Micro to macro levels in therapy. Dev Disabil Spec Interest Section Q 22(2), June 1999, pp 1–4.

228. Rie ED: Soft signs in learning disabilities. In Tupper DE: Soft Neurological Signs. New York, Grune & Stratton, 1987.

229. Rie HE: Definitional problems. In Rie HE, Rie ED (eds): Handbook of Minimal Brain Dysfunctions: A Critical View. New York, John Wiley & Sons, 1980.

230. Public Law 94–142: Education for All Handicapped Children Act. November 29, 1975. U.S. Congress (Section 5B–4).

231. Roberts TDM: Neurophysiology of Posture Mechanisms, 2nd ed. Boston, Butterworth, 1978.

232. Rourke BP: Brain-behavior relationships in children with learning disabilities: A research program. Am Psychol 30:911, 1975.

233. Rourke BP (ed): Neuropsychology of Learning Disabilities: Essentials of Subtype Analysis. New York, The Guilford Press, 1985.

234. Rourke BP: Socioemotional disturbances of learning disabled children. J Consult Clin Psychol 58:801–810, 1988.

235. Rourke BP, Telegdy GA: Lateralizing significance of WISC verbal-performance discrepancies for older children with learning disabilities. Percept Mot Skills 33:875, 1975.

236. Rourke BP, et al: The relationship between WISC verbal-performance discrepancies and selected verbal, auditory-perceptual, visual-perceptual and problem solving abilities in children with learning disabilities. J Clin Psychol 27:475, 1971.

237. Routh DK, Mesibov GB: Psychological and environmental intervention: Toward social competence. In Rie HE, Rie ED (eds): Handbook of Minimal Brain Dysfunctions: A Critical View. New York, John Wiley & Sons, 1980.

238. Royeen CB, DeGangi GA: Use of neurodevelopmental treatment

as an intervention: Annotated listing of studies, 1980–1990. Percept Mot Skills 75:175–194, 1992.

239. Rutter M, Yule W: The concept of specific reading retardation. J Child Psychol Psychiatry 16:181–187, 1976.

240. Rylander P: The ATNR in eight and twelve year old LD and normal boys. Master's Thesis, Sargent College, Boston University, 1977.

241. Sabari JS: Motor learning concepts applied to activity-based intervention with adults with hemiplegia. Am J Occup Ther 45:523–529, 1990.

242. Sage G: Motor Learning and Control: A Neurophysiological Approach. Dubuque, IA, W.C. Brown, 1984.

243. Sahler OJ, et al: Learning disorders and the hyperactive child: The pediatrician's role. In Smith DH, Hoekelman RA (eds): Controversies in Child Health and Pediatric Practice. New York, McGraw-Hill, 1981.

244. Sandler AD, Watson TE, Footo M, et al: Neurodevelopmental study of writing disorders in middle childhood. J Dev Behav Pediatr 13:17–22, 1992.

245. Satz P, et al: An evaluation of a theory of specific developmental dyslexia. Child Dev 42:2009, 1971.

246. Schaffer, et al: A study of children with learning disabilities and sensorimotor problems. Phys Occup Ther Pediatr 9:101–117, 1989.

247. Schoemaker MM, Kalverboer AF: Social and affective problems of children who are clumsy: How early do they begin? Adapted Phys Activity Q 11:130–140, 1994.

248. Schwartz SE, Budd D: Mathematics for handicapped learners: A functional approach for adolescents. In Meyer E, Vergason GA, Whelan BP (eds): Promising Practices for Exceptional Children—Curriculum Implications. Denver, Love Publishing, 1983.

249. Semmes J: Hemispheric specialization: A possible clue to mechanism. Neuropsychologia 6:11, 1968.

250. Shafer S, et al: Ten year consistency in neurological test performance of children without focal neurological deficit. Dev Med Child Neurol 28:417, 1986.

251. Shaw L, Levine M, Belfer M: Developmental double jeopardy: A study of clumsiness and self-esteem in children with learning problems. J Dev Behav Pediatr 3:191, 1982.

252. Shaywitz SE, Shaywitz BA: Attention deficit disorder: Current perspectives. Pediatr Neurol 3:129–135, 1987.

253. Shumway-Cook A, Horak F, Black FO: A critical examination of vestibular function in motor impaired learning disabled children. Int J Pediatr Otorhinolaryngol 14:21–30, 1987.

254. Shumway-Cook A, Woollacott M: Motor Control: Theory and Practical Applications. Baltimore, Williams & Wilkins, 1995.

255. Siegel LS, Metsala J: Subtypes of learning disabilities. In Singh NN, Beale IL (eds): Learning Disabilities: Nature, Theory, and Treatment. New York, Springer-Verlag, 1992.

256. Siegel LS, Ryan EB: The development of working memory in normally achieving and subtypes of learning disabled children. Child Dev 60:973–980, 1989.

257. Silver AA, Hagin RA: Disorders of Learning in Childhood. New York, John Wiley & Sons, 1990.

258. Silver S: Psychologic aspects of pediatrics: Postural and righting responses in children. Pediatrics 41:493, 1952.

259. Singh NN, Beale IL: Learning Disabilities: Nature, Theory, and Treatment. New York, Springer-Verlag, 1992.

260. Smyth TR: Abnormal clumsiness in children: A defect of motor programming? Child Care Health Dev 17:283–294, 1991.

261. Smyth TR, Glencross DJ: Information processing deficits in clumsy children. Aust J Psychol 38(1):13–22, 1986.

262. Sparrow S: Dyslexia and laterality: Evidence for a developmental theory. Semin Psychiatry 1:270, 1969.

263. Sparrow S, Satz P: Dyslexia, laterality, and neuropsychological development. In Bakker BJ, Satz P (eds): Specific Reading Disabilities: Advances in Theory and Method. Rotterdam, University of Rotterdam, 1970.

264. Stewart MA, et al: Hyperactive children as adolescents: How they describe themselves. Child Psychiatr Hum Dev 4:3, 1973.

265. Strauss AA, Lehtinen LE: Psychopathology and Education of the Brain-Injured Child. New York, Grune & Stratton, 1947.

266. Sugden D, Keogh J: Problem and Movement Skill Development. Columbia, SC, University of South Carolina Press, 1990.

267. Sugden D, Wann C: The assessment of motor impairment in children with moderate learning difficulties. Br J Educ Psychol 57:225–236, 1987.

268. Tarnopol L, Tarnopol M: Brain Function and Reading Disabilities. Baltimore, University Park Press, 1977.

269. Taylor HG: Learning disabilities. In Mash EJ, Barkley RA (eds): Treatment of Childhood Disorders. New York, The Guilford Press, 1989.

270. Thompson S: The Source for Nonverbal Learning Disorders. East Moline, IL, LinguiSystems, 1997.

271. Thompson S: Nonverbal learning disorders. The Gram: Newsletter of the East Bay learning disabilities association, 1998, www.ldaca.org/gram/thompson.htm

272. Tiffin J: Purdue Pegboard Test. Lafayette, IN, Lafayette Instrument Co, 1968.

273. Touwen BCL, Prechtl HFR: The Neurological Examination of the Child with Minor Nervous Dysfunction. Philadelphia, JB Lippincott, 1970.

274. Touwen BCL, Sporrel T: Soft signs and MBD. Dev Med Child Neurol 21:528, 1979.

275. Towbin A: Neuropathologic factors in minimal brain dysfunction. In Rie HE, Rie ED (eds): Handbook of Minimal Brain Dysfunctions: A Critical View. New York, John Wiley & Sons, 1980.

276. Tseng MH, Cermak SA: The evaluation of handwriting in children. Sensory Integration Q 19(4):1–6, 1991.

277. Tseng MH, Cermak SA: The influence of ergonomic factors and perceptual-motor abilities on handwriting performance. Am J Occup Ther 47:919–926, 1993.

278. Tupper DE: The issues with "soft signs." In Tupper DE: Soft Neurological Signs. New York, Grune & Stratton, 1987.

279. Tupper DE: Soft Neurological Signs. New York, Grune & Stratton, 1987.

280. US Department of Special Education. Assistance to states for education for handicapped children: Procedures for evaluating specific learning disabilities. Federal Register, 42:250, 62, 082–62, 085, 1977.

281. VanSant A: Motor control, motor learning, and motor development. In Montgomery PC, Connolly BH: Motor Control and Physical Therapy: Theoretical Framework and Practical Application. Hixton, TX, Chattanooga Group, 1991.

282. Walton JN, Ellis E, Court DM: Clumsy children: A study of developmental apraxia and agnosia. Brain 85:603, 1963.

283. Weiss G: MBD: Critical diagnostic issues. In Rie HE, Rie ED (eds): Handbook of Minimal Brain Dysfunctions: A Critical View. New York, John Wiley & Sons, 1980.

284. Whitmore K, Bax M: What do we mean by SLD? A historical perspective. In Whitmore K, Hart H, Willems G (eds): A Neurodevelopmental Approach to Specific Learning Disorders. London, MacKeith Press, 1999.

285. Willis AG, Hooper SR, Stone BH: Neuropsychological theories of learning disabilities. In Singh NN, Beale IL (eds): Learning Disabilities: Nature, Theory, and Treatment. New York, Springer-Verlag, 1992.

286. Willoughby C, Polatajko HJ: Motor problems in children with developmental coordination disorder: Review of the literature. Am J Occup Ther 49:787–789, 1995.

287. Wilson BN, Kaplan B: Follow-up assessment of children receiving sensory integration treatment. Occup Ther J Res 14:4, 1994.

288. Witelson SF: Developmental dyslexia: Two right hemispheres and none left. Science 195:309, 1977.

289. Wolff PH, Gunnoe CE, Cohen C: Associated movement as a measure of developmental age. Dev Med Child Neurol 25:417, 1983.

290. World Health Organization: The ICD-10 Classification of Mental Health and Behavioral Disorders: Clinical Descriptions and Diagnostic Guidelines. Geneva, World Health Organization, 1992.

291. Zinkus PW: Behavior and emotional sequelae of learning disorders. In Gottlieb MI, et al (eds): Current Issues in Developmental Pediatrics: The Learning Disabled Child. New York, Grune & Stratton, 1979.

292. Ziviani J: Qualitative changes in dynamic tripod grip between seven and 14 years of age. Dev Med Child Neurol 25:778–782, 1983.

293. Ziviani J, Elkins J: Effect of pencil grip on handwriting speed and legibility. Educ Rev 38:247–257, 1986.

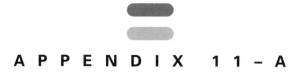

A Summary of Standardized Motor Tests

Bruininks-Oseretsky Test of Motor Proficiency

Movement Assessment Battery for Children (Movement-ABC)

Peabody Developmental Motor Scales (PDMS)

Quick Neurological Screening Test (QNST)

Miller Assessment for Preschoolers (MAP)

FirstSTEP

Tests for Motor Proficiency of Gubbay

Sensory Integration and Praxis Tests (SIPT)

Bender Gestalt Test for Young Children

Developmental Test of Visual-Motor Integration (VMI)—4th revision

Test of Visual-Motor Skills—Revised

Evaluation Tool of Children's Handwriting (ETCH)

Purdue Pegboard Test

BRUININKS-OSERETSKY TEST OF MOTOR PROFICIENCY (1978)[44]

Author: Robert H. Bruininks, PhD
Source: American Guidance Service, Inc., Circle Pines, MN 55014
Ages: 4 to 14 years
Administration: Individual; 45 minutes to 1 hour
Equipment: Test kit needed
Description: The Bruininks-Oseretsky Test of Motor Proficiency is the most recent revision of the Oseretsky Tests of Motor Proficiency first published in Russia in 1923. The Oseretsky Tests were first adapted by Doll in 1946 and then by Sloan in 1955 as the Lincoln-Oseretsky Motor Development Scale. As with the earlier versions, the Bruininks-Oseretsky Test yields an age equivalency score, but standard scores and percentile ranks also are available. The test assesses motor functioning in eight areas, each with standard score information:

1. Running speed and agility: Runs 15 yards, picks up blocks, and returns
2. Balance: Eight items ranging in difficulty from standing on one leg to stepping over object on a balance beam
3. Bilateral coordination: Seven items that require use of upper and lower extremities simultaneously or in sequential movement (e.g., tapping feet and fingers, and jumping and clapping). Final item requires pencil use with both hands simultaneously
4. Strength: Three items: standing broad jumps, sit-ups, and push-ups
5. Upper-limb coordination: Five items that involve catching and throwing balls and an additional four items assessing precise finger movements
6. Response speed: Requires a quick catch of falling stick
7. Visual motor control: Eight pencil, paper, and scissor items
8. Upper-limb speed and dexterity: Eight items that range from putting pennies in a box to making dots in circles

Construction and Reliability: The Bruininks-Oseretsky Test has been carefully standardized on 765 subjects from differing geographical regions and community size. Test-retest reliability coefficients for the subtests ranged from 0.50 to 0.89, and that of the total battery was 0.87 for second graders and 0.86 for sixth graders. With the exception of "response speed," the subtests differentiated significantly between normal children and children with learning disabilities.
Comment: The Bruininks-Oseretsky Test of Motor Proficiency appears to be one of the better standardized tests of motor performance. A short form, taking 15 to 20 minutes, can be used for screening. In testing children with motor dysfunction, careful attention must be paid to performance on individual items. For example, a child who compensates for poor proprioceptive postural control with vision can score in the normal range on the balance subtest, even though he or she fails the single item of balance with eyes closed. A problem with finger sequencing in the upper limb coordination subtest could be masked by good ball skills. These kinds of problems could result in not identifying a child's deficit. Another problem with the subtests is that a single item has a disproportionate effect on a child's age equivalence. Nevertheless, this is an excellent test for monitoring the motor development of a dysfunctioning child.

MOVEMENT ASSESSMENT BATTERY FOR CHILDREN (MOVEMENT-ABC) (1992)[126]

Authors: S. E. Henderson and D. Sugden
Source: Psychological Corporation
Ages: 4 to 12 years
Administration: Individual; 20 to 30 minutes
Equipment: Test kit required
Description: The Movement-ABC is a revision and expansion of the Test of Motor Impairment (TOMI)—Henderson Revision. The Movement-ABC includes three aspects: *Screening and Evaluation:* The Movement-ABC Checklist provides classroom assessment of movement difficulties, screening for at-risk children, and monitoring of treatment programs; *Assessment:* The Movement-ABC Test (similar to the TOMI) provides a more comprehensive assessment and includes both normative and qualitative measures of movement competence. The test is divided into four age bands: for children 4–6 years; 7–8 years; 9–10 years; and 11–12 years. *Treatment:* The manual provides guidelines for organizing intervention programs. The Movement-ABC Test includes eight categories, with a single item for each age in each category:

1. Manual dexterity 1: Speed and sureness of movement by each hand
2. Manual dexterity 2: Coordination of two hands for a single task
3. Manual dexterity 3: Hand-eye coordination using the preferred hand
4. Ball skills 1: Ball task emphasizing aiming at a target
5. Ball skills 2: Ball task emphasizing catching a ball
6. Static balance: Balance task
7. Dynamic balance 1: Balance task emphasizing spatial precision

8. Dynamic balance 2: Balance task emphasizing control of momentum

Construction and Reliability: Standardization of the test was done in the United States, whereas work on the checklist was based in the United Kingdom. Normative data on the test were gathered on 1234 children in the United States. The sample was approximately representative of the general population of children in the United States in terms of gender, region, and ethnic origin. Test-retest reliability for consistency of individual item scores with children ages 5, 7, and 9 showed a median percentage of agreement between test and retest from 80% to 90%. Percent agreement for total impairment score ranged from 73% for age 9 to 97% agreement for age 5.

Comment: This revision offers several advantages: (1) the checklist helps teachers identify children with movement problems; (2) information is provided for a cognitive-motor approach to intervention; and (3) the qualitative component of the test is more clearly defined and incorporated on the record form, and the scoring systems have been refined.

PEABODY DEVELOPMENTAL MOTOR SCALES (PDMS): REVISED EXPERIMENTAL EDITION (1983)[88]

Authors: M. Rhonda Folio and Rebecca R. Fewell
Source: DLM Teaching Resources, P.O. Box 4000, One DLM Park, Allen, TX 55002
Ages: Birth to 7 years
Administration: Individual (birth to 3 years) and/or individual or group (4 to 7 years); 40 to 60 minutes (test items may be scored by direct observation or by parent or teacher report)
Description: The PDMS were designed for use with children who show delay or disability in fine and gross motor skills. Test items are similar to those on other developmental scales, but only motor items are included. Items are scored on a three-point scale: 0 for unsuccessful, 1 for partial, and 2 for successful performance. Age-equivalent, motor quotients, percentile rankings, and standard scores are provided.

The following skill categories are tested in the Gross Motor Scale (170 test items). These tasks are considered to require precise movements of large muscles of body:

1. Reflexes (12 items): Includes items such as turning head in response to sound, aligning head on pull to sit, asymmetrical tonic neck reflex, protective reaction, and kicking
2. Balance (33 items): Includes propping and levels of sitting and standing, as well as higher-level items such as standing on one foot, beam walking, and walking on tiptoes
3. Nonlocomotion (42 items): Includes items such as head control, rolling, and weight bearing, as well as higher-level tasks such as jumping and situps
4. Locomotion (58 items): Examples include creeping, cruising, walking, stairs, hopping, tricycle riding, running, and jumping hurdles
5. Receipt and propulsion (25 items): Catching, throwing, and kicking balls

The Fine Motor Scale has 112 test items considered to require precise movements of small muscles. The following skill categories are included:

1. Grasping (22 items): Includes reflex grasping and voluntary grasping with the hands and with the fingers as well as crayon grasp
2. Hand use (26 items): Includes a variety of items ranging from maintaining hands closed to hand preference and including the manipulation of cubes, pegs, and other objects
3. Eye-hand coordination (46 items): Early items include visual fixation and tracking; later items building, and copying forms
4. Manual dexterity (18 items): turning and includes screwi

Construction and Reliabil
the normative sample rang
with samples beginning at 2
1-year intervals in older children.
majority having 30 or fewer children. Sa
reflect socioeconomic status and rural-urban c
test-retest reliability of 0.95 for the Gross Motor Sca
0.80 for the Fine Motor Scale was reported based on a sam
of 38 children. Validity was demonstrated by the significantly lower scores of 104 children with developmental deviations on all but the 0- to 5-month-old children. Another study of 43 children established a low but significant correlation (0.37) between the PDMS Gross Motor Scale and the Bayley Psychomotor Index and a moderately high correlation (0.78) between the PDMS Fine Motor Scale and the Bayley Mental Scale.

Comment: The PDMS are primarily useful for children with mild to moderate motor deficits, such as a child with learning disabilities or a child with developmental delay. The test does not discriminate among children with moderate to severe motor disability, because they fall far below the standard scores given. The standardization sample is small, especially in the age subgroups. The Fine Motor Scale has a high cognitive element, as demonstrated by the high correlation with the Bayley Mental Scale. The skill categories are unevenly distributed and have too few items at some age levels to be meaningful. Despite their drawbacks, the PDMS are probably the most valuable motor scales currently available for preschool children.

QUICK NEUROLOGICAL SCREENING TEST (QNST) (1978)[201]

Authors: M. A. Mutti, H. M. Sterling, and N. V. Spalding
Source: Academic Therapy Publications, 20 Commercial Boulevard, Novato, CA 94947
Ages: 5 years and older
Administration: Individual; 20 minutes
Equipment: None
Description: The QNST was developed as a screening device to identify children who have possible learning disabilities. The tasks are adapted from pediatric neurological examinations as well as from developmental assessments. The test is made up of the following fifteen subtests:

1. Hand skill: Writing his or her name and a sentence
2. Figure recognition and production: Naming, then drawing, five geometric forms
3. Palm form recognition: Recognizing numbers written on the palm by examiner with his or her finger
4. Eye tracking: Following pencil back and forth and up and down
5. Sound patterns: With hands on knees and eyes closed, imitating patterns demonstrated by the examiner
6. Finger to nose test: Includes observation
7. Thumb and finger circle: Forming circle with thumb and each of the fingers; laterality also observed
8. Double simultaneous stimulation of hand and cheek with eyes closed: Child must identify hands and cheeks touched by examiner in various combinations simultaneously
9. Rapid reversing, repetitive hand movements: Observation of diadochokinesis
10. Arm and leg extension: With eyes closed, extending legs, arms, and tongue for 1 to 15 seconds
11. Tandem walk: Walking straight line, heel to toe, forward and backward

on one leg: Balancing first on one leg, then on the
[...], 10 seconds each; eyes open, then closed; right-left
[...]erentiation observed
[...]kip: Skipping across the room
Left-right discrimination: Scored from subtests 6, 7, and 12
Behavior irregularities: General observation for behaviors
such as distractibility, perseveration, defensiveness, and hyperactivity

The test is scored based on careful observation and requires
a subjective evaluation of performance. The manual provides
ages at which 75% of neurologically intact children pass each
test as well as total scores indicative of probable neurological
dysfunction.
Construction and Reliability: The QNST has been used in
numerous research studies of normal children and of children
with suspected learning disabilities. Although the manual reported these studies, the test has not been formally standardized. Reliabilities on the whole test on children with learning
disabilities of 0.81 and 0.71 are reported, but the data are
incomplete. Ages at which 25%, 50%, and 75% of normal
children pass each subtest are given based on a compilation
of subjects from many studies. Norms for the total test are
not given.
Comment: The QNST is a screening device that identifies
children with possible neurological dysfunction. It is not, and
should not be, used as a standardized test but rather as an
adjunct to clinical observation. It is important to realize that the
test is primarily of motor function. It does not include language
tests and, therefore, will not identify all children with learning
disabilities. The test does screen for possible minimal brain
dysfunction or motor deficits.

MILLER ASSESSMENT FOR PRESCHOOLERS (MAP) (1988)[187, 191]

Author: Lucy Jane Miller
Source: Psychological Corporation, 555 Academic Court, San
Antonio, TX 78204-0952
Ages: 2 years, 9 months to 5 years, 8 months
Administration: Individual; 20 to 30 minutes including scoring
Equipment: The MAP Test Kit
Description: The MAP was designed to identify children who
exhibit mild to moderate developmental delays. The MAP is a
developmental assessment intended for use by educational and
clinical personnel to identify those children in need of further
evaluation and remediation. It can also be used to provide a
comprehensive, clinical framework that would be helpful in
defining a child's strengths and weaknesses and that would
indicate possible avenues of remediation. The test is made up
of 27 items and a series of structured observations. The test
items are divided into five performance indices:

1. Foundations: Items generally found on standard neurological
examinations and sensory integrative and neurodevelopmental tests
2. Coordination: Gross, fine, and oral motor abilities and articulation
3. Verbal: Cognitive language abilities, including memory, sequencing, comprehension, association, following directions,
and expression
4. Nonverbal: Cognitive abilities such as visual figure-ground,
puzzles, memory, and sequencing
5. Complex tasks: Tasks requiring an interaction of sensory,
motor, and cognitive abilities

Construction and Reliability: The MAP has been well standardized on a random sample of 1200 preschool children. The
sample was stratified by age, race, sex, size of residence, community, and socioeconomic factors. Data were collected nationwide in each of nine U.S. Census Bureau regions. Reported
reliabilities are good. In a test-retest on 90 children, 81% of the
children's scores remained stable. The coefficient of internal
consistency on the total sample was 0.798. Interrater reliability
on 40 children was reported as 0.98.
Comment: The MAP was developed by an occupational therapist and provides information that is of particular relevance to
therapists. it is carefully standardized and fills a need for early
identification of learning and motor deficits in children. Several
articles have now been published supporting the validity of this
test as a screening instrument.[188–190, 196] Reviews of the MAP in
the *Ninth Mental Measurements Yearbook* have described it as
"the best available screening test for identifying preschool children with moderate preacademic problems"[68] and "an extremely
promising instrument which should find wide use among clinical
psychologists, school psychologists, and occupational therapists
in assessing mild to moderate learning disabilities in preschool
children."[184] A more complete review of this test is provided by
King-Thomas and Hacker.[156]

FIRSTSTEP (SCREENING TEST FOR EVALUATING PRESCHOOLERS) (1993)[193]

Author: Lucy J. Miller, PhD
Source: The Psychological Corporation, San Antonio, TX
Ages: 2 years, 9 months to 6 years, 2 months
Administration: Individual; 15 minutes
Equipment: Test kit needed
Description: The FirstSTEP is a quick screening test for identifying developmental delays in all five areas defined by IDEA
(Individuals with Disabilities Education Act) and mandated
by PL 99–457: cognition, communication, physical, social/
emotional, and adaptive functioning. Twelve subtests assess
cognitive, communication, and motor domains. An optional
Social-Emotional Scale includes 25 items from five areas (task
confidence, cooperative mood, temperament and emotionality,
uncooperative antisocial behavior, and attention communication
difficulties) that are scored based on behaviors observed by
the examiner during the test session. The Adaptive Behavior
Checklist is an optional measure completed by parent interview
to assess the child's self-help and adaptive living skills. The
Parent/Teacher Scale provides additional information about the
child's typical behavior.

Cognitive Domain

Money Game (Quantitative Reasoning)

Description: The child is asked a series of questions about
coins, regarding quantity, amount, comparisons, size, and nu-
meration. This subtest requires cognitive understanding of simple arithmetic concepts.

What's Missing Game (Picture Completion)

Description: The child is asked to identify what is missing
from the pictures of common objects or events by naming or
pointing. This subtest measures visual figure-ground as well as
gestalt closure abilities.

Which Way? Game (Visual Position in Space)

Description: The child is asked to look at a stimulus figure
that is turned in a specific direction. The child then selects
the response figure that matches. This subtest measures visual
discrimination and the ability to visually perceive directionality.

Put Together Game (Problem Solving)

Description: The child is asked to select the pieces that best fit a certain space. The subtest requires abstract thinking.

Language Domain

Listen Game (Auditory Discrimination)

Description: This two-part activity requires the child to listen as the examiner names and points to three similar-sounding pictures. Then the child chooses the pictures that represent the words. The second part requires the child to discriminate between words that are the same and words that are different. This task taps phoneme discrimination and requires good auditory processing skills.

How Many Can You Say? Game (Word Retrieval)

Description: The child's linguistic fluency and word-finding skills are measured by asking the child to count, recall animals, and recite rhyming words.

Finish Up Game (Association)

Description: The child is asked to complete a phrase that is initiated by the examiner. The subtest requires the child to demonstrate an understanding of the association between concepts (e.g., big and little).

Copy Me Game (Sentence and Digit Repetition)

Description: The child is asked to repeat a series of meaningful verbal stimuli and then a series of numbers. This subtest measures verbal memory, grammatical abilities, and verbal expression skills.

Motor Domain

Drawing Game (Visual-Motor Integration)

Description: The child is presented with paper and pencil tasks. This subtest requires the integration of fine motor and visual-perceptual abilities.

Things with Strings Game (Fine Motor Planning)

Description: The child is asked to perform a series of motor movements with the upper extremities using a wooden cube and a string. These items tap the ability to plan and execute a series of motor actions and measures fine motor planning or praxis.

Statue Game (Balance)

Description: The child is asked to assume a series of increasingly more difficult positions that require the child to balance with eyes open and vision occluded. The subtest taps the abilities needed to maintain equilibrium and screens for proprioception, vestibular perception, and/or visual processing difficulties.

Jumping Game (Gross Motor Planning)

Description: The child is asked to imitate the examiner through a series of increasingly more difficult tasks that involve jumping in specific patterns. Gross motor and motor planning abilities are measured.

Construction and Reliability: The FirstSTEP is norm referenced and was standardized on 1,433 children. Norms are provided in 6-month intervals for each of seven age groups. Standardization sample closely matches demographic characteristics provided by the U.S. Census Bureau. Scores are reported in standard scores as well as a three-category color-coded risk status to indicate whether the child is functioning in the normal or delayed range. The FirstSTEP is a highly reliable instrument. Overall test reliability (Split half) is 0.90, with individual domains ranging from 0.71 to 0.87. Test-retest reliability indicated a high degree of consistency in the classification of a child's performance across two test sessions (90% agreement for composite score; 85% to 93% for individual domain scores). Results also indicated a high level of interrater agreement (r = 0.94 on composite scores).

Comment: The FirstSTEP is a new test that shows exceptional promise as a screening instrument. A Spanish version, Primer Paso, will be published in the near future. The FirstSTEP was developed by the occupational therapist who also developed the MAP (The Miller Assessment for Preschoolers); and, like the MAP, the test provides information that is of particular relevance to therapists. Although individual items on the FirstSTEP differ from the MAP, many are derived from the MAP, and the test is based on the same theoretical framework as the MAP.

Initial validity studies of the FirstSTEP appear highly promising and indicate that FirstSTEP has good construct, content, and discriminant validity. The FirstSTEP can effectively identify children with developmental delays. A study of 900 children demonstrated that children with delays perform 1.5 to 2 standard deviations below the mean in all domains.

With regard to the Motor Domain of the FirstSTEP, which taps motor skills, the results of a concurrent validity study suggest that the Motor Domain measures constructs similar to those measured by the Bruininks-Oseretsky Test of Motor Proficiency and support the use of the Motor Domain of the FirstSTEP as an indicator of the child's motor functioning.

TESTS OF MOTOR PROFICIENCY OF GUBBAY (1975)[108]

Author: Sasson S. Gubbay
Source: In Gubbay SS: The Clumsy Child. Philadelphia, WB Saunders, 1975
Ages: 8 to 12 years
Administration: Individual; 5 minutes
Equipment: Described in book, must be purchased or constructed
Description: Gubbay's Tests of Motor Proficiency make up a quick screening instrument for the identification of developmental dyspraxia. The battery is made up of eight items that best discriminate between clumsy and normal children in a study of 1,000 schoolchildren:

Whistle through pursed lips
Skip forward five steps
Roll ball with foot around objects
Throw tennis ball, clap hands, then catch tennis ball
Tie one shoelace with double bow
Thread 10 beads
Pierce 20 pinholes in graph paper
Posting box: fit six shapes in appropriate slots

The first two items are scored pass or fail; the score for the fourth item is the number of claps, and the other items are timed. Percentile values at each age level from 8 to 12 years are reported.

Comment: Gubbay's tests were devised as a rapid screening to be used together with teacher questionnaires to identify clumsy children in a school program. They are valuable if used as intended. One or more of the items could be incorporated into an evaluation protocol using a cutoff based on normative data given. However, this is not a fully standardized test, and further normative data as well as validity and reliability studies are required.

THE SENSORY INTEGRATION AND PRAXIS TESTS (SIPT) (1989)[24]

Author: A. Jean Ayres
Source: Western Psychological Services, 12031 Wilshire Boulevard, Los Angeles, CA 90025
Ages: 4 years to 8 years, 11 months
Administration: Individual; 1 hour; examiner certification highly recommended
Equipment: SIPT Test Kit
Description: The SIPT are a major revision and restandardization of the Southern California Sensory Integration Tests.[22] Four new tests of praxis were added, five tests underwent major revisions, eight tests underwent minor revisions, and four tests were deleted. The tests are designed to identify sensory integration and praxis deficits in children with learning disabilities. There are 17 tests, described as follows:

1. Space visualization: Select from two blocks the one that will fit into a form board; it is necessary to mentally manipulate the forms to arrive at the correct choice on the more difficult test items.
2. Figure-ground perception: The child selects from six pictures the three that are superimposed or embedded with other forms on the test plates.
3. Manual form perception: Part I: a geometric form is held in the hand and the counterpart is selected from a visual display. Part II: a geometric form is felt with one hand while its match is selected from several choices with the other hand.
4. Kinesthesia: With vision occluded, the child attempts to place his or her finger on a point at which this finger had been placed previously by the examiner; a separate recording sheet is provided for each child.
5. Finger identification: With hands screened from view, the examiner touches the child's finger, the shield is removed, and the child then points to the finger touched.
6. Graphesthesia: The examiner uses his or her finger to draw a design on the back of the child's hand, without the child looking; the child then reproduces the design.
7. Localization of tactile stimuli: With vision occluded, the child touches the spot on his or her hand or arm that was touched by the examiner with a specially designed pen.
8. Praxis on verbal command: The examiner verbally describes a series of body movements and the child executes them.
9. Design copying: Part I: The child copies a design by connecting dots on a dot grid. Part II: The child copies a design without the use of a dot grid; both process and product are scored.
10. Constructional praxis: Working with blocks, the child attempts to duplicate two different block structures; in the first structure, the child observes the examiner building the model; the second structure is preassembled.
11. Postural praxis: The child imitates unusual body positions demonstrated by the examiner.
12. Oral praxis: The child imitates movements of the tongue, lips, and jaw demonstrated by the examiner.
13. Sequencing praxis: The child imitates a series of simple arm and hand movements demonstrated by the examiner.
14. Bilateral motor coordination: The child imitates a series of bilateral arm and foot movements demonstrated by the examiner.
15. Standing and walking balance: The subtest consists of 15 items in which the child assumes various standing and walking postures.
16. Motor accuracy: The child traces a printed, curved black line with a red, nylon-tipped pen, first with the preferred hand and then with the nonpreferred hand.
17. Postrotatory nystagmus: The child is rotated first counter-clockwise and then clockwise on a rotation board and the duration of postrotatory nystagmus, a vestibuloocular reflex, is observed.

In addition to these 17 tests, a series of clinical observations aids in interpreting the SIPT. These clinical observations include the following:

Eye dominance

Eye movements

Muscle tone

Co-contraction

Postural background movements

Postural security

Equilibrium reactions and protective extension

Schilder's arm extension posture

Supine flexion

Prone extension

Asymmetrical tonic neck reflex

Hyperactivity, distractibility

Tactile defensiveness

Ability to perform slow motions

Thumb-finger touching

Diadochokinesis

Tongue-to-lip movements

Hopping, jumping, skipping

Construction and Reliability: The construction of the SIPT was based on a theoretical model developed from observation of children with learning disabilities and supported by factor analytical and cluster analysis studies. Interpretation follows a clinical model based on patterns of scores rather than a poor score on any one test.

The SIPT was nationally standardized on 1,997 children from across the United States and Canada. Sex, geographical location, ethnicity, and type of community are represented in proportion to the 1980 U.S. census.

Test-retest reliability was evaluated in a sample of 41 dysfunctional children and 10 normal dysfunction and ranges from moderate to high. As a group, the praxis tests had the highest reliabilities. Interrater reliability is excellent, with most correlations between raters at 0.90 or higher.

Comment: The SIPT is computer scored and interpreted, and a full eight-color profile (WPS Chronograph) is provided that summarizes major SIPT testing and statistical results in a clear manner. Initial validity studies of the SIPT indicate a good ability to discriminate between normal and dysfunctional groups and across ages. The SIPT is the most comprehensive assessment of sensory integration and praxis; however, it requires specialized training for administration and interpretation, and the test kit and scoring of protocols are expensive.

BENDER GESTALT TEST FOR YOUNG CHILDREN (1963)[163]

Author: E.M. Koppitz
Source: Grune and Stratton, Inc., New York, NY

Ages: 5 to 10 years
Administration: Individual; 7 to 15 minutes; special training required
Description: The Bender Gestalt Test for Young Children is an adaptation of the Bender Visual Motor Gestalt Test, which is an individually administered test of performance in copying designs. The test consists of nine designs that are printed on separate cards and presented one at a time to the child. The child is given unlimited time to copy each successive design on a sheet of paper. The developmental scoring system for young children to age 10 was developed by Koppitz.[163] The Bender Gestalt is used by psychologists to assess visual motor functions and possible neuropsychological impairment, and it is also used with the Koppitz scoring system to evaluate perceptual-motor maturity and emotional adjustment. The reproduced design is scored for distortion, rotation, perseveration, method of reproduction, and other factors. The Koppitz scoring system yields an estimate of the child's developmental age.
Construction and Reliability: The Bender Gestalt Test is a widely used and heavily researched test of neuropsychological impairment following brain injury in adults. The Koppitz version, standardized for children, makes possible similar diagnoses with children. Test-retest reliability for the Koppitz scoring of the Bender Visual Motor Gestalt test is moderate, ranging from 0.60 to 0.66. Interscorer agreement is 93%.
Comment: The Bender Gestalt Test yields more information about a child's deficit than simpler tests of geometric form reproduction, but it requires special skills for interpretation. Inability to copy geometric forms may occur for several reasons: faulty visual-perceptual discrimination, poor motor ability, or, more likely, problems in the translations of the perception of the form to its reproduction.

DEVELOPMENTAL TEST OF VISUAL-MOTOR INTEGRATION (VMI), 4TH REVISION (4R) (1997)[32]

Author: K. Berry
Source: Modern Curriculum Press, 13900 Prospect Road, Cleveland, OH 44136
Ages: 3 years to adult (standard scores to 17 years, 11 months)
Administration: Individual or group; 10 to 15 minutes
Equipment: Protocol booklets (test forms)
Description: The VMI tests the ability to copy geometric forms. A booklet is provided with 24 designs in an age-graded sequence. A shorter format including the first 15 forms is available for children aged 3 to 7 years. The child copies each design in a space directly below it. The first three items are presented twice and may be demonstrated for imitation. Items are judged pass or fail on criteria given in the manual. One point is awarded for each passed item, with a total of 27 possible points
Construction and Reliability: Additional specificity was added for the scoring of some items in the 1989 revision. The VMI manual contains information relating to ages at which forms are passed based on Gesell and other researchers. Developmental drawing trends are illustrated. Age equivalences, standard scores, percentile equivalents, and T scores are based on a sample of over 6,000 children. This reflects normative samples from 1964, 1981, and 1989. Various studies of reliability and validity are reported in the manual. Studies of test-retest reliability were reported for groups of children of all ages and range from 0.63 (7-month interval) to 0.92 (2-week period), with a median of 0.81. There are no reports of reliability at individual ages. Split-half reliability was 0.88, and interscorer agreement was 0.94.
Comment: The VMI provides a quick and easy method to assess the development of a child's ability to copy geometric

forms. It is useful as an adjunct to other assessments of the child with learning disabilities. When the test is presented to the child, he or she is told that the booklet must remain parallel to the edge of the table. This prevents some of the problems of other tests, such as the child turning the individual paper on which designs are reproduced. However, the structured format does not allow the assessment of overall organization of copying forms, as can be done when the child copies forms on a blank sheet of paper (e.g., Bender Gestalt Test). Therefore, overall organization also should be tested.

TEST OF VISUAL-MOTOR SKILLS—REVISED (TVMS-R) (1995)[93]

Author: Morrison F. Gardner
Source: Children's Hospital of San Francisco, Publication Department OPR-110, P.O. Box 3805, San Francisco, CA 94119
Ages: 3 to 13 years
Administration: Individual or group; 3 to 6 patients
Equipment: Protocol booklet
Description: The TVMS-R consists of a series of 23 forms to be copied by the child. Each form is on a separate page of the booklet. The booklet contains some forms commonly used in visual-motor tests (e.g., lines and circles), but many forms are unique to this test. Care was taken to avoid forms that resemble language symbols. The revision of the TVMS has updated norms, standardization, and scoring criteria.

Two different scoring methods are now available. Modifications in scoring the TVMS-R include a classification system to characterize errors in one of eight categories. The eight classifications are closure, angles, intersecting and overlapping lines, size of design, rotation or reversals, line length, over or under penetration, and modification of design. Scoring of each design is completed through following a definitive criterion with errors and strengths identified. The examiner can identify specific areas of strength and weakness in visual-motor integration based on the number of errors and accuracies recorded. Standard scores, scaled scores, percentile ranks, and stanines are available for both weaknesses and strengths. An alternative scoring method (ASM) was also designed to allow a straight point system designation to each form. The forms are scored on a 0- to 3-point scale. A score of 0 indicates that the child is unable to copy the form with any degree of motor accuracy. Scores of 1 and 2 indicate various visual-motor errors for which criteria are both written and illustrated. A score of 3 demonstrates precision in execution. Age equivalents, standard scores, scaled scores, percentile ranks, and stanines are provided.
Construction and Reliability: The Test of Visual-Motor Skills—Revised was administered to 1,484 children in the San Francisco Bay area from age 3 years to 13 years, 11 months. The overall sample was 51.9% male and 48.1% female. Cronbach's coefficient alpha was used to determine the internal consistency of the test. These reliability coefficients ranged from 0.72 to 0.84 over the age ranges, with a value of 0.90 for the sample as a whole. Test-retest reliability was not reported in the manual, but the author noted the need for research in that area.
Comment: The TVMS-R is a companion test to the Test of Visual-Perceptual Skills (TVPS), which is a motor-free test of form perception. Using the tests together can determine whether the child's form reproduction reflects incorrect visual perception or whether the problem is in motor execution. The TVMS-R places greater expectations on motor precision than do other visual-motor tests. For example, a line must touch an intersecting line without crossing over it. Therefore it should be used only when motor control and constructive abilities are important.

EVALUATION TOOL OF CHILDREN'S HANDWRITING (ETCH) (1995)[8]

Author: Susan J. Amundson
Source: O.T. Kids, P. O. Box 1118, Homer, AK 99603
Ages: First through sixth grades (6 to 11 years)
Administration: Individual
Equipment: Protocol booklet, task sheets and wall charts, stop watch
Description: The ETCH is designed to evaluate manuscript and cursive writing for components of legibility and speed. Specific components of the child's handwriting including letter formation, spacing, size, and alignment are included for assessment. Tasks are presented in order and are as follows:

1. Lower case alphabet letters (from memory)
2. Upper case alphabet letters (from memory)
3. Numeral writing (from memory)
4. Near point copying (visual model)
5. Far point copying (visual model)
6. Dictation (verbal)
7. Sentence composition (independent)

A quick reference card is included with standardized directions and timing criterion. Written and illustrated scoring criteria have been designed to assist the evaluator in determining the legibility of letters and numbers. The primary focus of scoring is whether the written material is readable.

Construction and Reliability: Pilots of the ETCH were designed using adaptations of written tasks from existing tools. Three editions of the ETCH have been sampled by practitioners working in school systems with feedback on the examiner's manual, ease of administration and scoring, item selection, scoring procedures, and face validity of the instrument. Normative data have not yet been collected on the ETCH tasks, although the author suggests that occupational therapists and classroom educators might collaboratively collect data. Eight studies of handwriting speed have been included for reference in the manual. No test-retest or internal reliability studies have been conducted. Interrater reliability ranged from 0.63 to 0.94 for individual manuscript items and 0.64 to 0.97 for cursive. Overall, the total word reliability is more stable than task scores, ranging from 0.90 to 0.98.

Comment: The ETCH assesses functional writing skills that are relevant to academic performance. The varied tasks allow you to identify areas of strength and weakness in written performance, including legibility components, speed, and composition models (visual, verbal, and memory). Information received from the ETCH is qualitative at this point because of the lack of normative samples. The author suggests that the ETCH be used in conjunction with observations of the child's writing activity in natural environments, such as classroom and home, as a determination of difficulties in functional written performance.

PURDUE PEGBOARD TEST (1948, 1968)[272]

Author: Joseph Tiffin, PhD
Source: Lafayette Instrument Co., P.O. Box 5728, Lafayette, IN 47903
Ages: 5 years through adult
Administration: Individual; 10 to 15 minutes
Equipment: Pegboard with pins, collars, and washers required
Description: This test of manual dexterity consists of four parts, each described as follows:

1. Right hand: Subject inserts small pegs into holes in pegboard using right hand for a 30-second trial
2. Left hand: Subject inserts pegs into pegboard with left hand for a 30-second trial
3. Both hands: Both hands pick up and insert pegs into board at same time for a 30-second trial
4. Assembly: Using hands cooperatively, subject assembles sequences of pins, collars, and washers for a 60-second trial

Construction and Reliability: This test has recently been standardized with 1,334 normal schoolchildren, ages 5 to 16, from New Jersey. Means, standard deviations, and percentile scores are presented as a function of age (6-month intervals) and gender. Reliability data on children are not presented in the test manual, although reliability with college students ranged from 0.60 to 0.71. A number of validity studies indicate that learning-disabled subjects perform more poorly than normal controls on this test. Additional normative data are presented in the manual for various age and diagnostic groups.

Comment: This test was originally designed for adults to assist in the selection of employees for manual industrial jobs. It has recently been standardized with school-aged children[94] and adolescents.[180]

Beyond the Central Nervous System: Neurovascular Entrapment Syndromes

BRADLEY W. STOCKERT, PhD, PT • LAURIE KENNY, MS, PT • PETER I. EDGELOW, MA, PT

Chapter Outline

PERIPHERAL NEUROANATOMY
MOBILITY OF THE PERIPHERAL
   NERVOUS SYSTEM

PATHOGENESIS OF PERIPHERAL
   NERVE ENTRAPMENT
ADAPTIVE RESPONSES TO PAIN

CLINICAL EXAMINATION AND
   TREATMENT
CASE STUDY

Key Words

– double crush injury

– neural irritability

– neural mobility

– neural sensitivity

– neurovascular entrapment

Objectives

After reading this chapter the student/therapist will:

1. Understand the concept of a mechanical interface as it applies to nerves.

2. Understand the changes that occur with intraneural and extraneural movements.

3. Understand the concept of tension points.

4. Be able to describe the mechanisms involved in the development of a double crush injury and neurovascular entrapment.

5. Be able to assess for the presence of neural sensitivity and irritability.

The purpose of this chapter is twofold. The first purpose is to emphasize the concept that the entire nervous system forms a continuous tissue tract. This concept is central to the idea that movements of the trunk and/or limbs can have a profound biomechanical and physiological impact on the peripheral and central nervous systems. The extraneural and intraneural mechanisms involved in the response of the nervous system to normal and pathological movements are discussed.

The second purpose is to develop in the reader an understanding of neurovascular entrapment syndrome. This is an underrecognized impairment present in patients with a wide variety of diagnoses (e.g., repetitive strain injury and cumulative trauma disorders). These patients frequently fail to respond to standard medical care. The theoretical mechanisms involved in the development of neurovascular entrapment are presented. Background information necessary to understand the syndrome is provided and the appropriate screening tools for assessment of the impairment are discussed. Treatment suggestions and a case study are presented at the end of the chapter.

PERIPHERAL NEUROANATOMY

The peripheral nervous system (PNS) is generally regarded as that portion of the nervous system that lies outside the central nervous system (CNS) (i.e., the brain and spinal cord).[18, 21] The major components of the PNS include motor, sensory, and autonomic neurons found in spinal, peripheral, and cranial nerves. Although this partitioning is valid from an anatomical perspective it often leads to a lack of appreciation of the truly continuous nature and integrative function of the nervous system as a whole. The concept that the entire nervous system is a continuous tissue tract reinforces the idea that limb and trunk movements can have a mechanical effect on the PNS and the CNS that is local and global.

The nervous system is composed of two functional tissue types. One type of tissue is concerned with impulse conduction. This functional category includes nerve cells and Schwann cells. The second functional tissue type provides support and protection of the conduction tissues (i.e., the connective tissues). Three levels in the organization of a peripheral nerve have been described[20, 21] (Fig. 12–1). At the innermost level the nerve fiber is the conducting component of a neuron (nerve cell). A connective tissue layer called the endoneurium surrounds each nerve fiber. The endoneurium surrounds the basement membrane of the neuron and plays an important role in maintaining fluid pressure within the endoneurial space. At the second level of organization, a collection of many nerve fibers (a fascicle) is surrounded by a layer of connective tissue called the perineurium. The perineurium acts as a barrier to diffusion, and it is the last connective

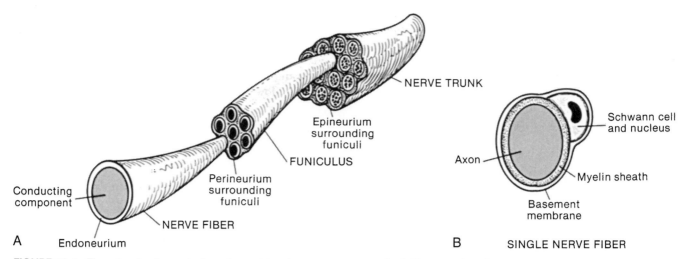

FIGURE 12–1. Three levels of organization of a peripheral nerve or nerve trunk. *A*, Nerve trunk and components. *B*, Microscopic structure of nerve fiber.

tissue layer to rupture in tensile testing of peripheral nerves.[24] The outermost connective tissue layer of a peripheral nerve is called the epineurium. The epineurium protects the fascicles and enhances gliding between them. All three connective tissue layers are interconnected; that is, they are not separate and distinct but are continuous tissue layers. Each of the connective tissue layers contains free nerve endings, making all three layers a potential source of pain. In addition, all three layers are continuous with the homologous connective tissue layers of the CNS (e.g., the dura mater and the epineurium).

The vascular supply for peripheral nerves is designed to provide uninterrupted blood flow regardless of the position of the trunk and limbs. Extrinsic vessels provide blood flow to "feeder" vessels, which in turn supply an extensive intrinsic (intraneural) vasculature within the nervous system. The feeder vessels branch off the extrinsic vessels and enter peripheral nerves in areas of low nerve mobility relative to the surrounding tissue. The intrinsic vasculature supplies all three connective tissue layers within the PNS, but only capillaries cross the perineurium.[2, 12]

Nerves are regularly subjected to stretch (elongation) and compression. The diameter of a nerve has been shown to decrease when a stretch is applied, and this will lead to an increase in the intraneural pressure. Compression, elongation, and/or an increase in intraneural pressure can decrease the diameter of the intrinsic blood vessels and lead to a reduction in blood flow within the nerve. Complete arrest of the blood flow has been shown to occur in the sciatic nerve of a rabbit at 8% elongation.[2] The changes in blood flow and intraneural pressure have the potential to interfere with neuronal conduction, metabolism, and axonal transport.

MOBILITY OF THE PERIPHERAL NERVOUS SYSTEM

Several types of tissues (e.g., bone, fascia, and muscle) surround peripheral nerves as they "travel" to target tissues. Peripheral nerves can be thought of as passing through a series of tissue tunnels composed of various biological materials. The composition of the tunnel changes during the passage of the nerve from the vertebral column (an osseous tunnel) to the target tissue (e.g., from osseous tunnel to a soft tissue and/or fibro-osseous tunnel). A "mechanical interface" exists at the junction between the nerve and the material adjacent to the nerve that forms the tissue tunnel. Movement of the trunk and/or limbs can cause two types of movement to occur in the peripheral nerves: sliding and elongation.[2]

Sliding can be defined as movement between the nerve and the surrounding tissues at the mechanical interface (extraneural movement). Sliding does not cause a significant amount of elongation or tension to develop within the nerve. *Elongation* of the nerve occurs when tension is applied and there is little or no movement at the mechanical interface. Elongation causes sliding to occur between the fascicles or between the neural elements and connective tissue layers (intraneural movement). Elongation results in a significant increase in the tension within the nerve and a decrease in the diameter of the nerve.[2]

Both extraneural and intraneural movements may occur when a body part is moved, but they may not be uniformly distributed within a nerve. When the body is moved some parts of the nervous system will undergo primarily extraneural movement with little or no development of tension whereas other areas will undergo intraneural movement (elongation), resulting in an increase in intraneural tension. As a consequence, some areas within a nerve develop little or no tension whereas other areas of the same nerve develop a significant amount of intraneural tension; that is, a "tension point" develops. In areas repeatedly exposed to high amounts of tension (e.g., the median nerve at the wrist) the nerves are found to contain a higher than average amount of connective tissue.[2] If one considers the entire nervous system as a continuous tissue tract, then the idea that movement and/or tension developed in one region of the nervous system can be distributed and dissipated throughout the entire nervous system becomes apparent.[8, 15] In contrast, the inability of a component within the nervous system to dissipate and/or distribute movement and tension will lead to abnormal force development elsewhere in the continuous tissue tract.[1]

PATHOGENESIS OF PERIPHERAL NERVE ENTRAPMENT

Seddon's classification of nerve injury is based on mechanical trauma.[22] Schaumberg[21] modified this paradigm into an anatomically based scheme containing three classes of injury (Table 12–1). Injuries in class II and III are due to macrotrauma that results in some disruption to the integrity of the nerve fiber. The following discussion of entrapment is focused on microtrauma in which there is no breach in the anatomical integrity of the nerve fiber (class I). Mechanical microtrauma resulting in nerve entrapment can occur with excessive or abnormal (1) friction, (2) compression, and/or (3) stretch (tension).[21]

Tissue tunnels, peripheral nerves, and the mechanical interfaces between them are all vulnerable to mechanical microtrauma (i.e., abnormal friction, compression, and/or tension).[2, 21] Some peripheral nerves are exposed to bony hard interfaces (e.g., the lower cords of the brachial plexus at the first rib) that are potential sources of abnormal friction. Inflammation and swelling within a tissue tunnel can produce compression of a nerve (e.g., the median nerve within the carpal tunnel). Abnormal tension can develop in nerves where excessive intraneural movement occurs and/or extraneural movement is restricted (e.g., tibial nerve in the popliteal fossa). The point(s) at which a nerve branches (e.g., brachial plexus) limit(s) the amount of gliding (extraneural movement) available at that site and increase(s) the amount of local intraneural tension developed with movement.[2, 21]

Microtrauma can produce an intraneural lesion.[2, 21] Conducting tissue injuries can result in a decrease in axoplasmic flow, demyelination, and/or hypoxia. If the lesion occurs in the connective tissues of the nerve, there may be inflammation, proliferation of fibroblasts, and scar formation (fibrosis). An intraneural scar will decrease the compliance of the nerve and increase the amount of tension generated with movement of the trunk and limbs.[15] These intraneural changes can impair or completely block the ability of the nerve to conduct action potentials.[2, 19, 21] Partial or complete conduction blocks can result in a loss of motor function and positive and/or negative sensory phenomena.

Microtrauma can produce an extraneural lesion.[2, 15, 19, 21] The damage in an extraneural lesion can occur in the tissue tunnel around the nerve or at the mechanical interface. Swelling within the tissue tunnel can produce compression of the nerve, leading to abnormalities in the conducting and connective tissues. Fibrosis can occur at the mechanical interface, leading to a decrease in sliding (extraneural movement) of the nerve at the mechanical interface. A decrease in the ability of a nerve to slide within a tissue tunnel will result in an abnormal increase in the tension (intraneural movement) within the nerve as elongation occurs with movement of the trunk and limbs. The increase in local intraneural tension will be distributed in an abnormal manner throughout the continuous tract of the nervous system.[2]

Friction, compression, and stretch can produce microtrauma that results in intraneural and extraneural pathology.[2, 21] For example, fibrosis can produce a combined pathological state that results in a substantial reduction in the ability of a nerve to slide within the tissue tunnel (extraneural movement) and a substantial increase in tension within the nerve (intraneural movement) as the compliance of the nerve is decreased. These changes result in an abnormal distribution of sliding and tension throughout the nervous system with movement of the trunk and/or limbs. The abnormal distribution of tension within a nerve increases the probability of a second injury or abnormality developing elsewhere within the nerve. This scenario has led to the use of the term *double crush injury*, first used by Upton and McComas[25] in 1973. (This term should be considered a misnomer because a "crush" does not necessarily occur.) For example, entrapment of the median nerve at the carpal tunnel can cause the development of abnormal tension in the cervical spinal nerves, resulting in fibrosis at a second site.

Sunderland[23] has advocated that a change in the normal pressure gradients within the compartments of the median nerve can lead to compression within the carpal tunnel. For proper nerve nutrition to occur, blood must flow into the tunnel, then into the nerve, and back out of the tunnel. The normal pressures within the compartments of the median nerve at the carpal tunnel must be the highest within the epineurial arterioles and become progressively less in the capillaries, fascicles of the nerve, and epineurial venules and least in the tunnel for normal blood flow to occur. Any increase in the pressure of a single compartment has the potential to disrupt the normal pressure gradients and impair the flow of blood within the tunnel. An increase in pressure within the carpal tunnel compartment can occur with thickening of tendons, synovial hyperplasia, and/or edema. Venous blood flow is impaired and venous stasis develops if pressure within the carpal tunnel compartment becomes greater than the pressure within the epineurial venules.

TABLE 12–1. Classification of Acute Traumatic Peripheral Nerve Injury

Anatomical Classification	Class I	Class II	Class III
Previous nomenclature	Neurapraxia	Axonotmesis	Neurotmesis
Lesion	Reversible conduction block resulting from ischemia or demyelination	Axonal interruption but basal lamina remains intact	Nerve fiber and basal lamina interruption (complete nerve severance)

Adapted from Schaumberg HH, Spencer PS, Thomas PK: Disorders of Peripheral Nerves. Philadelphia, FA Davis, 1983.

Sunderland[23] has proposed that venous stasis will lead to local hypoxia, resulting in abnormal impulse conduction within the nerve fibers and a deterioration of the capillary endothelium. A breakdown of the capillary endothelium causes the formation of a protein-rich edematous fluid in the interstitial space. This fluid (1) stimulates proliferation of fibroblasts resulting in fibrosis and (2) intensifies the abnormal pressure gradients present, producing more hypoxia. Fibrosis will decrease compliance of the nerve and result in an abnormal increase in the tension within the nervous system. This set of circumstances may be more appropriately referred to as a *neurovascular entrapment*, and it has the potential to cause the development of problems elsewhere in the system (i.e., a double crush injury). Because all nerves essentially travel within tissue tunnels the potential exists for this scenario to occur elsewhere in the continuous tissue tract of the nervous system.[2, 7, 24]

ADAPTIVE RESPONSES TO PAIN

A thorough discussion of the pain associated with peripheral nerve entrapment is beyond the scope and intent of this chapter. The topic of pain is discussed in Chapter 29 of this book. However, there are a couple of issues related to the pain associated with peripheral nerve entrapment that need to be discussed.

"Normal" or physiological pain occurs when peripheral nociceptors are subjected to a stimulus that is at or above the threshold. "Abnormal" or pathological pain can occur when there is a change in the sensitivity (threshold) of the somatosensory system.[26] A change in the sensitivity can occur in several ways.[6] First, the threshold of the peripheral nociceptors can be decreased; that is, there is an increase in the sensitivity of the nociceptors. The sensitization of the nociceptors allows weak subthreshold stimuli to activate the nociceptors, resulting in abnormal pain. Second, under certain conditions peripheral nerves develop the capacity for ectopic impulse generation that can lead to pathological pain.[6, 11, 15, 26]

Devor[6] has written: ". . . the crucial pathophysiological process triggered by nerve injury is an increase in neuronal excitability." Axons that become hypoxic and/or demyelinated from nerve injuries can enter a hyperexcitable state.[6, 21] A nerve in a hyperexcitable state can begin to discharge spontaneously, become mechanosensitive, and/or develop a sustained rhythmic discharge after stimulation, all of which can result in the production of pathological pain.[6, 11] A hyperexcitable state can occur with the mechanical microtraumas normally associated with peripheral nerve entrapments (e.g., compression, tension, friction, and inflammation).[6, 11, 21]

The dorsal root ganglion appears to play a significant role in the pain associated with peripheral nerve entrapment.[26] Pathological amounts of compression, tension, inflammation, and/or other injuries to peripheral nerves can cause the dorsal root ganglion to become hyperexcitable (sensitized), as described earlier. The change in sensitivity (threshold) allows what were weak subthreshold stimuli to evoke pain and suprathreshold stimuli to evoke exaggerated pain. This change in sensitivity reflects a change in the physiology of the nerve and may become a chronic state.[26]

As stated previously, the peripheral and central nervous systems represent a continuous tissue tract. The pain and symptoms associated with musculoskeletal injury and/or peripheral nerve entrapment can include changes that are the result of an alteration in the autonomic nervous system, which is considered part of the continuous tissue tract of the nervous system.[14, 21] Wyke[27] demonstrated that stimulation of nociceptors in spinal joints resulted in reflex changes in the cardiovascular, respiratory, and endocrine systems. Feinstein[9, 10] showed that injecting saline solution into the thoracic paraspinal muscles caused pallor, diaphoresis, bradycardia, and a drop in the blood pressure. These changes are often associated with an alteration in the output from the autonomic nervous system.[7, 13, 14] Some clients who are treated for musculoskeletal injuries show signs that may be related to autonomic dysreflexia. These "autonomic" signs include excessive vasoconstriction that leads to cold pale skin, hyperactive flexor withdrawal reflexes, and paradoxical breathing patterns that rely on excessive use of the scalene muscles.[7] Autonomic dysreflexia is often used synonymously with the term *hand-shoulder syndrome* described in individuals after stroke. A better appreciation of the contribution of the autonomic nervous system to the pathology and symptomatology present in some clients with musculoskeletal injuries could enhance the effectiveness of their treatment.

CLINICAL EXAMINATION AND TREATMENT

To effectively evaluate a client, the "whole person" must be addressed, and the patient must be involved in the evaluation and treatment processes. This philosophy requires the therapist to become the evaluator, teacher, and guide for the patient. Whenever possible the testing procedures should be performed by the patients so that they can learn to assess their status before and after treatment procedures. In some cases if the therapists use their hands it may be detrimental to the patient in a lifelong sense. The concept of patients gaining control of their problem(s) is fundamental and must be integrated into the initial patient contact to develop an effective self-management approach. Without an effective self-management strategy patients are at risk for recurrent problems and development of a chronic condition.

The standard musculoskeletal evaluation centered on a biomechanical model of the musculoskeletal and nervous systems is adequate for patients who present with straightforward symptoms that appear to be of biomechanical origin. However, a biomechanical approach is inappropriate for patients who present with severe or irritable signs and symptoms that may be neurological and/or vascular in origin. Patients with neurovascular entrapment often present with severe, irritable symptoms.

First, a subjective evaluation is conducted in a patient with a potential neurovascular entrapment problem to determine how the objective examination should proceed. The history of the condition is discussed with the patient.

Key components that should be discussed with the patient include a history of trauma, repetitive activities, sustained static or tension postures (e.g., computer keyboard work), and/or physical activities performed with a high level of cognitive demand (e.g., playing the piano). The history should include a discussion of any potentially significant medical conditions (e.g., asthma or diabetes) and the general health of the individual. Phase 1 of the differential diagnosis (medical screening; see Chapter 2) should be completed to guarantee that the patient is an appropriate candidate for potential evaluation and intervention.

A discussion of the patient's symptoms and complaints should include questions that determine if the neural and/or vascular systems are potential sources of the problem. Sensory disturbances relevant to the potential problem of neurovascular entrapment include complaints of fullness, swelling, tingling, pain, cold, numbness, and/or dropping things. In addition, the progression of the symptoms/complaints and the level of irritability should be determined. If pain is a major factor, then a functional pain questionnaire should be completed (see Chapter 29). Motor changes of relevance to the potential problem of neurovascular entrapment include complaints of dropping things, weakness, and/or an inability to perform a motor task that was done previously without difficulty. The level of neural irritability and the presence of peripheral or central sensitization should be determined by asking the patient what activities aggravate and ease the symptoms. Irritability may be indicated when an extended period of time is required for symptoms to ease after provocation. Sensitization is indicated when minor mechanical or normally nonnoxious stimuli (e.g., clothing on the skin) provoke pain. Vascular complaints relevant to the potential problem of neurovascular entrapment include complaints of fullness, swelling, abnormal skin color, and/or cool skin temperatures. A change in the vascular symptoms with a change in limb position is particularly significant.

In a biomechanical evaluation model (Table 12–2) the therapist examines the quantity and quality of active movements to determine if there is pain, spasm, and/or resistance at an "end feel." In clients with neurovascular entrapment this procedure may evoke a significant flare and worsening of symptoms. In these patients the "feel" of involuntary muscle tension can be the first sign of abnormality in assessing movement. This tension is often subtle and may occur earlier in the range of motion than where traditional symptoms and/or the end feel normally occurs. Moving into the range of motion to the initial point of tension minimizes the risk of provoking adverse neurological and/or vascular consequences.

The client presenting with severe or irritable symptoms should be examined initially for neurological sensitivity and irritability. Neurological testing should include the use of (1) upper limb tension tests for various components of the brachial plexus, (2) a straight-leg raising test for the components of the lumbosacral plexus, and (3) neck and/or trunk flexion with the extremities placed in various functional positions. These tests are used to assess the ability of the various peripheral nerves to tolerate normal extraneural and intraneural movement with movements of the trunk and extremities. All of the neurological tension tests should be done to the onset of tension when the client has a severe and irritable condition. Tinel's sign can be used at several locations in the extremity (e.g., the carpal tunnel, Guyon's canal, cubital tunnel, and the supraclavicular region in the upper extremity) to assess for neural sensitivity.[17]

The next essential step in the examination of patients with an upper quadrant dysfunction is to assess motor function in the thumb adductor and flexor carpi ulnaris. If there is weakness in one or both of these muscles, the patient is shown how to use a self–cervical traction technique (Fig. 12–2). The strength of the two muscles is reassessed immediately after the application of cervical traction. A selectively directed minimal stress is then applied to the neck to determine if this results in a decrease in the strength of the same muscles. If traction augments the strength and the application of a selectively directed minimal stress to the neck diminishes the strength, then the patient is considered to be "Kabat positive." Herman Kabat, a physician involved in the early development of proprioceptive neuromuscular facilitation, developed this clinical examination and self-treatment procedure.[16] A positive test result may be a sign of dural irritability rather than a cervical disk lesion as originally postulated by Kabat. Patients who have positive results on this testing procedure are taught a specific self-treatment program to maintain strength of the affected muscle groups.[16]

The next portion of the examination involves evaluating the integrity of the vascular system in the extremities. This involves inspecting the hands and/or feet for discoloration and assessing the skin temperature in each of the peripheral nerve territories present. Cool, cyanotic skin can be an indication of arterial insufficiency or sympathetic dysreflexia in the area, whereas swelling can be an indication of venous insufficiency or inflammation. An Adson test and the elevated arm stress test (EAST) are

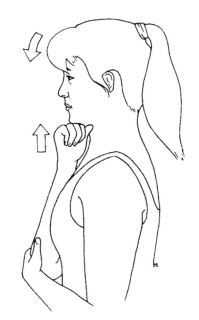

FIGURE 12–2. Self–cervical traction. Traction is applied by supplying upward pressure from one upper extremity onto the chin.

● T A B L E 1 2 – 2. Suggested Modifications to a Standard Biomechanical Evaluation

Observation

Cervical/thoracic: WNL _____ kyphosis _____ flat _____

Scapula: equal _____ high R/L _____ low L/R _____

Lumbar: WNL _____ lordosis _____ flat _____

Hands and feet: swelling _____ discoloration _____

other _____

Active Range of Motion
(for a patient with upper quadrant symptoms)

Cervical
Flexion: _____° causes/increases symptoms

Extension: _____° causes/increases symptoms

Rotation (R): _____° causes/increases symptoms

Rotation (L): _____° causes/increases symptoms

Lateral flexion (R): _____° causes/increases symptoms

Lateral flexion (L): _____° causes/increases symptoms

Shoulder Flexion
Right with elbow extension: _____° causes/increases symptoms

Left with elbow extension: _____° causes/increases symptoms

Right with elbow flexion: _____° causes/increases symptoms

Left with elbow flexion: _____° causes/increases symptoms

Shoulder Internal Rotation—reaching behind back
(functional tension test with radial nerve bias)
Right position: causes/increases symptoms
Left position: causes/increases symptoms

Neural Examination

Brachial Plexus Tension Test[61]
Right position: causes/increases symptoms
Left position: causes/increases symptoms

Lumbosacral Plexus Tension Test[15]
(straight-leg raising test or Laségue's test)
Right: _____° causes/increases symptoms

Left: _____° causes/increases symptoms

Tinel's Sign[15]
(Normal = 0; Mild = 1+; Moderate = 2+; Severe = 3+)
Supraclavicular region: Right _____ Left _____

Elbow: Right _____ Left _____

Wrist: (Median) Right _____ Left _____

(Ulnar) Right _____ Left _____

Kabat Tests[67]

Strength Tests[67]
Flexor carpi ulnaris (FCU): (R) _____ /5 (L) _____ /5

Adductor pollicis (AP): (R) _____ /5 (L) _____ /5

Cervical Traction[67]
(temporary strengthening of the FCU and AP)
no/yes—which muscles are affected and by what amount

Vascular Integrity

Temperature of Hands
(ambient room temperature _____°)
Right: (index) _____° (digiti minimi) _____°

Left: (index) _____° (digiti minimi) _____°

Adson's Test[15] (change in pulse pressure)
Right after: 1 minute _____ 2 minutes _____

3 minutes _____

Left after: 1 minute _____ 2 minutes _____

3 minutes _____

EAST[15] (change in pulse pressure)
Right after: 1 minute _____ 2 minutes _____
3 minutes _____

Left after: 1 minute _____ 2 minutes _____
3 minutes _____

Sensation[16]
(localization, stereognosis, graphesthesia, and others)

Breathing Pattern
(ability to relax the scalene muscles with quiet breathing)
Normal or dysfunctional pattern

Palpation Findings (tenderness)
normal = 0; mild = 1+; moderate = 2+; severe = 3+)
Scalene: Right _____ Left _____

Subclavius: Right _____ Left _____

Pectoralis minor: Right _____ Left _____

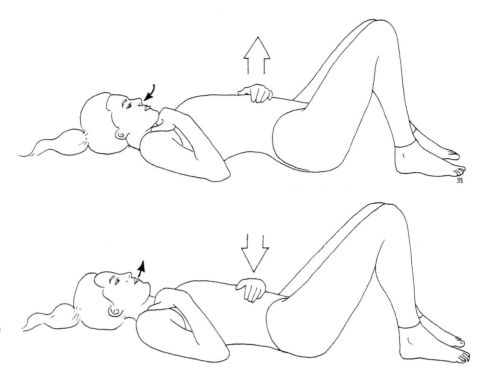

FIGURE 12–3. Diaphragmatic breathing. As the client inhales, the stomach should rise and the lordosis in the low back should increase. During exhalation the stomach should fall and the back flatten against the floor.

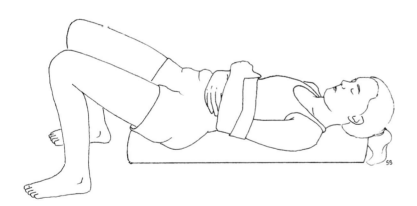

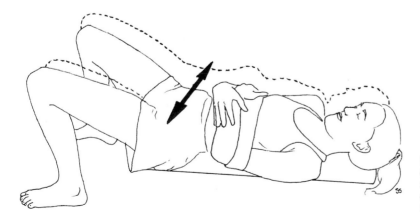

FIGURE 12–4. Foam roller exercise for mobilization of the spine. The roller is placed underneath the spine with the client in the supine position. The client gently rolls from side to side to increase mobility of the spine.

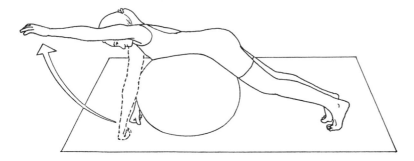

FIGURE 12–5. Patient in a quadruped position on a therapy ball with the chin tucked and the neck straight. The patient can lift an upper or lower extremity to provide a challenge to the muscles that stabilize the spine.

used to evaluate vascular integrity (i.e., does the pulse pressure decrease with a change in the position of the limb?).[17] The Adson test and the EAST should be performed on both upper extremities and the pulse pressure evaluated at 1, 2, and 3 minutes.

The patient is evaluated for potential sensory changes after the vascular assessment. Sensory changes may be subtle, and they are not always accompanied by obvious motor dysfunction. The most common complaint with neurovascular entrapment in the upper extremity is that "I drop things," and yet standard tests of strength, light touch, and two-point discrimination may be normal. Therapists often think of this problem as motor until the standard tests fail to demonstrate motor dysfunction. Subtle changes in the higher sensory cortex can occur as a consequence of repetitive motions, particularly when performed under conditions of intense concentration and/or in the presence of pain.[3–5] Byl[4] observed severe degradation in the representation of the hand in the somatosensory cortex of owl monkeys that were trained in a behavior of rapid, active opening/closing of the hand under conditions of high cognitive drive. In addition, Byl[3] found a significant difference in the response on some sensory integration and praxis tests in human subjects with diagnoses of tendinitis and focal dystonia. Byl has postulated that similar changes can be identified in humans with repetitive strain injuries using Ayer's tests of sensory localization, stereognosis, and graphesthesia.

The next portion of the examination involves an assessment of the patient's breathing pattern at rest and palpation of the subclavius, pectoralis minor, and scalene muscles. The normal breathing pattern at rest is primarily diaphragmatic (Fig. 12–3). However, patients with neurovascular entrapment often demonstrate a breathing pattern at rest that relies predominantly on the scalene muscles. The scalene breathing pattern mechanically narrows the thoracic outlet area, thus increasing the risk of neurovascular entrapment. The scalene breathing pattern may be a sign of protective posturing. Palpation is used to determine if tenderness and/or tightness is present. Findings on palpation of the subclavius, pectoralis minor, and scalene muscles are significant because of the relationship these muscles have with the subclavian vein, brachial plexus components, and subclavian artery, respectively. The results of the palpation should be correlated with the neurological and vascular changes found elsewhere in the extremity.

At the conclusion of this phase of the examination process a therapist must determine if intervention will involve a direct "hands on" treatment approach or a more indirect method using the self-treatment approach

discussed earlier. If the neurological, vascular, sensory, and motor examinations are found to be normal, then a biomechanical examination of the musculoskeletal system can be performed. (See the list of references provided in the suggested reading section for more information on how to conduct this type of examination.) If results of the preliminary examination are not normal, then biomechanical examination and treatment techniques should be deferred until the sensitivity and irritability of the nervous system are improved.

Treatment must follow the same principles that guide the evaluation. The patient is taught self-assessment techniques and strategies so that he or she has control of the progression of treatment and activities of daily living. The patient may use any of the following self-assessment techniques, as appropriate, to guide the course of treatment: a pain scale, a thermometer to test skin temperature, a neural tension test, or a Kabat strength test. Any treatment or activity that increases symptoms, protective posturing, and/or tension is modified or discontinued.

The goals of treatment are to:

1. Restore normal relaxed diaphragmatic breathing at rest and in functional positions.
2. Restore the normal sensitivity of the entire nervous system.
3. Restore strength and endurance to the muscles throughout the body.
4. Do the above without increasing symptoms.
5. Do the above without loss of strength in the thumb or wrist flexors (if the patient is Kabat positive).

Treatment is begun using sensorimotor integration with an emphasis on functional skills (e.g., breathing, balance, and hand function) in a manner that does not cause irritation of the patient's condition. The patient is guided through a series of breathing exercises designed to improve the circulation to the extremities, calm the nervous system, and retrain the scalene muscles, if appropriate. The breathing exercises are progressed through the use of foam rollers (Fig. 12–4). These are used to increase the mobility of the spine and rib cage. The breathing exercises are combined with functional movements of the trunk and extremities in a manner that mobilizes the nervous system. Once the patient is able to manage his or her symptoms the treatment can progress to stabilization exercises using a gym ball (Fig. 12–5). If the patient has vestibular, balance, or sensory integration deficits, then specific techniques for balance or sensory retraining can be added.

PATIENT DESCRIPTION

The patient is a 35-year-old right-handed legal secretary who has worked at her present job for 16 years. About 2 years ago her office switched to software applications requiring increased use of the computer mouse. She reports a 2-year history of right arm pain of gradual onset that worsened and has been constant for the past 4 months. She has been off work for 4 months because of the symptoms in her right arm. Her recreational activities include aerobics and softball but she has done neither for several months because of her arm symptoms. She has experienced sensations of numbness and tingling on the dorsal surface of both hands, as well as "tension" in her neck. She has had "4 or 5" cortisone injections in the elbow, participated in physical therapy for "stretching and strengthening," and switched to a trackball pointing device at her computer workstation without significant benefit. Ten days before the current physical therapy evaluation she had right elbow surgery (débridement). The sutures were removed 4 days ago. She reports her current symptoms as a constant "throb" at the elbow of 3/10 intensity at rest on a 0 to 10 pain scale. The neck tension is still present, but the hand numbness has not been present since surgery. She states her arm pain increases with trying to take a shirt off over her head or if she does any task that involves gripping with the right hand. She is avoiding using her right arm.

Her significant history includes a meat cutter accident at age 5 that resulted in the amputation of fingertips 2 and 3 on the right hand. She reports no residual limitation in function from that injury. Five years ago she fell, injuring her right wrist and left ankle. The wrist symptoms resolved without intervention, and the ankle recovered after 1 month of physical therapy. One year ago she fell while playing softball, resulting in a sore neck for 1 day.

She reports no general health problems. She denies use of anticoagulant and corticosteroid medications. She reports normal sensation in both feet and denies any dizziness. She is currently able to sleep through the night. Her medications include Vicodin and Tylenol with codeine.

CLINICAL REASONING

Hypothesis/diagnosis based on the subjective examination includes:

1. *Potential soft tissue edema* in the forearm extensor muscles 10 days after surgery.
2. *Potential adverse neural tension* based on the:
   a. duration of symptoms
   b. pattern of symptoms that do not fit isolated tendonitis (neck tension and bilateral numbness/tingling)
   c. lack of response to multiple interventions

PHYSICAL EXAMINATION

In this patient the nervous system is considered a potential source of dysfunction. (See Table 12–2 for suggested modifications to a biomechanically based musculoskeletal examination.) The referring physician specified a precaution of "no resistive exercises of the right upper extremity until 6 weeks post op"; therefore, no strength tests or Kabat tests were done.

The incision at the right lateral epicondyle area was well healed with mild ecchymosis. The right upper extremity otherwise had normal skin color and temperature. Girth measurements at 2 inches were +1.9 cm below the olecranon and +1.3 cm at the olecranon on the right versus the left. The patient sat with a mild forward head posture and a flat upper thoracic kyphosis while she held the right arm at her side with her elbow flexed.

The patient was instructed to complete active movement testing just to the point of feeling tension or resistance to movement. This precaution is meant to minimize the potential for a significant flare of symptoms from provocation testing of potentially irritable neurovascular structures while still providing a repeatable measurement for reassessment. The patient moved through full cervical flexion and bilateral rotation without report of tension or symptoms. Cervical extension at 45 degrees produced a feeling of neck stiffness. On further investigation, left lateral flexion at 75% range produced vague soreness in her right arm that was similar to, but less intense than, her present symptoms. Right lateral flexion was 100% and did not provoke symptoms. Isolated right upper-extremity movements were done without provocation of her symptoms and included elbow flexion, 120 degrees; extension, −10 degrees; pronation, 80 degrees; and supination, 70 degrees. Passive neural provocation testing was performed to the onset of tension or a change in symptoms (Table 12–3). The upper-limb tension test (ULTT) was the only passive neural provocation test performed because of the patient's suspected nervous system irritability. (See Suggested Readings at the end of this chapter for a more complete description of how to perform this and other ULTTs.) On palpation, the scalene muscles were noted to be active during breathing at rest.

CLINICAL REASONING

Diagnosis/hypothesis based on physical examination includes:

1. *Postoperative edema in forearm extensor muscles* confirmed by circumferential measurements
2. *Adverse neural tension* based on the presence of:
   a. reproduction of elbow pain with cervical movement

(Continued)

b. early onset of protective muscle tension and reproduction of symptoms with ULTT (indicator of possible neurovascular entrapment)
c. scalene breathing pattern (indicator of possible adaptive response to chronic pain)

INTERVENTION

The patient was instructed to perform active range of motion exercises for the upper extremity in "out of tension" positions, that is, in positions that allowed for minimal tension on neural structures and did not provoke symptoms. For example, she was able to do relaxed right wrist flexion/extension as long as she was lying on her left side with her right arm supported on her body and the elbow flexed. This position did not result in abnormal tension-related symptoms and probably provided her with a minimal amount of tension on the brachial plexus. She was instructed in relaxed diaphragmatic breathing in the supine position. She was issued a foam roller and instructed in spine mobilization exercises (see Fig. 12–4). She was instructed to walk daily, supporting her right arm as needed. Use of ice and of edema reduction measures for the right upper extremity was reviewed. A trial of cervical traction using a towel was found to increase cervical range in left lateral flexion without producing forearm symptoms. The patient was instructed in the towel traction technique for symptom management (Fig. 12–6).

TABLE 12–3. Changes Observed in the Upper Limb Tension Test

Shoulder

Depression	Abduction	External Rotation
(R) neutral	80°	neutral
(L) neutral	full	full

Forearm

Supination
(R) 70° without symptoms
(L) full without symptoms

Wrist

Extension
(R) 40° without symptoms
(L) full without symptoms

Elbow

Extension
(R) deferred
(L) −10°

Cervical

Lateral Flexion
(R) increase in forearm symptoms
(L) full with no symptoms

At her second visit she was instructed in self-assessment techniques to evaluate her response to activity. If she had a negative response to an exercise or activity of daily living, as evidenced by an increase in symptoms or a decrease in the range of her upper-limb tension screening test, she was instructed to modify or discontinue the activity and perform a self treatment that restored her tension-free range. The techniques that she found successful in restoring her mobility were diaphragmatic breathing (see Fig. 12–3) and supine cervical traction.

At 4 weeks after her elbow surgery the surgeon gave the approval to start light resistive exercises. At this stage the patient no longer demonstrated signs of neural irritability. Treatment was progressed with the addition of foam roller exercises to improve spinal mobility (see Fig. 12–4). The patient was started on gentle strengthening for the wrist extensors. Neural mobilization exercises progressed from active exercise in tension-free range to active exercise into mild resistance (i.e., to a feeling of "stretch" in the ULTT position). Once full mobility was gained in the standard ULTT, then the radial nerve biased test position was examined and determined to be restricted. The radial nerve–biased ULTT was taught to the patient as a treatment technique to restore mobility in the branches of the radial nerve that cross the extensor surface of the forearm. The patient was placed prone on fists and knees and prone on a therapy ball to perform exercises that promote scapular stabilization, postural strengthening, and progressive weight bearing through the wrist and elbow joints (see Fig. 12–5).

Final treatment sessions focused on problem solving related to symptom management and postural training with simulated work tasks and recreational activities. Diaphragmatic breathing and cervical traction techniques were adapted to the upright position so that the patient could manage symptoms while performing work tasks. Emphasis was placed on continued self-assessment of the response of the nervous system to the progression of activity.

OUTCOME

At the first follow-up visit 2 days after the initial evaluation the patient reported a significant reduction in symptoms after walking for 1 hour. Her girth measurements at the right elbow were improved by 1 cm, indicating a reduction in edema. The right ULTT was performed to the onset of tension: shoulder depression (neutral), abduction (90 degrees), external rotation (80 degrees), forearm supination (85 degrees), wrist extension (60 degrees), and elbow extension (−70 degrees), indicating a significant improvement in tension-

Continued

CASE STUDY *Continued*

free range (compare with Table 12–3). The patient was able to objectively see and experience the benefit of the activities that were prescribed. The intent of the treatment program was to improve function in the vascular, neural, and lymphatic systems without provoking a protective tension response. The early success with self-guided treatment set the stage for teaching the patient to evaluate the effect of any activity, manage symptoms with one or two easing techniques, and ultimately progress her own activity level. This approach gave the patient control of her problem.

The patient received a total of nine treatments at the time of discharge (3 months after surgery). Grip strength was equal bilaterally at 75 pounds. At this point she was working full time at her regular job with ergonomic improvements to her workstation. She reported a residual symptom of spot pain at the elbow that she could control with exercise. Through trial and error and self-assess-

ment she determined that her aerobic exercise class was a consistent irritant so she switched her aerobic activity to walking.

DISCUSSION

This case illustrates the importance of evaluating the role of the nervous system in patients with chronic and/or irritable symptoms. Sensitization[26] and possible processing changes in the central nervous system[3-5] necessitate evaluation of the nervous system as a potential source of symptoms in patients with chronic and/or irritable symptoms (e.g., cumulative trauma disorder). If the issues of nervous system irritability and sensitization are not addressed during evaluation and throughout treatment, then the risk for increasing the patient's symptoms and continuing the cycle of nervous system hypersensitivity is high.

The indicators that this patient may have had a

(Continued)

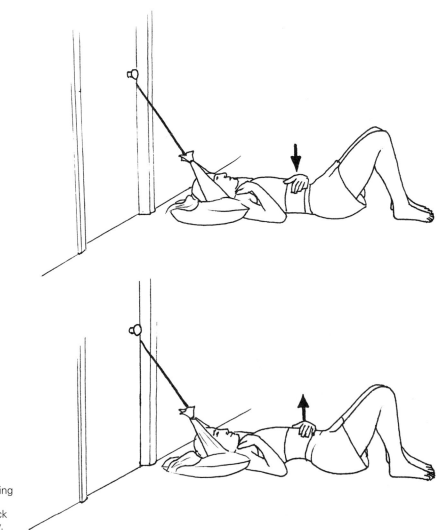

FIGURE 12–6. Towel traction unit. By arching the low back the amount of traction is increased slightly. By flattening the low back the amount of traction is decreased slightly.

CASE STUDY *Continued*

nervous system dysfunction were her history of repetitive work, prior trauma, pattern of symptoms, and lack of response to standard medical care. The indicators on physical examination were the restricted ULTT, the reproduction of symptoms with selected neck movements, and the altered breathing pattern. Other objective indicators that were not assessed initially that may have further guided the treatment include Kabat testing and sensory testing of localization and graphesthesia. A key concept to keep in mind is the role of education in treating patients with a chronic problem such as repetitive strain injury. Teaching patients a self-assessment tool restores their control, allowing them to guide their own treatment and to be more responsible for their own well-being.

REFERENCES

1. Breig A: Adverse Mechanical Tension in the Central Nervous System. Stockholm, Almqvist & Wiksell International, 1978.
2. Butler DS: Mobilization of the Nervous System. Edinburgh, Churchill Livingstone, 1991.
3. Byl N: Sensory dysfunction associated with repetitive strain injuries of tendonitis and focal hand dystonia: A comparative study. J Orthop Sports Phys Ther 23(4):234, 1996.
4. Byl N: A primate model for studying focal dystonia and repetitive strain injury: Effects on the primary somatosensory cortex. Phys Ther 77(3):269, 1997.
5. Byl N, Melnick M: The neural consequences of repetition: Clinical implications of a learning hypothesis. J Hand Ther 10:160, 1997.
6. Devor M: The pathophysiology of damaged peripheral nerves. *In* Wall PD, et al (eds): Textbook of Pain, 3rd ed. Edinburgh, Churchill Livingstone, 1994.
7. Edgelow PI: Neurovascular consequences of cumulative trauma disorders affecting the thoracic outlet: A patient-centered treatment approach. *In* Donatelli RA (ed): Physical Therapy of the Shoulder, 3rd ed. New York, Churchill Livingstone, 1997.
8. Elvey RL: The investigation of arm pain. *In* Grieve GP (ed): Modern Manual Therapy of the Vertebral Column. Edinburgh, Churchill Livingstone, 1986.
9. Feinstein B, Langton JNK, Jameson RM, et al: Experiments on pain referred from deep somatic tissues. J Bone Joint Surg Am 36:981, 1954.
10. Feinstein B: Referred pain from paravertebral structures. *In* Buerger AA, et al (eds): Approaches to the Validation of Manipulative Therapy. Springfield, IL, Charles C Thomas, 1981.
11. Gifford L: Fluid movement may partially account for the behavior of symptoms associated with nociception in disc injury and disease. *In* Shadlock M (ed): Moving in on Pain. Sydney, Butterworth-Heinemann, 1995.
12. Gilliatt RW: Physical injury to peripheral nerves. Mayo Clin Proc 56:361, 1981.
13. Grieve GP: Referred pain and other clinical features. *In* Grieve GP (ed): Modern Manual Therapy of the Vertebral Column. Edinburgh, Churchill Livingstone, 1986.
14. Grieve GP: The autonomic nervous system in vertebral pain syndromes. *In* Grieve GP (ed): Modern Manual Therapy of the Vertebral Column. Edinburgh, Churchill Livingstone, 1986.
15. Grieve GP: Common Vertebral Joint Problems, 2nd ed. Edinburgh, Churchill Livingstone, 1988.
16. Kabat H: Low Back and Leg Pain from Herniated Cervical Disc. St. Louis, Warren H. Green, 1980.
17. Magee D: Orthopedic Physical Assessment, 2nd ed. Philadelphia, WB Saunders, 1992.
18. Mather LH: The Peripheral Nervous System: Structure, Function and Clinical Correlations. Reading, Addison-Wesley Publishing Co, 1985.
19. Ochoa J, Fowler TJ, Gilliatt RW: Anatomical changes in peripheral nerves compressed by a pneumatic tourniquet. J Anat 113:433, 1972.
20. Pratt NE: Neurovascular entrapment in the regions of the shoulder and posterior triangle of the neck. Phys Ther 66:12, 1986.
21. Schaumberg HH: Disorders of Peripheral Nerves. Philadelphia, FA Davis, 1983.
22. Seddon HJ: Three types of nerve injury. Brain 66:237, 1943.
23. Sunderland S: The nerve lesion in carpal tunnel syndrome. Neurol Neurosurg Psychiatry 39:615, 1976.
24. Sunderlund S: Nerves and Nerve Injuries, 2nd ed. Baltimore, Williams & Wilkins, 1978.
25. Upton ARM, McComas AJ: The double crush injury in nerve entrapment syndromes. Lancet 2:359, 1973.
26. Woolf CF: The dorsal horn: State-dependent sensory processing and the generation of pain. *In* Wall PD, et al (eds): Textbook of Pain, 3rd ed. Edinburgh, Churchill Livingstone, 1994.
27. Wyke BD: The neurological basis of thoracic spinal pain. Rheum Phys Med 10:356, 1970.

SUGGESTED READINGS

Butler DS: Mobilization of the Nervous System. Edinburgh, Churchill Livingstone, 1991.
Edgelow PI: Neurovascular consequences of cumulative trauma disorders affecting the thoracic outlet: A patient-centered treatment approach. In Donatelli RA (ed): Physical Therapy of the Shoulder, 3rd ed. New York, Churchill Livingstone, 1997.
Grieve GP: Common Vertebral Joint Problems, 2nd ed. Edinburgh, Churchill Livingstone, 1988.
Grieve GP (ed): Modern Manual Therapy of the Vertebral Column. Edinburgh, Churchill Livingstone, 1986.
Kabat H: Low Back and Leg Pain from Herniated Cervical Disc. St. Louis, Warren H. Green, 1980.
Magee D: Orthopedic Physical Assessment, 2nd ed. Philadelphia, WB Saunders Co, 1992.
Sunderland S: The nerve lesion in carpal tunnel syndrome. Neurol Neurosurg Psychiatry 39:615, 1976.
Wall PD, et al (eds): Textbook of Pain, 3rd ed. Edinburgh, Churchill Livingstone, 1994.
Upton ARM, McComas AJ: The double crush injury in nerve entrapment syndromes. Lancet 2:359, 1973.

Neuromuscular Diseases

ANN HALLUM, PhD, PT

Key Words

- amyotrophic lateral sclerosis (ALS)

- disuse atrophy

- Duchenne muscular dystrophy (DMD)

- Guillain-Barré syndrome (GBS)

- overwork damage

- polyradiculoneuropathy

Objectives

After reviewing this chapter the student/therapist will:

1. Describe the basic pathology and medical treatment of amyotrophic lateral sclerosis, Guillain-Barré syndrome, and Duchenne muscular dystrophy.

2. Describe the current goals and treatment program for each condition.

3. Describe the "safe" exercise windows related to disuse atrophy and exercise (overwork) damage.

4. Be able to apply treatment concepts discussed in this chapter to other neuromuscular diseases.

This chapter traces the connections between the central nervous system (CNS) and muscle using three disorders: amyotrophic lateral sclerosis (ALS), which damages upper and lower motor neurons; Guillain-Barré syndrome (GBS), which affects the peripheral nervous system; and Duchenne muscular dystrophy (DMD), which impairs muscle function. The upper motor neurons that are affected in ALS originate in the motor cortex of the brain (Betz cells). These upper motor neuron axons descend by means of the corticobulbar and corticospinal tracts to synapse with lower motor neurons (primary motor neurons) in the brain stem and spinal cord (anterior horn cells). From the lower motor neuron, the axon runs within the peripheral nerve, which includes motor and sensory fibers, to synapse with muscle fibers. Depending on the site of the pathology, neuromuscular diseases can be classified as neurogenic or myopathic. ALS and GBS are neurogenic disorders; DMD is a primary myopathy (Fig. 13–1).

AMYOTROPHIC LATERAL SCLEROSIS

Pathology and Medical Diagnosis

ALS, commonly known in the United States as "Lou Gehrig's disease," is a relentless, degenerative, terminal

Neuromuscular diseases

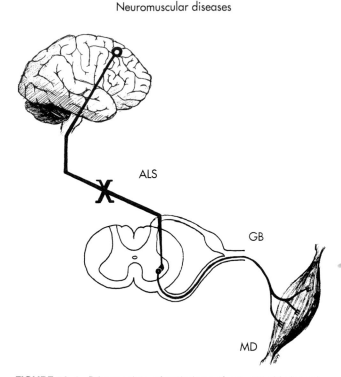

FIGURE 13–1. Primary sites of pathology of amyotrophic lateral sclerosis (ALS), Guillain-Barré syndrome (GB), and Duchenne muscular dystrophy (MD).

disease affecting both upper and lower motor neurons. Massive loss of anterior horn cells of the spinal cord and the motor cranial nerve nuclei in the lower brain stem results in muscle atrophy and weakness (amyotrophy). Demyelination and gliosis of the corticospinal tracts and corticobulbar tracts caused by degeneration of the Betz cells in the motor cortex result in upper motor neuron symptoms (lateral sclerosis). Diagnosis of ALS depends primarily on the identification of a constellation of motor system changes. Little is known about the early changes occurring in the motor neurons; however, histologically, there is extensive neuronal loss with astrocytic gliosis. Some neurons seem to remain intact, whereas others show nonspecific cytoplasmic and nuclear shrinkage associated with the accumulation of lipofuscin.[40, 68, 105]

The etiology of ALS is unknown; however, numerous theories have been proposed. Toxic theories related to increased lead and aluminum levels and abnormalities in calcium and magnesium levels have been suggested.[40] More recently, research has focused on possible causes associated with a deficiency of nerve growth factor, an excess of extracellular glutamate in the CNS, and an autoimmune process.[148] These hypotheses have led to specific treatment protocols currently in the clinical trial stages. Most recently, a viral origin for ALS has been proposed. Berger and associates, using new molecular techniques, identified traces of a virus in the spinal cord tissue of 15 of 17 patients who died of ALS, but of only 1 of 29 patients who died of other causes.[22]

ALS is the most common form of motor neuron disease, with an incidence of approximately 1 to 2 cases per 100,000 persons. Mean age at onset is 57 years[22] with two thirds of patients being between 50 and 70 years old at time of onset. Men are affected one and one-half to two times more frequently than women.[40] Ninety to 95% of cases are classified as sporadic, with 5% to 10% of cases classified as a familial form of ALS caused by a mutation in the superoxide dismutase-1 gene located on chromosome 21.[181] The clinical presentation of the familial form is identical to that of the patients with a sporadic form of ALS.[156] ALS occurs about as often as muscular dystrophy and is three times more common than myasthenia gravis.[8]

Clinical Presentation

The World Federation of Neurology has developed suggested diagnostic criteria (suspected, possible, probable, and definite) for patients with ALS entering clinical research trials. Essentially, a patient with "definite" ALS must show concomitant upper motor neuron and lower motor neuron signs in three spinal regions or in two spinal regions with bulbar signs. Either upper or lower motor signs must also be evident in other regions of the body.[34, 182] Exclusionary criteria are the presence of sensory and autonomic nervous system (ANS) dysfunction, sphincter control problems, oculomotor nerve pathway abnormalities, and significant movement disorder patterns or cognitive deterioration.[19, 35] Although a consistent diagnostic criterion for ALS has been the absence of sensory involvement, Mulder and Kurland[153] have reported that 20% of their patients show signs of sensory dysfunction. Several investigators have shown possible dysfunction in somatosensory evoked potentials transmitted in the posterior columns.[153, 214] In addition to the possible sensory deficits, subclinical abnormalities of the ANS, both sympathetic and parasympathetic, have also been identified in a sample of 74 patients using a quantitative sudomotor axon reflex test (sweat testing) and parasympathetic vascular reflex testing of heart rate change during a Valsalva maneuver and deep breathing. Thirty-eight percent of patients showed symptoms of autonomic dysfunction. The authors suggested that the problems appear to be associated with atrophy and bulbar changes. Progression of signs and symptoms is essential for a confirmed diagnosis, and patients with ANS dysfunction seemed to have a faster rate of progression.[55] (See also Rowland[182] and Belsh[19] for succinct reviews of the differential diagnosis for ALS.)

No single laboratory test is currently available to confirm a diagnosis of ALS, although creatine phosphokinase levels are elevated in about 70% of patients.[68] Genetic testing to identify the mutation in the superoxide dismutase-1 gene is available if there is a family history of ALS. Other laboratory tests, such as identification of biochemical markers in the blood and cerebrospinal fluid, and neuroimaging techniques are used to exclude other neurological diseases. Electromyography (EMG) and nerve conduction studies can be very helpful to confirm the presence of widespread lower motor neuron disease without peripheral neuropathy or polyradiculopathy. Nerve conduction velocities are usually within normal limits. EMG studies typically show spontaneous fibrillations and fasciculations with giant or large unit spikes with voluntary activity.[19, 40, 230] Because of the absence of clear laboratory markers of ALS, the clinical diagnosis must be based on recognition of a pattern of observed and reported symptoms and behaviors supported with inclusionary and exclusionary diagnostic testing.

Fatigue or the loss of exercise tolerance is the most common complaint of patients presenting for diagnosis.[213] The earliest clinical markers of ALS are fasciculations (especially unequivocal fasciculation in the tongue), muscle cramps, fatigue, weakness, and atrophy.[182, 213] In 90% of patients, weakness occurring in any striated muscle or group of muscles is the primary complaint. Because the onset of ALS is insidious, most patients are not aware of the strength changes or they have adjusted to the changes until they have difficulty with a functional activity, such as tying shoes or climbing stairs. Physical examination usually demonstrates more widespread weakness and atrophy than reported by the patient.[8, 40, 153] By the time most patients complain of weakness, they have lost approximately 80% of their motor neurons in the areas of weakness. This demonstrates the plasticity of the nervous system and its drive to adapt to meet functional goals. The weakness spreads over time to include musculature throughout the body. Succeeding symptoms of weakness in other muscle(s) depend on the continued loss of motor neurons to the 20% threshold needed for perception of weakness.[37, 201] A typical, but not absolute, pattern of motor progression is early distal involvement followed by proximal limb involvement. In some cases, bulbar symptoms herald the onset of ALS, but more commonly, bulbar symptoms occur later in the disease. Flexor muscles tend to be weaker than extensor muscles.[30]

Although the atrophy and weakness component of ALS is most obvious, 80% or more of patients show early clinical evidence of pyramidal tract dysfunction (i.e., hyperreflexia in the presence of weakness and atrophy, spasticity, and Babinski and Hoffman reflexes).[153, 182] Although in some cases the upper motor neuron signs may be absent clinically, Chou[47] has shown on autopsy that significant involvement may be present despite the lack of clinical evidence.

The pattern of ALS onset is highly varied, with several patterns identified by primary area of onset. Lower-extremity onset is slightly more common than upper-extremity onset, which is more common than bulbar onset. Some patients show initial symptoms in distal musculature of upper and lower extremities. A significant diagnostic feature of the pattern of disease is the asymmetry of the weakness and the sparing of some muscle fibers even in highly atrophied muscles. For example, a patient may present with weakness of the right intrinsics and shoulder musculature or weakness of the left anterior tibial muscles. Bulbar symptoms are heralded by tongue fasciculations and weakness, facial and palatal weakness, and swallowing difficulties, which result in dysphagia and dysarthria. Oculomotor nuclei are almost always spared.[40] Despite the pattern of onset, however, the eventual course of the illness is similar in most patients, with an unremitting spread of weakness to other muscle groups leading to total paralysis of spinal musculature and muscles innervated by the cranial nerves. Death is usually related to respiratory failure.[174]

In a multisite study of 167 patients with ALS, subjects were followed for 2 years on a monthly basis with 42 strength and functional assessments. Data confirmed findings of other studies that showed a more rapid loss of strength in the upper extremities than in the lower extremities. There was no difference between men or women in the rate of progression. In contrast to other studies, results indicated that older patients did not show a faster rate of deterioration, although they did enter the study in a weaker, more debilitated state, which may be related to their apparent shorter disease course.[174] In an ongoing study using monthly questionnaires, direct patient interviews, record reviews, physician interviews, and family member interviews, Brooks and coworkers[37] followed 702 patients with ALS. Their findings suggest that spread of neuronal degeneration occurred more quickly to adjacent areas than to noncontiguous areas. The spread to adjacent areas was more rapid at the brain stem, cervical, and lumbar regions. Limb involvement after bulbar onset was more aggressive in men than in women.[37]

Several studies have focused on developing methods to assess the natural history of the progression of ALS so that medical and supportive treatment planning and interventions can be instituted.[11] Hillel and co-workers[103] have developed an Amyotrophic Lateral Sclerosis Severity Scale for rapid functional assessment of disease stage. Their 10-point ordinal scale allows clinicians and therapists to score patients in four categories of function: speech, swallowing, lower extremity, and upper extremity (see the box on pages 366–368).

A five-point scale of severity is currently being used in ALS clinical drug trials. Patients in stage 1 (mild disease) have a recent diagnosis and are functionally independent in ambulation, activities of daily living (ADL), and speech. Stage 2 (moderate) identifies patients with a mild deficit in function in three regions or a moderate to severe deficit in one region and mild or normal function in two other regions. Stage 3 (severe) defines a patient who needs assistance because of deficits in two or three regions; for example, the patient needs assistance to walk or transfer and/or needs help with upper-extremity activities and/or the patient is dysarthric/dysphasic. Stage 4 identifies patients with nonfunctional use of at least two regions and moderate or nonfunctional use of a third area. Stage 5 is death.[36] (See Brooks and associates[34] and Pradas and colleagues[169] for information on the natural history of ALS and its importance in the design of clinical treatment trials.)

Prognosis

In almost all cases, ALS progresses relentlessly and leads to death from respiratory failure. The rate of progression seems to be consistent for each patient but varies considerably among patients. Patients with an initial onset of bulbar (dysarthria, dysphagia) and respiratory weakness (dyspnea) tend to have a more rapid progression to death than patients whose weakness begins in the distal extremities.[174] Caroscio[40] reported that in a study of 397 patients with ALS, the median survival time was 4.08 years after onset of symptoms with a shortening of median survival time with increasing age at onset. A small number of

AMYOTROPHIC LATERAL SCLEROSIS SEVERITY SCALE: LOWER EXTREMITY, UPPER EXTREMITY, SPEECH, SWALLOWING

Lower Extremities (Walking)

Normal

10	Normal ambulation	Patient denies any weakness or fatigue; examination detects no abnormality.
9	Fatigue suspected	Patient experiences sense of weakness or fatigue in lower extremities during exertion.

Early Ambulation Difficulties

8	Difficulty with uneven terrain	Difficulty and fatigue when walking long distances, climbing stairs, and walking over uneven ground (even thick carpet).
7	Observed changes in gait	Noticeable change in gait; pulls on railings when climbing stairs; may use leg brace.

Walks with Assistance

6	Walks with mechanical device	Needs or uses cane, walker, or assistant to walk; probably uses wheelchair away from home.
5	Walks with mechanical device and assistant	Does not attempt to walk without attendant; ambulation limited to less than 50 ft; avoids stairs.

Functional Movement Only

4	Able to support	At best, can shuffle a few steps with the help of an attendant for transfers.
3	Purposeful leg movements	Unable to take steps, but can position legs to assist attendant in transfers; moves legs purposely to maintain mobility in bed.

No Purposeful Leg Movement

2	Minimal movement	Minimal movement of one or both legs; cannot reposition legs independently.
1	Paralysis	Flaccid paralysis; cannot move lower extremities (except, perhaps, to close inspection).

Upper Extremities (Dressing and Hygiene)

Normal Function

10	Normal function	Patient denies any weakness or unusual fatigue of upper extremities; examination demonstrates no abnormality.
9	Suspected fatigue	Patient experiences sense of fatigue in upper extremities during exertion; cannot sustain work for as long as normal; atrophy not evident on examination.

Independent and Complete Self-Care

8	Slow self-care	Dressing and hygiene performed more slowly than usual.
7	Effortful self-care performance	Requires significantly more time (usually double or more) and effort to accomplish self-care; weakness is apparent on examination.

Continued

AMYOTROPHIC LATERAL SCLEROSIS SEVERITY SCALE:
LOWER EXTREMITY, UPPER EXTREMITY, SPEECH, SWALLOWING *Continued*

Intermittent Assistance

6 Mostly independent

Handles most aspects of dressing and hygiene alone; adapts by resting, modifying (electric razor) or avoiding some tasks; requires assistance for fine motor tasks (e.g., buttons, tie).

5 Partial independence independent

Handles some aspects of dressing and hygiene alone; however, routinely requires assistance for many tasks such as make-up, combing, shaving.

Needs Attendant for Self-Care

4 Attendant assists patient

Attendant must be present for dressing and hygiene; patient performs the majority of each task with the assistance of the attendant.

3 Patient assists attendant

The attendant directs the patient for almost all tasks; the patient moves in a purposeful manner to assist the attendant; does not initiate self-care.

Total Dependence

2 Minimal movement

Minimal movement of one or both arms; cannot reposition arms.

1 Paralysis

Flaccid paralysis; unable to move upper extremities (except, perhaps to close inspection).

Speech

Normal Speech Processes

10 Normal speech

Patient denies any difficulty speaking; examination demonstrates no abnormality.

9 Nominal speech abnormalities

Only the patient or spouse notices speech has changed, maintains normal rate and volume.

Detectable Speech Disturbance

8 Perceived speech changes

Speech changes are noted by others, especially during fatigue or stress; rate of speech remains essentially normal.

7 Obvious speech abnormalities

Speech is consistently impaired; affected are rate, articulation, and resonance; remains easily understood.

Intelligible with Repeating

6 Repeats message on occasion

Rate is much slower, repeats specific words in adverse listening situation; does not limit complexity or length of messages.

5 Frequent repeating required

Speech is slow and labored; extensive repetition or a "translator" is commonly used; patient probably limits the complexity or length of messages.

Speech Combined with Nonvocal Communication

4 Speech plus nonverbal communication

Speech is used in response to questions; intelligibility problems *need* to be resolved by writing or a spokesman.

3 Limits speech to one-word responses

Vocalizes one-word responses beyond yes/no; otherwise writes or uses a spokesperson; initiates communication nonvocally.

Continued

AMYOTROPHIC LATERAL SCLEROSIS SEVERITY SCALE:
LOWER EXTREMITY, UPPER EXTREMITY, SPEECH, SWALLOWING *Continued*

Loss of Useful Speech

2	Vocalizes for emotional expression	Uses vocal inflection to express emotion, affirmation, and negation.
1	Nonvocal	Vocalization is effortful, limited in duration, and rarely attempted; may vocalize for crying or pain.
X	Tracheostomy	

Swallowing

Normal Eating Habits

10	Normal swallowing	Patient denies any difficulty chewing or swallowing; examination demonstrates no abnormality.
9	Nominal abnormality	Only patient notices slight indicators such as food lodging in the recesses of the mouth or sticking in the throat.

Early Eating Problems

8	Minor swallowing problems	Complains of some swallowing difficulties; maintains essentially a regular diet; isolated choking episodes.
7	Prolonged times/smaller bite size	Meal time has significantly increased and smaller bite sizes are necessary; must concentrate on swallowing thin liquids.

Dietary Consistency Changes

6	Soft diet	Diet is limited primarily to soft foods; requires some special meal preparation.
5	Liquefied diet	Oral intake adequate; nutrition limited primarily to liquefied diet; adequate thin liquid intake usually a problem; may force self to eat.

Needs Tube Feeding

4	Supplemental tube feedings	Oral intake alone no longer adequate; patient uses or *needs* a tube to supplement intake; patient continues to take significant (greater than 50%) nutrition orally.
3	Tube feeding with occasional oral nutrition	Primary nutrition and hydration accomplished by tube; receives less than 50% of nutrition orally.

No Oral Feeding

2	Secretions managed with aspirator and/or medications	Cannot safely manage any oral intake; secretions managed with aspirator and/or medications; swallows reflexively.
1	Aspiration of secretions	Secretions cannot be managed noninvasively; rarely swallows.

Adapted with permission from Hillel AD, et al: Amyotrophic lateral sclerosis severity scale. Neuroepidemiology 8:142–150, 1989.

patients have lived for 15 to 20 years after onset. Although time of onset is determined primarily by the patient's recognition of the disease manifestations, autopsies of patients who have died of respiratory failure soon after diagnosis have shown evidence of more widespread disease in the skeletal musculature even though there was no clinical evidence of skeletal muscle involvement.[153] Years of survival after diagnosis may change as increasing numbers of patients elect mechanical ventilation treatment options as opposed to palliative care.

Medical Management

There is no known cure and no definitive treatment for ALS. Recently, however, several multicenter drug treatment trials with riluzole have shown slight evidence of positive effect on length of survival (several months), although the effect is marginal.[44, 57, 132] Riluzole, a drug that inhibits the presynaptic release of glutamate, is the first drug approved by the U.S. Food and Drug Administration (FDA) for use with ALS. Other drug therapies under investigation are gabapentin (to decrease the synthesis of glutamate); supplemental doses of tocopherol (vitamin E), an antioxidant and free-radical scavenger; and insulin-like growth factors (rhIGF-1). Using viral vectors to introduce gene products into the CNS is also under investigation. The reader is referred to the work of Eisen and Weber[65] for a comprehensive discussion of pharmaceutical interventions.

The popular press has reported on nutritional cures for ALS. To date, however, nutritional therapy has not been found effective in clinical trials. Norris and Denys[155] reported on a number of studies to determine the effectiveness of several nutrients, including tocopherol (vitamin E), octacosanol (long-chain alcohols reported by the ALS Society of America as helping some patients), and intravenous amino acids. They concluded that nutritional deficiencies are not related to the onset of ALS and that dietary supplements have no effect on the course of the disease. They also caution that national publicity and unwarranted anecdotal claims about improvement in function are based on a placebo effect, in keeping with the uneven progression of the disease in some patients.

Because of the apparent hopelessness of the diagnosis, many physicians, especially those not associated with major medical centers having neuromuscular disease units, do not refer patients with ALS for services. In a survey of ALS patients, 90% stated that their referring neurologists made no referrals or follow-up appointments. Most patients had been told to expect death within 1 to 3 years, although evidence shows that the median life span is approximately 4 years. Some physicians are concerned that providing aggressive treatment will only increase or prolong the patient's distress.[108] Other physicians, however, believe that withholding care and symptom relief seriously impairs the patient's quality of life.[133] The fact is that supportive medical and therapy interventions are available.[136]

Muscle Spasms and Pain

Some patients experience muscle cramps and spasms related to the upper motor neuron changes. Although most spasms can be relieved with stretching or increased movement, some patients require medications such as quinine or baclofen to relieve symptoms (see Chapter 32). In addition to muscle spasms, patients report nonspecific aching and muscle soreness, probably related to immobility and trauma to paralyzed muscles during caregiving procedures. However, many patients do not receive adequate pain medication, or if they were on pain medication, the pain was not controlled.[79] Because many patients have compromised respiratory function, the physician must take great care when prescribing pain medication, especially opiates. Patients should be instructed to keep a daily reporting log of the effectiveness of the medication so that the dosage can be adjusted.[155]

Dysphagia

Dysphagia accounts for considerable misery in the patient with advanced ALS, and it must be dealt with aggressively.[41, 137] Patients with dysphagia present with both nutritional and swallowing problems associated with weakness of the lips, tongue, palate, and mastication muscles.[231] Although dietary treatment is not effective in changing the course of the disease, a nutritious diet to meet caloric, fluid, vitamin, and mineral needs must be maintained. Seventy-three percent of patients with ALS have difficulty bringing food to the mouth, making them dependent on others for their dietary needs. Because of the time it takes to be fed, many patients decrease their intake. As the progressive loss of swallowing develops, patients are also at extreme risk for aspiration. Most patients with dysphagia also have severe problems with management of their saliva (sialorrhea). Normal average flow is about 1 mL/min from the parotid, submaxillary, sublingual, and minor salivary glands. With stimulation, this amount can increase to 8 mL/min. If a patient has difficulty transporting saliva back to the oropharynx for swallowing, choking and drooling are common. This is very disconcerting to the affected person, who must constantly wipe the mouth or have someone do it for him or her.

In addition, secretions are often thickened because of dehydration. With pooling of the thickened saliva, the possibility of aspiration is increased. Viscosity of saliva can best be treated by hydration and in some cases with papaya tablets or papase, the enzyme in meat tenderizer. Drugs such as decongestants, antidepressant drugs with anticholinergic side effects, and atropine-type drugs have been used to help control the amount of saliva, provided the patient is well hydrated.[189]

All patients with dysphagia should be referred for a dietary consultation to determine the choice and progression of solid and liquid foods and supplements. With mild aspiration problems in a patient who is still able and wants to eat, dietary changes and instruction in swallowing techniques by speech, occupational, and/or physical therapists can be very helpful. Techniques as simple as changing the eating position, head position, or the temperature, texture, or viscosity of the food may lengthen the time that the patient can enjoy eating safely.[121] Appel and colleagues[9] describe nutritional plans to maintain nutrition and hydration in patients with motor neuron diseases. The ALS Association also publishes manuals on dealing with swallowing problems.[6]

Patients with bulbar symptoms and severe dysphagia who are no longer able to consume nutrients orally because of motor control problems and aspiration may need feedings through nasogastric or jejunostomy tubes or percutaneous endoscopic gastrostomy (PEG), depending on the patient's wishes for long-term care.[193]

Aspiration can be the cause of sudden death in the patient with ALS, although it is not common. In extreme cases of recurrent aspiration pneumonia, various surgical procedures, such as ligation of the salivary gland ducts, severing the parasympathetic supply to the salivary glands, and excision of the salivary glands, have been used effectively.[101, 102, 104]

Dysarthria

Speech impairments are the initial symptom in majority of patients with bulbar involvement secondary to progressive weakness and/or spasticity of the oral and laryngeal muscles. Speech intelligibility is compromised by dysarthria, hypernasality, abnormalities of speed and cadence of speech, and reduced vocal volume. Speech is further compromised by inadequate breath volumes for normal phrasing. Most patients, however, are able to phonate to some degree even in relatively advanced stages of ALS.

Respiratory Management

Progressive respiratory failure is related to primary diaphragmatic, intercostal, and accessory respiratory muscle weakness; decreased pulmonary compliance; a weak cough; and bulbar symptoms such as a decreased gag reflex with aspiration.[109] Physiological factors indicating respiratory failure are vital capacity and maximum voluntary inspiratory and expiratory ventilation of 30% of predicted or less, hypoxemia, mild hypercapnea, and acidosis. Clinical signs are dyspnea with exertion or lying supine, hypoventilation, weak or ineffective cough, increased use of auxiliary respiratory muscles, tachycardia (also a sign of pulmonary infection with fever and tachypnea), changes in sleep pattern, daytime sleepiness and concentration problems, mood changes, morning headaches, and diffuse pain in the head, neck, and extremities. Chronic respiratory insufficiency should be assessed with tests of standing and supine forced vital capacity, or transcutaneous nocturnal oximetry may be necessary to determine oxygen saturation levels. Scheduled, serial evaluations of respiratory status are essential so that the patient and the treatment team can make informed decisions about appropriate treatment relative to both acute illnesses and progressive respiratory difficulties.[27, 109, 157]

Approximately half the patients with ALS experience dyspnea as a secondary symptom of an acute respiratory illness. Concurrent infection and disease that may respond to medication or short-term respiratory support measures must be ruled out and treatment or nontreatment, as desired by the patient, should be initiated. Early involvement of respiratory or pulmonary physical therapists is very advantageous. Physical therapists may be involved in the treatment of gradual respiratory failure by providing postural drainage with cough facilitation (suctioning if necessary), especially during acute respiratory illnesses. The patient and care providers should also be taught breathing exercises, chest stretching, and incentive spirometry techniques.[109] An assessment of the home environment is imperative to identify sleeping positions and energy conservation techniques that can be incorporated into the patient's daily life.

Within the past 10 to 15 years, respiratory management of the patient with ALS has changed dramatically. Today, despite quadriplegia and respiratory muscle paralysis, patients can choose long-term mechanical ventilation to prolong life. Although in the initial stages of ALS most patients indicate that they would not want prolonged respirator dependence at home, patients may change their minds as they adapt to the disease restrictions.[152] Oliver states that when counseling patients about outcome and treatment options, the "aim should be to avoid inappropriate treatment, which could cause harm to the patient, may merely prolong a poor quality of life and could lead to further distress."[157 (p 15)] In a more recent study of 121 patients, Albert and associates[4] determined that patients with slower disease progression tended to choose technological interventions less often than patients with more aggressively progressive disease. In their study, preferences stated early after diagnosis predicted later treatment decisions; however, only a few patients expressed a preference for any specific intervention.

Decisions about long-term respirator use should be made by the patient and involved family members, friends, or partners, with input from the interdisciplinary team caring for the patient. Discussions of preferred long-term care options should be revisited as the patient's condition changes. However, lurking in the decision-making process are ethical considerations, especially those related to the relationship between patient autonomy or self-determination and justice or the secondary family and societal effects associated with any decision about long-term technological interventions. (See Russell[184] for references on studies of ethical issues in the treatment of ALS.)

Physicians and health care workers who have input to the patient and family must be aware of their own feelings and beliefs about prolonging life. For example, a healthy physician or therapist who values control and an active lifestyle may envision a life on a ventilator as intolerable and pass that value on to the patient, who may or may not have the same needs. The patient's decision, or change in decision, must be respected by the medical team involved in care.[43] In medical centers using a team approach, patients and families may find support by meeting with counselors or peers with ALS who are making or have made decisions about long-term ventilator care.

If a patient decides that home ventilation is a reasonable option, it can be helpful for those involved to visit another patient who is using in-home mechanical ventilation.[159] Because the decision for home mechanical ventilation (HMV) affects the life not only of the patient but also of the patient's spouse, children, and extended family who may be responsible for some aspects of home care, or whose lives may be affected by the presence of in-home nurses or attendants, the decision for HMV should not be taken lightly. Extensive preparation, ongoing support, and respite options for caregivers are necessary if HMV is to be successful. Success of HMV also depends on such variables as third-party payment for home care equipment and nurse/attendant staffing, working status of the partner/spouse, age and physical fitness of spouse and children, pre-ALS family psychosocial interactions, and financial factors. HMV should be viewed as long-term, often extending for more than 1 year. In a Kaiser Foundation Hospital program from 1987 to 1992, 34 patients with ALS were discharged to HMV. On average, the patients were on the ventilator[158] 23 hours per day and needed 24-hour, 7-day-a-week care (at least three trained caregivers per week). Eighty-seven percent of the patients were alive at the end of 1 year, 58% at 3 years, and 33% at the end of 5 years. Less than 25% of the ALS patients in the Kaiser study had elected HMV in advance of the decision to begin ventilator assistance.[159]

With chronic respiratory insufficiency, the patient and family must be involved in the long-term care decisions related to instituting mechanical assistance under either emergency situations or in response to gradual deterioration. This discussion should occur before the patient develops respiratory failure (see Chapter 7). Acute respiratory failure can be so frightening, however, that few patients or family members are prepared to forego intubation and artificial ventilation during the emergency. If patients have stated that they do not want mechanical ventilation, appropriate use of medications such as morphine can markedly control the person's sense of air hunger[157] during the dying process.

As respiratory symptoms increase, oxygen at 2 L/minute or less can be used intermittently at home. When hypoventilation with a decline in oxygen saturation becomes common during sleep, resulting in morning confusion and irritability, noninvasive mechanical ventilation can be instituted if the patient elects to use mechanical support. Negative pressure devices, such as a cuirass respirator (external chest unit providing intermittent negative pressure) or a pneumowrap (an airtight chest suit sealed at the neck, shoulders, and hips), may be helpful.[27, 40, 159] Noninvasive, positive-pressure units are useful for some patients with ALS. Examples are intermittent nasal ventilation[97] and the more common bilevel positive airway pressure (BiPAP) unit, which provides greater inspiratory pressure than expiratory pressure to decrease the effort of breathing. Patients electing BiPAP can use either mask or contoured nasal delivery systems. Another, more difficult to use positive-pressure device that requires lip closure is the insufflation-exsufflation unit, which delivers and sucks out air to assist with coughing to remove mucus plugging.[27]

There is some evidence that noninvasive ventilation may increase survival by several months and improves the quality of life for the patient, with possible financial consequences and increased burden of care. However, when a patient can no longer benefit from noninvasive ventilation, a decision must be made about initiating ventilation by tracheostomy or palliative care.[149] (See the work of Miller and associates[146] for an excellent discussion of practice parameters in the decision-making process related to ventilatory support.)

Therapeutic Management of Impairments and Disabilities

When determining therapeutic goals and treatment, one must consider the rate of the patient's disease progression, the extent and areas of involvement, and the stage of illness. This is particularly important today considering the increasing number of patients choosing noninvasive ventilation that may extend life span. Patients with severe respiratory and bulbar complications may not benefit as greatly from active exercise programs. The goal in the end stages, however, is to optimize health and increase the quality of life. With guidance and environmental adaptations, patients with slowly progressing weakness may be able to continue many of their ADL for an extended number of years. In the final stages of the disease when the patient is bedridden, physical therapy interventions, such as stretching, may not effectively control contractures. The patient may benefit, however, from range of motion (ROM) exercises to decrease muscle and joint pain related to immobility. The efficacy of therapeutic interventions is also related to the timing of interventions, the motivation and persistence of the patient in carrying out the program,[221] and support from family members.

Evaluation

The extent of the therapeutic evaluation of a patient with ALS may depend on whether the therapist is working as a member of a neuromuscular team or as an independent or clinic-based therapist receiving a referral to evaluate and treat. Physical and occupational therapists working as team members may have a more circumscribed role related to gross motor function and ADL, with other consultants focusing on bulbar, respiratory, and environmental adjustments. The therapist working in a facility without a neuromuscular disease clinic or in a community or rural environment, however, should be aware of the need to carry out a broad-based assessment. In addition to the standard neuromuscular, musculoskeletal, and functional level examinations, the therapist should also evaluate the patient's stated or observed functional problems relative to bulbar and respiratory impairments, environmental blocks to independence, and caregiving demands.

Before the patient's initial visit, the therapist should contact the patient and request that he or she keep an activity log for 5 days. If an early contact is not possible, the therapist can assign that task during the initial session. The log should include 15-minute time increments in which the patient or caregiver can record what he or she was doing during a specific time period. Space also should be included to indicate whether the patient was experiencing fatigue or pain during the activity and how the patient perceived his or her respiratory status. An example of an activity log and how it is used is shown in Figure 13–2.

The evaluation will vary depending on the patient's situation; however, a typical initial assessment may include:

• Review of the patient's medical and activity record.
• Discussion of the patient's lifestyle, ADL tasks, hobbies

Name: _J. Costello_   DATE: _5-10-00_
                                       DAY: _Saturday_

DAILY ACTIVITY LOG

Instructions: 1) In column I write in what you are doing during the 24 hour period. You may draw a line or an arrow to indicate when the activity occurs for more than one 15 minute time period.

2) In column II indicate whether you are lying down, sitting, standing, or moving actively (walking, etc.) during the activity.

3) In column III on a 10 point scale, indicate how fatigued you feel while performing the activity (No fatigue = 0, extreme fatigue = 10.)

4) In column IV indicate where you feel pain if any and score the intensity on a 10 point scale (No pain = 0, extreme pain = 10.)

Try to fill out your log three or four times a day so you don't forget what you have been doing. An example is shown below.

	I	II	III	IV	
	What are you doing?	What position are you in	Fatigue level	Pain	
	Type of activity	(lying, sitting, standing, moving)	0 – 10	Location	Intensity 0 – 10
5:30 AM	Sleep	lying	0		
45					
6:00					
15					
30	Bathroom	Standing	2	neck	3
45	Shave, etc				
7:00					
15	Breakfast	sitting	3	neck	3
30					
45					
8:00	Reading	sitting	3	neck	3
15				shoulder	
30					
45	walk	standing, walking	4	neck	2
9:00					
15	nap				
30		lying	2	neck	4
45				hips	
10:00	Reading / TV	sitting	4	neck	3
15				hips	
30					
45	walk	standing, walking	5	hips	3
11:00					

FIGURE 13–2. Example of a log for monitoring activity level of patients with amyotrophic lateral sclerosis.

or interests, work focus, respiratory status, fatigability, safety issues, psychosocial support issues (family and agencies), and patient concerns and goals.
- Baseline testing of muscle strength (manual muscle testing or dynamometer testing if standards are clear and can be replicated) and ROM assessment.
- Evaluation of functional activity level. (It is preferable to use one of the standardized tests or see the previous box listing the components of the ALS Severity Scale.)
- Evaluation of pain (type, site, and intensity; use body chart and subjective pain scale). Identify what makes pain worse or better.
- Evaluation of bulbar and respiratory function. (For an in-depth evaluation of bulbar function, the patient should be referred to an ear, nose, and throat clinic or communications disorders clinic unless full evaluation is available in a comprehensive ALS clinic.) See Table 13–1 for bulbar and respiratory evaluation suggestions.

Intervention Goals

Treatment goals and the recommended exercise/activity program must be based on the patient's personal goals. Intervention goals are often a difficult area for physical therapists to discuss with the patient because both know that the disease is progressive despite interventions. It is common for the patient, therapist, and physicians to assume that because nothing can be done to "cure" the disease, it is kinder not to make additional demands on a patient who is already coping with daily loss. Some believe that exercise programs may create false hopes that exercise will delay progression. The literature on rehabilitation in neuromuscular disorders, however, suggests that patients with ALS can benefit from carefully designed exercise and activity programs.

The general, broad goals for both patient and therapist are related to maintaining maximal independence in daily living and a positive quality of life for as long as possible. More specific therapeutic goals are (1) maintenance of maximal muscle strength within limits imposed by ALS and (2) prevention and minimization of secondary consequences of the disease such as contractures, thrombophlebitis, decubitus ulcers, and respiratory infections.[106, 221]

Therapeutic Considerations

To prevent more rapid functional loss than expected by the natural history of the disease, both the patient and therapist must delicately balance the level of activity between the extremes of inadequate exercise and excessive exercise. Two major factors must be considered when planning and implementing an activity or exercise program for patients with ALS: (1) prevention of disuse atrophy and (2) prevention of overuse injury.

Disuse Atrophy. The first consideration for the therapist working with a patient with ALS is to prevent further deconditioning and disuse atrophy beyond the level caused specifically by the disease process. Although no studies have shown a relationship between disability and disuse atrophy in persons with ALS, there are a number

of reasons why it would be plausible. Because ALS is a disease of older adults, the patients may not have maintained their aerobic fitness or muscle strength before the onset of their neuromuscular problem.[123] It is also common for newly diagnosed patients to report that they had markedly decreased their activity level in the months before diagnosis because of a sense of fatigue or increasing clumsiness. If the patient had led a sedentary lifestyle before diagnosis, the additional decrease in activity level after the onset of ALS can lead quickly to marked cardiovascular deconditioning and disuse weakness.[139, 154] The disuse weakness lowers muscle force production and reduces muscle endurance.[10] Disuse atrophy in combination with pathological weakness and spasticity of specific muscle groups contributes to poorly coordinated, less efficient movements that require more energy expenditure. Disuse atrophy, therefore, contributes to the patient's level of functional loss and disability.

Exercise or Overwork Damage. The second, and perhaps more critical, consideration in designing an intervention program is to "do no harm." Anecdotal evidence that muscle activity or overwork exercise can lead to a loss of muscle strength has been reported since the poliomyelitis epidemic of the 1940s and 1950s.[205] During that epidemic, physicians and therapists noted that patients with poor and fair grade muscles who exercised repeatedly or with heavy resistance after reinnervation often lost the ability to contract the muscle at all.[20]

Reitsma[172] noted that vigorous exercise damaged muscles with less than one third of motor units functional. If more than one third of the motor units remained, exercise led to hypertrophy. Therefore, the extent of strengthening attained seems to be proportional to the number of intact or undamaged motor units. Exercise at a level to elicit a training effect in normal muscle, however, may cause overwork damage in weakened, denervated muscle. Because of the concerns about damage from stressing an abnormal neuromuscular system, Sinaki and Mulder[196] suggested that patients not engage in any vigorous exercise and focus instead on exercise associated with walking and daily activities. Later, several researchers demonstrated that repeated maximal eccentric contractions in normal muscle damaged muscle fibers, resulting in muscle weakness of several weeks' duration. Although normal muscle eventually adapts to repeated eccentric exercise, it is uncertain whether the reparative effect is possible in patients with neuromuscular diseases.[49]

In contrast, Sanjak and others[186] suggested that muscle damage does not necessarily result from resistance exercise testing or training, although fatigue occurs more easily during both anaerobic and aerobic exercise. Exercise energy requirements during bicycle ergometry testing were greater than expected, possibly because of motor inefficiency secondary to weakness. Work capacity and maximum oxygen consumption were decreased, but heart rate, respiratory responses, and blood pressure were within normal limits. In addition, patients in several case studies had lowered responses in force production and oxygen use related to their decreased muscle mass. Milner-Brown and Miller[147] found that mild progressive resistance exercise was helpful if the patient had muscle

T A B L E 1 3 – 1. Common Physical Findings in Bulbar Amyotrophic Lateral Sclerosis

Anatomical Site	Innervation	Method of Evaluation	Progression of Findings	Progression of Symptoms
Group 1				
Tongue	XII	Inspect for fasciculations at rest	Fasciculations evident	Dysarthria (disturbance of lingual-alveolar consonants "t," "d," "l," etc.)
		Range of motion	Slow, incomplete lateral movements Loss of lateral force Unable to reach palate with mouth open	Inability to clear buccal sulcus of food Marked dysarthria (slow rate and slurring of consonants)
		Protrusion	Unable to protrude beyond lips	Oral transport difficulties Dietary changes
		Perform rapid lateral motion	Unable to protrude beyond incisors Atrophy evident Paralysis	Speech intelligibility problems
Lips	VII	Suck on gloved finger Smile or curl lips over teeth Hold seal and blow out cheeks	Lack of suction Inability to complete a seal Inability to purse lips	Inability to whistle Inability to use a straw Dysarthria (loss of bilabial consonants "p" and "b") Drooling
Group 2				
Palate	V, X, XI	Visual examination during phonation and stimulation of gag Puff out cheeks to check for nasal air leak (hold lips closed if necessary)	Unsustained or slow palatal elevation Soft palate fails to reach Pasavant's ridge Absence of palatal movement	Dysarthria (hypernasal speech) Inability to use a straw Nasal air emission during speech Nasopharyngeal reflex on swallowing
Muscles of mastication				
Masseter/ temporalis	V	Palpate during bite Visual inspection for wasting	Noticeable wasting Unable to palpate contraction	Chewing fatigue Elimination of specific, tough foods from diet Dietary changes (soft foods and liquids) Mouth breathing and drying of secretions
Pterygoids		Move jaw from side to side	No observable lateral jaw movement	Unable to use dentures
Group 3				
Neck and shoulder	XI			
Trapezius		Hold arm in coronal plane, hand externally rotated, as patient elevates arm against resistance while the trapezius is palpated	Progressive inability to raise the arm (often asymmetrical weakness)	Inability to comb hair Inability to perform facial grooming
Sternocleido-mastoid or mounted head support		Turn the head against resistance applied to opposite side of patient's chin	Progressive weakness in turning the head against resistance (often asymmetrical)	Inability to lift head when supine Inability to support head while sitting. Wears neck collar, has weakness
Vocal cords	X	Mirror or fiberoptic laryngoscopy	Progressive loss of abduction of vocal cords: mild abductor weakness, near-midline paralysis Paradoxical vocal cord movement	Strained-strangled voice Short of breath (stridor usually not present due to impaired respiratory function)
Group 4				
Extraocular muscles	III, IV, VI	Assessment of extraocular movements	Limitation of extraocular movement	Limitation of gaze
Respiratory group				
Diaphragm	C$_{3, 4, 5}$	Pulmonary function test or hand-held respirometer for vital capacity	Diminishing vital capacity: 1.5–2.0 liters	Shortness of breath during exertion if patient has remained active
Intercostal	C$_7$–L$_3$			
Accessory muscles of respiration	VII, XI, XII, C$_{5-8}$	Cough Sustain a vowel Blow against a tissue	1.0–1.5 liters	Weak cough Change in speech phrasing (5–10 syllables per breath)
			0.5–1.0 liter	Speech produced in syllable-by-syllable fashion (if vocal) Shortness of breath on swallowing

Adapted with permission from Hillel AD, Miller RM: Bulbar amyotrophic lateral sclerosis: Patterns of progression and clinical management. Head Neck 11(1):51–59, 1989. Copyright 1989. Reprinted by permission of John Wiley & Sons, Inc.

strength in the good (4) to normal (5) range. Based on their work, they determined that patients should begin their exercise program early because strength training of muscles with less than 10% of normal function was generally not effective. In more recent studies, Chan and Sinaki[45] have suggested that patients follow a program of six maximal isometric contractions held for 6 seconds and isotonic elastic band exercises at submaximal levels to maintain and improve muscle strength.

In general, impairments in muscle strength, the presence of spasticity, and decreases in ROM are clearly associated with decreases in functional abilities—hence the interest in correlating changes in level of impairment with level of functional loss. Although some research has shown improvements in muscle force production with strengthening and endurance training, functional improvements were not clear.[187] Jette and colleagues[114] calculated the percentage of predicted normal maximal isometric force (%PMF) relative to four walking levels: unable to walk, walking within the home only, walking in the community with assistance, and independent walking in the community. Although they found great variation in muscle force production between and within the different levels of walking for each patient, they demonstrated that relatively small changes in force production were associated with losses of functional levels.

For example, on average, when an independent ambulator began to need assistance in the community, the lower extremity %PMF dropped to below 54%. When the patient became an in-home ambulator only, the average %PMF dropped to about 37%, and it was approximately 19% when the patient was no longer able to walk. Jette and others[114] acknowledge that there are many factors that need to be considered when interpreting their work. However, their study is valuable to therapists because it relates functional skills to isometric muscle force production, which by itself is not sufficient evidence to predict functional status. Many studies focus on the impact of exercise on muscle strength; however, knowledge of impairments does not necessarily correlate directly with functional status. One must also consider factors such as spasticity, age at onset of ALS, prior levels of fitness and activity, and psychological factors, including past responses to extremely challenging situations and satisfaction with social support.

Most recently, Kilmer and coworkers[124] and Wright[235] found positive physiological effects of directed exercise programs and aerobic walking programs, respectively. The positive effects of focused exercise programs can have a positive psychological effect on a patient's coping strategies.[53] Kilmer and Aitkens,[123] in an excellent review of the literature on exercise for patients with neuromuscular disorders, developed seven exercise prescription recommendations[123 (p 263)]:

1. To improve compliance, consider both a formal exercise program and enjoyable physical activities.
2. Include activities with opportunities for social development and personal accomplishment.
3. Strengthening programs should emphasize concentric rather than eccentric muscle contractions.
4. High-resistance strengthening programs probably have no benefit over moderate-resistance programs.

5. Muscles with less than antigravity strength have little capacity to improve; the program should focus on stronger muscles.
6. Periodically monitor muscle strength to assess for possible overwork weakness, particularly in unsupervised programs.
7. Activity modifications should include periods of physical activity with rest.

Vignos[221] suggests that for a patient to make any gain in function, a therapist (or physician) should be prepared to accept the possible consequences of overwork weakness when establishing an exercise program. The therapist should carefully monitor the patient's exercise or activity program to ensure that any decrement in strength is related to the progression of the disease rather than excessive overwork of weakened muscles. When determining the possible detrimental effects of exercise, a distinction must be made between the transient muscle fatigue that most of us feel from moderate heavy work and the prolonged, persistent decrease in muscle strength and endurance after excessive exercise of weakened muscles.[20] If a patient shows evidence of significant, persistent weakness after institution of an exercise program or persistent morning fatigue after exercise on the previous day, the therapist must carefully redesign the patient's exercise program and activity level and increase the frequency of monitoring the patient's home program. Because the possible positive and negative effects of resistive exercises are not clear, the therapist must take an assertive yet cautious approach to exercise. Although the therapist cannot determine the number of intact motor units available to a patient or whether the patient is evoking maximal motor unit recruitment during activities, the therapist must make decisions about underwork and overwork and adjust the patient's program based on his or her response to exercise. The program must be adjusted as the disease progresses to prevent possible damage from excessive overwork and fatigue. Figure 13–3 is a diagram showing the appropriate exercise "window" for use in working with a patient with a neuromuscular disorder.

Therapeutic Interventions

Maintenance of strength and endurance requires daily activity and repetitive muscle contractions. In normal persons, absence of muscle contraction can result in 3% to 5% decreases in muscle strength per day. If the patient's exercise level requires less than 20% of the maximal voluntary contraction of the muscles, a decrease in strength will occur,[154] yet overwork must be monitored. A summary of the literature on strength training in neuromuscular disease is presented in Table 13–2.

When designing an intervention program, the therapist should know what the patient has been told about the disease process and the expected course of symptom development. If diagnostic and prognostic information is not explicit, neither therapist nor patient will be able to make appropriate goal and treatment plans. Before finalizing an intervention plan based on patient goals, the therapist must consider the following:

• The typical rate of the patient's disease progression
• Distribution of weakness and spasticity, respiratory fac-

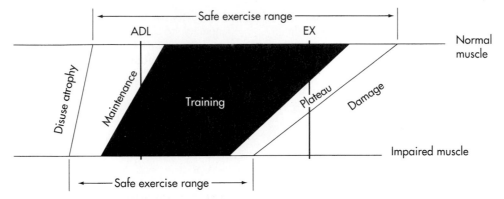

FIGURE 13–3. Exercise window for normal and damaged or denervated muscles. (From Coble NO, Maloney FP: Effects of exercise on neuromuscular disease. In Maloney FP, Burks JS, Ringel SP [eds]: Interdisciplinary Rehabilitation of Multiple Sclerosis and Neuromuscular Disorders. New York, JB Lippincott, 1985.)

tors leading to hypoxemia, and easy fatigability and bulbar involvement
• Phase of the disease

Sinaki[195] has described three phases and six substages of ALS with recommended exercise levels. Although therapists should not assume that all patients will fit precisely within the stages as described, the stages do provide

suggestions for interventions based on degree of impairment, functional limitations, and level of disability. Therefore, in the following section staging patterns are used as the framework for therapy interventions. Staging information is particularly helpful to therapists who do not have the opportunity to work with large numbers of patients with ALS. See the box on pages 377 and 378 for an adapted version of the Sinaki phases and substages.

TABLE 13–2. Summary of Strength Training Studies in Neuromuscular Disease (NMD)

Author	Study Population and Sample Size	Duration of Training	Training Modality	Training Protocol	Response(s)
Vignos & Watkins, 1966[223]	Various NMDs (24)	12 months	Weight training (multiple muscle groups)	Unspecified, but based on 10-repetition maximum (RM)	Strength increased; % increase correlated with initial strength
Milner-Brown & Miller, 1988[147]	Various NMDs (12)	>12 months (variable)	Weight training (elbow flexion and knee extension)	Initially 1 set of 10 reps based on 15 RM performed on alternate days; gradually increased to a maximum of 5 sets 4 days/wk; protocol individualized	Strength increased significantly when the initial degree of strength loss was not severe (<10%)
McCartney et al., 1988°	Various NMDs (12)	9 weeks	Weight training (arm curl and leg press)	3 days/wk; initially 2 sets of 10–12 reps at 40% max.; gradually progressed to 3 sets of 10–12 reps (1 set at 50%, 60%, and 70% max.); contralateral arm control	Strength and muscular endurance increased; considerable intersubject variability
Aitkens et al., 1993†	Slowly progressive (12 wk). NMD (27) and able-bodied controls (14)	12 weeks	Weight training (elbow flexion, knee extension, grip)	3 days/wk; submaximal exercises	Significant improvement in most strength measures (not grip) in both groups; cross-training effect
Kilmer et al., 1994[124]	Slowly progressive NMD (10) and able-bodied controls (6)	12 weeks	Weight training (elbow flexion, knee extension)	3 days/wk; high resistance exercise	Results mixed; some increased in leg strength coupled with decrease in arm strength in NMD
Lindeman et al., 1995‡	NMD (33) and HMSN (29); non-exercise control group	24 weeks	Weight training (knee extension and flexion, hip extension and flexion)	3 days/wk; initially 3 sets of 25 reps at 60% of 1 RM; progressed to 3 sets of 10 reps at 80% of 1 RM	In NMD group, no change in strength In HMSN group, increased strength of knee extensors

°McCartney, et al: The effects of strength training in patients with selected neuromuscular disorders. Med Sci Sports Exerc 20(4):362–368, 1988.
†Aitkens, et al: Moderate resistance exercise program: its effect in slowly progressive neuromuscular disease. Arch Phys Med Rehabil 74(7):711–715, 1993.
‡Lindeman, et al: Strength training in myotonic dystrophy and hereditary motor and sensory neuropathy: a randomized clinical trial. Arch Phys Med Rehabil 76(7):612–620, 1995.
Modified by A. Hallum, October 5, 2000.

EXERCISE AND REHABILITATION PROGRAMS FOR PATIENTS WITH ALS ACCORDING TO STAGE OF DISEASE

Phase I (independent)
Stage 1:

Patient Characteristics:

Mild weakness

Clumsiness

Ambulatory

Independent in ADL

Treatment:

Continue normal activities or increase activities if sedentary to prevent disuse atrophy.

Begin program of ROM exercises (stretching, yoga, tai chi).

Add strengthening program of gentle resistance exercises to all musculature with caution not to cause overwork fatigue.

Provide psychological support as needed.

Stage 2:

Patient Characteristics:

Moderate, selective weakness

Slightly decreased independence in ADL; examples:
difficulty climbing stairs
difficulty raising arms
difficulty buttoning clothing

Ambulatory

Treatment:

Continue stretching to avoid contractures.

Continue cautious strengthening of muscles with manual muscle test grades above $F+$ $(3+)$. Monitor for overwork fatigue.

Consider orthotic support (i.e., ankle-foot, wrist, thumb splints).

Use adaptive equipment to facilitate ADL.

Stage 3:

Patient Characteristics:

Severe selective weakness in ankles, wrists, and hands

Moderately decreased independence in ADL

Easily fatigability with long-distance ambulation

Ambulatory

Slightly increased respiratory effort

Treatment:

Continue stage 2 program as tolerated. Caution not to fatigue to point of decreasing patient's ADL independence.

Keep patient physically independent as long as possible through pleasurable activities, walking.

Encourage deep breathing exercises, chest stretching, postural drainage if needed.

Prescribe wheelchair, standard or motorized, with modifications to allow eventual reclining back with head rest, elevating legs.

Phase II (partially independent)
Stage 4:

Patient Characteristics:

Hanging-arm syndrome with shoulder pain and sometimes edema in the hand

Wheelchair dependent

Severe lower-extremity weakness (with or without spasticity)

Able to perform ADL but fatigues easily

Treatment:

Heat, massage as indicated to control spasm.

Preventive antiedema measures.

Active assisted passive ROM exercises to the weakly supported joints—caution to support, rotate shoulder during abduction and joint accessory motions.

Encourage isometric contractions of all musculature to tolerance.

Try arm slings, overhead slings, or wheelchair arm supports.

Motorized chair if patient wants to be independently mobile. Adapt controls as needed.

Continued

EXERCISE AND REHABILITATION PROGRAMS FOR PATIENTS WITH ALS ACCORDING TO STAGE OF DISEASE *Continued*

Stage 5:

Patient Characteristics:

Severe lower-extremity weakness

Moderate to severe upper-extremity weakness

Wheelchair dependent

Increasingly dependent in ADL

Possible skin breakdown secondary to poor mobility

Treatment:

Encourage family to learn proper transfer, positioning principles, and turning techniques.

Encourage modifications at home to aid patient's mobility and independence.

Electric hospital bed with antipressure mattress.

If patient elects HMV, adapt chair to hold respirator unit.

Phase III (dependent)

Stage 6:

Patient Characteristics:

Bedridden

Completely dependent in ADL

Treatment:

For dysphagia: soft diet, long spoons, tube feeding, percutaneous gastrostomy.

To decrease flow of accumulated saliva: medication, suction, surgery.

For dysarthria: palatal lifts, electronic speech amplification, eye pointing electronic.

For breathing difficulty: clear airway, tracheostomy, respirator if patient elects HMV. Medications to decrease impact of dyspnea.

ADL, activities of daily living; ROM, range of motion; HMV, home mechanical ventilation.

Adapted with permission from Sinaki M: Exercise and rehabilitation measures in amyotrophic lateral sclerosis. In Yase Y, Tsubaki T (eds): Amyotrophic Lateral Sclerosis: Recent Advances in Research and Treatment. Amsterdam, Elsevier Science, 1988.

Most patients need specific guidance about what type of activities and exercises they should do.[221] Although many physicians may suggest to patients that they increase their activity level, their suggestions are seldom specific. Examples of exercise advice patients have recalled are "Try to move around as much as possible," "Walk some more," and "Be active, but don't overdo it." Because it is difficult for most patients to change their typical exercise pattern even when they know it is important, referral for a physical therapy consultation can be very helpful.

Phase I: Stages 1 to 3. The first step in working with a patient in phase I, stages 1 to 3 (independent), of ALS is to determine the patient's current activity level. A program to increase activity must be designed specifically with input from the patient about willingness to participate and with knowledge of the patient's environmental situations and social support systems. In the early stages of the disease, patients should be encouraged to continue as many prediagnosis activities as tolerated. For example, a golfer should continue to golf as long as possible. Walk-

ing the course should be encouraged if it is not too fatiguing. When walking or balance becomes difficult on uneven terrain, the golfer can use a golf cart, decrease the number of holes played, move to a par 3 course, or hit balls at a driving range. If upper-extremity weakness is a major problem that interferes with swinging the club for distance shots, the player can continue playing the greens or on putting courses. Some golfers may need adaptations to club handles with nonskid material such as Dycem or Scoot Guard to prevent the club from rotating on impact.

Older patients with newly diagnosed ALS who have had a sedentary lifestyle before diagnosis should be encouraged to increase their activity level. This may include activities that require muscular effort within or around the home such as sharing household and gardening tasks or beginning a walking program around the neighborhood. After diagnosis, some patients begin searching for in-home exercise devices such as bicycles and rowing machines. As with healthy persons who start an exercise program after the purchase of exercise equipment, it is unlikely that patients with ALS will use the equipment consistently. The search for a "perfect" exercise machine may reflect the patient's desperation to do something tangible. Without taking away the patient's motivation to exercise, therapists can encourage participation in exercise programs that do not require expensive equipment, such as walking or working out to specific exercise videos. A clever therapist can make a videotape for each patient that includes stretching and gentle exercise programs that elicit muscle contractions from all functional muscle groups (using inexpensive elastic bands or small weights) with follow-up breathing, "warm down," and relaxation exercises. As mentioned earlier, Chan and Sinaki[45] have suggested that patients follow a program of six maximal isometric contractions held for 6 seconds and isotonic elastic band exercises at submaximal levels to maintain and improve muscle strength. It is best if patients exercise for short periods several times a day rather than attempting to exercise all muscle groups in one session.

In general for most patients in the early stages of ALS, it is best to "prescribe" pleasurable, natural activities such as swimming, bowling (if shoulder strength is not yet a problem), walking, bicycling (three-wheeler may be needed), and yoga. Some patients prefer to exercise alone, whereas others will gain confidence and companionship by joining a group activity. It is important to listen to the patient's desires related to group activities. Among those who have been pressured to participate, the dropout rate is high. Some spouses or family members are supportive of the patient's activity needs and will join the patient in his or her regimen. If possible, the spouse and family members should be engaged in the treatment planning process.[200]

The therapist must observe the patient completing his or her entire recommended activity program. It is essential to monitor the patient's response to the program because fatigue from exercise sessions can interfere with the ability to carry out other normal daily activities. If the patient becomes too exhausted at the end of a session, he or she may learn to fear exercise and may become depressed about the decreased activity status. This depression may lead to decreased activity and deconditioning.[106]

Phase II: Partially Independent. During phase II (partially independent), the goal of physical therapy intervention should be to help the patient adapt to limitations imposed by weakness and spasticity, an increasingly compromised cardiorespiratory status, and possible pain from stress related to weakness or muscle imbalance. This transition stage is often frightening for patients because the decrease in function and independence becomes clear. If possible, the patient should be seen for a comprehensive physical therapy reevaluation at this time. The first step in the reassessment is to ask the patient about his or her current activity level and to identify what the patient can and can no longer do. After a full physical assessment of the patient's motor status similar to the initial evaluation, the patient, family members, and the therapist (include occupational and speech therapists if a team approach is possible) should discuss treatment options and adaptive devices that can help the patient remain as independent as possible.

During late phase I, stage 3, and during phase II, stages 4 and 5, many patients show significant weakness of both upper- and lower-extremity musculature, but each patient has his or her own pattern and rate of progression of weakness and onset of spasticity, bulbar, and respiratory symptoms. A typical patient at this time may have marked weakness of the intrinsic muscles, shoulder muscle weakness (in some cases "hanging arm" syndrome) with shoulder pain, and generalized lower-extremity weakness (in some cases more severe distally). Patients may be able to walk within the home environment, but many patients have precarious balance and fall easily because of muscle weakness. At this stage, most patients complain of fatigue with minimal work and have to rest frequently when carrying out ADL tasks.[194]

Because Mr. Turner in Case 13–1 (pages 383–385) was cared for in a neuromotor disease clinic, he benefited from input from multiple specialists working as a team to help him maintain his independence. Unfortunately, many patients do not have the benefit of such a coordinated treatment environment. Therefore, when necessary, the therapist must be in a position to provide input on adaptive and safety devices and bulbar issues if specialist input is not available. Therapists working in smaller communities and rural areas most likely need to be chameleon-like to play many therapeutic roles when working with the patient with ALS.

Phase III: Dependent. Physical and occupational therapists are usually less involved in the care of the patient in phase III, stage 6 (dependent), and nursing personnel become more active. During this phase, therapists make home visits to support caregivers and respond to questions about pain control, bed mobility, positioning, ROM, and equipment adaptations. Therapists should be sure to teach all caregivers some basic body mechanics to use during lifting and patient care activities. If possible, caregivers should be taught how to safely move the person with ALS from the bed to a reclining wheelchair or neuro-chair during specific times of the day so that the person can continue to be part of the family activities. However, the ease of caregivers in transferring and caring for the person in the wheelchair must also be considered. Although some patients want to be in the midst of family activities even when dependent on HMV, other patients feel uncomfortable with their dependency and appearance and are reasonably content to stay in their room with television and visits from family members. This very personal decision by patients must be respected. The therapist should review ROM procedures with family and professional caregivers and provide splinting or positioning devices if spasticity or paralysis leads to caregiving difficulties (e.g., excessive adductor tone and contractures interfering with hygiene and bowel care) or tissue damage and pain. If nursing care providers do not give advice on pressure relief beds or mattresses, therapists should be prepared to do so. Unfortunately, many insurance providers and Medicare may not fund special mattresses, and they can be very costly. Therapists may also need to review postural drainage techniques with caregivers.

By phase III most patients have severe problems eating

and maintaining nutrition, although these problems may manifest in earlier stages. These problems are best handled medically, and the aggressiveness of treatment intervention depends on the patient's preference and whether he or she still wants to attempt any oral feeding (e.g., syringe feeding, oral gastric tubes) or wishes to have a PEG or another alternative to oral feedings implemented.

Of greatest importance at phase III, and sometimes in earlier stages, is the patient's ability to communicate. In the earliest manifestation of dysarthria, therapists train patients to slow the speech rate and cadence, exaggerate lip and tongue movements, and manage phrasing through breath control.[74] Some patients with hypernasality benefit from using an orthodontic palatal appliance. Patients with a tracheostomy may benefit from use of the Passy-Muir speaking valve tracheostomy tube (Passy-Muir Inc, Irvine, CA). These devices need to be recommended by communication specialists. As speech quality deteriorates and sound projection wanes, the spouse or caregiver can use an electronic speech amplifier to magnify the patient's speech. Speech pathologists and therapists will have information on commercially available amplifying devices that are often used by persons with hearing problems but can be used by hearing people to amplify the speech of a person with severe weakness of phonation.

Although spouses and caregivers can often interpret their partner's or patient's severely dysarthric speech, most patients who use noninvasive or invasive ventilation for a prolonged periods need to find nonoral methods to communicate. If severe bulbar impairments precede extremity paralysis, paper and pencil, alphabet/word boards, and adapted computer keyboards can be used with minimal upper-extremity or finger control for pointing. When no extremity movement is possible, subtle neck movements or pressures, eye gaze, eye blink, upper facial movements, and electroencephalographic activity can be harnessed to operate communication devices.[51, 120]

When selecting a communication device, therapists must work closely with the patient and family members to ensure that the system is compatible with patient skills and communication needs and preferences. It is common for very expensive systems to lie unused because of simple factors such as lack of proximity to the patient, interference of the unit with personal care, increased caregiver workload to manage the unit, and slowness of communication processing. The best systems are tailored to the precise needs of the patient; however, many patients do not have the financial or insurance support to purchase the device, and many patients in the end stages of ALS do not have the time to wait for systems designed for their specific needs. Therefore, commercially manufactured systems may be most appropriate. (See Table 9.6 in *Augmentative and Alternative Communication Systems* by Cook and Hussey[51] for a comprehensive list of communication devices and control interfaces.)

Some patients and caregivers learn to communicate very effectively with simple eye gaze, eye blinking, and clicking techniques using Morse code or self-developed codes. At minimum, patients with no ability to communicate or move, and their caregivers, must have some system to communicate emergency needs, such as, looking to the right means "help" and looking to the left means "pain." Therapists should help patients develop alternative modes of communication before intelligible speech becomes impossible. (See also Cobble for information on language impairments.[50]) In addition to communication systems, environmental control systems can be programmed to turn on and off television, lights, and other electronic units using the same type of switching units used for communication (e.g., eye blink, infrared beam, head movement pressure). Unfortunately, these devices are often very expensive and may not be available to all patients. (See Cook and Hussey[51] for a comprehensive review of environmental control systems.) Financial support is often not extended for "high tech" equipment by third-party payers because of the patient's limited life expectancy. The ability to communicate and to call for help, however, is of paramount importance with totally dependent patients.

Psychosocial Issues

Giving the bad news of a terminal diagnosis is difficult for even the most experienced clinician. In dealing with the diagnosis of ALS, most physicians now believe that the diagnosis, prognosis, and possible patterns of progression should be shared with the patient and family or partners and caregiving friends. Only by knowing the truth can patients and families deal openly with each other and make plans for the future.[28, 157] All information need not be given at the time of diagnosis. Rather, the patient and family can be exposed to more in-depth information over a number of sessions when they have the opportunity to ask questions that occur during the assimilation process. However, information should be delivered to patients and families in time to make thoughtful decisions rather than having to make decisions during a time of crisis, for example, during a respiratory crisis or arrest. Care should also be taken to respect the cultural and spiritual views of the patient and family. Preferably, patients and family members will prepare an advance medical directive that should be reviewed with the physician at least every 6 months.[146] If patients are referred to a specialty clinic from a rural area, it is absolutely imperative that patients be contacted regularly at home by phone after the initial diagnosis to allow follow-up questions and to make appropriate support referrals if needed.

Patients will progress through the diagnostic process with different responses and at different rates on a continuum from taking a very cognitive approach by asking many questions and reviewing the most current research to the extreme of marked denial and disinterest in participating in any medical or therapeutic recommendations. Although some degree of denial can be a useful coping strategy, Oliver and Cardy[158] have found that most patients with motor neuron disease want to talk about their prognosis and future. The opportunity to express fears and concerns is essential. The overall goal of helping the patient and family members express themselves is to provide a forum for self-reflection and insight[170] about the process of living while dying. Nevertheless, the view by some health care workers that patients and families cannot deal with the disease effectively unless they express complete acceptance may be as faulty as hiding the diagnosis from the patient.

Purtilo and Haddad[170] identify four major fears of the patient who has a terminal condition: fear of isolation, fear of pain, fear of dependence, and fear of death itself. Patients with progressive diseases often see their social contacts decrease. Mr. Turner in Case 13–1 was very concerned when he was no longer able to join his colleagues in the company cafeteria. After he received his motorized wheelchair he was able to continue his social contacts until his bulbar symptoms progressed to a point that he chose not to eat in public. When Mr. Turner lost the ability to speak and had to use his computerized speech system, he noticed that fewer colleagues stopped by his office to talk because of the slowness of the communication process. Although he understood the problem, Mr. Turner mourned considerably about his loss of friendship and his loss of standing as a competent computer expert. Because of his need for social contact, Mr. Turner continued to work until he could no longer tolerate the sitting position (see Goldstein and colleagues).[82] His fear of isolation increased when he became homebound. Although colleagues came for visits regularly at first, as Mr. Turner progressed to a near locked-in state only a few close friends came by for brief visits. Mr. Turner's greatest fear was being separated from his family and abandoned to hospital care with the usual inconsistent staffing patterns. Fortunately, in his community, Mrs. Turner was able to set up visitations from several church members, clerics, and hospice volunteers.

Fear of uncontrolled pain is common among persons with terminal diseases. Patients need assurance that their pain will be controlled. Many patients can recall the postsurgical horrors of being in severe pain but being told they had to wait another 2 hours for their next medication. Fortunately, today pain medications can be administered in many forms, dosages, and frequencies that can be tailored to the patient's specific needs. Because many patients are routinely undermedicated for pain, patients with ALS and their families need to be assertive about pain management.[79] Keeping a pain log of intensity, type, location, and time of pain may provide the physician with information necessary to best prescribe dosages. Although sensory systems of patients with ALS are essentially normal and are not the cause of pain, many patients do experience significant pain from musculoskeletal sources, persistent spasms, or spasticity and pressure sores. Most of these problems can be handled with appropriate pain medications, muscle relaxants, careful positioning, frequent ROM, and tissue massage.

A major concern of patients with ALS is the dependence for ADL associated with late phase II and phase III of the disease. Because the process is gradual, most patients have the opportunity to make adjustments. The dependency issues and resulting privacy issues are more uncomfortable for some patients than for others, especially the person who has always valued self-control and

independence. Some patients are concerned about their increasing dependence because of the consequences or increasing burden of care on spouses or other caregivers. That concern for others sometimes causes patients to choose hospital or nursing home care over home care during the terminal stage of the disease. (See Damiano and associates[54] for information on measurement of health-related quality of life.)

Not all patients with terminal illness react the same way during the dying process. Throughout the process, patients and family members may cycle and recycle through a range of different reactions, such as the stages described by Kübler-Ross: depression, anger, hostility, bargaining, and acceptance/adaptation (order is not implied).[170] How the patient coped with life's difficulties before the illness and his or her prior relationship patterns often direct how the patient will deal with the terminal illness. In one study, patients adjusted most successfully to the changes in their functional status if they did not look back to the past and compare their losses to their future.[80]

Health care providers and family members often have great difficulty coping with a patient who is depressed, and they make repeated efforts to "talk the person out of" the depression. Smith[197] reminds us to distinguish between depression that can be destructive and the mourning or grieving that is a necessary and vital response to dealing with loss. In both states, the person may feel a level of withdrawal, sadness, apathy, loss of interest in activities, and cognitive distortions. In a depressive state, however, the patient experiences an accompanying loss of self-esteem. A person in mourning rarely experiences that loss of self-esteem essential to a diagnosis of depression. The grieving person's feelings are congruent with the degree of loss experienced.[151]

Complicating the issue of depression is pseudobulbar affect of emotional lability (inappropriate laughing and crying), which is manifested by approximately 50% of patients with ALS. This emotional lability is not under complete control of the patient and is often misunderstood by family members and caregivers. Although current treatment is antidepressant medications, there may or may not be underlying clinical depression that would respond to higher doses of antidepressant medication and/or counseling.[146]

Because overt grieving or emotionality causes observers discomfort, some professional caregivers try to rush the patient and family into formal counseling as soon as mourning occurs. This option should be offered, but other recommendations such as guidance from a cleric, support groups, hospice volunteers, and informal support from friends are also invaluable resources for the person uncomfortable with formal counseling situations.

With today's pressure to express oneself and talk about one's feelings, patients are often pressed to "talk out" their problems and feelings. Although it is important for a caregiver to give a patient the opportunity to talk about dying and to feel comfortable with the topic, each patient's personal style in talking about death must be respected. For example, some persons are not comfortable sharing feelings with a professional counselor or psychologist. This is especially true for older patients or those who were raised with the view that one should maintain the appearance of control or that seeking emotional help shows weakness or defect. Pressuring a patient to see a mental health worker can lead to loss of trust. Therefore, occupational and physical therapists and other persons involved in the care of a dying patient should feel comfortable talking with their patients about death and be prepared to suggest various options if the patient expresses the need for emotional support.

Caregiver Issues

Often in the concern for the patient's needs, professionals pay little attention to the effect a person's degenerative illness has on other members of the family. ALS significantly affects the person's extended family because the patient gradually becomes increasingly dependent on family members, partners, or caregiving friends for physical care, social arrangements, cognitive stimulation, and emotional support. For some families, the spouse may have to take on additional work, return to work, or, in the case of some older women, join the work force for the first time to deal with the financial stresses that occur when chronic illness invades the family unit. Family members must absorb the former family duties of the dependent person. For example, a husband may have to handle all the cooking and cleaning tasks; older children may have to take on the total care of younger siblings, increase household chores, or work to help support the family. All family members may have to become involved in the physical care of the increasingly dependent person with ALS.

Families have differing levels of long-term care coverage. Some families are fortunate to have excellent coverage that provides extensive home nursing support, whereas other families are unable to cope with the financial stresses and must accept public assistance during the final stages of the person's disease. For example, the Springer family, consisting of the father with ALS (age 61), mother (age 59), and son (age 25), was forced to live on a combination of Supplemental Security Income, general assistance, and food stamps after the father became ill. The family had little savings and catastrophic insurance coverage that did not cover any long-term care. Mrs. Springer returned to work full-time and cared for her husband all evening. When he reached the point of needing full-time care, the wife had to quit work to care for her husband because she did not make an adequate salary to pay for nursing care and maintain the family finances. Because the son had to care for his own family of four, he was not able to help out the family financially, although both he and his wife provided several half-days of respite care for their mother so she could do shopping and spend some time out of the home. The process of "going on welfare" was very upsetting to the family. After numerous discussions about options for home care, Mr. Springer decided that continuing his life was too great a burden on his family and he requested that his life be terminated. Because that was not considered an option, his family and primary physician worked out a plan to allow a peaceful death without placing Mr. Springer on any artificial feeding, respiration, or antibiotics. He died at home 3 months after the decision was made.

In another case, a young single woman who lived alone and had no family found that she could not rely on friends for her care even though they were supportive and visited her often. When she was no longer able to care for herself safely she was admitted to a nursing home, where she died 2 years later.

Children of patients with ALS also have to deal with major changes in their lifestyle. Although they may love their parent who is sick, at some level most are very frustrated with factors such as the need to provide physical care to parents. This is a very difficult problem for children who have not had a positive relationship with that parent. Children living in the home of a parent who is dying of ALS also express frustration about the lack of privacy in their home when nursing personnel and attendants are present, interruptions in family and personal life plans, embarrassment because of the parent's appearance and dependency, lack of attention from the caregiving-working parent, and fear of financial crises (e.g., possible loss of home, no financial support for college).

The entire family is affected by the sick person's increasing dependency and impending death.[42] The changes the family must make to anticipate and deal with the dependent person's needs have a significant emotional overlay. Anger, helplessness, frustration, sadness, or mourning for an impending loss; guilt; and remorse commonly occur and recur at different stages as the sick person and family try to adjust to the progression toward death. Weariness and exhaustion from day-to-day caregiving and frequent interactions with health and social agencies can try the soul of the most adaptable persons.[225] In a small study of 11 family caregivers, many caregivers felt frustrated and resentful because their lives were consumed with the caregiving responsibilities. Most caregivers had adjusted to some degree after 2 to 4 years. Caregivers who adjusted most successfully learned to take time for themselves without guilt and to tap their social support systems for help.[80] In a study of 40 caregivers of young adults with severe disabilities, caregivers reported being overwhelmed by the physical requirements of daily care and felt a severe loss of spontaneity in their lives. They also reported a sense of isolation from everyday social interactions. Although they highly valued their social support systems, they expressed frustration that few people offered instrumental or direct service support, such as respite care or help with medical appointments, housekeeping, or shopping.[91]

Fortunately, most families manage to cope with the process—the major contributing factor being the coping ability of families before the illness. To be really effective, the therapist working with the patient with ALS must be prepared to help families and caregivers find appropriate ways of coping with the emotional, social, and physical stress of caregiving.

Mr. Turner is a 45-year-old man diagnosed 2 years ago with ALS. He lives at home with his wife, who works full-time, and two teenaged children. Mr. Turner is a computer programmer for an engineering firm in the area. Since his diagnosis, Mr. Turner has been able to continue his full-time work schedule, although he states that he is no longer able to touch type and can type with the index fingers only. He has noticed that his shoulders and neck hurt after an hour at the computer. In the last 2 weeks he has found it very fatiguing to walk to the cafeteria for lunch, and he fears that he will be knocked down when walking in crowds. He dropped his tray last week, which was very embarrassing, so he decided to eat in his office even though he misses the socialization and opportunity to discuss work issues with this colleagues.

Mr. Turner has been able to continue most of his nonwork activities, although he is no longer able to operate his sailboat independently and is having trouble maintaining his balance when golfing. He states that his wife and children are supportive and that they have made some changes in the home environment to accommodate his increasing weakness. He also revealed, however, that his children seem frustrated with him because he is so much slower than he was before the illness.

On assessment, Mr. Turner showed marked wasting of hand intrinsics. He was unable to abduct or flex either shoulder past 90 degrees. His right shoulder showed considerable atrophy, especially of the deltoid and supraspinatus muscles. All other upper-extremity movements were weakened but in the G− (4−) range. His neck posture was forward (neck extension is F+ (3+), neck flexion is G− (4−). Scapular winging was noted bilaterally. No spasticity was evident in the upper extremities.

Lower-extremity musculature showed generalized weakness at about the F (3) to F+ (3+) range, with left musculature weaker than right, marked wasting of the foot intrinsics, and a cavus foot position bilaterally. Spasticity of the hip adductors and hamstrings was noted on passive motion. Most obvious during gait was inadequate dorsiflexion for heel strike and no propulsion during heel-off. He showed bilateral corrected gluteus medius pattern on weight bearing. He needed to pause to lock each knee during weight bearing and at times he pushed his knee into extension with his hand. He had great difficulty ascending and descending steps in his home. There were no stairs to negotiate at work.

Until this appointment, Mr. Turner had not been willing to discuss the use of adaptive equipment or to use a wheelchair. During prior clinic visits his decisions were supported and he was told that when he was ready, therapists would work with him and his family to help with equipment decisions. It is important that therapists present but not press adaptive equipment options to patients when they first start to show impairment in functional ability. If shown how the equipment will help them maintain independence, most patients are receptive to its use. Even when presented in a positive way, however, a wheelchair or adaptive devices may be resisted long after the adaptations would facilitate mobility and ADL. Therapists must be very attentive to patients' feelings and fears at this time because use of a wheelchair heralds to many patients the beginning of the end.

Mr. Turner also showed some early bulbar signs. He noted that he sometimes had to catch drool when working intensely, and that his pillow was moist in the morning. Food sometimes got stuck in his cheek area and he could not move it out with his tongue. Swallowing was still adequate for eating all foods; however, he had had a few coughing episodes when drinking coffee and wine. He showed increased use of accessory musculature when breathing but had no complaints of respiratory distress. His cough was adequate to clear secretions.

With input from the therapist, Mr. Turner and his wife identified the following general goals:

1. Increase mobility
2. Control fatigue and pain of upper extremities and neck during computer work
3. Maintain maximal muscle strength and ROM (patient complained that he felt stiff)
4. Identify safety issues within the home and work environment and adjust household and work environment to prepare for the time when Mr. Turner could not ascend and descend stairs safely

A treatment plan was discussed to achieve the following:

1. **Increase mobility.** Because of his increased walking difficulties, Mr. Turner decided to use a front-wheeled walker with a seat attachment at home. Because of his hand grip weakness, he felt most stable using attached forearm troughs. For his worksite, he selected a motorized wheelchair so that he could maintain his independence at work. Although he found that he could push an ultralight manual chair, it was clear that his upper extremity strength was decreasing. To prevent overworking and further damaging weakened musculature, he was discouraged from self-propelling a manual chair because of the repetitive pushing action and the effort necessary to cope with inclines. Although most patients will need a motorized device, such as a wheelchair or scooter, to maintain independent mobility, some homes would need adaptations to allow electric wheelchair access. Some patients are initially horrified at the "appearance of disability" when using a motorized wheelchair and prefer the electric scooter, which is more socially accepted. The scooter,

Continued

however, does not provide adequate support for the patient in the later stages of the disease. Therefore, its purchase should be discouraged unless the patient has adequate financial resources to make the transition later to a motorized chair.

Factors to consider include: extent of insurance coverage or financial assistance programs for purchase of wheelchair (some policies or programs may provide only one type of wheelchair or only one wheelchair, either motorized or manual); transportability of motorized chair from home to community and work (few motorized wheelchair brands fold for stowing in car trunk and few families can afford to purchase a van that will allow patient to drive or be driven while in motor chair); reclining potential of chair back and head rest (preferably electric) to allow the patient to shift weight and rest while in the chair during later stages of the disease; removable arm rests for ease of transfer; potential for head rest attachment or extension; potential mounting area for portable respirator equipment if needed; ease with which caregiver can help patient with chair mobility transfers. Because Mr. Turner's insurance and Medicare would not fund an additional manual chair and because the family had no way to transport the electric wheelchair, the ALS Society loaned the family a manual wheelchair for home use. Although not ideal it was functional. Mr. Turner's son made some inexpensive adjustments to adapt the chair for a head rest and his daughter and grandchildren repainted the chair to his specifications.

Because Mr. Turner wanted to keep as active as possible and use his walker within the home, he was fitted with bilateral ankle-foot orthoses (AFOs) with a flexible ankle joint and pretibial shell to facilitate knee extension. Straps were simple overlap style because Mr. Turner had poor thumb and grasp control.

2. **Decrease fatigue and pain of upper extremities.** Mr. Turner was taught some simple self-ROM exercises of the neck and arms to carry out every half hour while working at the computer. In a simulated work environment, the therapist noted that Mr. Turner had a very forward head position when working at a computer similar to his workstation. The height of the computer was adjusted to decrease his neck strain, and the desk height was adjusted to allow his wheelchair to fit under the desk so that his arms could rest fully on the surface. He felt immediate relief with the adaptations. He wasalso fitted for a soft neck collar to wear when he felt he needed more neck support. (As his condition worsened, he learned to rest his head on the headrest of his chair and recline slightly for a few minutes every 15 minutes.)

3. **Maintain maximal muscle strength and ROM.** Mr. Turner was taught as many self-ranging maneuvers as possible, which he was encouraged to do in small segments frequently throughout the day. For example, his series of motions included neck rotations, side bends, and flexion and extension within strength limits, upper-extremity motions with the exception of shoulder flexion and abduction past 90 degrees, hip flexion, abduction and rotations, full knee extension, and all ankle motions. When using the walker, Mr. Turner was encouraged to extend each hip fully and to stretch his heel cords. Mrs. Turner and their adult children were taught to administer full ROM exercises, including trunk rotations, with special attention to ranging of the shoulder to prevent impingement. Simple massage techniques were also taught to all family members who felt comfortable with the task.

Maintaining maximal muscle strength is difficult because any program must be designed to prevent disuse activity *and* prevent overwork damage. No exercise program should be recommended that would cause enough fatigue to require extensive periods of postexercise rest or interfere with his participation in normal ADL. Mr. Turner had been active before the onset of ALS and he liked to exercise. Therefore, he rented a portable pedaling unit to attach to a chair at home. He pedaled two to four times a day, with no additional resistance, to the point at which he felt fatigue (usually 3 to 5 minutes at this stage). He carefully monitored his soreness and fatigue level after exercise and increased and decreased his pedaling depending on how he felt immediately and several days after exercise. Mr. Turner felt invigorated by this exercise, which he usually did while watching television. He was also taught a series of simple elastic band exercises, with tensile strength adjusted according to his ability to contract his muscles without fatigue. Mr. Turner was also shown a series of isometric exercises for all muscle groups to do throughout the work day. Because he had some foot and ankle edema, he was encouraged to wear lightweight pressure stockings while sitting. Mr. Turner also had access to a swimming pool, and he was encouraged to carry out walking and upper-extremity exercises provided another adult was with him in the water at all times.

4. **Assess environment of home and work.** Occupational therapy input was requested to help with ADL aids such as reachers, utensil adaptors to facilitate grip, rubber pen grippers, key adaptors to permit turning, and thumb abduction splints to assist in pincer grasp. Mr. Turner's occupational therapist made several visits to his worksite and home to identify adapta-

Continued

tions of the environment for safety and independence. His wheelchair was eventually adapted with universal joint arm troughs to decrease his effort during self-feeding and basic upper body hygiene. Ramps were recommended for home entry, and nonpermanent safety rails were placed in the bathroom. Mr. Turner was able to assist with transfer to a shower chair and the shower head was replaced with a handheld unit.

A speech pathology consultation was also requested. Using information from the physical therapist's Manual Muscle Test (MMT), the speech pathologist carried out a thorough bulbar evaluation and provided information about swallowing techniques. The speech therapist focused on ways to decrease drooling and ways to cope with food "pocketing" (tongue mobility was impaired) using techniques such as hand pressure on the cheek to push food back to the center of the mouth. The therapist also instructed Mr. Turner and his wife how to prepare foods with textures that were easily swallowed and manipulated. Mr. Turner had lost 5 pounds during the last 6 months so he was also referred to the dietitian for information about how to maintain nutritious calorie intake.

Mr. Turner had great difficulty adjusting to his physical dependence. Because of his very slow onset of dysphagia and his augmented communication system, he was able to continue control over his expressive, cognitive, and emotional life until the last 5 or 6 months of his life. Initially, Mr. Turner angrily resisted his wife's attempts to help him with eating and dressing tasks. This began to alienate her and the children until a family meeting was held with their medical social worker and physical and occupational therapists. All family members had the opportunity to express their frustrations. A major irritation to the children was what they perceived to be their constant waiting for their father to complete a task. Mrs. Turner was most irritated when Mr. Turner yelled at her when she attempted to help even though he frequently expressed anger about his clumsiness. Mr. Turner sadly admitted that he was having increasing difficulty with his ADL and was sometimes too tired after dressing to participate in family activities. At the end of the meeting, the family had worked out a compromise plan. Mr. Turner would continue to do as much as possible for himself. He would specifically ask for help from Mrs. Turner when he wanted it so she did not get caught in his anger about needing help. He preferred that the children not have to take any role in his care at this point, but realized that he might need their help later. Visiting nurse support was requested twice a week to help with bathing, and the occupational therapist was requested to make another home visit to help with toileting needs. Mr. Turner felt comfortable with his wife and children carrying out ROM. A therapy home visit was arranged to review the exercise/positioning program as well as respiratory exercises and postural drainage techniques.

As Mr. Turner became totally dependent, he needed 24-hour care. Professional nurses were provided through his insurance contract 14 hours a day from 6:30 AM to 8:30 PM. Family members provided care until midnight. Initially, Mr. Turner was able to activate a bell at night to call for help. His wife and children followed a schedule to turn him every 3 hours throughout the night. When Mr. Turner became respirator dependent and was no longer able to call for help, it became clear that the nighttime responsibilities were taking a heavy toll on his wife, who worked full-time, and the children, who were in high school and college. Fortunately the family was able to pay for a nurse assistant to remain at Mr. Turner's bedside throughout the night, although the family members all felt that they had no privacy. Although the family was committed to having Mr. Turner remain at home until his death, all agreed that they needed respite. Thus, several week-long hospitalizations were made to give the family a break in the constant care needs.

Although Mr. Turner had elected HMV, he also had signed a Durable Power of Attorney for Health Care, indicating that he did not want treatment for infections and that palliative care for comfort should direct his treatment. He had a strong lust for life, but he had come to accept his impending death. He did not have a strong religious view of life, but he had talked with all his caregivers and therapists about his concerns related to death. He freely expressed his fear of "non-being." Because his caregivers and therapists were willing to talk about his and their own feelings, Mr. Turner came to believe that he would live on in the minds, hearts, and behavior of those he had known. This idea seemed to give him great comfort. He particularly liked to talk to others about special times they had had together and how their interactions had affected each other. To help Mr. Turner process his death, his family, friends, and medical team put together an album of pictures and statements about their time together. Mr. Turner frequently liked to have his wife read through the book with him. His family continued to carry out his ROM exercises and massage because Mr. Turner had indicated that the treatments provided him physical comfort and the spiritual closeness he needed with his family. His primary treatment during the last few days consisted of morphine to decrease his respiratory discomfort. After 5 to 6 months totally dependent for all care and respiratory function, Mr. Turner died at home in his sleep after a respiratory illness.

DEMYELINATING INFLAMMATORY POLYRADICULONEUROPATHIES

Pathology and Medical Diagnosis

In the past 15 years a broad spectrum of demyelinating inflammatory polyradiculoneuropathies has been identified. Guillain-Barré syndrome (GBS), or acute inflammatory demyelinating polyradiculoneuropathy, is the most common form of the disease that affects nerve roots and peripheral nerves leading to motor neuropathy and flaccid paralysis.[89] The incidence of GBS is 1 to 2 cases per 100,000 persons. A variant form is acute motor axonal neuropathy, which like GBS has a good prognosis. Less common forms are acute motor and sensory axonal neuropathy, which has a less positive prognosis (which some consider to be a distinct type of peripheral neuropathy) and Miller-Fisher syndrome with primarily cranial nerve symptoms, ataxia, and areflexia.[161]

Approximately 27% of patients with GBS have no identified preceding illness. Although no consistent predisposing factors are known, 49% had a preceding respiratory infections; 3%, pneumonia; 3%, infection due to Epstein-Barr virus; and 10%, a gastrointestinal illness.[178] Two infections have been clearly implicated in the GBS process—Campylobacter jejuni infection and cytomegalovirus (CMV) infection. Patients with preceding C. jejuni and CMV infections tended to have the axonal forms of the disease.[164] Other researchers have suggested that axonal polyneuropathies are most often related to toxic and metabolic causes such as diabetes, alcohol abuse, and, less commonly, chronic exposure to heavy metals and household or industrial toxins.[173]

Recent studies into the complex pathogenesis of the demyelinating inflammatory polyradiculoneuropathies have demonstrated significant associations with autoimmune reactions, such as autoantibodies against myelin constituents, and against gangliosides and glycolipids of axonal and myelin membranes. (See Steck and others[207] for a comprehensive review of the pathogenesis of inflammatory demyelinating diseases.)

Peripheral nerve biopsies are seldom indicated in GBS, but when performed they show mononuclear inflammatory cells, primarily lymphocytes, infiltrating the interstitium and perivascular spaces with deterioration of the myelin sheath. Patchy areas of demyelinization occur along peripheral nerves and nerve roots with the axons spared except in severe cases. Inflammatory processes can also be seen in the dorsal roots and autonomic ganglia. Within 2 to 3 weeks of the acute demyelinization process, Schwann cells proliferate, the inflammation resolves, and remyelinization begins.[60, 164] Cerebrospinal fluid protein is often elevated after several days or within the second week of illness.[179]

Because of damage to the myelin sheath, saltatory propagation of the action potential is disturbed, resulting in slowed conduction velocity, dyssynchrony of conduction, disturbed conduction of higher frequency impulses, or complete conduction block.[143] In axonal neuropathies, the conduction velocity is within normal limits, but the number of functional motor units is decreased (Fig. 13-

4). For a very readable review of reactions of neurons and peripheral nerves to injury see Kandel and others[117] and refer to Chapter 12. See Hartung and others[94] and Trojaborg[219] for reviews of GBS and other forms of inflammatory, immune-mediated neuropathies such as chronic inflammatory demyelinating polyradiculoneuropathy and acute motor axonal neuropathy.

The diagnostic criteria for GBS are detailed in the box on page 387.

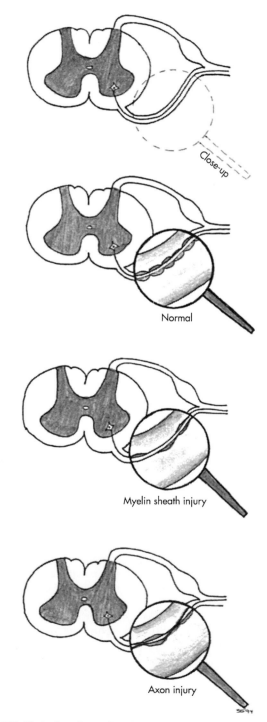

FIGURE 13–4. Drawings of peripheral nerve showing axonal degeneration and demyelination.

COMMON DIAGNOSTIC FEATURES OF GUILLAIN-BARRÉ SYNDROME

A. Motor weakness
1. Progressive symptoms and signs of motor weakness that develop rapidly
   a. Relative symmetry of motor involvement
   b. Usual progression of weakness from distal to proximal; self-limiting to distal limbs of upper and/or lower extremities or may extend to full quadriplegia with respiratory and cranial nerve involvement
2. Areflexia of, at least, distal tendon responses

B. Mild sensory symptoms or signs, particularly paresthesias and hypesthesias

C. Autonomic dysfunction such as tachycardia and arrhythmias, vasomotor symptoms

D. Absence of fever at onset of symptoms; history of flulike illness common

E. Laboratory tests nonspecific but may have elevation of cerebrospinal fluid protein; cerebrospinal fluid cells at 10 or fewer mononuclear leukocytes per cubic millimeter of cerebrospinal fluid

F. Electrodiagnostic testing, nerve conduction velocities usually abnormal

G. Recovery usually begins 2 to 4 weeks after plateau of disease process

Clinical Presentation

GBS in both children and adults is characterized by a rapidly evolving, relatively symmetrical ascending weakness or flaccid paralysis. Motor impairment may vary from mild weakness of distal lower-extremity musculature to total paralysis of the peripheral, axial, facial, and extraocular musculature. Tendon reflexes are usually diminished or absent. Twenty to 30% of patients may require assisted ventilation because of paralysis or weakness of the intercostal and diaphragm musculature. Impaired respiratory muscle strength may lead to an inability to cough or handle secretions and to decreased vital capacity, tidal volume, and oxygen saturation. Secondary complications such as infections or organ system failure lead to death in approximately 5% of patients with GBS.[171] Approximately 50% of patients develop some cranial nerve involvement, primarily facial muscle weakness, although patients may also develop oropharyngeal and oculomotor involvement.[164]

ANS symptoms are noted in about 50% of patients. Low cardiac output, cardiac dysrhythmias, and marked fluctuations in blood pressure may compromise management of respiratory function and can lead to sudden death. Other typical ANS symptoms may result in peripheral pooling of blood, poor venous return, ileus, and urinary retention.[238]

Sensory symptoms such as distal hyperesthesias, paresthesias (tingling, burning), numbness, and decreased vibratory or position sense are common but not progressive or persistent. The sensory disturbances often have a stocking-and-glove pattern rather than the dermatomal distribution of loss. Although the sensory problems are seldom disabling, they can be very disconcerting and upsetting to patients, especially during the acute stage.[117, 177, 178]

Pain was identified as a significant symptom in the original articles describing GBS.[75] In 1949, 1963, and 1984 studies of 50, 35, and 29 patients with GBS, respectively, approximately 55% of patients reported pain preceding their illness or early during onset. Seventy-two percent reported pain at some time during the full course of the disease process. When pain was prominent, patients spontaneously revealed its presence during a medical history. Therefore, patients who present with the onset of low back pain not associated with known injury or stress and complaints of paresthesias and vibratory or decreased tendon reflexes should be evaluated or monitored for possible GBS.[48, 165]

The most common description of pain was of muscle aching typically associated with vigorous or excessive exercise. Pain was usually symmetrical and reported most frequently in the large-bulk muscles such as the gluteals, quadriceps, and hamstrings, and less often in the lower leg and upper-extremity muscles. Some pain reported during late stages of the illness was described as "stiffness." Pain was consistently more disturbing at night.[165] Some patients experience severe burning or hypersensitivity to touch or even air movement, which can interfere with nursing care and limit therapy interventions.

Based on the absence of clinical sensory or electrophysiological abnormalities, Ropper and others[178] stated that GBS pain is not "neuritic" pain and that nerve or spinal ganglia inflammation is not responsible for the perceived pain. The serum creatine kinase level was elevated in 10 of 13 patients with pain and in only one of eight patients without pain. This finding suggests that changes in muscle related to neurogenic origin may be the cause of pain.

Prognosis

Although some patients have a fulminating course of progress with maximal paralysis in 1 to 2 days, 50% of patients reach the nadir (the point of greatest severity) of the disease within 1 week, 70% by 2 weeks, and 80% by 3 weeks.[164] In some cases, the process of increasing weakness continues for 1 to 2 months. Onset of recovery is varied, with most patients showing gradual recovery of muscle strength 2 to 4 weeks after progression has stopped or the condition has plateaued. Although 50% of the patients may show minor neurological deficits (i.e., diminished or absent tendon reflexes) and 15% may show persistent residual deficits in function, approximately 80% become ambulatory within 6 months of onset of symptoms. The most common long-term deficits are weakness of the anterior tibial musculature, and less often weakness of the foot and hand intrinsics, quadriceps, and gluteal musculature. Five percent of patients die of secondary cardiac, respiratory, or other systemic organ failures.[179, 233]

Until studies in the mid to late 1980s, it was difficult to

determine which patients will have a complete recovery. A clear relationship between nerve conduction velocities and prognosis has not been found.[141] More recently, several researchers have identified a subgroup of patients diagnosed with GBS who present with primary axonal degeneration as opposed to demyelinization. Those patients tended to show a prolonged recovery period with persistent disability.[38] In contrast, when a group of Chinese patients with a pattern typical of axonal GBS was compared with a group of patients with demyelinating GBS, no difference was shown in recovery pattern. Factors related to a poor prognosis have been identified as rapidity of onset and progression to quadriplegia, respirator dependence, severity of disease at nadir, failure to show improvement within 3 weeks of plateau,[62, 233] and prodromal C. jejuni infection.[94]

Medical Intervention

Medical treatment depends on the rate and degree of ascending paralysis. Because most patients return to their prior functional status, excellent supportive care during the acute stage is imperative. Respiratory compromise should be expected and all patients, including those with limited paralysis and sensory dysfunction, must be closely monitored for the rapid onset of pulmonary and cardiac decompensation or cardiac arrhythmias secondary to dysautonomia. Because of the possibility of sudden respiratory failure, patients with evidence of GBS must be hospitalized so that immediate cardiorespiratory support can be given if vital capacity falls below 20 mL/kg or oxygen saturation falls below 75%.[171] Patients who progress to respiratory paralysis must be treated in an intensive care environment where adequate respiratory function can be maintained, secondary infections can be prevented or limited, and metabolic functions can be carefully monitored. The patient should be intubated if the forced vital capacity falls below 12 mL/kg or if the patient is increasingly dyspneic even if forced vital capacity is above the cutoff level.[15, 164] After extubation, aspiration can be a serious complication because of oral muscle weakness and dysphagia.

In addition to the intensive supportive care required, two specific drug-based treatments are under investigation for their ability to decrease the duration of respirator dependence and the time to onset of improvement. Because humoral factors and an autoimmune response are thought to be involved in the process of GBS,[84, 160, 218] several studies have focused on the value of plasma exchange as a moderator of disease severity. Since the initial studies in 1984,[84, 160] two large clinical trials (see French Cooperative Group[75] and Guillain-Barré Syndrome Study Group[90]), carried out in the United States and France, have shown that patients undergoing plasmapheresis (removal of plasma from withdrawn blood with retransfusion of the formed elements back into the blood) had shorter periods on mechanical ventilation and walked earlier than subjects who did not undergo exchange.

In the North American study, time to independent walking was 53 days in the treated group and 85 days in the untreated group. Treatment effect was particularly strong for patients treated within the first week of hospitalization and those with more severe disease. Plasma exchange started later than 2 weeks into the illness did not result in any clear benefit to the patient. Plasma exchange, however, has some serious possible complications that relate to an increased incidence of hypotension and arrhythmias, which makes it unsuitable for GBS patients with autonomic instability. The need for multiple infusion lines increases the possibility of septicemia and thrombosis. The technique is also expensive and requires highly skilled personnel and equipment.[29]

Intravenous immunoglobulin (IVIG) also has a positive impact in the treatment of chronic inflammatory polyneuropathy. A randomized controlled trial of IVIG and plasmapheresis was conducted with 150 patients. Results indicated that IVIG was at least as effective as plasma exchange. More recently, a study comparing plasma exchange and IVIG demonstrated that the outcome measures did not differ between the two groups, although the incidence of complications was slightly higher in the plasma exchange group. The relapse rates were similar in the two groups.[30] Therefore, evidence supports the use of either intervention provided that it is initiated within the first 1 or 2 weeks of treatment.[164] Although corticosteroids were used to decrease the inflammatory process in GBS beginning in the 1960s, a clinical study of corticosteroid effectiveness in 1993 suggested that corticosteroids were not useful in the treatment of GBS,[112] although they may have some place in the treatment of other chronic demyelinating polyneuropathies.[150, 236]

Therapeutic Evaluation

A comprehensive therapeutic evaluation of the patient with GBS includes factors shown in the box on page 389.

Motor Evaluation

The extent of the evaluation depends on the patient's condition and his or her ability to participate in the assessment. In many situations, therapists carry out manual muscle testing (MMT) procedures by testing functional muscle groups. In GBS, however, it is important to test muscle strength and ROM as specifically as possible so that the patient's course of progression or improvement can be tracked, possible patterns leading to contractures can be predicted and prevented, and the appropriate level of exercise can be implemented. Because one cannot complete full MMT every week with a debilitated patient, it is most common to select a few specific muscles (i.e., sternocleidomastoids, deltoids, triceps, flexor carpi ulnaris, lumbricals, iliopsoas, gluteus medius, anterior tibialis, flexor hallucis longus) to test weekly.

More complete testing should be performed once the acute stage is over or for major evaluations only. Patients who report considerable pain during handling or active movement may not tolerate testing or may be unwilling or unable to cooperate with muscle testing. Therefore, the therapist may wish to track the patient's level of pain on a pain scale to help determine weakness related to pathology or apparent weakness secondary to pain. Changes in the patient's condition should be monitored with serial MMT, ROM assessments, sensory testing, and

---

FACTORS TO CONSIDER IN EVALUATION OF PATIENT WITH GUILLAIN-BARRÉ SYNDROME

History

Patterns and sequence of symptom onset

Recent illness, injury, prior episodes of sensorimotor problems

Motor Function

Visual inspection to identify symmetry of muscle bulk and function

Myotatic reflexes, rule out tonic reflexes

Manual muscle testing carefully identifying pattern of weakness (testing should be as muscle specific as possible rather than assessing muscle groups only) (use form for serial recording)

Presence of muscle fasciculations

Cranial nerves

Range of motion (use form for serial recording)

Equilibrium reactions sitting and standing (if testable)

Current functional status (ADL including bowel and bladder function, ambulation)

Sensory System

Identify pattern of sensory loss or changes (use body chart)

Identify specific type of sensory change (i.e., paresthesias, anesthesias, hypesthesias [use body chart])

Identify pain type and location (use body chart). What makes it better, what makes it worse?

Identify pressure points or areas that might lead to pressure sores

Autonomic System

Blood pressure resting and immediately after activity (prone, sitting, standing, if possible)

Heart rate resting and immediately after activity, dysrhythmias

Body temperature stability

Bowel and bladder control

Psychosocial Systems

Identify patient and family concerns in acute circumstances and concerns about long-term issues that may affect patient and family. Assessment need not be extensive if referral can be made for social service evaluation of patient and family financial concerns, day-to-day living problems (e.g., transportation, child care), support systems, and coping strategies.

Electrodiagnostic Testing

Nerve conduction velocity. (Physician will order these studies to be performed by a clinician skilled in the procedures. This may be a physical therapist, physician, or technician depending on facility.)

---

functional status evaluations (see Karni and associates[118] and Lewis and Bottomley[128] for suggestions on serial functional assessments). Care should be taken not to fatigue the patient in any single evaluation session.

Respiratory and Dysphagia Evaluation

Therapists are usually involved early in the care of patients with GBS. For patients with respiratory and/or bulbar paralysis, the physical therapist's initial contact may be in the intensive care unit. Although most hospitals have fully equipped intensive care units (ICUs), a therapist working in rural or smaller community hospitals may be the first person to note a patient's changing respiratory status during an evaluation and treatment session for muscle weakness. Therefore, the therapist must be prepared to advise nursing and medical staff about the need to test oxygen saturation levels and vital capacity. Thera-

pist attention to respiratory complications is particularly important in the managed care environment, which discourages hospitalization if presenting symptoms are not life endangering.[92] Pascuzzi and Fleck[164] recommend a simple estimate of forced vital capacity that can be done at bedside. If after taking a large breath the patient can count only to 10, the forced vital capacity is about 1 L and intubation should be considered. Complete information on the physical therapist's evaluation of patients in acute respiratory failure is provided by Humberstone.[109]

Patients with severe oral-motor problems and dysphagia should be evaluated thoroughly and treated by a therapist skilled in oral-motor dysfunction and feeding. This may be a speech therapist, occupational therapist, or physical therapist, depending on the facility. Patients with a feeding tube should receive their feedings in a relatively upright position and should remain in that position for 30 to 60 minutes after feeding to decrease the chance of aspiration. According to Longemann,[130] about 40% of patients receiving bedside swallowing assessments have undetected aspiration. Therefore, the bedside evaluation should be considered only a preliminary step in the diagnostic process. In addition to careful evaluation of oral-motor control, some clinicians recommend cervical auscultation to listen to swallowing sounds, particularly during the acute phase of the illness.

With evidence of swallowing difficulties and possible aspiration, the patient should be referred for comprehensive testing with videofluoroscopy. Swallowing also can be assessed using techniques such as fiberoptic endoscopy, ultrasound, electroglottography to determine laryngeal movement, and scintigraphy, which involves scanning a radioactive bolus during swallowing.[202]

Intervention Goals

Goals for the care of the patient with GBS include the following:

- Facilitate resolution of respiratory and dysphagia problems
- Minimize pain
- Prevent contractures, decubitus ulcers, and injury to weakened or denervated muscles
- Introduce a graduated program of active exercise while monitoring overuse and fatigue

Therapeutic Interventions

Respiratory and Dysphagia Dysfunction

Depending on the facility, physical therapists may be involved in the respiratory care of patients with GBS. Goals of treatment are related to increasing ventilation or oxygenation, decreasing oxygen consumption, controlling secretions, and improving exercise tolerance. Readers should refer to *Cardiopulmonary Physical Therapy*[109] for coverage of treatment programs and techniques for the GBS patient with acute or residual respiratory dysfunction. Chapter 15[109] in that book provides a thorough review of postural drainage, positioning and secretion control techniques, and breathing exercises to minimize oxygen consumption and improve exercise tolerance. Chapter 17[92] details how to work with the patient with acute respiratory failure, and Chapter 18[107] provides extensive coverage in working with the respirator-dependent patient.

In many facilities, speech pathologists or occupational therapists are responsible for establishing a dysphagia treatment program. Therapists responsible for treatment of patients with dysphagia and swallowing problems should refer to Langmore and Longemann's classic text on the evaluation and treatment of swallowing disorders.[125] Basic treatment goals are the prevention of choking and aspiration and the stimulation of effective swallowing and eating. The act of chewing and swallowing is complex and requires coordinated reflexive and conscious action. Treatment is focused on positioning, head control, and oral-motor coordination (i.e., sucking an ice cube,

stimulating the gag response, facilitating swallowing with pressure on neck and thyroid notch timed with intent to swallow). A conscious swallowing technique is introduced with thick liquids and progressed to thinner liquids after the patient's oral-motor coordination response is enough to control movement of fluids. Once the patient has good lip closure, fluids should be introduced one sip at a time from a straw cut to a short length to minimize effort. Gradually, semi-soft moist foods are introduced (pasta, mashed potatoes, squash, Jell-O). Any crumbly or stringy foods (coffee cakes, cookies, snack chips, celery, cheeses) should be avoided, and the patient should not attempt to talk or be interrupted during eating until choking does not occur and swallowing is comfortable and consistent.[183] Feeding training should occur during frequent, short sessions to prevent fatigue. Therapists should be prepared to use the Heimlich maneuver if choking occurs.

Pain

If pain seems to be a major factor in limiting the patient's passive or active motion, the treatment team should determine the best approach to alleviating pain. According to one study, patients with GBS did not seem to show a consistent response to any specific pain medication, although 6 of the 13 patients seemed to have a positive response to codeine, oxycodone, and acetaminophen (Percocet) or oxycodone and aspirin (Percodan).[177] Some patients may find relief with medications used to treat neurogenic pain, such as the tricyclic antidepressants. For patients who do not respond to conventional analgesics or tricyclics, a short course of high-dose corticosteroids can lead to pain relief.[164]

In several studies,[129, 142, 216] some patients with neuropathies have had decreased pain after using transcutaneous electrical nerve stimulation (TENS) (see Chapters 28 and 29). Although there is no study related to the effect of TENS specifically on pain associated with GBS, it might be a treatment option in patients whose pain is not controlled with passive movement or pain medications. (*Note:* Some patients who experience extreme sensitivity to light touch, such as from movement of sheets, air flow, and intermittent touch contact, benefit from a "cradle," which will hold the sheets away from the body. Some find relief if the limbs are wrapped snuggly with elastic bandages, which provide continuous low pressure while warding off light, intermittent stimuli.)

Contractures, Decubitus Ulcers, and Injury to Weakened or Denervated Muscles

Positioning. To prevent pressure sores, the physical therapist needs to be involved within the first few days of hospitalization, especially for the patient who has complete or nearly complete paralysis. A positioning program for the dependent patient is the first line of defense. The therapist should arrange for a special mattress or unit that constantly changes the pressure within the mattress or shifts the patient's position or is designed to spread pressure over wide surfaces. For patients who are slender with prominent bony surfaces, the therapist may need to fashion foam "doughnuts" or pads or use sheepskin-type protection for pressure relief. Patients who are experiencing muscle pain may prefer to have their hips and knees flexed. In these cases, it is imperative to position the patient out of the flexed position for part of each hour.

As part of a complete positioning program, therapists should consider how to best maintain the physiological position of the hands and feet. Research has shown that mild continuous stretch maintained for at least 20 minutes is more beneficial than stronger, brief stretching exercises.[210] Therefore, use of splints for prolonged positioning is superior for maintaining functional range to use of short bursts of intermittent manually applied passive stretching. Although some facilities still use a footboard to control passive ankle dorsiflexion, most therapists now use moldable plastic splints, which can be worn when the patient is in any position. Because ankle-foot splints often prevent visual inspection of the heel position, however, care must be taken to ensure that the heel is firmly down in the orthosis and that the strapping pattern is adequate to secure the foot. The strap system must be simple enough to be positioned properly by all staff and family members caring for the patient. The ankle-foot splint should extend slightly beyond the end of the toes to prevent toe flexion and skin breakdown from the toes rubbing on sheeting. Care should be taken not to compress the peroneal nerve with the splint as it crosses the fibula.[178] Wrist and hand splints may be prefabricated resting-style splints or molded to meet the patient's specific needs. Because increased tone is not a problem in the patient with GBS, a simple cone or rolled cloth may be adequate to maintain good wrist, thumb, and finger alignment.

Another concern is regaining tolerance to the upright position. A review of the literature on dysautonomia found that between 15% and 50% of patients with GBS have problems with hypotension[238] secondary to prolonged immobility in supine position. Most patients must be placed on a graduated program to regain tolerance to the upright position. A program to improve tolerance to upright position can be started in the intensive care environment if the patient is on a circle electric or Nelson "standing bed." If a standing bed is not available, a sitting program can be initiated as soon as it is tolerated. A progressive standing program can be instituted when the patient's respiratory and autonomic nervous systems are no longer unstable and the patient can be moved to a tilt table. Caution should be taken to fully stabilize the patient to maintain alignment and to limit activity in muscles below the fair range. When beginning training, some patients benefit from using an abdominal binder or foot-to-thigh compression stockings if tolerated. Because of the relationship between poor hydration and hypotension, it is essential for therapists to make sure their patient is well hydrated before beginning upright or standing tolerance programs.[143]

Range of Motion. The onset of connective tissue shortening in response to immobilization is very rapid.[3] To be effective, the ROM program must include both accessory and physiological motions to increase circulation, provide lubrication of the joints, and maintain extensibility of capsular, muscle, and tendon tissue.

ROM can usually be maintained with standard positioning and ROM programs. Nevertheless, some patients, especially those who have complained of severe extremity and axial pain early during the disease process and those who have been quadriplegic and respirator dependent for prolonged periods, may develop significant joint contractures despite preventive interventions.

Soryal and colleagues[203] reported on three patients who had marked residual contractures that limited function after strength improved. None of the patients had radiological signs of erosive arthopathy or inflammatory joint disease. Soryal and colleagues hypothesized a number of possible mechanisms for the limitations in ROM: (1) therapists and nurses may have been reluctant to take patients who complained of marked pain during passive movement through the full ROM; (2) the contractures may have been secondary to pain or damage caused by inappropriate excessive passive movement of hypotonic and sensory impaired joints and muscles; (3) the paralysis may have resulted in lymphatic stasis with accumulation of tissue fluid in tissue spaces and nutritional disturbances; and (4) vasomotor disturbances resulting from autonomic neuropathy may have led to adhesions and fibrosis. Although the authors found few reports describing contractures as a significant residual problem, they suggested that ROM programs must be defined precisely as to frequency and duration, particularly for patients complaining of early joint pain.

Some patients will continually position their limbs so muscle and tendons are in the shortened range in an attempt to decrease muscle pain. This may lead to capsular contractures. The therapist should be aware of changes in "end feel" over time when testing ROM of each joint to determine if capsular and ligamentous structures are also becoming more restricted as the muscle and tendon tissue shortens. Patients who have intact sensation of pain and temperature may respond positively to the use of heat to decrease muscle pain and to facilitate tissue elongation before stretching. Several basic studies of the relationship between load and heat, using rat tail tendon, have shown that it is possible to attain permanent length increases in collagenous tissue using a combination of heat and stretch.[127, 215, 227, 228]

Based on these studies, Warren[226] suggests that stretch be combined with the highest tolerable therapeutic temperature (approximately 45°C [113°F]). He also recommends that the application of stretch should be of long duration, that moderate forces should be used, that tissue temperature should be elevated before stretching, and that elongation of tissue should be maintained for at least 8 to 10 minutes while the tissue is cooling. (*Caution*: Heat should not be used on a patient with a sensory deficit, particularly an inability to distinguish differences in temperature.) Because heating of deep tissue is not possible with patients, Warren's[226] suggestions may be relevant only for superficial muscle/tendon groups. (Heating muscle and tendon tissue before sustained stretching, however, was a mainstay in prevention of contractures caused by muscle spasms secondary to poliomyelitis, and it may have a place in treatment of muscle spasm and contractions in GBS provided there is no sensory impairment.[204])

Because denervated or weakened muscles can be injured easily, it is the therapist's responsibility to ensure that joint structures are not damaged and that ROM is done with appropriate support of the limb to prevent sudden overstretching. This is particularly true at the shoulder because many caregivers, especially those with minimal or no training in ROM, do not know to carefully rotate the shoulder externally during abduction to prevent impingement and capsular damage.[122] Caution also should be taken when "ranging" or stretching the ankle into dorsiflexion to ensure that the subtalar joint is in neutral or locked position so that the Achilles tendon is effectively elongated and the midfoot structures are not overstretched. In hospitals where the patient is treated by a changing therapy or nursing staff or by family members, a positioning schedule with diagrams, a splinting plan, and ROM recommendations should be presented in poster form at the patient's bedside to provide consistent treatment.

ROM stretching of all involved joints should be performed at least twice a day and more frequently if the patient has no active movement. Patients should be encouraged to move actively when they can do so without causing pain or fatigue. They should be observed carrying out their active range to determine whether change has occurred in the quality of movement that may be related to decreasing strength. If the patient cannot complete ROM through full range independently, the therapist or nursing staff must carefully assist the patient in moving to the end range. This may not be easy if the patient experiences pain with motion. Knowing whether to "push through the pain" or stay within the limits of pain is often a great dilemma for the therapist. The therapist needs to find a balance between working for full joint range and reacting to the patient's complaints of pain.

Based on evidence that continuous passive motion (CPM) is effective in maintaining joint range in both rabbits and humans,[185] Mays[138] described a case study of a patient with GBS (quadriplegia with 7 days of mechanical ventilation) who had persistent pain and stiffness of the upper extremities and fingers approximately 3 months after the onset of GBS. Therefore, CPM of the hands and fingers was added to a program of occupational therapy that included ROM, splinting, and ADL. The author reported an increase in the rate of recovery of finger range and a decrease in pain after use of CPM. Numerous other studies have reported the value of CPM in maintaining or increasing ROM after hip and knee surgery. It may be a very useful adjunct to traditional therapy for patients with GBS, especially those who continue to develop contractures with intermittent ROM programs.

Massage also may play a positive role in maintaining muscle tissue mobility and tissue nutrition. A study of crush injuries of muscle in rats reported that massage may lessen the amount of fibrosis that develops in immobilized, denervated, or injured muscle.[99] The use of massage in patients with GBS has not been reported; however, it makes intuitive sense that it may be a useful adjunct to ROM exercises in patients who do not have marked hypersensitivity to touch, dysesthesias, or muscle pain.

Progressive Program of Active Exercise While Monitoring for Overuse and Fatigue

Although most patients with GBS recover from the paralysis, the course and rate of recovery may vary significantly between patients. Strength usually returns in a descending pattern—opposite of the pattern noted during onset of the disease. *The most important concept to remember in designing an exercise program is that exercise will not hasten or improve nerve regeneration, nor will it influence the reinnervation rate during the rehabilitation process.*[208] The major goal of therapeutic management, therefore, must be to maintain the patient's musculoskeletal system in an optimal "ready" state, to prevent overwork, and to pace the recovery process to obtain maximal function as reinnervation occurs.

The rule in developing an exercise program for patients with GBS is that muscle fatigue must be avoided and rest periods must be frequent.[98, 210] Bensman[21] reported on eight patients who had stabilized after acute polyradiculoneuritis (among them patients with GBS). All eight patients experienced a temporary loss of function after strenuous physical exercise. Three patients apparently had significant decreases in strength. All patients were then placed on a program of passive ROM and an increase in muscle strength was noted. Recurring episodes of a temporary loss of function appeared to be related to strenuous exercise and fatigue. Studying the effect of exercise on rat muscle after nerve injury, Herbison and colleagues[98] identified a loss of contractile proteins during initial reinnervation. After reinnervation the same amount of exercise resulted in muscle hypertrophy. Reitsma[172] noted that vigorous exercise damaged muscles if fewer than one third of motor units were functional. If more than one third of the motor units remained, exercise led to hypertrophy. Therefore, the amount of strengthening attained seems proportional to the number of intact or undamaged motor units. Exercise at a level to elicit a training effect in normal muscle may cause overwork damage in damaged muscle. Because the therapist cannot determine the number of intact motor units available to a patient, the therapist must be cautious when initiating exercise with any patient who is undergoing reinnervation.

It is important to remember that the safe exercise range differs for normal and impaired muscle, with the therapeutic window being smaller for muscles undergoing reinnervation. (See the section on overwork damage in patients with ALS and Figure 13–3 for a graphic example of the exercise "window" for normal and damaged or denervated muscle.)

Bensman[21] recommended that once the patient has stabilized, active exercise may begin as follows:

- Short periods of nonfatiguing exercise appropriate to the patient's strength
- An increase in activity or exercise level only if the patient improves or if there is no deterioration after 1 week
- A return to bed rest if a decrease in function or strength occurs
- A program of exercise directed at strengthening for function rather than strength itself

- A limit of fatiguing exercise for 1 year with a gradual return to sport activities and more strenuous exercise

Steinberg[208] suggested that patients be allowed to exercise to the first point of fatigue or muscle ache. Abnormal sensations (tingling, paresthesias) that persist for prolonged periods of time after exercise may also indicate that the exercise or activity level was excessive.

When neural recovery begins, the initiation of active exercise must be implemented with a clear understanding that excessive exercise during early reinnervation, when there are only a few functioning motor units, can lead to further damage rather than to the expected exercise-induced hypertrophy of muscle.

Based on that information, a graduated exercise program can be viewed as a pyramid with passive ROM at the base, antigravity and specific, functionally focused, resistive exercises in the middle levels with integrated, coordinated, and functional exercises and activities at the top.[166] During the initial stages of exercise, the repetitions per exercise period should be low and the frequency of short periods of exercise should be high.[210] As reinnervation occurs and motor units become responsive, the early process of muscle reeducation exercise used by the therapist may be similar to that used during the polio era. To encourage active contraction of the muscle the therapist should carefully demonstrate to the patient the expected movement. The therapist then passively moves the patient's limb while the patient observes. After gaining a clear picture of what movement is expected, the patient is encouraged to contract his or her muscle(s). Facilitatory techniques such as skin stroking, brushing, vibration, icing, and tapping may be used in conjunction with the muscle reeducation process. The patient is taught to reassess his or her movements and to make corrective responses. As the patient gains strength, the movements are translated into functional activities.[98]

Functionally directed exercise should be initiated judiciously, and the activities should be appropriate for the muscle grade of that muscle or muscle group. For example, if the patient's deltoid muscle receives a poor (2) grade (full range of motion with gravity eliminated), the patient should be cautioned not to repeatedly attempt to elevate his or her arm against gravity (e.g., to shave or do one's hair). Exercises should be developed to allow the patient to exercise in the gravity-free position (overhead slings, powder boards, pool exercises) that allow the patient to move actively through a full range until he or she can take resistance in the gravity-eliminated position. Many younger patients have to be reminded to pace their activity so they do not overly fatigue and possibly injure their recovering muscles. Children, teenagers, or adults with impaired judgment often need a strict schedule of rest and activity. Patients and staff also need to be reminded that prolonged sitting in bed or in a wheelchair, even when supported, may tax the axial musculature and a program of gradual sitting should be instituted, with the final goal being independent, unsupported sitting with functional adaptive reactions. In busy hospitals a schedule of sitting and activity should be posted in clear view at the patient's bedside.

As reinnervation progresses and strength and exercise tolerance increase, the therapist may choose to use facilitative exercise techniques such as proprioceptive neuromuscular facilitation (PNF), which intentionally recruits maximal contraction of specific muscle groups. Although PNF techniques are excellent for eliciting maximal contraction, care must be taken not to overwork the weaker components of the movement pattern. A positive aspect of PNF techniques is that they can be tied in with functional patterns such as rolling, which is necessary for bed mobility, transitions to quadruped, kneeling, sitting, and standing stability, and gait. (The reader is also referred to the works of Blei and colleagues,[25] Bushbacher,[39] and Fielding and Bean.[70])

Because patients with GBS are being transferred from acute care facilities to rehabilitation, skilled nursing, or home environments more quickly than in the past, therapists must be very careful to document any serial negative changes or plateaus in motor, sensory, or respiratory impairments or functional status that may herald a relapse.[143] Standard measures of impairment, MMT, ROM, and sensory tests should be completed before and after discharge from the acute setting as well as assessments of functional status or disability, such as the Functional Independence Measure (FIM) or Barthel Index (BI). See also the work of Guccione[88] and van der Putten.[220] In addition, before discharge from the hospital or rehabilitation unit, therapists should complete an assessment of the patient's home environment so that appropriate safety and adaptive equipment can be in place in time for the patient's return home. Schmitz[200] has written a comprehensive review of home assessment protocols.

Although 65% to 75% or more of patients with GBS show a return to clinically normal motor function, between 2% and 5% of patients have a recurrence of symptoms similar in onset and pattern to the original illness. The recurrence differs from a chronic inflammatory demyelinating polyneuropathy.[83] In addition, there is anecdotal and empirical evidence that some patients continue to show deficits during strenuous exercises that require maximal endurance. Four soldiers who were considered clinically recovered from GBS (normal motor power with or without reappearance of reflexes and the absence of sensory impairment) were unable to pass the Army Physical Fitness Test (APFT), which is designed to measure a minimal acceptable age-related level of physical fitness (maximal effort to challenge respiratory and muscular endurance, strength, and flexibility). Before onset of GBS, the four patients had all exceeded the APFT standards. None was able to pass the APFT as long as 4 years after the illness, indicating that the sustained effort required in the fitness testing unmasked a significant, persistent deficit that interfered with their ability to continue their military careers.[38] Therefore, the possibility of long-term endurance deficits should be considered when patients appear to have reached full recovery but report difficulty when returning to work or activities that require sustained maximal effort.[119]

Cardiovascular fitness may also be compromised after recovery from GBS. This may be due to altered muscle function but is also related to deconditioning from an imposed sedentary lifestyle. Several studies have attempted to determine the effect of endurance exercise training after GBS. In one case study a 23-year-old woman with a chronic-relapsing form of GBS (usually a slow-onset polyneuropathy with a remitting-relapsing course and persistent slowing of nerve conduction velocities) with onset at age 15 was placed on a walking and cycling program at 45% or less of her predicted maximal heart rate reserve. The low-intensity exercise program was selected to prevent possible fatigue-related relapse. After the program, the subject had increased her walking time 37%, her walking distance approximately 88%, and her cycle ride time more than 100%. Although no standardized or formalized recording of functional level was recorded before and after the exercise program, the patient reported that her energy level for ADL was a "little higher" and that stair walking was easier.[119]

In another single-subject study of a 54-year-old man 3 years after onset of GBS with residual weakness, the authors demonstrated similar improvements in cardiopulmonary and work capacities, as well as in leg strength, after a 16-week course of a three-times-a-week aerobic exercise program. The subject also reported expanded ADL capabilities. The authors suggested that their training regimen may disrupt the cycle of inactivity after recovery from GBS that leads to disuse atrophy and further deconditioning in patients with mild residual weakness.[168] Of future research and clinical interest is the long-term consequences of GBS and how the normal aging process will affect patients who have some mild residual—for example, whether some patients will develop increasing weakness over time similar to persons with postpolio syndrome.[143] For an example of treatment progression during the acute stage from week 1 through week 12, see the box on page 395.

Adaptive Equipment and Orthoses

Judicious use of orthotic devices and adaptive equipment should be considered an integral part of the rehabilitation process. The purpose of the orthotic and adaptive devices is twofold: (1) to protect weakened structures from overstretch and overuse and (2) to facilitate ADL within the limits of the patient's current ability. Orthotic devices and adaptive equipment should be introduced and discontinued based on serial evaluations of strength, ROM, and functional needs. For example, a hospitalized patient who has poor (2) middle deltoid strength may practice upper-extremity activities such as eating while using suspension slings. A thumb position splint may be used temporarily to aid thumb control in grasping tasks.

Most patients will need a wheelchair for several months until strength and endurance improve. As strength returns, patients recovering from severe paralysis may need to change from use of a wheelchair with a high, reclining back with head rest to use of a lightweight, easily maneuverable chair. A quandary for the therapist is to predict how long a wheelchair will be necessary and whether it should be rented or purchased as the patient progresses through different stages of recovery. While moving from wheelchair mobility to independent ambulation, patients will usually progress from parallel bars, to a walker with a seat to allow frequent resting, and then to crutches or a cane. Because wheelchairs, walkers, crutches, and canes,

especially custom appliances, are very expensive and are not always included in insurance coverage, the therapist should carefully consider the cost to the patient during the recovery process.

Although most patients with GBS have a complete functional recovery, many show a more prolonged residual weakness of calf and, most commonly, anterior compartment musculature, requiring the use of an ankle-foot orthosis (AFO). The decision whether to use a prefabricated orthosis or custom appliances is not always simple. Several temporary orthotic measures can be considered. For example, if the patient shows good gastrocnemius-soleus strength with mild weakness of the dorsiflexors, a simple elastic strap attached to the shoelaces and a calf band may be sufficient to prevent overuse of the anterior compartment muscles. An old-fashioned, relatively inexpensive spring wire brace, which can be attached to the patient's shoes to facilitate dorsiflexion, is a good choice for patients who complain of sensory hypersensitivity when wearing a plastic orthosis.

Most therapy units today have access to varied sizes of plastic, fixed-ankle AFOs that can be used until a decision is made to have the patient fitted with custom AFOs. A newer system of prefabricated AFOs with adjustable ankle motion cams has been developed that allows the therapist to limit plantarflexion and dorsiflexion to the specific needs of the patient. For patients with reasonable control of plantarflexion and dorsiflexion, but with lateral instability because of peroneal weakness, a simple ankle stirrup device such as the Aircast Swivel-Strap stirrup splint (Aircast, Inc., Summit, NJ) can be used temporarily to provide lateral ankle stability. Although very few patients with GBS need knee-ankle-foot orthoses (KAFOs) on a long-term basis, inexpensive air splints or adjustable long-leg metal splints to control knee position are sometimes helpful when working on standing weight bearing and during initial gait training. See Chapter 31 for additional information on orthotics.

Psychosocial Issues

Although most patients with GBS have a complete recovery, the acute stage of the disease can be very frightening, especially to patients who progress to complete paralysis and respiratory failure. Nancy, in Case 13–2 on page 396, reported that she was terrified during the time she was totally paralyzed (including eyelid movement) and on a respirator. She said that nurses, doctors, and hospital staff seemed to assume she could not hear because she was unable to respond in any manner. In her words,

They acted like I was already dead, and I thought I would be from the way they were talking. The thing I hated the most was when the night nurses from the registry would come in and ask how to make the ventilator work! I felt panicked. Can you imagine having your life depend on a machine and knowing that the person who was supposed to make it work had no idea what to do if a tube came unconnected? They were always worried about my blood pressure. Who wouldn't have high blood pressure in that situation! The thing I liked about my therapists was that they told me what they were going to do even when I couldn't respond. They didn't just start doing things or pulling on me like other people did.

MEDICAL STATUS OF PATIENTS WITH GBS AND POSSIBLE TREATMENT OUTLINE

Medical Status

Tracheostomy

Respirator dependent

Complete cranial nerve paralysis

Quadriplegia

Respirator set on intermittent mandatory ventilation

Weaning to respirator at night by end of week 7

No active muscle contractions except eye opening and lip movements

Dysphagia

Palpable muscle activity in neck, trunk, proximal musculature of upper and lower extremities

Treatment: (Depends on rate of recovery)

Week 1:

Postural drainage every 3 hours around the clock

Passive ROM to all joints

Splinting (molded plastic) of hands and feet to maintain functional position

Positioning, splinting, and ROM program schedule posted at bedside

Weeks 2–5:

Postural drainage decreased to two times each shift (every 8 hours)

Passive ROM, physiological and accessory motions, gentle stretching of intercostal musculature, trunk rotations

Continue splinting and positioning program

Family education: family members taught gentle physiological ROM techniques, with attention to correct shoulder patterns and simple massage techniques

Weeks 6–7:

Postural drainage two times each shift (every 8 hours)

Continue ROM program, splinting, and positioning

Begin to build tolerance of upright sitting with good trunk alignment

Begin facilitation of active facial/tongue muscle activity in patterns necessary for swallowing, eating, and speaking; speech pathology, occupational therapy consultation for dysphagia training

Family members active in care, helping with ROM, splinting, and positioning schedule as they choose

Weeks 8–12:

Postural drainage one time each shift

Chest stretching, breathing exercises

Dysphagia program in collaboration with speech consultant

Muscle reeducation program with EMG biofeedback progressing to gravity-eliminated exercises using suspension slings attached to bed

Tilt table standing program to increase tolerance to upright (wearing positioning splints if necessary)

Collaborate with occupational therapy for treatment in wheelchair with suspension slings to facilitate active arm motion in gravity-limited position

Exercise, rest, positioning schedule posted

Family, patient educated about stimulating activity level to prevent fatigue, overuse of reinnervating muscles

---

ROM, range of motion; EMG, electromyography.

CASE 13–2   Nancy

Nancy, a 16-year-old girl with a history of repeated hospitalizations for asthma, was admitted to the hospital with tingling in the hands and feet and mild respiratory distress. Because staff thought there was a significant emotional component to her asthma attacks, her repeated complaints of paresthesias, muscle pain, and weakness were largly ignored or attributed to anxiety attacks. The day after admission, Nancy began staggering while walking and became extremely agitated and hysterical, screaming that she was dying and could not breathe. A medical assessment showed evidence of wheezing with a normal chest radiograph and decreased vital capacity. She was uncooperative during strength testing, although strength was estimated to be within normal limits except for approximately Fair+ (3+) strength of the dorsiflexors and everters and Good (4) strength of the plantarflexors. She became extremely upset when her feet were touched.

Because of her psychological history, she was referred for psychiatric assessment and was placed on an anxiolytic medication. Two hours later she suffered a full respiratory arrest and was intubated and maintained on mechanical ventilation. Over the next 3 days she developed flaccid quadriplegia and within 5 days she had complete cranial nerve involvement. She was weaned from the respirator after 29 days following several episodes of pneumonia. Postextubation, she had swallowing and speech problems that resolved by time of discharge at 3 months after onset. During the acute stage, she was catheterized because of urinary retention and was treated for a bowel obstruction. Sensation was normal for perception of temperature changes and deep pressure.

Proprioception was diminished at the ankle, knee, and fingers. Paresthesias and hypesthesias, aggravated by light touch, were present in a glovelike pattern of both hands and feet.

Nancy's physical therapy treatment began in the intensive care unit (ICU). Although her postural drainage treatment was performed using respiratory therapy techniques in conjunction with aerosol medication by intermittent positive pressure, physical therapists began a course of chest stretching techniques in coordination with a fastidious ROM program performed twice a day by a therapist and on the evening and night shifts by a nurse. A pressure relief mattress was ordered for her bed. To prevent contracture development, an occupational therapist fabricated bilateral wrist and finger splints; a physical therapist molded ankle splints to maintain 90 degrees of dorsiflexion with neutral eversion-inversion. A positioning and ROM schedule in poster form with pictures of positions and ROM patterns was posted at Nancy's bedside.

Because Nancy complained of severe hypersensitivity to light touch or to any passive movement of her limbs, a cradle was placed on the bed to prevent sheets from touching her and to prevent air flow changes from irritating her skin. She was fitted for above-knee light pressure stockings, which seemed to decrease her sensitivity to light touch.

Progression of the GBS process seemed to plateau at approximately 15 days after onset with a very gradual return of respiratory function complicated by infections. Weaning from the respirator was difficult and the physical therapist played a major role in instructing Nancy, the staff, and her family in appropriate breathing exercises to be performed every 1 or 2 hours. Because her parents wanted to be involved with her care, they were taught ROM techniques with special attention to correct shoulder ROM techniques. The physical therapists continued to follow Nancy twice a day to ensure that accessory motions were completed with the physiological motions. Moist hot packs similar to those used during the polio era were used effectively before ROM for 1 week during which Nancy complained of severe muscle pain.

As part of her positioning program, Nancy was placed in supported semisitting position while on the respirator. As muscle control returned, a muscle reeducation program was initiated, which focused initially on head and trunk and then on upper and lower extremities. Exercise periods were limited to 15 minutes twice a day. Ideally, she would have benefited from more frequent short sessions; however, this was not possible. Therefore, her parents were shown how to cautiously guide her active exercise program so that she was able to exercise more frequently at low repetitions. When each muscle group reached an MMT grade of Fair+ (3+) or greater, Nancy was allowed to use the muscles in functional activities with very proscribed limitations in activity duration. When she was able to tolerate upright sitting and had some bed mobility, Nancy was transferred to a Nelson bed in which she could begin a gradual standing weight-bearing program.

A speech therapist worked with Nancy in the ICU to help her relearn safe swallowing patterns and to reintroduce her to different-textured foods. A dietitian had been working with Nancy throughout her hospitalization to ensure adequate nutrition while intubated, and she worked closely with the speech therapist to progress Nancy's diet as she became able to handle liquids and solids.

After being weaned from the respirator and transferred to the general floor, Nancy was brought to the physical therapy department for treatment, which was frequently done in conjunction with occupational therapy. As strength in-

Continued

CASE 13–2 Nancy *Continued*

creased, she began a program of resisted exercise. Trunk and upper- and lower-extremity PNF patterns were used as the primary exercise technique; however, great caution was used to avoid overworking weak muscle groups evoked during use of the PNF pattern. A full mat program with rolling and coming to sitting was also instituted. Occupational therapists focused on graduated use of Nancy's upper extremities, first using overhead slings attached to a wheelchair and later using a lap board to support her weakened shoulder musculature while practicing hand activities.

After 2 months of hospitalization, Nancy was discharged home to return for daily outpatient rehabilitation. Because Nancy appeared to be regaining strength well, she was provided with an ultralight rental wheelchair through her insurance for use until a final determination was made for long-term need. Nancy was also fitted with prefabricated adjustable AFOs, which were purchased through the physical therapy department. After 4 to 6 months a determination would be made about expected return of her persistently weakened dorsiflexors. If it appeared that Nancy would need AFOs for a prolonged period, a set of specifically molded AFOs would be ordered. At discharge, both the physical and occupational therapists

made a home visit with the hospital social worker and parents to determine what home adaptations and support services would be necessary.

Follow-up of Nancy's outpatient therapy showed that she continued to make gradual recovery over the next 1½ years. She initially returned to school, 3 months after discharge, using a wheelchair. She graduated to a walker, then to forearm crutches, and finally to independent ambulation. She refused to be seen using a walker at school so she continued to use the wheelchair at school until she was independent on crutches. She continued to wear bilateral AFOs but was weaned from full-time use approximately 14 months after discharge. During the weaning process, Nancy wore her AFOs at school while walking and for any walking distance over four city blocks or if she heard her feet begin to slap from fatigued dorsiflexors. By 14 months, Nancy showed no evidence of overuse weakness following her regular activities, although she had difficulty with endurance activities in her physical education classes. When hiking, she carried her AFOs to use when she expected a long downhill trek to prevent overwork from eccentric muscle activity. By age 19, Nancy had returned fully to her normal activity level.

In a nursing study of patient experiences in the ICU, researchers found that patients often felt anxious, apprehensive, and fearful. The patients expected ICU nurses to be experienced and technically adept, but those who felt most secure despite the traumatic ICU experiences felt that the nurses were vigilant to their needs and offered personalized care,[110] a point clearly made by Nancy. Although one might expect ICU staff to be carefully tuned-in to patient needs, the highly technically nature of modern ICUs may attract personnel less focused on individual patient care or it may prevent caring staff from attending to the "little kindnesses" that are so comforting to critically ill patients.

Nancy also recalled the long-term psychological consequences of her ICU experiences. Hunt[110] also identified issues related to longer-term psychological consequences. With our current understanding of posttraumatic stress disorder, one might also assume that some patients, like Nancy, have recurrent "flashbacks" of their ICU experiences that may need to be dealt with during or after their rehabilitation experiences or after they return to school or work.

In summary, the rehabilitation program for a person with GBS must be graded carefully according to the stage of illness. In the acute care environment when respiratory deficits are present, the initial emphasis is directed toward support of maximal respiratory status through postural drainage, chest stretching, and breathing exercises. Because of prolonged bed rest and immobility related to

weakness, accessory and physiological ROMs must be maintained with around-the-clock efforts. Splinting or positioning devices are recommended to maintain functional positions during prolonged periods of immobility. A gradual program to increase upright tolerance is begun when respiratory and autonomic functions have stabilized. Adaptive equipment and orthoses should be used as needed to protect weakened muscles, facilitate normal movement, and prevent fatigue during the reinnervation process.

MUSCULAR DYSTROPHY

Pathology and Medical Diagnosis

Muscular dystrophy refers to a group of hereditary myopathies characterized by progressive muscle weakness, deterioration, destruction, and regeneration of muscle fibers. During the process, muscle fibers are gradually replaced with fibrous and fatty tissue. Each of the inherited myopathies (i.e., Beckers dystrophy, myotonic dystrophy, limb-girdle dystrophy, and facioscapulohumeral) has its own unique genetic and phenotypic characteristics. (For comprehensive reviews of muscular dystrophies and myopathies see references 26, 61, 67, 76–78, 81, and 211.)

Because Duchenne (pseudohypertrophic) muscular dystrophy (DMD) is one of the most commonly known forms of the dystrophies, it will be used as a model for discussion of treatment implications for therapists. DMD is a disease of progressive muscle weakness leading to total paralysis and early death in the late teens or young adulthood. It has an incidence of between 13 and 33 cases per 100,000 live births and a new mutation rate of approximately 1 in 10,000 (i.e., one third or more cases occur in families without a family history of DMD). In the past few years the abnormal gene for DMD has been detected on the X chromosome at band Xp21, which encodes for dystrophin, a 427-kD cytoskeleton protein in the membrane. Because it has an X-linked, recessive pattern, the disease affects males almost exclusively. In almost 100% of patients with DMD, immunoblotting or immunostaining techniques show complete absence of dystrophin from muscle tissue. An early abnormality during the process of muscle fiber destruction is the breakdown of the muscle fiber plasma membrane. The membrane destruction results in an influx of calcium-rich extracellular fluid and complement components into the muscle fibers. In addition, there is activation of intracellular proteases and complement, with the ultimate removal of necrotic fibers by macrophages.[116, 232, 236]

Laboratory studies show serum creatine kinase (CK) elevated more than 100 times normal in early stages of the disease. These CK levels decrease over time with loss of muscle mass. Elevated CK is evident at birth long before symptoms are evident. Muscle biopsy specimens show degeneration with gradual loss of fiber, variation in fiber size, and a proliferation of connective and adipose tissue. Histochemical studies indicate loss of subdivision into fiber types, with a tendency toward type I fiber predominance. EMG studies show patterns of low amplitude, short duration, polyphasic motor unit action potentials. Cardiac involvement is universal, although clinically significant cardiomyopathy is not common and death caused by cardiac dysfunction occurs in only about 10%

of patients. Typically, the posterobasal area of the left ventricle is scarred, producing electrocardiographic patterns with tall right precordial R waves and deep left precordial Q waves in 90% of patients.[236] Weakness of the respiratory muscles is usually evident by the tenth or twelfth year, although the diaphragm remains functional longer than do the intercostal and accessory muscles. A progressive, sometimes severe scoliosis may contribute to respiratory compromise. Pure respiratory failure or respiratory failure secondary to infection is the usual cause of death, most commonly between the ages of 18 and 25. Other less common causes of death include gastric dilation and aspiration.[232]

The average intelligence quotient (IQ) of boys with DMD is approximately 85, with one third of the boys testing below 75. A specific deficit of verbal intelligence and verbal memory has been identified.[23, 24] Although the relationship between lower IQ and DMD was initially thought to be related to limited life experience caused by the disease, recent studies have shown that dystrophin is also found in brain tissue. This suggests a possible relationship between the gene defect, which may cause decrease in dystrophin in brain tissue, and impaired IQ. In contrast to the progressive pattern of muscle deterioration, intellectual impairment is not progressive.[24, 232]

Clinical Presentation

Although histological studies have indicated that DMD may be identified in the fetus as early as the first trimester, symptoms are seldom noted until the child is between 2 and 5 years of age. When recalling the child's early development, parents often state that the affected child was more placid and less physically active than expected.[7] The earliest obvious manifestations of DMD, however, may be the delay of early developmental milestones, par-

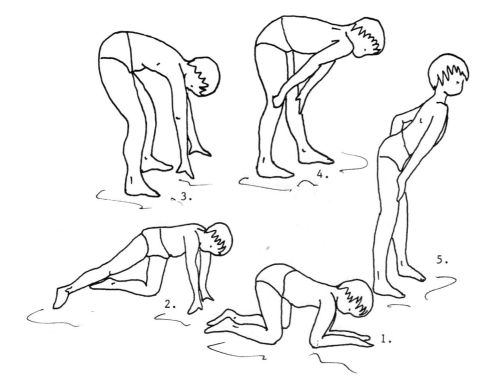

FIGURE 13–5. Child demonstrating Gowers maneuver necessary to achieve upright posture because of pelvic and trunk weakness due to DMD.

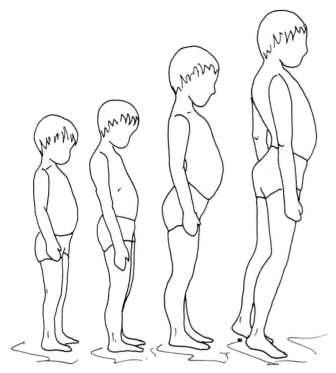

FIGURE 13–6. Pattern of progression of muscle imbalance affecting trunk and lower extremities in DMD.

ticularly crawling and walking. In many cases the onset is very gradual. Parents or teachers may first identify a problem because the boy is noted to have difficulty keeping up with peers during normal play activities and to be somewhat clumsy with frequent falling when attempting to run, jump, climb structures, or negotiate uneven terrain. By age 5 years, symmetrical muscle weakness can usually be clearly identified with MMT. Deep tendon reflexes may be absent by 8 to 10 years or earlier. Sensation is normal.[33]

The typical progression of weakness is symmetrical from proximal to distal, with marked weakness of the pelvic and shoulder girdle musculature preceding weakness of the trunk and extremity muscles. Muscles innervated by cranial nerves (except the sternocleidomastoids) are not involved, and bowel and bladder function is usually spared. Progression of weakness is slow but persistent. Marked weakness of the legs and anterior neck musculature affecting functional activities, including head control, usually precedes upper-extremity muscle weakness affecting functional activities. A typical child will continue walking until about age 12, at which time use of a wheelchair becomes imperative. A rapid decrease in strength may occur after prolonged periods of immobilization secondary to illness, injury, or surgery.[60]

Progression of Lower-Extremity Weakness

Before age 5, hypertrophy of the calf muscles is frequently noted. Pseudohypertrophy is evident as the muscle tissue is replaced by fat and fibrous tissue.[7] Even in the early stages of the disease, few boys with DMD walk with a normal gait pattern. Because of early pelvic girdle muscle weakness, most young boys retain a developmen-

tally immature, wide-based gait pattern. An early distinctive feature of DMD is Gowers maneuver, in which the child gets up from the floor by using his arms to crawl up his own legs (Fig. 13–5).

Muscle imbalance occurs in typical patterns secondary to weakness and contractures. As the posterior hip muscles weaken, the child must arch his back when standing and retract his shoulder girdle to maintain the center of gravity behind the hip joint. This creates a pattern of lumbar lordosis with protrusion of the abdomen. As the quadriceps weaken, the child must maintain his knees in hyperextension to place the axis of rotation posterior to the line of gravity. At this point, mild equinus contractures caused by a muscle imbalance between the plantar and dorsiflexors may help the child maintain knee control because the gastrocnemius-soleus group provides a torque opposing knee flexion. If plantarflexion contractures become severe, however, the child will not be able to maintain standing balance because his base of support is too small and his ankle adaptive strategies are nonfunctional.

Once the child stops weight bearing, development of severe equinovarus deformities is common. Figure 13–6 shows a pattern of progression of muscle imbalance affecting the trunk and lower extremities in stance. Note the increasing lordosis and plantarflexion as the boys attempt to maintain their center of gravity posterior to the hip joint and anterior to the knee joint.

Progression of Gait Pattern Changes

The typical changes in gait pattern over time are identified in Figure 13–7. Age alone is not an adequate index

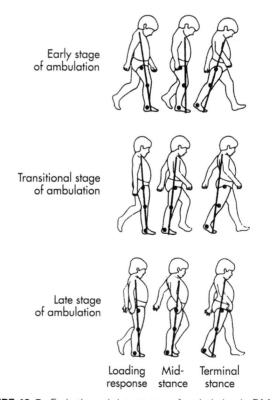

FIGURE 13–7. Early through late stages of ambulation in DMD demonstrating changes in alignment at loading response, mid stance, and terminal stance phases of gait. (From Hsu JD, Furumasu J: Gait and posture changes in the Duchenne muscular dystrophy child. Clin Orthop Rel Res 288[Mar]:122–125, 1993.)

of predicted gait pattern. Many factors influence how long a child will be able to ambulate. Contributing factors are rate of progression of weakness; severity of contractures (hip flexion, external rotation, abduction, knee flexion, and plantarflexion-inversion contractures occur as disease progresses); influence of body weight; degree of respiratory compromise; type of treatment interventions such as bracing, surgery, and exercise; extent of family support; and the child's personal motivation to ambulate. (For an extensive analysis of changes in gait pattern see the work of Sutherland and colleagues.[212]) When the child can no longer ambulate functionally, a wheelchair must be ordered to fit the specific needs of that child within his home and community environment.

Progression of Upper-Extremity Weakness

The upper-extremity pattern of weakness is similar to that in the lower extremities, with proximal musculature being affected before distal musculature. Functional changes related to weakness of upper extremity musculature, however, usually lag behind those in the lower extremities by 2 to 3 years. The early weakness of the scapular stabilization muscles interferes with controlled movement of the arms and hands during reaching. Gradually, the boy loses biceps and brachioradialis function, followed by contin-

ued deterioration of triceps and more distal musculature. The marked instability of scapular musculature is clearly evident when the child tries to elevate his trunk with his arms (e.g., when attempting to use crutches) or when he is lifted from under the shoulders.[5, 33] A classic test of scapular stability is the test for the Meryon sign, in which the child slips from the examiner's grip as the child is being lifted from under the arms (Fig. 13–8). Typical progression of upper-extremity weakness is shown by use of the reaching test (Fig. 13–9).

By the time the child reaches stage 3 of the reaching test, he needs considerable help with eating, hair care, and oral hygiene. Because of major trunk involvement and marked lower-extremity weakness, the child will also be dependent for most ADL tasks, such as hygiene, dressing, and transferring. Typical functional stages in DMD are identified in the box below.

Medical Intervention

Treatment of Primary Pathology

There is no cure. Some clinicians suggest that until an effective treatment can be found, the best way to decrease the number of children with DMD is through genetic counseling. Statistical tables are available to determine the risk of a mother or daughter with an affected

---

FUNCTIONAL TRANSITIONS IN PATIENT WITH MUSCULAR DYSTROPHY

1. Ambulates with mild waddling gait and lordosis. Can run with marked effort, gait problems magnified. Can ascend, descend steps, curbs.
2. Ambulates with moderate waddling gait and lordosis. Cannot run. Difficulty with stairs and curbs. Rises from floor using Gowers maneuver. Rises from chair independently.
3. Ambulates with moderately severe waddling gait and lordosis. Rises from chair independently but cannot ascend or descend curbs or stairs, or rise from floor independently.
4. Ambulates with assistance or in some cases with bilateral knee-ankle-foot orthoses. May have had surgical release of contractures. May need assistance with balance. Needs wheelchair for community mobility. Propels manual chair slowly. Independent in bed and self-care, although may need help with some aspects of dressing and bathing because of time constraints.
5. Transfers independently from wheelchair. Unable to walk independently, but can bear and shift weight to walk with orthoses if supported. Can propel self in manual chair but limited endurance. Motorized chair more functional. Independent in self-care with transfer assist for bath or shower.
6. Wheelchair independence in motorized chair. May need trunk support or orthosis. Needs assistance in bed and with major dressing. Can perform self-

grooming but dependent for toileting and bathing. May need alternating pressure relief mattress.
7. Wheelchair independence in motorized chair but may need to recline intermittently while in chair. Dependent in hygiene and most self-care requiring proximal upper-extremity control.
8. As for No. 7 and will use two hands for single-hand activities—one hand supports working arm. May perform simple table-level hand activities, some self-feeding with arm support.
9. Sits in wheelchair only with trunk support and intermittent reclining or transfer to a supine position. Boys attending school may need to be on gurney for part of day. May benefit from night-time ventilatory support or intermittent daytime positive pressure breathing. (Some patients may have had an elective tracheostomy and need ventilatory support unit attached to wheelchair.) May have some hand control if arms supported. Will need help with turning at night.
10. Totally dependent. Unable to tolerate upright position, may elect home ventilatory support. Tracheostomy necessary for prolonged ventilation. Tracheostomy may be adapted for speech if oral musculature adequate. Needs 24-hour care. If around-the-clock home care cannot be arranged, patient must be hospitalized.

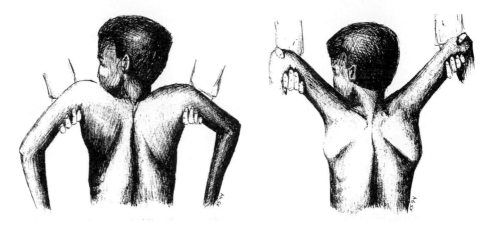

FIGURE 13–8. Meryon sign shows lack of scapular stability as the child slips from the examiner's grip when lifted from under the arms.

son or brother. The risk factor is determined by calculating the number of normal males in the family and the CK level of the female and her mother. Serum CK is elevated in the female carriers, although its level is cyclic, with a peak level occurring in the few months after the carrier's birth and then decreasing until age 4 years. Another peak in carrier CK level occurs at age 10 years; the level falls again at age 40 years, when it begins to rise again. Genetic molecular probes of possible carriers are now available to identify deletions within the Xp21 region (the short arm of the X chromosome) at a 95% accuracy level. Of course, some families may have belief systems that do not allow consideration of pregnancy termination to prevent having a boy with possible DMD. Those views

must be respected. Prenatal diagnosis of DMD for women without a family history of the disease is not yet practical.[192]

Despite much effort an effective pharmaceutical agent has not been identified to treat DMD. Research was initiated in the 1980s to determine if the growth hormone inhibitor mazindol would slow weakness and contracture in DMD; however, no evidence was found to support that hypothesis.[86] In some cases, oral corticosteroids are effective to prolong ambulation,[32, 58, 69] although the results have been questioned because of possible problems with research bias.[96] Researchers have also attempted to implant the normal precursor muscle cells or myoblasts directly into dystrophic mice and, in several cases, into

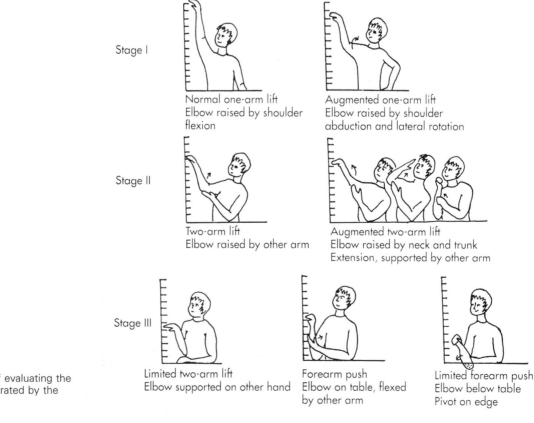

Stage I

Normal one-arm lift
Elbow raised by shoulder flexion

Augmented one-arm lift
Elbow raised by shoulder abduction and lateral rotation

Stage II

Two-arm lift
Elbow raised by other arm

Augmented two-arm lift
Elbow raised by neck and trunk Extension, supported by other arm

Stage III

Limited two-arm lift
Elbow supported on other hand

Forearm push
Elbow on table, flexed by other arm

Limited forearm push
Elbow below table
Pivot on edge

FIGURE 13–9. Method of evaluating the working hand as demonstrated by the reaching test.

children with DMD to precipitate the proliferation of normal donor muscle cells into the host muscles of dystrophic subjects, but results have not led to significant improvement.[163] Most recently, researchers have been working on recombinant adenovirus vector–mediated dystrophin gene transfer to DMD patients.[167] Although no cure for DMD looms in the immediate future, the functional status of the patient, quality of life, and life expectancy can be influenced with thoughtful, functionally based treatment and supportive care.

Treatment of Cardiopulmonary Factors

Respiratory failure is the cause of death in 70% to 80% of patients with DMD. Cardiac and other causes account for the remaining deaths.[96] Because of limited activity, the cardiorespiratory fitness of children with DMD is impaired early in the disease process. Once the child becomes wheelchair dependent, his cardiorespiratory fitness deteriorates markedly. With increasing weakness of the respiratory musculature and the development of scoliosis, physicians must be vigilant in their treatment of respiratory infections. Physical therapy interventions, such as postural drainage and breathing exercises, are invaluable in preventing early death from respiratory failure (see *Cardiopulmonary Physical Therapy*[113] and recommendations for respiratory physical therapy in the ALS and GBS sections of this chapter). Sleep hypoxia is common in the later stages of DMD. In some cases, intermittent positive-pressure ventilation (IPPV) by nasal mask has been effective in controlling oxygen desaturation at night.[192, 194, 198] Nighttime mechanical ventilatory support seems to provide relief for symptoms such as insomnia, progressive drowsiness, morning headaches, dyspnea, and anxiety.[17, 126, 175]

Several options for sustaining life in the final stages of DMD other than nasal or mouthpiece-delivered IPPV are the use of a cuirass chest respirator, iron lung, and tracheostomy with mechanical ventilation. Tracheostomy care becomes increasingly important when the patient has marked bulbar muscle weakness.[52] External ventilation support is used initially at night and then intermittently throughout the day until respiratory support is required at all times. As with patients with ALS, many significant treatment and ethical decisions must be made by the patient, family, and health care providers when submitting to prolonged HMV.[145, 199]

Cardiomyopathy, frequently associated with DMD, seldom becomes symptomatic because the child's decreased activity level does not stress the weakened heart muscle. In later stages of the disease, however, cor pulmonale with right-sided heart failure may occur. Medical treatment of any cardiac symptoms generally follows the conventional interventions. Some boys with a severe scoliosis that creates cardiac compression may require correction by spinal fixation.[144]

Treatment of Orthopedic Factors

Scoliosis is a frequent complication of DMD, with incidence being reported from 49% to 93%. In a retrospective study of 88 patients with DMD, Lord and associ-

ates[131] showed that scoliosis was age related, being identified in 30% of boys in the 8- to 14-year age group, 92% in the 15- to 20-year age group, and 64% in boys older than age 20 years. The decrease in the number of boys with scoliosis older than age 20 suggested that boys without scoliosis have greater longevity, although the evidence was not conclusive. Figure 13–10 presents an example of a boy with a moderate scoliosis affecting sitting posture. Note the pelvic asymmetry that would seriously affect sitting alignment.

Scoliosis tends to occur in two basic patterns: the early-onset form (seen in approximately 23%), which becomes evident before the child becomes wheelchair dependent, and the late-onset form, which develops, on average, 4 years after wheelchair dependency. In the early-onset form the curve usually becomes severe and progressive, leading to pulmonary compromise and structural-based pain. In the late-onset form the course is usually mild. The traditional view of scoliosis development has been that the child's increasing weakness leads to abnormal sitting postures, which in turn leads to severe kyphoscoliosis. Unfortunately, attempts to control sitting posture through the use of spinal orthosis and wheelchair seating inserts (i.e., inserts that place the child in lumbar lordosis to lock facets, thereby preventing rotation and lateral collapse or, more commonly, lumbar and thoracic lateral supports) have been disappointing.[131] Although DMD is generally thought to have a symmetrical pattern of weakness, recent evidence suggests an asymmetrical paraspinous involvement, which may be the cause of the severe scoliosis seen in some boys.[209] Bach[13] states that thoracolumbar bracing is never indicated to slow scoliosis development in DMD and it cannot substitute for surgical correction.

Miller and coworkers[144] reported on 68 patients with DMD who underwent posterior spinal fusion with instrumentation for severe scoliosis. (Over the course of the study, several different forms of fixation were used.) Although they found that the boys who underwent spinal fixation were more comfortable in their later years and were easier to care for, deterioration of pulmonary func-

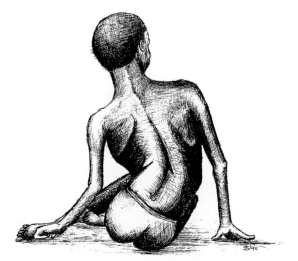

FIGURE 13–10. Moderate scoliosis affecting sitting stability.

tion was not slowed after surgery. The average age at death of the boys in the study was 18.3 years. This was the same as the average age at death reported for another similar group of boys who did not have spinal surgery.

In interviews with 42 end-stage patients who underwent scoliosis surgery or with their caregivers, 35 believed that the instrumentation was beneficial, 6 believed that it was not, and 1 was uncertain.[145] Of 15 patients interviewed, all thought that the surgery was helpful. Seventeen percent of the boys had pulmonary complications after surgery. Based on their experience, the authors suggest that a forced vital capacity of at least 35% of normal is necessary before surgery can be performed. They recommend that spinal stability is best achieved with segmental fixations rather than with Harrington rods because the segmental fixation systems allow immediate postoperative mobilization of the patient, which is essential to prevent marked disuse deterioration. Attention must also be given to how the spine is positioned with fixation. If the curve cannot be completely corrected, the curves should be balanced to create a horizontal pelvis. Maintenance of some lumbar lordosis (45 degrees) and thoracic kyphosis (25 degrees) is essential because it allows the boy to keep his head in a forward position to compensate for severely weakened anterior neck muscles. Physical therapists must play an aggressive role in treatment of children with DMD after spinal fixation. Other orthopedic interventions to prolong ambulation are discussed with the therapeutic interventions.

Nutritional Concerns

Excessive weight gain that impairs functional ability is a frequent and difficult problem for children with DMD and their families. The typical active child needs about 2,400 calories daily to maintain weight and grow. The child with DMD who is more sedentary or is wheelchair dependent may need 1200 or fewer calories to maintain weight. Because of decreased esophageal and intestinal motility, exacerbated by weak or absent abdominal muscle strength, a healthy low-fat diet should be encouraged with adequate bulk foods, stool softeners, and fluids to facilitate bowel function and motility. Problems with obesity are often related to the family's typical pattern of eating and nurturing. It is not uncommon for the child and family members to "feed" their anxiety or depression about the disease.[192] In many cases family members and friends feel that the child's only pleasure may be eating. Although this may seem true, caring for a totally dependent obese teenager or young adult can become problematic for both the child and the caregivers. Before obesity becomes an issue, the child and his family should be referred for comprehensive nutritional advice from a specialist experienced in dealing with childhood obesity. Suggestions for adapting eating behavior and food choices will not be followed if they are too restrictive or unreasonable for the child's social situation.[63, 85]

As the disease progresses, some children develop problems swallowing. To decrease the possibility of aspiration, careful attention must be paid to food textures and chewing and swallowing functions (see section on ALS for information on dealing with bulbar symptoms). De-

pending on the patient's and family's decisions about prolongation of life, some patients choose to supplement or receive their nutrition by means of a nasogastric or orogastric tube or elect to have a permanent percutaneous endoscopic gastrostomy placed.

Therapeutic Management

Therapeutic Evaluation

Ideally, a team of specialists should be involved in the long-term care of a child with DMD and his family. The therapist's primary role is twofold: to perform serial evaluations of the child's movement capabilities and to adjust the child's intervention program accordingly to maximize function and quality of life as the disease progresses. A typical therapy evaluation should include assessment of muscle strength and ROM impairments with a comprehensive assessment of functional status and level of disability. In some facilities the therapist also collects data on the child's pulmonary status (see Chapter 15 in *Cardiopulmonary Physical Therapy* for assessment information[113]).

Manual Muscle Testing. MMT is a reasonably reliable technique for measuring muscle strength of children with DMD if consecutive evaluations are made by the same rater. Reliability of scores in the gravity-eliminated position was highest.[71] In DMD, there is a linear pattern of decreased muscle strength without marked changes in the rate of deterioration in strength over time. The rate of actual muscle weakness is not influenced by bracing programs or wheelchair use,[5] although functional status may change. MMT after prolonged periods of immobility, however, may reflect increased weakness from disuse atrophy rather than the disease progress. Therefore, marked, precipitous decreases in MMT scores may reflect a transitory situation that will respond to increased activity and exercise.

Range of Motion. As with MMT, serial ROM evaluations should be completed by the same therapist because intrarater reliability is higher than interrater reliability.[162] Careful tracking of ROM is imperative because the development of contractures of the hip, knee, and ankle caused by muscle imbalance is a more common reason for early loss of ambulation than actual muscle weakness.[191] Particular attention should be given to the accuracy of measuring hip ROM. Rideau and associates[176] recommend the "dangling leg" test, in which the child is placed supine with his lower legs hanging over the end of the table. An inability to bring the thighs to midline indicates a contracture of the iliotibial band and hip abductors. One can quantify the contracture by measuring the distance of the thigh from the midline and from the surface of the table. Additionally, the therapist should note pelvic obliquity, preferably with serial photographs taken in the sitting and supine positions.

Functional Status. The child's functional status continues to be relatively stable for some time even when MMT indicates that the child is losing strength. Because the weakness is gradual, many children develop remarkably adaptive adjustments in movement patterns to cope with the loss of strength. Brooke and coworkers[31] describe a functional scale for determining the child's status and for predicting appropriate care (see also the work of Vignos and colleagues[222]). As part of the patient's assessment, adaptive behaviors should be noted. For example, a child may not be able to lift his arm overhead, but he may use his fingers (strength often remains intact even after respiratory support is necessary) to "crawl" up his chest to reach his head or he may lean forward to approximate his chest to his hand or use his other arm or a lever system to assist with activities.[13]

Respiratory Function. The physical therapist's role in evaluating respiratory status in children with DMD will vary depending on the facility and area of the country in which the therapist works. For information on a full evaluation see *Cardiopulmonary Physical Therapy*, Chapter 15,[109] and refer to the section on ALS in this chapter. At a minimum, the therapist should evaluate bulbar function, cough effectiveness, and vital capacity (a simple spirometer available in most clinics is adequate). For more sophisticated testing, the child should be seen by a pulmonary function specialist. In addition, the therapist may find it helpful to test the child's energy cost during ambulation using the Energy Expenditure Index described by Rose and coworkers,[180] which divides walking heart rate minus resting heart rate by walking speed (EEI = WHR − RHR/D/T). By determining the child's work efficiency using this simple method, it may be possible for clinicians to help the child, family, and treatment team to determine when it may be best to make the transition to a wheelchair. Additionally, in late stages, the therapist may need to assess the child's bulbar function to prevent swallowing and aspiration problems secondary to tongue and oral-facial muscle weakness. (See section on dysphagia treatment in ALS.)

Therapeutic Goals

The basic goals for a therapeutic program are very straightforward: (1) to prevent contractures that can lead to further disability and pain, (2) to maintain maximal strength/prevent disuse atrophy, (3) to facilitate maximal functional abilities using appropriate adaptive equipment, (4) to maintain maximal respiratory muscle strength and movement of secretions, and (5) to foster realistic child and family expectations within the context of the environment. These broad-based goals, however, may not be adequate for today's third-party payers, and the therapist may need to write more specific, time-oriented goals.

Therapeutic Interventions

In today's health care environment, therapists act primarily in the role of consultant rather than direct service provider. Much of the child's exercise program must be carried out at home by caregivers. Because both parents often work today, or because the child lives in a single-parent home with a working parent, compliance with home programs is problematic. As many exercise activities as possible should be encouraged within the child's school day so that parents can focus on parenting, nurturing,

general caregiving, and simple positioning and bedtime exercises. Under the supervision of a consulting therapist, the child's therapy often can be provided in some form at the child's school if on-site therapists, personal attendants, or adaptive physical education teachers are available.

Respiratory and Dysphagia Care. In the school therapy environment where most children with DMD are followed, the therapist should be prepared to provide the child and family with methods to improve breathing efficiency. In the early stages of the disease, the child and family can be taught simple breathing exercises stressing diaphragmatic breathing, full chest expansion, air shifts, and rib cage stretching. Most children enjoy playing with hand-held incentive spirometer units and playing blowing games (e.g., bubbles, pinwheels). Once the child begins to have difficulty clearing secretions, the family should be taught postural drainage and coughing techniques such as "huffing" and manual coughing assists (see *Cardiopulmonary Physical Therapy*, Chapter 25, for information on techniques that can be adapted for DMD).[229] These techniques should be reviewed and used aggressively whenever the child is bedbound for more than 1 or 2 days and before and after all surgical procedures.

Respiratory muscle exercises increase strength and endurance in subjects with and without pulmonary disease.[12] Preliminary evidence suggests that respiratory endurance can be improved in children with DMD.[59] More recently, in a study of 18 boys with DMD to determine the efficacy of respiratory endurance and strength training programs, the investigators found improvement in ventilatory muscle endurance but not in respiratory muscle strength.[135] Although respiratory exercise cannot reverse the process of respiratory failure, attention to pulmonary hygiene and breathing exercise can help the child cope more effectively with respiratory infections and the discomfort accompanying respiratory compromise.

In end stages of DMD when the child is dependent, it is imperative to deal with oral-motor problems that may interfere with eating and swallowing. Techniques such as positioning, increased sensory input (texture, temperature), and volume changes in foods may improve the child's swallowing and allow the child to continue taking food orally.[217] The interventions are similar to those described in the section on ALS and are clearly documented in most occupational and speech therapy manuals and texts. The Muscular Dystrophy Association also publishes manuals dealing with both respiratory and dysphagia problems.[9]

Prevention of Contractures. The two-joint muscles are most prone to developing significant contractures. Early in the course of the disease process, a home program must be instituted to include ROM, stretching, and positioning. Both parents and the child must be educated about the expected changes in muscle balance and how they can play an active role in preventing or limiting the impact of contractures secondary to muscle imbalance.

Initially, the child should be encouraged to move his own limbs actively through full range. At the first sign of loss of end ROM, the therapist should adjust the child's program to include specific stretches. As active ROM becomes more difficult, parents will need to assist the child to move his limbs to the end ranges of all motions to stretch the muscles and periarticular structures. The stretching program should use static stretching techniques with prolonged, mild tension to impact both the viscoelastic and plastic properties of the muscle.[237] Although studies to show the best length of time to stretch muscles with contractures have not been performed, a stretch of 15 seconds increased ROM in persons with normal muscle tissue.[134] If the child can actively contract the affected muscle, hold-relax or contract-relax PNF techniques may be useful to increase ROM. Joint mobilization techniques should be included in the treatment program before capsular contractures occur. Intuitively, one would expect that to decrease contractures, the length of stretching time should be prolonged and the increased range should be maintained with positioning or bracing. The best approach to contractures, however, is to prevent them.[140] (See the work of Grossman and colleagues[87] for a review of the effect of immobilization on muscle and appropriate therapy interventions.)

Because the development of contractures follows a predictable pattern, a positioning program should be started before contractures are evident. For example, the child can be encouraged to watch television while lying prone with legs aligned out of the common "frog leg" pattern. Once a child has significant hip flexor or iliotibial band contractures, stretching techniques must be very specific because simple prone positioning can force the lumbar spine into excessive lordosis. Although difficult to accomplish in some mainstreamed school environments, positioning the child in a standing frame during several class periods helps provide prolonged stretch to hip, knee, and ankle musculature. Some children will tolerate night splinting to control plantarflexion contractures; however, few children will tolerate wearing long-leg splints at night to prevent knee flexion contractures or to align the hips (additional bar between legs to control rotations). Research supports the view that the combination of stretching, positioning, and splinting should begin before contractures exist. If night ankle splints are worn consistently in combination with stretching, the rate of progression of contractures can be minimized.[33] In a prospective study of prevention of deformity in DMD, Scott and co-workers[190] found that boys who had consistent treatment with AFOs (splints) and daily stretching were able to continue walking longer than boys who did not have a stretching and splinting program.

Exercise and the Maintenance of Maximal Functional Level. Ideally, the child with DMD should be as active as possible to prevent disuse weakness not directly related to the disease process. Elder[66] reports on studies related to the value of active exercise on dystrophic muscles. In animal studies, dystrophic mice trained on a treadmill showed increased damage to muscle tissue whereas forced swimming in dystrophic mice had no adverse effect. In a more recent study of endurance training of dystrophic hamsters, Elder[66] concluded that increased contractile activity associated with treadmill exercise had no detrimental effect on developing muscle and may have had a beneficial effect in young animals by improving fiber hypertrophy, increasing maximal tetanic force, and decreasing fiber degeneration.

Studies of humans with muscular dystrophy have also shown mixed results. In a case review of three generations of patients with facioscapulohumeral muscular dystrophy (seven cases and one suspected case), Johnson and Braddom[115] noted asymmetrical weakness of the upper extremities. They related the weakness to patterns of overuse (dominant side or side used most often in work activities). Based on their information and additional evidence that muscle-derived enzymes (CK and myoglobin concentrations in blood) were markedly elevated in patients with DMD after prolonged exercise,[72] they suggested that endurance exercise may be contraindicated.

In another study, boys exercised one quadriceps isokinetically for 6 months. The contralateral leg was used as a control. At the end of the study, no evidence of overwork weakness was noted. There was a nonsignificant increase in muscle strength of the exercised quadriceps over the nonexercised contralateral muscle, which was maintained for 3 months after cessation of exercise. The authors concluded that submaximal exercise did not negatively affect muscle tissue, but it may be of limited value in increasing strength.[56]

Other research has shown that judicious exercise may have a positive effect on function. For example, Vignos and Watkins,[223] in 1966, compared two groups of boys with DMD. One group participated in a 12-month home strengthening program using graduated weights for maximal resistance. The control group continued their normal activities but did not participate in the exercise program. The muscle strength of both groups had showed a decline during the year before the study. At the end of the study, the control group showed continued decline. The exercise group, however, showed a small increase in strength as measured by MMT. They noted that the initial strength of the muscles before the program was initiated was positively related to improvement in strength. Therefore, the authors suggested that the exercise program should be started during the initial stages of the disease rather than waiting until the child has quit ambulating.

In addition to active and resistive exercise programs, Scott and coworkers[190] completed a small study of the effect of intermittent chronic low-frequency electrical stimulation on dystrophic anterior tibialis muscles. They demonstrated a significant increase in mean voluntary contraction force and suggested that electrical stimulation can have a beneficial effect if used with children whose muscles are not already markedly weakened.

Overall, the data from animal and human studies suggest that submaximal exercise is not harmful and it may be helpful in maintaining maximal movement function if the patient does not exercise into marked fatigue. Hasson,[95] in his review of exercise studies of patients with muscular dystrophy, concluded that exercise consisting of brief periods of low- or high-intensity activity can improve strength for patients with minimal to moderate weakness. However, exercise programs have no effect on strength of muscles already severely weakened. Oxygen consumption also improved with endurance training, although it is not clear whether repetitive endurance training at moderate or high intensity (70% of Vo_2max) may cause muscle damage. Increased recruitment of motor units from training effects also may improve muscle coordination and reduce disuse atrophy. Figure 13–11 is a graphic example of responses of normal and impaired muscle to exercise. (See also the ALS section for a review of disuse atrophy and overwork damage that may influence intervention decisions for children with DMD.)

Ideally, the child's exercise needs can be incorporated into pleasurable activities adapted for children with movement and weakness-related balance problems. Because endurance is a problem, aerobic-type programs are not appropriate in most cases, with the exception of respiratory endurance programs previously noted.[59] Many ambulatory children, however, enjoy ball activities, walking-based simple obstacle courses, parachute games, table tennis, cycling (preferably tandem), and especially swimming. Swimming is an excellent exercise for children with DMD because they often are quite buoyant because of their increased fat/muscle ratio. Many children can continue to float or swim independently on their backs well into the time they are able to move only distal muscle. All activity programs should have structured rest periods. A safe indicator of extent and intensity of exercise is that the patient should recover from exercise fatigue after a night's rest. An active exercise program did not benefit patients who were in later, dependent stages of DMD.[95] (See also the case studies cited in the sections on ALS and GBS.)

Maintenance of Ambulation. As the DMD progresses, the child's posture and gait pattern abnormalities become extreme and he must work harder to maintain balance while walking. Most children gradually discontinue walking about a year after they lose their ability to deal with stairs or when daily ambulation time decreases to less than 30 minutes per day.[223] Toward the end of the child's independent walking stage, he has a marked anterior pelvic tilt with lordosis and a protuberant abdomen. His shoulders are retracted and he may hold his hands behind his hips or elevated in a mid-guard position to stabilize his hips. He has a severe waddling gait with a shortened stride, and he must carefully lock his knees at each step. He falls frequently. Figure 13–12 shows the typical walking pattern of a boy with DMD who is being considered for release of contractures and bracing.

If the child and his family have followed an aggressive ROM, positioning, and activity program, the child's walking time may be extended by months. In most cases, however, the contractures from muscle imbalance continue relentlessly and the child begins to need support when walking.[176] When contractures at the hip, knee, and ankle show evidence of interfering with the child's ability to stabilize each joint during stance, most children are referred for surgery to restore functional joint motion.

Bach and McKeon[16] studied 13 boys with DMD who

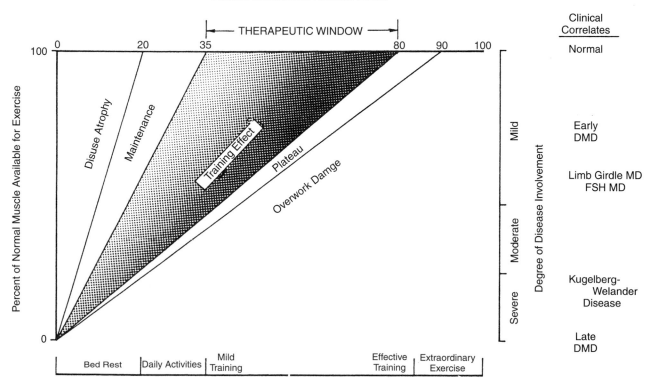

FIGURE 13–11. Idealized response of normal and impaired muscle to exercise. The therapeutic window of safe exercise narrows progressively. Activities (lower X axis) causing normal exercise effects in normal muscle (upper X axis) correlate with different effects in impaired muscle. (From Coble NO, Maloney FP: Effects of exercise on neuromuscular disease. *In* Maloney FP, Burks JS, Ringel SP [eds]: Interdisciplinary Rehabilitation of Multiple Sclerosis and Neuromuscular Disorders. New York, JB Lippincott, 1985.)

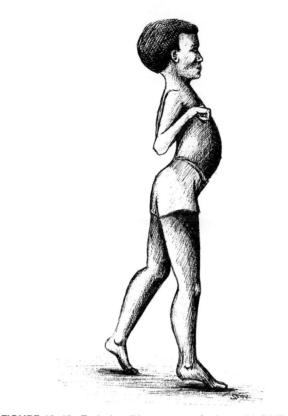

FIGURE 13–12. Typical walking pattern of a boy with DMD who is being considered for release of contractures and bracing.

had surgery to release lower-extremity contractures. Seven boys were ambulating independently before surgery (early surgery group), and six boys were preparing to use or had begun using a wheelchair before surgery (late surgery group). Depending on the contracture patterns, the boys underwent surgical procedures that typically included subcutaneous release of the Achilles tendons and hamstring muscles and fasciotomy of the iliotibial bands. Four patients had rerouting of the posterior tibialis to the dorsal surface of the second or third cuneiform to balance the foot and prevent the often severe varus position of the foot. Boys in the late surgical group required more extensive inpatient rehabilitation, whereas boys in the early surgical group were treated as outpatients after a short hospitalization.

Physical therapy was started on the second postoperative day. The program consisted of general conditioning exercises of the trunk and extremities (i.e., rolling, trunk stabilization, neck and head control), stretching exercises, and intensive weight bearing in standing while wearing bilateral long-leg casts or below-knee casts, depending on the surgery. One child participated in a pool therapy program.

Based on their results, Bach and McKeon[16] suggest that early surgery for contractures followed by intensive physical therapy can prolong brace-free ambulation. The number of falls experienced by the boys decreased markedly after the surgery and rehabilitation period. Boys in the early intervention groups benefited from the surgical interventions more than the boys in the later intervention groups. All patients and their families in the early surgery

group thought that the procedures were helpful. Boys in the late surgery group, however, stated either that they would not have had the surgery if they had a chance to decide again or that they had no opinion.

In current standard treatment protocols for children with DMD, bilateral KAFOs are used in conjunction with surgical release of contractures.[18] Surgery is followed by an aggressive therapy program. The main criterion for the surgery-bracing program is the child's impending loss of ability to walk independently. When this occurs, the child has usually lost about 60% of his muscle mass[204] and he has a pattern of contractures that magnifies the effect of the weakness. Ideally, the KAFOs should be measured and fitted in final form before the surgery so the child can begin upright weight bearing in the KAFOs the day after surgery. The KAFOs are commonly fabricated of molded plastic thigh units (ischial weight-bearing quadrilateral socket) with metal joints at the knee (drop locks) and ankle (or a flexible plastic ankle component)[111] (Fig. 13–13). If the orthoses are not immediately available, the child can begin the standing program in long-leg casts.

In the hospital, standing in bilateral KAFOs can be initiated on a tilt table. Most children are quite fearful after surgery and complain of significant pain when their legs are moved or if they are placed upright. For therapy to be successful during this early standing stage and during passive ROM exercises, the child must have adequate pain medication. If the child is not properly medicated in the first few days after surgery, the therapist may have to deal with very difficult, resistant behaviors of

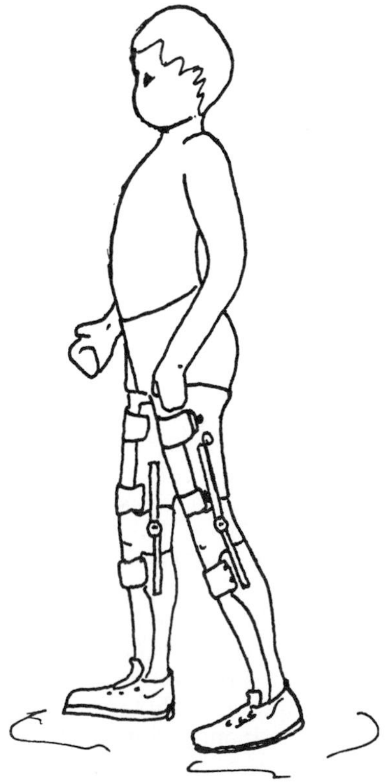

FIGURE 13–13. Example of boy walking in knee-ankle-foot orthoses showing ischial weight–bearing quadrilateral socket, knee drop locks, and plastic ankle component.

the child, which persist long after the pain should have subsided. Pain protocols must be discussed before the child's surgical procedures. The child should be medicated at least 30 minutes before the therapist's visit.

Gait training is usually begun within 48 hours after surgery. Initial work focuses on helping the child regain his sense of standing balance because his old patterns of equinus, lordosis, and shoulder retraction may no longer be adaptive. The child should be allowed to find his own best center of balance, and he should be allowed to use compensatory gait deviations necessary to allow the best mobility and stability. Depending on the child's upper-extremity strength and control, he may progress from parallel bars for balance assist, to pushing a wheelchair or weighted walker, to balance assist from a therapist using a safety strap to prevent falls. Some children who seem to need a walker for balance transition do best if they use a walker with forearm rests and vertical hand grips, which seems to help them stabilize their arms more effectively than a standard walker. Fortunately, most children do learn to walk independently without support again after surgery, although they are unable to negotiate steps or inclines or rise from the floor independently.[93]

Hyde and associates[111] reported that 24 of 30 boys treated with KAFOs were able to achieve functional ambulation again. In another study, 15 of 17 boys with DMD who had ceased walking were able to ambulate again after release of contractures followed by use of KAFOs and physical therapy. Even though the children's walking speed was decreased after bracing and the children were not able to rise from the floor or negotiate stairs, the children's ability to move about independently at home or around the classroom was considered invaluable for their independence.[223] Vignos and colleagues[224] report in a review of long-term treatment of DMD that a combination of operative procedures combined with orthotics, stretching, and a program of standing and walking extended walking until a mean age of 13.6 years and standing for 2 years after that. With the early use of surgery and bracing procedures to maintain ambulation, the expected deterioration in muscle strength and function, secondary to becoming sedentary in a wheelchair, is deferred.[175]

Unfortunately, none of the studies on bracing included formalized evaluations of the children's level of satisfaction with the surgical treatment, bracing, and rehabilitation process. In addition to providing gait training, the therapist should work with the child to help him learn to fall as safely as possible. Even though practice falls do not duplicate the sudden crash from unexpected falls, most children develop a stronger sense of confidence if they have worked on falling techniques.

Because most children with DMD today are discharged home within a few days after surgery, physical therapists must provide options for continuing the standing within the home. Standing frames are often available through the child's school district or therapy unit. If they are not, the therapist can help the family build a simple standing frame for home. This frame often can be made from a piece of plywood, or a gluteal strap system can be attached to a table at home. If possible the child should be positioned just forward of the line of gravity to encourage back extension with facet stability and to allow the

child better head control (remember the weak anterior neck muscles). Use of swivel walkers has been recommended by some therapists and physicians because the child does not need upper-extremity control for support. Although the concept of hands-free walking seems logical, boys with DMD had more difficulty using the walkers when compared with children with paraplegia because of the more delicate postural adjustments needed by children with dystrophy and their greater sensitivity to the motion restriction of the swivel walker. Some therapists have reported success using the ORLAU VCG (variable center of gravity) walker[206]; however, support for its use is not widespread.

Transition to Wheelchair. Although surgical and orthotic interventions may prolong ambulation within the home and classroom past the predicted time for cessation of independent walking (8 to 12 years), most children begin to use a wheelchair for community mobility and long distances before this time. When children begin to spend more time in their chair, the rate of development of contractures, disuse weakness, and obesity increases.[111, 204] Because of this more rapid deterioration in the child's functional skills, professionals and parents often discourage the child from using a chair for mobility. Children, however, tend to welcome use of the chair because they have more energy for their social interactions and learning tasks.[111]

Selection of the appropriate wheelchair is often difficult for the patient and family because of the multiple decisions that must be made. Few children with DMD can propel a manual wheelchair for more than a few years because of their increasing upper-extremity weakness. In addition, their propulsion speed in their manual chair is seldom adequate to keep up with their peers. Eventually, the child will need a motorized chair. Although this provides tremendous freedom for the child, a motorized chair presents problems to many families because transporting the chair requires a van and lift unit, which is seldom funded by insurance or donations. Ideally, the child should have both a manual and a motorized chair; however, in today's health policy climate, parents often have to engage in protracted efforts to obtain adaptive equipment for their child.

An important consideration when purchasing a wheelchair is the trunk support system. Traditionally, boys with DMD are thought to develop a gravity collapse of the spine related to their functional sitting posture. To control the collapsing spine, spinal orthosis and seat inserts to lock the spine in extension (to prevent lateral bending and rotation) are frequently recommended. Unfortunately, the effectiveness of positioning devices to control the development of scoliosis has been disappointing.[131] Although Drennan[60] suggests that spinal fixation is necessary to control scoliosis, all children are not candidates for surgery. The therapist, therefore, should work with the child, family, and the orthopedist to determine the best system to maintain optimal spinal alignment and trunk stability as the child weakens. In addition, as the child becomes more physically dependent, the chair may need to be fitted with a pressure relief molded seat and trunk cushions, elevating leg rests, and a reclining back with a head rest.[64] The Tilt-in-Space chair (La Bac Systems, Inc, Denver) is a good example of a chair that can be motorized to allow mobility as well as maximal adjustment of seat position using mouth control systems. It can also be adapted for respirator attachment. The decision about the type of power chair necessary in the later stages of disease progression takes considerable thought. Therapists, the patient, and the parents or caregivers must review environmental constraints, access issues, social goals, and work and recreational needs.

Because of the problems associated with increased wheelchair use, the therapist must work closely with the family, and any school-based personnel, to design a realistic plan to prevent rapid deterioration in strength and independent function. If possible, the child's standing program in KAFOs should be continued at school and at home as long as possible, with a goal of 3 to 5 hours of standing per day. With mainstreaming, however, continuing a standing program at school is sometimes difficult because attendants and equipment are not available, the child may need to move from room to room for different classes, and the child may not like being singled out for special treatment. It is helpful to caregivers if the child continues to wear his KAFOs when using the chair until he is totally dependent for transfers and can no longer be pivoted from chair to another surface.

If the child uses a motorized wheelchair, directional control systems must be adapted to each child's needs. Most young people with advanced DMD do well for years with a hand control system; however, some young people need control systems that can be operated by head, tongue, or breath movements. A patient using a respiratory support system will need his wheelchair adapted to accommodate the ventilation unit. When the child can no longer tolerate the sitting position, some children have continued to attend school on a gurney.

Once the person with DMD is no longer able to attend school or work, the home environment will need to be adapted for maximal self-direction despite significant physical dependence. Both low- and high-technological environmental control systems are more readily available today than 10 years ago. Television control units, voice-activated telephones, switch-activated bed controls, and page turners are among the low-technological systems. Sip-N-puff, blink-operated, and voice-activated control units can be adapted to operate most electronic devices. Occupational and physical therapists can provide invaluable support to the person with DMD and the caregivers by making several home visits to suggest modifications and adaptive devices and systems. (See Cook and Hussey[51] for detailed information on assistive technology systems and Hicks[100] for rehabilitation management of myopathies.)

Psychosocial Issues

Psychosocial issues related to DMD are family issues. At the time of the child's diagnosis, the parents are often emotionally devastated and cycle back and forth through many phases of denial, anger, sadness, and active coping. This process tends to recur when the child does not meet expected normal physical and social milestones or when he reaches predicted stages of deterioration, such as the transition to a wheelchair. Early in the child's life, the family should be guided to encourage the child's independence and to discourage overprotection. Therapists can play an important role in helping the child and family identify realistic goals for independence. In addition, therapists can be instrumental in extending independence and the sense of self-direction by anticipating patient needs for adaptive equipment and identifying appropriate assistive devices and environmental control systems that empower the person with DMD and provide relief for caregivers from the constant attention required by a totally dependent person.

Psychosocial support should be made available to the child and family during predictable times of crisis. Major times of crisis occur around the age of 5 years when the child begins to realize his differences, between the ages of 8 to 12 years when the child loses the ability to walk independently, during the adolescent years when social interactions become restricted, and around the time of high school graduation when the child and family must face vocational limitations[73] and almost certain death within the next decade. Transition times are often accompanied by depression, withdrawal, and anxiety in the child and family members. Parents had a marked preoccupation with their sons and a diminished expression of enjoyment.[64, 234]

In a pilot study, 43 boys with DMD between the ages of 4 and 15 years completed human figure drawings (HFDs). HFDs have been used for 75 years as a projective tool to identify emotional factors that may not be verbalized clearly by the child. Using the process, the authors found that the children's drawing were characterized by emotional indicators suggesting physical inadequacy, body inadequacy, immaturity, and insecurity. Adolescents with DMD felt significantly isolated from the mainstream of life.[234] Predictably, the integrity, strength, and intragenerational and intergenerational function and coping styles of the child's family contribute a great deal to the way the family responds to the child's progressive deterioration. Extended periods of anxiety and depression should be treated vigorously with cognitive interventions, support groups, respite care, and, when appropriate, short-term anxiolytics and antidepressants. Parents and the child should be given the opportunity to discuss the impending death in an accepting environment with persons who are experienced dealing with degenerative diseases. Because the child and family have long anticipated the child's death and have made transitions through many levels of grieving, the process of separation and mourning may have occurred before the child's death. Each child and family member, therefore, should be helped to deal with the process according to his or her own pace and in response to individual needs.

The child's death is sometimes considered a welcome relief.[46] This feeling of relief, however, is often accompanied by survivor guilt and a tremendous sense of loss of life focus for the family members whose lives have been so intertwined with that of the child's. Ideally, arrangements should be made for the family to meet with the professionals with whom they feel most comfortable several weeks after the child's death and again several

CASE 13–3   Jeremy

Jeremy was 3 years old when he was diagnosed with DMD. He lived at home with his mother and a 5-year-old sister. There was no known family history of DMD, although family lore suggested that a cousin died very young from pneumonia and a "wasting disease." Jeremy was referred for a medical evaluation when a playground supervisor at his preschool noted that he was very clumsy when running and that he had difficulty on the playground climbing equipment and the slide. He also had difficulty rising from the ground and needed to hold onto a railing when stepping up a stair.

During a medical history, Jeremy's mother said that she had noticed that he was "slow to develop" but was not worried because she thought he was just a "late bloomer." A muscle biopsy was positive for a diagnosis of DMD. A physical therapy evaluation 3 months after diagnosis showed ROM to be within normal limits for all joints. Muscle weakness was evident on MMT with G− (4−) hip abduction and extension and quadriceps strength bilaterally. Hip flexion, knee flexion, dorsiflexion, and toe extension were in the G (4) range. Plantarflexion was G+ (4+) with evident hypertrophy. Shoulder abduction and flexion was in the G (4) range, although he had difficulty sustaining abduction for more than 5 seconds.

Jeremy had a moderate head lag when moving from supine to sitting due to G− (4−) anterior neck muscles. The therapist made an on-site school visit to help the teachers identify obstacles to Jeremy's full integration with his classmates. The school custodian built some ramps to help Jeremy use the playground equipment.

Jeremy ambulated independently until age 8 years. His gait pattern was typical of late stage ambulation (marked equinus, knee hyperextension during stance, bilateral Trendelenburg on stance, marked lordosis with a protuberant abdomen with arms held posterior to hips). He had 40-degree hip flexion contractures with iliotibial band tightness, no knee contractures, and 25-degree plantarflexion contractures. MMTs showed the expected decrease in strength, with pelvic and shoulder girdle muscles being weaker than more distal musculature, except that the anterior tibialis and the peroneals were F+ (3+). He was unable to rise independently from the floor and needed assistance with stairs. Because his gait pattern was very slow and he needed to rest frequently when walking more than 20 feet at school, Jeremy had been using a manual wheelchair for long-distance mobility since the age of 7 years.

On the recommendation of orthopedist consultants, Jeremy underwent bilateral percutaneous hip flexor lengthenings, iliotibial band fasciotomies, and heel cord releases. Bilateral KAFOs had been fitted before surgery, and Jeremy was placed in the braces after surgery. No casting was done. Despite his complaints, he was gradually brought to the full weight-bearing standing position by late afternoon on the day after surgery. Adjustments were made in his pain medication schedule to allow him to tolerate the process more comfortably. By the third hospital day, Jeremy participated in two therapy sessions per day and was standing in the parallel bars where he was taught lateral and anteroposterior weight shifting in preparation for ambulation. Active assisted and passive ROM exercises were performed without the KAFOs twice a day. On the fourth hospital day, Jeremy began to take short steps using the parallel bars for balance. His mother was also taught his exercises so that Jeremy could have more than two therapy sessions a day. On the fourth day, he practiced walking for 10 minutes six times a day with full physical therapy treatment twice a day.

Because Jeremy was from a rural area and daily physical therapy would not be available on discharge, he was kept in the hospital for 3 additional days for intensive rehabilitation. An occupational therapist worked with Jeremy to provide adaptive equipment for reaching, self-care, and eating (he was unable to raise his arms above 45 degrees and needed his left arm to assist the right when reaching). He was discharged home on the eighth day. An Elks Traveling Therapist arranged to visit the family once a week for the next month to continue ambulation training and to guide the mother in a home positioning and ROM program. The therapist also helped the mother adapt the home environment and his school to adjust expectations of Jeremy so he was less prone to falling and excessive fatigue.

The family was lost to follow-up, but by report, Jeremy continued to ambulate in his KAFOs for approximately 9 months after surgery when he chose to use his wheelchair full-time. A motorized wheelchair was recommended; however, his mother felt that it was easier to handle Jeremy in his manual chair. The Muscular Dystrophy Association loaned Jeremy a motorized wheelchair for school use. He had developed a moderate scoliosis, but did not complain of pain. He refused to wear a molded spinal corset, but the padded thoracic pads fitted to his chair increased his comfort. By age 15, Jeremy was dependent for all care except feeding. He was able to sit with support in a large living room chair and he enjoyed watching television and playing card games with a few friends who visited his home. He was disinterested in continuing school and missed more days than he attended. He was not cooperative with his home-based teacher.

During his fifteenth year, Jeremy had repeated

Continued

CASE 13-3 Jeremy *Continued*

episodes of chest congestion and difficulty handling stringy foods. The visiting therapist taught his mother some postural drainage and breathing exercises for Jeremy; however, the mother did not follow through with the recommendations. Because his mother had to work full time, a public agency provided in-home care during the days when Jeremy was not at school or after he re-

turned from school. The mother refused in-home nursing care, preferring to continue with the attendant, who was not comfortable carrying out Jeremy's exercises or pulmonary care. The family refused counseling or support from parents of other children with disabilities, Jeremy died at home after a brief bout with pneumonia.

months later so that the family (and caregivers) can deal with their thoughts and feelings. See Alhstrom and Gunnarsson[1] and Ahlstrom and Sjoden[2] for further information on coping and quality of life of patients with muscular dystrophy. (See Case 13–3 and also the caregiver section under ALS.)

SUMMARY

Three very different diseases have been described to depict the varied effects of neuromuscular pathology on a person's day-to-day function. Amyotrophic lateral sclerosis is an adult-onset degenerative disease of the upper and lower motor neurons; Guillain-Barré syndrome is an inflammatory process affecting the peripheral nervous system of children and adults; and Duchenne muscular dystrophy is an inherited degenerative disease presenting in childhood that affects muscle tissue.

In all three conditions, the therapist is challenged to design a therapy program that will provide the patient with the impetus to become or remain as active as possible without causing possible muscle damage from excessive exercise demands or overwork.

Therapists must also be aware of their own feelings and reactions to patients with severe neuromuscular diseases. Working with patients with GBS is usually a positive experience because the majority of patients attain full recovery despite their often severe disability during the acute illness and long recovery period. Working with patients with degenerative terminal diseases, however, draws deeply on the therapist's emotional and spiritual strength.

A typical response of health care professionals is to view these patients' conditions as hopeless and to assume that the patients must also perceive their existence as hopeless, depressing, and without value. Research does suggest that there is an increased incidence of depression and demoralization in patients with degenerative, terminal diseases when compared with nonaffected populations. Other research, however, has indicated that many patients perceive their own life satisfaction much more positively than professionals would believe.[14] Therefore, therapists must tap into patients' positive energy to design treatment programs that respect patients' goals and life plans within the context of their environments.

After reading this chapter, therapists will realize that there is not an extensive literature documenting the most

appropriate exercise and therapeutic intervention programs for patients with progressive neurological diseases. In addition, there is some concern that patients with a history of severe GBS may show age-related changes in muscle strength similar to those in patients with postpolio syndrome. Because few medical-clinical facilities see a large enough sample of patients, it is imperative that therapists align with their professional organizations to institute nationwide, multisite research studies that will provide clear information about appropriate therapy programs.

REFERENCES

1. Ahlstrom G, Gunnarsson L: Disability and quality of life in individuals with muscular dystrophy. Scand J Rehabil Med 28:147–157, 1996.
2. Ahlstrom G, Sjoden P: Coping with illness-related problems and quality of life in adult individuals with muscular dystrophy. J Psychosom Res 41:365–376, 1996.
3. Akeson WH, et al: The connective tissue response to immobility: An accelerated aging response? Exp Gerontol 3:289, 1968.
4. Albert SM, et al: A prospective study of preferences and actual treatment choices in ALS. Neurology 53:278–283, 1999.
5. Allsop KG, Ziter FA: Loss of strength and functional decline in Duchenne dystrophy. Arch Neurol 38:406, 1981.
6. ALS Association: Adjusting to swallowing and speech difficulties: Diet. In Living with ALS Manuals. ALS Association. http://www.alsa.org/serving/lib_manuals.
7. Appel SH: The muscular dystrophies. Neurol Clin 1(1):7, 1979.
8. Appel SH, Smith GR: Can neurotrophic factors prevent or reverse motor neuron injury in amyotrophic lateral sclerosis? Exp Neurol 124:100, 1993.
9. Appel V, et al: Meals for Easy Swallowing. Tucson, AZ, Muscular Dystrophy Association, 1986.
10. Appell HJ: Muscular atrophy following immobilization. Sports Med 10:42–58, 1993.
11. Armon C, Moses D: Linear estimates of rates of disease progression as predictors of survival in patients with ALS entering clinical trials. J Neurol Sci 160(Suppl 1):S37–S41, 1998.
12. Asher MI, et al: The effects of inspiratory muscle training in patients with cystic fibrosis. Am Rev Respir Dis 126:855, 1982.
13. Bach JR: Therapeutic interventions and habilitation considerations: A historical perspective from Tamplin to robotics for pseudohypertrophic muscular dystrophy. Semin Neurol 15:38–45, 1995.
14. Bach JR, Campagnolo DI, Hoeman S: Life satisfaction of individuals with Duchenne muscular dystrophy using long-term mechanical ventilatory support. Am J Phys Med Rehabil 70:129–135, 1991.
15. Bach JR, Ishikawa Y: Letters to the Editor: GBS respiratory complications revisited. Arch Phys Med Rehabil 79:115–116, 1998.
16. Bach JR, McKeon J: Orthopedic surgery and rehabilitation for the prolongation of brace-free ambulation of patients with Duchenne muscular dystrophy. Am J Phys Med Rehabil 70(6):323, 1991.
17. Bach JR, et al: Management of end stage respiratory failure due to late stage Duchenne muscular dystrophy. Arch Phys Med Rehabil 10:177, 1987.

18. Bakker JPJ, et al: Prescription pattern for orthoses in The Netherlands: Use and experience in the ambulatory phase of Duchenne muscular dystrophy. Disability Rehabil 19:318–325, 1997.

19. Belsh JM: Diagnostic challenges in ALS. Neurology 53(Suppl 5):S26–S30, 1999.

20. Bennett RL, Knowlton GC: Overwork weakness in partially denervated skeletal muscle. Clin Orthop 12:22, 1958.

21. Bensman A: Strenuous exercise may impair muscle function in Guillain-Barré patients. JAMA 214:468, 1970.

22. Berger M, et al: Detection and cellular localization of enterovirus RNA sequences in spinal cord of patients with ALS. Neurology 54(1):20–25, 2000.

23. Billard C, et al: Cognitive functions in Duchenne muscular dystrophy: A reappraisal and comparison with spinal muscular atrophy. Neuromuscul Disord 2:371–378, 1992.

24. Billard C, et al: Reading ability and processing in Duchenne muscular dystrophy and spinal muscular atrophy. Dev Med Child Neurol 40:12–20, 1998.

25. Blei ML, Fall AM, Kushmerick MJ: Energy balance for muscle function: Principles of bioenergetics. In Frontera WR, Dawson DM, Slovik DM (eds): Exercise in Rehabilitation Medicine. Champaign, IL, Human Kinetics, 1999, pp 3–22.

26. Bonnemann CG: Limb-girdle muscular dystrophies: An overview. J Child Neurol 14(1):31–33, 1999.

27. Borasio GD, Gelinas DF, Yanagisawa N: Mechanical ventilation in amyotrophic lateral sclerosis: A cross-cultural perspective. J Neurol 245(Suppl 2):S7–S12, 1998.

28. Borasio GD, Sloan R, Pongratz DE: Breaking the news in amyotrophic lateral sclerosis. J Neurol Sci 160(Suppl 1):S127–S133, 1998.

29. Bouget J, et al: Plasma exchange morbidity in Guillain-Barré syndrome: Results from the French prospective, double-blind, randomized, multi-center study. Crit Care Med 21:651–658, 1993.

30. Bril V, et al: Pilot trial of immunoglobulin versus plasma exchange in patients with Guillain-Barré syndrome. Neurology 46:100–103, 1996.

31. Brooke MH, et al: Clinical investigations in Duchenne muscular dystrophy: II. Determination of the "power" of therapeutic trials based on the natural history. Muscle Nerve 6:91, 1983.

32. Brooke MH, et al: Clinical investigation of Duchenne muscular dystrophy: Interesting results in a trial of prednisolone. Arch Neurol 44:812, 1987.

33. Brooke MH, et al: Duchenne muscular dystrophy: Patterns of clinical progresison and effects of supportive therapy. Neurology 39:475, 1989.

34. Brooks BR: El Escorial World Federation of Neurology criteria for the diagnosis of amyotrophic lateral sclerosis. J Neurol Sci 124(Suppl):96–107, 1994.

35. Brooks BR: Introduction: Defining optimal management of ALS: From first symptoms to announcement. Neurology 53(Suppl 5):S1–S3, 1999.

36. Brooks BR: What are the implications of early diagnosis? Maintaining optimal health as long as possible. Neurology 53(Suppl 5):S43–S49, 1999.

37. Brooks BR, et al: Design of clinical therapeutic trials in amyotrophic lateral sclerosis. In Rowland L (ed): Advances in Neurology, vol 56. New York, Raven Press, 1991.

38. Burrows DS, Cuetter AC: Residual subclinical impairment in patients who totally recovered from Guillain-Barré syndrome: Impact on military performance. Milit Med 155:438, 1990.

39. Bushbacher L: Rehabilitation of patients with peripheral neuropathies. In Braddom RL: Physical Medicine and Rehabilitation. Philadelphia, WB Saunders, 1995, pp 972–989.

40. Caroscio JT: Amyotrophic lateral sclerosis: The disease. In Caroscio JT (ed): Amyotrophic Lateral Sclerosis. New York, Thieme Medical, 1986.

41. Carpenter RJ, McDonald TJ, Howard FM: The otolaryngologic presentation of amyotrophic lateral sclerosis. ORL 86:479, 1978.

42. Carter JH, Nutt JG: Family caregiving: A neglected and hidden part of health care delivery. Neurology 51:1245–1246, 1998.

43. Carver AC, et al: End-of-life care: A survey of US neurologists' attitudes, behavior, and knowledge. Neurology 53(2):284–293, 1999.

44. Cashman NR: Do the benefits of currently available treatments justify early diagnosis and announcement? Arguments for. Neurology 53(Suppl 5):S50–S52, 1999.

45. Chan CW, Sinaki M: Rehabilitation management of the ALS patient. In Belsh JM, Schiffman PL (eds): Amyotrophic Lateral Sclerosis: Diagnosis and Management for the Clinician. New York, Futura, 1996.

46. Childress J: The dying child. In Kruger DW (ed): Rehabilitation Psychology. Rockville, MD, Aspen Publishers, 1984.

47. Chou SM: Pathology of intraneuronal inclusions in ALS. In Tsubaki T, Toyokura Y (eds): Amyotrophic Lateral Sclerosis. Baltimore, University Park Press, 1979.

48. Clague JE, MacMillan RR: Backache and the Guillain-Barré syndrome: A diagnostic problem. BMJ 293:325, 1986.

49. Clarkson PM, Nokasa K, Braun B: Muscle function after exercise-induced muscle damage and rapid adaptation. Med Sci Sports Exerc 24:512–520, 1992.

50. Cobble M: Language impairment in motor neurone disease. J Neurol Sci 160(Suppl 1):S47–S52, 1998.

51. Cook AM, Hussey SM: Augmentative and Alternative Communication Systems. New York, CV Mosby, 1995.

52. Corrado A, Gorini M, DePaola E: Alternative techniques for managing acute neuromuscular respiratory failure. Semin Neurol 15:84–89, 1995.

53. Dal Bello-Haas V: Physical therapy for a patient through six stages of amyotrophic lateral sclerosis. Phys Ther 78:1314–1324, 1998.

54. Damiano AM, et al: Measurement of health-related quality of life in patients with amyotrophic lateral sclerosis in clinical trials of new therapies. Med Care 37:15–26, 1999.

55. Daube JR, et al: Classification of ALS by autonomic abnormalities. In Tsubaki T, Yase Y (eds): Amyotrophic Lateral Sclerosis. Amsterdam, Elsevier Science Publishers, 1987.

56. de Lateur BJ, Giaconi RM: Effect on maximal strength of submaximal exercise in Duchenne muscular dystrophy. Am J Phys Med 58(1):26, 1979.

57. Desai J, Sharief M, Swash M: Riluzole has no effect on motor unit parameters in ALS. J Neurol Sci 160(Suppl 1):S69–S72, 1998.

58. De Silva S, et al: Prednisolone treatment in Duchenne muscular dystrophy. Arch Neurol 44:818, 1987.

59. Di Marco AF, et al: Respiratory muscle training in muscular dystrophy. Clin Res 30:427, 1982.

60. Drennan JC: Neuromuscular disorders. In Morrissy RT (ed): Pediatric Orthopaedics, 3rd ed. Philadelphia, JB Lippincott, 1990.

61. Dubowitz V: Forty years of neuromuscular disease: A historical perspective. J Child Neurol 14(1):26–28, 1999.

62. Eberle E, et al: Early predictors of incomplete recovery in children with Guillain-Barré polyneuritis. J Pediatr 86:356, 1975.

63. Edwards RHT: Weight reduction in boys with muscular dystrophy. Dev Med Child Neurol 26:384, 1984.

64. Eggers S, Zatz M: Social adjustments in adult males affected with progressive muscular dystrophy. Am J Med Genet 81:4–12, 1998.

65. Eisen A, Weber M: Treatment of amyotrophic lateral sclerosis. Drugs Aging 14(3):173–196, 1999.

66. Elder GCB: Beneficial effects of training on developing dystrophic muscle. Muscle Nerve 15:672, 1992.

67. Emery AEH: Fortnightly review: The muscular dystrophies. BMJ 317:991–995, 1998.

68. Felice KJ, North WA: Creatine kinase values in amyotrophic lateral sclerosis. J Neurol Sci 160(Suppl 1):S30–S32, 1998.

69. Fenichel G, et al: Long-term benefit from prednisone therapy in Duchenne muscular dystrophy. Neurology 41:1874, 1991.

70. Fielding RA, Bean J: Physiological adaptations to dynamic exercise. In Frontera WR, Dawson DM, Slovik DM (eds): Exercise in Rehabilitation Medicine. Champaign, IL, Human Kinetics, 1999, pp 41–54.

71. Florence J, et al: Intrarater reliability of manual muscle test grades in Duchenne muscular dystrophy. Phys Ther 72:115, 1992.

72. Fowler WM, et al: The effect of exercise on serum enzymes. Arch Phys Med 49:554, 1968.

73. Fowler WM, et al: Employment profiles in neuromuscular diseases. Am J Phys Med Rehabil 76:26–37, 1997.

74. Francis K, Bach JR, DeLisa JA: Evaluation and rehabilitation of patients with adult motor neuron disease. Arch Phys Med Rehabil 80:951–963, 1999.

75. French Cooperative Group on Plasma Exchange in Guillain-Barré Syndrome: Efficiency of plasma exchange in Guillain-Barré syndrome: Role of replacement fluids. Ann Neurol 22:753, 1987.

76. Fukuyama Y: Congenital muscular dystrophies: An update. J Child Neurol 14(1):28–30, 1999.

77. Gabreels F: Mitochondrial myopathies. J Child Neurol 14(1):37–38, 1999.
78. Gabreels-Festin A: Hereditary neuropathies in childhood: Morphologic hallmarks and pathophysiologic mechanisms. J Child Neurol 14:52–53, 1999.
79. Ganzini L, Johnston WS, Hoffman WF: Correlates of suffering in amyotrophic lateral sclerosis. Neurology 52(7):1434–1440, 1999.
80. Gelinas DF, O'Connor P, Miller RG: Quality of life for ventilator-dependent ALS patients and their caregivers. J Neurol Sci 160(Suppl 1):S134–S136, 1998.
81. Goebel H: Congenital myopathies: The current status. J Child Neurol 14(1):30–31, 1999.
82. Goldstein LH, et al: The psychological impact of MND on patients and careers. J Neurol Sci 160(Suppl 1):S114–S121, 1998.
83. Grand'Maison F, et al: Recurrent Guillain-Barré syndrome. Brain 115:1093–1106, 1992.
84. Greenwood RJ, et al: Controlled trial of plasma exchange in acute inflammatory polyradiculoneuropathy. Lancet 1:877, 1984.
85. Griffith R, Edwards RHT: A new chart for weight control in Duchenne muscular dystrophy. Arch Phys Med Rehabil 63:1256, 1988.
86. Griggs RC, et al: Randomized, double-blind trial of mazindol in Duchenne dystrophy. Muscle Nerve 13:1169–1173, 1990.
87. Grossman MR, Sahrmann SA, Rose SJ: Review of length associated changes in muscle: Experimental evidence and clinical implications. Phys Ther 62:1799, 1982.
88. Guccione AA: Functional assessment. In Physical Rehabilitation: Assessment and Treatment. Philadelphia, FA Davis, 1994, pp 193–207.
89. Guillain G, Barré JA, Strohl A: Sur un syndrome de radiculo-névrité avec hyperalbuminose du liquide cephalorachidien sans réaction cellulaire: Rémarques sur les caractères cliniques et graphiques des réflexes tendineux. Bull Mem Soc Med Hop Paris 40:1462, 1916.
90. Guillain-Barré Syndrome Study Group: Plasmapheresis and acute Guillain-Barré syndrome. Neurology 35:1096, 1985.
91. Hallum A, Krumboltz JD: Parents caring for young adults with severe physical disabilities: Psychological issues. Dev Med Child Neurol 35:24–32, 1993.
92. Hammon WE: Physical therapy for the acutely ill patient in the respiratory intensive care unit. In Irwin S, Tecklin JS (eds): Cardiopulmonary Physical Therapy. St. Louis, CV Mosby, 1990.
93. Harris SE, Cherry DB: Childhood progressive muscular dystrophy and the role of physical therapy. Phys Ther 54(1):4, 1974.
94. Hartung HP, van der Meche FGA, Pollard JD: Editorial review: Guillain-Barré syndrome, CIDP and other chronic immune-mediated neuropathies. Curr Opin Neurol 11:497–513, 1998.
95. Hasson SM: Progressive and degenerative neuromuscular disease and severe muscular dystrophy. In Hasson SM: Clinical Exercise Physiology. St. Louis, CV Mosby, 1994.
96. Heckmatt J, et al: Management of children: Pharmacological and physical. Br Med Bull 45:788, 1989.
97. Heckmatt J, Loh L, Dubowitz V: Night-time nasal ventilation in neuromuscular disease. Lancet 335:579–582, 1990.
98. Herbison GJ, et al: Exercise therapies in peripheral neuropathies. Arch Phys Med Rehabil 64:201, 1983.
99. Hertling D, Jones D: Relaxation. In Kessler RM, Hertling D (eds): Management of Common Musculoskeletal Disorders: Physical Therapy Principles and Methods. Philadelphia, Harper & Row, 1983.
100. Hicks JE: Role of rehabilitation in the management of myopathies. Curr Opin Rheumatol 10:548–555, 1998.
101. Hillel AD, Miller RM: Management of bulbar symptoms in amyotrophic lateral sclerosis. In Cosi V, et al (eds): Amyotrophic Lateral Sclerosis. Therapeutic, Psychological and Research Aspects. New York, Plenum Press, 1987.
102. Hillel AD, Miller RM: Bulbar amyotrophic lateral sclerosis: Patterns of progression and clinical management. Head Neck 11(1):51–59, 1989.
103. Hillel AD, et al: Amyotrophic lateral sclerosis severity scale. Neuroepidemiology 8:142, 1989.
104. Hillel AD, et al: Presentation of ALS to the otolaryngologist/head and neck surgeon: Getting to the neurologist. Neurology 53(Suppl 5):S22–S25, 1999.
105. Hirano A: In pursuit of the early pathological alterations in ALS. In Tsubaki T, Yase Y (eds): Amyotrophic Lateral Sclerosis. Amsterdam, Elsevier Science, 1988.
106. Hoberman M: Physical medicine and rehabilitation: Its value and limitations in progressive muscular dystrophy. In Proceedings of the Third Medical Conference of the Muscular Dystrophy Association of America, 1954, pp 109–115.
107. Holtacker TR: Physical rehabilitation of the ventilator-dependent patient. In Irwin S, Tecklin JS (eds): Cardiopulmonary Physical Therapy. St. Louis, CV Mosby, 1990.
108. Houpt JL, Gould BS, Norris FH: Psychological characteristics of patients with amyotrophic lateral sclerosis. Psychosom Med 39:299, 1977.
109. Humberstone N: Respiratory assessment and treatment. In Irwin S, Tecklin JS (eds): Cardiopulmonary Physical Therapy, 3rd ed. Philadelphia, CV Mosby, 1995.
110. Hunt JM: The cardiac surgical patient's expectations and experiences of nursing care in the intensive care unit. Aust Crit Care 12:47–53, 1999.
111. Hyde SA, et al: Prolongation of ambulation in Duchenne muscular dystrophy by appropriate orthoses. Physiotherapy 68(4):105, 1982.
112. Irani DN, et al: Relapse in Guillain-Barré syndrome after treatment with human immunoglobin. Neurology 43:872, 1993.
113. Irwin S, Tecklin JS (eds): Cardiopulmonary Physical Therapy. St. Louis, CV Mosby, 1990.
114. Jette DU, et al: The relationship of lower-limb muscle force to walking ability in patients with amyotrophic lateral sclerosis. Phys Ther 79:672–681, 1998.
115. Johnson EW, Braddom R: Over-work weakness in facioscapulohumeral muscular dystrophy. Arch Phys Med Rehabil 52:333, 1971.
116. Jones KJ, North KN: Recent advances in the diagnosis of the childhood muscular dystrophies. J Paediatr Child Health 33:195–201, 1997.
117. Kandel ER, et al (eds): Principles of Neural Science, 3rd ed. East Norwalk, CT, Appleton & Lange, 1991.
118. Karni Y, et al: Clinical assessment and physiotherapy in Guillain-Barré syndrome. Physiotherapy 70:288, 1984.
119. Karper WB: Effects of low-intensity aerobic exercise on one subject with chronic-relapsing Guillain-Barré syndrome. Rehabil Nurs 16:96, 1991.
120. Kazandjian NS: Communication intervention. In Kazandjian NS (ed): Communication and Swallowing Solutions for the ALS/MND Community. San Diego, Singular Publishing Group, 1997.
121. Kelly JH, Buccholz DW: Nutritional management of the patient with a neurologic disorder. Ear Nose Throat J 75(5):293–300, 1996.
122. Kessler RM: The shoulder. In Kessler RM, Hertling D (eds): Management of Common Musculoskeletal Disorders: Physical Therapy Principles and Methods. Philadelphia, Harper & Row, 1983.
123. Kilmer DD, Aitkens S: Neuromuscular disease. In Frontera WR, Dawson DM, Slovik DM (eds): Exercise in Rehabilitation Medicine. Champaign, IL, Human Kinetics, 1999, pp 253–266.
124. Kilmer DD, et al: The effect of a high-resistance exercise program in slowly progressive neuromuscular disease. Arch Phys Med Rehabil 75:560–563, 1994.
125. Langmore SE, Longemann JA: After the clinical bedside swallowing examination: What next? Am J Speech Lang Pathol 1:13, 1991.
126. Leger P, et al: Home positive pressure ventilation via nasal mask for patients with neuromuscular weakness or restrictive lung or chest-wall disease. Respir Care 34:73, 1989.
127. Lehmann JF, et al: Effect of therapeutic temperature on tendon extensibility. Arch Phys Med Rehabil 51:481, 1970.
128. Lewis CB, Bottomley JM (eds): Geriatric Physical Therapy: A Clinical Approach. East Norwalk, CT, Appleton & Lange, 1994.
129. Long DM, et al: Transcutaneous electrical stimulation for relief of chronic pain. Adv Pain Res Ther 3:593, 1979.
130. Longemann J: Evaluation and Treatment of Swallowing Disorders. San Diego, College-Hill Press, 1983.
131. Lord J, et al: Scoliosis associated with Duchenne muscular dystrophy. Arch Phys Med Rehabil 71:13, 1990.
132. Ludolph AC, Riepe MW: Do the benefits of currently available treatments justify early diagnosis and announcement? Arguments against. Neurology 53(Suppl 5):S46–S49, 1999.
133. Mackin GA: Optimizing care of patients with ALS: Steps to early detection and improved quality of life. Postgrad Med 105(4):141–158, 1999.

134. Madding SW, et al: Effect of duration of passive stretch on hip abduction range of motion. J Orthop Sports Phys Ther 8:409–416, 1987.

135. Martin AJ, et al: Respiratory muscle training in Duchenne muscular dystrophy. Dev Med Child Neurol 28:314, 1986.

136. Matheron L, Barrau K, Blin O: Disease management: The example of amyotrophic lateral sclerosis. J Neurol 245(Suppl 2):S20–S28, 1998.

137. Mayberry JF, Atkinson M: Swallowing problems in patients with motor neuron disease. J Clin Gastroenterol 8:233–234, 1986.

138. Mays ML: Incorporating continuous passive motion in the rehabilitation of a patient with Guillain-Barré syndrome. Am J Occup Ther 44:750, 1990.

139. Mazzini L, et al: The natural history and the effects of gabapentin in amyotrophic lateral sclerosis. J Neurol Sci 160(Suppl 1):S57–S63, 1998.

140. McDonald CM: Limb contractures in progressive neuromuscular disease and the role of stretching, orthotics and surgery. Phys Med Rehabil Clin North Am 9:187–211, 1998.

141. McLeod JG: Electrophysiological studies in the Guillain-Barré syndrome. Ann Neurol 9(Suppl):20, 1981.

142. Melzack R: Prolonged relief of pain by brief, intense, transcutaneous somatic stimulation. Pain 1:357, 1975.

143. Meythaler JM: Rehabilitation of Guillain-Barré syndrome. Arch Phys Med Rehabil 78:872–879, 1997.

144. Miller F, Moseley CF, Koreska J: Spinal fusion in Duchenne muscular dystrophy. Dev Med Child Neurol 34:775, 1992.

145. Miller JR, Colbert AP, Schock NC: Ventilator use in progressive neuromuscular disease: Impact on patients and their families. Dev Med Child Neurol 30:200–207, 1988.

146. Miller RG, et al: Practice parameter: The care of the patient with amyotrophic lateral sclerosis (an evidenced-based review). Neurology 52:1311–1323, 1999.

147. Milner-Brown HS, Miller RG: Muscle strengthening through high-resistance weight training in patients with neuromuscular disorders. Arch Phys Med Rehabil 69:14–19, 1998.

148. Milonas I: Amyotrophic lateral sclerosis: An introduction. J Neurol 245(Suppl 2):S1–S3, 1998.

149. Mitsumoto H: Patient choices in ALS: Life-sustaining treatment versus palliative care. Neurology 53:248–249, 1988.

150. Molenaar DSM, de Haan R, Vermeulen M: Impairment, disability, or handicap I peripheral neuropathy; analysis of the use of outcome measures in clinical trials in patients with peripheral neuropathies. J Neurol Neurosurg Psychiatry 59:165–169, 1995.

151. Moore MJ, Moore PB, Shaw PJ: Mood disturbances in motor neurone disease. J Neurol Sci 160(Suppl 1):S53–S56, 1998.

152. Moss AH, et al: Home ventilation for amyotrophic lateral sclerosis patients: Outcomes, costs and patient, family and physician attitudes. Neurology 43:438, 1993.

153. Mulder DW, Kurland LT: Amyotrophic lateral sclerosis (motor neuron disease): Four clinical questions. In Tsubaki T, Yase Y (eds): Amyotrophic Lateral Sclerosis. Amsterdam, Elsevier Science, 1987.

154. Muller EA: Influence of training and of inactivity on muscle strength. Arch Phys Med Rehabil 51:449, 1970.

155. Norris FH, Denys EH: Nutritional supplements in amyotrophic lateral sclerosis. In Cosi V, et al (eds): Amyotrophic Lateral Sclerosis. Therapeutic, Psychological and Research Aspects. New York, Plenum Press, 1987.

156. Norris FH, Smith RA, Denys EH: The treatment of amyotrophic lateral sclerosis. In Cosi V, et al (eds): Amyotrophic Lateral Sclerosis. Therapeutic, Psychological and Research Aspects. New York, Plenum Press, 1987.

157. Oliver D: Ethical issues in palliative care—an overview. Palliat Med 7(Suppl 2):15, 1993.

158. Oliver D, Cardy P: Motor Neuron Disease: Death and Dying. North Hampton, Motor Neuron Disease Association, 1991.

159. Oppenheimer EA: Decision-making in the respiratory care of amyotrophic lateral sclerosis: Should home mechanical ventilation be used? Palliat Med 7(Suppl 2):49, 1993.

160. Osterman PO, et al: Beneficial effects of plasma exchange in acute inflammatory polyradiculoneuropathy. Lancet 2:1296, 1984.

161. Ouvrier R: Update on acute and chronic inflammatory polyneuropathy. J Child Neurol 14:53–57, 1999.

162. Pandya S, et al: Reliability of goniometric measurements in patients with Duchenne muscular dystrophy. Phys Ther 65:1339, 1985.

163. Partridge TA: Myoblast transfer: Possible therapy for inherited myopathies. Muscle Nerve 14:197, 1991.

164. Pascuzzi RM, Fleck JD: Acute peripheral neuropathy in adults. Neurol Clin 15:529–547, 1997.

165. Pentland B, Daonald SM: Pain in the Guillain-Barré syndrome: A clinical review. Pain 59:159–164, 1994.

166. Petajan JH, White AT: Recommendations for physical activity in patients with multiple sclerosis. Sports Med 27:179–191, 1999

167. Petrof BJ: Respiratory muscles as a target for adenovirus-mediated gene therapy. Eur Respir J 11:492–497, 1998.

168. Pitetti KH, et al: Endurance exercise training in Guillain-Barré syndrome. Arch Phys Med Rehabil 74:761, 1993.

169. Pradas J, et al: The natural history of amyotrophic lateral sclerosis and the use of natural history controls in therapeutic trials. Neurology 43:751, 1993.

170. Purtilo R, Haddad A: Health Professional and Patient Interaction, 5th ed. Philadelphia, WB Saunders, 1996.

171. Rees J: Guillain-Barré syndrome: The latest on treatment. Br J Hosp Med 50:226, 1993.

172. Reitsma W: Skeletal muscle hypertrophy after heavy exercise in rats with surgically reduced muscle function. Am J Phys Med 48:237, 1969.

173. Ringel SP, Cooper WH: Classification of neuromuscular disorders. In Maloney FP, et al (eds): Interdisciplinary Rehabilitation of Multiple Sclerosis and Neuromuscular Disorders. Philadelphia, JB Lippincott, 1985.

174. Ringel SP, et al: The natural history of amyotrophic lateral sclerosis. Neurology 43:1316, 1993.

175. Rideau Y, et al: Prolongation of life in Duchenne's muscular dystrophy. Acta Neurol 38:118, 1983.

176. Rideau Y, et al: Early treatment to preserve quality of locomotion for children with Duchenne muscular dystrophy. Semin Neurol 15:9–16, 1995.

177. Ropper AH, et al: Pain in Guillain-Barré syndrome. Arch Neurol 41:511, 1984.

178. Ropper AH, et al: Severe acute Guillain-Barré syndrome. Neurology 36:429, 1986.

179. Ropper AH: The Guillain Barré syndrome. N Engl J Med 326:1130–1136, 1992.

180. Rose J, et al: The energy expenditure index: A method to quantify and compare walking energy expenditure for children and adolescents. J Pediatr Orthop 11:571, 1991.

181. Rosen DR, et al: Mutations in Cu/Zn superoxide dismutase gene are associated with familial amyotrophic lateral sclerosis. Nature 362:59–62, 1993.

182. Rowland LP: Diagnosis of amyotrophic lateral sclerosis. J Neurol Sci 160(Suppl 1):S6–S24, 1998.

183. Ruttenberg N: Assessment and treatment of speech and swallowing problems in patients with multiple sclerosis. In Maloney FP, et al (eds): Interdisciplinary Rehabilitation of Multiple Sclerosis and Neuromuscular Disorders. Philadelphia, JB Lippincott, 1985.

184. Russell J: Ethical considerations in disease management of amyotrophic lateral sclerosis: A cross-cultural, worldwide perspective. J Neurol 245(Suppl 2):S4–S6, 1998.

185. Salter R: Clinical application of basic research on continuous passive motion for disorders and injuries of synovial joints: A preliminary study. J Orthop Res 1:325, 1984.

186. Sanjak M, Reddan W, Brooks BR: Role of muscular exercise in amyotrophic lateral sclerosis. Neurol Clin 5:251, 1989.

187. Sanjak M, et al: Physiologic and metabolic response to progressive and prolonged exercise in amyotrophic lateral sclerosis. Neurology 37:1217–1220, 1987.

188. Schmitz TY: Environmental assessment. In Physical Rehabilitation: Assessment and Treatment. Philadelphia, FA Davis, 1994, pp 209–223.

189. Scott A, Heughan A: A review of dysphagia in four cases of motor neurone disease. Palliat Med (Suppl 2):41, 1993.

190. Scott OM, et al: Responses of muscles of patients with Duchenne muscular dystrophy to chronic electrical stimulation. J Neurol Neurosurg Psychiatry 49:1427, 1986.

191. Scott OM, et al: Prevention of deformity in Duchenne muscular dystrophy. Physiotherapy 67(6):177, 1981.

192. Siegel IM: Update on Duchenne muscular dystrophy. Comp Ther 15(3):45, 1989.

193. Silani V, Kasarskis EJ, Yanagisawa N: Nutritional management in amyotrophic lateral sclerosis: A worldwide perspective. J Neurol 245(Suppl 2):S13–S19, 1998.

194. Simonds AK, et al: The impact of nasal ventilation on survival in hypercapnic Duchenne muscular dystrophy. Thorax 53:949–952, 1998.

195. Sinaki M: Exercise and rehabilitation measures in amyotrophic lateral sclerosis. *In* Yase Y, Tsubaki T (eds): Amyotrophic Lateral Sclerosis: Recent Advances in Research and Treatment. Amsterdam, Elsevier Science, 1988.

196. Sinaki M, Mulder DW: Rehabilitation techniques for patients with amyotrophic lateral sclerosis. Mayo Clin Proc 53:173–178, 1978.

197. Smith EWL: A gestalt therapist's perspective on grief. *In* Stern EM (ed): Psychotherapy and the Grieving Patient. New York, Harrington Park Press, 1985.

198. Smith PEM, Calverly PMA, Edwards RHT: Hypoxia during sleep in Duchenne muscular dystrophy. Am Rev Respir Dis 137:884, 1988.

199. Smith PEM, et al: Practical problems in the respiratory care of patients with muscular dystrophy. N Engl J Med 316:1197, 1987.

200. Smith PS: Maintaining quality of life: To the Editor. Phys Ther 79:423, 1999.

201. Sobue G, et al: Degenerating compartment and functioning compartment of motor neurons in ALS: Possible process of motor neuron loss. Neurology 33:654, 1983.

202. Sonies BC: Instrumental procedures for dysphagia diagnosis. Semin Speech Lang 12:185, 1991.

203. Soryal I, et al: Impaired joint mobility in Guillain-Barré syndrome: A primary or a secondary phenomenon? J Neurol Neurosurg Psychiatry 55:1014, 1992.

204. Spencer GE, et al: Bracing for ambulation in childhood progressive muscular dystrophy. J Bone Joint Surg 44–A(2):234, 1962.

205. Spencer WA: The Treatment of Acute Poliomyelitis. Springfield, IL, Charles C Thomas, 1954.

206. Stallard J, et al: The ORLAU VCG (variable centre of gravity) swivel walker for muscular dystrophy patients. Prosthet Orthop Int 16:46, 1992.

207. Steck AJ, Schaeren-Wiemers N, Hartung HP: Demyelinating inflammatory neuropathies, including Guillain-Barré syndrome. Curr Opin Neurol 11:311–318, 1998.

208. Steinberg JS: Guillain-Barré Syndrome (Acute Idiopathic Polyneuritis): An Overview for the Lay Person. Wynnewood, PA, The Guillain-Barre Syndrome Support Group International, 1987.

209. Stern LM, Clark BE: Investigation of scoliosis in Duchenne dystrophy using computerized tomography. Muscle Nerve 11:775, 1988.

210. Stillwell GK: Rehabilitative procedures. *In* Dyck PJ, et al (eds): Peripheral Neuropathy, 2nd ed. Philadelphia, WB Saunders, 1984.

211. Stubgen JP, Stipp A: Limb girdle muscular dystrophy: A prospective follow-up study of functional impairment. Muscle Nerve 20(4):453–460, 1997.

212. Sutherland DH, Olshen R, Cooper L: The pathomechanics of gait in Duchenne muscular dystrophy. Dev Med Child Neurol 23:3, 1981.

213. Swash M: Early diagnosis of amyotrophic lateral sclerosis/motor neuron disease. J Neurol Sci 160(Suppl 1):S33–S36, 1998.

214. Tashiro K, et al: Sensory findings in amyotrophic lateral sclerosis. *In* Tsubaki T, Yase Y (eds): Amyotrophic Lateral Sclerosis. Amsterdam, Elsevier Science, 1988.

215. Taylor DC, et al: Viscoelastic properties of muscle-tendon units: The biomechanical effects of stretching. Am J Sports Med 18:300, 1990.

216. Thorsteinsson G, et al: Transcutaneous electrical stimulation: A double blind trial of its efficacy for pain. Arch Phys Med Rehabil 58:8, 1977.

217. Tilton AH, Miller MD, Khoshoo V: Nutrition and swallowing in pediatric neuromuscular patients. Semin Pediatr Neurol 5:106–115, 1998.

218. Toyka KV, Heininger K: Humoral factors in peripheral nerve disease. Muscle Nerve 10:222, 1987.

219. Trojaborg W: Invited review: Acute and chronic neuropathies: New aspects of Guillain-Barré syndrome and chronic inflammatory demyelinating polyneuropathy, an overview and an update. Electroenceph Clin Neurophysiol 107:303–316, 1998.

220. van der Putten JJ, et al: Measuring change in disability after inpatient rehabilitation: Comparison of responsiveness of the Barthel Index and the Functional Independence Measure. J Neurol Neurosurg Psychiatry 66:480–484, 1999.

221. Vignos PJ: Physical models of rehabilitation in neuromuscular disease. Muscle Nerve 6:323, 1983.

222. Vignos PJ, Spencer GE, Archibald KC: Management of progressive muscular dystrophy of childhood. JAMA 184:89, 1963.

223. Vignos PJ, Watkins MP: The effect of exercise in muscular dystrophy. JAMA 197(11):843–848, 1966.

224. Vignos PJ, et al: Evaluation of a program for long-term treatment of Duchenne muscular dystrophy. J Bone Joint Surg Am 78:1844–1852, 1996.

225. Vine P: Families in Pain. New York, Pantheon Books, 1982.

226. Warren CG: The use of heat and cold in the treatment of common musculoskeletal disorders. *In* Kessler RM, Hertling D (eds): Management of Common Musculoskeletal Disorders: Physical Therapy Principles and Methods. Philadelphia, Harper & Row, 1983.

227. Warren CG: Elongation of rat tail tendon: Effect of load and temperature. Arch Phys Med Rehabil 52:465, 1971.

228. Warren CG, et al: Heat and stretch procedures: An evaluation using rat tail tendon. Arch Phys Med Rehabil 57:122, 1976.

229. Wetzel JL, et al: Respiratory rehabilitation of the patient with a spinal cord injury. *In* Irwin S, Tecklin JS (eds): Cardiopulmonary Physical Therapy. St. Louis, CV Mosby, 1990.

230. Wilbourn AJ: Clinical neurophysiology in the diagnosis of amyotrophic lateral sclerosis: The Lambert and the El Escorial criteria. J Neurol Sci 160(Suppl 1):S25–S29, 1998.

231. Willig TN, et al: Nutritional rehabilitation in neuromuscular disorders. Semin Neurol 15:18–23, 1995.

232. Wilson J, et al (eds): Harrison's Principles of Internal Medicine, 12th ed. New York, McGraw-Hill, 1991.

233. Winer JB, et al: Prognosis in Guillain-Barré syndrome. Lancet 1:1202–1203, 1985.

234. Witte RA: The psychosocial impact of a progressive physical handicap and terminal illness (Duchenne muscular dystrophy) on adolescents and their families. Br J Med Psychol 58:179, 1985.

235. Wright NC, et al: Aerobic walking in slowly progressive neuromuscular disease: Effect of a 12-week program. Arch Phys Med Rehabil 77:64–69, 1996.

236. Wyngaarden JB, et al (eds): Cecil Textbook of Medicine, 19th ed. Philadelphia, WB Saunders, 1992.

237. Zachazewski JE: Improving flexibility. *In* Scully RM, Barnes MR (eds): Physical Therapy. Philadelphia, JB Lippincott, 1989.

238. Zochodne DW: Autonomic involvement in Guillain-Barré syndrome: A review. Muscle Nerve 17:1145–1155, 1994.

Traumatic Brain Injury

PATRICIA A. WINKLER, MS, PT

Key Words

- anticipatory responses
- knowledge of results
- learning theory
- motor control
- motor learning
- motor skill
- plasticity
- synergy
- systems theory
- traumatic head injury

Objectives

After reading this chapter the student/therapist will:

1. Have an understanding of current concepts in motor control and motor learning theories.

2. Understand the meaning of impairment, disability, and handicap and their interrelationships.

3. Be knowledgeable in methods of assessing, evaluating, and treating head-injured clients based on impairment and disability analysis.

4. Be able to differentiate between development of basic movement patterns and motor skills.

5. Understand the role of synergy formation, synergy selection and modification, and anticipatory <u>and</u> feedback information as used in motor skills.

6. Be familiar with the learning concepts of knowledge of results, whole-task practice, and breaking tasks into natural subtasks.

The National Head Injury Foundation provides the following definition of traumatic head injury[88, 89]:

Traumatic head injury is an insult to the brain, . . . caused by an external physical force, that may produce a diminished or altered state of consciousness, which results in impairment of cognitive abilities or physical functioning. It can also result in the disturbance of behavioral or emotional functioning. These may be either temporary or permanent and cause partial or total functional disability or psychological maladjustment.

OVERVIEW OF BRAIN INJURY

Epidemiology of Traumatic Brain Injury

Every 5 minutes in the United States one person dies and another becomes disabled as a result of a traumatic brain injury (TBI). One million people with brain injuries are treated in emergency departments every year, 230,000 with injuries severe enough to require hospitalization. Fifty thousand people die yearly of TBI, 80,000 injuries result in disabilities, and 5.3 million people are living with permanent disabilities from TBI. Brain injury is the leading killer and disabler of children and young adults.[26] Motor vehicle crashes cause 50% of all TBIs, falls cause 21%, violence causes 12% (the majority from firearms), and sports and recreation account for 10%. Child abuse accounts for 64% of infant brain injuries. Fifty thousand children sustain bicycle-related brain injuries, and 400 of these die.[29] Two thirds of firearm-related TBIs are suicidal. Falls are the leading cause of TBI in people aged 65 and older, with 11% proving fatal.[26]

Population of Brain-Injured Clients

The incidence of brain injuries is higher for males than for females by more than 2:1. The majority of those injured are between 15 and 24 years old.[26]

Cost

The estimated lifetime cost for each severely brain-injured individual exceeds $4 million. Annual costs for all TBIs in the United States exceed $48 billion dollars.[26]

Mechanisms of Injury

External forces impacting the brain cause TBI. Injuries include those with skull fracture and those without skull fracture (closed head injuries).

Direct blows to the head can cause coup injuries (at the site of impact) and contrecoup injuries (distant from the site of impact). Penetrating objects cause direct cellular and vascular damage. Injuries to the face and neck can cause brain injury by damaging the blood supply to the brain.[56]

Pathophysiology of Injury

Acceleration, deceleration, and rotational forces as well as penetrating objects act to cause tissue laceration, compression, tension, shearing, or a combination resulting in primary injury.

Primary Damage

Contusions and lacerations of the brain can occur with or without skull fractures. Either an object hits the head, neck, or face, or the head hits an object. Damage suffered can be to any area of the brain. Occipital blows are more likely to produce contusions than are frontal or lateral blows. Areas in which the cranial vault is irregular, such as on the anterior poles, undersurface of the temporal lobes, and undersurface of the frontal lobes, are commonly injured. Lacerations of blood vessels within the brain itself or of blood vessels that feed the brain from the neck or face can be injured and reduce the flow of blood carrying oxygen to the brain.

Contusions and lacerations can also injure the cranial nerves. The most commonly injured are the optic, vestibulocochlear, oculomotor, abducens, and facial nerves. Lacerations of dura and/or arachnoid may cause cerebrospinal fluid to discharge from the nose (cerebrospinal fluid rhinorrhea in which discharge increases with neck flexion, coughing, or straining[67]).

Diffuse axonal injury, or shearing injuries, may be one of the most common types of primary lesions in patients with brain trauma.[1, 119] Unequal acceleration, deceleration, or rotation of contingent tissues, which differ in structure, causes diffuse axonal injury. Severing of the axons may be severe enough to result in coma. In milder forms, more spotty lesions are seen, including deficits such as memory loss, concentration difficulties, decreased attention span, headaches, sleep disturbances, and seizures. Damage often involves the corpus callosum,[67, 119] basal ganglia, brain stem, and cerebellum.

Penetrating objects with high velocities, such as bullets, can cause additional damage remote from the areas of impact secondary to shock waves. Foreign objects such as sticks and sharp toys cause low-velocity injuries, directly damaging the tissues they impact.

Secondary Damage

Secondary injuries are mainly due to a lack of oxygen in the high-oxygen–demanding brain. Secondary problems may result from the following:

1. *Increased intracranial pressure* (due to swelling or intracranial hematoma). Swelling of the brain causes distortion because the brain is held in the skull, a rigid, unyielding structure. The resultant increased intracranial pressure can lead to herniation of parts of the brain. The most often seen herniations include cingulate herniation under the falx cerebri, uncus herniation, central (or transtentorial) herniation, and herniation of the brain stem through the foramen magnum.[48]

   Acute hydrocephalus occurs when blood accumulates in the ventricular system, expanding the size of the ventricles and causing increased pressure on brain tissue being compressed between the skull and the fluid-filled ventricles. The increased pressure can then result in changes in Pco_2, which is also harmful to nervous tissue.

   Increased intracranial pressure has been correlated with poorer outcomes and higher mortality rates.[113]
2. *Cerebral hypoxia or ischemia* (occurring when blood vessels are ruptured or compressed). Hypoxia can occur from a lack of blood to the brain or from lack of oxygen in the blood secondary to airway obstruction or chest injuries.
3. *Intracranial hemorrhage,* causing hypoxia to tissues fed by the hemorrhaging blood vessels as well as adding pressure and distortion to brain tissue. Metabolic products from damaged cells and blood bathe the brain. Cell death occurs within minutes after injury from ischemia, edema, necrosis, and the toxic effects of blood on neural tissues.
4. *Electrolyte imbalance and acid-base imbalance.* Secondary cell death occurs either by swelling and then bursting of the cellular membrane (necrosis) or by destruction from within the cell through changes in the DNA (apoptosis). Cell death can occur days, weeks, or months after injury.[17]

5. *Infection secondary to open wounds.* Infection in brain tissue may cause swelling and cell death.
6. *Seizures due to pressure or scarring.* Seizures are most common immediately after injury and between 6 months and 2 years after injury. The seizures can cause additional brain damage owing to high oxygen and glucose requirements.

Physiological, Cognitive, and Behavioral Changes After Brain Injury

Autonomic Nervous System Changes. These may include changes in pulse and respiratory rates and regularity, temperature elevations, blood pressure changes, and excessive sweating, salivation, tearing, and sebum secretion.[24]

Motor, Functional, Sensory, and Perceptual Changes. Motor abnormalities after severe head trauma are common. The terms "decorticate rigidity" and "decerebrate rigidity" are often used to denote abnormal posturing. Decerebrate rigidity denotes extension in all four limbs. Decorticate posturing includes flexion of the upper extremities and extension of the legs. These postures are not always well defined in clients, and a description of the abnormalities is preferred.

Common motor abnormalities include monoplegia or hemiplegia and abnormal reflexes. Great variability exists. Initial flaccidity can gradually become spasticity or rigidity. Abnormal extensor responses in upper and lower extremities, abnormal extensor responses in the upper extremities with flaccidity or weak flexor responses in the lower extremities, absence of motor responses (flaccidity), or a mixture of these can occur. Change can be bilateral or unilateral. Furthermore, a client can initially display flexor responses in the arms that can later change to extensor responses. These shifts possibly reflect the physiological effects of changes in the amount of tissue compression or irritation.[95] Daily changes in tone can be stimulated by internal irritants as well as by external stimuli. Motor disturbances of timing, sequencing, and coordination can occur when trauma is to the cerebellar areas. Combinations of asymmetrical cerebellar and pyramidal signs and of bilateral pyramidal and extrapyramidal signs have all been reported.[97] The specific manifestations can include a wide range of deficits, such as loss of selective motor control, balance, and sensation. Primitive reflexes can return, and the presence of abnormal tone may be noted.

Aphasia, dysarthria, dysphagia, and visuospatial and perceptual motor difficulties can occur because of focal lesions.

Cranial nerve involvement is common. Abnormalities in pupil size, shape, and light reflexes can be manifested unilaterally or bilaterally. Eye movements can be abnormal, as can the oculocephalic and oculovestibular reflexes. In coma, brain stem responses may include grimacing to pain, which is frequently associated with a flexor or localizing motor response. The pharyngeal reflex may also be absent; the implications of this are obvious. There may be facial paralysis, loss of hearing or balance, abnormal palate and tongue movements, and loss or distortion of taste.

More severe head injuries tend to manifest more persistent physical problems.[67] In at least two studies[67, 97] a quarter of the cases had no neurophysical sequelae.

Changes in Consciousness/Coma. Changes in consciousness including coma result from conditions in which there are diffusely extensive and bilateral cerebral hemispheric depression of function, direct depression or destruction of the brain stem–activating system that is responsible for consciousness, or a combination of the two. In moderate or severe head injury, unconsciousness can be prolonged.

Plum and Posner's definitions[95] of various stages of acutely altered consciousness are briefly presented, intermingled with some insights from the descriptions offered by Gilroy and Meyer.[48] Plum and Posner[95] do not equate the presence or absence of motor responses with the depth of coma. These authors point out that the neural structures regulating consciousness differ from and are more anatomically distant from those regulating motor function.

In mild concussion, the loss of consciousness lasts a relatively short time and there is little or no retrograde amnesia. The client may be irritable or distractible and have difficulty with reading and memory. There may be complaints of headache, fatigue, dizziness, and changes in personality and emotional disposition. This group of symptoms constitutes what is called posttraumatic syndrome. The effects of repeated concussions are cumulative.[106]

Coma is defined as a complete paralysis of cerebral function, a state of unresponsiveness. The eyes are closed, and there is no response to painful stimuli. Within 2 to 4 weeks, nearly all clients in coma begin to awaken. Oculomotor and pupillary signs are valuable in assisting with the diagnosis, localizing brain stem damage, and determining the depth of coma.[95]

Stupor is a condition of general unresponsiveness. However, the client, who is usually mute, can be temporarily aroused by vigorous and repeated stimuli. *Obtundity* describes the condition of a client who sleeps a great deal and who, when aroused, exhibits reduced alertness, disinterest in the environment, and slow responses to stimulation. *Delirium* is often observed in recovery from unconsciousness after severe brain injury. Disorientation, fear, and misinterpretation of sensory stimuli characterize this state. The client is frequently loud, agitated, and offensive. *Clouding of consciousness* is a state of quiet confusion, distractibility, faulty memory, and slowed responses to stimuli.

Recovery of consciousness, if it occurs, includes a gradual return of orientation and recent memory.[95] The duration of each of these stages is variable and can be prolonged. Improvement can be arrested at any point.

Finally, no discussion of changes in consciousness would be complete without mention of those unfortunate enough to remain in a "persistent vegetative state." This state is characterized by a wakeful, reduced responsiveness with no evident cerebral cortical function. The vegetative state can result from diffuse cerebral hypoxia or from severe, diffuse white matter impact damage. The brain stem is usually relatively intact. Clients may track with their eyes and show minimal spontaneous motor activities that even appear purposeful, but they do not speak, nor do they respond to verbal stimulation.[65] Life expectancy can be weeks, months, or years.[66, 101] Brain-injured clients who remain vegetative for 3 months rarely achieve an independent outcome. However, the term "persistent" should not be added to "vegetative state" until the injury has stabilized or the state has lasted for approximately 1 year.[10]

Cognitive, Personality, and Behavioral Changes. Temporary or permanent disorders of intellectual function and memory are frequent. Uncontrolled anger, irritability, memory loss, shortened attention span, concentration problems, perseveration, reduced problem-solving skills, lack of initiative, loss of reasoning, poor abstract thinking, and inappropriate social behaviors all can be secondary effects of TBI.

Cognitive and behavioral sequelae can result from generalized or focal brain injuries. Memory impairments are an aftermath of generalized lesions.

Two types of amnesia are frequently associated with brain injury: retrograde and posttraumatic.[41] Cartlidge and Shaw[24] define retrograde amnesia as a "partial or total loss of the ability to recall events that have occurred during the period immediately preceding brain injury." The duration of the retrograde amnesia may progressively decrease.

Posttraumatic amnesia is defined "as the time lapse between the accident and the point at which the functions concerned with memory are judged to have been restored."[24] The duration of posttraumatic amnesia is considered a clinical indicator of the severity of the injury.[24] An additional deficit can be the inability to form new memory, referred to as anterograde memory. The capacity for anterograde memory is frequently the last function to return after recovery from loss of consciousness.[102]

The client's inability to develop ongoing short-term memory can be quite frustrating for the rehabilitation team as well as the client because memory is an important component of learning.[116] There are two types of memory: declarative and procedural. Memory in which the client can recall facts and events of a previous experience is called declarative memory. Explicit learning, a conscious, verbal learning, is based on declarative memory. However, many clients who cannot reproduce memories through conscious recollection do have learning skills.

Implicit learning, a noncognitive type of learning in which clients can show changes in performance after prior experience, is based on procedural memory. Clients can show the ability to change motor, perceptual, or cognitive behaviors with practice or training but may lack declarative memory. That procedural memory may be present without declarative memory in clients with TBI has been demonstrated in several studies.[41]

Many clients with brain injury suffer injuries to the frontal lobe areas of the brain that control executive functions. Executive functions are those that affect how behavior is regulated. Lezak[79] outlined four functions: (1) choosing a goal, (2) developing a plan, (3) executing a plan, and (4) evaluating the execution of the plan.

Deficits in attention are also common. Clients show impulsiveness, hyperactivity, and difficulty sustaining attention.

Emotional changes may be seen with lesions in the orbitofrontal areas. Behavior may be excessive and disinhibited. Also, euphoria, irritability, intolerance, inappropriate sexual behavior, and generally inappropriate social and interpersonal behaviors occur with lesions in this area. Septal area lesions result in rage and overall irritability. Pseudobulbar injuries can result in emotional lability of involuntary laughing or crying not associated with feelings of emotions.

Behavioral changes can be present even without cognitive and physical deficits. Although actual psychoses can be sequelae, they appear to be neither common nor definitively related to the brain injury. The social consequences of inappropriate behavior can be disastrous and a stumbling block to achieving therapy goals. A correlation between preinjury personality and postinjury changes has not been established.[67] It does seem reasonable, however, that factors within an individual's psychological makeup may affect reaction to the injury. Head trauma frequently happens to adolescents—an age group fraught with its own problems that may be aggravated by the injury.

Depression occurs frequently after brain injury and can alter functional outcome. It appears that a combination of neuroanatomical, neurochemical, and psychosocial factors are responsible for the onset and maintenance of the depression.[100]

Other Complications. A list of the complications that may accompany brain injury would be limitless. In addition to any concomitant injuries, some of the diagnostic, monitoring, and therapeutic procedures themselves carry hazards. So does prolonged bed rest. Catheters, nasogastric tubes, and tracheotomies can cause iatrogenic injuries. Infections, contractures, skin breakdown, thrombophlebitis, pulmonary problems, heterotopic ossification, and surgical complications are but a few risks. Posttraumatic epilepsy is also a possible sequela. See the box on page 420 for additional information.

Examination

The selection of tests depends on the availability of the special equipment required for testing and on the perceived need for the tests. The results of some of these procedures may secondarily aid the therapist in the selection of intervention strategies. Conversely, other monitoring procedures may restrict the choice of therapeutic approaches.

Testing depends on the client's particular dysfunctions. Computed tomography (CT),[114] magnetic resonance imaging (MRI), cerebral angiography, positron emission tomography (PET), radioisotope imaging, ventriculography, echoencephalography, electroencephalography (EEG), monitoring of intracranial pressure, measurement of cerebral blood flow and metabolism, monitoring of cardiorespiratory and cardiovascular function, and cerebrospinal fluid and other biochemical studies all provide good information. Changes in electrocerebral potentials that occur in response to specific stimuli also are studied. Visual, auditory, and somatosensory evoked potential examina-

FACTORS THAT CAN INFLUENCE MANAGEMENT AND RECOVERY AFTER A TRAUMATIC HEAD INJURY

Preinjury Characteristics

A. Cognitive factors
   1. Intelligence°
   2. Memory
   3. Level of education

B. Behavioral factors
   1. Personality°
   2. Psychological status

C. Social factors
   1. Vocational skills
   2. Avocational skills
   3. Interpersonal skills
   4. Family/friends support systems

D. Physical factors
   1. Age°
   2. General health and physical fitness
   3. Existing physical deficits
   4. Morphology
   5. Level of **motor skill** development and capacity for motor learning

Postinjury Characteristics

A. Static factors
   1. Trauma factors (neurological)
      a. Location(s) and extent of injury
      b. Cause and type of injury°
      c. Immediacy of injury°
   2. Cognitive factors
      a. Ultimate duration of retrograde amnesia (RA)°
      b. Ultimate duration of posttraumatic amnesia (PTA)°
   3. Physical factors: extracranial injuries

B. Dynamic factors
   1. Trauma factors (neurological)
      a. Depth and duration of coma°
      b. Secondary brain damage
      c. Brain stem reflexes
      d. Special investigations (radiological and laboratory tests)
   2. Cognitive factors
      a. Rate of recovery of intellectual and memory functions°
      b. Quality of recovery of intellectual and memory functions°
      c. Communication disorders
   3. Behavioral factors
      a. Primary personality changes°
      b. Secondary personality changes°
      c. Psychological status
   4. Social factors
      a. Opportunity to reenter occupation/school
      b. Avocational reintegration abilities
      c. Reaction to family/friends
      d. Family adjustment and support capabilities°
   5. Physical factors
      a. Pattern and quality of sensorimotor recovery°
      b. Rate of recovery of sensorimotor function°
      c. Range of motion and muscle flexibility
      d. Cranial nerve deficits
      e. Concomitant disabilities
   6. Environmental factors
      a. Staff/facilities/equipment available
      b. Attitude of health care providers
      c. Expertise of health care providers
      d. Room/housing and treatment settings

°Discussed in the text.

tions are used with brain-injured clients but are more effective when combined with other examinations.[135] These examinations make it possible to observe the presence, evolution, and resolution of a lesion.[67]

With the possible exception of the diagnosis and, hence, prognosis of diffuse white matter impact damage,[148] the Glasgow study[64] and other studies[75, 148] indicate that prediction of outcome should not be based on CT or MRI alone.

Evoked potential studies may aid in prognosis[55, 95]; however, the usefulness and significance of evoked potential studies with these clients are still being investigated (see Chapter 28 for additional information).

A third of the clients hospitalized with brain injuries have extracranial injuries, which are explored with a physical examination and appropriate special tests.[67]

Reflex motor responses in unconscious clients are tested by applying a noxious stimulus, such as pressure on a nail bed using a pencil or supraorbital pressure, and observing the response. Most responses generally fall into three categories: appropriate, inappropriate, or absent.[95] The Glasgow Coma Scale (see box on page 421) is used to grade coma severity.

Testing for cognitive and behavioral functions is usually done by neuropsychological tests. In some circumstances, previous tests including IQ tests, achievement tests, and Armed Forces tests may be available for comparison.

Differentiating changes in cognitive and behavioral functions caused by brain injury from posttraumatic stress syndrome, conversion or hysterical reactions, malingering, depression, and anxiety is extremely important.

Early Hospitalization

On the client's admission to the hospital, a neurosurgeon usually assumes initial and primary responsibility for the client. The first priority in medical care is resuscitation, after which baseline assessments are made and a history obtained. Immediate surgery may or may not be indi-

GLASGOW COMA SCALE

Eye opening	**E**
Spontaneous	4
To speech	3
To pain	2
Nil	1
Best motor response	**M**
Obeys	6
Localizes	5
Withdraws	4
Abnormal flexion	3
Extensor response	2
Nil	1
Verbal response	**V**
Oriented	5
Confused conversation	4
Inappropriate words	3
Incomprehensible sounds	2
Nil	1
Coma Score (E + M + V) = 3 to 15	

From Jennett B, Teasdale G: Management of Head Injuries. Philadelphia, FA Davis, 1981.

cated. Surgery is indicated in cases where blood and necrotic tissue are present in the cranial vault.

Early concerns may include the management of respiratory dysfunction, cardiovascular monitoring, treatment of raised intracranial pressure by means of pharmacological, mechanical, or surgical procedures,[24] and general medical care. Examples of general medical care are familiar: maintenance of fluid and electrolyte balance, nutrition, eye and skin care, prevention of contractures, postural drainage, and safety considerations.[67] The need for this type of care gradually lessens as the client responds, or it may continue if unconsciousness persists.

Pharmacological Interventions

Fulop and colleagues[43] recently reviewed pharmacological interventions after brain injury. Their article separates the medications by symptoms to be treated as follows:

1. *Drugs that decrease intracranial pressure.* When intracranial pressure (ICP) increases, changes in P_{CO_2} are seen. A P_{CO_2} between 30 and 40 appears most appropriate. Osmotic agents such as mannitol are used to pull fluid from brain tissue back into the blood system, thus lowering intracranial pressure.

   Intracranial pressure has, in the past, been lowered by intentional hyperventilation, which causes an increase in blood P_{CO_2} resulting in vasoconstriction of the central vessels and reduced cerebral blood flow. However, Muizelaar and colleagues[85] as well as information from the traumatic coma data band[45] showed that dramatically reducing a client's P_{CO_2} in this manner resulted in a worse outcome than that in clients managed with medication. Therefore, hyperventilation is currently used only for nonresponsive cases and for short durations. Glucocorticoids have been used to treat cerebral edema (dexamethasone [Decadron], methylprednisolone [Solu-Medrol]), but most studies show no long-term changes in outcome.[33] Finally, barbiturates have been used to lower intracranial pressure but carry a high mortality rate.[17] See Chapter 32 for additional information.

2. *Drugs that control blood pressure.* Blood pressure control is important in brain-injured clients. In a study of 717 clients with TBI, systolic blood pressure below 90 mm Hg during resuscitation was a predictor of poor outcome.[16] Cerebral perfusion pressure[27] or adequate blood pressure to maintain cerebral blood flow against increased intracranial pressure is calculated by subtracting the ICP from the mean arterial pressure. If fluid management cannot keep the blood pressures elevated, then vasopressor drugs such as phenylephrine (Neo-Synephrine) are used. They constrict peripheral vessels but not the vessels of the brain.

3. *Drugs to treat the physiological injury.* Experimental substances that have been useful in animals are currently being tried in humans to prevent secondary damage and promote nervous system recovery or regeneration. Free radical–scavenging compounds such as vitamin E (alpha-tocopherol), superoxide dismutase, dimethyl sulfoxide (DMSO), and *Ginkgo biloba* preparations have been shown to speed recovery after brain damage in animals.

   The brain produces neurotrophic agents such as nerve growth factor in response to damage. These neurotrophins are thought to prevent neuronal death[58] and are being added to TBI regimens in a few cases. Substances that affect glial cell function are also being investigated. Endogenous glycolipid ganglioside (GM_1) has improved function in rats but has not been successful in humans.

4. *Drugs that affect the motor, behavioral, and cognitive functions* (see Chapter 32). Medications also may be prescribed for motor abnormalities involving increases in tone. Baclofen is now used more frequently with brain-injured clients; however, baclofen also can produce lethargy, confusion,[147] and reduction in attention span[51] in some clients. These effects are greatly reduced with implantation of a pump to deliver the baclofen. Dantrolene sodium is another medication used to decrease spasticity and rigidity. This drug works directly at the muscle level and therefore is less likely to cause cognitive disturbances but more likely to cause generalized weakness.[146] Botulinum toxin type A (Botox) is now widely used to inject into specific muscles, such as the finger flexors, biceps, or gastrocnemius, to decrease that muscle's tone. Diazepam (Valium) initially was the drug most commonly administered for spasticity or high tone. However, diazepam also promotes drowsiness and decreased respon-

siveness and can increase muscle weakness and ataxia.[147] These side effects actually hinder rather than assist in rehabilitation. Glenn and Wrobewski[51] conclude that "rarely, if ever, are the benefits of diazepam's antispasticity effect great enough to justify its use in the brain-injured population."

Drugs to treat behavioral or cognitive dysfunction have not been particularly successful. Antidepressive drugs as well as carbamazepine (Tegretol) and propranolol (Inderal) have been used to treat aggression and agitation. There have been several reports that carbamazepine reduced agitation or aggression in brain-injured clients.[86]

Sedative drugs prescribed in an attempt to control delirium may add to the client's confusion[67] and may also contribute to a decreased responsiveness. Later in the rehabilitative process, various antidepressants may be used to treat aggressive and disruptive behaviors. These, too, may have deleterious side effects. Antidepressents other than the tricyclics are apparently the most effective for treating depression.[1]

Traumatically acquired neuroendocrine dysfunctions, such as hyperphagia and thermal regulation, also may be treated with pharmacological agents.[50]

Severe, intractable pain may be present in clients who have suffered injury to the thalamus. In these cases, some of the antiseizure drugs appear to be more effective, including phenytoin (Dilantin) and gabapentin (Neurontin). Late seizure control is usually through valproic acid (Depakote or Depakene).

Other pharmaceutical agents are prescribed as an adjunct to care for a variety of reasons. Antibiotics may be used with respiratory complications or with compound fractures.

Prognostic Indicators

Numerous problems are encountered in trying to predict outcome. Included among these problems are the reliability of the tests used, the uniform implementation and interpretation of predictive factors, the percentage of error in prediction, the possible effects of intervention strategies and bias in treatment based on predictions, and, finally, the definition of what constitutes a "successful" outcome. Understanding these problems is imperative because the therapist can provide persuasive suggestions as to the type and intensity of rehabilitative care after injury. Accordingly, the following discussion of prediction includes some possible prognostic indicators.

If, indeed, there are factors or tests that have predictive value, then they need to be identified or administered, respectively, and the data compared and interpreted uniformly. The differences in operational definitions, types and sizes of populations, and length of time after injury when outcome assessment was made contribute to the lack of consistency in studies of predictive factors. For example, several authors have found that clients younger than age 20 usually recover[8, 76, 117]; however, even this has not been uniformly confirmed.[47]

Another concern is the percentage of error in prediction. If prediction is 80% or even 90% accurate, there are still 10% to 20% of the clients with head trauma whose outcome may be predicted incorrectly. Even if the statistics are significant, one may feel very differently if the client whose future is misinterpreted is a family member.

Van der Naalt and coworkers[127] report a positive correlation between outcomes of clients with mild to moderate brain injury and lesions on CT and also in patients with cerebral edema. Lesions in the frontal regions found on early MRI were predictive of outcome. Late MRI showing focal atrophy in the frontotemporal regions was also predictive of outcome. MRI in 80 adult patients (6 to 8 weeks after injury)[70] was predictive of nonrecovery from persistent vegetative states at 12 months when the client had corpus callosum and dorsolateral brain stem lesions.

One study of the Glasgow Coma Scale[64] indicates that this scale is a simple and consistent outcome predictor. A study of 67 patients[128] with a Glasgow Coma Scale score between 9 and 14 (mild to moderate brain injury) on admission were studied 12 months after injury. Outcome correlated with duration of posttraumatic amnesia and Glasgow Outcome Scale (see the box on page 423) related to time in coma or stupor[118] ($r = 0.46$) but not with Glasgow Coma Scale score ($r = 0.19$).[95] Eighty-two percent of brain injuries had good recovery according to the Glasgow Outcome Scale. Other studies,[82, 126] however, have not confirmed the scale's reliability and suggest that the criteria may not be applied in standard fashion.

Several studies have reported that absence of substance abuse, absence of previous TBI,[27] a higher level of educational achievement, and stable work history also are positive preinjury variables for better prognosis.[39]

The Wechsler Adult Intelligence Scale (WAIS)—Revised IQ test may correlate with prognosis according to some studies.[39]

Outcomes (Management Results)

Motor disturbances resulting from brain injury generally have a good prognosis.[24] Of the physical deficits encountered, dysfunctions in the cerebral hemispheres and of the cranial nerves are the most common disorders, and these may partially resolve. In one Glasgow study, some degree of hemiparesis was present 6 months after injury in 49% of the 150 clients who regained consciousness after severe brain injury.[67]

Absence of brain stem reflexes usually indicates a poorer prognosis, but this is not necessarily a predictor of ultimate outcome.[24] Interpretation can be difficult, partially because of the variety of influences on these signs.[67]

As already mentioned, damage to one or more cranial nerves is not uncommon. Recuperation tends to occur, except that with hearing, vestibular function, and smell, complete recovery is rare. Losses of these functions can be more permanent,[24, 48] especially without skilled rehabilitation interventions.

Psychosocial outcomes vary after severe brain injury.[14] Psychosocial variables that significantly increased life satisfaction for persons with TBI were total family satisfaction, being employed, being married, having memory and bowel independence, and not blaming oneself for the injury. Those who do not blame themselves show a greater number of functional activities as indicators for their self-satisfaction.[131]

CONCEPTUAL FRAMEWORK FOR THERAPEUTIC INTERVENTION

Motor Control Theory

Motor control and learning theories try to explain how the central nervous system (CNS) accomplishes the miracle of coordinated, meaningful movement.

Motor control theory and factors affecting effectiveness and speed of motor learning are reviewed here in this section and are discussed in detail in Chapters 4 and 5. This chapter's examination, evaluation, and intervention techniques sections are based on that framework. A quick review of basic principles follows.

Synergistic Organization

Synergies, or motor patterns, were seen by Bernstein[9] as the basis of movement. The need for the brain to use synergistic organization comes from the infinite number of movement combinations that are available. By use of synergies, flexibility of response is maintained but speed and efficiency are added. Force (amplitude) of contraction, velocity, and timing can be changed to meet task demands.

Research suggests that synergies are shaped through experience and that they develop before birth (innate) and after birth (learned).

Early experiments on motor learning demonstrate how synergies may develop. Payton and Kelley[93] showed that, with practice of a novel motor task, movements become more organized. In learning a new skill, movement begins with a "gross approximation" of the movement that includes agonist/antagonist co-contraction. As movement is refined, reciprocal movement replaces co-contration.[107] In electrophysiological studies of skill acquisition, less electrical activity is seen on electromyography (EMG) and less time to peak activation of the muscle is noted in motor tasks after they are better learned. Additionally, fewer muscles are recruited for the same movement.[22] PET scans have confirmed these EMG findings, demonstrating decreasing areas of brain activity after skill acquisition.

Neuronal changes brought about through long-term potentiation and long-term depression are a basis for learning new tasks and developing synergies and behavioral changes.[32] As neurons are repetitively fired at the same time, networks develop. These neuronetwork or cell assemblies are formed with increasing complexity and self-organization. The more they are used, the stronger and more permanent are the changes that occur. Finally, specific stimulus now provokes a learned or skilled response. The output of the networks is not a summation of individual functions but has "emergent properties" that are more than the sum of the output of individual neurons.

The best understood synergies are the balance and reaching patterns. Both appear to be basic innate synergies. Quiet standing in humans is maintained by somatosensory, visual, and vestibular inputs. It requires the coordination of many muscles, especially those of the hips, knees, and ankles, to maintain the body's center of gravity over its base of support. This complex coordination of muscle control is accomplished by sequences of stereotyped patterns mediated through the brain stem, cerebellum, and spinal cord. Somatosensory input during body sway stimulates the response in which posture is stabilized by small changes in the angle between the foot and the leg. For example, when length, force of contraction, or movement velocity of the calf muscles exceeds a preset threshold, somatosensory signals to the brain initiate rapid postural readjustments by triggering a synergistic response to decrease sway. For small center of gravity movements, these synergies are sequenced in a distal to proximal manner. The direction of sway determines the particular synergy elicited to correct for the shift in the center of gravity. In forward losses of balance the posterior extensor muscles of the legs and trunk respond at about 100 ms. In backward losses, the anterior muscles respond including anterior tibialis, hip flexors, and abdominals. The timing between muscle contractions and the proximal to distal sequence are preset. The amplitude of contraction varies with the environmental demands and the amount and velocity of sway. In greater losses of balance, a different synergy is used in which the person may bend at the hips and knees. If the balance loss is great enough, the person takes a step to maintain upright balance.[87] (For additional information see Chapter 21 on balance and vestibular dysfunction.)

In gait, weight shifts from one leg to the other and stability after the weight shift are other aspects of dynamic balance performed through synergies. The movement pattern of the swing leg in gait is limited in number of degrees of freedom at each joint and sequence of movement by synergies. There is also a specific coordination and timing of swing leg movement in relation to the stance leg movement (interlimb timing and coordination).

In walking, the sequence of contraction of the leg muscle from ankle to hip, the time of onset of the contraction of each muscle, and a ratio of force for each muscle are all preset in the motor control program of the brain or spinal cord. If an increase in speed is needed, force can be increased within the synergy, but the basic synergies, or motor patterns, are what give identity to a gait pattern. Whether the person is walking fast or slow, there is an individually recognizable pattern.

In the reaching and grasping pattern, three components have been identified: the reaching portion (transport), the grasping or prehension portion, and the maintenance of balance. The reaching and maintenance of balance are synergies.[46, 53] The target determines the reaching pattern. Again, there is a distal to proximal sequence of firing. Movement is in a straight line and the velocity curve is always bell shaped.[83]

The characteristics of hand control differ from control of many other parts of the body. Hand control is not a synergistic movement. Unlike in many motor acts, the motor/sensory cortex helps with force production and selection of muscles[40] during hand movement. This may be why more severe deficits are seen in the hand after cortical injury.

Anticipatory and Adaptive Responses

To meet the motor task (external) requirements, synergies are used and modified through a feedforward and feedback system of control. The brain adapts synergies to environmental constraints, such as obstacles, by modifying the basic synergies' velocity, intensity, and/or duration of contractions before the movement even begins.

Feedforward, or anticipatory response (often from vision and past memory of successful movements), is used for the initial movement. Feedback is used to check the effectiveness of the response and modify it, if needed. A final check is made to determine that the motor pattern matched the original "planned" pattern after movement occurred. These adaptive responses allow modification for environmental changes and are usually mediated through sensory system feedback.

Sensory information helps fine tune the subsequent steps in the walking example. When movement of the head occurs, the visual array moves in the peripheral visual field, the joints and muscles move, and the semicircular canals' hair cells fire. These sensory impulses result in motor system adaptations to the environment. In the reaching/prehension pattern, target location is coded by the visual system. Both the spatial and temporal conditions are present before the movement begins. Once the hand is at the target, the hand has already been shaped for prehension. Initially, grip is determined by the visual system (anticipatory response) and past memory (learning) of the characteristics of the object to be picked up. Tactile input from the finger tips (feedback) is then used to make adjustments in grip force if the initial grip was not effective.[68] Once movement occurs, there is a final comparison of the original planned pattern with the executed pattern to see if they match.

Another example of an anticipatory response is the backward shift triggered by gastrocnemius firing that occurs before a forward reach occurs.[62]

Dynamic Pattern Theory

The dynamic pattern theory[71, 111] addresses problems of when motor behavior changes and also uses concepts of basic patterns of movement. This theory states that certain patterns are very stable or unstable and that transition between patterns or to a new pattern depends on pattern stability. (See Giuliani[49] for a summary of this theory.)

The challenge for therapists is to identify what makes these "stuck" behaviors become more unstable and perhaps amenable to change. Patterns that are very "set" are much more difficult to change than those that are more variable. In fact, phase transitions between old and new patterns are noted by periods of increased variability. The client appears to vacillate between the old and the new behaviors during transition phases and before new behavior establishment points. Repetition is important to develop more consistent motor patterns and new establishment points.

Intervention Efficacy

Bach-y-Rita[3, 4] states that long-term rehabilitation is key to improved motor control and that recovery can continue to occur as long as the brain is challenged.

The concept that structural neural changes are influenced by the external environment is basic to physical and occupational therapy intervention; that is, activities in which a client participates change brain structure and organization.

Evidence that mammalian brain anatomy and function are modifiable by environmental factors was first irrefutably demonstrated by Wiesel and Hubel,[63, 136, 137] who described the importance of environmental experience on functional development of brain cells in the visual cortex of kittens. These experiments showed that visual experiences determine the synaptic organization of neurons in the visual cortex.

Devor[35] and many others have demonstrated plasticity in other sensory systems.

That physical intervention makes a difference in recovery after brain injury has been shown in many studies. Black and associates[11] showed an 82% recovery in monkeys that had early physical training and only a 67% recovery in those whose training did not start for 4 months after creation of their brain lesions. In the kitten sight deprivation studies of Mitchell and coworkers,[84] recovery occurred in the sutured eye only if the animal was forced to use that eye. Wolf and colleagues[142] and Taub and associates[122] showed that function in hemiplegic upper extremities is improved by forced use of the involved arm when the uninvolved arm was constrained. Tower[125] demonstrated that when brain lesions caused limb dysfunction, monkeys did not use the involved limb, but if the remaining useful limb was restrained, the monkeys used the original "useless" limb for climbing and other activities.

Active participation is also important in motor learning as Held's[60] experiments demonstrated. Plasticity in the normal CNS is well established. The neurophysiological mechanisms thought responsible for CNS recovery[69] after injury are discussed in earlier chapters.

Knowledge of Results

Interventions are designed to produce a task-oriented behavioral change that becomes permanent without continued therapist help or intervention. When this does not happen, the client performs well during therapy but does not seem to carry the improved performance outside the clinic. This difference between performance and learning is discussed by Schmidt[109, 110] (see Chapter 4).

Many therapy techniques that improve a client's performance inhibit learning because they are based on the external controls and support provided by the therapist's manipulations. The type of feedback and the method in which it is provided are critical to learning new motor skills. For example, when the hip stabilization component of walking is externally provided by the therapist during gait training, the client has no need to develop his or her own hip stabilization patterns, and feedback lacks a basic component of gait.

Knowledge of results, that is, information on how successful the movement was in meeting the task goals, is also basic to learning. Knowledge of results consists of extrinsic information over and above that proved by the task itself.[110] During the practice portion of most taks, increasing any type of feedback appears to improve task performance.[90] But long-term learning may occur better with knowledge of results provided less often. The relative frequency with which knowledge of results is provided in relation to the number of trials is important in learning. Bandwidth knowledge of results, in which information is given about trials falling outside a certain range, and a random schedule of feedback appear to be the most effective for learning. Delaying knowledge of results also improves learning.[110]

Changing Motor Function with Adaptive and Part-Task Training

The commonly used techniques of teaching a task by practicing at a slower speed or practicing a part of a motor task has not been shown to be effective. For example, to make walking easier, a therapist may have the client practice the stepping component of gait while providing balance support for the client. Weight shifting is often practiced as a component of gait before walking is initiated. In a study by Man and others,[81] a complex task was broken down into adaptive training methods (e.g., slower motions) and part-task training (on components of the task). Those practicing the whole task did as well as or better than either experimental group. This may explain why Winstein and others[141] found no carryover of successful weight shift training in standing to weight shift in walking in a group of hemiplegic clients. A finding that practicing small components of a task does not make one better at the whole task is not too surprising. Many of us can jump, have good shoulder power, and can throw overhead but cannot, without practice, put this together to play basketball. A minimum basic amount of strength, range of motion (ROM), and interlimb sequencing is necessary to play basketball but is not adequate to play without the actual practice of the sport.

Practicing other than the whole task may be possible. Using the same task as that used by Man and co-workers,[81] Newell and colleagues[91] showed that part-task training was effective when it was conducted in natural subtasks of the whole. These subtasks are part of the whole task but are distinguished by changes in speed or direction. This area of skill acquisition has not been studied adequately to identify subtasks of most common movements.

To review, the conceptual framework for the evaluation of and intervention in clients with TBI is based on distributed motor control theory that states movement is task or goal oriented and a result of combined systems working together to produce synergistic movement. Synergistic movement has an anticipatory component and is matched with sensory feedback and previous experience to contribute to task refinement, adaptation, and accomplishment. Changes in motor behavior may be determined by how "set" patterns (dynamic pattern theory) are influenced by the type of practice, knowledge of the effectiveness of the results, and how the motor skills are broken down for practice.

EXAMINATION, EVALUATION, AND INTERVENTION

The World Health Organization's International Classification of Impairment, Disability and Handicap (ICIDH)[144] can be useful for evaluation. In the ICIDH model, impairment is the result of disease at the organ level, disability is the result of impairment at the functional or skill level, and handicap is the consequence of impairment at the societal level.

Currently, many health care entities place more emphasis on disabilities than on impairments. There is much debate by the insurance industry, case managers, and therapists about a client's right to have a therapist reestablish normal movement and/or functional skill. Until societies truly accept people whose physical movements vary from "normal," however, there will be deficits in the handicap area, even for those who have no functional deficits. Societies have been unable to accept people with physical disabilities such as paralysis, ataxia, and dysarthria as fully capable.

Most of this section describes motor function; however, motor function is only a small part of the problem of the brain-injured client. Social and family problems will likely be the most devastating in the long term. Motivation, attention skills, emotional instability, memory, learning, and social deficits are all cognitive processes that prevent or retard clients' progress in the therapy program as well as in home and work environments. Working with professionals who specialize in these areas will improve the client's chances to escape deficits that are permanently handicapping.

The purpose of the evaluation and diagnosis is to determine what prevents the client from performing in a functional, acceptable manner as identified by the client, the therapist, and the society. For the *components of examination*, see the accompanying box.

Examination Tools for Cognitive Deficits

Figure 14–1 depicts the close association of cognitive, behavioral, and physical functioning soon after injury. The

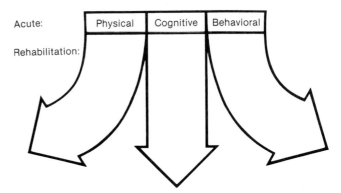

FIGURE 14–1. Schema representing the close association of cognitive, behavioral, and physical functioning soon after injury. The three domains gradually become more distinguishable in the later stages of recovery.

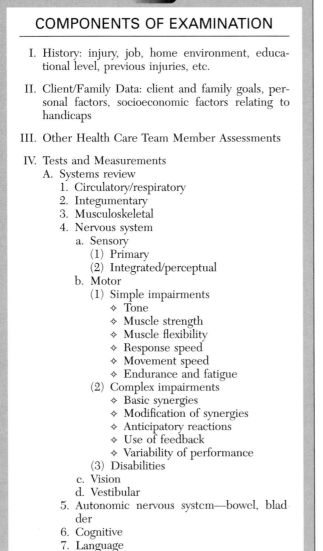

COMPONENTS OF EXAMINATION

  I. History: injury, job, home environment, educational level, previous injuries, etc.

 II. Client/Family Data: client and family goals, personal factors, socioeconomic factors relating to handicaps

III. Other Health Care Team Member Assessments

 IV. Tests and Measurements
   A. Systems review
     1. Circulatory/respiratory
     2. Integumentary
     3. Musculoskeletal
     4. Nervous system
       a. Sensory
         (1) Primary
         (2) Integrated/perceptual
       b. Motor
         (1) Simple impairments
           ◇ Tone
           ◇ Muscle strength
           ◇ Muscle flexibility
           ◇ Response speed
           ◇ Movement speed
           ◇ Endurance and fatigue
         (2) Complex impairments
           ◇ Basic synergies
           ◇ Modification of synergies
           ◇ Anticipatory reactions
           ◇ Use of feedback
           ◇ Variability of performance
         (3) Disabilities
       c. Vision
       d. Vestibular
     5. Autonomic nervous system—bowel, bladder
     6. Cognitive
     7. Language
     8. Emotional

three domains gradually become more distinguishable in later stages of recovery and can be assessed more independently; however, their interrelationships remain exceedingly complex.

Cognition includes many aspects of function, including memory, learning, information processing, attention span, motivation, and initiation. Cognitive impairment was the primary contributor to disability in the majority of brain-injured subjects who scored moderate to severe on the Glasgow Outcome Scale.[59]

Testing of cognitive function is usually performed by neuropsychologists, speech pathologists, and occupational therapists. These tests may include word association, written word fluency, figural fluency, and card sorting tests. Attention can be tested with tests such as the digit span and arithmetic tests on the WAIS[134] as well as serial counting by 7. Information processing is reflected in reaction time tests and digit symbol tests. Choice reaction time is an indicator of information processing and a common residual cognitive problem in brain-injured clients.[25]

Testing of intellectual functions is with the WAIS. However, formal testing of intellectual function can be hampered by inadequate perceptual, visual, and motor performance.

Memory can also be tested with the WAIS. Testing of declarative memory can also be done with the Mini-Mental State Exam[42] or the Galveston Orientation and Amnesia Test (GOAT).[78]

Language and cognitive problems are examined by speech pathologists and neuropsychological tests using naming tests, aphasia examinations, and tests of auditory comprehension and speed of comprehension.

A widely used system of cognitive function at the disabilities level is based on numerous observations of clients with brain injuries at Rancho Los Amigos Hospital. This has resulted in a descriptive categorization of various stages of "cognitive function," as shown in the box on page 427.

Structure for Examination and Evaluation

The American Physical Therapy Association has published levels of client management leading to optimal out-

RANCHO LOS AMIGOS HOSPITAL SCALE OF COGNITIVE FUNCTION

I. No response

II. Generalized response

III. Localized response

IV. Confused–agitated

V. Confused–inappropriate

VI. Confused–appropriate

VII. Automatic–appropriate

VIII. Purposeful–appropriate

comes.[57] The Association's *Guide to Physical Therapy Practice* uses examination, evaluation, diagnosis, prognosis, intervention, and outcomes as its basis.

Examination establishes a baseline by which to judge future improvement or lack thereof. This baseline should be quantified to permit measurement of the effectiveness of the intervention strategies.

Evaluation identifies the problems that can be managed by the therapist and serves to "tease" out those factors that influence or restrict the choice of therapeutic approaches. Evaluation provides a qualitative means of determining reasons why a problem is present. It includes considerations of testing, motivation, and psychosocial areas. The evaluation thus determines intervention goals.

Diagnosis examines the various possible causes of the problem to determine which are most critical. The therapist has a multilevel task that includes (1) identification of the components that compose a complex task or disability; (2) evaluation of the degree to which a component's deficit contributes to impairment, disability, or handicap; and (3) evaluation of the ability of the client to recover the necessary improvement in a component and the need to provide substitutions.

Prognosis is used to determine the optimal level of improvement that may be attained.

The interventions are provided by skilled professionals to treat the impairments, disabilities, and handicaps to achieve optimal outcomes.

An example of examination, evaluation, and diagnosis would be as follows. A client falls several times a week. Examination reveals impairments of decreased strength and ROM, increased tone, and poor balance strategies. Evaluation conclusions were that the 20-degree hip flexion contracture and 2+ ankle strength together prevent the client from using normal ankle strategies, resulting in balance losses and falling. This evaluation or diagnosis is based on many facts, including ankle strategies that require hip extension to be effective; research by Perry and coworkers[94] shows that for normal walking velocity a strength level of 3 is necessary in the ankle muscles. Intervention is performing exercises to achieve neutral hip extension and ankle strength at the 4 level through strengthening of the gastrocnemius and anterior tibialis and passive and dynamic stretching of the hip flexors. The prognosis would be for a significant improvement in balance because strength and ROM, major contributors to balance, are impaired in this client. Outcomes would be a decrease in falling and establishment of ankle strategies.

The method of examination should lead to understanding the underlying causes of the disabilities and should be the basis of the treatment program. Starting examination at the disability level might be most useful. Once disabilities are determined, the impairments in strength, speed, ROM, sensation, timing, sequencing, velocity, and endurance can be identified and evaluated for their contribution to the disability.[69, 73] For example, a paretic disability may be the result of multiple impairments, but certain critical components appear to have more influence on a function. In gait disabilities in children with cerebral palsy, Olney and coworkers[92] demonstrated that poor force output by ankle plantarflexors during the late stance and toe-off (terminal swing) phase of gait was the most important factor in their poor gait performance. Therefore, weakness in the gastrocnemius area may be considered a critical impairment in these clients that affects the major disability of gait dysfunction. In deficient standing balance, breakdown in the sequencing of lower-extremity muscle contractions may be the crucial impairment. In grasping activities, arm movement, prehension, and maintenance of balance constitute the task. Deficiencies of timing, strength, or sequencing can contribute to poor hand function. Sensory deficits at the hand level, however, may be the critical impairment related to poor manipulation skills. Additionally, impairments in the circulatory, respiratory, integumentary, and musculoskeletal systems can account for disability in the brain-injured client (Fig. 14–2).

The therapist's evaluation and diagnosis[103] therefore determine relative contributions of the impairments to disability, which then focuses the intervention program.

When resolving problems at the impairment level is not possible, the ICIDH system helps the therapist identify substitutions that can achieve the same functional goals (e.g., use of a wheelchair for the client who will not be able to walk or use of a feeding cuff for a client who will not develop adequate motor function in the hand for feeding).

Examination of Motor Performance in the Brain-Injured Client

Disabilities

Disabilities in brain-injured clients range over the entire spectrum of problems. They include loss of mobility in bed; loss of household and community ambulation; loss of activities of daily living (ADL) such as dressing, toileting, and feeding; and loss of instrumental ADL such as shopping and driving.

Disability can be assessed with formal measurement tools. Wade[130] provides an in-depth presentation of examinations for this level. The Barthel Index is an example of a very simple tool for gross measurement of overall disability.[80] It simply asks whether functional skills can be

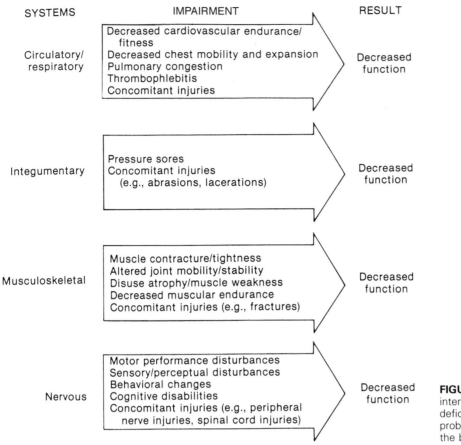

SYSTEMS   IMPAIRMENT   RESULT

Circulatory/   Decreased cardiovascular endurance/   Decreased
respiratory   fitness   function
                   Decreased chest mobility and expansion
                   Pulmonary congestion
                   Thrombophlebitis
                   Concomitant injuries

Integumentary   Pressure sores   Decreased
                   Concomitant injuries   function
                     (e.g., abrasions, lacerations)

Musculoskeletal   Muscle contracture/tightness   Decreased
                   Altered joint mobility/stability   function
                   Disuse atrophy/muscle weakness
                   Decreased muscular endurance
                   Concomitant injuries (e.g., fractures)

Nervous   Motor performance disturbances   Decreased
                   Sensory/perceptual disturbances   function
                   Behavioral changes
                   Cognitive disabilities
                   Concomitant injuries (e.g., peripheral
                     nerve injuries, spinal cord injuries)

FIGURE 14–2. Therapists develop intervention strategies to deal with functional deficits that may result from a variety of problems occurring primarily in one or more of the body systems depicted.

performed within a reasonable time limit. However, its usefulness sometimes is limited, because the clients must make large changes to show improvement in their scores. The Functional Independence Measure (FIM)[54] has six categories that evaluate independence. Twelve items relating to swallowing, community functions, and cognition (Functional Assessment Measure [FAM][44]) have been added to the FIM to make it useful for TBI clients. The combined tests are the FIM + FAM. The Disability Rating Scale[96] is also widely used.

Upper-extremity movement patterns and function can be examined using functional tests such as the Nine-Hole Peg Test,[133] Frenchy Arm Test,[34] or the arm portion of the Motor Assessment Scale (MAS).[23]

These types of indexes should be chosen to address what abilities the client can accomplish and are not treatment tools. Their sole purpose is to identify disabilities. Additionally, many are not effective in measuring changes in the higher level functioning client.

Impairments

Impairment at Basic Component Level of Performance. Breaking motion down to its most basic components may be helpful, but two caveats are necessary. First, improvement in abnormal components may not lead to improvement in disabilities. Second, treating the individual impairments will not necessarily result in learning a skill. Skills result from an organization of many motor functions together. Conversely, not having a critical com-

ponent, such as arm strength, may be the one factor preventing a person from learning to perform a skill (e.g., enough force cannot be generated to throw a ball 5 feet in the air to hit a basket).

Many examinations address the impairment level. These include muscle strength tests, flexibility (ROM) tests, and speed of motion, reaction time, sensation, vision, vestibular, tone, and proprioceptive examinations (see Chapter 3).

Strength or Force Production. Evidence consistently shows that traditional strengthening programs lead to functional improvements in clients with neurological injuries.[20]

Weakness may occur in any muscle affected by paralysis. Individuals with brain damage show atrophy in motor units, as well as motor units that fatigue easily.[36, 38] Disuse, cast immobilization, joint dysfunction, improper nutrition, drugs, and aging can cause differential weakness with altered morphological, biochemical, and physiological characteristics within the muscle.[98] EMG studies by numerous investigators[99, 120] suggest that reduced activity alters motor unit properties, discharge frequency, and recruitment patterns. Loss of motor units also has been reported.[36]

Changes in muscle length affect strength. In clients with a cerebrovascular accident, shortened muscles tend to be strong in short ranges and lengthened muscles are strongest in lengthened ranges but weak in shorter positions when compared with the strength-length curves of normal muscles.[104]

Strength or force at the component level may be examined functionally (e.g., the client has enough strength to lift the arm overhead, out to the side, and up to the mouth and being able to stand from sitting). In some cases, such as those in which the client is unable to perform balance reactions or has been on extended bed rest, testing individual muscles may be important. Traditional manual muscle testing, using force transducers, or strength testing with isokinetic testing[132] throughout the range provides good strength information. The level of testing chosen should be consistent with the deficit and the therapist's knowledge of its importance in contributing to disability.

Flexibility. Flexibility at the muscle and joint level is important. Evaluations should determine the contribution of both tone and tissue factors in limiting flexibility. Active and passive motion should be compared because stiffness (not contracture) often prevents good function. For example, active dorsiflexion is often limited in clients who have full passive ROM because stiffness begins at neutral dorsiflexion. The functional result is footdrop or toe catch in the swing phase of gait because the anterior tibialis muscle cannot generate adequate strength to overcome the stiffness. This restriction also may limit forward movement of the body over the foot during the stance phase of gait, resulting in hip retraction or an apparent balance loss. Knee hyperextension also can result from lack of forward motion of the tibia.

Flexibility measurements are done with goniometers, motion analysis systems, tape measures, inclinometers, photographs, or electronic devices. Taking both passive and active measurements is critical in identifying treatment approaches.

Tone. In the motor learning theories of today, many of the behaviors and resulting motor patterns after brain injury are seen as attempts by the CNS to compensate for loss. For example, spasticity may be the result of an attempt to compensate for the client's inability to increase force. When the amplitude of a contraction cannot be increased due to injury, the CNS may increase the length of time the muscle fires or may recruit muscles not normally used in a particular pattern of movement; both are characteristics seen in spasticity.

Whatever the cause of increased tone, the physical therapist can evaluate tone at two levels: is it interfering with function, and, if so, can it be changed? Spasticity is not a single problem.° It includes:

- Changes in response to stretch
- Lack of force production
- Increased latency of activation
- Inability to rapidly turn off muscles
- Loss of reciprocal inhibition between spastic muscles and their antagonists
- Changes in the intrinsic properties of the muscle fibers
- Inability to generate enough antagonist power to overcome spastic muscles

Examination begins with identifying whether there is increased or decreased muscle tension at rest. If it is increased, is the tension at the muscle level (stiffness or

sarcomere involvement) or the neurological level? Muscle stiffness secondary to tissue changes is common in the brain-injured client. If there is increased tone during movement, EMG may be beneficial to determine the nature of the tone. Is it a problem of co-contraction of agonist and antagonist at a joint? Is it a problem of prolonged contraction? Or is it poor sequencing, either temporally or spatially, of other muscles involved in the movement?

Spatial sequencing of movement involves the contraction of a preset group of muscles. Temporal sequencing involves muscles contracting in a fixed sequence. EMG and videoanalysis provide additional depth of information regarding the sequence and timing of movement patterns (Fig. 14–3). For example, is the normal temporal sequencing in the distal to proximal manner present in the upper extremity during a reaching task? In a balance reaction, are the ankle, hip, and back extensors (spatial sequencing) all contracting in response to a forward perturbation? (See section on intervention for a discussion of modifying tone-related components.)

The most commonly used tool in examination of tone is the Ashworth scale or Modified Ashworth scale[13] (see the box on page 430). Testing of deep tendon reflexes identifies problems with stretch reflexes, and surface EMG can determine the presence of co-contraction, prolonged contraction, sequence and timing problems, and increases in latencies.

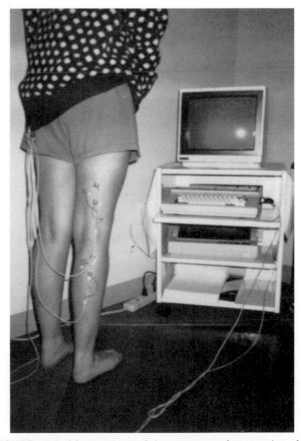

FIGURE 14–3. Measurement of the sequence of contraction of gastrocnemius and hamstring in forward perturbation using dual-channel electromyographic surface electrodes.

°See references 15, 31, 37, 38, 72, 98, 99, 105, 120, and 121.

MODIFIED ASHWORTH SCALE

Grade	Description
0	No increase in muscle tone
1	Slight increase in muscle tone, manifested by a catch and release or by minimal resistance at the end of the ROM when the affected part(s) is moved in flexion or extension
1+	Slight increase in muscle tone, manifested by a catch, followed by minimal resistance throughout the remainder (less than half) of the ROM
2	More marked increase in muscle tone through most of the ROM, but affected part(s) easily moved
3	Considerable increase in muscle tone; passive movement difficult
4	Affected part(s) rigid in flexion or extension

Reprinted from Bohannon R, Smith M: Interrater reliability of a modified Ashworth scale of muscle spasticity. Phys Ther 67:207; 1987, with permission of the American Physical Therapy Association.

Speed of Motion. Research shows that seemingly very different movements may actually be spatially the same (same muscles involved) but appear different because of pauses within the movements, velocity, or speed.[52] Movement speed or velocity can be a primary indicator of change in units of movement or help define subtasks of a movement or skill.

Measurements include how quickly a joint can be moved. Recording the number of repetitions of a movement in a specific time frame provides an easy clinical measurement. Instruments can measure partial- and whole-extremity motion speed. Speed of movement at each joint in a synergistic movement (videotaped or movement analysis systems) can help to analyze function. Is poor performance due to speed of movement problems in just one part of the synergy or in all parts?

Computerized motion analysis techniques can also help examine speed of motion relationships between and among limb segments, which is particularly useful in assessing upper limb movements such as reaching and grasping activities.

Reaction Time. How fast can the client begin motion? This parameter can be measured by EMG or with other computerized equipment.

Simple reaction time examination gives insight into the time for neurological processing. It is the measurement of time from a stimulus to a response. Quick reaction time may be critical for more automatic patterns, such as balance responses, to be effective.

Endurance. Muscle endurance refers more to the ability at the muscle level to produce the same level of contraction over time. It may be measured by repeating muscle testing before and after using the muscle for a set time or by EMG using medium-frequency analysis. Studies show that endurance may be a large component of dysfunction.

Cardiovascular endurance determines how effectively the body can use oxygen and how soon fatigue sets in. This type of endurance can be measured with several bicycle tests[2, 145] and with treadmills using a Bruce[19] protocol or a branching protocol for clients with less endurance. A simple test is heart rate before and after activity; the less change and more rapid the return to resting rate, the better is the fitness level.

Fatigue, which is separate from impaired endurance, may result from increased energy requirements resulting from less efficient motor patterns or more CNS activity.

Sensory Function. Various sensations can be impaired. Problems in the sensory system are often reflected in the motor system, creating distorted movement through faulty information in the feedforward or feedback processes.

Two broad categories of sensations can be defined based on type of information: primary sensations and cortical (or integrative) sensations. This arbitrary division is useful functionally but is not anatomically based. Primary sensations include exteroception and proprioception. The exteroceptors of smell, sight, and hearing are sometimes referred to as teloreceptors. Vision, hearing, olfaction, gustation, pain, touch, temperature, position sense, and kinesthesia are commonly checked primary sensations. Sensations cannot be tested definitively clinically without client participation. Further evaluations of sensation are provided in specific systems.

Proprioception, Light Touch, Two-Point Discrimination, and Stereognosis. Traditional evaluations of proprioception include the ability to distinguish motion and motion direction at each joint. Some clients who cannot distinguish direction or movement still function well. They may have proprioceptive function at the unconscious level (e.g., cerebellar) while not perceiving the input at the parietal (cortical) level.

Proprioception may be tested by having the client close his eyes and then placing one of his limbs in a specific position and asking the client to copy the position with the other limb. It may also be tested by asking the client to close his eyes and identify when small movements of a joint are passively presented by the therapist while the client indicates specific direction of movement.

Light touch is tested with a brush for localization and quality of sensation. For more definitive light touch discrimination, especially on the hands, Van Frey fibers can be used. Two-point discrimination can be tested using instruments specifically designed to measure how far apart two separate spots of contact need to be to identify them as distinct.

Stereognosis, the ability to identify objects placed in the hand without visual assistance, may be critical to normal hand use.

Vision and Visual Perception. Vision is critical in recovery of many motor functions because it is responsible for much of the feedforward or anticipatory control of movement. For example, balance can be maintained through the visual system by modifying synergy before surface change occurs. Feedback through the peripheral field by array movement can also trigger balance synergies. Some clients are able to use their hands for grasp and release in spite of severe somatosensory deficits when able to use vision to guide the motion.

General visual functions can be screened by the physical or occupational therapist as follows:

1. Tracking is assessed through the whole visual field, observing for any nystagmus or multiple saccades. Eye muscle paralysis can be observed during tracking when the client cannot move the eye(s) laterally, up, down, or medially.
2. Focus or accommodation can be checked by observing constriction and dilation of the pupil, which should occur as an object is moved to and from the nose.
3. Binocular vision is controlled through feedback when vision is blurred or doubled. This reflex signals whether the eyes and fovea are focused on a single point or target; do the images in both eyes fall on the same retinal points? A "cover test" can screen for binocular vision. The client stares at an object at about 18 inches from the nose. The therapist covers one eye. If there is movement to adjust the remaining uncovered eye back to the object, both retinas may not be focusing on the same point. Observing whether light reflections fall on exactly the same place on both pupils is also useful in evaluating binocular eye focus.
4. Visual fields can be grossly tested by having the client look forward at a point (observer sits in front of the client to be sure client remains focused on a point; Fig. 14–4). The client indicates when he or she first sees an object coming into the peripheral field from behind or a "spotter" notes when the client looks toward the object.
5. Visual interactions with the vestibular system are assessed through the vestibulo-ocular reflex. This reflex maintains a fixed gaze on a target as the head moves.
6. Peripheral visual movement receptors are stimulated with an optokinetic drum. This may provide insight into the peripheral visual field's perception of movement.
7. Perceptual tests that evaluate how visual information is used include visual memory tests, cancellation tests, and figure-ground tests.

Neuro-optometrists and neuro-ophthalmologists are appropriate referrals for clients needing in-depth visual workups, especially when visual perception is involved. See Chapter 27 for additional information on vision and visual testing.

Vestibular System. The vestibular system monitors position of the head in space and helps distinguish when the body is moving from when the visual surround is moving. Vertigo, dizziness, eye/head incoordination, and postural and balance complications occur as a result of problems in the vestibular-cerebellar systems.

Vestibular tests can be performed at the screening level, to note dizziness with body, head, or eye motions. A practical division includes testing head movement in lying, sitting, and standing positions. Positive tests in these positions include symptoms of dizziness or nausea occurring when the head is fixed with eyes moving, eyes fixed with head moving, head on body motions, body on body motions, or body moving in space.

Symptoms occurring only with specific head positions can be an indicator of problems in the semicircular canals. In-depth evaluation tools may be used when clients are symptomatic. (See Chapter 21 for additional information on balance and vestibular dysfunctions.)

Impairment at Complex Task Level. Once the basic components of performance have been evaluated, the task is to determine which aspects of poor performance are associated with that impairment and which aspects are related to the use of these components in combined manners or synergies. Complex task evaluation asks different questions from those covered in component examination and requires extensive knowledge of abnormal and normal movement.

Complex task evaluation may be considered from the point of view of motor control theory as follows:

1. *Are basic motor patterns available, accessible, and used appropriately?* Are basic reflexes intact? Do movement patterns show basic synergies such as in standing and reaching? Are swallowing, eye tracking, smiling, withdrawal reflexes, and the ability to voluntarily move the trunk, head, and limbs present? Does the client appear to have the ability to coordinate motions (decrease the degrees of freedom)? Injury at this level may most affect basic synergy production and sequencing. The kinetic system involving the basal ganglia is presently most associated with these functions.
2. *Are the basic synergies being selected or modified to*

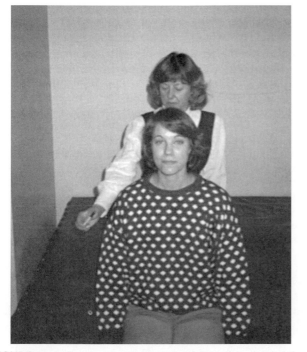

FIGURE 14–4. Testing of peripheral visual fields from behind the client.

meet specific task requirements? These functions are presently associated with the synergistic or cerebellar functions, which provide tone, timing, coordination, and amplitude of motions. The synergistic system smoothes out the motor program and provides adaptability. Is the client able to use the basic synergies in a useful manner? Is the client able to modify and then accomplish activities such as walking and ball catching? Is there good interlimb coordination? Does the client respond correctly to environmental changes or stimuli? When synergies are used, are they appropriate for the stimulus? For example, many clients inappropriately use the hip strategy in response to all losses of balance.

3. *Does the client show anticipatory reactions*? These reactions are dependent on learning. Anticipatory reactions require combining past information with present information to make motor responses appropriate to internal and external needs. Counterforces to our movements that must be anticipated are almost always necessary. For example, does the gastrocnemius contract before forward-reaching activities? Does the client step over objects or shape the hand for picking up objects? Almost all motor functions have an anticipatory component. The sensory systems modify performance at this level of functioning. Component examination of visual, vestibular, and somatosensory systems may lead to understanding deficits at this level.

4. *Does the client use feedback correctly*? Feedback is used to modify and fine tune responses. Is activity corrected to meet changing environmental conditions? When not successful at task performance, does the client use this information to modify or adapt subsequent responses? Is the adaptation appropriate, or does it result in poorer performance?

5. *Does the client show variability of performance*? The plastic nervous system can adapt and change its motor output to meet different requirements. VanSant[129] showed that children and adults vary in the way they stand from supine, even under the same environmental conditions. She states that the most striking observation in normal individuals is this variability of performance. The lack of variability has been suggested by many[108] as a sign of system damage. When assessing the brain-injured client, one should look for variability of performance in basic motor acts. Can the client accomplish the same task in several ways? Can the client adapt to different task demands? As the complex task is being performed, keep in mind that the extent of deficit is important. To what extent is the observed motor behavior involved? Is the behavior totally absent? Is it deficient, or are there signs of substitution of function or adaptation?

Consider assessment of walking as an example of the examination process. The activity requires three complex elements: postural control, balance, and extensor strength.[123]

In complex task analysis, postural control requires the client to be able to support the body in an upright position from the head down. Is there coordination between body segments? Is the head righted to the body or to gravity, as is normal in adults? Balance uses basic synergies to control sway. These synergies can be impaired after CNS injury.[5, 31, 36, 62] Is the client using balance synergies with a temporal sequence of distal to proximal contraction in the lower extremities during small perturbations? Or is the client co-contracting, indicating a temporal or spatial sequencing problem in disrupting the synergy? Does the client use only the appropriate muscles in balance responses (spatial sequence)? Does he or she appropriately use an ankle strategy in stance? Is there efficient movement in the swing leg? Does it move in a straight line and is foot placement on the floor appropriate (coordinated movement)? If not, does closing the eyes change the character of the movement? If it does, the client may be dominated by the visual system and may be having difficulty using somatosensory input for movement. Is interlimb timing good? Does the client step over a small object (anticipatory and adaptation)? If not, was it because the client misjudged the height of the object (visual anticipatory responses) or misjudged the distance to move the leg (modification of the locomotion synergy at the amplitude level)? Or is movement too disorganized to clear the object (problem with control of the degree of freedom, timing, or perhaps a lack of basic locomotor synergy)?

Tools for Examination of Gait and Balance. Many gait or walking examinations exist. At the impairment level, the Rancho Los Amigo Observations Gait Analysis analyzes kinematic aspects of the patterns of upper extremity, trunk, pelvis, and lower extremities in each phase of gait. The Bartel Index,[80] FIM,[54] Tinniti,[124] Gait Assessment Rating Scale,[143] and MAS[23] also examine different components of gait but at more of the disability level. Speed of walking for functional activities such as crossing a street at a stoplight and endurance can be measured by distance and a stopwatch. Endurance can be measured using a 6-minute walk test.[21]

Outcome

Leahy,[77] in a discussion of brain-injured adults, suggested a general categorization of clients for prognosis as follows: cognition as low, moderate, or high level and physical dysfunction as severely impaired, moderately impaired, or minimally impaired. The therapist may use the Glasgow Outcome Scale and the Rancho Los Amigos Hospital Scale of Cognitive Function to determine the categories. This system provides a means of predicting return of functional skills as well as long-term disability. As Leahy points out, clients with higher-level physical skills and moderate-level or low-level cognition skills are often the most difficult to reintegrate into the family and society. Therefore, they may have the higher levels of handicaps remaining after rehabilitation because family and co-worker expectations are high based on motor function, but it is the cognitive functions that make one more successful in society.[25] These clients need aggressive help in the behavioral and cognitive areas early on. Neuropsychologists and counselors can suggest interventions that help with cognitive functions, especially techniques to deal with memory problems, attention span decreases, and inappropriate behavior. These programs can make a difference. Brotherton and associates[18] documented long-term social behavior improvement in four severely brain-injured clients who had undergone traditional social skills training programs.

Clients with low-level motor skills and higher-level cognitive skills do better because there are available adaptive devices for these clients that help substitute for their loss of motor functions. These include head-, mouth-, or hand-controlled electric wheelchairs, computerized communications systems, electric lifts for vans, and hand controls for driving, books on tape, and numerous upper- and lower-extremity devices to help with hand control and ADL. (See Chapter 16 on spinal cord injury for all types of substitution devices.)

Intervention

Multiple problems may occur after brain injury. A partial list of the most common are in the accompanying box.

Motivation

The motivational aspect of TBI may be one of the most difficult for the therapist to deal with. Clients' initiation and practice of movement are dependent on the internal control of the client and not easily dealt with from the external environment.

Working on client goals helps to establish motivation. Client goals that seem unrealistic should not be dismissed as inappropriate. The high school athlete who wants to play football next week and presently has no postural control can focus on how he will learn to sit, stand, walk, and run in order to play. Most clients who go through rehabilitation programs begin to assess their own potential more appropriately once they have worked through part of their program. Many clients and their families believe that the brain heals like any other part of their body and expect full recovery provided a client tries hard enough.[115] Sometimes giving clients time out of therapy to experience everyday life at home and work helps them determine and readjust goals and skills and then to set new

---

PROBLEMS AFTER TRAUMATIC BRAIN INJURY

- Impaired affect
- Impaired arousal and attention
- Impaired expressive or receptive communications
- Impaired motor function, including oculomotor and oral motor
- Altered muscle elastic properties
- Impaired respiratory function
- Impaired autonomic nervous system
- Impaired cognition
- Impaired learning
- Impaired sensory integrity and perception
- Impaired balance and anticipatory reactions

---

priorities. The client who couldn't see doing "silly exercises" comes back asking to learn ADL. In many cases it is the families who need help understanding their family member's social and behavioral changes.

Nearly as difficult to work with are alterations in attention span. The neuropsychological evaluation becomes crucial for treatment in the client with a short attention span. Early on, techniques to increase attention span will probably include removing distracting stimuli from the client's environment, including auditory, tactile, and visual distractions. But slowly, distracting stimuli need to be reintroduced and attention maintained. (See Chapter 7 for additional information.)

Because the therapist can identify a deficit during the examination does not mean the deficit can be fixed. Based on evaluation, two levels of treatment are likely to be ongoing. At the impairment level, basic components of performance that are faulty and are contributing to lack of motor performance can be addressed. Loss of complex movements and synergies also will be part of the rehabilitation targets. At the disability level, substitutions for loss of function such as bracing, wheelchairs, functional electrical stimulation, and ambulation devices and environmental changes such as ramps, chairs, bath benches, padding for skin care, and reachers provide immediate change and improve the disability almost immediately.

Although debate is ongoing as to whether many of the abnormalities seen after brain injury result from loss of functions or from an attempt to compensate for the lost functions, the goal of intervention is the same: to help a client work in the environment to produce movements that are efficient, successful, and to some extent socially acceptable.

Using the ICIDH model of impairment, disability, and handicap, the therapist determines whether improvement is possible at the level of impairment and then addresses these specific impairments. For example, for a client who is both weak and has contractions and is therefore unable to roll over, strengthening, stretching, and casting may be done. In the client with a permanent contracture or paralysis, a cloth loop may be provided to allow rolling over by pulling with the arm.

An example of the ICIDH treatment model for walking is presented in the box on page 434.

Whether brain-injured clients can relearn motor skills as those who do not have brain injuries can is controversial, and evidence to direct us to better approaches is lacking. One difference may be that basic components of movement such as strength and ROM may contribute significantly to loss of the motor function in brain-injured clients and impede their ability to relearn functional skills. To develop skill in an activity, many, many repetitions must be performed. Knowledge of results and feedback are also important in motor practice.[139]

Attention span and motivation factors alone can impede skill acquisition.

The ability to "fix" an impairment does not depend solely on the therapist's skills but includes inherent properties within the client such as the amount of physical damage, cognition, family support, and motivation. Just as critical are external constraints, for example, the availability of treatment devices such as electromyographs

DISABILITY: NOT ABLE TO WALK

Impairment: P + Lower-Extremity Extensor Strength

Can improve	Use weights, resistive exercises, antigravity work, etc.
Cannot improve (significantly)	Address at disability level; use wheelchair, cane, walker, bracing, etc.

Impairment: Disrupted Sequence of Muscle Contraction

Can improve	Use exercises to sequence muscles distally to proximally; use electromyography feedback, etc.
Cannot improve	Use bracing, electrical stimulation for bracing, wheelchair

for biofeedback, stimulation devices, pools, and other equipment; travel to and from treatment; availability of qualified providers of care; and financial constraints on treatment.

Component Level Treatment of Impairment

At the component level are numerous and well-known approaches to treatment. A quick review of some of the current basis of component treatment and more nontraditional approaches may be useful.

Disability Level of Intervention

Mobility and prehension are the two most frequent disability losses after brain injury. In clients who will not be able to reestablish walking or prehension skills, functional devices are provided for substitution of the lost skills. This level also teaches functional tasks such as transfers, cooking, and self-care with assistive devices and modified techniques.

Retraining programs with emphasis on cognitive function, endurance, or social interactions are also available in larger communities.

Strength. Muscle tension is increased and decreased by the number of motor units firing (spatial summation) and the rate at which they are fired (temporal summation).

Improvements in strength are usually speed specific, so use of resistance at different speeds is critical. Body position in space may also be related to differences in force production. Current thought is that the brain uses different spatial maps for movement; therefore, use of the

extremities and trunk in multiple positions is important to address all different types of patterns of muscle activation.

Consideration of very weak muscles is important. Weak muscles sometimes fail to respond as rapidly if overworked. Treatment in the pool or decreasing the number of repetitions and weight during strengthening may lead to more efficient strengthening. Production and practice of eccentric contractions are important in controlling speeds of movement and achieving accuracy of movement, especially in gait and upper-extremity reaching tasks. Using functional tasks for strengthening is often effective. For example, practicing sit to stand will help strengthen the hips and knees.

Flexibility. Loss of sarcomeres and tissue shortening can occur rapidly in muscle and joints when clients are less active and in those with high levels of muscle tone. Flexibility can be addressed with traditional orthopedic techniques, including joint mobilization, stretching, and dynamic splinting as well as serial casting. Additionally, electrical stimulation[6, 7] is extremely effective in improving flexibility, especially in dorsiflexion. For example, a small spot electrode placed over the peroneal nerve at the fibular head and a 2-inch-square electrode medial to the lateral hamstring 2 to 3 inches above the knee works well. Using this technique 10 to 20 minutes twice a day is usually adequate (Fig. 14–5). Wrist flexor tightness has

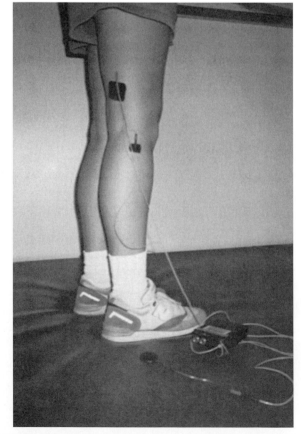

FIGURE 14–5. Placement of electrical stimulation electrodes for peroneal nerve to attain dorsiflexion for stretching a tight gastrocnemius or for electrical bracing when used with a heel switch.

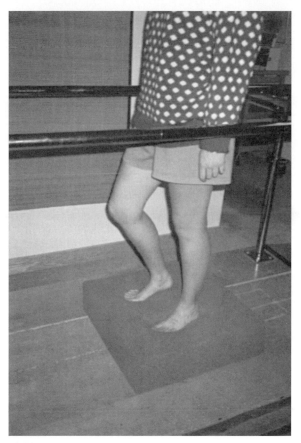

FIGURE 14–6. Foam block to improve speed of motion and reaction time.

been treated with electrical stimulation with good results. However, electrical stimulation in the unconscious client with increased ICP or one who is agitated is usually contraindicated because noxious stimuli can increase these problems.

Speed of Movement. Speed of movement may be trained with isokinetic equipment, manually during resistive exercises, or with computerized equipment such as force platforms. Varying speed is important with activities. Many gait studies show that disability becomes most apparent when the speed of gait is increased.

Reaction Time. Reaction time training also can be done on force platforms with the client sitting or standing. In a pilot study by Winkler,[138] exercise performed while standing on foam pads (10 inches thick and of medium density, Fig. 14–6) significantly improved reaction times during weight shifting to a visual stimulus in a group of eight clients with neurological deficits. Work on compliant surfaces may require that the client make faster corrections to avoid falling.

Endurance. Use of repetitions, increasing duration, and intensity can improve endurance. Upper-extremity ergometry can enhance cardiovascular conditioning in clients who are unable to walk or ride bicycles.

Sensory. Incorporating sensory function into movement is critical. Clients with poor tactile function can perform activities such as manipulation of objects, first in view and then out of view (nuts and bolts of different sizes are useful); picking out objects by tactile discrimination from other objects (e.g., safety pins in a bowl of rice) is also challenging. These tasks help the system to concentrate on and interpret information through sensory systems. To isolate the proprioceptive and muscle force feedback system, gloves can be used on the hands while performing grasp and release tasks with and without visual guidance. Difficulty of task can be increased by initiating treatment with vision and then removing all visual cues or by giving verbal cues and then removing verbal cues. Light, thin gloves can be changed for heavier, thicker gloves. Changing the surface of the objects that are manipulated from rough to increasingly smoother and slipperier also increases difficulty. Activities can progress from one-handed to two-handed tasks for interlimb coordination. Proprioceptive work at the shoulder and elbow can be done by using a marking pen in the involved hand (a utility cuff may be required for securing) and then having the client practice writing and drawing on paper or a blackboard while sitting or standing. Lower-extremity sensory retraining can also use targets with and without vision and with shoes on and off.

Tone. As previously discussed, problems with tone are due to a variety of issues. Problems in spatial and temporal sequencing seem better addressed with multiple-channel surface EMG (Fig. 14–7). The client can see both the

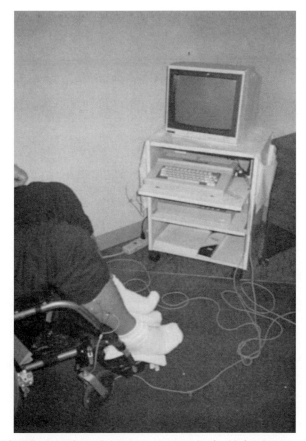

FIGURE 14–7. Superficial electromyography for biofeedback to shape contraction at onset and offset.

level of muscle recruitment and the sequence in which the muscles function if dual channels are used (see Fig. 14–3). Co-contraction can be decreased during functional activities such as gait or reaching using EMG biofeedback. Activation of muscles omitted in the gait or reaching patterns can be enhanced and ability to "turn off" muscles with prolonged contractions are also effectively treated by surface EMG. In clients unable to use EMG biofeedback information to make changes, functional electrical stimulation may achieve some of the goals (see Fig. 14–5). For example, gait training using an electrical stimulator on the dorsiflexor and/or plantarflexor nerves can achieve more normal activation patterns of the foot while providing some internal feedback information about sequencing. A heel switch and unit with separate channel controls and ramp adjustment are necessary. Using electrical stimulation on the gastrocnemius and hamstrings, with a slight delay of hamstring activation, has been effective in assistance with ankle strategy retraining. The second channel current can be ramped slightly to delay its onset for hamstring contraction. The goal is to slowly remove the "artificial" assistance over time. Strengthening exercises may also assist in improving central control of muscles and therefore improve tone control.

Vestibular System. Basic research has indicated good response to treatment, especially for peripheral vestibular dysfunction.[74, 112] Clients with sensory mismatches may require treatment that enhances input from the two normally functioning systems to adapt or retrain the faulty vestibular system. For example, the client who is dizzy when moving the head may need increased somatosensory input to provide information of the specific body motion that is occurring. The client can perform head motion while supine or sitting with feet and arms well supported (proprioceptive and tactile input) and eyes open. Progress in treatment occurs by decreasing the additional input as symptoms decrease so that the client is finally in standing position and increasing the amount of movement without dizziness or imbalance occurring. Visual cues can be altered by adding movement in visual areas (movement in the visual surround). This causes the visual system to perceive body motion when there is none and forces the use of the somatosensory and vestibular systems to determine the real motion. Wearing bicycle glasses or taping the medial or lateral aspects of glasses can reduce peripheral visual input, enhancing vestibular and somatosensory input in clients with dizziness caused by visual movement or visual-vestibular conflicts. In clients whose vestibular systems no longer function, enhancing visual and proprioceptive information is critical. Working on the motor aspect of balance using soft or inclined surfaces and narrow beams to facilitate hip strategies (see Figs. 14–6 and 14–8) and using small perturbations and quick stops to facilitate ankle strategies are important.

Many brain-injured clients who have vertigo have benign positional vertigo and will need a canalith repositioning maneuver for effective treatment (see Chapter 21 for more in-depth discussion of treatment).

Visual System. The visual system can have losses in the oculomotor areas of tracking, convergence/diver-

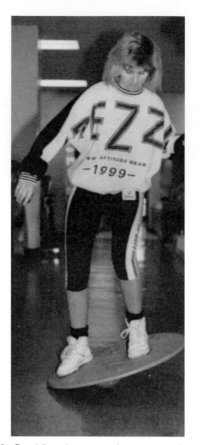

FIGURE 14–8. Providing the appropriate sensory input is critical to stimulating the correct movement synergy or balance response. Although treatment of mechanoreceptive balance problems requires using flat, firm surfaces, visual and vestibular balance problems are best treated on irregular, compliant, or moving surfaces, such as the multidimensional balance disk shown. The client should not be permitted to hold onto the therapist or to assistive devices because use of the arms changes the balance responses.

gence, vestibulo-ocular reflex, saccadic motion, and so on. These can be treated with oculomotor exercises, such as looking from a near object to a far object or tracking while the client watches his or her own thumb for increased proprioceptive feedback, with eyes fixated on a target during head movement.

Occipital lobe injuries generally result in more perceptual problems, those of making sense of the visual environment. These are more difficult to treat and usually handled best by professionals specializing in this type of problem.

The visual system has separate pathways for movement, color, and form. Therapy can enhance visual input by increasing contrast between objects, such as light objects or print on dark backgrounds. Colors also can assist in easier object identification. Red is often a strongly recognized color in deficient systems. Moving visual targets are easier to perceive than stationary ones. Finally, objects with sharp edges and vertical or horizontal lines are easier to perceive than objects with less distinct or curved lines. (See Chapter 27 for more information on visual problems and treatments.)

Complex Level Treatment of Impairment

Synergies. In clients who have available the basic component function, basic synergy or skill acquisition should be based on whole-task and natural subtask work. As stated earlier, using subtasks of a whole task improves performance. Identifying natural subtasks is difficult. Winstein[140] suggests that "natural breaks in the resultant velocity profile of a multisegment movement may signify the end of one subunit and may identify natural subtasks of a movement."

The variability shown in the task performance by normal subjects also may help elucidate subtasks. Assessment of a task, as done by VanSant[129] in her supine to stand studies, may provide a model to identify subtasks. In VanSant's study, the upper-extremity patterns varied in six ways: push and reach to bilateral push, asymmetrical push, symmetrical push, symmetrical reach, asymmetrical push with thigh push, and push and reach to bilateral push with thigh push. The head and trunk movement patterns varied in five ways: full rotation abdomen down, full rotation abdomen up, partial rotation stomach down, partial rotation stomach up, and partial rotation; and the lower extremity patterns varied in five ways: kneel, jump to squat, half kneel, asymmetrical squat, and symmetrical squat.

A subtask exercise program to teach a client to get up from supine might work as follows: Upper-extremity patterns of asymmetrical push with the trunk in partial rotation is practiced until successful; then lower-leg patterns are added; and finally whole-task training is used.

Natural subtask work probably will be more effective if performed in the environment in which the pattern is normally used.

Sit to stand practice is outlined in other chapters in detail. Sliding the hips forward and coming to partial standing appears to be a subtask unit and may be practiced.

Ambulation training requires working in the upright position. Many clients are impaired in walking because the more involved leg is slowed in swing phase. This not only decreases the total knee flexion but also affects clearance of the toe and increases time on the stance leg. This task may be broken down into more natural subtasks of gait, for example, working on half a gait cycle by stepping from the fully extended position (toe-off) to the initial contract position. Practicing pulling the thigh forward rapidly and changing speeds of thigh flexion can also be helpful.

Whole-task practice of gait in the brain-injured client leads to the question of safety. How does the therapist allow a client who cannot walk without falling to practice walking in light of research indicating that holding onto or using assistive devices changes the very skill the therapist is trying to teach? If the deficit is in balance, then walking without assistance may be critical to progress. The best the therapist may be able to do is to change the environment. Allowing a client to walk between parallel bars increases the likelihood he or she will either catch himself or herself or that the therapist can catch the client during falls. Walking on mats may allow both for environmental stimulus for soft, uneven surface work and

for safer falling. Falling may be critical in relearning ambulation. Little research is available in this area, but in a study by Cintas,[28] children who performed more daring gait activities fell more often (more problem-solving experiences?) but gained better gait skills.

Functional electrical stimulation, as described earlier, has been shown more effective than kinetic joint training in clients with cerebrovascular accidents.[12]

Goal-oriented tasks are mandatory in working with upper-extremity losses (Fig. 14–9). Many clients with minimal function can pick up and carry boxes. Often grip, but not release, is present. Again, EMG biofeedback is useful in helping develop release.[30] Functional release in clients with grip can be achieved by using an electrical stimulator on the finger extensors and using a hand switch. Some clients respond to a continuous low-level stimulation of the finger extensors and can learn to release by relaxing their grip. These activities are practiced while grasping and releasing objects. Feeding can be performed with this technique, as can other ADL tasks such as hair combing and opening doors.

The upper extremity also appears to use specific synergies for hand use in different positions. Clients often can open their hands in forward-reaching position but not with the elbow bent. Many clients with minimal functioning can be fitted with a utility cuff to hold writing instruments and write on boards or on tables while standing. This technique assists the shoulder in producing appropriate movement sequences for hand use but does not facilitate hand function. The treatment, however, does provide whole-task practice even though some basic com-

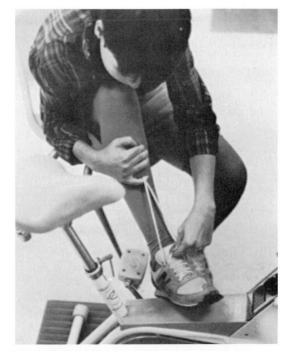

FIGURE 14–9. Most clients seem to respond to functional activities such as dressing. Sitting and leaning forward (as to put on shoes) simulates the inverted position and actively involves the client in the treatment. This is also an example of integrating components of movement into a meaningful activity and using the same activity to further develop motor components.

ponents are compensated through substitution. The therapist also may consider using a restraining device on the uninvolved side (with the client's permission) to force use of the involved extremity.

The use of whole-task practice at each treatment session is critical for two reasons. First, it is the only legitimate feedback of performance. For example, when teaching a throwing motion for basketball, if practice of the arm motion and ball throwing is without a target, feedback may indicate that ball release is adequate. The skill of shooting the ball into the basket is placing the ball at a specific point in space. The feedback that the ball hit the target determines the accuracy of the motion. Throwing the ball into the air is not the same task and uses different motor and sensory information than that needed for basket shooting. Second, the forced use studies of Wolf and coworkers[142] and Taub and colleagues[127] demonstrate that motor skills improve better with functional use (whole-task practice). When they restrained the unaffected arm in clients with a cerebrovascular accident and monitored improvement in the involved arm, they found significant improvement in function in clients who had previous traditional arm rehabilitation.

Reversing tasks in some clients allows them to develop increased control but requires modifying a task or synergy as well as working muscles both eccentrically and concentrically. For example, slowly lowering a spoon from the mouth may improve lifting the spoon to the mouth by improving motor control of the biceps during eccentric contractions. Wrist weights can be added to improve somatosensory feedback. Changing control by having clients stop and start at different points in an activity or changing directions also develops improved responses as well as flexibility. The client is asked to stop without taking another step, to turn right, or to step backward during ambulation. These techniques provide external influences on motor activities, helping to establish flexibility into responses.

Adding objects to the environment to avoid and/or manipulate and exposing the client to changing environments also develop adaptations and modifications to synergies.

Anticipatory Responses. More complex activities such as postural stability require work at the anticipatory response level as well as at the stability level. Moving the extremities (Fig. 14–10), adding weights to extremities during forward movement, and changing motion speeds are effective techniques. Pulling and pushing activities require an anticipatory set. More dynamic movement may be practiced with ball activities. Using punching, catching, throwing, and kicking activities with weighted balls as well as regular balls will change the force and speed involved, requiring the client to adapt responses to the changing environmental demands. Treadmills help clients to adapt their motion to environmental changes and to make anticipatory responses. But remember, treadmills cause sensory conflicts because the somatosensory system and vestibular systems report movement but the visual system reports no forward movement.

Variability. VanSant[129] also stated that variability of performance in her study had "some to do with body size,

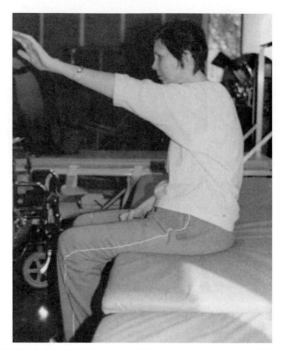

FIGURE 14–10. Anticipatory trunk movements are essential to provide postural stability immediately before some extremity movements. For example, spinal extension and an anterior pelvic tilt usually accompany elevating an arm overhead. However, brain-injured clients frequently lack adequate preparatory movements and typically maintain trunk flexion while attempting this activity.

strength and ROM." Because force production (strength) and ROM may be critical components in variability, work in water or with weight to change force production and ROM may also enhance different responses. It is important to build environmental constraints so clients can perform functional movements in alternative ways.

Learning, Practice, and Feedback. According to Winstein,[140] knowledge of results research presently suggests a need to reexamine intervention approaches that advocate performance accuracy, strong guidance (either manual, tactile, or verbal), frequent and continuous feedback, and avoidance of errors or "abnormal movements." The knowledge of results research findings are consistent with the motor control model that requires the client to be actively involved in problem solving through trial and error and adapting to new environmental situations. The higher-level client needs help to solve his or her own motor problems and thus less physical support but expanded environmental experiences.

Conversely, the client with minimal motor function or the client who is in an early recovery state may require a great deal of external help with basic components of movement before learning how to access or develop basic synergies and skill. Assisting movement is appropriate for the level of this client's functioning. For example, in training upper-extremity reaching patterns, this client may need trunk support intermittently, and then slowly decreasing the support will help develop the balance component necessary for successful reaching.

Handling techniques using righting reflexes may help with rolling and coming to sit or stand in clients who have lost basic synergies.

Because feedback is so critical to learning and improving motor performance, especially at the higher levels of functioning, the method of treating clients by assisting motion comes into question. Normal movement is unique in that it will change depending on the context in which it is performed and on the task constraints. The client being assisted in ambulation will not be making balance responses if the therapist is providing balance support.

The same problems may be inherent in using assistive devices such as canes and walkers. For example, Horak[61] showed that using a cane for balance disrupts the normal distal to proximal sequence in the lower extremities, and much of the balance responses are transferred to the arm, shoulders, and trunk. One might suspect the same to be true of many externally guided motions. The therapist must provide the client with opportunities to practice all parts of the complex motor tasks, or the task requirements are not the same. Practice needs to be task specific, but flexibility of response can be built in by changing environmental and task constraints.

Summary of Treatment Concepts

In general, lower-level-functioning clients (those with losses of basic synergies, component impairments, or cognitive changes) need more hands-on help from the therapist while trying to develop basic motor programs. Treatment may need to focus at the component level, establishing strength, flexibility, timing, and sequencing of movements. In lower-level clients, assistive devices such as braces, neck supports, and postural seating systems are often used to substitute for missing components of function. Forced use may also play a role in higher-level clients who are able to accomplish complex-level work. For clients who cannot manage multiple tasks, such as balance, coordination of synergies, and anticipatory reactions, the therapist may choose to work in subtasks. For example, body positioning and stabilization may be critical for developing adequate head stabilization and mobility in sitting. Additional requirements of balance can be added later. When head control is emerging, it may be appropriate to work on anticipatory reactions by requiring the client to move the head and not fall over. Visual control of head motion can be used. When possible, the whole-task practice of sitting unsupported can be added.

Many higher-level clients benefit from high-level functional activities. Square dancing, line dancing, karate, tai chi, handball, and other sports often promote additional progress in balance, sequencing, and speed of movement. The clever therapist will tease out those components of the activities that best address the deficits in the client and structure enjoyable activities that provide specific training for the deficits in balance, gait, upper extremity use, and so on.

No matter at what level the client is, the teaching of functional skills is critical. The lowest-level client may learn to roll over and assist with eating or other ADL tasks by using assistive devices. Modern equipment can enhance all types of function. Computers communicate for those with severe dysarthria, and power wheelchairs with switches to run lights, television, and so on are available. These devices assist clients in their societal interactions and reduce handicaps. Remember, the main purpose of motion is for exploration and getting the brain to a place it can be used!

SUMMARY

The following concepts summarize the theory, research, and intervention concepts presented in this chapter.

1. Treatment is based on the nervous system's ability to learn through environmental influences.
2. The client's goals must be addressed to provide motivation and persistence in exercise and practice.
3. As a starting point, examination and evaluation are done at the disability level.
4. Impairments that are the major contributors to the disability are identified.
5. Interventions for contractures and muscles tightness due to loss of muscle fiber and so on need to begin early to prevent progression and loss of function.
6. Strength or force production is critical in movement, and loss of this ability contributes significantly to disability; therefore, strengthening exercises are important.
7. Changing speed of motion and varying the context and environment are necessary for thorough skill reacquisition.
8. Once components of movement are in place, the use of synergies or skill learning should be stressed through repetition of functional activities.
9. Treatment should be performed with the goal of the movement incorporated into the treatment.
10. Practice is necessary in multiple environments and conditions.
11. The client should be allowed to problem solve.
12. Assistance by the therapist to clients with moderate and minimal levels of disability should be kept to a minimum.
13. Variability in performance is normal.
14. Surface EMG biofeedback, functional electrical stimulation, and isokinetic methods, as well as kinematic feedback, should be used to modify responses that appear more resistant.
15. Environmental situations that cause changes in responses should be identified.
16. Feedback should be provided randomly and as a summary rather than on a continous basis.
17. Substitution devices, assistive devices, and environmental changes should be provided for those clients who will not recover from their impairments.
18. Remember that the therapist's uniqueness lies in the ability to do evaluation and effective intervention.

QUALITY OF LIFE

A life has been saved. The job of the rehabilitation team is to help improve the quality of that life. But what is quality of life? Family members knew the client before injury. The "rehabilitated" client may be dramatically dif-

Text continued on page 444

CASE 14–1   MRS. E.K.

Mrs. E.K. is a 60-year-old woman who sustained a brain injury in a fall. Injury to the cerebellum and midbrain resulted in left-sided body involvement. Mrs. E.K. walks with circumduction during swing phase on the left side with minimal knee bend and slowed dorsiflexion. The left arm is held tightly against her chest with the elbow in flexion and the hand in full supination. Client goals included being able to sew again and to square dance with her club.

Examination

I. Unsafe walking with frequent falls
  A. Impairments—component
    1. Strength: F+ left hip extensor, hamstring, and gastrocnemius; otherwise within normal limits in lower extremities.
    2. Flexibility: left rectus femoris tight at 100 degrees in prone.
    3. Tone: modified Ashworth level 3 left quadriceps.
    4. Reaction time to weight shift delayed in the left leg.
    5. Speed of motion slowed in left knee extension and flexion and left foot dorsiflexion.
  B. Impairments—complex
    1. Synergies are poor in trunk. There is no trunk rotation during walking and a proximal to distal balance response during small perturbations (EMG). Visual-vestibular control of balance is poor; she cannot stand on 12-inch thick foam pad without balance loss and cannot maintain narrow-base stance with eyes closed.
    2. Anticipatory responses are poor on soft and irregular terrain.
    3. Feedback from lower-extremity proprioceptors is generally ignored in balance and gait.

Evaluation and Diagnosis: Poor walking and balance secondary to decreased use of proprioceptive information, weakness in the hip extensors and gastrocnemius, and increased tone in the quadriceps.

II. Poor reaching and manipulation skills in the left upper extremity
  A. Impairments—component
    1. Tone—co-contraction of anterior and posterior deltoid and biceps and triceps in forward reaching
    2. Poor sequencing and timing of movement; tremor of high frequency in the scapular stabilizers, especially the external rotators at rest and with movement; there are lower-frequency tremors of larger amplitude in the wrist flexors and extensors during voluntary motion.
  B. Impairments—complex
    1. Modification of synergies is poor for upper-extremity reaching. Amplitudes of movement are far too large for tasks. During walking, if the left arm is placed at the left side it flails wildly, knocking Mrs. E.K. off balance secondary to loss of walking synergy, trunk component.

Evaluation and Diagnosis: Upper extremity is not being used functionally owing to tremor and large amplitude, poor sequencing, and timing of motion coming mainly from the scapular and shoulder muscles during activities. The arm is held in co-contraction during walking and other activities to decrease the instability in balance caused by large movements and loss of synergy with gait.

Handicap: Decreased social interaction with friends

Interventions. Mrs. E.K. lived 70 miles from the treatment clinic. Most of her treatment consisted of a home program. She was seen in the clinic once every 3 weeks for 3 months and then once a month for a year.

The initial home program focused on the basic impairments of reducing quadriceps tightness and increasing hip extensor and gastrocnemius strength in the lower extremity. To reestablish some control of amplitude of motion in the left arm, gross movement activities using the hand with the elbow stabilized and a wrist splint were initiated for the left upper extremity and included drawing large circles with a pen in a fisted hand and pulling yarn through some large holes. She also used her left elbow to stabilize paper while writing.

Outcomes. Strength and flexibility improved to within normal limits.

The remaining program focused on hand-guided movement activities such as sewing with yarn on a large (1-inch squares) mat, writing, combing hair, molding clay, playing the organ, and so on. These activities were first performed with the elbow stabilized and a wrist splint, then with the elbow not stabilized, and finally without the wrist splint.

Surface electromyography was used to reestablish the basic walking synergies coordinating trunk and lower-extremity control. Lower-extremity work included trying to improve the use of proprioceptive function. Standing exercises with the eyes intermittently closed and open and wearing glasses that had Vaseline on them were used to decrease visual inputs. She also practiced identifying objects with her feet (e.g., pen, checker, modeling clay). Quickness of motion was promoted through rapid walking while the client's husband told her to stop abruptly and the client tried not to take a

Continued

CASE 14–1   MRS. E.K. *Continued*

second step after the command. Speed of dorsiflexion was facilitated through use of a rocker board (without holding on), jumping on foam, and walking with a longer step on the right.

As the amplitude of arm motion decreased with use, Mrs. E.K. was able to walk with her hands clasped behind her back and worked on trunk rotation coordinated with gait. When this was accomplished, she was able to allow her arm to hang freely at her side and had a natural trunk rotation

in walking. A videotape with beginning line dancing was used at home for higher-level balance exercises and for enjoyment.

At discharge, Mrs. E.K. had good synergies and improved pattern of motion in the left lower extremity. An articulated ankle-foot orthosis was used for long walks or when she was very fatigued. She was able to sew and use the left arm for most activities, although a much smaller tremor persisted with volitional movement.

CASE 14–2   P.H.

P.H., a 21-year-old woman, was in an automobile accident and sustained a severe brain injury and fractures of the left scapula, left radius, right ankle (fused), and jaw. She developed heterotopic ossification in the right elbow. P.H. was in a coma for 1 month and a stupor for 2 more months.

Expressive language was minimal with severe aphasia. The few words said were dysarthric. P.H. appeared to understand well, following directions and nodding appropriately to questions.

Behavior was immature. For example, she continuously hugged and kissed her boyfriend when he was in the room. P.H. was easily frustrated by difficult tasks. At these times she became extremely agitated and scratched herself to the point of bleeding.

Mobility was by wheelchair. P.H. was independent in transfers. She could roll and come to sit independently, but she needed moderate assistance to kneel and come to stand and maximal assistance to walk.

Examination

I. Unable to do self-care, to perform personal grooming hygiene, or to dress
   A. Impairments—components
      1. Strength—right arm fairly normal strength; left arm—not able to actively abduct shoulder but able to actively hold if placed at 90 degrees; external rotation and flexion—fair; active elbow flexion and extension through available range; wrist extension through half range and flexion through full range; gross and fine finger control present. Head was held in extreme forward position with neck flexed; normal head position could be maintained only 2 to 3 seconds. Trunk was in flexed position, and normal extension also held no longer than 2 to 3 seconds.
      2. Flexibility—left shoulder limited to 120 degrees of flexion and abduction; 45 degrees of external rotation; left forearm supination 10 degrees; right elbow 90 degrees of flexion; 20 degrees of extension.
      3. Tone—cervical hypotonia; left biceps, triceps, wrist flexor, and finger flexors are 3 (modified Ashworth scale). The tone in the left arm was of a co-contraction nature at the elbow; there was poor spatial sequencing throughout the limb.
      4. Speed of movement was extremely delayed throughout the left upper extremity and normal in the right extremity.
      5. Reaction time was decreased in all left arm movements and normal in right arm movements (using a touch plate).
      6. Endurance—cervical and trunk extensors and the left scapular muscles had poor muscular endurance with decreasing active range after three to five contractions. Cardiovascular fitness was poor; P.H.'s heart rate was 135 beats per minute after mild exercise of 5 minutes.
      7. Sensory—light touch was intact in both upper extremities; proprioception was within normal limits in both arms except for the left hand where movement was perceived correctly but direction was not consistent. P.H. identified 4 of 10 objects placed in the hand. The visual system showed lateral deviation to the left in the left eye and a dilated left pupil. Visual tracking was poor; P.H. stopped tracking at midline, going toward the left. She did not use saccadic motion when trying to read and had intermittent diplopia.
      8. Vestibular function appeared intact except for possible abnormality in perception of vertical (this did not appear as a

Continued

CASE 14–2   P.H. *Continued*

visual problem because eyes closed did not change off vertical position).
  B. Impairments—complex
    1. Synergies appear intact except in the cervical area, where the head is not held upright to maintain the eyes level.
    2. Modification of synergies is poor in the left arm, where movement patterns were gross and poorly refined and interlimb coordination was poor.
    3. Anticipatory responses were present in the trunk in sitting and reaching forward; they were not present during grasp of objects; hand size and grip were not matched to objects being picked up.
    4. Variability of performance—P.H. was able to reach and grasp as well as bend in many different ways with the right arm but had mainly an adducted, internal rotation pattern with elbow flexed on the left.

Evaluation and Diagnosis: Poor motor manipulation and prehension synergies in the left upper extremity resulted in nonuse of the left hand. Precision in grip was impaired by poor feedback from the fingers. Contributing to the lack of use of the hand was poor strength in the scapular stabilizers secondary to the scapular fracture and injury. Lack of adequate elbow ROM secondary to heterotopic ossification in the right elbow prevented grooming, personal hygiene such as teeth brushing, and applying makeup with the right arm, which had fairly normal function. Prolonged bed rest had resulted in poor trunk postural muscle endurance and a forward lean when standing. Visual and synergy dysfunctions resulted in flexed-forward head position. Perception of vertical was abnormal, perhaps from vestibular-cerebellar dysfunction.

II. Unable to Walk
  A. Impairments—components
    1. Strength—fair to good strength in left leg except poor in the gastrocnemius; good strength in right leg except fair in the right gastrocnemius; trunk extensors were fair.
    2. Flexibility—trunk flexion is limited to about half-normal lumbar flexion by tight back extensors; gastrocnemius is tight at neutral on the left. Fusion of right ankle at +5 degrees of dorsiflexion.
    3. Tone—modified Ashworth 3 in the left quadriceps and gastrocnemius.
    4. Reaction time in gastrocnemius and dorsiflexors was significantly delayed (force platform).

    5. Speed of left dorsiflexion was poor in swing phase dorsiflexion.
    6. Endurance was poor in trunk and lower extremity muscles; there was a reduction in amount of resistance tolerated after approximately 10 repetitions using isolated muscle testing.
    7. Sensory systems—light touch and proprioception were intact in the right lower extremity; proprioception was decreased (needs larger movement for accuracy) in the left lower extremity. Vision and vestibular systems were addressed under the disability.
  B. Impairments—complex
    1. Synergies—appear intact in the right lower extremity, but ankle strategy is absent in the left.
    2. Modification of synergies—right lower extremity shows a poor ability to modify walking patterns, resulting in large-amplitude movements at the hip and knee during walking. The left lower extremity shows modification of the hip strategy for different surfaces. Interlimb coordination in the lower extremities is poor.
    3. Anticipatory responses were generally absent in the left lower extremity and trunk during standing when right leg lifting.
    4. Anticipatory reactions did occur in the right leg when lifting the left leg forward. Use of feedback was evident when feedback occurred through the tactile or auditory systems. Use of visual feedback was poor in modification of walking or standing in both lower extremities. There appeared to be poor ability to vary the movement pattern in the right lower extremity during balance and walking (in the parallel bars). Variability of response was present depending on verbal cues but not spontaneously present in response to environmental cues. Pattern was fairly fixed and of a steppage-type gait.

Evaluation and Diagnosis: P.H. appears unable to walk without moderate to maximum assistance owing to lack of higher-level balance synergies and lack of anticipatory responses to movements of her center of gravity. Poor gastrocnemius strength also probably contributes to lack of ankle strategy. Poor quality of movement in the right leg is secondary to inability to modify underlying synergies.

Continued

CASE 14–2 P.H. *Continued*

III. Postural disability—unable to hold head up, stands with weight on right leg leaning about 15 degrees to the right
   A. Impairments—components
      1. Strength is fair in the extensors of the mid and lower trunk muscles and poor in cervical extensors.
      2. Flexibility—forward flexion is limited to 50% of normal by tightness in the lumbar extensors. The left lumbar extensors have above-normal tone and often elicit an extensor spasm during forward bending.
      3. Sensory—right tilt off vertical 15 degrees.
   B. Impairments—complex
      1. Balance synergies show proximal to distal firing beginning in the trunk flexors and extensors during small perturbations in normal standing. Occluding vision during normal standing does not change balance and only slightly degrades balance when on foam.
      2. Modification of upright balance is poor with the visual and/or proprioceptive feedback.

Evaluation and Diagnosis: P.H. has problems perceiving the vertical position in sitting and standing secondary to visual and proprioceptive losses. She has poor muscular endurance secondary to prolonged bed rest, slowed movement, and decreased activity level over months. Walking is with hip strategy of knees and hips bent owing to poor production of torque on floor by the gastrocnemius muscles and delayed responses to movement. Anticipatory responses for ambulation are minimal and secondary to lack of accurate visual input.

Handicap: Immature behavior resulting in loss of friends and inability to hold a job.

Long-term goals were independent ambulation without an assistive device at home and with a cane in the community and independence in all self-care and ADL. Behavior modification was initiated.

Intervention. Initial goals included addressing those impairments in the basic component level that did not allow higher levels of functioning. These were improvements in neck and trunk strength and endurance, left scapular and shoulder muscle strength and flexibility, and gastrocnemius strength and flexibility; visual skills, particularly in gaze stabilization and tracking; and awareness of vertical. P.H.'s attention span was slightly shorter than normal.

Functional electrical stimulation to the posterior cervical muscles, intermittent use of a supportive collar to take the extensor muscles off stretch, and eye fixation exercises to focus on a single point were used to encourage visual control of head position.

Complex neck activities to encourage basic synergy use and modification included seated activities in which P.H. wore a "hat" with a flat top from which she tried to prevent an object from falling off (first flat stable objects and later more rounded objects). This exercise was performed first on a firm, flat-seated surface and progressed to sitting on an exercise ball. The ball promoted automatic neck muscle synergies in which the body moves and the head is kept upright and still.

Traditional basic left upper-extremity strengthening exercises included use of Theraband. Functional activities that required scapular use such as emptying the dishwasher with the left hand were assigned homework.

Electrical stimulation twice a day for 15 minutes to the right triceps gained 20 degrees of extension and 100 degrees of flexion. Active extension exercises were also given. In the clinic, P.H. worked on picking up and manipulating objects of different sizes and shapes, throwing balls at targets, two-handed carrying, and so on. She sorted different-sized objects by retrieving them from a bucket also containing marble-sized balls with her vision occluded to force use of stereognosis.

P.H. enjoyed cooking, so tasks were given that used right elbow extension, such as rolling cookie dough. Exercises such as washing the dishes with hands in soapy water for proprioceptive feedback and practice of slip grip for enhancement of feedback through the finger tips were used. Setting the table with the left hand helped establish better functional use (plastic dishes).

Complex functions in manipulation with the left arm were facilitated by doing two-hand activities. P.H. used large mats to hook a small rug, and she had a list, as mentioned earlier, of chores to do that required lifting and manipulating with both hands. When able, she began trying two-hand typing. Two of the most motivating activities were applying makeup and inserting contact lenses.

Visual treatment used exercises that required visual fixation at different points in space and at different distances using letters and objects, with the goal of seeing only one image. These exercises advanced to include moving objects and head moving with a fixed object and progressed to both the object and head moving while maintaining a single image. Finally, full body movement with eyes fixed on moving object was accomplished.

Improved use of vestibulocerebellar function was promoted through use of foam, standing on narrow beam, and walking on ramps and grass,

Continued

CASE 14–2   P.H. *Continued*

activities that require the use of the visual and vestibular systems.

Spasticity was addressed with exercises to promote less co-contraction and distal to proximal sequencing in both the left leg and left arm. Electromyographic biofeedback with a two-channel setup on the triceps/biceps and wrist flexors/wrist extensors was used to teach decreased co-contraction during activities such as reaching and lifting. This was carried over to the home program.

P.H. used a Nordic Track machine for general cardiovascular fitness work. The gliding motion with toe loops allowed her to keep her feet near the ground when moving forward, and the arm work encouraged free movement of the trunk in rotation.

In the lower-extremity program, gastrocnemius strengthening concentrated on standing exercises such as heel lifts and toe walking along. Speed of motion exercises were performed with left foot back and pulling forward quickly and exercises moving on foam, including walking.

Exercises were not popular. The goal P.H. had when first starting therapy was "to dance with my boyfriend." To encourage functional use of postural and balance synergies, dancing was used. She started first with slow dancing with her boyfriend. Gradually, she was able to dance to faster music without being held, by using trunk and arm motion and a side-stepping motion. Finally, forward-backward movements and turning and bending were added. Additionally, P.H. agreed to model in the brain injury association fashion show, which provided motivation to walk independently.

Balance exercises such as swaying around the ankles, getting from kneeling to standing, and working on a force platform for attaining and feeling vertical were successful. A video camera recording from behind was used to teach P.H. to lift her foot so that "she could see her sole on the left foot"; this approach resulted in increased left knee flexion in her gait pattern. Walking was started with a full step program on each foot. Goals were to keep the light worn at her waist from moving more than 2 inches side to side. This was also facilitated by moving the parallel bars extremely close together and asking P.H. not to touch the bars with either hip as she practiced stepping.

Exercises to promote trunk and anticipatory responses early on used a Gymnastik ball, as well as weighted and reaching exercise, ball kicking to a goal, ball catching, and ball throwing to a target. P.H. practiced walking over and around various objects.

A behavioral modification program was established so that P.H. was given control to stop activities that were too stressful for her; and she participated in a volunteer program on a farm feeding and watering animals two to three times a week on a fixed schedule to establish personal responsibility and provide a positive learning environment.

P.H. reached the goals of independent household ambulation and community ambulation with a cane. She had normal posture and good assistive and gross independent use of the left hand and arm. Tone in the left arm and left quadriceps was at a level 2 at discharge.

---

ferent from their expectation. The rehabilitation team members, who can contrast the client's progress only since injury, may be quite pleased. Is quality measured by past performance, past potential, present performance, or future potential? Clients themselves may or may not have insight into past, present, or future performance and potential. What is the standard by which quality of life is measured? Is it income, reduction of dependency, contribution to society, or social interaction? Each of these indicators has been used as a standard. Ultimately, the determination of successful rehabilitation relies on the answer to these questions. Jennett and Teasdale[67] suggest six aspects of living: ADL, mobility and life organization, social relationships, work or leisure activities, present satisfaction, and future prospects. Most of these factors, although important, cannot be quantitatively measured, and they do not entirely answer the question of what is quality of life. However one estimates the quality of life, those who have chosen to help rehabilitate clients with brain injury continue to pursue an ideal of quality for each life that has been saved and may, by doing so, enhance the quality of their own.

ACKNOWLEDGMENT

Thank you to Susan Smith, PhD, PT, the author of this chapter in the previous edition, for information included in this chapter.

REFERENCES

1. Adams JH, Graham DI, Murray LS, Scott G: Diffuse axonal injury due to non-missile head injury in humans: An analysis of 45 cases. Ann Neurol 12:557–563, H1982.
2. Astrand P: Quantification of exercise capacity and evaluation of physical capacity in man. Prog Cardiovasc Dis 19(1):51–67, 1976.
3. Bach-y-Rita P: Brain plasticity as a basis for therapeutic procedures. *In* Bach-y-Rita P (ed): Recovery of Function: Theoretical Considerations for Brain Injury Rehabilitation. Baltimore, University Park Press, 1980.
4. Bach-y-Rita P: Brain injury. Wall Street Journal, October 12, 1993.
5. Badke MB, Duncan PW: Patterns of rapid motor response during postural adjustment when standing in healthy subjects and hemiplegic patients. Phys Ther 63:13, 1983.
6. Baker LL, Parker K: Neuromuscular electrical stimulation for the head injured patient. Phys Ther 63:1967–1974, 1983.
7. Benton L, et al: Functional Electrical Stimulation: A Practical Clinical Guide. Downey, CA, Rancho Los Amigos Rehabilitation Engineering Center, 1981.

8. Berger MS, et al: Outcome from severe head injury in children and adolescents. J Neurosurg 62:194, 1985.

9. Bernstein N: Coordination and Regulation of Movements. New York, Pergamon Press, 1967.

10. Berrol S: Evaluation and the persistent vegetative state. Head Trauma Rehabil 1:7, 1986.

11. Black P, et al: Recovery of motor function after lesions in motor cortex of monkey. In Black P: Outcome of Severe Damage to the Central Nervous System. New York, Elsevier, 1975, pp 65–83.

12. Bogatry U, Gros N, Kljajic M, et al: The rehabilitation of gait in patient with hemiplegia: A comparison between conventional theory and multi functional electrical stimulation. Phys Ther 75:490, 1995.

13. Bohannon R, Smith M: Interrater reliability of a modified Ashworth scale of muscle spasticity. Phys Ther 67:206–207, 1987.

14. Bond MR: Assessment of psychosocial outcome of severe head injury. Acta Neurochir 34:57, 1976.

15. Bourbonnais D, et al: Abnormal spatial patterns of elbow activation in hemiparetic human subjects. Brain 112:85, 1989.

16. The Brain Foundation Report. Guidelines for cerebral perfusion pressure. J Neurotrauma 12:693–697, 1996.

17. The Brain Foundation Report. The use of barbiturates in the control of intracranial hypertension. J Neurotrauma 13:711–714, 1996.

18. Brotherton J, et al: Social skills training in the rehabilitation of patients with traumatic closed head injury. Arch Phys Med Rehabil 69:827, 1988.

19. Bruce RA: Exercise testing of patients with coronary artery disease. Ann Clin Res 3:323, 1971.

20. Buchner D, deLatuer B: The importance of skeletal muscle strength in physical function in older adults. Ann Behav Med 13:12–21, 1991.

21. Butland J, Pang J, Gross E: Two-six and 12 minute walking tests in respiratory diseases. BMJ 284:1607–1608, 1982.

22. Carey J, Allison J, Manudale M: Electromyographic study of muscular overflow during precision handgrip. Phys Ther 63:505–511, 1983.

23. Carr J, Shepard RB: Investigation of new motor assessment scale for stroke patients. Phys Ther 65:175–180, 1985.

24. Cartlidge N, Shaw DA: Head Injury. London, WB Saunders, 1981.

25. Cecchini A: Functional assessment after traumatic brain injury. Neurol Rep 22(4):136–143, 1998.

26. Centers for Disease Control and Prevention: Atlanta, April 1999.

27. Chesnut R, Marshall L, Klauber M: The role of secondary brain injury in determining outcome from severe head injury. J Trauma 34:216–222, 1993.

28. Cintas H: The relationship of motor skill level and risk-taking during exploration in toddlers. Pediatr Phys Ther 165:59–63, 1992.

29. Colorado Head Injury Foundation, Inc. Brochure, 1993.

30. Cozean C, et al: Biofeedback and functional electric stimulation in stroke rehabilitation. Arch Phys Med Rehabil 69:401, 1988.

31. Craik R: Abnormalities of motor behavior. In Lister M (ed): Contemporary Management of Motor Control Problems. Alexandria, VA, American Physical Therapy Association, 1991.

32. Deadwyler S, Hampson R: The significance of neural ensemble codes during behavior and cognition. Annu Rev Neurosci 20:217–244, 1997.

33. Dearden N, Gibson J, McDowall D: Effects of high-dose dexamethasone on outcome from severe head injury. J Neurosurg 64:81–88, 1986.

34. DeSouza L, Langton T, Miller S: Assessment and recovery of arm control in hemiplegic stroke patients: Arm Function Test. Int Rehab Med 2:3–9, 1984.

35. Devor M, et al: Dorsal horn neurons that respond to stimulation of distant dorsal roots. J Physiol (London) 270:519, 1977.

36. Dietz V, et al: Motor unit involvement in spastic paresis: Relationship between leg muscle activation and histochemistry. J Neurol Sci 75:89, 1986.

37. Dietz V, Berger W: Interlimb coordination of posture in patients with spastic paresis: Imperial functions of spinal reflexes. Brain 107:965, 1984.

38. Edstrom L, et al: Correlation between recruitment order of motor units and muscle atrophy pattern in upper motorneurone lesion: Significance of spasticity. Experimentia 29:560, 1973.

39. Evans R: Predicting outcome following traumatic brain injury. Neurol Rep 22:144–148, 1998.

40. Evarts EV: Role of motor cortex in voluntary movements in primates. In Brookhart JM, et al (eds): Handbook of Physiology, the Nervous System—Motor Control. Bethesda, MD, American Physiological Society, 1981.

41. Ewert J, Levin H, Watson M: Procedural memory during post-traumatic amnesia in survivors of severe closed head injury. Arch Neurol 46:911–916, 1989.

42. Folstein M, Folstein S, McHugh P: Mini-mental: A practical method for grading the cognitive state of patients for the clinician. J Psychiatr Res 12:189–198, 1975.

43. Fulop Z, Wright D, Stein D: Pharmacology of traumatic brain injury: Experimental models and clinical implications. Neurol Rep 22(3):100–109, 1998.

44. Functional assessment measure. J Rehabil Outcome Measurement 1(3):63–65, 1991.

45. Gentry R: Imaging of closed head injury. Radiology 191:1–17, 1994.

46. Georgopolous AP: On reaching. Annu Rev Neurosci 9:147, 1986.

47. Gilchrist E, Wilkinson M: Some factors determining prognosis in young people with severe head injuries. Arch Neurol 36:355, 1979.

48. Gilroy J, Meyer J: Medical Neurology, 3rd ed. New York, Macmillan, 1979.

49. Guliani C: Theories of motor control. In Lister M (ed): New Concepts for Physical Therapy in Contemporary Management of Motor Control Problems. Alexandria, VA, American Physical Therapy Association, 1991.

50. Glenn MB: Update on pharmacology: Antispasticity medications in the patient with traumatic brain injury: I. J Head Trauma Rehabil 3:87, 1988.

51. Glenn MB, Wrobewski B: Update on pharmacology: antispasticity medications in the patient with traumatic brain injury. J Head Trauma Rehabil 1:71, 1986.

52. Golani I, Fentress JC: Early ontogeny of face grooming in mice. Dev Psychobiol 18:529, 1985.

53. Gordon J: Anticipatory guidance from a motor control perspective. Presented at Annual Sensorimotor Integration Symposium, San Diego, July 10–12, 1992.

54. Granger C, Hamilton B, Keith R: Advances in functional assessment for medical rehabilitation. Topics Geriatr Rehabil 1:59–71, 1986.

55. Greenberg R, et al: Prognostic implications of early multimodality evoked potentials in severe head injury patients: A prospective study. J Neurosurg 55:227, 1981.

56. Groswasser Z, et al: Closed cervical cranial trauma associated with involvement of the carotid and vertebral arteries. Laryngoscope 81:1381, 1971.

57. Guide to physical therapy practice. Phys Ther 77:1180, 1997.

58. Hagg T, Vahlsing H, Manthorpe M: Nerve growth factor infusion into the denvervated adult rat hippocampal formation promotes cholinergic reinnervation. J Neurosci 10:3087–3092, 1990.

59. Heinemann A: Functional states and therapeutic intervention during rehabilitation. Am J Phys Med Rehabil 74:315–326, 1995.

60. Held R: Plasticity in sensory-motor systems. Sci Am 213:84, 1967.

61. Horak FB: Determinants of movement in central nervous system damage: Implications for assessment and treatment of children and adults. Presented at Symposia, Denver, July 27–29, 1984.

62. Horak FB, et al: The effects of movement velocity, mass displaced, and task certainty on associated postural adjustments made by normal and hemiplegic individuals. J Neurol Neurosurg Psychiatry 47:1020, 1984.

63. Hubel DH, Wiesel TN: The period of susceptibility to the physiological effects of unilateral eye closure in kittens. J Physiol 206:419, 1970.

64. Jennett B, Bond M: Assessment of outcome after severe brain damage: A practical scale. Lancet 1:480, 1975.

65. Jennett B, Plum F: Persistent vegetative state after brain damage: A syndrome in search of a name. Lancet 1:734, 1972.

66. Jennett B, Teasdale G: Aspects of coma after severe head injury. Lancet 1:878, 1977.

67. Jennett B, Teasdale G: Management of Head Injuries. Philadelphia, FA Davis, 1981.

68. Johansson RS, Westling G: Signals in tactile afferents from the fingers eliciting adaptive motor responses during precision grip. Exp Brain Res 66:14, 1987.

69. Johnson D, Almi CR: Age, brain damage and performance. In

Finger S (ed): Recovery from Brain Damage. New York, Plenum Press, 1978.

70. Kampfi A, Schmutzhard E, Franz G, et al: Prediction of recovery from post-traumatic vegetative state with cerebral magnetic-resonance imaging. Lancet 351:1763–1767, 1998.

71. Kelso J, Schoner G: Self-organization of coordinative movement patterns. Hum Move Sci 7:27, 1988.

72. Knutsson E, Martensson A: Dynamic motor capacity in spastic paresis and its relationship to prime motor dysfunction, spastic reflexes and antagonistic coactivation. Scand J Rehabil Med 12:93, 1980.

73. Kondraske GV, et al: Human performance measurement: Some perspectives. IEEE Eng Med Biol Soc Mag 7:11, 1988.

74. Konrad H, et al: Rehabilitation therapy for patients with disequilibrium and balance disorders. Otolaryngol Head Neck Surg 107:107, 1992.

75. Lanksch W, et al: Correlations between clinical symptoms and computed tomography findings in closed head injuries. In Frowein RA, et al (eds): Advances in Neurosurgery, 5th ed. Berlin, Springer-Verlag, 1978.

76. Leahy BJ, Lam CS: Neuropsychological testing and functional outcome for individuals with traumatic brain injury. Brain Injury 12(12):1025–1035, 1998.

77. Leahy P: Head trauma in adults: Problems, assessment, and treatment. In Contemporary Management of Motor Control Problems. Proceeding of II Step Conference. Foundation for Physical Therapy (ed): Fredericksburg, VA, Brookcrafters, 1991, pp 247–252.

78. Levin H, O'Donnell V, Grossman R: The Galveston Orientation and Amnesia Test: A practical scale to assess cognition after head injured. J Nerv Ment Dis 167:675–684, 1979.

79. Lezak M: Neuropsychological assessment. In Executive Functions and Motor Performance. New York, Oxford Press, 1983.

80. Mahoney FI, Barthel DW: Functional evaluation: The Barthel Index. Md State Med J 14:61, 1965.

81. Man AM, et al: Adaptive and part-whole training in the acquisition of a complex perceptual-motor skill. Acta Psychol (Amsterdam) 71:179, H 1989.

82. Marrubini MB: Classification of coma. Intens Care Med 10:217, 1984.

83. Martenicuk RG, et al: Constraints on human arm movement trajectories. Can J Psychol 41:365, 1987.

84. Mitchell DE, et al: Recovery from the effects of monocular deprivation. J Comp Neurol 176:53, 1977.

85. Muizelaar J, Marmarou A, Ward JD: Adverse effects of prolonged hyperventilation in patients with severe head injury: A randomized clinical trial: J Neurosur 75:731–739, 1991.

86. Mysiw WJ, Sandel ME: The agitated brain injured patient. Part 2: Pathophysiology and treatment. Arch Phys Med Rehabil 78:213–220, 1997.

87. Nashner LM: Organization and programming of motor activity during posture control. Prog Brain Res 50:177, 1979.

88. National Brain Injury Association, 1999. http://www.biausa.org.

89. National Head Injury Foundation, Annual Report, 1985–1986.

90. Newell KM: Knowledge of results and motor learning. J Motor Behav 4:235, 1974.

91. Newell KM, et al: Whole-part training strategies for learning the response dynamics of microprocessor driven simulator. Acta Psychol (Amsterdam) 71:197, 1989.

92. Olney S, et al: Mechanical energy patterns in gait of cerebral palsied children with hemiplegia. Phys Ther 67:1348, 1987.

93. Payton O, Kelley D: Electromyographic evidence of the acquisition of a motor skill: A pilot study. Phys Ther 52:3:261, 1987.

94. Perry J, Ireland M, Gronley J, Hoffer M: Predictive value of manual muscle testing and gait analysis in normal ankles by dynamic electromyography. Foot Ankle 6:254–259, 1986.

95. Plum F, Posner JB: The Diagnosis of Stupor and Coma, 3rd ed. Philadelphia, FA Davis, 1980.

96. Rappaport M, et al: Disability rating scale for severe head trauma: Coma to community. Arch Phys Med Rehabil 63:118, 1982.

97. Roberts AH: Long-term prognosis of severe accidental head injury. Proc R Soc Med 69:137, 1976.

98. Rose SJ, Rothstein JM: Muscle mutability: I. General concepts and adaptations to altered patterns of use. Phys Ther 62:1773, 1982.

99. Rosenfalck A, Andreassen S: Impaired regulation and firing pattern of single motor units in patients with spasticity. J Neurol Neurosurg Psychiatry 43:907, 1980.

100. Rosenthal M, Christensen BK, Ross TP: Depression following traumatic brain injury (review). Arch Phys Med Rehabil 79:90–103, 1988.

101. Rosin AJ: Very prolonged unresponsive state following brain injury. Scand J Rehabil Med 10:33, 1978.

102. Russell WR: Cerebral involvement in head injury: A study based on the examination of two hundred cases. Brain 55:549, 1932.

103. Sahrmann SA: Diagnosis by the physical therapist—a prerequisite for treatment: A special communication. Phys Ther 68:1703, 1988.

104. Sahrmann SA: Posture and muscle imbalance: Faulty lumbar-pelvic alignment and associated musculoskeletal pain syndromes. In Post-graduate Advances in Physical Therapy: A Comprehensive Independent Learning Office Study Course. Alexandria, VA, American Physical Therapy Association, 1987.

105. Sahrmann SA, Norton BJ: The relationship of voluntary movement to spasticity in the upper motor neuron syndrome. Ann Neurol 2:460, 1977.

106. Salcido R, Costich J: Recurrent traumatic brain injury. Brain Injury 11:391–402, 1997.

107. Sale D: Influence of exercise and training on motor unit activation. Exer Sports Sci Re 15:95–151, 1987.

108. Schmidt RA: A schema theory of discrete motor learning. Psychol Rev 82:225, 1975.

109. Schmidt RA: Motor Control and Learning: A Behavioral Emphasis. Champaign, IL, Human Kinetics, 1988.

110. Schmidt RA: Motor learning principles for physical therapy. In Lister M (ed): Contemporary Management of Motor Control Problems. In Proceeding of the II Step Conference, Norman, OK, American Physical Therapy Association, 1991.

111. Schoner G, Kelso JAS: Dynamic pattern generation in behavioral and neural systems. Science 239:1513, 1988.

112. Shepard N, Telian S: Vestibular and balance rehabilitation therapy. Ann Otol Rhinol Laryngol 102:198–205, 1993.

113. Signorini DF, Andrews PJ, Jones PA, et al: Adding insult to injury: The prognostic value of early secondary insults for survival after traumatic brain injury. J Neurol Neurosurg Psychiatry 66:26–31, 1999.

114. Snoek J, et al: Computerized tomography after recent severe head injury in patients without acute intracranial hematoma. J Neurol Neurosurg Psychiatry 42:215, 1979.

115. Springer J, Farne J, Bower D: Common misconceptions about traumatic brain injury among family members of rehabilitation patients. J Head Trauma Rehabil 12(3):41–50, 1997.

116. Squire L: Memory: Neural organization and behavior. In Mountcastle VB, Plum E, Gaiger S (eds): Handbook of Physiology, Vol V, The Nervous System, Higher Functions of the Brain. Bethesda, MD, American Physiological Society, 1987, pp 295–370.

117. Stewart WA, et al: A prognostic model for head injury. Acta Neurochir 45:199, 1979.

118. Stover S, Zeiger HE: Head injury in children and teenagers: Functional recovery correlated with the duration of coma. Arch Phys Med Rehabil 57:201, 1976.

119. Strich SJ: Lesions in the cerebral hemispheres after blunt head injury. J Clin Pathol 23(Suppl 4):154, 1970.

120. Tang A, Rymer WZ: Abnormal force–EMG relations in paretic limbs of hemiparetic human subjects. J Neurol Neurosurg Psychiatry 44:690, 1981.

121. Tardieu C, et al: For how long must the soleus muscle be stretched daily to prevent contracture? Dev Med Child Neurol 30:3, 1988.

122. Taub E, et al: Technique to improve chronic motor deficit after stroke. Arch Phys Med Rehabil 74:247, 1993.

123. Thelen E: Evolving and dissolving synergies in the development of leg coordination. In Wallace SA (ed): Perspectives on the Coordination of Movement. New York, Elsevier, 1991.

124. Tinniti M: Performance oriented assessment of mobility: Problems in elderly patients. J Am Geriatr Soc 34(2):119–126, 1986.

125. Tower SS: Pyramidal lesions in the monkey. Brain 63:36, 1940.

126. Van Den Berge JH, et al: Interobserver agreement in assessment of ocular signs in coma. J Neurol Neurosurg Psychiatry 42:1163, 1979.

127. Van der Naalt J, Hew JM, van Zomeren AH, et al: Computed tomography and magnetic resonance imaging in mild to moderate head injury: Early and late imaging related to outcome. Ann Neurol 46(1):70–78, 1999.

128. Van der Naalt, van Zorneren AH, Sluiter WJ, Minderhoud JM:

One year outcome in mild to moderate head injury: The predictive value of acute injury characteristics related to complaints and return to work. Neurol Neurosurg Psychiatry 66:207–213, 1999.

129. VanSant A: Rising from a supine position to erect stance: Description of adult movement and a developmental hypothesis. Phys Ther 68:185, 1988.

130. Wade D: Measurement in Neurological Rehabilitation. New York, Oxford University Press, 1992.

131. Warren L, Wrigley J, Yoles W, Fince P: Factors associated with life satisfaction among a sample of persons with neurotrauma. J Rehabil Res Dev 33(4):404–406, 1996.

132. Watkins MP, et al: Isokinetic testing in patients with hemiparesis: A pilot study. Phys Ther 64:184, 1984.

133. Weber K, Kashner L: Adult norms in nine hole peg test of finger dexterity. Occup Ther J Res 5:24–37, 1986.

134. Wechsler D: Wechsler Memory Scale—Revised. San Antonio, Psychological Corporation, 1987.

135. Wedekind C, Fischbach R, Pakos P, et al: Comparative use of magnetic resonance imaging and electrophysiologic investigation for the prognosis of head injury. J Trauma Injury Infect Crit Care 47(1):44–49, 1999.

136. Wiesel TN, Hubel DH: Single-cell responses in striate cortex of kittens deprived of vision in one eye. J Neurophysiol 26:1003, 1963.

137. Wiesel TN, Hubel DH: Comparison of the effects of unilateral and bilateral eye closure on cortical unit responses in kittens. J Neurophysiol 28:1029, 1965.

138. Winkler P: Use of the Sandune in exercise of multiple sclerosis patients. Unpublished data, 1994.

139. Winstein C: Designing practice for motor learning. In Lister M (ed): Clinical Implications in Contemporary Management of Motor Control Problems. Proceedings of the II STEP Conference, Alexandria, VA, American Physical Therapy Association, 1991.

140. Winstein C: Knowledge of results and motor learning: Implications for physical therapy. In Movement Science, a monograph of the American Physical Therapy Association. Alexandria, VA, APTA, 1991.

141. Winstein CJ, et al: Standing balance training: Effect on balance and locomotion in hemiparetic adults. Arch Phys Med Rehabil 70:755, 1989.

142. Wolf SL, et al: Forced use of hemiplegic upper extremities to reverse the effect of learned nonuse among stroke and head-injured patients. Exp Neurol 104:125, 1989.

143. Wolfson L, Whipple R, Amernan P, Tobin J: Gait assessment in the elderly: A gait abnormality rating scale and its relationship to falls. J Gerontol 45:m12–m19, 1990.

144. World Health Organization: International Classification of Impairments, Disabilities and Handicaps. Geneva, Switzerland, World Health Organization, 1980.

145. World Health Organization: The 3-step ergometer test. In The Future Fitness Measurement Guide. Geneva, Switzerland, World Health Organization, 1972.

146. Young RR, Delwaide PJ: Drug therapy: Spasticity: Part I. N Engl J Med 304:96, 1981.

147. Young RR, Delwaide PJ: Drug therapy: Spasticity: Part II. N Engl J Med 304:96, 1981.

148. Zimmerman RA, et al: Computed tomography of shearing injuries of the cerebral white matter. Radiology 127:393, 1978.

Congenital Spinal Cord Injury

JANE W. SCHNEIDER, PhD, PT • KRISTIN J. KROSSCHELL, MA, PT

Key Words

- Chiari malformation
- crouch-control AFO
- diastematomyelia
- hydrocephalus
- lipomeningocele
- myelodysplasia
- myelomeningocele
- reciprocating gait orthosis (RGO)
- sacral agenesis
- spina bifida cystica
- spina bifida occulta
- standing A-frame
- tethered spinal cord

Objectives

After reading this chapter the student/therapist will:

1. Understand the various types of spina bifida.

2. Understand the incidence and etiology of spina bifida.

3. Identify the clinical manifestations of myelomeningocele, including neurological, orthopedic, and urological sequelae.

4. Comprehend medical management in the newborn period and beyond.

5. Determine physical and occupational therapy evaluations, including manual muscle testing, range of motion, sensory testing, reflex testing, developmental/functional assessments, and perceptual/cognitive evaluations.

6. List the major physical and/or occupational therapy goals and appropriate therapeutic management for each of the following stages: (a) before surgical closure of sac, (b) after surgery during hospitalization, (c) preambulatory, (d) toddler through preschool age, and (e) primary school through adolescence.

7. Understand psychological adjustment to congenital spinal cord injury.

A spinal cord injury is a complex disability. When a spinal cord lesion exists from birth, an additional complexity is added. This congenital condition predisposes that many areas of the central nervous system (CNS) may not develop or function adequately. In addition, all areas of development (physical, cognitive, and psychosocial) that depend so heavily on central functioning will likely be impaired. The clinician therefore must be aware of the significant impact this neurological defect has not only on motor function but also on a variety of related human capacities.

A developmental framework has been used to aid in understanding the sequential problems of the child with spina bifida. The developmental model, however, must always stay in line with the functional model for adult trauma, because the problems of the congenitally involved child grow quickly into the disabilities of the injured adult. With concentration on the present but with an eye to the future, appropriate management goals can be achieved.

OVERVIEW OF CONGENITAL SPINAL CORD INJURY

A congenital spinal cord lesion occurs in utero and is present at the time of birth. To understand how this

449

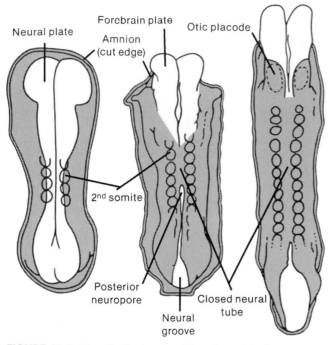

FIGURE 15–1. Neural tube forming. (From Stark GD: Spina Bifida Problems and Management. London, Blackwell Scientific, 1977.)

malformation develops, one needs an appreciation of normal nervous system maturation.

The nervous system develops from a portion of embryonic ectoderm called the neural plate. During gestation, the neural plate develops folds that begin to close, forming the neural tube (Fig. 15–1). The neural tube differentiates into the CNS, which is composed of brain and spinal cord tissue.[98]

In the normal embryo, neural tube closure begins in the cervical region and proceeds cranially and caudally. Closure is generally complete by the twenty-sixth day.[98]

Types of Spina Bifida

In spina bifida there is a defect in the neural tube closure and the overlying posterior vertebral arches. The extent of the defect may result in one of two types of spina bifida: occulta or cystica.

Spina bifida occulta is characterized by a failure of one or more of the vertebral arches to meet and fuse in the third month of development. The spinal cord and meninges are unharmed and remain within the vertebral canal (Fig. 15–2A). The bony defect is covered with skin that may be marked by a dimple, pigmentation, or patch of hair.[120] The common site for this defect is the lumbosacral area, and it is usually associated with no disturbance of neurological or musculoskeletal functioning.[87]

Spina bifida cystica results when the neural and overlying vertebral arches fail to close appropriately. There is a cystic protrusion of the meninges or of the spinal cord and meninges through the defective vertebral arches.

The milder form of spina bifida cystica, called meningocele, involves protrusion of the meninges and cerebrospinal fluid (CSF) only into the cystic sac (see Fig. 15–2B). The spinal cord remains within the vertebral canal, but it

may exhibit abnormalities.[82] Clinical signs vary (according to spinal cord anomalies) or may not be apparent. This is a relatively uncommon form of spina bifida cystica.

A more severe form of spina bifida cystica, called myelocele or myelocystocele, is present when the central canal of the spinal cord is dilated producing a large skin-covered cyst. The neural tube appears to close normally but is distended from the cystic swelling. The CSF may ceaselessly expand the neural canal. Prompt medical attention is mandatory. This form of spina bifida is also rare.[46]

The more common and severe form of the defect is known as myelomeningocele, in which both spinal cord and meninges are contained in the cystic sac (see Fig. 15–2C). Within the sac, the spinal cord and associated neural tissue show extensive abnormalities. In incomplete closure of the neural tube (dysraphism), abnormal growth of the cord and a tortuous pathway of neural elements make normal transmission of nervous impulses abnormal. The result is a variable sensory and motor impairment at the level of the lesion and below.[120] In an open myelomeningocele, nerve roots and spinal cord may be exposed with dura and skin evident at the margin of the lesion.

Although spina bifida cystica can occur at any level of the spinal cord, myelomeningoceles are most common in the thoracic and lumbosacral regions. Two thirds of open lesions involve the thoracolumbar junction.[120] Because myelomeningocele occurs in 94% of the cases of spina bifida cystica, therefore, the terms *spina bifida, myelodysplasia,* and *myelomeningocele* are frequently used interchangeably.[82]

Other forms of spinal dysraphism include diastematomyelia, lipomeningocele, and sacral agenesis. Diastematomyelia is present in 30% to 40% of patients with myelomeningocele and is secondary to partial or complete clefting of the spinal cord.[18] Lipomeningocele, another form of spina bifida cystica, is usually due to a vertebral defect associated with a superficial fatty mass (lipoma or fatty tumor) that merges with the lower level of spinal cord. There is no associated hydrocephalus, and neurological deficit is generally minimal; however, problems with urinary control and motor control of the lower extremities may be noted.[105] Neurological tissue invasion may be secondary to a tethered spinal cord; therefore, early lipoma resection is indicated not only for cosmesis but also to minimize neurological sequelae. Lumbosacral or sacral agenesis may occur and is due to an absence of the caudal part of the spine and sacrum. Children with this form of dysraphism may present with narrow flattened buttocks, weak gluteal muscles, and a shortened intergluteal cleft. The normal lumbar lordosis is absent, although the lower lumbar spine may be prominent. Calf muscles may be atrophic or absent. The pelvic ring is completed with either direct apposition of the iliac bones or with interposition of the lumbar spine replacing the absent sacrum. These children may have scoliosis, motor and sensory loss, and visceral abnormalities including anal atresia, fused kidneys, and congenital heart malformations. Management is started early and is symptomatic for each system.[28]

Failure of fusion of the cranial end of the neural tube results in a condition known as anencephaly. In this condition, some brain tissue may be evident, but forebrain

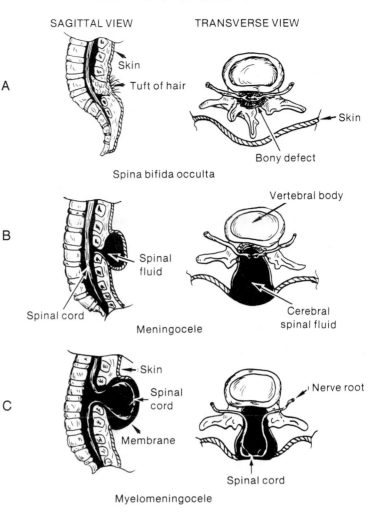

SAGITTAL VIEW   TRANSVERSE VIEW

A

Skin

Tuft of hair

Skin

Bony defect

Spina bifida occulta

B

Vertebral body

Spinal cord

Spinal fluid

Meningocele

Cerebral spinal fluid

C

Skin

Spinal cord

Membrane

Nerve root

Spinal cord

Myelomeningocele

FIGURE 15–2. Types of spina bifida. *A,* Spina bifida occulta. *B,* Meningocele. *C,* Myelomeningocele. (From McLone DG: An Introduction to Spina Bifida. Chicago, Children's Memorial Hospital, Northwestern University, 1980.)

development is usually absent.[87] Because sustained life is not possible with this neural tube defect, anencephaly is not discussed further.

Incidence and Etiology

Statistics about the incidence of spina bifida vary considerably in different parts of the world. In the United States the incidence is approximately 2 per 1,000 births.[62] This is about midrange in world statistics, considering a spina bifida birth rate of 0.3 per 1,000 in Japan and 4.5 per 1,000 in certain parts of the British Commonwealth.

There is some evidence of seasonal variation, suggesting a positive relationship between the occurrence of spina bifida and conceptions in March to May.[13, 113, 120]

Spina bifida is thought to be more common in females than in males, although some studies suggest no real sex difference.[2, 58, 82, 120] The incidence of spina bifida is higher in those of Celtic origin and lower in blacks and Asians.[13, 69] A study of the association of race and gender with different neurological levels of myelomeningocele reported the proportions of whites and females to be significantly higher in thoracic level patients.[46] A significant relationship also has been noted between social class and spina bifida: the lower the social class, the higher the incidence.[91, 92]

Genetic factors seem to influence the occurrence of

spina bifida. The chances of having a second affected child are between 1% and 2%, whereas in the general population the percentage drops to one fifth of 1%.[65, 71] While these factors are related to the incidence of spina bifida, the cause of this defect remains in question. Environmental conditions, such as hyperthermia in the first weeks of pregnancy, or dietary factors, such as canned meats, potatoes, or tea, have been implicated but not substantiated.[13, 55, 56] In addition, nutritional deficiencies, such as folic acid and vitamin A, have been implicated as a cause of primary neural tube defect.[72, 117] Genetic considerations, such as an Rh blood type, a specific gene type (HLA-B27), and an X-linked gene, have been implicated, but not conclusively.[5, 16, 100] It appears that environmental factors combined with genetic predisposition may trigger the development of spina bifida, although definitive evidence is not available to support this claim.[69, 120]

The incidence of spina bifida has declined with the advent of amniocentesis. The presence of significant levels of alpha-fetoprotein in the amniotic fluid has led to the detection of large numbers of affected fetuses.[44] Currently, maternal serum alpha-fetoprotein levels have been effective in detecting approximately 80% of neural tube defects.[34] Prenatal screening can be most effective when a combination of serum levels, amniocentesis/amniography, and ultrasonography is used.[19, 47] Although this screening is not yet performed routinely, it is suggested for those at risk for the defect. Knowledge of the defect allows for preparation for cesarean birth and immediate postnatal care. This includes mobilization of the interdisciplinary team who will continue to care for the child. For parents who decide to carry an involved fetus to term, their adjustment to their child's disability can begin before birth, which includes mobilizing their own support system. Education from an integrated team regarding what will follow after delivery and neurosurgical closure is imperative to aid families in decision making and to allow families to assess and understand the child's disability and future care options.

Other advances in the field of prenatal medicine that impact spina bifida management and outcome include the in utero treatment of hydrocephalus and the in utero surgical repair to close the myelomeningocele. It has been shown that treatment such as this, in conjunction with prenatal diagnosis, has had a positive impact on the incidence and severity of complications associated with spina bifida.[83, 128]

Clinical Manifestations

The most obvious clinical manifestation of myelomeningocele is the loss of sensory and motor functions in the lower limbs. The extent of loss, while primarily dependent on the degree of the spinal cord abnormality, is secondarily dependent on a number of factors. These include the amount of traction or stretch resulting from the abnormally tethered spinal cord, the trauma to exposed neural tissue during delivery, and postnatal damage resulting from drying or infection of the neural plate.[120] Specific clinical impairments that commonly lead to functional limitations for the child with spina bifida are addressed in this section.

Sensory Impairment

Children with spina bifida present with impaired sensation below the level of the lesion. The loss often does not match exactly the level of the lesion and needs to be carefully assessed. Sensory loss includes kinesthetic, proprioceptive, and somatosensory information. Because of this, children will often have to rely heavily on vision and other sensory systems to substitute for this loss.

Musculoskeletal Impairment

Weakness/Paralysis. The previous factors indicate that determining neurological involvement is not as straightforward as it would seem. At birth, two main types of motor dysfunction in the lower extremities have been identified. The first type involves a complete loss of function below the level of lesion, resulting in a flaccid paralysis, loss of sensation, and absent reflexes.[13, 120] The extent of involvement can be determined by comparing the level of lesion with a chart delineating the segmental innervation of the lower limb muscles. Orthopedic deformities may result from the unopposed action of muscles above the level of lesion. This unopposed pull leads commonly to hip flexion, knee extension, and ankle dorsiflexion contractures.

When the spinal cord remains intact below the level of lesion, the effect is an area of flaccid paralysis immediately below the lesion and possible hyperactive spinal reflexes distal to that area.[13, 120] This condition is very similar to the neurological state of the severed cord seen in traumatic injury. This second type of neurological involvement again results in orthopedic deformities, depending on the level of the lesion, the spasticity present, and the muscle groups involved.

Orthopedic Deformities. The orthopedic problems seen in myelomeningocele may be the result of (1) the imbalance between muscle groups; (2) the effect of stress, posture, and gravity; and (3) associated congenital malformations. Decreased sensation and neurological complications also may lead to orthopedic abnormalities.[132]

Besides the obvious malformation of vertebrae at the site of the lesion, hemivertebrae and deformities of other vertebral bodies and their corresponding ribs also may be present.[13, 110, 132] A lumbar kyphosis may be present as a result of the original deformity. In addition, as a result of the bifid vertebral bodies, the malaligned pull of the extensor muscles surrounding the deformity, as well as the unopposed flexor muscles, contribute further to the lumbar kyphosis. As the child grows, the weight of the trunk in the upright position also may be a contributing factor.[13, 110] Scoliosis may be present at birth because of vertebral abnormalities or may become evident as the child grows older. There is a low incidence of scoliosis in low lumbar or sacral level deformities.[90, 110] Scoliosis may also be neurogenic, secondary to weakness or asymmetrical spasticity of paraspinal muscles, tethered cord syndrome, or hydromyelia.[128] Lordosis or lordoscoliosis is often found in the adolescent and is usually associated with hip flexion deformities and a large spinal defect.[13, 82, 110] Many of these trunk and postural deformities exist at birth but are exacerbated by the effects of gravity as the child grows. They can compromise vital functions (cardiac and respiratory) and therefore should be closely monitored by the therapist and the family.

As has been alluded to previously, the type and extent of deformity in the lower extremities depend on the muscles that are active or inactive. In a total flaccid paralysis, in utero deformities may be present at birth, resulting from passive positioning within the womb. Equinovarus (clubfoot) or "rocker-bottom" deformity are two of the most common foot abnormalities. Knee flexion and extension contractures also may be present at birth. Other common deformities are hip flexion, adduction, and internal rotation, usually leading to a subluxed or dislocated hip.[13] Although many of these problems may be present at birth, it is of utmost importance to prevent positional deformity (such as the frog-leg position), which may result from improper positioning of flaccid extremities.[41]

Osteoporosis. Because the paralyzed limbs of the child with spina bifida have increased amounts of unmineralized osteoid tissue, they are prone to fractures, particularly after periods of immobilization.[30, 103] Early mobilization and weight bearing can aid in decreasing osteoporosis.[110] Fortunately, these fractures heal quickly with appropriate medical management.

Neurological Impairment

Hydrocephalus. Hydrocephalus develops in 80% to 90% of children with myelomeningocele.[69, 71] Hydrocephalus results from a blockage of the normal flow of CSF between the ventricles and spinal canal. The most obvious effect of the buildup of CSF is abnormal increase in head size, which may be present at birth because of the great compliance of the cranial sutures in the fetus or may develop postnatally.[78] Other signs of hydrocephalus include bulging fontanelles and irritability. Internally, there is usually a concomitant dilation of the lateral ventricles and thinning of the cerebral white matter. Without reduction of the buildup of CSF, increased brain damage and death may result.

Chiari Malformation. Patients with myelomeningocele have a 99% chance of having an associated Chiari II malformation.[18] This malformation is a congenital anomaly of the hindbrain in which there is herniation of the medulla and at times the pons, fourth ventricle, and inferior aspect of the cerebellum into the upper cervical canal. The herniation usually occurs between C1 and C4 but may extend down to T1.[18] Not all Chiari II malformations are symptomatic. Secondary to a symptomatic Chiari malformation, problems with respiratory and bulbar function may be evident in the child with spina bifida.[13, 69, 120] Paralysis of the vocal cords occurs in a small percentage of patients and is associated with respiratory stridor. Apneic episodes also may be evident, although their direct cause remains in question. Children with spina bifida also may exhibit difficulty in swallowing and have an abnormal gag reflex.[120] Problems with aspiration, weakness and cry, and upper-extremity weakness also may be present in children with a symptomatic Chiari II malformation.[85, 129] Thus, depending on the orthopedic deformities present and the neurological involvement, there is a potential from both sources for severe respiratory involvement in the affected child. These symptoms may be due to significant compression of the hindbrain structures or to dysplasia of posterior fossa contents, which can also occur in patients with Chiari II malformation.[18, 94] This complex hindbrain malformation is a common cause of death in children with myelomeningocele despite surgical intervention and aggressive medical management.[76] Other common neurological problems for children with spina bifida include hydromyelia and tethered cord.

Hydromyelia. Between 20% and 80% of patients with myelomeningocele may present with hydromyelia.[1, 18, 22] Hydromyelia signifies dilation of the center canal of the spinal cord as hydrocephalus signifies dilation of the ventricles of the brain. The area of hydromyelia may be focal, multiple, or diffuse extending throughout the spinal cord. The hydromyelia may be a consequence of untreated or inadequately treated hydrocephalus with resultant transmission of CSF through the obex into the central canal, with distention secondary to increased hydrostatic pressure from above.[18] The increased collection of fluid may cause pressure necrosis of the spinal cord, leading to muscle weakness and scoliosis.[20] Common symptoms of hydromyelia include rapidly progressive scoliosis, upper-extremity weakness, spasticity, and ascending motor loss

in the lower extremities.[18, 50] Aggressive treatment of hydromyelia at the onset of clinical signs of increasing scoliosis is mandatory and may lead to improvement in or stabilization of the curve in 80% of cases. Surgical interventions may include revision of a CSF shunt, posterior cervical decompression, or a central canal to pleural cavity shunt with a flushing device.[18, 94]

Tethered Cord. Tethered spinal cord is defined as a pathological fixation of the spinal cord in an abnormal caudal location. This fixation produces mechanical stretch, distortion, and ischemia with daily activities, growth, and development.[104] The presence of tethered cord syndrome should be suspected in any patient with abnormal neurulation (including patients with myelomeningocele, lipomeningocele, dermal sinus, diastematomyelia, myelocystocele, tight filum terminal, and lumbosacral agenesis). Presenting symptoms may include decreased strength (often asymmetrical), development of lower-extremity spasticity, back pain at the site of sac closure, early development of or increasing degree of scoliosis (especially in the low lumbar or sacral level child), or change in urological function.[39, 76, 111] This clinical spectrum may be primarily associated with these dysraphic lesions or may be secondary to spinal surgical procedures.[104] The cord may be tethered by scar tissue or by an inclusion epidermoid or lipoma at the repair site.[18] Surgery to untether the spinal cord (tethered cord release) is done to prevent further loss of muscle function, to decrease the spasticity, to help control the scoliosis, or to relieve back pain.[74]

The effectiveness of a tethered cord release may be demonstrated by an increase in muscle function, relief of back pain, and stabilization or reversal of scoliosis. Spasticity, however, is not always alleviated in all patients.[77] Selective posterior rhizotomy has been advocated for patients whose persistent or progressive spastic status after tethered cord repair continues to interfere with their mobility and functional independence.[122, 123]

Bowel and Bladder Dysfunction. Because of the usual involvement of the sacral plexus, the child with spina bifida must commonly deal with some form of bowel and bladder dysfunction. Besides various forms of incontinence, incomplete emptying of the bladder remains a constant concern because infection of the urinary tract and possible kidney damage may result.[3] Regulation of bowel evacuation must be established so that neither constipation nor diarrhea occurs.

Cognitive Impairment and Learning Issues. The last major clinical manifestation resulting from the neurological involvement of myelomeningocele is that of impaired intellectual function. Although children with spina bifida without hydrocephalus may show normal intellectual potential, children with hydrocephalus, particularly those who have shunt infections, are likely to have below-average intelligence.[13, 14, 79, 102, 120] These children often demonstrate learning disabilities and poor academic achievement. Even those with a normal IQ show moderate to severe visual-motor perceptual deficits.[69] This inability to coordinate eye and hand movements not only affects learning but also may interfere with activities of daily living (ADL), such as buttoning a shirt or opening a lunch box.[42] Difficulties with spatial relations, body image, and development of hand dominance may also be evident.[42, 120] Children with myelomeningocele demonstrate poorer hand function than age-matched peers. This decreased hand function appears to be due to cerebellar and cervical cord abnormalities, rather than hydrocephalus or cortical pathology.[89] (See Chapter 11 on learning disabilities.)

Prenatal studies have shown that the CNS as a whole is abnormally developed in fetuses with myelomeningocele.[6] The impairment of intellectual and perceptual abilities has been linked to damage to the white matter caused by ventricular enlargement.[13, 120] This damage to association tracts, particularly in the frontal, occipital, and parietal areas, could account for the often severe perceptual-cognitive deficits noted in the child with spina bifida. Lesser involvement of the temporal areas may account for the preservation of speech, whereas the semantics of speech, dependent on association areas, is impaired. It is easy to be fooled by the "cocktail party speech" of children with spina bifida, because they generally use well-constructed sentences and precocious vocabulary.[13] A closer look, however, reveals a repetitive, inappropriate, and often meaningless use of language certainly not associated with higher intellectual functioning.

Integumentary Impairment

Latex allergy and sensitivity has been noted with increasing frequency among children with myelomeningocele, with frequent reports of intraoperative anaphylaxis.[7, 43, 114, 116] It has also been reported that these same children have a higher than expected prevalence of atopic disease.[8] A 1991 Food and Drug Administration Medical Bulletin estimated that 18% to 40% of patients with spina bifida demonstrate latex sensitivity.[41] Within latex is 2% to 3% of residual-free protein material that is thought to be the antigenic agent.[114] Frequent exposure to this material results in the development of the IgE antibody. Children with spina bifida are more likely to develop the IgE sensitivity due to repeated parental or mucosal exposure to the latex antigen.[115] Because of the risk of an anaphylactic reaction, exposure to any latex-containing products such as rubber gloves, therapy balls, or Thera-Band should be avoided. Latex-free gloves, therapy balls, treatment mats, and Thera-Band are now widely available and should be considered for standard use in all clinics treating children with spina bifida.

The presence of paralysis and anesthetic skin places the child with spina bifida at major risk for pressure sores and decreased skin integrity. Various types of skin breakdown have occurred in 85% to 95% of all children with spina bifida by the time they reach young adulthood.[112] A pressure sore may result from excessive skin pressure that can cause reduced capillary flow, tissue anoxia, and eventual skin necrosis. Excessive pressure may manifest itself early as reactive hyperemia, a blister, and later as an open sore or overt necrosis. Chronic untreated sores may lead to osteomyelitis and eventual sepsis.[8] Pressure sores often result in loss of time at school and work and can lead to financial hardship secondary to medical treatment and hospitalizations. These negative consequences can largely be prevented with attention to education and instruction of the child and family. The goal of such education is to foster an understanding of the causes of skin breakdown and the necessary meticulous attention to skin care that must be carried out on a regular basis.

Growth and Nutrition

Nutritional intake and weight gain and/or loss have been found to be problematic in children with myelomeningocele. Early on, infants with spina bifida may present with feeding issues secondary to an impaired gag reflex, swallowing difficulties, and a high incidence of aspiration.[120, 129]

Altered oral-motor function has been attributed to the Chiari II malformation.[66] These impairments may lead to nutritional issues and delayed growth and weight gain. Speech, physical, and occupational therapy are often needed to address these issues as a team.

Conversely, obesity can be a significant issue for children with spina bifida. This problem is complex and multifactorial. Mobility limitations and decreased energy expenditure results in lower physical activity levels. In addition, decreased lower limb mass diminishes the ability to burn calories, which leads to weight gain. Decreased caloric intake as well as a lifelong engagement in rewarding and physically challenging physical activities are both necessary to enhance weight control and control obesity.

It is widely reported that children with myelomeningocele are short in stature. Growth in these children may be influenced by growth-retarding factors secondary to neurological deficit such as tethered cord.[109] Endocrine disorders and growth hormone deficiency have also been found to contribute to short stature in this population.[126] Secondary to complex CNS anomalies (midline defects, hydrocephalus, Arnold-Chiari malformation) these children are at risk for hypothalamopituitary dysfunction leading to growth hormone deficiency.[127] Recent treatment with recombinant human growth hormone has proven successful in fostering growth acceleration in these children.[66, 127]

Psychosocial Issues

Considering all the clinical manifestations resulting from this congenital neurological defect, there is no doubt that social and emotional difficulties will arise for these children and their families. These will be considered as appropriate when discussing the stages of recovery and rehabilitation from birth through adolescence.

The preceding discussion concerning the clinical problems of the child with spina bifida was intended to inform, not overwhelm, the clinician. With a firm understanding of the difficulties to be faced, evaluation and intervention can be more efficient and effective.

Medical Management

At or before birth, the myelomeningocele sac presents a dynamic rather than static disability. The residual neuro-

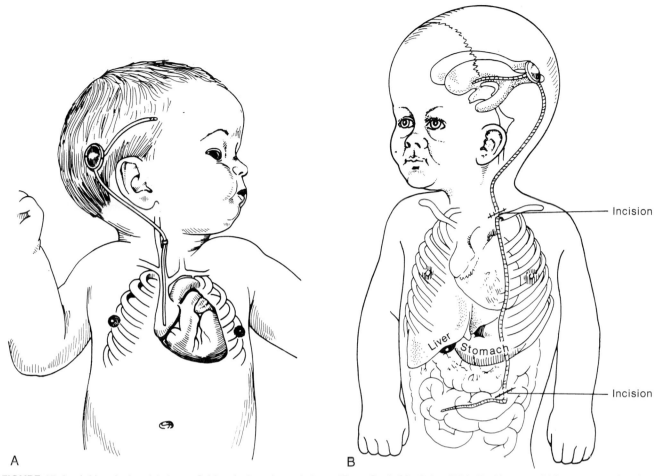

FIGURE 15–3. *A,* Ventriculoatrial shunt. *B,* Ventriculoperitoneal shunt. (From Stark GD: Spina Bifida Problems and Management. London, Blackwell Scientific, 1977.)

logical damage will be contingent on the early medical management that the fetus and/or newborn receives.

Since the early 1960s the presence of a myelomeningocele has been treated as a life-threatening situation, and sac closure now most often takes place within the first 24 to 48 hours of life.[99, 120] However, recent advances in treatment have led to investigational treatment in utero to repair the defect before birth.[83] The aim of this surgery is to replace the nervous tissue into the vertebral canal, cover the spinal defect, and achieve a watertight sac closure.[75] This early management has decreased the possibility of infection and further injury to the exposed neural cord.[69, 73, 75, 80]

Progressive hydrocephalus may be evident at birth in a small percentage of children born with myelomeningocele. A greater majority, however, develop hydrocephalus 5 to 10 days after the back lesion is closed.[70, 72, 75, 121] With the advent of computed tomography (CT), early diagnosis of hydrocephalus can be made in the newborn without the need for clinical examination.

Although clinical signs are not always definitive, hydrocephalus may be suspected if (1) the fontanelles become full, bulging, or tense; (2) the head circumference increases rapidly; (3) there is a palpable separation of the coronal and sagittal sutures; (4) the infant's eyes appear to look downward only, with the cornea prominent over

the iris (sun-setting sign); and (5) the infant becomes irritable or lethargic and has a high-pitched cry, persistent vomiting, difficult feeding, or seizures.[52, 71, 78]

If the results of CT confirm hydrocephalus, a ventricular shunt is indicated. This procedure involves diverting the excess CSF from the ventricles to some site for absorption. In general, two types of procedures—the ventriculoatrial (VA) and ventriculoperitoneal (VP) shunt—are currently used, the latter being the most common[113] (Fig. 15–3). The shunt apparatus is constructed from Silastic tubing and consists of three parts: a proximal catheter, a distal catheter, and a one-way valve.[36] As CSF is pumped from the ventricles toward its final destination, back flow is prevented by the valve system. In this manner intercranial pressure is controlled, CSF is regulated, and hydrocephalus is prevented from causing damage to brain structures.

Unfortunately for children with spina bifida, their problems do not end after the back is closed and a shunt is in place. Shunt complications occur frequently and require an average of two revisions before age 10.[9, 69] The most common causes of complications are shunt obstruction and infection.[13, 120] Obstructions can be cleared by revising the blocked end of the shunt. Infections may be handled by external ventricular drainage and courses of antibiotic therapy followed by insertion of a new shunting system.[120]

The problem of separation of shunt components has been largely overcome by the use of a one-piece shunting system. The single-piece shunt decreases the complications of shunting procedures.

Prophylactic antibiotic therapy 6 to 12 hours before surgery and 1 to 2 days postoperatively is effective in controlling infection for both sac repair and shunt insertion.[23, 69] This brief course of antibiotics has not led to resistant organisms. The main cause of death in children with myelomeningoceles remains increased intercranial pressure and infections of the CNS.[69] With the use of antibiotics, shunting, and early sac closure, the survival rate has increased from 20% to 85%.[79]

Initial newborn workup should include a urological assessment. It is the aim of the urology team to preserve renal function and to promote efficient bladder management.[71] Initially, a renal and bladder ultrasound is done to assess those structures.[60] Radiographic tests such as the voiding cystourethrograms or a cystometregram can be performed to determine any blockage in the lower urinary tract. Functioning of the bladder outlet and sphincters, as well as ureteric reflux, also can be evaluated.[13, 71, 120] These tests, plus clinical observations of voiding patterns, help the urologist classify the infant's bladder function. If the bladder has neither sensory nor motor supply, there will be a constant flow of urine. In this case infection is rare, because the bladder does not store urine and the sphincters are always open.[20]

If there is no sensation but some involuntary muscle control of the sphincter, the bladder will fill, but emptying will not occur properly. Overflow or stress incontinence results in dribbling urine until the pressure is relieved. Because of constant residual urine, infection is a potential problem and kidney damage may be the sequela.[20] When some voluntary muscle control but no sensation is present, the bladder will fill and empty automatically. The child can eventually be taught to empty the bladder at regular intervals to avoid unnecessary accidents.

Regardless of the type of bladder functioning, urine specimens are taken to check for infection, and blood samples are taken to determine the kidney's ability to filter the body's fluids. Based on clinical findings, the urologist will suggest the appropriate intervention.

A program of clean intermittent catheterization (CIC) done every 3 to 4 hours prevents infection and maintains the urological system.[3, 29] Parents are taught this method and can then begin to take on this aspect of their child's care. At the age of 4 or 5 years, children with spina bifida can be taught CIC. By doing so, they have become independent in bladder care at a young age. Achieving this form of independence adds to the normal psychological development of these children. Some children may require urinary diversion through the abdominal wall (ileal conduit) or other less common methods such as intravesical transurethral bladder stimulation to handle their urinary problems.[3] Although CIC is not possible for all children with spina bifida, it remains the method of choice for bladder management.

Orthopedic management of the newborn with a myelomeningocele will generally concentrate on the feet and hips. Soft tissue releases of the feet may take place during surgery for sac closure. Casting the feet also has been effective in reducing clubfoot deformities (Fig. 15–4). Early aggressive taping for clubfoot also is effective in the management of clubfoot deformities.[53] Short-leg posterior splints (ankle-foot orthoses [AFOs]) may be used to maintain range and prevent foot deformities (see Fig. 15–4).

The orthopedist also will evaluate the stability of the hips. In children with lower-level lesions, attempts to prevent dislocation are made by using a hip abductor brace (Fig. 15–5A) or a total-body splint (see Fig. 15–5B) for a few months after birth. With higher-level lesions, dislocated hips are no longer treated, because they do not appear to have an effect on later rehabilitation efforts.[3, 32, 33, 52, 63] Orthopedic management needs to be ongoing throughout the child's lifetime with continued assessment of orthopedic deformities and need for surgical intervention.

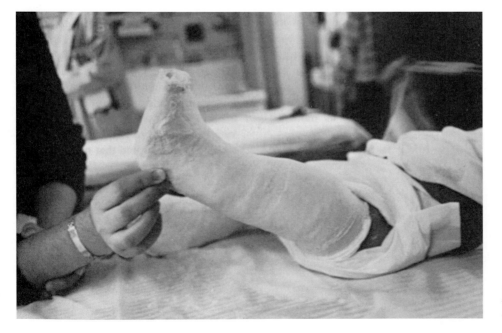

FIGURE 15–4. Plaster cast of the foot and ankle to reduce clubfoot deformities.

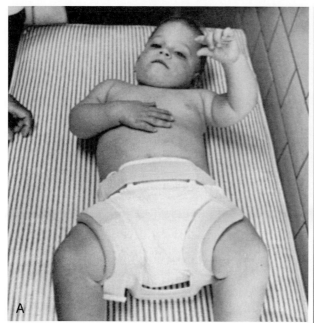

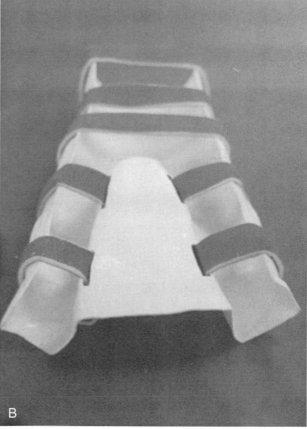

FIGURE 15–5. *A,* Hip abductor brace. *B,* Total body splint.

EVALUATIONS

In attempting to evaluate the child with spina bifida, there are any number of evaluations from which to choose, each designed to test specific, yet perhaps unrelated, components of function. The following section discusses those test procedures or specific standardized tests that would best define the complexity of the problem.

Manual Muscle Testing (MMT)

The first and most obvious request for evaluation may be to determine the extent of motor paralysis. In the newborn, testing may be done in the first 24 to 48 hours before the back is surgically closed. In this case, care must be taken not to injure the exposed neural tissue during testing. Prone and side lying to either side offers the most convenient and safe position for evaluation during this time. Subsequent testing is done soon after the back is closed and as indicated throughout childhood.

The traditional form of MMT is not appropriate or possible for the infant or young child. The following is a discussion of how muscle testing can and must be adapted for this age group.

In evaluating the newborn, the importance of state is paramount. A sleeping or drowsy infant will hardly respond appropriately during the evaluation. It is essential that the infant be in the alert or crying state to elicit the appropriate movement responses. There is an advantage to testing hungry or crying infants, because they are likely to demonstrate more spontaneous movements in these behavioral states.

The cumulative effect of a variety of sensory stimuli may be more effective in alerting the infant than using one made in isolation. For example, the infant may be picked up and rocked vertically to allow maximum stimulation to the vestibular system and to help bring the child to an alert state. In addition, the therapist may talk to the child to help him or her fixate visually on the therapist's face. Tactile stimuli above the level of the lesion further add to the child's level of arousal, thus contributing to more conclusive test results. In this way, the CNS receives an accumulation of information from a variety of sensory systems, rather than relying on transmission from one system that may be weak or inefficient.

As the child is aroused, spontaneous movements can be observed and muscle groups palpated. Additional methods to stimulate movement may be necessary. For example, "tickling" the infant generally produces a variety of spontaneous movements in the upper and lower extremities. Passive positioning of children in adverse positions may stimulate them to move. For example, if the legs are held in marked hip and knee flexion, the infant may attempt to use extensor musculature to move out of that position. If the legs are held in adduction, the child may abduct to get free. Holding a limb in an antigravity position may elicit an automatic "holding" response from a muscle group when spontaneous movements cannot be obtained in any other way.[134]

In grading muscle strength, it is important to differentiate between spontaneous, voluntary movement and reflexive movement. After severing of a spinal cord, distal segments of the cord may respond to stimuli in a reflexive manner. This results from the preservation of the spinal reflex arc and is known as distal sparing. If distal sparing of the spinal cord is present, the muscles may respond to stimulation or muscular stretch with reflexive, stereotypical movement patterns. The quality of this reflexive movement will be different from that of spontaneous movement and must be distinguished when testing for level of voluntary muscle functioning.

Muscle strength is generally graded for groups of muscles and can be graded by using either a numerical (1–5) or alphabetical designation (Fig. 15–6) or simply by noting presence or absence of muscular contraction by a plus or a minus on the muscle test form. Initially, this latter method may be sufficient, but as the child matures a more definitive muscle grade should be determined.

By using an MMT form that lists the spinal segmental level for each muscle group, one can determine an approximate level of lesion from the test results (see Fig. 15–6). Because the spinal cord is often damaged asymmetrically, MMT does not always reflect the level of lesion accurately. If reflex activity is also noted on the form, the presence of distal sparing of the spinal cord can be determined. Muscle testing of the newborn gives the clinician not only an appreciation of muscle function and possible potential for later ambulation but also an awareness of possible deforming forces. For example, if hip extensors or abductors are not functioning, then the action of hip flexors and adductors must be countered to prevent future deformities.

Muscle testing of the toddler or young child may require some of the techniques described previously. In addition, developmental positions can be used to assess muscle strength in an uncooperative youngster. For example, strength of hip extensors and abductors can be assessed as a child attempts to creep up steps or onto a low mat table. By adding resistance to movements, fairly accurate muscle grades can be determined. To elicit hip flexors in sitting, if an interesting toy or object is placed on the child's ankle or between the toes the child will often lift the leg spontaneously to reach for it. Ingenuity and creativity are certainly prerequisites for muscle testing in the young child.

By the age of 4 or 5 years, muscle grades can generally be determined through traditional testing techniques, although the reliability of the test results will increase with the age of the child.

Muscle testing is indicated before and after any surgical procedure and at periodic intervals of 6 months to 1 year to detect any change in muscle function. The level of innervation should not decrease throughout the life of the child with spina bifida. In the growing child or adolescent, an increasing weakness resulting from shunt malfunction, tethering of the spinal cord, or hydromyelia frequently can be substantiated by a muscle test of the lower extremities.

Sensory Testing

Sensory testing of the infant and young child is simplified to determine the level of sensation as accurately as possible, with a minimum amount of testing. Full sensory tests are not possible until the child has acquired sufficient cognitive and language abilities to respond appropriately to testing.

In the newborn, sensory testing can best be done if the child is in a quiet state. Beginning at the lowest level of sacral innervation, the skin is stroked with a pin or other sharp object until a reaction to pain is noted. Although none of these methods are fail safe, they may be helpful in adapting a muscle test to a newborn or young infant. Repeated evaluation may be necessary to get an accurate picture of muscle function.

Because of dermatome innervation the pin is usually drawn from the anal area, across the buttocks, down the posterior thigh and leg, then to the anterior surface of the leg and thigh, and finally across the abdominal muscles. Reactions to be noted are a facial grimace or cry, which indicates that the painful sensation has reached a cortical level. Care must be taken to see that each sensory dermatome has been evaluated. Results can be recorded by shading in the dermatomes where sensation is present (Fig. 15–7).

The therapist may be called on to evaluate the newborn before surgical closure of the spinal meningocele. Although sensory and motor levels can be determined as previously described, it is important to consider the infant's general condition when interpreting test findings. Any medication taken by the mother during labor and delivery may influence the neonate's performance and thus should be noted. In addition, the physiological disorganization normally seen in all infants during the first few days after birth may also affect testing.[12] At best, this presurgical evaluation establishes a tentative baseline, but significant changes in the infant's neurological status in the first few weeks of life should not be surprising to the clinician.

In the young child from 2 to 7 years of age, light touch sensation and position sense can be tested in addition to pain sensation. Again, the ingenuity of the therapist will be called forth to elicit an appropriate response and reliable test results. Using games, such as "Tell me when the puppet touches you," may be more effective for the young child than traditional testing methods.

From age 7 years through adolescence, additional sensory tests of temperature and two-point discrimination may be added. Usually, traditional methods are sufficient to ensure reliable testing, but a more behavioral approach may be indicated, depending on the individual's cognitive functioning.

After testing, a survey of the sensory dermatome chart should indicate whether sensation is normal, absent, or impaired.

Range of Motion Evaluation

A complete range of motion (ROM) evaluation of the lower extremities is indicated for the newborn with spina bifida. The therapist must be aware of normal physiological flexion that is greatest at the hip and knees. In the normal newborn these apparent "contractures" of up to 35 degrees are eliminated as the child gains more control

THE CHILDREN'S MEMORIAL HOSPITAL
PHYSICAL / OCCUPATIONAL THERAPY

MUSCLE EXAM - MM

PATIENT NAME _____ M.R. # _____

ATTENDING M.D. _____ PT. D.O.B. _____

DIAGNOSIS _____
_____

DATE:_____

P.T. NAME: _____

	*	LEFT	RIGHT	*	COMMENTS: (Include ROM limitations, spasticity, reflexive movements, etc.)
ILIOPSOAS (L₁ - 2)					
SARTORIUS (L₁ 3)					
HIP ADDUCTORS (L₂ - 4)					
TENSOR FASCIA LATA					
GLUTEUS MEDIUS (L₄ - S₁)					
GLUTEUS MAXIMUS (L₅ - S₁)					
QUADRICEPS (L₂ - 4)					
MEDIAL HAMSTRINGS (L₄ - S₂)					
LATERAL HAMSTRINGS (L₄ - S₁)					
ANTERIOR TIBIALIS (L₄ - L₅)					
POSTERIOR TIBIALIS (L₄ - L₅)					
PERONEUS LONGUS (L₅ - S₁)					
PERONEUS BREVIS (L₅ - S₁)					
GASTROC - SOLEUS (S₁ - S₂)					
EXT. HALLUCIS LONGUS (L₅ - S₁)					
FLEX. HALLUCIS LONGUS (S₁ - S₂)					
EXT. DIGITORUM LONGUS (L₄ - S₁)					
EXT. DIG. B. (L₄ - S₁)					
FLEX. DIGITORUM LONGUS (L₄ - S₁)					
FLEX. DIG. B. (L₄ - S₁)					
LUMBRICALES					

*INDICATE INCREASE (↑) OR DECREASE (↓) IN STRENGTH IN COMPARISON TO PREVIOUS TEST DATED _____

PLEASE NOTE ANY SIGNIFICANT INFORMATION ON OTHER MUSCLE GROUPS UNLISTED ABOVE (i.e., EHB; Flex. HB; Internal or External Rotators)

X	PRESENT	UNABLE TO BE GRADED
N	NORMAL	COMPLETE RANGE OF MOTION AGAINST GRAVITY WITH FULL RESISTANCE
G	GOOD	COMPLETE RANGE OF MOTION AGAINST GRAVITY WITH MODERATE RESISTANCE
G-	GOOD MINUS	COMPLETE RANGE OF MOTION AGAINST GRAVITY WITH SOME RESISTANCE
F+	FAIR PLUS	COMPLETE RANGE OF MOTION AGAINST GRAVITY WITH SLIGHT RESISTANCE
F	FAIR	COMPLETE RANGE OF MOTION AGAINST GRAVITY
F-	FAIR MINUS	INCOMPLETE (GREATER THAN 1/2 WAY) RANGE OF MOTION AGAINST GRAVITY
P+	POOR PLUS	LESS THAN 1/2 WAY AGAINST GRAVITY OR FULL ROM GRAVITY ELIMINATED PLUS SL RESISTANCE
P	POOR	COMPLETE RANGE OF MOTION WITH GRAVITY ELIMINATED
P-	POOR MINUS	INCOMPLETE RANGE OF MOTION WITH GRAVITY ELIMINATED
T	TRACE	CONTRACTION IS FELT BUT THERE IS NO VISIBLE JOINT MOVEMENT
O	ZERO	NO CONTRACTION FELT IN THE MUSCLE

FORM 354042790

FIGURE 15–6. Muscle examination form using alphabetical designation. (Courtesy of Josefina Briceno, PT, Children's Memorial Hospital Chicago.)

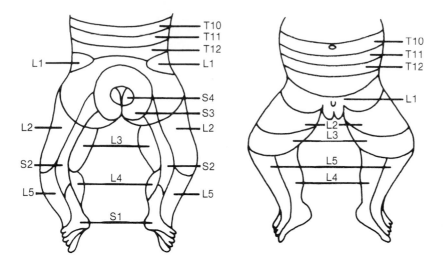

FIGURE 15–7. Lower limb dermatomes. (From Brocklehurst G: Spina bifida for the clinician. Clin Dev Med 57:53, 1976.)

of extensor musculature and kicks more frequently into extension.

In the child with spina bifida, contractures may be evident at birth because of unopposed musculature. Hip adduction should not be tested beyond the neutral position to avoid dislocation of hips that are often unstable. Range should be done slowly and without excessive force to avoid fractures so often experienced in paralytic lower extremities. ROM should be checked with the same frequency as muscle testing.

Active ROM of the upper extremities can be assessed by observation and handling the infant. A formal ROM evaluation for the upper extremities is not usually indicated. A baseline ROM and tone assessment of the upper extremities should be completed.

Reflex Testing

The purpose of reflex testing is twofold: to check for the presence of normal reflex activity and to check for the integration of primitive reflexes and the establishment of more mature reactions.[36] In the newborn, for example, one would expect strong rooting and sucking reflexes. In the child with spina bifida, because of possible involvement of the CNS as described previously, these reflexes may be depressed or absent. Because these reflexes play an integral part in obtaining nutrients for the infant, their value is obvious.

On the other hand, primitive reflexes, which persist past their expected span, also may indicate abnormality. For example, if the asymmetrical tonic neck reflex persists past 4 months, it will limit the infant's ability to bring the hands to midline for visual and tactile exploration.

As the primitive reflexes (initially needed for survival and to experience movement) become integrated, they are replaced by more mature and functional reactions. The righting and equilibrium reactions help the child attain the erect position and counteract changes in the center of gravity. Because these reactions depend on an intact CNS, as well as a certain level of postural control, they may be delayed, incomplete, or absent in the child with spina bifida. For example, a child with a low thoracic

spinal cord lesion may show an incomplete equilibrium reaction in sitting. This may be caused by the lack of a stable postural base or by lack of initiation of the reaction centrally. Both the neurological and muscular components of these reactions must be considered.[37]

Reflex testing for the child with spina bifida may not be as intensive as that for a child with cerebral palsy. It may, however, provide a check on the progress of normal development and as such reflect the integrity of the CNS.

Developmental/Functional Evaluations

Besides being aware of a child's sensory and motor levels, it is also important to assess the functional level. Two important questions need to be asked: "Does the child show normal components of posture and movement synergies?" and "What is the child's level of mobility?"

Several developmental and/or functional evaluations can be adapted for the child with spina bifida. The following are some suggestions for evaluation approaches or specifically designed tests to assist in assessment of this area.

Initially, a developmental sequence may be used to assess how a child is functioning. In each position used, both posture and movement will be evaluated. The goals in using this type of assessment are to determine what a child can and cannot do, the quality of the action, and what is limiting the child. The progression would begin in the supine position, rolling to prone, prone-on-elbows, prone-on-hands, up-to-sitting, hands-knees, kneeling, half-kneeling, standing, and walking. Both the ability to attain and the ability to maintain the positions should be assessed.

It is not merely the accomplishment of the task that must be evaluated but, simultaneously, the way in which it is accomplished. For example, in rolling, is head righting sufficient to keep the head off the supporting surface? From the hands-knees position, can reciprocal crawling be initiated without the lower extremities being held in wide abduction? Can the child pull to stand easily by using trunk rotation? Assessing the quality of the child's abilities will assist the clinician in determining where therapeutic measures should begin and what the goals of such intervention will be.[23]

If a standardized assessment is desired, the Alberta Infant Motor Scale (AIMS) would be appropriate.[101] The AIMS is designed to measure motor development from birth to 18 months of age. It is a 58-item observational test of infants in supine, prone, sitting, and standing positions. For each item there are detailed descriptions of the weight-bearing surface, the infant's posture, and antigravity movements expected of the infant in that position. The AIMS requires minimal handling of the infant and can be completed in 20 to 30 minutes. The test was normed on a cross-sectional sample of 2,200 infants in Alberta, Canada. Interrater and test-retest reliability is high (0.95–0.99), as is concurrent validity with the Peabody Developmental Motor Scales (PDMS) (0.99) and the Bayley Scales of Infant Development (0.97). Predictive validity of the AIMS is being studied and appears to be fair.[25] For the child with spina bifida, the AIMS could be used to assess current motor development and to track progress in motor development over time.

The Milani-Comparetti motor development screening test may also be useful in assessing the functional level of the child with spina bifida. This screening examination is designed to evaluate motor development from birth to 2 years of age (Fig. 15–8).[84] It requires no special equipment and can be administered in 4 to 8 minutes. The test evaluates both spontaneous behavior and evoked responses. Spontaneous behavior includes postural control of the head and body in various positions, as well as a sequence of active movement patterns. Primitive reflexes, righting, and equilibrium reactions comprise the evoked responses. The Milani was normed on a sample of 312 children from Omaha. Interrater rater reliability percent of agreement was 89% to 95%. Test-retest reliability percent agreement was 82% to 100%. Predictive validity of the Milani has not been well established. The Milani-Comparetti test should assist the clinician in evaluating each child's underlying postural mechanisms and his or her ability to attain the erect position. The reader is referred to the test manual for special examination procedures and scoring.[84]

The PDMS[38] is another standardized assessment that may prove helpful in evaluating a child with congenital spinal cord injury. The PDMS consists of gross and fine motor scales from birth through 83 months. The two scales allow a comparison of the child's motor performance with a normative sample of children at various age levels. A stratified sample of 617 children throughout the United States was used to develop PDMS test norms. Test-retest and interrater reliability are high (0.95 to 0.99). Content, construct, and concurrent validity have been well established. Although the disabled child would not be expected to pass many of the gross motor items at the later age levels, the scale still serves as a reminder of expected gross motor performance at each age. The fine motor scale offers a chance to assess fine motor performance of children with congenital spinal cord injury. This area has been frequently overlooked with children with myelomeningocele. Fine motor development, however, may be affected because of congenital abnormalities in brain development associated with myelomeningocele or related to tethering of the spinal cord that can result in fine motor paresis. In addition, the PDMS offers guidelines for administering the test to children with disabilities.[38]

The Bruininks-Oseretsky Test of Motor Proficiency can be used to evaluate the higher level child with spina bifida. Fine motor subtests of response speed, visual-motor control, and upper-limb speed and dexterity can be used to assist in evaluating areas of fine motor control and coordination difficulties. This test has been standardized on a large sample of children from 4 through 14 years of age.[15]

Finally, the Pediatric Evaluation of Disability Inventory (PEDI)[49] is a comprehensive assessment of function in children aged 6 months to 7 years. The PEDI measures both capability and performance of functional activities in three areas: (1) self-care, (2) mobility, and (3) social function. Capability is a measure of the functional skills for which the child has demonstrated mastery. Functional performance is measured by the level of caregiver assistance needed to accomplish a task. A modifications scale provides a measure of environmental modifications and equipment needed in daily functioning. The PEDI has been standardized on a normative sample of 412 children from the New England area. Some data from clinical samples (N = 102) are also available. Interrater reliability of the PEDI is high (ICCs = 0.96 to 0.99). Concurrent validity of the PEDI with the Wee-FIM (child's version of the Functional Independence Measure) was also high (r = 0.80 to 0.97). The PEDI can be administered in about 45 minutes by clinicians or educators familiar with the child or by structured interview of the parent. The PEDI should provide a descriptive measure of the functional level of the child with myelomeningocele as well as a method for tracking change over time.

Perceptual/Cognitive Evaluations

When evaluating a child with spina bifida, it is important to include some assessment of perceptual/cognitive status. The appropriate assessment depends largely on the age of the child. The assessment may be performed by the physical, occupational, or speech therapist, depending on the setting.

For the newborn from 3 to 30 days old, the Brazelton Neonatal Behavioral Assessment scale may be adapted to assess the infant's organization in terms of physiological response to stress, state control, motoric control, and social interaction.[12] Ideally, the infant should be medically stable and free from CNS-depressant drugs before evaluation. Generally, this evaluation will occur after the back lesion is closed and a shunt is positioned to relieve the hydrocephalic condition.

Although test results may not have prognostic value because of the plasticity of the nervous system at this young age, they supply the clinician with information concerning the current status of the child. This information can be conveyed to the infant's caregivers—both medical personnel and parents—so that strengths can be appreciated and weaknesses anticipated and handled

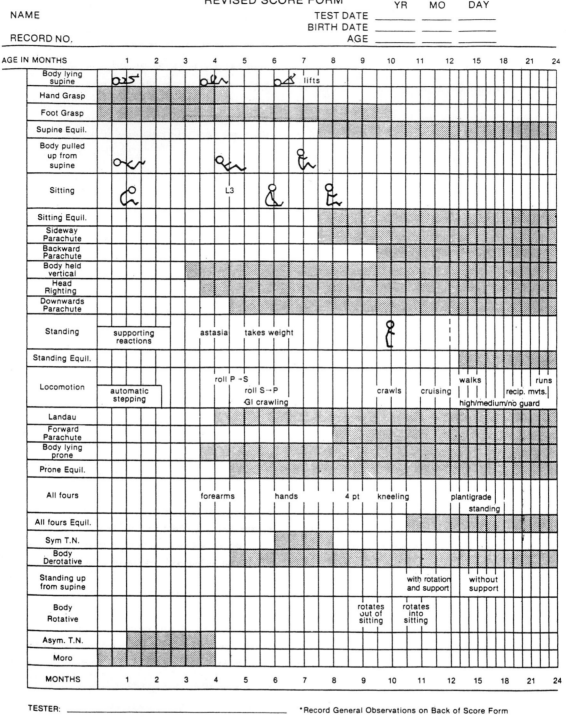

FIGURE 15–8. Milani-Comparetti Motor Development Screening Test Revised score form.

appropriately. Helping parents to identify that their infant has his or her own unique characteristics and assisting them in dealing with these characteristics does a great deal to strengthen already precarious parent/infant bonding.

Repeated administration of the Brazelton Neonatal Behavioral Assessment scale in the first month of life may help monitor the infant's progress in organization and reflect the curve of recovery. Although the manual for this behavioral assessment is quite complete, proper administration scoring and interpretation require direct training with someone already proficient in using the scale.[12] Excellent training films for the Brazelton Neonatal Behavioral Assessment scale are available for purchase or through your local university's learning resource center (see Appendix 15–A at the end of the chapter).

A full developmental evaluation appropriate for the infant and toddler with spina bifida is the Bayley Scales of Infant Development—2nd edition (BSID-II).[9] The Bayley Scales, consisting of a mental and motor scale and a behavioral rating scale, can be used to test children from age 1 month to 42 months. The test provides information on gross motor, fine motor, language, personal-social, and cognitive development.

The BSID-II is well standardized and reliable and takes about 45 minutes to administer. It is not an easy test to learn and would initially require supervision of an experienced tester. The new edition provides new normative data, extended age range, expanded content coverage, and improved psychometric qualities.

The BSID-II will provide the clinician with a broader view of the child's total development. The gross motor information from this developmental assessment will not be specific enough for a therapist evaluating a child with spina bifida. The additional information on fine motor, language, personal-social, and cognitive development, however, is sufficient and will be most important in planning a comprehensive intervention program.

Various tests are available as screening tools to test visual-motor integration and perception. The Developmental Test of Visual-Motor Integration (VMI) is an early screening tool to aid in diagnosis of learning problems in children. It assesses integration of visual perception and motor control of children from 2 years, 6 months to 19 years of age. The test takes 10 to 15 minutes to complete and requires the child to be able to copy designs. The VMI is norm referenced and was standardized on a large sample chosen from throughout the United States.[10]

Because children with spina bifida often exhibit upper-extremity weakness a non–motor-perceptual test is often desired. The Motor-Free Visual Perception Test—Revised (MVPT-R) and the Test of Visual Perceptual Skills (TVPS) can be used to determine the child's visual perceptual processing skills based on a nonmotor assessment of these skills. Both tests evaluate visual discrimination, visual memory, spatial relations, figure-ground, and visual closure. The TVPS also evaluates form constancy and sequential memory. The MVPT-R can be used with children from 4 to 11 years of age, and the TVPS can be used with children from 4 to 12 years of age. Both tests are easy and quick to administer (less than 15 minutes), and, based on the examiner's experience and training, interpretations can be made with prescription for remediation. The MVPT-R was standardized on a sample of 912 children in Georgia and northern California.[25] The test-retest reliability of the MVPT-R was 0.81. Performance on the motor-free test has been shown to be independent of the degree of motor involvement when compared with other tests of visual perception. The TVPS was standardized on a sample of children in San Francisco.[24, 40]

With a firm database provided by a thorough physical/occupational therapy evaluation with referrals to other professionals as appropriate, a reasonable treatment plan can be developed and updated as necessary.

TREATMENT PLANNING AND REHABILITATION RELATED TO SIGNIFICANT STAGES OF RECOVERY

Newborn to Toddler (Preambulatory Phase)

Stage 1: Before Closure of Myelomeningocele—Newborn

Physical therapy management of the infant in stage 1 is limited by his or her medical condition (Table 15–1). Attempts can be made, however, to prevent deformity and to maintain ROM while giving stimulation to provide as normal an environment as possible.

In addition to evaluation, the therapist may begin some early intervention measures that can be continued and expanded postsurgically. ROM and positioning in prone or side lying may be initiated to prevent or decrease contractures in the lower extremities. If clubfeet are present, soft tissue stretching may be indicated. Stretching begins distally on the soft tissue of the forefoot and proceeds proximally toward the calcaneus. This is done to take advantage of the pliability of soft tissue structures and to minimize fixed deformity later. In addition, taping may be used to maintain optimal ROM and alignment between periods of stretching.[53] When treating the newborn before surgery, great care must be taken to avoid contaminating an open sac, which is usually covered with a sterile dressing and kept moist with a saline solution.[69]

Stage 2: After Surgery, During Hospitalization—Newborn to Infant

Therapeutic intervention during stage 2 will be more aggressive than before surgery but will often be limited by the infant's neurological and orthopedic status. A major goal during this stage is to prevent contracture and to maintain ROM.

Traditional ROM can be taught to nursing staff and family. It also can be carried out while the child is being held at the adult's shoulder or prone over the adult's lap. These positions allow closeness between the caregiver and infant, thus encouraging maximum relaxation and interaction between them.

Because of their medical conditions, hospitalized infants often experience early separation from their parents. Teaching the family to handle the child as just described may enhance parent/infant bonding. Adequate bonding is essential for normal psychosocial development to occur.

When the child is not being handled, resting positions can be used to maintain ROM and enhance development. The prone position is the most advantageous, because it prevents hip flexion contractures and encourages development of extensor musculature as the child lifts his or her head. Side lying, which allows the hands to come to midline and generally encourages symmetrical posture, can be used for alternating positioning. As much as possible, the supine position should be avoided because the child is most dominated by primitive reflexes and the

TABLE 15-1. Summary of Treatment Planning and Rehabilitation Related to Significant Stages of Recovery

Stage of Recovery	Major Physical Therapy Goals	Physical Therapy Management
Newborn to Toddler (Preambulatory Phase)		
Stage 1: before surgical closure of myelomeningocele—newborn	Prevent contractures and deformity	ROM, positioning
	Encourage normal sensorimotor development	Graded auditory and visual stimuli
Stage 2: after surgery during hospitalization—newborn to infant	Prevent contracture and deformity	ROM taught to hospital personnel and family
		Positioning in prone and side-lying
		Providing toys of various colors, textures, and shapes
	Encourage normal sensorimotor development	Graded auditory and visual stimuli—music boxes, squeaky toys, brightly colored objects
		Therapeutic handling to encourage good head and trunk control
Stage 3: condition stabilized—infant to toddler	Encourage normal development sequence	Work in sitting on head righting and equilibrium reactions
		Eye-hand coordination activities
		Early weight bearing on lower extremities
		Encourage prone progression
		Weight shifting in standing frame
		Comprehensive home program
Toddler Through Adolescent (Ambulatory Phase)		
Stage 4: toddler through preschool	Begin ambulation	Choose appropriate orthotic device
		Gait training
		Development and strengthening of righting and equilibrium reactions
	Continue development in cognitive and psychosocial areas	Consider placement in 0-3 stimulation group
		Public preschool program
		Continue home program
	Collaborate goals with other team members	Open communication with other team members
Stage 5: primary school through adolescence	Reevaluate ambulation potential	Replace orthotic device as necessary
		Wheelchair prescriptions as necessary
	Maintain present level of functioning	Teach locomotion activities
		Maintain strength in trunk and extremities
	Prevent skin breakdown as child becomes more sedentary	Teach skin care
	Promote independence in self-care skills	Work with team members to teach dressing, feeding, hygiene, and bowel and bladder care
	Remediate any perceptual-motor problems	Provide program/activities for sensorimotor integration
	Provide appropriate adaptive devices	Check for fit and proper use of adaptive devices
	Promote self-esteem and social-sexual adjustment	Collaborate with other team members in counseling efforts

effects of gravity in this position. For example, for the child with spina bifida with CNS involvement in addition to the spinal cord lesion, the effects of the tonic labyrinthine reflex combined with paralytic lower extremities make movement from the supine position extremely difficult.

A normal sensory experience should be presented to the child in spite of the hospital setting. Toys of various colors, textures, and shapes should be available. Musical mobiles held low enough for the child to reach provide a variety of sensory experiences. Stimuli such as squeaky toys or the human face and voice can be used to encourage visual and auditory tracking. Controlled stimulation relevant to the infant's neurological state, rather than overstimulation, should be the rule. Depending on the age of the child, appropriate learning situations must be presented to provide the child with as normal an environment as possible for perceptual and cognitive growth.

A major therapeutic goal will be to guide the child through the developmental sequence, ultimately prepar-

ing him or her to assume the upright posture. In this immediate postsurgical stage, primary emphasis will be on attaining good head and trunk control and eliciting appropriate righting reactions. For example, the child can be seated on the therapist's lap, facing the therapist, and alternately lowered slowly backward and side-to-side. This will help to stimulate head righting and strengthen neck and abdominal muscles. Weight shifting in the prone-on-elbows position is another good activity for enhancing development of head and trunk control. Unfortunately, developmental handling may be limited by frequent shunt revisions that require the infant to be kept flat for days.

This second stage ends as the child is discharged from the hospital. The child will be followed closely by the rehabilitation team, which may include a neurosurgeon, an orthopedist, a urologist, a nurse clinician, a physical therapy/occupational therapy (PT/OT) team, and a social worker. Before discharge, a definitive home program as well as referral to a local PT/OT/0-3 program should be given to the family, because the child will most likely require ongoing therapy.

Stage 3: Condition Stabilized—Infant to Toddler

In this stage of rehabilitation, the major emphasis is on preparing the child mentally and physically for walking. Goals of preventing contractures and maintaining ROM will remain throughout the child's life. Unless this is done, ambulation not only becomes more difficult but often impossible. If possible, prone positioning during play and sleeping assists greatly in stretching tight musculature. Resting splints for the lower extremities or a total-body splint (TBS) can be used as necessary to position and maintain ROM and alignment.

Assuming that the child has previously gained good head and trunk control, the next step would be development of sitting equilibrium reactions. As sitting balance improves, fine motor and eye-hand coordination activities should be introduced. Upper-extremity functioning is often overlooked in the child with spina bifida, whose problems appear to be concentrated in the lower extremities. Because most children with spina bifida show decreased fine motor coordination,[69] this problem should be addressed as developmentally appropriate. The normal infant begins to reach and grasp by 6 months of age[23]; therefore, the child with spina bifida must be given ample opportunities to practice and to perfect these skills at an early age. Referral to and consultation with other therapists at this age is highly recommended.

Early weight bearing is also of utmost importance, both physiologically and psychologically.[111] The upright position has beneficial effects on circulation and renal and bladder functioning, as well as on the promotion of bone growth[48] and density.[108] Psychologically, weight bearing in an upright posture allows a normal view of the world and contributes to more normal perceptual, cognitive, and emotional growth. One way to achieve this weight bearing is in the kneeling position. This is developmentally appropriate, because children 8 to 10 months old frequently use kneeling as a transition from all fours to standing.

Because young infants are frequently held in the standing position and bounced on their parents' laps, it is appropriate to introduce this form of weight bearing on the lower extremities from birth onward. Failure to do so will deprive the spina bifida child of the normal experience of standing at a very early age. When standing these children, however, care must be taken to see that the lower extremities are in good alignment and that undue pressure is not exerted on them (Fig. 15–9). In this way the risk of fractures is minimized and a normal weight-bearing experience is provided.

Following a normal developmental sequence, the child with spina bifida will usually begin some form of prone progression as trunk and upper-extremity stability improve. This is a significant phase of development, because it allows for the development of a sensorimotor base as the child expands environmental horizons.[62] During this phase of high mobility, anesthetic skin must be checked for injury frequently and often protected by heavier clothing. This may help to prevent any major skin breakdown, which could significantly delay the rehabilitation process.

For some children with high-level lesions where prone mobility is not safe or practical for long distances, a caster

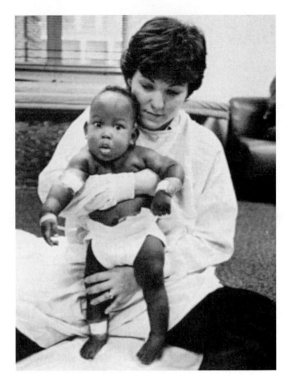

FIGURE 15–9. Assisted standing with normal postural alignment.

cart (Fig. 15–10) may be used.[62] This provides the child with a means of exploring the environment safely but independently.

Emphasis on head and trunk control and strengthening exercises in a variety of sitting postures are very important in this early preambulatory phase. Development of adequate strength and motor control for trunk righting, equilibrium reactions, and protective reactions will ultimately lead to improved sitting balance. Hands-free sitting with

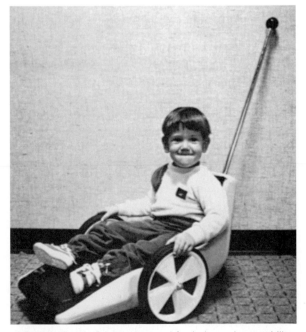

FIGURE 15–10. Caster cart used for independent mobility.

good balance is the optimal goal in this stage to allow for independence and freedom in play skills. In addition, hands-free sitting is a necessary precursor to ambulation with lower-extremity bracing and often is the determinant in deciding if a child will use a standing frame or will become a functional ambulator.

Also in this phase of preambulation, transitions from one position to another should be assessed and facilitated. Teaching the child strategies for transitions will enhance his or her optimal functional independence. Compensations may be taught to substitute for weakened musculature.

When the child attempts to pull to a standing position or would be expected to do so normally (at 10 to 12 months of age), the use of a standing device is indicated. Generally, a standing A-frame is the first orthosis chosen.[62] This is a relatively inexpensive tubular frame to which adjustable parts are attached (Fig. 15–11). Because it is not custom made, it can be fitted fairly quickly, although adjustments may be necessary to accommodate spinal deformities. This standing device offers support of the trunk, hips, and knees and leaves the hands free for other activities. Time spent in the standing frame should be increased gradually. This will allow the child to adjust to the upright position in terms of muscle strength, endurance, blood pressure, and pressure on skin surfaces.

After children have built up a tolerance for standing, they may be taught to move in the device by shifting their weight from side to side. Initial shifting of weight onto one side of the body is necessary to allow the other side to move forward. This preliminary weight shift is also a prerequisite for developing equilibrium reactions in the standing position and thus will prepare the child for later ambulation. As the child shifts weight, the trunk

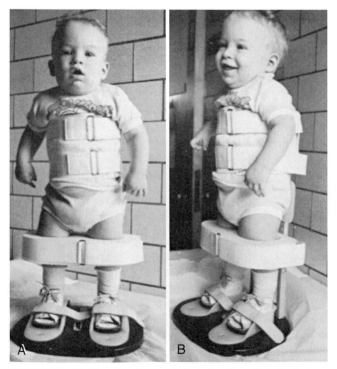

FIGURE 15–11. Standing frame. *A,* Anterior view. *B,* Lateral view.

musculature on the weight-bearing side should elongate and shorten on the non–weight-bearing side as muscle strength allows. This normal reaction to weight shifting also includes righting of the head and should be monitored closely by the therapist for completeness.

A therapy program must be designed to meet the individual's needs in each area. Age alone does not determine the appropriate therapeutic goals. Goals that are not suited for the child's cognitive and emotional needs, in addition to physical needs, will be doomed to failure before they are attempted. For example, an 18-month-old may have the physical capabilities to ambulate independently with crutches and braces. The child may not, however, have the cognitive skills necessary to learn a four-point gait or be ready emotionally to separate from his or her mother for intensive therapy sessions. A more realistic goal may be to let the child walk, holding onto furniture (cruising) while a wheeled walker for more independent ambulation is slowly introduced. Another alternative to using a conventional walker is to encourage the child to play with push-toys such as grocery carts and baby buggies.

During this preambulatory stage therapy goals may be accomplished through a comprehensive home program, with frequent checks to note progress or problems and to change the program accordingly. For the more involved child, increased frequency of direct intervention may be indicated to achieve optimal developmental progress.

The program often must be reevaluated and goals changed, if conditions such as shunt malfunctions or fractures occur. The warning signs for shunt dysfunctions are generally those previously described for suspected hydrocephalus. In addition, swelling along the shunt site may indicate a malfunction. Swelling and local heat or redness of a limb are the usual signs of a fracture. The limb may also look malaligned. Fever may accompany a fracture. As mentioned previously, these fractures generally heal quickly with proper medical intervention and interrupt rehabilitation efforts minimally.

Toddler Through Adolescent (Ambulatory Phase)

Stage 4: Toddler Through Preschool

This period in development marks the end of infancy and the beginning of childhood. For the normal child who has developed a strong sensorimotor foundation, physical development will be marked by increased coordination and refinement of movement patterns. In addition, a great variety of motor skills will be achieved as the normal child learns to throw, catch, run, hop, and jump. This is also a period of great cognitive growth, as children's use of mental imagery and physical knowledge of their environments expand. Concepts of size, number, color, form, and space are all developing. Emotionally, most children are becoming more independent and begin to break away from the sheltered environment of the home. They are now more interested in interacting with others and become social beings to a greater extent.

All of these changes in physical, cognitive, and emotional development will be evident in the child with spina

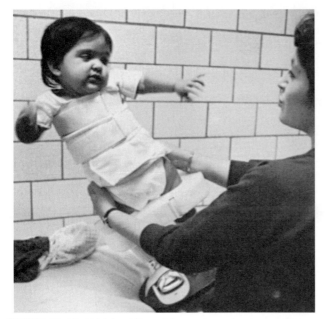

FIGURE 15–12. Weight shift and forward rotation in standing frame.

bifida, although the degree depends on the extent of the disability. It is of utmost importance to be aware of the characteristics of normal development, so that they can be nurtured and enhanced in the child with spina bifida.[95]

Goals for this as for any other stage must address not only physical but also cognitive and emotional development. The most obvious goal at this stage is to help the child who is already standing to progress to an ambulatory status. Even the child with a low thoracic lesion can usually manage some form of ambulation.

Thus far, the child has learned to shift weight in the standing frame. By rotating the trunk toward the weighted side, the non–weight-bearing side can be shifted forward (Fig. 15–12). By reversing the weight shift, the opposite side can be moved forward and a type of "pivoting-forward" progression can be accomplished. To maintain balance while shifting, the child may initially use a two-wheeled walker. The therapist may help initiate weight shift and trunk rotation by alternately pulling the arms forward.[45]

Once the child has gained this form of mobility, the type of permanent bracing chosen will depend on the level of the lesion. For thoracic and high-level lumbar lesions, a parapodium is often chosen. The parapodium was developed by the Ontario Crippled Children's Center in 1970 and is similar to the standing frame, except that hinges at the hips and knees allow for sitting and standing.[45] It, too, can be adjusted for growth and can accommodate orthopedic deformities. As with the standing frame, proper alignment of the parapodium is critical. The therapist, in conjunction with the orthotist, should check for correct standing alignment. The prevention of additional orthopedic deformities, development of good muscular control, and normal body image depend on a good-fitting orthosis.

After a pivoting gait is learned with the parapodium, a swing-to or swing-through gait can be attempted. By 4 to 5 years of age, a swing-through gait, with the child using Lofstrand crutches, can usually be accomplished.[45]

Variations of the parapodium are appearing that allow for easier locking and unlocking of hip and knee joints.[14] A swivel or pivot walker also may be attached to the foot plate to allow for crutchless walking.

Another type of orthosis for the child with a thoracic or high lumbar lesion is the Orlau swivel walker. It consists of modular design similar to the standing frame, with a chest strap and knee blocks attached to swiveling foot plates.[17] Rather than the whole base moving forward, as when weight is shifted in the parapodium, in the swivel walker each foot plate is spring loaded and is able to swivel forward independently. This allows for independent balance on one foot and therefore crutchless ambulation. The Orlau swivel walker is manufactured in Shrewsbury in the United Kingdom, and kits to be assembled may be obtained from there (see Appendix 15–B).[119]

Both the parapodium and swivel walker have had some problems with instability, ease of application, and cosmesis. New designs attempt to correct these problems. Nevertheless, existing limitations in the parapodium and swivel walker, particularly energy cost of walking, slow rate of locomotion, and cosmesis, have limited their use, primarily to the younger child.[107] These devices, however, remain an effective means of preventing musculoskeletal deformities caused by long-term sitting, wheelchair positioning, and general immobility. They also enhance social-emotional development gained from the upright position.[17] Another option for the higher-level child with good sitting balance is the reciprocating gait orthosis (RGO).[31] This brace consists of bilateral long-leg braces with a pelvic band and thoracic extension, if necessary. The hip joints are connected by a cable system that can work in two ways: If the child has active hip flexors, he or she can activate the cable system by shifting weight and flexing the non–weight-bearing extremity. This brings the weight-bearing extremity into relative extension in preparation for the next step. Without hip flexors, the child extends his or her trunk over one extremity, thus positioning it in relative extension. By virtue of the cable system, the non–weight-bearing extremity moves into flexion, thus initiating a step.[60] Several types of the RGO are in use, including the dual-cable LSU or the single-cable Jim Campbell type.[88]

Most recently the Isocentric Reciprocal Gait Orthosis (I-RGO) has been used for children with high-level spina bifida. It has a more cosmetic and efficient design as compared with the LSU or dual-cable type RGO. This "cable-less" brace has two to three times less friction and therefore is more energy efficient. The brace stabilizes the hip, knee, and ankle joints and balances the person, enabling him or her to stand "hands free" without the use of crutches or a walker. The I-RGO was designed by Wallace Motloch Company and is manufactured in Redwood City, California, at the Center for Orthotics Design, Inc. (Fig. 15–13).[88]

A more common means of maintaining the upright position has been through the use of long- or short-leg metal braces. In the 1970s conventional metal bracing was largely replaced by polypropylene braces. These plastic orthoses are considerably lighter than metal bracing and

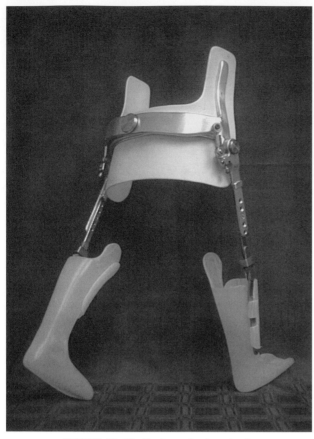

FIGURE 15–13. Reciprocal gait orthosis.

therefore reduce the energy cost of walking for the child with spina bifida.[64] They allow close contact and can be slipped into the shoe rather than being worn externally, thus affording the patient a better fitting, more cosmetic orthosis. These polypropylene braces are generally most effective with lower lumbar lesions where only short-leg bracing is required. Although these braces cannot be worn by everyone, they have greatly improved the rehabilitation potential of those able to use them.

The type of orthosis chosen (long-leg, with or without pelvic band, or short-leg) depends on the level of the myelomeningocele and the muscle power within that level. Because lesions are frequently incomplete, muscle strength must be assessed accurately before bracing is prescribed. Independent sitting balance with hands free also is a prerequisite for use of long- or short-leg braces. Even children with L3–L4 lesions, who demonstrate incomplete knee extension, may be able to use a short-leg brace with an anterior shell rather than requiring long-leg bracing.[26] This crouch-control AFO (CCAFO) will prevent a "crouch" gait pattern by improving knee extension during gait[11] (Fig. 15–14). The physical therapist must work in conjunction with the orthopedist and orthotist to have each child fitted with the minimum amount of bracing, which allows for joint stability and a good gait pattern (see Chapter 31).

Children with lower-level lesions (L5–S1) that utilize below-knee bracing often develop the ability to or choose to ambulate without assistive devices. However, recent studies have shown that crutch use may decrease excessive pelvic motion, which results in reducing abnormal joint forces.[130]

Children ambulating with AFOs often show excessive rotation at the knee because of the lack of functioning lateral hamstrings. Rather than going to a higher level of bracing, a twister cable can be added, which often decreases the rotary component during gait.[26] Twister cables can be heavy-duty torsion or more flexible elastic webbing depending on function. Typically, the young child who is just beginning to pull to stand and remains reliant on floor mobility as the primary means of mobility should have elastic twisters prescribed to allow for ease of creeping and transitions. The older and more active child will require heavy-duty torsion cables.

For children with a low lumbar or sacral lesion, often a polypropylene shoe insert to control foot position is the only bracing needed. These inserts fit snugly inside the shoe and help to control calcaneal and forefoot instabilities.[62] Even though a child may be able to ambulate without an assistive device or bracing, consideration must be given to the stresses that occur at the joints that over time may lead to orthopedic deformity. The greatest risk of joint instability often occurs at the knee. Barefoot walking versus use of an AFO has shown increased instability, joint stress and pain at the hip and knee as well as increased energy expenditure in the barefoot walking condition.[96, 125, 130] Even though children may be able to ambulate without the use of crutches, comparison of gait kinetics and kinematics of walking with crutches has shown a significant decrease of valgus forces at the knee and better overall alignment of the lower extremities.[131]

Gait training, begun as the child first starts to stand, can now continue in a more formalized manner. Using

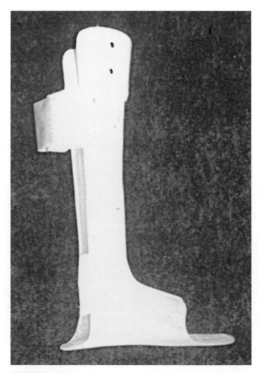

FIGURE 15–14. Crouch control ankle foot orthosis.

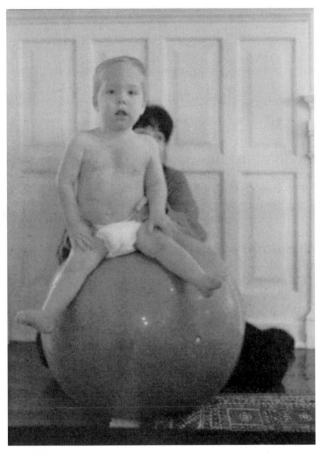

FIGURE 15–15. Balance and strengthening exercises done on a movable surface.

the appropriate orthosis and assistive devices (walker, crutches, or cane), each child must be helped to achieve the most efficient and effective gait pattern possible. As a part of gait training, the child should be taken out of the bracing and "challenged" so that righting and equilibrium reactions can be developed to their maximum. For example, having a child maintain balance while sitting on a ball or other movable surface (tilt board, trampoline) requires the participation of all available musculature, especially abdominal and trunk extensor muscles (Fig. 15–15). Strengthening available musculature is a primary objective in this phase of treatment. Often slow gains in muscle strength are the result of continued emphasis on strengthening during physical therapy. In addition to trunk muscles, the gluteus medius, gluteus maximus, and quadriceps are often targeted. Prone activities such as picking up toys while over a Swiss ball or moving around while prone on a scooter board will require use of these muscles while providing an enjoyable "exercise" for the child. These unconventional "gait-training" techniques can be used to improve muscle strength in general and to improve the gait pattern when bracing is reapplied. Regardless of the strengthening activities chosen, the pediatric therapist has the special task of using creativity to involve the child in therapeutic "play" activities. The ideas for creative activities are limitless but essential for combining therapy with age-appropriate cognitive abilities.

Sensory limitations may impede progress during early ambulation training. Because of limited kinesthesia and proprioception it is imperative that we augment available sensory systems and teach them to substitute with nonimpaired sensory systems. Impaired kinesthesia in children with myelomeningocele impedes their ability to anticipate changes in terrain and poses a safety problem. Vision may be the most relevant system to allow them to scan and preplan for changes in their walking environment.

Gait training and muscle strengthening are not the only consideration of the therapist. How cognitive and psychosocial development can be enhanced during this stage of the child's development is also important. One appropriate solution is to place the child in a 0- to 3-year developmental program. Although these programs may vary in the services they provide, most usually include age-appropriate play activities and some type of parental counseling. In addition, many offer therapeutic intervention from physical, occupational, and speech therapists. This intervention may occur in groups or individually.

Besides the socialization that 0- to 3-year programs provide for the child with myelomeningocele, they also teach the child age-appropriate ADL, such as dressing and undressing. At this age ADL skills are more appropriately taught in a group setting than individually. For many children the 0- to 3-year program, along with individualized therapy, is sufficient to enhance development in the physical, cognitive, and psychosocial realms.[133]

Presently, when children reach age 3, public school education becomes available to them. The preschool program continues to offer the same fundamental benefits as the 0- to 3-year program. It is the role of the hospital-based therapist to communicate the specific needs of each child entering the public school system. In this way continuity in the child's rehabilitation program is preserved.

The rehabilitation team, usually headed by a pediatrician or clinical nurse specialist, continues to follow the child closely during this stage. The neurosurgeon will check shunt functioning and perform revisions as necessary. The orthopedist will supervise bracing efforts to prevent and correct deformities in the spine and lower extremities. Well-child care and general medical treatment is the responsibility of the pediatrician on the team. The urologist continues to monitor renal functioning while keeping the child dry and free of infection. At this stage, bowel and bladder training will usually be taught to the child and family by the clinical nurse specialist. This clinician generally initiates this training following age-appropriate developmental guidelines.

Bladder training usually consists of transferring the job of intermittent catheterization from the parents to the child. Children as young as 3 years, but certainly by the age of 5, can learn CIC in a short period of time.[2] Children may first practice on dolls with male and female genitalia. Next, using mirrors to understand their own genitalia anatomy, they are able to accomplish the technique on themselves. CIC in conjunction with pharmacotherapy is useful in achieving continence in spina bifida children.[3] Another method of bladder training recently being used in the United States is intravesical transurethral bladder stimulation. This technique has allowed children with neurogenic bladder to rehabilitate their bladder function so that they can detect bladder fullness and generate effective destrusor contractions leading to improved continence.[60, 61]

Bowel training can be achieved through proper diet, regular evacuation times, and appropriate use of stool softeners and suppositories.[60, 71] Constipation (and resulting bypass diarrhea) can be prevented by proper habit training and use of fiber supplements. Stool softeners (not laxatives and enemas) and suppositories should be used to keep the stools soft and to help stimulate evacuation. Finally, toilet training, which amounts to scheduled toileting in time with the stool stimulants, usually achieves bowel continence. Consistency at each step along the way is the key to successful bowel training. A therapist may be called on to assist the parents and child in obtaining independence in this ADL activity.

Other members of the team, such as a psychologist, pedodontist, social worker, and dietitian, continue to function in their appropriate roles, interacting with the child and family as necessary. Physical and occupational therapists, as members of the team, must be sure that their treatment plans collaborate with the efforts of other team members.

Stage 5: Primary School Through Adolescence

This stage of development is marked by less rapid growth than earlier childhood but ends with a period of rapid physiological growth.[95] Children in the 6- to 10-year age group are interested in a wider variety of physical activities as they challenge their bodies to perform. The adolescent, however, is going through a period of great sexual differentiation as primary and secondary sexual characteristics develop more fully.

Cognitively, children are able to solve problems in a more sophisticated manner, although they revert to illogical thinking with complex problems. As they reach adolescence, they become capable of hypothetical reasoning and their thought processes approach that of adults.[95]

Emotionally, the 6- to 10-year-old is in a period of relative calm. Children are very interested in schoolwork and are eager to produce. During this period, they are building the skills of the future, preparing them for adult work. This is a prime time to introduce and teach new skills.

Adolescence is a stormy emotional period. Adolescents remain in turmoil as they seek their identities through sexual, social, and vocational activities. As their value systems develop, they feel less ambivalence between remaining as children or striving for independence. For the child with myelomeningocele, adolescence is not the optimum time to introduce learning new skills leading toward self-care and independence.[57]

As the energy cost of walking becomes too high, it often becomes appropriate for the adolescent to use a wheelchair for locomotion. To a teenager whose emotional needs include a strong peer identity, being confined to a wheelchair may be devastating. Appropriate alternatives may be to delay the decision to use a wheelchair full-time or to limit ambulation to short distances or to those places most important to the child. Again, goals

must be tailored to the child's needs and encompass his or her whole being.

In accordance with the child's growth spurts, frequent adjustment or reordering of bracing will be necessary. Continual reevaluation of orthotic needs may reveal that the level of bracing may decrease as the child grows and becomes stronger; the opposite development is also a possibility.

Usually during this stage, if it has not occurred previously, the evaluation of future ambulation potential will occur. This evaluation is frequently requested by the child whose larger size and limited abilities make ambulation more difficult each day. It must be remembered that strength does not increase in the same proportion as body weight.[99] Ambulation, although possible for the young child, may be impossible for that same person as a young adult.

Although no guidelines will include every patient, generally children with thoracic-level lesions are rarely ambulators by the late teens.[32, 62, 69] Those with upper lumbar lesions may be household ambulators with long-leg bracing but will require wheelchairs for quick mobility as adults. With low lumbar lesions, most adults can become community ambulators. Patients with sacral-level lesions are usually able to ambulate freely within the community. Many require minimal bracing and ambulate without assistive devices.[32, 62, 69] It must be remembered that ambulatory status is not determined by level of the lesion alone. The muscle power available, degree of orthopedic deformity, age, height, weight of the patient, and, of course, motivation are also determining factors.[26, 35, 62, 63, 111]

Because a large number of older spina bifida children will become wheelchair dependent, potential problems connected with a sedentary existence must be explored. Skin care, always a concern for the child with spina bifida, becomes a priority for the constant sitter. Mirrors may be used for self-inspection of the skin twice daily.[52] Well-constructed foam, gel, or air cell seat cushions are essential for distributing pressure evenly. Children should be taught frequent weight shifting within the chair to relieve pressure areas. Clothing should not be constricting but heavy enough to protect sensitive skin from wheelchair parts. Children must also be taught to avoid extremes of temperature and environmental hazards, such as radiators, sharp objects, and abrasive surfaces.[52] The therapist must reinforce the importance of skin care to prevent setbacks in the rehabilitation process that may result when skin breakdown develops.

Children with higher-level lesions may need spinal support to prevent deformities. Polyethylene body jackets can be used to provide this support and, hopefully, prevent the progression of any paralytic deformities.[62] Whatever type of device or wheelchair padding is used, the therapist must check to see that weight is distributed equally through both buttocks and that the spine is supported as necessary.

Part of the therapeutic intervention will be to provide strengthening exercises or activities to be done out of the supporting orthosis. This is necessary to maintain existing trunk strength and to preserve the child's present level of functioning.

Generally, in late childhood or early adolescence, orthopedic deformities that have been gradually developing require surgical intervention. Progressive scoliosis or kyphosis may require internal fixation when conservative methods fail.[81] Often sectioning of contracted muscles at the hip and knee is required.[32] The iliopsoas, adductors, and hamstrings are frequently the offending muscles. These surgeries, followed by strengthening exercises and gait training, often add to the ambulatory life of the child with spina bifida. For example, in a child who displays an extreme lordotic posture, hip flexors may be contractured and require surgery to lengthen them. A postoperative therapeutic program might include periods of prone lying to prevent future contractures and strengthening of hip extensors and abdominals that were previously overstretched by the lordotic position.

Of primary importance during this stage is preparing the child for independence in ADL, which may be broken down into self-care, locomotion-related, and social interaction activities.[118]

In conjunction with the nurse, physical therapist, and occupational therapist, self-care skills of dressing, eating and food preparation, general hygiene, and bowel and bladder care can be addressed. Because the adolescent is so concerned with achieving independence, he or she is more likely to comply with a regimen of strengthening exercises if shown how they relate to functional independence. A creative therapist may, for example, incorporate trunk stability and upper-extremity strengthening work in activities such as gourmet cooking or getting ready for a dance.

Locomotion activities should include all gait-related skills, such as falling down, getting up, or ambulation on various terrains. Transfers of all types are also included in locomotion activities. Again, a creative therapeutic program helps to make achievement of skills more palatable. For example, school-aged children may enjoy a competitive relay race situation, where each child falls, gets up, walks across the room, and sits down in a chair safely. This type of activity combines gait-training activities with group socialization and may meet a variety of goals (motor and psychosocial) at the same time.

Achievement of independence in ADL for the child and adult with spina bifida does not depend solely on the level of paralysis.[110] Also important are psychosocial and environmental factors. Mean ages for the achievement of various ADL activities have been developed and may assist the therapist in establishing realistic therapeutic goals in this area.[118]

Often during this stage of recovery, the therapist may be asked to assist in assessing cognitive functioning. The perceptual/cognitive evaluations referred to earlier may be administered and the results interpreted for parents and school personnel.

As previously discussed, children with spina bifida have a general perceptual deficit,[29] which can be manifested in a variety of ways. First, the child may have difficulty recognizing objects and the relationships that they have to each other. They may therefore perceive their world in a distorted manner, thus making their reactions unstable and unpredictable. These perceptual difficulties will most likely affect academic learning and may associate failure with the learning process. Difficulties in attaining

independence in ADL activities are also linked to perceptual problems. Finally, emotional disturbances may be attributed in part to the perceptual difficulties of the child with spina bifida.[42]

Remedial programs, such as the Frostig Program for the Development of Visual Perception, have been effective in improving the visual perception of spina bifida children.[42] Programs of this type are most effective when remediation begins early, preferably at or before the time the child enters school.

Children requiring programs for sensorimotor integration should be referred to a therapist certified in this area. If one is not available, many appropriate activities for sensorimotor integration may be adapted from Ayres[4] or Montgomery and Richter.[86]

Regardless of the school setting chosen for the child, the therapist should be able to serve the classroom teacher as a consultant. Advice on adaptive seating and therapeutic goals appropriate for the classroom will help ensure that the rehabilitation process will continue in the classroom, as well as promoting optimal conditions for learning.

When a child is going from a special to a regular school setting, the support of the therapeutic team is essential and invaluable. Teachers in the public school setting have had little exposure to handicapped children.[54] The teacher's expectations, as created by the therapist regarding the spina bifida child's special needs and abilities, often spell the difference between success and failure of this attempt at integration both academically and psychosocially. Even though the child may no longer require direct therapeutic intervention, periodic checks, including site classroom visits, are recommended to prevent minor problems from erupting into major ones. For example, bowel and bladder accidents can be avoided by scheduling regular times for toileting. The teacher may be able to make minor adjustments in the teaching schedule to accommodate for this scheduling. Also, full-control braces (from hip to ankles) may seem overwhelming to the layperson. If the teacher is shown how the braces lock and unlock to allow the child to sit or stand to walk, he or she may feel more at ease if ever called on to assist the child.

Therapeutic goals in this stage will be colored by the psychological perspective of the child. As the child nears adolescence, these psychosocial aspects become of paramount importance. While the therapist should not take on the role of the psychologist, collaborative efforts in the area of counseling will be necessary. Questions will arise many times during the physical/occupational therapy sessions, requiring factual answers that the therapist can and should provide.

Adolescents with spina bifida show great concern about self-esteem and social-sexual adjustment.[51] These concerns appear directly related to efficient bowel and bladder management.[67] Strategies to cope with bowel and bladder difficulties, as previously outlined, combined with appropriate emotional support from family and medical personnel will help to alleviate this concern.

Although great advances in medical management of children with myelomeningocele have occurred, there is a contrasting lack of improvement related to sexual func-

CASE 15–1 MICHAEL

Michael was a full-term baby, delivered via planned cesarean section with a prenatal diagnosis of myelomeningocele. The diagnosis was made during the second trimester after fetal ultrasound evaluation and amniocentesis. The family met with the neurosurgeon before delivery and prenatal counseling occurred after diagnosis.

Michael underwent myelomeningocele repair 24 hours after delivery. An orthopedic, urological, neurosurgical, and physical therapy examination occurred at 1 day of age before back closure. Presurgical MMT showed the presence of hip and knee musculature (L1–L4/5), but no muscle activity was noted below the knees. Three days after closure Michael required ventriculoperitoneal shunt insertion to control hydrocephalus. Postoperative MMT findings at 7 days of age were identical to preoperative results. Michael was discharged at 8 days of age. Before discharge Michael's parents were instructed in ROM exercises, positioning, and developmental handling. Developmental handling exercises included ways to increase head, trunk, and lower-extremity strength as well as appropriate play positions. Michael was discharged home with a referral for physical therapy and follow-up in a myelomeningocele clinic.

At 6 months of age Michael was readmitted to the hospital secondary to a shunt malfunction requiring ventriculoperitoneal shunt revision (VPSR). After 2 weeks at home Michael returned to the clinic for postoperative follow-up. There were no medical concerns, but it was discovered that Michael had not yet begun to roll over and to this point had not had physical therapy. The lack of physical therapy was due to serious health problems in another family member. Because of this situation, home physical therapy was initiated. A total-body night splint was fabricated to maintain hip alignment and prevent contracture of lower extremities.

Michael received weekly therapy through 3 years of age. Therapy focused on developmental exercises to promote mobility, sitting and standing balance activities, strengthening available lower-extremity musculature, and orthotic assessment and gait training. The family was instructed in home activities to complement the weekly therapy program. He sat and began belly crawling at 1 year of age. Michael began walking with AFOs and a forward walker at 30 months. Before this he used an A-frame for standing at 10 months and began gait training at 15 months.

Michael progressed to independent ambulation with Lofstrand crutches and AFOs over the next several years. At age 6 he entered school and was fully mainstreamed. An increase in falling was noted shortly after entering school. At the same time, his 6-month routine MMT showed increasing weakness in the left leg. In addition, some increased muscle tone was noted in the same leg. Magnetic resonance imaging revealed a tethered cord, and a tethered cord release was performed. Two months after tethered cord release, Michael was again independent in ambulation and had progressed to stair climbing with a rail. His next routine MMT showed a return of strength to the level before his tethered cord.

Michael's physical conditioning continued to progress, and from ages 7 to 10 he participated in adaptive sports activities in his community. Swimming had become a favorite activity since he had been swimming to increase strength from toddlerhood at the suggestion of his physical therapist. Because of his activity level and independence in most functional activities routine physical therapy had been discontinued with only biannual clinic visits. Michael and his family continued with an intensive stretching and prone positioning program that they had been performing independently since Michael was a toddler. At his 10-year-old visit, an area of skin breakdown was noted on the left lateral malleolus and decreased weight bearing on this side was noted during gait. There was no change in his manual muscle test or orthopedic examination. A brace check noted that the AFO was too small and needed to be replaced. The physical therapist reviewed skin care and brace fit with Michael and his family.

At age 13 Michael had gained a significant amount of weight that was limiting his endurance for long-distance ambulation. Michael was referred to a nutritionist for counseling. The physical therapist in conjunction with the physician discussed with Michael's parents the possibility of using a wheelchair for long-distance travel. After much discussion and initial resistance by Michael, Michael and his family decided to try a wheelchair. At age 16 Michael continues to be an independent community ambulator and uses a wheelchair for long distance only. He continues to be followed on an annual basis or as needed if problems arise. Michael's physical therapy has encouraged and continued to motivate Michael to maintain his participation in sports activities during his teenage years.

---

tion and reproductive issues. Five factors have contributed to delayed social and sexual growth in these adolescents: (1) severity of the mental handicap, (2) poor manual dexterity, (3) lack of education, (4) overprotective parents, and (5) difficulty of health care personnel to address sexuality with physically disabled patients and their families.[59] Questions about sexuality may be brought up by either the parents or the child. Parents of children with spina bifida realize the need to teach their children about sexuality, but they often feel inadequate about doing so and are reluctant to bring up questions to health care professionals.[97] The therapist must be open, informed, and able to provide resources to both parents and children.

Generally, the sexual capacity of the female with spina bifida is near normal; that is, she has potential for a normal orgasmic response, is fertile, and can bear children.[21, 56, 69] The pregnancy, however, may be considered high risk, depending on existing orthopedic abnormalities. Affected males are frequently sterile and have small testicles and penises. Their potential for erection and ejaculation will depend on the level of the lesion.

In many cases psychological problems may be a primary cause of sexual failure.[69] It must be remembered that sexuality is not merely a process involving the genitalia but depends on a positive body image and a feeling of self-esteem that is nurtured from birth.[27, 52]

PSYCHOSOCIAL ADJUSTMENT TO CONGENITAL CORD LESIONS

The previous sections on goal setting and rehabilitation of the child with spina bifida have covered birth through adolescence. After adolescence, rehabilitation can be handled in much the same manner as an adult spinal cord injury. It will be important, however, to keep in mind the global effects of spina bifida on the growing child as he or she approaches adulthood.

Because of the congenital nature of spina bifida, psychological adjustment will be somewhat different than adjustment to a traumatic spinal cord injury. The psychological adjustment to this congenital disability must be considered from the perspective of the parents, the family, and, of course, the child.

A longitudinal study concerning the psychological aspects of spina bifida shows that the parents go through a series of steps in the adjustment process. From birth to about 6 months of age, the parents experience shock and bewilderment. Information given during this time may be rejected or misinterpreted. Health care professionals therefore must be ready to repeat the same information to parents on several occasions during the first few years of the rehabilitation process.

The period of 6 to 18 months of the child's life may be the most stressful on parents. Frequent hospitalizations during this time place increased pressure on the whole family. Parents, now able to fully comprehend the implications of their child's disability, begin to worry about the future and the impact of the disability on the rest of the family structure.

The period from age 2 years through the preschool years is relatively peaceful. The parents are more concerned with toilet training, social acceptability, and general information on child rearing. They seem less aware of their child's mental limitations as he or she continues to develop into a relatively happy, well-adjusted child.

By the age of 6 years children are becoming more aware of their disabilities and parents are concerned about problems that may arise as their children enter primary school. The child's psychological adjustment will depend not on the severity of the disability but primarily on the attitude of the parents and family and on the environmental conditions to which he or she is exposed.[67, 93, 106]

Some evidence indicates that children with spina bifida may grow up in extreme social isolation.[99] Being placed in special schools, they have little interaction with normal children their own age. Because of their disabilities, they are often denied small tasks or chores that promote a sense of responsibility in the growing child.[51, 99] To promote emotional growth and psychological well-being, caregivers must be persuaded to "let go." Children with spina bifida must develop responsibility and independence by being given the chance to interact and even compete with their peers. As they approach adulthood, concerns of independent living situations and vocational placement must be addressed. With a foundation of strong support systems fostering emotional maturity, the future can be bright for the child with congenital spinal cord injury.

ACKNOWLEDGMENT

The authors wish to acknowledge the contribution of Kathryn L. Gabriel to the writing of the previous edition of this chapter.

REFERENCES

1. Alexander MA, Steg NL: Myelomeningocele: Comprehensive treatment. Arch Phys Med Rehabil 70:637–641, 1989.
2. Altshuler A, et al: Even children can learn to do clean self-catheterization. Am J Nurs 77:97–101, 1977.
3. American Academy of Pediatrics, Action Committee on Myelodysplasia, Section on Urology: Current approaches to evaluation and management of children with myelomeningocele. Pediatrics 63:663–667, 1979.
4. Ayres AJ: Sensory Integration and the Child. Los Angeles, Western Psychological Services, 1979.
5. Baker DA, Sherry CJ: Spina bifida and maternal Rh blood type. Arch Dis Child 54:567, 1979 (letter).
6. Bannister CM, Russell SA, Rimmer S: Prenatal brain development of fetuses with myelomeningocele. Eur J Pediatr Surg 8(Suppl I):15–17, 1998.
7. Banta JV, Benanni C, Prebluda J: Latex anaphylaxis during spinal surgery in children with myelomeningocele. Dev Med Child Neurol 35:540–548, 1993.
8. Banta JV, et al: The team approach in the care of the child with myelomeningocele. J Prosthet Orthot 2:263–273, 1990.
9. Bayley N: Manual for the Bayley Scales of Infant Development, 2nd ed. San Antonio, TX, The Psychological Corporation, 1993.
10. Beery KE: The Developmental Test of Visual-Motor Integration. Cleveland, Modern Curriculum Press, 1989.
11. Berard C, et al: Anticalcaneus carbon fibre orthosis for children with myelomeningocele. Rev Chir Orthop 76:222–225, 1990.
12. Brazelton TB: Neonatal Behavioral Assessment Scale, 2nd ed. In Clinics in Developmental Medicine, vol 88. Philadelphia, JB Lippincott, 1984.
13. Brocklehurst G: Spina bifida for the clinician. In Clinics in Developmental Medicine, vol 57. Philadelphia, JB Lippincott, 1976.
14. Brown JT, McLone DG: The effect of complications on intellectual function in 167 children with myelomeningocele. Z Kinderchir 34:117–120, 1981.
15. Bruininks RH: Bruininks-Oseretsky Test of Motor Proficiency Examiner's Manual. Circle Pines, MN, American Guidance Service, 1987.
16. Burn J, Gibben D: May spina bifida result from an X-linked defect in a selective abortion method. J Med Genet 16:210–214, 1979.

17. Butler PB, et al: Use of the Orlau Swivel Walker for the severely handicapped patient. Physiotherapy 88:324–326, 1982.

18. Byrd SE, Radkowski MA: The radiological evaluation of the child with a myelomeningocele. J Natl Med Assoc 83:608–614, 1991.

19. Carstens C, Niethard FU: The current status of prenatal diagnosis of myelomeningocele—results of a questionnaire (German). Geburtshilfe Frauenheilkd 53:182–185, 1993.

20. Cash J: Neurology for physiotherapists, 2nd ed. Philadelphia, JB Lippincott, 1977.

21. Cass AS, et al: Sexual function in adults with myelomeningocele. J Urol 136:425–426, 1986.

22. Charney EB, Melchionni JB, Antonucci DL: Ventriculitis in newborns with myelomeningocele. Am J Dis Child 145:287–290, 1991.

23. Colangelo C, Bergen AS, Gottlieb L: A normal baby: The sensory-motor processes of the first year, 2nd ed. Valhalla, NY, Valhalla Rehabilitation Publications, 1986.

24. Colarusso RP, Hammill DD: Motor-free visual perception test manual, revised. Novato, CA, Academic Therapy Publications, 1995.

25. Darrah J, Piper M, Watt MJ: Assessment of gross motor skills of at-risk infants: Predictive validity of the Alberta Infant Motor Scale. Dev Med Child Neurol 40:485–491, 1998.

26. De Souza LJ, Carroll N: Ambulation of the braced myelomeningocele patient. J Bone Joint Surg Am 58:1112–1118, 1976.

27. Dorner S: Sexual interest and activity in adolescents with spina bifida. J Child Psychiatry 18:229–237, 1977.

28. Dounes E: Sacrococcygeal agenesis: A report of four new cases. Acta Orthop Scand 49:475–480, 1978.

29. Drago JR, et al: The role of intermittent catheterization in the management of children with myelomeningocele. J Urol 118:92–94, 1977.

30. Drummond DS, et al: Post-operative neuropathic fractures in patients with myelomeningocele. Dev Med Child Neurol 23:147–150, 1981.

31. Durr-Fillaver Medical, Inc—Orthopedic Division: LSU Reciprocating Gait Orthosis: A Pictorial Description and Application model. Chattanooga, TN, 1983.

32. Feiwell E: Surgery of the hip in myelomeningocele as related to adult goals. Clin Orthop 148:87–93, 1980.

33. Feiwell E, et al: The effects of hip reduction on function in patients with myelomeningocele. J Bone Joint Surg Am 60(2):169–173, 1978.

34. Ferguson-Smith MA, et al: Avoidance of anencephalic and spina bifida births by maternal serum alpha-fetoprotein screening. Lancet 1:1330–1333, 1978.

35. Findley TW, et al: Ambulation in the adolescent with myelomeningocele: I. Early childhood predictors. Arch Phys Med Rehabil 68:518–522, 1987.

36. Fiorentino MR: Normal and Abnormal Development: The Influence of Primitive Reflexes on Motor Development. Springfield, IL, Charles C Thomas, 1972.

37. Fiorentino MR: Normal and Abnormal Development: The Influence of Primitive Reflexes on Motor Development, 2nd ed. Springfield, IL, Charles C Thomas, 1980.

38. Folio MR, Fewell RR: Peabody Developmental Motor Scales and Activity Cards. Allen, TX, DLM Teaching Resources, 1983.

39. Gabrieli AP, et al: Tethered cord syndrome in myelomeningocele: surgical treatment and results. Chicago, IL, International Spina Bifida Symposium, May 1990.

40. Gardner MF: Test of Visual-Perceptual Skills (Non-Motor) Manual. San Francisco, Health Publishing, 1988.

41. Gelb LN (ed): Food and Drug Administration medical bulletin, July 1991.

42. Gluckman S, Barling J: Effects of a remedial program on visual-motor perception in spina bifida children. J Genet Psychol 136:195–202, 1980.

43. Gold M, et al: Intraoperative anaphylaxis: An association with latex sensitivity. J Allergy Clin Immunol 87:662–666, 1991.

44. Goldberg MF, Oakley GP Jr: Interpreting elevated amniotic fluid alpha-fetoprotein levels in clinical practice: Use of the predictive value positive concept. Am J Obstet Gynecol 133:126–132, 1979.

45. Gram MC: The Paradigm: Adjunct to the Habilitation of the Child with Spina Bifida. Woodbridge, IL, MM Therapeutics, 1991.

46. Greene WB, et al: Effect of race and gender on neurological level in myelomeningocele. Dev Med Child Neurol 33:110–117, 1991.

47. Griscom NT, et al: Amniography in second trimester diagnosis of myelomeningocele. AJR 133:1151–1156, 1979.

48. Guttman L: Spinal cord injuries: Comprehensive Management and Research, 2nd ed. Oxford, Blackwell Publisher, 1976.

49. Haley SM, et al: Pediatric Evaluation of Disability Inventory (PEDI): Development, Standardization and Administration Manual. Boston, New England Medical Center Hospitals and PEDI Research Group, 1992.

50. Hall P, et al: Scoliosis and hydrocephalus in myelomeningocele patients: The effect of ventricular shunting. J Neurosurg 50:174–178, 1979.

51. Hayden PW, et al: Adolescents with myelodysplasia: Impact of physical disability on emotional maturation. Pediatrics 64:53–59, 1979.

52. Hendry J, Geddes N: Living with a congenital anomaly. Can Nurse 74(6):29–33, 1978.

53. Hensinger RN, Jones E: Neonatal Orthopedics. New York, Grune & Stratton, 1981.

54. Hunt GM: Spina bifida: Implications for 100 children at school. Dev Med Child Neurol 23:160–172, 1981.

55. Hyperthermia and meningomyelocele and anencephaly. Lancet 1:769–770, 1978 (letter).

56. Hyperthermia and the neural tube. Lancet 2:560–561, 1978 (editorial).

57. Ito JA, et al: A qualitative examination of adolescents and adults with myelomeningocele: Their perspective. Eur J Pediatr Surg 7 (Suppl 1):53–54, 1997.

58. James WH: The sex ratio in spina bifida. J Med Genet 16:384–388, 1979.

59. Joyner BD, McLorie GA, Khoury AE: Sexuality and reproductive issues in children with myelomeningocele. Eur J Pediatr Surg 8:29–34, 1998.

60. Kaplan WE: Management of the urinary tract in myelomeningocele. Prob Urol 2:121–131, 1988.

61. Katona F, Berenyi M: Intravesical transurethral electrotherapy in meningomyelocele patients. Acta Paediatr Hung 16(3–4):363–374, 1975.

62. Kupka J, et al: Comprehensive management in the child with spina bifida. Orthop Clin North Am 9:97–113, 1978.

63. Lee EH, Carroll NC: Hip stability and ambulatory status in myelomeningocele. J Pediatr Orthop 5:522–527, 1985.

64. Lindseth RE, Glancy J: Polypropylene lower-extremity braces for paraplegia due to myelomeningocele. J Bone Joint Surg Am 56:556–563, 1974.

65. Lippman-Hand A, et al: Indications for prenatal diagnosis in relatives of patients with neural tube defects. Obstet Gynecol 51:72–76, 1978.

66. Mathisen BA, Shepherd K: Oral-motor dysfunction and feeding problems in infants with myelodysplasia. Pediatr Rehab 1:117–122, 1997.

67. McAndrew I: Adolescents and young people with spina bifida. Dev Med Child Neurol 21:619–629, 1979.

68. McCall RE, Schmidt WT: Clinical experience with reciprocal gait orthosis in myelodysplasia. J Pediatr Orthop 6:157–161, 1986.

69. McLaughlin JF, Shurtleff DB: Management of the newborn with myelodysplasia. Clin Pediatr 18:463–476, 1979.

70. McLaurin RL: Myelomeningocele. New York, Grune & Stratton, 1977.

71. McLone DG: An Introduction to Spina Bifida. Chicago, Children's Memorial Hospital Myelomeningocele Service, 1980.

72. McLone DG: Results of treatment of children born with a myelomeningocele. Clin Neurosurg 30:407–412, 1983.

73. McLone DG: Treatment of myelomeningocele: Arguments against selection. Clin Neurosurg 33:359–370, 1986.

74. McLone DG: Spina bifida today: Problems adults face. Semin Neurol 9:169–175, 1989.

75. McLone DG, Dias MS: Complications of myelomeningocele closure. Pediatr Neurosurg 17:267–273, 1991–1992.

76. McLone DG, Knepper PA: The cause of Chiari II malformation: A unified theory. Pediatr Neurosci 15:1–12, 1989.

77. McLone DG, Naidich TP: Tethered cord. In McLauren RL, et al (eds): Pediatric Neurosurgery: Surgery of the Developing Nervous System, 2nd ed. Philadelphia, WB Saunders, 1989.

78. McLone DG, et al: An Introduction to Hydrocephalus. Chicago, Children's Memorial Hospital, 1982.

79. McLone DG, et al: Neurolation: Biochemical and morphological studies on primary and secondary neural tube defects. Concepts Pediatr Neurosurg 4:15–29, 1983.

80. McLone DG, et al: Central nervous system infections as a limiting factor in the intelligence of children with myelomeningocele. Pediatrics 70:338–342, 1982.

81. Menelaus MB: Orthopaedic management of children with myelomeningocele: a plea for realistic goals. Dev Med Child Neurol 6 (Suppl 37):3–11, 1976.

82. Menelaus MB: The Orthopedic Management of Spina Bifida Cystica, 2nd ed. New York, Churchill Livingstone, 1980.

83. Meuli M, et al: The spinal cord lesion in human fetuses with myelomeningocele: Implications for fetal surgery. J Pediatr Surg 32:448–452, 1997.

84. The Milani-Comparetti Motor Development Screening Test: Test Manual, 3rd ed revised. Omaha, NB, University of Nebraska Medical Center, Meyer Children's Rehabilitation Institute, 1992.

85. Milerad J, Logercrantz H, Johnson P: Obstructive sleep apnea in Arnold Chiari malformation treated with acetazolamide. Acta Pediatr 81:609–612, 1992.

86. Montgomery MA, Richter E: Sensorimotor Integration for Developmentally Delayed Children: A Handbook. Los Angeles, Western Psychological Services, 1977.

87. Moore KL: Before We Are Born: Basic Embryological and Birth Defects, revised reprint. Philadelphia, WB Saunders, 1974.

88. Motloch W: Isocentric Reciprocal Gait Orthosis (I-RGO). Handout from the Center for Orthotics Design, Inc, Redwood City, California.

89. Muen WJ, Bannister CM: Hand function in subjects with spina bifida. E UR J Pediatr Surg 7(Suppl I):18–22, 1997.

90. Muller EB, Nordwall A: Prevalence of scoliosis in children with myelomeningocele in western Sweden. Spine 17:1097–1102, 1992.

91. Nesbit DE, Ziter FA: Epidemiology of myelomeningocele in Utah. Dev Med Child Neurol 21(6):54–57, 1979.

92. Nevin NC, et al: Influence of social class on the risk of recurrence of anencephalus and spina bifida. Dev Med Child Neurol 23:155–159, 1981.

93. Nielsen HH: A longitudinal study of the psychological aspects of myelomeningocele. Scand J Psychol 21:45–54, 1980.

94. Oakes WJ: Developmental anomalies and neurosurgical diseases in children: Chiari malformations, hydromyelia, syringomyelia. In Wilkins RH, Rengachary SS (eds): Neurosurgery. New York, McGraw-Hill Book Co, 1984.

95. Papalia DE, Olds SW: Human Development. New York, McGraw-Hill, 1981.

96. Park BK, et al: Gait electromyography in children with myelomeningocele at the sacral level. Arch Phys Med Rehabil 78:471–475, 1997.

97. Passo S: Parents' perceptions, attitudes and needs regarding sex education for the child with myelomeningocele. Res Nurs Health 1(2):53–59, 1978.

98. Pearson PN, Williams CE: Physical Therapy Services in Developmental Disabilities. Springfield, IL, Charles C Thomas, 1976.

99. Perspectives in spina bifida (editorial). BMJ 2:909–910, 1978.

100. Pietrzyk JJ, Turowski G: Immunogenetic bases and congenital malformations: Association of HLA-B27 with spina bifida. Pediatr Res 13:879–883, 1979.

101. Piper MC, Darrah J: Motor Assessment of the Developing Infant. Philadelphia, WB Saunders, 1994.

102. Raimondi AJ, Soare P: Intellectual development in shunted hydrocephalic children. Am J Dis Child 127:664–671, 1974.

103. Ralis ZA, et al: Changes in shape, ossification and quality of bones in children with spina bifida. Dev Med Child Neurol 18(6: suppl 37):29–41, 1976.

104. Riegel DH: Diagnoses and surgical treatment of tethered cord. Allegheny General Hospital, Pittsburgh, PA. Presented at the International Spina Bifida Symposium, Chicago, May 1990.

105. Riegel DH: Lipomeningocele, surgical indications and results. Allegheny General Hospital, Pittsburgh, PA. Presented at International Spina Bifida Symposium, Chicago, May 1990.

106. Rogers BM: Comprehensive care for the child with a chronic disability. Am J Nurs 79:1106–1108, 1979.

107. Rose GK, Henshaw JT: Swivel walkers for paraplegics—considerations and problems in their design and application. Bull Prosthet Res 10(20):62–74, 1973.

108. Rosenstein BD, et al: Bone density in myelomeningocele: The effects of ambulatory status and other factors. Dev Med Child Neurol 29:486–494, 1987.

109. Rotenstein D, Riegel DH, Lucke JF: Growth of hormone-treated and nontreated children before and after tethered spinal cord release. Pediatr Neurosurg 24:238–241, 1996.

110. Schaffer MF, Dias LS: Myelomeningocele: Orthopedic Treatment. Baltimore, Williams & Wilkins, 1983.

111. Schopler SA, Menelaus MB: Significance of the strength of the quadriceps muscles in children with myelomeningocele. J Pediatr Orthop 7:507–512, 1987.

112. Shurtleff DB: Decubitus formation and skin breakdown. In Shurtleff DB (ed): Myelodysplasias and Exstrophies: Significance, Prevention and Treatment. Orlando, FL, Grune & Stratton, 1986, pp 285–298.

113. Singer HA, et al: Spina bifida and anencephaly in the cape. S Afr Med J 53:626–627, 1978.

114. Slater JE: Rubber anaphylaxis. N Engl J Med 320:1126–1130, 1989.

115. Slater JE, et al: Rubber specific IgE in children with spina bifida. J Urol 146:578–579, 1991.

116. Slater JE, et al: Type 1 hypersensitivity to rubber. Ann Allergy 65:411–414, 1990.

117. Smithells RW, et al: Apparent prevention of neural tube defects by periconceptional vitamin supplementation. Arch Dis Child 56:911–918, 1981.

118. Sousa JC, et al: Developmental guidelines for children with myelodysplasia. Phys Ther 63:21–29, 1983.

119. Stallard J, et al: Engineering design considerations of the Orlau Swivel Walker. Eng Med 15:3–8, 1986.

120. Stark GD: Spina Bifida: Problems and Management. Boston, Blackwell Scientific Publications, 1977.

121. Stein SC, Schut L: Hydrocephalus in myelomeningocele. Childs Brain 5:413–419, 1979.

122. Storrs B: Selective posterior rhizotomy for treatment of progressive spasticity in patients with myelomeningocele. Pediatr Neurosci 13:135–137, 1987.

123. Storrs BB, McLone DG: Selective posterior rhizotomy in treatment of spasticity associated with myelomeningocele. In Marlin AE (ed): Concepts Pediatr Neurosci 9:173–177, 1989.

124. Tappit-Emas E: Spina bifida. In Tecklin JS (ed): Pediatric Physical Therapy. New York, JB Lippincott, 1989.

125. Thomson JD, et al: The effects of ankle-foot orthoses on the ankle and knee in persons with myelomeningocele: Evaluation using three-dimensional gait analysis. J Pediatr Ortho 19:27–33, 1999.

126. Trollmann R, Strehl E, Dorr HG: Growth hormone deficiency in children with myelomeningocele (MMC)—effects of growth hormone treatment. Eur J Pediatr Surg 7(Suppl 1):58–59, 1997.

127. Trollmann R, et al: Arm span IGF-1 and IGFBP-3 levels as screening parameters for the myelomeningocele—preliminary data. Eur J Pediatr 157:451–455, 1998.

128. Tulipan N, Bruner JP: Myelomeningocele repair in utero: A report of three cases. Pediatr Neurosurg 28:177–180, 1998.

129. Vandertop P, et al: Surgical decompression for symptomatic Chiari II malformation in neonates with myelomeningocele. J Neurosurg 77:541–544, 1992.

130. Vankoski SJ, et al: Characteristic pelvic, hip and knee patterns in children with lumbosacral myelomeningocele. Gait Posture 3:51–57, 1995.

131. Vankoski SJ, et al: The influence of forearm crutches on pelvic and hip kinematics in children with myelomeningocele: Don't throw away the crutches. Dev Med Child Neurol 39:614–619, 1997.

132. Wescott MA, et al: Congenital and acquired orthopedic abnormalities in patients with myelomeningocele. Radiographics 12:1155–1173, 1992.

133. Wolf L: Development of self-care assessment tool for children with meningomyelocele. Dev Disabil 10(2):2–6, 1987.

134. Zausmer E: Evaluation of strength and motor development in infants. Phys Ther Rev 33:621–628, 1953.

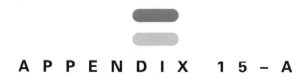

APPENDIX 15 – A

Audiovisual Resources

Brazelton Neonatal Behavioral Assessment (16-mm films)
Part 1 Introduction
Part 2 Self-scoring exam
Part 3 Variations in Normal Behavior
  Educational Development Center
  55 Chapel Street
  Newton, MA 02160

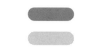

APPENDIX 15 – B

Orlau Swivel Rocker Distributors

UK

J Stallard
Technical Director
ORLAU
Orthopaedic Hospital
Oswestry
Shropshire, SY107AG
UK

US

Mopac Ltd
206 Chestnut Street
Eau Claire, WI 54703
715-832-1685

Traumatic Spinal Cord Injury

MYRTICE B. ATRICE, BS, PT • SARAH A. MORRISON, BS, PT • SHARI L. McDOWELL, BS, PT
• BETSY SHANDALOV, BS, OTR/L

Chapter Outline

Objectives

After reading this chapter, the student/therapist will:

1. Describe the etiology and demographics of spinal cord injury (SCI).
2. Discuss the pharmacological, acute medical management, and surgical stabilization of the SCI client.
3. Describe the secondary complications of SCI, the appropriate interventions, and the impact of complications on the rehabilitation process.
4. Identify the basic components of the examination process.
5. Identify problems based on the examination, set appropriate goals, and plan an individualized treatment program to reach the goals.
6. Describe adaptive equipment available to increase function.
7. Discuss client progression and the process of discharge planning throughout the rehabilitation process.
8. Describe functional expectations for individuals with complete SCIs.
9. Identify equipment needs for a given SCI lesion.

Spinal cord injury (SCI) is a catastrophic condition that, depending on its severity, may cause dramatic changes in the victim's life. The effects of SCI have an impact not only on the lives of the client and family but also on society as a whole. SCI usually happens to active, independent people who at one moment are in control of their lives and in the next moment are paralyzed, with loss of sensation and loss of bodily functions and dependence on others for their most basic needs. Clients need a well-coordinated, specialized rehabilitation program consisting of a team of physicians and health care professionals to provide the tools necessary to develop a satisfying and productive postinjury lifestyle.[14, 107]

The successful rehabilitation process is comprehensive. It includes prevention, early recognition, inpatient care, outpatient care, and community reintegration. The comprehensive rehabilitation team for SCI is composed of many health care professionals, including the physicians, case manager, occupational therapist, physical therapist, therapeutic recreation specialist, prosthetist/orthotist, nurse, speech-language pathologist, dietitian, assistive technologist, respiratory care practitioner, psychologist, social worker, vocational counselor, engineer, and chaplain.[30, 35, 80]

Persons with SCI are best treated at tertiary care facilities that have a direct link to emergency medical services, including full trauma team availability, spine traumatologists, neurourologists, and on-site consultation by the staff of an accredited SCI rehabilitation program. A coordinated system of care shortens hospital stays and improves efficiency of functional gains made during rehabilitation.[3, 38, 42, 58]

In this chapter a general overview is provided of the management of the client with SCI within the acute, rehabilitation, and postrehabilitation phases. The information is intended to aid health care professionals in the treatment of individuals with SCI by providing guidelines to maximize effective intervention. These guidelines must be modified with each client's input for the rehabilitation program to be truly successful in meeting individual needs.

SPINAL CORD LESIONS

SCI occurs when the spinal cord is damaged as a result of trauma, disease processes, or congenital defects. The clinical manifestations of the injury vary depending on the extent and location of the damage to the spinal cord.

Tetraplegia

Tetraplegia (quadriplegia) refers to impairment or loss of motor and/or sensory function due to damage of the cervical segments of the spinal cord. Function in the upper extremities, lower extremities, and trunk is affected.[91]

Paraplegia

Paraplegia refers to impairment or loss of motor and/or sensory function due to damage of the thoracic, lumbar, or sacral segments of the spinal cord. Depending on the level of the damage, function may be impaired in the trunk and/or lower extremities. This term does not refer to lumbosacral plexus lesions.[91]

Complete and Incomplete Lesions

In a complete lesion, there is total absence of sensory and/or motor function in the lowest sacral segment (S4–S5).[91] Complete injuries often damage the nerve root in the foramen.[41] Function of this root originating from the proximal intact cord can be expected to return within 6 months.[41]

With incomplete lesions there is partial preservation of sensory and/or motor function below the neurological level and in the lowest sacral segment. Sensation in the anal mucocutaneous junction, as well as deep anal sensation, must be present for a lesion to be referred to as incomplete.[91]

Spinal shock occurs 30 to 60 minutes after spinal trauma and is characterized by flaccid paralysis and absence of all spinal cord reflex activity below the level of the spinal cord lesion.[57] This condition can last for a few hours to several weeks. The completeness of the lesion cannot be determined until spinal shock is resolved. The signs of spinal shock resolution are controversial; however, the return of reflexes may be a good indication.

MECHANISMS OF INJURY

The majority of SCIs occur as a result of trauma. The degree and type of force that are exerted on the spine at the time of the trauma determine the location and severity of damage that occurs.[57] Injuries to the vertebral column can be classified biomechanically as pure flexion or flexion-rotation injuries, hyperextension injuries, and compression injuries.[36] Penetrating injuries to the cord are usually the result of gunshot or knife wounds.[36]

Spinal cord damage also can be caused by nontraumatic mechanisms. Circulatory compromise to the spinal cord resulting in ischemia causes neurological damage at and below the involved cord level. Compression of the spinal cord can be caused by degenerative bone diseases, by prolapse of the intervertebral disk into the neural canal, and by various tumors and abscesses of the spinal cord or surrounding tissues. Congenital malformation of the vertebral canal, such as spina bifida, also can damage the spinal cord. Diseases that result in compromise of the spinal cord include Guillain-Barré syndrome, transverse myelitis, amyotrophic lateral sclerosis, and multiple sclerosis.

ASSOCIATED INJURIES

The incidence of multiple trauma in the client presenting with a traumatic SCI is 55.2%.[93] The most common injuries are fractures (29.3%) and loss of consciousness (28.2%).[93] Traumatic pneumothorax/hemothorax are reported in 17.8% of persons with SCI. Traumatic head injuries of sufficient severity to affect cognitive and/or emotional functioning are reported in 11.5% of all cases.[93] Skull and facial fractures, along with traumatic head injuries and vertebral artery and esophageal disruptions, are common in cervical injuries.[85] Limb fractures and intrathoracic injuries (rib fractures and hemopneumothorax) are frequent in thoracic injuries, whereas intraabdominal injuries to the liver, spleen, and kidneys are associated with lumbar and cauda equina injuries.[85]

DEMOGRAPHICS

The incidence of traumatic SCI in the United States is approximately 10,000 new cases per year.[90] Approximately 3,000 new cases of spinal cord impairment secondary to disease and congenital anomalies occur each year.[111] The number of people living in the United States today with SCI is between 183,000 and 230,000.[90] Fifty-six percent of SCIs occur in persons between 16 and 30 years of age, with a mean age of 31.7 years and the most common age of 19 years.[32, 33, 90] Persons older than 60 years of age at injury have increased from 4.7% in the 1970s to 9.7% in 1990. This trend explains the increase in the median age during this same time period from 27.9 years to 33.1 years. Table 16–1 lists additional demographics.

In 1997, the average length of inpatient stay was 60 days (14 days in an acute care unit and 46 days in a rehabilitation unit). The average yearly health care and living expenses vary according to severity of injury. In the

T A B L E   1 6 – 1. SCI Demographics

Mean age at injury[90]	31.7 years
Most common age at injury[93]	19.0 years
Sex	
Male	81.8%
Female	18.2%
Causes of injury	
Motor vehicle accident	37.2%
Violent acts	26.8%
Falls	21.0%
Sports injuries	7.1%
Other	7.9%
Neurological categories at discharge (F&F)	
Incomplete tetraplegia	29.6%
Complete paraplegia	28.1%
Incomplete paraplegia	21.5%
Complete tetraplegia	18.6%
No deficits	0.7%
Unknown	0.7%
Common injury sites[93]	
C5	15.7%
C4	12.7%
C6	12.6%
T12	7.6%
C7	6.3%
L1	4.8%

first year individuals with high tetraplegia spend $529,675, whereas individuals with paraplegia spend an average of $193,543. Today, 91.7% of persons with SCI are discharged to a noninstitutional residence.[90]

CLINICAL SYNDROMES

Some incomplete lesions have a distinct clinical picture with specific signs and symptoms. An understanding of the various syndromes can be helpful to the client's team in planning the rehabilitation program. Figure 16–1 depicts the anatomy of the spinal cord.[36, 41] This basic anatomy of the spinal cord can be referred to as the various syndromes are described. These syndromes are addressed in other chapters of this book.

Central Cord Syndrome. Hyperextension injuries usually result in a central cord syndrome.[36] This injury causes bleeding into the central gray matter of the spinal cord, resulting in more impairment of function in the upper extremities than in the lower extremities.[36] The majority of incomplete lesions result in this syndrome.[41] Approximately 77% of clients with central cord syndrome will attain ambulatory function, 53% bowel and bladder control, and 42% hand function.[11]

Anterior Spinal Artery Syndrome. This syndrome is usually caused by flexion injuries in which bone or cartilage spicules compromise the anterior spinal artery.[36] Motor function and pain and temperature sensation are lost bilaterally below the injured segment.[36] The prognosis is extremely poor for return of bowel and bladder function, hand function, and ambulation.[11]

Brown-Séquard Syndrome. Occasionally, as a result of penetrating injuries (gunshot or stab wounds), only one half of the spinal cord is damaged. The Brown-Séquard syndrome is characterized by ipsilateral loss of motor function and position sense and contralateral loss of pain sensation several levels below the lesion.[36] The prognosis for recovery is good. Nearly all clients attain some level of ambulatory function, 80% regain hand function, 100% have bladder control, and 80% have bowel control.[11]

Posterior Cord Syndrome. Posterior cord syndrome is very rare, resulting from compression by tumor or infarction of the posterior spinal artery. Clinically, proprioception, stereognosis, two-point discrimination, and vibration sense are lost below the level of the lesion.[36]

Cauda Equina Syndrome. Damage to the cauda equina occurs with injuries at the L1 vertebral level and below, resulting in a lower motor neuron lesion, which is usually an incomplete lesion. This lesion results in flaccid paralysis with no spinal reflex activity present.[57, 91]

Conus Medullaris Syndrome. Injury of the sacral cord and lumbar nerve roots within the neural canal results in a clinical picture of lower-extremity motor and sensory loss and an areflexic bladder and bowel.[104]

MEDICAL MANAGEMENT

Acute medical treatment includes pharmacological management to prevent neurological trauma and enhance neural recovery and anatomical realignment and stabilization interventions.

Pharmacological Management

Neurological damage due to SCI may be a result of (1) physical disruption of axons traversing the injury site, (2) local infarction as a result of ischemia or hypoxia, or (3) prevention of impulses by microhemorrhages or edema within the spinal cord at the injury site.[45, 46] The initial trauma alone rarely causes anatomical transection of the spinal cord, even when there is a complete loss of sensory and motor function below the level of the injury.[46]

The injury usually causes damage more centrally in the gray matter, with lesser damage occurring to the surrounding white matter.[46] This central contusion is believed to lead to secondary damage 24 to 72 hours after the injury. Investigators believe that secondary injuries to surrounding tissues can be lessened by pharmacological agents, specifically methylprednisolone and monosialotetranexxosylylganglioside (GM$_1$) ganglioside.

The National Acute SCI Study (NASCIS)[2] used high doses of methylprednisolone and showed significant improvements in sensory and motor function 6 months after injury.[12] Young and Flamm[114] showed that methylprednisolone enhances the flow of blood to the injured spinal cords, preventing the typical decline in white matter, extracellular calcium levels, and evoked potentials. This acts to prevent progressive posttraumatic ischemia.[45, 53, 54]

GM$_1$ is a complex acidic glycolipid found at high levels in cell membranes in the mammalian central nervous system (CNS). Evidence suggests that GM$_1$ augments neurite growth in vitro, induces regeneration and sprout-

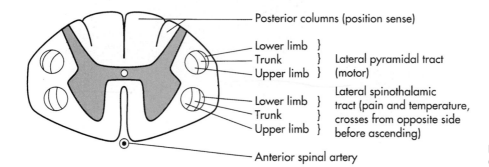

FIGURE 16–1. Cross-sectional anatomy of the spinal cord.

Posterior columns (position sense)

Lower limb }
Trunk } Lateral pyramidal tract
Upper limb } (motor)

Lower limb } Lateral spinothalamic
Trunk } tract (pain and temperature,
Upper limb } crosses from opposite side
before ascending)

Anterior spinal artery

ing of neurons, and restores neuronal function after injury in vivo.[46] The significant improvements in clients who received GM$_1$ were manifested in approximately 1 year, with some clinical changes seen as early as 1 day after receiving the drug. Motor function recovery was noted predominantly in the lower extremities. It is thought that neurological return was seen primarily in the lower extremities because GM$_1$ enhances the function of the surrounding white matter tracks to the lower extremities but not of the gray matter at the injury site.[45]

Theoretically, it may be more beneficial to combine the administration of these two drugs. Methylprednisolone would allow for initial survival of injured neurons, and GM$_1$ would enhance recovery in this larger number of surviving neurons.[46] Improvement of as few as one motor level could prove to be functionally relevant to the individual with SCI and may result in the difference between independence and dependence.

Surgical Stabilization

One of the first interventions after acute SCI is stabilizing the spine to prevent further cord or nerve root damage. In the emergency department, diagnostic studies reveal the severity of the spinal injury as well as the type and degree of the instability. Based on these findings, the physician, client, and family decide on treatment. Many options must be considered regarding the optimal operative strategy. Indications for surgical intervention include, but are not limited to, signs of progressive neurological involvement, type and extent of bony lesions, and degree of spinal cord damage.[20] The following discussion includes nonsurgical and surgical interventions.

Cervical Spine

At the scene of the accident, emergency medical technicians use extreme caution to immobilize the injured client and prevent excessive movement at the unstable spinal site. If there is compression of neurological tissue, vertebral fracture, or dislocation, reduction must occur to minimize ischemia and edema formation.[43] In the emergency department reduction is accomplished by cervical traction, with the goal of immediate and proper alignment of bone fragments and decompression of the spinal cord until further stabilization.[20, 78, 110] The most widely used traction is Gardner-Wells tongs (Fig. 16–2), which are inserted into the skull. Weights are added at approximately 5 pounds of traction per level of injury to achieve reduction of the dislocation and to maintain alignment.[78]

Certain precautions must be considered during therapy to prevent unnecessary movement at the injury site. The traction rope must be kept in alignment with the long axis of the cervical spine, and the weights must be allowed to hang freely. Cervical rotation must be prevented. In addition, care must be taken to ensure that continued traction is maintained at all times.

When surgical stabilization is indicated, common surgical protocols include posterior and anterior approaches. Unstable compression injuries are usually managed by a posterior procedure (Fig. 16–3) except when there is a deficient anterior column. Anterior approaches are used more for decompression of the spinal cord or when more bony support is needed for the anterior column.[43]

After cervical surgical stabilization, a hard collar such as a Philadelphia collar (Fig. 16–4) or sternal-occipital-mandibular immobilizer (SOMI) brace is used until a solid bony fusion has developed. The solid bony fusion usually takes 6 to 8 weeks. Postoperatively, care must be taken to protect the bony fusion.

When surgery is not indicated, an external device can be used. The best available device is halo traction. The halo traction device consists of three parts: the ring, the uprights, and the jacket (Fig. 16–5). The ring fits around the skull, just above the ears. It is held in place by four pins that are inserted into the skull. The uprights are attached to the ring and jacket by bolts. The jacket is usually made of polypropylene and lined with sheepskin. This equipment is left in place for 6 to 12 weeks until bony healing is satisfactory.[80] The advantage of using the halo device is the ability to mobilize the client as soon as the device has been applied without compromising spinal

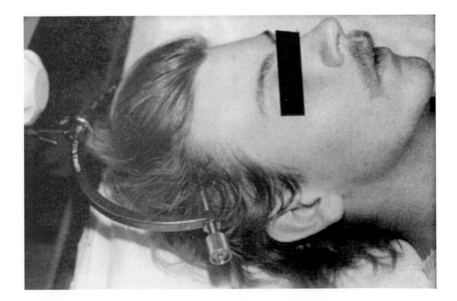

FIGURE 16–2. Gardner-Wells tongs. Reduction is accomplished through weights attached to the traction rope. (Courtesy of Dr. H. Herndon Murray, Assistant Medical Director, Shepherd Spinal Center, Atlanta, GA.)

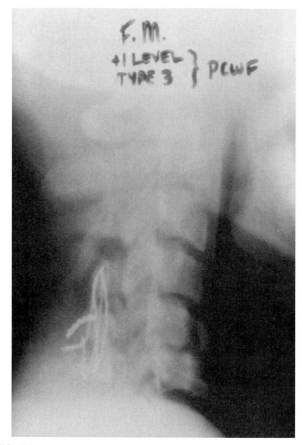

FIGURE 16–3. Radiograph of posterior cervical wiring and fusion. (Courtesy of Dr. H. Herndon Murray, Assistant Medical Director, Shepherd Spinal Center, Atlanta, GA.)

alignment. This allows the rehabilitation program to commence more rapidly. It also allows for delayed decision making regarding the need for surgery.

The disadvantage of the halo device is that pressure and friction from the vest or jacket may lead to altered skin integrity.[41] Special attention must be given to ensure that the skin remains intact. During more active phases of the rehabilitation process, the halo device may slow functional progress because of its added weight and its interference with the middle to end range of upper-extremity movement. In a small percentage of clients, there are complications of dysphagia and temporomandibular joint dysfunctions associated with wearing the halo device.[41]

Thoracolumbar Spine

Internal fixation of the thoracolumbar region is necessary when stability and distraction cannot be maintained by other means.[106] The most widely used fixation devices for thoracolumbar stabilization are Harrington rod instrumentation and fusion (Fig. 16–6), transpedicular screws (Fig. 16–7), and Contre-Dubousset instrumentation.

Postoperatively, an external trunk support is necessary to limit excessive vertebral motion and to maintain proper thoracic and lumbar alignment.[57, 106] This may be achieved by a custom thoracolumbosacral orthosis (Fig. 16–8) or a

Jewett brace (Fig. 16–9). Initially, the client's activity may be limited to allow for a complete fusion to take place and to minimize the possibility of rod displacement. All spinal limitations should be discussed with the surgeon postoperatively.

The goal of the operative procedures at any spinal level discussed is to reverse the deforming forces, to restore proper spinal alignment, and to stabilize the spine.[40] All of these procedures have advantages and disadvantages. The surgeon, client, and family must be involved in the decision-making process to select the most appropriate method of treatment. This will allow the therapeutic rehabilitation process to begin.

THERAPEUTIC REHABILITATION — CONTINUUM OF CARE

The therapeutic rehabilitation process is best described as a continuum of care. The continuum of care gives a framework for how a client may progress through rehabilitation.

Rehabilitation teams may use one of three models: multidisciplinary, interdisciplinary, and transdisciplinary.[30] As evidenced by standards set forth by the Commission on Accreditation for Rehabilitation Facilities (CARF), the interdisciplinary model of team structure is supported in the rehabilitation.[92]

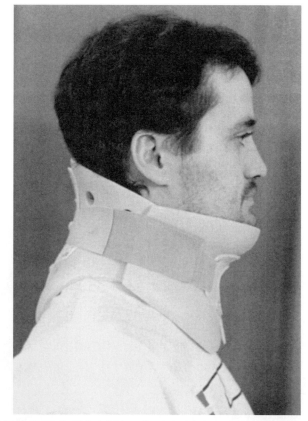

FIGURE 16–4. Philadelphia collar. It is fabricated of polyethylene foam with rigid anterior and posterior plastic strips, it is easily applied via Velcro closures, and it limits flexion, extension, and rotary movements of the cervical spine.

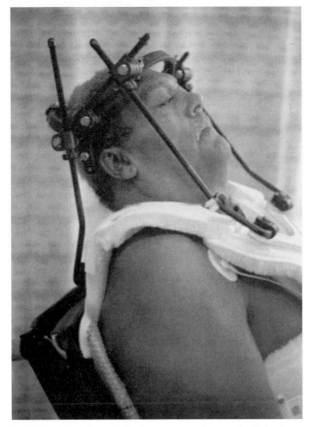

FIGURE 16–5. Halo vest. Basic components are the halo ring, distraction rods, and jacket.

The continuum of care may be divided into several phases, which include acute medical management (already addressed), early rehabilitation, inpatient rehabilitation, and outpatient rehabilitation/community reintegration. The progression of a client through the rehabilitation process will vary greatly from one client to the next. The client may move back and forth throughout the continuum of care.

Early Rehabilitation

Early rehabilitation includes all therapeutic interventions during the critical and acute care stages of rehabilitation. The primary emphasis of early rehabilitation is to lessen the adverse effects of neurotrauma and immobilization. This phase may last from a few days to several weeks, depending on the severity and level of injury and other associated injuries. Although therapeutic intensity may be limited, clients may begin out-of-bed activities. Goals during this phase should address prevention of secondary complications. The treatment team must begin discharge planning and family training in this phase.

Inpatient Rehabilitation

During inpatient rehabilitation, out-of-bed activities are tolerated for longer periods of time and the client begins to work toward specific long-term goals. In accordance with Medicare guidelines for rehabilitation, the client is able to participate in therapeutic programs a minimum of 3 hours a day.[19] The intensity of therapy may continue to be limited owing to unresolved medical issues.

As medical issues resolve and endurance improves, the client will progress to a higher and more active level of participation. During inpatient rehabilitation, the client gains varying levels of independence in specific skills. The client may be taught advanced skills in performance of activities of daily living (ADL), transfers, and mobility skills. Community outings may be scheduled to refine advanced skills, identify further needs, and foster community reintegration. The following will be completed unless otherwise noted: (1) family training, (2) home modification recommendations, (3) vocational testing/planning, (4) delivery and fitting of discharge equipment, (5) instruction of home management, (6) instruction in home exercise programs, (7) referrals for continued services, and (8) driving evaluation. Discharge planning largely encompasses activities aimed at a smooth transition to home.

Outpatient Rehabilitation and Community Reentry

Because of the shortened lengths of hospitalization, services provided after discharge are becoming increasingly important. Postinpatient discharge services may include day programs, single-service outpatient visits, and routine follow-up visits/services. The primary purpose of these services is to provide a coordinated effort for the client

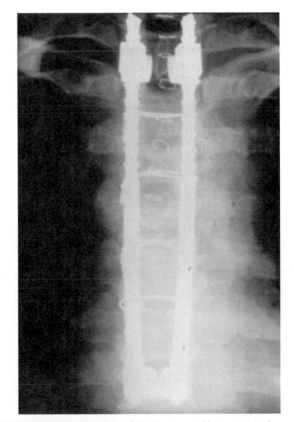

FIGURE 16–6. Radiograph of Harrington rod instrumentation. (Courtesy of Dr. H. Herndon Murray, Assistant Medical Director, Shepherd Spinal Center, Atlanta, GA.)

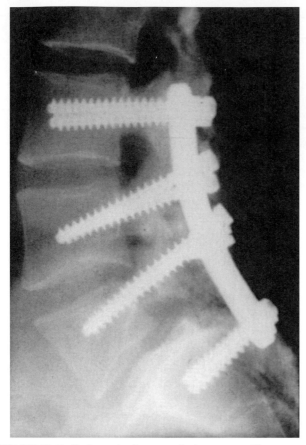

FIGURE 16–7. Radiograph of transpedicular screws. (Courtesy of Dr. H. Herndon Murray, Assistant Medical Director, Shepherd Spinal Center, Atlanta, GA.)

to reintegrate into the community. The goal is for the client to return to work or school and to resume family responsibilities.

EXAMINATION

Regardless of where the client begins in the rehabilitation process, an examination is completed on admission. The examination will assist in establishing the diagnosis and the prognosis of each client as well as determine the appropriate therapeutic interventions. The client/caregivers participate by reporting activity performance and functional ability.[52] Any pertinent additions to the history stated by the client should be described. The client's statement of goals, problems, and concerns should be included.

The main areas of the examination are outlined here.

History

A review of the medical record is the first step toward the examination because it provides the background information and identifies medical precautions. The history should include general demographics, social history, occupation or employment, pertinent growth and development, living environment, history of current condition, functional status and activity level, completed tests and measures, medications, past history of current condition if applicable, past medical and surgical history, family history, reported client/family health status, and social habits.[52]

Systems Review

The physiological and anatomical status should be reviewed for the cardiopulmonary, integumentary, musculoskeletal, and neuromuscular systems. In addition, communication, affect, cognition, language, and learning style should be reviewed.[52]

Tests and Measures

Depending on the data generated during the history and systems review, the clinician performs tests and measures to help identify impairments, functional limitations, and disabilities and establish the diagnosis and prognosis of each client. Tests and measures that are often used for persons with SCI may include the following.

Aerobic Capacity and Endurance

Because of possible autonomic nervous system (ANS) dysfunction and deconditioning that may have occurred during the preoperative period, aerobic capacity and en-

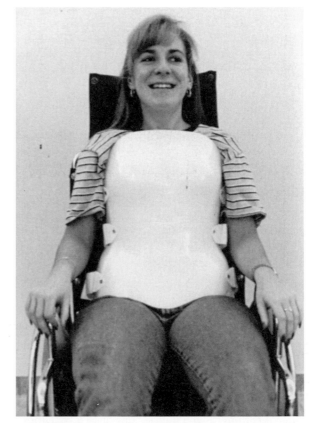

FIGURE 16–8. Custom thoracolumbosacral orthosis. This molded plastic body orthosis has a soft lining on the interior. It controls flexion, extension, and rotary movements until healing of the bone occurs.

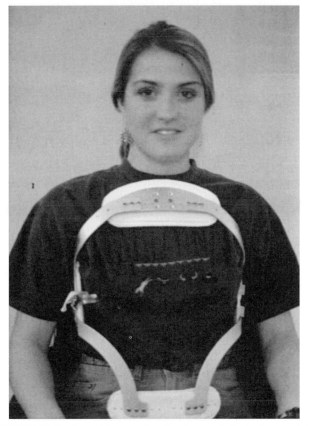

FIGURE 16–9. Jewett hyperextension brace. A single three-point force system is provided via sternal pad, suprapubic pad, and thoracolumbar pad. Forward flexion is restricted in the thoracolumbar area.

durance are important to examine. Assessments of aerobic capacity and endurance should include (1) autonomic responses to positional changes; (2) perceived exertion, dyspnea, or angina during activity using rating-of-perceived-exertion (RPE) scales, dyspnea scales, pain scales, or visual analog scales; (3) vital signs; (4) thoracoabdominal movements and breathing patterns; and (5) pulse oximetry. Monitoring responses at rest and during and after activity is recommended. Caution is advised because heart rate and blood pressure responses to exercise may be altered in persons with SCI.[48]

Anthropometric Characteristics

Assessments of anthropometric characteristics may include (1) activities and postures that aggravate or relieve edema, lymphedema, or effusion; (2) edema through palpation and volume and girth measurements, (3) assessment of height, weight, length, and girth of trunk and extremities; and (4) observation and palpation of trunk, extremity, or body part at rest and during and after activity.[52] Anthropometric measurements are particularly important when prescribing equipment (i.e., wheelchairs and orthoses).

Assistive and Adaptive Devices

Clients with acute, traumatic SCI may not have assistive devices on admission; however, these devices are often

critical to the functional success of each client. When assistive devices are received, assessments of assistive adaptive devices may include (1) effects and benefits of the device during client use; (2) analysis of the potential to reduce impairment, functional limitation, or disability through the use of the device; and (3) safety during use of the device.[52]

Community and Work Integration or Reintegration

The clinician assesses the client's preparedness to enter the premorbid community and/or work roles and determines when and how such integration might occur. To determine this, the clinician may assess (1) adaptive skills, (2) functional capacity, and (3) physiological responses during community, work, and leisure activities.[52]

Environmental, Home, and Work Barriers

Environmental barriers may prevent clients with SCI from functioning optimally in their surroundings. To ensure safety and accessibility, the assessment should include (1) analysis of physical space using photography or videotape, (2) assessment of current and potential barriers, and (3) questionnaires and interviews with the client and others as appropriate. Before performing these measures, a good understanding of all assistive devices required should be considered.[52] For example, knowledge of the height and width of a wheelchair is necessary before making recommendations on door width and table height.

Gait, Locomotion, and Balance

Assessment of gait, locomotion, and balance includes (1) analysis with and without the use of assistive, adaptive, orthotic, protective, supportive, or prosthetic devices or equipment; (2) analysis on various terrains and in different physical environments; (3) analysis of wheelchair management and mobility on various terrains and in different physical environments; and (4) assessment of safety while ambulating or propelling a wheelchair.

Integumentary Integrity

When assessing integumentary integrity clinicians should consider activities, positioning, posture, and assistive and adaptive devices that may result in trauma. In the event of altered skin integrity, the assessment should include (1) presence/absence of hair growth; (2) presence/absence of infection; (3) assessment of wound contraction, drainage, location, odor, shape, size, depth, tunneling, and undermining; and (4) assessment of wound tissue, including epithelium, granulation, necrosis, slough, and texture. It is recommended that the clinical guidelines from the Agency for Health Care Policy and Research[8] be used for examination and treatment for pressure sores.

Joint Integrity and Mobility

The clinician uses the joint integrity and mobility tests and measures to determine whether there is excessive or limited motion of the joint. Tests and measures for joint integrity and mobility include (1) assessment of soft tissue swelling, inflammation, or restriction and (2) assessment of joint hypermobility and hypomobility.[52]

Motor Function

Assessment of motor function includes (1) head, trunk, and limb movement; (2) posture during sitting, standing, and locomotion activities; and (3) dexterity, coordination, and agility.

Muscle Performance

Assessment of muscle performance allows for specific diagnosis of the level and completeness of injury. Tests and measures may include (1) muscle strength and power and endurance of the head, trunk, and limbs; (2) muscle tone; and (3) electromyography and nerve conduction velocity. The examination of muscle performance includes each specific muscle and identifies substitutions from other muscles.

A six-point scale is used to describe procedures for manual muscle testing[27, 61]:

0 = no visible or palpable contraction is detected
1 = muscle contraction is palpable, but no limb movement is detected
2 = full movement of limb with gravity eliminated
3 = full movement of limb against gravity
4 = full movement with moderate resistance through range
5 = normal strength

Along with the strength of each muscle, the presence, absence, and location of muscle tone should be described. The Modified Ashworth scale is a common tool used to describe tone.[60]

Orthotic, Protective, and Supportive Devices

Anticipated equipment needs are described. If the client already owns equipment, its appropriateness, general condition, need for repairs, rehabilitation technology supplier, funding source, and age of equipment are documented. Positioning of bilateral upper and lower extremities is noted. Some clients may benefit from an orthotic device, cast, or splint to prevent deformity or to position the extremity for increased function. Other considerations for orthotic prescription include muscle strength, mobility/stability of joints, sensation, palmar creases and web space, prehension patterns, tone, client acceptance, caregiver support, and funding.

Pain

Pain tests and measures determine the intensity, quality, and characteristics of any pain the client experiences.

Any devices and/or modalities and their effectiveness to control pain should be noted.

Posture

Posture is evaluated in the sitting and, if able, standing positions. Obtaining and maintaining good posture while sitting is essential to prevent secondary complications.[52]

Range of Motion

Adequate range of motion (ROM) is valuable for optimal performance of functional skills as well as for injury prevention. Clients with an SCI are at risk for joint contractures. This occurs due to hypotonicity, asymmetry in muscle groups, spasticity, and decreased passive and/or active range of motion (PROM, AROM).[69] Specific attention is noted for all upper-extremity mobility. In the lower extremities, straight-leg raise, ankle dorsiflexion, and hip flexion/extension are important to examine.[52]

Reflex Integrity

Clinicians use reflex integrity tests and measures to determine the excitability of the nervous system and the integrity of the neuromuscular system. Tests of the deep tendon reflexes indicate whether the SCI is an upper motor neuron lesion (injuries above T12) or a lower motor neuron lesion (injuries at or below T12). For example, the presence or absence of the bulbocavernosus reflex is helpful in choosing the most appropriate bowel program for the client.

Self-Care and Home Management

The Functional Independence Measure (FIM)[55] is recommended by the American Spinal Injury Association (ASIA) to describe the impact of the SCI on the client's function. The FIM evaluates different areas of function using a seven-point scale that describes the amount of assistance the client requires. The FIM includes areas such as self-care, sphincter control, mobility, locomotion, communication, and social cognition (Fig. 16–10). It is recommended that additional functional skills be examined because the FIM assesses only a limited number of skills.

Sensory Integrity

Clinicians use the results of sensory integrity tests and measures to determine the extent and severity of the SCI. The client's sensation is described by dermatome. The recommended tests include (1) sharp-dull discrimination or temperature sensitivity to test the lateral spinothalamic tract, (2) light touch to test the anterior spinothalamic tract, and (3) proprioception or vibration to test the posterior columns of the spinal cord. Sensation is indicated as intact, impaired, or absent per dermatome. A dermatomal map is helpful and recommended for ease of documentation.

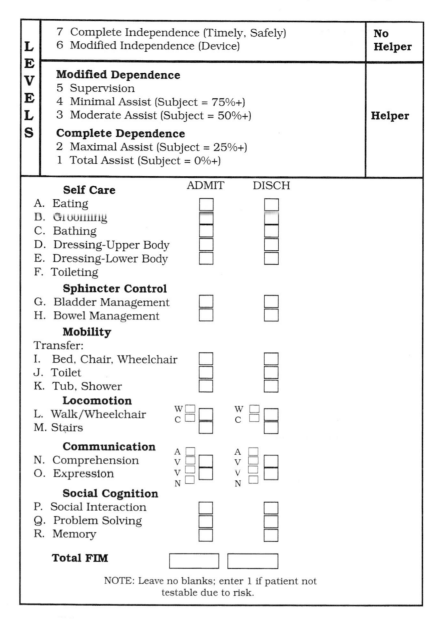

L	7 Complete Independence (Timely, Safely) 6 Modified Independence (Device)	**No** **Helper**
E **V** **E** **L** **S**	**Modified Dependence** 5 Supervision 4 Minimal Assist (Subject = 75%+) 3 Moderate Assist (Subject = 50%+) **Complete Dependence** 2 Maximal Assist (Subject = 25%+) 1 Total Assist (Subject = 0%+)	**Helper**

Self Care   ADMIT   DISCH
A. Eating
B. Grooming
C. Bathing
D. Dressing-Upper Body
E. Dressing-Lower Body
F. Toileting
        Sphincter Control
G. Bladder Management
H. Bowel Management
        Mobility
Transfer:
I. Bed, Chair, Wheelchair
J. Toilet
K. Tub, Shower
        Locomotion
L. Walk/Wheelchair   W   W
M. Stairs   C   C
        Communication
N. Comprehension   A   A
O. Expression   V   V
                        V   V
                        N   N
        Social Cognition
P. Social Interaction
Q. Problem Solving
R. Memory

Total FIM

NOTE: Leave no blanks; enter 1 if patient not
testable due to risk.

FIGURE 16–10. Functional Independence Measure. Guide for the Uniform Data Set for Medical Rehabilitation (Adult FIM^SM) Version 4.0, Buffalo, NY 14214: State University of New York at Buffalo, 1993.

Ventilation, Respiration, and Circulation

All clients should be screened for developing ventilatory compromise. Arterial blood gases are noted, and the vital capacity is measured. The breathing expansion pattern is described, as well as the use of accessory muscles. Artificial breathing devices, along with the use of supplemental oxygen, are documented. Cough strength and productivity, the need for assistive coughing and/or suctioning, and the use of an abdominal binder and antiembolism stockings are noted.

Diagnosis of Impairments/Disabilities

In addition to all of the tests and measures stated previously, it is highly recommended that the ASIA standards for assessing and classifying clients with SCI be completed. This is to facilitate more accurate communication between clinicians and investigators.[91] By systematically

examining the dermatomes and myotomes, one can determine the cord segments affected by the SCI. The ASIA neurological examination consists of sensory (Fig. 16–11) and motor (Fig. 16–12) examinations, which are used to determine the neurological levels as well as the completeness of the SCI. Once the examination and diagnosis have been completed, this information is used to establish goals.

GOAL SETTING

Goal setting is a dynamic process that directly follows the examination. Each problem identified should be addressed with specific short- and long-term goals.[41] The clinician must interpret new information continuously, which leads to ongoing reevaluation and revision of goals.[81] Goals are always individualized and should be established in collaboration with the treatment team, the

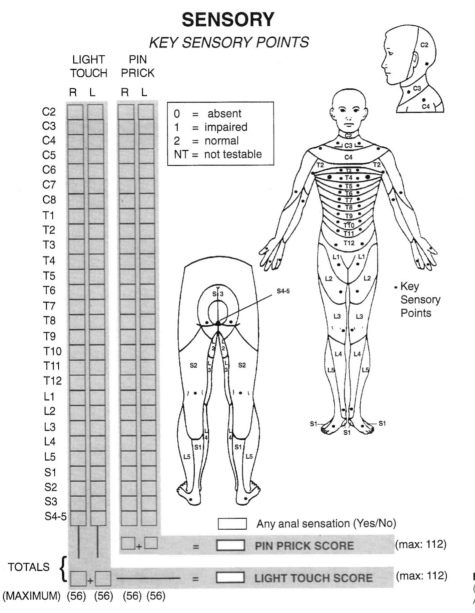

SENSORY
KEY SENSORY POINTS

		0 = absent
		1 = impaired
		2 = normal
		NT = not testable

Key Sensory Points

Any anal sensation (Yes/No)

PIN PRICK SCORE (max: 112)

LIGHT TOUCH SCORE (max: 112)

TOTALS

(MAXIMUM) (56) (56) (56) (56)

FIGURE 16–11. ASIA sensory form. (Courtesy of American Spinal Injury Association International, Atlanta, GA.)

MOTOR
KEY MUSCLES

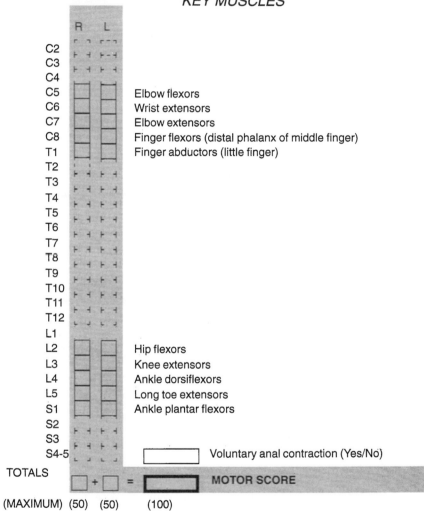

	R	L	
C2			
C3			
C4			
C5			Elbow flexors
C6			Wrist extensors
C7			Elbow extensors
C8			Finger flexors (distal phalanx of middle finger)
T1			Finger abductors (little finger)
T2			
T3			
T4			
T5			
T6			
T7			
T8			
T9			
T10			
T11			
T12			
L1			
L2			Hip flexors
L3			Knee extensors
L4			Ankle dorsiflexors
L5			Long toe extensors
S1			Ankle plantar flexors
S2			
S3			
S4-5			Voluntary anal contraction (Yes/No)

TOTALS   ☐ + ☐ = ☐   MOTOR SCORE

(MAXIMUM) (50) (50)   (100)

FIGURE 16–12. ASIA motor form. (Courtesy of American Spinal Injury Association International, Atlanta, GA.)

client, and the caregiver, and with realistic consideration of anticipated needs on return to the home environment.

Long-term goals for the rehabilitation of clients with SCI reflect functional outcomes and are based on the strength of the remaining innervated musculature. Short-term goals identify components that interfere with functional ability and are designed to "address these limiting factors while building component skills"[41] of the desired long-term goals.[94]

Factors that must be considered in the goal-setting process because they may limit functional outcomes include age, body type, medical problems, additional orthopedic injury, cognitive ability, psychological problems, spasticity, endurance, strength, ROM, funding sources, and motivation.

General Goals

Specific long-term goals are appropriate for all rehabilitation clients regardless of their level of SCI. Partial or limited success in attaining these goals directly affects the degree to which more functionally oriented goals are achieved.[81] When established for each patient the goals in the following box should be stated in measurable and objective terms.

GOALS

- Client will achieve/maintain full ROM in all joints.
- Client will achieve maximal strength in all intact muscle groups for functional activities of daily living and mobility.
- Client will achieve maximal respiratory capacity.
- Client will tolerate upright sitting without complication.
- Client will achieve maximal sitting tolerance without skin compromise.
- Client will have intact skin throughout.
- Client will attain level of maximum cardiovascular endurance.
- Client/caregiver will be independent, with a home exercise program.
- Client/caregiver will satisfactorily complete education classes and demonstrate ability to direct and/or perform client's care as appropriate.
- Client/caregiver will demonstrate appropriate understanding of all equipment operation and maintenance.
- All home modification recommendations will be issued in a timely manner.
- Appropriate outpatient referrals will be completed before discharge.

Functional Expectations

Functional goals are established in the following areas: bathing, bed mobility, bladder and bowel control, commu-

nication, environmental control/access, feeding, dressing, gait, grooming, home management, ROM/positioning, skin care management, transfers, transportation/driving, wheelchair management, and wheelchair mobility (Table 16-2). Information presented in Table 16-2 must be recognized as general guidelines because variability exists. These guidelines are most usefully applied to clients with complete SCI. Goal setting for individuals with incomplete SCI is often more challenging given the greater variability of client presentations and the uncertainty of neurological recovery. As with any client, ongoing reevaluations provide keys to functional limitations and potential and thereby direct the goal-setting process.

Rehabilitation teams may elect to hold a goal-setting or interim conference for each client during which team members, including the client, have the opportunity to discuss the long-term goals that have been established. It may be useful to request that the client sign a statement acknowledging understanding of and agreement to all long-term goals.

EARLY REHABILITATION AND COMPLICATION PREVENTION

Early rehabilitation of the client with SCI begins with prevention. Preventing secondary complications speeds entry into the rehabilitation phase and improves the possibility that the client will become a productive member of society.

Table 16-3 describes an overview of the primary complications that can arise due to an SCI. In this table, incidence is reviewed along with any known etiology. Tests and measures used to determine/diagnose the complication as well as the recommended medical and therapeutic interventions are covered. Because of their high incidence and potential effect on long-term outcomes, the following complications require further discussion: skin compromise, loss of ROM or joint contractures, and respiratory compromise after SCI.

Preventing and Managing Pressure Ulcers and Skin Compromise

After SCI and during the period of spinal shock, clients may be at greatest risk for developing pressure ulcers.[76, 109] The use of backboards at the emergency scene and during radiographic procedures contributes to potential skin compromise.

Preventive skin care begins with careful inspection. Areas with a bony prominence are at greatest risk for acquiring a pressure sore.[73] Key areas to evaluate include the sacrum, ischia, greater trochanters, heels, malleoli, knees, occiput, scapulae, elbows, and prominent spinous processes. Turning at regular intervals is initiated immediately. The client's position in bed should be initially established for turns to occur every 2 to 3 hours.[109] This interval is gradually increased to 6 hours with careful monitoring for evidence of skin compromise. Turning positions include prone, supine, right and left side lying, semiprone, or semisupine.[1, 89] Secondary injuries such as

Text continued on page 494

TABLE 16-2. Functional Expectation for Complete SCI Lesions

Functional Component	Outcome Potential	Anticipated Equipment to Achieve Outcomes
C1–4 Tetraplegia		
Sitting tolerance	80 degrees for 10 hours per day	
Communication		
Mouthstick writing	Minimal assist	Mouthsticks and docking station
ECU	Setup	ECU
Page turning	Minimal assist	Book holder
Computer operation	Minimal assist	Computer
Call-system use	Setup	Call-system and/or speaker phone
Cuff-leak speech	Up to 2 hours	
Feeding	Dependent, but verbalizes care	
Grooming	Dependent, but verbalizes care	
Bathing	Dependent, but verbalizes care	Reclining shower chair
Dressing	Dependent, but verbalizes care	
Bowel management	Dependent, but verbalizes care	
Bladder management	Dependent, but verbalizes care	
Bed mobility:		
Rolling side/side	Dependent, but verbalizes care	Four-way adjustable hospital bed to assist
Rolling supine/prone	Dependent, but verbalizes care	caregiver with care
Supine to/from sitting	Dependent, but verbalizes care	
Scooting	Dependent, but verbalizes care	
Leg management	Dependent, but verbalizes care	
Transfers:		
Bed	Dependent, but verbalizes care	Hydraulic lift and slings or overhead lift system
Tub/toilet	Dependent, but verbalizes care	
Car	Dependent, but verbalizes care	
Floor	Dependent, but verbalizes care	
Power wheelchair mobility		
Smooth surfaces	Modified independent	Power wheelchair with power recline/tilt system
Ramps	Modified independent	Lap tray
Rough terrain	Modified independent	Armrests and shoulder support
Curbs	Dependent, but verbalizes	
Manual wheelchair mobility		
Smooth surfaces	Dependent, but verbalizes	Manual reclining wheelchair with same options as
Ramps	Dependent, but verbalizes	the power wheelchair
Rough terrain	Dependent, but verbalizes	
Curbs	Dependent, but verbalizes	
Stairs	Dependent, but verbalizes	
Skin		
Weight shift	Modified independent with power wheelchair	Recline/tilt wheelchair and wheelchair cushion
Padding/positioning	Dependent, but verbalizes	Pillow splints/resting splints/pillows
Skin checks	Dependent, but verbalizes	Mirror
Community ADL		
Position at computer station	Maximal to moderate assist	Modified van
Dependent passenger eval.	Maximal to moderate assist	
ROM to scapula, upper extremity, left extremity, and trunk	Dependent, but verbalizes	
Exercise program	Independent for respiratory and neck exercises	Portable ventilator (C1–3)
		Bedside ventilator (C1–3)
C5 Tetraplegia		
Sitting tolerance	80 degrees for 10 hours per day	
Communication		
Telephone use	Modified independent	Telephone adaptations
ECU	Setup	ECU
Page turning	Setup	Book holder
Computer operation	Supervision	Computer
Writing/typing	Setup	Long Wanchik brace
Feeding	Minimal to setup assist	Mobile arm support or offset feeder; may need extended silverware
Grooming		
Wash face	Minimal assist	Mobile arm support or offset feeder
Comb/brush hair	Minimal assist	
Oral care	Minimal assist	
Bathing	Dependent, but verbalizes care	Upright shower chair
Dressing	Dependent, but verbalizes care	
Bowel management	Dependent, but verbalizes care	
Bladder management	Dependent, but verbalizes care	Automatic leg bag emptier

Table continued on following page

TABLE 16 – 2. Functional Expectation for Complete SCI Lesions *Continued*

Functional Component	Outcome Potential	Anticipated Equipment to Achieve Outcomes
Bed mobility:		
Rolling side/side	Maximal assistance to dependent and verbalizes care	Four-way adjustable hospital bed to assist caregiver with care
Rolling supine/prone	Maximal assistance to dependent and verbalizes care	
Supine to/from sitting	Maximal assistance to dependent and verbalizes care	
Scooting	Maximal assistance to dependent and verbalizes care	
Leg management	Maximal assistance to dependent and verbalizes care	
Transfers:	Maximal assistance to dependent and verbalizes care; may be able to assist with parts of the transfer	Hydraulic lift and slings or overhead lift system Possible transfer board
Bed	Dependent, but verbalizes. May assist some	
Tub/toilet	Dependent, but verbalizes. May assist some	
Car	Dependent, but verbalizes. May assist some	
Floor	Dependent, but verbalizes. May assist some	
Power wheelchair mobility		
Smooth surfaces	Modified independent	Power wheelchair with power recline/tilt system; recommend lap tray
Ramps	Modified independent	Armrests and shoulder support
Rough terrain	Modified independent	
Curbs	Dependent, but verbalizes	
Manual wheelchair mobility		
Smooth surfaces	Dependent, but verbalizes	Upright or reclining wheelchair with special back and trunk supports. Not recommended primary mode of locomotion owing to shoulder musculature imbalance
Ramps	Dependent, but verbalizes	
Rough terrain	Dependent, but verbalizes	
Curbs	Dependent, but verbalizes	
Stairs	Dependent, but verbalizes	
Skin		
Weight shift	Modified independent with power wheelchair	Recline/tilt wheelchair and wheelchair cushion
Padding/positioning	Dependent, but verbalizes	Pillow splints/resting splints
Skin checks	Dependent, but verbalizes	Mirror
Community ADL	Moderate assist	Modified van
Prepare snack	Maximal to moderate assist	
Position at computer station	Maximal to moderate assist	
Dependent passenger eval.	Maximal to moderate assist	
ROM to scapula, upper extremity, left extremity, and trunk	Dependent, but verbalizes	
Exercise program		
Upper extremity and neck	Minimal assistance	Airsplints and/or light cuff weights; E-stim unit
C6 Tetraplegia		
Sitting tolerance	80 degrees for 10 hours per day	
Communication		
Telephone use	Modified independent	Telephone adaptations
Page turning	Modified independent	Tenodesis splint
Writing/typing/keyboard	Modified independent	Short opponens splint
Feeding	Modified independent	Adaptive ADL equipment
Grooming	Modified independent	Various grooming equipment Tenodesis splint
Bathing		
Upper body	Minimal assist	Upright shower chair
Lower body	Moderate assist	Various bathing equipment
Dressing		
Upper body	Modified independent	Various dressing equipment
Lower body (bed)	Moderate to minimal assist	
Bowel management	Moderate assist	Dil stick
Bladder management	Male with minimal assist Female with moderate assist	Tenodesis
Bed mobility:		
Rolling side/side	Minimal assist to modified independent	Four-way adjustable hospital bed or regular bed with loops/straps
Rolling supine/prone	Moderate assist	
Supine to/from sitting	Minimal assist	
Scooting	Minimal assist	
Leg management	Minimal assist to modified independent	
Transfers:		
Bed	Minimal assist	Transfer board
Tub/toilet	Moderate assist	
Car	Moderate to maximal assist	
Floor	Dependent, but verbalizes procedure	
Power wheelchair mobility		Power upright wheelchair
Smooth surfaces	Modified independent	
Ramps	Modified independent	
Rough terrain	Modified independent	
Curbs	Dependent, but verbalizes	

TABLE 16-2. Functional Expectation for Complete SCI Lesions *Continued*

Functional Component	Outcome Potential	Anticipated Equipment to Achieve Outcomes
Manual wheelchair mobility		Upright wheelchair
Smooth surfaces	Modified independent	May need adaptations to facilitate more efficient
Ramps	Modified independent	propulsion (i.e., push pegs, plastic-coated hand
Rough terrain	Moderate to minimal assist	rims)
Curbs	Dependent, but verbalizes procedure	
Stairs	Dependent, but verbalizes procedure	
Skin		
Weight shift	Modified independent	Upright wheelchair with push handles
Pad/positioning	Moderate to minimal assist	Mirror
Skin checks	Moderate to minimal assist	
Community ADL		
Light home management	Minimal assist	Various ADL equipment
Heavy home management	Moderate assist	Modified vehicle
Driving vehicle	Modified independent	
ROM to scapula, upper extremity,		Leg lifter to assist with lower-extremity ROM
lower extremity, and trunk	Minimal assist	
Exercise program	Minimal assistance	Cuff weights
		E-stim unit
C7–8 Tetraplegia		
Sitting tolerance	80 degrees for 10 hours per day	
Communication		
Telephone use	Modified independent	
Page turning	Modified independent	
Writing/typing/keyboard	Modified independent	
Feeding	Modified independent	Adaptive feeding equipment
Grooming	Modified independent	Various grooming equipment
Bathing		
Upper body	Modified independent	Upright shower chair
Lower body	Modified independent	Various bathing equipment
Dressing (upper and lower body)	Modified independent	Various dressing ADL equipment
In bed	Minimal assist for lower body dressing	
In wheelchair	Modified independent for upper body dressing	
Bowel management	Modified independent	Dil stick
Bladder management		
Bed	Male/female with modified independence	
Wheelchair	Male with modified independence; female with moderate assist	
Bed mobility:		
Rolling side/side	Modified independent	
Rolling supine/prone	Modified independent	
Supine to/from sitting	Modified independent	
Scooting	Modified independent	
Leg management	Modified independent	
Transfers:		
Bed	Modified independent	Transfer board
Tub/toilet	Modified independent	May not need transfer board for even surfaces
Car	Minimal assist for loading WC	
Floor	Maximal assist	
Power wheelchair mobility		Power upright wheelchair
Smooth surfaces	Modified independent	
Ramps	Modified independent	
Rough terrain	Modified independent	
Curbs	Dependent, but verbalizes	
Manual wheelchair mobility		Upright wheelchair
Smooth surfaces	Modified independent	
Ramps	Modified independent	
Rough terrain	Modified independent	
Curbs	Minimal to moderate assist	
Stairs	Maximal assist	
Skin		
Weight shift	Modified independent	Upright wheelchair with push handles
Pad/positioning	Minimal assist to modified independent	
Skin checks	Minimal assist to modified independent	Mirror
Community ADL		
Light home management	Modified independent	Various ADL equipment
Heavy home management	Moderate assist	
Driving vehicle	Modified independent	Modified vehicle

Table continued on following page

TABLE 16–2. Functional Expectation for Complete SCI Lesions *Continued*

Functional Component	Outcome Potential	Anticipated Equipment to Achieve Outcomes
ROM to scapula, upper extremity, lower extremity, and trunk	Modified independent	Leg lifter to assist with lower-extremity ROM
Exercise program	Modified independent	Cuff weights and/or E-stim unit
Paraplegia		
Sitting tolerance	80 degrees for 10 hours per day	
Communication	Independent	
Feeding	Independent	
Grooming	Independent	
Bathing		
Upper body	Independent	Upright tub chair
Lower body	Modified independent	Long-handled sponge and hand-held shower hose
Dressing (upper and lower body)		
In bed	Modified independent	Various dressing ADL equipment
In wheelchair	Modified independent	
Bowel management	Modified independent	Dil stick if + bulbocavernosus reflex (BCR) Suppositories if − BCR
Bladder management	Modified independent	
Bed mobility:		
Rolling side/side	Modified independent	
Rolling supine/prone	Modified independent	
Supine to/from sitting	Modified independent	
Scooting	Modified independent	
Leg management	Modified independent	
Transfers:		
Bed	Modified independent	
Tub/toilet	Modified independent	
Car	Modified independent	
Floor	Modified independent	
Uprighting wheelchair	Modified independent	
Manual wheelchair mobility		Upright wheelchair
Smooth surfaces	Modified independent	
Ramps	Modified independent	
Rough terrain	Modified independent	
Curbs	Modified independent	
Stairs (3–4)	Moderate assist to modified independent	
Ambulation		
Smooth surfaces	Depends on level of injury; modified independent	Appropriate orthotics and assistive device(s)
Ramps	for T12 and below injuries; will vary with higher	
Rough terrain	thoracic injuries	
Curbs		
Stairs		
Skin		Mirror for skin checks
Weight shift	Modified independent	
Pad/positioning	Modified independent	
Skin checks	Modified independent	
Community ADL		Hand controls for vehicle
Light home management	Modified independent	
Heavy home management	Moderate assist	
Driving vehicle	Modified independent	
ROM to lower extremity and trunk	Modified independent	Leg lifter to assist with lower-extremity ROM
Exercise program	Modified independent	Cuff weights

fractures and the presence of vital equipment, such as ventilator tubing, chest tubes, and arterial lines, should be considered when choosing turning positions.

Pillows or rectangular foam pads are used to pad around the bony prominence and relieve potential pressure. Padding directly over a prominent area with a firm pillow or pad may only increase pressure. For clients who are not appropriate for rigorous turning schedules (e.g., clients with unstabilized fractures) specialty low-air-loss beds and flotation systems are available.[67] While sitting, a pressure relief (weight shift) schedule is established and strictly enforced.

Although pressure ulcers are one of the most prevalent causes of skin compromise, other forces may lead to problems, including friction, shearing, excessive moisture or dryness, infection, and bruising or bumping during activities. This is especially true of clients with SCI, because they have altered thermoregulation, changes in mobility status, and incontinent bowel and bladder function. As clients begin to learn functional skills, they may have poor motor control and impaired balance and must be carefully monitored to avoid injury.

Should skin compromise occur, the first line of intervention is to remove the source of the problem. Modifi-

Text continued on page 498

TABLE 16–3. Complications After SCI

Complication	Incidence	Etiology	Diagnostic Test and Measures	Medical Treatment or Intervention	Therapeutic Intervention
Cardiopulmonary					
Pneumonia Atelectasis	41.5%[2] Leading cause of death after 12 years[31]	Bacterial or viral infection, prolonged immobilization, prolonged artificial ventilation, general anesthesia	Radiographic studies, diagnostic bronchoscopy	Antibiotics, bronchodilator therapy; therapeutic bronchoscopy; suctioning	Chest physical therapy: percussion, vibration, postural drainage; mobilize the client; inspiratory breathing exercises
Ventilatory failure	40.5%[2]	Weakness or paralysis of the inspiratory muscles, unchecked bronchospasm	Pulmonary function tests (PFTs); arterial blood gases (ABGs), end-tidal CO_2 monitoring, pulse oximetry	Artificial ventilation and supportive therapy, management of underlying cause (i.e., pneumonia), oxygen therapy	Airway and secretion management treatment as above, early mobilization once stabilized, biofeedback to assist with ventilator weaning as appropriate
Deep vein thrombosis (DVT)[a]	12%–64%[103]	Venous status, activation of blood coagulation, pressure on immobilized lower extremity, and endothelial damage[49, 74, 77]	Doppler studies, leg measurements, extremity visual observation and palpation, low-grade fever of unknown origin	Subcutaneous heparin[30, 37] Prophylactic anticoagulation can decrease incidence to 1.3%[35] Vena cava filter for failed anticoagulant prophylaxis	Early mobilization and ROM for prevention, centripetal massage for prevention, compression garments, education about smoking cessation, weight loss, and exercise; avoid constricting garments and monitor overly tight leg bag straps and pressure garments (Paralyzed Veterans of America DVT guidelines)
Pulmonary embolus	5%–15% in persons with DVT[43] Leading cause of death within first year[31]	Dislodging of DVT	Ventilation/perfusion lung scan, signs and symptoms including chest pain, breathlessness, apprehension, fever and cough	Vena cava filter Anticoagulation therapy	None
Orthostatic hypotension	Unknown, but common	Vasodilation and decreased venous return, loss of muscle pump action in dependent lower extremities and trunk[49]	Monitor blood pressure with activity and changes in position, observation/signs and symptoms	Medications to increase blood pressure, fluids in the presence of hypovolemia	Gradient compression garments: Ace wraps, abdominal binders, appropriate wheelchair selection to prevent rapid changes in position early in rehabilitation
Apneic bradycardia	Unknown	True etiology unknown; believed to be caused by sympathetic disruption resulting in vagal dominance in response to a noxious stimuli or hypoxia[10]	Electrocardiogram Heart rate Respiratory rate	Hyperventilation	Remove noxious stimulus
Integumentary System					
Pressure ulcers	30%–56%[24]	Prolonged external skin pressure exceeding the average arterial or capillary pressure[24]	Wound measurements staging classification, nutritional assessment[8]	Nutritional support as needed, surgical or enzymatic debridement, surgical closure, muscle flap, skin flap or graft, antibiotics as appropriate	Irrigation and hydrotherapy, dressing management, electrotherapy[8]
Shearing	Unknown	Stretching and tearing of the blood vessels that pass between the layers of the skin[41]	See pressure ulcers	See pressure ulcers	Add protective padding during functional activities, skill perfection, correct handling techniques

Table continued on following page

T A B L E 16–3. Complications After SCI *Continued*

Complication	Incidence	Etiology	Diagnostic Test and Measures	Medical Treatment or Intervention	Therapeutic Intervention
Moisture	Unknown	Excessive sweating below the level of injury, urinary and bowel incontinence, poor hygiene	See pressure ulcers	See pressure ulcers, treat possible urinary tract infection, medications for bladder incontinence	Protective barrier ointments and powders, establish effective bowel and bladder programs, educate for improved hygiene, and refine ADL skills
Neuromuscular					
Spasticity	33.3%[3]	Upper motor neuron lesion[70,113]	Ashworth or Modified Ashworth scale; Deep tendon reflex spasticity scale evaluation	Antispastic pharmacological agents: baclofen, diazepam (Valium), dantrolene[113]; surgical intervention: myelotomy, rhizotomy, peripheral neurotomy[70]; Botox injection[22,70,77]; Baclofen pump insertion	Prolonged stretching; inhibitive positioning/casting; Cryotherapy, weight-bearing exercise and aquatic therapy
Flaccidity	Associated with clients with low paraplegia	Lower motor neuron lesion[36,41] Most often in injuries at L1 level and below	Deep tendon reflexes (would be absent)	None	None for treating flaccidity; however, secondary treatments that need to be considered include positioning to improve postural support, education for skin protection and bracing and splinting to maintain joint integrity
Neurogenic bowel†	Unknown	Refer to bowel management	Positive bulbocavernosus reflex: indicates reflexic bowel	Oral laxative, suppositories, and enemas	Establish a comprehensive bowel program
Autonomic dysreflexia	8.9%	Triggering of an uncontrolled hyperactive response from the sympathetic nervous system by a noxious stimulus[41]; noxious stimuli may include bowel or bladder distention, urinary tract infection, ingrown toenail, tight clothing, and pressure sore	Sudden rise in systolic blood pressure of 20–40 mm Hg above baseline[10] Observation of signs and symptoms: Sweating above the level of injury Goose bumps Severe headache Flushing of skin due to vasodilation above the level of injury[10]	Catheterization of the bladder, irrigation of indwelling catheter, pharmacological management if systolic blood pressure is greater than 150 mm Hg Remove ingrown toenail if present	Immediately position the client in the upright position, identify and remove noxious stimuli, check clothing and catheter tubing for constriction, and perform bowel program if fecal impaction is suspected

Other

Problem	Incidence/Prevalence	Description	Assessment	Treatment	Management/Education
Thermoregulation problems	Unknown; more prevalent with higher SCI injuries	Interruption between the communication with the autonomic nervous system and the hypothalamus / Lack of vasoconstriction and inability to shiver or perspire[10]	Body temperature	Cooling or warming blanket if extreme	Education about risk and proper protection from the elements; behavior modification, education for proper hydration and appropriate clothing
Pain	One third to one half of all SCI	Radicular pain originating from the injury[41,75], kinematic or mechanical pain, direct trauma, referred pain	Pain scales functional assessment	Immobilization and rest, pain medications; injections for pain or antiinflammatory measures	Restore ideal alignment and posture; thermal and electromodalities; manual therapy; improve movement patterns
Urinary tract infections	80.4%[2]	Presence of excessive bacteria in urine	Urinalysis, urine culture and sensitivity, temperature	Antibiotics	Monitor fluid intake and educate for proper technique during bladder care
Contractures	4.5% during acute stage overall; tetraplegia incidence is 8.4%[2]	Muscle imbalance around a joint; prolonged immobilization, unchecked spasticity, pain	Goniometric measurements	Tendon release; Botox injection for isolated spasticity	ROM functional use of extremity, casting or splinting, achieving and maintaining optimal postural alignment
Heterotopic ossification (HO)	5%–20% of males develop HO twice as often[108]	Unknown	Alkaline phosphatase levels (increase after 6 weeks)[95]; observation for sudden loss of ROM, local edema, heat, erythema, nonseptic fever	Etidronate disodium (Didronel): use prophylactically or during the inflammatory stage / Surgical resection	Maintain available ROM; avoid vigorous stretching during inflammatory stage; achieve and maintain optimal wheelchair positioning
Osteoporosis and degenerative joint changes	Unknown	Bone demineralization[44]	Bone scan	None; calcium supplement for prevention	Weight-bearing techniques: amount and type unknown specific to SCI
Spinal deformities	Unknown	Muscle imbalance or weakness around spinal column; poor postural support, asymmetrical functional activities	Posture evaluation, seating evaluation	If severe: surgical fixation, thoracic orthosis	Restore postural alignment, avoid repetitive asymmetrical activities, control spasticity
Gastroduodenal ulcers/gastrointestinal bleeding	22%[86] / Approx. one third of persons with complete lesions experience chronic bowel problems[7]	Acute: disruption of central nervous system, abdominal trauma or stress response to neuroendocrine system[86] / Chronic: impairment of the autonomic nervous system[41]	Hematocrit and hemoglobin; observation of gastrointestinal fluid;	Surgical intervention; restore normal gastrointestinal function	Establish effective bowel program, establish a high-fiber diet, provide education and stress management
Metabolic/endocrine	Unknown	Impairment of autonomic nervous system	Observe for fatigue, malaise; undesirable weight gain[81]	None known	Education, exercise, and weight control

*Consortium for Spinal Cord Medicine Clinical Practice Guidelines. Prevention of Thromboembolism in Spinal Cord Injury. Paralyzed Veterans of America, February 1997.
†Consortium for Spinal Cord Medicine Clinical Practice Guidelines. Neurogenic Bowel Management in Adults with Spinal Cord Injury. Paralyzed Veterans of America, March 1998.

cations to the seating system or changing to a more pressure-relieving sleep system may be necessary. Examination and treatment will then need to focus on healing the wound and preventing other secondary complications that may occur because of the potential immobility and delayed physical rehabilitation. The reader is encouraged to refer to *Pressure Ulcer Treatment: Clinical Practice Guideline* developed by the Agency for Health Care Policy and Research (AHCPR) for examination tools, including the classification of pressure ulcers.[8]

Treatment interventions may include hydrotherapy, speciality wound dressing changes, electromodalities, and thermomodalities to increase circulation.[8] Mechanical, chemical, or surgical débridement may be necessary to obtain and maintain a viable wound bed. If the wound does not heal, surgical interventions with skin flaps or muscle flaps may be necessary for closure. Tedious return-to-sit programs or protocols after such medical interventions are necessary to prevent opening of the surgical site. Such surgical procedures are costly and significantly delay functional rehabilitation.

After closure and healing of the wound, education becomes a priority. The client must adhere to a more rigorous skin check program, and rehabilitation should continue, with special attention to the area in question. Prevention of skin compromise is critical and cannot be stressed enough to health care providers, clients, and caregivers.

Prevention and Management of Joint Contractures

The development of a contracture may result in postural malalignment and/or impede potential function. Daily ROM exercises and proper positioning help prevent contractures.[109] Clients exhibiting spasticity may require more frequent treatments.[109, 112] Contracture prevention includes the utilization of splints for proper joint alignment, techniques such as weight-bearing, and functional exercises.

Although isolated joint ROM should be normal for all clients, allowing adaptive shortening or lengthening of particular muscles is recommended to enhance the achievement of certain functional skills.[89, 105] Likewise, unwanted shortening or lengthening of muscles should be prevented. The following reviews a few examples of these concepts as they relate to SCI.

Tenodesis is described as the passive shortening of the two-joint finger flexors as the wrist is extended. This action creates a grasp, which assists performance of ADLs (Fig. 16–13).[89, 101] A client with mid to low tetraplegia may rely on adaptive shortening of these long finger flexors to replace active grip.[89] If the long finger flexors are stretched across all joints during ROM exercises, some functional goals may not be achieved. ROM to the finger flexors should only be performed while the wrist is in a neutral position.

Clients with complete paraplegia who are candidates for ambulation require normal ROM in the lower extremities. If the hip flexors and/or knee flexors are allowed to adaptively shorten, achieving standing and ambulation goals will be difficult.

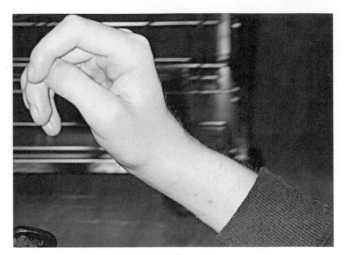

FIGURE 16–13. Tenodesis grasp.

The combination of lengthened hamstrings and tight back extensor muscles provides stability for balance in the short- and the long-sitting positions. This aids in the efficiency of transfers and bowel and bladder management. Balance in long sitting assists with lower-extremity dressing and other ADLs. Hamstrings should be lengthened to allow 110 degrees to 120 degrees of straight-leg raising without overstretching back extensor muscles.

In the presence of weak or paralyzed triceps, adaptive shortening of the elbow flexors impairs ADL and transfer skills.[41, 89] A contracted elbow flexor in a client with a C6-level SCI can cost this client his or her independence.

The rotator cuff and the other scapular muscles should be assessed for their length/tension relationships and their ability to generate force. Normal length of these muscles should be maintained. For example, achieving external rotation of the shoulder (active and passive) is critical for clients with low-level tetraplegia. Shortening of the subscapularis and other structures can quickly result in a decrease in this motion, limiting bed mobility, transfers, feeding, and grooming skills.

If a joint contracture occurs despite preventive measures, more aggressive treatments are necessary. This includes utilization of plaster or fiberglass casting techniques. The client with minimal ROM limitations may require only one cast. Most commonly, the client has a significant limitation and requires serial casts. Several casts would be applied and then removed over a period of weeks to increase extensibility in the soft tissues surrounding the casted joint.[26] The joint to be stretched would be placed at, or near, the end range and casted in that position for a few days until the deformity is resolved. The final cast is bivalved so that the cast can act as a positioning device yet be easily removed. Casting contraindications are skin compromise, heterotopic ossification, edema, decreased circulation, severely fluctuating tone, and inconsistent monitoring systems. Casting clients with SCI often takes two staff members to fabricate one cast over a 30-minute to 1-hour period.

The elbow, wrist/hand, and finger joints are the most common joints casted for clients with SCI. Casting for most of these clients may be the last resort to regain increased ROM before a client can begin feeding, grooming, and/or communication skills. Long-arm casts are used when elbow and wrist contractures must be managed simultaneously. If evaluation of the upper extremity reveals a pronation or supination contracture, a long-arm cast would also be the cast of choice. Dropout casts are used with severe elbow flexor or extensor contractures, but the patient should be in a position where gravity can assist. If the client must remain supine for extended periods of time, this would not be the cast of choice.

Wrist/hand and finger casts are indicated for contractures that prevent distal upper-extremity function. Most commonly, a client will have a wrist flexion/extension contracture and/or have finger flexor/extensor tone and will require a cast to use the tenodesis or individual fingers for fine motor skills. Sometimes wrist casts with finger shells or resting hand extensions on casts are needed to ensure that the hand, fingers, and web space are maintained in a position of optimal function. Casting can be a very expensive and labor-intensive treatment modality, but if indicated and used appropriately it can assist a client in regaining lost joint ROM needed for increased independence and function.

Prevention and Management of Respiratory Complications

Early management must focus heavily on preventing pulmonary complications and enhancing available pulmonary function. A client's ability to breathe effectively must be established before asking the client to do work.

The clinician should determine which ventilatory muscles are impaired. The primary ventilatory muscles of inspiration are the diaphragm and the intercostals. The diaphragm, which separates the thoracic and the abdominal cavities, is innervated by the phrenic nerve at C3 through C5. The intercostals are innervated by the intercostal nerves and are positioned between the ribs. If the diaphragm is weak or paralyzed, its descent will be lessened, reducing the client's ability to ventilate.[18, 23, 71, 79]

Accessory muscles of ventilation are primarily located in the cervical region.[31] In normal persons, the accessory muscles are used to augment ventilation when the demand for oxygen increases, as during exercise. Accessory muscles may also be recruited to generate an improved cough effort.[109] The most commonly cited accessory muscles are the sternocleidomastoids, the scalenes, the levators scapulae, and the trapezoids.[23, 71] The erector spinae group may assist by extending the spine, thus improving the potential depth of inspiration.[41, 71]

The primary muscles used for forced expiration in such maneuvers as coughing or sneezing are the abdominal muscles. The latissimus dorsi, the teres major, and the clavicular portion of the pectoralis major are also active during forced expiration and cough in the client with tetraplegia.[28] Alterations in the function of these muscles will impact the client's ability to clear secretions and produce loud vocalization and may actually impact the function of the inspiratory muscles.

Gravity plays a crucial role in the function of all ventilatory muscles.[71] Neural input to the diaphragm increases in the upright position in persons with intact nervous systems. As one moves into an upright position the resting position of the diaphragm drops as the abdominal contents fall.[71] The diaphragm is effectively shortened, which makes generating a strong contraction more difficult. With intact abdominal musculature, however, a counterpressure is produced and adequate intraabdominal pressure is maintained, allowing the diaphragm to perform work.[80] If weakness or paralysis of the abdominal wall is present, the client may need a binder or corset to maintain the normal pressure relationship.[18, 21, 72, 89] Unless the SCI has affected only the lowest sacral and lumbar areas, some degree of ventilatory impairment is present and should be addressed in therapeutic sessions.

Many treatment techniques are available to address the myriad of what may cause ventilatory impairment. Decreased chest wall mobility and the inability to clear secretions should always be addressed. Interventions may include inspiratory muscle training, chest wall mobility exercises, and chest physical therapy.[47, 79, 84, 89, 105]

Inspiratory Muscle Training

Inspiratory muscle training is used to train the diaphragm and the accessory muscles that are weakened by partial paralysis, disuse from prolonged artificial ventilation, or prolonged bed rest. In general, the inspiratory muscles should be trained initially in the supine position[21, 84, 105] and progressed to the sitting position. When training a moderately weak diaphragm, gentle pressure during inspiration may be used to facilitate the muscle (Fig. 16–14). Accessory muscle training may be facilitated with the client in the supine position while a slight stretch is placed on these muscles.[105] The stretch is accomplished by shoulder abduction and external rotation, elbow extension, forearm supination, and neutral alignment of the head and neck. A more challenging position incorporates upper thoracic extension. The clinician's hands are placed directly over the muscle to be facilitated. The client is instructed to breathe into the upper chest (Fig. 16–15). As the treatment progresses, the diaphragm may be inhibited for short training periods by applying pressure over the abdomen in an upward direction. Care must be taken to avoid excessive pressure to prevent occlusion of vital arteries.

As the inspiratory muscles strengthen, resistive inspiratory devices may be used. The diaphragm also may be trained using weights on the abdominal wall. Derrickson and co-workers[30a] concluded that both inspiratory muscle training devices and abdominal weights were effective in improving ventilatory mechanics. Muscle trainers, however, appear to promote more of an endurance effect than the use of abdominal weights.

Phrenic Nerve Pacing

When the primary inspiratory muscles are no longer volitionally active due to SCI, phrenic nerve pacing may be used to cause the diaphragm to contract. This may be indicated when the lesion is at or above the C3 level.[15, 68, 102] Electrical stimulation may be applied directly or indirectly through a vein wall or the skin or directly to the phrenic nerve. Family and clients must receive extensive educa-

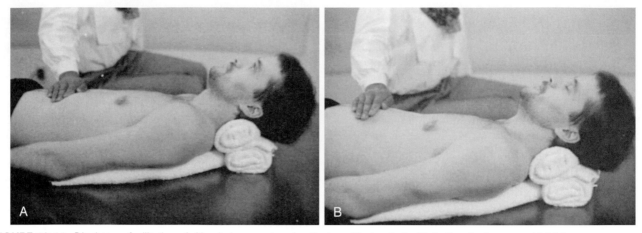

FIGURE 16–14. Diaphragm facilitation. *A*, Hand placement and patient positioning to facilitate the diaphragm and inhibit accessory muscle activity. *B*, Firm contact is maintained throughout inspiration. The lower extremities are placed over a pillow in flexion to prevent stretching of the abdominal wall.

tion to learn equipment management and emergency procedure plans in the event of pacer failure. Tolerance to phrenic nerve pacing is gradually increased. Most clients will still require some mechanical ventilation even after maximal tolerance is achieved so as not to overfatigue the phrenic nerve.

Glossopharyngeal Breathing

Glossopharyngeal breathing is another way of increasing vital capacity in the presence of weak inspiratory muscles.[21, 79, 84] By moving the jaw forward and upward in a circular opening and closing manner, air is trapped into the buccal cavity. A series of swallowing-like maneuvers forces air into the lungs, increasing the vital capacity. This technique has been reported to increase vital capacity by as much as 1 L.[105] Although this technique is rarely used to sustain ventilation for long periods of time,[6] it may be used in emergency situations and to enhance cough function. The client with high tetraplegia should attempt to master this skill.

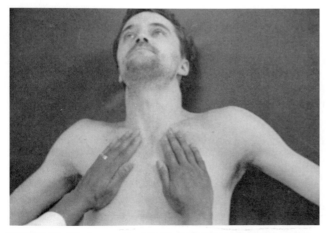

FIGURE 16–15. Accessory muscle facilitation. Hand placement and patient positioning.

Secretion Clearance

Ventilatory impairment occurs when the client is unable to clear secretions.[18, 104] Factors such as artificial ventilation and general anesthesia hamper secretion mobilization. With artificial ventilation, clients may require an artificial airway.[9, 104] The presence of this airway in the trachea poses an irritant, and the client subsequently produces more secretions.[6] A description of various types and parameters of ventilation is beyond the scope of this chapter. Clinicians working with clients requiring artificial ventilation, however, are referred to other publications.[50, 104]

Secretions are most commonly removed by tracheal suctioning, unassisted coughing, or assisted "quad" coughing. More recently, in-exsufflation is being used to remove secretions. In-exsufflation uses a set amount of inspiratory pressure followed by immediate reversal to rapid expiratory pressures, resulting in secretion removal. To date, conclusive research determining which single technique or combination of techniques achieves the best outcome is not available. Postural drainage, percussion or clapping, and shaking or vibration are used to assist with moving secretions toward larger airways for expectoration.[57, 89, 97]

Quad coughing is a term used to describe assisted coughing for a person unable to generate sufficient effort.[84] The assistant places both hands firmly on the abdominal wall. After a maximal inspiratory effort, the client coughs and the assistant simply supports the weakened wall. A gentle upward and inward force may be used to increase the intra-abdominal pressure, yielding a more forceful cough (Fig. 16–16).[84, 105] Excessive pressure over the xiphoid process should be avoided to prevent severe injury.

Clients may learn independent quad coughing. In preparation for a cough, the client positions an arm around the push handle of the wheelchair, which enhances inspiratory effort. The other arm is raised over the head and chest during inspiration. This procedure is followed by a breath hold, strong trunk flexion, and then a cough (Fig. 16–17).[84] Another technique for independent quad coughing is accomplished by placing the forearms over

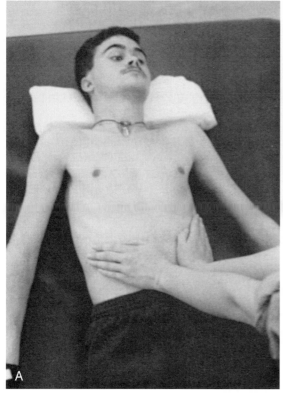

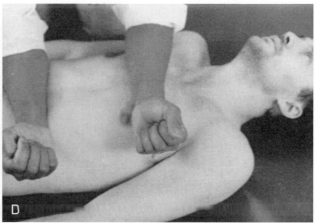

FIGURE 16–16. Quad coughing. *A*, Hand placement for the Heimlich-like technique. *B*, Anterior chest wall quad coughing. The inferior forearm supination promotes an upward and inward force during the cough.

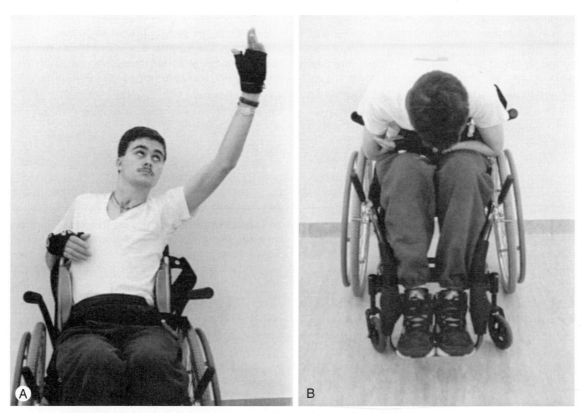

FIGURE 16–17. Self quad coughing. *A*, Full inspiratory position. *B*, Expiratory/cough position.

the abdomen and delivering a manual thrust during cough. This technique is more difficult and may not provide an inspiratory advantage.

Early Mobilization

Getting the client upright as soon as possible promotes self-mobility and should be planned carefully. An appropriate seating system for pressure relief and support should be chosen. Most clients require a reclining wheelchair with elevating footrests when they are first acclimating to the upright position.[84, 89, 105]

The client is transferred initially to a reclining position and progressed to an upright position as signs and symptoms of medical stability allow. The client should be monitored for evidence of orthostatic hypotension. Dizziness or lightheadedness is most common. Ringing in the ears and visual changes also may occur. Changes in mental function may indicate more serious hypotension, and the client should be reclined immediately. Assessing blood pressure before and during activities provides an objective measurement of the client's status.

Because the abdominal wall is not supporting the internal contents, abdominal binders or corsets should be applied to all clients with lesions above T12 to assist in venous return[72, 84, 105] and to enhance ventilatory function. If the client has a history of vascular insufficiency or prolonged bed rest, wrapping the lower extremities with elastic bandages while applying the greatest pressure distally may be beneficial.

Abdominal binders and corsets are fitted so that the top of the corset lies just over the lower two ribs.[105] They should not be placed too high or allowed to ride up, which may occur in the obese client, because this may impair ventilation by restricting chest wall excursion. The bottom portion is placed over the anterior iliac spine and figure crest (Fig. 16–18). The corset or binder should be adjusted slightly tighter at the bottom to assist in elevating the abdominal contents.[84, 89, 105]

The client can be transferred initially with a manual or mechanical lift. Lift systems may be advantageous, be-

cause they allow total control of the client and give the assistant more time to ensure that monitoring devices, lines, or tubes attached to the client remain intact. Lift systems may be freestanding hydraulic lifts, electronic devices, or those mounted on the ceiling.

Once the client is out of bed, a weight shift or pressure relief schedule is immediately established. Initially, weight shifts are performed at 30-minute intervals and modified according to skin tolerance.[73] A timer may be issued to ensure reminders for weight shifts. This is particularly important if the client has cognitive deficits. The skin is inspected thoroughly before and immediately after out-of-bed activities. Total sitting time is progressed according to tolerance.

REHABILITATION: ACHIEVING FUNCTIONAL OUTCOMES

Once secondary complications are managed and the client is able to tolerate out-of-bed activities, more aggressive rehabilitation begins. The following will address special considerations for functional progression as they relate to SCI.

Optimal neck, shoulder, and upper-extremity strength and ROM are important factors when achieving functional outcomes. Neck musculature is typically painful and restricted in cervical injuries. Most clients will have a collar in place to prevent rotation and flexion/extension. The client may be so tight that correcting their forward head posture with stretching and proper positioning is the first goal. Soft tissue massage and manual therapy may be beneficial. Once cleared by the physician the client can begin neck isometric exercises.

Key muscle groups in the shoulder to consider are the scapular stabilizers and movers, which allow for humeral flexion, adduction/abduction, and shoulder internal and external rotation and scapular movements. Clients with high cervical injuries have the potential to develop tight upper trapezius muscles. Upper trapezius inhibitory and/or scapular taping to relax the tight muscles and facilitate the weak scapular musculature is beneficial. In injury levels above C6, the scapular musculature may not be fully innervated and thus positioning in the proper alignment and strengthening the innervated musculature is essential. Findings from the manual muscle test and goniometric examination will determine the appropriate stretching/strengthening program. Clients may need to begin with gravity-eliminated exercises using an airsplint, bilateral slings, skateboards, functional electric stimulation (FES), and side-lying exercises.

Activities of Daily Living

Activities of daily living include skills such as communication, feeding, grooming, bathing, dressing, bladder management, bowel management, and home management. Depending on the level and severity of the SCI, clients will achieve varying levels of independence. Clients with high-level tetraplegia (C1–C4) will be dependent in most activities of daily living but will be able to verbalize how to safely perform all skills. Clients with low-level

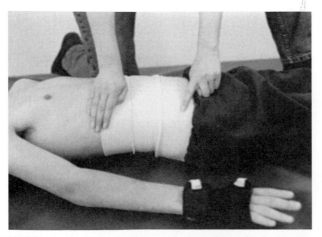

FIGURE 16–18. Abdominal binder. Correct placement is over the anterior-superior iliac spine and at the level of lower rib cage. Custom corsets may be used if an elastic binder does not provide adequate support to enhance vital capacity.

tetraplegia (C5–C8) may achieve some level of independence, but this will vary according to the amount of intact musculature. The ability of these clients to achieve maximum independence in all areas of ADL may be accomplished only through the use of appropriate orthoses or adaptive equipment. See Table 16–2 for functional expectations and Table 16–4 for orthotic indications.

Clients with C5 or C6 SCI are especially challenging in this area of rehabilitation. These clients must have good biceps and elbow ROM before any ADL goals can be achieved. Elbow positioning devices such as pillow splints, casts, and/or resting splints enhance alignment. Appropriate wheelchair positioning with lap trays, armrests, wedges, or lateral trunk supports maximizes function. To achieve these goals, clients also need to work toward simultaneous extension of the shoulder, elbow, and wrist for body weight–supported activities.

Clients with paraplegia usually obtain total independence with communication, feeding, and grooming. These clients may need adaptive equipment to perform some of these skills; however, they should be able to be performed without assistance from another person. Orthoses and adaptive equipment are discussed in each section.

Endurance is a major concern for client's independence while performing ADL. Some skills require a considerable amount of time and effort. If endurance becomes a factor, clients should choose to perform some activities while receiving assistance for other skills that are too challenging and/or time consuming.

Communication

Communication includes utilization of a call system, environmental control unit (ECU), telephone, and computer and the ability to perform writing, typing, and page turning. All levels of SCI can be independent with these skills after setup. Call systems, ECUs, and computers can be programmed to use pneumatic control (sip 'n' puff) for independence from bed and the wheelchair (Fig. 16–19). There are switches that can be activated with head or eye control, allowing clients with little movement the ability to communicate. Clients with C1 to C4 injuries can also use equipment such as mouthsticks for communication from the bed and the wheelchair (Fig. 16–20). Clients with C5 injuries begin to use their biceps and deltoid strength in communication. Adaptive splinting for support at the wrist can allow these clients to use their upper arms in writing, typing, page turning, and computer use (Fig. 16–21). Clients with wrist function but no finger function can use cuffs on speakerphones or use their natural tenodesis in a wrist-driven hand brace to grasp objects (Figs. 16–22 and 16–23). For injuries at the C7 level and below, communication in all areas should be independent.

Feeding

Clients with C1 to C4 tetraplegia are dependent in feeding but can verbalize this skill. Clients with weak shoulder and biceps musculature require a dynamic orthosis to support the upper extremity during feeding. The most common orthoses used are the mobile arm support (Fig. 16–24) and the offset feeder (Fig. 16–25). Clients with low-level tetraplegia may not have weakness in their shoulder that would affect feeding, but they may have weak wrist function. A cuff can be purchased and worn on the hand to support feeding utensils (Fig. 16–26). The client with no finger function can use a wrist-driven tenodesis brace to hold a feeding utensil (Fig. 16–27).

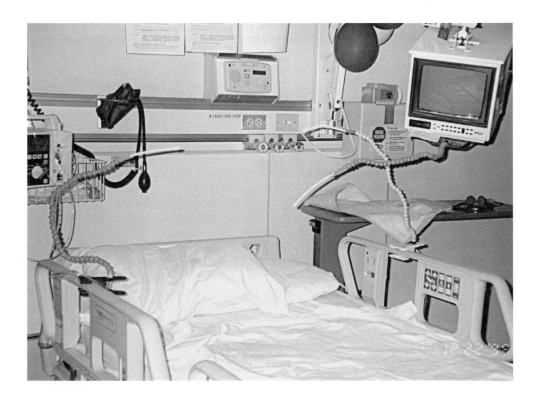

FIGURE 16–19. Sip 'n' puff bedside setup for call light, television, and telephone.

T A B L E 1 6 – 4. Upper-Extremity Orthotics

Level of Spinal Cord Injury	Splint	Rationale
Dynamic Orthotics		
Weak C5, incomplete injuries Also indicated with shoulder external rotator muscle grades 2− to 3− and bicep/supinator muscle grades of at least 2−.	Mobile arm support (ball bearing and swivel arm use, allowing gravity to assist)	• Assists in reaching maximum range and use in horizontal and vertical planes • Increases range of motion and strength • Independent feeding, hygiene after setup • Teaches correct movement patterns • Wheelchair trunk supports required for maximum benefit
C5, incomplete injuries Also indicated with shoulder external rotator muscle grades 3− to 3 in addition to biceps and supinator muscles grades of 3 or better.	Offset feeder (sling suspension with trough support for the forearm)	• Increases range of motion and strength throughout • Independent feeding and hygiene after setup • Teaches correct movement patterns • Adjunct device for functional ADL training • Lateral wheelchair trunk supports may be required
C5, incomplete injuries Also indicated with shoulder external rotator grades 3 to 3+ but client fatigues and/or biceps grades of 3 or better	Overhead rod and sling (supports the upper extremity with cuffs at elbow and wrist while attached to a spring overhead)	• Increases range of motion and strength • Can be used for driving wheelchair if shoulder strength is an issue • Independent for feeding and hygiene after setup • Lateral trunk supports may be required
16 Static Upper-Extremity Splints		
C1–C3	Resting hand	• Position • Prevents joint deformity • Cosmetic appearance
C4	Resting hand	• Position • Prevents joint deformity • Cosmetic appearance
C5	Resting hand	• Same as above • Preserves the web space • Preserves a balance between extrinsic and intrinsic musculature • Provides joint support at rest and prevents deformity
C5	Pillow (elbow)	• Position • Prevents elbow contractures from mild tone or muscle imbalance • Prevention of skin compromise
C5	Rolyan tap (tone and positioning) splint (prefab)	• Position • Prevents supination/pronation contracture • Provides constant low-level stretch • Use with mild to moderate tone • Best with incomplete clients, gravity can assist to promote elbow extension
C5	Elbow extension	• Position • Prevents skin compromise • Prevents elbow contractures from tone and/or muscle imbalance
C5	Economy wrist support	• Function (slot for utensils, etc.) • Position • Prevents severe wristdrop • Prevents ulnar deviation initially • Not enough support long term (clients often develop ulnar deviation and some wristdrop) • If position is needed long term, consider permanent splint made by an orthotist
C5	Long opponens	• Position • Can be dorsal or volar • Prevents wristdrop • Preserves the web space and promotes proper thumb positioning • Function (with slot) • Prevents ulnar deviation and wristdrop • If position is needed long term, consider more permanent splint made by an orthotist
C5	Wrist cockup	• Position • Supports or stabilizes wrist in extension • Allows for finger movement (incomplete injuries) • Preserves the web space
C6	Short opponens	• Position • Thumb in opposition for functional activities • Improves prehension by providing a stable post against which the fingers can pinch during tenodesis • Preserves palmar creases and web space • Function (wear underneath wheelchair push gloves) • Consider permanent metal splint made by orthotist for long term

⬤ **T A B L E   1 6 – 4. Upper-Extremity Orthotics** *Continued*

Level of Spinal Cord Injury	Splint	Rationale
C6	Tenodesis	• Wrist-driven function • Enhances natural tenodesis action of the wrist, allows for 3 jaw chuck or lateral pinch • Rehabilitation Institute of Chicago has pattern, or for more permanent metal splint consider an orthotist to fabricate • Enhances writing, feeding, money, and catheter management
C6	Resting hand	• Same as that for C5 • Usually worn only at night • Critical that wrist is supported and thumb and web space are well positioned for functional use
C6	Thumb abduction strap	• Position • Thumb in opposition for functional activities • Easy to put on • Doesn't take up much space • Can be worn underneath wheelchair gloves
C7	Resting hand Short opponens	• Same as C5, C6 • Same as C6
C8, T1 (weak)	Metaphalangeal block	• Position • Can also be used for strengthening finger flexors • Prevents "claw hand" by blocking metaphalangeals • Protects weak intrinsic muscles • Joint stability

Grooming

The components of grooming are washing the face, combing/brushing hair, oral care, shaving, and applying make-up. Individuals with C1 to C4 tetraplegia are dependent but can verbalize these skills. Clients with C5 injuries perform these skills with some assistance but may require the help of the mobile arm support or offset feeder for shoulder support and a splint for wrist support. Clients with low-level tetraplegia may need cuffs or built-up grips on razors, brushes, and toothpaste to be independent (Fig. 16–28). Proper bathroom setup for optimal wheelchair positioning is important for all clients. Clients with tetraplegia often rely on the support of their elbows as an assist, so sink height should be considered. The proper positioning and adaptive equipment will be the difference between independence and dependence in these skills (Figs. 16–29 and 16–30).

Bathing

Bathing includes washing and rinsing the upper and lower extremities and the trunk. Clients with C1 to C5 tetraplegia are dependent in bathing but are instructed to verbalize this skill. Clients with low-level tetraplegia bathe with moderate assistance to total independence using adaptive devices. Clients with paraplegia are independent in bathing but may need adaptive devices. After examination of the client's upper-extremity strength, balance, spasticity, body type, endurance, and home accessibility, the therapy team can determine the appropriate bathing equipment and setup for the client (Fig. 16–31). Clients with limited

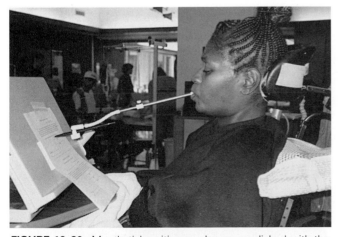

FIGURE 16–20. Mouthstick writing can be accomplished with the client upright in the wheelchair and with the support of a bedside table and bookstand.

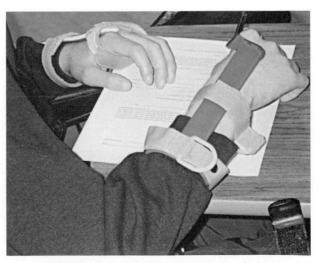

FIGURE 16–21. Long Wanchick writing device.

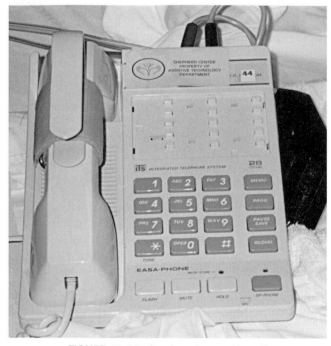

FIGURE 16–22. Speaker phone with cuff.

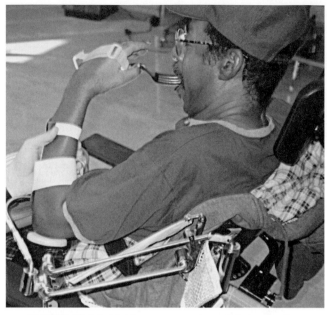

FIGURE 16–24. Mobile arm support used during feeding.

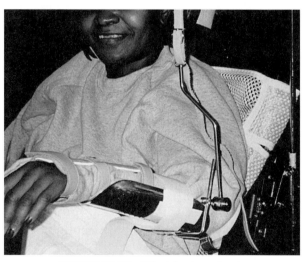

FIGURE 16–25. Offset feeder orthosis.

upper-extremity and trunk strength may need straps to assist with trunk support and adaptive cuffs to control the hand-held shower. Basic bathing safety should be taught to all clients. Bathing safety includes checking the water with a known area of intact sensation, skin checks before and after bathing, and skin protection during the transfers. These precautions are necessary to prevent burns and skin breakdown during the bathing process.

Dressing

Dressing includes dressing and undressing the upper and lower extremities. Clients with C1 to C5 tetraplegia are dependent, but they can verbalize safe techniques to perform all the dressing skills. Independence in this skill for clients with low tetraplegic and paraplegic injuries

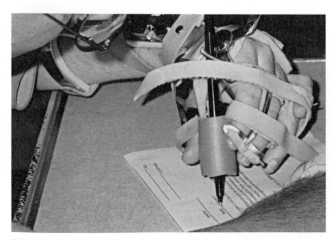

FIGURE 16–23. Tenodesis brace writing using a pen with a built-up grip.

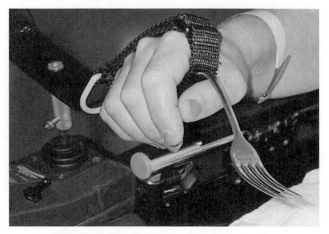

FIGURE 16–26. Universal cuff used for feeding.

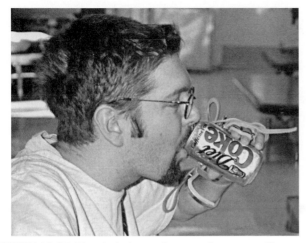

FIGURE 16–27. Tenodesis braces have varying grasps. The largest grasp position allows the client to hold a soda can.

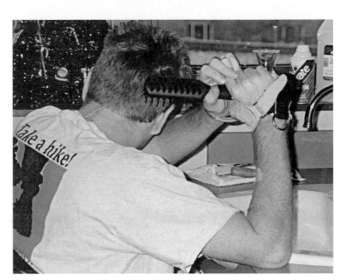

FIGURE 16–30. Sink height can be important in assisting this client with C6 spinal cord injury to brush his hair.

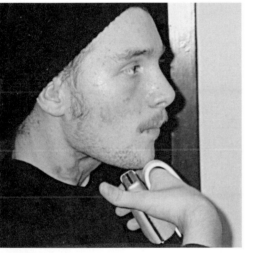

FIGURE 16–28. Client with a C5 spinal cord injury uses an electric razor with a wrist cuff.

may depend on where the skill is performed. Clients with low-level tetraplegia can perform upper body dressing/undressing independently with equipment such as a button hook (Fig. 16–32), Velcro, or adapted loops. Lower body dressing is usually performed in bed (Fig. 16–33) versus the wheelchair secondary to endurance, strength, and body type issues. Clients with paraplegia are expected to dress with total independence in the bed, but they may need equipment such as a leg lifter or a long-handled shoehorn for dressing in the wheelchair (Fig. 16–34).

Bladder Management

Bladder management includes determining and performing the program, clothing management, body positioning, setup/cleanup of equipment, and disposal of urine and cleanup of self. Water/video urodynamic studies are performed to determine the client's bladder status and

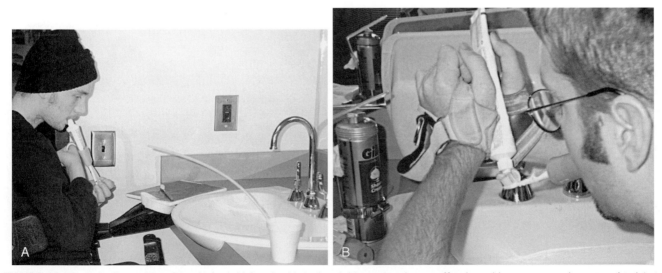

FIGURE 16–29. *A,* A client with a C5 spinal cord injury is able to brush his teeth using a cuff, adapted long straw, and proper wheelchair positioning at the sink. *B,* Client with C6 spinal cord injury uses bilateral tenodesis to support toothpaste while holding a toothbrush in his mouth.

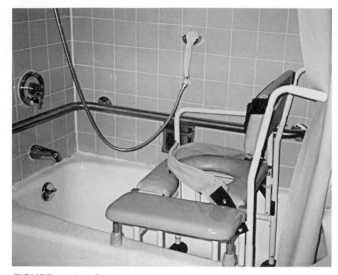

FIGURE 16–31. Bathroom setup with shower/commode chair and hand-held shower.

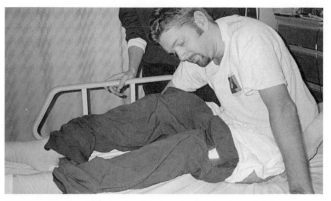

FIGURE 16–33. Client with low-level tetraplegia maintains balance while performing lower-extremity dressing in bed.

the most optimal bladder training program. Clients often enter the rehabilitation program with an indwelling catheter as their bladder management program. The indwelling catheter should be removed as soon as possible because it is a risk for chronic urinary tract infections.[87]

Based on the injury level, clients either have a reflex bladder (upper motor neuron lesions) or a nonreflex bladder (lower motor neuron lesions).[89] The reflex bladder reflexively empties when the bladder is full. The therapeutic goals for managing the reflex bladder include low-pressure voiding and low residual urine volumes.

The nonreflex bladder will not empty reflexively and needs to be manually emptied at regular intervals. The goals for managing the nonreflex bladder include establishing a regular emptying schedule and continence between emptying. Management of a nonreflex bladder includes performance of intermittent catheterizations.

Clients with C1 to C5 tetraplegia are typically dependent in their bladder programs. There are automatic leg-bag emptiers that can assist with just the elimination component of the bladder skill; however, the client will

still be dependent in all of the other components of bladder management. Clients with limited hand function may need adaptive devices such as orthoses to assist with catheter insertion, adaptive scissors to open bladder packages, leg bags with flip-top openers, and leg bag loops (Fig. 16–35). Women will most likely need to perform their training in bed with a mirror to obtain the most ideal position. Generally, clients with a nonreflex bladder are injured at, or below, the T12 level and will not require adaptive equipment.

Bowel Management

As described under bladder management, clients either have a reflex bowel or a flaccid bowel.[89] If the client has a positive bulbocavernosus reflex, this is indicative of a reflex bowel. With a reflex bowel, tone of the internal and external anal sphincter is present. Reflex bowel programs are most often managed through the use of a suppository

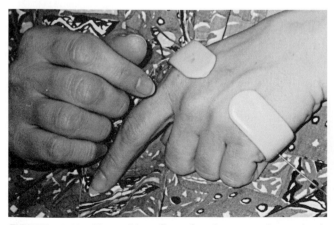

FIGURE 16–32. Client with no finger function uses a button hook for dressing.

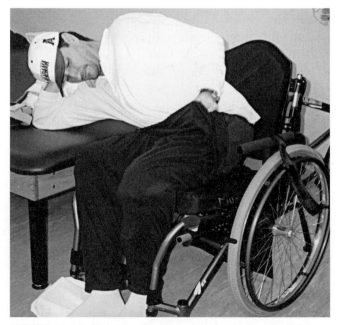

FIGURE 16–34. Early practice when dressing in the wheelchair may involve leaning on a surface to assist with this skill.

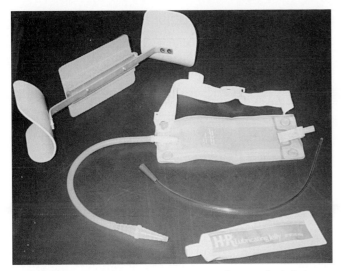

FIGURE 16–35. Bladder management supplies may include knee spreader with mirror, leg bag with tubing and adapter, catheter, and lubricating jelly.

followed by a 20-minute rectal digital stimulation program.

Flaccid bowel programs are much more difficult to regulate because there is no internal or external anal sphincter tone. Timing and diet are critical for the success of this program. A suppository may be required to assist with the process, and in this situation the rectum should be emptied before suppository insertion.[62] If the established bowel program is not followed consistently, involuntary bowel movements can occur during any strenuous activity.

Bowel management training must begin as soon as the patient is medically stable. The components of bowel management include clothing management, body positioning, setup/cleanup of equipment, performing the actual bowel program, disposing of feces, and cleanup of self. To establish the most effective bowel training program, the interdisciplinary team must work together. The team will need to discuss client medications that may affect the bowels, the time of day the client plans to perform the program, and all equipment that will be used.

Clients with injury levels above the C6 level will be dependent in performing the bowel program; however, they should be independent in the verbalization of the technique. Clients with limited hand function may require a dil stick and a suppository inserter with an adapted cuff (Fig. 16–36). In addition, a roll-in-shower chair or upright shower/commode chair with a cutout in the seat will allow the client to reach the buttock area to perform the stimulation. For this level of injury it may be advantageous to perform the bowel program in conjunction with the shower to conserve energy with transfers. For individuals with paraplegia, full independence is expected for completion of all bowel management skills. These programs are typically performed on a padded, raised toilet seat.

To increase the effectiveness of the bowel program the client should follow the guidelines identified in the following box:

GUIDELINES FOR BOWEL PROGRAM

1. Perform the bowel program at the same time each day.
2. Follow a diet high in fiber.
3. Drink at least 8 glasses of water per day.
4. Drink a hot liquid 30 minutes before initiating the bowel program.
5. Perform the bowel program in an upright position.
6. Consider premorbid bowel schedule.

Home Management

Home management may be divided into two components: light home management and heavy home management. Light home management includes money management, preparing a snack in the kitchen, laundry, and making the bed. Heavy home management includes grocery shopping, preparing a complex meal in the kitchen, dusting, and vacuuming. The clinician should discuss the role the client would like to assume at home. The client may want to resume previous home management roles or want to discuss changing roles with a family member or caregiver to have energy for other skills.

Clients with C1 to C5 tetraplegia will be dependent in home management. Clients with limited or no hand function will need adaptive kitchen devices, adapted utensils, and adapted cleaning equipment. Preplanning activities may be essential for independent function. Clients with hand function may require extended handles on equipment and must incorporate energy conservation techniques.

Mobility

Bed Mobility

The components of bed mobility include rolling side to side and supine to prone, coming to sit, and scooting in

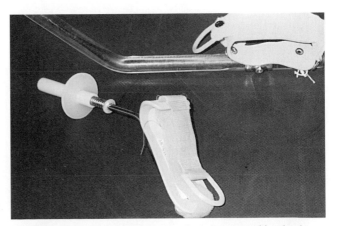

FIGURE 16–36. Dil stick and suppository inserter with adaptive cuffs.

all directions. Initial training for bed mobility is usually conducted on the mat, because movement on a firm surface is easier and leads to a more successful outcome. The client with high-level tetraplegia is dependent with these activities and is taught to instruct others.

Bed mobility is a challenging skill to learn for clients with tetraplegia owing to the limited strength in their upper extremities (Fig. 16–37).[41, 81] However, because of the functional upper-extremity strength of the client with paraplegia, bed mobility skills are often learned quickly and easily.

Pressure Relief in the Upright Position

The client with high tetraplegia achieves independent pressure relief in the wheelchair through appropriately prescribed specialty controls. For example, a pneumatic control switch may be used to activate the recline mode of a power wheelchair (Fig. 16–38). When the client is unable to operate a specialty switch, an attendant control is used. When powered options are not feasible because of cognitive deficits, financial limitations, or other reasons, a manual recliner (Fig. 16–39) or tilt wheelchair is used. When clients are dependent in performing pressure relief, they are taught to instruct others in this skill. Clients with mid- and low-level tetraplegia are taught to perform a side or forward lean technique for pressure relief if the shoulder musculature is within functional limits (Figs. 16–40 and 16–41). The client with paraplegia is usually taught to perform a push-up (depression) for pressure relief (Fig. 16–42).

Appropriate time to maintain the change in position is usually 60 seconds at intervals of 30 to 60 minutes. The treatment plan should include instructing the client in ways to ensure that the schedule for pressure relief is maintained in all settings. The use of watches, clocks, timers, and attendant care may be necessary.

Wheelchair Transfers

The physical act of moving oneself from one surface to another is described as a transfer. Wheelchair transfers may be accomplished in many different ways. The type of transfer used by a client is determined by the injury level, assistance needed, client preference, and safety of the transfer. When performing transfers, both the client and the person assisting must give attention to the use of appropriate body mechanics.

Dependent transfers may be accomplished with a hydraulic lift, manual pivot, transfer board, or manual lifts, which require two or three people. The use of a hydraulic lift may be desirable to decrease wear on the part of the caregiver. On the other hand, the hydraulic lift may not be the method of choice because the lift is bulky, difficult to store, and awkward to transport. Pivot transfers or manual lifts may be taught because of client or caregiver preference or when clients are smaller in stature.

Assisted and independent transfers include the use of

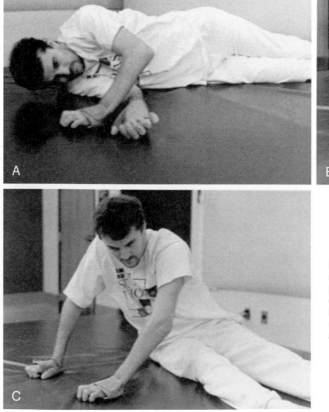

FIGURE 16–37. Bed mobility. *A*, The patient gains enough strength to effectively roll from supine to side lying. *B*, He progresses to supporting his weight through the downside elbow and shoulder. *C*, The third step is shifting his upper body weight onto the upper extremity that is topside and using the head and shoulders to direct the position of the body as he performs a side pushup into the upright sitting position.

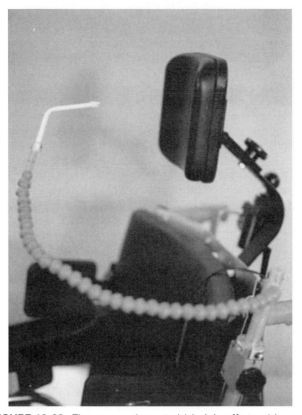

FIGURE 16–38. The pneumatic control (sip 'n' puff straw) is usually ordered on a power reclining wheelchair. The straw is removable, and several are supplied with the wheelchair. The straw is attached to a flexible arm so that it is adjustable to different heights and angles to fit the needs of the patient.

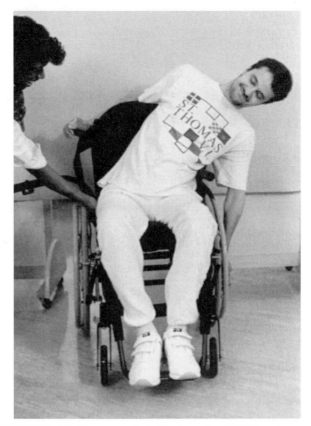

FIGURE 16–40. Pressure relief: side lean. The C6/C7-level tetraplegic patient may use a side lean to achieve pressure relief over the ischial tuberosities. The patient hooks one upper extremity around the push handle of the wheelchair on one side and leans away from the hooked upper extremity until the ischium on the hooked side is clear of the wheelchair cushion. The position is maintained for 1 minute and repeated on the other side.

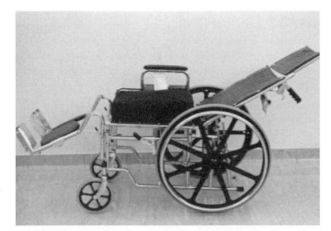

FIGURE 16–39. The manual reclining wheelchair is a piece of durable medical equipment that is prescribed on a temporary or a permanent basis. The back of the wheelchair fully reclines and the legrests elevate to allow for effective pressure relief while out of bed. Other features of the wheelchair are desk armrests, which may be adjustable in height; a removable headrest; and removable legrests. The wheelchair folds and may be transported in the trunk of a car.

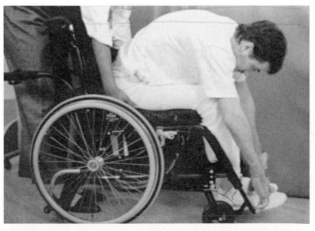

FIGURE 16–41. Pressure relief: forward lean. The forward lean method of pressure relief is used for many different injury levels. The subject must have adequate range of motion at the hips and in the lumbosacral spine to allow the ischia to clear the wheelchair cushion at the end range position.

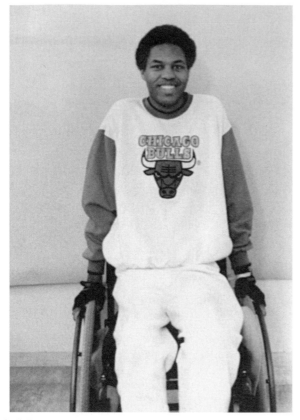

FIGURE 16–42. Pressure relief: depression. This method of pressure relief is consistent with a full pushup in the wheelchair. Most paraplegic and some low tetraplegic patients are able to perform this method of pressure relief.

transfer boards, depression-style transfers, and stand pivot transfers. The mechanics of teaching an assisted transfer to a client with C7 tetraplegia is depicted in Figure 16–43. The client is taught to position the wheelchair, position the transfer board, use correct body mechanics to get the best leverage to effect movement in the desired direction, remove the board, and position his/her body appropriately.[41, 81]

Wheelchair transfers are performed on many different surfaces. The training procedure begins with the easiest transfer and progresses to the more difficult transfer. Instructions for wheelchair transfers usually begin on level surfaces and progress to uneven surfaces as individual strength and skill allow.[41, 81] Given these two principles, the list below is an example of how one might proceed with transfer training:

1. Mat transfer
2. Bed transfer
3. Toilet transfer
4. Bath transfer
5. Car transfer (Fig. 16–44)
6. Floor transfer (Fig. 16–45)
7. Other surfaces (e.g., armchair, sofa, theater seat, pool)

Wheelchair Mobility Skills

Instructions in the safe and appropriate use of the wheelchair begin before getting the client out of bed. The client is oriented to the wheelchair and its component parts.

Ideally, a power reclining or tilt wheelchair is supplied for clients with C1 to C5 tetraplegia to promote maximal independence. A client with mid- to low-level tetraplegia may be instructed in the use of both power and manual upright wheelchairs. The client with paraplegia is instructed only in the use of a manual upright wheelchair unless there are extenuating circumstances. For example, a power wheelchair is appropriate for a client who is 50 years old and has severe rheumatoid arthritis.

Both power and manual wheelchair mobility training begins on level surfaces. Training progresses toward more difficult skills as follows:

1. Mobility in open areas
2. Setup for transfers
3. Mobility in tight spaces
4. Mobility in crowded areas
5. On/off elevators
6. Up/down ramps (Fig. 16–46)
7. In/out doors
8. Wheelies (Fig. 16–47)
9. Negotiation of rough terrain
10. Up/down curbs and steps (Figs. 16–48 and 16–49)

Ambulation

"Will I ever walk again?" is a question often asked during SCI rehabilitation. The team must be empathetic toward and acknowledge the client's goals for ambulation, and the subject should be discussed openly. The professionals must be careful not to take hope away from the client. Hope is important to maintain positive survival skills in SCI rehabilitation. Clients who are not candidates for ambulation should receive an explanation of why these goals are not feasible. It is imperative that the rehabilitation team be made aware of all discussions regarding ambulation so that the team may support both the client and the involved team member.

When ambulation is an appropriate goal, the treatment program may be short and relatively uncomplicated for some and laborious for others. Treatment techniques may include therapeutic exercise, biofeedback, neuromuscular stimulation, balance training, standing, and pregait and gait activities. The clinician must consider the postdischarge environment and include those surfaces in training.

Equipment

In SCI rehabilitation, the use of equipment is necessary to achieve the expected outcomes. Clinicians work closely with the physician and other team members, including the rehabilitation technology supplier, to determine the most appropriate equipment to meet individual needs. It is important to have access to trial equipment so the client has the opportunity to practice with equipment similar to that which is prescribed. The rehabilitation technology supplier should be accessible to the rehabilitation team to allow for necessary adjustments to the equipment. Additionally, rehabilitation technology suppliers should be knowledgeable and responsible for educating rehabilitation professionals regarding new products.

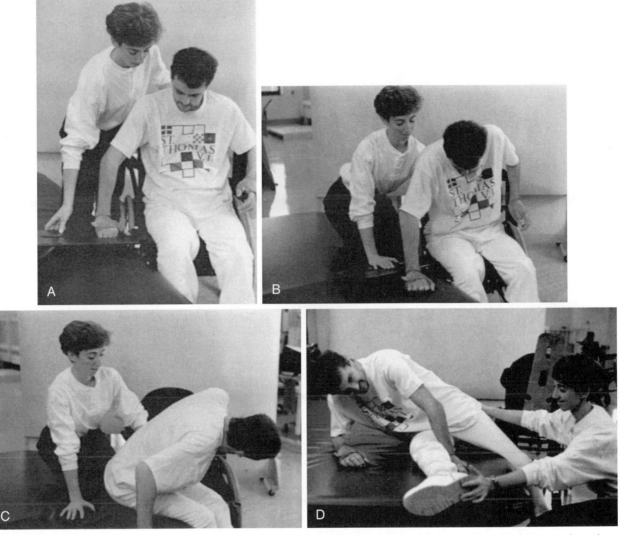

FIGURE 16–43. Wheelchair transfer using a transfer board. *A,* The client positions the wheelchair at a 20- to 30-degree angle to the surface to which he is transferring and positions the board with assistance. *B,* The client positions the trailing hand close to the trailing hip and the lead hand on the transfer board or on the surface in a diagonal line. *C,* To achieve the appropriate mechanical leverage, the client is instructed to twist the upper body and look over the trailing shoulder as he pushes and lifts to effect movement across the board. *D,* When the client has achieved a safe position on the transferring surface, the transfer board is removed and the client is assisted to get his feet onto the surface.

When possible, all equipment should be ordered from a single supplier to reduce confusion when the need for repairs arises. To ensure that the most appropriate piece of equipment is prescribed, the following must be considered: durability, function, transportability, comfort, cost, safety, cosmesis, and acceptance by the user.[81] Generally, the higher the injury level, the more costly the equipment owing to the technology involved. Table 16–5 lists equipment according to injury level.

Ideally, equipment should be ordered as soon as possible so the client can be fitted before discharge. Shorter lengths of stay make early equipment ordering difficult. For example, a client may not have ⅗ wrist extension to be fit with a tenodesis brace but with strengthening over time would be an excellent candidate. The clinicians need to negotiate with the funding source that equipment may be ordered in the outpatient setting. Equipment required for the SCI population is costly, requiring extensive re-

view by third-party payers before funding is approved or denied. Many health care policies do not cover the funding of needed equipment. As a result of these factors, many clients are discharged without the equipment they need. Lack of appropriate equipment may result in (1) a feeling of loss of control, (2) contractures and postural deformities, (3) skin breakdown, (4) a loss of skills learned in rehabilitation, (5) a feeling of poor self-image, and (6) increased dependence on others.

Education

Education of the client and caregivers is an integral part of the rehabilitation process. Formal education includes group and individual instruction and family/caregiver training. Clients and caregivers are taught preventive skin care, bowel and bladder programs, safe ways to perform all ADL tasks, nutritional guidelines, thermoregulation

Text continued on page 518

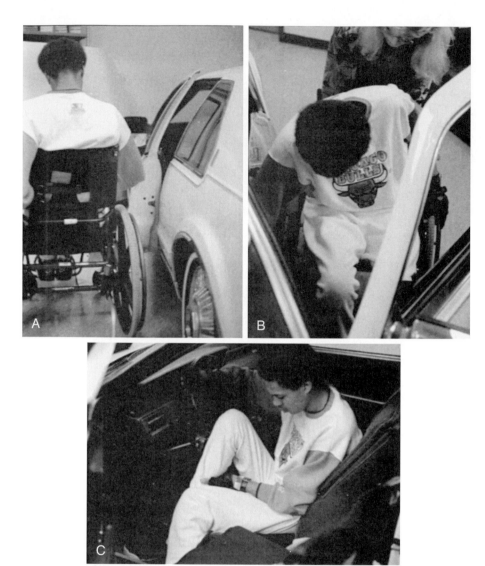

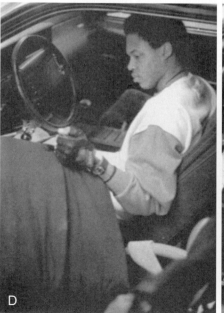

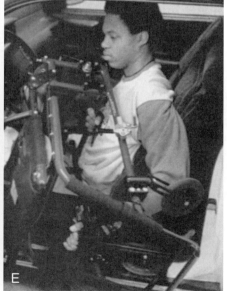

FIGURE 16–44. Car transfer. Most paraplegic patients are independent (no equipment needed) in the performance of a car transfer. The client *(A)* approaches the car on the driver's side and opens the door, *(B)* positions the wheelchair and does a depression-style transfer onto the seat of the car, *(C)* positions his lower extremities, and *(D)* prepares to get the cushion and wheelchair into the car. Depending on the make/model of the automobile and the model of the wheelchair (folding vs. rigid) *(E)*, the wheelchair is placed on the back seat or transferred across the patient and onto the passenger seat. Transferring out of the car is the reverse process, beginning with the wheelchair.

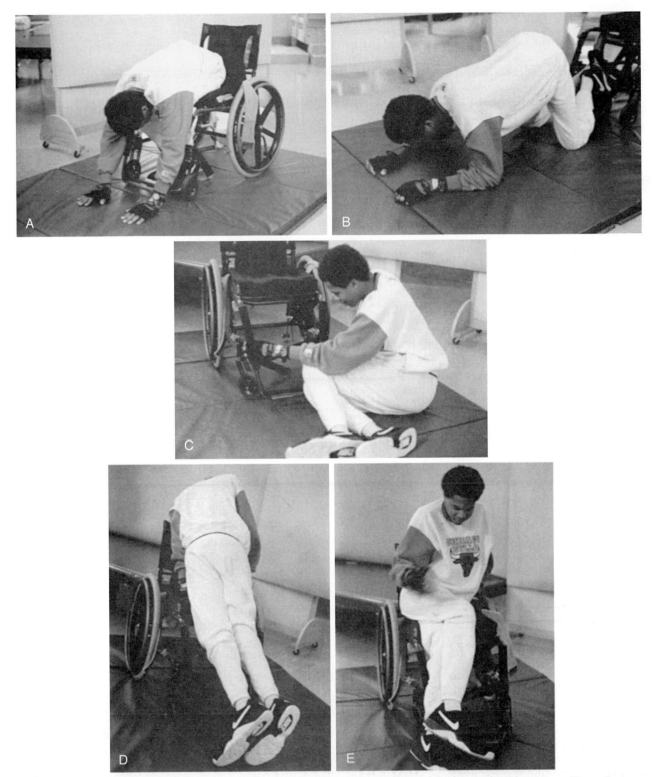

FIGURE 16–45. Floor transfer. The independent performance of a floor transfer is a goal for most paraplegic patients. The patient may use different techniques to get onto the floor. *A,* Here the patient positions his feet off the footrest and moves forward onto the front edge of his cushion. *B,* He reaches for the floor with both hands, lowers his knees to the floor, and advances his hands forward until his body is clear of the wheelchair. *C,* To get back into the wheelchair he approaches the wheelchair in a forward position and *(D)* uses the front frame, seat, and/or back of the wheelchair to push himself up into the wheelchair *(E),* turning simultaneously to assume the balanced sitting position.

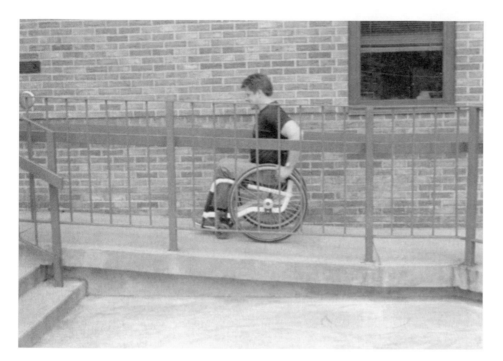

FIGURE 16–46. Ascending a ramp. It is necessary to have forward momentum to ascend a ramp efficiently. Forward momentum is achieved when the client leans slightly forward and away from the back of the wheelchair while performing an even pushing stroke for propulsion of the wheelchair. The client must be instructed in safety issues relative to the wheelchair and the percent of incline of the ramp.

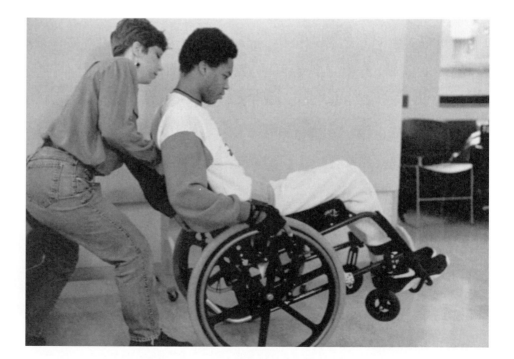

FIGURE 16–47. A wheelie is a functional mobility skill that enhances functional independence. The performance of a wheelie is a precursor to negotiating steep ramps, curbs, steps, and rough terrain.

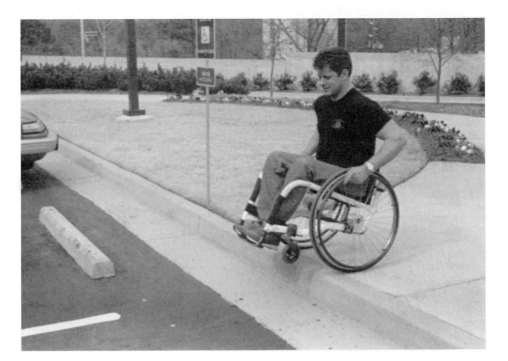

FIGURE 16–48. Descending a curb is an advanced wheelchair mobility skill. This male T7 paraplegic assumes the balanced wheelie position and approaches the curb in a forward position. The wheelie position is maintained as he rolls off the curb.

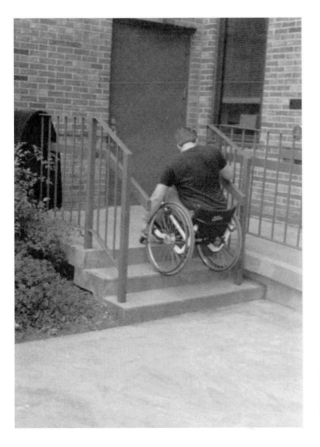

FIGURE 16–49. Descending steps using one handrail. This T7 paraplegic person approaches the steps backward and, using the handrail on his right side and the hand rim of the wheelchair on his left side, lowers himself down three steps. This is one of several methods that may be used to negotiate steps.

TABLE 16-5. Equipment Needs Correlated with Injury Level

Injury Level	Equipment	Cost (in dollars)
C1 to C3	Ventilator (bedside)	14,000
	Ventilator (portable for wheelchair)	14,000
	Power tilt/recline wheelchair	13,000–18,000
	Manual recline wheelchair for transport	2,000–4,000
	Lap tray	250–500
	Wheelchair cushion	400–500
	Reclining commode/shower chair	1,500–2,500
	ECU	1,500–6,000
	Call system	500–600
	Bedside table	150
	Fully electric hospital bed	1,500–2,200
	Communication devices	300–1,500
	Hydraulic lift for transfers	1,000–1,375
C4 to C5	Power tilt/recline wheelchair	13,000–18,000
	Manual wheelchair for transport	2,000–4,000
	Lap tray	250–500
	Wheelchair cushion	400–500
	Bedside table	150
	ECU	1,500–6,000
	Fully electric hospital bed	1,500–2,200
	Commode/shower chair	1,300–2,000
	Communication devices	300–1,500
	ADL equipment	300–1,200
	Hydraulic lift for transfers	1,000–1,375
C6	Power upright wheelchair	5,000–7,000
	Manual wheelchair	1,000–3,000
	Wheelchair cushion	400–500
	Bedside table	150
	ECU	1,500–6,000
	Electric hospital bed	1,500–2,200
	Specialized mattress	500–5,000
	Commode/shower chair	1,300
	ADL equipment	300–1,200
	Tenodesis splint	1,500
	Transfer board	80–100
	Hand control for car	500–700
	Bowel/bladder equipment	50–250
	Transfer board	80
C7 to C8	Power upright wheelchair	6,000–8,000
	Manual wheelchair	1,500–2,000
	Wheelchair cushion	400–500
	Bedside table	150
	ECU	200–700
	Electric hospital bed	1,500–2,200
	Specialized mattress	500–5,000
	Commode/shower chair	1,300
	Hand control for car	500–700
	ADL equipment	300–800
	Transfer board	80–100
	Bowel/bladder equipment	50–250
Paraplegia	Manual upright wheelchair	1,800–3,000
	Wheelchair cushion	400–500
	Raised/padded commode seat (cutout)	150
	Tub bench	200
	Hand control for car	500–700
	ADL equipment	100–300
	Bowel/bladder equipment	50–250
	Lower-extremity orthotics (if ambulation is a goal)	2,500–4,000

Based on 1999 Atlanta, GA, retail prices.

precautions, pulmonary management, cardiopulmonary resuscitation, management of autonomic dysreflexia, equipment management and maintenance, transfer techniques, wheelchair mobility, ambulation, proper body positioning, ROM exercises, ADL basics, and leisure skills.

Home programs are taught to maintain or increase strength, endurance, ROM, and function. Energy conservation techniques and proper body mechanics are incorporated into all aspects of training.

Clients are formally tested on their knowledge, and remedial instruction should be provided in deficient areas. During family training, caregivers are formally evaluated on their abilities to safely provide care to the client. Supervised therapeutic outings and passes allow the client, caregivers, and the team to identify problem areas and provide additional education in those areas.

Psychosocial Issues

The immediate reaction to the onset of SCI is physical shock accompanied by anxiety, pain, and fear of dying. The response to such an injury varies greatly and depends on the extent of the injury, premorbid activity level, style of coping with stress, and family and financial resources. There may be great sensory deprivation due to immobilization, neurological impairment, and the monotony of the hospital routine. Several psychological theories have been proposed to describe responses and coping mechanisms.[76] The process of coping with these changes is referred to as adjustment (see Chapter 7).

Rehabilitation personnel are becoming more aware of the need not only to teach functional skills but also to teach psychosocial and coping skills to the client and significant others. Education in the following areas facilitates the adjustment process: creative recreation, financial planning, negotiating community barriers, social skills, managing an attendant, creative problem solving, accessing community resources, fertility and child care options, assertiveness, sexual expression, vocational planning/training, and the use of community transportation. These skills may be introduced in the inpatient rehabilitation setting but will be developed further in the home and community environments. True adjustment and adaptation begin after discharge from rehabilitation.[98, 99]

Sexual Issues

Altered sexual function is of concern to the SCI population.[116] The injury may result in impairment of erection, ejaculation, orgasm, male fertility, and vaginal lubrication.[39] Table 16–6 lists the relationship of level of spinal injury to sexual function. Formal sexual counseling and education are indicated before discharge from a rehabilitation center. The educational program includes group sessions to address general issues as well as individual sexual function evaluations.[116] Sexual counseling, educational programs, and medical management provide opportunities to address the areas of sexual dysfunction, alternative behaviors, precautions, and other related areas.[39]

Treatment of sexual dysfunction is a coordinated effort between the client, significant other, psychologist, and urologist. Options may include surgical implantation of a penile prosthesis, vacuum erection devices, intracorporeal injection therapy, and the use of lubricants.[88] See Selected References at the end of this chapter for additional references regarding sexual function after SCI.

● **T A B L E   1 6 – 6. Relation of Level of Spinal Injury to Sexual Function**

Injury Level	Sexual Function
Cauda equina/conus	Males: 　Usually no reflex erections 　Rare psychogenic erection 　Ejaculation occasionally occurs Females: 　Vaginal secretions often absent 　Patients generally fertile
Thoracic/cervical	Males: 　Reflex erections predominate (usually 　　short duration) 　Psychogenic erections generally absent 　Ejaculation occasional Females: 　Vaginal secretions present as a part of 　　genital reflex 　Fertility preserved 　Sensation of labor pain absent

Discharge Planning

Discharge planning begins from the time the client is admitted and continues through the rehabilitation program. It is a continuous process that includes the client, family, treatment team, and community resources, with the goal being successful community reintegration and a perceived good quality of life. The rehabilitation team must identify the specific needs of the client and structure the program necessary to enhance the chance of success. Lengths of stay are getting shorter in response to pressure from third-party payers to contain costs. This requires the discharge planning process to be expedited so that procurement of needed equipment, completion of architectural modifications, and referrals to outpatient and community resources occur in a timely manner.

Architectural Modifications

Architectural barriers in the home, transportation system, workplace, or school may prevent access to opportunities. The architectural changes required by the person with SCI for independence in the home and community depend on the degree of impairment, financial resources, and client/family acceptance of modifications and/or equipment. The clinician should discuss equipment options with the client/family based on the degree of modification they plan to make to their home.

Many available resources describe the dimensions of the basic wheelchair and specifications for making homes and facilities accessible to wheelchair users. See Selected References at the end of this chapter for resources on architectural modification.

Return to Work or School

Successful reintegration after SCI may include returning to work or school. Public school systems have a legal obligation to provide an appropriate school setting for a disabled child. Less than 25% of individuals with SCI are employed 5 years after injury.[2, 90] Rehabilitation programs must emphasize returning to work throughout the process to improve a client's successful return to work and facilitate adjustment to SCI.

Many individuals can return to their previous jobs after SCI.[5, 65] The Americans with Disabilities Act (ADA) of 1990 (PL 101–336) prohibits businesses with 25 or more employees (effective July 26, 1992) and 14 to 24 employees (effective July 26, 1994) from discriminating against "qualified individuals with disabilities" with respect to the terms, conditions, or privileges of employment.[51] Some situations may require modifications to the job site or a change in responsibilities. For those who are unable to perform previous jobs or who were unemployed before injury, many programs exist for training in vocational skills. The Department of Rehabilitation Services (DRS) evaluates clients for skills and functional abilities and provides funding for those qualifying for job training, job site modification, and the purchase of essential equipment. Services offered by DRS vary from state to state. Each state agency has a list of resources available in the community, such as rehabilitation technology, independent living centers, and job training and placement programs. Individuals should refer to their state DRS for assistance with employment.

Outpatient Referral

When clients are unable to reach all of their goals as inpatients, a referral to an outpatient facility with experience in the treatment of SCI is necessary. The need for referral to outpatient care should be anticipated early in the rehabilitation program so that therapeutic intervention can continue without interruption. An outpatient follow-up appointment should be scheduled before the client's discharge to reevaluate medical and functional status and make any program changes before complications can occur.

OUTPATIENT SERVICES

Discharge from an inpatient rehabilitation program marks only the beginning of the lifelong process of adjustment to disability and community reintegration. Inpatient rehabilitation provides an environment best suited for learning self-care skills, yet "the implications of living in the community with SCI can scarcely be anticipated accurately by the newly injured individual or the able-bodied staff" (p 324).[56] Comprehensive outpatient services have traditionally been available for routine follow-up assessments, medical care, psychological services, vocational planning/training, and continued therapy services.

Common outpatient therapy treatment programs have included advanced transfer training, advanced wheelchair mobility training, gait training, upgraded ADL training, and upgraded home exercise program instruction. Outpatient therapy, however, is used increasingly for functional training, which traditionally was a part of the inpatient rehabilitation. This is a direct result of cost-containment efforts resulting in shortened length of stay. A direct consequence of this shift results in outpatient treatment of clients who present with more acuity, greater care needs, and fewer skills attained in the inpatient rehabilitation program before entry into the outpatient arena.

The "day program" concept has emerged to meet the demand for more cost-saving rehabilitation services. Clients who are medically stable, do not require skilled nursing services during the night, tolerate 3 hours or more of therapy per visit, need a coordinated approach for two or more services, and have a discharge plan in place are good candidates for this type of program. A day program offers the same rehabilitation services as inpatient rehabilitation but is performed in an outpatient setting. It offers more coordinated services than the traditional single-service outpatient programs. The focus is not only on performance of functional skills but also on the transference of these skills into the community.

ADDITIONAL CLINICAL CONSIDERATIONS

Orthoses

SCI splinting and upper-extremity orthotic philosophy remains fairly constant among rehabilitation centers. The evaluation and the rationale for determining the appropriate splint per injury level are agreed upon. One area that has generated debate is how early a splint or orthosis should be fabricated and if permanent orthoses enhance long-term function. Shorter lengths of stay and decreased communication among therapists across the continuum make it difficult to prescribe an orthosis because of time and/or funding. Early splinting for positioning to prevent deformity has proven to be effective with all injury levels (see Table 16–4).

Deformity prevention is the first goal for splinting.[63] Clients with spinal cord injuries may have no innervated musculature in their wrists or hands. Other clients that have some innervation will have muscle imbalances. If the wrist and hand are not supported, function will be limited.

Clients with C1 to C4 tetraplegia require resting hand splints to assist with proper positioning and maintain the support of the wrist and web space (Fig. 16–50).[25] Clients with tetraplegia at the C5 level can be independent with communication, feeding, and hygiene only with the assistance of an orthosis. They must have joint stability and support at the wrist and the hand to perform these skills. Usually the splint will also include a utensil slot or cuff so that the client can effectively perform the just-mentioned skills.

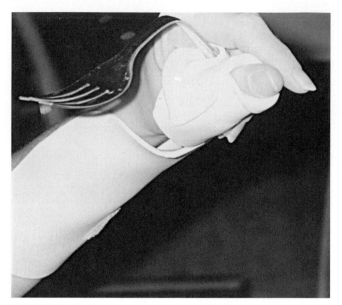

FIGURE 16–51. Long opponens splint with fabricated utensil holder.

As mentioned previously, clients with injuries at the C6 level can use their wrists for a tenodesis grasp.[59, 97, 101] Critical components of the splint assessment for these clients are the positioning of the thumb, web space, and index finger observed during the grasp. Clients who are not splinted may not have the proper positioning to pick up objects because their tenodesis is "too tight" or "too loose." The client may want to have a more defined three-jaw chuck grasp and not be limited to a lateral grasp.[97]

Clients who are not strong enough to use their wrists for tenodesis may require splinting to support their wrists until they can use their wrists against gravity. Long opponens splints can be used to position the thumb for function but support the weak wrist (Fig. 16–51). Once the wrist strengthens, the long opponens splint can be cut down to a hand-based short opponens to maintain proper web space and thumb positioning and maximize tenodesis.

There is controversy over shortening of the flexor tendons. Some clinicians argue that the client can develop a fixed flexion contracture of the proximal interphalangeal joints, which could interfere with future surgical attempts to restore finger function.[25] However, if only used for tenodesis education the splints may be discontinued and the client could resume daily stretching exercises if finger movement is in question.[25]

Clients with C8 to T1 injuries or clients who have incomplete injuries where finger extensor musculature is stronger than finger flexor musculature may experience "clawing."[96, 101] Fabricating a metacarpophalangeal block splint to block the metacarpophalangeal joints and promote weak intrinsic muscle function can prevent this. These splints can be used during function or only worn at night, depending on the extent of the imbalance.

Cost, time, material, and education are important considerations. It may be that a prefabricated splint can be as effective as a splint fabricated in the clinic. Prefabricated splints may not fit the client as well as a splint made by

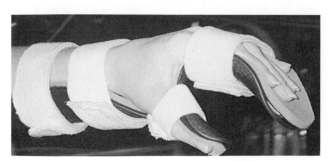

FIGURE 16–50. Resting hand splint.

the clinician. One way to maximize time in fabrication of splints is to use a good pattern and premade straps. Finally, educating the client on the splint-wearing schedule, skin checks, and splint care are very important in preventing skin breakdown.

Studies have not conclusively determined the long-term effects of permanent orthotics. Permanent orthoses are recommended if the client with an SCI has the appropriate funding and if the orthotics will enhance function and/or prevent deformity. In clients with a C6 level of injury, the development of a strong tenodesis pinch through the use of an orthosis may be an acceptable option to surgery if reimbursement is restricted.[34] The future is still uncertain about how proper positioning of extremities through orthoses could open doors for the client using the latest technology.

The philosophy regarding the use of orthoses for ambulation for individuals with complete paraplegia varies greatly among rehabilitation centers. Some facilities encourage ambulation for these individuals, whereas others strongly discourage it, given that only a small percentage of these clients continue to use orthotics after training has been completed.[13, 83]

When the philosophy of the rehabilitation center is to brace clients who are motor complete, criteria should be established so that both the client and the professional staff are consistent in the approach to ambulation. This gives the client specific information and clarifies goals to be attained, ensuring the most positive outcome.

CRITERIA FOR AMBULATION TRIAL

- Expressed desire for ambulation with appropriate goals
- Body weight not to exceed 10% of ideal
- ROM: hip extension 5 degrees, full knee extension, ankle dorsiflexion 5 to 15 degrees, passive straight-leg raise 110 degrees
- Intact skin
- Stable cardiovascular system
- Controlled spasticity
- Independent function at the wheelchair level

The ambulation trial gives the team and the client an opportunity to preview what the use of orthoses will be like. If the decision is made to order orthoses, specific goals are set. Goals range from standing and exercise ambulation to community ambulation. Most persons with complete injuries above the L2 level achieve only exercise ambulation because of the energy necessary for functional ambulation.

According to research performed at Rancho Los Amigos Hospital, the energy cost of ambulation for individuals with complete lesions at T12 or higher is above the anaerobic threshold and cannot be maintained over time. This study also concluded that ambulation for these individuals using a swing-through gait pattern is equivalent to "heavy work" or a variety of recreational and sporting activities.[17, 83] Consequently, it is easy to understand why lower-extremity orthoses may end up in the closet unused.

The energy cost for ambulation is highest for persons with complete paraplegia who use a swing-through gait pattern and lowest for persons who use bilateral ankle-foot orthoses (AFO) or a combination of an AFO and a knee-ankle-foot orthosis (KAFO). Even individuals requiring only bilateral AFOs have a gait efficiency of less than 50% of normal, underscoring the importance of the hip extensor and abductor muscles required for normal ambulation. These muscles are severely or completely paralyzed in this population.

Given intact upper extremities, the energy cost of ambulation is progressively reduced when more residual motor function is present in the lower extremities. Conversely, the person with incomplete tetraplegia has higher energy costs for ambulation despite spared lower-extremity function because of upper- and lower-extremity weakness.[17, 83]

FOUR CATEGORIES OF AMBULATION[29]

1. Standing only
2. Exercise—ambulates short distances
3. Household—ambulates inside home or work, uses wheelchair much of the time
4. Community—independent on all surfaces, does not use the wheelchair

---

LOWER-EXTREMITY ORTHOSES

Hip-Knee-Ankle-Foot Orthoses (HKAFOs)

  Reciprocating gait orthosis (RGO) (Fig. 16–52)

  Bilateral KAFOs with pelvic band

Knee-Ankle-Foot Orthoses

  Scott-Craig KAFOs (Fig. 16–53)

  Conventional KAFOs

  Polypropylene KAFOs (Fig. 16–54)

  New England Rehabilitation KAFOs

Ankle-Foot Orthoses

  Conventional AFOs

  Metal custom polypropylene AFOs

  Solid ankle (Fig. 16–55)

  Custom polypropylene AFOs, articulated ankle (Fig. 16–56)

University of California Biomechanics Lab (UCBL)

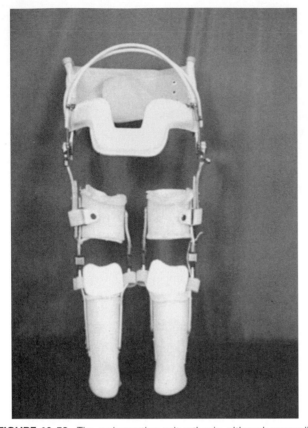

FIGURE 16–52. The reciprocating gait orthosis, although generally used with children, is also used with the adult population. Its main components are a molded pelvic band, thoracic extensions, bilateral hip and knee joints, polypropylene posterior thigh shells and ankle-foot orthosis sections, and cables connecting the two hip joint mechanisms.

Factors that affect brace selection are cost, experience and bias of the clinician, injury level, residual motor function, and client acceptance. Generally, the HKAFO is used when selected motions of the hip need control or benefits of the reciprocating gait orthosis are desired, as is the case with the pediatric population. Use of a KAFO is indicated when the quadriceps muscle strength is less than ⅗. AFOs are indicated in the presence of ankle instability and weakness and to prevent hyperextension of the knee joint. See Table 16–7 for correlation of complete injury levels and orthotic disposition.

Orthotic disposition of clients with incomplete SCI is more challenging owing to the complexity of problems and varying degrees of impairment. These clients may present with pain, ROM limitations, weakness, and spasticity. These problems sometimes preclude ambulation. Asymmetries such as muscle shortening on the stronger side and lengthening on the weaker side may lead to pelvic obliquity and scoliosis. An orthotic team approach is desirable for all orthotic dispositions but is extremely useful and considered a requirement to meet the needs of clients with incomplete SCI. Even if orthotic devices enable these clients to become independent, the energy and joint costs on normal joints and muscles over the life expectancy of each individual need to be considered.

Functional Electrical Stimulation

The NeuroControl Freehand System is an implanted medical device that uses electrical stimulation to replace the brain's original nerve impulses when SCIs interrupt the neural pathway. This system allows clients with tetraplegia to regain the use of their paralyzed hands by using neural prosthetics with conventional reconstructive hand surgery. The system was approved by the Food and Drug Administration (FDA) in 1997. The system enables appropriately selected clients with SCI (C5–C6) to flex and extend the thumb, fingers, and elbow, allowing a useful pinch and grasp. Clients who otherwise required equipment to perform ADL can now perform these same skills with no equipment, using their own hands. Electrodes are attached to muscles in the hands and forearms, and a pacemaker-type stimulator is surgically implanted in the chest. Signals come from the stimulator to the electrodes and cause muscles to contract and the hand to open and close. Externally, a transmitting coil is worn on the skin and the client uses simple shoulder movements to initiate hand function through a shoulder position sensor. An external controller is attached to the wheelchair as the power supply.

The application of FES for standing and stepping is referred to as neuroprosthetics. Initial work using surface

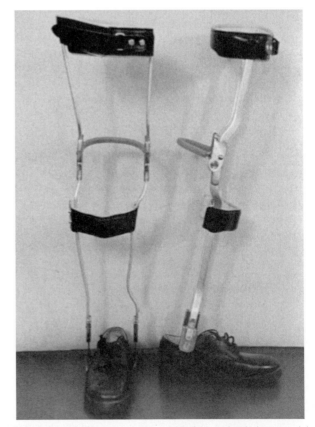

FIGURE 16–53. Scott-Craig knee-ankle-foot orthosis is a special design for spinal cord injury. The orthosis consists of double uprights, offset knee joints with pawl locks and bail control, one posterior thigh band, a hinged anterior tibial band, an ankle joint with anterior and posterior adjustable pin stops, a cushion heel, and specially designed longitudinal and transverse foot plates made of steel.

T A B L E   1 6 – 7. Correlation of Complete Injury Levels and Orthotic Disposition

Injury Level	Muscles Present	Orthoses	Goals	Bracing Recommended
Above T2	Partial upper-extremity function	Standing frames RGOs	Standing ?? Exercise ambulatory	No
T2 to T6	Complete upper-extremity function	Standing frames RGOs KAFOs w/spreader bar	Standing ? Exercise ambulatory	No
T7 to T10	Partial function of trunk muscles	RGOs KAFOs w/spreader bar	Standing Exercise ambulatory	
T11 to T12	Almost complete function of trunk	RGOs KAFOs w/spreader bar	Exercise ambulatory	Sometimes
L1	Complete trunk function	RGOs KAFOs w/spreader bar	Exercise ambulatory Sometimes household	Usually
L2	Hip flexors	KAFOs	Exercise ambulatory Household ambulatory	Usually
L3	Quadriceps	Combination KAFO/AFO Bil. AFOs	Household ambulatory Community ambulatory	Yes
L4 and below	Quadriceps Partial hamstrings Partial ankle Partial hips	AFOs UCBL	Community ambulatory	Yes

electrodes was performed in the 1970s and 1980s.[64] Principles developed by Slovenian investigators have formed the foundation for most of the ongoing research in this field.[82, 100] The first system to gain FDA approval was the Parastep II system developed by Sigmedic, Inc.[100]

These types of systems generally use 2 to 12 channels of stimulations. The system in its simplest form places one set of electrodes over the quadriceps muscle and another set over the sural, saphenous, or peroneal nerve. The systems consist of a computer control box, lead wire, electrodes, and a cable connected to a walking device that houses the command switch(es) for step function.

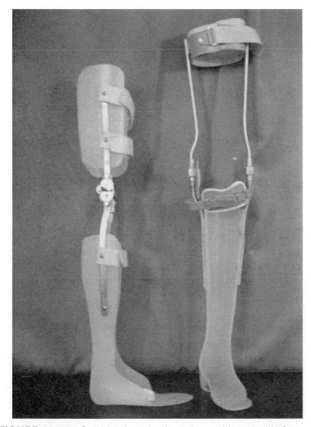

FIGURE 16–54. Combination plastic and metal knee-ankle-foot orthoses.

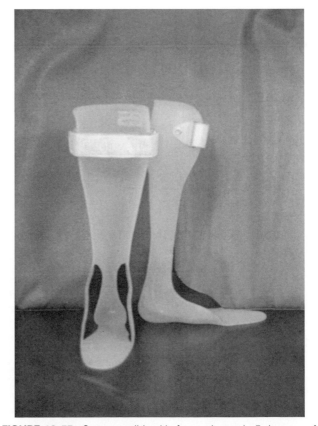

FIGURE 16–55. Custom solid ankle-foot orthoses in 5 degrees of dorsiflexion with full footplates.

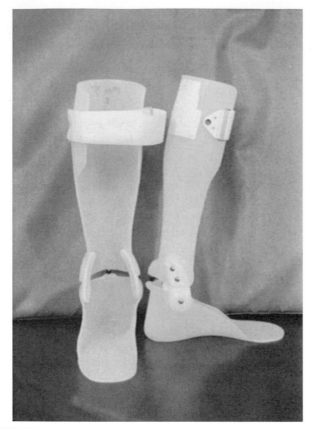

FIGURE 16–56. Custom articulated ankle-knee orthoses with adjustable Oklahoma ankle joints.

Other systems that use implanted electrodes are being investigated at this time, but none are FDA approved. The most promising work is being done at the Veterans Administration Medical Center and Case Western Reserve University in Cleveland. Both FES systems, the surface electrode system and the implanted system, in their present state show promise for the future. However, these systems currently do not present a viable alternative to wheelchair use because of the high-energy requirement.[100]

Hybrid FES orthosis systems are orthotic systems that incorporate FES. Usually the FES is a simple configuration of approximately four channels and uses surface stimulation. One such system is utilized with the RGO and was developed by Roy Douglass and Associates at the Louisiana State University Medical School. Systems such as this offer the advantage of increased energy efficiency when compared with the use of only orthoses or only FES. Conversely, the bulkiness of the systems impedes the completion of some ADL, and donning and doffing is more difficult.[96, 100] (See Chapter 28 for additional information on electrical stimulation intervention and Chapter 31 on orthotics.)

Seating Principles

Many individuals spend 8 hours or more per day in their wheelchairs after SCI. Consequently, proper seating of these clients may be the most important intervention

clinicians provide. The seating process should be addressed on admission, continually throughout the rehabilitation program, and regularly after discharge to help prevent and minimize complications.[41, 66] The wheelchair is an integral part of the client's self-image and in many ways will help define personal lifestyle.[81] Goals for seating the client with SCI are identified in the following box.

GOALS FOR SEATING THE CLIENT WITH SCI

1. Maximize functional independence
2. Optimize pressure distribution and relief of pressure
3. Optimize comfort
4. Enhance the quality of life
5. Optimize good postural alignment
6. Compensate for fixed deformities
7. Maximize ease of transportation of the seating system

The following are basic seating concepts of proper postural alignment:

Neutral pelvic alignment

Symmetrical alignment of the trunk and neck

Neutral head positioning over the pelvis

Maintenance of a horizontal gaze

Maintenance of a 90-degree angle at the hips, knees, and ankles

Maintenance of the thighs in neutral abduction

Neutral shoulder positioning to avoid shoulder elevation, protraction, or retraction and to provide adequate upper-extremity support.[66, 115]

Every seating session begins with a thorough examination, as described earlier. Trial simulations are essential to determine how the client will function and maintain posture over time in the seating system. Simulations help to avoid costly mistakes. The client must be involved in the decision-making process to ensure that the seating system will work.

The seating process may be complicated by impairment or loss of sensation and mobility. Great care must be taken to reduce pressure over bony prominences and to distribute pressure over as large an area as possible.[66] Presure-relieving cushions should be evaluated clinically and with pressure-sensing devices to determine the optimal wheelchair cushion for each individual.[66, 115]

Many clients with muscle paralysis of the trunk find that the effects of gravity in a sitting position pull their heads over their laps, resulting in a long kyphosis or a C-curved posture (Fig. 16–57).[115] Two resulting problems are increased weight-bearing on the bony sacrum and

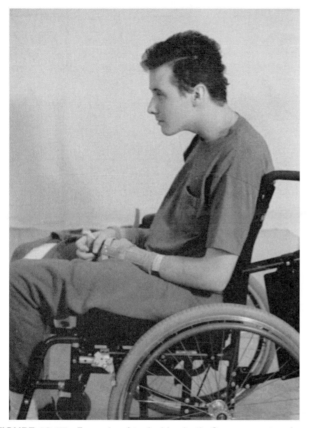

FIGURE 16–57. Example of typical kyphotic C-curve posture in the patient with tetraplegia.

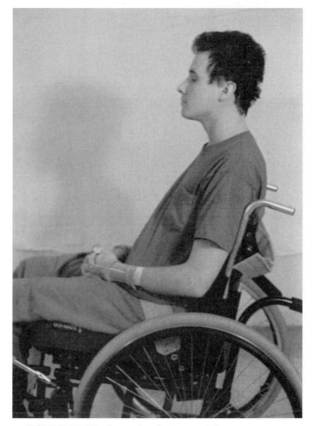

FIGURE 16–58. Example of corrected C-curve posture.

development of a thoracic kyphosis, leading to neck hyperextension in an effort to maintain a horizontal gaze.[4] Unfortunately, this poor seating posture is quickly learned and difficult to correct.[7] This posture can often be prevented by tilting the wheelchair slightly backward while maintaining a fixed seat-to-back angle (Fig. 16–58).[66] In that position, the effects of gravity augment sitting balance and facilitate good spinal alignment. The use of a sacral block, a firm wheelchair seat and back, and properly applied seat belts also aid in preventing the C-curved posture.[66]

Asymmetrical muscle strength, asymmetrical spasticity, and power wheelchair propulsion using predominantly one upper extremity often result in poor trunk alignment. The use of lateral trunk supports and lateral thigh bolsters combined, with properly applied seat belts and shoulder harnesses, may aid in maintaining symmetrical trunk posture.

Strong muscle spasms, combined with the effects of gravity, may cause the person with severely impaired mobility to slide down in the wheelchair, resulting in increased pressure on the sacrum and shearing of the skin. For these clients, a wheelchair with a fixed seat-to-back angle that tilts backward to allow for the performance of pressure relief may help to reduce this problem (Fig. 16–59).

The size, weight, and portability of the seating system affect the individual's lifestyle. The client's home or work environment must be evaluated closely for accessibility so

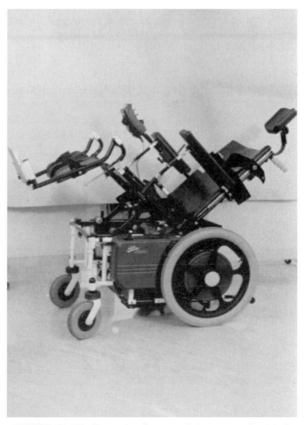

FIGURE 16–59. Example of power-tilt-in-space wheelchair.

CASE 16–1   C5–C6 Fracture

The client, a 24-year-old man, was drag racing while unrestrained on a country road. He had consumed several beers and lost control of his car. The car rolled several times and he was thrown approximately 20 feet from the vehicle. When the emergency medical services personnel arrived at the scene, the client was conscious and complaining of neck pain. He had a laceration across the left temporal area. A cervical collar was applied, and he was placed on a spine board for transportation to the closest emergency medical center.

On arrival, the client was reevaluated and the head laceration was cleaned and stitched. The physician ordered radiographs of the spine, skull, and chest, which revealed a C5–C6 fracture/subluxation and rib fractures laterally at ribs 4, 5, and 6 on the left; a skull fracture was ruled out. Physical examination revealed the following: client awake and alert, absent deep tendon reflexes (indicative of spinal shock), absent sensation below the nipple line, and no volitional movement in the upper or lower extremities except for shoulder shrugs and elbow flexion.

Within 2 hours of the initial injury, methylprednisolone, 30 mg/kg, was administered intravenously. Additional emergency department treatment consisted of starting an intravenous catheter, inserting a Foley catheter, administering oxygen by means of a nasal cannula, and continuing immobilization in the cervical collar. Arrangements were made for transfer to a model SCI center.

On admission to the SCI center, the client was taken to the intensive care unit and evaluated by the attending physician. Confirmation of the previously established C5 motor level was made, and the sensory picture had improved, with impaired light touch present in the lower extremities and sacral dermatomes. The diagnosis of incomplete C5 tetraplegia was determined. The client was immediately placed in cervical traction via Gardner-Wells tongs and was transferred to the computed tomographic (CT) scanner for imaging of the abdomen, cervical spine, and skull. CT scans of the skull and the abdomen were negative. CT scans of the cervical spine and the chest confirmed the initial diagnosis of fractures. A decision was made to manage the client with external fixation using halo traction. The client was placed on deep vein thrombosis prophylaxis, and the methylprednisolone protocol was continued.

Referrals were made to the rehabilitation team, including dietary services, occupational therapy, physical therapy, psychological services, respiratory therapy, social services, speech therapy, therapeutic recreation, and vocational counseling. The nursing staff initiated strict turning times with appropriate padding and positioning to prevent pressure ulcers and pulmonary complications.

All team members made initial contact with the client within 2 days of admission. The therapy evaluations were completed within 24 hours of admission and revealed the following neurological findings: the biceps and wrist extensors were 5/5; the triceps were a trace bilaterally; all other key muscles of the upper extremity were absent; a strong isometric contraction was noted in the trunk musculature (unable to fully test secondary to the halo vest; the hip flexor and extensor muscles were 2/5; knee extensors were 3/5; knee flexors were 1/5; ankle dorsiflexors were 1/5 bilaterally. The motor neurological level was C6 bilaterally, and the ASIA impairment scale had improved to a classification of C (incomplete motor).

The client's vital capacity was 1200 mL, and he complained of left chest wall pain during inspiration. His cough was weak but productive. There was evidence of spasticity with sustained clonus in the right ankle. The Ashworth score was 2 on the left and 3 on the right. Initial treatment consisted of ROM exercises, deep breathing exercises, and a positioning program to prevent adaptive shortening. Out-of-bed orders were received on day 3 and inpatient rehabilitation began when the client tolerated 3 hours of therapy daily. All team members established rehabilitation goals with the client and family.

As the client's rehabilitation progressed, functional strength of the triceps returned and weak hand intrinsics were noted. The lower extremities improved to functional strength on the left side; on the right there was weakness in the gluteal, hip flexor, and ankle musculature. He had normal bowel function. The client's bladder program was self-voiding; however, he performed intermittent catheterization for residual volume checks using a short opponens brace with a pincer grasp to assist.

The client was prescribed a rental hemiheight manual wheelchair in the seating clinic and was modified independent with propulsion on smooth surfaces and over rough terrain. He was evaluated in the brace clinic and began gait training on the parallel bars with the use of a right KAFO. He was independent in all transfers. The client required minimal assistance in meal preparation and was able to eat using utensils with built-up handles. He was able to dress his upper and lower extremities using a button hook and zipper pull. He was modified independent in all grooming and bathing skills. A tub bench was necessary during bathing to address balance and endurance deficits, and a long-handled sponge allowed access to hard-to-reach areas. The client was modified independent in written communication skills with adapted writing equipment (built-up pens/pencils or short Wanchik splint). A driving evaluation was completed, and the client was able to drive with minor modifications. The psychologist counseled the client and his wife on sexuality and sexual functioning.

Continued

CASE 16–1   C5–C6 Fracture *Continued*

The home assessment was completed and recommendations were made to accommodate the wheelchair yet leave flexibility for increased ambulation function. The client's work site, a car repair business, was also evaluated to ensure accessibility and safety. At the time of discharge from inpatient rehabilitation, the client was unable to perform his preinjury work duties as an auto mechanic because of hand weakness and the inability to lift heavy objects. The case manager contacted the vocational rehabilitation counselor to investigate other work opportunities at the client's present place of employment. Although the client's personal goal was to return to his previous duties, he would require a vocational evaluation following outpatient rehabilitation to determine the appropriateness of this goal.

At the time of discharge, the client and his family had completed family training and demonstrated appropriately the performance of all functional skills. The physical and occupational therapist provided the client with home exercise programs specific to his strengthening needs. The therapeutic recreation specialist enrolled him in a fitness program. Physical and occupational therapy outpatient referrals were made for gait and balance training, endurance training, upper-extremity strengthening to become independent in all ADL skills, and hand rehabilitation.

After 6 weeks of outpatient therapy, the client's endurance and balance had improved, allowing full-time ambulation. The rental wheelchair was discontinued. The client was discharged from outpatient physical therapy with a revised home exercise program. The patient had achieved independence with all dressing and grooming skills. He could complete home management skills with modified independence and planned to continue only with hand rehabilitation. Follow-up assessments from all other team members occurred at 8 weeks after discharge from inpatient rehabilitation. He was scheduled for a 6-month evaluation to determine his return to work goals.

---

that the seating system can be used effectively in those environments. The buildings must be structurally sound and spacious to accommodate heavy power wheelchair systems. The means of transportation of the wheelchair (car vs. van) determines whether a fixed or folding wheelchair frame is indicated and possibly whether a portable power wheelchair is the best choice.

The wheelchair must be as easy as possible to propel to reduce stress on upper-extremity joints. Many manual wheelchairs are lightweight (less than 35 pounds) and have multiple adjustments and choices of tires and casters that make manual wheelchair propulsion more efficient. The correct rear tire size reduces shoulder musculature fatigue. Rear tire size should be selected so that when the wheelchair user is seated with hands resting on the top of the push rims, there is 60 degrees of elbow flexion and no shoulder elevation.[16] In addition, shifting the distribution of the user's weight back over the rear axle (usually accomplished by moving the rear wheel axle forward) reduces the percentage of weight on the front casters, making propulsion more efficient.[16]

Distributing pressure over as large a surface area as possible without endangering function should be considered when taking wheelchair measurements. The width of the seat (wheelchairs are made with the same seat and back width) should be slightly more than that of the widest body part. The seat depth should come to within 1 inch of the popliteal fossae. The height of the back should reflect the client's motor function and be no lower than the presence of functional musculature to provide appropriate trunk support. If the back height is too high, it can restrict functional activities such as wheelchair propulsion and wheelies. Clients with tetraplegia who use the push handles of the wheelchair to hook while performing functional activities may require custom modification of the wheelchair back (Fig. 16–60).

Finally, the impact of the wheelchair on the individual's self-image must be considered. The entire focus of the rehabilitation process is successful community reintegration. An attractive seating system is an integral tool for the client's success.

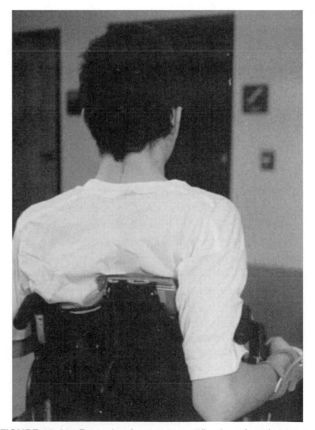

FIGURE 16–60. Example of custom modification of a wheelchair back to allow a patient with tetraplegia to hook the push handle with one upper extremity.

CONCLUSION

Comprehensive treatment of the individual with SCI continues to be a challenge to the rehabilitation team and to society as a whole. Health care reform issues force the rehabilitation team to explore new cost-efficient options to provide quality rehabilitation. New medical interventions improve the prognosis for return of function to a greater extent for the incomplete versus complete lesions. Additionally, the aging of this population presents new problems that require intervention and cause the team to examine past rehabilitation goals and treatment strategies. Passage of the ADA points out that community reintegration of individuals with disabilities is a responsibility of society. These and other issues will present many challenges for individuals with SCI in the future.

REFERENCES

1. Abruzzesse R: Pressure sores: Nursing aspects and prevention. In Lee B, et al (eds): The Spinal Cord Injured Patient: Comprehensive Management. Philadelphia, WB Saunders, 1991.
2. Annual reports 9 and 10 for the Model Spinal Cord Injury Care Systems, The National Spinal Cord Injury Statistical Center, University of Alabama, Birmingham, AL, 1992.
3. Apple DF, Hudson LM, (eds): Spinal cord injury: The model. In Proceedings of the National Consensus Conference on Catastrophic Illness and Injury—the Spinal Cord Injury Model: Lessons Learned and New Applications, December 1989. Atlanta, The Georgia Regional Spinal Cord Injury Care System, Shepherd Spinal Center, 1990.
4. Atrice M, et al: Acute physical therapy management of individuals with spinal cord injury. Orthop Clin North Am 2:53–70, 1993.
5. Axelson P, et al: Spinal Cord Injury: A Guide for Patient and Family. New York, Raven Press, 1987.
6. Bach JR: New approaches in the rehabilitation of the traumatic high level quadriplegic. Am J Phys Med Rehabil 70:13–19, 1991.
7. Banwell JG, et al: Management of the neurogenic bowel in patients with spinal cord injury. Urol Clin North Am 20:517–525, 1993.
8. Bergstrom N, Bennett MA, Carlson, et al: Pressure Ulcer Treatment. Clinical Practice Guideline. Quick Reference Guide for Clinicians, No. 15. Rockville, MD, US Department of Health and Human Services, Public Health Service, Agency for Health Care Policy and Research. AHCPR publication No. 95-0653. December 1994.
9. Biering-Sorensen M, Biering-Sorensen F: Tracheostomy in spinal cord injured: Frequency and follow up. Paraplegia 30:656–660, 1992.
10. Bloch RF: Autonomic dysfunction. In Bloch RF, Basbaum M (eds): Management of spinal cord injuries. Baltimore, Williams & Wilkins, 1986.
11. Bosch A, et al: Incomplete traumatic quadriplegia: A 10-year review. JAMA 216:473–478, 1971.
12. Bracken MB: Pharmacological treatment of acute spinal cord injury: Current status and future projects. J Emerg Med 2:43–48, 1993.
13. Bromley I: Rehabilitation: Some thoughts on progress. Paraplegia 30:70–72, 1992.
14. Brown DJ: Spinal cord injuries: The last decade and the next. Paraplegia 30:77–82, 1992.
15. Brownledd S, Williams S: Physiotherapy in the respiratory care of patients with high spinal injury. Physiotherapy 73:3, 1987.
16. Brubaker C: Ergonometric considerations. JRRD 2(suppl):37–48, March 1990.
17. Bunch W, et al: Atlas of Orthotics: Biomechanical Principles and Application, 2nd ed. St. Louis, CV Mosby, 1985.
18. Carter RE: Medical management of pulmonary complications of spinal cord injury. Adv Neurol 22:261–269, 1979.
19. CCH Business Law (ed): Medicare and Medicaid Guide 1993. Chicago, Commerce Clearing House, 1993.
20. Cervical Spine Research Society: The Cervical Spine, 2nd ed. Philadelphia, JB Lippincott, 1989.
21. Clough P, et al: Guidelines for routine respiratory care of patients with spinal cord injury. Phys Ther 66:1395–1402, 1986.
22. Coffey RJ, et al: Intrathecal baclofen for intractable spasticity of spinal origin: Results of a long-term multicenter study. J Neurosurg 78:226–232, 1993.
23. Crane LD: Functional anatomy and physiology of ventilation. In Zadai CC (ed): Clinics in Physical Therapy: Pulmonary Management in Physical Therapy. New York, Churchill Livingstone, 1992.
24. Curry K, Casady L: The relationship between extended periods of immobility and decubitus ulcer formation in the acutely spinal cord injured individual. J Neurosci Nurs 24(4):185–189, 1992.
25. Curtin M: Development of a tetraplegic hand assessment and splinting protocol. Paraplegia 32:159–169, 1994.
26. Cusick BD: Serial Casts. Tuscon, AR, Therapy Skill Builders, 1988.
27. Daniels L, Worthingham C: Muscle Testing: Techniques of Manual Examination, 5th ed. Philadelphia, WB Saunders, 1986.
28. De Troyer A, Estenne M: Review article: The expiratory muscles in tetraplegia. Paraplegia 29:359–363, 1991.
29. Decker M, Hall A: Physical therapy in spinal cord injury. In Bloch RF, Basbaum M (eds): Management of Spinal Cord Injury. Baltimore, Williams & Wilkins, 1986.
30. DeLisa JA, Martin GM, Currie DM: Rehabilitation medicine: past, present, and future. In DeLisa JA (ed): Rehabilitation Medicine: Principles and Practice. Philadelphia, JB Lippincott, 1988.
30a. Derrickson J, et al: A comparison of two breathing exercise programs for patients with quadriplegia. Phys Ther 72(11):763–769, 1992.
31. DeVivo MJ, Black KJ, Stover SL: Causes of death during the first 12 years after spinal cord injury. Arch Phys Med Rehabil 74:248–254, 1993.
32. DeVivo MJ, et al: Spinal cord injury rehabilitation adds life to years. West J Med 154(S):602–606, 1991.
33. DeVivo MJ, et al: Trends in spinal cord injury demographics and treatment outcomes between 1973 and 1986. Arch Phys Med Rehabil 73:424–430, 1992.
34. DiPasquale-Lehnerz P: Orthotic intervention for development of hand function with C6 quadriplegia. Am J Occup Ther 48:138–143, 1994.
35. Dollfus P: Rehabilitation following injury to the spinal cord. J Emerg Med 11:57–61, 1993.
36. Donovan WH, Bedbrook G: Comprehensive management of spinal cord injury. Clin Symp 34:2, 1992.
37. Donovan WH, Cutler HW: Traumatic spinal injuries: Cervical, thoracic, lumbar. In Hochschuler SH, Cutler HB, Guyer RD (eds): Rehabilitation of the Spine: Science and Practice. St. Louis, CV Mosby, 1993.
38. Donovan WH, et al: Incidence of medical complications in spinal cord injury: Patients in specialized compared with nonspecialized centers. Paraplegia 22:282–290, 1984.
39. Ducharme S, et al: Sexual functioning: Medical and psychological aspects. In DeLisa JA (ed): Rehabilitation Medicine: Principles and Practice. Philadelphia, JB Lippincott, 1988.
40. Errico TJ, Bauer RD: Spinal Trauma. Philadelphia, JB Lippincott, 1991.
41. Finkbeiner K, Russo SG (eds): Physical Therapy Management of Spinal Cord Injury: Accent on Independence. Fisherville, VA, Woodrow Wilson Rehabilitation Center Project SCIENTIA, 1990.
42. Frost FS: Role of rehabilitation after spinal cord injury. Urol Clin North Am 20:549–559, 1993.
43. Frymoyer JW: The Adult Spine—Principles and Practice, vol 2. New York, Raven Press, 1983.
44. Garland DE, et al: Osteoporosis after spinal cord injury. J Orthop Res 10:371–378, 1992.
45. Geisler FH: GM-1 ganglioside and motor recovery following human spinal cord injury. J Emerg Med 2:49–55, 1993.
46. Geisler FH, Dorsey FC, Coleman PW: Recovery of motor function after spinal cord injury: A randomized, placebo-controlled trial with GM-1 ganglioside. N Engl J Med 324:1829–1838, 1993.
47. Giffin J, Grush K: Spinal cord injury treatment and the anesthesiologist. In Lee B, et al (eds): The Spinal Cord Injured Patient: Comprehensive Management. Philadelphia, WB Saunders, 1991.
48. Glaser RM: Physiological responses to maximal effort wheelchair and arm ergometry. J Appl Physiol 48:1060–1064, 1980.

49. Green D, et al: Deep vein thrombosis in spinal cord injury: Summary and recommendations. Chest 102:633S–635S, 1992.

50. Grenvik A, et al (eds): Mechanical Ventilation and Assisted Respiration: Contemporary Management in Critical Care. New York, Churchill Livingstone, 1991.

51. Gross GR: What your company could be doing now to implement Title I of the ADA. Small Business News, May 1992.

52. Guide to Physical Therapy Practice. Alexandria, VA, American Physical Therapy Association, 1997.

53. Hall ED: The neuroprotective pharmacology of methylprednisolone: A review article. J Neurosurg 56:106–113, 1982.

54. Hall ED, Wolf DL, Baughler JM: Effects of a single large dose of methylprednisolone sodium succinate on experimental post traumatic spinal cord ischemia—dose response and time-action analysis. J Neurosurg 61:124–130, 1984.

55. Hamilton BB, Fuhrer MJ: Rehabilitation outcomes: Analysis and measurement. Baltimore, Brooks, 1987.

56. Hammell KR: Psychological and sociological theories concerning adjustment to traumatic spinal cord injury: The implication for rehabilitation. Paraplegia 30:317–326, 1992.

57. Hanak M, Scott A: Spinal Cord Injury: An Illustrated Guide for Healthcare Professionals. New York, Springer Publishing Co, 1983.

58. Heinemann AW, et al: Functional outcome following spinal cord injury: A comparison of specialized spinal cord injury centers vs general hospital acute care. Arch Neurol 46:52–59, 1989.

59. Hill JP: Spinal Cord Injury: A Guide to Functional Outcomes in Occupational Therapy. Rockville, MD, Aspen Publishers, 1986.

60. Katz RT, et al: Objective quantification of spastic hypertonia: Correlation with clinical findings. Arch Phys Med Rehabil 73:339–347, 1992.

61. Kendall FP, McCreary EK: Muscle Testing and Function, 4th ed. Baltimore, Williams & Wilkins, 1993.

62. Kraft C: Bladder and bowel management. In Buchanan LE, Nawoczenski DA (eds): Spinal Cord Injury: Concepts and Management Approaches. Baltimore, Williams & Wilkins, 1987, pp 81–98.

63. Krajnick SR, Bridle MJ: Hand splinting in quadriplegia: Current practice. Am J Occup Ther 46:149–156, 1992.

64. Kral A, Bajd T: Functional electrical stimulation: Standing and walking after spinal cord injury. Boca Raton, FL: CRC Press, 1989.

65. Krause JS, Kjorsvig JM: Mortality after spinal cord injury: A four-year prospective study. Arch Phys Med Rehabil 73:558–563, 1992.

66. Kreutz DL: Seating and positioning for the newly injured. Rehab Management, December 1993, pp 67–75.

67. Krouskop T: The role of mattresses and beds in preventing pressure sores. In Lee B, et al (eds): The Spinal Cord Injured Patient: Comprehensive Management. Philadelphia, WB Saunders, 1991.

68. Lee B: Deep vein thrombosis. In Lee B, et al (eds): The Spinal Cord Injured Patient: Comprehensive Management. Philadelphia, WB Saunders, 1991.

69. Lehmkuhl LD, et al: Multimodality treatment of joint contractures in patients with severe brain injury: Cost, effectiveness, and integration of therapies in the application of serial/inhibitive casts. J Head Trauma Rehabil 5(4):23–42, 1990.

70. Lewis KS, Mueller WM: Intrathecal baclofen for severe spasticity secondary to spinal cord injury. Ann Pharmacother 27:767–774, 1993.

71. Luce JM, Culver BH: Respiratory muscle function in health and disease. Chest 81(1):82–90, 1982.

72. McCool FD, et al: Changes in lung volume and rib cage configuration and abdominal binding in quadriplegia. J Appl Physiol 60:1198–1202, 1986.

73. Madsen B, Barth P, Vistnes L: Pressure sores: Overview. In Lee B, et al (eds): The Spinal Cord Injured Patient: Comprehensive Management. Philadelphia, WB Saunders, 1991.

74. Mammen EF: Pathogenesis of venous thrombosis. Chest 102:640S–644S, 1992.

75. Mariano AJ: Chronic pain and spinal cord injury. Clin J Pain 8(2):87–92, 1992.

76. Mawson AR, et al: Risk factors for early occurring pressure ulcers following spinal cord injury. Am J Phys Med Rehabil 67:123–127, 1988.

77. Merli GJ, et al: Mechanical plus pharmacological prophylaxis for deep vein thrombosis in acute spinal cord injury. Paraplegia 30:558–562, 1992.

78. Meyer RR: Surgery of Spine Trauma. New York, Churchill Livingstone, 1989.

79. Morgan M, Silver J: The respiratory system of the spinal cord patient. In Bloch RF, Basbaum M (eds): Management of Spinal Cord Injuries. Baltimore, Williams & Wilkins, 1986.

80. Nickel VL: The rationale and rewards of team care. In Nickel VL, Botte MJ (eds): Orthopaedic Rehabilitation, 2nd ed. New York, Churchill Livingstone, 1992.

81. Nixon V: Spinal Cord Injury: A Guide to Functional Outcomes in Physical Therapy Management. Rockville, MD, Aspen Systems Corporation, 1985.

82. O'Keefe M: Walking programs—rehab or razzle dazzle? Spinal Network Extra, Winter 34–40, 1992.

83. Perry J: Gait Analysis: Normal and Pathological Function. Thorofare, NJ, Slack, 1992.

84. Rinehart M, Nawoczenski D: Respiratory Care. In Buchanan L, Nawoczenski D (eds): Spinal Cord Injury: Concepts and Management Approaches. Baltimore, Williams & Wilkins, 1987.

85. Ryan M, Klein S, Bongard F: Missed injuries associated with spinal cord trauma. Am Surg 59:371–374, 1993.

86. Seaton T, Hollingworth R: Gastrointestinal complications in spinal cord injury. In Bloch RF, Basbaum M (eds): Management of Spinal Cord Injuries. Baltimore, Williams & Wilkins, 1986.

87. Shepherd AM, Blannin JP: The role of the nurse. In Mandelstam D (ed): Incontinence and its management, 2nd ed. Dover, NH, Croom Helm, 1986, pp 160–163.

88. Smith EM, Bodner DR: Sexual dysfunction after spinal cord injury. Urol Clin North Am 20:535–541, 1993.

89. Somers MF: Spinal Cord Injury: Functional Rehabilitation. East Norwalk, CT, Appleton & Lange, 1992.

90. Spinal Cord Injury: Facts and Figures at a Glance. Birmingham, AL, University of Alabama, National Spinal Cord Injury Statistical Center, 1990.

91. Standards for Neurological and Functional Classification of Spinal Cord Injury, Ditunno JF, chairman. Chicago, American Spinal Injury Association, revised 1996.

92. Standards Manual for Organizations Serving People with Disabilities. Tucson, AR, Commission on Accreditation of Rehabilitation Facilities, 1993.

93. Stover SL, DeLisa IA, Whiteneck GG: Spinal cord injury: Clinical outcomes from the model systems. Gaithersburg, MD, Aspen Publications, 1995.

94. Stover SL: Functional independence. Arch Phys Med Rehabil 70:509, 1989.

95. Stover SL: Heterotopic ossification after spinal cord injury. In Bloch RF, Bashaum M (eds): Management of Spinal Cord Injuries. Baltimore, Williams & Wilkins, 1986.

96. Sykes L, Campbell IG, Powell ES, et al: Energy expenditure of walking for adult patients with spinal cord lesions using the reciprocating gait orthosis and functional electrical stimulation. Spinal Cord 34:659–665, 1996.

97. Tenney CG, Lisa JM: Atlas of Hand Splinting. Boston, Little, Brown & Co, 1986.

98. Trieschmann RB: Psychosocial research in spinal cord injury: The state of the art. Paraplegia 30:58–60, 1992.

99. Trieschmann RB: Spinal Cord Injuries: Psychological, Social and Vocational Rehabilitation, 2nd ed. New York, Demos Publications, 1988.

100. Triolo RJ, Bogie K: Lower extremity application of functional neuromuscular stimulation after spinal cord injury. Topics Spinal Cord Injury Rehabil 5(1):44–65, 1995.

101. Trombly CA: Occupational Therapy for Physical Dysfunction. Boston, Boston University, Sargent College of Allied Professions, 1995.

102. Vincken W, Corne L: Improved arterial oxygenation by diaphragmatic pacing in quadriplegia. Crit Care Med 15:872–873, 1987.

103. Weingarden SI: Deep vein thrombosis in spinal cord injury: Overview of the problem. Chest 102:636S–639S, 1992.

104. West JB: Pulmonary Pathophysiology: The Essentials, 4th ed. Baltimore, Williams & Wilkins, 1992.

105. Wetzell JL, et al: Respiratory rehabilitation of the patient with a spinal cord injury. In Irwin S, Tecklin JS (eds): Cardiopulmonary Physical Therapy, 2nd ed. St. Louis, CV Mosby, 1990.

106. White AH, Rothman RH, Ray CD: Lumbar Spine Surgery Techniques and Complications. St. Louis, CV Mosby, 1987.

107. Whiteneck GG, et al: Mortality, morbidity, and psychosocial outcomes of persons spinal cord injured more than 20 years ago. Paraplegia 30:617–630, 1992.

108. Wittenberg RH, Peschke U, Botel U: Heterotopic ossification after spinal cord injury. J Bone Joint Surg Br 74:215–218, 1992.
109. Yarkony G: Spinal cord injury rehabilitation. In Lee B, et al (eds): The Spinal Cord Injured Patient: Comprehensive Management. Philadelphia, WB Saunders, 1991.
110. Yashon D: Spinal Injury, 2nd ed. Norwalk, Conn, Appleton-Century-Crofts, 1986.
111. Young JS, Northrup NE: Statistical information pertaining to some of the most commonly asked questions about SCI (monograph). Phoenix, AR, National Spinal Cord Injury Data Research Center, 1979.
112. Young R, Shahani B: Spasticity in spinal cord injured patients. In Bloch RF, Basbaum M (eds): Management of Spinal Cord Injuries. Baltimore, Williams & Wilkins, 1986.
113. Young RR, Delwaide PJ: Drug therapy, spasticity. New Engl J Med 304:28–33, 1981.
114. Young W, Flamm ES: Effect of high-dose corticosteroid therapy on blood flow, evoked potentials, and extracellular calcium in experimental spinal injury. J Neurosurg 57:667–673, 1982.
115. Zarcharkow D: Wheelchair Posture and Pressure Sores. Springfield, IL, Charles C Thomas, 1984.
116. Zigler JE: Rehabilitation of acute spinal cord injury. In Hochschuler SH, Cotler HB, Guyer RD (eds): Rehabilitation of the Spine: Science and Practice. St. Louis, CV Mosby, 1993.

SELECTED REFERENCES

Sexual Issues

Althof SE, Levine SB: Clinical approach to the sexuality of patients with spinal cord injury. Urol Clin North Am 20:527–534, 1993.
Berard EJ: The sexuality of spinal cord injured women physiology and pathophysiology: A review. Paraplegia 27(2):99–112, 1989.
Charlifue SW, et al: Sexual issues of women with spinal cord injuries. Paraplegia 30(3):192–199, 1992.
Drench ME: Impact of altered sexuality and sexual function in spinal cord injury: A review. Sex Disabil 10(1):3–14, 1992.
Farrow J: Sexuality counseling with clients who have spinal cord injuries. Rehabil Couns Bull 33:251–259, 1990.
Kettl P, et al: Female sexuality after spinal cord injury. Sex Disabil 9:287–295, 1991.
Lemon MA: Sexual counseling and spinal cord injury. Sex Disabil 11:73–97, 1993.
Lloyd LK, Richards JS: Medical and psychological considerations regarding the surgical or pharmacological treatment of impotence in males with spinal cord injury. J Rehabil Res Dev 28:419–420, 1991.
Nygaard I, Bartscht KD, Cole S: Sexuality and reproduction in spinal cord injured women. Obstet Gynecol Surg 45:727–732, 1990.
Robbins KH: Traumatic spinal cord injury and its impact upon sexuality. J Appl Rehabil Couns 16:24–27, 1985.
Sipski ML, Alexander CJ: Sexual activities, response and satisfaction in women pre- and post-spinal cord injury. Arch Phys Med Rehabil 74:1025–1029, 1993.
Tepper MS: Sexual education in spinal cord injury rehabilitation: Current trends and recommendations. Sex Disabil 10(1):15–31, 1992.
Trieschmann RB: Spinal cord injuries: Psychological, Social, and Vocational Rehabilitation, 2nd ed. New York, Demos Publications, 1988.
White MJ, et al: Sexual activities, concerns and interests of men with spinal-cord injury. Am J Phys Med Rehabil 71:225–231, 1992.

Architectural Modification

Accessibility in Georgia: A Technical and Policy Guide to Access in Georgia. Raleigh, NC, Georgia Council on Developmental Disabilities, 1986.
An Accessible Bathroom. Madison, WI, Design Coalition, 1980.
An Accessible Entrance: Ramps. Madison, WI, Design Coalition, 1979.
Handbook for Design: Specially Adapted Housing. VA pamphlet 26–13. Washington, DC, Department of Veterans Benefits, Veterans Administration, April 1978.
Harber L, et al: UFAS Retrofit Guide: Accessibility Modifications for Existing Buildings. New York, Van Nostrand Reinhold, 1993.
Lebrock C, Behar S: Beautiful Barrier-Free, A Visual Guide to Accessibility. New York, Van Nostrand Reinhold, 1993.
Mace RL: The Accessible Housing Design File. New York, Van Nostrand Reinhold, 1991.

CHAPTER 17

Inflammatory and Infectious Disorders of the Brain

REBECCA E. PORTER, PhD, PT

Key Words

- brain abscess
- encephalitis
- functional activities
- hypertonicity
- hypotonicity
- intervention goals
- meningitis
- postural control

Objectives

After reading this chapter the student/therapist will:

1. Understand the terminology for classifying different types of inflammatory and infectious disorders within the brain.

2. Discuss the range of neurological sequelae that occur.

3. Discuss the components of the comprehensive evaluation process and their interrelationships.

4. Structure the evaluation process to gather the information required to generate an intervention plan.

5. Discuss the general goals of the intervention process.

6. Plan the intervention process to meet the needs of the client.

7. Locate resources (both within this book and in other sources) to assist with ideas for the intervention program.

The diversity of neurological sequelae that may occur after an inflammatory disorder in the brain (brain abscess, encephalitis, or meningitis) provides a range of challenges to the rehabilitation team. The therapist must identify the problems underlying the individual's movement dysfunctions without the template of the cluster of "typical" problems available with some other neurological diagnoses. Each client presents a combination of problems that is unique to that client and that requires the creative design of an intervention program. The following discussion of the therapeutic management of individuals recovering from an inflammatory disorder in the brain focuses on the process of designing an intervention plan to address the specific dysfunctions of the individual client. Because the management of the clinical problems is built on an understanding of the underlying pathology and because therapists may not be as familiar with these disease processes, an overview of the inflammatory disorders of the brain is presented.

OVERVIEW OF INFLAMMATORY DISORDERS IN THE BRAIN

Categorization of Inflammatory Disorders

Inflammatory disorders of the brain can be categorized based on the anatomical location of the inflammatory process and the cause of the infection, as shown below:

A. Brain abscess
B. Meningitis (leptomeningitis)
  1. Bacterial meningitis

2. Aseptic meningitis (viral)
C. Encephalitis
  1. Acute viral
  2. Parainfectious encephalomyelitis
  3. Acute toxic encephalopathy
  4. Progressive viral encephalitis
  5. "Slow virus" encephalitis

In most individuals the defense mechanisms of the central nervous system (CNS) provide protection from infecting organisms. Compromises of the protective barriers can result in CNS infections as complications of common infections. The response of the CNS to the infection depends on several factors, including the type of organism, its route of entry, the CNS location of the infection, and the immunological competence of the individual. CNS infections occur with greater frequency and severity in individuals who are very young or elderly, immunodeficient, or antibody deficient.

The inflammatory process may be a localized, circumscribed collection of pus; may involve primarily the leptomeninges; may involve the brain substance; or may involve both the meninges and the brain substance. The infecting agents may be bacterial, fungal, viral, protozoan, or parasitic. The most common agents producing meningitis are bacterial; the most common agents producing encephalitis are viral. However, bacterial encephalitis and viral meningitis also are disease entities. The following overview of the inflammatory processes within the brain is organized based on the anatomical location of the infection. More comprehensive discussions based on specific infecting organisms can be found in the references at the end of the chapter. The site of the infection will determine the signs and symptoms of the CNS infections whereas the infecting organism determines the time course and severity of the problems.[9]

Brain Abscess

Brain abscesses occur when microorganisms reach brain tissue from a penetrating wound to the brain, by extension of local infection such as sinusitis or otitis, or by hematogenous spread from a distant site of infection. The route of infection influences the CNS region involved. The extension of a local infection tends to produce a solitary brain abscess in an adjacent lobe. Multiple abscesses may originate from the spread of microorganisms through the blood. The introduction of microorganisms by a penetrating trauma may result in an abscess soon after the trauma or several years later. As with the disorders presented in the subsequent discussions, circumstances that result in a compromised immune system (chronic corticosteroid or other immunosuppressive drug administration, administration of cytotoxic chemotherapeutic agents, or human immunodefiency virus [HIV] infection) may predispose the individual to develop opportunistic infections.

Whereas the site and size of the abscess influence the initial symptoms, evidence of increased intracranial pressure, a focal neurological deficit, and fever is described as the classic presenting triad[4]; however, the classic triad occurs in less than 50% of patients.[13] Most individuals experience an alteration of consciousness. In 47% of the cases, the frontal, parietal, or temporal lobe is involved.[13] Medical management of the abscess typically consists of antibiotic therapy (depending on the infecting agent and size and site of the abscess) and, often, surgical aspiration or excision. Bharucha and others[4] describe neurological sequelae in 25% to 50% of the survivors, with 30% to 50% having persistent seizures, 15% to 30% with hemiparesis, and 10% to 20% with disorders of speech or language.

Meningitis

Meningitis (synonymous with leptomeningitis) denotes an infection spread through the cerebrospinal fluid (CSF) with the inflammatory process involving the pia and arachnoid maters, the subarachnoid space, and the adjacent superficial tissues of the brain and spinal cord. Pachymeningitis denotes an inflammatory process involving the dura mater. Meningitis can be caused by a wide variety of organisms, some of which cross the blood-brain barrier and the blood-CSF barrier. The CSF can also become contaminated by a wound that penetrates the meninges as a result of trauma or a medical procedure such as implantation of a ventriculoperitoneal shunt. Once the organism compromises the blood-brain and blood-CSF barriers, the CSF provides an ideal medium for growth. All of the body's typical major defense systems are essentially absent in the normal CSF. The blood-brain barrier may impede the clearance of infecting organisms by leukocytes and interfere with the entry of pharmacological agents from the blood. The infecting organism is disseminated throughout the subarachnoid space as the contaminated CSF bathes the brain. Entry into the ventricles occurs either from the choroid plexuses or by reflux through the exit foramen of the fourth ventricle. The spread of the organism through the CSF circulation accounts for the differences in the variety and extent of the neurological sequelae that can result from meningitis.

Bacterial Meningitis

Clinical Problems. The diagnostic categorization of meningitis depends on the infecting agent (e.g., *Haemophilus influenzae* meningitis, *Streptococcus pneumoniae* meningitis, and viral meningitis) and on the acute or chronic nature of the meningitis (acute, subacute, or chronic meningitis). The term *acute bacterial meningitis* denotes infections caused by aerobic bacteria (both gram-positive and gram-negative).[34] The most common infecting organism producing acute bacterial meningitis varies according to the age of the population. During the neonatal period and in the older adult, infections by gram-negative enterobacilli, especially *Escherichia coli*, and group B streptococci occur most frequently. Typical causative agents in children include *H. influenzae, Neisseria meningitidis,* and *S. pneumonia.*[23] *S. pneumoniae, N. meningitidis,* and *H. influenzae* are the most common causes of community-acquired meningitis.[23, 24] Individuals with conditions such as sickle cell anemia, alcoholism, or diabetes mellitus and individuals who are immunosuppressed are at increased risk.[10]

An example of an organism that uses a typical systemic

route of bacterial infection is the *H. influenzae* organism that is a normal flora of the nose and throat. During an upper respiratory tract infection, the organism may gain entry to the blood. The route of transmission of the organism from the blood to the CSF is not well established.

The circulation of CSF spreads the infecting organism through the ventricular system and the subarachnoid spaces. The pia and arachnoid maters become acutely inflamed, and as part of the inflammatory response a purulent exudate forms in the subarachnoid space. The exudate may undergo organization, resulting in an obstruction of the foramen of Monro, the aqueduct of Sylvius, or the exit foramen of the fourth ventricle. The supracortical subarachnoid spaces proximal to the arachnoid villi may be obliterated, resulting in a noncommunicating or obstructive hydrocephalus as a result of the accumulation of CSF. As the CSF accumulates, the intracranial pressure rises. The increased intracranial pressure produces venous obstruction, precipitating a further increase in the intracranial pressure. The rise in the CSF pressure compromises the cerebral blood flow, which activates reflex mechanisms to counteract the decreased cerebral blood flow by raising the systemic blood pressure. An increased systemic blood pressure accompanies increased CSF pressure.

The mechanism producing the headaches that accompany increased intracranial pressure may be the stretching of the meninges and pain fibers associated with blood vessels. Vomiting may occur as a result of stimulation of the medullary emetic centers. Papilledema may occur as intracranial pressure increases.

Other routes of bacterial infection may involve a local spread as the result of an infection of the middle ear or mastoid air cells. Meningitis may occur as a complication of a skull fracture, which exposes CNS tissue to the external environment or to the nasal cavity. Fractures of the cribriform plate of the ethmoid bone producing CSF rhinorrhea provide another route for infection. Meningitis may be a further complication to the clinical problems of a traumatic head injury (see Chapter 14).

Clinical features of acute bacterial meningitis include fever, severe headache, altered consciousness, convulsions (particularly in children), and nuchal rigidity. Nuchal rigidity is indicative of an irritative lesion of the subarachnoid space. Cervical flexion is painful because it stretches the inflamed meninges, nerve roots, and spinal cord. The pain triggers a reflex spasm of the neck extensors to splint the area against further cervical flexion; however, cervical rotation and extension movements remain relatively free.

Several clinical tests are utilized to demonstrate nuchal rigidity. The Kernig test consists of flexion of the cervical area with the client supine. Signs of pain indicate a positive test.[16] The Kernig sign refers to a test performed with the client supine in which the thigh is flexed on the abdomen and the knee extended. This pulls on the sciatic nerve, which pulls on the covering of the spinal cord, causing pain in the presence of meningeal irritation. The same results are achieved with passive hip flexion with the knee remaining in extension. This is the same procedure described by Hoppenfeld[16] as the straight-leg raising test for determining pathology of the sciatic nerve or tightness

of the hamstrings. Passive hip flexion with knee extension can be painful because of meningeal irritation, spinal root impingement, sciatic nerve pathology, or hamstring tightness. Roos advocates performing the test for the Kernig sign with the individual sitting.[23] The Brudzinski sign refers to the flexion of the hips and knees elicited when cervical flexion (the Kernig test in supine) is performed.[23] These signs will not be present in the deeply comatose client who has decreased muscle tone and absence of muscle reflexes. The signs may also be absent in the infant or elderly patient.

The diagnosis of bacterial meningitis can be established based on blood cultures and a sample of CSF obtained by a lumbar puncture. CSF pressure is consistently elevated. The CSF sample in bacterial meningitis typically reveals an increased protein count and a decreased glucose level.

The type and severity of the sequelae of acute bacterial meningitis relate directly to the area affected, the extent of CNS infection, the age and general health of the individual, the level of consciousness at the initiation of pharmacological therapy, and the pathological agent involved. Some of the common CNS complications include subdural effusions, altered levels of consciousness, seizures, involvement of the cranial nerves, and increased intracranial pressure.

Medical Management. Medical management of bacterial meningitis consists of the initiation of the antimicrobial regimen appropriate to the infecting organism and procedures to manage the signs and symptoms of meningitis that have been described in the preceding paragraphs. Medical intervention strategies in both these areas change with the development of new pharmacological agents. The reader is encouraged to review recent literature for additional information on current aspects of the medical management of the client with meningitis.

Potential Neurological Sequelae. Even with optimal antimicrobial therapy, bacterial meningitis continues to have a finite mortality rate, which varies with the infecting organism, age of the individual, and time lapse to initiation of treatment, and has the potential for marked neurological morbidity. Neurological sequelae occur in 20% to 50% of the cases.[10] Bacterial meningitis is considered a medical emergency; delays in initiation of antibacterial therapy increase the risk of complications and permanent neurological dysfunction.[10]

Reports of the long-term outcome of individuals with bacterial meningitis indicate that up to 20% of them have long-term neurological sequelae.[4] The sequelae may be the result of the acute infectious pathological condition or subacute or chronic pathological changes. The acute infectious pathological condition could result in sequelae such as inflammatory or vascular involvement of the cranial nerves or thrombosis of the meningeal veins. Cranial nerve palsies, especially sensorineural hearing loss, are common complications. The risk of an acute ischemic stroke is greatest during the first 5 days.[10] Weeks to months after treatment, subacute or chronic pathological changes may develop, such as communicating hydrocephalus, which presents as difficulties with gait, mental status changes, and incontinence.[22] Approximately 5% of the survivors will have weakness and spasticity.[34] Focal cerebral signs that may occur either early or late in the course of bacterial meningitis include hemiparesis, ataxia, seizures, cranial nerve palsies, and gaze preference.[26]

Damage to the cerebral cortex can result in numerous expressions of dysfunction. Motor system dysfunction may be the observable expression of the damage within the CNS, but the location of the damage may include sensory and processing areas as well as those areas typically categorized as belonging to the motor system. Perceptual deficits or regression in cognitive skills may present residual problems. Cranial nerve involvement is most frequently expressed as dysfunction of the eighth cranial nerve complex and produces auditory and vestibular deficits.

Aseptic Meningitis

Aseptic meningitis refers to a nonpurulent inflammatory process confined to the meninges and choroid plexus usually caused by contamination of the CSF with a viral agent, although other agents can trigger the reactions. The symptoms are similar to acute bacterial meningitis but typically are less severe. The individual may be irritable, lethargic, and complain of a headache, but cerebral function remains normal unless unusual complications occur.[14] Aseptic meningitis of a viral origin usually has a benign and relatively short course of illness.[3, 18]

A variety of neurotropic viruses can produce aseptic (viral) meningitis. The enteroviruses (echoviruses and the coxsackieviruses), herpesviruses and HIV are the most common causes.[23, 25] The primary nonviral causes of aseptic meningitis are Lyme *Borrelia* and *Leptospira*.[27] The diagnosis of this type of aseptic meningitis may be established by isolation of the infecting agent within the CSF or by other techniques. Although the glucose level of the CSF in bacterial meningitis is usually depressed, the glucose level in viral meningitis is normal.[9]

Treatment of aseptic meningitis consists of management of symptoms. The condition does not typically produce residual neurological sequelae, and full recovery is anticipated within a few days to a few weeks.

Encephalitis

Clinical Problems. Encephalitis refers to a group of diseases characterized by inflammation of the parenchyma of the brain and its surrounding meninges. Although a variety of agents can produce an encephalitis, the term usually denotes a viral invasion of the cells of the brain and spinal cord.

Different cell populations within the CNS vary in their susceptibility to infection by a specific virus. (For example, the viruses responsible for poliomyelitis have a selective affinity for the motor neurons of the brain stem and spinal cord. Viruses such as coxsackieviruses and echoviruses typically infect meningeal cells to cause the benign viral meningitis discussed in the previous section.) In acute encephalitis, neurons that are vulnerable to the specific virus are invaded and undergo lysis. Viral encephalitis presents a syndrome of elevated temperature, headache, nuchal rigidity, vomiting, and general malaise

(symptoms of aseptic or viral meningitis) with the addition of evidence of more extensive cerebral damage such as coma, cranial nerve palsy, hemiplegia, involuntary movements, or ataxia. The difficulty in differentiating between acute viral meningitis and acute viral encephalitis is reflected in the use of the term *meningoencephalitis* in some cases.

The pathological condition includes destruction or damage to neurons and glial cells resulting from invasion of the cells by the virus, the presence of intranuclear inclusion bodies, edema, and inflammation of the brain and spinal cord. Perivascular cuffing by polymorphonuclear leukocytes and lymphocytes may occur as well as angiitis of small blood vessels. Widespread destruction of the white matter by the inflammatory process and by the thrombosis of the perforating vessels can occur. Increased intracranial pressure, which can result from the cerebral edema and vascular damage, presents the potential for a transtentorial herniation. The likelihood of residual impairment of neurological functions depends on the infecting viral agent. Patients with mumps meningoencephalitis have an excellent prognosis, whereas 55% of the individuals with herpes simplex encephalitis treated with acyclovir have some neurological sequelae.[34] Because of the slow recovery of injured brain tissue, even in patients who recover completely, return to normal function may take months.[8]

Plum and Posner[21] discuss viral encephalitis in terms of five pathological syndromes. Acute viral encephalitis is a primary or exclusively CNS infection. An example would be herpes simplex encephalitis, in which the virus shows a predilection for the gray matter of the temporal lobe, insula, cingulate gyrus, and inferior frontal lobe. Also included are the mosquito-borne viruses. Parainfectious encephalomyelitis is associated with viral infections such as measles, mumps, or varicella. Acute toxic encephalopathy denotes an encephalitis that occurs during the course of a systemic infection with a common virus. The clinical symptoms are produced by the cerebral edema in acute toxic encephalopathy, which results in increased intracranial pressure and the risk of transtentorial herniation. Reye's syndrome is an example. Global neurological signs such as hemiplegia or aphasia are usually present rather than focal signs. The clinical symptoms of the previous three syndromes may be very similar. Specific diagnosis may be established only by biopsy or autopsy.

Progressive viral infections occur from common viruses invading susceptible individuals, such as those who are immunosuppressed or during the perinatal to early childhood period. Slow, progressive destruction of the CNS occurs as in subacute sclerosing panencephalitis. The final category of encephalitis syndromes consists of "slow virus" infections by unconventional agents (the prion diseases) that produce progressive dementing diseases such as Creutzfeldt-Jakob disease and kuru.[20]

Medical Management. The medical management of virally induced encephalitis has been, and with many infecting agents remains, primarily symptomatic. In some cases, intensive, aggressive care is necessary to sustain life. Pharmacological interventions are available to treat some viral infections, such as herpes encephalitis. The probability of neurological sequelae differs according to the infecting agent. Aggressive management of increased intracranial pressure is required because persistently elevated intracranial pressure is associated with poor outcome.[29] Further information concerning the clinical features, medical management, and potential for neurological sequelae of a specific type of encephalitis should be sought in the literature based on the infecting agent.

Clinical Picture of the Individual with Inflammatory Disorders of the Brain

An individual within the acute phase of meningitis or encephalitis or with residual neurologic dysfunction from these disorders may demonstrate signs and symptoms similar to generalized brain trauma, tumor disorder, or other identified abnormal neurological state. The variability in the clinical picture is reflected in the inclusion of the category of "infectious diseases that affect the central nervous system" in the *Guide to Physical Therapist Practice*: pattern A (Impaired Motor Function and Sensory Integrity Associated with Congenital or Acquired Disorders of the Central Nervous System in Infancy, Childhood, and Adolescence), pattern B (Impaired Motor Function and Sensory Integrity Associated with Acquired Nonprogressive Disorders of the Central Nervous System in Adulthood), and pattern G (Impaired Arousal, Range of Motion, Sensory Integrity, and Motor Control Associated with Coma, or Vegetative State).[15]

In the acute phase, the inflammatory process may result in impairments in arousal and attention, which range from an individual who is nonresponsive to an individual who is in an agitated state. The degree of agitation may range from mild to severe depending both on the client's unique CNS characteristics and on the degree of inflammation. The agitated state may be the result of alterations in the processing of sensory input, with the consequence of inappropriate or augmented responses to sensory input. The client may respond to a normal level of sound as though it were an unbearably loud noise. Low levels of artificial light may be perceived as extremely bright.

Perceptual and cognitive impairments may be present, resulting in a variety of functional limitations and disabilities. Clients may have distortions in their perception of events as well as memory problems. As their memory returns, accuracy of time and events may be distorted, leading to frustration and anxiety for both the client and those family and friends who are interacting within the environment.

In addition to alterations in mentation, the individual may demonstrate impaired affect such as a hypersensitivity or exaggerated emotional responses to seemingly normal interactions. For example, when upset about dropping a spoon on the floor, a client may throw the tray across the table. When another individual was told his girlfriend would be a little late for her afternoon visit, the client became extremely upset and stated his intent to kill himself because his girlfriend did not love him anymore.

Because of the variety of pathological problems after acute inflammation, the client may have residual problems manifested as generalized or focal brain damage.

The specifics of these impairments cannot be described as a typical clinical picture because they are extremely dependent on the individual client. These variations require the therapist to conduct a thorough examination and evaluation process to develop an appropriate individualized intervention program. Although content from the *Guide to Physical Therapist Practice* has been incorporated into the discussion of the examination, evaluation, and intervention processes, the model presented provides a structure that can accommodate the specific disciplinary expertise of both occupational and physical therapists.

EXAMINATION AND EVALUATION PROCESS

Just as the medical intervention with clients who have an inflammatory disorder of the CNS is, to a large extent, symptomatic, so is the intervention by therapists. Designing an individualized intervention program based on the client's problems necessitates a comprehensive initial and ongoing evaluation to define the impairments, functional limitations, and disabilities and to note changes in them. Although the discussion of examination procedures is separated from the discussion of intervention strategies, it must be recognized that the separation is artificial and does not reflect the image of practice. The evaluation process should be considered in relationship to both the long-term assessment of the individual's changes and the short-term within-session and between-session variations. For example, documentation of the level of consciousness of a client on day one of intervention will provide a starting point for calculation of the distance spanned at the time of discharge. Perhaps more critical to the final outcome is determination of the level of consciousness before, during, and after a particular intervention technique to determine its impact on the individual's level of arousal and ability to interact with the environment. The evaluation process is a constant activity intertwined with intervention. The observations and data from the process are periodically recorded to establish the course of the disease process and the success of the therapeutic management of the client.

Observation of Current Functional Status

The evaluation process should be conceptualized as a decision-making tree that requires the therapist to actively determine which components are to be included in a detailed examination and which can be eliminated or deferred. The first step in this process is the observation of the client's current functional status. If the client is comatose and nonmobile, the focus of the initial session might be an assessment of the stability of physiological functions, level of consciousness, responses to sensory input, and joint mobility. If the client is an outpatient with motor control deficits, the initial session might focus on defining motor abilities and components contributing to movement dysfunctions with a more superficial assessment of physiological functions and level of consciousness. The therapist must be alert to indications of the need for a more detailed evaluation of perceptual and cognitive function (e.g., the client cannot follow two-step commands, indicating the need to assess cognitive skills).

Some of the components discussed in the evaluation process may be assessment skills that are more typically possessed by other professions (e.g., assessment of emotional/psychological status). The inclusion of these items is not meant to suggest that the therapist must complete the formal testing. The items are included to indicate factors that will affect goal setting for the client and that will have an impact on the intervention strategy. Although the therapist may not be the health care team member who has primary responsibility for evaluation of these areas, he or she should recognize these areas as potential contributors to movement dysfunctions.

Observation of the current functional status of the client provides the therapist with an initial overview of the client's assets and deficits. This provides the framework into which the pieces of information from the evaluation of specific aspects of function can be fit. The therapist must not allow assumptions made during the initial observation to bias later observations. The therapist might note that the client is able to roll from the supine to the side-lying position to interact with visitors in the room. When the same activity is not repeated on the mat table in the treatment area, the therapist, knowing the client has the motor skill to roll, might conclude that the client is uncooperative, or apraxic, or has perceptual deficits. The therapist may have failed to consider that the difference between the two situations is the type of support surface or the presence or absence of side rails, which may have enabled the client to roll in bed by pulling over to the side-lying position. It is characteristic of human observation skills that we tend to "see" what we expect to see. The therapist must attempt to observe behaviors and note potential explanations for deviations from normal without biasing the results of the subsequent observations.

The following discussion of the specific considerations within the evaluation process does not necessarily represent the temporal sequence to be used during the examination data collection process. As different items are discussed, suggestions for potential combinations of items will be made. The sequence of the process is best determined by the interaction of therapist and client. Figure 17–1 outlines the components that should be considered during the evaluation process and provides a synopsis of the following discussion.

Evaluation of Physiological Responses to Therapeutic Activities

It is assumed that the therapist enters the initial interaction with a client after reviewing the available background information. This may provide the therapist with information on the baseline status of the client's vital physiological functions. Any control problems in these areas should be particularly noted. Until the therapist determines that the vital functions such as rate of respiration, heart rate, and blood pressure vary appropriately with the demands of the intervention process, these factors should be moni-

tored. The monitoring process should include consideration of the baseline rate, rate during exercise, and time to return to baseline. The pattern of respiration and changes in that pattern also should be noted.

Other tests and measures of the status of ventilation, respiration, and circulation may be indicated in specific individuals. Individuals with limited mobility or motor control of the trunk or individuals with cranial nerve dysfunctions may demonstrate difficulty with functions such as moving secretions out of the airways. Inactivity during a prolonged recovery period may result in cardiovascular adaptations that compromise endurance and contribute to increases in the perceived exertion during activities.

Autonomic nervous system dysfunctions may be expressed as inappropriate accommodations to positional changes such as orthostatic hypotension. Clients with depressed levels of consciousness may display temperature regulation dysfunctions. One mechanism for assessing the client's ability to maintain a homeostatic temperature is to review the nursing notes. The events surrounding any periods of diaphoresis should be examined. If no causative factors have been identified, then interventions, which involve thermal agents as discussed in Chapter 4, should be used judiciously.

Evaluation of Cognitive Status

Because the evaluation process encompasses the stages of recovery from the critical acute phase through discharge from therapy, a range of aspects are included under the evaluation of cognitive status. As indicated previously, the observation of current functional status will direct the therapist toward the appropriate component tests and measures.

Acute bacterial meningitis and various forms of viral encephalitis may result in changes in the client's level of consciousness. *Consciousness* is a state of awareness of one's self and one's environment.[21] *Coma* can be defined as a state in which one does not open the eyes, obey commands, or utter recognizable words.[17] The individual does not respond to external stimuli or to internal needs. The term *vegetative state* is sometimes used to indicate the status of individuals who open their eyes and display a sleep-wake cycle but who do not obey commands or utter recognizable words. DeMeyer[11] presents a succinct description of the neuroanatomy of consciousness and the neurological examination of the unconscious patient. Plum and Posner[21] also provide extensive information in this area.

Several scales have been developed to provide objective guidelines to assess alterations in the state of consciousness. Jennett and Teasdale[17] developed the Glasgow Coma Scale, which assesses three independent items— eye opening, motor performance, and verbal performance. The scale yields a figure between 3 (lowest) and 15 (highest) that can be used to indicate changes in the individual's state of consciousness (see Chapter 14). The evaluation format is simple, and the scale demonstrates both interrater and intrarater reliability. The therapist can use assessment tools such as the Glasgow Coma Scale to determine if the intervention program has resulted in any

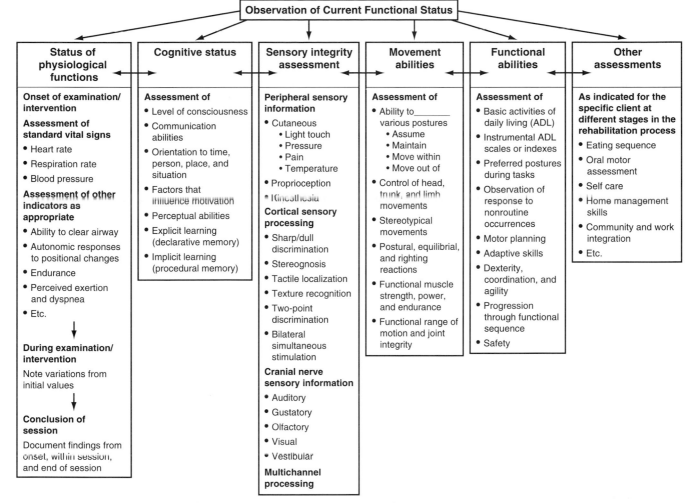

FIGURE 17–1. Flow chart of components of the evaluation process.

recordable changes in the client's level of consciousness. Ideally, the client with decreased levels of consciousness will be monitored at consistent intervals to determine changes in status. Any carryover or delayed effects of the intervention could then be noted. The record of the client's level of consciousness might also display a pattern of peak awareness at a particular point in the day. Scheduling an intervention session during the client's peak awareness time may maximize the benefit of the therapy.

In conjunction with the assessment of the client's state of consciousness is the determination of the individual's orientation to person, time, place, and situation. Because the individual's level of orientation (documented as oriented times 3 for person, time, and place) is frequently recorded by multiple members of the rehabilitation team, the information in the medical chart may provide insights into fluctuations over the course of a day or a week.

Gross assessment of the individual's ability to communicate—both the expressive and receptive aspects of the process—is an important component of the examination. If a dysfunction is present in the client's ability to communicate, the client should be evaluated by an individual with expertise in this area so that strategies for dealing with the communication deficit can be developed. Evaluation of the movement abilities of the client with

communication deficits requires creative planning on the part of the therapist but usually can be accomplished if generalized movement tasks are used. With the client who cannot comprehend a verbal command to roll, the therapist should use an alternate form of communication such as manual cueing or guidance. The therapist could structure the situation to elicit the desired behavior by activities such as placing the client in an uncomfortable position or positioning a desired object so that it can be reached only by rolling.

As the therapist progresses through the examination and intervention process, ongoing data collection should be occurring on factors that influence the motivation of the individual. Individuals with damage to certain areas within the frontal lobe will have difficulty with committing to long-term projects and may not be motivated to work during an individual therapy session by an explanation detailing the relationship of the current activity to the larger goal of returning home. In these situations, the therapist must discover appropriate immediate rewards such as a 2-minute rest break after completion of a specific movement task.

Deficits in cognition may be evident as problems in the area of explicit (declarative) or implicit (procedural) learning. Explicit learning is used in the acquisition of knowledge that is consciously recalled. This is information that can be verbalized in declarative sentences such as the sequential listing of the steps in a movement sequence. Implicit or procedural learning is used in the process of acquiring movement sequences that are performed automatically without conscious attention to the performance. Procedural learning occurs through repetitions of the movement task. Because explicit and implicit learning utilize different neuroanatomical circuits, implicit learning can occur in the individuals with deficits in the components underlying explicit learning (awareness, attention, higher-order cognitive processes).

The emotional and psychological aspects of the client as discussed in Chapter 7 and the higher-order cognitive and retention skills of the client should be evaluated informally by the therapist, with referral to appropriate professionals if dysfunction in these areas is suspected. A coordinated team approach is necessary for clients with emotional and psychological, cognitive, perceptual, or communication problems or a combination of these problems. A consistent strategy used by all team members eliminates the necessity of the client to try to cope with different approaches by different people in an area in which he or she already has a deficit. The impact of cognitive deficits on the process of learning motor skills is further discussed in the next section on movement assessment. The assessment of the impact of perceptual dysfunctions is incorporated within the evaluation of sensory channels.

Evaluation of Sensory Channel Integrity and Processing

The examination process must include an assessment of the channels for sensory input. Knowledge gained in the assessment of the sensory systems will be used in the program-planning process to select the intervention strategies that have the highest probability of success. Although movements can be performed (and in some cases even learned) in the absence of typical sensory feedback, the presence of altered sensory function creates more challenges for both the client/learner and the therapist/teacher. The therapist assesses both the client's ability to perceive the sensory stimulus and the appropriateness of the response to the stimulus. Tactile input could result in an appropriate activation of underlying muscles or a maladaptive increase of muscle activity in a stereotyped distribution.

Variations in the interpretation of sensory input may occur in some clients. Gentle tactile contact may be perceived by the person as a noxious input. Some individuals will have difficulty processing and discriminating information with high levels of one type of sensory input (e.g., the noisy clinic area) or with multiple simultaneous inputs (e.g., talking to the therapist while walking down a hallway with people moving toward the individual). The therapist should be alert to indications of substitution of sensory feedback channels. The client with impaired proprioception tends to compensate through the use of visual information. Although this compensation may be functional within the constraints of isolated tasks, prob-

lems arise when vision is required to monitor other items such as objects in the walking path.

During the evaluation process, the therapist must note the sensory inputs that elicit maladaptive behaviors so that these inputs can be either avoided within the intervention sequence or appropriately incorporated to progress toward an adaptive response.

The therapist should develop a systematic approach to the initial cursory screen of the sensory systems. Deficits identified in the initial examination will provide structure for scheduling more comprehensive evaluation of deficits in specific systems. The therapist must also monitor changes in the status of physiological vital functions during sensory input, especially if the client has a history of instability of heart rate, blood pressure, or rate of respiration.

Based on the information from the screen, the therapist will organize the components of the more detailed examination. Components to be considered include the integrity of the peripheral sensory circuits, the cortical level processing of the sensory information, the integrity of the cranial nerve sensory circuits, and the processing of multichannel input.

Cutaneous input has several aspects that must be assessed. Some of the inflammatory diseases of the brain may result in cutaneous distributions in which sensation is absent or diminished. These areas should be routinely evaluated for changes in distribution of level of sensation. Tests of light touch, pressure, and pain can be used if the client can communicate reliably. In most cases, inclusion of assessment of differentiation of hot and cold will not add appreciably to the information needed for treatment planning unless thermal modalities are a consideration.

A gross assessment of the intactness of the touch system can be made in the noncommunicative client by introducing a mildly adversive (not painful) stimulus, such as a light scratch, while monitoring the client for changes in facial expression, posture, or tonus. The possibility of a spinal-level reflex response should be kept in mind when interpreting the results of such a gross assessment.

Assessment of the client's response to proprioceptive input is incorporated within the assessment of the client's movement abilities and is intertwined with the intervention process because a variety of intervention techniques are based on proprioceptive input (see Chapter 4). Evaluation of the proprioceptive channels can be conducted through assessment of the client's static position sense and dynamic kinesthesis. These tests allow the therapist to make inferences concerning the client's cognitive abilities to interpret proprioceptive information. Inherent in the successful completion of these tests is the necessity for the client to be able to understand directions and to be able to communicate data to the therapist. Because information input, processing, and output are involved in these tests, failure to comply with the test instructions cannot be definitively attributed to dysfunction of the proprioceptive system. The therapist also should consider information obtained from watching the client move before drawing a conclusion concerning the intactness of the proprioceptive channels. Some of the factors to consider include disregard of an extremity and variations in quality of performance between visually directed and nonvisually directed movements. Although tests of position sense and kinesthetics provide one aspect of the evaluation of the proprioceptive system, the therapist also must be involved constantly in assessing the client's response to the intervention techniques that are part of the treatment plan. This again illustrates the intermingling of assessment and intervention. Intervention places a demand for movement on the client. As the movement occurs, the therapist assesses the quality of the movement. If the quality is not appropriate, the therapist initiates intervention to improve the quality. If the technique does not produce the desired result, a second technique can be tried and the cyclic process continues.

In addition to determining the integrity of the peripheral sensory pathways and recognition of the input, it is important to assess the individual's ability to process more complex presentations of cutaneous input. Difficulties in the cortical level processing of cutaneous stimuli are identified through tests of sharp and dull discrimination, stereognosis, tactile localization, texture recognition, two-point discrimination, and bilateral simultaneous stimulation.

Assessment of the integrity of the cranial nerve sensory channels is typically incorporated within the standard cranial nerve examination. Review of the physician's notes may provide sufficient information; however, the therapist may need to complete more specific tests before considering certain intervention techniques.

The olfactory channels are unique among the sensory input routes because the primary olfactory pathway directly synapses with the olfactory cortex within the limbic system before going to the thalamus. Olfactory inputs may provide a mechanism to elicit arousal in an otherwise unresponsive individual. The discussion in Chapter 4 is on the procedure for administering olfactory input as a component of evaluation and intervention regimens. Because of the potential hypersensitivity of any or all input systems, it is best to elicit arousal with pleasant odors rather than noxious odors, which may elicit a flight-or-fight response.

Gustatory sensory information is not typically an input channel used by therapists. In the client who is not receiving any gustatory stimulation because of prolonged tube feeding or in the client who demonstrates dysfunction of the oral musculature, the gustatory avenue of sensory input should not be overlooked. Various tastes can be incorporated in the evaluation of the effects of sensory inputs on clients with depressed levels of consciousness. Gustatory input can be incorporated into an intervention plan with the goal of facilitating movement of the oral and facial musculature. The gustatory/tactile input of a small amount of peanut butter placed on the corner of the client's mouth may elicit tongue protraction with lateral deviation to remove the morsel. Introduction of a slightly sour taste may facilitate a pucker response of the orbicularis oris. The possibility of achieving desired goals through the inclusion of gustatory input should be considered during the evaluation process.

The complex functions of the vestibular system can be assessed through a variety of avenues. The integrity of the connections underlying a vestibularly induced nystagmus response is assessed by physicians through the caloric test (warm and cold water or air introduced into the ear channel to induce nystagmus). Therapists have used the Ayres Post-Rotatory Nystagmus Test[1,2] and variations of the test to gain information on the postrotatory nystagmus response. Although the postrotatory nystagmus tests provide information on the response of the extraocular muscles to vestibular input, they should not be overinterpreted as yielding insight about the integrity of the vestibular connections underlying postural responses.

Located in the utriculus and sacculus are the maculae, which record changes in the relationship of the head to the pull of gravity (position detectors) and changes in linear acceleration. This end organ is responsible for the tonic labyrinthine reflexes. By manipulating the position of the client's head in relation to the pull of gravity, the therapist can evaluate this aspect of the vestibular system by noting changes in the distribution of muscle activity. The effect of rapid linear accelerations and decelerations can be evaluated as potential activating mechanisms increasing the level of consciousness or level of muscle activity. Slow, rhythmical reversals of linear movements may have a calming effect on the client's behavior or level of muscle activation. Linear movements in all planes and diagonals should be explored.

Auditory and visual channels can be grossly assessed by the therapist. More detailed information on the intactness of the sensory channels can be obtained from other health care team members. The types of information available from other health care team members can vary from the assessment of brain stem evoked potentials in response to auditory and visual inputs in the comatose individual to the identification of visual or auditory acuity deficits. Because the auditory and visual systems provide the therapist with a primary means of communicating with the client and because they can be used to augment performance in the event of deficits in other sensory channels, these systems should be incorporated in the therapist's evaluation process. Simple visual system tests, such as identification of field deficits, assessment of tracking abilities, and a gross evaluation of visual acuity, can be performed quickly. Neurology textbooks can be consulted on the techniques for administering these tests. Simple tests for assessing auditory thresholds can include such techniques as rubbing fingers by the individual's ear, placing a ticking watch to the client's ear, or assessing the presence of a startle response to sounds in the client with altered states of consciousness. Although these quick tests of the visual and auditory systems will not yield quantifiable information, they should provide the therapist with the necessary data to design an intervention plan that accounts for the presence of the deficits or that can use the intact system to compensate for input missing from an impaired system. See Chapter 27 for additional information regarding the visual-perceptual system.

During the evaluation of the client as well as during intervention with the client, the therapist must be aware of the potential to bombard the client with sensory input and overload his or her ability to respond discriminatively to it. If the therapist detects that the client has difficulty in appropriately responding to sensory input, such as the client in a lowered state of consciousness or an agitated state or the client demonstrating tactile defensiveness, sensory input should be used selectively during the initial examination or intervention sessions. If multiple sensory inputs are used, the positive or negative effects cannot be attributed to a specific input or necessarily to the series of inputs. Evaluation as well as intervention with sensory inputs should proceed in a controlled fashion. Inclusion of additional sensory modalities in the intervention plan should occur systematically.

The individual's response to multichannel sensory conflict input is typically assessed as a component of higher-level balance assessment and locomotor abilities. The reader is referred to Chapter 21 for more details on this aspect of the "sensory" assessment. The therapist should apply these concepts during the evaluation of all motor tasks. Consider the following example. A client who relies on visual input to supplement vestibular and somatosensory information is performing the task of sitting on the edge of the mat table. She remains relatively steady until someone walks directly toward her from across the clinic. This change in the environmental context of the performance requires her to assess whether she is moving toward the individual or the individual is moving toward her. Without reliable vestibular and somatosensory check points, the client may activate a postural response to the incorrect assessment. As this example demonstrates, the evaluation of the sensory channels is intertwined with the evaluation of the person's movement abilities.

Evaluation of Movement Abilities

The initial assessment of the individual's movement abilities is conducted by observing as he or she moves through a sequence of functional postures. The therapist determines the functional postures to be examined for a specific client, ranging from bed mobility activities (assessment of movement in prone and supine) through upright ambulation. The medical status of the individual, the extent of involvement, the intervention setting, and the age of the individual are considerations in determining the appropriate functional postures to be examined. The therapist gathers information on the movement abilities of the individual as the individual moves into, moves within, and moves out of the position.

The assessment focuses on both the quantity and quality of motor performance. The quantitative aspect of the movement assessment refers to the number of different functional postures the individual can use. The quality of the movement abilities is assessed within the posture as well as in the process of moving between postures. For example, the therapist should assess the quality of the head, trunk, and extremity control demonstrated throughout the movement sequences. The utilization of stereotypical movement patterns should be noted because their presence may limit the adaptability of movements required to accomplish functional tasks.

A number of additional items relating to the client's movement abilities are assessed during this process.

Indications of abnormal ranges of movement of all joints can be obtained. The range may show a limitation of movement or an indication of joint instability. Once the gross deviations are identified, these joints can be examined to determine the source of the problem—joint capsular, ligamentous, bony, skin, or muscular and fascial

dysfunction. Conducting the gross assessment of range while the client is moving eliminates the time spent in performing a joint-by-joint goniometric evaluation on articulations with normal excursions.

As the individual is moving (either independently or with the therapist assisting), an assessment of the distribution and fluctuations in muscle activity can be made providing information on functional muscle strength, power, and endurance. The timing, accuracy, and sequencing of muscle activation within the movement should be noted. The therapist can identify the postures that will be the most conducive to optimal motor performances and those that should be avoided. As the client is moving through various postures, the function of specific musculature can be examined. Muscle groups should be examined concerning their ability to function in stability (distal segment fixed) situations and in mobility (distal segment free) situations. Because numerous demands are being placed on each muscle group, therapists can assess their ability to perform isometric and isotonic (concentric and eccentric) contractions. Each different posture introduces a new set of variables; therefore, the performance of a muscle group must be reexamined as each new movement pattern is performed.

The therapist can identify the reflexes and reactions influencing each posture, particularly noting the presence or absence of the postural, equilibrial, and righting reactions. The reflexes and reactions should be categorized as supporting or interfering with the posture and movement patterns. Assessing the influence of the reflexes and reactions in each of the functional postures provides a more realistic picture of their influence than conducting a reflex inventory test, which considers only one posture. Integration of the tonic reflexes may appear to have occurred in the lower-level postures, whereas the reflex continues to influence movement at higher-level or more complex postures. Monitoring the influence of the reflexes and reactions as the client progresses through a sequence of postures and movements provides the more comprehensive assessment of the problems to be dealt with in therapy.

Within each posture, the therapist must examine the control the client displays over the posture. Because the assessment takes place as a part of a dynamic sequence, the therapist can assess the client's ability to assume the posture. If the posture cannot be achieved independently, the therapist assesses the factors interfering with achieving the position, the type of assistance necessary to facilitate assumption of the posture, and the effect of the various intervention techniques used to assist the client in achieving the position. Once the client is in the posture, his or her ability to maintain the posture is examined. Factors that interfere with the performance are noted. The client's ability to move within the posture is identified. Movement demands placed on the client should include aspects of both static and dynamic equilibrium. Static equilibrium in the sitting position (such as sitting on the side of the bed) could be demonstrated by the individual matching the strength of a force attempting to displace him backward and maintaining the position when the force is suddenly released.

The presence of dynamic equilibrium of the upper

torso in the sitting position could be demonstrated by the individual reacting to a quick sideways displacement force administered to the shoulder by activating the trunk lateral flexors to compensate for the displacement. Equally important is the individual's ability to demonstrate appropriate equilibrium responses to self-imposed perturbations.

The final stage in examining the individual's movement abilities explores the individual's ability to move out of the posture. The client should have the ability to move out of the posture to a lower-level posture and to a higher-level posture before mastery of the posture is considered to have been achieved.

Many aspects of the client's performance are analyzed simultaneously. When the therapist assists the client in moving to a new posture, an analysis of the influence of facilitation and inhibition techniques is being conducted. The individual's response to these handling techniques cues the therapist in projecting the client's response to an intervention program. The therapist is constantly monitoring the client for changes in physiological functions or changes in the level of consciousness. Anything that results in expressions of pain by the client should be noted. Intervention programs should be a learning experience for clients. If they are attending to pain, they cannot attend to learning. The factor(s) producing the pain should be identified and measures instituted to eliminate the factor(s). If the factors producing the pain cannot be resolved, the intervention program should be designed to avoid triggering the pain (see Chapter 29, Pain Management).

Evaluation of Functional Abilities

As indicated in the introduction to the evaluation of clients with inflammatory and infectious disorders of the brain, the examination process is not compartmentalized. As the therapist is examining the movement abilities of the individual through the format described in the previous section, the therapist is also collecting information of the functional abilities of the individual. The components underlying the movement abilities of the client can be examined within the framework of the basic or instrumental activities of daily living (ADL) depending on the functional level of the person. The treatment setting and documentation requirements within that setting will determine if the data on basic ADL and instrumental ADL skills are recorded using a formal scale or index or are gathered through an individualized process.

The introduction of specific tasks provides the therapist with the opportunity to observe the preferred posture used to accomplish the different tasks. The therapist should construct situations that require the individual to respond to unexpected occurrences to provide some insight into the person's ability to adapt to the unexpected. Throughout the process of examining the individual's movement abilities and functional abilities, the therapist is assessing the individual's awareness of safety considerations and judgment in attempting tasks.

The presence of motor planning dysfunctions can be noted as the client attempts a movement sequence or a functional task. The therapist may have to cue the client physically to initiate the sequence, which then flows smoothly. The therapist may observe that the client has the correct components to a movement sequence but that the sequence of the components is incorrect. Or the client may demonstrate the ability to produce a movement sequence under one set of conditions but not another. Indications of these types of motor planning problems can be observed during the initial interactions with the client. Similarly, the therapist also should be aware of indications of problems with dexterity, coordination, agility, as well as signs of cerebellar dysfunctions (see Chapter 24).

Another aspect of the evaluation process that can be integrated in the observations of movement abilities is identification of perceptual deficits. Aspects of the client's motor performance can provide indications for detailed perceptual testing to classify the deficits. This testing should be conducted by the health care team member qualified in the area of perceptual testing. During the general evaluation procedures, the therapist can screen the client for signs of perceptual deficits. Clients' abilities to cross their midlines with their upper extremities can be demonstrated in movement sequences such as moving from the supine to the side-sitting to the sitting position (Fig. 17-2). The quality of the integration of information from the two sides of the body can be indicated by the symmetry or asymmetry of posture in positions that should be symmetrical. The therapist may suspect that the client has a deficit in body awareness or body image by the poor quality of movement patterns that are within the motor capability of the individual. Spontaneous comments by the client as to how he or she feels when moving ("my leg feels so heavy") also add to the therapist's assessment of the client's body image. Problems with verticality can be seen with the client who lists to one side when in an upright posture. When the therapist corrects the list to a vertical posture, clients may express that they now feel that they are leaning to one side. Individuals who cannot appropriately relate their positions to the position of objects in their environments may have a figure-ground deficit or a problem with the concept of their position in space. When approaching stairs, these clients may fail to step up or may attempt to step up too soon. These examples should provide an indication of the observations that can indicate the need for detailed perceptual testing. See Chapters 11 and 27 for additional discussion of perceptual deficits.

The preceding aspects of evaluation of movement abilities have focused on facets of motor performance. Within this process, the therapist should intertwine an appraisal of the individual's ability to learn motor tasks (or elements of the task). The therapist attempts to determine whether the client can maintain a change in the ability to perform a movement throughout a therapy session and into the next session. The client's ability to capture and integrate changes into the movement repertoire is fundamental to the success of the intervention program. The program can focus on the learning of movement sequences and the generalization of these sequences to movements within other contexts. Individuals with lowered levels of consciousness (typically Rancho Los Amigos Stages 1–3) will be unable to learn or have difficulty learning and

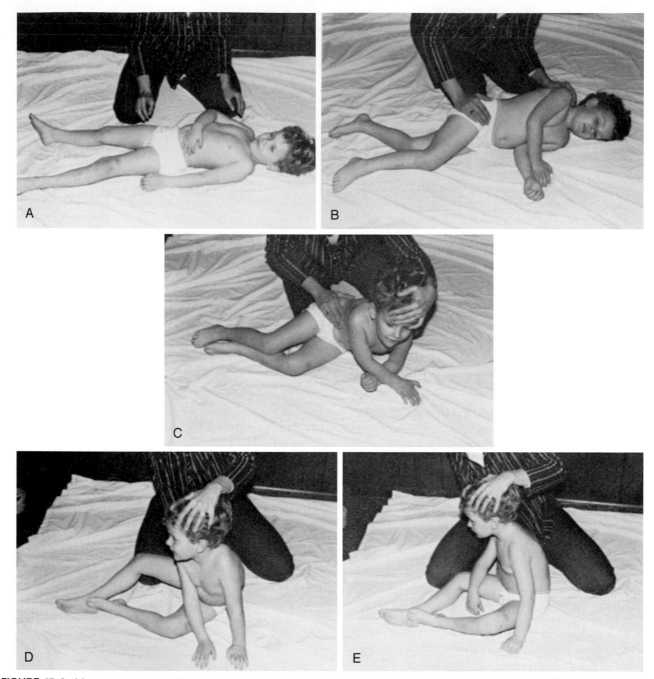

FIGURE 17–2. Movement sequence from the supine to side-sitting to sitting positions. *A*, Supine position. *B*, Handling to side lying. *C*, Handling toward side sitting; arm positions are important. *D*, Side sitting; note propping patterns with arms. *E*, Handling to symmetrical sitting.

generalizing new motor skills. Therapy sessions may be more successful if the focus remains on the performance of motor tasks that were previously "overlearned" and automatic. Although the therapist may be able to manually guide the individual in coming to sitting on the edge of the bed, until the individual demonstrates a higher level of processing, it may be unrealistic to expect that the person will consistently reposition the legs without cuing before attempting the movement sequence.

The general philosophy in the evaluation of the client with neurological deficits as a result of brain inflammation is a whole-part-whole approach. General observations of

the client's performance provide a general description of the client's abilities while indicating deficits in his or her performance. The cause(s) of the deficits (impairments) are explored to provide the pieces of data defining his or her performance. These pieces of data then are arranged within the framework provided by the general observation to define the whole of the client's assets and deficits. As the whole picture is established (with the realization that it will be constantly adjusted), the process of goal setting is initiated. The process presented for refining evaluation data into an intervention plan is applicable whether the client's neurological dysfunction is the result of a bacterial or viral infection, cerebrovascular accident, trauma, or other factors.

PROGNOSING AND GOAL SETTING

Ideally, the process of establishing the prognosis and setting the goals for a client is a coordinated effort that involves all members of the health care team, including the client (if feasible) and family. If the therapist is not functioning in a setting where involvement of many disciplines is viable, the therapist can progress through the goal-setting process in the context of his or her role in the client's care.

Having collected data from the examination process, the first steps are to establish two lists—one dealing with specific problems (impairments, functional limitations, and disabilities) the client is encountering and one dealing with his or her assets. Formulating an asset list focuses on the positive data elicited from the evaluation process and is critical for prognosing outcomes. Items on the asset list could be observations, such as the client being able to assume the position of sitting on the side of the bed with set up assistance only, improved head control in this posture being facilitated by approximation (see Chapter 4), and controlled weight shifting being elicited by alternated tapping (see Chapter 4). The asset list provides a reference defining the postures and intervention techniques that are effective. This reference is used to develop the intervention goals and plan. Formulating and recording a problem list and an asset list can be completed relatively quickly as one gains familiarity with the process. Whereas novice therapists will benefit from generating a written asset list, experienced clinicians may formulate a mental asset list while completing the written evaluation format required by the facility. Just as the evaluation process is ongoing, so are the steps involved in goal setting. The asset and problem lists are redefined as the client's status changes.

Having identified assets and problems, the next step is to establish the expected outcomes from this episode of care and is considered the prognosis. These outcome statements represent the general objectives toward which the intervention process is oriented. They identify the end point of the intervention process and are the exit criteria for terminating the episode of care.

The *Guide to Physical Therapist Practice* views outcomes in relationship to "minimization of functional limitations, optimization of health status, prevention of disability, and optimization of patient/client satisfaction" while goals "relate to the remediation (to the extent possible) of impairments."[15, pp1-7] The breadth of acceptance of these definitions with the neurorehabilitation professions remains to be determined.

Measurable, interim objectives should be established in relationship to the outcome statements. To determine if the objective has been achieved, the objective should be measurable either in terms of producing a numerical indicator of performance, such as time span, number of repetitions, distance covered, or accuracy of performance, or in terms of a precise description of the target motor behavior. The appropriate objective indicator must be carefully selected. Performing a movement more quickly may indicate that the individual is performing it with more normal control and therefore greater ease of movement, or it may indicate that the individual has become more skilled in using an abnormal pattern based on inappropriate muscle activation. If it is not appropriate to formulate the objective in terms of a numerical indicator, the objective can be formulated in terms of an observable behavior. The therapist can precisely describe body segment movements based on the component method of movement analysis presented by VanSant.[31, 32] For example, the task of coming to standing from supine can be described in terms of the upper-extremity component, axial component, and lower-extremity component. Formulation of an appropriate short-term objective could specify use of the upper extremities in a push and reach pattern during the task of coming to standing from supine. The interim objectives should be constructed so that observing the client's behavior will allow the therapist to state whether the criteria of the short-term objective were achieved. Table 17–1 gives an example of some

---

T A B L E 1 7 – 1. Examples of Short-Term Objectives Relating to Mastery of Functional Activities in Sitting*

	Condition Variables†	Activity	Criteria
1. When sitting on a mat	a. using the upper extremities for support	The client will maintain the posture	For ___ seconds.
2. When sitting on the edge of a mat table	b. using one upper extremity for support c. without using the upper extremities for support		
3. When sitting in a chair	d. with the therapist displacing the position of the: pelvis shoulders head lower extremities	The client will make postural adjustments of the head and trunk	Appropriate to the degree of displacement.
	e. leaning forward and returning to erect sitting	The client will bring the right foot to left knee (as if to put on a shoe)	

*Outcome: The client will master functional activities in sitting. Short-term objective: Select one phrase from each column.
†Therapist needs to consider all aspects of each variable, i.e., 1—a, b, c, d, e; 2—a, b, c, d, e; 3—a, b, c, d, e.

components of short-term objectives leading to mastery of functional activities in sitting.

The outcome statements define the client's destination. The interim objectives define the mileposts. The therapist then uses the asset list to design the intervention program, which is the vehicle to get the client to his or her destination. From the asset list, the therapist knows the intervention techniques that have the highest probability of success. Adopting this process simplifies the task of outlining the strategy for intervention.

As the therapist considers the appropriate outcomes and goals for the client, a decision must be made as to whether the format of the intervention will focus on a "training" approach or a "motor learning" approach. During the assessment process, if the therapist concludes that the individual's level of cognitive function precludes the development of insight into movement errors (both the detection and correction of an incorrect performance) or the ability to retain the insight over time, then the therapist should delineate the outcomes and intervention plan to accommodate this limitation. The "training" approach requires more structure and repetition of activities within that structure. If it is more appropriate to design the intervention plan according to motor learning considerations, the therapist must consider the appropriate schedule and environmental context for the practice, the type and schedule for the feedback provided, and techniques to promote the generalization of the learning beyond the specific practice session.

General Goals for the Intervention Process

While the goal-setting process described earlier results in specification of the outcomes, goals, and objectives for a specific client, the general goals for the intervention process can be delineated to guide the process. As described in the overview of inflammatory disorders at the beginning of this chapter, the extent of the neurological sequelae may range from a single discrete problem to a devastating clinical picture composed of compromised functions in multiple areas. The goals for the intervention process address the problem areas that (1) jeopardize the efficiency and effectiveness of functional activities and (2) are the primary or secondary results of compromised neurological function. The listing of goals does not directly include consideration of secondary problems (such as decreases in joint range of motion [ROM], cardiovascular fitness, and endurance). The therapist should integrate these considerations in the overall assessment of the components of the movement problems.

The following goals are written as outcomes of the intervention process and not as goals for a specific client. Because of the broad nature of the goals, other professions also will contribute to the attainment of the goals. The goals of the therapeutic intervention program for clients with inflammatory CNS disorders are as follows:

Goal 1: Postural control is optimized as demonstrated by the ability to maintain a position against gravity and the ability to automatically adjust before and continuously during movement.

Goal 2: Selective, voluntary movement patterns within functional activities are optimized.

Goal 3: Performance of functional activities is enhanced.

Goal 4: Integration of sensory information is fostered.

Goal 5: Cognitive status and psychosocial responses are optimized.

Each of these goals is discussed in conjunction with the general therapeutic intervention procedures that can be used to achieve the goal.

GENERAL THERAPEUTIC INTERVENTION PROCEDURES IN RELATION TO INTERVENTION GOALS

• *Postural control is optimized as demonstrated by the ability to maintain a position against gravity and the ability to automatically adjust before and continuously during movement.*

Because it is assumed that functional abilities are built on the base of the ability to control postures, the intervention goal of promoting optimal postural control underlies the ability to make selective, voluntary movement patterns (goal 2) and the performance of functional activities (goal 3). Optimalization of postural set includes the concepts of decreasing muscle activity that is too high to allow performance of movement sequences as well as augmenting activation that is too low to support the accomplishment of a movement sequence. The postural set of a client can fluctuate between degrees of hypertonicity and hypotonicity; the desired outcome is to achieve the optimal postural set for a particular movement. Intervention techniques to achieve this goal demand that the therapist constantly monitor the client's performance so that appropriate interventions are added when needed and continued only as long as they are needed.

Optimal postural control is defined by two elements. The client should have the ability to maintain a posture or a position against gravity and in the presence of external perturbations. Automatic adjustments in the postural set should occur in anticipation of and continuously during movements (internal perturbations). Both elements should be performed with minimal physical or cognitive effort on the part of the client.

Readers who are acquainted with the concept of the normal postural reflex mechanism introduced by the Bobaths[5] will recognize familiar constructs. This discussion, however, will not incorporate the assumption that dysfunction of postural control is based on problems with specific righting and equilibrium reactions, the presence of associated reactions, the effect of released asymmetrical tonic neck reflex activity, or the effect of released positive supporting reactions.[5] Although one or more of these elements may be present, it will not be assumed to be the causal factor. Clients with neurological sequelae may exhibit "primitive" reflexes—stereotypical motor responses that resemble the reflex responses that are present in the process of the typical development sequence but whose influence is suppressed as maturation proceeds. Typically, the motor responses demonstrated as the result of neurological dysfunction are of a greater magnitude and display less variation than the normal developmental reflexes.

The utilization of stereotypical reflexes as part of the intervention techniques for clients who have a limited ability to perform motor responses is controversial. These reflex linkages can be used to augment a response such as turning the head to the right to augment an extension response of the right upper extremity (asymmetrical tonic neck reflex [ATNR]). The potential problem with this approach is that the client may be learning a behavior that reinforces the limited stereotypical pattern and blocks the process of learning to make appropriate postural adjustments and selective muscle activation.

The reflex linkages can be useful to elicit a movement response, but they should be used only when other tools are not effective. If the movement response is elicited through a primitive reflex, the therapist should immediately attempt to elicit the response without the reflex input. Shaping the sequence in this manner promotes the learning of the desired response and not reinforcement of an undesired stimulus to achieve the response. If the ATNR is used to elicit triceps function, the head then should be returned to the neutral position and function augmented by other means such as tapping or other proprioceptive inputs. Once the triceps response is achieved with the head in the neutral position, the head should be rotated away from the side of the triceps. This final stage promotes a functional response against the influence of a sensory trigger for the stereotypical pattern.

Basing a decision on the needs of the client, the therapist must decide whether to use the influence from these reflexes to augment the initial response despite their potential negative effects. Regardless of this initial decision, the intervention should progress from movement with neutral support from the stereotypical response to movement against the influence of the reflex. As the client progresses to functionally higher level (and more stressful) postures, the influence of the stereotypical linkages may again be expressed. The process of developing selective control may require repetition in several positions and activities.

The client's ability to demonstrate optimal postural control may be restricted by the presence of hypertonicity or hypotonicity in various muscle groups. These states may be relatively static or may fluctuate with the demands of a particular situation. Inappropriately high levels of muscle activity may be present in a stereotypical muscle distribution in the extremities, whereas the activity of the trunk musculature may be too low to support an antigravity posture. The therapist must design the interventions creatively to meet the shifting responses of the demands of a particular activity.

A saying attributed to the Bobaths is "First make it possible, then make it happen." Although some contend that this philosophy shifts too much of the responsibility away from the client, it also can be interpreted as directing the therapist to create changes in the internal and external environments to afford the person the opportunity to formulate and execute a movement response that

otherwise would not be possible. The therapist also must consider structuring the situation so that the client can learn to make the response within a variety of environmental constraints.

Being cognizant of the fact that spasticity is a reaction to initial peripheral instability, treatment needs to be selected that deals with the fact that as spasticity is modified, weakness or hypotonicity may be present. Inappropriately high levels of activity in a muscle group or groups may limit the client's ability to demonstrate optimal postural control (and optimal selective movements as addressed in the second goal). The therapist can select intervention techniques that are mediated through any of the sensory channels functional for that client. The choice of which channel or combination of channels to use for the input is based on the therapist's initial and continuing evaluation of the client's response to specific types of sensory input (see Chapter 4).

The therapist must address the hypertonicity influencing postural control as a generalized problem before demanding selective voluntary activation of specific muscle groups. Vestibular input that is slow and rhythmical may promote a generalized relaxation of skeletal muscle activity. In some clients, the trunk remains "stiff" in movement sequences in which a segmental response between the upper and lower trunk should occur. Repetitions of rhythmical movements side lying in which the therapist gently and progressively stretches the client's pelvis in one direction around the body axis while moving the shoulder girdle in the opposite direction and then reverses the movement may effectively alter the biomechanical and neurological contributions to the stiffness (Fig. 17–3).

For some clients, changing the dynamics of a spastic extremity may permit the emergence of more optimal levels of postural control. The appropriately designed ankle-foot orthosis (AFO) may alter the individual's need to rigidly control the position of the pelvis to remain upright (see Chapter 31). Use of a soft webbing thumb loop to alter the resting position of the first metacarpal may change the overactivity of musculature throughout the upper extremity and allow appropriate adjustment of the shoulder girdle as part of postural responses.

For some of the more involved clients, the therapist may need to use handling techniques to change the alignment relationship of body segments before attempting to elicit automatic postural adjustments. Bobath[5] discusses

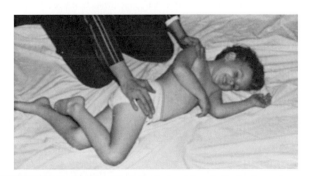

FIGURE 17–3. Counterrotation of shoulder girdle backward (retraction) and the pelvis forward. Hand placement of therapist is important so that shoulder and hip movements can occur freely.

the use of proximal and distal key points of control to influence the client's distribution of muscle activity. The therapist must remember that the static imposition of control will not help the client learn to move. The therapist imposes control so that the client can move. As the client moves and gains control of the movement, the therapist lessens the amount of control. The therapist's goal should be to remove his or her hands from controlling the client's responses.

In Chapter 4 some of the potential combinations of techniques that can produce the desired postural responses are discussed. The therapist may need to systematically alter the techniques until the desired response is achieved. Interventions should be withdrawn systematically to move the client toward responding appropriately and independently to the demands of a situation.

If the client is sufficiently alert so that attending to and understanding directions is a possibility, the therapist should direct the person to focus on the effects of the movement responses rather than focusing attention on the movement of the body.[20a] As the person begins to appreciate the consequences of what is transpiring, he or she should be asked to assist in maintaining the changes that promote the more skillful movement response. Unless otherwise indicated by the client's status, interventions must actively involve the individual in the process of planning, initiating, completing, and evaluating the movement. Although the therapist may manipulate the environment (internal and external) in which the response is made, the client must be an active participant for learning to occur.

Although some clients will demonstrate a pattern of generalized overactivity of the postural muscles of the trunk, many will have difficulty generating sufficient activity in the appropriate groups to sustain a posture or to permit movement in the posture. As presented in Chapter 4, several intervention techniques are available depending on how the individual responds.

With generalized hypotonia, temporary improvement in postural responses may occur by providing vestibular input that is characterized by rapid and irregular changes. The labyrinths should be stimulated by quick stops and starts with changes in direction. The program should include the introduction of movements in all planes. Approximation can be effective in developing appropriate postural activity from a state of either hypertonicity or hypotonicity. Empirically, it seems that more force is applied to increase the postural response than to decrease the response. Approximation appears to elicit a response in all the muscles surrounding a joint as preparation for responding to the demands to the erect posture or the demands of weight bearing. Approximation lends itself to combination with other proprioceptive techniques, such as quick stretch or tapping. Although the changes evoked by these techniques may be of short duration, the alterations can evoke movement components that would not otherwise occur and thereby provide the opportunity for the individual to learn from the movement.

As the therapist applies various techniques in an attempt to elicit a specific response, the therapist must evaluate the desired response in relationship to the environmental context. If the client is sitting on the edge of a mat table, the activity of the trunk musculature will vary depending on whether the feet are flat on the floor, whether the client is engaged in an activity, whether the client is leaning on one arm for support, or whether the client is resting between activities. The client who slouches in sitting when fatigued, bored, or overwhelmed by the sensory input may present a different clinical picture when the appropriate factors are altered.

• *Selective, voluntary movement patterns within functional activities are optimized.*

The concept of the influence of the environment on the quality of a movement response, discussed in relation to the first goal of the intervention process, is also incorporated in the second goal. Quality, selective, voluntary movement patterns are sought within the framework of functional activities rather than as isolated and abstract movements. Optimalization of the selective movement patterns may require a decrease in the stereotypical linkages of certain muscle groups, an increase in the ability to selectively activate certain muscle groups, the development of the ability to execute the movement in different postures, or a number of other variations.

Performance of functional activities requires that the individual have the capability of performing both mobility and stability patterns with the extremities. Mobility patterns are open kinetic chain movements in which the distal segment is free. These patterns are necessary for placing the extremities (e.g., swing phase of gait or reaching for a doorknob).

Clients who exhibit stereotypical posturing of the upper extremity with a restricted repertoire of available movement patterns require intervention to change the initial position of the extremity before movements are attempted. The influence of the spasticity that interferes with the repositioning of the extremity can be reduced by applying approximation through the long axis of the extremity. Preferably, the therapist's manual contacts for the application of the approximation force are on the weight-bearing surfaces of the hand. If the flexed position of the wrist prohibits application of the force to the heel of the palm, the approximation can be applied gradually through the fisted hand. As the resistance to passive movement diminishes, the wrist can be moved toward the neutral position so that the therapist can then apply the approximation through the heel of the palm (Fig. 17–4). The therapist is moving the extremity toward an alternative resting position so that a new movement sequence can be attempted. It is important to use an intervention technique such as approximation to reduce the level of the spasticity before passive movement is attempted so that a more appropriate position can be assumed without inappropriately stretching the spastic muscles.

The client is asked to assist the therapist with the movement with the person being cued to do so with a minimum of effort. Too often, clients attempt to make a selective movement through a massive effort and overactivation of the muscle groups, which compounds the underlying spasticity. Clients should be encouraged to make easy movements—movements that they are instructed to perform with reduced effort so that they can relearn

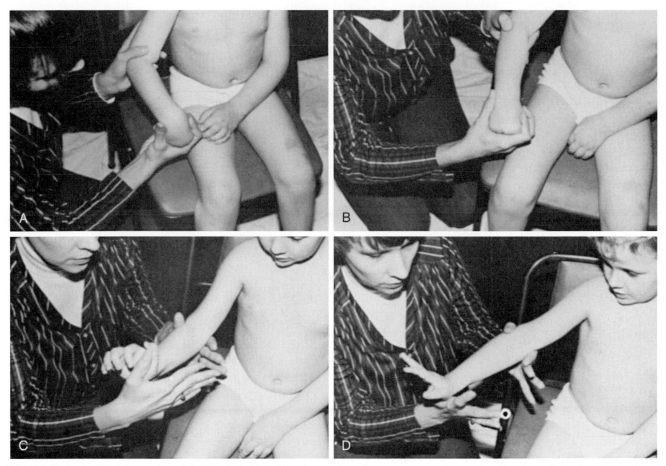

FIGURE 17–4. Facilitating opening of the hand. *A,* Fisted hand; stretch to the extensors and approximation through hand, wrist, and elbow is applied. *B,* Approximation is continued; some resistance to the extensors may be applied. *C,* Approximation is applied to thenar eminence to further facilitate extensor tone. *D,* Full extension is achieved; approximation is maintained.

selective activation of motor units rather than mass firing patterns.

Electrical stimulation can be used as an adjunct to facilitate performance of a particular component of a mobility pattern. The wrist extension component of the proprioceptive neuromuscular facilitation (PNF) pattern of flexion, abduction, and external rotation can be reinforced by using a portable electrical stimulation unit with an adjustable surge duration. The electrical stimulation elicits the correct movement so that the client could learn from the feel of the correct pattern. Adjusting the practice schedule so that the pattern is performed with and without the electrical stimulation support of the movement avoids the potential problem of reliance on the device to produce the movement. Electromyographic (EMG) biofeedback can be a useful adjunct to achieve activation of specific muscle groups or to guide the client's attempts to reduce the level of activity of a muscle group (see Chapter 28).

Mobility patterns in the upper extremity have as their foundation the freedom of the scapula to appropriately adjust to the position of the humerus. The mobility of the scapula can be addressed through techniques that result in a general decrease in muscle activity and diagonal movement patterns of the scapula. The scapular stabilizers, such as the rhomboids, trapezius, and serratus ante-

rior, must be capable of allowing appropriate adjustment of the scapula as well as providing the fixation base on which humeral elevation can occur.

In stability patterns, the distal segment of the extremity is fixed (closed kinetic chain). These patterns are used in the weight-bearing components of the functional activities, such as the stance phase of gait or creeping. The components of the stability patterns are enhanced by proprioceptive input such as approximation. During the performance of both stability and mobility patterns, the therapist should control the situation so that the client learns the appropriate movement patterns and not patterns imposed on top of inappropriate muscle activation.

As the client performs mobility and stability patterns as components of functional activities, all categories of muscle contractions should be elicited from each muscle group. If a particular type of contraction poses a problem for a muscle group, the therapist can select an alternate posture in which to build in the ability of the muscle group to perform that type of contraction. For example, if the client has problems with eccentric hamstring control during the swing phase of gait, the pattern can be worked on as a component of the rolling sequence from the supine to the prone position (Fig. 17–5). Once the client gains control of the pattern within one movement context, the therapist must design activities to promote generaliza-

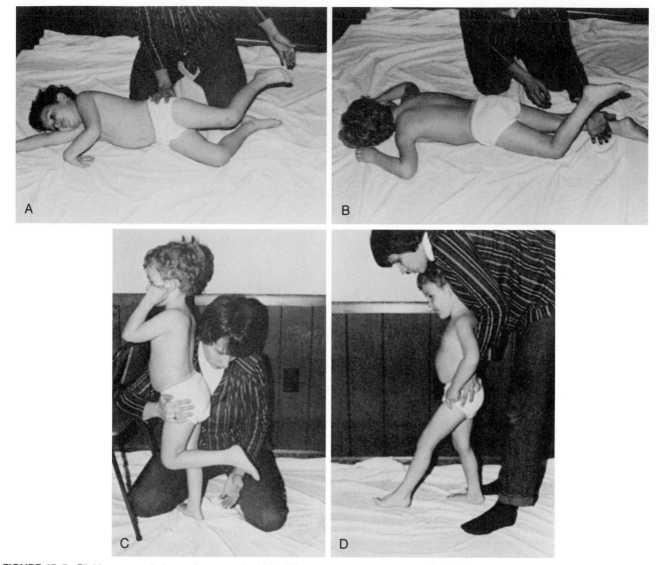

FIGURE 17–5. Eliciting eccentric hamstring control within different movement contexts. *A,* Roll from the supine to side-lying position (beginning sequence). *B,* Roll from the side-lying to prone position with controlled lengthening of the hamstrings. *C,* Standing eccentric hamstring contraction. *D,* Controlled hamstring activity during swing phase of gait.

tion of the pattern to other movement contexts to counter the specificity of strength training. The client who has difficulty with the co-contraction stability pattern of the upper extremity in the all-fours position may have more success with a forward propping position in sitting, which may allow more control of the amount of weight being supported by the upper extremity. After gaining control in the forward propped sitting, attempts can be made to generalize the response to positions such as side sitting and all fours.

Performance of movement patterns should progress toward an ability to easily reverse the direction of the movement. This can be promoted by incorporating rhythmical movements within a posture or between postures as early as possible in the intervention sequence. The end point at which the reversal is required should vary. In preparation for mastering the movements required to move from supine to sitting on the edge of the mat table, the client might be asked to move from the supine

position to side sitting and back to supine; then the client could move from the supine position to side lying propped on one elbow (the halfway point in the overall movement), then reverse to supine. Incorporating reversal of movement patterns within the intervention program prepares the client to deal with situations that mandate unexpected adjustments in the movement sequence.

Clients who demonstrate problems with the sequencing of movements, such as those with motor dyspraxia, frequently perform better if the movement is performed at a speed that is close to normal. Clients who had normal movement sequences before the brain infection seem to be able to trigger better movement responses at normal speeds than at slower speeds. The slower movement speeds appear to disrupt the typical flow of the movement. In working with clients with sequencing problems, all team members should provide the same, consistent sensory cues to elicit a movement pattern. For example, the therapist may establish a coupling of the verbal cue "roll" with a quick stretch to the ankle dorsiflexors to elicit a rolling pattern. These same cues can be used by other team members to assist the client in changing positions in bed or in performing dressing activities. The consistency of cues may elicit a consistent response from the client. Once the pattern is well established, the intervention program can be designed to include an extinction process for the cues progressing toward the ability of the client to perform the activity in response to the demands of the situation rather than to externally imposed cues.

The flow of a movement pattern may be disrupted by problems categorized as incoordination. The origin of the coordination problems could be dysfunction of the visual-perceptual system (see Chapter 27) or vestibular systems (see Chapters 11 and 21), dyspraxia (see Chapter 11), or dysfunction caused by cerebellar damage (see Chapter 24). If possible, the factors involved in producing a lack of coordination should be identified.

• *Performance of functional activities is enhanced.*

As the client develops more appropriate postural control and the ability to perform selective movement patterns within functional activities, he or she is developing the basis to perform increasingly challenging functional activities. The movement patterns (and the postural control that underlies them) provide the building blocks for mastering an expanding variety of activities.

As the therapist designs the expansion of activities within the intervention program, the demands of each new functional activity and posture must be scrutinized. The client's ability to meet these demands was examined in the evaluation process. The intervention strategy must focus on the quality of the client's ability to assume a posture, maintain the posture, move within the posture (static and dynamic equilibrium responses to both self-generated and external perturbations), and move out of the posture. The therapist will change the sequence of this progression of activities to meet the needs of the client. The client may achieve independence in maintaining a posture while still requiring assistance in assuming the posture.

This progression should be grounded within the context of functionally relevant activities. Unless the individual has difficulty tolerating change, activities should be practiced within different environments to enhance generalization of learning. The creative therapist can design a variety of functionally relevant activities that require similar movement components.

With infants, the therapist may choose to use the developmental sequence as a general model for the functional activities progression. Progression through the developmental sequence should be viewed as a dynamic process so that the intervention incorporates movement both within and between postures. For individuals through the remainder of the life span, the focus should be on the age-appropriate functional activities essential to the individual's daily life such as bed mobility, sit to stand, stand to sit, ambulation, reaching, and manipulation.

Samplings of handling techniques that can be adapted to enhance the individual's progression through the sequence of functional activities can be found in the works of Bobath,[5] Carr and Shepherd,[6, 7] Duncan and Badke,[12] Levitt,[19] Ryerson and Levit,[28] Sullivan and Markos,[30] and Voss and colleagues,[33] as well as throughout this book. These authors can provide the therapist with ideas for ways to enhance the client's performance within a specific activity.

• *Integration of sensory information is fostered.*

At the same time that the therapist addresses the previous intervention goals, the goal of fostering integration of sensory input must be considered. Unless the therapist has advanced knowledge of sensory integration theories, this goal may be secondary rather than primary; nevertheless, it cannot be ignored.

The potential for an exaggerated and inappropriate response to sensory input was discussed as part of the clinical picture. Before the therapist expects the client to exhibit adaptive behavior to the potential bombardment of input from combinations of cutaneous, proprioceptive, auditory, and visual input, the therapist must assess the client's ability to respond to multisensory inputs. The ability to respond adaptively progresses from a response to a single sensory system input, to a response to the input in the presence of multiple system input, and then to an adaptive response based on inputs from two or more sources. The therapist must be sure that adding more sensory inputs augments an adaptive response rather than detracts from it. The client may respond to handling techniques providing proprioceptive and cutaneous cues but may demonstrate a deterioration of performance when auditory input is added. When verbal cues are added, the therapist should follow the philosophy that verbal commands should be concise, sparse, and appropriately timed.[33]

All sensory inputs should evoke the correct response on the part of the client rather than cause him or her to sift through the jumble of inputs to recognize the appropriate inputs to which a response should be made. At the highest level, the client will demonstrate cross-modal learning in which input from one sensory system will evoke a response based on input previously obtained through a different system. Recognition of a comb by touch is based on the precept of "combness" usually obtained initially by visual input. If the therapist recognizes the hierarchy in the process of integrating sensory input, intervention situations that require too high a level of performance from the client can be avoided. The client who can respond adaptively to input from only one source will not be expected to perform in a crowded treatment area that presents extraneous visual and auditory input. The therapist will also recognize the need to include in the intervention plan situations that involve the controlled introduction of sensory inputs so that the client progresses toward the ability to deal with multiple inputs. Carr and Shepherd[7] discuss some general principles that can be used during the training of motor tasks in the presence of somatosensory and perceptual-cognitive impairments.

Dysfunctions in perceptual integration are addressed as the client moves through functional sequence activities. Although these movement activities would not provide the total program for an individual with a specific perceptual integration dysfunction, goals in this area can be addressed if the therapist is aware of indications of dysfunctions. The therapist must critically observe the performance of a movement sequence to identify substitute actions to compensate for problems such as inability to cross the midline. The therapist must then attempt to redesign the demands of the situation to elicit the desired behavior. The client who moves from the supine to the side sitting to the long sitting positions without the upper extremities crossing the midline could be required to side sit to the left and transfer objects with the right hand from the left side of the body to the right side (Fig. 17–6). The therapist must determine whether the client is truly crossing the midline or rotating the midline of the body to continue to avoid crossing it.

Therapists may be most aware of disturbances in the client's ability to integrate sensory information into an appropriate response when this dysfunction disrupts balance. The ability to maintain and move in upright postures requires successful processing of information from the equilibrial triad—the visual, vestibular, and somatosensory systems. When one component is missing, unreliable, or discrepant with the other two, the person is at risk for loss of balance. During the ongoing evaluation process, the therapist gathers information on the integrity of each system and any evidence of central processing difficulties. Incorporated within the practice of activities to develop postural control, to promote selective move-

ments with functional activities, and to develop mastery of increasing difficult functional activities is the simultaneous practice of integrating sensory information so that a successful response can be generated.

Clients who are performing at higher levels can be challenged to maintain balance when one element of the equilibrial triad is missing (e.g., vision occluded) or altered (e.g., sitting, standing, or walking on a soft, compliant surface). Successful maintenance of balance outside the protective environment of the therapy clinic requires the ability to switch the primary information source to any one of the three systems. Walking in the dark requires the person to rely on vestibular and somatosensory input. Standing on a moving bus looking out a window requires resolution of the conflict between visual input (the external world is moving), vestibular input (you are moving), and somatosensory input (you are stationary). Movement experiences within the therapy program should foster practice of this sensory integration process (see Chapter 21).

- *Cognitive status and psychosocial responses are optimized.*

In addition to attending to the factors directly related to motor performance, the therapist also must attend to the client's psychosocial and cognitive responses. Although the therapist does not have primary responsibility in this area, a goal of the intervention process should be to enhance the individual's psychosocial and cognitive responses.

Particularly in the agitated state that may be a component of the response to the inflammatory process, the client may demonstrate exaggerated and inappropriate emotional responses to events. Dealing with these emotional fluctuations can become a major determinant in goal attainment in the other areas. Maintaining a positive, nonthreatening interaction allows the client to use the therapist as a reference for judging the appropriateness of emotional responses.

If the client's state of agitation is interfering with the intervention program, the therapist may alter the program to include techniques that have a calming effect. For example, the individual can be wrapped in a cotton sheet blanket and rocked in a slow, rhythmical, repetitive manner to decrease the individual's agitation. Auditory and visual input should be controlled to avoid overloading sensory processing mechanisms.

In Chapter 7, Burton discusses the psychosocial adjustment that occurs in the process of recovering from a neurological disability. The therapist must be aware of how the client's regression in affective and cognitive domains affects the intervention process. The therapist should seek assistance from the health care team members responsible for intervention in these areas to deal with the client constructively. The therapist must remember that both the family members and the client are in the process of adjusting to the client's changed and, it is hoped, changing status. Family members may be an asset or a liability to the client's recovery process. During the therapist's interactions with the family members in activities such as instructions in the client's home program, the therapist should be prepared to deal with expressions of

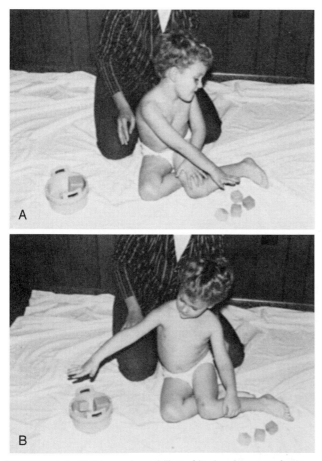

FIGURE 17–6. Child crossing midline of body when transferring objects from left to right. *A*, Beginning act on contralateral side. *B*, Ending sequence by crossing midline and placing objects on ipsilateral side.

the individual's difficulty in adjusting to the situation. The therapist also should be prepared to assist family members in identifying appropriate sources to help them deal with their problems.

Changes in mentation, perception of events, and memory losses present challenges to both the client and the therapist. Repetition in the recounting of past events may help reorder past knowledge. Use of brief verbal or visual cues may assist the client in recalling safety instructions or the components of the exercise program. The therapist should try to generate a nonstressful environment when working on these deficits so that attention and recall are not overshadowed by emotional pressure.

As the therapist works with the client on an intervention program, situations arise that require problem solving to determine a way to accomplish a task. If the task is to accomplish an independent transfer from a wheelchair into a bathtub, decisions must be made concerning the sequence of movements. Therapists can approach this situation in two ways. They can instruct clients step by step in what to do, or they can involve clients to the extent possible in the process of deciding what to do. If the therapist instructs the client step by step, the client may master the task but may not be able to perform it under different conditions. If the therapist involves the client in the decision-making process, the client may be learning not only how to accomplish the specific task but also how to accomplish the task under varied conditions. The intervention process should lead to the ability to respond to the demands of a situation, and involvement of clients in the problem-solving process helps prepare them for independence. The therapist must structure the client's role in decision making to the level of the client's ability to participate so that the experience is not frustrating. Although the client's participation may initially increase the time required to complete a task, it promotes skills that may lead more quickly to independence of function.

INTERACTION WITH OTHER PROFESSIONALS

The therapist needs to design an intervention program that is articulated with that of other members of the health care team. The recovery process of the client should be facilitated by a care plan in which each team member reinforces the goals of the other team members. The care of the person must be a collaborative effort. Each client deserves an intervention process that considers him or her as a whole person, not as a set of fragmented problems.

SUMMARY

This chapter has presented a brief discussion of the pathology and medical management of various inflammatory processes that affect the brain. The process of assessment, the role of assessment in designing an intervention program, the goals of the intervention process, and the means to meet those goals were presented to assist the reader

in more effective management of clients with these diagnoses.

Although the problem-solving process presented in this chapter for assessment, prognosis and goal identification, and treatment planning is not limited to clients with inflammatory supraspinal disorders, its application in the presence of typical neurological sequelae has been described. When dealing with inflammatory disorders of the brain, the variability of neurological sequelae is examined based on the anatomical location of the inflammatory process and the cause of the infection.

Although the neurological disorders discussed in this chapter are life threatening, many clients recover and return to their previous lifestyles. Clients will vary within the spectrum of minimal to severe involvement and specific to generalized CNS dysfunction and will demonstrate little to full recovery after the acute distress. Prognosis for recovery depends on the type of infecting organism and the extent of involvement. The therapist must remain flexible and willing to adjust every aspect of therapeutic intervention to meet the specific needs of each client.

REFERENCES

1. Ayres JA: Sensory Integration and Learning Disorder, Los Angeles, Western Psychological Services, 1972.
2. Ayres JA: Southern California Postrotatory Nystagmus Test. Los Angeles, Western Psychological Services, 1975.
3. Bhabha SK, Bharucha NE, Bharucha EP: Viral infections. In Bradley WG, et al (eds): Neurology in Clinical Practice, vol 2. Boston, Butterworth-Heinemann, 1996.
4. Bharucha NE, Bharucha EP, Bhabha SK: Bacterial infections. In Bradley WG, et al (eds): Neurology in Clinical Practice, vol 2. Boston, Butterworth-Heinemann, 1996.
5. Bobath B: Adult Hemiplegia: Evaluation and Treatment, 3rd ed. London, William Heinemann Medical Books, 1990.
6. Carr JH, Shepherd RB: Movement Science—Foundations for Physical Therapy in Rehabilitation. Rockville, MD, Aspen Publishers, 1987.
7. Carr JH, Shepherd RB: Neurological Rehabilitation—Optimizing Motor Performance, Boston, Butterworth Heinemann, 1998.
8. Cassady KA, Whitley RJ: Pathogenesis and pathophysiology of viral infections of the central nervous system. In Scheld WM, Whitney RJ, Durach DT (eds): Infections of the Central Nervous System, 2nd ed. Philadelphia, Lippincott-Raven, 1997.
9. Davis LE: Central nervous system infections. In Weiner WJ, Goetz CG (eds): Neurology for the Non-neurologist, 4th ed. Philadelphia, Lippincott Williams & Wilkins, 1999.
10. Davis LE: Infections of the central nervous system: Acute bacterial meningitis. In Weiner WJ, Shulman LM (eds): Emergent and Urgent Neurology. Philadelphia, Lippincott Williams & Wilkins, 1999.
11. DeMeyer W: Technique of the Neurological Examination. 4th ed. New York, McGraw-Hill, 1994.
12. Duncan PW, Badke MB: Stroke Rehabilitation—The Recovery of Motor Control. St. Louis, CV Mosby, 1987.
13. Fritz DP, Nelson PB: Brain abscess. In Roos KL (ed): Central Nervous System Infectious Diseases and Therapy, New York, Marcel Dekker, 1997.
14. Gluckman SJ, DiNubile MJ: Infections of the central nervous system: Acute viral infections. In Weiner WJ, Shulman LM (eds): Emergent and Urgent Neurology. Philadelphia, Lippincott Williams & Wilkins, 1999.
15. Guide to Physical Therapist Practice. Alexandria, VA, American Physical Therapy Association, 1999.
16. Hoppenfeld S: Physical examination of the spine and extremities. New York, Appleton-Century-Crofts, 1976.
17. Jennett B, Teasdale G: Management of Head Injuries, Philadelphia, FA Davis, 1981.
18. Johnson RT: Viral Infections of the Nervous System, 2nd ed. Philadelphia, Lippincott-Raven, 1998.

19. Levitt S: Treatment of Cerebral Palsy and Motor Delay, 2nd ed. London, Blackwell Scientific, 1982.

20. McCarthy M, Weber T, Berger JR: Central nervous system diseases caused by unconventional transmissible agents and chronic viral infections. In Bradley WG et al (eds): Neurology in Clinical Practice, vol 2. Boston, Butterworth-Heinemann, 1996.

20a. McNevin NH, Wulf G, Carlson C: Effects of attentional focus, self control, and dyad training on motor learning: implications for physical rehabilitation. Phys Ther 80:373–385, 2000.

21. Plum F, Posner JB: The Diagnosis of Stupor and Coma, 3rd ed. Philadelphia, FA Davis, 1980.

22. Pruitt AA: Infections of the nervous system. Neurol Clin 16:419–447, 1998.

23. Roos KL: Meningitis. London, Arnold, 1996.

24. Roos KL: Bacterial meningitis. In Roos KL (ed): Central Nervous System Infectious Diseases and Therapy. New York, Marcel Dekker, 1997.

25. Roos KL: Viral meningitis and aseptic meningitis. In Roos KL (ed): Central Nervous System Infectious Diseases and Therapy. New York, Marcel Dekker, 1997.

26. Roos KL, Bonnin JM: Acute bacterial meningitides. In Mandell GL (ed): Atlas of Infectious Diseases, Vol 3, Central Nervous System and Eye Infection. Philadelphia, Churchill Livingstone, 1995.

27. Rotbart HA: Viral meningitis and the aseptic meningitis syndrome. In Scheld WM, Whitney RJ, Durach DT (eds): Infections of the Central Nervous System, 2nd ed. Philadelphia, Lippincott-Raven, 1997.

28. Ryerson S, Levit K: Functional movement reeducation: A contemporary model for stroke rehabilitation. New York, Churchill Livingstone, 1997.

29. Schooley RT: Encephalitis. In Roper AH (ed): Neurological and neurosurgical intensive care, 3rd ed. New York, Raven Press, 1993.

30. Sullivan PE, Markos PD: Clinical Decision Making in Therapeutic Exercise. Norwalk, CT, Appleton & Lange, 1995.

31. VanSant AF: Analysis of movement dysfunction: Usefulness of a component approach. In Proceedings of the 13th Annual Eugene Michels Researchers' Forum, Section on Research, American Physical Therapy Association, Alexandria, VA, 1993.

32. VanSant AF: Rising from a supine position to erect stance—description of adult movement and a developmental hypothesis. Phys Ther 68:185–192, 1988.

33. Voss DE, Ionta MK, Myers BJ: Proprioceptive Neuromuscular Facilitation, 3rd ed. Philadelphia, Harper & Row, 1985.

34. Weiner WJ, Goetz CG: Neurology for the Non-neurologist, 4th ed. Philadelphia, Lippincott Williams & Wilkins, 1999.

Human Immunodeficiency Virus (HIV) Infection: Living with a Chronic Illness

MARY LOU GALANTINO, PhD, PT

Key Words

– AIDS

– human immunodeficiency virus (HIV)

– psychoneuroimmunology

Objectives

After reading this chapter the student/therapist will:

1. Appreciate the role of the immune system in chronic HIV disease.

2. Know the neuropathology of HIV infection and understand potential neurocognitive and neuropsychological alterations that may occur.

3. Understand the various systems (integumentary, musculoskeletal, cardiopulmonary, and neurological) that affect function in HIV-infected adult and pediatric patients.

4. Appreciate the role of psychoneuroimmunology in HIV rehabilitation management.

5. Establish safe exercise parameters in the HIV-positive population.

IDENTIFICATION OF THE CLINICAL PROBLEM

Initially recognized in 1982, acquired immunodeficiency syndrome (AIDS) has been the leading cause of death among young adults in the United States for much of the 1990s. It has had a devastating impact on people in the developing world.[23, 116] Since the mid 1990s, the epidemiology of HIV disease has changed the industrial world in the United States. For the first time in the history of the epidemic there has been a decrease in the annual national incidence and a decline in AIDS deaths.[24, 25, 108] Most epidemiologists and clinicians attribute these findings to the impact of new, highly active antiretroviral therapies (HAARTs). Because this has fostered longevity, HIV infection has become a chronic disease. This has great impact on rehabilitation medicine because multisystem involvement progresses slowly throughout the life span. Potential return to work may be fostered through vocational rehabilitation.

Adults and adolescents older than 13 years of age have accounted for almost 99% of the total AIDS cases. Less than 2% (1.3%) have occurred in children younger than 13 years of age. The newer HAARTs have slowed the progression from HIV infection to AIDS and from AIDS to death.[24] Perinatally acquired AIDS incidence has declined significantly as a result of policy changes and the administration of zidovudine (azidothymidine [AZT]) and other antiretroviral therapies.[26]

The clinical and pathological information about this disease is constantly increasing. Certainly, our understanding of the disease process and advances in drug regimens will change between the writing and the publication of this book. Changes in terminology reflect this

TABLE 18-1. Quality of Life Issues for HIV Disease Stages

Stage	CD4⁺ Category	Physical Indicators	Moderators of Quality of Life	General Quality of Life Issues
Asymptomatic HIV infection	≤500 µL	May have persistent generalized lymphadenopathy	*Appraisals:* Anticipatory grieving, catastrophizing, and other cognitive distortions; changed expectations of future; identity and self-esteem issues *Coping:* Dealing with present and future uncertainties; at risk for denial, disengagement, substance abuse, risky sex, suicidality; issues of eliciting social support	*Emotional functioning:* Depression, anxiety, anger, often increasing at diagnosis and diminishing and recycling as individual confronts realities of living with HIV disease *Role functioning:* Often able to work; possible decrements in job mobility and career opportunities; job loss *Social functioning:* Fear, isolation, issues of trust in relationships; stigmatization; changes in social support networks due to deaths; relationship and sexual changes; isolation, withdrawal *Physical functioning:* Normal but may be altered due to depression or anxiety; may have hypervigilance regarding all physical symptoms *Spiritual functioning:* Opportunity to direct attention inward, thus yielding to contemplation of life's meaning, reassessment of spiritual and existential issues
Symptomatic HIV infection	201–499 µL	Emergence of symptoms such as thrush, night sweats, low-grade fevers, oral hairy leukoplakia, peripheral neuropathy; commonly taking antiretroviral drugs and/or *Pneumocystis carinii* prophylaxis	*Appraisals:* Anticipatory grieving, catastrophizing, and other cognitive distortions; changed expectations of future; identity and self-esteem issues related to threats to occupational and functional abilities *Coping:* Dealing with present and future uncertainties; at risk for denial, disengagement, substance abuse, and risky sex	*Emotional functioning:* Depression, anxiety, anger, often increasing on emergence of symptoms and then fluctuating with challenges and threats to present and future functioning *Role functioning:* Often able to work; may take on new roles as part of HIV support-related network *Social functioning:* Changes in social support networks due to deaths, isolation, withdrawal, relationship and sexual changes, and stigmatization *Physical functioning:* May have reduced energy levels; moderate symptomatology; possible cognitive deficits; pain; wasting *Spiritual functioning:* Anticipatory grieving, sense of relatedness to something greater than the self, unavoidable confrontation with one's own mortality
AIDS	<200 µL	Opportunistic infections such as extensive candidiasis, cryptococcal meningitis; Kaposi's sarcoma; tuberculosis; *Pneumocystis carinii* pneumonia; lymphomas; commonly taking antiretroviral drugs, chemotherapy, antibiotics, etc.	*Appraisals:* Facing chronic illness and death; grieving about current and anticipated losses; catastrophizing and other cognitive distortions; reassessment of spiritual and existential issues *Coping:* Coping strategies may be overwhelmed in dealing with current difficulties such as financial losses, medical costs, treatment and side effects, housing; may lose some traditional coping strategies such as recreational outlets	*Emotional functioning:* Depression, anxiety, anger may cycle according to fluctuations in disease status and appraisals; relief from uncertainty *Role functioning:* Diminished capacity for work; role changes—often need care instead of being a caretaker *Social functioning:* May have diminished social networks due to lack of mobility, illness, as well as deaths among friends *Physical functioning:* Self-care difficulties; fatigue; wasting; much time spent in medical care; debilitation from infection and treatments; possible cognitive deficits *Spiritual functioning:* Essential worth is to provide a framework from which to pose and seek responses to metaphysical questions generated by the presence of a life-threatening disease; integration and transcending of one's biological and psychosocial nature, which gives access to nonphysical realms as prophecy, love, artistic inspiration, completion and, healing actions

evolution of clinical knowledge. The definitions used throughout this chapter reflect current use.

The virus thought to be responsible for the transmission of AIDS was identified as HIV (human immunodeficiency virus) in July 1986 at the International Conference on AIDS in Paris. A second virus, HIV-2, was identified in western Africa. Infection due to this second subtype, less widely distributed, has since been established in Europe and in South, Central, and North America. Both HIV-1 and HIV-2 have resulted in AIDS, but evidence suggests that HIV-2 may be less virulent than HIV-1. In addition to these subtypes, several strains of HIV-1 have been identified. Different strains reflect variations in cellular affinities and resistance to medications. The context of discussion for the purpose of this chapter will be HIV-1, herein discussed as HIV.

In 1993 the Centers for Disease Control (CDC) revised its definition of AIDS and classification system of HIV infection. To reflect current scientific knowledge, the new system elucidates the importance of T-helper (CD4) cell counts as indicators for pharmacological disease management. The changed definition of AIDS now includes HIV infection and CD4 counts below 200/mm^3, regardless of the status of opportunistic or concomitant disorders. In addition, three clinical conditions—pulmonary tuberculosis, recurrent pneumonia, and invasive cervical cancer—were added to the existing list of 20 AIDS-defining diseases.[28] The entire spectrum of illness from initial diagnosis to AIDS can be covered by the term *HIV infection*. The terms HIV asymptomatic, HIV symptomatic, and HIV advanced disease (AIDS) are used throughout this chapter because this delineates the progression of HIV disease. Table 18–1 presents the various modifiers of quality of life throughout the various stages of HIV disease.

Epidemiology

HIV infection has assumed the title of the leading cause of death in the world, according to the World Health Organization's (WHO) World Health Report.[145] The WHO estimates that in 1998 there were approximately 2.3 million AIDS-related deaths in the world, accounting for 4.2% of all deaths.

HIV infection is the fourth leading cause of disability-adjusted life-years (DALYs) lost, a measure that assesses the impact of disease on both length and quality of life. Only perinatal diseases, acute respiratory infections, and diarrheal diseases cause more premature loss of life and function than that due to AIDS.[30]

Tuberculosis (TB), the former leading microbial killer, was estimated to have killed 1.8 million people in 1998, but 400,000 of these deaths were in HIV-infected individuals, and the WHO credited these deaths to AIDS rather than to TB. HIV infection is now responsible for more than 20% of all deaths in people with TB.[30]

Normal Immunity

The immune system is complex and dynamic, comprising a multitude of components and subsystems, all of which interact continuously. The normal immune system has two main components or lines of defense against illness (Fig. 18–1). The first is the innate, or inborn, component that includes the skin, the cilia and mucosal linings of the respiratory and digestive systems, the gastric fluids and enzymes of the stomach, and the phagocyte cells. This innate component of the immune system keeps pathogens out of the body by creating barriers against them, by ejecting them, or by enveloping them and eliminating them. The second, the acquired component of the immune system, develops defenses against specific pathogens, starts in utero, and continues throughout life. It is acquired (or antibody) immunity that is most pertinent to understanding HIV infection and its progression.

Acquired Immunity

Acquired immunity is divided into humoral and cell-mediated responses. Humoral immunity depends on the production of antibodies. This response is effective for dispatching free-floating or cell-surface pathogens. The

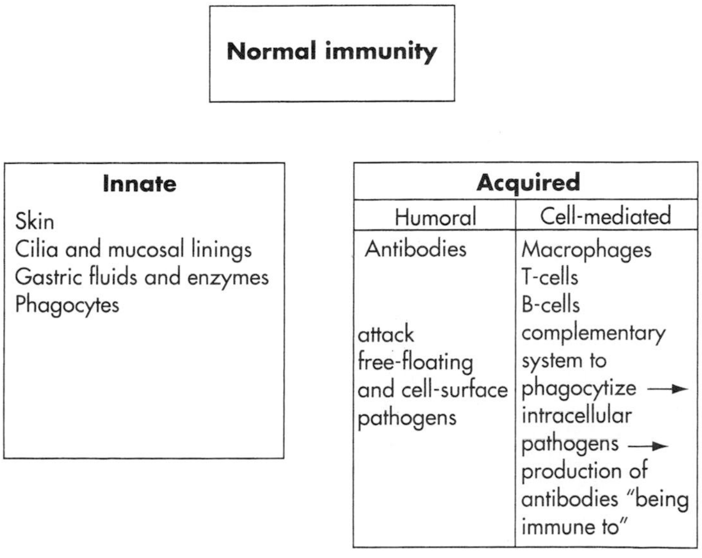

Normal immunity

Innate
Skin
Cilia and mucosal linings
Gastric fluids and enzymes
Phagocytes

Acquired	
Humoral	Cell-mediated
Antibodies	Macrophages
	T-cells
	B-cells
attack	complementary
free-floating	system to
and cell-surface	phagocytize →
pathogens	intracellular
	pathogens →
	production of
	antibodies "being
	immune to"

FIGURE 18–1. Main components of immunity.

cell-mediated response is required to destroy infected cells, those with intracellular pathogens. Cell-mediated immunity is essential for destroying pathogens responsible for the opportunistic infections and neoplasms that are associated with AIDS.[31, 32]

For the study of HIV pathology, it is important to consider three types of immune system cells: macrophages, T lymphocytes (T cells), and B lymphocytes (B cells). Macrophages originate in the bone marrow and then migrate to the organs in the lymphatic system. Macrophages recognize and then phagocytize, antigens—substances deemed foreign to the body. All but a fragment of the antigen is digested by the macrophage. This remaining portion protrudes from the cellular surface, where it is recognized by T and B cells.[93]

Both of the lymphocytes originate in the bone marrow. Their differentiation into T and B cells depends on where they develop immunocompetence. T cells migrate to the thymus to perform this task. B cells complete it before leaving the bone marrow. T cells then travel to lymph nodes, the spleen, and connective tissue, where they wait to phagocytize the antigens in the manner previously described. B cells function in the same way against free-floating blood-borne pathogens.[93]

There are at least eight types of T cells with various functions. Two relevant types are helper T cells (CD4) and suppressor T cells (CD8). These cells are regulatory and complementary. On recognition of an antigen, CD4 cells chemically stimulate production and activation of other lymphocytes to destroy the foreign material. When the action of the T and B cells is sufficient, CD8 cells stop this action, thus preventing destruction of noninfected cells.

In the process of identifying and destroying these antigens, the acquired immune system also retains a memory of the antigen, which allows it to respond more rapidly and effectively to the pathogen if it is reintroduced into the body. Herein lies the pertinence of vaccination and the phenomenon of being immune to an illness.[93]

Psychoneuroimmunology: Prevention and Wellness in HIV Infection

Psychoneuroimmunology is that field that investigates the interrelationships among psychological constructs (e.g., stressors and mood states) of the neuroendocrine and immune systems. Even though all the precise mechanistic links among these varied components of psychoneuroimmunology are not yet fully elucidated, psychoneuroimmunology does offer a very useful framework to our understanding of how stressors play a role in immunomodulation. These effects may have a profound influence on the occurrence and progression of ill health in chronic diseases such as HIV infection/AIDS.

Psychoneuroimmunological findings show that it may be useful to evaluate the influence of behavioral factors on immune functioning and disease progression among HIV-infected individuals.[1, 79, 80] Behavioral interventions with immunomodulatory capabilities may help restore competence and thereby arrest HIV disease promotion at the earliest stages of the infectious continuum.

A growing body of literature indicates that many different stressors have deleterious effects on the immune system.[68] These stressors in the case of people living with HIV infection may be attenuated by an exercise training program. Research indicates that continued aerobic exercise training may result in increased CD4 cell counts, heightened immune surveillance, and a potential for a slowing of disease progression.[80] Other researchers have demonstrated similar benefits of exercise for individuals infected with HIV who are at more advanced stages of disease. However, these are studies conducted on traditional modes of exercise. Exercise within the context of psychoneuroimmunology appears to be a very promising approach to the treatment of illness and promotion of health in chronic HIV disease.

PATHOGENESIS OF HIV INFECTION

HIV belongs to a class of viruses known as retroviruses, which carry their genetic material in the form of RNA rather than DNA. HIV primarily infects the mononuclear cells, especially CD4 and macrophages, but B cells also are infected.[35] HIV binds to the receptor sites on the surface of the lymphocytes, eventually fusing with and then entering the cells. Reverse transcriptase released from the HIV allows a DNA copy of the virus to be made within the host cell, which can then become integrated into the host cell genome. The lymphocyte becomes a "virus factory," as replicated virions bud out of the cell to infect others.

Within days of HIV infection, lymph nodes become sites of rampant viral replication, during which the individual remains asymptomatic. This time of seroconversion usually occurs within 3 months, but it can take 12 months. In retrospect, many affected people describe nonspecific and self-limited flulike symptoms: fever, diarrhea, myalgias, and fatigue. An asymptomatic period follows in which the individual tests seropositive. The interim stages of HIV infection are marked by generalized swelling of the lymph nodes followed by an extended period when the infected person will not necessarily develop further symptoms, but laboratory tests may reveal immune dysfunction: a decline in CD4 cells and an elevated viral load. The staging of HIV infection includes (1) early stage or asymptomatic (CD4 count >500/mm³), (2) middle stage or symptomatic (CD4 count 200–500), and (3) late stage or advanced disease (CD4 count <200).

Medical Management

Cell Counts, Viral Load, and Prophylaxis

Pharmacological interventions to combat the opportunistic infections associated with HIV infection are beyond the scope of this chapter, but a simplified summary of clinical information is pertinent. Medical management of HIV infection is most often guided by the CD4 cell count and viral load.

For the healthy non–HIV-infected adult, the average CD4 cell count is approximately 1000 cells/mm³. However, counts may vary widely and range from 500 to 1500 cells/mm³.[117]

A CD4 cell count of 200 cells/mm³ marks a critical point in the course of an HIV-infected individual. Multiple serious opportunistic infections occur once this level of immune depletion is attained.[34, 95, 111]

Exercise, stress, season, serum cortisol, and the presence of acute or chronic illness have all been reported to affect CD4 cell counts. Thus, the initial CD4 lymphocyte numbers should be confirmed by repeat testing. Caution should be exercised to avoid overinterpreting small changes in CD4 lymphocyte test results. The overall trend of CD4 counts is more important than any single value. Additionally, the frequency of testing is four times annually with CD4 counts around 300 cells/mm³. When counts are less than 50 CD4 cells/mm³ there is no need for additional testing. When patients are on HAART and stable, CD4 lymphocyte counts are generally measured every 3 months.

Currently, CD4 cell directives are as follows: CD4 counts above 500/mm³ usually indicate no need for antiretroviral therapy, because individuals are generally asymptomatic. CD4 counts between 200/mm³ and 500/mm³ indicate the need for antiretroviral therapy. CD4 cell counts below 200/mm³ direct preventive *Pneumocystis carinii* pneumonia (PCP) and toxoplasmosis measures. Persons with counts below 100/mm³ may also receive prophylactic agents against PCP and toxoplasmosis as well as cytomegalovirus (CMV) infection, infection with *Mycobacterium avium* complex (MAC), and fungal infections such as cryptococcosis and candidiasis.[31] Table 18–1 presents quality of life issues for HIV disease stages. Table 18–2 is a summary of common pharmacological agents prescribed to combat opportunistic infections and, most pertinent to rehabilitation, their potential side effects.

Viral Load Measurement

Testing for the amount of HIV in plasma by measuring viral RNA has become a standard component of the management of HIV-infected patients.[22]

There are important prognostic implications for the amount of viral load in persons with HIV disease.[97] In patients with higher viral loads, disease progression is more rapid, both immunologically in terms of the rate of CD4 cell count decline and clinically in terms of developing AIDS-defining illness. Additionally, the plasma levels in HIV pregnant women directly correlate with the risk of perinatal transmission.[37] Viral load is an important useful marker for judging the effectiveness of various antiretroviral drug interventions.[63, 94]

There are several assays available for testing HIV for resistance to antiretroviral agents. Genotypic and phenotypic testing have recently been implemented, and it is important that medication not be discontinued before resistance testing. Like genotypic testing, phenotypic testing may not detect small subpopulations of resistant HIV.[60]

Now that a viral etiology has been established with some certainty, researchers are concentrating on developing effective HAART and safe vaccines. The primary goal of antiretroviral therapy is to achieve prolonged suppression of HIV replication.[22, 57] In 1987, zidovudine (AZT) was approved by the U.S. Food and Drug Administration (FDA). Since that time several more antiretroviral therapies have been approved and include didanosine (ddI), zalcitabine (ddC), D4T, and 3TC. Each one inhibits the HIV enzyme reverse transcriptase.[83]

Additional drugs—nevirapine, delavirdine, and efavirenz—also inhibit the viral reverse transcriptase enzyme but they are not nucleoside analogs. These agents bind to the enzymatic binding pocket of the reverse transcriptase gene and block binding by nucleosides.[135]

Another drug target for anti-HIV agents is the viral protease enzyme. Protease inhibitors are structurally different from nucleoside analogs and include agents such as ritonavir, indinavir, nelfinavir, and saquinavir.[43]

Current medication regimens can significantly reduce the HIV level not only in the peripheral blood but also in the lymphoid tissue and the central nervous system.[126] In an effort to reduce the plasma HIV burden to levels below the threshold of detection by available assays, a series of HAART may be necessary. The challenge, however may arise quickly because resistance to one drug in a class of agents may induce partial or complete resistance with other agents, depending on the specific mutations involved.[4, 60] In a field that is rapidly changing, specific recommendations for antiretroviral therapy are difficult to make. The major therapeutic decisions include (1) when to initiate therapy and (2) when to change therapy and to which drugs. With the advent of protease inhibitors, the mortality rate of HIV-infected patients and incidence of opportunistic infections has dropped, both most likely due to the increased use of combination HAART.[109] The role of drugs with immunomodulating activity for use in combination with HAART is also undergoing extensive research.[75, 81] Drug regimens for HIV disease are dynamic, and clinical practice guidelines are consistently updated; many changes in the approach to drug interventions can be expected as HIV infection continues to be a chronic disease.[62]

Vaccines

HIV-positive individuals respond less well than noninfected persons to many vaccines. The degree of immunodeficiency present at the time of vaccination has impact on the response to hepatitis A or B, pneumococcal, and influenza A and B vaccines.[102] Those who have a CD4 count of more than 200 cells/mm³ respond the best. Patients should be informed that the extent and duration of the protective efficacy of these vaccines are still uncertain.

Vaccination for HIV is likely the best hope of controlling disease progression. The first human immunizations with potential AIDS vaccine took place in 1986 in healthy seropositive volunteers in France and Zaire. Low levels of both humoral and cell-mediated immune responses resulted. One conclusion of this study is that booster vaccinations could be effective.[74]

Genetic mutation of the virus further complicates attempts to disable it. It is thought that genetically similar but distinguishable strains of HIV can exist in one individual. Furthermore, drug-resistant strains of HIV have been identified.[137]

TABLE 18–2. Common Opportunistic Diseases in HIV Infection

Disease/Pathogen	Sites of Infection	Symptoms	Medications and Side Effects	Disease-Specific Precautions
Pneumocystis carinii pneumonia (PCP)/*Pneumocystis carinii*, a protozoan found in air, water, and soil, carried by domestic animals, and possibly latent in most people	Lungs, sometimes spreads to the spleen, lymph nodes, and blood	Fever, cough, shortness of breath, chills, chest pain, sputum production in late disease	Trimethoprim-sulfamethoxazole: rash, itching, Stevens-Johnson syndrome, extreme fatigue, dysphagia, fever, leukopenia, sore throat, thrombocytopenia, hepatitis, hematuria, diarrhea, dizziness, headache, anorexia, nausea, vomiting IM or IV pentamidine isethionate: azotemia, serum creatinine elevations, pain and induration at intramuscular sites, abscess or necrosis at injection sites, elevated liver function tests, leukopenia, nausea, vomiting, hypotension, syncope, blood sugar imbalances Aerosolized pentamidine isethionate: investigational Dapsone: nausea, vomiting, abdominal pain, vertigo, blurred vision, tinnitus, insomnia, fever, headache, phototoxicity, lupus, anemia Sulfadoxine-pyrimethamine: allergic skin reactions, nausea and vomiting, glossitis, stomatitis, headache, peripheral neuritis, mental depression, fatigue, weakness	None
Toxoplasmosis/*Toxoplasma gondii*, a protozoan found in air, water, soil, and some cats and other animals. Most often acquired by ingestion of uncooked infected lamb or pork, unpasteurized dairy products, raw eggs or vegetables. Mothers can give it to unborn children. Other human-human transmission does not occur.	Produces lesions in the central nervous system; may also involve heart and lungs	Fever, chills, headache, visual disturbances, lethargy, confusion, hemiparesis, seizures	Sulfadiazine: same as for trimethoprim-sulfamethoxazole Pyrimethamine: anorexia, vomiting, megaloblastic anemia, leukopenia, thrombocytopenia, glossitis	None
Cryptosporidiosis/*Cryptosporidium*, a protozoan primarily acquired through oral contact with feces of an infected animal, or oral sexual contact with an infected person	Gastrointestinal tract	Copious diarrhea, abdominal pain, anorexia, nausea, vomiting, dehydration, weight loss, weakness, fever	Spiramycin: nausea, vomiting, diarrhea, abdominal pain Eflornithine: investigational	Gloves and gown/apron when handling feces. Private room when patient has poor hygiene.
Isosporiasis/*Isospora belli*, a protozoan primarily acquired through eating uncooked beef or pork or through oral sexual contact with an infected person	Gastrointestinal tract	Diarrhea, abdominal pain, nausea, vomiting, anorexia, weight loss, weakness, fever	Trimethoprim-sulfamethoxazole: see under *Pneumocystis carinii*	Gloves and gown/apron when handling feces. Private room when patient has poor hygiene.
Mycobacterium avium-intracellulare (MAI) infection/*Mycobacterium avium-intracellulare*, a bacterium found in soil, water, animals, eggs, and unpasteurized dairy products and other foods. MAI infection is atypical and noncommunicable.	Disseminated	Fever, malaise, night sweats, anorexia, diarrhea, weight loss	Isoniazid: paresthesia and peripheral neuropathy, elevated liver function test values, anorexia, nausea, vomiting, fatigue, malaise, weakness Rifabutin: hepatotoxicity, neutropenia, nausea, vomiting, diarrhea, rash, itching Clofazimine: reddish-brown discoloration of skin, conjunctiva, sweat, hair, urine, and feces; abdominal pain, diarrhea Ethambutol: reversible blurring of vision, anaphylaxis, skin irritation, nausea, vomiting, fever Cycloserine: convulsions, drowsiness, headache, tremor, other central nervous system disturbances Ethionamide: nausea, vomiting, peripheral and optic neuritis, mental depression, postural hypotension, rash Rifampin: urine discoloration, heartburn, nausea, vomiting, abdominal cramps, headache, drowsiness, fatigue Streptomycin: nausea, vomiting, vertigo, numbness of the face, rash, fever, itching, elevated white blood cell count	Gloves and gown/apron when handling wound drainage.

TABLE 18–2. Common Opportunistic Diseases in HIV Infection *Continued*

Disease/Pathogen	Sites of Infection	Symptoms	Medications and Side Effects	Disease-Specific Precautions
Candidiasis/*Candida albicans,* a fungus that inhabits the oropharynx, vagina, large intestine, and skin, causing no harm as long as immunity remains undamaged; may occur as a secondary infection in conjunction with herpes simplex virus lesions	Anywhere skin or mucous membrane is damaged, including IV therapy and pressure monitoring sites, etc.	Thrush, esophageal, perianal irritation, vaginitis, proctitis; inflammation around fingernails can be disseminated.	Clotrimazole: abdominal pain, diarrhea, nausea, vomiting Nystatin: diarrhea, nausea, vomiting, stomach pain Ketoconazole: hepatitis, gynecomastia, nausea, vomiting, decreased libido, diarrhea, dizziness, drowsiness, photophobia, rash, itching, sleepiness Amphotericin B	None
Cryptococcosis/*Cryptococcus neoformans,* a fungus found in air, water, soil, raw fruits and vegetables, and pigeon droppings and found on window ledges and nesting places; acquired by inhalation	Central nervous system, lungs; can be disseminated	Altered cognition, low-grade fever, headache, nausea, vomiting, meningeal signs	Amphotericin B Ketoconazole: see under Candidiasis	None
Cytomegalovirus (CMV) infection/cytomegalovirus, an organism found in saliva, semen, cervical secretions, urine, feces, blood, breast milk. It causes problems only when immunity is compromised.	Disseminated	Fever, profound fatigue, muscle and joint aches, night sweats, impaired vision, cough, dyspnea, abdominal pain, diarrhea	Ganciclovir: leukopenia, bone marrow, depression, elevated liver enzymes, edema, nausea, muscle aches, headaches, anorexia, disorientation, rash, phlebitis	Private room if the patient has enteritis and poor hygiene. Gloves and gown/apron for handling excretions and secretions if soiling is likely.
Herpes simplex virus (HSV) infection/herpes simplex virus 1 is spread by contact with infected oral secretions. Herpes simplex virus 2 is spread by contact with infected genital secretions. Patient can spread either variety by touching lesions, then touching other body parts.	Mouth, perianal area; can be disseminated	Painful burning, itching vesicular lesions; sometimes colitis, pericarditis, esophageal infection	Acyclovir: rash, diarrhea, light-headedness, headache, nausea, vomiting, thirst, fatigue	Gloves and gown/apron for handling secretions from lesions. Private room if infection is disseminated or severe.
Progressive multifocal leukoencephalopathy (PML)/ JC virus; transmission routes unclear	Brain	Impaired speech, vision, and thought; ataxia and limb weakness; advanced disease can cause profound dementia	No known effective treatment	None

Another difficulty with vaccination development is a lack of animal models. Chimpanzees replicate simian immune deficiency virus (SIV), a similar but not identical disease. In addition, an average of 12 years and $231 million is required for a new drug to gain FDA approval. Many major pharmaceutical companies seem wary of the immense research expenses and potential liability risks linked to vaccine development. The result is that smaller biotechnology companies with fewer resources are assailing the complicated problems of HIV infection.[31] It is estimated that a vaccine will not be readily available for another 5 to 10 years. This vaccine will ideally induce both humoral and cellular immune responses and have no toxic effects. It will protect against initial infection and retard disease onset in infected individuals.

Nutrition

Involuntary loss of more than 10% of baseline body weight and chronic diarrhea or unexplained weakness and fever constitute HIV wasting syndrome.[29] Retrospective demographic research in the United States found that 17.8% of individuals with AIDS experienced wasting syndrome.[45, 100] The ensuing malnutrition contributes to further immunosuppression.[58] It is important to have nutritional consultation not only for patients presenting with wasting syndrome but also for prevention of disease and enhancement of the immune system.

Systemic Manifestations

Integumentary System

There are three AIDS-defining malignancies: Kaposi's sarcoma (KS), non-Hodgkin's lymphoma (NHL), and cervical cancer. KS can involve almost every part of the body, but the most common site of initial KS presentations is the skin or mucous membranes.[77] The disorder presents as cutaneous purple nodular lesions or as rife visceral lesions. AIDS-KS has been intimately associated with the lymphatic system, specifically, deficient lymphatic transport, nodal dysfunction, and tumors, which contribute to lymphedema that clinicians observe as swollen extremities.[143]

In KS there is a broad therapeutic spectrum from cryotherapy to systemic chemotherapy.[16] In NHL early therapeutic intervention is necessary because of the fast progress of the tumor.[12] The cervical cancer in HIV-infected women seems to be more aggressive than in non–HIV-infected women and also needs early therapeutic intervention.[91] The cancer incidence in HIV patients is reported to be higher among nonblacks.[66]

There are several other tumors that occur with people with HIV infection: anorectal cancer, lung cancer, malignant testicular tumor, Hodgkin's lymphoma, basal cell carcinoma, and even malignant melanoma.[12, 118] It is beyond the scope of this chapter to detail all aspects of cancer and dermatological concerns; however, the therapist needs to be aware of the importance of differential diagnosis because the skin is the first line of defense of the immune system and further workup may be warranted.

Musculoskeletal System

Musculoskeletal manifestations of HIV infection are not as common as manifestations seen in other parts of the body, including the central nervous system, pulmonary system, and gastrointestinal tract. They tend to occur in advanced HIV infection. Knowledge of the different abnormalities that may occur in the musculoskeletal system is crucial to patient management and affects morbidity and mortality. Primary abnormalities present as osseous and soft tissue infections, polymyositis, and arthritis. Secondary musculoskeletal complications are often due to the various compensatory patterns of gait as a result of HIV-related peripheral neuropathy syndrome or the change in biomechanics of the foot and ankle due to KS and NHL.[47] This leads to potential spinal changes and back pain.

HIV-infected patients with polymyositis typically present with proximal and less commonly distal muscle weakness and elevated creatine kinase levels.[136] Patients may have initial symptoms of difficulty with basic activities of daily living (ADL), such as rising from a chair.

Arthritis in HIV-infected persons has a wide spectrum of presentations ranging from mild arthralgias to very severe joint disability.[122] Arthritides seen in AIDS patients have been classified into five groups based on clinical presentation: (1) painful articular syndrome, (2) acute symmetrical polyarthritis, (3) spondyloarthropathic arthritis (Reiter's syndrome, psoriatic arthritis), (4) HIV-associated arthritis, and (5) septic arthritis.[134]

Cardiopulmonary System

Pulmonary diseases continue to be important causes of illness and death in patients with HIV infection, but changes in therapy and demographics of HIV-infected populations are changing their manifestations. The risk of developing specific disorders is related to the degree of immunosuppression, HIV risk group, area of residence, and use of prophylactic therapies.[120] Sinusitis and bronchitis occur frequently in the HIV-infected population, more so than in the general public. The increasing population of HIV-infected drug users is reflected in the increasing incidence of TB and bacterial pneumonia.

Anti-*Pneumocystis* prophylaxis has reduced the incidence of and mortality due to PCP. The PCP-causing organism is usually acquired in childhood, and between 65% and 85% of healthy adults possess PCP antibodies. Reactivation of latent infection is responsible for the recurrent fever, dyspnea, and hypoxia that characterize PCP.[9, 72] Adjunctive corticosteroid therapy has improved the outlook for respiratory failure.[120]

Mycobacterial infections in HIV-infected individuals usually present as either MAC infection or TB.[5] Steadily increasing incidence of infection by *M. tuberculosis* is likely the result of two factors: better medical management of HIV as a whole and the development of multidrug-resistant strains of mycobacteria.

MAC infection tends to present late in the course of HIV infection. Initial infection involves the gastrointestinal and pulmonary tracts and eventually disseminates throughout the body. This disorder probably is due not to latent reactivation of the organism but rather to primary infection by ingestion or inhalation.[71] Signs and symptoms of MAC infection include pneumonia, fever, weight loss, malaise, sweats, anorexia, abdominal pain, and diarrhea.

As in many other infections, initial signs and symptoms of TB include fever, weight loss, malaise, cough, lymph node tenderness, and night sweats. Pulmonary involvement accounts for between 75% and 100% of cases of TB infection in HIV-infected patients, but extrapulmonary infection, especially in lymph nodes and bone marrow, occurs in up to 60% of these individuals as well.[9, 71, 72, 113] Other less common areas of infection include the central nervous system (CNS) and cardiac and mucosal tissues.

TB is communicable, preventable, and treatable. Tuberculin skin testing should be available and routinely offered to individuals at HIV testing sites. Individuals at highest risk for concomitant HIV and TB infections include the homeless, intravenous drug users, and prisoners.[9, 113] The risk of infection to health care personnel as well as to the general public is a concern. Isolation rooms that provide negative pressure, nonrecirculated ventilation, and specific air filters and air exchange rates offer the best protection to health care providers exposed to TB-infected individuals. Properly fitted face masks that filter droplet nuclei should be worn. Monitoring of personnel who work with these populations will identify the need for necessary preventive therapy.[9]

CMV can affect the gastrointestinal and respiratory tracts but primarily targets optic structures. CMV infection also appears to be latent. Between 40% and 100% of healthy adults possess CMV antibodies.[76] Predominant consequences of HIV/CMV co-infection are unilateral or bilateral deficits in visual acuity, visual field cuts, and blindness.

Although most other organ system involvement has been extensively described in studies and reviews, cardiac complications related to HIV infection have remained less characterized. Most studies have described cardiac problems as postmortem findings, although some clinical series have been reported. It is now clear that cardiac involvement in people living with HIV infection is quite common. Pericardial effusion and myocarditis are among the most commonly reported cardiac abnormalities. Cardiomyopathy, endocarditis, and coronary vasculopathy have also been reported. It is now apparent that HIV infection itself, the medical management of HIV disease, and secondary opportunistic infections can all affect the myocardium, pericardium, endocardium, and blood vessels.[53, 146]

Over the past 2 years, body fat changes and lipid abnormalities have been reported in individuals with HIV/AIDS.[55] A number of cases of body fat and metabolic changes have been connected to protease inhibitor use.[18] These body fat changes may have strong implications for patients who receive rehabilitation intervention.

Signs and symptoms of the syndrome vary, and not all need to be present in any particular patient. However, in both males and females, three main components of the syndrome have emerged. These include changes in body shape, hyperlipidemia, and insulin resistance. Clinically, distinct body shape changes are apparent. The most prevalent include increased abdominal growth, dorsocervical fat pad, benign symmetrical lipomatosis, lipodystrophy, and breast hypertrophy in women.[85, 98] The increased abdominal growth is characterized by a redistribution and accumulation of fat in the central visceral areas of the body.[36, 98] Corresponding symptoms include gastrointestinal discomfort, bloating, distention, and fullness.[36]

In addition to visible signs and symptoms, adverse changes in lipids, glucose, and insulin have also been reported.[59] A number of studies revealed that hyperlipidemia was present in HIV-positive patients, many but not all of whom were on protease inhibitor therapy.[138]

To date, the exact cause of "lipodystrophy" has not been determined, but two main theories have been hypothesized. Each is still in the process of being studied.[19, 55] As individuals live longer with HIV disease, they are at greater risk for developing cardiac disease. Therapists need to be apprised of various changes in laboratory results and signs and symptoms of cardiac disease when designing an exercise program and facilitating return to function.

Neurological System

The neurological manifestations of HIV disease are numerous and they involve the autonomic nervous system (ANS), CNS, and peripheral nervous system (PNS).[8] Significant progress in understanding and treating the neurologically involved HIV patient has been made over the past 5 years.[142] However, HIV continues to affect every division of the human nervous system (see the accompanying box). Unfortunately, neurobehavioral dysfunction in early pediatric AIDS remains unchanged after therapy. Some adult patients develop dementia in spite of the multidrug therapies, and others develop subtle neurobehavioral changes that diminish the quality of their prolonged lives. Thus, HIV infection of the CNS remains an important clinical concern. Although much is known about neuropathology of HIV infection, major questions about neuropathogenesis remain. What is the neurotropism of HIV? What causes neuronal damage and loss? Is the CNS a reservoir of HIV?[142]

Autonomic Nervous System. Dysfunction of the ANS

NEUROPATHOLOGY OF HIV INFECTION

Central Nervous System

Mechanism of CNS infection is unclear, but HIV seems unable to cross blood-brain barrier alone. It probably crosses in macrophages and T cells and most directly affects subcortical structures (basal ganglia, thalamus, brain stem).

AIDS dementia complex (ADC), a subcortical dementia, is different from cortical dementia such as Alzheimer's disease.

Estimated 70% of infected → cognitive, motor, and behavioral constellation that is ADC.

Peripheral Nervous System

Sensory—In early and middle stages, distal lower extremities are largely involved, with paresthesia and decreased temperature sensitivity. In advanced stages, the patient has decreased ankle and knee reflexes, diminished temperature and vibration sensitivity and proprioception, and hyperesthesia.

Motor—Most closely resembles Guillain-Barré syndrome (progressive muscle weakness → paralysis, decreased deep tendon reflexes). Splints and ankle-foot orthoses may prevent deformities.

Autonomic Nervous System

Arrhythymias—especially tachycardia

Abnormal blood pressure—orthostasis and with isometric exercises

Autonomic nervous system involvement has been associated with dementia, myelopathy, and peripheral sensory neuropathies.

---

has been associated with HIV infection. This has implications for overall function and the design of a rehabilitation program for people living with HIV disease. In one study, individuals with the greatest ANS involvement also had dementia, myelopathy, and sensory peripheral neuropathy. Variations in heart rate, including resting tachycardia, were common. Abnormal blood pressure readings were identified in response to isometric exercise and positional changes (sit to stand and tilting).[44]

Central Nervous System. It is not possible in this context to discuss the neuropathology of each of the many secondary infections and neoplasms of HIV illness. It is important to realize, however, that the clinical manifestations of these pathological processes overlap with one another, as well as with the signs and symptoms of primary HIV infection of the CNS; lesions of the CNS can be the site of more than one opportunistic disease process simultaneously. In Table 18–2 a wide variety of organisms and/or conditions responsible for the neurological manifestations associated with HIV infection are listed. These include primary and secondary viral, protozoan, fungal, and *Mycobacterium* infections, as well as neoplasms and iatrogenic conditions.

Thirty to 40% of healthy adults have contracted toxoplasmosis, caused by *Toxoplasma gondii*.[43, 61] Unchecked by the immune system, toxoplasmosis results in CNS dysfunction, namely, altered cognition, headache, focal neurological deficits, encephalitis, and seizures. Cerebellar disorders associated with HIV infection are typically the result of discrete cerebellar lesions resulting from opportunistic infections such as toxoplasmosis and progressive multifocal leukoencephalopathy or primary CNS lymphoma.[139]

Recently, the relationship between stroke and AIDS was reported.[112, 119] The most common cause of cerebral infarction in both clinical and autopsy series was nonbacterial thrombotic endocarditis. Intracerebral hemorrhages were usually associated with thrombocytopenia, primary CNS lymphoma, and metastatic KS.

HIV-related pathology in the spinal cord includes not only HIV myelitis, opportunistic infections, and lymphomas but also vacuolar myelopathy, which affects predominantly the dorsolateral white matter tracts. The cause of vacuolar myelopathy is not understood, and it has not been unequivocally linked with HIV infection.[7] Unless treated with effective antiretroviral therapy, many AIDS patients develop vacuolar myelopathy of the spinal cord associated with moderate clinical disability.[127]

Treatment for CNS impairments include an eclectic blend of rehabilitation strategies. Neuromuscular disturbances may first appear as movement disorders. Subtleties of altered movement can be detected early and during subsequent treatment phases. A neurological examination can be performed to provide a diagnosis and prognosis. This may include the level of the lesion, neuromuscular deficits, need for assistive devices, ADL, and functional abilities. Various quality of life assessments used with the HIV population can be found in Table 18–3.

Peripheral Nervous System. Distal symmetrical polyneuropathy (DSP) is the most common form of neuropathy in HIV infection. The most frequent complaints in DSP are numbness, burning, and paresthesias in the feet. These symptoms are typically symmetrical and often so severe that patients have contact hypersensitivity and gait disturbances. Involvement of the upper extremities and distal weakness may occur later in the course of DSP. Neurological examination shows sensory loss to pain and temperature in a stocking-glove distribution, increased vibratory thresholds, and diminished ankle reflexes compared with knee reflexes.[129, 130] Patients with AIDS frequently have concurrent CNS disorders and neuropathy, characterized by hyperactive knee reflexes and depressed ankle reflexes.

The incidence of DSP increases with advancing immunosuppression, in parallel with decreased CD4 counts.[128]

Thirty-five percent of patients with AIDS may present with electrophysiological or clinical abnormalities.[133] Furthermore, pathological evidence of DSP is present in almost all patients who die of AIDS.[51] Various theories regarding the mechanism of DSP have been proposed. It was formerly thought that direct HIV invasion of the nervous system caused DSP[61]; however, most investigators now believe that this is not the case.[128] A "dying-back" neuropathy affecting all fiber types, with prominent macrophage infiltration of the peripheral nerve, has been described.[51] Cytokines, tumor necrosis factor, and interleukin-1 have been identified in peripheral nerves of patients with AIDS.[52]

Balance and Postural Mechanisms. Balance disturbances may be seen with HIV involvement of either the CNS or the PNS. Polyneuropathy due to zidovudine (AZT polyneuropathy) and CMV, which is a common pathogen in AIDS (inflammatory polyneuropathy), may manifest in the form of a generalized asymmetrical demyelination and chronic denervation of muscles.[99] Demyelination and denervation of nerves that supply postural muscles may weaken such muscles and result in balance problems (e.g., distal pain, paresthesia, or numbness). It is also possible that apart from muscle demyelination and denervation, the pathological process, which also includes macrophage infiltration of neural structures, could spread to affect the vestibular neural complex of the inner ear, which is very important in the maintenance of both static and dynamic balance. Our clinical experience shows that sensory changes are common in the lower limbs of neuropathic HIV/AIDS patients. The balance problems of these patients are likely to be connected to a lack of adequate proprioception from the legs during stance, and it is well known that diminished sensory information makes gait control more difficult.

Peripheral neuropathy weakens the neuromuscular system and causes a limitation in functional activities. These effects on the neuromuscular system manifest in disturbances of postural control. An appropriate posture should be regarded as the starting position for a functional activity. However, compromise of the postural pattern is so characteristic of HIV peripheral neuropathy that it is diagnostic for HIV-1 infection.[110] The neurological abnormality resulting from peripheral neuropathy in HIV/AIDS patients produces postural disturbances[2] that may take various forms that exacerbate with the severity of the neuropathy[10] and compromise functional activity at various levels. This means that as the condition of HIV/AIDS patients deteriorates, balance deficits may increase.

According to Husstedt and associates,[64] peripheral neuropathy in HIV disease progresses much more rapidly than that associated with diabetes or hereditary polyneuropathies. Again, as the HIV infection progresses, distal symmetrical peripheral neuropathy (DSPN) increases, resulting in a depression of certain motor functions such as gait and manual dexterity, and a worsening of the condition is due to demyelination.[64] There is therefore a need to treat HIV neuropathy as soon as it is diagnosed to avoid complications.

Our group[47] has identified peripheral neuropathy and its complications as causes of functional derangement in

TABLE 18-3. Quality of Life Assessments in HIV Disease

Instrument	Author	Dimensions	Length	Administration
AIDS Health Assessment Questionnaire (AIDS-HAQ)	Lubeck and Fries (1991–1992)	Physical function, mental health, cognitive function, social health, energy/fatigue	30 items	Self-administered (5 minutes)
AIDS Specific Functional Assessment (ASFA)	Rapkin, et al. (1991–1993)	Evaluates the usefulness of functional assessment	Varies	Self-administered, care provider
Individualized Functional Status Assessment (IFSA)	Rapkin, et al. (1991–1992)	Patient-generated activities associated with the pursuit of the following goal types: a. achievement b. problem-solving c. avoidance-prevention d. maintenance e. disengagement	75 items	Self-administered
Medical Outcomes Study HIV Instrument (MOS-HIV)	Wu, et al. (1991)	Health, pain, physical functioning, role functioning, social functioning, mental health, fatigue, energy, health distress, cognitive functioning, health transition, general quality of life	30 items	Self-administered (5 minutes)
HIV Patient-Reported Status and Experience (HIV-PARSE)	Berry, et al. (1991)	Physical health, mental health, general health	38 items	Self-administered (5 minutes)
Multidimensional Functional Evaluation of People with HIV	Marazzi, et al. (1992)	I ADL (4) Self-Care (8)	12 items	Self-administered
Neuropsychiatric AIDS Rating Scale (NARS)	Boccellari, et al. (1992)	Assesses patient's orientation, memory motor ability, behavioral changes, problem-solving ability, and ADL	Varies	Health care provider
HIV Overview of Problems Evaluation Systems (HOPES)	Schag, et al. (1992)	Global, physical, psychosocial, medical interaction, significant others, sexual	139 items	Self-administered (15 minutes)
HIV-Related Quality-of-Life Questions (HIV-QOL)	Cleary, et al. (1993)	Mental health, energy/fatigue, fever, limitations of basic ADL and intermediate ADL, disability days, all symptoms, sleep symptoms, neurological symptoms, memory symptoms, pain	30 items	Self-administered (5 minutes)
HIV-Quality Audit Marker (HIV-QAM)	Holzemer, et al. (1993)	Captures the nurse data collector's judgment of the status of the patient based on observations, interviews, and recorded interviews	Varies based on duration of interview	Nurse
HIV Visual Analog Scale	Nokes, et al. (1994)	Rates HIV-related symptom severity and general well-being	Varies	Nurse Self-administered
HIV Assessment Tool (HAT)	Nokes, et al. (1994)	Physical symptoms related to HIV disease, social/role functioning psychological well-being, and personal attitudes related to well-being	34 items	Self-administered
Multidimensional Quality of Life Questionnaire for Persons with HIV (MQOL-HIV)	Avis & Smith (1994)	Mental health, physical health, physical functioning, social functioning, social support, cognitive functioning, financial status, partner intimacy, sexual functioning, medical care	40 items	Self-administered (10 minutes)

HIV/AIDS patients. A patient who, for instance, has balance derangement resulting from peripheral neuropathy may not function effectively in ADL. It is well known that functional limitation is an important factor that takes people out of employment. The case is true for people with HIV/AIDS peripheral neuropathy. Pain may be the limiting factor in the ability to return to work. Any intervention that would reduce functional limitation should be applied.

Pain

Another factor closely related to the neuropathy of the HIV/AIDS patients is pain. Most AIDS patients require various pain treatment interventions. DSPN has been shown to be the most common peripheral neuropathy complaint in patients with HIV-1 infection.[11] Peripheral neuropathy is one of the most common types of pain suffered by HIV-infected men,[131] and peripheral neuropathies occur in as many as 40% to 60% of patients with HIV disease. When neuropathy results in distal painful paresthesia, imbalance in stance and gait may result from compensatory measures aimed at relieving pain in dynamic standing activities. Postural compensations may further exacerbate musculoskeletal, cervical, thoracic, or low back pain.

Pain management is a critical part of the overall care of individuals with HIV disease. Pain is the second most common reason for hospitalization of AIDS patients.[82] A study of 72 AIDS patients found 97% had pain related to their disease process.[103] Newshan and Wainapel, who surveyed 100 patients with pain associated with AIDS, showed that the two reported pain types were abdominal and neuropathic pain. In a longitudinal study of HIV-infected men, painful peripheral neuropathy was one of the most common types of pain suffered by these men.[131]

DSP exhibits painful paresthesia that may be resistant to pharmacological treatment. Our clinical experience shows that conventional transcutaneous electrical nerve stimulation may exacerbate peripheral pain in HIV/AIDS patients. Another consideration for treatment is low-voltage electroacupuncture.[46] Manual therapy to improve ankle and foot range of motion along with other compensatory areas is recommended for pain management and return to function.

Psychopathology

Medical and neuropsychiatric sequelae of HIV infection present a spectrum of diagnostic and treatment challenges to health care practitioners. Both HIV infection and the various opportunistic infections that manifest in patients due to an immunocompromised state also can affect the CNS. Therefore, therapists need to be familiar with the diagnosis and management of HIV infection–related medical and psychiatric disorders. This has great impact on the outcomes of rehabilitation.

Careful consideration of psychological function is warranted during clinical encounters with HIV-infected persons. AIDS-related psychopathologies mimic many previously described consequences of primary HIV infection, opportunistic infections, and drug side effects. These psychiatric complications can be affective or organic. Indicators include disturbances in sleep and appetite patterns, diminished memory and energy, psychomotor retardation, withdrawal, apathy, and emotional liability. Anxiety disorders (particularly posttraumatic stress disorder), adjustment reactions, reactive and endogenous depressions, and obsessive disorders frequently result.[41, 65, 107]

Using the American Psychiatric Association's *Diagnostic and Statistical Manual of Mental Disorders*, third edition revised, one study found Axis I disorders (excluding substance abuse) in 61.9% of the subjects.[132] Indeed, the virus' affinity with subcortical structures of the CNS that regulate affect and mood support research indicate a prevalence of manic episodes that is 10 times higher than that in the general population.[87] Manic syndrome has been identified at all stages of the disease process: initial HIV seropositivity, AIDS, and in response to zidovudine therapy.[35, 45, 125] When associated with HIV infection, mania appears to be secondary to structural CNS changes.[39, 73] Described manic episodes generally respond well to psychiatric medications and may not recur.[15, 45, 96, 105]

Analyses of new-onset psychosis among HIV-infected individuals yielded the following information. Psychotic episodes are preceded by a period (days to months) of affective and behavioral changes.[54] Admitting diagnoses to psychiatric units included "undifferentiated schizophrenia, schizophreniform disorder, 'reactive psychosis,' atypical psychosis, depression with psychotic features and mania." Some psychiatric diagnoses were revised during the course of hospitalization to "AIDS encephalitis, cryptococcal meningitis, or 'organic psychosis.'"[56] Eighty-seven percent of the subjects in one study displayed delusions that were usually persecutory, grandiose, or somatic. Affective disturbances were present in 81% of the subjects. Hallucinations and thought process disorders were each prominent in 61%. Several subjects received the diagnosis of AIDS during their psychiatric hospitalization.[56]

Remarkable progress was made in recent years in the therapeutics of HIV-associated dementia. Viral replication in and outside the CNS has been reduced by HAART. This has resulted in partial repair of cellular immune function with improvement in, and the prevention of, neurological deficits associated with HIV disease.[17]

Extensive use of protease inhibitors is associated with dramatic declines in overall mortality and morbidity, including HIV-associated dementia.[21, 109]

Neuropathological abnormalities seen in the brain tissue of patients with HIV-associated dementia are usually diffuse and predominantly localized to the white and deep gray matter regions. Myelin pallor and inflammatory infiltrates composed of macrophages and multinucleated giant cells are the hallmarks of this disease process, although a spectrum of lesions has been identified from encephalitis to leukoencephalopathy.[14, 84] The characteristic clinical feature of HIV-associated dementia is disabling cognitive impairment, often accompanied by behavioral changes, motor dysfunction, or both.[84] Degrees of impairment have been recorded, and a five-part staging system was subsequently developed.[101, 115] Motoric manifestations of AIDS dementia complex include gait disturbances, intention tremor, and abnormal release of reflexes.

Differentiation between psychiatric and physiological manifestations is complicated. Psychiatric and organic disorders are initially indistinguishable on the basis of behavior, and they may exist concurrently. Furthermore, other primary disease processes and drug reactions imitate psychopathologies. Differentiation is nonetheless essential, because many disorders respond well to established therapies, both psychological and pharmacological, once differential diagnoses are established. Awareness of the intricate interplay of all factors is essential for competent rehabilitative efforts for those infected with HIV.

Pediatric HIV Infection

The prediction of 6 million pregnant women and 5 to 10 million children infected with HIV-1 by the year 2000[124] may have been an underestimate. An accurate understanding of the timing of HIV transmission from mother to fetus is very important for the design of intervention strategies. The ACTG076 trial that included treatment from the fourteenth week of gestation in women with CD4 counts of more than 200/mm^3 prompts other considerations.[27] Onset of HIV-1 infection in children has a wide spectrum of clinical manifestations.[40]

In the first year of life severe immunodeficiency develops in 15% to 20% of pediatric patients with serious recurrent infections or neurological dysfunction, whereas in school-age children the disease progresses more slowly and the risk of developing HIV-related encephalopathy becomes less.[89] Some infants present with features of severe immunodeficiency, whereas others have nonspecific findings, such as hepatosplenomegaly, failure to thrive, unexplained fever, parotitis, and recurrent gastroenteritis. Adenopathy is common, and salivary gland enlargement occurs more frequently than in adults. Otitis media and measles, despite immunization, are also more frequent complications in children.[12, 59] Cardiac involvement in children with HIV infection is a well-known entity and occurs clinically more often in patients with advanced disease.[114]

Children are susceptible to disorders seen in adults—herpesvirus infection, pneumonia, toxoplasmosis, meningitis, and encephalitis. HIV encephalopathy is noted to have the most serious side effects because of its progressive deteriorating pattern and associated CNS abnormalities,[3] although static encephalopathy can be characterized by severely delayed cognitive functioning and neuromotor skills without deterioration.[13] Manifestations in children include cerebral atrophy, ataxia, rigidity, hyperreflexia, and the inability to achieve or sustain developmental milestones. Although the HIV-neurodevelopmental involvement cause a prognostic worsening, most studies about pediatric cases of neuro-AIDS demonstrate that an early diagnosis followed by adequate antiretroviral therapeutic regimens can lead to significant, even if temporary, improvement.[89]

Rehabilitation of the pediatric patient requires a multidisciplinary approach to meet the medical, emotional, and psychosocial needs of these children and their families. Children are encouraged to give form to their psychological experiences through play, writing or telling stories, and creating works of art.[90]

REHABILITATION INTERVENTIONS

The examination procedures for HIV illness are broadly outlined below. Of course, each case varies and the evaluation process is individualized according to the specific needs of the client (see the accompanying box).

What is the relationship of the person with HIV infection to the environment, both at present and in the future? The rehabilitation therapist should keep this question in mind throughout the examination process. In this context, the term *environment* is meant to include not only the physical aspects of surroundings but also the psychological and emotional climate in which the individual functions (see Table 18–1).

The examination process has a different focus for different stages of the disease. If the client is in the early stages of the disease, the therapist should determine whether he or she is still managing in accustomed life roles. Important issues may include new or adapted vocational and leisure skills. During advancing stages, the focus may change to more basic daily functional concerns. The therapist must remember, however, that the client may place more importance on participation in avocational interest than on independent self-care. This choice not only is valid but must be respected and supported by health care professionals. Another crucial determination to be made during the evaluative process is whether the

---

EVALUATION PROCEDURES FOR HIV ILLNESS

A. Baseline data (premorbid functional level)
   1. Accustomed life roles

B. Stage in disease process

C. Psychosocial issues
   1. Coping mechanisms
   2. Social support system

D. Cognitive/perceptual status
   1. Reality orientation
   2. Memory
   3. Organizational skills
   4. Visual perception
   5. Motor planning
   6. Safety awareness
   7. Judgment

E. Communication
   1. Oral language
   2. Written language

F. Sensorimotor status
   1. Balance
   2. Gait
   3. Coordination
   4. Sensation/pain
   5. Muscle tone
   6. Strength

G. Activities of daily living
   1. Grooming/hygiene
   2. Feeding
   3. Bathing
   4. Dressing
   5. Housework
   6. Community management
   7. Other self-care regimens (e.g., medications)
   8. Avocational interests
   9. Activity tolerance

---

person is to be discharged to home or some other supervised setting. In either case, it is critical to determine what kind of community-based support networks are available to the individual.

Astute evaluative questions about the psychosocial status of the client include the following:

- Does the client's perception of his or her status and prognosis agree with that of the treatment team?
- What is the client's predominant coping style?
- Who are the client's caregivers?
- What is the social support system?

The support system can be a critical issue for many people with HIV infection who are part of the high-risk groups of homosexual and bisexual men and intravenous drug users.[33] Many of these people have traditional networks of family, spouse, and friends; a significant number have equally strong nontraditional support systems. Some will be lacking in the kinds of support needed to cope with the devastating effects of the disease.

It is possible to use models developed for oncology and progressive neurological disorders, for HIV involvement of the CNS and PNS. An orthopedic approach may be taken when pain is a presenting factor or biomechanical alterations are a result of other disease processes. Functional fluctuations that characterize HIV infection and secondary infections must be understood; therefore, the therapist must appreciate the effects that HIV infection has on various systemic complications.

The neurorehabilitation evaluation of HIV infection should include standard cognitive, perceptual, and motor components of function. The idiosyncratic nature of the disease may necessitate more detailed evaluation of these specific areas. Recommended cognitive and perceptual evaluations are both formal and observational. Safety, judgment, and money management need to be assessed. In addition to the organicity of HIV-associated dementia evaluation of the systemic complications of HIV infection is necessary for optimal rehabilitative planning and treatment team efficacy.

The ADL evaluation is best made within the context of the immediate and projected life roles of the individual. Maximal independent functioning is the goal of rehabilitation, whatever the stage of illness. If the person is at home or is being discharged to home, a crucial component of the ADL examination is the assessment of community management skills. Consider access to transportation, socialization opportunities, shopping, and banking; ability to negotiate health care and insurance systems; and community involvement. Many people with HIV infection and their caregivers have little experience with disability because of their age or social status. This, combined with the stressors of illness, can create unrealistic expectations and unnecessary frustrations.

Treatment Process

The neuromuscular rehabilitation treatment procedures for HIV infection and an overview of treatment techniques for opportunistic infections are presented in the boxes here and on page 567.

Cognitive deficits in attention, concentration, and memory require consistency, structure, and environmental cues to minimize confusion. Safety and judgment deficits can be countered by environmental adaptations. Lethargic clients benefit from sensory enhancement. Maintenance of endurance and strength and passive and active range of motion are important components of any motor function treatment plan. Neuromuscular facilitation and inhibition, positioning, and splinting are feasible modalities to normalize tone as needed. Gait training, the use of ambulatory aids, training in motor planning, and balance and endurance exercises may be appropriate.

In addition to techniques and modalities, active listening, empathy, and unconditional positive regard are important aspects of one's therapeutic use of self. The clinician must set aside personal biases and beliefs to accurately hear the perspective of the individual client. The use of expressive modalities facilitates the development of coping skills while providing appropriate explora-

---

NEUROMUSCULAR REHABILITATION TREATMENT PROCEDURES FOR HIV INFECTION

A. Psychosocial intervention
   1. Facilitation of the expression of grief
   2. Validation and education of caregivers

B. Cognitive/perceptual intervention
   1. Rehabilitation
   2. Maintenance
   3. Compensation (including communication)

C. Sensory/motor intervention
   1. Sensory stimulation
   2. Maintenance of strength, range of motion, and endurance
   3. Tone normalization
   4. Functional mobilities (including ambulation equipment)

D. Pain control
   1. Psychological modalities
   2. Behavioral modalities
   3. Physical modalities

E. Training in Activities of Daily Living
   1. Leisure or avocational skill development
   2. Community management skills
   3. Transfer training
   4. Recommendations for adaptive equipment
   5. Self-care retraining
   6. Energy conservation
   7. Work simplification

F. Continuity of care
   1. Discharge planning
   2. Community linkages

---

tion and release of powerful emotions. Human touch can counter the powerful and isolating effect of fear of contagion. Rehabilitation therapists can demonstrate and educate caregivers about the safety and benefit of touch.

Motoric manifestations of AIDS dementia complex include gait disturbances, intention tremor, and abnormal release of reflexes.

Pain management is best approached with a behavioral and a physical approach. Pain reduction is achieved through training in breathing techniques, visualization, progressive muscle relaxation, autogenics, music, meditation, and engagement in meaningful activities. Electroacupuncture, ultrasonography, and manual therapy are also therapeutic tools. (See Chapters 4 and 33 for additional treatment ideas.)

The impact of HIV infection can be evident in cerebral, emotional, psychosocial, and other physical domains, affecting the patient infected with HIV and those around him or her. The prognosis and psychological and physical consequences of HIV infection are associated with significant emotional distress and clinical syndromes, such as adjustment disorders, depression, and anxiety in some patients.[42] Increasing focus is being placed on the poten-

MOST COMMON OPPORTUNISTIC INFECTIONS AND REHABILITATION INTERVENTIONS IN HIV-INFECTED PATIENTS

Pneumocystic carinii pneumonia (PCP)—most common opportunistic infection. Infectious agent unclear but probable latent infection; 65% to 85% healthy adults possess PCP antibodies. Fever, dyspnea, and hypoxia → <u>diaphragmatic breathing, energy conservation.</u>°

Candida albicans—present in healthy people, immunocompromised status → yeast infections of oral, esophageal, and vaginal mucosal tissues → <u>teach good oral care with soft brush, bland diet, salt water rinses.</u>

Cryptococcus neoformans—also a yeast but manifests in CNS as abscesses and meningitis. Headache, altered mental states, nausea, vertigo, somnolence, seizures, and coma → <u>pain management, safety and gait training, cognitive and sensory stimulation.</u>

Cryptosporidiosis—infects gastrointestinal tract → chronic diarrhea and malabsorption, contributes to wasting syndrome → <u>nutritional and hydration strategies.</u>

Wasting syndrome—involuntary loss of 10% of baseline body weight, weakness, chronic diarrhea, and unexplained fever. <u>Nutrition, hydration, energy conservation.</u>

Toxoplasmosis—affects CNS in 30% to 40% of cases; headache, altered cognition, encephalitis, seizures, focal deficits → <u>imposed structure, concrete tasks, pain management.</u>

Cytomegalovirus (CMV)—present in 40% to 100% of healthy adults. Can affect gastrointestinal and respiratory tracts, but most often affects ocular structures → unilateral or bilateral decreased visual acuity, field cuts and blindness → <u>compensatory skills, safety tasks and mobilities, home evaluation, supportive service referrals.</u>

Mycobacterial infections—Two are most pertinent: *M. avium-intracellulare complex* (MAC) and *M. tuberculosis* (causes TB). MAC affects 18% to 56%, but autopsies reveal this is a low estimate. MAC infection is not latent but is a primary infection. It appears late in HIV infection, begins in gastrointestinal or respiratory tract, and then disseminates. Pneumonia, fever, weight loss, malaise, sweats, anorexia, abdominal pain, diarrhea may occur. TB appears early, with latent reactivation in 90% of HIV-infected patients. Pulmonary TB estimates 75% to 100% in HIV-infected persons infected with the TB bacillus. It also infects lymph nodes and bone marrow in 60% of these, and it also infects CNS, cardiac, and mucosal tissues. Fever, weight loss, malaise, cough, lymph node tenderness, and night sweats → <u>energy conservation, nutrition and hydration, and caregiver and patient education in safe management of infection. Is communicable; wear a mask, follow respiratory isolation protocol.</u>

AIDS-Kaposi's sarcoma (AIDS-KS)—Frequent neoplasm and most frequent in homosexual men; it is rare in women and intravenous drug users. There are purple skin or visceral lesions. Associated are deficient lymphatic transport, nodal tumors, and lymph edema → swollen, painful lower extremities. <u>Nutrition, pain management, task simplification, mobility and ADL training.</u>

°Underlined components identify potential treatment procedures recommended for the specific problem.

---

tial impact of HIV infection–related stress on the course of infection because of the observed and postulated relationship between psychosocial stress, neuropsychological functioning, and immune status.[144] Minimizing stressful events throughout the management of chronic HIV infection can be approached in various ways, such as meditation, relaxation, and various forms of exercise.

Exercise

A review of all available literature in HIV and exercise reveals: (1) no decline in CD4 cell counts seen in any of

the studies, regardless of the initial stage of disease, level of CD4 cells, or symptomatology; (2) a trend toward an increase in the number of CD4 cells in all but one study, with the more significant increases seen in those subjects at earlier stages of the disease; and (3) the importance of homogeneous study samples when investigating the effects of exercise in a dynamic disease such as HIV/ AIDS.[78, 80] From a psychoneuroimmunological perspective, psychological stress has been implicated among the cofactors contributing to the immunological decline in HIV disease. Good evidence supports the stress management role of exercise training as a means to explain a buffering of these suppressive stressor effects, thereby facilitating a return of the CD4 cells. Early intervention with exercise, in compliance with guidelines, is most prudent to stave off opportunistic infections throughout the spectrum of HIV disease.

Precautions and Concerns During Exercise

It is important to address any orthopedic or neurological concern before embarking on an exercise or movement therapy program. If musculoskeletal problems exist or other pain symptoms are present, a concerted effort to modulate pain is necessary for the successful completion of an exercise regimen.[48] If HIV-related peripheral neuropathy exists, it is important to implement proper foot care and supportive shoes when performing weight-bearing activities.[47, 50]

There is some concern about aerobic exercise increasing the body's metabolic rate and thus increasing additional muscle loss. However, with a balanced high-calorie diet and incorporating a sound nutritional program, this should not pose a problem for the asymptomatic person with HIV disease. If wasting is present, the etiology needs to be addressed and treatment rendered.[100] One study determined the contribution of total energy expenditure to weight changes in individuals with HIV infection–related wasting. The researchers observed a significant positive relation between total energy expenditure and the rate of weight change. During rapid weight loss, total energy expenditure fell from an average 2750 kcal/day to 2189 kcal/day. The key determinant of weight loss in HIV infection–related wasting they concluded was reduced energy intake, not increased energy expenditure.[88]

Before beginning any exercise regimen, a differential diagnosis for fatigue must be made, including anemia, low testosterone levels, or specific vitamin deficiencies. Proper caloric intake must set the standard for each type of exercise to meet the energy expenditure required for the activity. Seeking the advice of a nutritionist is recommended for proper guidance.

Evidence of autonomic neuropathy on provocative testing is common in HIV infection, with estimates of incidence ranging from 30% to 60%.[121, 191] Underlying cardiac parasympathetic dysfunction may need to be assessed throughout the course of HIV disease. One method described by Mallet and colleagues[92] is the use of 4-s exercise test (4-SET), which consists in pedaling an uploaded ergometer at maximal individual speed from the fourth to the eighth second of a 12-s maximal inspiratory apnea. From an electrocardiogram, vagal activity is estimated through a ratio. In their study, subjects were submitted to the respiratory sinus arrhythmia, which is a valid method to detect vagal dysfunction. They found that there was a tendency for lower values of vagal function test in HIV-infected subjects. Vital sign monitoring is most prudent throughout any exercise regimen.

A supervised training program should be consistent with recommendations by the American College of Sports Medicine. Guidelines have been established for the spectrum of the three stages of HIV disease.[80] Exercise is safe and beneficial for most individuals with HIV disease; however, caution is warranted in stages 2 and 3. Stage 1, or asymptomatic, disease has no limitations on maximum graded exercise testing. In this stage, all metabolic parameters are within normal limits for most individuals. In stage 2, or symptomatic, disease, there may be reduced exercise capacity, VO_2 max, and O_2 pulse max. There may also be elevated heart rate reserve and breathing reserve. Patients with stage 3 disease, or AIDS, present with dramatically reduced exercise capacity, reduced vital capacity, VO_2 max, and O_2 pulse max. Elevated heart rate and breathing reserve persists in this stage. Therefore, careful monitoring of the stage and various other opportunistic infections is an important factor in comprehensive exercise management.

Complementary Therapies in HIV Infection

There is substantial evidence to suggest that traditional exercise, particularly aerobic exercise, can provide notable physiological and psychological benefits for most individuals, and especially those with chronic diseases. However, the mode, duration, and intensity of many traditional standardized exercise programs may not always be entirely appropriate during chronic illness. The stage of disease and the type of illness itself may preclude these more strenuous exercise activities at various times. During times like these, less traditional movement therapies may prove to be more appropriate and efficacious. In fact, movement therapy includes a number of similar constructs used in physical therapy and can be quite complementary to an individual's program of more traditional exercise.[49]

The HIV epidemic has witnessed an increasing utilization of alternative therapies, some more traditional than others.[123] The exploration outside the medical model has fostered investigations by the Office of Alternative Medicine at the National Institutes of Health.[106] Eisenberg reported that prayer and exercise combined to account for over 60% of all alternative therapies utilized.[38] Other therapies include relaxation techniques (13%), massage (7%), imagery (4%), and spiritual healing (4%). Traditional exercise such as aerobic and weight training are incorporated in the medical model through exercise physiology and rehabilitation. However, various movement therapies (such as martial arts) are often viewed as less traditional and outside the established medical model. In a recent study by Bastyr University (1998) various movement therapies were used by people living with HIV disease. This study evaluated the use of alternative therapies within the past 6 months. Yoga was used by 15.5%, tai chi by 4.8%, and qigong by 3.6% of the participants. Recent research[49] demonstrated beneficial physiological and psychological effects of the use of tai chi and aerobic exercise (see Chapter 33).

Social Interactions and the Association with Disease Management

The process of grieving is often mistakenly associated solely with the death of another. It is a natural reaction to loss, including the loss of one's own health and diminished independence. Loss of abstract human qualities, such as perceived attractiveness and productivity, results in grief. Such emotions are often difficult for a client to articulate. It is the therapist's responsibility to be sensitive to the client's individualized grief pattern (see Chapter 7).

Placement issues accompany discharge planning from acute health care facilities. The rehabilitation professional is often called on to make recommendations regarding the level of assistance the client will need. All of the previously discussed areas of cognitive/perceptual, sensorimotor, and ADL management combined with available psychosocial and practical support influence these recommendations. Options include a return to independent living and work, assisted independent living by a loved one, home with supportive services (often supplied by community-based AIDS organizations), home with hospital-based home care, hospice, and extended care facility.

Literature on long-term survivors with AIDS is replete with anecdotal evidence linking survival to one or more of the following: (1) holding a positive attitude toward the illness, (2) participating in health-promoting behaviors, (3) engaging in spiritual activities, and (4) taking part in AIDS-related activities.[69, 86, 104] Positive relationships have been demonstrated between hardiness and perception of physical, emotional, and spiritual health and participation in exercise and the use of special diets.[6, 20, 70]

Research provides support for the hypothesis that interpersonal relationships influence patterns of physiological functions. Data from experimental studies have shown that social contact can serve to reduce the physiological stress responses.[67, 140] Community-based studies have also shown negative associations between reported levels of support and physiological parameters such as serum cholesterol, uric acid, and urinary epinephrine levels.[140] Studies of immune function have demonstrated that social relationships have both positive and negative impacts on immune function. Loss of a partner to cancer or HIV infection, family caregiving for Alzheimer's patients, and divorce or poor marital quality all show negative associations with immune function, whereas more supportive relationships are associated with better immune function.[68]

Exercise and movement therapy in a group context may provide the socialization necessary to foster these physiological changes and adherence to an exercise regimen. Another area of potential socialization is the workplace. The quality of life issues of people with HIV/AIDS are becoming more complicated as more people with the disease achieve higher CD4 counts and lower viral load levels. Improvement in health status is directly related to the improved effectiveness of newer treatment regimens, and many individuals are improving enough to consider reentering the work force. Exercise and movement therapy may augment the stress and fatigue that may be associated with the adjustment to the workplace.

SUMMARY

Research and resultant treatments are extending lives so that more people require rehabilitative services that maximize function and quality of life. Medical management has focused on the treatment of reducing viral load, preventing the secondary illnesses, and improving the immunological status of chronic HIV disease. Neuromuscular rehabilitation evaluation and treatment for HIV infection are similar to those for other progressive neuromuscular disorders. The final stage of the syndrome, AIDS, can be addressed like other diseases such as cancer, but with an emphasis on cognitive and perceptual function. Rehabilitation treatment focuses on specific impairments, disabilities, and psychosocial ramifications of infection. Compensation, mobility, ADL retraining, pain control, and community management skills constitute a well-developed treatment plan.

The epidemic is a major challenge on a personal as well as a professional level because of the continued natural fear of contagion. The illness originally appeared in subcultures that are often disenfranchised. Social, racial, and economic status and controversial behaviors contribute to prejudice, fear, and limited access to health care. Rehabilitation professionals have responded significantly to this challenge. Continued advocacy and compassion combined with professional enlightenment will, in a small way, alter the course of the disease.

Future Directions for Research

The issue of HIV disability warrants a careful investigation into our present health care system. Long-term survivors of HIV disease who formerly received disability ranking are potentially ready to return to work. However, their grave concern about the long absence from work reflected on their resume and fears about potential opportunistic infections while on the job require specific strategies. Vocational rehabilitation and on-the-job counseling are necessary for optimal return to work. The systemic issues of acquisition of disability and the loss of all benefits when one relinquishes disability are quite complicated and overwhelming. The diagnosis of AIDS is the determining factor for disability, and many people living with HIV disease with CD4 counts less than 200/mm^3 have experienced considerable improvement in their immunological status with a concomitant drop in viral load. Prognosis for these individuals has great variability. Promoting quality of life may be greatly enhanced through the use of complementary therapies. An integral aspect of one's perception of oneself is often the role played in society. The workplace affords individuals a sense of identity and a self-sustaining purposefulness. Therefore, our health and governmental systems need to conduct further research on return-to-work outcomes, with ease of transition and on-the-job accommodations when necessary. Future directions in the AIDS epidemic as we see people living longer will be the full return to function in all domains of ADL and return to productive work.

CASE STUDIES

Four case studies are presented to help the reader understand and identify various stages of this clinical problem and how each stage may require a different therapeutic focus.

CASE 18–1   Early Stage

Ruby is a 23-year-old African American/Hispanic woman. She has a history of intravenous drug use and learned of her HIV-positive status at the time of her AIDS diagnosis 9 months ago. At that time Ruby was also diagnosed with *Pneumocystis carinii* pneumonia and pulmonary tuberculosis. Ruby is without an address or a job. She lives on the streets with other addicts or in transient hotels. Her social contacts revolve around obtaining and using drugs. She is not part of the welfare system.

Ruby was admitted to the acute psychiatric unit of a hospital after a hotel resident telephoned the police to report a woman was running through the halls, pounding on doors, shouting, and threatening to "get those children!"

Ruby's agitation and delusions responded well to neuroleptics. During her hospitalization, Ruby received methadone to counter narcotic withdrawal symptoms. An abscess on her left anterior deltoid was present on admission. Pain caused decreased left shoulder strength to poor (3/5), as opposed to normal (5/5) in her right shoulder.

Rehabilitation focused on left upper-extremity range of motion, one-handed ADL, dressing changes, and HIV infection prevention (needle sterilization). She was discharged with a limited supply of medication and a referral to community mental health services at the end of the week for follow-up medication and monitoring. Ruby was issued a voucher for a city-paid transient hotel, but she did not stay there. Most patients report feeling unsafe in them. Ruby returned twice for outpatient therapy to maintain her left shoulder range of motion.

CASE 18–2   Middle Stage

John is a 51-year-old white man who tested HIV positive in 1987. He received a diagnosis of AIDS in 1992 after his initial (and ongoing) struggle with cytomegalovirus retinitis. Additional significant medical history includes two bouts of *Pneumocystis carinii* pneumonia and a left cerebrovascular accident with mild residual right-sided weakness. Evaluation at this hospitalization also identified the presence of toxoplasmosis.

John has worked as a front office manager for a large hotel chain for 13 years. He transferred to his newest position in a large city 5 years ago. This job demanded that he often work more than 50 hours a week. Accrued vacation time has helped John combat illness while maintaining his job. His supervisors and coworkers are aware of, and generally supportive of, his condition. In the past 10 months John has been delegating more duties to his assistant to limit his work to between 30 and 40 hours a week. Four weeks before this hospitalization, John took a medical leave of absence from work.

John was admitted to the hospital after having fallen (with loss of consciousness) to the floor of his apartment, where he lay for 24 hours. He was severely dehydrated and confused. John lives with a roommate who is not a significant other but is willing to assist in home management for both of them. However, the roommate is uncomfortable with providing more personal assistance for John.

Rehabilitation services found John to have poor static and dynamic balance with decreased insight, safety, and judgment about his status. Although he was able to identify some of his limitations, he was unable to exercise problem-solving skills to ameliorate them. For example, after he repeatedly fell to the side while attempting to don his sock, John's solution was to state, "I have lousy balance." John was unable to demonstrate independent management of his 11 different medications or to sequence a 5-step simple meal preparation process, despite written instructions. John insisted on his capacity for independent self-care despite such problems. Physical therapy was able to improve John's ambulation from the level of moderate assist to contact guard with a front-wheeled walker. Occupational therapy was able to adapt John's home environment by rearranging furniture and installing assistive equipment that increased John's safety. Visual cues and structured routines were incorporated into his environment to compensate for cognitive deficits. Rehabilitation team collaboration resulted in John's return to home with 24-hour light supervision that included his roommate in the evenings. Referrals were made to existing community services for daily meal delivery.

CASE 18–3   Late Stage

Lorenzo is a 37-year-old man born in Ecuador. He has lived in the United States for 25 years. He has been married for 10 years. Lorenzo and his wife have a 9-year-old daughter. Lorenzo is an associate professor of history at a university. He is currently on sabbatical. He tested positive for HIV in 1987 and was diagnosed with AIDS in 1991. Lorenzo's wife and daughter know of his AIDS diagnosis and are supportive of all medical interventions on his behalf. Lorenzo's wife reports a negative HIV test result. The family fears discrimination and reprisal based on his HIV status. Consequently, none of his coworkers and few (three) friends know. Lorenzo's wife is his primary caregiver.

Lorenzo has experienced relatively few opportunistic infections associated with HIV infection. In 1993 he was diagnosed with AIDS-Kaposi's sarcoma, AIDS wasting syndrome, and anemia. Cachexia, generalized weakness, and frequent headaches have been tolerated by Lorenzo since that time. Lorenzo described a marked decrease in strength with more severe headaches in the past 3 weeks.

This hospitalization resulted from acute left-sided neurological dysfunction. He fell twice, without loss of consciousness or seizure, on the day before admission. On examination, Lorenzo reported anorexia, insomnia, dizziness, and left-sided sensory and motor impairment. Both right extremities were within normal limits for sensorimotor function. Severe pain in both left extremities precluded active or passive range of motion. Moderate spasticity and hyperreflexia were noted in both left extremities. Muscle strength in these were poor (2/5); he was unable to move them against gravity. Left elbow flexor and heel cord contractures were present. Decreased left-sided

coordination and numbness also were present. Sensation was intact for light touch, vibration, and proprioception. Lorenzo was alert and oriented times 4. No changes in mentation were reported by either Lorenzo or his wife, except for an ongoing depressed mood without suicidal ideation. During this hospitalization, some days he was somnolent and lethargic, responding with one-word answers. On other days he easily engaged in conversation and self-care. The diagnosis yielded by evaluation at this hospitalization was acute bacterial meningitis. A persistent cough throughout his 3-week stay resulted in a diagnosis of *Pneumocystis carinii* pneumonia. His CD4$^+$ cell count was 38/mm^3.

The physical therapist was unable to complete her examination because of the client's severe pain and hyperesthesia. The necessity for physical therapy to touch and urge movement, along with Lorenzo's poor prognosis, resulted in discontinued physical therapy in this case. The occupational therapist found Lorenzo to be bedridden and to require setup and moderate assistance to perform bed-level ADL. Yet Lorenzo expressed motivation to maintain independence. Interventions included a multidisciplinary team approach to provide comfort care for Lorenzo, emotional support for his family members, and community service connections. After family meetings with all disciplines, discharge plans were made for home-based hospice care rather than extended-care facility placement. Rehabilitation considerations were for quality of life issues; equipment needs; nonpharmaceutical pain control through relaxation training; and the use of meaningful activities, energy conservation training, environmental adaptations, and caregiver training.

CASE 18–4   Entire Diagnostic Process

Age/Language/Race/Sex. A 34-year-old African American male was referred for treatment of toxoplasmosis. He had complaints of headaches, disequilibrium, and difficulty walking and managing at work over the past 2 weeks. He has been HIV positive for 10 years and presented with right-sided weakness.

History of Present Illness. The patient had a gradual onset of balance problems and right-sided weakness over the past 2 weeks. He is a construction worker and has had difficulty coordinating his movements and operating heavy equipment. He simply attributed this to his overtime work. He also complains of "pins and needles" in his feet and attributed this to his job demands. The past medical history is also significant for herpes zoster.

Past Medical History/Surgery History. This is significant for appendectomy at age 18 but otherwise unremarkable.

Medications. HIV medications include stavudine (Zerit), didanosine (Videx), and saquinavir (Invirase).

Other medications included Prilosec (for gastrointestinal problems), megestrol (Megace), and acyclovir (Zovirax).

The patient takes a multivitamin including the B-complex vitamins. He also takes St. John's wort, echinacea, and valerian root.

Lab/Tests. Magnetic resonance imaging showed a ring-enhancing lesion at the left temporoparietal region. The facial nerve appeared to be symmetri-

Continued

cal and normal. He had decreased light touch sensation on the midportion of the face to cotton and along all distributions of the right hemibody.

Neurological findings revealed right hemiparesis with slight footdrop.

Family History/Growth and Development. This was noncontributory.

Work/Play History. Married, he lives in an apartment with his wife and one child. He works full-time as a construction manager. His insurance coverage is through a unionized construction company. His HMO provides six visits for return to full function and back to work.

Functional Status/Activity Level. He is independent and active in the community parent-teacher association and drives to and from work and social functions independently. He is the primary caretaker responsible for his wife and one 3-year-old boy (who is HIV negative). This primary role as a caretaker includes household chores and primary household income.

Social Habits/History/Living Environment. The client lives with his wife and son in a 2-bedroom apartment on the third floor. He smokes, occasionally drinks an alcoholic beverage, and is involved with community activities, doing volunteer work with people living with HIV/AIDS.

Systems Review
Cardiovascular: Vital signs are stable. Heart rate is regular.
Musculoskeletal: Slight right shoulder subluxation (one fingerdepth). Right slight footdrop noted during ambulation.
Pulmonary: Lungs were clear to auscultation.
Neuromuscular: Patient presented with a right hemibody weakness.
Integumentary: Skin is intact.
Psychosocial: Patient was very concerned about his job and family because his work is the primary income and he cannot afford to lose his position because of the importance of his health care benefits.

Tests and Measures
Temperature: 99.2 degrees
Height: 6'1"
Weight: 220 pounds
Girth: Not tested
Arousal, Attention, Cognition: Patient was oriented to place, person, and time.

Ventilation/Circulation: Arterial blood gases were within normal limits. Vital signs were stable.
Integumentary: Skin is intact. Herpes zoster scar is noted at T12 dermatomal level; right appendectomy scar is well healed.
Posture: Patient attempts to maintain upright posture with great difficulty. He feels as though his right arm and leg are "too heavy" to keep in alignment.
Joint Integrity and Mobility: Except for slight right shoulder subluxation this is within normal limits.
Range of Motion: Cervical range of motion is limited by 5% in side bending and rotation to the left. Passive range of motion was within normal limits.
Muscle Performance: Extremity strength is 5/5 throughout left extremities. Right upper extremity is 3+/5; right lower extremity is 4/5 proximally and 3+/5 distally.
Neuromotor Development and Sensory Integration: This was not tested.
Reflex Integrity: Upper motor neuron signs are present. Brisk reflexes are present throughout except for bilateral Achilles tendon reflexes. Romberg sign is positive.
Motor Function: Patient is able to respond to requests for all transfers.
Gait, Locomotion, and Balance: A narrow base of support, decreased trunk rotation, and slow gait with right foot slap and inversion are noted. Balance is decreased, and patient scored 48 on Berg Balance Scale.
Pain: There were no specific complaints of pain, except for right upper quarter achiness.
Self-Care Tests: The patient is independent in ADL except for concerns about driving. He reported driving with his left foot on occasion.

Diagnosis. Patient presents with neurological opportunistic infections that affect balance and safety in ADL and ambulation. Right hemiparesis and footdrop warrent potential use of MAFO, therapeutic exercise and gait training.

Prognosis. Since patient is now on medication to address his neurological central nervous system (CNS) problem, the rehabilitation prognosis is good. Caution, however, is necessary to consistently conduct differential diagnosis for CNS versus peripheral nervous system involvement of opportunistic infections. Patient's support system contributes to a positive rehabilitation outcome.

ACKNOWLEDGMENT

I would like to acknowledge Laura LeCocq, Johnny Bonck, and Anne MacRae, the authors of this chapter in the previous edition, for setting the foundation to this chapter and enlightening the readership through their case studies. Mostly, I wish to acknowledge those living with HIV disease who teach me so much through the many changing facets of the epidemic.

REFERENCES

1. Antoni MH, et al: Psychoneuroimmunology and HIV-1 (review). J Consult Clin Psychol 58:38–40, 1990.
2. Arendt G, et al: Control of posture in patients with neurologically asymptomatic HIV infection and patients with beginning HIV-1–related encephalopathy. Arch Neurol 51:1232–1235, 1994.
3. Armstrong FD, Seidel JF, Swales TP: Pediatric HIV infection: A neuropsychological and education challenge. J Learn Disabil 26:92–103, 1993.
4. Arts EJ, Wainberg MA: Mechanism of nucleoside analog antiretroviral activity and resistance during human immunodeficiency virus reverse transcription. Antimicrob Agents Chemother 40(5):27–40, 1996.
5. Barnes PF, et al: Tuberculosis in patients with human immunodeficiency virus infection. N Engl J Med 324:1644, 1991.
6. Belcher AE, Dettmore D, Holzemer SP: Spirituality and sense of well-being in persons with AIDS. Holistic Nurse Pract 3(4):16–25, 1989.
7. Bell JE: The neuropathology of adult HIV infection. Rev Neurol 154:816–829, 1998.
8. Berger J: Neurological complications of HIV disease. PAAC Notes 3:236–240, 1992.
9. Bernard EM, et al: Pneumocystis. Med Clin North Am 76:107, 1992.
10. Boucher P, et al: Postural stability in diabetic polyneuropathy. Diabetes Care 18:638–645, 1995.
11. Bradley WG, Venna A: Painful vasculitic neuropathy in HIV infection: Relief of pain with prednisone therapy. Neurology 47:1446–1451, 1996.
12. Brockmeyer NH, Pohl G, Mertins L: Combination of chemotherapy and antiviral therapy for Epstein-Barr virus–associated non-Hodgkin's lymphoma of high-grade malignancy in cases of HIV infection. Eur J Med Res 2:133–135, 1997.
13. Brouwers P, Belman AL, Epstein LG: Central nervous system involvement: Manifestations and evaluation. In Pizzo PA, Wilfert CM (eds): Pediatric AIDS: The Challenge of HIV Infection in Infants, Children and Adolescents. Baltimore, Williams & Wilkins, 1991, pp 318–335.
14. Budka H: HIV-associated neuropathology. In Gendelman HE, Lipton SA, Epstein L, Swindells S (eds): The Neurology of AIDS. New York, Chapman & Hall, 1998, pp 241–260.
15. Buhrich N, Cooper DA, Freed E: HIV infection associated with symptoms indistinguishable from functional psychosis. Br J Psychiatry 152:649, 1988.
16. Cai J, et al: Treatment of epidemic (AIDS-related) Kaposi's sarcoma. Curr Opin Oncol 9:433–439, 1997.
17. Carpenter CJ, et al: Antiretroviral therapy for HIV infection in 1998: Updated recommendations of the International AIDS Society—USA panel. JAMA 280:78–86, 1998.
18. Carr A, Cooper D: Lipodystrophy associated with an HIV protease inhibitor. N Engl J Med 339:1296, 1998.
19. Carr A, et al: Pathogenesis of HIV-1 protease inhibitor associated peripheral lipodystrophy, hyperlipidemia and insulin resistance. Lancet 351:1881–1883, 1998.
20. Carson VB: Prayer, meditation, exercise and special diets: Behaviors of the hardy person with HIV/AIDS. J Assoc Nurses AIDS Care 4(3):18–28, 1993.
21. Centers for Disease Control and Prevention: HIV/AIDS Surveill Rep 9:1–44, 1997.
22. Centers for Disease Control and Prevention: Report of the NIH panel to define principles of therapy of HIV infection and guidelines for the use of antiretroviral agents in HIV-infected adults and adolescents. MMWR Morb Mortal Wkly Rep (RR-5)47:1–83, 1998.
23. Centers for Disease Control and Prevention: Update: Acquired immune deficiency syndrome—United States 1994. MMWR Morb Mortal Wkly Rep 44:64–67, 1995.
24. Centers for Disease Control and Prevention: Update: Trends in AIDS incidence, deaths, and prevalence—United States, 1996. MMWR Morb Mortal Wkly Rep 46:165–173, 1997.
25. Centers for Disease Control and Prevention: Update: Trends in AIDS incidence—United States, 1996. MMWR Morb Mortal Wkly Rep 46:861–867, 1997.
26. Centers for Disease Control and Prevention: Update: Perinatally acquired HIV/AIDS—United States, 1997. MMWR Morb Mortal Wkly Rep 46:1086–1092, 1997.
27. Centers for Disease Control: Zidovudine for the prevention of HIV transmission from mother to infant. MMWR Morb Mortal Wkly Rep 43:285–287, 1994.
28. Centers for Disease Control: Projections of the number of persons diagnosed with AIDS and the number of immunosuppressed HIV-infected persons—United States, 1992–1994. MMWR Morb Mortal Wkly Rep 41 (RR-18), 1992.
29. Centers for Disease Control: Revision of the CDC surveillance case definition for acquired immunodeficiency syndrome. MMWR Morb Mortal Wkly Rep (suppl 2S), 1987.
30. Chaisson RE: HIV becomes world's leading infectious cause of death. In The Hopkins HIV Report. vol 11, No. 4. The Johns Hopkins University AIDS Service, p 1, July, 1999.
31. Clerici M, Shearer GM: A $TH_1 \rightarrow TH_2$ switch is a critical step in the etiology of HIV infection. Immunol Today 14(3):107–111, 1993.
32. Cohen S, et al: A National HIV community cohort: Design, baseline and follow-up of the AmFar Observational Database. American Foundation for AIDS Research Community-Based Clinical Trials Network. J Clin Epidemiol 51(19):779–793, 1998.
33. Cohen S, Syme SL: Social Support and Health. Orlando, Academic Press, 1994.
34. Crowe SM, et al: Predictive value of CD4 lymphocyte numbers for the development of opportunistic infections and malignancies in HIV-infected persons. J Acquir Immune Defic Syndr Hum Retrovirol 4:770–776, 1991.
35. Dauncey K: Mania in early stages of AIDS. Br J Psychiatry 152:716, 1988.
36. Di Perri G, DelBravo P, Concia E: Protease inhibitors. N Engl J Med 339:773–774, 1998.
37. Dickover RE, et al: Identification of levels of maternal HIV-1 RNA associated with risk of perinatal transmission: Effect of maternal zidovudine treatment on viral load. JAMA 275:599–605, 1996.
38. Eisenberg DM, Kessler RC, Foster C: Unconventional medicine in the United States: Prevalence, costs and patterns of use. N Engl J Med 328:246–252, 1993.
39. El-Mallakh RS: Mania in AIDS: Clinical significance and theoretical considerations. Int J Psychiatry 21:383, 1991.
40. European Collaborative Study: Children born to women with HIV-1 infection: Natural history and risk of transmission. Lancet 337:253–60, 1991.
41. Fernandez F: Neuropsychiatric syndromes and their treatment in HIV infection. In A Psychiatrist's Guide to AIDS and HIV Disease. Washington, DC, American Psychiatric Association, 1990.
42. Fitzgibbon ML, Cella DF, Humfleet G: Motor slowing in asymptomatic HIV infection. Percept Motor Skills 68:1331–1338, 1989.
43. Flexner C: HIV protease inhibitors. N Engl J Med 38:1281–92, 1998.
44. Freeman R, et al: Autonomic function and human immunodeficiency virus infection. Neurology 40:575, 1990.
45. Gabel RH, et al: AIDS presenting as mania. Compr Psychiatry 27:251, 1986.
46. Galantino ML, Eke-Okoro ST, Findley T, Condolucci D: Use of noninvasive electroacupuncture for the treatment of HIV-related peripheral neuropathy: A pilot study. J Altern Comp Ther 5(2):135–142, 1999.
47. Galantino ML, Jermyn RT, Tursi FJ, Eke-Okoro S: Physical therapy management for the patient with HIV: Lower extremity changes. Clin Podiatr Med Surg 15:329–346, 1998.
48. Galantino ML: Clinical Assessment and Treatment in HIV Disease: Rehabilitation of a Chronic Illness. Thorofare, NJ, Slack, 1992.
49. Galantino ML, Findley T, Krafft L, et al: Blending traditional

and alternative strategies for rehabilitation: Measuring functional outcomes and quality of life issues in an AIDS population. Proceedings of the 8th World Congress of International Rehabilitation Medicine Association. Monduzzi Editore 1:713–716, 1997.

50. Galantino ML, Pizzi M, Lehmann M: Interdisciplinary management of disability in HIV infection. In O'Dell MW (ed): HIV-Related Disability: Assessment and Management. Philadelphia, Hanley and Belfus, 1993.

51. Griffin JW, Crawford TO, Tyor WR, et al: Predominantly sensory neuropathy in AIDS: Distal axonal degeneration and unmyelinated fiber loss. Neurology 41(Suppl 1):374, 1991.

52. Griffin JWI, Wesselingh S, Oaklander AL, et al: MRNA fingerprinting of cytokines and growth factors: A new means of characterizing nerve biopsies (abstract). Neurology 43(Suppl 2):A232, 1993.

53. Grody WW, Cheng L, Lewis W: Infection of the heart by the human immunodeficiency virus. Am J Cardiol 66:203–206, 1990.

54. Halstead S, et al: Psychosis associated with HIV infection. J Br Psychiatry 153:618, 1988.

55. Hanna L: Body fat changes: More than lipodystrophy. Bull Exp Treat AIDS 5:32–35, 1999.

56. Harris MJ, et al: New-onset psychosis in HIV-infected patients. J Clin Psychiatry 52:369, 1991.

57. Havlir DV, Richman DD: Viral dynamics of HIV; Implications for drug development and therapeutic strategies. Ann Intern Med 124:984–994, 1996.

58. Hellerstein MK, et al: Current approach to the treatment of human immunodeficiency virus–associated weight loss: Pathophysiologic considerations and emerging management strategies. Semin Oncol 17(6, Suppl 9):17, 1990.

59. Henry K, Melroe H, Heubsch J, et al: Severe premature coronary artery disease with protease inhibitors. Lancet 351:1328, 1998.

60. Hirsch MS, Conway N, D'Aquila RT, et al: Antiretroviral drug resistance testing in adults with HIV infection: Implications for clinical management. JAMA 279:1984–1989, 1998.

61. Ho HH, Chung C, Liu T, et al: A randomized controlled trial on the treatment for acute partial ischemic stroke with acupuncture. Neuroepidemiology 12:106–113, 1993.

62. Holtzer CD, Roland M: The use of combination antiretroviral therapy in HIV-infected patients. Ann Pharmacother 33:198–209, 1999.

63. Hughes MD, Johnson VA, Hirsch MS, et al: Monitoring plasma HIV-1 RNA levels in addition to CD4 lymphocyte count improves assessment of antiretroviral therapeutic response. Ann Intern Med 126:939–945, 1997.

64. Husstedt I, Grotemeyer K, Heiner B, et al: Progression of distal-symmetrical polyneuropathy in HIV infection: A prospective study. AIDS 7:1069–1073, 1993.

65. Jacobsberg LB, Perry S: Psychiatric disturbances. Med Clin North Am 76:99, 1992.

66. Johnson CC, Wilcosky T, Kvale P, et al: Cancer incidence among an HIV cohort: Pulmonary complications of HIV Infection Study Group. Am J Epidemiol 146:470–475, 1997.

67. Kamarck TW, Manuck SB Jennings JR: Social support reduces cardiovascular reactivity to psychological challenge: A laboratory model. Psychosom Med 52:42–58, 1990.

68. Keicolt Glaser JK, Glaser R: Stress and immune function in humans. In Ader R, Felten DL, Cohen N (eds): Psychoneuroimmunology, 2nd ed. New York, Academic Press, 1991, pp 849–867.

69. Kendall J: Promoting wellness in HIV-support groups. J Assoc Nurses AIDS Care 3(1):28–38, 1992.

70. Kendall J: Wellness spirituality in homosexual men with HIV infection. J Assoc Nurses AIDS Care 5(4):28–34, 1994.

71. Kerlikowske KM, Katz MH: *Mycobacterium avium* complex and *Mycobacterium tuberculosis* in patients infected with the human immunodeficiency virus. West J Med 157(2):44, 1992.

72. Kessler HA, et al: AIDS Part II. Dis Mon 38(10):691, 1992.

73. Kieburtz K, et al: Manic syndrome in AIDS. Am J Psychiatry 148:1068, 1991.

74. Koff WC, Glass MJ: Future directions in HIV vaccine development. AIDS Res Hum Retroviruses 8(8):1313, 1992.

75. Kovacs JA, Vogel S, Albert JM, et al: Controlled trial of interleukin-2 infusions in patients infected with the human immunodeficiency virus. N Engl J Med 335:1350–1356, 1996.

76. Krech U: Complement-fixing antibodies against cytomegalovirus in different parts of the world. Bull World Health Organ 49:103, 1973.

77. Krown SE: Acquired immunodeficiency syndrome–associated Kaposi's sarcoma. Med Clin North Am 81:471–494, 1997.

78. LaPerriere A, Antoni M, Fletcher MA, Schneiderman N: Exercise training programs for health maintenance in HIV-1. In Galantino ML (ed): Clinical Assessment and Treatment in HIV: Rehabilitation of a Chronic Disease. Thorofare, NJ, Slack, 1992.

79. LaPerriere A, Fletcher MA, Antoni MH, et al: Aerobic exercise training in an AIDS risk group. Int J Sports Med 12(Suppl 1):S53–S57, 1991.

80. LaPerriere A, Ironson G, Antoni MH, et al: Exercise and immunology. Med Sci Sports Exer 26(2):182–190, 1994.

81. Lederman NM: Host-directed and immune-based therapies for human immunodeficiency virus infections. Ann Intern Med 122:218–227, 1995.

82. Lewis M, Warfield C: Management of pain in AIDS. Hosp Pract 30:51–54, 1990.

83. Lipsky JJ: Antiretroviral drugs for AIDS. Lancet 348:800–803, 1996.

84. Lipton SA, Gendelman HE: Dementia associated with the acquired immunodeficiency syndrome. N Engl J Med 332:934–940, 1995.

85. Lo J, Mulligan K, Tai V, et al: Body shape changes in HIV-infected patients. J Acquir Immune Defic Syndr Hum Retrovirol 19:307–308, 1998.

86. Lutgendorf S, Antoni MH, Schneiderman N, Fletcher MA: Psychosocial counseling to improve quality of life in HIV infection. Patient Educ Counsel 24:217–235, 1994.

87. Lyketsos CG, et al: Manic syndrome early and late in the course of HIV. Am J Psychiatry 150:326, 1993.

88. Macallan DC, Noble C, Baldwin C: Energy expenditure and wasting in human immunodeficiency virus infection. N Engl J Med 333:83, 1995.

89. Maccabruni A, Caselli S, Astori G, et al: Evaluation of a protocol for the early diagnosis of HIV-related neurologic dysfunction. Int Conf AIDS 12:1129, 1998 (abstract No. 60697).

90. MacDougall DS: Pediatric HIV: Evaluation, management and rehabilitation. J Int Assoc Physicians AIDS Care 4(5):16–25, 1998.

91. Maiman M, Fruchter RG, Clark M, et al: Cervical cancer as an AIDS-defining illness. Obstet Gynecol 89:76–80, 1997.

92. Mallet AL, Soares PP, Nobrega AC, et al: Cardiac parasympathetic function in HIV-infected humans. Int Conf AIDS 8(3):104, 1992 (abstract No. 7333).

93. Marieb EN: Human Anatomy and Physiology. Redwood City, CA, Benjamin/Cummings, 1989.

94. Marschner IC, Collier AC, Coombs RW, et al: Use of changes in plasma levels of human immunodeficiency virus type 1 RNA to assess the clinical benefits of antiretroviral. J Infect Dis 177:40–47, 1998.

95. Masur H, Ognibene FB, Yarchoan R, et al: CD4 counts as predictors of opportunistic pneumonias in HIV infection. Ann Intern Med 111:223–231, 1989.

96. Maxwell S, et al: Manic syndrome associated with zidovudine treatment. JAMA 259:3406, 1988.

97. Mellors JW, Munoz A, Giorgi JV, et al: Plasma viral load and CD4 lymphocytes as prognostic markers of HIV-1 infection. Ann Intern Med 126:946–954, 1997.

98. Miller K, Jones E, Yanovski J, et al: Visceral abdominal-fat accumulation associated with the use of indinavir. Lancet 351:871–875, 1998.

99. Morgello S, Simpson DM: Multifocal cytomegalovirus demyelinative polyneuropathy associated with AIDS. Muscle Nerve. 17:176–182, 1994.

100. Nahlen BL, et al: HIV wasting syndrome in the United States. AIDS 7:183, 1993.

101. Navia BA, Jordan BD, Price RW: The AIDS dementia complex: I. Clinical features. Ann Neurol 19:517–524, 1986.

102. Neilson GA, Bodsworth NJ, Watts N: Response to hepatitis A vaccination in human immunodeficiency virus infected and uninfected homosexual men. J Infect Dis 176:1064–1067, 1997.

103. Newshan G, Wainapel S: Pain characteristics and their management in persons with AIDS. J Assoc Nurses AIDS Care 4(2):53–59, 1993.

104. Nunes JA, Raymond SJ, Nicholas PK, Leuner J: Social support,

quality of life, immune function, and health in persons living with HIV. Holistic Nurs 12(2):174–198, 1995.

105. O'Dowd MA, McKegney KP: Manic syndrome associated with zidovudine. JAMA 260:3587, 1988.

106. Office of Alternative Medicine: Functional Description of the Office. Bethesda, MD, National Institutes of Health, 1993.

107. Ostrow DG: Psychiatric Aspects of Human Immunodeficiency Virus Infection. Kalamazoo, MN, Upjohn Pharmaceuticals, 1990.

108. Palella F, Moorman A, Delaney K, et al: Dramatically declining morbidity and mortality in an ambulatory HIV-infected population. In Abstracts of the 5th Conference on Retroviruses and Opportunistic Infections, Chicago, February 1–5, 1998, abstract 198.

109. Palella FJ, Delaney KM, Moorman AC, et al: Declining morbidity and mortality among patients with advance human immunodeficiency virus infection. N Engl J Med 338:853–860, 1998.

110. Petiot P, Vighetto A, Charles N, et al: Isolated postural tremor revealing HIV-1 infection. J Neurol 240:507–508, 1993.

111. Phair JP, Munoz A, Detels R, et al: The risk of *Pneumocystis carinii* pneumonia among men infected with human immunodeficiency virus type 1. N Engl J Med 322:161–165, 1990.

112. Pinto AN: AIDS and cerebrovascular disease. Stroke 27:538–543, 1996.

113. Pitchenik AE, Fertel D: Tuberculosis and nontuberculous mycobacterial disease. Med Clin North Am 76:121, 1992.

114. Plein D, VanCamp G, Coysyns B, et al: Cardiac and autonomic evaluation in a pediatric population with human immunodeficiency virus. Clin Cardiol 22:33–36, 1999.

115. Price R, Brew B: The AIDS dementia complex. J Infect Dis 158:1079–1083, 1988.

116. Quinn TC: Global burden of the HIV pandemic. Lancet 348:99–106, 1996.

117. Reichert T, DeBruyere M, Deneys V, et al: Lymphocyte subset reference ranges in adult Caucasians. Clin Immunol Immunopathol 60:190–208, 1991.

118. Remick SC: The spectrum of non-AIDS defining neoplastic disease in HIV infection. J Invest Med 44:205–215, 1996.

119. Roquer J, Palomeras E, Pou A: AIDS and cerebrovascular disease (letter). Stroke 27:1694, 1996.

120. Rosen MJ: Overview of pulmonary complications. Clin Chest Med 17:621–631, 1996.

121. Ruttimann S, Hilti P, Spinas GA, Dubach UC: High frequency of human immunodeficiency virus–associated autonomic neuropathy and more severe involvement in advanced stages of human immunodeficiency virus disease. Arch Intern Med 152:485–501, 1991.

122. Rynes R: Painful rheumatic syndromes associated with human immunodeficiency virus infection. Rheum Dis Clin North Am 17:83, 1991.

123. Sande MA, Volberding PA: Alternative therapies in HIV. In Medical Management of AIDS, 4th ed. Philadelphia, WB Saunders, 1995.

124. Scarlatti G: Paediatric HIV infection. Lancet 348:863–868, 1996.

125. Schmidt U, Miller D: Two cases of hypomania in AIDS. Br J Psychiatry 152:839, 1988.

126. Schrager LK, D'Souza MP: Cellular and anatomical reservoirs of HIV-1 in patients receiving potent antiretroviral combination therapy. JAMA 280:67–71, 1998.

127. Shepherd EJ, Brettle RP, Liberski PP, et al: Spinal cord pathology

128. Simpson DM, Olney RK: Peripheral neuropathies associated with human immunodeficiency virus infection. In Dyck PJ (ed): Peripheral Neuropathy. Philadelphia, WB Saunders, 1994.

129. Simpson DM, Tagliati M, Grinell J, Godbold J: Electrophysiological findings in HIV infection: Association with distal symmetrical polyneuropathy and CD4 level (abstract). Muscle Nerve 17:1113, 1994.

130. Simpson DM, Tagliati M: Neurologic manifestations of HIV infection. Ann Intern Med 121:769–785, 1994.

131. Singer E, Zorilla C, Fahy-Chandon B, et al: Painful symptoms reported by ambulatory HIV-infected men in a longitudinal study. Pain 54:15–19, 1993.

132. Snyder S, et al: Prevalence of mental disorders in newly admitted medical inpatients with AIDS. Psychosomatics 33:166, 1992.

133. So YT, Holtzman DM, Abrams DI, Olney RK: Peripheral neuropathy associated with acquired immunodeficiency syndrome: Prevalence and clinical features based on a population-based survey. Arch Neurol 45:945–948, 1988.

134. Solomon G, Brancato L, Winchester R: An approach to the human immunodeficiency virus patient with a spondyloarthropic disease. Rheum Dis Clin North Am 17:44–52, 1991.

135. Spence RA, Katz WM, Anderson KS, Johnson KA: Mechanism of inhibition of HIV-1 reverse transcriptase by non-nucleoside inhibitors. Science 267:988–993, 1995.

136. Steinbach L, Tehranzadeh J, Fleckenstein J, et al: Musculoskeletal manifestations of human immunodeficiency virus (HIV) infection. Radiology 186:833–838, 1993.

137. Stine GJ: Acquired Immune Deficiency Syndrome: Biological, Medical, Social and Legal Issues. Englewood Cliffs, NJ, Prentice-Hall, 1993.

138. Sullivan A, Nelson M, Moyle G, et al: Coronary artery disease occurring with protease inhibitor therapy. Int J STD AIDS 9:711–712, 1998.

139. Tagliati M, Simpson D, Morgello S, et al: Cerebellar degeneration associated with human immunodeficiency virus infection. Neurology 50:244–251, 1998.

140. Thomas PD, Goodwin JM, Goodwin JS: Effect of social support on stress-related changes in cholesterol level, uric acid level and immune function in an elderly sample. Am J Psychiatry 142:735–737, 1985.

141. Villa A, Foresti V, Confalonieri F: Autonomic nervous system dysfunction associated with HIV infection in intravenous heroin users. AIDS 6:85–89, 1992.

142. Vitkovic L, Tardieu M: Neuropathogenesis of HIV-1 infection: Outstanding questions. C R Acad Sci Paris 321:1015–1021, 1998.

143. Witte MH, Witte DL, Way MF: AIDS, Kaposi's sarcoma and the lymphatic system: Update and reflections. Lymphology 23:73, 1990.

144. Wolf TM, Dralle PW, Morse EV: A biopsychosocial examination of symptomatic and asymptomatic HIV-infected patients. Int J Psychiatry Med 21:263–279, 1991.

145. World Health Report, 1999. Geneva, WHO, 1999.

146. Yunis NA, Stone VE: Cardiac manfestations of HIV/AIDS: A review of disease spectrum and clinical management. J Acquir Immune Defic Syndr Hum Retrovirol 18:145–154, 1998.

The Postpolio Syndrome

LAURA K. SMITH, PhD, PT • CAROLYN KELLY, MS, PT

Key Words

– poliomyelitis

– postpolio muscular atrophy

– postpolio sequelae

– postpolio syndrome

– postpoliomyelitis

Objectives

After reading this chapter the student/therapist will:

1. Describe the pathological lesion occurring in poliomyelitis.

2. List three physiological processes that are the basis for recovery of muscle strength after the acute phase of poliomyelitis.

3. List five impairments commonly seen in people who have postpolio syndrome.

4. Describe the difference between fatigue in postpolio syndrome and normal fatigue.

5. Describe the most likely etiology of new muscle weakness in postpolio syndrome.

6. State the goals for clinical management of the postpolio syndrome.

7. State four musculoskeletal objectives designed to achieve these goals.

8. Explain why energy conservation techniques play such an important role in the management of postpolio syndrome.

9. State why exercises designed to strengthen polio-involved muscles can cause further weakness and pain.

10. Describe three common styles used by people with postpolio to cope with their impairments.

OVERVIEW

Poliomyelitis, or infantile paralysis, is an endemic disease of humans first recorded in Egypt in 1300 BC.[82] It is an acute infectious disease caused by an enteric virus with worldwide distribution.* Transmission is by human contact, and most of the population ingest the virus. Few persons, however, develop the paralytic form of acute poliomyelitis because they have developed immunity from breast feeding, subclinical infections, clinical infections without paralysis, and now vaccines. In the paralytic form, the virus selectively attacks the motor neuron cell bodies in the spinal cord and the brain with resulting flaccid muscle paresis or paralysis.

As sanitation levels increased in industrialized countries in the first half of the twentieth century and formula feeding was being advocated, acute poliomyelitis escalated to epidemic proportions. Frightening epidemics swept across North America and Europe from 1910 to 1959. In 1921, New York City recorded 9,000 cases with 2,000 deaths.[15] Franklin Roosevelt contracted poliomyelitis at that time. In 1937, when Roosevelt was president of the United States, he founded the March of Dimes (The National Foundation for Infantile Paralysis). An unprecedented outpouring of public funds occurred to provide treatment, research, and professional education. The results were spectacular. In just 20 years the "war on polio" was won with the introduction of the inactivated vaccine (Salk, 1955) and the live attenuated oral vaccine (Sabin, 1960). Polio was promptly forgotten as medicine and rehabilitation turned attention to other pressing disabilities. The surviving polio victims went on with their lives to compensate, compete, and become productive citizens.

In the 1970s and 1980s increasing numbers of people with a history of poliomyelitis began to have new weakness in both their polio muscles and muscles that they thought were unaffected by the poliovirus. Most people turned to exercise programs only to find that they were not getting stronger but rather weaker and more fatigued. They had what was called the late effects of poliomyelitis, postpolio sequelae, or postpolio muscular atrophy. Now the condition is usually referred to as postpolio syndrome (PPS).

IDENTIFICATION OF THE CLINICAL PROBLEM: PATHOLOGY

The Postpolio Syndrome

Postpolio syndrome is a complex combination of primary and secondary impairments resulting in neuromuscular, musculoskeletal, and psychosocial problems. Those who have swallowing or respiratory muscle involvement or severe scoliosis may have cardiopulmonary problems as

well. Primary impairments include flaccid muscle paresis and paralysis and excessive or limited range of motion (ROM). PPS adds the secondary impairments of a unique type of fatigue, deep muscle pain, and frightening new muscle weakness.[24] These problems may lead to further functional limitations in daily activities and disability in work, family, and social activities. Other physical problems may include muscle cramps and fasciculations, cold intolerance, swallowing difficulties, hypoventilation, and sleep disorders (Table 19–1). These new impairments occur after a long period of stability with the median time of approximately 35 years from the onset of acute poliomyelitis.[36]

The incidence of PPS is not well known because there is a lack of records. Based on the 1987 survey of the National Center for Health Statistics, Halstead[34] estimated that there are 600,000 people now living in the United States who were previously diagnosed as having paralytic poliomyelitis. He estimated 20% to 40%, or 120,000 to 420,000, of these people are experiencing PPS symptoms. The cause of the syndrome is not specifically known either, but most evidence points to metabolic overload on the limited capacity of the neuromuscular system. PPS is directly related to the impairments caused by the virus in the acute phase and to the relative level of physical activity during the stability phase.

Acute Poliomyelitis

In most instances the widely prevalent polioviruses were destroyed in the stomach or excreted through the intestinal tract without clinical infection, or they entered the bloodstream and produced a flulike infection with recovery and development of immunity. These people would be classed as having had nonparalytic poliomyelitis. If the virus crossed the blood-brain barrier, it attacked almost all of the motor nerve cells in the brain, brain stem, and spinal cord. Symptoms during this 2-week febrile illness included headache, sore throat, elevated temperature, severe meningismus, severe muscle pain to touch and

● **T A B L E   1 9 – 1.** Most Common New Health Problems in 132 Confirmed Postpolio Individuals with a Diagnosis of Postpolio Syndrome

	No.	%
Health problems		
Fatigue	117	89
Muscle pain	93	71
Joint pain	93	71
Weakness		
Previously affected muscles	91	69
Previously unaffected muscles	66	50
Cold intolerance	38	29
Atrophy	37	28
ADL problems		
Walking	84	64
Climbing stairs	80	61
Dressing	23	17

Adapted from Halstead L, Wiechers D (eds): Research and Clinical Aspects of the Late Effects of Poliomyelitis. White Plains, NY, March of Dimes, 1987, p 17.

---

*In 1988 the World Health Assembly resolved to eradicate acute poliomyelitis throughout the world. Progress toward this goal includes the Americas and the Western Pacific, which have been free from polio since 1991 and 1997, respectively. Europe is free from polio except for southeastern Turkey. Efforts to complete the eradication of polio in African and southern Asian countries are being intensified.[69]

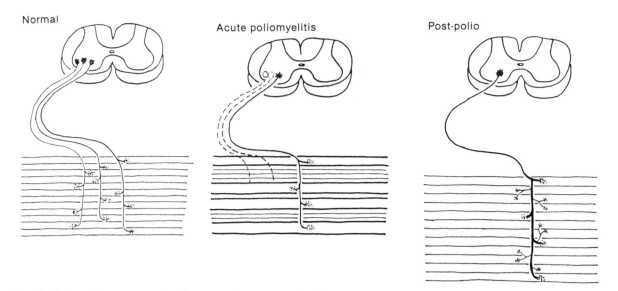

FIGURE 19–1. Schematic representation of motor units to a muscle. *Normal* represents the 100 to 1,000 motor neurons of a muscle and the 5 to 1,500 muscle fibers each axon innervates. *Acute poliomyelitis* depicts viral destruction of some of the anterior horn cells with atrophy of denervated muscle fibers. *Postpolio* represents axon sprouting by recovered nerve cells with reinnervation of the orphaned muscle fibers and subsequent hypertrophy.

stretch, and flaccid muscle paresis or paralysis (signs and symptoms of severe life-threatening poliomyelitis are outlined by Spencer).[82, 83] Many motor neurons fought off the virus and recovered, but many were destroyed. In animal studies, Bodian[11] found only 4% of the anterior horn cells histologically normal at 2 to 6 days from onset, but by 14 days the neurons were either destroyed or of normal appearance. Clinically, there was not a clear-cut distinction between those people with truly normal muscle strength and those with slight muscle weakness. Many people with mild paralytic poliomyelitis were diagnosed as nonparalytic.

Physiological Processes of Recovery of Muscle Strength

After approximately 2 weeks of febrile illness a motor neuron with its 5 to 1,500 muscle fibers could be unaffected, recovered, or destroyed with resulting denervation of the muscle fibers (Fig. 19–1). The 100 to 1,000 motor neurons to a particular muscle would be unaffected or recovered; all of the motor neurons to a muscle could be destroyed; or the muscle could be partially denervated with combinations of recovered and destroyed motor neurons. Diagnostic electromyography (EMG) at this time would show fibrillation potentials indicating recent denervation of muscle fibers.

In convalescent poliomyelitis, muscle strength in partially denervated muscles increased to a maximum over a 2-year period, with 50% of the muscle strength recovery occurring in the first 3 months after onset and 75% in the first 6 months (Fig. 19–2). The rate and magnitude of the recovery, however, could be compromised by injudicious treatment, overactivity, and excessive exercise.[9, 43, 82, 83] Muscle strength recovery and increase in functional ability occurred by four physiological processes:

1. Recovered neurons develop terminal axon sprouts to reinnervate orphaned muscle fibers[35, 85, 93] (see Fig. 19–1). It is estimated that a single motor neuron can reinnervate up to five or more times its normal complement of muscle fibers. Electromyographically, the action potentials of the single motor units are polyphasic with large amplitudes and are called giant motor units.

2. Innervated muscle fibers can be hypertrophied by intensive exercise and activity during the rehabilitation phase. This increase in muscle fiber size has been referred to as denervation hypertrophy.

3. Increased functional ability by neuromuscular learning whereby practice of an exercise or an activity leads to increased skill and performance without necessarily increasing muscle strength.[77]

4. Increased recruitment of the giant motor units for the task with use of the muscles at high levels of their already reduced capacity.

Such extensive compensatory physiological processes mask the profound neurological deficits caused by the disease. This was demonstrated by Sharrard,[78] who counted the number of anterior horn cells for each muscle in the spinal cord of individuals with postpolio who died of other causes. He compared the percentage of cells present with previous manual muscle test grades. Muscles graded 5(N) could have lost up to 60% of their anterior horn cells; muscles previously graded 4(G) had lost 60% to 90% of their motor neurons; and muscles of grades 3 to 1(FPT) lost 90% to 98%. It is truly remarkable how much the polio survivors accomplish with so few motor units.

Functional Compensation

Many convalescent polio clients in the early epidemics were encouraged to exercise for years and to use heroic compensatory methods for function. These compensa-

Percent chance of severely involved muscles recovering to "good" or "normal" eventual strength:

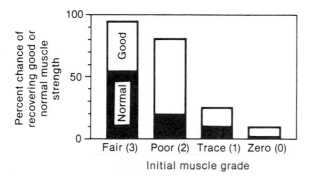

Rate of muscle recovery irrespective of the initial or final strength:

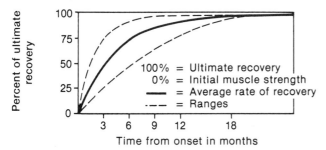

FIGURE 19–2. The rate and extent of increase in manual muscle test scores in postacute poliomyelitis. Muscles showing some strength on initial examination will increase in strength unless they are overworked, in which case they may plateau or lose strength. The grade of Normal (5) is a clinical definition and not an indication of preillness strength. This grade can be recorded with loss of 60% of the anterior horn cells to a muscle. (Adapted from Spencer WA: Treatment of Acute Poliomyelitis. Springfield, IL, Charles C Thomas, 1956.)

tions include use of muscles at high levels of their capacity, substitution of stronger muscles with increased energy expenditure for the task, and use of ligaments for stability with resulting hypermobility. Figure 19–3 shows a boy who had acute poliomyelitis several years before this picture was made. He appears to have a flail right lower extremity with nonfunctional muscle test grades of 3(F) to 0 and functional muscle strength of 5(N) or 4(G) in the rest of his body. His walking shows excessive vertical and lateral movements of the center of gravity of the body, arm swings, and muscle contractions of the left leg leading to abnormally high energy expenditure for the task. In an EMG study of walking in clients with PPS, Perry and co-workers demonstrated overuse and substitution activity of the vastus lateralis, biceps femoris, and gluteus maximus muscles when the soleus is nonfunctional.[62] In the long term, however, such substitution and overcompensation lead to microtrauma of ligaments and joint structures and exhaustion of neuromuscular units.

Etiology of the Postpolio Syndrome

The etiology of the new weakness and atrophy is unknown. Several theories have been proposed and are reviewed in detail by Jubelt and Cashman.[41] There is little current evidence to implicate reactivation of the poliovirus or an autoimmune response. Normal aging, with loss of neurons occurring after age 60, may be a factor in the older individuals with PPS because the loss of a few neurons from an already markedly depleted neuronal pool could result in a significant decrease in strength.[86] It has been suggested that the neurons that showed histological recovery from the virus may not have been physiologically normal and may be subject to premature aging and failure.[50]

Most of the theories as to the cause of PPS point to an increased metabolic demand on the giant motor units, with pruning of the axon sprouts to reduce the number of muscle fibers innervated by the motor nerve cell (Fig. 19–4). The sprouting and pruning process has evidently been going on since the convalescent stage of polio as a mechanism to maintain as many denervated fibers as possible. In time the theory proposes that more pruning than sprouting occurs, with downsizing of the number of muscle fibers in the motor units leading to muscle weakness and fatigue.[51, 52, 72, 73] Recent macro EMG studies

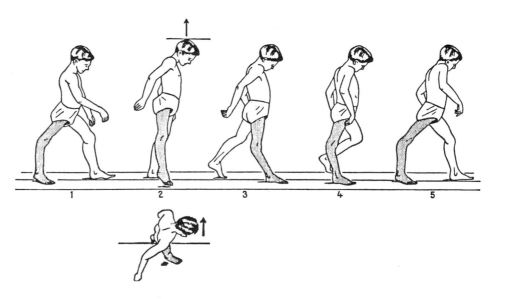

FIGURE 19–3. The functional compensations of a boy with paralysis of the right lower extremity show increased energy expenditure and progressive ligamentous laxity. (Adapted from Ducroquet R, et al: Walking and Limping—a Study of Normal and Pathological Walking. Philadelphia, JB Lippincott, 1968.)

POST-POLIO SYNDROME

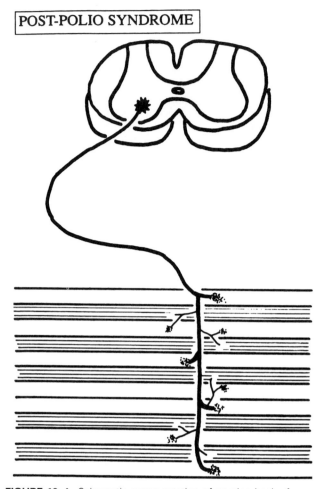

FIGURE 19–4. Schematic representation of pruning back of axon sprouts in postpolio syndrome resulting in reduced numbers of muscle fibers per motor unit and atrophy of the orphaned muscle fibers.

that measure the size of individual motor units do not support this theory.[71] Weaker muscles contained larger median macro EMG amplitudes than stronger muscles, and there was an increased amplitude of the macro EMG over the years rather than a decrease. Some muscle biopsies are suggestive of new denervation of muscle fibers.[18, 19] These findings suggest that there may be loss of individual motor units rather than just muscle fibers in the motor unit.

The second area of dysfunction in the giant motor units is at the neuromuscular junction. Single-fiber EMG studies show instability or failure of transmission of the nerve impulse at the axon terminal. This problem may be the cause of fatigue and decreased endurance.

MANAGEMENT

Diagnosis

The criteria most commonly used for establishing a diagnosis of PPS were developed by Halstead[36]: (1) a confirmed history of paralytic polio; (2) partial to complete muscle strength and functional recovery; (3) a period of

at least 15 years of neurological and functional stability; (4) onset of two or more new health problems listed in Table 19–1; and (5) no other medical conditions to explain these new health problems. Although localized joint pain is present in almost all people with PPS, joint pain is not used as a diagnostic criterion for PPS because the pain is an injury phenomenon from local abnormal joint and muscle forces. On the other hand, the deep muscle pain, PPS fatigue, and new muscle weakness are generalized to extremities or the whole body.

The manifestations of the late effects of polio are nonspecific and seem to be similar to symptoms of many other conditions. A comprehensive interdisciplinary evaluation is essential to confirm the original diagnosis of poliomyelitis because 10% to 15% of people who thought or were told they had polio did not, and many people with mild weaknesses were diagnosed as nonparalytic.[33, 36, 82] Individuals with mild weakness and excellent recovery from acute poliomyelitis usually have no primary disability. They may have, however, severe cases of PPS, with multiple secondary disabilities. The people who have PPS can also have any of the other physical and psychosocial health problems that may occur in the age ranges of 20 to 90 years. The current diagnoses need to be established and the differential diagnosis of PPS made by exclusion.[32, 36, 54]

Diagnosis of PPS may be difficult and time consuming, with examinations taking from 3 or 4 hours to several days. Some clinics require a diagnostic EMG, and others use the EMG when the muscle pattern or history is not typical. Polio typically causes muscle paralysis or paresis in a spotty and asymmetrical pattern with normal sensation and normal to absent tendon reflexes. There are no two people with polio who have the same muscle pattern.

Therapeutic Examinations and Evaluations

In the postacute and convalescent stages of polio the manual muscle test, goniometry, and the activities of daily living (ADL) test formed the basis of the daily intervention plan. In the chronic phase these tests are used to identify primary and secondary impairments and the need for interventions. The pattern of the definitive manual muscle test also is used to help in the confirmation of initial polio (flaccid, spotty, and asymmetrical muscle paresis or paralysis). Therapeutic examinations and evaluations should include the following:

1. History (or availability) including orthopedic surgeries.
2. Manual muscle testing of the entire body. Many persons who had polio when they were children do not know what is normal. They often think that a stronger extremity has not been affected by polio, and they expect to place heavy loads on it. Also years of substitution can cover up the involvement of muscles if only gross movement testing is done. For example, testing the motion of ankle dorsiflexion can cause the examiner to miss a weak or absent anterior tibialis muscle.
3. Measurement of hypermobile or hypomobile joints and contractures.
4. History and analysis of physical activity by type, time,

and intensity: in the home, at work, in travel, in community activities, in avocations, on vacations, in recreation, and with exercise. If these areas are not pursued in depth, such as how many steps are in the home or office and how many times a day does the person go up and down them, many of the causes of the muscle pain and fatigue will be missed.

5. Detailed evaluation of habitual sleeping, sitting, standing, and walking postures.
6. Modified spinal and upper lower-quarter evaluations according to problems presented.
7. Evaluation of needs for orthotic and assistive equipment interventions.

INTERVENTIONS

The long-term goal for interventions at the PPS stage is to provide the person with principles and methods for self-management of his or her body and to make lifestyle changes that will reduce the excessive metabolic load on the muscles. Most of the people with PPS have excellent knowledge of their body and what it can and cannot do. Many even remember the names of their muscles. They do not, however, know about what has happened to the body, because they were children when they caught polio and there was little patient or family education in the first part of the twentieth century. The most important aspect of the intervention program is client and family education on the pathology caused by the poliovirus, the processes of muscle strength recovery, and the effects of long term compensations. This information along with the conservation of energy focus is opposite to what the people with PPS have been brought up on. It takes time for the clients to assimilate the information and make meaningful changes. They need patience and written and verbal information and to talk to others with similar problems. Extensive information and resources will be found in *Managing Post-polio* by Halstead[34] and at the Gazette International Polio Networking Institute.[30]

GENERAL MUSCULOSKELETAL GOALS FOR INTERVENTIONS

1. Alleviate and prevent the causes of pain.
2. Decrease the abnormally high workload of muscles relative to their limited capacity.
3. Minimize postural and gait deviations mechanically.
4. Maintain and increase function, safety, and the quality of life.

Pain

Muscle Pain

Pain was found to be the predominant problem of reporting people who had PPS. There was an incidence of 85% in those walking without orthotic assistance and 100% in those using crutches or manual wheelchairs for locomotion.[81] The types and causes of pain are multiple. One type of pain is diffuse and generalized and often described as "bone pain" or "like having the flu." This pain occurs both in known weak muscles and particularly in extremities that have been thought to be normal. Most people report that this type of pain is unaffected by medications or physical modalities and that it is increased by physical activity and decreased by rest. The pain or fatigue is unusual because it usually does not occur at the time of the activity but rather 1 or 2 days later. Treatment should be directed to nonfatiguing functional activities, energy conservation techniques,[95] more frequent rest periods, and pacing of activities by interspersing rest periods or change of activity.[3]

Examples of some of the lifestyle changes that are recommended include avoiding stairs, low chairs, and deep knee bends and encouraging use of elevators, elevated chairs, bathtub bench or shower stool, reserved parking, and weight control. Recommendations for the neck and upper extremities include seating and workstation corrections, support of books and newspapers for reading, use of rolling carts for carrying, telephone headsets, and computer wristrests. Decreasing workloads on the muscles may require eliminating unessential walking, using an orthosis or a personal mobility vehicle (motorized cart or electric wheelchair), avoiding strengthening and aerobic exercises, and, in some cases, disability retirement.

Recovery from the diffuse muscle pain takes many months and depends on the severity, duration, and the client's compliance with treatment recommendations. Peach and Olejnik[61] found that muscle pain was resolved in 28% and improved in 72% of people who complied with recommendations. In those who were noncompliant, muscle pain was improved in 14%, unchanged in 57%, and increased in 29%.

Joint Pain

More localized pain such as joint pain is caused primarily by long-term microtrauma from abnormal biomechanical forces, as well as by injuries from falls. Joint pain may accompany PPS, but joint pain by itself is usually a repetitive injury and not a symptom of PPS. Common conditions include osteoarthritis,[92] sacroileitis, trochanteric bursitis, ligamentous laxity of the knee and ankle, patellar-femoral tracking problems, shoulder impingements, lateral epicondylitis (humerus), and carpal tunnel syndrome. Neck, shoulder, and back pain radiating to the hip and leg were reported by over 65% of those with PPS.[81] This pain should be expected because the incidence of major postural abnormalities and gait deviations is also high, as shown in Table 19–2. Interventions are complicated by the presence of osteoporosis, lack of compensatory substitutions to rest the injured part, and often poor response to exercise.

Local pain and dysfunction can be treated as athletic injuries from overuse, but they require major modifications and careful monitoring of performance, pain, and fatigue. Many joint pain problems can be relieved and controlled by a home program. Interventions include

TABLE 19-2. Major Postural Abnormalities in Sitting, Standing, and Walking in 111 Confirmed Postpolio Clinic Clients

Posture (N)	Abnormal Deviation	No.	%
Sitting (N = 111)	Absent lumbar curve	64	54
	Forward head (loss of cervical curves)	50	45
	Uneven pelvic base°	29	26
	Structural scoliosis	38	34
Standing (N = 76)	Absent lumbar curve	52	68
	Uneven pelvic base°	40	53
	Weight-bearing on stronger leg	29	38
Walking (N = 76)	Abnormal gait deviations	76	100
	Major lateral trunk oscillations	33	43
	Obvious forward lean	40	53

°Pelvic asymmetry was ½ inch or more.

Adapted from Smith L, McDermott K: Pain in post-poliomyelitis: Addressing causes versus effects. In Halstead L, Wiechers D (eds): Research and Clinical Aspects of the Late Effects of Poliomyelitis. White Plains, NY, March of Dimes, 1987.

methods to rest the injured part, mechanical postural corrections, cold packs (6 to 10 times a day), nonsteroidal antiinflammatory drugs, orthotics, and ROM exercises. The ROM exercises are passive, high-repetition, pain-free motions to maintain and then increase pain-free ROM. As the pain decreases, these motions can become assistive and then active according to the muscle strength present.

Successful intervention into joint pain, however, requires identification and elimination of the cause of the pain. These goals frequently are difficult to achieve because the person with PPS may not have the strength in other parts of the body to compensate and carry out an essential function, or the person may be unable or unwilling to make necessary lifestyle changes. Most clients and a family member can benefit from a short course of outpatient therapy to learn how to carry out needed interventions. This could include techniques for inhibiting muscle spasm, stretching fascia and muscles, decreasing edema and increasing nutrition in joint structures, and mobilizing or stabilizing joints.[12] At some point relaxation, meditation, modified tai chi (see Chapter 33), underwater exercise, or body awareness techniques such as Feldenkrais[74] may be helpful.

Although there is no radiological evidence that McConnell taping changes actual alignment of bone, individuals (nonpolio) have experienced a 50% to 78% reduction in patellofemoral pain during activities.[12, 68] In The Institute for Rehabilitation and Research, Houston, Texas (TIRR) Postpolio Clinic these taping techniques relieved anterior knee pain for several months at a time in all persons with PPS who were selected to receive the taping. This relief occurred even though their ability to strengthen surrounding muscles was limited or impossible. The therapy program also should include, as needed, assisting the client in carrying out the home program and lifestyle changes, along with the development of an ongoing program of appropriate exercises.

Other Types of Pain

Many persons who had poliomyelitis underwent extensive orthopedic surgery, and some experience pain or hyper-

sensitivities at these sites. Hypersensitivities can be decreased and even eliminated with desensitization exercises if the client is willing to devote the necessary time. The most frequent sites of pain at old surgical sites are in the trunk from surgery for scoliosis and the ankle near a subtalar arthrodesis, or in the foot with hypermobility of the transverse tarsal joint. In most instances, stabilization of the ankle and foot in a custom-made ankle-foot orthosis (AFO) and use of a rocker-bottom shoe has relieved the pain and permitted weight-bearing and walking.[65] Custom-made corsets and trunk supports in chairs have helped some people control the pain at previous surgical sites in the trunk. A few clients find transcutaneous electrical nerve stimulation helpful and continue to use it to control pain (see Chapters 28 and 29). Most individuals, however, stop using these devices because masking the pain permits them to physically overdo, leading to further injury to their bodies.

Static magnetic fields have become a popular alternative medicine for treatment of athletic injuries as well as persons with PPS who have localized pain. In a double-blind randomized clinical trial, Vallbona applied active (300–500 Gauss) and placebo magnets in a group of 50 subjects with PPS and chronic pain. The magnets were applied to the palpable pain pressure point for 45 minutes. There was a significant ($P < .0001$) and prompt decrease of pain in the group receiving the active magnets compared with those who received the placebo.[89] Some clients say that their pain literally "melts away" with a 30- to 45-minute application of magnets.

Temporary alleviation of chronic pain is not particularly difficult with people who have PPS, but correction of the causes and teaching the client to control and prevent pain are indeed challenges.

Abnormal Fatigue

Abnormal fatigue is reported by almost 90% of the clients with PPS as a new problem (see Table 19–1). This is a profound fatigue that may not seem to be related to a particular activity. The PPS fatigue may not appear at the time of the activity, and recovery does not occur with usual rest periods. In one study, subjects with PPS described their fatigue as increasing loss of strength during exercise, increasing weakness, and heavy sensation of muscles. These were significantly different descriptors than those used by a nonpolio control group.[10]

This fatigue also has been described as a sudden and total wipeout. In a few instances headaches and sweating appear suggestive of autonomic nervous system overload.[80] Often the fatigue occurs at the same time each day, usually in the early afternoon.

This PPS fatigue causes people to decrease activities and permit their world to become smaller. These individuals may develop excuses to avoid participation in social activities, shopping, family outings, and vacations. As the fatigue becomes worse the person is tired all the time and gets up in the morning fatigued and worn out. Many individuals go into a cycle of getting up to go to work, coming home to go to bed, getting up to go to work, and spending weekends in bed.

Abnormal fatigue is treated similarly to muscle pain

and new muscle weakness. In fact, Maxwell titles the entire treatment program for PPS as "learning to manage and control fatigue."[53] The general program may include using nonfatiguing daily activities and energy conservation techniques, breaking activities up into parts with frequent rest periods,[1] and advising daily rest periods including a nap if possible.[95] The client needs help in relaxation or meditation exercises and in gaining permission to rest. Short-term sick leave of 4 to 6 weeks with a major decrease in activity may relieve the fatigue, and work can then be resumed with modifications. If the fatigue shows some improvement, a second period to try to eliminate the fatigue may be a consideration. With uncontrollable fatigue problems, disability retirement is needed. The results of the sick leaves can be used to justify the need for retirement.

Recovery from this type of fatigue takes 3 to 12 months, depending on the severity of the problem and compliance with recommendations. Peach and Olejnik found on reevaluation that fatigue was resolved or improved in the group who complied and was unchanged or increased in the group who did not.[61]

New Muscle Weakness

New muscle weakness occurs in extremities known to have polio involvement and frighteningly in stronger extremities not thought by the client to have been affected. Weakness is primarily noticed in repetitive and stabilizing contractions rather than with single maximum efforts. The problem may be in decreased ability of the muscles to recover rapidly after contracting. Recovery of quadriceps muscle strength after fatiguing exercise was significantly less in symptomatic PPS subjects compared with nonsymptomatic and control subjects.[70] Decreases in strength do not usually show up on the manual muscle test because it is a single-effort maximum contraction. The two grades 5 (normal, "N") and 4 (good, "G") contain all of the resistive force, and the four other grades are nonresistive and mostly nonfunctional; and few examiners are now tested for reliability.[39] In a 1-year follow-up using quantitative muscle force testing no differences were found in muscle strength, work capacity, endurance capacity, or recovery from fatigue of the quadriceps in either nonsymptomatic or symptomatic groups with PPS.[2] Nevertheless, there is at best a slow decline in functional ability, which clients describe as loss of muscle strength.

Other signs relating to new muscle involvement include fasciculations, muscle cramps, atrophy, and elevation of muscle enzymes in the blood. Fasciculations are seen in muscles at rest and during contraction, and they tend to persist even when muscle pain and fatigue have been resolved. Muscle cramps are commonly found in fatigued muscles and are alleviated by decreased activity. New postpolio muscular atrophy of muscles is sometimes reported and is most noticeable when it occurs in the gastrocnemius or the anterior tibialis. Elevation of muscle enzymes, indicative of muscle damage, has been found in people with PPS and has been related to the intensity of work.[60, 90, 91]

Overuse of muscles for their limited capacity has long been associated with these new problems.[9, 60, 64] New weakness and atrophy have been attributed to metabolic overload of the giant motor units, with more pruning of muscle fibers than axon sprouting.[88, 93] Muscle overload occurs from use of muscles at high levels of their capacity for a long period. To perform the same activity with weak muscles, the muscles need to contract at a higher percentage of their capacity than is normally required. For example in walking, clients with PPS contract their muscles at both higher intensities and for prolonged or even continuous periods in the gait cycle.[64] Energy expenditure for the task is increased, and the prolonged contractions keep the capillaries compressed to limit needed muscle nutrition. Postpolio clients are often observed using nearly maximum voluntary contractions to perform a daily activity. Like elite athletes, the muscles of people with PPS cannot continue to maintain these high levels indefinitely.

To determine whether the cause of the new weakness is overuse or possibly disuse, a detailed assessment is required of home, work, recreational, and community activities.[95] If the client is merely asked what his or her activity level is, the answer usually will be something like, "I don't do anything anymore." This response leads the investigator to assume that weakness is from disuse. With specific questioning, one usually finds that the client is doing an extraordinary amount of physical activity. There are few "couch potatoes" in this group. What the client means by not doing anything is relative to the previous higher level of activity. It is important to establish a total picture of the client's activities in sitting, standing, walking, lifting, carrying, climbing stairs, using a telephone or a computer, as well as activities such as cooking, vacuuming, mowing the lawn, playing tennis, singing in a choir, or taking care of grandchildren.

The goal of treatment of overuse weakness is to slow the rate of progression by decreasing the workload on the muscle. This may include lifestyle changes with use of nonfatiguing functional activities, energy conservation techniques, pacing of activities with frequent rest periods, weight control or reduction, orthoses, and motorized assistance.

Generalized weakness from disuse is seen in clients who have had infections, fractures, surgery, and other illness requiring bed rest or immobilization. Treatment requires a modified conditioning program with careful monitoring of response (see the discussion on exercise later in the chapter).

Environmental Cold Intolerance

The involved extremities in people with PPS are frequently abnormally cold. This condition is due to sympathetic nerve cell involvement leading to decreased vasoconstriction and venoconstriction with heat loss to the environment. The impairment may become worse with PPS. Most people have learned to control the heat loss as best as they can with clothing.

Cold intolerance can cause a problem with the use of cold in the treatment of injuries. Most people with PPS do not want to use local cold on any part of the body. They use heating pads and hot water, which feels good at the time but may perpetuate or increase the edema, inflammation, and pain. Local cold is often more effective and is well tolerated by most people with PPS. Successful application of cold requires more client education about the use of cold and demonstration of the effects.

Sleep Disturbances

Over 50% of reporting individuals with PPS have been found to have sleep disturbances.[27] These disturbances may be caused by pain, stress, hypoventilation, or obstructive apnea.[5, 38, 79] The role of the therapist is primarily in the area of pain. A history of pain or numbness that is worse at night or on rising points to sleeping surfaces that are too firm or sleeping with joints in close packed positions (usually the neck and shoulders). These problems are correctable with foam mattress covers or the new air pressure mattresses, cervical pillows, and modification of sleeping postures.

Life-Threatening Conditions

Life-threatening conditions such as hypoventilation, dysphagia, and cardiopulmonary insufficiency require management by medical specialists.[5, 6, 82] These problems occur in people with previous bulbar poliomyelitis who may or may not be using ventilatory assistance and in those with severe kyphosis or scoliosis. The role of the therapist is to modify activities and teach glossopharyngeal breathing, manually assisted coughing, or bronchial drainage as indicated.[17, 23] If trunk supports are considered, vital capacity should be checked with and without an abdominal binder to determine the effect on breathing. The therapist's attention should also be directed toward prevention of problems that may occur from bed rest and maintaining as much function as can be permitted.

Decreasing the Workload of Muscles

Energy Conservation Techniques

Energy conservation techniques provide the easiest way to decrease the work of muscles without loss of function. A therapy program to assist the person in analysis of all activity by type, time, distance, and intensity is valuable. Such an inventory forms the basis for setting priorities and determining where and how individuals wish to use their limited neuromuscular capacity.[95]

Questions to be addressed include the following:

1. Can one trip do for two or three?
2. Can the activity be performed in a less strenuous way, such as by sitting or using a rolling basket?
3. Are there easier ways to perform the activity with modern comforts and technology, including motorization and electronics?
4. Can the activity be broken up into parts with change of activity or rest?
5. Are there other people who can perform some of the physical aspects of the activity?

Weight Reduction

Weight reduction is the single most effective way to decrease the muscle workload, but it is one of the most difficult. Weight loss is slow without exercise, but it can be accomplished. Weight control needs to be incorporated as a permanent modification of nutritional habits rather than achieved in a short-term diet. Dietetic counseling and support groups are important components of this difficult lifestyle modification.

Locomotion

Asymmetrical or abnormal gait patterns, crutch walking, or propelling manual wheelchairs for several decades are frequently the major sources of the pain, weakness, and fatigue in people with PPS. For example, the incidence of pain in a group of 114 patients with confirmed PPS increased from 84% in those who were ambulatory without orthotics to 100% for those who used crutches or wheelchairs for locomotion.[81] The high prevalence of osteoarthritis in patients with PPS was documented in the hand and wrist by radiography.[92] Over twice the number of PPS subjects had osteoarthritis of the wrist or hand than would be expected in a normal population of the same age. The risk factor was significantly increased with lower-extremity muscle paralysis and use of assistive devices.[92] Despite severe difficulties with locomotion, changes or modifications are hard for polio survivors to consider. As locomotion becomes more arduous or painful, many begin to limit outside activities rather than modify individual methods of locomotion. They find more and more reasons to avoid activities at work, with the family, and in the community. Resistance to lifestyle changes is common in the PPS population and leads to needless suffering and functional decline.[61]

Prevention of this spiraling disability and restoration of lost function requires marked decrease in the amount of walking or propelling a chair and a change to methods of locomotion that do not cause pain, weakness, and fatigue. Those who have been walking without assistive devices or with inadequate assistance may need to use a cane, forearm crutches, trunk support, shoe corrections, or new orthoses. Clients who have been walking for years with crutches with or without orthoses develop shoulder, elbow, and wrist injuries, as well as new muscle weakness, muscle pain, and fatigue. They need to use personal mobility vehicles (motorized carts) for distance locomotion or as their primary form of locomotion, with walking reserved for transfers and short distances only. Lightweight manual wheelchairs only perpetuate the problems and create new ones. Those propelling manual wheelchairs develop shoulder, elbow, wrist, and hand injuries. These people need to obtain electric wheelchairs or motorized carts if suitable. Manual wheelchairs at best only postpone problems.

Increased use of motorized vehicles for locomotion should be considered by almost all individuals with PPS to decrease unessential loads on muscles. Some require only occasional use of these vehicles, such as in airports, grocery stores, convention centers, and theme parks. All-terrain vehicles, riding lawn mowers, tractors, and golf carts can be used to permit continuing participation in farm, ranch, seashore, hunting, camping, fishing, and other outdoor activities. Some people need motorized locomotion only at work, home, or in the community, whereas others may use motorization as their primary form of locomotion. To transport the motorized carts and electric wheelchairs, hoists or ramps are required to place the vehicles into and out of autos, trucks, or vans.

The purposes of the changes in methods of locomotion are to increase safety and prevent costly falls, to reduce energy expenditure and decrease fatigue, to prevent further injury and pain, and, most importantly, to increase function and quality of life. Those who do make these difficult changes in their methods of locomotion seem to undergo a metamorphosis from pain and dysfunction to renewed activity and increased function. They enthusiastically state that they wished they had made these changes earlier.

Correction of Posture and Gait Deviations

In addition to sitting in poorly supporting chairs, sofas, auto seats, and wheelchairs, the individual with PPS may have trunk muscle paresis or asymmetries of the pelvic base and may spend up to 16 hours per day in the seated position. The typical posture is slumped hanging on posterior vertebral ligaments with loss of lumbar and cervical curves. Neck, shoulder, and back pain are common. Mechanical restoration of the lumbar curve in all seating at home, during meals, at work, in automobiles, in wheelchairs, at church, in meetings, and at social events can correct the problem if contractures do not limit motion. This can be accomplished by use of properly fitted clerical chairs, ergonometric chairs, anterior tilt seats, gluteal pads, and the many types of lumbar rolls, back supports, and seating systems.

Persons with abdominal muscle paralysis benefit from custom-made thoracolumbar corsets, with the posterior rigid stays bent to produce a normal standing lumbar curve. Paretic or paralyzed neck muscles can be rested and supported by soft foam collars or the more supportive microcellular neck collars. Those with neck muscle weakness should be advised to wear neck supports when driving or riding in automobiles as a protection against injury.

People with severe trunk muscle paralysis or scoliosis with or without spinal fusion often support their trunk or relieve pain by pushing down with their hands or elbows on chairs, tables, and on their hips (Fig. 19–5). In time, such self-traction results in pain and weakness in their arms. Chair inserts and fixed supports as well as custom-made corsets, back braces, and molded body jackets should be considered. The rigid trunk supports, however, take away mobility used for function. Usually such supports can be worn for part of the day in activities where trunk mobility is not essential.

STRETCHING

People with PPS may have limitation of joint motion from muscle contractures and from shortening of ligamentous joint structures. Before even attempting to stretch these contractures the physicians and therapists should carefully evaluate the functions the survivor will lose if a gain in ROM can be achieved. They then should evaluate what functions would be gained and what the cost would be. Fortunately after 20 to 40 years these contractures resist any significant elongation.

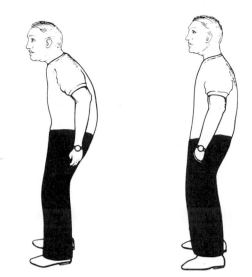

FIGURE 19–5. Polio paralysis of the erector spinae (and abdominal) muscles with inability to sit or stand erect. Erect posture is frequently achieved by causal-appearing activities such as pushing down on the body and chairs.

Sometimes in the convalescent stage of polio selective tightness was allowed to give some stability to joints with paralyzed muscles. In addition, the body in function may develop useful contractures. An excellent example can be seen in people who contracted polio as children. They had muscle involvement primarily in one lower extremity and a decrease in growth of that extremity because of diminished forces. If the survivor has at least a G− (4−) manual muscle test grade in the plantarflexors, the person will walk on the toe (in some plantarflexion) to decrease large drops in the center of gravity and increased energy expenditure for walking. Over the years a plantarflexion contracture develops that can provide up to 3 to 4 inches for weight-bearing on the shortened extremity. With a custom-made shoe the gait is similar to walking in a high-heeled shoe. This can be far more energy efficient than if motion were permitted to have dorsiflexion ROM.

On the other hand, *gentle* myofascial release can be beneficial for recent secondary impairments of muscles to decrease pain and muscle spasms, increase nutrition to the area, and slightly lengthen muscles.

Orthotics

Unlike most rehabilitation clients, people with PPS have strong and usually negative feelings about orthotics. Most individuals long ago discarded their braces and have relied on body compensations for walking (see Fig. 19–3). If an orthosis was essential for walking it has become a part of the body image, and the client does not want any changes. Some have already tried plastic orthoses and found them painful and of no use. Thus, it is difficult to get the person with PPS to consider orthoses or an orthotic change.

To gain the client's respect, the therapist must respect the client's knowledge of how his or her extremities function and give every one specific useful reasons to use the orthoses. Some of these reasons include preventing falls and potential fractures, limiting joint motion and preventing pain, restoring weight-bearing on the weak leg to decrease the work of the strong leg in standing, gaining erect posture and decreasing back pain, and decreasing energy expenditure and fatigue.

In some cases both the upper (talocrural) and the lower (subtalar) ankle joints were fused surgically. To walk, the subject places abnormal forces on the posterior structures of the knee and/or the transverse tarsal joint. In time, hypermobility and pain occur in these areas. Motion for walking can be restored by wearing rocker-bottom shoes. Pain in the transverse tarsal joint can be decreased by stabilizing the ankle and foot in an AFO. Pain at the knee may require a knee-ankle-foot orthosis (KAFO).

AFOs are needed for dorsiflexor weakness resulting in dropfoot or slapfoot, for plantarflexor weakness with absent heel rise, and for mediolateral instability. The reason that people with PPS have so much difficulty with plastic AFOs is that they are usually made in 5 to 10 degrees of dorsiflexion and are then placed in a shoe with a slight positive heel, increasing the angle of the posterior shell to the floor. In standing and walking this causes a knee flexion torque, with buckling of the knee if the quadriceps muscle is weak. Pain occurs because the client tries to straighten the knee by pushing back against the posterior shell of the AFO. If this is the problem, AFOs should be made in slight plantarflexion so that the tibia is perpendicular to the floor in the shoes the client is going to wear. This is the normal position of the ankle for toe and heel clearance.[59] In case of a plantarflexion contracture, more plantarflexion is required in the AFO. Most jointed AFOs are of limited value because they are heavier and bulkier, require a larger shoe than those with metal joints, and do not control the ankle. The advantage of jointed AFOs is their ability to adjust to find the best angle in function.

The floor reaction AFO prohibits all ankle motion and can place forces to control the knee.[48, 75, 94] The orthosis prevents dropfoot, promotes heel rise, provides an extension torque on the proximal tibia to supplement weak quadriceps muscles, and can limit hyperextension of the knee. This orthosis requires precision in fabrication to have the knee extension torque occur only when the tibia is perpendicular to the floor in the gait cycle. When this orthosis is used with rocker-bottom shoes to give back motion, a person with a flail foot can walk with a normal gait pattern. Subjects with ligamentous laxity of the knee, excessive tibial torsion, or paralysis of the quadriceps muscles are poor candidates for this type of AFO.

Heel lifts, shoe inserts, molded foot orthoses, and some normal footwear can provide a number of unobtrusive corrections. Positive heel shoes with a broad base, such as cowboy boots, stacked or Cuban heels, or the Swedish clog,[65] decrease the amount of dorsiflexion and plantarflexion motion and work needed in the gait cycle. Rocker-bottom soles provide mechanical heel rise to assist the calf muscles and are available commercially or can be added to shoes. Work boots, dress boots, or basketball shoes may provide needed ankle stability.

People with unilateral lower-extremity paralysis or pain stand with weight on the stronger limb, which must perform continuous, high-level isometric contractions (Fig. 19-6). Unloading the stronger leg requires restoration of

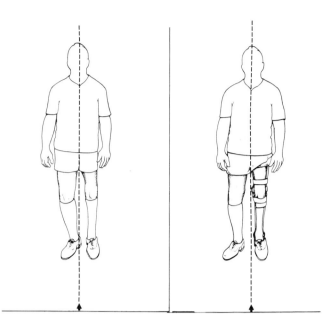

FIGURE 19–6. This man has paralysis of the left lower extremity with severe fatigue, low-back pain, pain and weakness in the right lower extremity, and decreased function. He can be seen to bear weight and stand on the right leg. Application of a left knee-ankle-foot orthosis with a free knee joint (with a drop lock for use in prolonged standing and walking on rough terrain) and a limited-motion ankle joint unloaded his right leg and permitted him to walk in an erect posture. His pain disappeared and he has regained function at work and in social activities.

weight-bearing on the more involved leg using a KAFO or, in some instances, an AFO that prevents advance of the tibia in the stance phase.[48, 75, 81, 94]

Fifty percent of ambulatory individuals with PPS walk with an obvious forward-leaning posture. This posture requires continuous contraction of the erector spinae muscles and leads to back pain, often radiating to the hip and leg. The forward-leaning posture is found in people with quadriceps muscle paresis and in those with ankle weakness. Those with quadriceps weakness must move the center of gravity of the body anterior to the knee axis to lock the knee and prevent knee flexion in stance. This posterior force also produces ligamentous instability and genu recurvatum (see Fig. 19–3). In some instances lightweight athletic knee braces allowing 10 to 15 degrees of hyperextension provide adequate control. More often a KAFO with an offset knee joint allowing necessary hyperextension is required.[14, 63, 66] People with dorsiflexor muscle paralysis or ankle instabilities walk in the forward-leaning posture to watch the floor and foot placement to avoid tripping and falling. Athletic ankle supports or boots may be sufficient to control some ankle instabilities. Molded and posted plastic AFOs with or without ankle joints are needed for more control. Flexible plastic AFOs and the dynamic spring dorsiflexion assists can correct simple dropfoot.[81] Once the need to walk in a forward-leaning posture is removed, the person can walk upright; and back pain may disappear in a few days.

Walking with lateral trunk shift in the stance phase (gluteus medius gait) produces abnormal forces and joint dysfunction from the spine to the foot (Fig. 19–7). These forces can be reduced by use of a forearm crutch or cane.

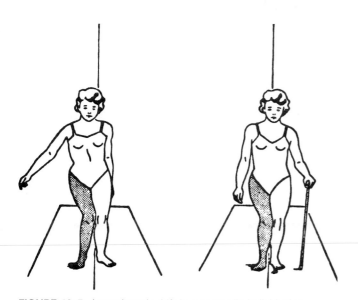

FIGURE 19–7. Lateral trunk shift in a postpolio individual to illustrate abnormal forces occurring in the back, knee, and ankle with resulting joint dysfunction and pain. Prevention of these abnormal forces and some correction can be provided by use of a cane or forearm crutch. (Adapted from Ducroquet R, et al: Walking and Limping—a Study of Normal and Pathological Walking. Philadelphia, JB Lippincott, 1968.)

People who are long-term crutch walkers with or without orthoses and those whose walking is slow, precarious, or labored should be guided to consider use of motorized vehicles as their primary form of locomotion. Orthotic corrections or applications may be indicated to improve transfers and short-distance walking.

Exercise

With the onset of new problems of weakness and fatigue, most people with PPS have been directed or are self-directed to engage in strengthening, aerobic, or sports exercise programs. Instead of correcting problems, these activities produce an increase in fatigue, muscle weakness, and pain.[4, 60] Exercise may cause increased problems because it is applied to motor units that are working at high levels of capacity and that may be in a state of decompensation. The initial objective of interventions is to reduce the load on the muscles, eliminate the pain and fatigue, and build a reserve capacity. Most clients with PPS are willing to stop exercise as part of lifestyle changes, at least on a trial basis. Later exercise can be evaluated for purpose, magnitude of energy expenditure relative to total energy expenditure, and the risk/benefit ratio to present and future muscle performance.

Exercises for stretching fascia and muscles, mobilizing joints, reeducating muscles to stabilize joints in activity, increasing joint nutrition, and decreasing edema are frequently used for the treatment of pain and injuries. For clients with PPS these exercises can be used safely with modification and careful monitoring. A beginning rule of thumb is for the therapist to estimate the intensity that the subject can tolerate and then apply one half, reduce the estimated repetitions to one half, and double the time of estimated rest periods. If fatigue does not last longer than 30 minutes or appear in the next 2 days and if pain does not increase, the program can be continued and gradually increased. Increased fatigue or pain is an indication for reevaluation of the exercise (and any other activities that the person may have engaged in) with consideration of decreasing the amount of exercise or activity.

The same modifications can be used in reconditioning exercises. Weakness of disuse may occur with fractures, illness, or surgery. If a pre-illness manual muscle test is not available, it is important to re-create with the client a gross picture of pre-illness muscle function. Individuals with PPS can relate what and to what extent they could move previously if the right questions are asked. It is important to obtain this information to avoid extensive efforts to try to strengthen muscles that are below functional strength and to identify new peripheral nerve lesions that may have occurred.

Many clients with PPS have excessive muscle tension (especially around the head and neck) and an inability to relax or to maximize rest periods. Initially, they may need treatment to alleviate pain, regain motion, and develop a home exercise program. Ongoing valuable exercise programs are critical but must be low-impact and low-energy activities.

Many recreational and sporting activities have important family and social purposes. These activities should be evaluated with the client for possible modifications that would reduce strenuous aspects but retain the client's ability to participate in the activity. Motorized carts, all-terrain vehicles, golf carts, snowmobiles, or trucks permit continued participation in outdoor activities such as camping, birding, fishing, playing golf, winter recreation, scouting, or coaching youth activities. Horseback riding can be continued if mounting and dismounting platforms are available. Those who enjoy the water should avoid competitive lap swimming but can participate in easy recreational and family fun activities. A few golfers are able to continue their sport in a modified manner, using a golf cart, longer clubs, and graphite shafts and by learning to swing the club using momentum rather than brute force. One mother hired a teenager to pick up toys, push swings, serve refreshments, and take children to the bathroom on the days when neighborhood friends came to play. This approach allowed the mother to be sedentary but interact with the children.

Individuals with PPS are exercise oriented from their early association of exercise and muscle strength recovery. Most of them again request exercises to make their muscles stronger, to lose weight, and to improve cardiorespiratory fitness. Unfortunately for the person with PPS, these types of strenuous, long-duration exercises are generally contraindicated. Exercise should be evaluated by the therapist in relation to the client's total activity and the risk/benefit ratio. Those who have asymptomatic PPS (and are in good health) should respond well to appropriate exercise programs. True gains in muscle strength will be limited because most people with PPS long ago achieved their maximum strength limits. Clients should know the signs of PPS and should exercise in moderation. Those who have PPS with muscle pain and fatigue are already getting too much exercise in their daily activities. These people need to further modify their lifestyles and avoid placing additional loads on decompensated muscles. When the muscle pain and fatigue are eliminated and a reserve capacity has been developed, additional activities and exercise can be considered. Most people will opt to increase nonfatiguing functional activities or social recreation rather than exercise in and of itself.

The General Guidelines for Activity and Exercise (see the following box) is read with the patient and family members. They also receive written recommendations specific to them, information on support groups, and two to three articles on PPS. "The patient's capacity to do work must always continue to exceed the demands placed upon him."[83]

POSTPOLIOMYELITIS

General Guidelines for Physical Activity and Exercise

■ Obtain a complete medical examination. The symptoms of the late effect of polio are similar and may be combined with the symptoms of other conditions. Self-diagnosis is dangerous.

■ Preserve and protect your limited muscle and joint capacities. Postpolio problems are caused by long-term overuse at high levels of capacity.

■ Control and reduce body weight by permanent modification of nutritional habits without use of exercise.

■ Make a detailed diary of your activities in type, time, and amount over days and averaged for a week or months. Analyze, set priorities, and use methods to conserve energy.

■ Maintain function by doing things the easy way. Take advantage of modern comforts and technology including motorization and electronics.

■ Correct injury producing abnormal postures in sleeping, SITTING, standing, and working using mechanical supports and assists.

■ Break up activities into parts with rest periods or change of activity. Incorporate frequent rest periods or a nap as needed.

■ Learn techniques of relaxation or imagery to maximize rest periods.

■ Avoid unessential physical activity such as walking, bicycling, or swimming laps and aerobic, "toning," body-building, or strengthening exercises.

■ Preserve muscle capacity for important function, work, family, and social activities.

■ LISTEN TO YOUR BODY! Build a reserve capacity and avoid facing every posture and activity with exhaustion or pain in muscles or joints.

Reprinted with permission of The Institute for Rehabilitation and Research Postpolio Clinic, Houston, TX.

A few exercise studies using quantitative measurements have been done with subjects with PPS. Aerobic testing using modified protocols to reduce fatigue has been used on the treadmill,[20] bicycle ergometer,[40] and arm ergometer.[44] There were no cardiorespiratory training effects in the first study, probably owing to the low intensity of the exercise, but the duration and distance of walking increased.[21] The two ergometry studies showed an increase in maximum oxygen consumption of 15% and 19%, which is a training effect comparable to normal values for age. There were, however, no changes in blood pressure or heart rate, particularly the expected decrease in resting heart rate that occurs with aerobic training. Although the intensity of the exercise protocols had to be reduced for some of the subjects, none had to terminate the exercise because of overuse symptoms, nor did these symptoms occur at the end of the studies. A problem in evaluating these studies is that it is not always clear whether the postpolio study subjects were asymptomatic, symptomatic (PPS), or mixed.

Isokinetic and isometric dynamometers have been used to record maximum muscle forces (or torques) in PPS subjects before and after resistive exercise programs designed to increase muscle strength. Two of the studies were of single cases,[31, 56] and two had 12 and 17 subjects.[22, 26] Both of the multisubject studies tested the quadriceps femoris. Einarsson and Grimby[22] reported an average gain of 29% in isometric strength and 24% in isokinetic strength over a period of 6 weeks. The same type of muscle contractions, however, were used for testing and training. Fillyaw and others[26] reported a strength gain of 8% over a 2-year period. An isometric contraction was used for testing, and concentric-eccentric contractions were used for the exercise. These results do not compare with the strength gains of 100% and higher made by normal subjects undergoing training but rather compare with serial testing when no exercise is done.[57, 58] For example, Munin and associates[57] measured the affected and nonaffected quadriceps muscle every 6 months over 3 years to document muscle weakness in persons with PPS. They reported increases in muscle strength up to 25%. In older persons without polio, test performance gains of the quadriceps increased an average of 174% in 90-year-old subjects[25] and 107% in 60- to 72-year-old men.[29] In these two studies, thigh muscle area (as documented by computed tomography) increased by 9% and 11%, respectively, indicating an increase in muscle bulk.

Because there are neural adaptations specific to the type of muscle contraction used for measurement and training, it is difficult to determine the differences in true increases in strength from the ability to increase a specific test performance. Another term for this phenomenon or increase in performance is motor learning (see Chapter 4). The theory states that the subject learns to perform the measurement or the exercise better without true gains in strength. This happens even with an apparently simple weekly maximum isometric contraction.[74] Evidence of this phenomenon can be seen when improvements are made in the opposite untrained muscle group (transfer of training), when the apparent strength gains are maintained for months after cessation of the training, and when there are no increases in the size of the muscle. The greatest increases in test performance occur when the muscle contraction is the same for both the test and the training. Smaller increases are seen when the measurement and training muscle contractions are different and when measures to decrease the effect of motor learning have been used.

The neural adaptation specific to the type of measurement or training is illustrated in the following study on older men.[29] Multiple tests to assess strength were performed. The training program required lifting and lowering 80% of the weight of one repetition maximum (1 RM), which was assessed weekly. After 12 weeks, there were average increases in quadriceps muscle strength of 104% for the 1 RM, 7% for maximum isometric, 8% for maximum isokinetic at 60 degrees per second, and 10% for isokinetic at 240 degrees per second. In addition, there was an increase in cross-sectional area of the quadriceps of 10% and muscle biopsy showed approximately 30% increase in muscle fiber size.[30] This study illustrates some of the complexities in designing or evaluating studies that attempt to measure changes in muscle strength.

PSYCHOSOCIAL CONSIDERATIONS

The psychosocial issues confronting persons with PPS often are more disruptive than the physical problems.[28, 36, 42, 45, 46, 87] To better understand this condition it is helpful to know about the background of those with PPS and a few of the myths that helped to shape their lives.

During the polio epidemics of the 1940s and 1950s, fear of the disease was rampant. Parents kept children out of public swimming pools in the summer, away from movies, and from congregating in groups. If children did get polio, many parents suffered feelings of guilt, which often were expressed later by encouraging the child to high levels of physical achievement. Approval and perks were gained by activities such as walking farther or faster and keeping up with or exceeding the performance of siblings and friends. The best treatment available was provided to all polio victims by the March of Dimes. To receive this treatment, polio patients were hospitalized for months at a time away from their families, friends, and communities. Many of the patients were children who felt abandoned, afraid, and totally dependent on strangers for their care and nurturing. The polio patient was expected to be a "good patient" and to "work hard." Indeed, they did work hard to reeducate weakened muscles and compensate for lost function.[13, 16, 32, 76] Later in the recovery process, parents made the decisions for children to undergo multiple surgical procedures so that the heavy braces could be eliminated and the children would look "normal and fit in." One can understand why clients react so negatively to the suggestion of orthotics.

One of the myths that flourished in the polio years was "don't wallow in self-pity." Courage, determination, and cheerfulness were attributes to be prized. The myth gained strength when polio patients' levels of disability were compared—"Look at him. He can't move. You should be grateful. It could be much worse!" The children were often shamed into silence and learned not to express feelings about their disability.

Coping Styles

Those with PPS developed several styles to cope with their disability. Maynard and Roller[55] described coping styles according to severity of muscular involvement. Those with little or no obvious physical involvement were able to hide atrophy with clothing, and they avoided activities that revealed the weakness. Many invested much energy in projecting normality to others and were so adept at denial that they disconnected themselves from the polio experience. Often spouses do not know of the history of polio. This group can develop the most severe cases of PPS. They do not identify with others with PPS and they are difficult to help. Those with obvious physical involvement such as a limp, an atrophied extremity, or use of an assistive device, usually have pushed themselves to function at a normal or supernormal level. Physical imperfections have been ignored by tuning out pain and discomfort brought about by their high levels of activity. They suffer tremendous pain before they will acknowledge the late effects of polio. The third group are the most severely impaired of the PPS groups. They usually require wheelchairs for mobility, and many have respiratory involvement. Attaining independence in self-care activities required great effort and persistence. This group integrated their disability into their self-image and have led active, productive lives. They are often involved in disabled rights and independent living movements.

The majority of polio survivors were adept at disguising their impairments and achieved high levels of productivity, enabling them to disappear into society.[87] The rate at which these individuals have been educated, employed, and married indicates their success at living "normal" lives. However, they have pushed themselves and lived with internal and external stresses similar to those persons with type A behavior.[13] Many polio survivors may have compensated for underlying low self-esteem and fear of losing control of their lives by exhibiting this excessive drive.

Response to New Diagnosis

When the client with PPS seeks help for new problems, the encounters with the medical community can be frustrating. Most health care professionals are unfamiliar with the late effects of polio and, as a consequence, the procedure for arriving at a diagnosis of PPS can take time and involve a series of physician consultations.[7, 13, 16, 37] Publicity by support groups has helped refer clients to PPS clinics or to specialists who have knowledge of PPS.[67]

The response to the diagnosis of PPS can vary from relief to despair. Relief occurs in those who have been searching for a diagnosis and those who have been told their symptoms were psychosomatic. Despair occurs as the treatment program of lifestyle changes is described. Most of the clients are distressed when diagnosed with PPS and are resistant to making changes in their lives. They have worked hard to accomplish their goals and are at the peak of their careers. They distrust the medical community because they are presented with management suggestions that are opposed to the ones they followed to recovery decades ago. They are being told that "use it or lose it" and "no pain, no gain" does not apply to them. Clients wonder whether the shift in philosophy is valid. They are disillusioned because their former medical heroes/heroines did not foresee their future problems.

The individual's feeling of pride and accomplishment about the initial recovery is often diminished, and he or she experiences a feeling of failure. These individuals fear the future for themselves and their loved ones. Some will not be able to hide physical problems and will have to admit their disability. They are anxious about the prospects of changing roles with their families, friends, and co-workers.[7, 16, 55] Many PPS clients experience the reemergence of repressed feelings. It is as if they are reliving the initial illness. The defenses and coping strategies they used successfully for so many years have broken down, and they experience overwhelming anxieties and conflicts.[7]

Most people who had polio never grieved their physical losses. They were sick for 2 weeks, and the following months and years were focused on muscle strength gains and improvements in function. There was no time for sadness and mourning necessary for emotional healing. To gain acceptance of their changing situation, these people need to grieve their physical losses both old and new.[7, 8, 37, 47, 49] Tate and colleagues[84] reported an association of feelings of depression with severity of physical symptoms in individuals with PPS who lacked appropriate coping behaviors. Some clients suffer from clinical depression and need treatment. Most clients could benefit from individual, group, or family psychotherapy during this period of emotional turmoil.

Compliance

A few clients readily accept suggestions for lifestyle changes and start making these changes immediately; a few clients refuse to consider any lifestyle modifications. Most clients, however, make needed changes but require support, patience, and time for processing and decision making.

Physical and occupational therapists can help clients in many ways to function while living with purpose and quality of life. First, it is important to respect their knowledge of their body and how it functions. Many of these people still remember the anatomical names of their muscles. They have developed their own unique methods of handling, transferring, walking, and performing activities. Attempts to "correct" their performance or do it another way can be disastrous and have resulted in unnecessary fractures. It is extremely important to follow each client's directions for transfers and other functional activities. Another important help is to allow clients to vent feelings about the new challenges, their past high levels of physical achievement, and their previous treatment.

Compliance of the client with PPS is markedly improved by the therapist's ability to provoke or alleviate pain in the initial evaluation and to suggest management strategies that are accepted as normal. Use of cold packs and lumbar pillows to relieve pain during the initial visit can markedly promote compliance. Recommendations for cervical pillows, ergonometric chairs, computer wristrests, or air pressure beds help pave the way for more emotionally charged suggestions such as orthoses, decreasing ambulation, or motorized carts. Therapists can be a source of information about PPS support groups.[67] People in these groups have faced their losses, and many have adopted new coping skills. The support groups eagerly share knowledge about every facet of living with PPS, and many of the members can be positive role models for the newly diagnosed individual.

Therapists can make recommendations in a way that helps clients view compliance as life enhancing and empowering and not as capitulation and failure. Polio survivors should be reassured that the resilience and ingenuity that helped them live successfully for so many decades will also enable them to face this new challenge.

CASE STUDIES

People with PPS usually have multiple problems and require multiple modifications and lifestyle changes to relieve or eliminate the fatigue, pain, and rate of progression of muscle weakness. Case histories are long and complex. To reduce the complexity, single problems and their solutions are presented. Remember that each one of these people is also working on other lifestyle changes and, in most cases, a program to manage their fatigue and perhaps another impairment.

CONCLUSION

The understanding of polio and acute treatment of this disease and of PPS and its management is still evolving. The therapist needs to update his or her understanding to provide the best treatment solutions for each individual.

CASE 19–1   J.R., W.N., M.B., J.S., J.W., P.N., M.M., A.B.

J.R. is a 53-year-old man who has chief complaints of pain and weakness in his previously strong right leg and low back pain. His disabilities include difficulty in meeting his work demands as an engineer and in playing golf. His primary functional limitation includes an inefficient gait and standing pattern, in that he avoided weight-bearing on his weak left leg (see Fig. 19–6). The muscles in the right leg were noted to be in a constant state of contraction. His impairments include severe weakness of the left leg (0/5 to 2/5) and new muscle weakness (4 to 4+/5) in what he considered a

(Continued)

CASE 19–1 J.R., W.N., M.B., J.S., J.W., P.N., M.M., A.B. *Continued*

"normal" right leg. He was also overweight. He was able to lose 20 pounds and accepted a left KAFO, subsequently reporting that all of his pain was eliminated.

W.N. is a 60-year-old woman who is having pain and weakness in her left hand and back pain that prevents her from sleeping through the night. She has been employed full time as a department head in a hospital for 30 years. She has almost total-body paralysis and is ventilatory dependent. She is able to use a motorized wheelchair, electronic feeder, computer, and telephone with a few muscles (3/5 or less) in her left hand. Functional evaluation showed that she used her hand muscles extensively for gestures as she talked. She was advised to avoid contracting these muscles except when needed for the essential tasks just listed. She did so, and the hand symptoms disappeared. Once positioned into bed, she is unable to make even small postural adjustments to increase her comfort. She purchased a mattress pad with magnets and reports that she has been able to sleep through the night for the first time in more than 15 years.

M.B. is a 48-year-old woman who has a primary complaint of low back pain that worsens when she walks. Her disabilities include difficulty in performing her job duties as a second-grade teacher and in going shopping. Her primary functional limitation is a bilateral dropfoot gait; she also displayed a forward lean to watch the floor. Her impairments were generalized weakness (2/5 to 4/5) in both of her legs. AFOs were recommended. With these she was able to walk in an erect position, and her back pain was eliminated.

J.S. is a 45-year-old man who is complaining of worsening bilateral shoulder pain. His disabilities include decreased ability to work as a teacher, to sleep, and to go on outings with his family. He has walked with bilateral long-leg braces and crutches for more than 30 years using a swing-through pattern; his shoulder pain limits this function. His impairments include paraplegia (0/5 to 1/5 throughout his legs), bicipital tendinitis, and painful arcs with shoulder flexion. He was advised to use a motorized scooter as his primary form of locomotion. He continued to walk with braces and crutches, and his physician recommended physical therapy for treatment of shoulder pain. His shoulder pain increased. When seen in a postpolio clinic, he again was advised to use a motorized scooter and to obtain a van with a lift to place him and the scooter into the van. He was advised to apply to agencies for financial help to supplement his resources for needed equipment. Physical therapy treatment was recommended to relieve and control shoulder pain. He followed these recommendations with total relief of pain. He is now independent in his community and particularly enjoys going to malls, theme parks, and sporting events with his family. He regrets that he did not accept motorized locomotion sooner.

J.W. is a 40-year-old single mother of two children. Her primary complaint was that of pain in the back of her pelvis. Her disabilities include her inability to perform her duties of mother and secretary because of increased pain with prolonged sitting, standing, or walking. Her functional limitations include a marked lateral trunk shift (gluteus medius gait) on right stance phase and dropfoot in right swing phase. She moves constantly from one position to another because of pain. Impairments include acute pain in the hips, radiating posteriorly to the knee and more severe on the right. The sacroiliac joints were painful to palpation. Compression of the ilia relieved the pain. She was advised to have outpatient therapy for treatment of sacroileitis, but because of financial, time, and transportation limitations, she requested alternatives. She was advised to obtain a sacroiliac belt, cane for use in the left hand, cold packs to apply to her sacroiliac joints six to eight times a day, and a right AFO. She was advised to correct her sitting posture with a lumbar support and a well-fitted clerical chair with armrests. She was taught how to stretch her piriformis muscles and to take nonsteroidal antiinflammatory medication. This regimen was quite rigorous to undertake without assistance, but she was able to comply with all the recommendations, and her pain was virtually eliminated. Perhaps the most important aspect of the program is that she gained control of the pain, and it has now become insignificant.

P.N. is a 46-year-old woman who works 40 to 50 hours a week as a nurse in an outpatient clinic; she has an additional 1-hour commute to work each way. She has a husband and two young children. Her disabilities include an inability to continue leisure and social activities with her family and friends. Her functional limitations include painful and inefficient gait and diffuse pain and fatigue throughout her body. Her impairments include severe weakness (3+ to 4/5) in her right lower extremity; limited but present passive ROM in right ankle dorsiflexion and plantarflexion because of an old joint fusion as a child, and severe pain in that ankle during terminal stance. She accepted an AFO designed to block the dorsiflexion that occurs in terminal stance and allow plantarflexion for weight acceptance in gait. She continues to have difficulty with her diffuse pain and fatigue. She hired a housekeeper, but she has been unable to make other domestic or work changes. She reports that her residual pain and fatigue are bearable now that her right ankle does not bother her.

(Continued)

CASE 19–1   J.R., W.N., M.B., J.S., J.W., P.N., M.M., A.B. *Continued*

M.M. is a 73-year-old woman with a history of falls and increasing diffuse aches. Her disabilities include not being able to leave her home more often than a trip to church and one to her hairdresser each week. Her functional limitations include a very steady and guarded gait with short step length bilaterally and wide base of support and diffuse muscle aches and fatigue throughout. Her impairments include generalized weakness throughout, with her right lower extremity weaker (2/5 to 4/5) than the left (3/5 to 4/5), her right lower extremity shorter than the left, muscle cramping in her left calf, low back and sacroiliac pain, numbness and tingling in both hands, and diffuse muscle aches and fatigue. She was reluctant to accept recommendations for bathroom equipment, a rolling walker, and a motorized scooter. She called requesting a scooter prescription after having fallen and broken her arm in her bathroom 2 weeks after her PPS clinic visit. She reported her confidence and balance had worsened since her fall and hospitalization. She had been chair- or bed-bound until she received her scooter.

A.B. is a 69-year-old woman with a history of increased difficulty with walking and severe pain in her knees and left shoulder. Disabilities included inability to leave her home other than once a week to church and once for volunteer activities at a nursing home. Her functional limitations were slowed gait with severe deviations, using a Lofstrand crutch in the right hand, frequent falling, and difficulty in rising from low surfaces. Her impair-

ments include severe bilateral lower-extremity weakness (quadriceps 0/5 on the right and 1/5 on the left); severe knee hyperextension during stance phase during gait bilaterally; bilateral upper-extremity weakness and limitations of passive ROM left more so than the right); and pain in both knees and left shoulder. She has used a scooter within her home part time for the past 7 years, but she has never taken it into the community because she does not have a lift for her automobile. She has not used any equipment to ease the energy requirements for bathing. Magnets were applied medial, proximal, and lateral to each patella, and her pain was reduced by two thirds within 30 minutes using the visual analog scale. Magnets, tub transfer bench, grab bar, hand-held shower head, and a scooter lift were prescribed for her. The recommendation was made for her to walk as little as possible and to use the scooter full time. Her son and husband questioned this recommendation with concerns of her becoming progressively weaker with less physical activity. Her falls and severe knee hyperextension with pain were emphasized to her family with the concern of trying to preserve what function she has left, decrease her pain, and improve her ability to continue to participate in the activities she enjoys. Two weeks after her clinic visit, she reported continued decrease in her knee pain with single use of the magnets within the clinic and a change in her daily activities.

ACKNOWLEDGMENT

The authors wish to acknowledge the contribution of Marsha G. Marbry to the writing of the version of this chapter in the previous edition.

REFERENCES

1. Agre JC, Rodriquez AA: Neuromuscular function in polio survivors. Orthopedics 14:1343–1347, 1991.
2. Agre JC, Rodriquez AA: Neuromuscular function in polio survivors at one-year follow-up. Arch Phys Med Rehabil 72:7–10, 1991.
3. Agre JC, Rodriquez AA: Intermittent isometric activity: Its effect on muscle fatigue in postpolio subjects. Arch Phys Med Rehabil 72:971–975, 1991.
4. Agre JC, Rodriquez AA, Tafel JA: Late effects of polio: Critical review of the literature on neuromuscular function. Arch Phys Med Rehabil 72:923–931, 1991.
5. Bach J, et al: Mouth intermittent positive-pressure ventilation in the management of postpolio respiratory insufficiency. Chest 91:859, 1987.
6. Bach JR, Alba AS: Pulmonary dysfunction and sleep disordered breathing as post-polio sequelae: Evaluation and management. Orthopedics 14:1329–1337, 1991.
7. Backman ME: The post polio patient: Psychological issues. J Rehabil 53(4):23–26, 1987.
8. Beisser A: Flying Without Wings. New York, Bantam, 1990.
9. Bennett RL, Knowlton GC: Overwork weakness in partially denervated skeletal muscle. Clin Orthop 12:22, 1958.
10. Berlly MH, Strauser WW, Hall KM: Fatigue in postpolio syndrome. Arch Phys Med Rehabil 72:115–118, 1991.
11. Bodian D: The virus, the nerve cell, and paralysis. Bull Johns Hopkins Hosp 83:1, 1948.
12. Bockrath K, Wooden C, Ingersoll CD: Effects of patella taping on patella position and perceived pain. Med Sci Sports Exerc 25:989–992, 1993.
13. Bruno RL, Frick NM: The psychology of polio as prelude to post polio syndrome: Behavior modification and psychotherapy. Orthopedics 14:1185–1193, 1991.
14. Clark D, Perry J, Lunsford T: Case studies—orthotic management of the adult post polio patient. Orthop Prosthet 40:43, 1986.
15. Cohn V: Four Billion Dimes. Minneapolis, MN, Minneapolis Star and Tribune, 1955.
16. Conrady L, et al: Psychological characteristics of polio survivors: A preliminary report. Arch Phys Med Rehabil 170:458–463, 1989.
17. Dail C: Clinical aspects of glossopharyngeal breathing: Report of its use by 100 post-polio patients. JAMA 158:445, 1955.
18. Dalakas MC, et al: Late effects of poliomyelitis muscular atrophy: Clinical, virologic and immunologic studies. Rev Infect Dis 6(Suppl):S562, 1984.
19. Dalakas MC, et al: A long-term follow-up study of patients with post-poliomyelitis neuromuscular symptoms. N Engl J Med 314:959, 1986.
20. Dean E, Ross J: Effect of modified aerobic training on movement energetics in polio survivors. Orthopedics 14:1243–1246, 1991.
21. Ducroquet R, Ducroquet J, Ducroquet P: Walking and Limping—a Study of Normal and Pathological Walking. Philadelphia, JB Lippincott, 1968.
22. Einarsson G, Grimby G: Strengthening exercise program in postpo-

lio subjects. *In* Halstead L, Wiechers D (eds): Research and Clinical Aspects of the Late Effects of Poliomyelitis. White Plains, NY, March of Dimes Birth Defects Series 23(4), 1987.

23. Fergelson C: Glossopharyngeal breathing as an aid to the coughing mechanism in patients with chronic poliomyelitis in a respirator. N Engl J Med 254:611, 1956.
24. Fetell MR, et al: A benign motor neuron disorder: Delayed cramps and fasciculations after poliomyelitis or myelitis. Ann Neurol 11:423, 1982.
25. Fiatarone MA, et al: High-intensity strength training in nonagenarians. JAMA 263:3029–3034, 1990.
26. Fillyaw MJ, et al: The effects of long-term nonfatiguing resistance exercise in subjects with post-polio syndrome. Orthopedics 14:1253–1256, 1991.
27. Fisher A: Sleep-disordered breathing as a late effect of poliomyelitis. *In* Halstead L, Wiechers D (eds): Research and Clinical Aspects of the Late Effects of Poliomyelitis. White Plains, NY, March of Dimes Birth Defects Series 23(4), 1987.
28. Frick N: Post-polio sequelae and the psychology of second disability. Orthopedics 8:851, 1985.
29. Frontera WR, et al: Strength conditioning in older men: Skeletal muscle hypertrophy and improved function. J Appl Physiol 64:1038–1044, 1988.
30. Gazette International Networking Institute/International Polio Network, 4207 Lindell Blvd. #10, St. Louis, MO 63118; (314) 534-0475; www.post-polio.org.
31. Gross MT, Schuch CP: Exercise programs for patients with post-polio syndrome: A case report. Phys Ther 69:72–76, 1989.
32. Halstead L: The residual of polio in the aged. Top Geriatr Rehabil 3(4):9–26, 1988.
33. Halstead L: Assessment and differential diagnosis for post-polio syndrome. Orthopedics 14:1209–1217, 1991.
34. Halstead L, Naierman N (eds): Managing Post-polio: A Guide to Living Well with Post-polio Syndrome. Washington, DC, NRH Press, 1998.
35. Halstead L, Wiechers D (eds): Late Effects of Poliomyelitis. Miami, Symposia Foundation, 1985.
36. Halstead L, Wiechers D (eds): Research and Clinical Aspects of the Late Effects of Poliomyelitis. White Plains, NY, March of Dimes Birth Defects Series 23(4), 1987.
37. Hanson B: Picking up the Pieces: Healing Ourselves after Personal Loss. Dallas, Taylor, 1990.
38. Hill R, et al: Sleep Apnea Syndrome After Poliomyelitis. Am Rev Respir Dis 127:129, 1983.
39. Iddings DM, Smith LK, Spencer WA: Muscle testing: II. Reliability in clinical use. Phys Ther Rev 41:249–256, 1961.
40. Jones DR, et al: Cardiorespiratory responses to aerobic training by patients with postpoliomyelitis sequelae. JAMA 261:3255–3259, 1989.
41. Jubelt B, Cashman N: Neurological manifestation of the post-polio syndrome. Crit Rev Neurobiol 3:199, 1987.
42. Kaufert J, Kaufert PA: Aging and respiratory polio. Rehabil Digest 13:15, 1982.
43. Kendall H, Kendall F: Orthopedic and physical therapy objectives in poliomyelitis treatment. Physiother Rev 27:2, 1947.
44. Kriz JL, et al: Cardiorespiratory responses to upper extremity aerobic training by postpolio subjects. Arch Phys Med Rehabil 73:49–54, 1992.
45. Laurie G, Raymond J (eds): Proceedings of Rehabilitation Gazette's Second International Post-Polio Conference and Symposium on Living Independently with a Severe Disability. St. Louis, Gazette International Networking Institute, 1984.
46. Laurie G, Raymond J (eds): Proceedings of Gazette International Networking Institute's Third Internation Polio and Independent Living Conference. St. Louis, Gazette International Networking Institute, 1986.
47. Leech P, Singer Z: Acknowledgement: Opening to Grief of Unacceptable Loss. Taytonville, CA, Wintercreek Publications, 1988.
48. Lehmann J, et al: Ankle-foot orthoses: Effect on abnormalities in tibial nerve paralysis. Arch Phys Med Rehabil 66:212, 1985.
49. LeMaistre J: Beyond rage: The Emotional Impact of Chronic Physical Illness. Oak Park, IL, Alpine Guild, 1985.
50. McComas A, Upton A, Sica R: Motor neuron disease and aging. Lancet 2:1474, 1973.
51. Martinez A, Ferrer M, Conde M: Electrophysiological features in

patients with non-progressive and late progressive weakness after paralytic poliomyelitis: Conventional EMG automatic analysis of the electromyogram and single fiber electromyography study. Electromyogr Clin Neurophysiol 24:469, 1984.
52. Martinez A, Perez M, Ferrer M: Chronic partial denervation is more widespread than is suspected clinically in paralytic poliomyelitis—an electrophysiological study. Eur Neurol 22:314, 1983.
53. Maxwell WC: Postpolio syndrome (video tape). 4011 West Plano Parkway, Plano, TX 75093.
54. Maynard F: Post-polio sequelae—differential diagnosis and management. Orthopedics 8:857, 1985.
55. Maynard FM, Roller S: Recognizing typical coping styles of polio survivors can improve re-rehabilitation. Am J Phys Med Rehabil 70(2):70–72, 1991.
56. Milner-Brown HS: Muscle strengthening in a post-polio subject through a high-resistance weight-training program. Arch Phys Med Rehabil 74:1165–1167, 1993.
57. Munin MC, et al: Postpoliomyelitis muscle weakness: A prospective study of quadriceps muscle strength. Arch Phys Med Rehabil 72:729–733, 1991.
58. Munsat TL, Andres P: Preliminary observations on long-term muscle force changes in the post-polio syndrome. *In* Halstead LS, Wiechers DO (eds): Birth Defects: Original Article Series 23:329–334, 1987.
59. Murray MP, Drought AB, Kory BC: Walking patterns of normal men. J Bone Joint Surg Am 46:335, 1964.
60. Peach PE: Overwork weakness with evidence of muscle damage in a patient with residual paralysis from polio. Arch Phys Med Rehabil 71:248–250, 1990.
61. Peach P, Olejnik S: Effect of treatment and noncompliance on post-polio sequelae. Orthopedics 14:1199–1203, 1991.
62. Perry J, Barnes G, Gronley JK: The postpolio syndrome: An overuse phenomena. Clin Orthop 233:145–162, 1988.
63. Perry J, Fleming C: Polio: Long-term problems. Orthopedics 8:877, 1985.
64. Perry J, Fontaine J, Mulroy S: Findings in post-poliomyelitis syndrome. J Bone Joint Surg Am 77:1148–1153, 1995.
65. Perry J, Gromley J, Lunsford T: Rocker shoe as a walking aid in multiple sclerosis. Arch Phys Med Rehabil 62:59, 1981.
66. Perry J, Hislop H (eds): Principles of Lower Extremity Bracing. Washington, DC, American Physical Therapy Association, 1967.
67. Post-Polio Directory—1993. St. Louis, International Polio Network, 1993.
68. Powers CM, Landel R, Sosnnick T, et al: The effects of patellar taping on stride characteristics and joint motion in subjects with patellofemoral pain. J Orthop Sports Phys Ther 26:286–291, 1997.
69. Progress toward global poliomyelitis eradication—1997–1998. MMWR Morbid Mortal Wkly Rep 48(20):416–421, 1999.
70. Rodriquez AA, Agre JC: Electrophysiological study of the quadriceps muscles during fatiguing exercise and recovery: A comparison of symptomatic and asymptomatic postpolio patients and controls. Arch Phys Med Rehabil 72:993–997, 1991.
71. Rodriquez AA, Agre JC, Todd MF: Electromyographic and neuromuscular variables in unstable postpolio subjects, stable postpolio subjects and control subjects. Arch Phys Med Rehabil 78:986, 1997.
72. Rosenheimer J: Effects of chronic stress and exercise on age-related changes in end-plate architecture. J Neurophysiol 53:1582, 1985.
73. Rosenheimer J, Smith D: Differential changes in the end-plate architecture of functionally diverse muscles during aging. J Neurophysiol 53:1567, 1985.
74. Ruth S, Kegerreis S: Facilitating cervical flexion using a Feldenkrais method: Awareness through movement. J Orthop Sports Phys Ther 16:25–29, 1992.
75. Saltiel J: A one-piece laminated knee locking short-leg brace. Orthop Prosthet 23:68, 1969.
76. Scheer J, Luborsky ML: The cultural context of polio biographies. Orthopedics 14:1173, 1181, 1991.
77. Schenck J, Forward E: Quantitative strength changes with test repetitions. Phys Ther 45:562, 1965.
78. Sharrard WJW: The distribution of permanent paralysis in the lower limb in poliomyelitis. J Bone Joint Surg Br 37:540, 1955.
79. Sleeper G, Kignman P, Armeni M: Nasal continuous positive pressure for at-home treatment of sleep apnea. Respir Care 30:90, 1985.
80. Smith E, Rosenblatt P, Limauro A: The role of the sympathetic nervous system in acute poliomyelitis. J Pediatr 34:1, 1949.

81. Smith L, McDermott K: Pain in post-poliomelitis: Addressing causes versus effects. *In* Halstead L, Wiechers D (eds): Research and Clinical Aspects of the Late Effects of Poliomyelitis. White Plains, NY, March of Dimes Birth Defect Series 23(4), 1987.

82. Spencer WA: Treatment of Acute Poliomyelitis. Springfield, IL, Charles C Thomas, 1956.

83. Spencer WA, Jackson RB: Poliomyelitis, acute. *In* Conn HF (ed): Current Therapy. Philadelphia, WB Saunders, 1957.

84. Tate DG, et al: Prevalence and associated features of depression and psychological distress in polio survivors. Arch Phys Med Rehabil 74:1056–1060, 1993.

85. Thompson W, Jansen JKS: The extent of sprouting of remaining motor units in partly denervated immature and adult rat soleus muscle. Neuroscience 2:523, 1977.

86. Tomlinson BE, Irving D: The numbers of limb motor neurons in the human lumbosacral cord throughout life. J Neurol Sci 34:213, 1977.

87. Trieschmann R: Aging with a Disability. New York, Demos Publications, 1987.

88. Trojan DA, Gendron D, Cashman N: Electrophysiology and electrodiagnosis of the post-polio motor unit. Orthopedics 14:1353–1361, 1991.

89. Vallbona C, Hazlewood C, Jurida G: Response of pain to static magnetic fields in postpolio patients: A double-blind pilot study. Arch Phys Med Rehabil 78:1200–1203, 1997.

90. Waring WP, Davidoff G, Werner R: Serum creatine kinase in the post-polio population. Am J Phys Med Rehabil 68:86–90, 1989.

91. Waring WP, McLaurin TM: Correlation of creatine kinase and gait measurement in the postpolio population: A corrected version. Arch Phys Med Rehabil 73:447–450, 1992.

92. Werner RA, Waring W, Maynard F: Osteoarthritis of the hand and wrist in the post poliomyelitis population. Arch Phys Med Rehabil 73:1069–1072, 1992.

93. Wiechers D, Hubbel S: Late changes in the motor unit after acute poliomyelitis. Muscle Nerve 4:524, 1981.

94. Yang C, et al: Floor reaction orthosis: Clinical experience. Orthop Prosthet 40:33, 1986.

95. Young G: Energy conservation, occupational therapy, and the treatment of post-polio sequelae. Orthopedics 14:1233–1239, 1991.

SELECTED READINGS

Carter NB: Of Myths and Chicken Feet: a Polio Survivor Looks at Survival. Omaha, NPSA Press, 1992.

Krauss P, Goldfischer M: Why Me? Coping with Grief, Loss, and Change. New York, Bantam, 1988.

Multiple Sclerosis

DEBRA FRANKEL, MS, OTR

Key Words

- autoimmune disease
- Avonex (interferon beta-1a)
- axonal damage
- Betaseron (interferon beta-1b)
- Copaxone (glatimer acetate)
- cytokines
- demyelination
- exacerbations and remissions
- experimental allergic
  encephalomyelitis (EAE)
- glial cells
- immunosuppression
- lesion
- myelin
- multiple sclerosis (MS)
- plaques
- relapse and remission
- T cells

Objectives

After reading this chapter the student/therapist will:

1. Be able to describe the medical basis of multiple sclerosis (MS), including epidemiology, etiology, signs and symptoms, diagnosis, and course.

2. Be able to cite current research strategies and findings.

3. Be able to identify options in the medical management of the MS patient.

4. Be able to identify the unique psychosocial and neuropsychological effects of MS.

5. Be able to list appropriate rehabilitation goals, formulate a rehabilitation plan, and develop rehabilitation strategies to maximize function and quality of life.

Multiple sclerosis (MS) is one of the most common neurological diseases of young adults. The disease was formally identified and established as a clinical pathological entity in 1868 by Jean Martin Charcot, a French neurologist. He called the disease "sclerose en plaques," describing the hardened patchlike areas found (on autopsy) disseminated throughout the central nervous system (CNS) of individuals with the disease.[8, 15, 37, 45]

In the normal human nervous system, impulses in many nerve fibers travel in excess of 200 mph. This remarkable velocity is achieved, to a large extent, by the insulation property of myelin, a complex of lipoprotein layers formed early in development by oligodendroglia in the CNS, which sheaths the axons.

Inflammatory lesions (plaques) characterize MS as distinct areas of myelin loss scattered throughout the CNS, primarily in the white matter (Fig. 20–1). These plaques of demyelination are accompanied by inflammation (or the accumulation of white blood cells and fluid around blood vessels that lie wihin the CNS). Demyelination

595

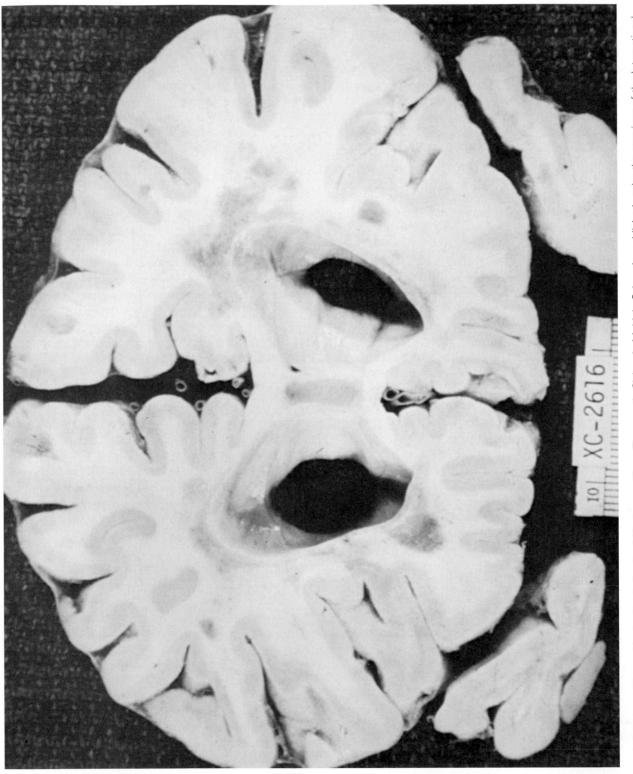

FIGURE 20–1. Photo of brain slice indicating MS plaques. (From Therapeutic Claims in Multiple Sclerosis, published under the auspices of the International Federation of Multiple Sclerosis Societies, 1982; photo courtesy of Cedric Raine, M.D., Albert Einstein College of Medicine, Yeshiva University, New York.)

results in impaired neurotransmission. Recent findings also indicate that axons become irreversibly damaged as a consequence of inflammation and may contribute to persistent neurological deficits and long-term disability in MS.[54] MS involves demyelination and axonal damage in the CNS only. CNS demyelination also occurs as a predominant finding in several other less common disorders, including acute disseminated encephalomyelitis and diffuse cerebral sclerosis.

OVERVIEW OF MULTIPLE SCLEROSIS

Epidemiology

MS is generally diagnosed between the ages of 20 and 40, with 85% occurring between the ages of 15 and 50 years; the majority of people are in their 30s at the time of diagnosis. It appears more predominantly in women, with a ratio of almost 2:1. MS is rare in some races (e.g., African blacks and Eskimos) and is most predominant in whites of northern European ancestry.

A number of studies have established geographical patterns of MS prevalence. MS appears more prominently in areas of the world farther from the equator (Fig. 20–2). A related observation is that the location where a person spends the first 15 years of life may determine a greater or lesser likelihood of developing MS as opposed to where he or she lives at the time of diagnosis. Some studies suggest that a person born in the north who moves to the south after age 15 brings with him or her the higher risk of a northerner.[1, 29, 37] The prevalence rate of MS in the northern United States is over 150/100,000, whereas in the southern United States it is about 50/100,000.

Epidemiological data collected from the Faroe, Orkney, and Shetland Islands (in the northern Atlantic Ocean) indicated a rise in recorded cases of MS for a 15- to 25-year period around World War II followed by a drop to prewar rates.[22] This rise and fall suggests that a viral agent may have been introduced by troops who occupied the islands during the war.

Also relevant to the epidemiological picture of MS is genetics. Family studies show a major genetic influence on susceptibility to MS. Five percent of people with MS have a sibling with MS, and about 15% have a close relative with the disease. The mode of inheritance and number of genes involved have not been determined, and it is clear from twin concordance data that an environmental trigger must also be at play.[10, 38, 57] Epidemiological studies have helped to identify MS as a disease that most probably has an environmental trigger and that occurs in genetically susceptible individuals. Approximately 300,000 people in the United States have MS, with a worldwide estimate of 1 million.

Etiology

Myelin damage is most likely to be mediated by the immune system. It appears that in genetically susceptible individuals there is an abnormality in the immune response that results in a widespread attack on the individual's own neural tissue—that is, an autoimmune response. A specific antigen has not yet been identified.

Researchers theorize that a virus is the responsible trigger. However, it may be a ubiquitous virus that infects a large number of people with only a few of the infected developing the secondary process (MS) or an unusual virus with a low rate of infection but a high rate of clinical expression.[38]

Some investigators suggest that the immune system mistakes a portion of myelin protein for a virus that is structurally similar and targets it for destruction (molecular mimicry). Others theorize that small amounts of myelin are released in the circulation after viral infection, resulting in autoimmunization.

Signs and Symptoms

Because of the great variability of the anatomical location, volume, and time sequence of lesions in people with MS, the clinical manifestations of the disease vary among individuals. Symptoms may develop quickly, within hours, or slowly over several days or weeks. Most commonly, symptoms develop over a day, although rapidity of onset and appearance of symptoms depend on the locus and size of the underlying lesion. The most common symptoms are fatigue, motor weakness, paresthesia, unsteady gait, double vision, tremor, and bladder/bowel dysfunction (see the box below).[2] Other types of onset, such as hemiplegia, trigeminal neuralgia, and facial palsy, are less common. In many individuals a history of vague functional impairment precedes definite symptoms. A comprehensive list of symptoms appears on page 599.

The subject of cognitive and affective changes that are mediated by the MS disease process has recently been addressed in a formalized way. It has been concluded that 50% to 70% of people with MS show evidence of some cognitive impairment. The majority of these individuals have mild impairment, with approximately 10% to 20% showing significant dysfunction. Research does not support the notion that the occurrence of cognitive symptoms

---

MOST FREQUENT SYMPTOMS OF MS*

Fatigue: 88%

Walking problems: 87%

Bowel and bladder problems: 65%

Pain and other sensations: 60%

Visual disturbances: 58%

Cognitive problems: 44%

Tremors: 41%

---

*From a study of 697 patients with MS.

From Aronson KJ, et al: Socio-demographic characteristics and health status of persons with multiple sclerosis and their care givers. MS Management 3(May):1–15, 1996.

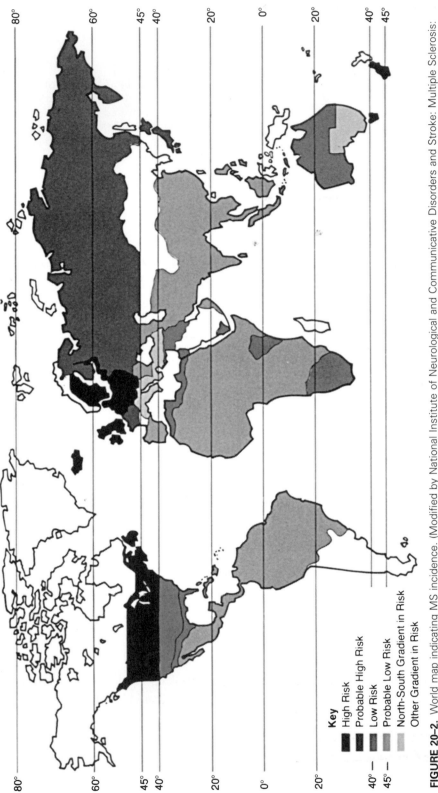

FIGURE 20-2. World map indicating MS incidence. (Modified by National Institute of Neurological and Communicative Disorders and Stroke: Multiple Sclerosis: Hope Through Research, publication No. 79–75, Washington, DC, 1981, National Institutes of Health; from McAlpine D, et al: Multiple Sclerosis, a Reappraisal. Edinburgh, E & S Livingstone, 1965.)

Key
High Risk
Probable High Risk
Low Risk
Probable Low Risk
North-South Gradient in Risk
Other Gradient in Risk

SUMMARY OF COMMON SIGNS AND SYMPTOMS

Motor Symptoms
Spasticity and reflex spasms
Weakness
Contractures
Gait disturbance
Fatigue
Cerebellar and bulbar symptoms
• Resultant swallowing/respiratory difficulties
• Nystagmus
• Intention tremor

Sensory Symptoms
Numbness
Pain (most often of musculoskeletal origin)
Paresthesia
Dysesthesia
Distortion of superficial sensation

Visual Symptoms
Diminished acuity
Double vision
Scotoma
Ocular pain

Bladder/Bowel Symptoms
Urgency
Frequency
Incontinence
Urinary retention
Constipation

Sexual Symptoms
Impotence
Diminished genital sensation
Diminished genital lubrication

Cognitive and Emotional Symptoms
Depression
Lability
Disorders of judgment
Agnosia
Memory disturbance
Diminished conceptual thinking
Decreased attention and concentration
Dysphasia

---

is related to severity of physical symptoms or to duration of the disease.[41, 43, 44, 49] Specifically, cognitive functions that seem most often affected are short-term memory, conceptual reasoning, and problem solving. Verbal fluency and speed of information processing are sometimes affected. It is rare to see widespread deterioration of intellectual function in MS.[43, 44, 53]

Depression appears more common in those with MS than in the general population or those with other medical conditions.[31–33] This finding probably results from a complex interaction of variables including the pathophysiology of the disease, the unique stressors that characterize MS, and the individual's particular circumstances.

A wide variety of symptoms are associated with the disease and should be understood by a therapist dealing with these problems.

Course and Prognosis

Overall prognosis is variable, and the course of the disease is unpredictable. The four categories currently used to describe the clinical course of MS are depicted in Figure 20–3. They are:

• Relapsing-remitting MS (characterized by clearly defined relapses—episodes of acute worsening—followed by recovery and disease stability) (A)
• Primary progressive MS (characterized by continuous worsening—steady progression—not interrupted by distinct relapses) (B)
• Secondary progressive (characterized by relapsing-remitting disease followed by progression with or without occasional relapse, minor remission or plateau) (C)
• Progressive relapsing (characterized by progressive disease from the onset with clear, acute relapses that may or may not resolve; periods between relapses are characterized by continued progression)[27] (D)

Efforts to identify factors that predict clinical course or long-term outcome have not been reliable, although the following factors may suggest a more favorable outcome: female sex, onset before 35 years of age, monoregional versus polyregional attack, and complete recovery after attacks. The following are associated with a less favorable outcome: male sex, brain stem symptoms (nystagmus, tremor, ataxia and dysarthria), poor recovery after exacerbations, and high frequency of attacks.[7, 37, 40]

Various factors have been associated with exacerbations or temporary worsening (pseudoexacerbation). These include excessive fatigue, trauma, and rise in body temperature because of fever, hot bath or shower, or hot weather conditions. However, no specific cause-effect relationship has been shown. For the most part, the course of MS is unpredictable.

Recent evidence has been presented by researchers that MS is actually active and progressive from its earliest

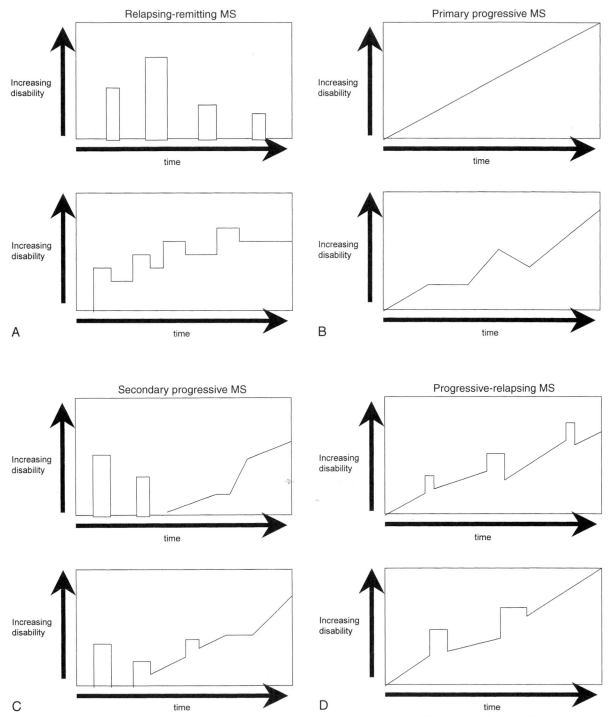

FIGURE 20–3. *A,* Relapsing-remitting (RR) MS. This type of MS is characterized by clearly defined acute attacks with full recovery *(top)* or with residual deficits after recovery *(bottom).* Periods between disease relapses are characterized by a lack of disease progression. *B,* Primary progressive (PP) MS. This type is characterized by progression of disability from the beginning without plateaus or remissions *(top)* or with occasional plateaus and temporary minor improvements *(bottom). C,* Secondary progressive (SP) MS. This type begins with a relapsing-remitting disease course, followed by progression *(top),* which may also include occasional relapses, and minor remissions and plateaus *(bottom). D,* Progressive relapsing (PR) MS. Progression occurs from the beginning but with clear acute relapses, with *(top)* or without *(bottom)* full recovery. (From Lublin F, Reingold S: Refining the course of multiple sclerosis, Neurology 46:907, 1996.)

stages. Until recently, MS was thought to be active only during acute exacerbations or periods of acute worsening of symptoms. Using gadolinium to enhance magnetic resonance (MR) images, scientists have shown that even when the patient's symptoms are stable, their MS can be active. Gadolinium enhances MR images to indicate new and active lesions.[30]

Diagnosis

The diagnosis of MS is largely clinical. The basic diagnostic criteria are:

- Evidence of multiple lesions in the CNS
- Evidence (clinical or paraclinical) of at least two distinct episodes of neurological disturbance in an individual between the ages of 10 and 59 years[20, 42]

Paraclinical evidence may include neuroimaging with magnetic resonance imaging (MRI) or computed tomography (CT), evoked potentials, or cerebrospinal fluid (CSF) analysis (see the box below).

MRI is currently the preferred method to detect MS lesions. Use of MRI has hastened the diagnosis in many cases; however, MS cannot be diagnosed solely on the basis of this test. About 5% of people confirmed to have MS based on other criteria show no lesions on MRI. Conversely, many other diseases may cause lesions that appear on the MRI, and many healthy individuals also may exhibit unidentified bright spots on MRI.[30, 58] Gadolinium, a chemical compound given during MRI that helps distinguish new (active) lesions from old, has been useful in monitoring disease activity. Studies using gadolinium enhancement indicate that the disease may be active even when functional status and neurological signs are stable.[30]

Evoked potentials may include visual evoked potentials (VEP), brain stem auditory evoked potentials (BAEP), and somatosensory evoked potentials (SSEP). These tests, which measure nerve conduction along visual, auditory, and sensory pathways, often provide evidence of altered nerve conduction that may not be apparent on neurological examination.

CSF examination is not routine in diagnosing MS but may provide additional clues in complicated cases. Elevated gamma globulin is found in many cases of MS, and about one fourth of persons with active MS may show white blood cells in the CSF.[37]

Psychosocial Considerations

The personality, history, and cultural background of the individual along with the family and community environment crucially affects the response to illness. The nature of the disability itself will also, of course, influence the emotional response.

MS is an emotionally challenging disease, and all members of the family feel its impact. Grief and anxiety accompany the diagnosis and may fluctuate with the disease course and the individual's particular circumstances.

Several clinical aspects of MS influence the psychosocial impact of the disease:

1. *Ambiguity of diagnosis.* Although MRI and increased knowledge about MS have hastened the diagnostic process, there is often a period of ambiguity during which the individual is experiencing symptoms without a clear explanation. During this time, individuals may harbor fantasies of life-threatening or debilitating illness or may not be taken seriously by physicians or friends. Once a confirmed diagnosis of MS is made, some individuals report feeling relief to have an explanation, even though the implications of the diagnosis remain ambiguous.

2. *Unpredictability of the course.* The course of MS is uncertain. The disease may remain benign for some but is severely disabling for others. An individual may be free of symptoms for months or years and then unexpectedly experience an exacerbation. Symptoms may even vary from morning to evening of the same day. This unpredictability and the accompanying sense of loss of control can frequently cause depression, anxiety, and fear. Planning for the future becomes difficult and has an impact on family, work, and social interactions and activities.

3. *Covert symptoms.* Many symptoms of MS, including fatigue, double vision, bladder dysfunction, and paresthesias, are not visible to others yet can be very disabling and disturbing to the individual. Many people find that they are misunderstood, are seen as lazy or lacking initiative, and find it difficult to explain the effect of these hidden symptoms to others. Some struggle with the decision to disclose their diagnosis to employers or friends. They fear job discrimination or alienating friends, but they may find that MS is a stressful and disturbing secret to keep.

Certainly, the stress of MS is in many ways like the stress of any kind of serious illness. A profound sense of fear, vulnerability, and exhausting self-concern underlies the coping process. The loss of a sense of control over one's body and lifestyle may precipitate an ongoing griev-

---

DIAGNOSTIC GUIDELINES FOR MULTIPLE SCLEROSIS

Definite MS

1. Two attacks and clinical evidence of two separate lesions
2. Two attacks, clinical evidence of one and paraclinical evidence of another separate lesion

Probable MS

1. Two attacks and clinical evidence of one lesion
2. One attack and clinical evidence of two lesions
3. One attack, clinical evidence of one lesion, paraclinical evidence for another separate lesion

From Poser C, et al: The Diagnosis of Multiple Sclerosis. New York, Thieme-Stratton, 1984.

ing process and a search to make some sense and give meaning to an otherwise confusing and purposeless event.

MEDICAL MANAGEMENT

Disease-Modifying Agents

In recent years, three disease-modifying agents have been approved by the U.S. Food and Drug Administration (FDA) for relapsing-remitting multiple sclerosis. These drugs are currently being evaluated for their effect on primary and secondary progressive disease. They are interferon beta 1a (Avonex), interferon beta 1b (Betaseron), and glatiramer acetate (Copaxone). All three agents are administered by injection (Avonex: weekly, intramuscularly; Betaseron: every other day, subcutaneously; Copaxone: daily, subcutaneously). All three drugs, in clinical trials, showed approximately a one third reduction in relapse rate. Additionally, Avonex trials also resulted in a 37% lower risk of progression of disability and Betaseron trials resulted in reduced severity of relapses. The interferon beta drugs are associated with flulike side effects that appear to lessen over time. Injection site reactions are associated with the subcutaneous injections of Betaseron and Copaxone. And a rare, seemingly benign reaction including anxiety, chest tightness, shortness of breath, and flushing may occur in patients taking Copaxone.

The development of the disease-modifying agents and the continued data collection on their effectiveness have made a significant impact on the treatment of MS. The availability of these agents has resulted in a reduction in disease activity and progression of disability for many people with MS. In September 1998, the National Multiple Sclerosis Society's medical advisors approved a statement regarding early intervention and access to these agents for patients with relapsing-remitting multiple sclerosis (see the following box). As a result, the drugs are becoming widely accepted as standard treatment for many patients with relapsing-remitting MS.

Treatment of Relapses and Symptoms

General medical management measures focus on the treatment of acute relapses, symptomatic management, improvement of function, and psychological support. Overall management calls for principles that will affect maximal health in general. These include ensuring adequate nutrition, encouraging balanced rest and exercise, avoiding exposure to infections, and preventing complications secondary to reduced activity (Fig. 20–4). It is also important to facilitate positive coping measures and to minimize family dysfunction, anxiety, and depression.

Treatment of Acute Relapses. Natural improvement of acute exacerbations frequently occurs within 4 to 12 weeks. The degree of improvement varies and most likely has to do with reduction in inflammation. For acute relapses, most neurologists prescribe high-dose intravenous corticosteroids such as methylprednisolone (Depo-Medrol) over 3 to 5 days. This high-dose intravenous course may be followed by a gradually tapering dose of oral corticosteroid (e.g., prednisone). Oral corticosteroids

---

NATIONAL MULTIPLE SCLEROSIS SOCIETY CONSENSUS STATEMENT

In September 1998, the National Multiple Sclerosis Society's medical advisors approved a statement regarding early intervention and access to therapy for patients with relapsing-remitting multiple sclerosis. The statement addresses the three immunomodulating agents approved for use in the United States. It does not address Rebif, which is approved in Canada but has not yet been approved for use in the United States.

Summary of Recommendations

The Medical Advisory Board of the National Multiple Sclerosis Society has adopted the following recommendations regarding use of the current MS disease-modifying agents: Betaseron (interferon beta 1b), Avonex (interferon beta 1a), and Copaxone (glatiramer acetate):

- Initiation of therapy is advised as soon as possible after a definite diagnosis of MS and determination of a relapsing course.
- Patients' access to medication should not be limited by the frequency of relapses, age, or level of disability.
- Treatment is not to be stopped during evaluation for continuing treatment.
- Therapy is to be continued indefinitely, unless there is clear lack of benefit, intolerable side effects, new data that reveals other reasons for cessation, or better therapy is available.
- All three agents should be included in formularies and covered by third-party payers so that physicians and patients may determine the most appropriate agent on an individual basis.
- Movement from one immunomodulating drug to another should be permitted.
- Most concurrent medical conditions do not contraindicate use of any of these therapies.

If a copy of the entire document is desired, please call 1-800-FIGHT-MS, and select option 1, or call the National Multiple Sclerosis Society at 1-212-986-3240 and ask for the Information Resource Center.

---

may also be used to treat a mild or moderate relapse, although intravenous methylprednisolone is usually prescribed for optic neuritis and retrobulbar neuritis. Although these antiinflammatory agents are used widely in acute attacks of MS, there is little evidence that they alter the extent of residual disability or the overall course of the disease.[17, 18, 50] Long-term side effects of corticosteroids (osteoporosis, hypertension, cataracts, muscle wasting) are not generally associated with short-term use; nevertheless,

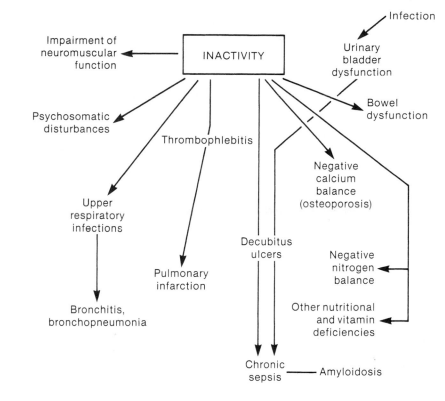

FIGURE 20–4. Inactivity chart. (From Bauer H: A Manual on Multiple Sclerosis, published under the auspices of the International Federation of Multiple Sclerosis Societies, 1977.)

side effects may include altered mood, epigastric distress, frequent urination, and blurred vision.

Symptomatic Management. Baclofen (Lioresol) and tinzanidine (Zanaflex) are the most commonly used medications to control *spasticity* in MS. Side effects such as increased weakness, lethargy, and fatigue may occur with baclofen. The surgical implantation of a pump to deliver a continuous dose of baclofen intrathecally is beneficial to many people with severe spasticity. The pump is implanted beneath the skin, usually on the lower abdomen, and the rate of drug delivery can be adjusted to meet individual need. Sodium dantrolene (Dantrium) may also be helpful, although it may induce weakness even at low doses. Diazepam (Valium) is also used, most frequently for spasms that occur at night. Cyclobenzaprine (Flexoril) is sometimes prescribed for back spasms and also may have an overall antispasticity effect. Carbamepazine (Tegretol) is generally used to control tonic spasms, and cortisone may also decrease overall spasticity but long-term use is not advocated. Phenol blocks or tendon release surgical procedures may be required if severe spasticity interferes with personal hygiene and other activities of daily living (ADL), although a combination of exercise, stretching, and medication can usually avoid these more extreme measures. Severe tremor is sometimes treated with drugs that have a sedative effect (e.g., clonazepam (Clonopin) and hydroxyzine (Vistaril). Propranolol (Inderal), a beta blocker, may be helpful in controlling some tremors. High doses of isoniazid, a drug used to treat tuberculosis, may also alleviate gross tremors that are influenced by posture.[9, 17, 18] Reducing spasticity generally results in improved mobility and function; however, a certain degree of spasticity may be beneficial to some individuals especially when it aids in the support of weak

legs. Physical and occupational therapy and a stretching regimen are also beneficial in reducing spasticity.

Fatigue is one of the most common symptoms of MS and may be very debilitating. Energy conservation, moderate exercise, rest, use of assistive devices, work simplification, and cooling may be effective in controlling fatigue in MS. Amantadine (Symmetrel) appears to be effective in managing MS fatigue in about 40% of cases, as are some stimulants such as pemoline (Cylert) and methylphenidate (Ritalin). These stimulants may cause sleeplessness or other side effects and must be monitored carefully. The experimental use of 4-aminopyridine, a nerve conduction enhancer, has shown improvement in fatigue, spasticity, and other symptoms in some patients.[17, 18] Depression may contribute to fatigue in some cases; and when the underlying depression is alleviated, fatigue levels improve. The Multiple Sclerosis Council of the Paralyzed Veterans of America has developed clinical practice guidelines of managing fatigue in MS patients. These present an evidence-based, systematic strategy for use by all health care providers and provide a framework for identifying appropriate care.[35]

Most *bladder symptoms* result from a neurogenic bladder; however, urinary tract infection must be considered because this may also cause changes in bladder function. Smooth muscle relaxants or nerve blockers such as propantheline (Pro-Banthine) and oxybutynin (Ditropan) may reduce urinary frequency and urgency. Urinary retention is frequently treated with bethanechol (Urecholine) or phenoxybenzamine (Dibenzyline). Credé technique and intermittent catheterization are used with the bladder that does not empty sufficiently. If a bladder problem cannot be solved with medication or intermittent catheterization, continuous catheterization using a Foley catheter may be necessary.[5] Bladder infections, secondary to urinary retention, are treated with an antibiotic specific to the bacteria present. Prevention of infection is the best approach by including acidifying agents to the diet. The Multiple Sclerosis Council of the Paralyzed Veterans Administration has developed clinical Practice Guidelines in bladder management that provide effective and widely used approaches to care.[34]

Absence of good bowel control may lead to constipation or incontinence. Bulk formers such as hydrophilic colloid (Metamucil) or stool softeners such as docusate (Colace) may be recommended. Laxatives such as milk of magnesia may be prescribed if expelling stool is the cause of the constipation. Rectal stimulants may also be effective such as glycerine or bisacodyl (Ducolax) suppositories. Frequent use of enemas should be avoided. A bowel program including dietary (adequate fluids and bulk) and drug regimens can usually control the constipation and incontinence of MS.

While *pain* is not a hallmark of MS, many people with the disease experience a variety of painful syndromes. Tic douloureux or trigeminal neuralgia, a sharp pain in the face stimulated by touch or facial movement, is most common. It is usually treated with carbamazepine (Tegretol), phenytoin (Dilantin), or baclofen (Lioresol). In extreme cases, surgical procedures may be used to sever the sensory root fibers of the trigeminal nerve. Many individuals with MS experience dysesthetic pain, frequently described as a burning sensation by those who experience it. This pain may be treated with the same drugs as trigeminal neuralgia. Pain frequently associated with MS is secondary to spasticity, poor posture, or abnormal use of muscles to compensate for loss of function. Physical and occupational therapy may play an important role in pain management of this type along with analgesics, nonsteroidal antiinflammatory agents (NSAIDs) and, in the case of back spasms, such drugs as cyclobenzaprine.

MS can affect *sexual function* directly by causing neurological impairment that results in erectile difficulties, orgasmic dysfunction, or decreased libido. Indirectly, such symptoms as fatigue, spasticity, depression, and bladder and bowel dysfunction may interfere with sexual expression and intimacy. Sexual aids, prosthetic devices, counseling, and medications such as sildenafil (Viagra), alprostadil (Muse), or prostaglandin injections for erectile dysfunction may improve function and satisfaction with sexual expression.

Dizziness and vertigo may accompany loss of balance. If vertigo is severe, medications such as meclizine (Antivert, Bonine) may be suggested. Physical therapy to address dizziness that is worsened by positional change may be useful (see Chapter 21).

Neuropsychological testing can assist in determining the degree of *cognitive impairment*. Treatment of cognitive problems usually involves retraining and teaching of compensatory strategies. Cognitive dysfunction may be a major disabling feature of MS. Symptoms may be exaggerated by underlying depression or may be confused by communication deficits.

There is a high incidence of *depression* among people with MS along with a suicide rate that one study identified as 7.5 times higher than the general population.[31, 32, 48]

Both organic and psychosocial factors contribute to depression and anxiety in MS. Counseling, support groups, and, in some cases, antidepressant medications and psychotherapy may be helpful in addressing these issues in MS.

In considering any therapy or treatment, one must keep in mind that a large percentage of persons with MS show improvement as a result of the natural history of the disease at various times regardless of treatment. Additionally, complementary therapies (e.g., acupuncture, massage, movement therapies, diets, vitamin supplementation) are gaining popularity among people with MS as in the general population. It is important to discuss any complementary therapies that are being used to be sure there are no contraindications or that no negative interactions result.

RESEARCH CONSIDERATIONS

MS is still a disease of unknown cause. It is generally accepted that MS occurs in genetically susceptible individuals. It is suspected that a viral infection is involved as well, yet efforts to culture a specific virus have not been successful, nor have efforts to transmit a virus to other mammals. The most widely accepted theory of the etiology of MS is that MS is an autoimmune disease of the CNS, triggered by an environmental agent in genetically susceptible individuals, which causes inflammation and ultimately destruction of myelin and damage to axons.

The search for the cause and cure of MS is the focus of efforts in the United States by both the National Multiple Sclerosis Society and the National Institutes of Health.[55] Internationally, work is being conducted in academic and scientific institutions worldwide. The International Federation of MS Societies (IFMSS) works to coordinate these efforts and to facilitate communication among investigators. Research efforts focus generally on four biomedical areas: immunology, genetics, virology, and biology of glial cells.

Immunology

Immune-modifying strategies have received considerable attention over the past several years. Global immunosuppressant therapies including cyclophosphamide, cyclosporine, azathioprine, methotrexate, total lymphoid irradiation, and plasmapheresis have undergone numerous clinical trials. The drawback to these global methods is that they leave the body open to serious infection, and their impact on the progression of MS is not conclusive. New mechanisms that target specific T cells such as monoclonal antibodies and synthetic peptides may be safer and have had some early success in blocking T-cell function in the animal model of MS, experimental allergic encephalomyelitis. Efforts to enhance immunological tolerance to myelin or its antigens include the use of oral tolerance therapy,[56] an area of investigation in which the natural immunological functions in the digestive tract are manipulated to block the autoimmune response. Initial clinical trials of an agent to use oral tolerance as a strategy proved disappointing, but additional research continues.

Also, continued research on the effects of disease-modifying agents on primary and secondary progressive disease will likely lead to FDA approval of these drugs for that purpose.

Genetics

A combination of several genes that determine immune function and control will most likely be implicated in MS susceptibility. Efforts to identify these genes are underway using families in which there are multiple cases of MS along with molecular genetics technology.

Virology

Dozens of viruses have been proposed as the trigger of MS, yet none has been shown to have a cause-and-effect relationship to the disease. Many researchers suspect that a single virus does not cause MS but that the problem lies in the way a genetically susceptible individual handles common viral infection in general. Recent studies have pointed to a role of the human herpesvirus as a precipitating factor in MS.[6] However, a definitive understanding of the role of viruses in MS has not yet been attained.

Glial Cell Biology

The study of oligodendrocytes, the glial cells that make and maintain myelin, offers the best hope for recovery of function. It is thought that astrocytes, another glial cell, produce toxic substances that damage myelin and create the nerve tissue lesions typical of MS. Efforts to transplant oligodendrocytes in mice and to manipulate the immune system to accelerate remyelination are showing promise in improving function.

Rehabilitation Research

Members from all branches of the health care community are embracing "evidence-based" management strategies to improve patient outcomes and enhance quality assurance. Evidence-based medicine refers to systematic weighting of health care practices according to research or scientific evidence supporting those practices. Where scientific evidence is lacking, practice guidelines are developed and/or evaluated based on expert opinion and consensus. This concept helps clinicians make treatment decisions informed by the best current evidence as opposed to relying solely on past experience, intuition, or anecdotal observation. Evidence-based practice closes the gap between research and clinical application.

The following summarizes some of the recent research in MS rehabilitation management. These findings will help inform the decisions made in determining rehabilitation goals, modalities, and techniques.

- Researchers[23] at William Beaumont Hospital in Royal Oak, Michigan, concluded that an interdisciplinary approach to MS rehabilitation (occupational and physical therapy) improved mobilization of the patient, minimizing such symptoms as spasticity and fatigue as well as reducing complications of inactivity.

- Researchers at the Institute of Neurology in London,[14] in a study to determine if the benefits of inpatient rehabilitation of MS patients carried over into the community, found that benefits were partly maintained although declined over time, reinforcing the need for continuity of care between inpatient settings and the community.

- Investigators at the Istituto Nazionale Neurologico in Milan, Italy,[52] concluded, in a study of the effects of physical rehabilitation in MS patients, that despite unchanging impairment, rehabilitation resulted in improvement of disability and had a positive impact on mental components of health-related quality of life measures.

- Granger and colleagues[16] evaluated functional assessment scales, determining that the Functional Independence Measure (FIM), Barthel Index, and Environmental Status Scale highly correlated with one another. And while each was predictive of physical care needs, the FIM was most useful. The FIM also contributed to predicting the patient's general satisfaction.

- Another study at the Institute of Neurology in London[24] attempted to identify the physical and cognitive variables affecting rehabilitation outcome in MS patients. The researchers concluded that verbal intelligence and cerebellar function are influential in determining rehabilitation outcomes.

- Therapists at the Jimmie Heuga Center in Edwards, Colorado, reported that physical fitness and emotional state improve in MS patients with exercise training despite increases in disability.[19]

- Neufeld[36] reported in preliminary findings that MS patients in an exercise- and skills-based wellness course, designed by an occupational therapist, showed gains in self-efficacy for self-management, increasing use of self-management behaviors and achievement of personal goals.

REHABILITATION MANAGEMENT

Although disease-modifying agents are now available to slow the progression of disability in MS, most people with the disease will continue to have limitations in their ability to manage daily living activities. Rehabilitation is directed toward maximizing function, preventing unnecessary complications, and empowering individuals to realize their highest potential and improving overall quality of life. Reducing "disablement," the World Health Organization's term that describes the consequences of disease or injury, is the primary goal of rehabilitation. Although rehabilitation interventions will not eliminate neurological damage in MS, they can reduce disablement and enhance functioning. From the time of diagnosis, even in the absence of obvious disablement, rehabilitation specialists can provide education and treatment to promote health and wellness and maximize overall fitness.[25]

The Rehabilitation Team and Setting

Involvement in a rehabilitation program may take several forms. From a practical point of view, fiscal considerations may dictate the frequency and duration of therapy visits as well as location, that is, whether the care is administered at home or on an inpatient or outpatient basis. Unfortunately, the availability of third-party payment for therapy is often conditional, with many individuals ineligible for reimbursement, particularly for maintenance and preventive therapies.

The place at which treatment is provided can often dictate the modalities used. An inpatient setting, for example, provides an opportunity for intensive therapies, a therapeutic community, multidisciplinary support, a comprehensive treatment environment, and easy availability of equipment and modalities. It is also important to realize that such a setting requires learning skills outside the home environment, transferring those skills after discharge, and adjusting psychologically to the home setting, where the client has the opportunity and responsibility to carry out his or her program.

Home-based treatment, as an alternative, provides a familiar environment; however, availability of equipment or modalities may be limited. The treatment environment selected needs to be based on the client's needs, the availability of resources, and cost.

Treatment focuses on helping the patient achieve optimal functional independence and is best carried out by an interdisciplinary team. Members of the team include the physician, occupational therapist, physical therapist, speech therapist, nurse, dietitian, social worker, recreation therapist, and, of course, the patient and his or her family. Not all members will be involved at all times, and financial realities may prohibit involvement of all team members; however, the team approach is the most comprehensive approach to management. The team uses a variety of methods to reduce disability and improve the quality of life for a person with MS: physical treatment, education, advocacy, environmental changes, compensation with adaptive equipment, and counseling. Table 20–1 indicates how the interdisciplinary team might collaborate on many common MS problems.[28]

Evaluation

The clinician must consider various factors when evaluating the individual with MS. Subjective perceptions of problems by the individual and family members may be of greater significance than objective measures. Functional assessment at times may not correlate with clinical measure; that is, MS lesions may be functionally silent in some cases yet in others significant functional impairment may result from apparently minimal clinical disease activity (as indicated by MRI). The individual with MS must be evaluated at intervals during the fluctuating course of the disease. Additionally, factors that influence performance such as heat and fatigue must be considered when the client is evaluated.

An assessment profile must be developed before establishing treatment goals. Ideally, a collaborative approach to assessment, pooling the various findings of the members of the rehabilitation team with the priorities of the individual, will provide direction to the rehabilitation process (see the following box).

Each patient serves as his or her own baseline because

ASSESSMENT PROFILE FOR MS

- Strength
- Tone
- Range of motion
- Balance
- Coordination
- Ambulation
- Fatigue/endurance
- Cardiovascular and respiratory status
- Bed mobility/transfers
- Bowel/bladder/sexual impairment
- Swallowing
- Speech/communication impairment
- Visual status
- Sensory impairment
- Activities of daily living
- Cognition
- Vocational and avocational status
- Psychosocial status (including family adjustment)
- Physical environment/community resources
- Medical stability

---

the course of MS and severity of symptoms are so variable.

Measurement Tools

A standardized profile such as the FIM or Barthel Index is often used in MS assessment. These tools help to develop a patient profile, can be compared with previous assessments, and help to develop functional goals.

The Kurtzke Scale[21] (see the box on page 609) is the standardized assessment of MS disability used widely by MS clinicians and researchers to quantify the degree of disability and provide a common language to describe patient status. The Kurtzke Scale is frequently used to measure the effectiveness of a particular treatment or as a criterion for participation in a clinical trial.

A tool specific to multiple sclerosis, the Multiple Sclerosis Quality of Life Inventory (MSQLI) is a standard measure used widely in MS research. It has significant value to the therapist as well in assessing the impact of MS on various aspects of daily life. Questions cover health status (SF-36), fatigue (Modified Fatigue Impact Scale [MFIS]), pain (Most Pain Effects Scale [PACE]), sexual function (Sexual Satisfaction Scale [SSS]), bladder function (Bladder Control Scale [BLCS]), bowel function (Bowel Control Scale [BWCS]), visual impairment (Impact of Visual Impairment Scale [IVIS]), cognitive deficits (Perceived Deficits Questionnaire [PDQ]), mental health status (Mental Health Inventory [MHI]), and social support (Modified Social Support Survey [MSSS]). The scale was developed with funding from the National MS Society, the MS Society of Canada, and the Consortium of MS Centers.[12]

TABLE 20-1. Examples of Team Interaction on Common MS Problems

Problem	Goals	Team*	Plan
Weakness	Strengthen disuse component Maintain fitness	MD/nurse/OT/PT†	Strengthening exercises, substitution, compensation, protective splints
Spasticity	Normalize tone without causing loss of support	MD/nurse/OT/PT	Medication, stretching, positioning, cold bath or spray, movement techniques, motor point block
Incoordination/tremor/impaired balance	Improve balance and control	MD/nurse/OT/PT	Medication, coordination/balance exercises, joint approximation, adaptive equipment, extremity weights, compensatory techniques, air splints, weighted canes/crutches, gait training
Impaired sensation	Enhance sensory awareness Teach precautions	MD/nurse/OT/PT	Education, visual compensation, developmental sequence exercises, joint approximation, tapping, brushing, weights
Pain	Decrease source of pain Decrease perception of pain	Biofeedback†/counselor/MD/nurse/OT/PT	Medication, improve posture, transcutaneous nerve stimulation, increase activity, stress management, muscle relaxation, diminish pain behavior
Visual impairment	Improve vision Compensate for loss	Blind services/MD/nurse/OT/PT ophthalmologist	Medication for acute optic neuritis, patch for double vision, compensatory techniques, talking books, home visit
Fatigue	Increase and conserve available energy	Biofeedback/counselor/MD/nurse/OT/PT	Teach energy conservation, treat depression, improve endurance, efficient compensatory techniques and equipment, stress management, have patient keep record of activities and readjustment, rest periods at onset of fatigue
Memory/cognitive impairment	Identify Compensate	Counselor/MD/OT/speech†/neuropsychologist	Evaluation, educate patient and family, teach compensatory techniques, alteration of home environment
Ambulation/transfers	Safe and efficient mobility	Nurse/OT/PT	Decrease spasticity, strengthen and improve balance, improve trunk stability, gait training, gaiting aids, practice on ward, evaluate environment (hospital, home, work) for safety, accessibility, wheelchair evaluation, training
Activities of daily living/community skills	Efficient and safe self-care Energy conservation Access to community	Driver education/nurse/OT/PT/recreation†	Transfers, balance, bed mobility, home equipment, new skills, adaptive equipment, energy conservation, and practice on ward, at home and on supervised recreational outing
Bowel dysfunction	Regularity without constipation, diarrhea, incontinence	Dietitian/MD/nurse/OT/PT	Diet, decrease constipating medications, manage bladder program, sitting balance, transfers, hand function, increase daily activity
Bladder dysfunction	Freedom from incontinence and infection	MD/urologist/nurse/OT/PT°	Evaluation, medication, teach bladder program, sitting/standing balance, transfers, hand function, treat infections
Sexual dysfunction	Compensation/education	Counselor/MD/urologist/OT/PT	Evaluation, education, mobility, balance, decrease spasticity, contractures, hand function, bowel and bladder control, compensatory techniques, prosthesis, support, self-image
Dysarthria	Improve communication Maintain functional communication Compensation Energy conservation	Nurse/OT/PT/speech	Retraining, teach others to listen, abdominal breathing exercises, oral exercises, decrease spasticity, practice on ward, communication boards, hand function for boards
Dysphagia	Nutrition Safety Energy conservation	Dietitian/MD/nurse/OT/speech	Diet, patient and family training and education, evaluation of alternative routes of nutrition if needed
Adjustment/motivation	Facilitate adjustment Appropriate independence/dependence Prevent isolation Stress management	Biofeedback/counselor/MD/nurse/OT/PT/recreation/speech	Supportive counseling, alternative goals, success at valued tasks, improved ability to communicate, antidepressant medication, biofeedback/relaxation, positive social/recreational experiences
Medical complication: decubitus ulcer	Prevent/treat	Dietitian/MD/nurse/OT/PT	Evaluate, educate patient and family, strengthen and position, decrease spasticity, improve nutrition, protective equipment, correct contractures
Medical complication: contractures	Prevent/decrease	MD/nurse/OT/PT/surgeon	Stretching, positioning, educate patient and family, equipment, strengthen, surgical release
Medical complication: nutrition	Maximize nutrition Avoid fads	Dietitian/MD/nurse/OT/PT	Evaluate, educate, train in swallowing, body position, hand control, treat depression, proper diet

Table continued on following page

T A B L E   2 0 – 1.   Examples of Team Interaction on Common MS Problems *Continued*

Problem	Goals	Team*	Plan
Medical complication: respiratory problems	Improve breath control Avoid respiratory illness	MD/nurse/PT	Breathing exercises, improve posture, increase activity, medical care if needed
Vocation Family adjustment Avocation Home-making	Best and most interesting job and recreation available Strengthen family Mobilize community resources	Counselor/MD/nurse/OT/ PT/recreation/speech/ vocation counselor	Physical skills, motivation, help to overcome environmental barriers, build bridges to community resources, counseling

°Team members are listed in alphabetical order.
†MD, physicians; OT, occupational therapist; PT, physical therapist; speech, speech/language phatologist; biofeedback technician; recreation, recreation therapist.
From Maloney FP: Interdisciplinary Rehabilitation of Multiple Sclerosis and Neuromuscular Disorders. Philadelphia, JB Lippincott, 1985.

Other generic measures can help provide a broad picture of functional and clinical status.[51] Many MS clinical centers have developed their own screening measures that draw from the various tools just indicated. The Consortium of MS Centers, representing MS Clinical Centers in the US and Canada, is an excellent resource to network with these MS centers. The consortium may be reached at (201) 837-0727 or on the worldwide web at www.cmsc.org.

Setting Goals

A statement from *A Manual on Multiple Sclerosis* summarizes important guidelines in setting goals[3, p34]:

In every rehabilitation program, the patient must be treated as a whole, the best physical and psychological condition under the circumstances must be achieved, complications eliminated as far as possible and realistic motivations exploited. This can only be accomplished by the well-coordinated teamwork of doctors, nurses, physiotherapists, occupational therapists, clinical psychologists, social workers, the patient and his family and friends, and organizations with a genuine interest and sense of responsibility for him.

The ideal rehabilitation model acknowledges the client's responsibility and resources. It recognizes both the client's and family members' priorities and values; it considers not only the home environment but also community resources, medical issues, history of the disease, and the cognitive and affective status of the individual. Frequently in MS, the therapist's role is one of support in helping the patient solve problems to improve the quality of his or her interactions with the environment as opposed to offering therapeutic activities designed to restore function or ability per se. Problem solving and education are key aspects of the rehabilitation process in MS, particularly since restoration of abilities and reversal of clinical symptoms may not be realistic expectations.

Therefore, the overriding principle in setting rehabilitation goals is to maximize independence, self-determination, and quality of life within the context of the individual's lifestyle and abilities (see the box on page 609).[28] Vital to achieving these goals, however, is concordance between the therapist's and patient's expectations. Unrealistic expectations and discrepancies between what "improvement" and "getting better" means to the therapist and

to the patient can lead to a disappointing rehabilitation experience.

Often, for more stable or clear-cut disabilities, goals are set according to a functional skill such as ambulatory or wheelchair level. This may not be appropriate for clients with MS. A large number may be ambulatory for short distances but require a wheelchair for more demanding tasks. Additionally, for periods of exacerbation, training in wheelchair mobility may be a temporary, yet important necessity. The variations in MS confirm the need for ongoing reestablishment of goals in response to therapy and to changes in the client's condition, home environment, patient priorities, and the family situation.

Fatigue

Fatigue is the most common MS symptom: 75% to 95% report experiencing fatigue, and 50% to 60% report fatigue as their worst symptom. It can cause significant disability, even in those with few other symptoms.[13] Fatigue is a major reason for unemployment in MS. Because of its impact on the workforce, fatigue is listed as a cause of MS disability in the Social Security Administration impairment guidelines. As an invisible symptom, friends, family, or employers frequently misunderstand fatigue. The pathophysiological basis for MS fatigue is not well understood and most likely has biological, emotional, environmental, pharmacological, and lifestyle origins.

The factors contributing to fatigue are fatigue due to sleep deprivation (sleep disturbance secondary to urinary frequency or muscle spasms is common in MS), fatigue due to poor diet, deconditioning fatigue (loss of aerobic capacity, endurance, and muscle tone secondary to inactivity), fatigue of handicap (more effortful and inefficient approaches to accomplishing daily activities secondary to ataxia, weakness, spasticity, and so on), fatigue associated with depression, neuromuscular fatigue (more energy consumption by demyelinated axons), and fatigue of MS (some researchers and clinicians describe a lassitude that is unique to MS that worsens as the day progresses and prevents sustained physical activity).

Rise in body temperature, as little as 0.1 degree Fahrenheit in body temperature during the course of the day, may affect nerve conduction velocity, resulting in increased fatigue. Emotional stress has also been cited as associated with worsening of fatigue.

SPECIFIC SCORING OF THE DISABILITY SCALE: KURTZKE SCALE (DSS)

0 = Normal neurological examination (all grade 0 in functional groups).

1 = No disability, minimal signs (Babinski, minimal finger-to-nose ataxia, diminished vibration sense) (grade 1 in functional groups).

2 = Minimal disability—slight weakness or stiffness, mild disturbance of gait, or mild visuomotor disturbance (1 or 2 functional grade 2).

3 = Moderate disability—monoparesis, mild hemiparesis, moderate ataxia, disturbing sensory loss, or prominent urinary or eye symptoms, or combinations of lesser dysfunctions (1 or 2 functional grade 3 or several grade 2).

4 = Relatively severe disability not preventing ability to work or carry on normal activities of living, excluding sexual function. This includes the ability to be up and about 12 hours a day (1 functional grade 4 or several grade 3 or less).

5 = Disability severe enough to preclude working, with maximal motor function walking unaided up to several blocks (1 functional grade 5 alone, or combination of lesser).

6 = Assistance (canes, crutches, braces) required for walking (1 functional grade 6 alone or combination of lesser).

7 = Restricted to wheelchair—able to wheel self and enter and leave chair alone (combinations with at least 1 above functional grade 4).

8 = Restricted to bed but with effective use of arms (combinations usually functional grade 4 or above in several functional groups).

9 = Totally helpless bed patient (combinations usually functional grade 4 or above in most functional groups).

10 = Death due to multiple sclerosis.

From Kurtzke JF: On the evaluation of disability in multiple sclerosis. Neurology 11:688, 1961.

---

to assess outcomes of intervention. Employing energy conservation techniques, using adaptive equipment and assistive technology, and planning exercise and rest activities may compensate for fatigue. Adapting the work environment for energy conservation often allows the MS patient to continue employment. In addition, exercise to increase general endurance, cardiovascular health, and overall conditioning may address this symptom. Pharmacological intervention includes amantadine, pemoline, and

ASPECTS OF QUALITY OF LIFE

Psychophysiological Equilibrium

- Understanding of the disease, the symptoms, and how to manage them
- Understanding of limitations and strengths; functioning up to but respecting limits
- Maintenance of function with minimum effort and maximum safety (balancing rest and activity appropriately)
- Functional improvement despite persistent neurological signs
- Return to preexacerbation physical status
- Altering environment to support independence, diminish disability
- Wellness lifestyle
- Mastery over potential uncertainty and loss of control

Interrelatedness

- Realistic expectations for patient and family
- Preservation of family unit
- Learning new ways to fulfill family/friendship roles
- Knowing and practicing how to be realistically independent—not being a burden—but also being able to communicate when and how help is needed
- Avoiding social isolation
- Knowing and appropriately using community resources

Productivity

- Developing alternative plans to already established vocational goals (job, education, other training)
- Establishing a productive life (paid or volunteer)

Creativity

- Developing problem-solving skills
- Developing avocational interests
- Reaching important life goals; focusing on remaining possibilities
- Developing an enjoyable, personally meaningful life (MS not being the focus of one's life)

Adapted from Maloney FP, et al: Interdisciplinary Rehabilitation of Multiple Sclerosis and Neuromuscular Disorders, Philadelphia, JB Lippincott, 1985.

Because MS fatigue is multidimensional, so, too, is the approach to fatigue management, addressing the various contributing factors. In 1999, the Multiple Sclerosis Council for Clinical Practice[35] developed an algorithm intended to guide clinicians in the evaluation and treatment of MS fatigue. The guidelines include several self-report measures, a daily activity log, and sleep questionnaire to guide assessment. The Modified Fatigue Impact Scale (MFIS), a component of the MSQLI,[12] is used

4-aminopyridine (AP) and 3,4-aminopyridine (DAP). Also, cooling may be beneficial in reducing fatigue and aerobic exercise may help to improve fatigue in some individuals.

Weakness

Decreased strength results from several causes: upper motor neuron weakness, fatigue, disuse, or overriding spasticity in an antagonistic muscle. To enhance function in weak muscles, active assistive exercise, active exercise, and/or resistive exercise should be incorporated into a daily program. Proprioceptive neuromuscular facilitation (PNF) techniques may increase the benefit of assisted, active, and resisted exercise. Although strengthening exercises will not alter neurological status, compensatory strengthening of nonaffected muscle groups, preventing weakness secondary to disuse, and strengthening agonistic muscles to overcome spasticity in antagonistic muscle groups may improve function.

If compensatory strengthening proves to be limited in improving mobility, bracing may be effective in reducing gait abnormalities and improve the individual's ability to function with less effort. Ankle-foot orthoses (AFOs) are used to stabilize the ankle and compensate for footdrop and are commonly used for MS gait problems. Other orthotics also may compensate for weakness in both upper and lower extremities. See the box below for general principles of a strengthening program.[46]

Spasticity

In managing spasticity, the therapist should consider reflex dominance, hypertonicity, and abnormal movement. A stretching routine may be beneficial and should allow for slow elongation of the muscle through relaxation. The application of cold has been useful in some cases in reducing hypertonicity, as have other inhibitory relaxation techniques, including joint approximation, slow rolling from supine to side, slow rocking, slow stroking of the paravertebral muscles, and pressure on the tendinous insertion of the spastic muscle (see Chapter 4).

Reflex-inhibiting movement patterns and positioning (side lying) may inhibit abnormal postural reflex mechanisms (e.g., asymmetrical tonic neck reflex or tonic labyrinthine reflex and abnormal movements). Additionally, the use of functional exercise and weight bearing performed in various spatial positions may be helpful in

---

GENERAL PRINCIPLES OF A STRENGTHENING PROGRAM

The following are common principles to remember while implementing a strengthening program:

1. Unaffected muscle groups should be maximally strengthened to allow maximal use of compensation techniques that involve unaffected limbs.
2. Use adaptive devices (i.e., canes and crutches) to allow the patient to remain ambulatory longer and maintain functional strength levels as long as possible.
3. Strengthening exercises must be safe and efficacious. Therapists must teach the patient a judicious balance between rest and exercise.
4. The patient should progress through the strengthening program very slowly. For example, if s/he is starting at 8–10 repetition (reps) of each exercise, s/he can increase 1–2 reps every 2–3 weeks, to 20–25 reps. One- to two-pound weights may then be added and the reps decreased to 8–10, with the progression starting over. This slow increase in progression accompanied by good compliance will lead to successful strengthening. A cool atmosphere allows for more efficient exercise, because MS patients are often highly sensitive to heat.
5. Home programs for these exercises are essential; the effectiveness of any exercise program depends on its being carried out on an ongoing basis.

6. Before strengthening, stretching exercises should be performed to decrease spasticity, increase flexibility, and increase blood flow to the area.
7. To improve functional strength, exercises should be performed at submaximal resistance with frequent repetitions.
8. Emphasis should be placed on proximal strengthening to decrease energy consumption during functional activities.
9. Large fluid movements to enhance coordination should be used.
10. If a patient has difficulty initiating movement, try starting with large body/trunk movements, then moving from proximal to distal.
11. Light weights may help stabilization if a patient has significant tremors.
12. Combining strengthening exercises with aerobic, balance, and/or spasticity-reducing exercises whenever possible will maximize benefits within the patient's exercise tolerance.
13. Avoid excessive fatigue of a muscle: 1–5-minute rest periods throughout the exercise session will facilitate recovery of neurotransmission.
14. Set realistic goals and expectations with the patient. Be creative, realistic, and simplistic. The more enjoyable the exercises, the better the compliance.

From Schapiro R: Multiple Sclerosis: A Rehabilitation Approach to Management, New York, Demos Publications, 1991.

normalizing movement. Daily active and passive range of motion (ROM) exercises will help maintain joint range. Training in self-ROM and encouragement of participation in functional tasks will aid in the prevention of contractures. Severe ROM limitations may require surgical intervention such as myotenotomy. Medications, as discussed earlier, may augment physical treatment. (For additional information see Chapter 32.)

Balance and Coordination

Cerebellar problems are common in MS and difficult to manage. Ataxia, incoordination, dysmetria, and tremor that becomes exaggerated with movement may be present in both the extremities and trunk. Treatment sequences in functional activities may help improve balance in various positions. Progress is made from a wide to narrow base of support, from static to dynamic activities, and from a low to a high center of gravity. Additionally, strengthening the fixation musculature, using visual cues, and biofeedback may improve balance and lessen tremor. For the most part, however, treatment is compensatory. Use of adaptive equipment in ADLs, weighted cuffs to reduce tremor, or weighted canes to reduce ataxia may prove useful. The use of weighted cuffs may increase the imbalance, however, and, once removed, exaggerate the problem. Also, increased fatigue related to the extra weights may contraindicate their use. Tremors of the head and neck may be controlled with a collar or brace. Tremors in MS are frequently exaggerated by stress. Drug treatment, as discussed earlier, may augment compensatory training techniques but frequently has an unwanted sedating effect.

Sensory Dysfunction

Impaired sensation is frequently a problem in MS. Treatment is aimed at compensating for the loss, maximizing safety, and increasing awareness of the sensory impairment. Inability to perceive temperature or pain must be attended to by training in visual compensation and safety techniques. Routine skin inspection, particularly where there is significant immobility, should be taught, appropriate wheelchair cushioning or mattresses provided, and pressure relief techniques taught. Unpleasant dysesthesias, such as burning or tight banding sensations, may respond to cold applications. Medication, such as corticosteroids, phenytoin (Dilantin), amitriptyline (Elavil), or carbamazepine (Tegretol), may be useful if sensations are painful or interfere with function.

Dysarthria and Dysphagia

Fatigue, weakness, tremors, incoordination, and abnormal tone may contribute to imprecise articulation, vocal harshness, slurring, changes in rate of speech, hypernasality, and other problems in oral communication. After evaluation, speech therapy generally focuses on compensating for dysfunction. Specific techniques of speech therapy include using pauses to improve speech that is slurred, rapid, and runs together; exaggerating articulation; reducing phrase length; increasing voice volume;

using oral exercise to maximize ROM and strength of oral musculature; and using augmentative communication devices including writing, computer-driven systems, communication boards, and pointing. Those who have motor difficulties, however, may be limited in the use of some of these methods. Frequently, a referral to a speech therapist is not made until severe dysarthria or dysphagia is present. Early intervention, as with all rehabilitation therapies, increases the potential for minimizing dysfunction.

Treatment for dysphagia focuses on body positioning (to prevent aspiration), style of eating "think swallow" (a conscious swallow as opposed to relying on reflexive swallowing), and food and liquid selection (semisoft, moist foods and thick liquids with progression to more challenging foods). Because fatigue can exacerbate swallowing problems, larger meals taken earlier in the day followed by smaller meals later may be easier to manage. Placement of feeding tubes may be required if a practical degree of swallowing cannot be achieved.

Ambulation and Mobility

Weakness, spasticity, impaired sensation, ataxia and proprioception, problems with balance, fatigue, visual problems, and incoordination influence gait in MS patients. In addressing ambulation, trunk control and balance should be addressed first, followed by normalization of tone and maximizing flexibility and ROM. Gait is often more functional when strength can be improved in the trunk and extremities. Some patients also may require a graduated sitting tolerance program, tilt-table routine, and graduated standing tolerance schedule before specific gait training. Using visual and tactile cues may help compensate for sensory and proprioceptive loss. Prescription of specific ambulation aids can improve safety, decrease energy expenditure, and improve endurance. Upper-extremity strength and motor control, cognitive status, and emotional response to using the device must be considered in prescription. Bracing to improve ambulation should follow the guidelines outlined in the box on page 612.[46]

In wheelchair prescription, the goal is proper positioning to be sure the pelvis, spinal column, and limbs are in correct alignment and the patient is secure in the chair. Seating may be modified by the use of foam inserts, clamp-on side supports, and customized contour seating systems. Footrests should be adjusted so that the thighs are parallel to the floor. A seat belt should be used for safety. Functional training should include propulsion, retropulsion, and maneuvering in narrow areas and on various terrains. Manipulation of armrests, legrests, footrests, brakes, and other wheelchair accessories must be included in wheelchair mobility training. A reclining chair may be most effective for those with head, neck, and trunk instability. Electric wheelchairs may be necessary when fatigue, weakness, or tremors make independent propulsion of a manual chair impossible. Three-wheel scooters are used frequently by people with MS with adequate trunk stability and upper-extremity function. The three-wheeler also offers greater ease of dismantling and loading into a car than a traditional electric wheel-

BRACING

The most common braces used to brace the lower extremities in MS are standard polypropylene AFOs and those with an articulated joint. The following guidelines may be helpful.

A standard AFO is indicated if the patient exhibits

1. Consistent footdrop or toe drag
2. Poor knee control (especially hyperextension)
3. Weakness of grade 2 or 3 at the ankle with dorsiflexion testing
4. Minimal-to-moderate spasticity
5. Poor endurance in gait
6. Poor proprioception and sensory sense

The advantages of an AFO are that it

1. Saves energy during gait because the patient does not work as hard to clear his/her toes during the swing-through phase of the gait
2. Improves footdrop or toe drag during the swing phase of gait
3. Improves general safety during walking by avoiding many falls due to the toe drag
4. Provides more knee control during mid-stance phase of gait by avoiding hyperextension of the knee
5. Provides greater ankle stability
6. Improves the overall gait pattern
7. Provides better cosmesis for the patient

The advantages of the AFO with an articulating joint are

1. All of the above listed for the standard AFO.
2. It allows some mobility at the ankle joint. This permits a more natural movement at the ankle during gait, which looks more normal. It allows the patient to drive while wearing the brace and allows more freedom for squatting down to reach objects on the floor.
3. It provides a plantarflexion stop to prevent the foot from further plantarflexion during swing phase of gait.

4. It still allows for dorsiflexion assist and can be set up to 5 degrees of dorsiflexion to clear the foot during the swing-through phase.

Relative contraindications for these types of braces are

1. Moderate or severe spasticity in the lower extremities
2. Severe foot edema
3. Severe weakness (muscles grades 2 or less) at the hips

A double upright metal brace can provide some of the same advantages listed above and usually provides more adjustments for the ankle and the knee. However, this brace is usually not the preferred choice due to its weight and poorer cosmetic appearance.

The polypropylene AFOs may be set in a few degrees of dorsiflexion to provide better knee control. If hyperextension is severe, a Swedish hyperextension knee cage may be useful. In some people this device may be quite helpful, but it is decidedly more bulky and often moves down the leg, which decreases its effectiveness. Custom bracing of the knee can be the answer to this problem, because effective orthotics may make up for instability of the joints, tendons, and ligaments. This usually requires the skills of a trained orthotist and is a topic beyond the scope of this book.

Some therapists have found rocker clog shoes to be of some help for those few people who need to have the plantarflexed position neutralized while the curved forefoot sole will initiate knee flexion. A skilled therapist should determine if this situation is present before purchase of this device is recommended.

For additional information on bracing refer to Chapter 31.

From Schapiro R: Multiple Sclerosis: A Rehabilitation Approach to Management. New York, Demos Publications, 1991.

---

chair. Many people with MS find that the three-wheeled scooter carries less of a stigma and is more convenient than a traditional wheelchair. Cushion prescription to minimize skin breakdown and discomfort should be made with regard to the patient's risk for developing these problems.

Cognitive Dysfunction

Cognitive problems in MS result from demyelination in the cerebral tracts that connect with primary sensory, motor, speech, and integration areas of the cerebrum.

This results in poor recognition of deficits as well as an inability to store and retrieve new information, a combination that may present a major impediment to rehabilitation.[43, 44, 48]

Rehabilitation strategies focus mostly on compensatory strategies, for instance using a memory book, electronic organizer, tape recorder, timers or alarms, or "ticker files." In therapy, deficits in judgment, logical analysis, reasoning, and self-monitoring may require the use of clear, written, sequenced steps for exercises or adapted methods of performing ADL, transfers, and ambulation. The therapist should be aware that what may appear to be low motivation or poor compliance in therapy may be the interference of cognitive deficits.

It is important to remember that people with MS are as varied as the population and that there is not an "MS personality." Additionally, age, severity of disability, and duration of illness are not good predictors of cognitive or affective changes.

Given this information, many with MS would derive benefit from a neuropsychological evaluation. Such an evaluation could be helpful in several ways:

- The person with MS as well as family members can gain a better understanding of the nature and extent of the illness.
- The evaluation can identify impaired and intact functions.
- The evaluation may assist the person in developing realistic vocational and other life goals.
- The results can clarify misconceptions on the part of others who may incorrectly attribute cognitive problems to uncooperative or oppositional behavior
- The results can suggest compensatory techniques.

General Conditioning and Fitness

A reduction in physical activity because of MS limitations may result in a general reduction in overall fitness. This reduction is characterized by the following[46]:

- Increased neuromuscular tension
- Increased pulse rate at rest
- Decreased adrenocortical reserve
- Decreased muscular strength
- Decreased vital capacity at rest
- Decreased maximal vital capacity
- Increased fatigue
- Increased anxiety
- Increased depression

A physical conditioning program is not likely to have an impact on the course of MS. It is likely, however, that enhanced overall health and fitness can improve a sense of well-being, reduce fatigue, improve mood, and reduce the other secondary effects of inactivity.[19] With attention to raising body temperature, incoordination, cycles of fatigue, and safety, a conditioning program geared to the individual can offer a sense of control over some aspects of health and improve the quality of life. Aerobic exercises such as swimming, walking, stationary bikes, and rowers may be appropriate for some patients. Swimming and other water exercise can be ideal for those with MS, especially if water temperature can be maintained to avoid overheating. All patients should have a cardiovascular examination by a physician before starting an aerobic program. This is an area that should be addressed even when there are no obvious signs of disability and should be modified according to ability thereafter.

Activities of Daily Living

Functional improvement or maintenance of functional independence is a key goal of the rehabilitation program. Carryover of therapeutic exercise, mat exercises, and am-

bulation training to ADL tasks is vital. In addition, specific training in techniques of dressing, bathing, toileting, personal hygiene, feeding, and bed mobility can improve or maintain independence in ADL. Adaptive equipment can be used to conserve energy and compensate for weakness and incoordination. For example, weighted silverware and plate guards can compensate for tremor and incoordination in self-feeding. Button hooks, reachers, stocking aids, and Velcro may improve independence in dressing. Transfer training should be incorporated into functional activities. The use of sliding board, hydraulic lift, or assistance from another individual must be geared to the client's ability and priorities regarding expenditure of energy.

Adapted tools for communication skills (i.e., writing or typing), such as built-up pencils, keyboard shield, adapted keyboard, or universal cuffs, may assist communication. Homemaking tasks and child care from a wheelchair level, ambulatory-assisted level, or ambulatory level can be practiced with the aid of assistive devices and energy conservation techniques.

Driving often presents problems for the individual with MS. Diplopia or blurred vision, decreased coordination, weakness, and spasticity may interfere with safe driving or require the use of hand controls or adapted vehicle. Perceptual and cognitive considerations must be made in a predriving evaluation or in driver training along with physical assessment.

Employment

It is estimated that 90% of people with MS have worked at some point in their lives and 65% were working at the time of diagnosis. However, only 25% to 35% remain in the workforce 5 to 10 years after diagnosis.[46] Many leave employment prematurely, perhaps under the advice of a health care provider or well-meaning family member during an acute exacerbation or for fear of disclosing their diagnosis at work, fear of asking for accommodation, or ignorance of their rights under the Americans with Disabilities Act. People who leave the workforce most commonly cite fatigue, cognitive dysfunction, visual problems, bowel and bladder dysfunction, and mobility problems as barriers to keeping working.[46] Often, the rehabilitation team can be of help in assessing how symptoms might be effectively managed at the workplace and accommodations made to help the individual retain employment. Common, reasonable accommodations for MS include part-time or flex-time schedule, work-at-home options, accessible work environment (e.g., bathrooms, desk), special transportation, memory aids (e.g., day planners, tape recorders), vision aids (e.g., voice recognition software, large print materials, voice mail), an office close to the elevator and/or restroom, hands-free telephone devices, air conditioning, wheeled carts for transporting files, and mobility aids (e.g., scooters, walkers, wheelchairs). The therapist can play an important role in both helping the individual to retain employment as well as to make decisions regarding retirement, career change, or temporary leave of absence.

Psychosocial Issues

The challenges of MS are formidable and ongoing. Despite new drug treatments, MS remains an incurable disease with an uncertain prognosis. While many individuals and families cope quite effectively with the disease, the incidence of depression is high, and the impact on family and marital relationships, finances, work life, and social activities of the individual is pervasive.

The meaning of illness or disability in a family relates to culture, religion, and personal values and beliefs. For some, disability is associated with personal weakness, imperfection, and asexuality. For others, illness may be seen as a growth-inspiring experience, one that provides new insights and awareness of priorities. We also are influenced strongly by the viewpoints of our friends, family, medical caregivers, and rehabilitation team members. The attitudes and beliefs of the therapist about disability are important to examine because therapists may communicate these beliefs in subtle ways to their patients.

Helping families cope with MS may involve an examination of their premorbid patterns of dealing with stress, conflict, and tragedy. Often, MS magnifies preexisting problems and tensions so that families who present "MS-generated" problems may have had these problems well before the diagnosis was made.

The relationship among attitude, psyche, and physical wellness or disease is well documented.[4, 39, 47] Although stress cannot be implicated in causing exacerbations per se, the ability to manage stress can positively influence overall health and well being. To treat the body without adequate consideration of the accompanying psychological, spiritual, and social issues would be an injustice.

SUMMARY

MS is a chronic and often progressive disease of the CNS, characterized by disseminated patches of demyelination in the brain and spinal cord, resulting in multiple and varied neurological symptoms and signs. Destruction of myelin, accompanied by edema and inflammation and followed by tissue scarring and axonal damage, appears to be the underlying cause that impedes or prevents neurotransmission.

The clinical diagnosis of MS depends on evidence of two or more distinct CNS lesions, of symptoms and signs that have appeared in distinct episodes or have progressed over time, and the exclusion of other neurological explanations. Laboratory and electrophysiological tests provide support of a clinical diagnosis; however, at the present time no test is pathognomonic for MS.

The course of the disease is characterized by an unpredictable course of exacerbations and remissions in some cases, progressive disability over time in other cases, or a combination of the two, often accompanied by periods of disease stability.

The etiology of MS appears to be an autoimmune process in which myelin is destroyed. The trigger of this abnormal immune response is unknown, although a viral cause is probable.

Treatment of MS has improved with the availability of several disease-modifying agents (Avonex, Betaseron, and Copaxone), which appear to reduce the relapse rate and slow progression of disability in some patients. Sympto-

matic therapies and treatment of acute MS exacerbations are also effective. Many other therapeutic agents are under investigation, and the future of MS treatment is bright. Rehabilitative measures, including physical, occupational, and speech therapy, do not appear to alter the underlying pathology of the disease. Therefore, the overriding principle in setting rehabilitation goals for a person with MS is to maximize functional independence, minimize complications and problems secondary to decreased mobility, compensate for loss of function, and maximize quality of life. Psychosocial adjustment, vocational disposition, and family issues merit significant attention by the treatment team, because MS generates tremendous need in these areas.

REFERENCES

1. Alter M, et al: Migration and risk of multiple sclerosis. Neurology 28:1089, 1978.
2. Aronson KJ, et al: Sociodemographic characteristics and health status of persons with multiple sclerosis and their caregivers. MS Management 3:1, 1996.
3. Bauer H: A Manual on Multiple Sclerosis. Vienna, International Federation of Multiple Sclerosis Societies, 1977.
4. Benson H: The Mind/Body Effect. New York, Simon & Schuster, 1979.
5. Catanzaro M: Nursing care of the person with MS. Am J Nurs 80(2):286, 1980.
6. Challoner PB, et al: Plaque-associated expression of human herpes virus 6 in multiple sclerosis. Proc Natl Acad Sci U S A 92:7440, 1995.
7. Cook S: Handbook of Multiple Sclerosis. New York, Marcel Dekker, 1990.
8. Dean G: The multiple sclerosis problem. Sci Am 223(1):40, 1970.
9. Dimitrijevuc MR, Sherwood AM: Spasticity—medical and surgical treatment. Neurology 30(7 pt 2):19, 1980.
10. Eastwood A: Genes and MS Susceptibility. NMSS Fact Sheet. New York, National Multiple Sclerosis Society, 1999.
11. Ellison GW, Myers LW: Immunosuppressive drugs in multiple sclerosis: Pro and con. Neurology 30(7 pt 2):28, 1980.
12. Fischer JS, et al: Recent developments in the assessment of quality of life in multiple sclerosis. Multiple Sclerosis 5:251, 1999.
13. Freal JF, et al: Symptomatic fatigue in multiple sclerosis. Arch Phys Med Rehabil 65:135, 1984.
14. Freeman JA, et al: In-patient rehabilitation in multiple sclerosis: Do the benefits carry over into the community. Neurology 52:50, 1999.
15. Giesser B: Hormones in Multiple Sclerosis. Fact Sheet. New York, National Multiple Sclerosis Society, 1999.
16. Granger CV, et al: Functional assessment scales: A study of persons with multiple sclerosis. Arch Phys Med Rehabil 71:870, 1990.
17. Halper J, Holland N: Comprehensive Nursing Care in Multiple Sclerosis. New York, Demos Vermande, 1996.
18. Halper J, Holland N: Multiple Sclerosis in 1998: An Interactive Teleconference. New York, National Multiple Sclerosis Society, December 9–10, 1998.
19. Hutchinson B, et al: Increased physical fitness and emotional state with increased disability in multiple sclerosis. Poster presentation. Kansas City, MO, Consortium of MS Centers, 1999.
20. Johnson KP: Cerebrospinal fluid and blood assays of diagnostic usefulness in multiple sclerosis. Neurology 30(2):107, 1980.
21. Kurtzke JF: On the evaluation of disability in multiple sclerosis. Neurology 11:686, 1961.
22. Kurtzke JF, Hyllested K: Multiple sclerosis in the Faroe Islands: I. Clinical and epidemiological features. Ann Neurol 5:6, 1979.
23. Laban MM, et al: Physical and occupational therapy in the treatment of patients with multiple sclerosis. Phys Med Rehabil Clin North Am 9:603, 1998.
24. Langdon DW, Thompson AJ: Multiple sclerosis: A preliminary study of selected variables affecting rehabilitation outcome. Multiple Sclerosis 5:94, 1999.
25. LaRocca N, Kalb R: Efficacy of rehabilitation in multiple sclerosis. J NeuroRehab 6:147, 1992.

26. Lisak RP: Multiple sclerosis: Evidence for immunopathogenesis. Neurology 30(2):99, 1980.
27. Lublin F, Reingold S: Defining the course of multiple sclerosis. Neurology 46:907, 1996.
28. Maloney FP, et al: Interdisciplinary rehabilitation of multiple sclerosis and other neuromuscular disorders. Philadelphia, JB Lippincott, 1985.
29. McAlpine D, et al: Multiple Sclerosis, 4th ed. Edinburgh, Churchill Livingstone, 1985.
30. Miller DH, et al: Serial gadolinium enhanced MRI in multiple sclerosis. Brain 111:927, 1988.
31. Minden SL, et al: Depression in multiple sclerosis. Gen Hosp Psychiatry 9:426, 1987.
32. Minden SL, Schiffer R: Affective disorders in multiple sclerosis. Arch Neurol 47:98, 1990.
33. Mohr D, et al: Depression, coping and neurological impairment in multiple sclerosis. Multiple Sclerosis 3:254, 1997.
34. Multiple Sclerosis Council for Clinical Practice Guidelines: Urinary dysfunction and multiple sclerosis: Evidence-based strategies for urinary dysfunction in multiple sclerosis. Washington, DC, Paralyzed Veterans of America, 1999.
35. Multiple Sclerosis Council for Clinical Practice Guidelines: Fatigue and multiple sclerosis: Evidence-based strategies for fatigue and multiple sclerosis. Washington, DC, Paralyzed Veterans of America, 1998.
36. Neufeld P: Wellness Course Efficacy with MS. Washington University School of Medicine poster presentation. Kansas City, MO, Consortium of MS Centers, 1999.
37. Paty DW, Ebers GC: Multiple Sclerosis. Philadelphia, FA Davis, 1998.
38. Paty DW, et al: Interferon beta-1b is effective in relapsing-remitting multiple sclerosis. Neurology 43:655, 1993.
39. Pelettier KL: Mind as Healer, Mind as Slayer. New York, Dell, 1977.
40. Percy AK, et al: MS in Rochester, Minn: A 60-year appraisal. Arch Neurol 25:105, 1971.
41. Peyser JM, et al: Cognitive function in patients with multiple sclerosis. Arch Neurol 37:577, 1980.
42. Poser C, et al: The Diagnosis of Multiple Sclerosis. New York, Thieme-Stratton, 1984.
43. Rao SM: Neuropsychology of multiple sclerosis: A critical review. J Clin Exp Neuropsychol 8:503, 1986.
44. Rao SM, et al: Cognitive dysfunction in multiple sclerosis. Arch Neurol 41:685, 1991.
45. Rolak R: The History of Multiple Sclerosis. New York, National Multiple Sclerosis Society, 1996.
46. Rumrill P: Employment Issues and Multiple Sclerosis. New York, Demos Publications, 1996.
47. Schapiro R: Multiple Sclerosis: A Rehabilitation Approach to Management. New York, Demos Publications, 1991.
48. Schapiro R: Symptom Management in Multiple Sclerosis, 3rd ed. New York, Demos Publications, 1998.
49. Schiffer RB, Slater RJ: Neuropsychiatric features of multiple sclerosis: Recognition and management. Semin Neurol 5:127, 1985.
50. Sibley W: Therapeutic Claims in Multiple Sclerosis. New York, Demos Publications, 1992.
51. Slater RJ, et al: Minimal Record of Disability for Multiple Sclerosis. New York, National Multiple Sclerosis Society, 1985.
52. Solari A, et al: Physical rehabilitation has a positive effect on disability in multiple sclerosis patients. Neurology 52:57, 1999.
53. Surridge D: Psychiatric aspects of multiple sclerosis. Br J Psychol 115:5245, 1969.
54. Trapp BD, et al: Axonal transection in the lesions of multiple sclerosis. N Engl J Med 338:278, 1998.
55. Waksman BH, et al: Research on Multiple Sclerosis, 3rd ed. New York, Demos Publications, 1987.
56. Weiner H, et al: Double blind trial of oral tolerization with myelin antigens in multiple sclerosis. Science 259:1321, 1993.
57. Williams A, et al: An investigation of multiple sclerosis in twins. Neurology 30:1139, 1980.
58. Yetkin FZ, et al: Multiple sclerosis: Specificity of MR for diagnosis. Radiology 178:447, 1997.

Balance and Vestibular Disorders

LESLIE ALLISON, MS, PT • KENDA FULLER, PT, NCS

Key Words

- anticipatory postural responses
- automatic postural responses
- balance
- base of support
- center of gravity (COG)
- disability
- impairment
- limit of stability
- motor learning stages
- sensory conflict
- sensory environment
- strategies
- systems model or systems approach
- volitional postural movements

Objectives

After reading this chapter the student/therapist will:

1. Understand the relationship between impairments and disabilities.

2. List common postural control impairments found in neurological clients.

3. Describe both central and peripheral sensory and motor components of the postural control system.

4. Understand the function of the vestibular system in balance activities.

5. List commonly used balance tests.

6. Understand how test results are used to identify impairments and disabilities.

7. Know the stages of motor learning.

8. Understand the interaction of individual, task, and environmental factors that affect balance.

9. Describe how to progress balance exercise programs to increase the use of, or compensation with, available sensory inputs.

10. Describe how to progress balance exercise programs to increase the control of center of gravity in upright postures.

11. Describe how to progress exercise programs to promote habituation to reduce dizziness.

12. Describe how to facilitate adaptation and central nervous system reorganization to regain control of balance and decrease dizziness.

No matter what the neurological diagnosis, a disease or injury that affects the nervous system is likely to compromise one or more of the postural control mechanisms. Clients with stroke, head trauma, spinal cord injury, peripheral neuropathy, multiple sclerosis, Parkinson's disease, cerebellar dysfunction, cerebral palsy, Guillain-Barré syndrome, and so on all experience disequilibrium problems. The common thread among all of these different diagnoses is the presence of balance impairments. Clients with different diagnoses may have the same balance impairments; clients with the same diagnosis may have different balance impairments, depending on which portions of the postural control system are involved.[2] To optimally understand and manage balance problems, an evaluation of each balance component and the interactive nature of the components is important. The traditional medical "diagnostic" model does not provide this information and is not the most beneficial model for balance rehabilitation interventions. The diagnosis is relevant: it is critical, for example, to know whether deficits are permanent or temporary or whether recovery or progressive decline is expected. This prognostic information will assist in goal setting and intervention planning.

An alternative model, which better explains balance disorders, is the concept of "impairment" and "disability" described by the World Health Organization (see Chapter 1, Fig. 1–1). This disablement model has been adopted by the American Physical Therapy Association and applied specifically to the rehabilitation of clients with neuromuscular disorders in "The Guide to Physical Therapist Practice,"[62] Impairments are problems that result from the diagnosis, such as the loss of strength, sensation, or flexibility that may follow a stroke. Disabilities are the functional limitations that result from the impairments (i.e., "unable to walk" or "needs moderate assistance to transfer"). Therapists perform functional tests (e.g., transfers, walking, lifting) to determine whether treatment is indicated and, if so, what tasks need to be learned. They also strive to identify neuromusculoskeletal problems through the assessment of strength, sensation, range of motion (ROM), and so on to discern what impairments are causing the reduced function. To improve the functional level of their clients, therapists treat both impairments and disabilities. For example, weakness of the quadriceps may interfere with the ability to rise from a chair; sufficient strength in the quadriceps will contribute to the independent achievement of standing. Treatment might include both strengthening exercises and practice of sit-to-stand tasks from different surfaces.

Balance impairments negatively affect function, leading to disability.[21] These impairments often restrict activity levels, produce abnormal compensatory motor behavior, and may require support from devices or assistance from others. When imbalance is severe, falls can result, leading to secondary injuries. To avoid these consequences and advance the functional status of their clients, therapists should understand both the demands that various environments and functional tasks place on postural control systems and the impairments that may diminish the ability of those systems to respond adequately.

VESTIBULAR DISORDERS

Within the larger overview of "balance deficits," vestibular disorders form a specific subset. Problems in this crucial system can have significant impact on function. Dizziness, vertigo (sensation of spinning), imbalance, visual fatigue, and headache are symptoms that should alert the clinician to potential vestibular involvement. Diagnosis and intervention plans are established through a specialized set of tests and measures particular to this population of clients. Understanding how the vestibular system works is critical for the examiner to determine which of these tests to perform and to know how to use the acquired information to establish the appropriate balance exercises.[25]

Lesions of the vestibular system can be broadly categorized according to the area of dysfunction: the end-organ, the vestibular nerve terminals, the connections of the end-organ to the brain stem, and the higher centers of the cerebellum and the cerebrum (Table 21–1). Vestibular disorders may occur independently or in conjunction with other neurological disease or injury. The causes of lesions are varied and include infections, vascular disease, neoplasia, trauma, metabolic disorders, toxic drugs, and diseases of unknown etiology.[13]

The most common cause of dizziness associated with a vestibular disorder is viral infections. The virus can be preceded by a systemic illness or an upper respiratory tract infection, or it can be an isolated virus affecting the labyrinths. This causes an acute, severe dizziness as the brain is suddenly provided with abnormal information coming from the involved vestibular end-organ. The result is loss of normal postural reactions (described later) and the sensation of spinning known as vertigo. Infection caused by bacteria can also cause damage and should be treated by antibiotics.[5]

Traumatic brain injury (TBI) can impact the vestibular system in several ways. It can cause direct damage to the vestibular end-organ (in the temporal bone), benign positional vertigo (BPV), and, in many cases, disruption of the integration of the vestibular nuclei (in the brain stem) and cerebellum. Sensorimotor disturbances are common with TBI involving the cerebellum or parietal lobe. Visual dysfunction results from damage to brain stem areas such as the pontine gaze centers or central damage in the medial longitudinal fasciculus. Frequently, the third, fourth, or sixth cranial nerves are damaged, and this affects the ability to move the eyes for conjugate gaze. In some extensive TBI cases, the brain loses its

---

● **TABLE 21–1. Vestibular Pathways**

End-organ (labyrinth sensory receptors) → Vestibular nerve (cranial nerve VIII) collaterals → Vestibular nuclei and cerebellum → Central sensory tracts → cerebral hemispheres

The end-organ mechanically responds to movement of the head. This mechanical firing is turned into signals carried by the vestibular nerve. At the level of the vestibular nuclei, the information is integrated with information from the visual and somatosensory systems. The cerebellum calibrates vestibular reflexes and modulates the vestibular ocular reflex. This information is then carried along the central sensory tracts to the cerebral cortex.

ability to use any of the three sensory systems accurately. Dizziness and imbalance are prevalent complaints from these clients because there are often situations in which they cannot acquire accurate sensory information. Each system should be evaluated individually for its function. In clients with TBI, the adaptation of the vestibular system occurs more slowly and with more effort than for other clients with vestibular deficits. The client with vestibular problems associated with TBI requires significantly more intervention, and the outcomes are not as high, as with other clients experiencing vestibular dysfunction.[65]

Ischemia in the areas of the vestibular system (brain stem, cerebellum, parietal-insular cortex) can cause dizziness and imbalance. Vertebral basilar artery insufficiency syndrome, for example, classically produces these problems. Ischemia is usually seen in individuals older than the age of 50, but it can also be associated with bleeding disorders such as leukemia. Migraine headache can cause intermittent dizziness from compromise of blood flow in the areas of the vestibular system.

Neoplasia can compromise vestibular function when it occurs near any part of the vestibular system. Schwannoma (also known as acoustic neuroma) can cause damage as it slowly grows on the sheath of the vestibular nerve. The schwannoma can grow into the pontocerebellar angle and cause symptoms typically associated with cerebellar lesions. Meningiomas growing in the area of the temporal lobe can cause pressure on the vestibular mechanism. In some cases, damage to the vestibular nerve occurs with surgical removal of the encapsulated tumor.

Vertigo and dizziness are often reported with metabolic disorders such as diabetes. Autoimmune diseases such as rheumatoid arthritis, lupus, and human immunodeficiency syndrome (HIV) infection can also cause symptoms when the disease process damages components of the vestibular system.

Aminoglycosides, antibiotics used in cases of massive or systemic infection, can be ototoxic (causing damage to the vestibular hair cells). Although this side effect is suffered by only a small percentage of users, it can affect both sides of the bilateral vestibular apparatus and cause significant disability. Often the client does not begin to experience the symptoms until the medication has been used for more than a week. Other medications that are known to be ototoxic are listed in Table 21–2.

Persons who suffer from allergies are often predisposed to episodes of dizziness. Foods, airborne allergens, and chemicals can trigger dizziness in these individuals.

Meniere disease will cause intermittent vertigo associated with changes of the membranous fluid pressure within the labyrinths. When the fluid pressure changes, the brain receives abnormal signals from one of the labyrinths and the result is the sensation of spinning. The episode can last from just a few minutes to a day. The use of diuretics can sometimes control the fluid changes and decrease the number and intensity of symptoms. The clinical diagnosis of Meniere disease is related to the fact that the person has normal balance when not in episode, and there is often concurrent permanent loss of hearing.[3] Over time there appears to be a gradual degradation of

TABLE 21–2. Potential Ototoxic Medications

Aminoglycoside Antibiotics
Gentamycin
Amikacin
Streptomycin
Kanamycin
Tobramycin
Dihydrostreptomycin

Antineoplastics
Cisplatin
Bleomycin
Vincristine
Vinblastine

Diuretics
Furosemide
Bumetanide
Mannitol

Environmental Toxins
Toluene
Mercury
Tin
Lead
Carbon monoxide

the vestibular system; individuals with Meniere disease typically lose some vestibular function. This results in symptoms associated with chronic unilateral vestibular loss. These clients often develop a diffuse dizziness and complain of imbalance. Therapeutic intervention can improve the chronic dizziness and imbalance, although it cannot remedy the disease itself.

BALANCE

Definitions of Balance

Balance is a complex process involving the reception and integration of sensory inputs, and the planning and execution of movement, to achieve a goal requiring upright posture. It is the ability to control the center of gravity (COG) over the base of support in a given sensory environment.[51, 52] The COG is an imaginary point in space, calculated biomechanically from measured forces and moments, where the sum total of all the forces equals zero. In a normal person standing quietly, it is located just forward of the spine at about the S2 level. With movement of the body and its segments, the location of the COG in space will change constantly. The base of support is the body surface that experiences pressure as the result of body weight and gravity; in standing, it is the feet, in sitting, it is the thighs and buttocks. The size of the base of support will affect the difficulty level of the balancing task. A broad base of support makes the task easier; a narrow base makes it more challenging. The COG can travel farther while still remaining over the base if the base is large. The "shape" of the base of support will alter the distance that the COG can move in certain directions.

With any given base of support, there is a limit to the distance a body can move without either falling (as the

COG exceeds the base of support) or establishing a new base of support by reaching or stepping (to relocate the base of support under the COG). This perimeter is frequently referred to as the "limit of stability" or "stability limit."[37, 51] It is the farthest distance in any direction a person can lean (away from midline) without altering the original base of support by stepping, reaching, or falling.

Environmental Context

This biomechanical task (keeping the COG over the base of support) is always accomplished within an environmental context, which is detected by the sensory systems. The sensory environment is the set of conditions that exist, or are perceived to exist, in the external world that may affect balance. Peripheral sensory receptors gather information about the environment, body position in relation to the environment, and body segment positions in relation to the self. Central sensory structures process this information to perceive body orientation and spatial position and to determine the opportunities and limitations present in the environment. Gravity is one environmental condition that must be reckoned with to remain stable. For all except the astronauts, it is a constant condition. Surface and visual conditions, however, may vary significantly and may be stable or unstable. Unstable surface conditions might include the subway, a sandy beach, a gravel driveway, or an icy parking lot. Common unstable visual conditions are experienced on mass transit, in crowds, or on a boat. Rapid head movements may render even a stable visual environment unusable for postural cues, and darkness may preclude the use of vision. The more stable the environment, the lower the demand on the individual for balance control. Unstable environments place greater demands on the postural control systems.

Balance is also affected by an individual's intentions to achieve certain goals and the purposeful tasks that are undertaken. Volitional balance disturbances are self-initiated almost constantly, such as shifting from foot to foot, reaching for the telephone, or catching an object that is falling from a high shelf. Even reactions to involuntary balance disturbances, such as a slip or trip, will be modified based on the immediate task. A man carrying a bag of groceries who slips may drop the bag to reach with both hands and catch himself. If he is instead carrying his infant child, he may reach with only one hand, or even suffer the fall if by doing so he can protect the infant from harm.

All of these variables—the location of the COG, the base of support, the limit of stability, the surface conditions, the visual environment, the intentions and task choices—are inconstant, producing changing demands on the systems that control balance. The integrity and interaction of postural control mechanisms allow a wide range of movements and functions to be achieved without loss of balance.

HUMAN CONTROL OF BALANCE

Early studies of postural control mechanisms using selectively lesioned cats and primates focused on reflexive and reactive equilibrium responses that are relatively "hard wired."[66] These valuable studies brought to light certain stereotypical motor responses to specific sensory stimuli, such as the "crossed extension" reflex or tonic neck reflexes. Earlier balance treatment methods based on this neurophysiological science sought to "inhibit" abnormal reflexes and "facilitate" normal responses.[12, 42] Controversy exists regarding the merit of these techniques, but recent research advances make it clear that this view of the nervous system and resultant scope of treatment are too narrow.[50, 74] Balance abilities are heavily influenced by higher level neural circuitry and by other systems (e.g., cognitive, musculoskeletal) as well.[37] In addition, it is now widely accepted that the nervous system is influenced by and responsive to the demands placed on it by the tasks being accomplished and the environments in which those tasks are performed.[28, 29, 35] More recent theory attempts to include all of these facets in a "systems model or systems approach" to dynamic equilibrium.[6, 63, 70] Contemporary testing and treatment methods based on this systems model have consequently evolved.[34, 63] Prior techniques have been modified and expanded to allow for a more comprehensive approach.[60]

The Systems Approach

The dynamic systems model for dynamic equilibrium recognizes that balance is the result of interactions between the individual, the task the individual is performing, and the environment in which the task must be performed. These interactions are represented in Figure 21–1. Within the individual, both sensory inputs and processing systems (left side of figure) and motor planning and execution systems (right side of figure) are critical. Both peripheral components (lower level of figure) and central components (upper level of figure) of the systems are involved in the cycle. The cycle is driven both by purposeful choices of the individual (task) and demands placed on the individual by the environment. Successful function of the sensory systems allows recognition of body position in relation to self and the world. The desired outcome from the motor systems is the generation of movement sufficient to maintain balance and perform the chosen task.

Peripheral Sensory Reception

The three primary peripheral sensory inputs contributing to postural control are the bilateral receptors of the somatosensory, visual, and vestibular systems.[6, 52] Somatosensory receptors located in the joints, ligaments, muscles, and skin provide information about muscle length, stretch, tension, and contraction; pain, temperature, pressure; and joint position. The feet, ankles, knees, hips, back, neck, and eye muscles all furnish useful information for balance maintenance. Visual receptors in the eyes perform dual tasks. Central (or focal) vision allows environmental orientation, contributing to the perception of verticality and object motion, as well as identification of the hazards and opportunities presented by the environment.[6] For example, a canoeist may see rocks in a stream as a hazard to be avoided, whereas a hiker who wants to

Dynamic equilibrium

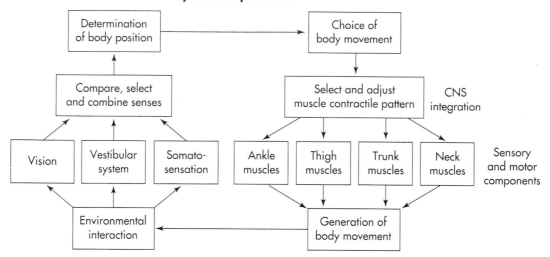

FIGURE 21–1. The systems model of postural control illustrates the constant cycle that occurs simultaneously at many levels. (Reprinted with permission from NeuroCom International, Inc.)

cross the stream may see the same rocks as a welcome opportunity. Peripheral (or ambient) vision detects the motion of the self in relation to the environment, including head movements and postural sway, whereas central visual inputs tend to receive more conscious recognition.[6] Both are normally used for postural control.[6] Orientation to the environment allows "feedforward," or anticipatory, actions; detection of head movement and body sway provides feedback for responsive actions.

Disease of, or damage to, any of the peripheral sensory receptors impairs or removes the detection capabilities of the system, rendering sensory information unavailable for use in postural control. Many patients with neurological diagnoses have peripheral sensory impairments. Peripheral somatosensory loss occurs after spinal cord injury, peripheral neuropathy, tabes dorsalis, amputation, and so on. Peripheral vision loss may result from diabetic retinopathy, cataracts, and glaucoma. Peripheral vestibular loss is experienced with temporal bone fracture, acoustic neuroma, Meniere disease and other disorders.[32]

VESTIBULAR FUNCTION

Each of the three sensory systems provides both unique and redundant information for postural control. The vestibular system provides the central nervous system (CNS) with information about the position and motion of the head in relation to gravity. The vestibular system is critical for balance, because it uniquely identifies self-motion as different from motion in the environment, provides stable vision while the head is moving, and serves as a "referee" when visual and somatosensory inputs conflict. It also contributes directly to postural stability through the activation of antigravity muscles.

The sensory component of the vestibular system consists of the labyrinths, a mechanical system designed to convert head motion into neural firing. This system includes the semicircular canals and the otoliths.[30] The semicircular canals are ring-shaped, fluid-filled structures containing hair cells that respond to the movement of the fluid when the head moves. The hair cell sits in a support-

ing surface called the crista ampularis and extends into the fluid-filled canal. When the hair cells are bent by the movement of fluid in the canal, the direction and speed of the deflection of the hair cell are converted to neural firing of the vestibular nerve (Fig. 21–2).

The semicircular canals sit at right angles to each other and are named according to their relationship to the head—thus, the anterior, lateral, and posterior canals. This relationship provides the CNS information regarding the direction of head movement in relationship to the level of stimulation recorded from each canal and compared with the others. The canals are arranged so that when the head moves, the direction and velocity in each canal are compared with a mutually perpendicular canal on the opposite side of the head. This provides for sensory redundancy, so that if there is damage to the vestibular system on one side the information can be captured by the intact canal on the opposite side.

The otoliths, located in the vestibule or central component of the labyrinth, also respond through hair cell deflections. In these compartments there are multiple hair cells attached to the walls and connected to the vestibular nerve. These hair cells are embedded in a gel-like substance called the macula. Sitting on top of the macula are crystals of calcium carbonate, known as otoconia. The purpose of the otoconia is to establish mass, so that the hair cells can measure the effects of gravity as well as movement. The otoliths respond to movement of the head by the shearing effect of the otoconia pressing on the macula and displacing the hair cell in the opposite direction of the movement. These signals from the otoliths are used to compare this motion with the resting tone established by gravity. There are two components of the otolith, the utricle and the saccule, which are oriented in different planes so that by working together they can detect both acceleration and tilt[5] (Fig. 21–3).

Head movement stimulates both sets of semicircular canals, so that the vestibular nerve on one side becomes inhibited while the other becomes excited. The vestibular nerve transports the information from the labyrinths to

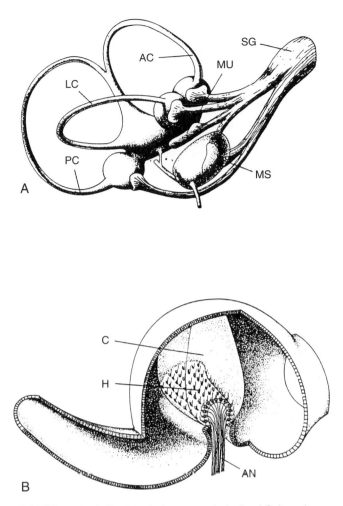

A

B

FIGURE 21–2. *A*, The labyrinth system, including LC, lateral or horizontal semicircular canal; AC, anterior semicircular canal; PC, posterior semicircular canal; MU, macula utriculi; MS, macula sacculi; SG, Scarpa's ganglion. *B*, Cross sectional view of the semicircular canal. C, cupula; H, hair cells; AN, afferent nerves. (Adapted from Barber HO, Stockwell CW: Manual of Electronystagmography. St. Louis, CV Mosby, 1976.)

inferior nucleus has connections to the other nuclei and the reticular formation.

Each side of the brain stem contains a set of nuclei as described earlier, and there are interconnections between the two sides that allow the information from each labyrinth to be assimilated at this level before being interpreted by the CNS. The connections from the nuclei to other structures of the brain are complex, with the major outflow going to the cerebellum. When the cerebellum is not functioning properly, the calibration of the vestibular reflexes is affected, and the ability to make corrective movements at the appropriate scale and speed is compromised.

Central Sensory Perception

The brain processes all of the environmentally available sensory information gathered by the peripheral receptors in varying degrees. This processing is usually referred to as sensory integration or sensory organization.[6, 52] Central sensory structures function first to compare available inputs between two sides and among three sensory systems. The somatosensory system alone is unable to distinguish surface tilts from body tilts. Also, the visual system by itself cannot discriminate movement of the environment from movement of the body.[32] Therefore, the brain needs information from all three senses to correctly distinguish motion of the self from motion in the environment. For example, with head movement, firing from one vestibular organ will increase, whereas in the other, firing will decrease proportionately. This is known as push-pull function, and the information is considered to "match." Using the same example, if the eyes are open while the head moves, the rate of the visual flow will be equal and the direction of the visual flow will be opposite to rate and

the CNS. The brain uses the relative change in firing from both sides to identify the direction of rotation. Pitch (neck flexion/extension), yaw (right/left head rotation), and roll (right/left neck side bending) are terms used to describe the angular accelerations experienced with head movements that are detected by the semicircular canals. Horizontal and vertical accelerations, such as riding in a car or an elevator, are detected by the otoliths[32] (Fig. 21–4).

VESTIBULAR PATHWAYS

The vestibular input is delivered to the vestibular nucleus at the pontomedullary junction. Each of the four nuclei is involved as a relay for specific functions of the vestibular system. The superior and medial nuclei drive eye movement to maintain gaze stability. The medial nucleus is involved in coordinated head and eye movements that occur together as well as some input for control of movement of the extremities and trunk. The lateral nucleus is primarily responsible for coordination of input to muscles of the extremities and trunk to maintain balance. The

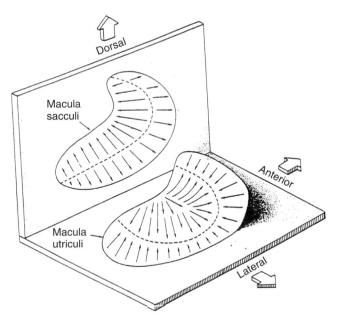

FIGURE 21–3. Polarization of hair cells on the otolith organs. The direction of arrows indicates the direction of hair deflection that excites hair cells in that region of the receptor surface. (From Barber HO, Stockwell CW: Manual of Electronystagmography. St. Louis, CV Mosby, 1976.)

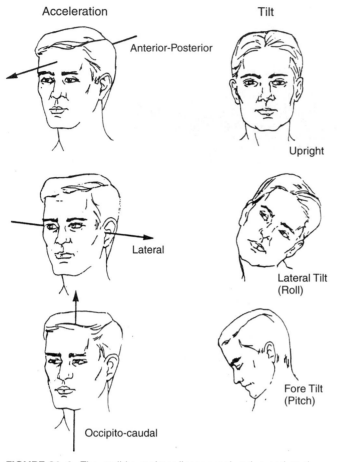

Acceleration

Anterior-Posterior

Lateral

Occipito-caudal

Tilt

Upright

Lateral Tilt
(Roll)

Fore Tilt
(Pitch)

FIGURE 21–4. The otoliths register linear acceleration and static tilt of the head. (From Hain TC, Ramaswany TS, Hillman MA: Anatomy and physiology of the normal vestibular system. *In* Herdman SJ (ed): Vestibular Rehabilitation. Philadelphia, FA Davis, 2000.)

direction information from the vestibular inputs. The inputs from the two systems are congruent. If both sides and all three systems provide compatible inputs, the process of organization is simplified.

Sensory conflict can arise when information between sides or between systems is not synchronous. Sensory organization processing then becomes more complex, because the brain must then recognize any discrepancies and select the correct inputs on which to base motor responses. The vestibular system is used as an internal reference to determine accuracy of the other two senses when they conflict. For example, a driver stopped still at a red light suddenly hits the brake when an adjacent vehicle begins to roll. Movement of the other car detected by the peripheral visual system is momentarily misperceived as self-motion. In this situation, the vestibular and somatosensory systems do not detect motion, but the forward visual flow is interpreted as backward motion. Because the brain failed to suppress the (mismatched) visual inputs, the braking response was generated.

When the brain recognizes that the information coming from one sensory input is inaccurate, as is the case when the vestibular system is sending abnormal signals of head acceleration or rotation, it will become dependent on the remaining senses (somatosensation and vision) to determine position in space. The brain then compares and uses information from senses it considers "accurate" (in the previous example, visual and somatosensory information) for balance. An individual with the problem just described may compensate for the loss of vestibular function by becoming visually dependent for balance during movement. If vision or somatosensation subsequently becomes disrupted, this individual may have loss of balance, dizziness, or both. Clients with this type of vestibular problem will limit head motion during walking and step with a flat foot.

Activities or environments that create sensory conflict become more difficult to manage when the vestibular system is deficient or underutilized. These situations, such as going down stairs, escalators, elevators, walking on uneven ground, and making quick turns, are often avoided. When the sensory conflict cannot be resolved rapidly, dizziness occurs.

Intrinsic central sensory processing impairments also can produce sensory conflict. An adult hemiplegic patient with pusher syndrome illustrates an inability to integrate visual, vestibular, and somatosensory inputs for midline orientation. Within a single system, discrepancies between the sides are also problematic. Unequal firing from opposite sides of the vestibular system, as in unilateral vestibular hypofunction, produces a "mismatch" that is subsequently interpreted as head rotation when there is no actual head movement. This spinning sensation is known as vertigo.[32] Vertigo is resolved if the brain is able to adapt to the mismatch.

Finally, the central processing mechanisms combine any available and accurate inputs to answer the question "Where am I?" This includes both an internal relationship of the body segments to each other (e.g., head in relation to trunk, trunk in relation to feet) and an external relationship of the body to the outside world (e.g., feet in relation to surface, arm in relation to handrail). CNS disease or trauma involving the parietal lobe may impair these processing mechanisms, so that even available, accurate sensory inputs are not recognized or incorporated into determinations of position and movement.[19, 38] Impairments of central sensory processing may occur after stroke, head trauma, tumors, or aneurysms; with disease processes such as multiple sclerosis; and with aging.

Central Motor Planning and Control

Whereas sensory processing allows the interaction of the individual and the environment, motor planning underlies the interaction of the individual and the task. Aside from reflexive activity such as breathing and blinking, most motor actions are voluntary and occur because some goal is to be achieved. That is not to say that reflexes occur separately from volitional movements; for example, the vestibuloocular reflex is active concurrently with tracking activity[32] but most actions occur because of some purposeful intent. These task intentions precede motor actions.[6, 17] Wrist and hand movements will vary depending on what is to be grasped (a cup vs. a doorknob); foot placement and trunk position will vary depending on what is to be lifted (a heavy suitcase vs. a laundry basket). The initiation of volitional motor actions depends on intention, attention, and motivation.[6, 64]

Once an objective ("Where do I want to be? What do I want to do?") has been chosen, the next step in motor planning is to determine how to best accomplish the goal given the many options that are potentially available. For example, when the task demands fine skills or accuracy, the dominant hand is preferred; when the task involves lifting a large or heavy object, both hands are preferred. In addition to which limbs, joints, and muscles will be used, motor planning also adjusts the timing, sequencing, and force modulation. This can be demonstrated in various reaching tasks. Reaching to remove a hot item from the oven will occur slowly, whereas reaching to put an arm through a sleeve will occur more quickly. Optimal motor plans are developed with knowledge of self (abilities and limitations), knowledge of task (characteristics of successful performance), and knowledge of the environment (risks and opportunities).[64]

The motor plan must be transmitted to the peripheral motor system to be enacted. A copy of the intended movement plan is sent to the cerebellum during the transmission. When the movement begins, incoming sensory inputs ("feedback") about the actual movements and performance outcome are compared with the intended movements and performance outcome. Movement errors (the difference between the intended and the actual movement) and performance errors (desired goal not achieved) are detected, and plans for correction are then formed and transmitted. This process of error detection and error correction is the foundation of motor learning.

Clients with CNS disorders often have central motor planning and control impairments. After a stroke, clients may have hypertonus; clients with head trauma may have difficulty initiating or ceasing movements; clients with Parkinson's disease exhibit bradykinesia, and those with cerebellar ataxia display modulation problems.[15]

Peripheral Motor Execution

Movement is accomplished through the bilateral joints and muscles. Normal ROM, strength, and endurance of the feet, ankles, knees, hips, back, neck, and eyes must be present for the execution of the full range of normal balance movements. Decreased ankle dorsiflexion ROM, for example, will restrict the forward limits of stability. Strength deficits are a primary cause of movement abnormalities in both central and peripheral nervous system disorders. In addition, weakness may be the result of force modulation deficits or disuse.[63] Balance is directly impacted by loss of strength. For example, weakness of the hip extensors and abductors will impede successful use of a hip strategy for upright trunk control. Initially adequate toe clearance may diminish with fatigue. Many neurological clients also develop stiffness and contractures as a result of persistent weakness or hypertonus. Restrictions in ROM also limit balance abilities.

The ability to achieve static postural alignment, although necessary for normal balance, is not sufficient to allow volitional functions. Adequate strength (to control body weight and any additional loads) through normal postural sway ranges is needed to permit dynamic balance

activities such as reaching, leaning, and lifting. Postural control demands are increased during gait because the forces of momentum and the relationships of recruitment, timing, and velocity also must be regulated.[57] Traditionally considered orthopedic problems, deficits in strength, ROM, and endurance have a great impact on balance abilities. Attention must be given to these musculoskeletal impairments in examination of and intervention for clients with neurological diagnosis.

Influence of Other Systems

Balance abilities also are influenced by other systems. Attention, cognition, and memory, often impaired in hemiplegic and head-injured clients, are critical for optimal balance function. Attentional deficits reduce awareness of environmental hazards and opportunities, interfering with anticipatory postural control.[70] Cognitive problems such as distractibility, poor judgment, and slowed processing increase the risk of falls. Memory loss may preclude recall of safety measures. Emotional lability, agitation, or denial of impairments also can increase the risks for loss of balance. In addition to having a direct impact on balance abilities themselves, these cognitive and behavioral problems impede motor learning processes, which are crucial for the relearning of balance skills.

Constant Cyclic Nature

The systems model of postural control presented previously illustrates the constant cycle that occurs simultaneously at many levels. Attention and intention allow feedforward processing for active sensory search of the environment and motor planning, both needed for anticipatory postural control. Movements are initiated and executed, with resultant sensory experiences and error detection, or feedback. Successful movements are repeated and refined; unsuccessful ones are modified. The nature of this cycle presents the clinician with opportunities for intervention. Through feedback and practice, balance abilities can improve.[60]

Motor Components of Balance

Reflexes

Many levels of neuromuscular control must be functioning to produce normal postural movements. At the most basic level, reflexes and righting reactions support postural orientation. The vestibuloocular reflex (VOR) and the vestibulospinal reflex (VSR) contribute to orientation of the eyes, head, and body to self and environment.[6]

When motion of the head is identified by the semicircular canals, it triggers a response within the oculomotor system called the angular VOR. This causes the eyes to move in the opposite direction of the head but at the same speed. Stimulation of the otoliths drives the eyes to respond to linear head movement. Quick movements of the head will trigger the VOR.

The VOR allows the coordination of eye and head movements. When the eyes are fixed on an object while the head is moving, the VOR supports gaze stabilization. Visuoocular responses often work concurrently with the VOR. They permit "smooth pursuit" when the head is fixed while the eyes move and visual tracking when both the eyes and the head move simultaneously.[6]

The VSR helps to control movement and stabilize the body. Both the semicircular canals and the otoliths activate and modulate muscles of the neck, trunk, and extremities after head movement to maintain balance. Abnormal muscular responses in the extremities are noted when there is an acute vestibular disorder. This can result in postural instability. Vestibular dysfunction can result in an unconscious lateral weight shift, most often to the side of the lesion. The VSR permits stability of the body when the head moves and is important for the coordination of the trunk over the extremities in upright postures. Righting reactions support the orientation of the head to the trunk and the head position relative to the ground and include labyrinthine head righting, optical head righting, and body-on-head righting.[6]

Automatic Postural Responses

At the next level, automatic postural responses operate to keep the COG over the base of support. They are a set of functionally organized, long-loop responses that act to keep the body in a state of equilibrium.[51, 52] Functionally organized means that the responses, although stereotypical, are matched to the stimulus in direction and amplitude. If the stimulus is a push to the right, the response is a shift to the left, toward midline. The larger the stimulus, the greater the response. Automatic postural responses always occur in response to a stimulus. Because they occur rapidly, in less than 250 ms, they are not under volitional control.

There are four commonly identified automatic postural responses, or strategies. Ankle strategy describes postural sway control from the ankles and feet. The head and hips travel in the same direction at the same time, with the body moving as a unit over the feet (Fig. 21–5A). Muscle contractile patterns are from distal to proximal (i.e., gastrocnemius, hamstrings, paraspinals). This strategy is used whenever sway is small, slow, and near midline. It occurs when the surface is broad and stable enough to allow

pressure against it to produce forces that can counteract sway to stabilize the body.

Hip strategy describes postural sway control from the pelvis and trunk. The head and hips travel in opposite directions, with body segment movements counteracting one another (Fig. 21–5B). Muscle contractile patterns are from proximal to distal (i.e., abdominals, quadriceps, tibialis anterior). This strategy is observed when sway is large, fast, and, nearing the limit of stability, or if the surface is too narrow or unstable to permit effective counterpressure.

Suspensory strategy describes a lowering of the COG toward the base of support by means of bilateral lower-extremity flexion or a slight squatting motion (Fig. 21–5C). By shortening the distance between the COG and the base of support, the task of controlling the COG is made easier. This strategy is often used when a combination of stability and mobility is required, as in windsurfing.

Stepping and reaching strategies describe steps with the feet or reaches with the arms in an attempt to reestablish a new base of support with the active limb(s) when the COG has exceeded the original base of support (Fig. 21–5D).

Whereas these strategies are stereotypical in humans, there is great individual variation in strategy selection from other influential factors. For example, an anxious person may reach or step much sooner than a relaxed person with similar physical deficits. It is also important to know that all of these strategies do *not* occur in sequence with every balance disturbance.[46, 48] In other words, we normally do not try ankle strategy and wait until it fails before trying hip strategy (although early learning may involve this exploration). Because these responses have to occur very rapidly to prevent balance loss, such a sequential approach would be inefficient. Instead, the normal response is the emergence of the single strategy best suited to the particular perturbation, the limitations of the individual, and the conditions in the environment.

Abnormal use of automatic postural responses is often observed in clients with vestibular deficits. There is typically a reliance on ankle strategy, which permits the head to remain aligned with the feet and reduces the need to resolve sensory conflict. Use of hip strategy may be modi-

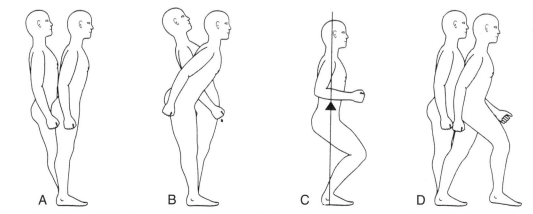

FIGURE 21–5. Automatic postural strategies. *A,* Ankle strategy. *B,* Hip strategy, *C,* Suspensory strategy. *D,* Stepping strategy. (From Hasson S: Clinical Exercise Physiology. St. Louis, CV Mosby, 1994.)

fied or limited because of difficulty in resolving the conflict created when the head is moving in an opposite direction as the COG. Activities that require use of hip strategy, such as standing in tandem or on one leg, can be a problem for clients with bilateral vestibular loss or an uncompensated vestibular lesion. However, there are some cases in which there is actually excessive use of hip strategy on a level surface.[36] Clinicians may also observe increased use of a stepping strategy when on a rotational or compliant surface.

Anticipatory Postural Responses

Anticipatory postural responses are similar to automatic postural responses, but they occur before the actual disturbance.[17] If a balance disturbance is predicted, the body will respond in advance by developing a "postural set" to counteract the coming forces. For example, if an individual lifts an empty suitcase thinking it is full and heavy, the anticipatory forces generated before the lift (to counter the anticipated weight) will cause excessive movement and brief instability. Failure to produce these anticipatory responses increases the risk of sudden balance loss, creating the need to use rapid, reactive automatic postural responses to prevent a fall.

Volitional Postural Movements

Volitional postural movements are under conscious control. Weight shifts to reach the telephone or put the dishes in the dishwasher, for example, are self-initiated disturbances of the COG to accomplish a goal. Volitional postural movements can range from simple weight shifts to complex balance skills of skaters and gymnasts. They can occur after a stimulus or be self-initiated. Volitional postural movements can occur quickly or slowly, depending on the goal at hand. The more complex or unfamiliar the task, the slower the response time. A broad variety of movements that might successfully achieve a goal is possible. Volitional postural movements are strongly modified by prior experience and instruction. Automatic and anticipatory postural responses allow the continuous unconscious control of balance, whereas volitional postural movements permit conscious activity.

CLINICAL ASSESSMENT OF BALANCE

Objectives of Testing

When present, disabilities need to be identified and measured: functional scales are usually used to determine the presence and severity of disabilities. From these functional tests, decisions can be made about whether to treat and, if so, what tasks need to be practiced. If treatment is indicated, clinicians must make judgments about what to treat. Further testing to identify and measure impairments is then necessary to know what systems are involved. A comprehensive evaluation of balance includes both functional and impairment tests.[70] *There is currently no one single test of balance that adequately covers the many multidimensional aspects of balance.*

There is no single, simple test for balance because balance is a complex sensorimotor process.[20] Many balance tests exist, but not all tests are appropriate for all clients. Different tests may be needed to answer specific questions. For example, several good tests have been developed to determine the risk for falls in elderly people. These would be totally insufficient to discern whether an injured dancer can resume practice or an injured roofer is ready to return to work. Clinicians should understand the advantages and limitations of different balance tests to be able to select appropriate evaluative tools.

In general, a balance test will not be useful unless it sufficiently challenges the postural control system being tested. Tests for stability ("static balance") are appropriate for clients who are having difficulty just finding midline and/or holding still in sitting or standing. They are of much less value for clients with higher-level abilities. Conversely, single-leg stance tests or sensory tests using a foam surface may be far too difficult for clients with lower-level abilities to perform.

A word of caution about interpreting test results is indicated. Most clinical tests rely on observations of motor behavior to arrive at some conclusion about impairments. There are many possible causes for abnormal motor behavior, and clinicians should be careful before concluding that an observed behavior is due to problems in a certain, single system. For example, the Romberg test is commonly assumed to test the use of vestibular inputs. Yet, during the test, both somatosensory and vestibular inputs are (normally) used for balance control. If balance control is impaired, is it certain that the vestibular system is the culprit? Could somatosensory system deficits also result in a poor test result? Or alternatively, because the Romberg test is performed with feet together, what effect would hip weakness have on the ability to stand with a narrowed base of support? When using a test whose results may be altered by problems in more than one system, any relevant system should be evaluated. If multiple system deficits exist, and they often do in neurological clients, then use caution in making "commonly assumed" conclusions based on clinical test results.

Because there are so many balance tests from which to choose, several questions must be asked to determine whether a test is appropriate for use.[20] For what purpose and population was the test designed? Is it appropriate to use that test for a different purpose or with a different population? Is it valid? Is it repeatable by different examiners or by the same examiner multiple times? Are results reliable? In what populations are they reliable? What is the threshold for this test; that is, how large must changes be before this test can detect them? Are there normative data for comparison? Most of these questions have not been answered yet as they relate to the clinical balance tests commonly used by therapists.

Types of Balance Tests

Balance tests can be grouped or classified by type. There is no single test that can adequately measure all the components of balance. Different types of tests measure different facets of postural control (Table 21–3). Quiet standing (static) refers to tests where the client is standing

TABLE 21-3. Types of Balance Tests

Type	Tests
Quiet standing	Romberg
	Sharpened Romberg/Tandem Romberg
	One-Legged-Stance Test (OLST)
	Postural Sway
	Nudge/Push
	Postural Stress Test
	Motor Control Test
Active standing	Functional Reach
	Limits of Stability
Sensory manipulation	Sensory Organization Test (SOT)
	Clinical Test for Sensory Interaction on Balance (CTSIB)
	Vertiginous Positions
	Hallpike-Dix Maneuver
	Nystagmus
	Semicircular Canal Function
	Visual-Vestibular Interaction
	Visual Acuity
	Oculomotor Tests
	Fukuda Stepping Test
Functional scales	Berg Balance Scale
	Get Up and Go/Timed Get Up and Go
	Tinetti Performance Oriented Assessment of Balance
	Tinetti Performance Oriented Assessment of Gait
	Gait Assessment Rating Scale (GARS)
	Dynamic Gait Index
Combination test batteries	Fregley-Graybiel Ataxia Test Battery
	Fugl-Meyer Sensorimotor Assessment of Balance Performance
	Speechley's Physical Therapy Checklist

and the movement goal is to hold still. Disturbances to balance, called perturbations, may or may not be applied. Active standing (dynamic) tests also position the patient standing, but the movement goal involves voluntary weight shifting. Sensory manipulation tests use various body and head positions, eye movements, or stepping to stimulate or restrict visual, vestibular, and somatosensory inputs. Functional balance, mobility, and gait scales involve the performance of whole-body movement tasks, such as sit-to-stand, walking, and stepping over objects. Finally, a few test batteries offer a combination of the preceding tests. A commonly accepted test for sitting balance in adults is not yet available, although clients with neurological problems may often need sitting balance retraining in early stages. Usually, clinicians modify standing tests or pediatric sitting tests to assess sitting balance in adult neurological clients. For example, the Functional Reach Test has been used to measure excursion in seated individuals with spinal cord injuries.[44]

Quiet Standing

The classic Romberg test was originally developed to "examine the effect of posterior column disease upon upright stance."[54] The client stands with feet parallel and together and then closes the eyes for 20 to 30 seconds. The examiner subjectively judges the amount of sway. Quantification of sway can be accomplished with a videotape or forceplate. Excessive sway, loss of balance, or stepping during this test is abnormal. The sharpened

Romberg,[54] also known as the tandem Romberg, requires the client to stand with feet in a heel-to-toe position and arms folded across the chest, eyes closed for 60 seconds. Often four trials of this test are timed with a stopwatch, for a maximum score of 240 seconds.

One-legged-stance tests (OLSTs) are commonly used.[9, 54] Both legs must be alternately tested, and differences between sides are noted. The client stands on both feet and crosses the arms over the chest, then picks up one leg and holds it with the hip in neutral and the knee flexed to 90 degrees. This test is scored with a stopwatch. Five 30-second trials are performed for each leg (alternating legs), with a maximum possible score of 150 seconds per leg. Normal young subjects are able to stand for 30 seconds, but this may not be a reasonable expectation for older clients.[54]

In both the Romberg test and the OLST, problems in sensory organization processes can be observed. To determine how much of the stability is achieved through visual stabilization, each test can be repeated with eyes closed. The client with visual dependency for balance will often have an immediate loss of balance when the eyes are closed. As noted earlier, the client with vestibular loss may have difficulty producing the hip strategy necessary to perform these tasks.

A battery of timed stance tests has been developed by Bohannon and colleagues.[10] This set of tests varies the foot position (apart, together, tandem, and single-leg) and the availability of visual information (eyes open and closed) to produce eight different combinations. Maintenance of balance in each condition is timed for a maximum of 30 seconds; the assigned score is the total number of seconds that balance could be maintained. The best possible score on this test is 240 seconds. This test is reliable, valid, and sensitive to change over time.[10]

Objective postural sway measures can be obtained through the use of computerized forceplates.[23, 49] The client is asked to adopt a standardized foot placement if possible (varies with manufacturer) and to stand quietly with arms at sides or hands on hips for 20 or 30 seconds. Sway with both eyes open and eyes closed is commonly measured. Graphic and numerical quantification is provided (Fig. 21–6). Normative data may be provided.

Automatic postural responses are assessed through the client's response to perturbations. The client is asked to stand quietly, and the examiner disturbs the balance, either manually or with equipment. Most commonly used are nudge/push tests.[69, 70] Although not totally valueless, these tests are not quantifiable or repeatable, and thus are not reliable measures. For this reason their use is discouraged. Should the examiner decide to use such tests, the client is given slight to moderate pushes backward at the sternum or pelvis and then forward between the shoulder blades or at the pelvis. The clinician subjectively notes any losses of balance and the use of recovery strategies (e.g., ankle, hip). Scoring involves rating the responses as normal, good, fair, poor, or unable. If used, these nudge/push tests should be performed both predictably (i.e., "Don't let me push you") to judge anticipatory postural control and unpredictably (no cues) to judge automatic postural responses.

The Postural Stress Test was developed to examine

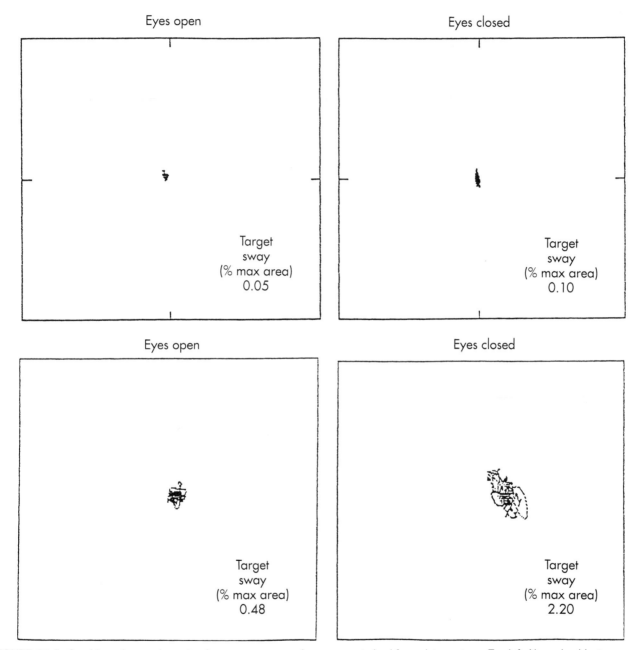

FIGURE 21–6. Graphic and numeric postural sway measures using a computerized forceplate system. *Top left*, Normal subject, eyes open. *Top right*, Normal subject, eyes closed. *Bottom left*, Client with Parkinson's disease, eyes open. *Bottom right*, Client with Parkinson's disease, eyes closed. (Reprinted with permission from NeuroCom International, Inc.)

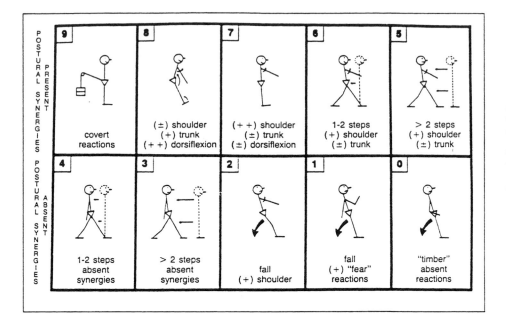

FIGURE 21–7. Ratings of balance strategies used by elderly subjects during the postural stress test after a backward postural perturbation. (+) and (+ +) symbols indicate very frequently visible and invariably visible synergistic responses, respectively. (±) refers to less frequently seen components. Frames 2 to 0 show essentially absent coordinated activity followed by a fall. (Reprinted from Whipple R, Wolfson LI: Abnormalities of balance, gait, and sensorimotor function in the elderly population. *In* Duncan P (ed): Balance: Proceedings of the APTA Forum. Alexandria, VA, American Physical Therapy Association, 1990.)

elderly people and determine risk for falls.[77] It is essentially a quantifiable, repeatable nudge/push test that is known to be reliable with trained raters.[31] The client stands wearing a waist belt attached posteriorly to a line that travels through a pulley and is attached on the other end to one of three weights. The weights are 1.5%, 3.0%, or 4.25% of the client's body weight. Each of these weights is dropped from a standard height, pulling the line that displaces the client backward. The expected response is a compensatory forward adjustment. Clients are videotaped, and the videotape is reviewed to assign scores to the balance responses (Fig. 21–7), from 0 (no response/fall) to 9 (appropriate response). If a videotape cannot be made, a second examiner may be asked to observe the responses during the test.

In the case of vestibular loss, the sense of body position in space can be lost. Postural reflexes triggered by a perturbation may not be appropriate for the actual circumstance and therefore cause destabilization. Clients with vestibular deficits often hold the COG in a posterior position during quiet stance. When perturbed, they reach the posterior limits of stability before appropriate postural adjustments can be made. This can result in a fall backward.

The Motor Control Test perturbs the client through surface displacement (Fig. 21–8).[51] The client stands on the forceplate, which is movable, with feet parallel and arms at sides. The support surface very rapidly rotates toes up or toes down or translates (slides) forward or backward. Both of these surface displacements result in a rapid shift in the relationship between the COG and the base of support. The expected responses are directionally specific (to the direction of the stimulus) forces generated against the surface to bring the COG back to the center. Response latencies and postural sway are measured. Normative data are available. This test can be used to look for abnormal stepping strategies when failure to select hip strategy occurs.

Active Standing

Volitional control of the COG is evaluated by asking the client to make voluntary movements that require weight shifting. The Functional Reach Test was developed for use with elderly people to determine risk for falls.[14] The client stands near a wall with feet parallel. Attached to the wall at shoulder height is a yardstick. The client is asked to make a fist and raise the arm nearest the wall to 90 degrees of shoulder flexion. The examiner notes the position of the fist on the yardstick. The client is then asked to lean forward as far as possible, and the examiner notes the end position of the fist on the yardstick (Fig. 21–9). Beginning position is subtracted from end position to obtain a change unit in inches. Three trials are performed. Normative data are available, and the test is reliable. However, the standard error of measurement for

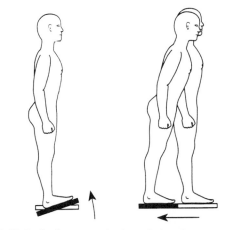

FIGURE 21–8. Surface perturbations during the motor control test using computerized dynamic posturography. Forceplate measures include latency and amount of response, and adaptation of the response to repeated perturbations. (From Hasson S: Clinical Exercise Physiology. St. Louis, CV Mosby, 1994.)

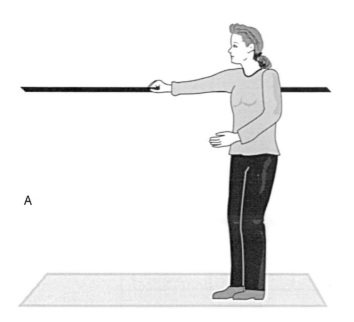

A

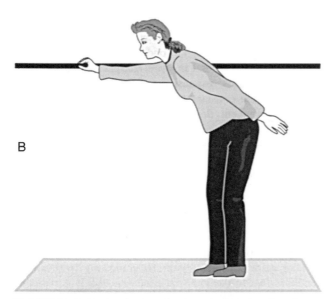

B

FIGURE 21–9. During the functional reach test, the client is asked to reach forward as far as possible from a comfortable standing posture. The excursion of the arm from start to finish is measured via a yardstick affixed to the wall at shoulder height. *A,* Functional reach—starting position. *B,* Functional reach—ending position.

this test may be as high as 2 inches, meaning that a change in score of less than 2 inches cannot be attributed to clinical improvement, because it may reflect only measurement error.

One serious limitation of the Functional Reach Test is that it measures sway in only one direction (forward). An expansion of this test has been devised to measure sway in four directions.[55] The Multi-Directional Reach Test is conceptually equivalent but measures sway anteriorly, posteriorly, and laterally to both sides. This test should provide a more comprehensive picture of volitional COG control limitations. However, because it is a new test, reliability is not known and normative data are not available.

The limits of stability test uses a computerized forceplate to measure postural sway away from midline in eight directions.[16, 23] Clients assume a standardized foot position and control a cursor on the computer monitor by shifting their weight. They are asked to move the cursor from midline to eight targets on the screen (Fig. 21–10). Measures include movement time, path sway (length of the trajectory of the COG), and accuracy of target achievement (COG position). This test should be performed once for familiarization, then a second time for scoring purposes. Second and subsequent tests are reliable. Normative data are available.

Vestibular pathology can produce an abnormal internal representation of self-position in space.[8] This may, in turn, cause the client's perceived limits of stability to be different from their actual physical limits of stability. Poor motor strategy selection may thus follow when the client attempts to perform this test. For clients with vestibular deficits, eye and head movements during this test may disturb equilibrium sense and lead to abnormal postural responses.

For vestibular signals, the head orientation relative to the trunk must be taken into account to control posture.[39] Orientation of the eyes appears to change the organization of the whole-body posture, as well as the integration of body space with extrapersonal space. When the CNS is unable to manage the input from each of the visual and vestibular systems, misperception of verticality may occur. In these clients, abnormal and inefficient postural adjustment for weight shift can be seen.[39]

Sensory Manipulation

Sensory inputs play a critical role in postural control, but tests to measure their use to produce a balance performance outcome have only recently been developed. The Sensory Organization Test (SOT) uses a computerized movable forceplate and movable visual surround to systematically alter the surface and visual environments.[51, 52] The client stands with feet parallel and arms at the sides on the forceplate and is asked to stand quietly. Three 20-second trials under each of six sensory conditions are performed (Fig. 21–11). In conditions one, two, and three the support surface (forceplate) is fixed. During conditions four, five, and six the support surface is sway-referenced to the sway of the client. In other words, the movement of the surface is matched to the movement of the client in a 1:1 ratio. This responsive surface movement maintains a near-constant ankle joint angle despite body sway, rendering the somatosensory information from the feet and ankles inaccurate for use in balance maintenance. Visual inputs are undisturbed in conditions one and four. Vision is absent (eyes are closed) in conditions two and five. The movable visual surround is sway-refer-

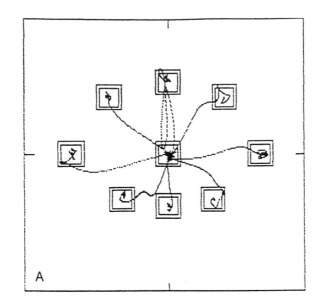

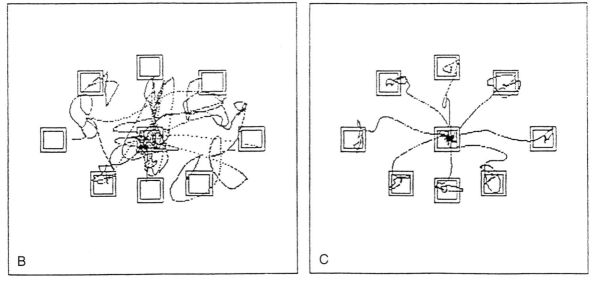

FIGURE 21–10. Graphic postural sway measures from the limit of stability test using a computerized forceplate system (numerical measures not shown). Clients are asked to move away from and return to midline. *A,* Normal subject. *B,* Hemiplegic client on initial evaluation. *C,* Hemiplegic client on discharge evaluation. (Reprinted with permission from NeuroCom International, Inc.)

enced in conditions three and six. This responsive visual surround movement maintains a near-constant distance between the eyes and the visual environment despite body sway, rendering visual inputs from the eyes inaccurate for balance maintenance in those two conditions.

Under condition one, all three senses (vision, vestibular, and somatosensory) are available and accurate. Body sway is measured by means of the forceplate; this initial measurement forms the baseline against which subsequent measures are compared (Fig. 21–12). Under condition two, the eyes are closed, so only somatosensory and vestibular cues remain. In a normal subject, the somatosensory inputs will dominate in this condition. By comparing sway during condition two to sway during condition one, it is possible to detect how well the client is using somatosensory inputs for balance control. Clients with somatosensory loss due to spinal cord injury, diabetes, and amputation have difficulty in condition two. Functional

situations with inadequate lighting or unusable visual cues (e.g., busy carpeting) are similar to condition two.

Under condition four, the support surface is sway-referenced (somatosensory cues are available but are inaccurate), so only visual and vestibular cues remain. In a normal subject, the visual inputs will dominate in this condition. Comparing sway during condition four to sway during condition one indicates how well the client is using visual inputs for balance control. Clients with visual loss due to diabetes, cataracts, or field loss have difficulty in condition four. Functional situations that correlate with condition four include compliant surfaces (beach, soft ground, gravel driveway) and unstable surfaces (boat deck, slipping throw rug).

Under condition five, the eyes are closed (visual cues are absent) and the support surface is sway-referenced (somatosensory cues are inaccurate), leaving the vestibular inputs as the only remaining sense that is both avail-

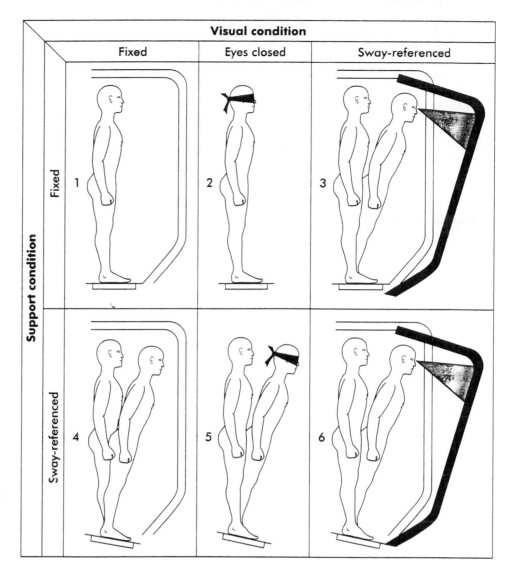

Visual condition

Fixed | Eyes closed | Sway-referenced

Support condition

Fixed — 1, 2, 3

Sway-referenced — 4, 5, 6

FIGURE 21–11. The six sensory organization test conditions. The SOT determines the relative reliance on visual, vestibular, and somatosensory inputs for postural control using computerized dynamic posturography. (From Hasson S: Clinical Exercise Physiology. St. Louis, CV Mosby, 1994.)

able and accurate. Comparison of sway during condition five to sway during condition one indicates how well the client is using vestibular inputs for balance control. Clients with vestibular loss due to head injury, multiple sclerosis, and acoustic neuroma may have difficulty with condition five. Many elderly clients also may be unstable in this condition. Functional situations where these clients may be at risk for falls would have both inadequate lighting and compliant or unsteady surfaces (i.e., walking on a gravel driveway or thick carpet in the dark).

Under both conditions three and six, the visual surround is sway-referenced (visual cues are available but inaccurate). By comparing sway during these two conditions to sway in the absence of vision (conditions two and five, with eyes closed), it is possible to determine how well the client can recognize and subsequently suppress inaccurate visual inputs when they conflict with somatosensory and vestibular cues. Some clients with CNS lesions (e.g., head injury, stroke, tumor) may have difficulty with this condition. Clients who cannot recognize and ignore inaccurate visual cues cannot distinguish whether they are moving or the environment is moving. If they perceive that they are moving (away from midline) when

in actual fact they are not, they may often actively generate postural responses to "right" themselves. These responses, invoked to bring the COG to midline, then result in movement away from the midline. The inaccurate perception leads to a self-initiated loss of balance. Functional situations that correlate with this test condition include public transportation, grocery and library aisles, and moving walkways.

The SOT is valid and reliable in the absence of motoric problems, which increase sway for reasons unrelated to sensory reception and perception. Normative data are available.

The Clinical Test for Sensory Interaction on Balance (CTSIB) is a clinical version of the SOT that does not use computerized forceplate technology.[67] The concept of the six conditions remains intact (Fig. 21–13). Instead of sway measures, the examiner uses a stopwatch and visual observation. A thick foam pad substitutes for the moving forceplate during conditions four, five, and six. A modified Japanese lantern substitutes for the moving visual surround in conditions three and six. The client is asked to stand with feet parallel and arms at sides or hands on hips. Five 30-second trials of each condition are per-

SENSORY ANALYSIS			
RATIO NAME	**TEST CONDITIONS**	**RATIO PAIR**	**SIGNIFICANCE**
SOM Somatosensory	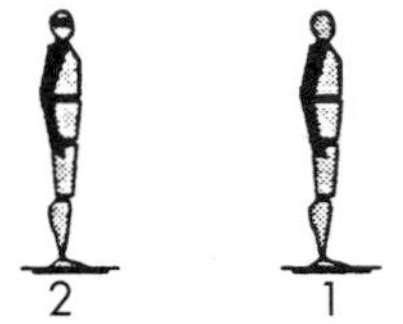 2 1	Condition 1 / Condition 2	Question: Does sway increase when visual cues are removed? Low scores: Patient makes poor use of somatosensory references.
VIS Visual	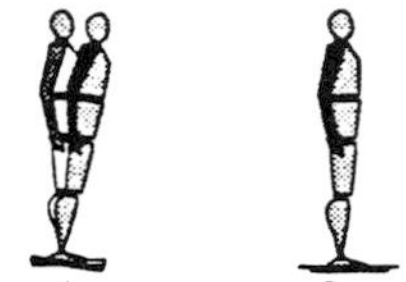 4 1	Condition 4 / Condition 1	Question: Does sway increase when somatosensory cues are inaccurate? Low scores: Patient makes poor use of visual references.
VEST Vestibular	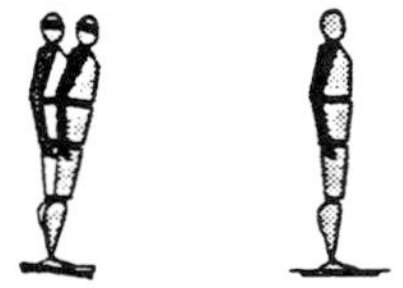 5 1	Condition 5 / Condition 1	Question: Does sway increase when visual cues are removed and somatosensory cues are inaccurate? Low scores: Patient makes poor use of vestibular cues, or vestibular cues unavailable.
PREF Visual Preference	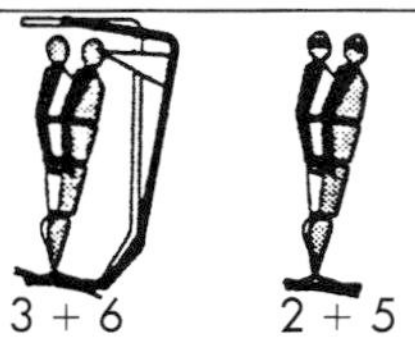 3 + 6 2 + 5	Condition 3 + 6 / Condition 2 + 5	Question: Do inaccurate visual cues result in increased sway compared to no visual cues? Low scores: Patient relies on visual cues even when they are inaccurate.

FIGURE 21–12. Postural sway measures from each of the six SOT conditions are compared and the ratios are used to identify impairments in the use of sensory inputs for postural control. (From Jacobson GP, Newman CW, Kartush JM: Handbook of Balance Function Testing. St. Louis, CV Mosby, 1993.)

formed.[19] The watch is stopped if the client steps, reaches, or falls during the 30 seconds. A maximum score for five trials of each condition is 150 seconds. Normal subjects are able to stand without loss of balance for 30 seconds per trial per condition. In normal subjects and clients with peripheral vestibular lesions, measures using foam correlate to moving forceplate measures.[76] Studies have not shown that measures using the Japanese lantern correlate with the moving visual surround measures. The CTSIB may not be a reliable measure in clients with hemiplegia.[18]

Tests of sensory integration or organization can be of benefit to the clinician working with clients with vestibular dysfunction, especially when used with other measures of vestibular dysfunction such as VOR. The clinician can use the information regarding client response within a variety of environmental conditions to determine intervention management strategies.[26] The SOT is also used to identify the individual with "aphysiological" balance disorders, when no physical cause for the dizziness and imbalance has been found. Aphysiological disorders are most often seen when secondary emotional reactions decrease the client's ability to compensate for mild to moderate dysfunction. Clients in this group perform more poorly than normal on the first three (easier) conditions of posturography and better than normal during the more challenging conditions (four, five, and six). More intertrial

variability is noted with the client with suspected aphysiological symptoms than with normal individuals or clients with known vestibular dysfunction.

Often individuals with compensated vestibular system deficiencies will select visual or somatosensory information as the primary input for balance, to decrease the sense of sensory conflict. Vestibular input does not appear to play its normal role during certain activities, and vestibular deficits may be difficult to detect. For example, when testing the individual with chronic vestibular insufficiency, standing balance on foam may appear normal with eyes open and a static head position but not when the head is quickly turned and visual inputs for balance are disrupted. The standard SOT and CTSIB tests do not take this component into consideration; however, having the individual perform head movements during these tests can indicate visual dependence (the need for gaze stabilization to maintain balance).

TESTS OF NYSTAGMUS

Assessment of eye movement control can help to diagnose dysfunction of the peripheral and central vestibular pathways through the medial longitudinal fasciculus. In particular, tests for a specific type of abnormal eye movement called nystagmus should be performed. Nystagmus is nonvoluntary, rhythmic oscillation of the eyes, with movement in one direction clearly faster than movement in the other

VISUAL CONDITIONS

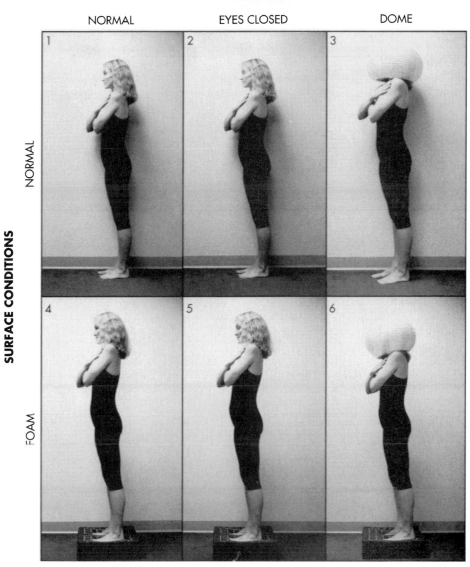

FIGURE 21–13. The clinical test for sensory interaction in balance uses foam and a Japanese lantern to replicate the six sensory conditions. A stopwatch is used to time trials.

direction. The client with nystagmus will also usually complain of vertigo. There is more than one type of nystagmus; identification of the particular type can direct the clinician toward the area of dysfunction.[32]

Spontaneous nystagmus results from imbalance in the vestibular signals through their transmission to the oculomotor neurons. This imbalance produces a constant drift of the eyes in one direction interrupted by brief fast movement in the opposite direction. Spontaneous nystagmus occurs after acute lesions and usually lasts about 24 hours. Peripheral versus central lesions may be distinguished by asking the patient to fix his or her gaze on a stable target. Nystagmus from peripheral vestibular lesions is easily inhibited with visual fixation. Nystagmus due to central lesions of the brain stem or cerebellum is not easily inhibited with visual fixation.

Positional nystagmus is induced by a change in head position. Paroxysmal nystagmus due to stimulation of the canals lasts only seconds and then dissipates. Central nystagmus due to central vestibular system damage lasts

minutes or longer before abating. Static nystagmus occurs with lesions to the otolith system through connections in the vestibular nuclei and cerebellum. It is provoked with change of head position in relation to gravity and continues as long as the position is maintained, although it can fluctuate in frequency and amplitude. Static nystagmus can be suppressed with visual fixation.

Gaze-evoked nystagmus occurs when clients shift their eyes from a primary central position to a second location. It is caused by the inability to maintain stable gaze position and the eye drifts back toward the center or primary position. Usually indicative of a CNS problem, it is common in multiple sclerosis, brain injury, and congenital lesions.

The head-shaking nystagmus test is performed by the examiner passively moving the client's head. Starting with the head anteriorly flexed to 30 degrees (placing the lateral canal parallel to the ground), the head is moved side to side 45 degrees in each direction for 30 cycles with a velocity of 360 degrees per second. Normal individuals do not have nystagmus after this stimulus, but nystagmus occurs in clients with vestibular dysfunction. It can be immediate or with latency (delay of onset; usually about 10 seconds) and lasts for 5 to 20 seconds. This test can be easily performed in the clinic and is an indicator of vestibular dysfunction.[73]

TESTS OF SEMICIRCULAR CANAL FUNCTION

Tests that attempt to stimulate the vestibular semicircular canals are usually called vertiginous positions tests because they move or place clients in various positions and monitor for vertigo, dizziness, nausea, and nystagmus.[32] No single list of positions is used consistently across sites, but in general most of these tests have 10 to 20 provoking movements that are performed from least to most disturbing (Fig. 21–14). A standardized method of scoring is not used across sites, but the examiner usually monitors the number of positions that induce symptoms (i.e., 10/16), the number of repetitions of the maneuver that can be performed before symptoms begin to increase, the intensity of the symptoms as rated by the client (i.e., 0 = no symptoms, up to 10 = severe symptoms with near vomiting), and the duration of the change in symptom level (e.g., client began at intensity level two and

symptoms increased with the positioning maneuver to a level seven; it took 26 seconds for the symptoms to return to a level two). If a canal is hyperresponsive to head motion, the canal that is affected will be activated and cause dizziness when the head moves in the direction of that canal. For example, if the head is tipped forward and to the right, the right anterior canal and the right posterior canal will be activated. The response will most often be vertigo and will be brief (less than 1 minute). If the dizziness is persistent, not decreasing over time, the disorder may be central in nature. In this case the complaint may be vertigo or diffuse dizziness. With a central disorder the examiner may observe nystagmus during the change of positions, or the complaint may come as the client returns to the starting point. When symptoms are due to canal hypersensitivity, improvement is noted by fewer provoking positions, a greater number of repetitions before symptom exacerbation, lower intensity of symptoms, and shorter duration of symptoms.[67]

The Hallpike-Dix maneuver is a vertiginous position test to stimulate the posterior semicircular canal (Fig. 21–15).[32] This test is used to determine if there are otoconia in the semicircular canal. A positive response (vertigo and nystagmus) on this test leads to a diagnosis

UNIVERSITY OF MICHIGAN VESTIBULAR TESTING CENTER HABITUATION TRAINING

NAME: _____ MRN: _____ AGE: _____ SEX: _____

DATE: _____	INTENSITY	DURATION	SCORE
BASELINE SYMPTOMS			
1. Sitting → Supine			
2. Supine → Left Side			
3. → → Right Side			
4. Supine → Sitting			
5. Left Hallpike			
6. → → Sitting			
7. Right Hallpike			
8. → → Sitting			
9. Sitting → Nose To Left Knee			
10. Sitting → Erect Left			
11. Sitting → Nose To Right Knee			
12. Sitting → Erect Right			
13. Sitting → Head Rotation			
14. Sitting → Head Flex. And Ext.			
15. Standing → Turn To Right			
16. Standing → Turn To Left			

INTENSITY: SCALE FROM 0 TO 5 (0=NO SX, 5=SEVERE SX)
DURATION: SCALE FROM 0 TO 3 (5-10 SEC=1 POINT, 11-30 SEC=2 POINTS, ≥30 SEC=3 POINTS)

MOTION SENSITIVITY QUOTIENT: $\dfrac{\text{POSITIONS} \times \text{SCORE}}{2048} \times 100 =$ _____ 28-12.

TOTAL

FIGURE 21–14. An example of a standardized list of vertiginous positions tests. Intensity of dizziness is rated by the client, and duration of dizziness is measured with a stopwatch. (Courtesy of the University of Michigan Vestibular Testing Center.)

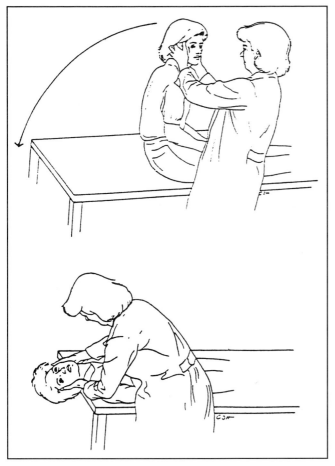

FIGURE 21–15. The Hallpike-Dix maneuver. Moving the patient rapidly from a sitting to a supine position with the head turned so that the affected ear is 30 to 45 degrees below the horizontal will stimulate the posterior canal and may produce vertigo and nystagmus. (From Herdman S: Treatment of benign paroxysmal positional vertigo. Phys Ther 70:381–388, 1990, with permission of the American Physical Therapy Association.)

of BPV. The client is positioned in long sitting on a mat or plinth such that, when supine, the head and neck extend over the upper edge of the surface. The examiner holds the head of the sitting client between both hands and then rapidly moves the client backward and down with the head turned to the side and the neck extended 30 to 45 degrees below the horizontal. The head is held in this position for 20 to 30 seconds. The examiner monitors for symptoms of vertigo and observes the eyes for nystagmus. If nystagmus occurs, the direction of the nystagmus indicates whether or not the otoconia are free floating or adherent. When the quick phase of the nystagmus is toward the ground (geotropic), the otoconia are free floating. If the otoconia are adherent to the hair cells, the quick phase of the nystagmus is away from the ground (ageotropic).[33] In cases of BPV, the involved side is distinguished by which ear is toward the ground when the symptoms occur. The critical hallmark of BPV is that the vertigo usually starts after 5 to 10 seconds and resolves or fatigues within 20 to 40 seconds. Benign positional nystagmus or vertigo is a common sequela of head concussion, viral labyrinthitis, and vascular occlusion of the

inner ear. It can also develop without a known external cause.[32]

BPV may involve any semicircular canal, although the posterior canal is most common due to its relationship to the otoliths when the person is in the recumbent position. However, the horizontal canal can collect otoconia and the result is horizontal nystagmus generated with head movement. Horizontal canal BPV is tested in the supine position with the head held in 30 degrees flexion to keep the lateral canal perpendicular to the ground or in the neutral position for ease of positioning. The head is then turned in each direction and the eyes observed for horizontal nystagmus. This must be distinguished from static positional nystagmus by the fact that the nystagmus will fatigue if it is due to movement of the otoconia but otherwise persists.[22]

VISUAL-VESTIBULAR INTERACTION

The VOR test examines the interaction of the visual and vestibular systems for eye and head orientation. The ability to hold the eyes fixed on a target while the head is moving is known as gaze stabilization. The client is asked to perform these tasks in horizontal, vertical, and diagonal planes (Fig. 21–16) and at the speed of 2 Hz. If the image blurs, the gain of the system is abnormal, meaning that the vestibular system is unable to move the eyes at the exact same speed in the opposite direction as the head movement. The ratio of eye velocity to head velocity is known as the gain of the VOR. The gain of an intact VOR is usually equal to one, which means movement of the eyes is equal to the movement of the head. The client with vestibular disorder has usually self-limited the speed of head movement to accommodate for the abnormal gain. In some instances, the client will not describe blurring (a lack of gaze stabilization) with testing but will complain of dizziness while performing the test procedure. This is most likely related to the blurring of the visual field beyond the target, which is interpreted as motion. Blurring of the image during head movement may also be the result of an oculomotor dysfunction that limits convergent gaze.

The ability to synchronize simultaneous eye and head movements in the same direction is associated with the ability of the brain to suppress the VOR and is known as VOR cancellation. If the central integration capabilities are abnormal, the client will not be able to override the reflex activity and cannot keep the eye and head moving at the same rate in the same direction.

VISUAL ACUITY TEST

Oculomotor tests are performed to determine the ability of the eyes to orient the head during movement.[32] Saccades, or the ability for the eyes to move suddenly to locate a point in space, are tested by asking the client (head fixed) to look at one target. The examiner then suddenly presents a second target on the opposite side of the visual field. The client must look at this second target as quickly as possible without moving the head. In normal subjects, a single rapid jump of the eyes occurs. Abnormal responses include an undershooting or overshooting of the visual target, which must be adjusted with subsequent smaller jumps. The examiner observes for these multiple

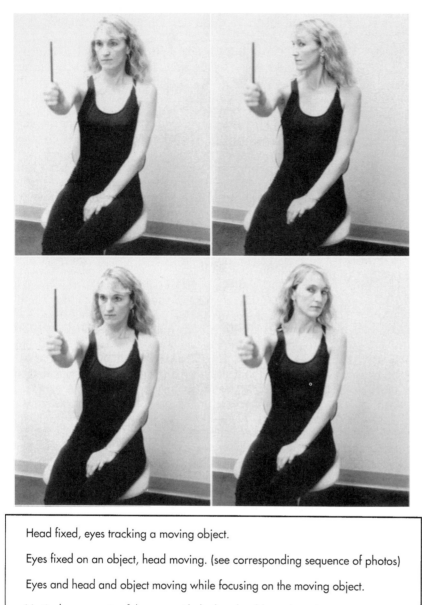

Head fixed, eyes tracking a moving object.

Eyes fixed on an object, head moving. (see corresponding sequence of photos)

Eyes and head and object moving while focusing on the moving object.

Vertical movements of the eyes with the head stable and moving.

Eyes diagonal with the head stable and moving.

Eye movements incorporated with trunk movements.

FIGURE 21–16. Eye and head motions are assessed to determine whether symptoms associated with the vestibular-ocular reflex mechanism are present. (From Whitney S: Dizziness and balance disorders. Clin Manage 11:42–48, 1991, with permission of the American Physical Therapy Association.)

attempts to exactly locate the visual target. Smooth pursuit, or the ability for the eyes to move at various speeds to follow a moving visual target, is tested by asking the client (head fixed) to follow a moving object held by the examiner. The examiner moves the object at different speeds and in different directions throughout the visual field and observes for any inability to follow the object. Normal subjects have no difficulty following the moving target (see Chapter 27).

The Fukuda stepping test was developed to assess labyrinth function.[54] A grid is drawn on the floor (Fig. 21–17) with two concentric circles (1 and 2 m in diameter, respectively) divided into 30-degree sections. The client is placed standing in the center of the circles, is blind-folded, and raises the arms outstretched to shoulder height. The examiner instructs the client to take 100 marching steps (knees high) in place, then observes for postural sway and deviations of position of the head, arms, and body. Once the client has stopped, the examiner quantitatively measures the angle of rotation, angle of displacement, and the distance of displacement. According to Fukuda, normal subjects are able to take 100 steps without traveling more than 1 m and without rotating more than 45 degrees, whereas clients with peripheral vestibular dysfunction deviate outside this range toward the side of the deficit. Individuals with a normal vestibular system and no symptoms can also test positive on this test, so it should be used for diagnostic purposes only in

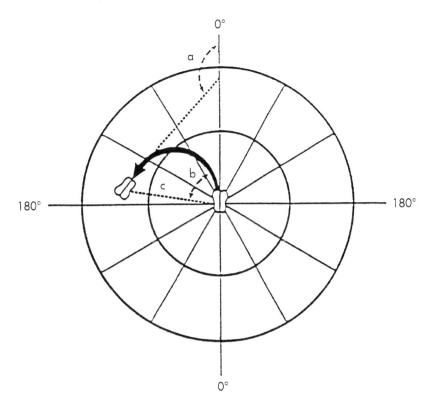

FIGURE 21–17. The Fukuda stepping test for peripheral vestibular clients uses a floor grid to detect the extend of drift that occurs during an eyes-closed stepping task. (From Newton R: Brain Injury 3:334, 1989.)

conjunction with other tests—never in isolation. Obviously, the client being tested must be motorically very high level to perform this test, and the examiner must be sure that any observed deviations are not due to motoric (versus vestibular) causes. The reliability of this test is poor, and its use is not recommended.[11]

Functional Scales

A comprehensive balance evaluation must include both impairment measures and disability measures. Functional scales help to address the latter. By asking the client to perform functional tasks that demand balance skills, the clinician can determine the presence of disabilities and identify the tasks that the client needs to practice. Three mobility scales and three gait scales focus on postural control; five of these were developed for the elderly population to determine risk for falls. Many clinicians also are using them to assess neurological clients, although their usefulness with neurological populations has not been formally evaluated.

The Berg Balance Scale is a list of 14 tasks that the client is asked to perform.[7] The examiner rates the client on each task using a scoring scale of 0 to 4, where 0 is unable to perform and 4 is able to perform without difficulty. Originally designed for assessing risk for falls in older adults, it has also been used (although not validated) with clients post stroke.[56] The original Get-Up-and-Go test is made up of seven items scored on a scale of 1 to 5, where 1 is normal, and 5 is severely abnormal.[47] This test has been modified to increase its objectivity and reliability. The Timed Get-Up-and-Go test eliminates the "standing steady" segment and uses a stopwatch to time the performance.[58] This test may be performed using an assistive device; however, the use of a device will alter the speed at which the task can be accomplished, and any retesting must be done with the same device to produce comparable results. The Tinetti Performance Oriented Assessment of Balance is a list of nine items scored on scales of either 0 to 1 or 0 to 2, with the higher numbers reflecting better (more normal) performance.[72] The best possible score is a 16. The score value is specific to the item. Most balance and mobility scales have been developed to assess risk for falls in the elderly. Many share similar items. See Table 21–4 for a summary of scale items.

The Tinetti Performance Oriented Assessment of Gait is a list of seven normal aspects of gait that are observed by the examiner as the client walks at a self-selected pace and then at a rapid but safe pace.[72] Scoring scales are again either 0 to 1 or 0 to 2, and higher numbers indicate better performance. Score values are specific to the item being observed (Table 21–5). The best possible score is a 12. When combined, the Tinetti balance and gait scales offer a best possible score of 28. The original Gait Assessment Rating Scale (GARS) is a list of 16 abnormal aspects of gait observed by the examiner as the client walks at a self-selected pace[77] (see Table 21–5). These abnormalities are commonly seen in elderly people who fall. The items are scored on a scale of 0 to 3, with lower numbers reflecting better (less abnormal) performance. The best possible score is 0. This gait scale provides some relative numerical indication of the quality of gait. A shorter, modified version of this test, the Modified GARS, has been developed and provides equivalent sensitivity while taking less time to perform.[75] These two gait scales were developed to assess risk for falls in the elderly. The Dynamic Gait Index is a more recently developed test spe-

TABLE 21-4. Balance and Mobility Scale Items

Activity	Berg Test	Dynamic Gait Index	Get Up and Go	Tinetti Balance
1. Sit unsupported	√			√
2. Sit-to-stand	√		√	√
3. Stand-to-sit	√		√	√
4. Transfers	√			
5. Stand unsupported	√		√	√
6. Stand with eyes closed	√			√
7. Stand with feet together	√			
8. Tandem stand	√			
9. Stand on one leg	√			
10. Trunk rotation while standing	√			
11. Retrieve object from floor	√			
12. Turn 360 degrees	√			√
13. Stool stepping	√			
14. Reach forward while standing	√			
15. Sternal nudge				√
16. Walk		√	√	
17. Abrupt stop		√		
18. Walk then turn		√	√	
19. Step over obstacle		√		
20. Stairs		√		
21. Walk at preferred and varied speeds		√		
22. Walk with horizontal and vertical head turns		√		
23. Step around obstacles		√		

● **T A B L E   2 1 – 5. Gait Scale Items**

Gait Activities	Tinetti Gait Scale	Gait Assessment Rating Scale
1. Initiation (hesitancy)	√	√
2. Step length	√	√
3. Step height	√	√
4. Step symmetry	√	√
5. Step continuity	√	√
6. Path deviation	√	√
7. Trunk	√	√
8. Walking-heel distance	√	
9. Staggering		√
10. Heel strike		√
11. Hip ROM°		√
12. Knee ROM°		√
13. Elbow extension°		√
14. Shoulder extension°		√
15. Shoulder abduction°		√
16. Arm-heelstrike synchrony		√
17. Forward head°		√
18. Shoulders held elevated°		√
19. Forward flexed trunk°		√

°During gait.
ROM, range of motion.

cifically designed to look at postural control during gait.[70] It includes eight items requiring changes in gait speed, walking with horizontal and vertical head turning, whole-body turns during gait, stepping over and around obstacles, and stair ascent and descent. Items on this test are scored on a scale of 0 to 3, with 3 being "normal" performance and 0 indicating "severe impairment." The best possible score on this test is a 24. The presence of head and whole-body turns in this test may help identify clients with potential vestibular dysfunction. The reliability of this test with neurological clients has not yet been demonstrated. The three tests listed above are distinct from traditional gait tests because they focus on elements of postural control during gait.

Combination Test Batteries

Because no single test can give a complete picture of a client's balance abilities, three commonly used test batteries combine several types of tests. The Fregley-Graybiel Ataxia Test Battery is a list of eight test items that the client must perform (Fig. 21–18).[54] Standing trials in tandem stance both off and on a rail with eyes open and closed are timed. Timed single-leg stance trials also are performed for each leg. Walking 10 steps with eyes closed is included. Five trials of each task are given. Trials are stopped if the client uncrosses the arms, opens eyes (during eyes closed trials), steps (during standing trials), or falls. Trials are judged on a pass/fail basis. This test battery is valid for use with clients who have peripheral vestibular dysfunction. Normative data are available from a normative database composed primarily of young men. As noted earlier, clients must be motorically very high level to perform these tasks: this test is a good choice for clients with higher level abilities because it does provide more demanding balance tasks. Interpretations regarding a client's use of sensory inputs when motor involvement is also present cannot be made with certainty.

The Fugl-Meyer Sensorimotor Assessment of Balance Performance is a subset of the Fugl-Meyer Physical Performance Battery, which was designed for use with hemiplegic clients (Fig. 21–19).[19] Three sitting and four standing balance activities are listed. The items are scored on a 0 to 2 scale, with score values specific to each item. Higher scores indicate better performance; the maximum (best) score is 14; however, a client could achieve this score of 14 and still not have normal balance.

The physical therapy checklist is a combination of risk factor items relating to the status of neuromuscular systems, foot problems, balance skills, and walking abilities (Fig. 21–20).[71] It was designed to assess risk for falls in elderly clients. Items are scored either normal (0) or abnormal (1) for neuromuscular and foot items and negative (0) or positive (1) for balance and gait problems. This test has not been validated. Normal subjects would receive the best possible score of 0.

The Dizziness Handicap Inventory (DHI) was developed to identify specific functional, emotional, or physical problems associated with an individual's reaction to imbalance or dizziness.[40, 41] The DHI assesses the client's perception of the effects of the balance problem and the client's level of emotional adjustment. It also looks at perceived physical limitations as a consequence of the disorder. There are 25 total items divided into three subscales in this self-assessment inventory. Included are a nine-item functional scale, a nine-item emotional scale, and a seven-item physical scale. Each item is assigned a value of four points for a "yes," two points for a "sometimes," and zero points for a "no." This inventory is reliable, is easy to administer, and can be used to evaluate treatment outcomes.[53] Changes in scores on the functionally based DHI correlate highly with changes in scores on the impairment-based SOT.[40]

Considerations in the Selection of Balance Tests

To determine the type and level of challenge of the tests to be used during the examination, a thorough subjective history is critical. In describing the symptoms and the situations that cause dizziness or imbalance, the client offers clues to possible deficits and thereby the measures that will help to identify them. Typical components of the

FREGLEY TEST

Condition	Trials				
	1	2	3	4	5
1. Sharpened Romberg, EC (60 sec; feet in tandem)					
2. Walk on Rail, EO (5 steps; best 3/5 trials)					
3. Stand on Rail, EO (3 trials; 60 sec/trial)				x	x
4. Stand on Rail, EC (3 trials; 60 sec/trial)				x	x
5. Stand on Right Leg, on Floor, EC (5 trials; 30 sec/trial)					
6. Stand on Left Leg, on Floor, EC (5 trials; 30 sec/trial)					
7. Walk on Floor, EC (3 trials; 10 steps each)				x	x
8. Stand sideways on rail (characterize sway)*					

*Added by the author to observe the movement strategy used by the individual
EO, eyes open; EC, eyes closed.

FIGURE 21–18. A combination of tasks (Romberg, OLST, walking) and environments (EO, EC, rail) are included in the Fregley-Graybiel ataxia test battery. (From Newton R: Review of tests of standing balance abilities. Brain Injury 3;33, 1989.)

FUGL-MEYER

Test	Scoring	Maximum Possible Score	Attained Score
1. Sit without support _____	0—Cannot maintain sitting without support 1—Can sit unsupported less than 5 minutes 2—Can sit longer than 5 minutes		
2. Parachute reaction, non-affected side _____	0—Does no abduct shoulder or extend elbow 1—Impaired reaction 2—Normal reaction		
3. Parachute reaction, affected side _____	Scoring is the same as for test 2		
4. Stand with support _____	0—Cannot stand 1—Stands with maximum support 2—Stands with minimum support for 1 minute		
5. Stand without support _____	0—Cannot stand without support 1—Stands less than 1 minute or sways 2—Stands with good balance more than 1 minute		
6. Stand on unaffected side _____	0—Cannot be maintained longer than 1–2 seconds 1—Stands balanced 4–9 seconds 2—Stands balanced more than 10 seconds		
7. Stand on affected side _____	0—Scoring is the same as for test 6		
	Maximum Balance Score		

FIGURE 21–19. The Fugl-Meyer Sensorimotor Assessment of Balance Performance includes both very low level and very high level tasks. (From DiFabio RP, Badke MB: Relationship of sensory organization to balance function in patients with hemiplegia. Phys Ther 70:20, 1990.)

PHYSICAL THERAPY CHECKLIST*

Item/Criteria		Scoring
Neuromuscular		Normal = 0
		Abnormal = 1
Shoulder strength/ROM		
Hand grip strength		
Hip flexion		
Knee flexion		
Knee extension		
Ankle dorsiflexion		
Ankle plantar flexion		
Foot problems		Absent = 0
		Present = 1
Grossly long nails		
Severe callouses		
Any bunions		
Any toe deformities		
Balance items		Negative = 0
		Positive = 1
Nudge	Subject standing at full height, examiner pushes gently on sternum three times. Positive score is staggering or struggling for balance.	
Single leg balance	Subject asked to balance on each leg for 5 seconds. Positive score is touching ground with other foot.	
360° turn	Subject asked to turn one complete revolution on the spot. Positive score is any unsteadiness.	
Chair sit	Subject asked to sit down in a firm armless chair. Negative score is safe smooth motion, else positive.	
Gait items		Negative = 0
		Positive = 1
Path deviation	Subjects asked to walk straight line over a 3 m course (or use of walking aid).	
Trunk sway	Subjects observed over 3 m straight course. Positive score is trunk sway, flexion of knees or back, abduction of arms, (or use of walking aid).	
Pick up speed	Subjects asked to walk at as fast a pace as they feel is safe. Positive score is inability to pick up speed.	
	Total (Max. = 18)	

* These items, derived from a variety of sources 1-4, 6-8, 11-13 are included because they have been both associated with falling and are potentially modifiable through physical therapy. This checklist may prove useful in identifying those who are at increased risk of falling because of deficits that may be remediable through physiotherapy.

Because this is not a validated scale, the score has no standard meaning. It is not recommended for use as a comprehensive risk assessment instrument.

FIGURE 21–20. Designed as a risk-for-falls screening tool for use with the elderly, Speechley and Tinett's physical therapy checklist covers both impairments (strength, ROM) and functional tasks (stand-to-sit, walking). (From Speechley M, Tinetti M: Assessment of risk and prevention of falls among elderly persons. Physiother Can 42:75, 1990.)

history to be included in the evaluation are listed in Table 21–6.

Many of the functional scales reviewed previously were designed to determine whether balance is abnormal in elderly clients who have no diagnosis—in other words, as screening tools. Clinicians working with clearly diagnosed neurological clients often do not need such tools to establish that balance skills are abnormal because the deficits are patently obvious. These tools can be useful, however, to identify disabilities, establish a baseline, monitor progress, and document outcomes.

Many clinical facilities have their own therapy evaluation forms that include a section on balance. Usually, items and scoring are defined by the facility. They are not standardized across sites as are published scales and are rarely tested for measurement quality such as validity and reliability. As rehabilitation professions evolve toward evidence-based practice, the use of nonstandardized tests with unknown measurement quality is no longer acceptable. Clinicians should use standardized, objective, quantifiable, valid tests with high reliability, sensitivity, and specificity whenever possible. Facilities with their own tests should conduct research to ensure that they are valid, reliable, and sensitive to change over time. It is important to use a functional balance rating scale in the evaluation of clients with neurological impairment. To be sensitive enough to measure changes in clients who clearly are not (and may never be) clinically normal, scales should have at least five, and perhaps seven, possible relative scores.

In addition, it is necessary to perform additional tests to assess the systems that may affect postural control to help identify and measure impairments (e.g., ROM, strength, sensation and sensory organization, motor planning and control). These types of measures should be sensitive, objective, and quantifiable. Unfortunately, there are some systems for which objective, quantifiable clinical measures have not been developed (e.g., motor planning, coordination). In these cases, clinicians must continue to use subjective rating scales.

Other factors to include when deciding what tests to use are the time it takes to perform the test, the number of staff who must be present, and the space and equipment needed. Clinicians must now weigh the potential benefits of technological tools (e.g., computerized electromyography, forceplates, isokinetics, motion analysis) against their cost and practicality (i.e., their cost-effectiveness). The test must be suitable for the client's level of

TABLE 21–6. Client History Reveals Provoking Activities

Activities commonly reported as a trigger for symptoms, associated with the probable area of vestibular dysfunction.

Otolith (linear acceleration)
Riding in elevators and escalators
Riding in a car
Lunges

Semicircular Canals (angular acceleration)
Bending forward
Tipping head back to look up or reach up
Rolling over
Quick head movement

Vestibular Ocular Reflex Dysfunction
Loss of gaze stabilization
Reading
Head movement with walking

Oculomotor Dysfunction
Reading
Looking quickly from target to target
Following a moving target
Convergence and divergence

Visual Dependency for Balance
Quick head turns
Reading
Looking at a computer screen
Fluorescent lights
Stimulating visual environments
Walking in crowds
Riding in a car
Riding an escalator
Standing or walking in the dark or with eyes closed

functioning (physical and cognitive). Many head-injured clients, for example, cannot initially participate in traditional forms of testing due to cognitive limitations.

PROBLEM IDENTIFICATION, GOAL SETTING, AND TREATMENT PLANNING

Clinical Decision Making

Treatment of clients with neurological diagnosis is based on the particular set of impairments and disabilities possessed by each individual. Remediation of balance deficits similarly must be specific to the involved systems and functional losses in each client. Clinicians should generate an overall problem list for each client; if imbalance is a listed problem, then a sublist of balance problems also can be developed (Fig. 21–21).

To direct and establish priorities for treatment, clinicians must review the problem list and ask themselves the following questions (Fig. 21–22): Which impairments are temporary and can be remedied? How much improvement can be expected? How soon will it occur? Which impairments are permanent and must be compensated for? What other systems can be counted on to substitute? What external compensations may be needed? For example, consider two clients, both with vestibular diagnosis. One client has unilateral peripheral vestibular

hypofunction. This situation may be temporary, or the contralateral vestibular organ may be able to compensate. In either case the use of vestibular inputs for balance control could improve, so exercises to stimulate the vestibular system are indicated. The other client has total bilateral vestibular loss secondary to neurotoxic medication. This condition is permanent, and no use of vestibular inputs is possible, so exercises must focus on improving the use of remaining inputs (somatosensory and visual).

With some clients with neurological impairments, it is often not possible to know whether a problem is permanent or temporary, as in recovery from a stroke or head injury. In others with progressive diseases such as Parkinson's disease or multiple sclerosis, the rate of decline is unknown and abilities may fluctuate. In these cases the clinician should consider the following issues: Would a consult provide me with the information I need to know? If so, referral is appropriate. Are there any contraindications to treatment? What are the risks and benefits of providing versus withholding treatment? Is some amount of functional improvement possible? If there are no contraindications, the benefits outweigh the risks, and there is an expectation of functional improvement, then a trial of treatment may be given if it cannot be known for certain whether the problem(s) will respond to the treatment. In these cases especially, a baseline must be established against which to measure any change. Change for the worse or no change after a reasonable trial period indicates that treatment should be altered or discontinued.

In some clients with vestibular impairments, the receptors or neurons that were damaged may recover. Spontaneous recovery after unilateral vestibular loss may occur as the resting tone of the system is reestablished and nystagmus is eliminated. Vestibular adaptation occurs when the vestibular system responds to facilitation and recovers function. This takes time and the appropriate stimuli. Appropriate stimuli include activities that will produce an error (mismatch) signal to provoke the brain to make the calibration changes necessary for adaptation. Habituation is a different process by which pathological responses to vestibular-provoking activities become controlled. Exercises to promote habituation are used primarily when the sensory mismatch is persistent and the system does not have the ability to adapt. They are often used for clients with positional dizziness, or when dizziness is related to self-limiting behavior.[65]

Using the Systems Model to Identify Postural Control Impairments

The systems approach is useful to develop a balance problem list because it can be applied to different diagnoses equally well and allows deficits in multiple systems to be recognized. Table 21–7 illustrates several examples of ways this framework is used to identify balance deficits in clients with different neurological diagnosis.

For each client, problems affecting postural control should be described in objective, measurable terms whenever possible. For example, writing "impaired vision" is too vague; "two-line drop on eye chart" is more specific. "Poor use of visual inputs for balance control" is an

EXAMPLE OF BALANCE PROBLEM LIST

General Problem List	Balance Problem List
1. Decreased strength (L) side	
2. Decreased ROM (L) shoulder	
3. Decreased endurance	
4. Impaired sensation (L) side	
5. Decreased balance	a. Decreased weight bearing on left (L) LE b. Unable to maintain midline orientation c. Extraneous sway with eyes closed d. Unable to stand on (L) LE e. Decreased limits of stability to 40/100% f. Unable to shift to (L) side g. Unable to establish stable base of support h. Unable to stand on unstable surface i. Unable to perform hip strategy
6. Increased tone (L) side	
7. Synergistic movement (L) side	
8. Min. assist transfers	
9. Mod. assist ambulation	

FIGURE 21–21. An example of a balance-specific problem list (as a subset of a general problem list), which should be developed to guide balance rehabilitation treatments.

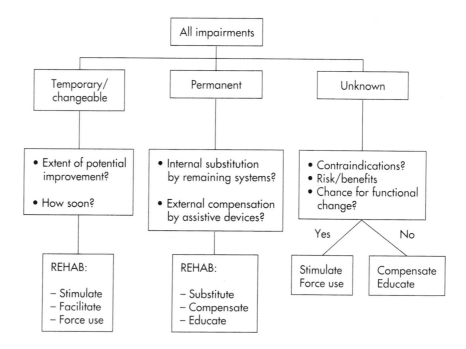

FIGURE 21–22. A clinical decision-making tree to illustrate the treatment-planning process in balance rehabilitation.

T A B L E 2 1 – 7. Examples of Impairments and Diagnosis

Impairments from Systems Model	Client with Diabetic Stroke	Client with Parkinson's Disease	Client with Incomplete Paraplegia
Peripheral Sensory			
Vision	Retinopathy	Cataracts	
Vestibular		Hair cell loss	
Somatosensory	Peripheral neuropathy	Slowed transmission time	Complete loss
Central Sensory			
Vision	Hemianopia	Vision dominant	Needs superior use to compensate
Vestibular	Failure to use inputs		Needs superior use to compensate
Somatosensory	Failure to use inputs	Failure to use inputs	
Strategy selection	Step dominant	Ankle dominant	Hip dominant
Perception of position in space	Midline shift with left neglect	Restricted limits of stability	
Central Motor			
Timing	Increased reaction time	Bradykinesia	
Sequencing	Disordered	Co-contraction	
Force modulation	Spasticity	Rigidity	
Error correction	Use right side only		
Peripheral Motor			
Range of motion	Knee hyperextension	Bilateral ankle plantarflexor contractures	Hip flexion contractures
Strength	Decreased left side	Decreased bilateral left extremity	Severe weakness bilateral lower extremities and trunk
Endurance	Severely impaired	Moderately impaired	Mildly impaired

interpretation; the objective result could be stated "Loss of balance after less than 15 seconds on 5/5 trials of standing on foam, eyes open." Documenting problems in this manner makes goal writing (and consequently, treatment planning) much easier.

Writing Goals Based on Impairments and Disabilities

Goals also should be stated in objective and measurable terms so that their achievement can be judged. "Improved balance" is open to anyone's interpretation, whereas "Able to stand on right leg for 30 seconds on 3/3 trials" and "Walks tandem entire length of balance beam without misstep 7/10 times" are measurable goals. These types of goals may be helpful to the clinician who understands the link between impairments and function, but they may seen nonfunctional (and therefore unnecessary) to others who read them (e.g., case managers, third-party payers). It is beneficial from their standpoint to incorporate into the impairment goal the functional task that will be affected positively by its achievement. For example: "Able to stand on right leg for _____ so that stairs can be ascended/descended step-over-step without railing," or "Walks tandem on balance beam _____ to demonstrate ability to avoid falls using hip strategy." By describing the impairment/function relationship in the treatment objectives, clinicians force themselves to focus on functional outcomes and illustrate for others why these goals are meaningful. The need for and validity of the treatment are then more likely to be perceived clearly.

If a problem cannot be alleviated and requires compensation, the goal(s) should reflect this as well. For example, a client with diabetes has progressive peripheral neuropathy with somatosensory loss and ineffective ankle strategy.

If the client's visual and vestibular sensory systems and proximal strength are relatively intact, however, then the goals might mention improved use of visual cues and successful substitution of hip and stepping strategies. Educational and environmental modification goals for safety also are appropriate in these situations.

Developing a Treatment Plan

Once the goals are listed and priorities are established, the treatment plan is developed. The most effective and efficient treatments will focus first on those problems with the greatest impact on function and address more than one problem at a time. Training balance on an unstable surface contributes not only to the use of visual and vestibular inputs but also (1) to the use of hip strategy, (2) to increased lower-extremity strength, and (3) to increased motor control (skill) on that type of surface. Training gait on a treadmill with eyes closed or head movement increases (1) the use of somatosensory and vestibular inputs, (2) endurance, and (3) lower-extremity strength. Creative clinicians develop comprehensive treatment plans with this type of multiproblem approach to maximize the time available with clients.

The clinician must thoughtfully choose environments and tasks that together stimulate and challenge the appropriate postural control systems. To stimulate one sensory system, the other systems must be placed at a disadvantage to force reliance on the targeted system. The environment is then structured to put the other systems at a disadvantage (i.e., training with eyes closed or in the dark puts vision at a disadvantage and forces the use of somatosensory and vestibular inputs). If one side or limb is significantly more affected, such as in hemiplegia, then the other side must be disadvantaged to force reliance on the targeted side. Tasks are then selected to disadvantage the less affected side. For example, placing the less affected leg up on a step or small ball makes it more difficult to use for balance and forces the transference of weight to the more affected leg. To achieve optimal function, however, all systems and all sides must be capable of working together, so training to improve balance impairments must be incorporated and interspersed with training functional tasks. For carryover of improvements into "real-life" situations, training tasks should be varied enough to promote motor problem solving on the part of the client.[59] For example, sitting balance and transfers should be taught to stable and unstable surfaces, of different heights and firmnesses, with and without armrests and back supports, or to both right and left sides. This technique may improve the client's abilities to perform safe sitting and transfers in new situations not previously practiced in therapy.[60]

Tables 21–8 through 21–10 illustrate the process of test choice, problem identification based on test results, goal setting based on impairments and disabilities, and treatment planning based on goals in three different types of clients. Note that for each client, only selected tests were performed. Goals were directly related to the problems that were identified by the tests, and treatment plans followed directly from the goals.

BALANCE RETRAINING TECHNIQUES

Motor Learning Concepts

Although it is not within the scope of this chapter to cover the principles of motor learning, it is not possible to approach balance retraining methods without some consideration of several motor learning concepts that must be incorporated into treatment. The clinician must remember that successful treatments address the interaction of the individual, the task, and the environment (Fig. 21–23).[60, 70]

Individual

Therapists should know their client's impairments: sensory and motor, peripheral, and central. Whenever possible, therapists should know which impairments can be rehabilitated and which will require compensation or substitution. Because of the nature of neurological insult, this includes an awareness of cognitive and perceptual impairments that may affect the ability to relearn old skills or develop new ones. Optimal learning of skilled movement requires that the client have (1) knowledge of self (abilities and limitations), (2) knowledge of the

---

TABLE 21–8. An Example of Test Selection, Problem Identification, Goal Setting, and Treatment Planning in a Client with Peripheral Vestibular Deficit

Patient Profile:
- 50-year-old woman
- DX: Uncompensated (R) unilateral peripheral vestibular deficit for 6–7 years
- ENT → Psychol → Neuro Otol → Outpatient PT

Test	Problems Identified	Goals Set	Treatment Plan
Visual acuity	Two-line drop on chart	Able to read chart with only one-line drop	Gaze stabilization exercises

Ocular motor
  Saccades
  Pursuit
  Nystagmus
	Positive nystagmus with Fresnel lenses		

Gaze stabilization
  Visual/vestibular interaction
  VOR cancellation
  Hallpike
	Unable to perform test
	↓ fixation with horizontal + vertical head movements after 5–10 sec
		Able to rotate head horizontally 2 minutes without problems
		Able to perform visual/vestibular interaction test
			Gaze stabilization exercises

Sensory Organization Test	Decreased use of somatosensory inputs 70/100 Decreased use of visual inputs 55/100 Absent use of vestibular inputs 0/100 Unable to resolve visual conflict 0/100	Somatosensory use 100/100 Vision use 90/100 Vestibular use 70/100 Visual conflict resolution 90/100	Sensory environment stimulation
Limits of stability	Restricted anteriorly and posteriorly to 35% limit of stability Slow movement time	Limits of stability expanded to 85% anterior and posterior at 5-second pacing	COG control training
ROM/strength	None		
Gait			
Eyes open	Weaves side to side	Walks in a straight line with eyes closed	Gait training
Eyes closed	Deviates to (R) with eyes closed		
Head turning	Dizzy with horizontal head turns	Walks with only slight deviation with eyes closed and head turning	
Pivots	Loss of balance and dizzy with (R) pivot		
Abrupt stops	Very unsteady with abrupt stop—feels "off"	Spins to (R), (L) with eyes closed Comes to abrupt stop steadily	

COG, center of gravity; (L), left; (R), right; ROM, range of motion; VOR, vestibuloocular reflex.
Reprinted with permission from NeuroCom International, Inc.

T A B L E   2 1 – 9. An Example of How Treatment Planning Flows from Test Results in an Elderly Client with Frequent Falls

Patient Profile:
- 72-year-old woman
- DX: Disequilibrium of aging, frequent falls
- Cardiologist → Neurologist → PT Outpatient

Test	Problems Identified	Goals Set	Treatment Plan
Peripheral sensory			
Somatosensory	Mildly decreased vibration sense bilateral lower extremity	Compensate for permanent sensory loss	Educate about safe surfaces and lighting
Vision	↓ Acuity-cataracts ↓ Depth perception		Home safety evaluation
Sensory Organization Test (SOT)	Absent use of vestibular inputs 0/100	Increase use of vestibular inputs to 30/100	Somatosensory and vestibular stimulation°
	Decreased use of somatosensory inputs 60/100	Increase use of somatosensory inputs to 75/100	
	Dependent on vision		
Static postural sway	Excessive sway—2 standard deviations outside normal range for age	Standing sway within normal limits for age	COG control training
Nudge/push test	No use of ankle or hip strategy Steps immediately	Survives 5/10 pushes with hip strategy	Hip strategy exercises°
Limit of stability (LOS)	No ankle strategy—all hip Sway to 45% LOS anterior, 35% LOS posterior Slow movement time	Uses ankle strategy to reach 40% LOS anterior/posterior Reaches 8/8 targets at 75% LOS using hip or ankle within 4 s	COG control training
Range of motion (ROM)	↓ Neck extension 0–10° ↓ Lumbar extension 0–15° ↓ Hip extension 0–5°	↑ Spinal extension neck 0–20° lumbar 0–20° ↑ Hip extension 0–10°	ROM exercises°
Strength	Flexion 4/5 (B) Hip abduction 3⁺/5, extension 3/5 (B) Knee extension 4⁺/5, flexion 4/5 (R) Ankle dorsiflexion 3⁻/5 (L) Ankle dorsiflexion 2/5 (B) Ankle plantarflexion 3⁺/5	↑ (B) Hip abduction/extension to 4/5 ↑ (B) Ankle dorsiflexion to 4⁻/5	Progressive resistive exercises, including bicycle°
Gait (GARS)	Score 25/51 Deviations Forward flexed trunk Double stance Bilaterally prolonged Short step length	GARS Scales 35/51 (I) Ambulation with walker in home/community	Gait training° 1—starts, stops, turns 2—treadmill 3—uneven surfaces, curbs, stairs, carpet, outdoors
Endurance	Fatigue after ambulating 60 ft	Ambulates > 200 ft without stopping	Gait training as above
Tinetti Balance Scale	6/16 score	Tinetti Balance score 10/16	Gait training as above
Tinetti Gait Scale	5/12 score Falls and catches self	Tinetti Gait score 8/12	Gait training as above

°Also included in Home Exercise program.
(B), bilateral; COG, center of gravity; (I) independent; (L), left; (R), right.
Reprinted with permission from NeuroCom International, Inc.

environment (opportunities and risks), (3) knowledge of the task (critical components), (4) the ability to use those knowledge sets to solve motor problems, and (5) the ability to modify and adapt movements as the task and environment change. To the extent that a client is missing these characteristics, the clinician should attempt to support their development, or even to supply them until they are present. Different types of clients will vary in which characteristics are likely to be missing. For example, a cognitively impaired head-injured client may lack awareness of self and environment, even though his or her physical abilities make it quite possible for him or her to modify and adapt movements. Conversely, a quadriplegic client may be very aware of his or her limitations, the environment, and the task demands but may initially have

limited experience to know how to solve a motor problem and limited physical ability to modify movements.

The clinician must also ask what motor learning stage the client is in for different tasks. Skill acquisition is the first stage. The objective is for the client just to "get the idea of the movement"[27] to begin to acquire the skill. In this stage, errors are frequent and performance is inefficient and inconsistent. Within the nervous system, only temporary changes are occurring. Skill refinement is the second stage. The goal is for the client to improve the performance, reducing the number and size of the errors, and increasing the consistency and efficiency of the movements. Skill retention is the final stage. The ability to perform the movements and achieve the functional goal has been accomplished, and the new objective is to retain

T A B L E   2 1 – 1 0.   An Example of How Treatment Planning Flows from Test Results in a Client with Right Hemiparesis

Patient Profile:
- 69-year-old woman
- DXL: Left CVA with right hemiparesis
- Acute Rehabilitation → Home Health → Outpatient Rehabilitation

Test	Problems Identified	Goals Set	Treatment Plan
Peripheral somatosensory	None		
Sensory Organization Test	Average overall stability 47/100 Absent use of vestibular inputs 0/100	Average stability 60/100 ↑ Use of vestibular inputs 15/100	Vestibular stimulation with forced use and head movements
Postural sway			COG control training
Functional reach	Forward lean restricted to 5 inches	Able to reach forward 8 inches	
Static	Weight shift asymmetry to left in static standing and medial/lateral sway, 25% LOS to left of midline	↑ Control of COG: Stands midline ↑ Forward LOS to 50% ↑ Right LOS to 50% ↓ Extraneous sway scores by 50%	
Limit of stability	Forward weight shift restricted to 25% LOS		
Rhythmic weight shift	Extraneous sway off desired path		
OLST	Unable on right leg 30 seconds on left leg	Stands on left leg, 10 seconds	COG control training
Nudge/push (motor strategy selection)	Switch from ankle to hip strategy noted but unable to withstand perturbation	Able to stand upright after mild perturbations 5/10 times Able to "catch" self by stepping/reaching 5/10 times	Hip and stepping strategy training
Range of motion	None		
Strength: right leg	4/5 Knee extension 3/5 Knee flexion 2/5 Ankle dorsiflexion 3/5 Ankle plantarflexion	↑ R.LE strength 5/5 Knee 4/5 Ankle	Progressive resistive exercises
Endurance	Standing tolerance less than 10 minutes	Able to stand unaided for 15 minutes	Standing tolerance tasks
Gait	↓ Step length—R.LE ↓ Step height—R.LE ↓ Heel strike—R.LE ↓ Toe off—R.LE	Symmetrical step height and length 5/10 times ↑ Heel strike R.LE 5/10 times	Gait training on treadmill
Tinetti Gait Scale	4/12 score Unable to turn, reach, or bend without loss of balance Falls: uneven surfaces low lighting head turning No community ambulation Requires cane Requires supervision for household ambulation	8/12 score No falls Gait independent without cane in household; with cane in community	Gait training on uneven surfaces, with head movements, with low lighting Safety education

COG, center of gravity; LOS, limit of stability; OLST, one-legged stance test; R.LE, right lower extremity.
Reprinted with permission from NeuroCom International, Inc.

the skill (across time) and transfer the skill to different settings. Retention and transfer are the hallmarks of true learning, where some relatively permanent changes have occurred within the nervous system. A client may have attained the skill retention phase for sitting balance tasks, be in the skill refinement stage for standing balance, tasks, and be in the skill acquisition stage for locomotor balance tasks.

Therapists use practice and feedback to teach motor skills. Repetition is necessary to develop skill; feedback is necessary to detect and correct errors. During skill acquisition, frequent repetition of a movement or task and frequent feedback are beneficial to help the client begin to be able to perform the desired movements and tasks. As the client progresses to the skill refinement stage (the clinician observes reduced errors and less variable performance), however, then practice should be varied and feeback briefly delayed. For example, the task of standing and reaching to one side to take an object from the therapist might initially be repeated to the same side and at the same height several times. Then the therapist should begin to gradually vary the task demands: reach

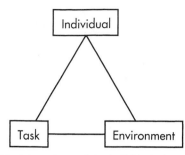

FIGURE 21–23. Interactions of the individual, the environment, and the task are critical to postural control skills. Although they may be isolated in the mind of the clinician for assessment purposes, they are never isolated in the function of the client.

farther, or faster; take different objects of various weights, shapes, and sizes; and take the object from higher and lower heights and reach to right and left sides alternately. This variation introduces a problem-solving demand for the client: modifications in timing, force, and sequencing are now necessary.[59]

Feedback, which is especially helpful for those with sensory reception or perception problems, initially may contain information to assist the client in detecting errors about the goal achievement (knowledge of results, i.e., "you did not lean far enough to reach this last time") or about a movement error (knowledge of performance, i.e., "you did not straighten your knee enough last time").[45] Early feedback also may contain cues about what to do better next time, such as "straighten your knee before you shift weight onto that leg." If feedback is always provided by an external source, such as the therapist, a mirror, or a computer monitor, then the client is not given the opportunity to develop internal error detection/ error correction mechanisms and will not be as likely to retain or transfer the skill. By delaying the feedback and asking the client to estimate or describe their own errors, and afterward providing the feedback, clients are allowed to compare their own developing internal frame of reference with the (correct) external frame of reference. By asking clients to suggest what might be done to correct the errors, the error correction process shifts from the external source to the clients, supporting motor problem-solving processes. As clients progress to the skill retention level, variations should increase (including task and environmental demands) and feedback delays should be longer. The clinician must develop a sense of how to therapeutically use practice variation and feedback delay to progress clients through the stages of motor learning. Too much variation and too little feedback early on impede skill acquisition; insufficient variation and excessive feedback later on hamper skill retention and transfer.

Task

Functional rating scales performed as a part of the evaluation yield information about what tasks, or functional activities, are limited by the postural control impairments. Bed mobility, sitting, sit-to-stand, transfers, standing, walking, working, and sports participation may be affected. Repeating the problematic tasks over and over is one approach; however, it is far more productive for the

clinician to analyze the problematic tasks to determine what postural control demands are placed on the client when undertaking those tasks. Does a task demand predominantly stability? mobility? both? For example, standing to take a photograph demands the ability to hold still, standing to move laundry from the washer to the dryer requires weight shifting, and standing to don a pair of pantyhose calls for both steadiness and movement. All three are standing tasks, but each places different postural control demands on the client. By using task analysis, the therapist may consciously select or design tasks to place specific demands on the client such that the postural control systems that need improvement will be challenged to respond.

Analysis of mobility tasks includes attention to timing, force, and duration of movements. Consider the different timing demands for weight shifting and reaching to (1) catch an item falling from a shelf, (2) take a hot casserole out of the oven, or (3) open a door. Compare the different amounts of force necessary to pick up a heavy suitcase, pick up a baby from a crib, or replace a ceiling light bulb. The duration of a balance demand may be brief, as in recovering from a trip, or extended, as in walking across an icy parking lot. Clinicians should choose tasks that vary these parameters to prepare clients for activities with various mobility demands. Activities that incorporate changing head positions will further challenge the individual with vestibular insufficiency.

Therapists also need to consider whether the elements of the task are predictable or unpredictable. In other words, will the postural control demand be a voluntary movement (e.g., sweeping the porch), an automatic postural response (e.g., missing the last step on a flight of stairs), or an anticipatory postural preparation (e.g., preceding a lift)? Clients need to learn to respond in all three conditions, which are often combined. For instance, lifting is a voluntary movement. Predicting the load to be lifted leads to anticipatory postural preparation. Counteracting the destabilizing force of a greater-than-predicted load requires an automatic postural response. If, during therapy, the clinician says "don't let me push you" before nudging the client, the demand is for anticipatory postural preparation. If the disturbance is provided without warning, the demand calls for automatic postural reactions. If the clinician requests a lean to the right, that is a voluntary postural adjustment. Activities that demand all three types of balance control, either one at a time or in combination, should be included in balance retraining programs.

Environment

Just as tasks can be purposefully selected to promote postural control responses, environmental conditions also must be included in the design of the therapy plan to stimulate the necessary systems. Gravity cannot be manipulated by the clinician, but the client needs to learn to counteract it at different speeds and from different positions, among other things. Familiarity with how gravity can aid movement, as in walking, is also important. The therapist can vary the surface conditions. They may be stable, even, and predictable (hospital hallway, sidewalk), unstable (boat, subway, gravel driveway), uneven (grass, curbs, stairs), or compliant (beach, padded carpeting). Visual conditions also may be manipulated. Visual cues may be available and accurate (daylight, fluorescent lighting), unavailable (darkness or poor lighting, or lack of environmental cues such as a busy carpet pattern on a stairway), unstable (moving crowd, public transportation), used for purposes other than balance (fixation on a ball in tennis), or dependent on head movements. Clinicians should help prepare their clients to function in the real world by training them to maintain balance under different combinations of surface and visual conditions. This includes situations where cues from the environment agree; that is, visual, somatosensory, and vestibular inputs are all sending the same message, so to speak, as well as in sensory conflict environments, where cues from one system may disagree (not match) with cues from the other sensory systems. Functional situations where sensory conflicts may exist include elevators, escalators, people movers, airplanes, and subways.

Treatment Progressions

To treat each problem that may contribute to a balance disorder individually would not be practical. The therapist must address several problems at a time, not just for efficiency, but because these systems should be able to function together to perform functional activities in real-world environments. Treatment then, is multi-impairment oriented, with tasks and environments selected to stimulate involved or compensatory systems.

Sensory Systems

In general, the less sensory information available, the more difficult the task of balancing. A treatment progression, then, might start with full sensory inputs (vision, somatosensory, and vestibular: 3/3) available in the environment and perhaps augmented feedback if intrinsic sensory channels are deficient, as with somatosensory loss or a vestibular disorder. Challenge is added by manipulating either visual or somatosensory inputs, so that equilibrium must be maintained using only two of three senses (vision and vestibular or somatosensory and vestibular). If both vision and somatosensory inputs are manipulated, then only the vestibular inputs are a reliable source of sensory information and balance is accomplished with only one of three senses.[68]

To stimulate the use of somatosensory inputs, environments are designed to disadvantage vision while providing reliable somatosensory inputs (stable surfaces). Having the client close the eyes, or practice in low lighting or darkness, removes or decreases visual inputs. For clients with an overreliance on visual input for balance, the somatosensory system needs to be facilitated while the visual system is disrupted. This can be accomplished by having the client sit or stand on a stable surface while performing quick head turns. For the client with self-limited head movement, the intervention may begin with head movement during quiet standing and progress to head movements during weight shifts and then walking.

Eyes-closed standing and weight shifting also increase the use of somatosensation for balance.

To stimulate the use of visual inputs, environments are designed to disadvantage somatosensation while providing reliable visual cues (stable visual field with landmarks). Somatosensation cannot be removed like vision, but it can be destabilized by sitting/standing on unstable surfaces (rocker board, BAPS board, randomly moving platforms) or confused by sitting/standing on compliant surfaces that "give way" to pressure, such as foam, space boots, or responsively moving platforms.

To stimulate the use of vestibular inputs for adaptation of the CNS, environments are designed to disadvantage both vision and somatosensation while providing reliable vestibular cues (detectable head position). Practicing on unstable or compliant surfaces, with vision either absent (eyes closed), destabilized (eye movements or head movements), or confused (i.e., optokinetic stimulation) provides challenging combinations. Adding neck extension and rotation to place the vestibular organ at a disadvantaged angle can increase difficulty.

Adaptation of the VOR is accomplished by having the client move his or her head while trying to maintain gaze stabilization (keeping a stationary object in clear focus).[4, 24] The speed of head movement is gradually increased, with the goal of achieving head movement at 2 Hz (cycles per second) without the object blurring. Initially, the client can focus on the thumb or a business card held at arm's length. The activity is progressed to a higher level of difficulty by adding background visual stimulus such as a television set or a visually complex environment. Gaze stabilization with head turns while standing on an uneven surface or while walking creates a higher-level challenge. Many clients have avoided head movement, so initially just turning the head may trigger dizziness. Head movements should be made in whichever directions provoke dizziness; these directions may differ from client to client.

The VSR is facilitated when the vestibular system is the primary input for balance, a relatively rare occurrence in a system with three redundant sensory sources. For this to occur, both somatosensory and visual inputs must be placed at a disadvantage as previously described. For example, the vestibular system becomes the primary input when the surface is compliant or the base of support is narrow (tandem or single-leg stance) and visual cues are unstable. Quick movements of the head, head tilts, or forward bending will trigger vestibular signals to add input to the system. Combining these types of activities can create progressively complex challenges. Standing on foam with eyes closed, weight shifts with eyes closed, and head and eye movement while walking all require vestibular input for successful performance.

Certain positions or movements of the head during upright activities can affect balance if there is an abnormal function of just one part of the vestibular system. If the otoliths are damaged or hypersensitive, a lateral tilt of the head can cause destabilization. Activities that require quick changes of position in a superior or inferior direction, such as a lunge or going up and down stairs, can be difficult when the otoliths are damaged. Good program components for otolith stimulation are activities involving up-and-down body movements. Examples include sit-to-stand, seated bouncing on a Swiss ball, and standing bouncing on a minitrampoline, all with eyes closed to eliminate use of vision for stability.

A vestibular adaptation program should challenge the patient at the limit of his or her ability. Clients will often choose to do the easiest exercise and avoid the more difficult exercises if they are not educated about the need to trigger the symptoms. Conversely, if the challenge is too far above the ability of the patient, the CNS will fail to adapt.

When the use of vestibular inputs has been minimized through self-limitation of head and eye movements to control symptoms of dizziness and imbalance, the visual system often becomes dominant for balance. To train the client to use vestibular input versus vision, activities such as watching a ball tossed from hand to hand while walking, walking backward, or walking with eye movements can be used. Clients with visual dependency will often complain of excessive fatigue after activity due to the strain of using vision for postural stability. When these clients are in situations where there is excessive visual stimulation, complaints of dizziness increase. The subtle eye movements associated with viewing a computer monitor will cause more fatigue for the individual with vestibular disorder. These individuals will also often avoid crowds as in a mall, grocery store, or airport. Often, attending church, where there is low lighting, visual stimulation, and the need to stand with eyes closed or to read a hymnal while singing challenges the vestibular system.

When the Hallpike-Dix test position indicates BPV, specific, highly effective procedures can be performed in the clinical setting to remediate the disorder.[22, 78] Canalith repositioning is a series of passive movements designed to move loose debris (otoconia) through the canal and back into the otolith (Fig. 21–24). The client is first brought down into the extended and rotated position that causes the nystagmus and vertigo (the positive Hallpike-Dix position). The head is held in that position until the symptoms fade completely or for 60 to 90 seconds. The head is maintained in extension and then slowly rotated toward the unaffected side and kept in that position for an additional 1 to 2 minutes to allow movement of the otoconia through the canal. The client then rolls so that he or she is side-lying and the head is turned to a 45-degree position relative to the ground. Often, this position will produce more vertigo and nystagmus as the otoconia continue to move through the canal. In the next movement, the head is tipped toward the chest and the client is assisted into the sitting position. The client must then follow specific instructions for 48 hours. These include avoiding forward, backward, or lateral head tilts or bending activities. It is also recommended that clients sleep with the head elevated to at least 30 degrees and that they avoid turning to the involved side.[26]

When the BPV is within the horizontal canal, dizziness or vertigo is reported when rolling, especially if the head is elevated on a pillow because that puts the canal in a position perpendicular to the ground. The symptoms are reported when the head is turned in either direction, but the side that triggers the worst symptoms is thought to be the side of the dysfunction.[5] The repositioning intervention begins with the client supine with the head turned toward the most affected ear. The head is then turned away from the affected ear and the client is slowly rolled 360 degrees (essentially staying in the same place) until the head is returned to the original position. The client sits back up with the head tucked. Side tilts of the head, as well as forward and backward movements of the head and trunk, are avoided for 2 days.

In cases of position-provoked dizziness that do not appear to be BPV, habituation exercises should be done to increase the client's tolerance to the provoking position(s). This involving having the client perform the provoking positions, repeating each position up to three times per session, to give the CNS the opportunity to adjust to the sensation that the position triggers. In addition to the exercise sessions, it is important to incorporate the provoking positions into daily activities.

Remember that each sensory system has two peripheral receptors. In cases where the sensory loss is unilateral and permanent, the other side should be stimulated to compensate for the loss. If the sensory loss is unilateral and temporary, however, the other side should be placed (temporarily), when possible, at a disadvantage to force reliance on the underused side. As the affected side improves, integration of the two sides and the three systems is the desired outcome.

In older clients, there is often dysfunction in all three sensory systems. Disease-related disruptions of the somatosensory or visual systems (e.g., a peripheral neuropathy or cataracts) are combined with age-related declines in the vestibular system. In some cases, therapy aimed at increasing vestibular function can have a significant impact on postural stability. If the vestibular system cannot adapt, the client is classified as having a multisensory balance disorder. If sensory loss is permanent or progressive, safe function may require the use of an assistive device.[43] Choosing an assistive device for these clients can be a challenge. A single cane often does not allow for compensation for changes in direction of an impending fall, and a standard aluminum walker does not provide support when changing directions because it must be lifted. The ideal walker has four rotating wheels and thus the ability to change direction without being lifted. This increases stability greatly, and the client usually describes a significant increase in confidence.

Many neurological clients have temporary difficulty with head control early on in their recovery, and others have chronic head control problems. Their ability to properly orient the vestibular organs, eyes, and neck proprioceptors is impaired, which negatively affects the ability to perceive internal and environmental cues that could assist in balance maintenance. Clients with spasticity or contractures of the ankles and feet who cannot place their feet in full contact with the floor are not only at a biomechanical disadvantage but also have difficulty receiving somatosensory inputs that could support postural control processes. The more accurate and reliable sensory information available, the greater the chances that the sensoriperceptual processes that contribute to balance can fulfill their role. Treatment progressions should include attention to increasing the client's ability to receive and process sensory information pertinent to balance control,

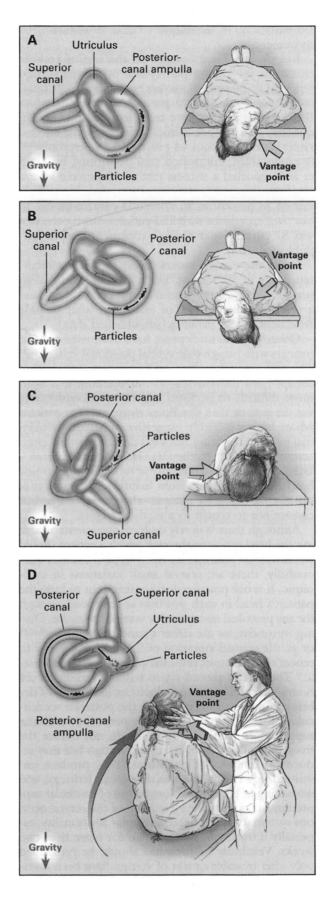

FIGURE 21–24. Canalith repositioning maneuver for the patient with posterior canal BPV. Figure represents procedure for right side BPV. Movement of particles through the canal is shown in each position. (From Furman JM, Cass SP: Benign paroxysmal positional vertigo. N Engl J Med 341:1590–1596, 1999. Copyright © 1999 Massachusetts Medical Society. All rights reserved.)

through oculomotor, head, and peripheral limb positioning and movement.

Control of the Center of Gravity

Effective control of the COG depends on accurate awareness of body position in space and the relationship between body parts (perception), as well as biomechanical and musculoskeletal systems (execution). Trunk and head control abilities are primary. For clients with paralysis or degenerative disease that limits the ability of arms and legs to assist with postural stability, head and trunk control may be the dominant means of balance. Both the head/neck and trunk need to be able to (1) achieve and hold a midline position, (2) rotate around this midline axis, and (3) move away from and return to the midline without loss of balance. The term "midline" here refers not to a line between right and left sides but to a point where right/left and forward/backward components are centered in all planes—medial/lateral, anterior/posterior, rotary, and side bending (shortening/elongation on either side).

SITTING BALANCE

In sitting, the pelvis and posterior thighs form the primary base of support, with additional stability provided by the feet in contact with the floor. The axis of anteroposterior movement rotates around the greater trochanter, and forward/backward leans are achieved through pelvic and trunk movement. Anterior pelvic tilt with upper trunk extension allows forward reaching and begins the sit-to-stand transition. Lateral weight shifts with trunk elongation precede right/left reaching and scooting. Lateral weight shifts with trunk rotation permit cross-midline reaching and begin the sit-to-supine progression. The use of arms to prop in sitting is an extension of the base of support.

In standing, the feet form the base of support. The axis of anteroposterior movement rotates around the medial malleolus. Weight shifts move the COG through space for reaching and lifting tasks as well as in preparation for stepping. Ankle strategy is most effective for movement of the COG through the limits of stability. As the COG nears the sway boundary, hip strategy works to restrict its travel. If this fails, stepping or reaching strategies are used to reestablish a new base of support. During gait, the COG follows a sinusoidal path as forward progression of the body mass combines with alternating lateral weight shifts to the stance foot (Fig. 21–25).[57] Each step creates a new base of support. Assistive devices such as canes, walkers, and crutches extend the base of support and thus reduce the demands on the intrinsic balance control system. In sitting, standing, and walking, control of the COG involves the ability to establish a stable base of support and to transfer weight over it. Treatment progressions for COG control then involve training to establish, maintain, and reduce the base of support and to produce automatic, anticipatory, and voluntary postural responses to restrict or produce weight shifts.

Early treatment progression for COG control includes neurodevelopmental sequence activities (e.g., prone on elbows, all fours, kneeling, right/left side sitting, half-kneeling), not for the purpose of "reflex development" in

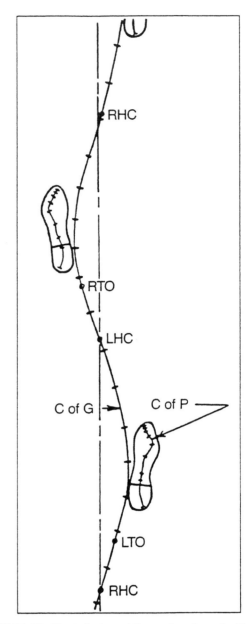

FIGURE 21–25. The trajectory of the center of gravity (C of G) and the center of pressure (C of P) during a gait cycle. RHC, Right heel contact; RTO, right toe off; LHC, left heel contact; LTO, left toe off. (From Palia AE, et al: Identification of age-related changes in the balance control system. *In* Duncan P (ed): Balance: Proceedings of the APTA Forum. Alexandria, VA, American Physical Therapy Association, 1990.)

the traditional sense but because the task demands are to balance with progressively less surface contact (i.e., shrinking the base of support). It also is useful for simultaneously addressing impairments such as lower-extremity extensor tone, trunk weakness and asymmetries, and head/neck extensor weakness. Functionally, bed mobility and floor-to-stand transfers are related to neurodevelopmental sequence exercises and should be practiced concurrently in low- and high-level clients, respectively.

Sitting balance can be progressed by (1) removing upper-extremity support (hands on firm surface—moveable surface [i.e., ball, bolster, rolling stool]; one hand free; both hands free); (2) making the seating surface less stable (mat–bed–rocker board–Swiss ball); and (3) removing the use of one foot by crossing the leg or of both feet by raising the height of the seat so they do not touch the floor. Tasks might include multidirectional weight shifts with the hands in contact with a bolster or ball, which is pushed/pulled to and fro, reaching or passing objects, upper body tasks (grooming, dressing), and managing socks/shoes and wheelchair armrests/footrests, and so on. Sitting activities can be the best place to start clients with vestibular dysfunction because there is less challenge and a lower demand for sensory integration.

SIT-TO-STAND AND TRANSFER BALANCE

Transitional movements such as sit-to-stand and transfers involve large COG excursions over a stable base of support. For sit-to-stand, the base of support must change from the seat to the feet. The feet begin to accept the weight first by downward pressure through the heels as the pelvis rolls anteriorly. The weight moves to the front of the feet as the trunk comes forward and the pelvis lifts from the surface, then backward toward midline as the trunk extends into standing. The COG stays near midline if both legs are participating equally, but it will often deviate to a preferred side during the transition in clients with hemiplegia. Training should include disadvantaging the preferred leg (perhaps by moving it a bit forward) to allow the more affected leg and foot to experience the weight transference. During transfers, a lateral weight shift is required in addition to the partial stand. The COG does not remain near midline, but instead it moves forward to load the feet and then laterally toward the side of the transfer. Progression of balance skills in sit-to-stand and transfer tasks may involve gradually lowering the height of the surface, removing armrests to preclude upper-extremity assist, and transfers to surfaces of different heights and firmnesses. Remember that velocity is a normal part of sit-to-stand movements, because the momentum is used to assist the weight transfer from seat to feet, so the clinician must allow some speed during this task. If the client is unsteady on arising (cannot dampen or slow the speed in a controlled manner), working gradually from stand-to-sit initially may be beneficial before progression to sit-to-stand. Practice of sit-to-stand with the eyes closed can be an effective way to train clients who are overdependent on vision for balance. Without the use of vision for stability, integration of vestibular and somatosensory systems can be facilitated.

STANDING BALANCE

Standing balance tasks also can begin with finding midline and becoming stable there. Controlled mobility (volitional) should be encouraged as soon as possible, at first on a stable surface with slow, small weight shifts. Challenge is added by increasing the distance traveled away from midline, moving toward restricted regions of the limits of stability, altering speed of sway, adding combined upper-extremity activities (e.g., dribbling a basketball, reaching), adding resistance (manual, Theraband), and so on. Narrowing the base of support (Romberg, tandem, single leg) makes control of the COG more demanding. Placing the feet in a diagonal stride position is more desirable for pregait weight shifting than symmetrical double stance. Attention should be given to the stance (loading) leg regarding pelvic protraction, hip and knee extension, and ankle dorsiflexion, with the tibia traveling forward over the foot. Focus on the swing (unloading) leg should include pelvic drop with knee flexion as the heel comes up and pressure through the ball of the foot and toes to maximally load the opposite leg. Standing balance exercises can be made more difficult by training on a less stable surface (carpet, foam, rocker board, BAPS board) and by adding combined head/eye movements tasks or closing the eyes. The goals for dynamic sitting and standing balance exercises are to increase the size and symmetry of the limits of stability and improve the ability to transfer weight to different body segments with control at different speeds and with varied amounts of force. To facilitate somatosensory and vestibular integration, the activities above can be performed with decreased or distorted visual cues. Closing the eyes, quick head turns, turning the lights down low, or wearing sunglasses will decrease the use of vision for stabilization.

STRATEGY TRAINING

Training ankle, hip, and stepping strategies begins in a voluntary manner but must progress to an automatic level of use to develop more normal balance and to prevent loss of balance. Before strategy training, the clinician should be sure that the client has the ability to develop the desired strategy(ies). The observed dominance of other strategies is appropriately compensatory, not dysfunctional, if a missing strategy cannot be effectively executed. Clients use these strategies to prevent loss of balance, so the clinician must take care not to reduce reliance on an effective strategy but to add additional strategies to the repertoire.

Ankle strategy should be practiced on a firm, broad surface. Clients can be asked to sway slowly in anterior/posterior, right/left, and diagonal directions, first to and from midline, progressing to passing midline, and finally progressing to sway toward the periphery without return to midline. Head and pelvis should be traveling in the same direction at the same time. Clients can practice standing near a wall with a table in front of them, swaying forward to touch the table with their stomach (leading with the pelvis) and backward to touch the wall with the back of their head. Cues are given not to "bow" to the table and not to touch the wall with the buttocks. As soon as the client begins to be able to perform this protocol, functional meaning should be added with maneuvers such as forward or lateral reaching tasks, hands over head to take things off shelves, and leaning backward to rinse hair in the shower. To improve anticipatory and automatic ankle strategy use, add slight perturbations to the body or the surface when midline, progress to gentle perturbation when away from midline, and finally progress from predictable to unpredictable perturbations.

Hip strategy is practiced on a narrow surface, such as standing sideways on a balance beam or a half-slice foam roller, or on an unstable surface such as foam or a rocker board. The head and pelvis travel in opposite directions to counterbalance each other, in a forward bow/backward bending motion for anterior/posterior sway. Rapid sway is requested in forward/backward, right/left, and diagonal directions. Using the wall and table setting mentioned previously, clients can be cued to bow to touch the nose toward the table while simultaneously touching the wall with the buttocks. Lateral hip strategy can be trained similarly, with the client standing sideways to the wall, touching the table with one hip and the wall with the opposite shoulder. Sway close to the edge of the client's limit of stability should produce a shift from ankle to hip strategy, so to enhance the use of hip strategy, the client should practice sway control as far away from midline as possible without stepping. As soon as the client demonstrates the ability to perform this strategy, it should be incorporated into functional tasks such as low reaching (e.g., trunk of car, laundry dryer). To promote anticipatory and automatic use of hip strategy, the client is in midline and given moderate, rapid perturbations to the body or the surface such that ankle strategy will be insufficient to counteract the force. Then the size of the disturbance is increased, and the client is positioned away from midline when the perturbation is given so that righting to midline is appropriate. The shift should be made from predictable ("Don't let me make you step or fall") to unpredictable perturbations.

Stepping strategy can be practiced first from atop a step, curb, or balance beam. Both legs should be included in training, because real-life situations such as a slip or trip often preclude the use of one limb and demand the use of the other. Progress is made by stepping on a level surface and then to stepping up onto a step or curb or over progressively larger obstacles (appliance cord, shoe, phone book). All directions should be practiced. Large, rapid perturbations are given such that ankle and hip strategies will be inadequate and stepping/reaching is demanded. Again, one should progress from predicted to unpredictable disturbances.

GAIT TRAINING

The initial focus for controlling the COG during gait is a stable base of support that can continually be reestablished quickly and reliably through stepping. The training is begun first in the forward direction, but also includes backward and sideways directions (sidestepping, braiding, or karaoke). Challenge can be added by narrowing the base of support (tandem) or reducing the foot/surface contact (walk on toes or heels). Unlike standing balance, where the base is stable and the COG moves over it, during locomotion the base is moving and the COG moves to stay over the base. Achieving a symmetrical, smoothly oscillating COG movement is the objective, with the forces of gravity and momentum being exploited. Speed assists in this process; excessively slow gait cannot take advantage of these forces. Treadmill training is gaining in popularity with neurological patients because the increased speed reduces some abnormal asymmetries.[61] Training to integrate postural control with locomotor skills is best accomplished not through continuous, steady pace walking, but by starting, stopping, turning, bending, varying the speed, and avoiding or stepping over obstacles. Difficulty is added by increasing the abruptness, frequency, and unpredictability of these types of tasks and by adding tasks such as carrying or reading while walking.

Altered surface conditions (carpets, ramps, curbs, stairs, grass, gravel) or reduced lighting conditions also heighten the challenge. Head and eye movements while walking should be added as the client improves. Walking quickly while reading signs on the wall or room numbers, for example, or looking toward and away from the therapist while walking makes it more difficult to use vision for stability. Walking in crowds or in busy, cluttered environments is also challenging.

Gait training for the individual with vestibular dysfunction is important because there is often a maladaptation of normal gait parameters. Because head movement causes visual disturbances and dizziness, the client with a vestibular disorder will significantly limit head movement while walking. When visual cues are used predominantly for balance, the client will try to keep the body in line with vertical and horizontal visual targets. This will decrease the small natural movements typically made during the gait cycle. Clients with permanent bilateral vestibular loss must use this compensatory strategy, but other clients with potentially recoverable vestibular function should be trained to walk with eye and head movements, trunk rotation and arm swing, and so on.

When the vestibular system does not accurately inform the client about the speed and direction of head movement, visual cues are used to determine movement speed and direction in relation to nonmoving objects. However, in environments where there is a lot of motion, or if someone approaches in the opposite direction, it becomes more difficult to determine speed and direction of self-movement. Clients will often complain of dizziness and imbalance in a crowd. Changing visual environments can trigger imbalance in the client with visual dependency. Often, walking into a darkened room, especially if the surface is uneven, as in a theater, can cause a fall or stumble. Clients with permanent vestibular loss should be educated about these potentially high-risk environments and taught compensatory strategies to ensure safe mobility. If improvement in vestibular function is anticipated, however, then progressive exposure to these busy environments is needed to prepare the client for real-world mobility.

To increase somatosensory input, clients with a vestibular disorder will often put the whole foot down at once to get better input on the position of the body relative to the ground. The normal heel-toe weight progression over the ball of the foot is diminished. This is often seen in conjunction with increased step width while walking. This compensatory strategy is acceptable in clients with permanent loss but should be discouraged in those clients who do not need to be overreliant on somatosensation for balance control during walking. Walking on uneven surfaces can be a challenge if the client is reliant primarily on somatosensory input and has poor visual-vestibular interaction. This is one reason why walking indoors is less of a problem than walking outdoors. Again, clients who are not expected to recover vestibular function should be educated about these potentially hazardous environments and encouraged to develop compensatory mechanisms to permit safe mobility. Gait training on progressively less stable surfaces is appropriate for clients who need to reduce overreliance on somatosensory cues and improve visual-vestibular interaction.

Other Considerations

Treatment Tools

Therapists use both high-technological and low-technological equipment in the remediation of balance deficits; each has advantages and disadvantages. High-technological options include forceplate systems with postural sway biofeedback, electromyographic biofeedback, optokinetic visual stimulation (from visual surround or moving lights), videotaping, and treadmills. Computerized systems allow advanced monitoring of progress and biofeedback, which supports motor learning.[1] Motorized systems provide the ability to manipulate the environment easily and efficiently and to safely graduate tasks and environmental challenges. Drawbacks to high-tech equipment include cost, space requirements, and operator training requirements. Low-technological options include mirrors, soft foam pads, hard foam rollers, rocker boards, BAPS boards, tilt boards, Swiss balls, mini-trampolines, and wedges/incline boards. All of these items are accessible (low cost, easy to obtain), portable, and easy to use. They do not provide novel feedback, objective scoring, or graphic recording; and clinicians must be skilled and creative in their use for appropriate gradation of task difficulty and environmental conditions.

Safety Education and Environmental Modifications

It is not always possible to remediate balance deficits, but it is the clinician's responsibility to ensure the safety of each client. When permanent deficits exist, the client and the family should be taught in what environments the client is at risk (e.g., a client with vestibular loss on a gravel driveway at night), what tasks are unsafe (e.g., ladder climbing, changing ceiling light bulbs), how the client can compensate (e.g., use a cane at night or in crowds), and what changes in the home or workplace are needed (e.g., night lights, stair stripes). Clinicians can ask the client (or family) to problem solve risky situations: What would the client do? Home evaluations should be followed by a recommendation list of safety modifications. Falls are frightening and dangerous; clinicians should do their utmost to see that they do not occur. If falls are likely, clients and families should be taught what to do if a fall occurs, including floor-to-stand or floor-to-furniture transfers. Home monitoring services such as LifeLine may be indicated if the client lives alone and is prone to falling.

Home Programs

Many balance exercises can (and should) be performed at home if safety and compliance can be ensured; however, unstable clients should always be supervised. Many standing tasks can be completed in a corner or near a countertop so that no other person is needed. The community setting is ideal for postural control training. Grocery or library aisles, public transportation, elevators, escalators, grass, sandboxes or beaches, ramps, trails, hills, and varied environmental conditions in general provide both challenge and functional relevance.

CASE STUDIES

CASE 21–1   ANDY

Andy is a 27-year-old man who sustained a severe closed-head injury in a skiing accident. He was hospitalized for 2 months, and at a long-term care facility for 6 months, before cranial surgery for removal of bilateral subdural hygromas and revision of a ventriculoperitoneal shunt. Postsurgically, he demonstrated marked improvement and was transferred to a rehabilitation unit. His initial physical therapy assessment revealed the following impairments, which had a negative effect on postural control:

1. Oculomotor deficits (difficulty tracking to the right and upward)
2. Disorientation
3. Very delayed and slow responses
4. Bilateral ankle plantarflexion contractures (1–10 degrees left, 1–15 degrees right); limited right shoulder flexion (0–100 degrees) and external rotation (0–20 degrees)
5. Hypotonic trunk (right, moderate; left, mild), hypertonic (extensor) lower extremities (right, moderate; left, mild), hypertonic right upper extremity, mild
6. Fair head control
7. Poor trunk control with right scapular atrophy, shortened right side, strength 3⁻/5
8. Left upper and lower extremity movement isolated and coordinated but slow, strength 4/5 at shoulder, 4⁺/5 elbow/wrist/hand, 4/5 hip and knee, 3⁺/5 ankle, able to place and hold for weight-bearing
9. Right upper extremity rests and moves in synergistic pattern but can move out of synergy with request or demonstration; strength 3⁻/5 at shoulder and 4⁻/5 distally; coordination is poor; can place and hold for weight-bearing if cued but not spontaneously
10. Left lower extremity moves in flexor/extensor pattern, grossly 3⁺/5 in hip and knee flexion, 2⁺ hip extension, 3⁺/5 knee extension, no isolated ankle movement, cannot place or hold for weight-bearing

Continued

CASE 21–1   ANDY *Continued*

Functional tests found the following disabilities:

1. Minimum assist supine-to-sit
2. Sitting balance, poor
3. Moderate assist sit-to-stand
4. Standing balance, unable
5. Moderate assist transfers
6. Nonambulatory

Impairment goals were the following:

1. Increase ROM to within normal limits throughout
2. Increase trunk tone to normal and strength to $4^+/5$
3. Decrease right-sided tone to normal
4. Increase spontaneous use, isolated movement and strength ($4^+/5$) in right extremities
5. Able to place and bear weight on right lower extremity

Short-term functional goals were the following:

1. Independent in all bed mobility
2. Independent in wheelchair transfers
3. Good static and fair dynamic sitting balance
4. Contact guard sit-to-stand
5. Minimum assist static standing balance. Ambulation goals were temporarily deferred because of the ankle contractures and balance deficits.

Early treatments included

1. Standing frame activities for head control, visual tracking, trunk control, reduced lower-extremity extensor tone, and heel cord stretching with ultrasound
2. Neurodevelopmental sequence activities for head and trunk control, trunk strengthening, decreased lower-extremity extensor tone, balance on all fours/heel-sitting/kneeling
3. Supine to-and-from sitting, especially over the right arm
4. Sitting balance with upper-extremity functional tasks (e.g., putting glasses on/off, taking shirt off/on, wiping nose with tissue), with focus on right visual tracking, right trunk elongation, and incorporation of right lower-extremity ground pressure for stability
5. Transfer training with incorporation of right upper extremity to push up, reach and grasp, and right lower-extremity placing and weight-bearing

As soon as Andy's ankle dorsiflexion ROM was near neutral on the right (was then 0 to 5 degrees on the left), neurodevelopmental activities were phased out and standing balance and pregait activities in the parallel bars were initiated with moderate assistance. He rapidly progressed to minimum assistance gait in the parallel bars, but with significant scissoring of the lower extremities. Gait outside the bars was begun with a quad cane on the left, but Andy was not able to organize the sequence for cane use and did not use it when loss of balance occurred, so it was discontinued. Gait without an assistive device required moderate assistance from the therapist for balance. A line drawn on the floor provided a visual cue to remind him to keep his feet apart; when walking without this cue, about 25% of his steps were close or crossed.

At discharge, 2 months after admission, Andy had good visual tracking; normal ROM with the exception of right lower-extremity dorsiflexion, which was limited to 0 to 5 degrees; normal tone in the left extremities; mildly increased tone in the right extremities with slight extensor patterning in the leg; good head and trunk control; and strength grossly $4^+/5$ throughout. Functionally, he was independent in bed mobility, wheelchair mobility, and sitting balance. He required supervision for safety in transfers and standing activities and minimum to moderate assistance for indoor ambulation without an assistive device, depending on his fatigue level.

CASE 21–2   DORIS

Doris is a 73-year-old woman with a long history of Parkinson's disease who had fallen four times within the 6 months before referral to physical therapy. As a result of her most recent fall, during which she hit her head, Doris developed ear pounding, light-headedness, and headaches. After referral to an otolaryngologist, she was diagnosed with unspecified peripheral vestibular dysfunction and referred to outpatient therapy. Her therapist found that Doris complained of increased light-headedness and dizziness, with anterior/posterior head movements, rolling in bed, sit-to-stand, and the Hallpike-Dix maneuver (worse to the right). Multiple impairments that could be contributing to her instability and falls, as well as symptoms related to the vestibular disorder, were also noted. Doris had mildly decreased ROM in her left ankle, shoulders, and neck; mild left-sided weakness and lack of coordination; marked bilateral upper-extremity tremor, and moderate forward flexed pos-

Continued

CASE 21–2 ● DORIS *Continued*

ture. She could not perform an ankle strategy at all and used hip strategy continually; she also used stepping strategy frequently with the least shift or sway. Static postural sway tests indicated that Doris had excessive sway when attempting to stand still and that she kept her COG slightly posterior and to the right of midline. Sway increased 10-fold with eyes closed. Doris could not perform repeated weight shifts in either anterior/posterior or medial/lateral directions. Her limits of stability were severely restricted to less than half of normal sway range anteriorly, and her movement time was very slow.

Functional testing revealed that Doris had several disabilities. She had to use a walker or have manual assistance to ambulate and could negotiate level surfaces only. Without her walker or handhold assistance, Doris could stand for less than 30 seconds and take a maximum of 10 steps. For community ambulation, Doris needed minimum assistance with her walker and could go only very short distances. She also required minimum assistance with bathing and household tasks.

Doris participated in therapy twice a week for 6 weeks and also performed a home exercise program daily. Her treatment plan included vestibular habituation exercises for the dizziness and balance retraining exercises for instability and falls. The habituation exercises she was given were designed to repeatedly provoke her symptoms and included head turning in supine and sitting (progressed to standing), rolling in bed, rocking in a rocking chair, and sit-to-stand practice. As her dizziness subsided, her home program was modified

to increase the number and rate of head movements. To improve her use of somatosensory and vestibular inputs, Doris also practiced standing on a firm surface with eyes closed (with family supervision). In the clinic, Doris did stretching, strengthening, and postural extension exercises to address her musculoskeletal limitations. Using postural sway biofeedback, she practiced achieving the midline position, controlled anterior and left-sided weight shifts at progressively faster speeds, and ankle strategy. Gait training included starts, stops, turns, and obstacle avoidance and progressed to community ambulation tasks such as curbs and ramps.

Despite her multiple problems, Doris was able to reduce the severity of her impairments and consequently improve her functional level. Her dizziness resolved completely. Although she still had excess sway during static standing, she was able to achieve and hold a midline position, and her sway with eyes closed reduced by more than half. Doris could shift her weight in both anterior/posterior and medial/lateral directions at moderate speeds using ankle strategy, without stepping. Her limits of stability were expanded from 35% to 80% of normal, and she was able to shift her weight much more quickly. Functionally, she could stand without the walker for 8 minutes and walk independently indoors on level surfaces without the walker for short distances. She was independent in community ambulation with the walker. At a 3-month follow-up visit, Doris reported that she had had no more falls.

CASE 21–3 ● SARAH

Sarah is a 20 year old with a history of cystic fibrosis. During an acute episode she was treated with gentamicin, an antibiotic in the aminoglycoside family. Approximately 6 days later, she lost her balance when getting out of bed. As she tried to get up, the room began to feel like it was moving. She was unable to regain her balance. Although previously functionally independent, she became reliant on her family to assist her for all of her mobility. Evaluation by a neurootologist determined that she had lost 70% of her vestibular function in one ear and 65% in the other.

On her initial physical therapy evaluation she was unable to maintain focus on her outstretched thumb while turning her head side to side or up and down. She could move her eyes from target to target, but it made her dizzy. She reported dizzi-

ness with smooth pursuit of the eyes and had difficulty maintaining focus as the speed of the moving target increased.

She had an increased base of support in quiet standing and was unable to keep her balance with her feet touching. Even with a wide base of support, she lost her balance when she moved her head. She could not stand with her eyes closed, even on a firm surface. She fell immediately when trying to stand on foam, and therefore she was not asked to try to close her eyes.

INITIAL TREATMENT

Because her ability to walk was so impaired, Sarah was given a cane to increase the somatosensory input and to further increase her base of support. She was able to walk with the cane without assistance on smooth surfaces, but she needed help

Continued

CASE 21–3   SARAH *Continued*

with stairs, curbs, and when walking on grass. Sarah was also given gaze stabilization exercises, one of which was to look at a business card and move her head only as fast as she could and keep the letters in focus. Each day she would try to move her head faster.

Sarah was instructed to stand in the corner, with her back about 4 inches away from the wall. She was told to close her eyes and count. Each time that she fell against the wall she was to right herself and start her count over. Her goal was to stand for 30 seconds without touching the wall. When she could stand for 30 seconds, she would try to move her feet closer together.

She was also instructed to stand in the corner and begin to move her head as she was looking at a nonmoving object.

To avoid the oscillopsia associated with turning her head while walking, she was instructed to turn her body in the direction that she wanted to turn while she was focused on a stable object. Then she would close her eyes as she turned her head, using her somatosensation to maintain balance. She would refocus to move forward. She was instructed to return in 3 weeks.

PROGRESSION
At her next visit Sarah could move her head at about 1 Hz and maintain focus. Her ability to use somatosensation for balance improved with both eyes closed and turning her head while standing on a firm surface. She could stand with her feet close together with her eyes open on a firm surface. Her program was progressed to include standing on foam in the corner and beginning to turn her head while looking at a stationary target. She was instructed to begin a gentle sway while standing on a firm surface with eyes closed. For her gait training, she was instructed to use visual targets to maintain stability as she began to slowly move her head (called "hanging on with your eyes"). She continued to use her cane for community mobility. She could now move around her house without use of the cane.

Three weeks later, she demonstrated gaze stabilization at 2 Hz. She was told then to start holding the card in front of the television while she turned

her head to further challenge the ability to maintain gaze stabilization.

She could easily stand in the corner with eyes closed but felt uneasy with weight shifts. She could move her head at about 1 Hz while walking on a firm surface with gaze stabilization. Standing on foam was easy with head turns.

To progress her program further, she worked on a Profitter to shift from side to side as she maintained gaze stability. She began doing the StairMaster with head turns. She started walking on the treadmill at 1.0 mph without upper-extremity support. She was encouraged to try to move outdoors as much as possible to be on uneven surface. She started to try reading while standing. She was given a ball to toss in the air and instructed to follow it with her eyes while maintaining her peripheral gaze on vertical and horizontal targets. Driving was addressed because she was hoping to return to school in the fall. Because she still demonstrated some oscillopsia and complained of dizziness with head turns, she was instructed to look in the rear-view mirror and then close her eyes as she moved her head back to the front of the car. This eliminated the blurred vision during head turns, and she could do it quickly enough to be safe. She was warned not to drive during inclement weather, when the snow or rain would disrupt her vision.

Three months later, she returned for a follow-up evaluation before returning to school. She had spent the summer babysitting for two small children and played outside throwing and catching the ball. She stated they loved it when she fell down, but for her it was good training to incorporate head movements and gaze stabilization on uneven surfaces. She was able to walk in the community without an assistive device. She described difficulty when the wind was blowing (disrupting visual cues), when there was glare, and when she had to walk in a dark theater.

Although the physician reported no increase in her vestibular function, she had made significant improvement in her ability to move through her environment and return to her normal activities.

ACKNOWLEDGMENT

Thanks to Janet Helminski, PhD, PT, Linda Horn, PT, NCS, and Pat Huston, MS, PT, for their significant contributions to the development of this chapter. Gratitude is also extended to Darcy Umphred, PhD, PT, and our families for their patience and support.

REFERENCES

1. Allison L: The role of biofeedback in balance retraining. Biofeedback 24:16, 1996.
2. Allison L: Imbalance following traumatic brain injury: Causes and characteristics. Neurol Rep 23:15, 1999.
3. Arenberg IK: Meniere's disease: Diagnosis and management of vertigo and endolymphatic hydrops. In Arenberg IK (ed): Dizziness and Balance Disorders. New York, Kugler, 1993.
4. Asai M, Wantanabe Y, Shimizu K: Effects of vestibular rehabilitation on postural control. Acta Otolaryngol (Stockh) 528:116, 1997.
5. Baloh R, Honrubia V: Clinical Neurophysiology of the Vestibular System, 2nd ed. Philadelphia, FA Davis, 1990.
6. Barnes ML, et al: Reflex and Vestibular Aspects of Motor Control, Motor Development, and Motor Learning. Atlanta, Stokesville Publishing, 1990.
7. Berg K, et al: Measuring balance in the elderly: Preliminary development of an instrument. Physiother Can 41:304, 1989.
8. Bisdorff A, Wolsley C, Anastasopoulos D, et al: The perception of body verticality (subjective postural vertical) in peripheral and central vestibular disorders. Brain 119:1523, 1996.
9. Bohannon RW: One-legged balance test times. Percept Mot Skills 78:801, 1994.
10. Bohannon RW, Leary KM: Standing balance and function over the course of acute rehabilitation. Arch Phys Med Rehabil 76:994, 1995.
11. Bohannon M, Newton R: Test-retest reliability of the Fukuda Stepping Test. Physiother Res Int 3:58, 1998.
12. Bobath B: Adult Hemiplegia: Evaluation and Treatment, 2nd ed. London, William Heinemann, 1978.
13. Britton B: Common Problems in Otology. St. Louis, Mosby–Year Book, 1991.
14. Chandler J, Duncan P: Balance and falls in the elderly: Issues in evaluation and treatment. In Guccione A (ed): Geriatric Physical Therapy. St. Louis, CV Mosby, 1993.
15. Charness A: Stroke/Head Injury: A Guide to Functional Outcomes in Physical Therapy Management. Rockville, MD, Aspen Publications, 1986.
16. Clark S, Rose DJ: Generalizability of the limits of stability test in the evaluation of dynamic balance among older adults. Arch Phys Med Rehabil 78:1078, 1997.
17. Cordo P, Nashner L: Properties of postural adjustments associated with rapid arm movements. J Neurophysiol 47:287, 1982.
18. Cromwell S, Held J: Test-retest reliability of three balance measures used with hemiplegic patients. Neurol Rep 17:24, 1994.
19. DiFabio RP, Badke MB: Relationship of sensory organization to balance function in patients with hemiplegia. Phys Ther 70:20, 1990.
20. Duncan P, et al: Is there one simple measure for balance? PT Magazine 1:74, 1993.
21. Fields J, et al: The disablement model: The relationships between and among impairment, functional limitation and disability in the elderly population. Issues on Aging 22:5, 1999.
22. Fife T: Recognition and management of horizontal canal benign positional vertigo. Am J Otol 19:345, 1998.
23. Flores AM: Objective measurement of standing balance. Neurol Rep 16:17, 1992.
24. Foster CA: Vestibular rehabilitation. Ballieres Clin Neurol 3:577, 1994.
25. Fuller K: Vestibular dysfunction. In Goodman C, Boissonnault B, (ed): Pathology: Implications for the Physical Therapist. Philadelphia, WB Saunders, 1998.
26. Furman JM, Cass SP: Benign paroxysmal positional vertigo. N Engl J Med 341:1590, 1999.
27. Gentile AM: A working model of skill acquisition with application to teaching. Quest 17:3, 1972.
28. Gibson JJ: The Senses Considered as Perceptual Systems. Boston, Houghton Mifflin, 1966.
29. Gordon J: Assumptions underlying physical therapy intervention: Theoretical and historical perspectives. In Carr JH, Shepherd RB, Gordon J (eds): Movement Sciences: Foundations for Physical Therapy in Rehabilitation. Rockville, MD, Aspen Publishers, 1987.
30. Hain T, Ramaswamy T, Hillman M: Anatomy and physiology of the normal vestibular system. In Herdman S (ed): Vestibular Rehabilitation, 2nd ed. Philadelphia, FA Davis, 2000.
31. Harburn KL, et al: Clinical applicability and test-retest reliability of an external perturbation test of balance in stroke subjects. Arch Phys Med Rehabil 76:317, 1995.
32. Herdman S: Vestibular Rehabilitation, 2nd ed. Philadelphia, FA Davis, 2000.
33. Herdman S, Tusa R: Assessment and treatment of patients with benign paroxysmal positional vertigo. In Herdman S (ed): Vestibular Rehabilitation, 2nd ed. Philadelphia, FA Davis, 2000.
34. Horak F: Clinical measurement of postural control in adults. Phys Ther 67:1881, 1987.
35. Horak F: Assumptions underlying motor control for neurologic rehabilitation. In Lister MJ (ed): Contemporary Management of Motor Control Problems: Proceedings of the II-STEP Conference, Alexandria, VA, Bookcrafters, 1992.
36. Horak F, Shupert C: Role of the vestibular system in postural control. In Herdman S (ed): Vestibular Rehabilitation, 2nd ed. Philadelphia, FA Davis, 2000.
37. Horak F, Shupert C, Mirka A: Components of postural dyscontrol in the elderly: A review. Neurobiol Aging 10:727, 1989.
38. Ingersoll C, Armstrong C: The effects of closed head injury on postural sway. Med Sci Sports Exerc 24:739, 1992.
39. Ivanenko Y, Grasso R, Lacquanti F: Effect of gaze on postural responses to neck proprioceptive and vestibular stimulation in humans. J Physiol 519:301, 1999.
40. Jacobson GP, et al: Balance function test correlates of the Dizziness Handicap Inventory. J Am Acad Audiol 2:253, 1991.
41. Jacobson GP, Newman CW: The development of the Dizziness Handicap Inventory. Arch Otolaryngol Head Neck Surg 116:424, 1990.
42. Knott M, Voss D: Proprioceptive Neuromuscular Facilitation: Patterns and Techniques, 2nd ed. New York, Harper & Row, 1968.
43. Lackner J, et al: Precision contact of the fingertip reduces postural sway of individuals with bilateral vestibular loss. Exp Brain Res 126:459, 1999.
44. Lynch SM, Leahy P, Barker SP: Reliability of measurements obtained with a modified functional reach test in subjects with spinal cord injury. Phys Ther 78:128, 1998.
45. Magill RA: Motor Learning: Concepts and Applications, 5th ed. Boston, McGraw-Hill, 1998.
46. Maki BE, McIlroy WE: The control of foot placement during compensatory stepping reactions: Does speed of response take precedence over stability? IEEE Trans Rehabil Eng 7:80, 1999.
47. Mathias S, Nayak U, Isaacs B: Balance in the elderly patient: The "Get Up and Go" test. Arch Phys Med Rehabil 67:387, 1986.
48. McIlroy WE, Maki BE: Age-related changes in compensatory stepping in response to unpredictable perturbations. J Gerontol A Biol Sci Med Sci 51:M289, 1996.
49. Moore S, Woollacott M: The use of biofeedback devices to improve postural stability. Phys Ther Pract 2:1, 1993.
50. Morris SL, Sharpe MH: PNF revisited. Physiother Theory Pract 9:43, 1993.
51. Nashner L: Evaluation of postural stability, movement, and control. In Hasson S (ed): Clinical Exercise Physiology. Philadelphia, CV Mosby, 1994.
52. Nashner L: Sensory, neuromuscular, and biomechanical contributions to human balance. In Duncan P (ed): Balance: Proceedings of the APTA Forum. Alexandria, VA, American Physical Therapy Association, 1990.
53. Newman C, Jacobson G: Balance handicap assessment. In Jacobson G, Newman C, Kartush J (eds): Handbook of Balance Testing Function. St. Louis, Mosby–Year Book, 1993.
54. Newton R: Review of tests of standing balance abilities. Brain Inj 3:335, 1989.
55. Newton RA: Balance screening of an inner city older adult population. Arch Phys Med Rehabil 78:587, 1997.
56. Niam S, et al: Balance and physical impairments after stroke. Arch Phys Med Rehabil 80:1227, 1999.
57. Patla AE, et al: Identification of age-related changes in the balance

control system. *In* Duncan P (ed): Balance: Proceedings of the APTA Forum. Alexandria, VA, American Physical Therapy Association, 1990.

58. Podsiadlo D, Richardson S: The Timed "Up and Go": A test of basic functional mobility for frail elderly persons. J Am Geriatr Soc 39:142, 1991.

59. Rose DJ: A Multilevel Approach to the Study of Motor Control and Learning. Boston, Allyn & Bacon, 1997.

60. Rose DJ, Clark S: Can the control of bodily orientation be significantly improved in a group of older adults with a history of falls? J Am Geriatr Soc 48:275, 2000.

61. Rose DK, Guiliani CA: A comparison of overground walking and treadmill walking in patients with cerebral vascular lesion. Neurol Rep 17:23, 1993.

62. Rothstein JM (ed): Guide to physical therapist practice: I and II. Phys Ther 77:1371, 1997.

63. Schenkman M, Butler RB: A model for multisystem evaluation, interpretation, and treatment of individuals with neurologic dysfunction. Phys Ther 69:538, 1989.

64. Schmidt RA, Lee TD: Motor Control and Learning: a Behavioral Emphasis, 3rd ed. Champagne, IL, Human Kinetics, 1999.

65. Shepard NT, et al: Vestibular and balance rehabilitation therapy. Ann Otol Rhinol Laryngol 102:198, 1993.

66. Sherrington C: The Integrative Action of the Nervous System. New Haven, CT, Yale University Press, 1961.

67. Shumway-Cook A, Horak F: Assessing the influence of sensory interaction on balance. Phys Ther 66:1548, 1986.

68. Shumway-Cook A, Horak F: Vestibular rehabilitation: An exercise approach to managing symptoms of vestibular dysfunction. Semin Hearing 10:194, 1986.

69. Shumway-Cook A, Horak F: Vestibular Rehabilitation, unpublished course syllabus, 1991.

70. Shumway-Cook A, Woollacott MH (eds): Motor Control: Theory and Practical Applications. Baltimore, Williams & Wilkins, 1995.

71. Speechley M, Tinetti M: Assessment of risk and prevention of falls among elderly persons. Physiother Can 42:75, 1990.

72. Tinetti M: Performance oriented assessment of mobility problems in elderly patients. J Am Geriatr Soc 41:479, 1986.

73. Tseng H, Chao W: Head-shaking nystagmus: A sensitive indicator of vestibular dysfunction. Clin Otolaryngol 22:549, 1997.

74. Van Sant AF: Should the normal motor developmental sequence be used as a theoretical model to progress adult patients? *In* Lister MJ (ed): Contemporary Management of Motor Control Problems: Proceedings of the II-STEP Conference, Alexandria, VA, Bookcrafters, 1992.

75. VanSwearingen JM, et al: The modified Gait Abnormality Rating Scale for recognizing the risk of recurrent falls in community-dwelling older adults. Phys Ther 76:994, 1996.

76. Weber P, Cass D: Clinical assessment of postural stability. Am J Otol 14:566, 1993.

77. Whipple R, Wolfson LI: Abnormalities of balance, gait, and sensorimotor function in the elderly population. *In* Duncan P (ed): Balance: Proceedings of the APTA Forum. Alexandria, VA, American Physical Therapy Association, 1990.

78. Wolf M, et al: Epley's manuever for benign paroxsymal positional vertigo: A prospective study. Clin Otolaryngol 24:43 1999.

Basal Ganglia Disorders: Metabolic, Hereditary, and Genetic Disorders in Adults

MARSHA E. MELNICK, PhD, PT

Key Words

– basal ganglia

– exercise

– Huntington's disease

– Parkinson's disease

– physical therapy

Objectives

After reading this chapter the student/therapist will:

1. Describe the circuitry of the basal ganglia.

2. Relate the anatomy and physiology of the basal ganglia to its role(s) in sensorimotor and cognitive processes.

3. Utilize the information on anatomy, physiology, and pharmacology to explain the signs and symptoms seen in the classic disease states; for example, Parkinson's disease and Huntington's disease.

4. Develop an evaluation plan for patients with diseases of the basal ganglia.

5. Develop a treatment plan for these patients with the rationale for intervention methods.

6. Determine treatment efficacy, especially in the case of degenerative disease.

7. Integrate the information in this chapter with the information provided in Section I of this book to develop treatment plans for patients with metabolic or toxic disorders.

This chapter considers the metabolic, hereditary, and genetic disorders that typically have their onset in adulthood, including Huntington's disease (HD), Wilson's disease, heavy metal poisoning, and drug intoxication. Because of the wide variety of diseases with a wide variety of causes, the concentration here is on understanding the clinical problems and commonalities that exist within this grouping. The predominant area of the brain affected by these disorders is the basal ganglia. For this reason Parkinson's disease (PD), a degenerative disease of the basal ganglia of unknown etiology, but perhaps caused by environmental toxins, is also included.

THE BASAL GANGLIA

The most commonly seen disorders affecting the basal ganglia include PD, HD, Wilson's disease, and dystonias, as well as drug-induced dyskinesias. All involve changes in muscle tone, a decrease in movement coordination, and the presence of extraneous movement. Taken together, these disorders now affect approximately 1 million people in the United States.[5, 210] To understand how one interrelated area of the brain can account for such a wide variety of symptoms, it is first necessary to understand the anatomy, physiology, and pharmacology of these structures.

Anatomy

The dorsal or sensorimotor basal ganglia are composed of three nuclei located at the base of the cerebral cortex—hence their name. These nuclei are the caudate nucleus, the putamen, and the globus pallidus. Two brain stem nuclei, the substantia nigra and the subthalamic nucleus, are included as part of the basal ganglia because they have a close functional relationship to the forebrain nuclei. Other parts of the basal ganglia, the ventral basal ganglia, are intimately related to the limbic system and are discussed in Chapter 6; they will not be considered in this chapter. (The anatomical location of the various parts of the basal ganglia is shown in Fig. 22–1.)

Embryologically, anatomically, and functionally, the caudate nucleus and the putamen are similar structures, and are often referred to together as the *neostriatum*—a term derived from *striate* and used to denote pathways from and to the caudate and putamen. The term *corpus striatum* refers to the caudate, putamen, and globus pal-

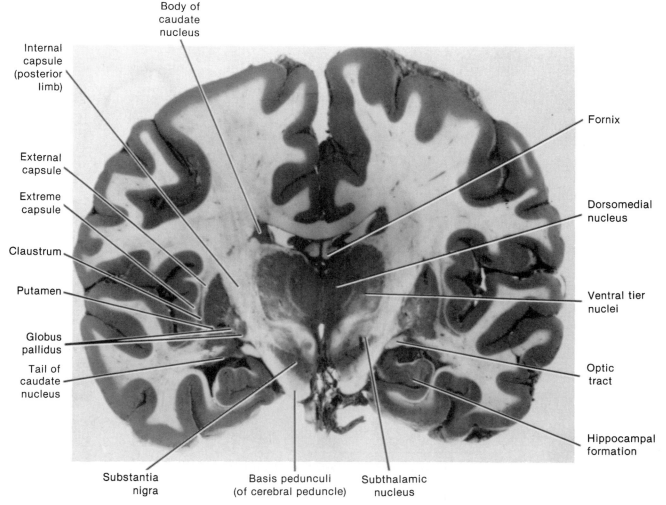

FIGURE 22–1. Anatomical location of various parts of the basal ganglia. (From Nolte J: The Human Brain: An Introduction to Its Anatomy. St Louis, Mosby, 1981.)

lidus. The various connections and interconnections of this system are discussed on the basis of these definitions.

Afferent Pathways

Functionally, the basal ganglia can be divided into an afferent portion and an efferent portion (Fig. 22–2). The afferent structures are the caudate and putamen. They receive input from the entire cerebral cortex, the intralaminar thalamic nuclei, and the centromedian-parafascicular complex of the thalamus, as well as from the substantia nigra and the dorsal raphe nucleus, both in the brain stem. The projections from the cortex are systematically arranged so that the frontal cortex projects to the head of the caudate and putamen and the visual cortex projects to the tail. The prefrontal cortex projects mainly to the caudate, whereas the sensorimotor cortex projects mainly to the putamen.[117] Those projections from the cortical regions that represent the proximal musculature and those from the premotor regions may be bilateral.[103, 116] hese very close and very profuse connections between the cortex and the basal ganglia are suggestive of a close interfunctional relationship between the cortex and the neostriatum. The projections from the thalamus to the caudate and putamen are also somatotopically arranged. The heaviest projections are from the centromedian nucleus, which also receives massive input from the motor cortex.[113, 117]

The somatotopic arrangement of the cortico-striatal-thalamic-cortical pathways is maintained throughout the loop. This finding has led to an important functional hypothesis, that the basal ganglia form parallel pathways subserving specific sensorimotor and associative functions.[4] The putamen is linked to the sensorimotor functions and the caudate to the associative functions.

As our knowledge of the circuitry of the basal ganglia

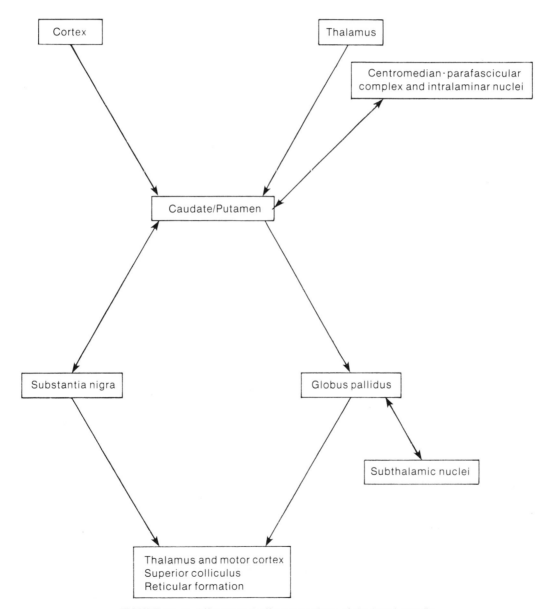

FIGURE 22–2. Afferent and efferent portions of the basal ganglia.

has advanced, so has knowledge regarding their microscopic structure. The caudate and putamen look somewhat homogeneous because of the predominance of one cell type. Careful analysis using precise staining methods has demonstrated the appearance of patches within these nuclei. Input can be segregated depending on whether the patches are innervated or the areas around the patches (matrix) are innervated.[73] The intrinsic structure of the caudate and putamen also suggests that at least nigral input occurs in a way that could immediately modulate the input coming from the cortex.[201]

Efferent Pathways

The input that has been processed in the caudate and putamen is then sent to the globus pallidus and substantia nigra, which constitute the efferent portion of the basal ganglia. The globus pallidus and substantia nigra are each divided into two regions. The globus pallidus has an external and an internal region; the substantia nigra consists of the dorsal pars compacta and the ventral pars reticulata. Embryologically and microscopically, the internal segment of the globus pallidus and the pars reticulata of the substantia nigra are very similar. These two regions are the primary efferent structures for the basal ganglia. The projections from the caudate and putamen to the globus pallidus and substantia nigra maintain the somatotopic arrangement. The caudate projects primarily to the rostral and dorsal third of the globus pallidus and the anterior portion of the substantia nigra. The putamen projects to the caudal and ventral portions of the globus pallidus and the caudal substantia nigra.[37, 61] Evidence suggests that the projection from the caudate and putamen are separate in the globus pallidus and substantia nigra.[103] From these structures the information is transmitted to the thalamus and then to the cortex. The globus pallidus projects to the lateral portions of the ventrolateral and ventroanterior nuclei of the thalamus. The substantia nigra projects to the medial portions of these nuclei. The superior colliculus, the pedunculopontine nucleus (PPN), and other less-defined brain stem structures (perhaps the reticular formation) also receive pallidal and nigral output. All output of the basal ganglia has then been processed through the globus pallidus or the substantia nigra, or both, before proceeding to other areas of the brain (see Fig. 22–2).

Pathways to the Motor System

Information processed in the basal ganglia can influence the motor system in several ways, but no direct pathway to the alpha or gamma motor neurons of the spinal cord exists. The first route is the projection to the ventroanterior and ventrolateral nuclei of the thalamus, which then projects predominately to the premotor cortex. Another pathway is through the superior colliculus and then to the tectospinal tract. There are also pathways from the globus pallidus and substantia nigra that terminate in areas of the reticular formation (e.g., the PPN) and then through the reticulospinal pathways. Anatomically, therefore, the basal ganglia are in good position to affect the motor system at many levels.

The basic circuitry of the basal ganglia comprises two loops.[3] The loops for the sensorimotor system are shown in Fig. 22–3. The direct loop is the loop that begins in the motor regions of the cortex and projects to the putamen and then directly to the globus pallidus internal segment, and on to the thalamus. The indirect pathway adds the subthalamic nucleus between the globus pallidus external segment, and the thalamus. The subthalamic nucleus also receives direct input from the premotor and motor cortex as well as from the globus pallidus.[81, 160] The black neurons represent inhibitory connections, and the shaded neurons represent excitatory connections. In general, the direct pathway, via disinhibition, activates the thalamocortical pathway; the indirect pathway inhibits the thalamocortical system. The role of these loops in normal and diseased states will become clearer as we discuss the physiology and pharmacology of the basal ganglia.

In summary, input from the motor cortex, all other areas of the cortex, parts of the thalamus, and the substantia nigra enter the basal ganglia through the caudate and putamen. Here they are processed and sent on to the globus pallidus and substantia nigra. The appropriate "gain" of the system is adjusted, for example, how large a movement is necessary, and how much postural stability

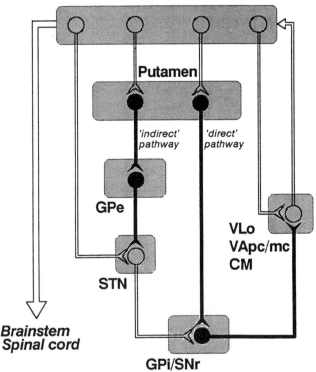

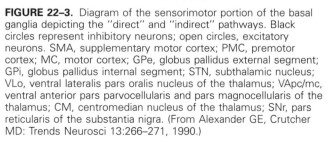

FIGURE 22–3. Diagram of the sensorimotor portion of the basal ganglia depicting the "direct" and "indirect" pathways. Black circles represent inhibitory neurons; open circles, excitatory neurons. SMA, supplementary motor cortex; PMC, premotor cortex; MC, motor cortex; GPe, globus pallidus external segment; GPi, globus pallidus internal segment; STN, subthalamic nucleus; VLo, ventral lateralis pars oralis nucleus of the thalamus; VApc/mc, ventral anterior pars parvocellularis and pars magnocellularis of the thalamus; CM, centromedian nucleus of the thalamus; SNr, pars reticularis of the substantia nigra. (From Alexander GE, Crutcher MD: Trends Neurosci 13:266–271, 1990.)

is needed. The information is sent to the muscles by way of the thalamus and motor cortex, the superior colliculus, or the reticular formation.

Physiology

Understanding of the physiology of the interactions among areas of the basal ganglia has greatly increased in the last decade. Initially, the prevalent view was that the basal ganglia exerted an inhibitory influence on the motor system. An early study by Mettler and colleagues[148] demonstrated an inhibition of cortically evoked movements following caudate stimulation. More recent studies show both excitatory and inhibitory influences.

The caudate and putamen are composed of neurons that fire very slowly, whereas the neurons in the globus pallidus fire tonically at fairly high rates. (The spontaneous activity of the caudate and putamen is therefore low, whereas that of the globus pallidus is high.) The low firing rates of neostriatal neurons are partially a result of the nature of thalamic synaptic inputs.[30]

Stimulation of the cortex, thalamus, and substantia nigra almost always produces excitatory postsynaptic potentials (EPSPs) followed by longer inhibitory postsynaptic potentials (IPSPs)—the EPSP-IPSP sequence. Further, input from the cortex seems to have priority over input from the thalamus and substantia nigra.[93] The data provide evidence that the cortex is instrumental in regulating the responsiveness of caudate neurons.[124–126]

Cortical recruiting responses have been demonstrated following caudate, putamen, and pallidal stimulation.[28, 29, 51]

especially over the area of the motor cortex. This led Dieckmann and Sasaki[54] to conclude that the neostriatum and globus pallidus have an important functional role in controlling the activity level of the cerebral cortex. The experiments of Hull and co-workers[91] suggested that basal ganglia input to the cortex might "enhance the magnitude of subsequent excitatory inputs." They also suggested that basal ganglia–cortical interactions might be important in tasks in which a response must be withheld until an appropriate stimulus occurs, for example, keeping the foot on the brake until the light turns green.[92] This is also similar to the hypothesis of Mink,[150] that the basal ganglia activate only the most necessary pathways and inhibit all unnecessary pathways (Fig. 22–4).

The physiology of the direct and indirect pathways adds further support for the basal ganglia's role in modifying input to the cortex. The neurons of the efferent portion of the basal ganglia respond with either phasic increases or phasic decreases in activity which in turn will affect the activity in the thalamus and hence the cortex. A decrease in activity of the globus pallidus internal segment removes inhibition to the thalamus and thus enables cortical activation. It is not yet known whether the two pathways are activated concurrently or whether different activities activate the two pathways separately. In the former possibility, the indirect pathway is seen as a "brake" on ongoing activity; if the latter, the indirect pathway would act to decrease all other patterns in a form of lateral inhibition.[3] In both cases, the basal ganglia would have a role in cortical activation and modulation. In fact, one of the current views in relationship to disease

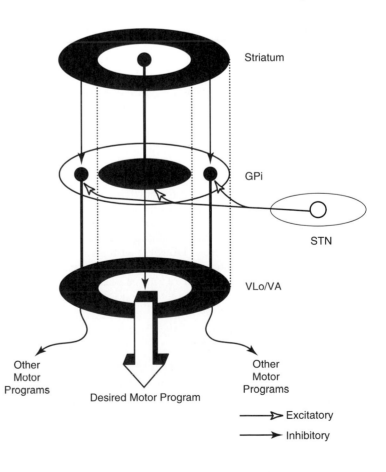

FIGURE 22–4. The figure illustrates the net effect of basal ganglia circuitry to produce an area of excitation (the desired program) surrounded by an area of inhibition (all other unnecessary programs). GPi, globus pallidus internal segment; STN, subthalamic nucleus; VLo/VA, ventral lateralis oralis/ventral anterior. (Adapted from Mink JW: The basal ganglia: Focused selection and inhibition of competing motor programs. Prog Neurobiol 50:381, 1996.)

Striatum

GPi

STN

VLo/VA

Other Motor Programs

Desired Motor Program

Other Motor Programs

⟶▷ Excitatory

⟶ Inhibitory

processes is that an underactive direct pathway or an overactive indirect pathway, or a combination of both, would lead to decreased activation of the cortex and hence bradykinesia and akinesia, whereas an overactive direct pathway or underactive indirect pathway, or a combination of these, would lead to the presence of extraneous movements[2, 76] (see Fig. 22–3).

How do these pathways relate to everyday function? (see Figs. 22–3 and 22–4). Rigidity could be explained by too much muscle activity, the akinesia, and bradykinesia of PD by not enough excitation or too many conflicting patterns of movement, as well as the increased extraneous movements that are characteristic of basal ganglia diseases. Mink's hypothesis[150] also fits with the role of the basal ganglia in selection of environmentally appropriate behaviors.[74]

Relationship of the Basal Ganglia to Movement and Posture

Lesion experiments, single-unit recording in awake, behaving animals, and careful observations of the sequelae of human disease processes have provided some answers regarding the precise role of the basal ganglia in movement and posture.

Automatic Movement

The earliest view of the basal ganglia came from Thomas Willis in 1664. He hypothesized that the corpus striatum received "the notion of spontaneous localized movements in ascending tracts. . . . Conversely, from here tendencies are dispatched to enact notions without reflection [automatic movements] over descending pathways."[227, p. 8] In his discussion of the signs and symptoms of basal ganglia disease, the reader will see that Willis possessed great insights. Magendie in 1841 demonstrated that removal of the striatum bilaterally produced compulsive movements, whereas removal of only one striatum produced no visible effect.[134] Studies by Nothnagel[166] demonstrated that destruction of the globus pallidus produced a twisting of the spine with the convexity toward the side of the lesion, whereas lesions of the substantia nigra tended to produce immobility. With the advent of the use of electrical stimulation in the late nineteenth century, further information on the function of the basal ganglia was gathered. Stimulation of the caudate nucleus did not (and does not) produce movement of muscles or limbs as occurs with stimulation of the motor cortex. However, at higher levels of current, total body patterns and postures were usually evoked. The earliest stimulation of the caudate nucleus produced an increase of flexion of the head, trunk, and limbs and tonic contraction of the facial muscles.[63]

Motor Problems in Animals

Contemporary experiments concerning lesions show a wide variety of motor problems in a variety of animals. Hypokinesia following the occurrence of lesions in the basal ganglia is one frequent result. Stern[206] observed that bilateral lesions of the substantia nigra produced poverty of movement and a tendency to assume fixed postures.

Monkeys with large lesions in the basal ganglia assume a "somersault" position; that is, the animal is flexed so that the head rests on the floor while the animal is standing.[51] Cooling of the putamen or globus pallidus in the monkey produces a slowing of movements as well as a tendency toward flexed postures.[87, 88] In one experiment, electromyogram (EMG) recordings of the biceps and triceps of monkeys demonstrated an increase in co-contraction of these muscles.[87] Although movement is still possible, it must be made with an abnormal starting position and a delay in appropriate activation of the prime movers.

Movement Initiation and Preparation

The hypothesis that the basal ganglia are involved in movement initiation and preparation also receives support from human experiments. Kornhuber[113] observed, while recording from the scalp in humans, a slow negative potential bilaterally just before movement. This *Bereitschaftspotential*, or "readiness potential," was not present in patients with PD. Kornhuber hypothesized that the generator for this readiness potential was not in the motor cortex but rather in subcortical structures.[113] More recent studies of the readiness potential continue to implicate the basal ganglia; however, deficits in this potential are more apparent in complex than in simple movements.

More precise investigations into how movements were programmed and initiated used the technique of single-unit recording in awake, performing animals: Evarts[60] in the motor cortex, DeLong[49] in the basal ganglia, Thach[214, 215] in the cerebellum, and Massion and Smith[138] and Strick[208] in the ventroanterior and ventrolateral nuclei of the thalamus. All these researchers found that units in these areas alter their activity before changes in the EMG activity of the muscles performing the task; that is, before arrival of sensory feedback information from the muscles, joints, and skin could modify the centrally generated movement program. These changes in neuronal activity occurred 50 to 200 ms before the EMG activity changes, and there was enough overlap of the onset of these changes so that no clear answer established which of these areas gave the command to move. However, these results do indicate that all of these brain sites are involved in movement generation. Experiments using cooling procedures demonstrated that cooling the ventrolateral thalamic nucleus,[17] the cerebellum, or basal ganglia[25, 88, 226] produced a delay in the onset of the movement, as well as a slowing in the velocity of the movement itself, again indicating that these structures are involved in the initiation and execution phases of movement.

Neafsey and colleagues[161, 162] and Melnick and co-workers[144] presented further evidence for the involvement of the globus pallidus, ventroanterior and ventrolateral nuclei, and motor cortex in the preparation of movement. Of the units recorded in the globus pallidus, ventroanterior and ventrolateral nuclei, and medical precruciate cortex of the cat, 30% to 70% changed their firing pattern more than 250 ms before changes in EMG activity. Neafsey and colleagues hypothesized that these early unit activity changes were the "neural correlate of the state of set,"[161, p. 712] or readiness that exists as a preparatory adjustment for performing a task, as proposed by Woodworth and Schlosberg.[230] Buchwald and associates have defined this preparatory activity as "response set," which entails "the ability to initiate and carry out smoothly and in proper sequence a set of movements that comprise a defined response."[30, p. 175] Denny-Brown,[51] in studying the effects of lesions of the basal ganglia on movement, also suggested that the basal ganglia participate in the "activating set." Denny-Brown and Yanagesawa defined this "set" as the "preparation of the mechanism preparatory to a motor performance oriented to the environment."[52] The difficulty in parkinsonism of initiating movements or in changing from one movement to another is an example of a disruption in this "response set" process.

As electrophysiological techniques have improved, there is more controversy regarding the onset of activity changes in the basal ganglia.[151] Some investigators did not find changes in activity in the basal ganglia prior to EMG changes and suggested that the basal ganglia are only involved in movement execution time. Some of the differences in results may be related to the experimental task. Investigators who have utilized movements made to external cues rather than internal cues find less activity associated with initiation of a movement. As is discussed later, it appears that the basal ganglia play a greater role in movements without external signals.

Postural Adjustments

The involvement of the basal ganglia in the initiation of movement may include a role in directing the postural adjustments necessary before distal movement can take place. In fact, in addition to the assumption of flexed, fixed postures, other postural abnormalities have been observed following lesions of the basal ganglia. In an experiment by Winkelmuller and Nitsch,[229] rats with bilateral lesions of the substantia nigra were unable to balance skillfully or correct imbalance by quick movements or by shifting their weight. In another experiment animals with caudate lesions had to move the entire body right and left for movement of the appropriate paw in a bar-pressing task, whereas normal animals were able to move their paws without moving the body.[168]

Similar postural deficiencies have been observed in monkeys with lesions of various parts of the basal ganglia.[52] Potegal[182] observed that animals with lesions in the anterior caudate were unable to guide their behavior by taking their own body position into account. He referred to this deficit as a breakdown in "egocentric localization." Studies of human disease processes support the hypothesis that the basal ganglia have a role in the postural mechanisms active before movement. Martin,[137] in his extensive studies of patients with PD, found that these patients, in addition to their akinesia, demonstrated severe disturbances in posture. He noted that especially when vision was occluded these persons were unable to make the normal postural shifts involved in equilibrium reactions. Melnick and colleagues[147] showed that there was a decrease in static postural adjustments in persons with PD and that these changes could be seen early in the disease process.

The exact role of the basal ganglia in postural stability is not known. The early unit activity changes seen in the basal ganglia are not related in a simple fashion to early EMG activity in the proximal and axial muscles.[144, 161, 162] Early neuronal activity is consistent with the theory of long-term biasing of the cortex discussed earlier. Stimulation of the caudate nucleus or globus pallidus can modify alpha and gamma motor responses evoked by motor cortex or pyramidal tract stimulation.[72, 163, 188] DeLong and Strick interpreted the changes in basal ganglionic activity preceding movement to be a faciliting discharge to "establish the climate for the performance rather than the detailed pattern of the movement."[50, p. 334]

Perceptual and Cognitive Functions

The basal ganglia's function is not solely in the initiation and control of movement and posture. Several studies demonstrate that the basal ganglia are involved in aspects of sensory integration. Lidsky and co-workers[129] found that neurons in the basal ganglia were related to the reward properties and particularly to the sensation of perioral stimulation. Their work and the work of Schneider and Lidsky[193] demonstrated that the basal ganglia were involved in modulating reflex responses about the face. Hore and co-workers[87, 88] and Brooks,[25] recording from the striatum during cooling, found that the animals had the greatest difficulty with performance of learned movements in the absence of vision. The studies of Crutcher and DeLong[45] found that movement-related cells in the putamen were also sensitive to proprioceptive input. Klockgether and Dichgans,[106] as well as Jobst and colleagues,[96] found that patients with PD likewise had impairments in kinesthesia and that these impairments increased with distance from the center of the body. Schneider and co-workers[194] found that animals made parkinsonian by a neurotoxin had deficits in operantly conditioned behavior. They suggested that the decrease in performance was due to a "defect in the linkage" between a stimulus and the motor output centers. These sensory difficulties may be important factors in evaluation and treatment of basal ganglia diseases, especially those associated with dystonia.

There is also evidence to show that the basal ganglia are involved in perceptual and cognitive functions. Following lesions of the basal ganglia, deficits appear in the performance of a variety of alternation tasks in rodents, carnivores, primates, and humans (see Teuber[213] for a review). One reason for these deficits is the animal's tendency toward perseveration of a previously reinforced cue. In learning a delayed spatial alternation task, the animal must learn the temporal sequence (i.e., the alternation of position) and must be able to remember the location and consequences of its last response.[131] Stimulation of the caudate nucleus immediately following movement to the goal prevents the acquisition of this task and also disrupts performance of the task once it is learned, but it does not affect motor ability. Livesey and Rankine-Wilson[131] concluded therefore that interference in caudate functioning at this time selectively disrupted the registration of information generated internally. Frontal cortical lesions also produce deficits in delayed spatial response tasks, but the cortex and the neostriatum appear to mediate separate aspects of delayed response behavior.[57, 131, 220]

Animals with basal ganglia lesions also show difficulties in performance of go/no-go tasks because of a difficulty in suppressing a response to the no-go cue.[12] Graybiel[74] used this information together with her anatomical and chemical studies to suggest that the basal ganglia are important in providing behavioral flexibility. She hypothesized that the basal ganglia are involved in procedural learning that leads to the development of habits. These habits become routine and are easily performed without conscious effort. Because these activities can proceed without thought, we are free to react to new events in our environment and to think. She and colleagues have performed electrophysiological experiments that explain this learning process and these studies demonstrate great plasticity in basal ganglia networks.[67] An elegant study by Brown and colleagues,[27] demonstrated a model of the basal ganglia that can reflect these cognitive and learning activities of the basal ganglia. Their model seems to integrate many of the functions of the basal ganglia with the physiology and pharmacology of the entire system.

Humans with basal ganglia disease also show problems in perceptual abilities. Bowen[24] found that these individuals exhibited deficits in a variety of tasks involving perception of interpersonal and intrapersonal space. In pursuit-tracking tests persons with PD had particular difficulties in correcting errors, which is consistent with Teuber's view that "the basal ganglia may play a role in the regulation of 'corollary' discharges, that is, in presetting of the motor system by sensory stimuli."[213, p. 164] If the motor system is inflexibly set, corrections can be made only by a complete reprogramming. Further, Bowen noted differential responses when persons with PD were categorized according to the side of their major neurological symptoms. She suggested that hemispheric specialization in humans may be affected by basal ganglia lesions.[24] It is interesting to note that children with learning disabilities frequently display deficits in the postural mechanisms thought to be mediated by the basal ganglia.[7]

Based on the literature indicating involvement of the basal ganglia in these complex behaviors, Buchwald and co-workers[30] have hypothesized that the basal ganglia are involved in "cognitive set" as well as "response set." They defined "cognitive set" as "the ability to discriminate a situational context and make an appropriate response to a given signal"[30, p. 175] The term "cognitive" was used for "situations where information has to be transferred across some period of time before a response is initiated."[30, p. 177] They further suggested that the basal ganglia were more involved in complex tasks than in simpler behaviors. Animal and human experiments seem to support this hypothesis as complex learned responses are the ones most affected by basal ganglia lesions.[54] These earlier ideas lend still more support to the hypothesis of Graybiel,[73, 74] that one of the principal functions of the basal ganglia is to provide variety and flexibility in motor programs. This enables the individual to select the proper movements in the proper environmental context.

The ability to perform cognitive activities involves integrating sensory information and, based on this information, making an appropriate response. The basal ganglia seem to have a sensory integrative function as evidenced by experiments that show a multisensory and heterotopic convergence of somatic, visual, auditory, and vestibular stimuli.[114, 139, 158] Segundo and Machne[195] observed unitary discharges of the basal ganglia to both somatic and vestibular stimuli. They hypothesized that the function of the basal ganglia was not in subjective recognition of the stimuli but rather in the regulation of posture and movements of the body in space and in the production of complex motor acts (see Potegal[182] for a similar hypothesis).

For movements to be properly controlled and properly sequenced, the two sides of the body need to be well integrated. Some anatomical evidence suggests some means of bilateral control for the basal ganglia. A lesion of one caudate nucleus or nigrostriatal pathway produces a change in the unit activity of the remaining caudate.[124, 131, 171] Studies of the dopaminergic pathway also indicate interactions between the two sides of the body.[124] For this reason one may find deficits in function even on the "uninvolved" side of an individual with disease of the basal ganglia. It is also possible that diseases of the basal ganglia may go unnoticed until damage is found bilaterally.

It is hoped that this summary of experimental results on the function of the basal ganglia illustrates several points. At least in some general way the basal ganglia are involved in the processes of movement related to preparing the organism for future motion. This may include preparing the cortex for approximate time activation, "setting" the postural reflexes or the gamma motor neuron system, organizing sensory input to produce a motor response in an appropriate environmental context, and inhibiting all unnecessary motor activity. The various parts of the basal ganglia may subserve different aspects of movement, which might account for the differences between an individual with PD and one with HD. In a clinical assessment one must carefully examine the loss of automatic postural adaptations appropriate for the task at hand. It is hoped that the day is approaching when it will no longer be necessary to say, "The exact nature and function of the large mass of basal grey matter known as the corpus striatum have hitherto constituted, it is no exaggeration to say, one of the unsolved problems of neurology."[228, p. 428] The therapist's job will certainly be easier. Until then it is crucial that clinicians carefully observe all aspects of movement (simple and complex) and postural tone during examination and treatment, as well as the responses to treatment. For additional information, see Chapter 5.

Neurotransmitters

Before a detailed analysis of the diseases of the basal ganglia can be considered, a brief description of the neurotransmitters of this region is necessary. The most prevalent diseases discussed in this chapter indicate a deficit in specific neurotransmitters. The pharmacological treatment of PD and, in the future, perhaps of HD, is based on these neurochemical deficits. The basal ganglia possess high concentrations of many of the suspected neurotransmitters: dopamine (DA), acetylcholine (ACh), γ-aminobutyric acid (GABA), substance P, and the enkephalins and endorphins. This discussion, however, includes only the first three neurotransmitters. A diagram of the basal ganglia pathways, which includes the neurotransmitters, is shown in Fig. 22–5.

DA is the major neurotransmitter of the nigrostriatal pathway. It is produced in the pars compacta of the substantia nigra. The axon terminals of these dopaminergic neurons are located in the caudate nucleus. For years a battle raged as to whether DA was excitatory or inhibitory. At present there is evidence that DA is both excitatory and inhibitory.[6, 37] DA appears to be excitatory to the neurons in the direct pathway (GABA and substance P neurons) and inhibitory to the neurons in the indirect pathway (GABA and enkephalin neurons).[2] This dual effect means that a loss of DA will lead to a loss of excitation in the direct pathway and an excess of excitation of the indirect pathway leading to a powerful decrease in activation of the thalamocortical pathway.

There are now five DA receptors; however, their chemical interactions permit the continued usage of D1 and D2 receptor classes.[6] There is some thought that the role of DA is to modulate the effects of other neurotransmitters such as glutamate. Many new drugs (called DA agonists) influence only one of these receptors. Recent experiments have been trying to determine which behaviors are mediated by which DA receptor in the hope that this research may lead to more effective drug treatment with fewer side effects.

Because various drugs and chemicals can act as agonists (similar to) and antagonists (block the action of) of DA, they are used in treating disease involving the basal ganglia. Agonists include amantadine, apomorphine, and a class of drugs called the ergot alkaloids (e.g., bromocriptine). Amphetamine, which prevents the reuptake of DA, can enhance the effect of any DA present in the system. Antagonists include haloperidol, clozapine, and antipsychotic drugs of the phenothiazine class. With time these drugs may deplete the basal ganglia of DA and thus cause PD or tardive dyskinesia. The DA agonists and antagonists are discussed again in the treatment of PD and the occurrence of drug-induced dyskinesia. Further information is provided in Chapter 32.

ACh is believed to be the neurotransmitter of the small interneurons of the caudate and putamen. It is presumed to inhibit the action of DA in this region and classically must be "in balance" with DA (and GABA). Dopaminergic axon terminals are found on cholinergic neurons. Substances that increase dopaminergic activity decrease release of ACh and vice versa.[165] The antagonists of ACh, such as belladonna alkaloids and atropine-like drugs, were one of the first classes of drugs used in the treatment of PD. ACh antagonists are still used as adjuncts to treatment in PD.

GABA is an inhibitory neurotransmitter that is found throughout the brain. In the basal ganglia it is synthesized in the caudate nucleus and transmitted to the globus pallidus and substantia nigra.[187] GABA in the basal ganglia may permit movement to occur by allowing a distribution of neuronal firing. It also may provide a means of feedback inhibition in the efferent parts of the basal ganglia so that the program of activity is not repeated unless needed (see reference 183 for a summation of the role of GABA). Individuals with HD have a deficiency of this chemical. Although agonists of GABA exist (e.g., muscimol and imidazole–acetic acid), a successful drug for the treatment of HD has not yet been found. This may be a result of either the ubiquitous nature of GABA or the very complex circuitry and interrelationships that exist among GABA, ACh, and DA.

In addition to the transmitters discussed, there may be cotransmitters in the basal ganglia. Two such cotransmitters are cholecystokinin and neurotensin. The interactions of these cotransmitters may alter the sensitivity of DA receptors. Fuxe and colleagues[66] suggested that the interactions of cotransmitters may alter the "set point" of transmission in synapses. They may therefore be important in one of the side effects of DA therapy, supersensitivity.

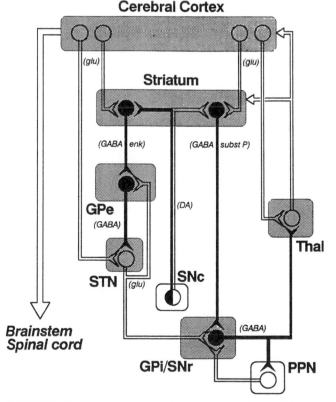

FIGURE 22–5. Diagram showing the neurotransmitters of the direct and indirect pathways of the basal ganglia. Black circles represent inhibitory neurons; shaded circles, excitatory neurons. glu, glutamate; GABA, gamma-aminobutyric acid; enk, enkephalin; subst P, substance P; DA, dopamine; Thal, thalamus; GPe, globus pallidus external segment; GPi, globus pallidus internal segment; STN, subthalamic nucleus; SNr, pars reticularis of the substantia nigra; PPN, pedunculopontine nucleus. (From Alexander GE, Crutcher MD: Trends Neurosci 13:266–271, 1990.)

SPECIFIC CLINICAL PROBLEMS ARISING FROM BASAL GANGLIA DYSFUNCTION

Parkinson's Disease

PD, first described by Parkinson in 1807, is characterized by rigidity, bradykinesia (slow movement), micrography, masklike facies, postural abnormalities, and a resting tremor. As might be suspected from the review of functional physiology of the basal ganglia, the postural abnormalities include assumption of a flexed posture; a lack of equilibrium reactions; especially of the labyrinthine equilibrium reactions; and a decrease in trunk rotation. PD is among the most prevalent of all central nervous system (CNS) degenerative diseases. Presently there are an estimated 800,000 people in the United States with this disease; the incidence is 4.5 to 20.5 and the prevalence is 31 to 347 per 100,000.[210] Incidence increases with advancing age and it is estimated that one in three adults over the age of 85 years will have this disease.[5] The personal and societal burden of PD is great and includes the costs of actual treatment, the burden of caregiving, and the costs of lost earnings in those patients under the age of 65.[226]

The pathology of PD consists of a decrease in the DA stores of the substantia nigra with a consequent depigmentation of this structure and the presence of Lewy bodies (intracellular inclusions).[95] It is DA that gives the substantia nigra its coloration (and hence its name); therefore the lighter the nigra, the greater the DA loss. It has been proposed that PD is an abnormal acceleration of the aging process.[140] DA shows an increase in concentration very early in life, followed by a rapid decrease from 5 to 20 years of age and a slow continuous loss from age 20 to 80 years. Carlsson[37] proposed that while a loss of or damage to the DA neurons early in life (because of, e.g., infection or toxicity) may be insufficient to precipitate PD, the additional loss of neurons with the natural physiological aging process may add cumulatively to that early loss, and the signs of PD are seen when some critical level is reached. Indeed the average age of onset for PD is 35 to 60 years. The disease affects men slightly more than women.

The exact cause of PD remains unknown. Calne and co-workers[36] suggested that, like pneumonia, PD may have several causes. A slow viral process or the long-term effects of early infection were implicated in postencephalitis parkinsonism. There is evidence that environmental factors are involved in the etiology and that the interaction of environment and aging leads to a critical decrease in DA. Several investigators have found a link between growing up in a rural area and PD; the important factors include pesticide use, insecticide use, and well water.[11, 32, 90, 110, 184] Genetics may also be a factor in PD. Although twin studies indicate that there may not be a single gene involved in PD, as in HD, a family history is an important risk factor.[32] Hubble and colleagues[90] also found that a history of depression was a risk factor for PD. The accumulation of free radicals, cell death from toxins to the excitatory neurons, and dysfunction of nigral mitochondria have been implicated from studies of a known neurotoxin (discussed later in this chapter); however, this has not been proved in idiopathic PD.

In view of possible treatment effects for parkinsonism, it is interesting that a study by Sasco and colleagues[190] found an inverse relationship, albeit small, between participation in exercise or sports and later development of parkinsonism. Most researchers agree that the etiology is an interaction of toxic exposure, genetics, and aging. The loss of DA from the substantia nigra leads to alterations in both the direct and indirect pathways of the basal ganglia, resulting in a decrease in excitatory thalamic input to the cortex and perhaps a decrease in inhibitory surround that leads to the symptomatology of PD.

Symptoms

BRADYKINESIA AND AKINESIA

Bradykinesia (a decrease in motion) and akinesia (a lack of motion) are characterized by an inability to initiate and perform purposeful movements. They are also associated with a tendency to assume and maintain fixed postures. All aspects of movement are affected, including initiation, alteration in direction, and the ability to stop a movement once it is begun. Spontaneous or associated movements, such as swinging of the arms in gait or smiling at a funny story, are also affected. Bradykinesia is hypothesized to be the result of a decrease in activation of the supplementary motor cortex, premotor cortex, and motor cortex.[176] The resting level of activity in these areas of the cortex may be decreased so that a greater amount of excitatory input from other areas of the brain would be necessary before movement patterns could be activated. In the person with PD, an increase in cortically initiated movement, even for such "subcortical" activities as walking, supports this hypothesis. These automatic activities are now cortically controlled, and each individual aspect seems to be separately programmed. Associated movements in the trunk and other extremities are no longer automatic. This means that great energy must be expended whenever movement is begun.

Bradykinesia and akinesia affect performance of all types of movements; however, complex movements are more involved than simple movements.[15, 16, 26, 219] This fact was demonstrated in a study showing that the readiness potential preceding gait was more abnormal than the same potential preceding single-joint ankle dorsiflexion performed in an open kinetic chain.[219] Additionally, patients with parkinsonism have increased difficulty performing simultaneous or sequential tasks, over and above that seen with simple tasks. Parkinsonian patients must complete one movement before they can begin to perform the next, whereas control subjects are able to integrate two movements more smoothly in sequence. This deficit has been shown in a variety of tasks, from performing an elbow movement and grip to tracing a moving line on a video screen. The parkinsonian patient behaves as if one motor program must be completely played out before the next one begins, and there is no advance planning for the next movement while the present movement is in progress.[15, 16, 26, 152, 172] Morris and Iansek[154] demonstrated a similar phenomenon in walking. Patients with parkinsonism were unable to perform walking while reciting a numerical sequence.

Sequential movements become more impaired as more movements are strung together; for example, a square is disproportionately slower to draw than a triangle; a pentagon, more difficult than a square.[1, 16] These results indicate that parkinsonian patients have difficulty with transitions between movements. Transitional difficulties are more impaired in tasks requiring a series of different movements than tasks requiring a series of repetitive movements. (This fact is important when determining a client's disability as well as in planning a comprehensive treatment program.)

Results of reaction time experiments are controversial. Some studies find that simple reaction time tasks (the direction and extent of movement are known) are more impaired than choice reaction time tasks (direction or extent of movement are not known)[76]; others find that choice tasks are more impaired than simple tasks[27]; still others find that they are equally impaired[93] These conflicting views may be hard to reconcile in the evaluation and treatment process; however, the task differences may be indicative of task-dependent impairments. Differences in results may involve differences in subject familiarity with the task, whether there is a warning cue, whether the cues involve many sensory systems, and whether the movement sequence must be represented internally. Those authors that find simple reaction time tasks are less impaired suggest that parkinsonian patients can use prior information to preplan movement[231]; those that find choice reaction time tasks more impaired suggest that parkinsonian patients are able to select the correct movement, but have difficulty in initiation only. Clinically, it is important to remember that there is agreement that programming of movements in parkinsonism is definitely task-dependent and that familiarity with the task and the use of multisensory systems improve performance.

It is important to remember that bradykinesia is not caused by rigidity or an inability to relax. This was demonstrated in an EMG analysis of voluntary movements of persons with PD.[77] Although the pattern of EMG agonist-antagonist burst is correct, these bursts are not large enough, resulting in an inability to generate muscle force rapidly enough. Even in slow, smooth movements, however, these persons demonstrated alternating bursts in the flexor and extensor muscle groups. This type of pattern, expected in rapid movements that require the immediate activation of the antagonist to halt the motion, interferes with slow, smooth, continuous motion. Other experimenters[75, 149, 212] have found an alteration in the recruitment order of single motor units. These alterations included a delay in recruitment, pauses in the motor unit once it was recruited, and an inability to increase firing rates. These persons therefore would have a delay in activation of muscles and an inability to properly sustain muscle contraction for movement, and a decreased ability to rapidly dissipate force.[75, 115, 149] Such changes may account for decreases in strength that are seen in persons with PD.

RIGIDITY

The rigidity of PD may be characterized as either "lead pipe" or "cogwheel." The cogwheel type of rigidity is a combination of lead pipe rigidity with tremor. In rigidity there is an increased resistance to movement throughout the entire range in both directions without the classic clasp knife reflex so characteristic of spasticity. Procaine injections can decrease the rigidity without affecting the decrease of spontaneous movements, confirming that rigidity is not the same phenomenon as bradykinesia.[181, 223]

Rigidity is not due to an increase in gamma motor neuron activity, a decrease in recurrent inhibition, or a generalized excitability in the motor system.[122] Long and middle latency reflexes are enhanced in parkinsonism, and the increase in long latency reflexes approximates the observable increase in muscle tone. Short latency reflexes (i.e., deep tendon reflexes), on the other hand, may be normal in persons with PD.

Tatton and colleagues[211] found differences in certain cortical long-loop reflexes in normal and drug-induced parkinsonian monkeys, which led them to speculate that the "reflex gain" of the CNS may lose its ability to adjust to changing environmental situations. For example, in normal persons the background level of motor neuron excitability is different for the task of writing compared with the task of lifting a heavy object; in persons with PD, motor neuron excitability would be set at the same level. Similarly, in the normal person there would be a difference in excitability if the environmental demands were for excitation or inhibition of a muscle; for the person with PD, there would be similar motor neuron excitability regardless of task demands. It is possible that the basal ganglia help to modulate the gain of proprioceptive feedback occurring through the motor cortex. Disease in these structures might then limit the range of this modulation so that all inputs are treated the same (no surround inhibition[150]), and the whole system is adjusted at a higher level of activity. This means that the person with parkinsonism may have the perception of moving farther than he or she is actually moving. It also means that there may be a decrease in system flexibility[74] and an inability to adjust to equilibrium perturbations.[19, 20]

An important aspect of rigidity is that it might increase energy expenditure.[138] This would increase the patient's perception of effort on movement and may be related to feelings of fatigue, especially postexercise fatigue.[65]

TREMOR

The tremor observed in PD is present at rest, it usually disappears or decreases with movement, and it has a regular rhythm of about 4 to 7 beats per second. Some people with PD may have a postural tremor. The EMG tracing of a person with such a tremor shows rhythmical, alternating bursting of antagonistic muscles. Tremor can be produced as an isolated finding in experimental animals that have lesions in various parts of the brain stem or that have been treated with drugs, especially DA antagonists. DA depletion, however, is not the sole cause of tremor. It appears that efferent pathways, especially from the basal ganglia to the thalamus, must be intact because lesions of these fibers decrease or abolish the tremor.[179] Poirier colleagues[179] proposed that tremor results from a combined lesion of the basal ganglia and cerebellar–red nucleus pathways. Because both the basal ganglia and the cerebellum project to the thalamus, a lesion of the thalamus can abolish the tremor regardless of the specific pathway(s). Although tremor may be cosmetically disabling, the tremor rarely interferes with activities of daily living (ADL).

POSTURAL INSTABILITY

Postural instability is a serious problem in parkinsonism that leads to increased episodes of falling and the sequelae of falls. Koller and co-workers[109] found that more than one third of all patients with parkinsonism fall and that over 10% fall more than once a week. They also found that the likelihood of falling increased as the length of duration of disease increased. Drug treatment is not usually effective in reducing the incidence of falls. Unilateral pallidotomy is also ineffective in altering postural disturbance.[147]

Although the cause of balance difficulties is not known, there are several hypotheses. One explanation for postural instability is ineffective sensory processing. Several investigators have found deficits in proprioceptive and kinesthetic processing.[96, 115] Martin,[137] for example, found that labyrinthine equilibrium reactions were delayed in parkinsonian patients. Studies of the vestibular system itself, however, have shown that this system functions normally. Pastor and co-workers[173] studied central vestibular processing in parkinsonian patients and found that the vestibular system responds normally and that patients can integrate vestibular input with the input from other sensory systems. This group hypothesized that the parkinsonian patients had an inability to adequately compensate for baseline instability. This theory is in partial agreement with studies by Beckley,[13] Bloem[19, 20] and their co-workers demonstrating that parkinsonian patients were unable to adjust the size of long and middle latency reflex responses to the degree of perturbation. These patients are therefore unable to activate muscle force proportional to displacement. Melnick and colleagues[147] found that subjects with PD were unable to maintain balance on a sway-referenced force plate. Glatt and associates[71] found that parkinsonian patients did not demonstrate anticipatory postural reactions and, in fact, behaved exactly as a rigid body with joints. Horak and co-workers[85] reported similar findings and found defects in strategy selection as well; parkinsonian patients chose neither a pure hip strategy nor a pure ankle strategy but mixed the two in an inappropriate and maladaptive response. These investigators[13, 19, 20, 86] found that antiparkinsonian medications could improve background postural tone but did not improve automatic postural responses to external displacements. Taken together, it appears that postural instability results from inflexibility in response repertoire, and an inability to inhibit unwanted programs, as well as the interaction of akinesia, bradykinesia, and rigidity with some disturbance in central sensory processing.

GAIT

Shortened stride, decreased speed, and increased cadence characterize the gait in PD.[155, 156] In many patients, especially as the disease progresses, there is also a progressive increase in speed and shortening of stride as if the individual is trying to catch up with his or her center of gravity; this is termed *festination*. Forward festination is called propulsion; backward festination is known as retropulsion. One hypothesis is that festinating gait is caused by the decreased equilibrium responses. If walking is a series of controlled falls and if normal responses to falling are delayed or not strong enough, then the individual will either fall completely or continue to take short, running-like steps. The abnormal motor unit firing seen with bradykinesia may also be the cause of ever-shorten-

ing steps. If the motor unit cannot build up a high enough frequency or if it pauses in the middle of the movement, then the full range of the movement would decrease; in walking this would lead to shorter steps. Festination may also be the result of other changes in the kinematics of gait.

The changes in gait kinematics include changes in excursion of the hip and ankle joints (Fig. 22–6). Instead of a heel-toe progression there may be a flatfooted or, with disease progression, a toe-heel sequence. It is as if the parkinsonian patient has lost the adult gait pattern and is using a more primitive pattern. The flatfooted gait decreases the ability to step over obstacles or to walk on carpeted surfaces. The use of three-dimensional (3-D) gait analysis has shown that there is a decrease in plantarflexion at terminal stance. Changes are also seen in hip flexion and these changes may alter ankle excursion. However, qualitative aspects of the timing of joint excursion appear intact. Figure 22–6 is an illustration of the joint angles in people with PD compared with normal adults. The patient in this example is 55 years old.

Gait and postural difficulties are the two impairments that cause the greatest handicap to persons with parkinsonism. They have been found to be the major elements of disability at home and work for these patients.[67]

PERCEPTION, ATTENTION, AND COGNITIVE DEFICITS

Especially in recent years, researchers have tried to address the cognitive and perceptual impairments of people with PD. Whereas the movement deficits are hypothesized to be due to a decrease in putamenal excitation of the cortex, the learning and perceptual deficits are hypothesized to be due to a decrease in cortical excitation from the caudate nucleus.[172] The deficits are of frontal lobe function and include an inability to shift attention, an inability to quickly access "working memory," and difficulty with visual-spatial perception and discrimination. Research attention has focused on the specific deficits of parkinsonian patients compared with patients with Alzheimer's disease, patients with frontal lobe damage, and those with temporal lobe damage. There appears to be an increase in these perceptual deficits with progression of the disease process. In general, patients have difficulty in shifting attention to a previously irrelevant stimulus,[169] learning when selective attention is necessary,[169] or selecting the correct motor response based on the sensory stimuli.[205] These impairments will affect treatment strategies.

Learning deficits also have been found in patients with parkinsonism; procedural learning has been particularly implicated. Procedural learning is learning that occurs with practice or, as defined by Saint-Cyr and colleagues, "the ability gradually to acquire a motor skill or even a cognitive routine through repeated exposure to a specific activity constrained by invariant rules."[189] In their tests, parkinsonian patients did very poorly on tests of procedural learning, but their declarative learning was within normal limits. Pascual-Leone and colleagues[172] studied procedural learning in more detail. They found that parkinsonian patients could acquire procedural learning but needed more practice than control subjects did. They also

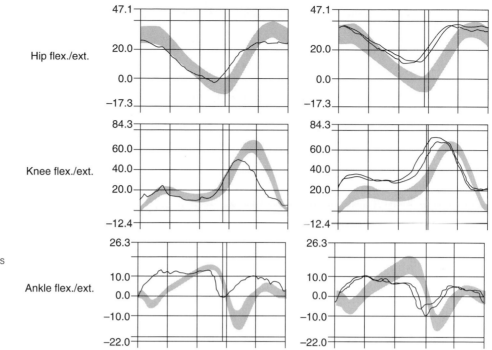

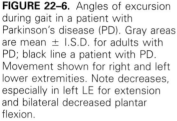

FIGURE 22–6. Angles of excursion during gait in a patient with Parkinson's disease (PD). Gray areas are mean ± 1.S.D. for adults with PD; black line a patient with PD. Movement shown for right and left lower extremities. Note decreases, especially in left LE for extension and bilateral decreased plantar flexion.

found that the ability to translate procedural knowledge to declarative knowledge was more efficient if it occurred with visual input alone rather than the combination of visual input with motor task. This may be a rationale for more therapy, not less.

Stages of the Disease

PD is a progressive disorder. Usually the initial symptom is a resting tremor or micrography (bradykinesia of the upper extremity) unilaterally. With time, rigidity and bradykinesia are seen bilaterally and then postural alterations begin to occur. This commonly starts with an increase in neck, trunk, and hip flexion, which, accompanied by a decrease in righting and equilibrium responses, leads to a decreasing ability to balance.

While these postural changes are occurring, there is also an increase in rigidity, which is most apparent in the trunk and proximal musculature. Trunk rotation is severely decreased. There is no arm swing in gait and no spontaneous facial expression, and movement becomes more and more difficult to initiate. Movement is usually produced with great concentration and is perhaps cortically generated, thereby bypassing the damaged basal ganglia pathways. This great concentration then makes movement tiring, which heightens the debilitating effects of the disease.

Eventually the individual becomes wheelchair-bound and dependent. In the late and severe stages of the disease, especially without therapeutic attention to movement, the client may become bedridden and may demonstrate a fixed trunk-flexion contracture no matter what position he or she is placed in. This posture has been called the "phantom pillow" syndrome because, even when lying supine, the person's head is flexed as if on a pillow.

Throughout this progressive deterioration of movement, there is also a decrease in higher-level sensory processing. In addition, the patient can perform only one task at a time. Reports of the prevalence of dementia in PD patients range from 30% to 93%.[99] However, there is no conclusive evidence of a loss in cognitive abilities.[25] It is generally thought that the appearance of dementia in parkinsonian patients is a result of the presence of extranigral or cortical changes similar to those seen in Alzheimer's disease. Frequently, the amount of dementia is related to the age of the patient, and these patients may represent a subset of PD. The presence of dementia with PD may indicate involvement of ACh or the noradrenergic mesolimbic system, or both. In this case, treatment with anticholinergic drugs may increase a tendency toward dementia, especially in older patients. Sometimes cognitive deficits are inferred because of slowed responses, spatial problems, sensory processing problems, and a masklike facies (see Chapter 32).

The most serious complication of PD is bronchopneumonia. Decreased activity in general, along with decreased chest expansion, may be contributing factors. The mortality rate is greater than in the general population, and death is usually from pneumonia.

Pharmacological Considerations and Medical Management

The knowledge that the symptoms of PD are caused by a decrease in DA led to the pharmacological management of this disease (see Chapter 32). As DA itself does not cross the blood-brain barrier, levodihydroxyphenylalanine (levodopa), a precursor of DA that does, has been used to treat PD since the late 1960s.[44, 89, 132] Usually an inhibitor of aromatic amino acid decarboxylation (carbidopa) is given with levodopa to prevent the conversion to DA before entering the brain. The decarboxylase inhibitor allows a reduction in dosage of levodopa itself, which helps decrease the cardiac and gastrointestinal side effects of DA.

Amantadine is another drug that has been effective in treatment of PD. Although the mechanism of action of this antiviral medication is unknown, it is thought to include a facilitation of release of catecholamines (of which DA is one) from stores in the neuron that are readily releasable. It is often administered in combination with levodopa.

Treatment of PD with levodopa in these various combinations is extremely helpful in reducing bradykinesia and rigidity. It is less effective in reducing tremor. Because PD involves the nigral neurons, the receptors and the neurons in the striatum (which are postsynaptic to DA neurons) remain intact and initially are somewhat responsive to DA.[62] With time, however, the receptors appear to lose their sensitivity, and the prolonged effectiveness (10 years or more) of levodopa therapy is questionable.[102, 135, 142] A further complication of levodopa therapy is the development of involuntary movements (dyskinesias) and the "on/off" phenomenon—a short-duration response resulting in sudden improvement of symptoms followed by a rapid decline in symptomatic relief and perhaps the appearance of dyskinesias or dystonias, or both.[167] With time the "on" effect becomes of shorter and shorter duration.[102] The effectiveness of levodopa does not appear to be closely correlated with the stage of the disease.

The use of levodopa alone or in combination with carbidopa has not provided a cure or even prevented the degeneration of PD. Therefore, many new drugs are being tested and tried. As scientists learn more about the DA receptors and their role in motor control, more effective medications may be found. Some of these "newer" drugs include bromocriptine and pergolide, both D2 receptor agonists. Low doses of bromocriptine seem to decrease the wearing-off phenomenon of levodopa and may also decrease the dyskinesia.[36] However, the side effects include hallucinations, nausea, and vomiting. Pergolide also appears to be effective in treatment; however, double-blind studies seem to indicate recovery with placebo as well.[49] It is quite likely that newer D2 or D2-D1 agonists will be developed. Other pharmacologic interventions also include drugs that prevent the breakdown (e.g., catechol-o-methyltransferase [COMT] inhibitors) or reuptake of DA. Entacapone, a COMT inhibitor, has now been approved for use.[100]

Another approach to pharmacological treatment of PD developed from research on a designer drug that contained the neurotoxin 1-methyl-4-phenyl-1,2,3,6-tetrahydropyridine (MPTP). It was found that the conversion of MPTP to the active neurotoxin MPP$^+$ could be prevented by monoamine oxidase inhibitors such as deprenyl and pargyline.[83] Deprenyl is now used before the initiation of, or in conjunction with, levodopa and carbidopa. Although its mechanism of action is still not fully understood, it may act as a neuroprotective agent.[39, 112] Neurotrophic factors such as brain-derived or glial-derived neurotrophic factors are also under investigation.

Stereotactic surgery is an old technique[102] that has made a comeback based on the new knowledge of basal ganglia connectivity and improvements in instrumentation. Three classes of surgery are presently under investigation and include lesions, deep brain stimulation with implanted electrodes, and neural transplantation. Lesions are made in specific areas of the globus pallidus and, in nonhuman primates, in the subthalamic nucleus. Following the appearance of these lesions, which are small in size and usually restricted to the posteroventral region of the globus pallidus, there is improvement in the rigidity, bradykinesia, and akinesia. Patients demonstrate associated reactions spontaneously. In many cases, the dyskinesias also improve. Thalamic lesions are made in cases in which tremor is the most disabling symptom. Deep brain stimulation is another surgical alternative. The advantage of this technique is that, unlike removal, it is reversible and safer for bilateral surgeries. Sites include the thalamus for tremor, the globus pallidus and subthalamic nucleus for other symptoms of PD. Thalamic deep brain stimulation for tremor relief has been approved by the Food and Drug Administration (FDA). The globus pallidus and subthalamic nucleus have also been recommended for approval. Deep brain stimulation of the globus pallidus and subthalamic nucleus or pallidotomy has been shown to decrease all symptoms, especially dyskinesias. The effects are greater for symptoms manifested in the "off state." Stimulation of the subthalamic nucleus often leads to a decrease in the amount of medication needed. Deep brain stimulation, especially of the subthalamic nucleus, is usually performed bilaterally. Although these results are promising, it is important to realize that to date the studies of surgical efficacy are based upon poorly controlled, largely nonrandomized studies. Therapists may find that prompt and intense treatment immediately following these surgeries may be able to take advantage of neural plasticity.[180]

Fetal transplantation of the substantia nigra to the caudate nucleus is presently under investigation. A blinded, controlled study is nearing completion and will provide the means by which this procedure can be evaluated. At this time, the American Academy of Neurology (AAN) had made no recommendations for use of fetal transplantation. The use of adrenal medulla transplantation is not recommended.[78]

Examination

Examination of the client with PD should focus on the degree of rigidity, bradykinesia, balance, and gait impairments and how far these symptoms interfere with ADL, that is, how the symptoms are influencing the client's handicap. These examinations should, of course, be as objective as possible. The most commonly used descriptor for the patient's level of involvement is the Hoehn and Yahr Scale[84] (see Case 22–1). The most prevalent and one of the most comprehensive physician examinations is the Unified Parkinson's Disease Rating Scale (UPDRS),[62] which measures cognitive and emotional status, ADL ability, motor function, and side effects of medication. This scale is helpful, but is not objective and has limited utility in planning a physical therapy plan of treatment. Nonetheless, the therapist who will treat many clients with PD should be familiar with the UPDRS. Another clinical scale is the Core Assessment Program for Intracerebral Transplantation (CAPIT), which includes timed tests as part of the examination. This scale, as its name implies, is more time-consuming and therefore tends to be used in research more than in the clinic.

In assessing the function of the client with PD, the therapist must note not only that the client can accomplish the activity but also how long it takes to do so. Gait can be assessed by general pattern and also by speed and distance. Forward and backward walking, as well as braiding, should be evaluated. Measurement of gait should include stride length, speed of walking, and cadence.[155, 156] During periodic examinations, the therapist should measure the ability of the client to alter gait speed. Similarly, the time it takes to complete transitional movements such as moving from sitting to standing, standing to sitting, and supine-lying to sitting and back again should be recorded. Handwriting should be periodically sampled. Additionally, active and passive range of movement (ROM) and general strength should be measured.

A careful analysis of equilibrium is imperative for the parkinsonian client. This must include assessment with and without vision and the difference in the two recorded. My own investigation also highlights the importance of assessing challenges to balance such as tandem walking or standing on foam, especially in the early stages of the disease. This may be the first sign of equilibrium impairment. Posturography is the most sensitive measure of postural instability, especially in the early (Hoehn and Yahr stages I and II) stages of disease.[147] A clinically useful tool to assess dynamic balance is the functional reach test and recent studies have shown this to be an effective, predictive tool in people with PD, as it is in the elderly.[203]

Another aspect of assessment would include the detailed observation of associated postural movements. For example in rising from a chair, does the patient move forward in the chair, place the feet underneath the knees, and lean forward before rising? Ideally, the evaluation format should also include the performance of simultaneous and sequential tasks. An assessment of chest expansion and vital capacity should also be included. This is important because of the complication of pneumonia. At present a complete and easy-to-use form for evaluation does not exist for PD.

General Treatment Goals and Rationale

As with all treatment, the general goals will be related to the findings on examination of each client. In the case of PD, it is important to remember that this is a degenerative disease and the prognosis and treatment plan must keep this in mind. Nonpharmacological and surgical interventions, especially therapy treatment, are especially important in the beginning of the disease.[111] In general, goals include increasing movement as well as ROM, maintaining or improving chest expansion, improving equilibrium reactions, and maintaining or restoring functional abilities. Increased movement may in fact modify the progression of the disease and prevent contractures.[57] It may further help to retard dementia. Although levodopa decreases the bradykinesia, it alone will not be effective in increasing movement or improving balance, and therefore aggressive intervention in the early stages is necessary. Increasing trunk rotation goes hand in hand with increasing ROM and motion in general. The longer clients are kept mobile, the less likely they are to develop pneumonia and the longer they can maintain independence in ADL.

Treatment Procedures

The person with PD will usually see a therapist for treatment of gait or balance disorder as well as difficulty in moving and "stiffness." Therapy is also effective in treating generalized fatigue. This discussion starts with general treatment ideas based on disease progression and level of handicap and then more details for each separate problem will be presented. Movement throughout a full ROM is crucial, especially early in the disease process, to prevent changes in the properties of muscle itself. In PD the contractile elements of flexors become shortened and those of the extensor surface become lengthened,[191] enhancing the development of the flexed posture traditionally seen. As with all other neurological diseases, early intervention is always better than late.

Treatment proceeds better if rigidity is decreased. Many relaxation techniques appear to be effective, including gentle, slow rocking, rotation of the extremities and trunk, and the use of yoga (see Chapter 4). With the parkinsonian client success in relaxation may be better achieved in the sitting position because rigidity may increase in the supine position.[9, 10] Further, because the proximal muscles are often more involved than the distal muscles, relaxation may be easier to achieve by following a distal-to-proximal progression. The inverted position may be used with care. Initially, this position facilitates some relaxation (increase in parasympathetic tone) and then increases trunk extension, which is important for the parkinsonian client. Relaxation may also be effective in reducing the tremor of PD.

Once a decrease in rigidity is achieved through relaxation, movement must be initiated. For the client with PD, this movement should be large and through the entire range. As with relaxation techniques it may be easier to start with distal motions first and gradually increase the movement, bringing in proximal and trunk muscles. Sitting is a good position from which to begin, starting perhaps with swinging the arms in ever-increasing amplitude. Because bilateral symmetrical patterns are easier than reciprocal patterns, they should be used first, and then followed by diagonal patterns. To add trunk rotation (which will also help decrease proximal rigidity),[21] proprioceptive neuromuscular facilitation (PNF) patterns and rhythmical initiation may be used.[107] Additionally, neurodevelopmental treatment (NDT) and mobilization techniques may be useful to increase scapular and pelvic mobility. The use of rhythm and auditory cues facilitates movement. Rhythm, especially as in a march, seems to enable the client to move continuously with alternating flexion and extension without becoming fixated. Clapping or music enhances this effect. At present, no explanation can be given for this phenomenon, but perhaps it diminishes cortical initiation and abnormal EMG activity (which was discussed earlier). Movement is thus accomplished in a more automatic, nonfragmented manner. Once the therapist has improved movement, functional activities should be practiced.

Exercise itself is important for the client with PD. There is a relationship between longevity and physical activity.[118] Those who exercised had a lower mortality rate. There is also some evidence to indicate that exercise may alter the generation of free radicals and other compounds linked to aging and to parkinsonism. Immunological function may also be improved with exercise.[190] Sasco and colleagues[190] demonstrated a link between lack of exercise and the development of parkinsonism. Finally, the role of aerobic fitness itself may be a factor in reducing dysfunction.[143, 209] Aerobic exercise may improve pulmonary function in parkinsonian patients because these functions appear to suffer from deficiencies in rapid force generation of the respiratory muscles,[48] similar to limb musculature. Exercise is most beneficial when it is begun early in the disease process and exercise is recommended in all books and pamphlets for the patient.[59] All research on the effects of exercise programs in parkinsonism buttresses this point. Hurwitz[94] found that patients who were still independently mobile at home and in the community benefited the most from a home program. Schenkman and Butler[191] also indicated that patients in the earlier stages of the disease had the best potential for improvement. If patients practice regular physical exercise in conjunction with disease-specific exercises, the ill effects of inactivity will not potentiate the effects of the disease process itself. Although most patients with parkinsonism can achieve an adequate exercise level, many clients have fitness levels that are poor or very poor prior to medical diagnosis.[136] We have found that exercise even once a week is effective in improving gait and balance in clients with PD.[146]

So far all but one study has found that exercise under the guidance of a therapist is effective. There are, however, few studies using random assignment with good controls.[10] A report by Palmer and co-workers[170] utilized precise, quantitative measures to assess motor signs, grip strength, coordination, and speed, as well as measurements of the long latency stretch reflex, following two exercise programs in parkinsonian patients. These two programs were the United Parkinson's Foundation program and karate training. Their results indicated improvement over 12 weeks in gait, grip strength, and coordination of fine motor control tasks but no change in a decline in movements requiring speed. The patients all reported an increase in general well-being. The results of this careful study indicate that more research and careful documentation of exercise programs are needed. A study by Comella and colleagues,[40] as well as one by Patti and colleagues,[174] also found decreases in parkinsonian symptoms with physical and occupational therapy. However, these studies found no long-term carryover of therapy. The authors did not explain the exercise program precisely or give the instructions provided for a home program.

Another study utilized "sports activities" in a twice-weekly program.[185] The program included exercises on land designed to improve gait and balance and exercises in the water to increase strength. These investigators reported significant improvements in the UPDRS, cognitive function, and mood in addition to ADL and motor scores during the 14-week program. Interestingly, they also found decreases in dyskinesia. The greatest changes with exercise appeared early and were maintained up to 6 weeks after cessation of the exercise program. Our program, utilizing dance and other weight-bearing exercise, demonstrated similar improvements in balance, especially in initiation of gait.[146]

Physical activity and movement appear to increase quality of life by decreasing depression, and improving mood and initiative. Group classes can serve as an extra support system for parkinsonian patients and their spouses.[67, 159] Intensive exercise is beneficial in the early stages of the disease.[189] A carefully structured low-impact aerobics program appears to be beneficial to patients, even those with long-standing disease.[146] One program begins with seated activities for the upper extremities (Fig. 22-7A) and then combination movements for warm-up (see Fig. 22-7B). The participants then progress to standing and marching activities that incorporate coordinated movements of arms and legs as well as balance and trunk rotation (Fig. 22-8). All movements are performed to music similar to that used in aerobics classes in any gymnasium or health spa. (The rationale for the use of external cues has been mentioned previously; the role of rhythm in gait training is discussed in subsequent paragraphs.) Heart rate should be monitored periodically. Many PD associations also have audiotapes for exercises (e.g., United Parkinson's Foundation).

Rhythmical exercise has been shown to decrease rigidity and bradykinesia and improve gait over time.[64, 67, 141, 146, 232] Ballroom dancing is a form of rhythmical therapy for parkinsonian patients which incoporates rhythmical movement, rotation, balance, and coordination. The waltz or fox trot is a good beginning dance as it is easy and somewhat slow (Fig. 22-9). Latin dances promote separation of the pelvis from the trunk and also increase coordination. A modified Charleston can be used to increase one-legged balance, as can modified tap-dancing. The use of dance also facilitates changing direction. Some of the group activities and possible exercises are depicted in Figures 22-7 through 22-10. We have found a decrease in the time it takes the client to respond to a go signal and walk 3 feet and continue walking 20 feet. There was a concomitant increase in stride length. Balance improved for those patients who could not stand on foam at the start of the program. We also found that clients with more severe PD (stages 3 and 4) also demonstrated improvement in gait following a 6-week session of group exercise.

The most successful exercise programs appear to be those that incorporate context-dependent responses and a varied environment, which ameliorate many of the dysfunctions associated with parkinsonism.[44, 46, 97, 146, 157, 170, 185] Examples of these activities are presented in the first box on page 679. Aerobic exercises that are not as effective in requiring context-dependent responses are presented in the second box on page 679. Research has shown the importance of adjusting the response to the specific task and has also demonstrated the importance of practice for the parkinsonian patient.[41, 97, 98, 205] The principles of motor

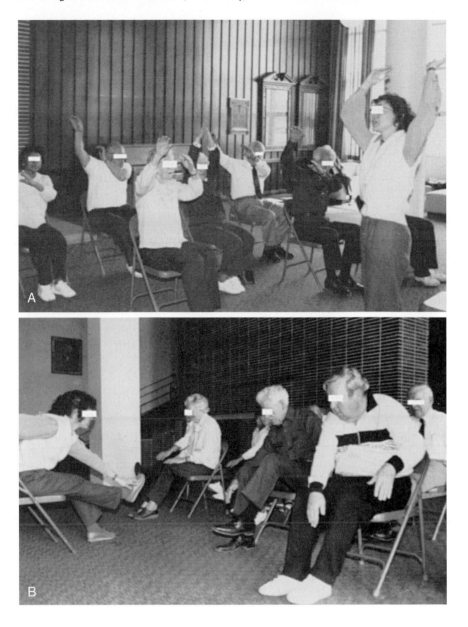

FIGURE 22–7. Seated aerobics or warm-up exercises. *A,* Clients are utilizing bilateral upper extremity patterns to facilitate trunk rotation. Instruction was to let the head follow the hands. *B,* This exercise encourages trunk rotation, large movements, and coordination of the upper and lower extremities. Clients are to reach with the arms and touch the opposite foot. This coordination is very difficult in Parkinson disease, and initially many clients could not move the arms and legs at the same time.

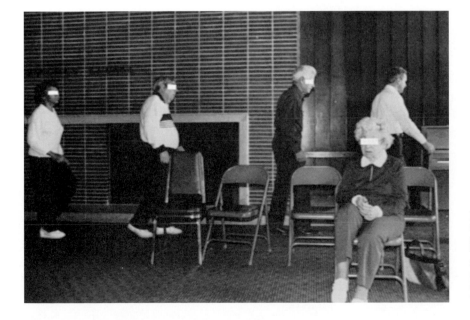

FIGURE 22–8. Initial warm-up in standing. Clients are to walk with the head up, back as straight as possible, and take large steps. When the group began, walking was the major aerobic activity and used to increase endurance and encourage movement. Nonambulatory patients march in place in the chair.

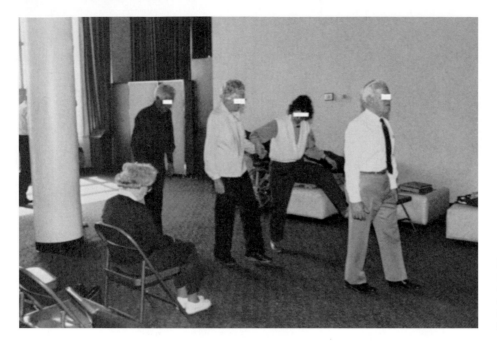

FIGURE 22–9. Walking in a "waltz rhythm" (slow, quick, quick) emphasizes a big step for the slow step. Note lack of automatic arm swing. Also note flexed posture of seated patient during rest period.

learning are of paramount importance in the treatment program of these patients. Random practice may enable the patient to learn the correct schema by which to regulate the extent, speed, and direction of the movement. Random practice also may be important in facilitating the ability of the patient to shift attention and to learn to access "working memory." The parkinsonian patient may benefit from visual instruction and mental rehearsal before performing the movement.[173, 205] Research on sensory systems in PD indicates effectiveness in the use of multisensory cuing.

Strengthening exercises have been advocated for the patient with PD. With disuse there is, of course, decreased strength. Weakness occurs with initial contraction and also with prolonged contraction. Manual muscle testing may not reveal losses in strength; however, most of the successful exercise programs mentioned above did include strength training as part of the program. In reviewing the literature, it seems that functional strength training is more effective than weightlifting.[185] An important part of any strengthening program is the trunk musculature. Spinal extensors need to be exercised and spinal flexibility likewise encouraged.[192]

As the disease progresses, intensive exercise programs may need to be revised or altered. By stage 2.5, gait disorders are the most common impairment for which the person with PD will see a therapist. There are many aspects of gait that are amenable to treatment. The problem that causes the biggest handicap is "freezing" and small steps. Both auditory and visual stimuli have been used in treatment of parkinsonian gait disorders. Thaut and colleagues[216] have demonstrated that use of a metronome or carefully synthesized music will improve stride length and speed and that these improvements remain

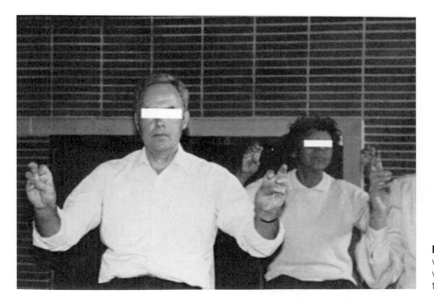

FIGURE 22–10. Cool-down period allows time to work on fine finger movements. Thumb abduction with rounded fingers and various rhythms are used to increase coordination. Note "masked face."

EXAMPLES OF EXERCISE REGIMENS THAT PROMOTE CONTEXT-DEPENDENT RESPONSES

1. Walking outdoors
2. Karate and other martial arts
3. Dancing (all forms)
4. All ball sports
5. Cross-country and downhill skiing
6. Well-structured, low-impact aerobics classes

This list is an example of activities; it should not be considered all-inclusive.

---

up to 5 weeks after cessation of the auditory stimulus. Melnick and co-workers have also demonstrated both immediate and longer-lasting improvements in gait following a rhythmical exercise program once a week in patients needing assistance to walk.[146]

It is well known that people with PD find it easier to climb stairs than to walk on a flat surface. This is because of the visual stimulation provided by the stairs. Visual stimuli have been effective in coping with freezing episodes. These include the use of lines on the floor and stair climbing. Martin[137] found that parallel lines were more facilitating than other lines and that the space between lines was also important; the lines cannot be too close together. The difficulty in the use of visual stimuli is that there is scant evidence of carryover. One client has utilized visual stimuli in special glasses. These glasses provide constant lines for the client to step over. At present these glasses are not commercially available. Dunne and colleagues[58] described a cane that could present a visual cue for the patient who has freezing episodes. I have found it especially useful for patients who fall because of freezing. If a specialized cane is not available, the client can turn his or her own cane upside down. Several of my clients have tried other visual stimuli to help in initiating movement after freezing. One patient tosses pennies ahead of him and steps over them. (He cautions that one should not bend to pick them up as this will again lead to freezing.) Another watches the movement of a person walking beside him, as just the movement of that person's feet will encourage his feet to move. Morris and others[156] have tried to increase carryover of visual stimuli by incorporating them into a program of visualization. Their clients practiced walking with lines until the steps were near normal in size and then the clients were to visualize the lines on the floor as they walked. Their visualization program met with initial success. Providing sensory cues from both auditory and visual cues has, as expected, met with excellent success. Additionally, improvements occurred in ADL. Improvements were seen in postural stability, as well as gait, in a study that added tactile cues to visual and auditory cues.[68, 157]

Gait rehabilitation must include walking in crowds, through doorways, and on different surfaces. Practice in walking slowly and quickly is important, as is walking with differing stride lengths. Although no controlled studies have yet been reported, the principles of motor learning presented in Chapter 4 appear to be very helpful for facilitating carryover of the therapeutic effects in our preliminary studies.

Balance disorder is another problem for which therapy is indicated, especially considering that drug and surgical treatment are ineffective. This problem is one that will eventually affect all persons with PD. If at all possible, the client should be instructed in practicing balance exercises at the early stages of the disease. Equilibrium reactions in all planes of movement and under different control should be encouraged. Rhythmical stabilization may be used if the use of resistance does not lead to an increase in truncal rigidity. The timing of the resistance must be very gradual, allowing the client time to develop force in one set of muscles before increasing resistance, and then switching directions. This alters the context of the environment and allows the client to practice a variety of variations of the original plan. If proper time is not allowed, the therapist may reinforce the already inefficient, ineffective patterns of motor activity. (See Chapter 21 for other procedures to improve balance.)

Rarely will the client with PD state that he or she has difficulty performing two tasks at once. Nonetheless, this becomes quite apparent when the client is asked to perform a very simple activity, such as counting backward and walking at the same time.[22, 156] One solution is to instruct the client to attend to only one task at a time. Another is to have the client practice doing two things at the same time and constantly alter activities in a random practice mode during treatment. Differences in the efficacy of these two approaches have not yet been studied.

Transitional movements pose great problems for the client, especially by stage 3. This is most likely because normal postural adjustments are no longer automatic and they become a sequential task. Practice is helpful with frequent review. Nicholson and associates[164] report improvement in moving from a seated to a standing position after practicing techniques designed to increase forward

---

EXERCISE REGIMENS THAT PROMOTE FITNESS AND INCREASE IN RANGE OF MOTION BUT NO CONTEXT-DEPENDENT RESPONSES

1. Walking on treadmill
2. Stationary bicycle
3. Strengthening machines and free weights (with low weights or low resistance)
4. Step exercises and stair climbers
5. Rowing machines
6. Swimming laps

This list is an example of activities; it should not be considered all-inclusive.

weight shift (e.g., lifting a chair while standing up). Visualization of this task demonstrated carryover. Rolling in bed and rising from the supine position also become difficult and need practice and increased emphasis on trunk rotation.

Bed mobility is another important consideration for parkinsonian patients. A firm bed may make getting in and out of bed easier. Most patients report that satin sheets with silk or satin pajamas make moving in bed far easier. This is true in both the early and later stages of the disease. Teaching the client to roll onto his or her side and lowering the hips off the bed facilitates getting out of bed; the client may not be using this method and so relearning this movement is important. Beds with a head that can be raised electrically may be helpful as the disease progresses, but while sleeping the patient should lower the head as close to horizontal as possible. If getting up from a chair becomes too difficult, chairs with seats that lift up have been used effectively.

Breathing exercises are crucial for the patient with PD. As stated previously, the most common cause of death is pneumonia. Chest expansion may be included in upper extremity activities, for example, incorporated with swinging the arm. The clinician may also have the client shout—especially some kind of rhythmical chant, even a simple "left, right," while walking. With disease progression, specific breathing exercises need to be incorporated. This is crucial for the patient who is no longer able to walk.

In addition to treatment in the therapy department, the parkinsonian client also should be given a home program. The home program should encourage making moderate, consistent exercise a part of the normal day. Periodic checks may enhance compliance. Fatigue should be avoided and the exercise graded to the individual's capability. The therapist should keep in mind that learned skills such as sports are sometimes less affected than automatic movements,[61] perhaps because these skills may rely on cortical involvement.

Fatigue is a frequent complaint of people with PD.[101] Although it has been correlated with disease progression, depression, and sleep disturbances, it also exists in a high percentage of those without depression or sleep difficulty (44% of patients in one study).[65] This fatigue is over and above that associated with the exertion of the exercise program and may be one reason those with PD no longer exercise. The client with PD frequently experiences postexercise fatigue. If the client is tired after exercise and cannot perform normal ADL, exercise will not become a part of his or her daily routine. There is a documented postexercise fatigue that is easily alleviated by extending a cool down period and making certain that the cooldown is gradual.

Patients frequently ask about the timing of medication and exercise. For any form of exercise in parkinsonism to be effective, movement must be possible, especially movement through the full arc of the joint. It seems plausible therefore that exercise should be performed during the "on" period. On the other hand, perhaps there would be a more long-lasting effect if the parkinsonian patient tried to exercise without medication. The question of the effects of exercise on DA agonist absorption were recently investigated by Carter and colleagues.[38] They concluded that the effect was variable from patient to patient; however, the response of each patient was consistent. It should be noted, however, that none of the patients exercised vigorously, which may have skewed the results. Reuter and her colleagues[185] interpreted the decrease in dyskinesia seen following their exercise program as indicative of more efficient DA absorption. Nevertheless, this study supports the concept that the patient needs to be "in tune" with his or her own response and to adjust medications and exercise to a schedule accordingly. Patients appear able to integrate their exercise and medication schedule well.

The therapist is also involved in the prescription of assistive devices. The use of assistive devices in gait for the parkinsonian patient is an area with no clear-cut guidelines. Because coordination of upper and lower extremities is often difficult, the ability to use a cane or walker is often lacking. The patient may drag the cane or carry the walker. Walkers with wheels sometimes increase the festinating gait, and the patient may fall over the walker. Nonetheless, four-wheel walkers with pushdown brakes appear to work best for many clients. For patients with a tendency to fall backward, a reverse walker may be helpful. Therefore, the reason for using the assistive device must be carefully assessed. Walkers or canes can be helpful for the person with postural instability and the ability to walk with a heel-toe gait. The height of the walker or cane should be adjusted carefully to promote extension and avoid an increase in trunk flexion. A survey by Mutch and colleagues[159] in Ireland found that nearly half of the patients responding used some type of assistive device. These devices included devices for walking and for reaching, and ADL. Parkinsonian patients may also benefit from assistive devices for eating or writing. For a few patients small cuff weights may decrease tremor when walking; however, for many patients cuff weights only exacerbate the tremor.

As PD progresses the patient may experience difficulty in swallowing and even in chewing. Therapy for oral motor control should be initiated, and a dietitian consult may be necessary to ensure adequate nutrition. A dietitian may also be beneficial in guiding the patient's protein intake. A high-protein diet may reduce the responsiveness of the patient to DA replacement therapy. Regulating the amount and timing of protein ingestion can improve the efficacy of drug treatment in some patients.

The resurgence of surgery as a treatment alternative in PD means that the therapist will face new and exciting challenges in treatment. Following a lesion, stimulation of deep brain sites, or fetal transplantation, the brain may have increased plasticity. Many researchers have shown that fetal cells do survive and connect to target cells. However, whether functional connections occur without motor learning interventions has not been proved conclusively. Intense physical therapy, especially incorporating complex motor skills, has been demonstrated to be effective in improving function following a lesion in animal studies.[98] Therefore, intense physical therapy following surgery may be necessary to maximize benefits from all surgeries in PD (and in HD and the dystonias). (See the discussion in Graybiel[74] for further justification.)

Finally, PD is a progressive, degenerative disease. Therapy and exercise may modify the progression but cannot halt or reverse it. Quality of life throughout the course of the disease may be enhanced, however, and the therapist can assist the client and family in coping with the constraints of this disease. As stated in one study of PD, the total cost of treatment must also include the cost to the spouse or other family members. (See Case 22–1 and Case 22–2 on page 682.)

There are several other disorders that are lumped together as the Parkinson-plus syndrome. Clients with these disorders usually do not respond to levodopa. The most common of these is progressive supranuclear palsy. These clients can be evaluated and treated in a manner similar to the client with PD. However, there is usually more cognitive impairment and the progression is more rapid. These syndromes are rarer than PD and far more variable, and there have been no studies of treatment efficacy.

Huntington's Disease

Huntington's disease (formerly Huntington's chorea) is another degenerative disease of the basal ganglia. It is the classic disorder representing hyperactivity in the basal ganglia circuitry. This disease gets its name from George Huntington, who first described it in 1872. HD is inherited as an autosomal dominant trait and affects approximately 6.5 per 100,000 people.[61] The defect is on the short arm of chromosome 4.[79] The altered genetic material has an increase in the CAG sequence; in normal people there are 11 to 34 CAG triple repeats, but in the person with HD there are 37 to 86 repeats.[56] The CAG repeat is related to glutamine. The target protein affected by the polyglutamine expansion has been named huntingtin. The length of the expansion is correlated with an earlier age of disease onset. Huntingtin combines with ubiquitin and induces intranuclear inclusions and interference with mitochondrial function. There is severe loss of the medium spiny neurons and preservation of the ACh aspiny neurons.[56] There are decreases in choline acetyltransferase (CAT), and ACh, as well as in the number of muscarinic ACh receptors, glutamic acid decarboxylase (GAD), and substance P. There is usually no de-

---

CASE 22–1   Mrs. T

Mrs. T is a 55-year-old woman who was diagnosed with PD 1 year ago. The disease began in her left arm and leg when she noticed increasing stiffness and difficulty moving. She complains of some instability in walking and recently has developed a slight resting tremor in the left hand. On initial evaluation she had full active and passive ROM in all extremities, neck, and trunk. There is a mild resting tremor present in the left hand. There is mild cogwheel rigidity in the left upper and lower extremity; there is some intermittent resistance to passive movement in the right upper extremity as well. Strength is grossly within normal limits throughout. Sensation is intact throughout. Equilibrium reactions are delayed, but the patient demonstrates an ankle strategy on a flat surface and a hip strategy when standing on the balance beam; there is no mixing of the synergies and her balance responses are appropriate to the degree of displacement.

The patient is able to stand in the sharpened Romberg position for 30 seconds with the eyes open and 20 seconds with the eyes closed. She can stand on the right leg for 30 seconds with the eyes open and 15 seconds with the eyes closed; she can stand on the left leg for 15 seconds with the eyes open and 10 seconds with the eyes closed. When walking, she has a heel-toe sequence, shortened stride length, and normal stride width. There is no arm swing on the left and a diminished arm swing on the right. There is no trunk rotation and very slight trunk flexion throughout the gait cycle. Speed is within normal limits for a 25-foot walk. The patient is able to turn freely. She has recently begun to suffer from a foot dystonia, which is worse with fatigue. It has interfered with her daily walking program and

her tennis, an activity she enjoys with her husband twice a week. Her only medication is deprenyl.

This patient is in Hoehn and Yahr stage I, with some beginning of bilateral symptoms and progression to stage II. She is young, employed full-time, and has been involved in regular exercise for the past 10 years. Her complaints are stiffness, slowed movements, and foot dystonia. Because her symptoms are mild at present and she has good balance in standing and walking, this patient should be encouraged to continue exercising regularly. She should try to continue playing tennis, as this requires complex, sequential, context-dependent movements. Although tennis involves motor responses to external cues, it does necessitate rapid force generation and anticipatory movements. This should encourage continued motor learning. Additionally, she should be encouraged to continue walking outdoors and practice alternating the speed of walking. The dystonia is more difficult to resolve. It may be tied to medication and differing medication schemes are being tried. She is also on a program of stretching and strengthening of the ankle, as well as a sensory stimulation program for the feet. Foam between the toes has helped to decrease dystonia early in the day.

Mrs. T has also been informed about the importance of maintaining chest expansion and monitoring her breathing. This will be important as the disease progresses. She attends a support group for young parkinsonian patients to increase her awareness of the disease and of new treatments. As the disease progresses, she will need a home program appropriate for her symptoms. The home program will be reassessed every 3 to 6 months.

CASE 22–2 ● Mr. R

Mr. R is a 68-year-old man with a 7-year history of PD. He now falls two or three times a day, has difficulty eating, and has noticed weakness in his right hand. He would like to return to full activity, including golf twice a week, swimming, and skiing. On evaluation he has moderate rigidity in all extremities; the right side is worse than the left. It is most marked in the right wrist, forearm, and hand. Shoulder flexion and abduction lack 15 degrees bilaterally. He has a 15-degree knee flexion contracture on the right; all other joints in the lower extremity have range within functional limits. Strength is grossly 4 to 4|m+ throughout, including grip strength. Sensation is within normal limits throughout. Static and dynamic sitting balance is good.

The patient sits with a posterior pelvic tilt, rounded shoulders, and flexed neck. On rising to a standing position, he does move forward in the chair, which positions his feet under his knees. He does not lean forward as he stands. He momentarily loses his balance upon rising from a chair. Static standing balance is fair; dynamic balance is fair. When pushed on the sternum, he takes one to two steps backward, even to a gentle push. When pushed from behind he takes several steps forward. He lost his balance and required assistance when trying to catch a large ball thrown to the side. His gait pattern is typical of a parkinsonian patient. There is a shortened step and a flatfooted foot contact. He complains of festination and of freezing, but neither were observed during the evaluation. He turns 'en bloc.' There is no arm swing and no trunk rotation. He walks slowly and was unable to increase his speed measurably in a 25-foot walk. He is taking levodopa with carbidopa and deprenyl. He tried another D2 agonist but experienced hallucinations. He was able to ski until last winter. At that time, he found that he could not stand up once he fell down, and sometimes he fell without realizing that he was falling. He stated that he "did not think it was safe to ski." He also no longer swims because he has difficulty breathing in the pool and coordinating his breathing with his strokes. He does not play golf because it takes him too long.

This patient needs to be encouraged to continue to exercise and to socialize while exercising. He has been encouraged to resume golf at times when the course is less crowded. Additionally, he has been given a home program consisting of activities performed in the seated and standing positions, which encourage trunk rotation and large movements and are coordinated with good breathing practices. He has been given some balance exercises that challenge his equilibrium in a safe environment. His home program is being monitored every 3 months because of the distance he must travel to come to the clinic. His wife was instructed to exercise with him and to exercise to music. He was referred to the speech pathologist for a swallowing evaluation and was given a joint program for speech and breathing. He is able to play golf once a week; he is not yet ready to resume swimming or skiing.

---

crease in DA, norepinephrine, or serotonin (5-HT), although more recent studies with single-photon emission computed tomography (SPECT) indicate that DA does diminish significantly in the later stages of the disease.[123]

HD is usually manifested after the age of 30 years, although childhood forms appear rarely. Death from this disease occurs about 15 years after the onset of symptoms. A marker for the HD gene has been localized.[79] If the family pedigree is known and the chromosomes of the parents can be obtained, it is now possible to detect presymptomatically which offspring have the faulty chromosome. As one might expect there are ethical and practical issues related to early detection of this disease. At present, although testing is available, it is not widely used. Further, testing for HD is typically only available to those over the age of 18. Despite these problems, localization of the gene and the repeat is promising and offers hope for improved means of treatment.

Symptoms

Some of the signs and symptoms of HD are similar to those of PD: abnormalities in postural reactions, trunk rotation, distribution of tone, and extraneous movements. Persons with HD, however, are at the other end of the spectrum; rather than a paucity of movement, they exhibit too much movement, which is evident in the trunk and face in addition to the extremities. The gait takes on an ataxic, dancing appearance (Gr. *choreia*, a choral dance), and fine movements become clumsy and slowed. As with the person with parkinsonism there is a decrease in associated movements (e.g., arm swing). The extraneous movements are of the choreoathetoid type, that is involuntary, irregular isolated movements that may be jerky and arrhythmical, as in chorea, to rhythmical and wormlike, as in athetosis. Usually, however, these occur in successive movements so that the entire picture is one of complex movement patterns. It is as if the "movement generator" aspects of the basal ganglia are continuously active, as would fit the hypothesis of a disruption in the indirect pathway. As the disease progresses, the choreiform movements may give way to akinesia and rigidity.

Gait patterns of the person with HD are in some ways similar to those of PD. Gait velocity and stride length are decreased. The decrease in velocity is correlated with progression. Unlike the person with PD, however, the person with HD has a decreased cadence as well.[108] There is an increase in the base of support (again unlike the pattern seen in PD). In addition, there is an increase in lateral sway along with great variability in distal movements.[186]

There are disruptions in movement of the person with HD that reflect the role of the basal ganglia in movement. For example, the person with HD, like the person with PD, has difficulty responding to internal cues.[70] Kinematic analysis of upper extremity complex tasks demonstrates that the person with HD must rely on visual guidance in the termination of a movement. This has been interpreted to indicate impairment in the development and fine-tuning of an internal representation of the task.[70] These clients have increasing difficulty with more complex movements in the absence of advanced cues.[69] The lack of internal cuing in the person with HD has been linked to the increased variability of response seen in these clients.[178]

In addition to the involvement of the motor systems, the client with HD also shows signs of dementia and emotional disorders that become worse as the disease progresses. The client may show lack of judgment and loss of memory, deterioration in speech and writing (i.e., severe decrease in ability to communicate), depression, hostility, and feelings of incompetence. There is a decrease in IQ, with performance measures decreasing more rapidly than verbal levels. There is also evidence of ideomotor apraxia, especially as the disease progresses.[197] Suicide is fairly common.

The movement disorders of HD are presumed to be related to degeneration of the striatal neurons, specifically the enkephalinergic neurons.[61] The dementia is associated with cortical destruction.[204]

The exact mechanisms producing choreoathetoid movements are unknown. Because these extraneous movements are part of a person's normal repertoire of movement patterns, it is possible that they are "released" at inappropriate times and without any modulation. A postmortem examination showed a decrease in GABA which was greater in the globus pallidus external segment than the globus pallidus internal segment.[207] This agrees with the previously described current model.[2] Recent use of positron emission tomography (PET) scans demonstrates loss of ACh and GABA neurons. A pattern, therefore, may be released before it is necessary, and inappropriate portions of the pattern cannot be inhibited. Petajan and colleagues[177] also found motor unit activity indicative of bradykinesia. Recordings of single motor units in the muscles indicate that persons with HD have a loss of control evidenced by an inability to recruit single motor units.[177] As the efforts at control increased, these individuals demonstrated an overflow of motor unit activity that resulted in full choreiform movements. Those in the earlier stages of the disease demonstrated what the experimenters termed "microchorea," small ballistic activations of motor units.[177] As in PD, difficulty occurs in modulating motor neuron excitability. Another finding in this experiment revealed motor unit activity indicative of bradykinesia. Yanagasawa[233] used surface EMG recordings to classify involuntary muscle contractions in HD patients with varying movement disorders, ranging from chorea to rigidity. He found brief, reciprocal, irregular contractions in those patients with classic chorea and tonic nonreciprocal

contractions in those patients with rigidity. The presence of athetosis or dystonia was associated with slow, reciprocal contractions. During sustained contractions, EMG activity demonstrated brief, irregular cessation of activity in the choreic patients. Thus patients with HD have interruption of normal motor function at rest and during sustained activity (e.g., stabilizing contractions).

The abnormal postural reactions of the person with HD may occur from a misinterpretation of sensory input, especially vestibular and proprioceptive (similar to the parkinsonian syndrome). However, the dementia of HD precludes further testing. Although it appears as if the thalamus also plays a role in the movement disorders of HD, the specifics are unknown at present.[51, 177]

Weight loss is also a common problem for persons with HD. A study by Pratley and co-workers[183] found that sedentary energy expenditure was higher in the patient population than in age-and sex-matched controls; however, the sleeping metabolic rate was not different from the controls. They also found that the HD group was less active than the control group. The increase in energy expenditure was related to the severity of the disease.

Stages of the Disease

HD is a progressive disorder. The initial symptoms are most often complaints of incoordination, clumsiness, or jerkiness. A classic test for eliciting choreiform movements in this early stage is a simple grip test. The client grips the examiner's hand and maintains that grip for a few seconds. The person with HD will display what is called the "milkmaid's sign"; there will be alternating increases and decreases in the grip, perhaps the equivalent of the EMG abnormalities seen during sustained contractions. Facial grimacing or the inability to perform complex facial movements also may be present very early.

In many cases the dementia and psychological symptoms of HD occur after the onset of the neurological signs. In cases in which very subtle personality changes occur first, the diagnosis may be more difficult. Such persons may appear forgetful or unable to manage appointments and financial affairs. They may be thought to have early senility, or they may show signs of severe depression or schizophrenia. Early diagnosis may be important, and SPECT shows promise for early detection of the disease.[80]

With time, the combination of psychological and neurological problems causes the individual to lose all ability to work and perform ADL. This person eventually can be cared for only in an extended care facility. By this time the choreiform movements have given way to rigidity, and the patient is bedridden. Figure 22–11 shows the stages of HD according to Shoulson and Fahn.[198]

Pharmacological Considerations and Medical Management

The great advances in pharmacological management of PD have led to a great deal of research to find appropriate drugs for the management of HD. At present, however, there is no fully effective medication for this disease.

The symptoms of HD indicate an increase in dopamin-

	Engagement in occupation		Capacity to handle financial affairs		Capacity to manage domestic responsibility		Capacity to perform activities of daily living		Care can be provided at	
		Score		Score		Score		Score		Score
Stage 1	Usual level	3	Full	3	Full	2	Full	3	Home	2
Stage 2	Lower level	2	Requires slight help	2	Full	2	Full	3	Home	2
Stage 3	Marginal	1	Requires major help	1	Impaired	1	Mildly impaired	2	Home	2
Stage 4	Unable	0	Unable	0	Unable	0	Moderately impaired	1	Home or extended care facility	1
Stage 5	Unable	0	Unable	0	Unable	0	Severely impaired	0	Total care facility only	0

From Shoulson and Fahn (1979).

FIGURE 22–11. Functional stages of Huntington's disease. (From Shoulson I, Fahn S: Huntington's disease: Clinical care and evaluation. Neurology 29:2, 1979.)

ergic effect. At autopsy there is a decrease in the number of intrinsic neurons of the striatum that contain the neurotransmitter GABA or ACh. Biochemical studies reveal a definite decrease in GABA concentration in addition to a decrease in ACh concentration in the basal ganglia. Therefore drug therapy depends on those drugs that are cholinergic or GABA-containing agonists and those that act as DA antagonists. To date the DA antagonists have been more effective in ameliorating neurological symptoms; however, these drugs have severe side effects, including PD and tardive dyskinesia.

In general, pharmacological treatment is not started until the choreiform movements interfere with function[200] because these drugs have side effects that may be worse than the chorea (see Tardive Dyskinesia). Perphenazine, haloperidol, and reserpine are still the most commonly used medications. The first two block the DA receptors themselves; reserpine depletes DA stores in the brain. Side effects include depression, drowsiness, a parkinsonian type of syndrome, or sometimes dyskinesia. Drugs such as choline, which would increase ACh concentrations, have produced only transient improvement.[198] There have been many efforts to find a GABA agonist that would reduce the symptoms of HD, but these have so far been unsuccessful.[18, 200] The problem with finding a medication to increase GABA is that such a drug will probably cause inhibition throughout the brain, not just in the basal ganglia. Thus the individual's level of alertness and ability to function might be reduced—something a person with HD can ill afford.[18] New medications are currently in clinical trials and include neurotrophic factors.[14]

Because management of the dementia and personality problems is not satisfactory with any present drug therapy, it becomes more difficult than the choreiform problem. Cortical degeneration is most certainly involved, but disruption of the heavy corticostriate projections also may be a factor in progression of this disease. Although alterations in DA have been implicated in psychotic problems such as schizophrenia, the role of the basal ganglia in thought processes is, at best, little understood.

At present the best hope for the person with HD lies in a better understanding of the genetic mechanisms causing destruction of the GABA-containing cells in the striatum, and cortical destruction. In the meantime correct and early diagnosis is important in providing the proper early intervention, which must include counseling.[105] The Commission for the Control of Huntington's Disease has set up several research centers, including a brain and tissue bank, in an effort to facilitate research into the causes of the disease.

Transplantation is also in clinical trials in HD. As with PD, the tissue does survive, but the results are even more preliminary than for the person with parkinsonism.

Examination

The standard medical evaluation is the United Huntington's Disease Rating Scale (UHDRS). This is a comprehensive evaluation that examines cognitive function as well as motor function. The physical or occupational therapy evaluation of a person with HD must assess the degree of functional ability and how the chorea interferes with function. Which extremities, including the face, are involved? Does the client have any cortical control of the chorea or any means of allaying extraneous movements? What exacerbates the symptoms? What lessens them? A simple rating scale is the capacity to perform ADL (see Fig. 22–11). A standard ADL form with space to write in how the client performs these activities or why she or he cannot perform them would be helpful.

Gait analysis can include a timed walk and cadence; stride length can then be calculated. A subjective assessment of variability and incoordination should also be made. Additionally, posture and equilibrium reactions should be tested. What associated reactions, if any, are present? In assessing posture, care should be taken to observe the posture of the extremities in addition to those of the trunk, head, and neck. Dystonic posturing should be carefully noted, especially if the client is taking medication. Any changes should be reported to the physician. A gross assessment of strength should be made with particular attention paid to the ability to stabilize the trunk and proximal joints. To reduce the effects of rigidity, ROM exercises become important as the disease progresses.

In the assessment of the client with HD, the stage of psychological involvement and mental state must be reliably assessed both during evaluation and treatment. SPECT and other computed tomography scans may give some clues to the amount of cortical and basal ganglia degeneration, which can assist in determining possible cortical functioning.

General Treatment Goals and Rationale

Maintaining an optimal quality of life is the most important goal for treatment of persons with HD and their families. This includes maintenance of functional skills and advice to the family on adaptive equipment. Techniques that reduce tone may also reduce choreiform movements. Increasing stability about the shoulders, trunk, neck, and hips will help maintain function. Again, it must be repeated that the evaluation results will dictate treatment procedures.

Treatment Procedures

The Commission for the Control of Huntington's Disease[199] has stated that these clients are underserved by physical and occupational therapy. Peacock[175] surveyed physical therapists in one state. Of the 585 therapists who responded, only 15.5% had worked with at least one patient with HD; 6.2% had worked with more than one patient, thus confirming the underutilization of physical and occupational therapy today. Hayden[82] and Peacock[175] have suggested that therapy can improve the quality of life. Yet there are few articles on treatment procedures. Theories as to which techniques may prove most beneficial are offered here with the warning that to date none have documented efficacy. (See also Chapter 4 for specific treatment techniques.)

The treatment of HD has some parallels with the treatment of cerebral palsy athetosis. These techniques, however, must be adapted to the adult. Of critical importance are the techniques for improving co-activation and trunk stability. The use of the pivot-prone and withdrawal patterns of Rood is helpful, and their benefit may be increased with the use of Theraband. Neck co-contraction and trunk stability may improve or at least maintain oral functions. Additionally, the techniques of rhythmical stabilization in all positions, as well as the heavy work patterns of Rood, should be helpful.[107] Yet movements practiced out of context may not carry over into functional activities; thus the practice of co-activation in functional patterns during treatment is recommended, if at all possible.

Relaxation aids in reduction of extraneous movements. In the early stages methods that require active participation of the client, such as biofeedback and traditional relaxation exercises, may be included. As dementia becomes more apparent, more passive techniques such as slow rocking and neutral warmth must be used. These techniques are also helpful in reducing the choreiform movements of the mouth and tongue, which may prove useful for the dentist and those responsible for proper nutrition of the client. In most cases of HD, the individual is quite thin (almost emaciated) and begins to age rapidly as the disease progresses. The extraneous movements, especially as they become more severe, increase metabolic demands, and nutrition therefore becomes increasingly important. Attention therefore must be paid to head, neck, and oral motor control. Increased pressure on the lips may aid in lip closure and facilitate swallowing. Special straws with a mouthpiece similar to a pacifier may be useful. A dietitian should be consulted for assistance in teaching the family how to prepare balanced and appetizing meals and snacks that are easy to swallow.

The degree of dementia influences treatment. Conscious efforts to control extraneous movements become more difficult as cognitive function decreases. Further, new memories and new patterns of movements become difficult to establish. The therapist therefore must use techniques that require subcortical control and keep in mind that the client can sometimes remember old, normal patterns of movement.

Peacock's study[175] suggested that group programs, including strength, flexibility, balance, coordination, and breathing exercises, may be successful, especially in the early stages of the disease. No amount of physical or occupational therapy, however, can prevent neuronal cell loss. Because HD is a progressive, degenerative disease, the client will get worse. Eventually, goals must be aimed at preventing total immobility, assisting caretakers in transfer techniques and advising them in the use of adaptive equipment. One aspect of treatment that cannot be measured but is important in my view is the degree of hope offered just by the fact that a health professional is providing ongoing care. This may lessen the client's degree of despair and depression and may help maintain the quality of life.

The gait disorder of HD has been shown to respond to rhythmical auditory stimuli.[217] The ability to respond decreased in those most severely involved, indicating that treatment in the later stages of the disease may not be amenable to rhythmical stimuli. Another finding was that cadence was a larger problem than stride length, especially at normal and fast speeds (compare this to the findings in PD). Interestingly, persons with HD were able to modulate gait to a metronome but had more difficulty with musical cues, even when the tempos were identical. Nevertheless, the subjects demonstrated short-term carryover of metronome auditory stimuli to gait without auditory stimuli. Although the long-term carryover was not studied, using a metronome in gait training may be helpful in clients with HD.

Wilson's Disease

Wilson's disease is a disease caused by faulty copper metabolism. The toxic effects of copper lead to degeneration of the liver and the basal ganglia, hence the noneponymous name, hepatolenticular degeneration. Wilson's disease, inherited as an autosomal recessive trait, affects a very small percentage of the population.

In Wilson's disease there is an increase in the amount of copper absorbed from the intestinal tract, a subsequent elevation in the amount of copper in the blood serum, and an increase in the amount of copper deposited in tissue.[224] There is a concomitant reduction in ceruloplasmin. The increase in tissue copper may interfere with various enzyme systems of particular cells. The connection of copper with DA metabolism may account for the basal ganglia involvement.

Neuronal degeneration is present in the globus pallidus and putamen and to a lesser extent in the caudate nucleus. There also may be atrophy in the gray matter of the cortex and the dentate nucleus of the cerebellum.

Symptoms

The deposition of excess copper in the cornea results in the classic diagnostic sign of Wilson's disease, the Kayser-Fleischer ring—a brownish-green or brownish-red ring found in the sclerocorneal junction.

Based on the constellation of signs and symptoms, there are several forms of Wilson's disease. One type entails only liver involvement and no neurological signs. A dystonic form is most common in those with an onset of the disease after the age of 20 years. The individual shows the same abnormal positioning of the limbs and trunk that characterizes the dystonia, rigidity, and bradykinesia seen in PD. Associated reactions and facial expressions are absent. There is a festinating gait and flexed posture. There may be a tremor of the hand, head, and body. If the onset of the disease occurs before age 20, choreoathetoid movements of the face and upper extremities are usually present. The gait resembles that of the individual with HD. This early-onset form is accompanied by very rapid deterioration.

Common to all forms of Wilson's disease that involve brain structures is difficulty in speaking and swallowing, incoordination, and personality changes. The personality changes are the first signs of the disease, especially emotional lability and impaired judgement. If the disease progresses, there is increased dementia, increased cirrhosis of the liver, and progressive decrease in motor function.

The term *dystonia* is used for involuntary movements with a sustained contraction at the end of the movement.[61] Usually these movements involve a twisting of the extremity. If the contraction at the end of the movement is prolonged, the term *dystonic posture* is used. A very peculiar aspect of dystonia is that it can be decreased with proprioceptive or tactile input.[61] Dystonia is usually seen with widespread involvement of the basal ganglia and intralaminar nuclei of the thalamus. The cerebellum also may be involved.[42] Dystonia, like bradykinesia and choreoathetosis, belongs on the continuum of extraneous movements present with basal ganglia involvement. The movement patterns are total and involve rotation of the limb. As in the other diseases of the basal ganglia discussed so far, there is also a decrease in the normal associated movements. As Wilson's disease progresses, the classic abnormal posture of increased flexion occurs, along with rigidity and, if severe enough, total inability to move. As with other diseases of the basal ganglia, there appears to be an imbalance or abnormal response in neurotransmitters; however, the precise imbalance is not yet known.

Stages of the Disease

The first symptom of Wilson's disease is usually a change in the individual's personality. When this becomes severe enough or when the movement disorder appears, a diagnosis can be made by the presence of the Kayser-Fleischer ring or by an analysis of copper metabolism. Because Wilson's disease is now treatable by chemical means, the full progression of this disease is usually not seen. If left untreated, the dystonia becomes worse and the person becomes more rigid. Additionally, muscle weakness can occur and progress, seizures may develop, and the dementia and personality disorder become worse.

Medical Management

Wilson's disease is usually one of the first diseases to be ruled out when a patient presents with movement disorders and behavioral problems, especially in the younger patient. Because the signs and symptoms of Wilson's disease are caused by an increased absorption of copper, treatment consists of drugs that will inhibit this absorption. Concomitantly, copper intake in the diet should be restricted. Penicillamine is the drug of choice, usually in combination with vitamin B_6.[61] There are some side effects of penicillamine, but these appear to be infrequent. If the copper imbalance is treated, the neurological signs do not progress.

Examination and Treatment Intervention

Because Wilson's disease is fully treatable and can be diagnosed early, it is possible that it will not concern the therapist. If the client is referred for therapy, treatment techniques should be wholly based on symptomatology.

Examination is similar to that of the parkinsonian or HD client. It consists of describing the type of extraneous movement present, when it is present, and factors that influence the degree of dystonia. Ease of movement also should be assessed, and it may be timed as for the parkinsonian client. Additionally, ROM and strength should be evaluated, especially if the disease is progressing.

Treatment will then be designed to alleviate the problems. Extraneous movements may be reduced by any technique that reduces tone. Positioning is important. If bradykinesia is the major sign, then treatment would be similar to that used in PD; if trunk stability is poor, the therapist proceeds as in HD. The client with Wilson's disease has knowledge of what normal movement feels like and usually has good cognitive abilities at the time treatment is started. Because of the emotional liability, which is one of the first symptoms in this disease, the treatment session should be well planned and quite structured.

Tardive Dyskinesia

Tardive dyskinesia is a drug-induced disorder and thus will be used to indicate the problems that can arise from drug intoxication. In particular, this section concentrates on the problems associated with drugs that affect DA metabolism, including amphetamine, haloperidol, and classes of drugs used in the treatment of psychotic disorders: the phenothiazines, butyrophenones, and thioxanthenes. As the use and misuse of drugs becomes more common, these types of disorders may become more frequent. (See Chapter 32 for additional information.)

The use of phenothiazines (one of the neuroleptics) has become a very effective and common treatment for schizophrenia. This treatment protocol has enabled many persons with schizophrenia to leave the mental institution. These drugs are DA antagonists and thus decrease the amount of DA in the brain. The exact site of the brain involved in schizophrenia itself is not within the scope of this chapter, but the neurological signs that occur will be discussed. As might be expected, they involve structures within the basal ganglia. Tardive dyskinesia is a gradual disease that occurs after long-term drug treatment. The most typical involvement is of the mouth, tongue, and muscles of mastication; therefore tardive dyskinesia may be called orofacial or buccolingual masticatory (BLM) dyskinesia.

Symptoms

Dyskinesia is defined as an inability to perform voluntary movements.[105] In practical terms, however, dyskinesia is usually a series of rhythmical extraneous movements. In tardive dyskinesia this typically begins with, or may be confined to, the region of the face. These extraneous movements may include choreoathetoid or dystonic movements. Because of abnormality in basal ganglia function, there are also accompanying abnormalities in postural tone and postural adjustments. Instead of the typical flexed posture of PD, clients with tardive dyskinesia show extension of the trunk with increased lordosis and neck flexion.[133] This description of the disease is rather broad, but the problems of drug-induced movement disorders are varied. They may take the form of drug-induced PD or dystonia. In tardive dyskinesia, akinesia and rigidity similar to that seen in parkinsonism may exist simultaneously with the choreoathetoid movements. The key factor in tardive dyskinesia is its slow onset after the ingestion of neuroleptic medications.

Etiology

Although many people take neuroleptic drugs, only a small percentage acquire tardive dyskinesia. Many factors may predispose an individual to movement disorders. One of these is age.[202] This might be expected because of the influence of aging processes on the concentration of DA. Sex may also be a factor. Women are more at risk for tardive dyskinesia.[133] The fact that sex can affect DA levels is supported in studies of animals with brain lesions. In one study, female rats had a lower concentration of DA after early brain lesion than did their male littermates.[196] The absolute amount of neuroleptic ingested may also be a factor, but to date definitive studies have not been completed. So far it appears that the length of time the individual takes medication is not a strong predisposing factor. As the biological abnormalities of schizophrenia become better understood, further understanding of the causes of tardive dyskinesia may be elucidated. It is hypothesized that the development of tardive dyskinesia is caused by supersensitivity.[8, 105] With the use of drugs that deplete the brain of DA, the brain becomes more sensitive to DA. And, in fact, in humans, withdrawal of neuroleptics tends to exacerbate the disease; essentially, withdrawal of the DA antagonist means that far more DA is able to act on these already sensitive terminals.[8, 31, 105]

Because of the effectiveness of long-term treatment for schizophrenia provided by neuroleptics, research into the underlying cause and therefore treatment of the major side effect of tardive dyskinesia, the motor disorders, has greatly increased. But as with PD and HD, animal models are difficult to produce. For one thing, the normal function of the basal ganglia in movement is obscure. However, experimental evidence indicates that the basal ganglia are involved in movements about the face, especially the mouth, and buccolingual dyskinesia is the most frequently encountered symptom in tardive dyskinesia.[129, 193] Lidsky and colleagues[130] hypothesized that sensory input about the face was involved in the high number of globus pallidus units responsive to licking. Further experiments showed that basal ganglia stimulation could alter the threshold of mouth reflexes.[119] The response of basal ganglia neurons to sensory input shows increasing localization of response with age; the region about the mouth becomes increasingly sensitive.[193] Further research along these lines, both in normal animals and those with lesions, may answer the question of what is happening at a neuronal level. This would facilitate drug and physical therapy intervention.

Pharmacological and Medical Management

One serious problem of tardive dyskinesia is that it is often irreversible. The withdrawal of medication, in fact, may increase the movement disorders. Or it may be that recovery takes even more time than the time required for the onset of the disease. It is a strange fact that sometimes the drug that caused the disease may be the drug that reduces the symptoms; that is, increasing the dose may lessen the movement disorder. This might be expected if supersensitivity to DA is involved. But again, with time the increased dose will also cause a reappearance of the symptoms.

The use of other drugs in conjunction with the neuroleptics has been tried in various animal models of the disease. As might be expected, anticholinergic drugs (which would worsen an imbalance between DA and ACh) worsen the dyskinesia. Lithium has been successful in one animal model of dyskinesia.[105] Some neuroleptic drugs seem to have less effect on movement than others; however, the side effects of one such drug, chlorpromazine, are life-threatening. More research is needed into both the mechanisms of schizophrenia and the mechanisms for the production of the abnormal movements.

Evaluation and Treatment Intervention

The effectiveness of therapy intervention in drug-induced dyskinesia is, as yet, not completely known. However, because the neuroleptics do provide an effective long-term treatment of schizophrenia, therapists need to become aware of the problem and offer some assistance.[104] Early drug holidays (time without use of drugs) may be of value in the treatment of tardive dyskinesia, and therefore early awareness of incipient changes in motor function may be of value. Assessment of patients receiving drug therapy could perhaps begin before treatment and then at prescribed intervals. The knowledge that postural adjustments are abnormal in most basal ganglia diseases means that analysis of posture, statically and in motion, might provide early clues to the development of movement disorders. The same would be true for equilibrium reactions and changes in tone with changes in position. Once movement disorders appear, an assessment of when and where the extraneous movements occur is important. (See Chapter 21 for tests of balance.)

General treatment is similar to that used in HD; oral treatment corresponds to that for the athetotic child with cerebral palsy. If hyperreactivity to sensory stimulus exists, then oral desensitization may be of value.

Ameliorating the oral grimacing, of course, would be helpful for the schizophrenic person who is trying to return to society. The effectiveness of physical and occupational therapy cannot be assessed until therapists become involved with these clients and record their results. In cases in which the parkinsonian-like symptoms are stronger than the dyskinetic movements, treatment would follow the plan for the client with PD.

Other Considerations

Other drugs besides neuroleptics may also produce movement disorders. Amphetamine, for example, has been shown to cause long-term changes in brain function, even with very small doses.[127, 128, 222] Adults who were hyperactive children sometimes show a decrease in the readiness potential.[23] Further research is under way to determine the role that medications such as methylphenidate (Ritalin), used in treating hyperactive children, might play in causing movement disorders. The problem of drug-induced movement disorders may become an ever-increasing one for the therapist.

In 1982 several young people were treated for rigidity and "catatonia" after the use of what they thought was heroin. Careful examination of these patients revealed that they had parkinsonian-like symptoms.[47, 121] The chemical responsible for the symptomatology was MPTP, a meperidine analog that was an impurity in the designer heroin. This discovery has enabled research in animals and clinical studies in humans. Although there are some differences among idiopathic Parkinson's disease, MPTP-induced Parkinson's disease, and MPTP-induced parkinsonism, there are important similarities: MPTP selectively damages DA cells in the substantia nigra, levodopa is effective in alleviating the symptoms, and the symptoms seen are irreversible and progressive. In animal studies, age does affect the degree of damage,[145, 221] and in humans, some of those who used MPTP are now beginning to show symptoms of parkinsonism.[120] This delay in appearance of symptoms fits a model of PD that suggests that an initial insult to the DA system may not result in disease until a critical level is reached. The critical level of DA depletion may occur with age because of a gradual loss of DA in the aging process. The real importance of the discovery of MPTP-induced parkinsonism is that it may enable better understanding of the pathogenesis and, in turn, of the treatment of the disease. One hypothesized cause of PD implicated environmental toxins (because some herbicides such as paraquat resemble the chemical structure of MPTP) and the involvement of the superoxide free radical.[10, 40, 112] Epidemiological studies are now under way to investigate PD in areas known for high herbicide usage, and α-tocopherol is under investigation as a protective agent.

The Dystonias

Dystonia is a movement disorder characterized by sustained muscle contraction in the extreme end range of a movement; frequently there is a rotational component. There are inherited dystonias that usually involve the entire body. These dystonias are most prevalent in those of European Jewish descent. There are also focal dystonias that involve just one joint, such as spasmodic torticollis or writing cramps. Full-body dystonia is a disease of the basal ganglia and the current view is that the focal dystonias also involve lesions of precise areas of the basal ganglia.

Symptoms

The person with generalized dystonia will begin a movement such as walking and then will experience a torsional contractions of the trunk; upper extremity, especially at the shoulder; and of the ankle, foot, and toes. These contractions may be so strong that further movement is impossible. For many patients there is pain as the muscles remain contracted for long periods of time.

Spasmodic torticollis is the most common focal dystonia. The person with this disorder will have involuntary contractions of neck muscles that result in head turning or head extension and flexion movements that are often sustained for long periods of time. Other common sites of focal involvement are the vocal cords; the tongue and swallowing muscles; the facial muscles, especially about the eye; the hand; and the toes. Writer's cramp is a task-specific dystonia, unlike other focal dystonias.

An interesting phenomenon of dystonia is the fact that many patients will develop a sensory or motor "trick" that will decrease the severity of the muscle contraction(s) and may even stop these movements.

In all cases of dystonia there is excessive co-activation of agonists and anatagonists that interferes with the timing, execution, and loss of independent joint motions. Rarely are there any abnormalities of muscle tone per se; that is, there is no increase in deep tendon reflexes nor is there rigidity. Muscle strength and ROM are usually within normal limits unless disuse leads to weakness.

Etiology

The etiology of full-body dystonia is predominantly genetic. The etiology of the focal dystonias is unknown. Some authors have suggested that focal dystonias may also be genetic; others speculate that it occurs following injury. In addition to the motor component of the disease there is also strong evidence that the sensory systems are involved. Byl and colleagues[34] found that subjects with focal hand dystonia had difficulty in discriminative sensory processing and frequently had an abnormal sensation of movement. Tinazzi and co-workers[218] found a significantly higher sensory evoked potential in subjects with dystonia which they thought might be indicative of decreased activity in the putamen and thought that poor processing of sensory information in the basal ganglia-thalamus-cortical loop could lead to the motor dysfunction. Focal dystonia has also been linked to repetitive movements produced under high cognitive constraints and attention.[34] It is thought that the rapid, high repetition might be interpreted because simultaneous contraction and a learned sensorimotor dysfunction ensue.[33] Byl and co-workers[35] have indeed developed an animal model of focal hand dystonia following repetitive movements and have demonstrated degradation in the sensory cortex following training. Whether these results can be generalized to other focal dystonias is unknown.

Pharmacological and Medical Management

The most common medical treatment for the focal dystonias is injection of botulinum toxin. This toxin binds with the ACh receptors on the muscle and prevents muscle contraction. The injections are made under EMG guidance so that only those motor units involved in the production of the extraneous movements are paralyzed. The treatment is not permanent, however, and so the patient must have these injections every 3 to 4 months. At present only botulinum A is approved by the FDA and only for blepharospasm. Some patients have developed antibodies to the toxin after which the toxin is no longer effective. Other botulinum strains (B and F) are under investigation.

Evaluation and Treatment Intervention

Evaluation of the person with full-body dystonia is similar to the evaluation of the person with tardive dyskinesia or HD. Evaluation of the person with focal dystonia must involve some other aspects of the disease manifestation. It is important to note the duration of the dystonia, the trigger, and the person's "trick," if any, to decrease the dystonia. Tricks are sensory in nature and help to relieve the pain often associated with extreme movement. (The Toronto Western Spasmodic Torticollis Rating Scale [TWSTRS] is one evaluation for the person with spasmodic torticollis.)

Several ADL should be examined. For example, the person with writer's cramp will have no difficulty holding a fork or a toothbrush, only with holding a pen for writing. Additionally, there is a position dependence so that writing in the prone position may not evoke the dystonia despite severe inability to hold the pen at a desk.[33]

In addition to the full extent of the motor abnormality, it is also important to test sensation, especially higher-level sensory processing such as precise localization of touch, graphesthesia, and kinesthesia. Recent evidence suggests that balance, particularly dynamic balance, should also be assessed in patients with torticollis.[153] These balance difficulties were not relieved with botulinum toxin.

Physical therapy interventions are only now being developed. One successful program utilizes sensory integration and relearning techniques performed with attention.[34] Practice is a crucial element of treatment and the client must be willing to practice the sensory tasks many, many times throughout the day to obtain benefit. The client practices cognitively demanding sensory discrimination tasks throughout the day as well as utilizing only normal, tension-free movements.[33]

Treatment of torticollis must include a relearning of midline before the person can begin to practice normal movement away from midline. The client may find this relearning process easier following the botulinum injection.

Other Considerations

Like other extraneous movements associated with basal ganglia disorders, relaxation can reduce the muscle contraction. However, I have found that the time to incorporate relaxation is prior to the full-blown development of the muscle contraction—a difficult task. Therefore, clients should practice relaxation on a regular basis. There is frequently a psychological aspect to the focal dystonias that may need the intervention of a psychiatrist or psychologist.

METABOLIC DISEASES AFFECTING OTHER REGIONS OF THE BRAIN

All alternations of metabolism, if allowed to continue, affect nervous system function. This includes alternations in sodium, water, sugar, and hormonal balance. Table 22–1 lists metabolic diseases that often have neurological sequelae. Proper treatment is usually medical management of the imbalance. Physical therapeutic intervention, if necessary, should address specific neurological symptoms. (See the chapters that discuss these individual problems.)

Ingestion of or exposure to heavy metals may also lead

TABLE 22–1. Neurological Complications of Metabolic Disorders

Metabolic Problem	Treatment	Neurological Complication
Decreased sodium (too much H_2O)	Restrict water intake	Muscle twitching, seizures, coma
Increased sodium	Rehydration, *slowly*	Cerebral edema, muscle rigidity, decerebrate rigidity
Decreased potassium (hypokalemia), often caused by aldosteronism	Restoration of calcium levels after assessing primary cause	Changes in resting potential of neuron; hyperpolarization; muscle weakness and fatigue with eventual total paralysis
Magnesium imbalance	Improved diet, intravenous magnesium	Mental confusion, muscle twitching, myoclonus, tachycardia, hyperreflexia, extraneous movements, seizures
Diabetes mellitus	Proper control of diabetes	Peripheral neuropathy, pseudotabes, possible seizures and coma
Hypoglycemia	Treatment of primary cause; diet adjustment	Anoxia of the brain, seizures, mental confusion
Hyperthyroidism	Thyroid-blocking agents; intravenous fluids, hydrocortisone, and propranolol if patient in thyroid crisis	Hyperkinesia, irritability, nervousness, emotional lability, symmetrical peripheral neuropathy
Hypothyroidism	Thyroid supplement	Sluggishness, mental and motor retardation, muscle weakness, sometimes muscle pain
Hypercalcemia	Treatment of primary cause, which is often hyperparathyroidism, vitamin D malignancy (therefore surgical removal)	Headache, weakness, fatigue, proximal neuropathy, rigidity, tremor, disorientation
Hypocalcemia	Intravenous administration of calcium (possible medical emergency)	Hyperexcitability of the peripheral and central nervous systems, which can lead to tetany and convulsions

● **T A B L E 2 2 – 2. Neurological Complications of Heavy Metal Poisoning**

Type of Metal	Treatment	Neurological Complication
Lead Source: lead paint, industrial (fumes of molten lead)	Elimination of source, reduction of fluids, intravenous urea or mannitol, use of chelating agents	Interstitial edema and hemorrhage (especially in cerebellum) in acute poisoning; all levels of central nervous system affected in chronic poisoning In children: seizures, mental retardation, behavior problems, hyperactivity In adults: spasticity, rigidity, dementia, personality changes Peripheral neuropathy may occur in adults and children
Arsenic Source: paint and insecticides	Removal of source, gastric lavage, intravenous fluids, maintenance of electrolyte balance; penicillamine used in acute poisoning	Demyelinization of peripheral nerves in all extremities
Manganese Source: industrial if manganese dust is not removed; symptoms appear 2–25 yr after exposure	Levodopa	Neuronal loss in basal ganglia, substantia nigra, and cerebellum Initially psychiatric disturbances, including nervousness, irritability, and a tendency toward compulsive acts Later, muscular weakness and parkinsonian-like symptoms
Mercury Rare, but may affect farmers and dental office workers	Penicillamine; function returns only with physical, occupational, and speech therapy	Loss of neurons, especially in cerebellum; also in cortex near calcarine fissure Alternating periods of confusion, drowsiness, and stupor with restlessness and excitability Ataxia, dysarthria, visual deterioration

to CNS disease. Table 22–2 describes the sequelae of these problems.

SUMMARY

This chapter has focused on the pathophysiology, evaluation, and treatment of genetic, hereditary, and metabolic diseases affecting adults. In all of these diseases the therapist is an important (though sometimes underused) part of the rehabilitation team. Knowledge of the possible mechanisms involved in the production of the varying movement disorders may make the appropriate evaluation and subsequent treatment more meaningful. Even with degenerative, progressive disorders the therapist plays an important role in maintaining quality of life and assists the client and family in coping with the disease. Throughout this chapter the importance of documentation and publication has been stressed. Both will assist in the development of improved therapeutic techniques and also may help researchers in planning and interpreting appropriate experimental studies.

REFERENCES

1. Agostino R, et al: Sequential arm movements in patients with Parkinson's disease, Huntington's disease and dystonia. Brain 115:1481, 1992.
2. Albin RL, et al: The functional anatomy of basal ganglia disorders. Trends Neurosci 12:366, 1989.
3. Alexander GE, Crutcher MD: Functional architecture of basal ganglia circuits: Neural substrates of parallel processing. Trends Neurosci 13:266, 1990.
4. Alexander GE, et al: Basal ganglia-thalamocortical circuits: Parallel substrates for motor, oculomotor, "prefrontal" and "limbic" functions. Prog Brain Res 85:119, 1990.
5. Aminoff MJ: Treatment of Parkinson's disease. West J Med 161:303, 1994.
6. Ariano MA, et al: D2 dopamine receptor distribution in the rodent CNS using antipeptide antisera. Brain Res 609:71, 1993.
7. Ayres AJ: Sensory Integration and Learning Disorders, Los Angeles, Western Psychological Services, 1972.
8. Baldessarini RJ, Tarsy D: Dopamine and the pathophysiology of dyskinesias induced by antipsychotic drugs. Annu Rev Neurosci 3:23, 1980.
9. Ball J : Demonstration of the traditional approach in the treatment of a patient with parkinsonism. Am J Phys Med 46:1034, 1967.
10. Ball J : Personal communication, 1983.
11. Barbeau A, et al: Ecogenetics of Parkinson's disease: Prevalence and environmental aspects in rural areas. Can J Neurol Sci 14:36, 1987.
12. Battig K, et al: Comparison of the effects of frontal and caudate lesions on discrimination learning in monkeys, J Comp Physiol Psychol 55:458, 1962.
13. Beckley DJ, et al: Impaired scaling of long latency postural reflexes in patients with Parkinson's disease. Electroencephalogr Clin Neurophysiol 83:22, 1993.
14. Bemelmans AP, et al. Brain-derived neurotrophic factor–mediated protection of striatal neurons in an excitotoxic rat model of Huntington's disease, as demonstrated by adenoviral gene transfer. Hum Gene Ther 10:2987, 1999.
15. Benecke R, et al: Performance of simultaneous movements in patients with Parkinson's disease. Brain 109:739, 1986.
16. Benecke R, et al: Disturbance of sequential movements in patients with Parkinson's disease. Brain 101:361, 1987.
17. Benita M, et al: Effects of ventrolateral thalamic nucleus cooling on initiation of forelimb ballistic flexion movements by conditioned cats. Exp Brain Res 34:435, 1979.

18. Bird ED: Biochemical studies on γ-aminobutyric acid metabolism in Huntington's chorea. *In* Bradford HF, Marsden CD (eds): Biochemistry and Neurology. London, Academic Press, 1976.

19. Bloem BR, et al: Altered postural reflexes in Parkinson's disease. A reverse hypothesis. Med Hypotheses 39:243–247, 1992.

20. Bloem BR, et al: Influence of dopaminergic medication on automatic postural responses and balance impairment in Parkinson's disease. Mov Disord 11:509–521, 1996.

21. Bobath B: Adult Hemiplegia: Evaluation and Treatment. London, Heinemann, 1976.

22. Bond JM, Morris ME: Goal-directed secondary motor tasks: Their effects on gait in subjects with Parkinson's disease. Arch Phys Med Rehabil 81:110, 2000.

23. Boop R, et al: Methylphenidate (MPH): Absence of readiness potential in patients with Parkinson's disease and in patients following long-term MPH treatment. Neurosci Abstracts 7:779, 1981.

24. Bowen FP: Behavioral alterations in patients with basal ganglia lesions. *In* Yahr MD (ed): The Basal Ganglia. New York, Raven Press, 1976.

25. Brooks VB: Roles of cerebellum and basal ganglia in initiation and control of movements. Can J Neurol Sci 2:265, 1975.

26. Brown J, et al: How the basal ganglia use parallel excitatory and inhibitory learning pathways to selectively respond to unexpected rewarding cues. J Neurosci 19:10502–10511, 1999.

27. Brown RG, et al: Response choice in Parkinson's disease: The effects of uncertainty and stimulus-response compatibility. Brain 116:869, 1993.

28. Buchwald NA, et al: The "caudate-spindle." III. Inhibition by high frequency stimulation of subcortical structures. Electroencephalogr Clin Neurophysiol 13:525, 1961.

29. Buchwald NA, et al: The "caudate-spindle." IV. A behavioral index of caudate-induced inhibition. Electroencephalogr Clin Neurophysiol 13:536, 1961.

30. Buchwald NA, et al: The basal ganglia and the regulation of response and cognitive sets. *In* Brazier MAB (ed): Growth and Development of the Brain. New York, Raven Press, 1975.

31. Burt DR, et al: Antischizophrenic drugs: Chronic treatment elevates dopamine receptor binding in brain. Science 196:326, 1977.

32. Butterfield PG, et al: Environmental antecedents of young-onset Parkinson's disease. Neurology 43:1150, 1993.

33. Byl NN, Melnick ME: The neural consequences of repetition: Clinical implications of a learning hypothesis. J Hand Ther 10:160, 1997.

34. Byl NN, et al: Sensory dysfunction associated with repetitive strain injuries of tendonitis and focal hand dystonia: A comparative study. J Orthop Sports Phys Ther 23:234, 1996.

35. Byl NN, et al: A primate genesis model of focal dystonia and repetitive strain injury: I. Learning-induced dedifferentiation of the representation of the hand in the primary somatosensory cortex in adult monkeys. Neurology 47:508, 1996.

36. Calne DB, et al: Bromocriptine in parkinsonism. BMJ 4:442, 1974.

37. Carlsson A: Some aspects of dopamine in the basal ganglia. *In* Yahr MD (ed): The Basal Ganglia. New York, Raven Press, 1976.

38. Carter JH, et al: The effect of exercise on levodopa absorption. Neurology 39(Suppl 1): 320, 1989.

39. Cohen G, Heikkila RE: The generation of hydrogen peroxide, superoxide radical and the hydroxyl radical by 6-hydroxy dopamine, dialuric acid and related cytotoxic agents. J Biol Chem 249:2447, 1974.

40. Comella CL, et al: Physical therapy and Parkinson's disease: A controlled clinical trial. Neurology 44:376, 1994.

41. Conner NP, Abbs JH: Task-dependent variations in Parkinsonian motor impairments. Brain 114:321, 1991.

42. Cooper IS: Involuntary Movement Disorders. New York, Harper & Row, 1969.

43. Corcos DM, et al: Strength in Parkinson's disease: Relationship to rate of force generation and clinical status. Ann Neurol 39:79, 1996.

44. Cotzias GC, et al: Modification of parkinsonism: Chronic treatment with L-dopa. N Engl J Med 280:337, 1969.

45. Crutcher MD, DeLong MR: Single cell studies of the primate putamen. II. Relations to direction of movement and pattern of muscular activity. Exp Brain Res 53:244, 1984.

46. Dam M, et al: Effects of conventional and sensory enhanced physiotherapy on disability in Parkinson's disease patients. Adv Neurol 69:551, 1996.

47. Davis CG, et al: Chronic parkinsonism secondary to intravenous injection of meperidine. Psychiatry Res 1:249, 1979.

48. deBruin PFC, et al: Effects of treatment on airway dynamics and respiratory muscle strength in Parkinson's disease. Am Rev Respir Dis 148:1576, 1993.

49. DeLong MR: Activity of basal ganglia neurons during movement. Brain Res 40:127, 1972.

50. DeLong MR, Strick P: Relation of basal ganglia, cerebellum and motor cortex units to ramp and ballistic limb movements. Brain Res 71:327, 1974.

51. Denny-Brown D: The Basal Ganglia and Their Relation to Disorders of Movement. Liverpool, UK, Liverpool University Press, 1962.

52. Denny-Brown D, Yanagesawa N: The role of the basal ganglia in the initiation of movement. *In* Yahr MD (ed): The Basal Ganglia. New York, Raven Press, 1976.

53. Diamond SG, Markham CH: One year trial of pergolide as an adjunct to Sinemet in the treatment of Parkinson's disease. Adv Neurol 40:537, 1984.

54. Dieckmann G, Sasaki K: Recruiting responses in the cerebral cortex produced by putamen and pallidum stimulation. Exp Brain Res 10:236, 1970.

55. DiFiglia M: Clinical genetics II. Huntington's disease from the gene to pathophysiology. Am J Psychiatry 154:104, 1997.

56. DiFiglia M, Sapp E, Chase KO, et al: Aggregation of huntingtin in neuronal intranuclear inclusions and dystrophic neurites in brain. Science 277:1990, 1997.

57. Divac I: Neostriatum and functions of perfrontal cortex. Acta Neurobiol Exp (Warsz) 32:461, 1972.

58. Dunne JW, et al: Parkinsonism: Upturned walking stick as an aid to locomotion, Arch Phys Med Rehabil 68:380, 1987.

59. Duvoisin RC: Parkinson's Disease: A guide for Patient and Family. New York, Raven Press, 1978.

60. Evarts EV: Pyramidal tract activity associated with a conditioned hand movement in the monkey. J Neurophysiol 29:1011, 1966.

61. Fahn S: The extrapyramidal disorders. *In* Wyngaarden JB, Smith LH (ed): Cecil Textbook of Medicine, 16th ed. Philadelphia, WB Saunders, 1982.

62. Fahn S, Elton RL: Unified Parkinson's disease rating scale. *In* Fahn S, et al (eds): Recent Developments in Parkinson's Disease, vol 2. NJ, MacMillan Healthcare Information, London, 1987.

63. Ferrier D: The Functions of the Brain. London, Smith, Elder, 1876.

64. Formisano R, et al: Rehabilitation and Parkinson's disease. Scand J Rehabil Med 24:157, 1992.

65. Friedman J, Friedman H: Fatigue in Parkinson's disease. Neurology 43:2016, 1993.

66. Fuxe K, et al: Heterogeneities in the dopamine neuron systems and dopamine cotransmission in the basal ganglia and the relevance of receptor-receptor interactions. *In* Fahn S, et al (eds): Recent Developments in Parkinson's Disease. New York, Raven Press, 1986.

67. Gauthier L, et al: The benefits of group occupational therapy for patients with Parkinson's disease. Am J Occup Ther 41:360, 1987.

68. Georgiou N, et al: Reduction in external cues and movement sequencing in Parkinson's disease. J Neurol Neurosurg Psychiatry 57:368, 1994.

69. Georgiou N, et al: Reliance on advance information and movement sequencing in Huntington's disease. Mov Disord 10:472, 1995.

70. Georgiou N, et al: Impairment of movement kinematics in patients with Huntington's disease: A comparison with and without a concurrent task. Mov Disord 12:386, 1997.

71. Glatt S, et al: Anticipatory and feedback postural responses in perturbation in Parkinson's disease (abstract). *In* Proceedings of the Society for Neuroscience, Phoenix, 1989.

72. Granit R, Kaada BR: Influence of stimulation of central nervous structures on muscle spindles in cat. Acta Physiol Scand 27:130, 1952.

73. Graybiel AM: Functions of the nigrostriatal system. Clin Neurosci 1:12, 1993.

74. Graybiel AM: The basal ganglia and chunking of action repertoires. Neurobiol Learn Mem 70:119, 1998.

75. Grimby L, Hannerz J: Disturbances in the voluntary recruitment order of anterior tibial motor units in bradykinesia of parkinsonism. J Neurol Neurosurg Psychiatry 37:47, 1974.

76. Hallett M: Physiology of basal ganglia disorders: An overview. Can J Neurol Sci 20:177, 1993.

77. Hallett M, et al: Analysis of stereotyped voluntary movements at the elbow in patients with Parkinson's disease. J Neurol Neurosurg Psychiatry 40:1129, 1977.

78. Hallett M, et al: Evaluation of surgery for PD: Report from AAN. Neurology 53:1910, 1999.

79. Harper PS: Localization of the gene for Huntington's chorea. Trends Neurosci 7:1, 1984.

80. Harris GJ, et al: Reduced basal ganglia blood flow and volume in pre-symptomatic, gene-tested persons at-risk for Huntington's disease. Brain 122:1667, 1999.

81. Hartmann-von Monakow K, et al: Projections of the precentral motor cortex and other cortical areas of the frontal lobe to the subthalamic nucleus in the monkey. Exp Brain Res 33:395, 1978.

82. Hayden MR: Huntington's Chorea. Berlin, Springer-Verlag, 1981.

83. Heikkila RE, et al: Protection against the dopaminergic neurotoxicity of MPTP by monoamine oxidase inhibitors. Nature 311:467, 1984.

84. Hoehn MM, Yahr MD: Parkinsonism: Onset, progression and mortality. Neurology 17:427, 1967.

85. Horak FB, et al: Postural instability in Parkinson's disease: Motor coordination and sensory organization (abstract). In Proceedings of the Society for Neuroscience, Anaheim, CA, 1984.

86. Horak FB, et al: Effects of dopamine on postural control in parkinsonian subjects: Scaling, set, tone. J Neurophysiol 75:2380, 1996.

87. Hore J, Vilis T: Arm movement performance during reversible basal ganglia lesions in the monkey. Exp Brain Res 39:217, 1980.

88. Hore J, et al: Basal ganglia cooling disables learned arm movements of monkeys in the absence of visual guidance. Science 195:584, 1977.

89. Hornykiewicz O: The mechanisms of action of L-dopa in Parkinson's disease. Life Sci 15:1249, 1974.

90. Hubble JP, et al: Risk factors for Parkinson's disease. Neurology 43:1693, 1993.

91. Hull CD, et al: Intracellular responses in caudate and cortical neurons. In Crane G, Gardener R (eds): Psychotropic Drugs and Dysfunctions of the Basal Ganglia. Washington, DC, US Public Health Service, 1969.

92. Hull CD, et al: Intracellular responses of caudate neurons to brainstem stimulation. Brain Res 22:163, 1970.

93. Hull CD, et al: Intracellular responses of caudate neurons to temporally and spatially combined stimuli. Exp Neurol 38:324, 1973.

94. Hurwitz A: The benefit of a home program exercise regimen for ambulatory Parkinson's disease patients. J Neurosci Nurs 21:180, 1989.

95. Jellinger K: Pathology of parkinsonism. In Fahr S, et al (eds): Recent Developments in Parkinson's Disease. New York, Raven Press, 1986.

96. Jobst E, et al: Sensory perception in Parkinson's disease. Arch Neurol 54:450, 1997.

97. Jog MS, et al: Building neural representations of habits. Science 286:1745, 1999.

98. Jones TA, et al: Motor skills training enhances lesion-induced structural plasticity in the motor cortex of adult rats. J Neurosci 19:10153, 1999.

99. Jordan N, et al: Cognitive components of reaction time in Parkinson's disease. J Neurol Neurosurg Psychiatry 55:658, 1992.

100. Kaakkola S, et al: Effect of entacapone, a COMT inhibitor, on clinical disability and levodopa metabolism in parkinsonian patients. Neurology 44:77, 1994.

101. Karlsen K, et al: Fatigue in patients with Parkinson disease. Mov Disord 14:237, 1999.

102. Kelly PJ, Gillingham FJ: The long-term results of stereotaxic surgery and L-dopa therapy in patients with Parkinson's disease: A 10-year follow-up study. J Neurosurg 53:332, 1980.

103. Kemp JM, Powell TPS: The connexions of the striatum and globus pallidus: Synthesis and speculation. Phil Trans R Soc Lond B Biol Sci 262:441, 1971.

104. Klawans HL: Therapeutic approaches to neuroleptic induced tardive dyskinesia. Res Publ Assoc Res Nerv Ment Dis 55:447, 1976.

105. Klawans HL, et al: Presymptomatic and early detection in Huntington's disease. Ann Neurol 8:343, 1980.

106. Klockgether T, Dichgans J: Visual control of arm movement in Parkinson's disease. Mov Disord 9:48, 1994.

107. Knott M, Voss D: Proprioceptive Neuromuscular Facilitation Patterns and Techniques, 2nd ed. New York, Harper & Row, 1968.

108. Koller WC, Trimble J: The gait abnormality of Huntington's disease. Neurology 35:1450, 1985.

109. Koller WC, et al: Falls and Parkinson's disease. Clin Neuropharmacol 12:98, 1989.

110. Koller W, et al: Environmental risk factors in Parkinson's disease. Neurology 40:1218, 1990.

111. Koller WC, Tolosa E: Current and emerging drug therapies in the management of Parkinson's disease. Neurology 50(Suppl 6):51, 1998.

112. Kopin IJ, et al: Mechanisms of neurotoxicity of MPTP. In Fahr S, et al (eds): Recent Developments in Parkinson's Disease, New York, Raven Press, 1986.

113. Kornhuber HH: Motor functions of cerebellum and basal ganglia: The cerebellocortical saccadic (ballistic) clock, the cerebellonuclear hold regulator, and the basal ganglia ramp (voluntary speed smooth movement) generator. Kybernetik 8:157, 1971.

114. Krauthamer GM, Albe-Fessard D: Electrophysiological studies of the basal ganglia and striopallidal inhibition of non-specific afferent activity. Neuropsychologia 2:73, 1964.

115. Kunesch E, et al: Altered force release control in Parkinson's disease. Behav Brain Res 67:43, 1995.

116. Kunzle H: Bilateral projections from precentral motor cortex to the putamen and other parts of the basal ganglia: An autoradiographic study in Macaca fascicularis. Brain Res 88:195, 1976.

117. Kunzle H: Projections from the primary somatosensory cortex to basal ganglia and thalamus in the monkey. Exp Brain Res 30:481, 1977.

118. Kuroda K, et al: Effect of physical exercise on mortality in patients with Parkinson's disease. Acta Neurol Scand 86:55, 1992.

119. Labuszewski T, Lidsky TI: Basal ganglia influences on brain stem trigeminal neurons. Exp Neurol 65:471, 1979.

120. Langston JW: MPTP neurotoxicity: An overview and characterization of phrases of toxicity. Life Sci 36:201, 1985.

121. Langston JW, et al: Chronic parkinsonism in humans due to a product of meperidine analog synthesis. Science 219:979, 1983.

122. Lelli S, et al: Spinal cord inhibitory mechanisms in Parkinson's disease. Neurology 41:553, 1991.

123. Leslie WD, et al: Clinical deficits in Huntington disease correlate with reduced striatal uptake on iodine-123 epidepride single-photon emission tomography. Eur J Nucl Med 26:1458, 1999.

124. Levine MS, et al: Pallidal and entopeduncular intracellular responses to striatal, cortical, thalamic and sensory inputs. Exp Neurol 44:448, 1974.

125. Levine MS, et al: The spontaneous firing patterns of forebrain neurons. II. Effects of unilateral caudate nuclear ablation. Brain Res 78:411, 1974.

126. Levine MS, et al: The spontaneous firing pattern of forebrain neurons. III. Prevention of induced asymmetries in caudate neuronal firing rates by unilateral thalamic lesions. Brain Res 131:215, 1977.

127. Levine MS, et al: Long-term decreases in spontaneous firing of caudate neurons induced by amphetamine in cats. Brain Res 194:263, 1980.

128. Levine MS, et al: Long-term behavioral and neurophysiological effects of neonatal lgd-amphetamine administration in kittens. Neurosci Abstracts 8:965, 1982.

129. Lidsky TI, et al: Pallidal and entopeduncular single unit activity in cats during drinking. Electroencephalogr Clin Neurophysiol 39:79, 1975.

130. Lidsky TI, et al: The effects of stimulation of trigeminal sensory afferents upon caudate units in cats. Brain Res Bull 4:9, 1979.

131. Livesey PJ, Rankine-Wilson J: Delayed alternation learning under electrical (blocking) stimulation of the caudate nucleus in the cat. J Comp Physiol Psychol 88:342, 1975.

132. Lloyd KG, et al: The neurochemistry of Parkinson's disease: Effect of L-dopa therapy. J Pharmacol Exp Ther 195:453, 1975.

133. MacKay AVP: Clinical controversies in tardive dyskinesia. In Marsden CD, Fahn S (eds): Movement Disorders. Boston, Butterworth, 1981.

134. Magendie M: Fonctions et maladies du système nerveux. Paris, Lecapalin, 1841. [English translation in Assoc Res Nerv Ment Dis 21:8, 1940.]

135. Markham CH, Diamond SG: Evidence to support early levodopa therapy in Parkinson disease. Neurology 31:125, 1981.

136. Markus HS, et al: Raised resting energy expenditure in Parkinson's disease and its relationship to muscle rigidity. Clin Sci 83:199, 1992.

137. Martin JP: The Basal Ganglia and Posture. London, Pitman Books, 1967.

138. Massion J, Smith AM: Activity of ventrolateral thalamic neurons related to posture and movement during contact placing responses in the cat. Brain Res 61:400, 1973.

139. Matsunami K, Cohen B: Afferent modulation of unit activity in globus pallidus and caudate neurons and changes induced by vestibular nucleus and pyramidal tract stimulation. Brain Res 91:140, 1975.

140. McGeer PL, et al: Aging and extrapyramidal function. Arch Neurol 34:33, 1977.

141. McIntosh GC, et al: Rhythmic auditory-motor facilitation of gait patterns in patients with Parkinson's disease. J Neurol Neurosurg Psychiatry 62:22, 1997.

142. Melmon KL, Morrelli HF: Clinical Pharmacology: Basic Principles in Therapeutics, 2nd ed. New York, Macmillan, 1978.

143. Melnick ME, Palmer G: Physical therapy. In Koller WC, Paulson G (eds): Therapy of Parkinson's Disease. New York, Marcel Dekker, 1990.

144. Melnick M, et al: Activity of forebrain neurons during alternating movement in cats. Electroencephalogr Clin Neurophysiol 57:57, 1984.

145. Melnick ME, et al: Comparison of behavioral effects of MPTP in young adult and year-old rats. In Markey SP, et al (eds): MPTP: A Neurotoxin Producing a Parkinsonian Syndrome. Orlando, FL, Academic Press, 1986.

146. Melnick ME, et al: The effect of rhythmic exercise on gait, balance and depression in people with Parkinson's disease. J Am Geriatr Soc 47:283, 1999.

147. Melnick ME, et al: Effects of pallidotomy on balance and motor function in patients with Parkinson's disease. Arch Neurol 56:1361, 1999.

148. Mettler FA, et al: The extrapyramidal system. Arch Neurol Psychiatry 41:984, 1939.

149. Milner-Brown HS, et al: Electrical properties of motor units in Parkinsonism and a possible relationship with bradykinesia. J Neurol Neurosurg Psychiatry 42:35, 1979.

150. Mink JW: The basal ganglia: Focused selection and inhibition of competing motor programs. Prog Neurobiol 50:381, 1996.

151. Montgomery EB, et al: Motor initiation versus execution in normal and Parkinson's disease subjects. Neurology 41:1469, 1991.

152. Montgomery EB, et al: Reaction time and movement velocity abnormalities in Parkinson's disease under different task conditions. Neurology 41:1476, 1991.

153. Moreau MS, et al: Static and dynamic balance function in spasmodic torticollis. Mov Disord 14:87, 1999.

154. Morris ME, Iansek R: Characteristics of motor disturbance in Parkinson's disease and strategies for movement rehabilitation. J Hum Mov Sci 3:9, 1996.

155. Morris ME, et al: The pathogenesis of gait hypokinesia in Parkinson's disease. Brain 117:1169, 1994.

156. Morris ME, et al: Stride length regulation in Parkinson's disease. Normalization strategies and underlying mechanisms. Brain 119:551, 1996.

157. Muller V, et al: Short-term effects of behavioral treatment on movement initiation and postural control in Parkinson's disease: A controlled clinical trial. Mov Disord 12:306, 1997.

158. Muskens L: The central connection of the vestibular nuclei with the corpus striatum and their significance for ocular movements and for locomotion. Brain 45:452, 1922.

159. Mutch WJ, et al: A pilot study of patient rated disability and the need for aids in Parkinson's disease. Clin Rehabil 3:151, 1989.

160. Nauta HJW, Cole M: Efferent projections of the subthalamic nucleus: An autoradiographic study in monkey and cat. J Comp Neurol 180:1, 1978.

161. Neafsey EJ, et al: Preparation for movement in the cat. I. Unit activity in the cerebral cortex. Electroenchephalogr Clin Neurophysiol 44:706, 1978.

162. Neafsey EJ, et al: Preparation for movement in the cat. II. Unit activity in the basal ganglia and thalamus. Electroencephalogr Clin Neurophysiol 44:714, 1978.

163. Newton RA, Price DD: Modulation of cortical and pyramidal tract induced motor responses by electrical stimulation of the basal ganglia. Brain Res 85:403, 1975.

164. Nicholson DE, et al: Sensory cueing improves motor performance and rehabilitation in persons with Parkinson's disease. Neurology Report 21:117, 1997.

165. Nieoullon A, et al: Interdependence of the nigrostriatal dopaminergic systems on the two sides of the brain in the cat. Science 198:416, 1977.

166. Nothnagel H: Experimentelle Untersuchungen über die Funktion des Gehirns. Virchows Arch 57:184, 1873. [English translation in Assoc Res Nev Ment Dis 21:8, 1940.]

167. Nutt JG, et al: The "on-off" phenomenon in Parkinson's disease: Relation to levadopa absorption and transport. N Engl J Med 310:483, 1984.

168. Olmstead CE, Villablanca JR: Effects of caudate nuclei or frontal cortical ablations in kittens: Bar pressing performance. Exp Neurol 63:244, 1979.

169. Owen AM, et al: Contrasting mechanisms of impaired attentional set-shifting in patients with frontal lobe damage or Parkinson's disease. Brain 116:1159, 1993.

170. Palmer SS, et al: Exercise therapy for Parkinson's disease. Arch Phys Med Rehabil 67:741, 1986.

171. Pan HS, Walters JR: Unilateral lesion of the nigrostriatal pathway decreases the firing rate and alters the firing pattern of the globus pallidus neurons in the rat. Synapse 2:650, 1988.

172. Pascual-Leone A, et al: Procedural learning in Parkinson's disease and cerebellar degeneration. Ann Neurol 34:594, 1993.

173. Pastor MA, et al: Vestibular induced postural responses in Parkinson's disease. Brain 116:1177, 1993.

174. Patti F, et al: Effects of rehabilitation therapy on Parkinson's disability and functional independence. J Neurol Rehabil 10:223, 1996.

175. Peacock IW: A physical therapy program for Huntington's disease patients. Clin Manage 7:22, 1987.

176. Pechadre JC, et al: Parkinsonian akinesia, rigidity and tremor in the monkey. J Neurol Sci 28:147, 1976.

177. Petajan JH, et al: Motor unit control in Huntington's disease: A possible presymptomatic test. Adv Neurol 23:163, 1979.

178. Phillips JG, et al: Bradykinesia and movement precision in Huntington's disease. Neuropsychologia 34:1241, 1996.

179. Poirier LJ, et al: Stereotaxic lesions and movement disorders in monkeys. Adv Neurol 10:5, 1975.

180. Polgar S, et al: Implications of neurological rehabilitation for advancing intracerebral transplantation. Brain Res Bull 44:229, 1997.

181. Pollock LJ, Davis L: Muscle tone in parkinsonian states. Arch Neurol Psychiatry 23:303, 1930.

182. Potegal M: The caudate nucleus egocentric localization system. Acta Neurobiol Exp (Warsz) 32:479, 1972.

183. Pratley RE, et al: Higher sedentary energy expenditure in patients with Huntington's disease. Ann Neurol 47:64, 2000.

184. Rajput AH, et al: Geography, drinking well water chemistry, pesticides and herbicides and the etiology of Parkinson's disease. Can J Neurol Sci 14:414, 1987.

185. Reuter I, et al: Therapeutic value of exercise training in Parkinson's disease. Med Sci Sports Exerc 31:1544, 1999.

186. Reynolds NC, et al: Analysis of gait abnormalities in Huntington disease. Arch Phys Med Rehabil 80:59, 1999.

187. Roberts E: Some thoughts about GABA and the basal ganglia. In Yahr MD (ed): The Basal Ganglia. New York, Raven Press, 1976.

188. Robertson C, Flowers KA: Motor set in Parkinson's disease. J Neurol Neurosurg Psychiatry 53:583, 1990.

189. Saint-Cyr JA, et al: Procedural learning and neostriatal dysfunction in man. Brain 111:941, 1988.

190. Sasco AJ, et al: The role of physical exercise in the occurrence of Parkinson's disease. Arch Neurol 49:360, 1992.

191. Schenkman M, Butler RB: A model for multisystem evaluation treatment of individuals with Parkinson's disease: Rationale and case studies. Phys Ther 69:932, 1989.

192. Schenkman M, et al: Exercise to improve spinal flexibility and function for people with Parkinson's disease: A randomized, controlled trial. J Am Geriatr Soc 46:1207, 1998.

193. Schneider JS, Lidsky TI: Processing of somatosensory information in striatum of behaving cats. J Neurophysiol 45:841, 1981.

194. Schneider JS, et al: Deficits in operant behavior in monkeys treated with MPTP. Brain 111:1265, 1988.

195. Segundo JP, Machne X: Unitary responses to afferent volleys in lenticular nucleus and claustrum. J Neurophysiol 19:325, 1956.
196. Shellenberger MK: Persistent alteration of rat brain monoamine levels by carbon monoxide exposure: Sex differences and behavioral correlation. Neurotoxicology 2:431, 1981.
197. Shelton PA, Knopman DS: Ideomotor apraxia in Huntington's disease. Arch Neurol 48:35, 1991.
198. Shoulson I, Fahn S: Huntington's disease: Clinical care and evaluation. Neurology 29:1, 1979.
199. Shoulson I, et al: Clinical care of the patient and family with Huntington's disease. In Commission for the Control of Huntington's disease and Its Consequences, vol 2. Washington, DC, National Institutes of Health, 1977.
200. Shoulson I, et al: Huntington's disease: Treatment with muscimol, a GABA-mimetic drug. Trans Am Neurol Assoc 102:124, 1977.
201. Smith AD, Bolam JP: The neural network of the basal gangila as revealed by the study of synaptic connections of identified neurones. Trends Neurosci 13:259, 1990.
202. Smith JM, Baldessarini RJ: Changes in prevalence, severity and recovery in tardive dyskinesia with age. Arch Gen Psychiatry 37:1368, 1980.
203. Smithson F, et al: Performance on clinical tests of balance in Parkinson's disease. Phys Ther 78:577, 1998.
204. Sotrel A, et al: Evidence for neruonal degeneration and dendritic plasticity in cortical pyramidal neurons of Huntington's disease: A quantitative Golgi study. Neurology 43:2088, 1993.
205. Stelmach GE, et al: Movement preparation in Parkinson's disease: The use of advanced information. Brain 109:1179, 1986.
206. Stern G: The effect of lesions in the substantia nigra. Brain 89:449, 1966.
207. Storey E, Beal MF: Neurochemical substrates of rigidity and chorea in Huntington's disease. Brain 116:1201–1222, 1993.
208. Strick PL: Anatomical analysis of ventrolateral thalamic input to primate motor cortex. J Neurophysiol 39:1020, 1976.
209. Sunvisson H, et al: Changes in motor performance in persons with Parkinson's disease after exercise in a mountain area. J Neurosci Nurs 29:255, 1997.
210. Tanner CM, Goldman SM: Epidemiology of Parkinson's disease. Neurol Clin 14:317, 1996.
211. Tatton WG, et al: Altered motor cortical activity in extrapyramidal rigidity. Adv Neurol 24:141, 1979.
212. Teasdale N, et al: Temporal movement control in patients with Parkinson's disease. J Neurol Neurosurg Psychiatry 53:862, 1990.
213. Teuber HL: Complex functions of basal ganglia. In Yahr MD, (ed): The Basal Ganglia. New York, Raven Press, 1976.
214. Thach WT: Discharge of cerebellar neurons related to two maintained postures and two prompt movements. I. Nuclear cell output. J Neurophysiol 33:527, 1970.
215. Thach WT: Discharge of cerebellar neurons related to two maintained postures and two prompt movements. II. Purkinje cell output and input. J Neurophysiol 33:537, 1970.
216. Thaut MH, et al: Rhythmic auditory stimulation in gait training for Parkinson's disease patients. Mov Disord 11:193, 1996.
217. Thaut MH, et al: Velocity modulation and rhythmic synchronization of gait in Huntington's disease. Mov Disord 14:808, 1999.
218. Tinazzi M, et al: Evidence for an abnormal cortical sensory processing in dystonia: Selective enhancement of lower limb P37–N50 somatosensory evoked potentials. Mov Disord 14:473, 1999.
219. Vidailhet M, et al: The Bereitschaftspotential preceding simple foot movement and initiation of gait in Parkinson's disease. Neurology 43:1784, 1993.
220. Villablanca JR, Marcus R: Effects of caudate nuclei removal in cats: Comparison with effects of frontal cortex ablation. In Buchwald NA, Brazier MAM (eds): Brain Mechanisms in Mental Retardation. New York, Academic Press, 1975.
221. Wagner GC, Jarvis MF: Age-dependent effects of MPTP. In Markey SP, et al (eds): MPTP: A Neurotoxin producing a Parkinsonian Syndrome. Orlando, FL, Academic Press, 1986.
222. Wagner GC, et al: Long-lasting depletions of striatal dopamine and loss of dopamine uptake sites following repeated administration of methamphetamine. Brain Res 181:151, 1980.
223. Walshe FMR: Nature of musculature rigidity of paralysis agitans and its relationship to tremor. Brain 47:159, 1924.
224. Walshe JM: Wilson's disease: The presenting symptoms. Arch Dis Child 37:253, 1962.
225. Wenger KK, et al: Impaired reaching and grasping after focal inactivation of globus pallidus pars interna in the monkey. J Neurophysiol 82:2049, 1999.
226. Whetten-Goldstein K, et al: The burden of Parkinson's disease on society, family, and the individual. J Am Geriatr Soc 45:844, 1997.
227. Willis T: Cerebri anatome: Cui accessit nervorum descriptio et usus. London, 1664. [English translation in Assoc Res Nerv Ment Dis 21:8, 1940.]
228. Wilson SAK: An experimental research into the anatomy and physiology of the corpus striatum. Brain 36:427, 1914.
229. Winkelmuller W, Nitsch FM: Quantitative registration of motor disorders following bilateral lesions of substantia nigra in the rat. Appl Neurophysiol 38:291, 1975.
230. Woodworth RS, Schlosberg H: Experimental Psychology. New York, Holt, Rinehart & Winston, 1961.
231. Worringham CJ, Stelmach GE: Practice effects on the preprogramming of discrete movements in Parkinson's disease. J Neurol Neurosurg Psychiatry 53:702, 1990.
232. Wroe M, et al: Parkinson's disease and physical therapy management. Phys Ther 53:849, 1973.
233. Yanagasawa N: The spectrum of motor disorders in Huntington's disease. Clin Neurol Neurosurg 94(Suppl):S182, 1992.

Brain Tumors

CORRIE J. CHRISTIANSEN, MS, PT • RACHEL O'HARA LOPEZ, MPT • KARLA M. PHILLIPS, BA, BSPT

Key Words

- astrocytoma
- biopsy
- chemotherapy
- Gamma knife
- glioblastoma multiforme
- hospice care
- Karnofsky performance status scale
- meningioma
- metastatic
- radiation therapy
- ventriculostomy

Objectives

Upon completion of this chapter the student/therapist will:

1. Identify the categories of primary brain tumors.

2. Recognize and interpret signs and symptoms of primary brain tumors specific to tumor location.

3. Understand current diagnostic tests used to detect brain tumors.

4. Understand the types of medical and surgical management for brain tumors.

5. Describe the side effects associated with the treatment of brain tumors and recognize their impact on therapeutic intervention.

6. Discuss the multiple considerations necessary to plan and execute an intervention program for the client with a brain tumor.

7. Recognize the emotional and psychosocial impact of the disease process on the client, the client's support system, and the interdisciplinary team.

AN OVERVIEW OF BRAIN TUMORS

The rehabilitation clinician serves many different populations, including clients with brain tumors. Despite the prognosis for limited survival associated with primary brain tumors, these individuals have shown progress in the rehabilitation setting similar to that noted in clients with diagnoses of stroke or traumatic brain injury.[29, 45, 55] Advances in medical and surgical treatment for clients with cancer have resulted in improved survival rates and longer life expectancy. However, individuals are often faced with progressive functional impairments resulting from the disease process.[45] These impairments can be physical or cognitive, or both, and require an interdisciplinary team approach to best facilitate the individual's return to a meaningful lifestyle. The clinicians must also

recognize the psychological and emotional needs of the individual given this diagnosis and be sensitive and flexible in accommodating these feelings. Improved quality of life, especially the opportunity to return home, remains the ultimate goal of the rehabilitation process.

The clinical presentation of clients with brain tumors mimics that of persons with other central nervous system (CNS) conditions. The location of the tumor or vascular accident determines the deficits the client will exhibit. However, in the brain tumor client, the burdensome effects of standard medical intervention and the aggressive nature of the disease course itself provide obstacles to therapeutic intervention. The client's probability of eventual physical and cognitive deterioration provides a challenge to the clinician attempting to formulate realistic goals and plan for future needs. Therefore, a thorough knowledge of the tumor's natural history, the complications and side effects of treatment, and the neurological deficit the client exhibits will assist the clinician in best developing a comprehensive, individualized plan of care.

Incidence and Etiology

The incidence of adult brain tumors is on the rise in the United States, with an estimated 35,519 new cases of primary benign or malignant brain tumors for 2001. Of these, 16,500 are expected to be malignant, resulting in 13,000 deaths. The statistics for children include 2,899 new cases of primary benign or malignant brain tumors for the same 12-month period.[64, 86]

The exact cause of the increase in incidence of brain tumors is not known. Studies suggest that the increase is the result of more tumors being diagnosed with improved tumor imaging, rather than an actual increase in the occurrence of malignant brain tumors.[14, 23]

Brain tumors typically afflict two distinct categories: (1) children aged 0 to 15 years and (2) adults in the fifth to seventh decades of life. In adults, white Americans have a higher incidence than black Americans, and in both pediatric and adult populations males are more frequently affected than females.[82, 86] In children, a primary brain tumor is the second most common cause of cancer death in the 0- to 15-year-old age group.[86]

The frequently occurring meningioma, typically benign, accounts for nearly 24% of all primary brain tumors. Glioblastoma multiforme, a malignant tumor, accounts for 22.6% of adult primary tumors[10] (Fig. 23–1). Pediatric tumors, unlike adult tumors, are unique in their histology and behavior and are rarely metastatic. The predominant tumors in children are typically infratentorial in location, most specifically, cerebellar astrocytoma, medulloblastoma, and fourth ventricular ependymoma.[67]

The etiology of brain tumors remains unclear. Theories suggest that heredity is a contributing factor, but studies show familial incidence can be explained by a common toxic or infectious exposure.[24, 41] Research indicates an association, but not a causal relationship, linking brain tumors to certain chemicals and materials (petrochemicals, organic solvents, rubber). These materials are frequently found in specific occupations, such as farming and manufacturing. Electromagnetic field exposure is associated with an increased incidence of brain tumor.[85] Ionizing radiation, used therapeutically in high doses to treat tumors, was found to have a causal relationship to the development of a second brain tumor.[3]

Continued investigation into possible causal relationships with potential risk factors is essential if the incidence and mortality rate associated with brain tumors is to decrease.

Classification of Tumors

The World Health Organization (WHO) first published a universal classification system for CNS tumors in 1979. This system classifies tumors according to their microscopic characteristics and has been accepted as the universal method for the classification of brain tumors.[32, 51]

Primary tumors originate in the CNS, whereas metastatic or secondary tumors spread to the CNS from systemic cancer sites outside the brain. Characteristics of the most common brain tumors are discussed in the following paragraphs with information provided regarding age, location, medical treatment, and prognosis.

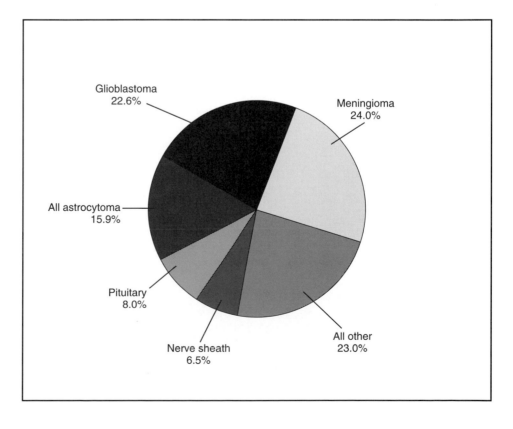

FIGURE 23–1. Distribution of all primary brain and central nervous system tumors by histology. (From CBTRUS: 2000 annual report. Chicago, Central Brain Tumor Registry of the United States, 2000.)

Gliomas are primary tumors that arise from supportive tissues of the brain and are frequently located in the cerebral hemispheres. These tumors may also present in the brain stem, optic nerve, and spinal cord. In children, the cerebellum is a primary location for gliomas.[13] Gliomas have four primary categories and are classified by their predominant cellular components: astrocytomas and oligodendrogliomas originate from glial cells, ependymomas from ependymal cells, and medulloblastomas from primitive cells.[66]

Astrocytomas are derived from astrocytes, which are star-shaped glial cells, and are the most common primary brain tumor in adults and children.[28] Astrocytomas vary in morphology and biological behavior, from those that are diffuse and infiltrate surrounding brain structures to those that are circumscribed with a decreased likelihood of progression. Astrocytomas are typically found in the cerebrum, originating in the frontal lobe in adults, and in the cerebellum in children. In adults the primary age at onset is typically in the third to fifth decades of life.[23, 32]

Astrocytomas are further classified into four grades: well-differentiated, low-grade (grades 1 and 2) tumors; anaplastic, mid-grade (grade 3) tumors; and glioblastoma multiforme, high-grade (grade 4) tumors. The higher the grade, the poorer the prognosis.[23]

Low-grade tumors grow slowly and are typically subtotally resected through surgery when accessible. Recurrence is common as a result of incomplete resection.[23] If these tumors recur, their morphology often changes to that of an anaplastic astrocytoma or glioblastoma.[66]

Anaplastic, mid-grade (grade 3) tumors grow rapidly, typically carry malignant cell traits, and routinely progress toward glioblastoma multiforme tumors.[32] Grade 4 tumors, glioblastoma multiforme, are discussed below.

Astrocytomas are typically treated with surgery, radiation therapy, and chemotherapy depending upon the grade, location of the tumor, age of the patient and Karnofsky performance scale score[13, 23, 31] (Table 23–1).

On average, patients with astrocytomas have a 5-year survival rate of 30%.[81] Patients with low-grade astrocytomas treated with radiation therapy and surgery have a 65% 5-year survival rate and a 40% 10-year survival rate.[77] Those with mid-grade astrocytomas have a 5-year survival rate of only 22% when treated similarly.[81]

Glioblastoma multiforme is the distinct name given to the highly malignant grade 4 astrocytoma. These tumors grow rapidly, invading nearby tissue, and contain highly malignant cells. Glioblastomas are predominantly located in the deep white matter of the cerebral hemispheres but may be found in the brain stem, cerebellum, or spinal cord. Fifty percent of these tumors are bilateral or occupy more than one lobe of a hemisphere. The typical age at onset is during midlife, with males having a 2:1 incidence rate over females.[13, 23, 32] The prognosis is poor for persons with glioblastoma: less than 20% survive more than 1 year and only 2% survive 5 years following diagnosis.[81] The most important prognostic variables are age, tumor histology, and postoperative Karnofsky performance status scale score. These tumors are treated by surgical resection, radiation therapy, stereotactic radiosurgery, and chemotherapy.[23]

Oligodendrogliomas are slow-growing, but progressive tumors that typically develop over a period of several years, with 50% involving multiple lobes. Fifty percent of these tumors occur in the frontal lobe, 42% in the temporal lobe, and 32% in the parietal lobe. Many clients have seizures as the only clinical manifestation of the tumor.[22, 32, 71] Oligodendrogliomas typically appear in the fourth to sixth decades of life, and the ratio of affected males to females is 2:1.[1] The prognosis with oligodendrogliomas varies considerably and is dependent upon age at diagnosis and tumor grade. Positive prognostic indicators have been age at onset of less than 40 years and a tumor grade of 1 or 2. These patients have a median survival of 9 years with a 5-year survival rate of 60% to 75% and 10-year survival rate of 46%.[46, 71, 81] Negative prognostic

● **T A B L E   2 3 – 1. Karnofsky Performance Status Scale**

Condition	Performance Status (%)	Comments
A. Able to carry on normal activity and to work. No special care is needed.	100	Normal. No complaints. No evidence of disease.
	90	Able to carry on normal activity. Minor signs or symptoms of disease.
	80	Normal activity with effort. Some signs or symptoms of disease.
B. Unable to work. Able to live at home, care for most personal needs. A varying degree of assistance is needed.	70	Care of self. Unable to carry on normal activity or to do active work.
	60	Requires occasional assistance, but is able to care for most of personal needs.
	50	Requires considerable assistance and frequent medical care.
C. Unable to care for self. Requires equivalent of institutional or hospital care. Disease may be progressing rapidly.	40	Disabled. Requires special care and assistance.
	30	Severely disabled. Hospitalization is indicated, although death not imminent.
	20	Very sick. Hospitalization necessary. Active supportive treatment necessary.
	10	Moribund. Fatal processes progressing rapidly.
	0	Dead.

From Karnofsky DA, Burchenal JH: The clinical evaluation of chemotherapeutic agents in cancer. *In* Macleod C (ed): Evaluation of Chemotherapeutic Agents. New York, Columbia University Press, 1949.

indicators include age at onset over 40 years, hemiparesis, and cognitive changes.[46] The 5-year survival rate decreases to 36% with anaplastic oligodendroglioma.[81] Treatment is dependent upon symptoms and ranges from observation and seizure control with anticonvulsant drugs to surgical resection followed by radiation and chemotherapy.[13, 22, 23, 66]

Ependymomas and *ependymoblastomas* are tumors arising from ependymal cells lining the ventricles which grow in the ventricles or in adjacent brain tissue.[13, 66] Sixty percent to 66% of ependymomas are located in the posterior fossa.[1, 23] Anaplastic ependymomas, also known as ependymoblastomas, are primarily located supratentorially, are more commonly seen in children, and have a tendency to metastatic spread via the cerebrospinal fluid (CSF).[1, 23, 32] For 40% of infratentorial tumors the age at onset is in the first decade of life, whereas for supratentorial tumors the age at onset is evenly distributed.[1] Ependymomas are primarily treated with surgical resection followed by radiation therapy, but chemotherapy is also used.[1, 13, 23, 66] These tumors frequently recur and prognosis is dependent upon the success of resection, with a 5-year survival rate ranging from 58% to 68%.[3, 26, 83]

Medulloblastomas are malignant tumors thought to arise from primitive cells in the granular layer of the cerebellum, but the exact cell of origin is unknown. These tumors are typically located in the posterior fossa, originating laterally in the cerebellar hemispheres in young adults and in the vermis in children.[32] Medulloblastomas typically grow into the fourth ventricle, blocking CSF flow, causing hydrocephalus and increased intracranial pressure (ICP).[23] These tumors primarily occur in children, accounting for 25% of childhood brain tumors.[13, 32] Five-year survival rates range from 30% to almost 70%.[23, 81] Systemic metastases occur in 5% of cases and bone metastases in 90%. Because of the increased incidence of metastases, the prognosis for children under the age of 4 years is poor.[23] Prognosis is better for children under 4 years of age, with tumors with complete resection, and with decreased metastases present. Treatment is surgery followed by radiation therapy and chemotherapy.[13]

Meningiomas are slow-growing tumors that primarily originate from cells located in the dura mater or arachnoid.[1, 13, 28] Frequently these tumors are found incidentally during imaging studies or at autopsy.[61] Approximately 25% are symptomatic when diagnosed.[12, 28, 61] The incidence increases with age and they occur in females in a 2:1 ratio over males.[12, 23, 28, 61] Resectable tumors are primarily treated by surgery and recurring tumors are treated with surgery, radiation therapy, or stereotactic radiosurgery.[66] Patients with nonmalignant meningiomas have a 5-year survival rate of 70% vs. a 5-year survival rate of 55% with malignant meningiomas.[48, 81]

Pituitary adenomas are benign epithelial tumors originating from the adenohypophysis of the pituitary gland and frequently invading the optic chiasm.[1, 32, 66] These tumors are characterized by hyper- or hyposecretion of hormones.[13, 23] Age at onset spans all ages but pituitary adenomas are rare before puberty.[23] The female-to-male ratio of incidence is 2.25:1. These tumors are primarily

treated by surgical resection and drug therapy.[13, 23, 66] Prognosis is related to size and cell type of the tumor.[23]

Schwannomas are encapsulated tumors composed of neoplastic Schwann cells that can arise on any cranial or spinal nerve.[13, 66] The eighth cranial nerve is the cranial nerve usually involved and a schwannoma here is called an *acoustic neuroma*.[32] Acoustic neuromas produce otologic or focal or generalized neurological deficits depending upon the location of the tumor. These tumors are typically located in the internal auditory canal but may extend into the cerebellopontine angle.[1, 23] These tumors are frequently treated by surgical resection, but stereotactic radiosurgery is increasing in popularity as an alternative method of treatment.[13, 44, 72] The prognosis for patients with these tumors is good, yet complications can result from treatment, including facial paralysis, deafness, and equilibrium impairments. Resulting neurological deficits after surgery vary depending on the size and location of the tumor. Currently, these tumors rarely result in death and with the increasing use of noninvasive procedures, the eighth cranial nerve is being preserved more frequently.[72]

Metastatic brain tumors are secondary tumors that have spread to the brain, typically through the arterial circulation, from a primary systemic cancer site elsewhere in the body.[23] The frontal lobe is the most common site for metastatic disease from primary systemic sources, including the lungs, breast, and kidneys, or from melanoma.[58] Approximately 20% to 30% of people with systemic cancer develop metastatic brain tumors.[87]

Treatment for these tumors is tailored to the individual and dependent upon the management of the systemic disease, the accessibility of the lesion, and the number of lesions present. The prognosis varies, with positive prognostic indicators including a Karnofsky performance scale score of 70 or greater, age 60 years or less, remission or resolution of the primary cancer, and metastases located in the brain only. Typically, an individual will survive approximately 1 month after diagnosis without treatment.[77, 87] With corticosteroids, survival increases to 2 months, and whole-brain radiation therapy extends survival to 3 to 5 months. Radiosurgery or microsurgical resection of single metastases has been shown to increase survival to 9 to 14 months.[4, 77, 87] Survival increases to 16 months when surgical resection and whole-body radiation are combined. In one study in which the systemic disease was controlled and solitary brain metastases occurred, a survival rate greater than 5 years was shown in 21% of cases.[76]

Signs and Symptoms

The clinical manifestation of a brain tumor can range from a decreased speed in comprehension or a minor personality change, to progressive hemiparesis or seizure, depending on the type and site of the tumor. Patients with brain tumors typically present with headaches, seizures, nonspecific cognitive or personality changes, or focal neurological signs.[1, 5] Some may present with a general sign, a specific neurological symptom, or a combination of both.

General Signs and Symptoms

General signs and symptoms of the presence of a brain tumor include headache, seizures, altered mental status, and papilledema. *Headache* is the presenting symptom in 30% of cases and develops during the course of the disease in 70% of cases. These headaches are generally dull, intermittent, and nonspecific, and are usually on the same side as the tumor. They are often difficult to distinguish from tension headaches. It is important to identify the specific nature of the headaches because certain features often indicate the presence of a brain tumor. These features include:

1. *The headache that interrupts sleep (10% to 32%) or is worse upon waking and improves throughout the day (15% to 36%)*
2. *The headache that is elicited by postural changes, coughing, or exercise (20% to 32%)*
3. *The headache of recent onset that is more severe or of a different type than usual*
4. *The new onset of headache in a previously asymptomatic person*
5. *The headache associated with nausea and vomiting (30% to 40%), papilledema, or focal neurological signs*[1, 5]

The mechanism of the headache is not clearly understood but may be related to local swelling, distortion of blood vessels, direct invasion of the meninges, and increased ICP. With increased ICP, a bifrontal or bioccipital headache is present regardless of the tumor location.[1, 53]

Seizure activity is the presenting symptom in one third of cases and is present in 50% to 70% of cases at some stage of the disease.[3, 5] Approximately 10% to 20% of adults with new-onset seizure activity have brain tumors. Half of the patients experience focal seizures and half experience general seizures. Frontal lobe gliomas produce seizures in 59% of all cases. The percentage of cases exhibiting seizures from gliomas in other lobes is as follows: parietal, 42%; temporal, 35%; and occipital, 33%.[5]

Altered mental status is the initial symptom in 15% to 20% of cases and is frequently present at the time of diagnosis. Mental status changes can range from subtle changes in concentration, memory, affect, personality, initiative, and abstract reasoning to severe cognitive problems and confusion.[5] Subtle changes may be incorrectly attributed to worry, anxiety, or depression.[1] Changes in mentation are common with frontal lobe tumors and in the presence of elevated ICP. Increased ICP causes drowsiness and decreased level of consciousness, which can progress to stupor or coma if treatment is not initiated.[5]

The incidence of *papilledema*, swelling of the optic nerve, is less frequent today because brain tumors are being diagnosed earlier with the use of sensitive imaging techniques. Papilledema is associated with symptoms of transient visual loss, especially with positional changes, and reflects evidence of increased intracranial hemorrhage transmitted through the optic nerve sheath. It is more common in children and with slow-growing tumors and posterior fossa tumors.[5] Other less common symp-toms are vomiting and frank positional vertigo, usually accompanying tumors found in the posterior fossa.[1]

Specific Signs and Symptoms

Certain clinical features are related to functional areas of the brain and thus have a specific localizing value when diagnosing a brain tumor.[5] In addition, it is essential that clinicians be familiar with the lobes of the brain and their distinct functions, to effectively manage the deficits resulting from the tumor (Fig. 23–2).

The *frontal lobe* is responsible for motor functioning, initiation of action, and interpretation of emotion, including motor speech, motor praxis, attention, cognition, emotions, intelligence, judgment, motivation, and memory.[20, 53] Therefore, frontal lobe tumors may result in hemiparesis, seizures, aphasia, and gait difficulties. Initially, the tumor may be clinically silent. As the tumor grows, however, there may be personality changes, including disinhibition, irritability, impaired judgment, and lack of initiative.[5, 63]

The *parietal lobe* processes complex sensory and perceptual information related to somesthetic sensation, spatial relations, body schema, and praxis. General symptoms of a parietal lobe tumor include contralateral sensory loss and hemiparesis, homonymous visual deficits or neglect, agnosias, apraxias, and visual-spatial disorders. If the dominant parietal lobe is involved, aphasia and seizures may be present. When the nondominant parietal lobe is involved, contralateral neglect and inability to recognize deficits may be apparent.[5, 20, 53]

The *occipital lobe* is the primary processing area of visual information. Therefore, lesions of the occipital lobe often result in disorders of eye movement and homonymous hemianopsia. If the parieto-occipital junction is involved, visual agnosia and agraphia are often present. Although less common, visual seizures may be present, characterized by lights, colors, and formed geometric patterns.[5, 20, 53]

The *temporal lobe* is responsible for auditory and limbic processing. Anterior temporal lobe lesions may be clinically silent until becoming quite large, resulting in seizures. If the lateral hemispheres are involved, auditory and perceptual changes may occur. When the medial aspects of the lobe are involved, changes in cognitive integration, long-term memory, learning, and emotions may be seen. When the dominant temporal lobe is involved, aphasia may be present. Anomia, agraphia, acalculia, and Wernicke aphasia, characterized by fluent, nonsensical speech, are specific to left temporal lobe lesions.[5, 20, 53]

The *cerebellum* is responsible for coordination and equilibrium.[20] The most common symptoms of cerebellar tumors in adults include headache, nausea, and vomiting in 40% of cases and ataxia in 25% of cases. Lesions of the midline cause truncal ataxia and lesions of the hemispheres cause appendicular ataxia. Lesions of either hemisphere may cause ipsilateral dysmetria, dysdiadochokinesia, and intention tremor. If the tumor involves the cerebellopontine angle, hearing loss, headache, ataxia, dizziness, tinnitus, and facial palsy may occur. If the tumor invades the meninges at the foramen magnum or increased ICP causes cerebellar tonsil herniation, nuchal

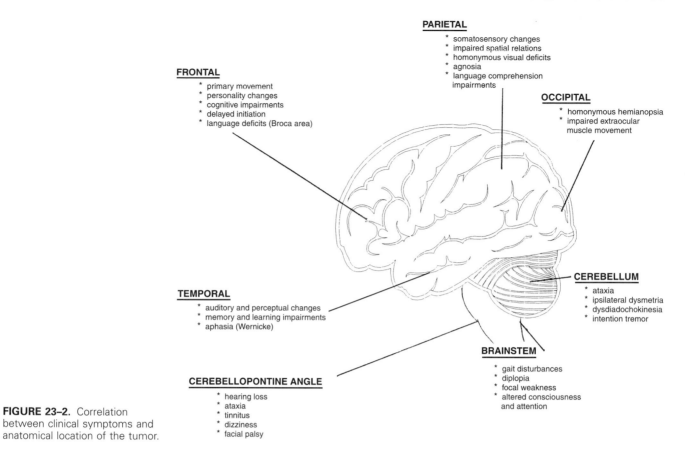

PARIETAL
* somatosensory changes
* impaired spatial relations
* homonymous visual deficits
* agnosia
* language comprehension impairments

FRONTAL
* primary movement
* personality changes
* cognitive impairments
* delayed initiation
* language deficits (Broca area)

OCCIPITAL
* homonymous hemianopsia
* impaired extraocular muscle movement

CEREBELLUM
* ataxia
* ipsilateral dysmetria
* dysdiadochokinesia
* intention tremor

TEMPORAL
* auditory and perceptual changes
* memory and learning impairments
* aphasia (Wernicke)

BRAINSTEM
* gait disturbances
* diplopia
* focal weakness
* altered consciousness and attention

CEREBELLOPONTINE ANGLE
* hearing loss
* ataxia
* tinnitus
* dizziness
* facial palsy

FIGURE 23–2. Correlation between clinical symptoms and anatomical location of the tumor.

rigidity and head tilt away from the lesion may be seen. Because the cerebellum is located in an extremely confined space, even minimal increases in pressure can cause death from cerebellar tonsil herniation.[5, 23, 34]

The *brain stem* communicates information to and from the cerebral cortex via fiber tracts and controls basic life functions. The reticular formation specifically controls consciousness and attention. Symptoms of a brain stem tumor have an insidious onset and may include gait disturbances, diplopia, focal weakness, headache, vomiting, facial numbness and weakness, and personality changes.[23] If the dorsal midbrain is involved, Parinaud syndrome, characterized by loss of upward gaze, pupillary areflexia to light, and loss of convergence, may be seen. If the reticular system of the pons and medulla is involved, symptoms of apnea, hypo- or hyperventilation, orthostatic hypotension, or syncope may occur.[23, 34]

Pituitary tumors are typically large and affect pituitary function by compressing its structure or hypersecreting hormones. An enlarging tumor causes the loss of pituitary function and decreases hormone secretion, resulting in pituitary disorders specific to the type of hormone involved (Cushing disease, hypothyroidism, Addison disease, diabetes, etc.). As the tumor enlarges it may invade or compress nearby structures. Lateral extension involving the third and fourth cranial nerves causes .diplopia, fifth cranial nerve involvement causes ipsilateral facial numbness, and internal carotid artery occlusion causes cerebral infarction. Upward extension is more common and may compress the optic chiasm, hypothalamus, or third ventri-

cle. Downward extension may compress the sphenoid sinus, typically without clinical signs.[23]

Diagnosis of Disease/Pathology

Advances in research and the development of sophisticated diagnostic equipment have greatly improved brain tumor diagnosis. When a physician suspects a brain tumor, there are many specialized tests used to gather clinical, radiological, pathological, and laboratory information to confirm the diagnosis.[5]

Clinical Diagnosis

A clinical diagnosis consists of information the physician gathers during a comprehensive evaluation. First, a thorough medical history, including the specific nature of signs and symptoms, must be obtained. A neurological examination is then performed to assess visual, cognitive, sensory, and motor function, and test reflexes.[34] If the presence of a brain tumor is suspected after the neurological examination, the next diagnostic step, tumor imaging, is warranted.[1]

Radiological Diagnosis

The modern era of CNS imaging began with the introduction of computed tomography (CT) in 1973 and with magnetic resonance imaging (MRI) in 1979.[23] The availability of sensitive imaging allows for earlier tumor detection and has revolutionized the diagnosis and management of brain tumors.[5, 9] Tumor imaging has continued to develop and can be classified into three categories: static imaging, dynamic imaging, and computer integration imaging.

Static Imaging. Static neurological imaging includes CT and MRI, which are noninvasive techniques that provide accurate anatomical and functional analysis of intracranial structures.[5] *Computed tomography*, which relies on the electron density and photon energy of tissues, was the first brain imaging technique to determine tumor size. Contrast enhancement helps to identify isodense tumor from surrounding parenchyma, hypodense lesions in edematous areas, and optimal sites for tumor biopsy.[5, 23] Following surgical intervention, CT can be used to confirm the proper tissue biopsy site and determine the success of tumor resection. However, caution should be exercised when relating contrast enhancement images to malignancy because some low-grade tumors display striking enhancement, whereas some large glioblastomas will display no contrast enhancement. Although MRI has become the preferred method, CT scanning offers lower cost, shorter scanning time, and a more sensitive method to detect calcification bony involvement.

Magnetic resonance imaging is the initial diagnostic imaging procedure of choice. It enables early detection of certain primary intracranial tumors that would be missed by CT.[23, 70] MRI is a more sensitive imaging modality than CT for identifying lesions and margin abnormalities, by providing greater anatomical detail with thin slices and multiplanar images. With MRI, different signal intensities differentiate between normal brain and tumor. Contrast enhancement with gadolinium sharpens the definition of a lesion.[1, 23, 53] Under certain conditions, MRI enhanced with gadolinium can distinguish between tumor and edema. However, not all high-grade astrocytomas enhance with gadolinium and MRI signals may imitate imaging abnormalities seen in low-grade astrocytomas or nonmalignant conditions. MRI also cannot accurately predict tumor type or grade of malignancy for which surgical biopsy is necessary.[5, 23]

Dynamic Imaging. Dynamic functional imaging includes positron emission tomography (PET), single-photon emission computed tomography (SPECT), magnetic resonance spectroscopy (MRS), and echo planar MRI. *Positron emission tomography* is a noninvasive technique utilizing a cyclotron and specific isotopes to obtain dynamic information about the metabolism and physiology of the brain tumor and the surrounding brain tissue. PET scans using fludeoxyglucose F18 ([18]FDG) to measure glucose metabolism can be useful in determining the grade of primary brain tumors and in differentiating tumor regrowth from radiation necrosis.[7, 53, 84] However, recent studies suggest that [18]FDG-PET actually has a limited ability to differentiate recurrent tumor from radiation necrosis.[30, 63] PET can also be helpful in studying the metabolic effects of chemotherapy, radiation therapy, and steroids on the tumor.[5] However, PET is less reliable in patients treated heavily with chemotherapy and radiation therapy.[1, 23]

Single-photon emission computed tomography is a functional imaging technique evolved from PET and utilizes infused thallium (Tl), which localizes in tumor but not in necrotic or normal brain tissue.[1, 5, 23] SPECT is used to distinguish between high- and low-grade tumors and between tumor recurrence and radiation necrosis.[5, 23] Along with [18]FDG-PET, SPECT is used preoperatively with static imaging to localize the highest metabolic area within tumor for biopsy. Although SPECT is a less sensitive method of obtaining physiological information on brain tumors, it is more readily available and less expensive.[23]

Magnetic resonance spectroscopy is a noninvasive technique used in conjunction with static MRI to measure the metabolism of brain tumors.[23] MRS has been proved to successfully differentiate normal brain from malignant tumor and recurrent tumor from radiation necrosis. It has also been used to document early treatment response and provide information regarding histological grade of astrocytomas.[52, 54] In the future, MRS targeting may enhance the diagnostic yield of brain biopsy and possibly be a noninvasive alternative to surgical biopsy.[27, 52]

Echo planar MRI, functional MRI, is a new technique using a conventional MRI scanner fitted with echo planar technology. This technique maps cerebral blood flow at the capillary level. Its intended purpose is to provide information regarding the diffusion of contrast into tumor, resulting in better resolution of tumor and edema.[23]

Modern computer technology allows for the two- and three-dimensional reconstruction of identical planes in cranial space by combining tumor images from different modalities, including CT, MRI, PET, and SPECT. *Computed integration imaging* involves the simultaneous display of images from different techniques in a single imaging system that is transposed to a reference stereotactic frame. This development has resulted in significant advances in stereotactic biopsy, interstitial radiotherapy, and laser-guided stereotactic resection.[23] By improving targeting and visualization of tissues, stereotaxis provides a safer, more accurate method of tissue acquisition and biopsy. A correct tissue diagnosis can be made in 95% of cases with this technique.[60]

Biopsy

Surgical biopsy is performed to obtain tumor tissue as part of tumor resection or as a separate diagnostic procedure.[3] Stereotactic biopsy is a computer-directed needle biopsy. When guided by advanced imaging tools, stereotactic biopsy yields the lowest surgical morbidity and highest diagnostic information. This technique is frequently used with deep-seated tumors in functionally important or inaccessible areas of the brain in order to preserve function.[43]

Laboratory Diagnosis

Laboratory testing is often used to further assess focal deficits during the diagnosis and management of brain tumors. Perimetry is the measurement of visual fields used when evaluating tumors near the optic chiasm. Electroencephalography (EEG) is used to monitor brain activity and detect seizures but has limited value during screening because EEG is often normal in clients with brain tumors.[5] Lumbar puncture analyzes CSF, which is useful in the diagnosis and detection of dissemination of certain brain tumors. However, lumbar puncture is risky in patients with increased ICP and in those cases should be avoided.[1, 5, 53] Audiometry and vestibular testing are useful for diagnosing tumors in the cerebellopontine angle. Endocrine testing is used to examine endocrine abnormalities with tumors in the pituitary gland and hypothalamus.[5]

Medical and Surgical Management

After diagnosis of a brain tumor is confirmed, specific treatment must be selected. The ultimate goals of tumor management are to improve quality of life and extend survival, by preserving or improving neurological function.[56] These goals are accomplished by removing, or decreasing the size of, the tumor. Treatment techniques are determined by histological type, location, grade, and size of tumor; age at onset; and medical history of the patient.[3, 23, 56, 66] Four types of treatment are discussed: (1) traditional surgery, (2) chemotherapy, (3) radiation therapy, and (4) stereotactic radiosurgery.

Traditional Surgery

The primary goal of traditional surgery is maximal tumor resection with the least amount of damage to neural or supporting structures.[23] Benign tumors, if accessible, are resected completely, whereas malignant tumors are typically partially resected secondary to location or size of the tumor.[23, 56] The *purposes* of surgery in the management of brain tumors include:

1. *Biopsy to establish a diagnosis*
2. *Partial resection to decrease the tumor mass to be treated by other methods*
3. *Complete resection of the tumor*
4. *Providing access for other treatment techniques*[13]

Biopsies are performed through open, needle, and stereotactic needle techniques. Open biopsies involve exposure of the tumor followed by removal of a sample through surgical excision. Needle biopsies involve insertion of a needle into the tumor through a hole in the skull and the excision of the tissue sample drawn through the needle. Stereotactic needle biopsies utilize computers and MRI or CT scanning equipment to assist in directing the needle into the tumor. This type of biopsy is useful for deep-seated or multiple brain lesions.[3, 23]

Partial and *complete resections* are accomplished through craniotomy. Craniotomy involves removal of a portion of the skull and separation of the dura mater to expose the tumor. Stereotactic craniotomy utilizes recent technology to create computed three-dimensional pictures of the brain to guide the neurosurgeon during the procedure. CT scanning and more recently MRI scanners are used to provide an evaluation of the tumor resection during the procedure.[3, 6, 23]

Preoperative Management. Prior to surgery clients are evaluated for general surgical risks and the possibility of tumors in additional locations. Unless medically contraindicated, steroids are administered before surgery if brain edema is present or if extensive manipulation will be occurring during surgery. Anticonvulsant medications are also administered preoperatively to prevent seizures during or after surgery.[23, 56]

Intraoperative Management. During surgery, precautions are taken to prevent an increase in edema or brain volume. Mannitol is utilized to shrink the surrounding brain tissue, thus providing easier access to the tumor. Steroid use is continued and antibiotics are administered to prevent infection. Hyperventilation, with a CO_2 level of 25 mEq/L, is also used to reduce brain volume.[23, 56]

Postoperative Management. Patients are observed in an intensive care unit for at least 24 hours for possible intracranial bleeding or seizures. Blood pressure is monitored continuously. Following surgery, patients are at risk for developing deep vein thrombosis or pulmonary embolism secondary to decreased muscle activity, but, because these patients are at risk for intracranial bleeding, anticoagulants cannot be given.[18] Steroids are tapered after surgery over 5 to 10 days. Anticonvulsant medications are continued after surgery with the length of time dependent on the presence of seizure activity before and after surgery.[23, 56] The primary limitations of traditional surgery include:

1. *Medical complications such as hematoma, hydrocephalus, infection, and infarction from the surgical procedure*
2. *Complications resulting from general anesthesia*
3. *Increased cost of hospital stay and surgical procedure*[56, 72, 77]

Chemotherapy

Chemotherapy is another treatment frequently used to manage brain tumors. It can be used independently or as an adjuvant to surgery or radiation. Chemotherapeutic drugs are not effective on all types of tumors. Certain tumors are known to be resistant to certain drugs, and other treatments are more effective for these tumors.

Chemotherapy drugs act on the DNA of the tumor cells, interfering with their ability to copy DNA and reproduce. Once the replicating capability of the tumor cell is disrupted it dies. In this way the tumor is prevented from growing and is destroyed at the cellular level.[3]

One of the challenges in delivering cytotoxic drugs to the brain is the blood-brain barrier (BBB). The BBB is the brain's natural protective barrier against transmission of foreign substances from the blood into the brain.[3] One class of drugs that does permeate the BBB is the *nitrosoureas*. These include BCNU (carmustine) and CCNU (lomustine) and are lipid-soluble and cell cycle–specific. These drugs are given in high doses and typically are used for glioblastoma multiforme and anaplastic astrocytoma.

Methotrexate is a highly toxic drug and is usually paired with a drug called an antidote drug to reverse the side effects on normal cells. Leucovorin is used to counteract high-dose methotrexate.[65] Typically, this drug is used to treat cancer outside of the CNS. Methotrexate has been found to produce a high degree of neurotoxicity when used in combination with radiation therapy.[59]

Other drugs used to treat brain tumors include cisplatin, procarbazine, vincristine, etoposide (VP-16), and a newer drug called temozolomide.[7] Often drugs are given in combination in order to target all cell types present within the tumor. Because different drugs have different modes of action and side effects, combined drug therapy often proves to be the most effective treatment.[3]

Hormones. Tamoxifen and mifepristone (RU-486) regimens are two hormone therapies that appear to inhibit tumor growth. These estrogen and progesterone antagonists, respectively, are currently being tested for efficacy in tumor treatment.[3]

Administration. Chemotherapy can be administered in a number of different ways. Most agents are given intravenously through a catheter such as a peripherally inserted central catheter (PICC), Groshong catheter, or Port-a-Cath. Other drugs are placed directly into the tumor bed or are given intramuscularly, orally, or by means of an implanted device.

Chemotherapy agents such as BCNU can be placed in the tumor area in the form of wafers that release the drug over time. Drugs are introduced directly into the CSF when an Ommaya reservoir is implanted under the scalp. The reservoir is filled by use of a syringe and the medication is then circulated through the ventricles to the brain.[3]

The drugs are typically given in a clinic setting by a registered nurse certified in chemotherapy administration. A patient's chemotherapy schedule varies depending on the drug given. An on/off cycle is used to allow the patient to recover from the toxic effects of the drug.

Radiation Therapy

Radiation therapy can be used alone or in conjunction with surgery or chemotherapy to treat malignant brain tumors. It is typically chosen as a treatment option for tumors that are too large or inaccessible for surgical resection and to eradicate residual neoplastic cells following a surgical debulking.

Radiotherapy consists of the delivery of high-powered photons, with energies in a much greater range than that of standard x-rays, as an external beam directly at the tumor site. The external beam is transmitted to the tumor through a linear accelerator or a cobalt machine that uses cobalt isotopes as the radiation source. External beam radiation is the most widely used form of radiation treatment.[23]

Conventional radiation therapy as described above is delivered in units called *fractions*.[3] This refers to the dose of radiation delivered at each treatment session. Often if a large fraction is to be delivered, the dose is divided and given more than once per day; this is called hyperfractionation. Hyperfractioned radiation therapy is believed to increase the efficacy and decrease the long-term side effects of radiation. More studies need to be completed

to know its exact benefits. This form of delivery is being used to treat malignant gliomas.[61]

Conformal radiation is the utilization of high-dose external beam radiation, produced by a linear accelerator, to precisely match or "conform" to the tumor shape. One such method of conformal radiation delivery is the Peacock system. This method attempts to deliver a uniform amount of radiation to the tumor and minimize irradiation of healthy brain tissue.[3]

Another type of radiation therapy is focal radiation. Two types of focal radiation exist: interstitial brachytherapy and radiosurgery. *Brachytherapy* refers to the placement of radioactive iodine 125 in or near the lesion. Patients who have poor access to medical care or who will not tolerate other forms of radiation or chemotherapy are candidates for such radiation. The iodine can be delivered through transcranial catheters or iodine seeds can be placed in the resected tumor bed. These implants can deliver low-dose radiotherapy for about 6 months.[23] Patients receiving this type of radiation are considered to be radioactive and precautions must be taken to protect others around them from radiation exposure. *Radiosurgery* involves the use of high-dose radiation beams directed at small tumor areas through the use of computer planning.[3] This type of treatment includes the Gamma knife procedure, which is discussed later.

The treatments described above are those most frequently used, but the following are several promising methods under continuous research. These methods are boron neutron capture therapy (BNCT), hyperthermia, and the administration of radiosensitizers or radioprotectors. BNCT uses a drug that concentrates in tumor cells and is activated by nonionizing radiation. The boron drug captures neutrons, becomes unstable, and disintegrates. The radiation activates the boron and the combined effect kills tumor cells. Interest in BCNT began more than 25 years ago but at that time the appropriate radiation beam had not yet been developed. Research continues to look for boron compounds that will concentrate in tumor cells only and have limited side effects.[3]

Hyperthermia is a method of heating tumor cells to make them more susceptible to radiation. Tumor cells sometimes are hypoxic, acidic, or poorly perfused, which makes them more prone to damage from heat. Normal cells are threatened by heat also; therefore, normal healthy brain tissue must be avoided during the heating process. Research continues into the different means of delivering heat to the tumor site.[86]

Certain drugs have been found to increase (radiosensitizers) or decrease (radioprotectors) the effects of radiation on normal cells and are administered prior to radiation delivery. Currently these drugs are being tested in adults undergoing conventional radiation therapy.[3]

The radiation oncologist determines the dosage, frequency and method of radiation delivery depending on tumor type, location, growth rate, and other medical issues for each client. A typical course of radiation therapy will last 6 weeks. Clients are irradiated for just 1 to 5 minutes 5 days a week. The radiation is intended to kill the malignant cells and preserve healthy cells, but certain rapidly growing cells, as in skin tissue and mucosa, are killed as well. The side effects experienced by those undergoing treatment are a result of this destruction of healthy cells.

Radiation therapy has considerable limitations and disadvantages. There is an accepted maximum lifetime dosage of radiation that the brain and body can tolerate. As doses come close to this limit, the risk of radiation necrosis increases. Because the brains of young children are particularly vulnerable to radiation, other therapies, such as chemotherapy, are used until the developing brain is more tolerant of radiation. Metastatic lesions have invaded multiple organs or body systems and a more systemic treatment such as chemotherapy is most effective for this type of brain cancer.[3]

Stereotactic Radiosurgery

Stereotactic radiosurgery is defined as delivery of a high dose of ionizing radiation, in a single fraction, to a small, precisely defined volume of tissue.[23, 56, 77, 78] The high-energy accelerators involved with stereotactic radiosurgery improve the physical effect of radiation by allowing energy to travel more precisely in a straight line and penetrate deeper, before dissipating.[78] The goal of stereotactic radiosurgery is to arrest tumor growth.[80] This technique has been shown to be most beneficial for treating centrally located lesions less than 3 cm in size and for patients with increased surgical risk factors.[77, 78] Advantages of stereotactic radiosurgery are as follows:

1. *Noninvasive procedure utilizing local anesthesia and sedation to place the stereotactic frame*
2. *Avoids risks of general anesthesia and immediate postoperative risk such as bleeding, CSF leak, or infection*
3. *Lowers treatment cost and shortens hospital stays*[23, 72, 78, 88]

Stereotactic radiosurgery is used to treat benign and malignant tumors, vascular malformations, and functional disorders.[56, 78] The primary modes of administration for stereotactic radiosurgery include the Gamma knife and linear accelerators.[23, 56, 66]

The *Gamma knife* (Fig. 23–3) was first introduced in Sweden in 1968 and is now used worldwide at 65 sites. The Gamma knife utilizes 201 discrete sources of cobalt 60 that are focused precisely to one point in three-dimensional space within the cranium.[16, 56, 77, 78] The Gamma knife is typically used for deeply embedded, small tumors that require precise delivery of radiation.[77]

MRI, CT scanning, or angiography is utilized to identify the exact location of the lesion to be treated after the stereotactic frame is placed on the client's head. The stereotactic frame is then fixed to the machine and attached to a collimator helmet containing 201 holes for the radiation to pass through. The patient is then locked into position. The prescribed dose is given over 20 minutes to 2 hours. After treatment the frame is removed, and the client is observed and is frequently discharged after 24 hours. Return to previous activity typically occurs within a few days.[16, 56, 72, 77]

With the Gamma knife the full dose of radiation is received only at the point where the 201 beams intersect, thereby giving only a minimal dose to uninvolved tissue when targeted accurately. Side effects are rare but headache and nausea may occur.[23] The primary limitations of the Gamma knife are the limited brain volume that can be treated with one dose and the cost of the Gamma knife machine.[23, 56]

Linear accelerators utilized for conventional radiation can be modified for stereotactic radiosurgery. The brain lesion to be targeted is stereotactically placed in the center of the arc of rotation of the machine. A single highly focused beam of radiation is delivered over multiple sweeps around the brain lesion. Linear accelerators can be used to treat larger tumors with precise shape while maintaining uniform dose. Because linear accelerators are used for conventional radiation, a quality check

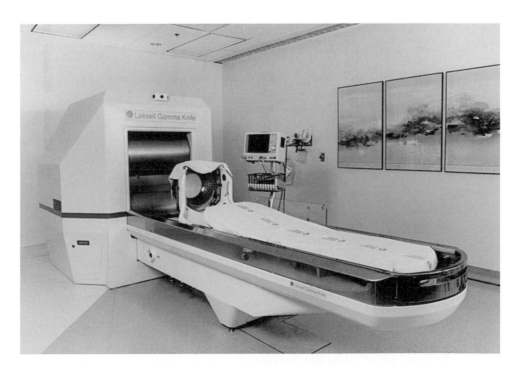

FIGURE 23–3. The Leksell Gamma Knife.

for beam accuracy is imperative before using the machine for stereotactic radiosurgery.[23, 56]

Several research studies have reported on the use of stereotactic radiosurgery, including the Gamma knife and linear accelerators, and compared this modality with microsurgery. In patients with brain metastases, the Gamma knife is typically indicated for small lesions that are centrally located. Surgical resection is indicated for superficial lesions greater than 3 cm in diameter, when a marked mass effect of the tumor exists, or if edema is present in the cranium.[77] The Gamma knife has been shown to achieve tumor control rates as high as those for surgery and whole-body radiation therapy combined, and to halt or reverse neurological progression in 78% of patients treated.[2, 37]

Microsurgical resection has shown a 90% cure rate for acoustic neuromas less than 3 cm in size. Stereotactic radiosurgery avoids the risk of an open procedure but the tumor is controlled rather than removed. Thus far, a 92% tumor control rate has been noted but the patients in this study have not had a 10-year follow up.[44, 72]

Research exists for both low- and high-grade gliomas, but large, controlled studies are few. With low-grade tumors, small studies have shown increased survival after stereotactic radiosurgery, but these studies are uncontrolled and limited by the small number of participants.[88] For high-grade tumors, recent studies found median survival rates ranging from 9.5 to 17 months with use of stereotactic radiosurgery.[8, 19, 47, 50] For recurrent malignant gliomas, survival after fractionated and nonfractionated stereotactic radiosurgery was shown to be 8 to 11 months.[18, 26, 36, 73] The addition of radiosurgery to surgery and radiation therapy produced only modest improvement when compared with surgery and radiation therapy alone.[88]

The preferred treatment for *meningiomas* is surgical resection if complete resection is possible. When surgery is not an option and the tumor is less than 3 cm in size, or 5 mm away from the optic nerve, stereotactic radiosurgery is indicated.[25, 33, 42] Four-year survival rates of 91% in benign meningiomas and 21.5% in malignant meningiomas have been demonstrated after use of the Gamma knife.[25, 33] In a survey taken 5 to 10 years after radiosurgery, 96% of patients believed radiosurgery had provided a satisfactory outcome.[33]

REHABILITATION

Overview

Rehabilitation is a key component in the management of the client with a brain tumor. With advances in technology and treatment intervention, survival rates of people with cancer have improved. Consequently, people are living longer with physical impairments resulting from the disease or its treatment, necessitating interdisciplinary therapeutic intervention.[45] Rehabilitation assists the client and family to appropriately address these impairments and determine a plan of action that will best facilitate the individual's transition to home or work and improve quality of life.

The most effective rehabilitation plan is flexible, to allow for increasing disability, and sensitive, to accommodate the highly emotional impact that accompanies the diagnosis of a primary brain tumor. The tumor's invasion is marked by complaints of pain and growing functional deficits with daily activities. These functional consequences of the disease process are the target of the rehabilitation team. In addition to the side effects of therapeutic intervention, functional progress may be affected by cerebral edema, hydrocephalus, tumor regrowth, infection, and radiation necrosis.

The management of a client with a brain tumor is different from that of other CNS disorders, despite a similar clinical presentation. In order to establish an appropriate plan of care, the clinician must understand the nature of the specific tumor, consider the client's fluctuating neurological status, and prepare for the likelihood of progressive decline. The preferred approach is wholistic, addressing quality of life issues such as physical, psychosocial, and emotional needs, incorporated into the systems model of motor control. Factors defining quality of life are unique to each individual and therefore clinicians should identify and utilize these factors to construct a meaningful treatment program.

Evaluation, clinical analysis, intervention, discharge planning, and psychosocial issues specific to the management of the client with a brain tumor are discussed in the following sections.

Evaluation

The evaluation process must include a comprehensive examination and assessment of all systems in order to establish an appropriate impairment/disability diagnosis, problem list, prognosis, and plan of care. Before a neurological assessment is performed, a thorough review of the client's medical history and an understanding of the medical diagnosis are necessary. The client's occupation, support system, personal goals, and role in the family are important psychosocial factors that should be identified in the evaluation. These factors, along with a thorough functional and neurological examination, assist the clinician through the diagnostic process. This process includes identification of clinical problems, establishment of realistic and appropriate goals, selection of the most effective intervention, and discharge planning.

Although the neurological examination yields important information regarding strength, reflexes, sensation, vision, and cognition, it is important not to rely solely on its finding to determine an appropriate intervention. Because multiple systems interact to produce normal movement, it is difficult to examine isolated systems and apply the findings accurately to movement patterns. Therefore, clinicians are encouraged to examine all systems through functional tasks to understand how the impaired neurological, musculoskeletal, and cognitive systems are affecting the client's movement. During the evaluation process, the clinician notes systems that are functioning normally, identifies abnormal components of movement, and determines appropriate interventions to optimize motor recovery.[17] The progressive nature of the disease necessitates ongoing evaluation followed by accommodating intervention.

Goal Setting

The functional deficits and objective neurological findings provide the clinician with valuable information to assess prognosis, establish goals, and determine a treatment plan. Despite the progressive nature of the disease, treatment goals should maximize the potential for function, introduce effective, task-oriented movement strategies, and offer multiple movement options.[17]

To set realistic and client-oriented goals, it is important for the clinician to envision where the patient will be at discharge based on present level of function, prognosis, and disease course, while considering client/caregiver personal goals. Appropriate goals range from comprehensive caregiver training to independent mobility with transition back to a work environment. Goals need to challenge the patient to attain an optimal level of function but must also allow for fluctuations in potential due to the disease process. Clients who have the potential to return to work may require additional intervention from neuropsychology, vocational rehabilitation, or a multidisciplinary day program, depending on the nature of their job and their deficits.

Functional Assessment

Because of the progressive nature of their disease, historically persons with primary malignant brain tumors have not been considered rehabilitation candidates. Physicians, health care providers, and third-party payers have questioned the efficacy of rehabilitation in this population because of poor prognoses and limited survival rates. However, advances in medical diagnosis and intervention are resulting in longer survival of people with multiple functional deficits that require rehabilitation. Functional assessment scales provide objective evidence that rehabilitation is effective and worthwhile for these clients.[55]

The functional assessment is a critical component in the development of the treatment intervention. It provides a method of analyzing deficits, compiling a problem list, developing a treatment plan, and measuring functional outcomes. The Functional Independence Measure (FIM) is a functional assessment tool used to measure degree of disability, regardless of underlying pathology, and burden of care to demonstrate functional outcomes of rehabilitation and assist clinicians with discharge planning.[18]

The use of functional outcome scales like the FIM provides a means of documenting the client's response to therapy intervention for clinicians, physicians, and third-party payers in the rehabilitation setting. Research utilizing FIM data demonstrates efficacy for inpatient rehabilitation of brain tumor clients similar to that noted in those with traumatic brain injury or stroke when matched by age, sex, and functional status on admission.[29, 45, 55]

Physicians utilize specific functional evaluation scales to measure the success of treatment. The Karnofsky performance scale, which rates patients' functional performance, is the tool most widely used in clinical research

and treatment decisions[31] (see Table 23–1). The client receives a score from 0 to 100 based on independence or level of assistance required for normal activity. The scale is used in research to evaluate an individual's physical response to treatment.[18, 31, 57, 79]

Side Effects and Considerations

Through advances in chemotherapy and radiation therapy, the ability to reduce tumor mass has greatly improved. Unfortunately, despite the often favorable long-term results of these treatments, the immediate effects create physical and psychological challenges for the client and clinician. Clients who are being treated aggressively during the rehabilitation phase will probably experience a decline in neurological or hematological status. These declines often limit the individual's tolerance for treatment intervention and increase client and caregiver feelings of depression and hopelessness. Clinicians have the opportunity to provide more than physical restorative services and should offer psychosocial support to enhance successful rehabilitation.[35]

The side effects and special considerations that arise with this population range from physical, to cognitive, to psychosocial and emotional. The following paragraphs relate the spectrum of complications and side effects the client may experience when undergoing medical treatment and the impact these may have on therapeutic intervention.

Not everyone undergoing chemotherapy or radiation treatment will experience physical side effects; the possibilities include hair loss, fatigue, nausea, skin burn or irritation, difficulty eating or digesting food, anorexia, and dry, sore mouth.[62, 65] The side effects are caused by the toxic effects the drugs have on healthy, rapidly dividing cells, including bone marrow cells, cells lining the mucosa, and hair cells.[3, 62]

The toxic effect chemotherapy has on bone marrow impairs the client's ability to produce red and white blood cells and platelets.[3] The client may develop anemia, infection, or a hemorrhage as a result of depressed hematological values.

The lining of the mouth, esophagus, and intestines may become inflamed and irritated and interfere with the ability to eat or digest food. The client may experience nausea, vomiting, diarrhea, or constipation, any of which will impair mobility and energy for daily activities.[65]

Hair loss is a common side effect of brain radiation and chemotherapy. This requires an especially difficult adjustment for most people because it causes a drastic change in appearance.[3]

Clinicians involved in the management of clients who are currently receiving radiation therapy or chemotherapy need to be mindful of these side effects when developing a plan of intervention. Fatigue, low blood count, and gastrointestinal complaints may limit a client's ability to fully participate in the planned therapy session or may call for a modification in activity or environment. Moreover, the clinician must utilize these factors to determine if the client's health or safety would be jeopardized by therapeutic intervention at any particular time. In addition, the clinician must be flexible in order to determine the optimal time when intervention is most effective and does not interfere with medications or meals.

Together with the physical side effects mentioned above, many clients with brain tumors have changes in cognition or personality as a result of the tumor's location. A patient with a frontal lobe tumor who was previously quiet and withdrawn may over time become loud and disinhibited as a result of tumor growth. Tumors that invade the speech language area cause communication and comprehension difficulties that create challenges for client and clinician. The client who has a left parietal tumor may be aphasic and not respond to verbal commands. In this case the clinician must engage in alternative means of communication or provide therapeutic facilitation with tactile cues only. An observant, critical analysis of the client's physical deficits and impaired communication, comprehension, and feedback mechanisms is essential in order to select an effective intervention plan that is client-specific.

Because of the emotionally charged nature of the disease process psychosocial and emotional issues frequently arise. Clinicians should be sensitive to fluctuations in temperament and mood that the diagnosis itself and subsequent treatment strategies create. Clinicians can offer psychosocial support and direct the client and family to resources that may give direction and guidance during difficult periods.

Intervention

The ultimate goal of rehabilitation is to achieve maximum restoration of function, within the limits imposed by the disease, in the client's preferred environment. The clinician must recognize that the physical, cognitive, and emotional status of these individuals is inconsistent and changing as a result of the disease process or medical intervention. Treatment plans must be flexible to effectively manage fluctuations in the client's presentation. A comprehensive rehabilitation plan is individualized to accommodate progressive changes in functional mobility and provides problem-solving experiences to prepare the client and caregiver for these situations. The rehabilitation process typically begins in the intensive care unit and continues throughout inpatient, outpatient, and home health settings.

In the intensive care unit, communication with nursing staff regarding the client's present medical status and an understanding of ICP, hemodynamic values, and monitoring devices is crucial to determining tolerance for therapy intervention (Fig. 23–4). For a ventriculostomy, a catheter is placed in the third ventricle to drain CSF and to monitor ICP. Mobilizing a patient with a ventriculostomy is possible, but nursing staff must close the drain prior to any positional change and should inform the clinician of appropriate treatment measures. A client's dependence upon these monitoring devices does not prevent therapeutic intervention, but the critical status of these individuals must be considered. The monitoring equipment provides constant feedback that assists the clinician in assessing the client's tolerance to activity and his or her ability to proceed with treatment.

As the client becomes more medically stable, the clinician upgrades mobility and prepares the client for the next stage of rehabilitation. Despite clients' decreased medical acuity in the rehabilitation setting, clinicians must continually reassess functional and neurological status and alert physicians to any changes. Clinicians spend many hours with clients during their rehabilitation stay. This day-to-day interaction gives the clinician the opportunity to connect with the client on a personal level and observe him or her in many settings. Intuitive therapists are often the first to notice physical, cognitive, and emotional changes. Communication to the physician of significant changes is imperative for appropriate follow-up procedures and referrals to provide optimal care.

In the inpatient rehabilitation setting, treatment focuses on optimizing functional capabilities to prepare the client and family for discharge. Integrating the client's personal goals and interests into therapeutic intervention invests the client and family in the rehabilitation process. The incorporation of these quality of life issues encourages the pursuit of a meaningful lifestyle upon discharge. If clinicians believe the client's goals are unrealistic, gentle redirection is necessary to channel energy toward achievable goals. Goals for inpatient rehabilitation range from returning the client to an independent lifestyle to training family to be caregivers in the home environment.

The restoration of previous functional movement patterns is desired. Literature reports increasing evidence that the CNS has dynamic properties, including neural

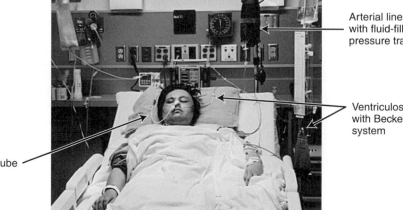

Arterial line with fluid-filled pressure transducer

Ventriculostomy with Becker drainage system

Duotube

FIGURE 23–4. A patient following a partial tumor resection. Labels indicate the equipment commonly seen in the neurological intensive care unit.

regeneration and collateral sprouting, which supports the concept of plasticity. Plasticity allows intact neural centers to recognize and assume functions of areas of the brain impaired or destroyed by the lesion or medical management.[39] The treatment focus may need to turn to compensatory strategies if the potential for motor recovery and learning is lacking. Once compensatory patterns are established, it is not clearly known whether recovery of normal movement will be achieved.[39] Compensatory techniques may be beneficial in increasing safety and efficiency with mobility and activities of daily living or in providing more independence for the client.[18] Increasing independence can assist in improving quality of life for the client and may permit return to work or participation in previous recreational activity.[18] For example, an avid golfer with right-sided hemiparesis and impaired standing balance can modify his clubs and return to the game at the wheelchair level.

The rehabilitation program should prepare the client and caregivers for an efficient transition from the structured care setting to the home. Utilizing motor learning principles to teach functional mobility will best produce transfer of learning from a constant environment to an unpredictable home environment. Repetitious practice of specific parts of a skill in fixed surroundings, with physical and verbal guidance throughout the movement, and frequent feedback during and following the completion of the task, is beneficial in teaching acquisition of a specific movement or activity.[11, 68, 69] Practicing the whole activity in a variable context, with irregular feedback and decreased physical and verbal guidance, expedites learning.[49, 09, 89]

Learning results in the ability to execute a task in any setting. Community outings and home passes naturally provide an environment that facilitates learning. The clinician can measure retention and transfer of learning by the client's performance in the community or at home. This information should be utilized to adjust the treatment plan and make recommendations for environmental modifications that minimize physical and cognitive demands on the client. A client whose individual treatment focus is transfers gains confidence when able to transfer from a wheelchair to a table chair in a crowded restaurant.

An interdisciplinary team approach is utilized for community reentry in order to provide a meaningful experience for the client. Recreational therapists play an integral part in identifying the individual's interests, reintegrating the client into the community, and modifying leisure activities to meet physical abilities. Activities addressed in daily therapy sessions are practiced in the community and feedback is provided to the appropriate clinician as well as the client. Initial reentry into the community can be intimidating to the client and may cause changes in the client's behavior which will affect mobility performance. Therefore, it is necessary for the clinician to be sensitive and recognize the issues the client may be experiencing.

In order for caregiver training and education to be successful a good rapport must be established between clinician, client, and the family members/caregivers. Caregiver training includes not only mobility training but edu-

cation regarding the effect the tumor may have on the client's present and future mobility. Instruction should be given based on present level of function, but the probability of progressive decline should not be overlooked. An intuitive clinician should offer effective techniques and problem-solving situations to address potential obstacles created by the disease process. For example, when performing transfer training the clinician may demonstrate a stand-pivot transfer, but may also suggest a squat-pivot transfer if physical or cognitive changes mandate increased assistance by the caregiver.

Discharge Planning

Discharge planning is initiated early, continues throughout the rehabilitation process, and must allow for changes in the client's functional status. Upon discharge from the rehabilitation setting, the client will make the transition to one of the following settings: home, skilled nursing facility, or hospice. The transition to home is typically preferred by the client, caregiver, and interdisciplinary rehabilitation team. If the client cannot be physically or medically managed at home, then placement in a skilled nursing facility may be necessary. The client may choose hospice care when medical treatment is no longer providing control of the tumor and the physical demands of the client are not manageable by the caregivers. The appropriate case management worker contacts insurance providers to determine coverage, and after conferring with the interdisciplinary team gives the client and family information regarding discharge options.

Client and caregiver training and education constitute an integral part of discharge planning. Prior to discharge, the client and caregiver should be instructed in functional mobility and activities of daily living, informed of equipment needs and vendor resources, and provided with community resources for support and education. During individual training, the clinician is able to provide feedback to the caregiver and client to facilitate an easier transition to home. Documentation of caregiver education and training should be included in the progress and discharge notes. A sample form for interdisciplinary documentation of education is provided in Figure 23–5.

Equipment necessary to assist the client and family with mobility and activities of daily living is recommended by the appropriate clinician. When ordering equipment, fluctuations in the client's present status, as well as the probable progressive decline in function, are considered. If the client is functioning without equipment at discharge, resources such as equipment vendors or local charitable organizations for future equipment needs should be provided.

Local community and national resources specific to brain tumors should also be provided before discharge. These resources can be found using the Internet, local phone book, or communication with previous patients, or other health care professionals familiar with these organizations. Support groups provide the caregiver and the client with an opportunity to share experiences and information, prevent isolation, foster hope, discover coping skills, and offer emotional support.[38] A study conducted to describe experiences and needs of clients with

**St. Joseph's Hospital
and Medical Center**
Mercy Healthcare Arizona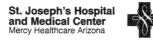

NEURO REHABILITATION UNIT

BRAIN TUMOR TEACHING GOALS

ADULT BRAIN TUMOR

* Please note: For the brain tumor patient who is able to completely or partially use his or her extremities and cognitive abilities, the emphasis on rehab is to maximize the patient's own ability to be independent. It is also to educate and teach the family or care giver appropriate care and safe assistance with the patient and his or her equipment. Efforts will be directed to facilitate the patient's return to home and to resume work (if able) in his or her community in the most efficient and practical manner possible for the patient and the family.

Initials = Full Name & Title

=	=	=
=	=	=
=	=	=

KEY

I	= Instructed	RD =	Return Demonstration	NI =	Not available for instruction
D	= Demonstrated	VD =	Verbally directs care	NA =	Not Applicable
C	= Comprehended	DC =	Discharge review		

FIGURE 23–5. Interdisciplinary education inventory for brain tumor teaching. (From Barrow Neurological Institute, St. Joseph's Hospital and Medical Center, Phoenix, AZ.)

PATIENT NAME: _____ DATE _____

NURSING

	PATIENT								CARE GIVER						
	I	D	C	RD	VD	DC	NI	NA	I	D	C	RD	DC	NI	NA

1. Anatomy and physiology of brain tumor
2. Application of braces-splints
3. Bowel elimination
4. Circulation
5. Depression / grieving
6. Family adjustment
7. Hydrocephalus
8. Medications
9. Nutrition
10. Safety
11. Seizures
12. Sensory stimulation
13. Skin integrity
14. Sexuality
15. Stress management
16. Tube feedings
17. Treatments
18. Urinary elimination
19. Other _____
20. Other _____

RESPIRATORY

	PATIENT								CARE GIVER						
	I	D	C	RD	VD	DC	NI	NA	I	D	C	RD	DC	NI	NA

1. CPR training
2. List emergency numbers
3. Suction (in hospital) - (in community)
4. Trach care
5. Other _____

OCCUPATIONAL THERAPY (OT)

UPPER EXTREMITY

	PATIENT								CARE GIVER						
	I	D	C	RD	VD	DC	NI	NA	I	D	C	RD	DC	NI	NA

1. R.O.M. - exercise
2. Positioning
3. Splinting

SELF CARE

	PATIENT								CARE GIVER						
	I	D	C	RD	VD	DC	NI	NA	I	D	C	RD	DC	NI	NA

1. Swallowing
2. Self-feeding
3. Hygiene

FIGURE 23–5 *Continued*

Illustration continued on following page

PATIENT NAME: _____ DATE _____

OCCUPATIONAL THERAPY (OT)

4. Bathing
5. Dressing
6. Adaptive equipment - vendors
7. Home management
8. Cooking

TRANSFERS

1. Toilet - Commode
2. Tub - Shower

PHYSICAL THERAPY (PT)

1. Range of motion exercise
2. Bed mobility
3. Bed transfers
4. Car transfers
5. Wheelchair mobility and management
6. Ambulation
7. Safety precautions
8. Equipment vendor resources
9. Other _____

SPEECH LANGUAGE PATHOLOGY

1. Aphasia
2. Dysarthria
3. Dysphagia
4. Cognitive deficits due to tumor- surgical area
5. Cognitive deficits (generalized)
6. Other _____

THERAPEUTIC RECREATION

1. Community re-entry skills

   _____
2. Community leisure referrals

   _____
3. Adapted recreation resources and or referrals

   _____
4. Community mobility skills

   _____

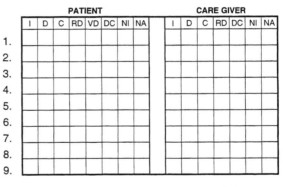

FIGURE 23–5 *Continued*

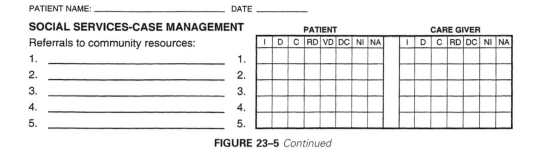

PATIENT NAME: _____ DATE _____

SOCIAL SERVICES-CASE MANAGEMENT

Referrals to community resources:

	PATIENT								CARE GIVER						
	I	D	C	RD	VD	DC	NI	NA	I	D	C	RD	DC	NI	NA
1.															
2.															
3.															
4.															
5.															

FIGURE 23–5 *Continued*

brain tumors found that "attendance and participation in a support group empowers people to seek the most out of life following a brain tumor diagnosis."[38] National organizations (see the accompanying box) can provide educational information and support to clients. These organizations can assist the client to find local resources unfamiliar to the clinician.

Hospice Care

A time may come when traditional tumor treatment is ineffective and local control is no longer expected. Patient and family must make a decision regarding the living environment and type of care desired. One option available is hospice care. In the United States, the hospice movement in health care has evolved to include specific standards, licensure requirements, and certification. Providing physical, emotional, and psychosocial support to patients and their families in their final days is the intent of hospice care.[71] The hospice recognizes the impact terminal illness has on a patient's family system, and the demands, both physical and emotional, it places on the caregiver.[15] The use of the hospice implies a wholistic approach that allows families the opportunity to be di-

rectly involved in the patient's care, and encourages the expression of grief, love, support, and acceptance.

Inpatient hospice facilities provide continuous nursing care in a structured, supervised environment. Hospice services in these facilities offer ongoing pastoral counseling and emotional support to patient and family. However, if patient and family prefer, hospice care can be provided in the patient's home, with home health aides and nursing giving limited physical care or providing respite care.

Typically, mobility and caregiver training for the hospice patient are addressed by a therapist earlier in the patient's disease process. However, positioning, range of motion, and pain relief are important to the patient's continued comfort throughout the course of the disease and in any setting.

PSYCHOSOCIAL CARE

With many clients with brain tumors living extended lives, it is important to measure the efficacy of treatment not only in terms of functional outcome but also in terms of its effect on quality of life. Quality of life is the individual's subjective sense of well-being as a whole and has been studied closely in the treatment of clients with brain tumor.[79] Quality of life is a multifaceted concept encompassing emotional and physical well-being, life satisfaction, material wealth, meaning of life, coping mechanisms, and social network. A single assessment to comprehensively evaluate a person's quality of life does not exist. Therefore, a multidimensional approach incorporating multiple assessment tools is necessary.[21, 79] Some of these tools include the Functional Living Index, the Karnofsky performance scale, the Index of Independence in Activity of Daily Living, the State-Trait Anxiety Inventory, and the Self-Rating Depression Scale.[21]

The development of a strong supportive relationship with client and caregivers is key to successful rehabilitation. This process begins with respecting the client's unique experience and involves continually evaluating and addressing his or her changing psychosocial needs.[40] The clinician must feel invested, demonstrate good communication skills, and exhibit self-confidence in discussing sensitive issues for a caring relationship to develop. By actively listening, the clinician can identify the client's true concerns and feelings and assist the client and family in coping with the cancer experience.[40] The clinician's consistent interaction with the client can foster a supportive and safe environment in which emotional and spiritual feelings can be shared. Once a trusting relationship is established, the clinician's empathy can help decrease

NATIONAL ORGANIZATIONS

The Brain Tumor Society
124 Watertown St., Suite 3-H
Watertown, MA 02472
(617) 924-9997
http://www.tbts.org
e-mail: info@tbts.org

American Brain Tumor Association
2720 River Rd.
Des Plaines, IL 60018
(847) 827-9910
http://www.abta.org
e-mail: info@abta.org

National Brain Tumor Foundation
414 Thirteenth Street, Suite 700
Oakland, CA 94612-2603
(510) 839-9777
http://www.braintumor.org
e-mail: nbtf@braintumor.org

common feelings of isolation and helplessness and support the client through the different stages of the disease.[40]

Hope is a key psychosocial need of the individual with cancer. It is an important coping strategy that can help clients with brain tumors face an uncertain and often fearful future. Hope gives the client something to look forward to each day. Clinicians can create a hopeful environment by encouraging clients to share their expectations, identify realistic short-term goals, and acknowledge hopes even if unrealistic. It is important to recognize that hope must be balanced with reality and honest disclosure regarding diagnosis and prognosis.[40, 75]

Psychological and social problems are not identified in 80% of physically ill persons possibly owing to clinicians' personal behaviors or beliefs. Clinicians may find it easier to focus on the physical aspect of care to avoid becoming emotional or experiencing the client's distress. Persons with cancer often experience feelings of powerlessness and isolation, which may be increased by distancing behaviors demonstrated by clinicians. Before offering support to clients, clinicians need to examine their own thoughts, feelings, and past experiences with death and dying. This awareness may prevent the clinician from internalizing the client's grief, from protecting the client and family members from the pain of grieving, and from allowing personal values to influence adversely their psychosocial support.[75]

By recognizing that psychosocial care involves wholistic healing, clinicians will be able to develop the best environment for interventions to successfully optimize multiple aspects of the client's quality of life.[75]

SUMMARY

It is important for the clinician involved in the treatment of a client with a brain tumor to anticipate the functional limitations that will develop as a result of the medical intervention or the tumor itself. These limitations provide the foundation for treatment planning and goal setting. Improved quality of life is the goal of the rehabilitation process. This means restoring the client to maximal functional capacity with the least amount of assistance from others. Regardless of the client's life expectancy, the rehabilitation process should enable the client to pursue a productive and meaningful life.

CASE STUDY 23–1   MEDICAL DIAGNOSIS: LOW-GRADE ASTROCYTOMA

Mrs. S is a 46-year-old woman diagnosed 9 years ago with a low-grade astrocytoma in the right posterior frontal lobe. Prior to this diagnosis, she had a 4-year history of seizures. She underwent a partial resection of a microcystic pilocystic astrocytoma. Postoperatively, medical management focused on controlling seizure activity, and radiation theapy or chemotherapy was not provided. Physically, she presented with resultant left foot weakness and minor seizures characterized by tingling numbness and tremors in the left foot. She was able to continue to work, but a career change was necessary owing to cognitive changes, including inability to perform fast calculations, impaired memory, and decreased recall.

Three years later scans revealed tumor enlargement and Mrs. S underwent Peacock radiation therapy. She remained independent for an additional 2 years. Two weeks ago, she presented with left facial weakness, progressive left hemiparesis, and hyperreflexia on the left side. MRI scans revealed a lesion in the right midcerebral hemisphere below the original tumor site. A stereotactic biopsy confirmed a diagnosis of glioblastoma multiforme. She then underwent a gross total tumor resection, received Gamma knife radiosurgery, and was subsequently treated with chemotherapy.

Mrs. S was admitted to the neurological rehabilitation unit for comprehensive rehabilitation. During the examination, it was noted that her speech was fluent and she tended to be hyperverbal, distractible, and perseverative. Manual muscle testing revealed functional strength in the right hemibody and 0/5 strength in the left hemibody except for hip flexion of 2−/5. Decreased sensation to light touch and proprioception in the left hemibody was noted. Because of left seventh cranial nerve involvement causing left homonymous hemianopsia, severe left-sided neglect and right gaze preference was noted. These visual-perceptual deficits greatly impaired her mobility. She was able to attend to the left side with maximal cues, but carryover was not observed.

Functionally, Mrs. S required moderate assistance to assume sitting on the edge of the bed, where she demonstrated fair sitting balance. Owing to poor standing balance, she required maximal assistance to stand and pivot to her wheelchair. In standing, her head was rotated to the right and flexed, her pelvis was rotated to the right, her hips were flexed, her left knee was buckled, and her left foot was inverted. She was able to ambulate 15 feet in the parallel bars with maximal assistance to address these postural impairments and to advance the left leg. She was able to propel her wheelchair with her right arm and leg with much assistance and encouragement.

Mrs. S refuses to use a wheelchair at home because her goal is to walk. She is married with three children and lives in a single-story house. Her husband works full-time, necessitating independent and safe mobility to return home. Mrs. S and her family demonstrate poor understanding of her prognosis and express unrealistic goals. They frequently refer to her previous return to independence following her first resection and expect a similar outcome this time.

(Continued)

CASE STUDY 23–1 MEDICAL DIAGNOSIS: LOW-GRADE ASTROCYTOMA *Continued*

The clinician, in consideration of the client's goal to walk, incorporated standing, pregait, and gait training into treatment sessions. However, Mrs. S was encouraged to propel her wheelchair as a means of independent mobility on the unit. A knee-ankle-foot orthosis (KAFO) was fabricated to provide stability in the left leg and assist her in walking again.

Two weeks into her rehabilitation program, Mrs. S began to demonstrate increased lethargy, decreased ability to participate in treatments, and increased weakness. She required more assistance with mobility. The clinician modified the treatment intervention to an appropriate yet challenging level. Sitting balance and transfers became the focus rather than standing balance and gait. The therapy team notified the physician of these changes and the client was transferred to acute care. She underwent additional surgery to drain a cyst and remove necrotic tissue within the tumor.

Upon her return to rehabilitation Mrs. S became more alert and able to participate in therapy sessions. She and her family express hope that this surgery will cure the tumor. The clinician expresses encouragement but gently reminds the client and family members that while the drainage of the cyst may allow for functional improvements, the tumor is still present. The client's strength continues to improve and functional gains are observed. In gait, her left leg is now able to stabilize during the stance phase; however, an Ace bandage is necessary to control footdrop. The client is able to ambulate household distances with minimal assistance.

The interdisciplinary team has provided the client and family with the appropriate resources to choose a facility where Mrs. S can continue her therapy and the family can easily visit. They have also been provided with referrals regarding support groups and hospice care if needed in the future. At the time of discharge, Mrs. S was delighted with her ability to walk but is disappointed that her left arm remains flaccid and that she is not returning home. The client and family continue to search for hope daily, but leave with a better understanding of the poor prognosis.

REFERENCES

1. Adams RD, Victor M, Ropper AH: Principles of Neurology, 6th ed. New York, McGraw-Hill Information Services, 1997.
2. Alexander M, Friedrich WK, Gerhard AH: Surgery and radiotherapy compared with Gamma knife radiosurgery in the treatment of solitary brain metastases of small diameter, J Neurosurg 91:35–43, 1999.
3. A Primer of Brain Tumors. Des Plaines, IL, American Brain Tumor Association, 1998.
4. Bindal RK, et al: Surgical treatment of multiple brain metastases. J Neurosurg 79:210–216, 1993.
5. Black P, Wen PY: Clinical, imaging and laboratory diagnosis of brain tumors. *In* Kaye AH, Laws ER (eds): Brain Tumors. New York, Churchill Livingstone, 1997.
6. Black PM, et al: Development and implementation of intra-operative magnetic resonance imaging and its surgical applications, Neurosurgery 41:831–845, 1997.
7. Brock CS, et al: Phase I trial of temozolomide using an extended continuous oral schedule. Cancer Res 58:4363–4367, 1998.
8. Buatti JM, et al: Linac radiosurgery for high grade gliomas: The University of Florida experience. Int J Radiat Oncol Biol Phys 32:205–210, 1995.
9. Byrne TN: Imaging of gliomas. Semin Oncol 21:162–171, 1994.
10. Cancer statistics 1998. CA Cancer J Clin 48:10–27, 1998.
11. Carr JH, et al: Movement Science: Foundations for Physical Therapy in Rehabilitation. Rockville, MD, Aspen, 1987.
12. Chang Y, Horoupian DS: Pathology of benign brain tumors. *In* Morantz RA, Walsh JW (eds): Brain Tumors: A Comprehensive Text. New York, Marcel Dekker, 1994.
13. Color Me Hope, 3rd ed. Boston, Brain Tumor Society, 1997.
14. Desmeules M, Mikkelson T, Mao Y: Increasing incidence of primary malignant brain tumors: Influence of diagnostic methods. J Natl Cancer Inst 84:442–445, 1992.
15. Enyert G, Burman M: A qualitative study of self-transcendence in caregivers of terminally ill patients. Am J Hospice Palliative Care 16:455–462, 1999.
16. Fiedler JA: Physical aspects of stereotactic radiosurgery. BNI Q 13:11–21, 1997.
17. Fisher B, Yakura J: Movement analysis: A different perspective. Orthop Phys Ther Clin North Am 2:1–4, 1993.
18. Freeman G: Brain tumors. *In* Umphred D (ed): Neurological Rehabilitation, 3rd ed. St. Louis, Mosby, 1994.
19. Gannett D, et al: Stereotactic radiosurgery as an adjunct to surgery and external beam radiotherapy in the treatment of patients with malignant gliomas. Int J Radiat Oncol Biol Phys 33:461–468, 1995.
20. Gillen G, Burkhardt A: Stroke Rehabilitation: A Function-Based Approach. St. Louis, Mosby, 1998.
21. Giovagnoli AR, Tamburini M, Boiardi A: Quality of life in brain tumor patients. J Neurooncol 30:71–80, 1996.
22. Grant R: Oligodendroglioma and oligoastrocytoma. *In* Gilman S, Goldstein G, Waxman S (eds): Neurobase. San Diego, Arbor Publishing Corporation, 1996.
23. Greenberg HS, Chandler WF, Sandler HM: Brain Tumors. New York, Oxford University Press, 1999.
24. Grossman SA, et al: Familial gliomas: The potential role of environmental exposures. Proc Am Soc Clin Oncol 14:149, 1995.
25. Hakim R, et al: Results of linear accelerator based radiosurgery for intra-cranial meningiomas. Neurosurgery 42:446–453, 1998.
26. Hall WA, et al: Stereotactic radiosurgery for recurrent malignant gliomas. J Clin Oncol 13:1642–1648, 1995.
27. Hall WA, et al: Brain biopsy using high-field strength interventional magnetic resonance imaging. Neurosurgery 44:807–813, 1999.
28. Hill JR, et al: Molecular genetics of brain tumors. Arch Neurol 56:439–441, 1999.
29. Huang ME, Cifu DX, Keyser-Marcus L: Functional outcome after brain tumor and acute stroke: A comparative analysis. Arch Phys Med Rehabil 79:1386–1390, 1998.
30. Kahn D, et al: Diagnosis of recurrent brain tumor: Value of 210T1 SPECT vs F-fluorodeoxyglucose PET. AJR Am J Roentgenol 163:1459–1465, 1994.
31. Karnofsky DA, Burchenal JH: The clinical evaluation of chemotherapeutic agents in cancer. *In* Macleod C (ed): Evaluation of Chemotherapeutic Agents. New York, Columbia University Press, 1949.
32. Kleihues P, Burger PC, Scheithauer BW: Histological Typing of the Tumours of the Central Nervous System. World Health Organization. Berlin, Springer-Verlag, 1993.
33. Kondziolka D, et al: Long term outcomes after meningioma radiosurgery: Physician and patient perspectives. J Neurosurg 91:44–50, 1999.
34. Kornblith PL, Walker MD, Cassady JR: Neurologic Oncology. Philadelphia, JB Lippincott, 1987.
35. Kuchler T, Wood-Dauphinee S: Working with people who have cancer: Guidelines for physical therapists. Physiother Cancer 43:19–23, 1991.
36. Laing RW, et al: Efficacy and toxicity of fractionated stereotactic

radiosurgery in the treatment of recurrent gliomas (phase I/II study). Radiother Oncol 27:22–29, 1993.

37. Lavine SD, Petrovich Z, Cohen-Gadol AA: Gamma knife radiosurgery for metastatic melanoma: An analysis of survival, outcome, and complications. Neurosurgery 44:59–64, 1999.

38. Leavitt MB, Lamb SA, Voss BS: Brain tumor support group: Content themes and mechanisms of support. Oncol Nurs Forum 23:1247–1256, 1996.

39. Levere TE: Recovery of function after brain damage: A theory of the behavioral deficit. Physiol Psychol 8:297–308, 1980.

40. Loney M: Death, dying and grief in the face of cancer. In Sigler B (ed): Psychosocial Dimensions of Oncology Nursing Care. Pittsburgh, Oncology Nursing Press, 1998.

41. Lossignol D, Grossman SA, Sheidler UR, et al: Familial clustering of malignant astrocytoma. J Neurooncol 9:139–145, 1990.

42. Lunsford LD: Contemporary management of meningiomas: Radiation therapy as an adjuvant and radiosurgery as an alternative to surgical removal? J Neurosurg 80:187–190, 1994.

43. Lunsford LD, Coffey RJ: Stereotactic surgery in the diagnosis and therapy of malignant intra-cranial gliomas. In Apuzzo MLJ (ed): Malignant Cerebral Glioma. Park Ridge, IL. American Association of Neurological Surgeons, 1990.

44. Lunsford LD, et al: Gamma knife stereotactic radiosurgery for acoustic neuromas: What we have learned. Neurosurgeons 14:164–169, 1995.

45. Marciniak CM, et al: Functional outcome following rehabilitation of the cancer patient. Arch Phys Med Rehabil 77:54–57, 1996.

46. Mark SJ, et al: Oligodendroglioma: Incidence and biological behavior in a defined population. J Neurosurg 63:881–889, 1985.

47. Masciopinto JE, et al: Stereotactic radiosurgery for glioblastoma: A final report of 31 patients. J Neurosurg 82:530–535, 1995.

48. McCarthy BT, et al: Factors associated with survival in patients with meningioma. J Neurosurg 88:831–839, 1998.

49. McCracken HD, Stelmach GE: A test of the schema theory of discrete motor learning. J Motor Behav 9:193–201, 1977.

50. Mehta MP, et al: Stereotactic radiosurgery for glioblastoma multiforme: Report of a prospective study evaluating prognostic factors and analyzing long term survival advantage. Int J Radiat Oncol Biol Phys 30:541–549, 1994.

51. Mennel H: Grading of intracranial tumors following the WHO classification systems. Neurosurg Rev 14:249–260, 1991.

52. Meyerand ME, et al: Classification of biopsy-confirmed brain tumors using single-voxel MR spectroscopy. AJNR Am J Neuroradiol 20:117–123, 1999.

53. Morantz RA, Walsh JW: Brain Tumors: A Comprehensive Text. New York, Marcel Dekker, 1994.

54. Norfray JF, et al: Clinical impact of MR spectroscopy when MR imaging is indeterminate for pediatric brain tumors. AJR Am J Roentgenol 173:119–125, 1999.

55. O'Dell MW, et al: Functional outcome of inpatient rehabilitation in persons with brain tumors. Arch Phys Med Rehabil 79:1530–1534, 1998.

56. Ojemann, RG: Surgical principles in the management of brain tumors. In Kaye AH, Law ER (eds): Brain Tumors. New York, Churchill Livingstone, 1997.

57. O'Toole DM, Golden AM: Evaluating cancer patients for rehabilitation potential. West J Med 155:384–387, 1991.

58. Patchell RA: Brain metastases. Neurol Clin 9:817–824, 1991.

59. Pizzo PA, Poplack DG, Bleyer WA: Neurotoxicities of current leukemia therapy. Am J of Pediatr Hematol Oncol 1:127–140, 1979.

60. Rabb CH, Apuzzo MLJ: Stereotaxis in the diagnosis and management of brain tumors. In Kaye AH, Laws ER (eds): Brain Tumors. New York, Churchill Livingstone, 1997.

61. Radhakrishman K, et al: The trends in incidence of primary brain tumors in the population of Rochester, Minnesota. Ann Neurol 37:67–73, 1995.

62. Radiation Therapy and You: A Guide to Self-Help During Treatment, revised ed. Bethesda, MD, National Cancer Institute, National Institutes of Health, 1993.

63. Ricci PE, et al: Differentiating recurrent tumor from radiation necrosis: Time for re-evaluation of positron emission tomography? AJNR Am J Neuroradiol 19:407–413, 1998.

64. Ries LG, et al (eds): SEER Cancer Statistics Review 1973–1996. Bethesda, MD, National Cancer Institute, 1999.

65. Rottenburg DA: Neurological Complications of Cancer Treatment. Boston, Butterworth-Heinemann, 1991.

66. Rowland LP: Merrit's Textbook of Neurology, 9th ed. Baltimore, Williams & Wilkins, 1995.

67. Salcman M: Epidemiology and factors affecting survival. In Apuzzo MLJ (ed): Malignant Cerebral Glioma. Park Ridge, IL. American Association of Neurological Surgeons, 1990.

68. Schmidt RA: A schema theory of discrete motor skill learning. Psychol Rev 82:225–259, 1975.

69. Schumway-Cook A, Woolcott MH: Motor Control Theory and Practical Applications. Baltimore, Williams & Wilkins, 1995.

70. Segall HD, et al: CT and MR imaging in malignant gliomas. In Apuzzo MLJ (ed): Malignant Cerebral Glioma. Park Ridge, IL. American Association of Neurological Surgeons, 1990.

71. Shaw EG, et al: Oligodendrogliomas: The Mayo Clinic experience. J Neurosurg 76:428–434, 1992.

72. Shetter AG: Gamma knife radiosurgery for the treatment of acoustic neuromas. BNI Q 13:30–36, 1997.

73. Shrieve DC, Alexander E, Wen PY: Comparison of stereotactic radiosurgery and brachytherapy in the treatment of recurrent glioblastoma multiforme. Neurosurgery 36:275–282, 1995.

74. Simpson DA, Pitorak E: Hospice or palliative care? Am J Hospice Palliative Care 15:122–123, 1998.

75. Sivesind DM, Rohaly-Davis JA: Coping with cancer: Patient issues. In Sigler B (ed): Psychosocial Dimensions of Oncology Nursing Care. Pittsburgh, Oncology Nursing Press, 1998.

76. Smalley SR, et al: Resection for solitary brain metastases. J Neurosurg 77:531–540, 1992.

77. Smith KA: Metastatic brain tumors: Gamma knife radiosurgery or microsurgical resection. BNI Q 13:22–29, 1997.

78. Speiser B: Gamma knife stereotactic radiosurgery: An overview. BNI Q 13:4–10, 1997.

79. Stewart-Amidei C, et al: Quality of life in the neuro-oncology patient: A symposium. J Neurosci Nurs 27:219–223, 1995.

80. Subach BR, Kondziolka D, Lunsford LD: Stereotactic radiosurgery in the management of acoustic neuromas associated with neurofibromatosis Type 2. J Neurosurg 90:815–822, 1999.

81. Surawicz T, et al: Brain tumor survival: Results from the National Cancer Data Base. J Neurooncol 40:151–160, 1998.

82. Surawicz T, et al: Descriptive epidemiology of primary brain and CNS tumors: Results from the Central Brain Tumor Registry of the US 1990–1994. J Neurooncology 41:14–25, 1999.

83. Sutton LN, et al: Prognostic factors in childhood ependymomas. Pediatr Neurosurg 16:57–65, 1990–1991.

84. Thomas GT, Gill SS, Wilson C: Current and future utilization of PET scanning in the evaluation and management of malignant cerebral glioma. In Apuzzo MLJ (ed): Malignant Cerebral Glioma. Park Ridge, IL. American Association of Neurological Surgeons, 1990.

85. Thomas T, Inskip P: Brain and other nervous system. In Cancer Rates and Risks, 4th ed. Publication No. 96-691. Bethesda, MD, National Cancer Institute, 1996.

86. United States Population Estimates by Age from Census Data 1992–1997. Chicago, Central Brain Tumor Registry of the United States, 2000.

87. Williams J, et al: Stereotactic radiosurgery for brain metastases: Comparison of lung carcinoma v. non-lung tumors. J Neurooncol 37:79–85, 1998.

88. Williams J, et al: Stereotactic radiosurgery for human glioma: Treatment parameter and outcome for low vs. high grade. J Radiosurg 1:3–8, 1998.

89. Winstein CJ: Knowledge of results and motor learning implications for physical therapy. Phys Ther 71:140–149, 1991.

Movement Dysfunction Associated with Cerebellar Problems

MARSHA E. MELNICK, PhD, PT • BARBARA OREMLAND, MEd, PT

Key Words

– cerebellum

– motor control

– movement dysfunction

– therapeutic examination

– therapeutic intervention

Objectives

After reading this chapter the student/therapist will:

1. Understand the anatomy, physiology, and function of the cerebellum.

2. Identify the signs and symptoms of cerebellar disorders.

3. Explain the physiology responsible for the clinical presentation of patients with cerebellar disorders.

4. Understand the relationship between the cerebellum and other parts of the brain and how the important feedback loops affect movement.

5. Select an appropriate treatment technique for the patient with a cerebellar disorder.

The signs of cerebellar disease are seen in specific diseases as well as in head trauma, cerebrovascular accidents, multiple sclerosis, and the like. All involve disorganization of movement, especially rapid movement, and a decrease in balance and central postural control. Cerebellar symptoms are also very common in the late stages of alcoholism and for this reason, alcoholism is discussed in this chapter. Additionally there is a loss of motor learning, perhaps the most devastating symptom. In this chapter, the anatomy, physiology, and common disorders of the cerebellum are presented, as well as examination and treatment suggestions for the specific symptoms of loss of cerebellar neurons and connections.

The word *cerebellum* means "little brain" and yet this region of the brain contains more neurons than all the rest of the brain put together. This "little brain" also has a large role in motor control and motor learning. Loss of the cerebellum or its connections with the remainder of

the brain results in many well-known motor problems that are often difficult for the therapist and the physician to treat.

OVERVIEW OF CEREBELLAR ANATOMY AND PHYSIOLOGY

The cerebellum is a highly organized, three-layered structure. Traditionally, it is divided into three parts: the vestibulocerebellum (archicerebellum), with connections predominantly to the vestibular system; the spinocerebellum (paleocerebellum), with connections predominantly to the ascending somatosensory tracts of the spinal cord; and the cerebropontocerebellum (neocerebellum), with connections to the cerebral cortex, primarily through the nuclei in the pons. Connections with lower structures are ipsilateral; those with the cortex and other brain struc-

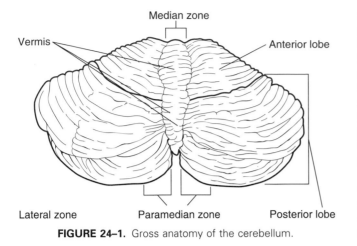

Median zone

Vermis

Anterior lobe

Lateral zone   Paramedian zone   Posterior lobe

FIGURE 24–1. Gross anatomy of the cerebellum.

tures are contralateral. Therefore the cerebellum affects the ipsilateral side of the body. The cerebellum communicates with the rest of the brain through three pairs of deep cerebellar nuclei: the fastigial, interposed, and dentate nuclei. The deep cerebellar nuclei are the structures that communicate with the rest of the brain. (This general organization is similar to the basal ganglia in that there is an afferent portion of the system and an efferent portion.) Connections between the cerebellum and the rest of the brain occur in three large bundles: the superior, middle, and inferior cerebellar peduncles. The gross anatomy of the cerebellum is presented in Figure 24–1. A magnetic resonance image (MRI) of the cerebellum is shown in Figure 24–2.

Input to the cerebellum is rapid; there are few synapses between the projection areas and the specific cerebellar location receiving the input. The cerebellum receives input regarding head, trunk, and extremity position and

movement, as well as extensive input from the cerebral cortex regarding the motor command. Its connections, therefore, allow it to compare ongoing movement with the motor command. Input to the cerebellum greatly exceeds output, which denotes that this is an integrative structure. Based upon the anatomical connections of the cerebellum, it is involved in balance and eye movements (vestibular and cerebropontocerebellum), integration of proprioceptive information (spinocerebellum) control of voluntary movement (cerebropontocerebellum and spinocerebellum), and learning (all areas).[52]

The cellular organization of the cerebellar cortex is very precise. There are three layers with only five neuronal types. There is only one neuron that leaves the cerebellar cortex, the large Purkinje cell, which is inhibitory to the deep cerebellar nuclei and to the vestibular nuclei. All input to the cerebellar cortex is excitatory and is through either climbing fibers from the inferior olivary complex in the medulla or via mossy fibers from everywhere else. The climbing fibers wrap around a Purkinje cell and form many synapses as they climb their way up the dendritic tree. A climbing fiber contacts only a few Purkinje cells (1 to 10) and each Purkinje cell receives input from only one climbing fiber. This unique relationship will be important as we discuss the motor learning and cognitive functions of the cerebellum. Anatomical research indicates that the interactions between the climbing fibers and the Purkinje cells are somatotopically arranged, as is the output of the Purkinje cells. Mossy fibers on the other hand are distributed to many thousands of Purkinje cells via parallel fibers. The circuitry of the cerebellum is such that a strip of Purkinje cells is activated as those on either side of it are inhibited. This lateral inhibition is provided by the interneurons in the cerebellar cortex.[52]

The Purkinje cells send inhibitory input to the deep

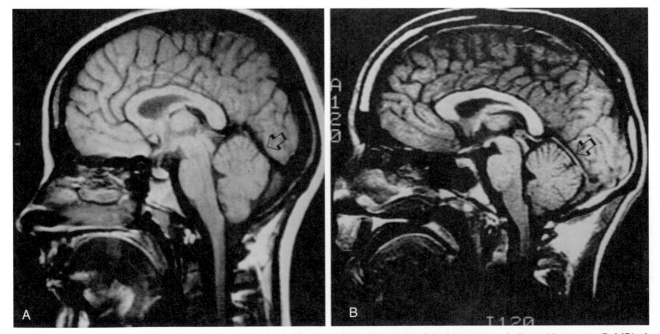

FIGURE 24–2. *A,* Magnetic resonance imaging (MRI) of normal cerebellum. Note full solid white area as indicated by arrow. *B,* MRI of spinocerebellar atrophy. Note dark and branching areas of cerebellum as indicated by arrow, which denotes atrophy.

cerebellar and vestibular nuclei. The output of the deep cerebellar nuclei is excitatory. The combinations of inhibition and excitation have led to the description of the cerebellum as a base 2 computer. It is exceedingly simple yet allows rapid information processing. We prefer the description of the cerebellum as a player piano, which can play complex music through the precise location and sequence of holes in the card.[52]

Physiological investigations support the functions of the cerebellum in movement and motor control. Recent studies of the activity of the cerebellum during movement also link the cerebellum with changes associated with plasticity of learning as well as emotions. The cerebellum is vital in environmental adaptation and if this structure is lost, it is likely that adaptation will be permanently lost or severely impaired. One hypothesis for the adaptive ability of the cerebellum comes from experiments by Llinas[63] who was able to demonstrate synchronous firing in Purkinje cells, and also in the olivary complex, that may enable cooperative behavior among Purkinje cells. These enclaves of cooperativity change as the motor behavior requires changes. Another important finding linking the cerebellum to learning is a process known as "long-term depression." In long-term depression there is a reduction in the response to subsequent excitatory input. Long-term depression appears to be very selective in the cerebellum[48] and also time-dependent, but it can last for hours. It is dependent upon a large influx of calcium which occurs with climbing fiber synapses. The specific anatomical areas of the cerebellum will now be discussed briefly with some indication of their clinical significance.

The vestibulocerebellum receives input from the inner ear, from both the semicircular canals and the utricle and saccule, and relays information to the vestibular nuclei. Outside of the deep cerebellar nuclei, the vestibular nuclei are the only areas in the brain to receive direct input from the Purkinje cells. Lesions of the vestibulocerebellum, as might be expected, lead to difficulty with maintenance of balance as well as inability to coordinate the eyes with head movements.[23] Movement in the distal parts of the extremities is difficult to execute without the ability to maintain balance. The person with dysfunction in the vestibulocerebellum is able to control the extremities in a supported (e.g., supine) position.

The spinocerebellum receives input from the spinal cord, especially from the proprioceptors within the muscles, namely the muscle spindle and Golgi tendon organs. The spinocerebellum also receives information from the cortex regarding the motor command. Input from the lower extremities is greater than that from the upper extremities. The input is somatotopically arranged and there are two maps of the body. In these maps the trunk is represented in the medial cerebellum; this portion projects to the fastigial nucleus and to the vestibular nuclei. These projections eventually make their way to the portion of the motor cortex that controls proximal musculature. Thus, the medial cerebellum is involved in control of posture and balance.[17] There is also limb control from the more lateral portions of the spinocerebellum, which project to the interposed nuclei (globose and emboliform in the primate) and then to the red nucleus and the motor cortex (via the thalamus). The input from

the spinal cord travels to the cerebellum via two pathways, the dorsal and ventral spinocerebellar tracts. The dorsal spinocerebellar tract relays precise information on individual muscle activity and provides sensory feedback during movements. The ventral spinocerebellar tract, on the other hand, appears to be more related to internally generated processes involved in rhythmical automatic movement such as walking and other centrally generated patterns of movement. The spinocerebellum is in a position to compare the ongoing movements (inputs from the muscles and joints) with the intended movements (input from the cortex), both rhythmical patterns and precise voluntary movements. Posture and gait disturbances are therefore seen when the function of the spinocerebellum is impaired.[17, 52]

Lesions of the spinocerebellum produce many of the symptoms seen in persons with cerebellar disease. One such problem is hypotonia. This is hypothesized to occur because of decreased excitation of the red nucleus and motor cortex and in turn a decreased activation of motor neurons excited by the rubrospinal and corticospinal pathways.

The interpositus nucleus is strongly related to properties of ongoing movement rather than those of intended movement.[12, 99, 101] A disruption of the interposed nuclei decreases the accuracy of reaching movements because of loss of control of the direction, extent, force, and timing of the movement. This is what is seen clinically as dysmetria.

Joint movements, especially multijoint movements, lose control in a way that movements tend to be curved instead of straight. This lack of precision and coordination is known as ataxia. Corrections of these imprecise or ataxic movements lead to further errors of timing and extent which increases the ataxia, further increasing the error, and so on. The result is an oscillation at the end of a movement, an intention tremor. Unlike the tremor of Parkinson disease, which occurs at rest, a cerebellar tremor occurs at the end of the movement. Oscillation at the end of movement is also seen in the deep tendon reflexes and although the response to a tendon tap may be normal, the limb moves in a pendular manner after the initial response.

The cerebropontocerebellum is involved in complex motor tasks as well as performance of perceptual and cognitive tasks. It is this region of the cerebellum that has undergone the largest phylogenetic growth. It receives input from the cortex through the pontine nuclei and projects back to the cortex, primarily the motor cortex, via the dentate nucleus and the ventrolateral nucleus of the thalamus. There is also a projection from the dentate to the red nucleus and inferior olive. Discharge of the dentate nucleus appears to be tightly related to properties of intended movements as well as to properties of ongoing movement.[12] Imaging of the brain indicates that these loops, especially the cerebellar-red nucleus-inferior olive-cerebellar loop, are especially active during the mental rehearsal of a movement.

Lesions of the cerebropontocerebellum lead to a decomposition of movement. As in lesions of the spinocerebellum, there is a disruption in the timing of movements. Instead of several aspects of the movement being sequenced together, each part of the movement is sequenced separately. These disturbances are especially important in hand function. Loss of the dentate nucleus also leads to a slowing of reaction time and delayed initiation of movement. Single-unit recording studies have shown that the dentate nucleus is active prior to activation of electromyographic (EMG) activity.[22, 93, 103, 104] There has been some thought that the cerebellum is especially important in initiation of rapid (i.e., ballistic) movements.

Timing of movements is but one of the deficits that occurs following cerebropontocerebellum lesions. The person's perception of timing is also impaired. A person with a lesion here is unable to determine which of two objects is moving faster, for example. This finding led to investigations to determine the role of the cerebellum in cognitive functions. Gao and colleagues[31] and Middleton and Strick[73] indicate that cerebellar processing is crucial to one's ability to solve spatial and temporal problems, as are needed, for example, in hitting a baseball with a bat.

THE CEREBELLUM AND MOTOR CONTROL

Understanding the contribution of the cerebellum to movement has come a long way from the original concept in 1839, that its only function was to maintain sexual potency.[28] Electrophysiological studies of the normal function and consequences of lesions of the cerebellum strongly suggest that the cerebellum controls the onset, level, and rate of force production by muscles. Based upon these findings and the anatomical connections of the cerebellum, it has been suggested that the cerebellum acts as a comparator between sensory input and motor output.[25, 26, 87] Remember, there are far more axons projecting to the cerebellum (from the vestibular and proprioceptive systems as well as the motor cortex) than leaving the cerebellum. For that reason, the cerebellum is in a good position to compare the voluntary command for movement with the sensory signals produced by the evolving movement. If the motor commands and evolving sensory signals are not appropriately matched, the cerebellum will provide corrective feedback to motor pathways capable of influencing the movement prior to the end of the movement.[26] Without such a function, movement will be inaccurate. To understand this concept, think about what a disaster it would be if NASA were unable to compare the location, speed, and trajectory of a rocket destined to land on the moon with the location and movements of the moon.

This idea of the cerebellum as a comparator has been refined in recent years. Rather than simply providing corrections to ongoing voluntary movement, the cerebellum is assumed to perform predictive compensatory modification of reflexes in preparation for movement.[66] The success of voluntary movement depends largely on the stability and adjustment of many different reflexes. For example, if the stretch reflexes of a limb are too sensitive, a high-speed movement may be impeded by the constant response to stretch. Thus muscle spindle activity will have to be reduced before and during such movement. In other circumstances the sensitivity of muscle spindles may have to be increased before movement. The cerebellum may be the initiator of such compensatory modification of the stretch reflex, as well as of many other reflexes.

A vital function of the cerebellum is its role in motor learning. Ito[47] proposed that the cerebellum acts as an adaptive feedforward control system, which programs or models voluntary movement skills based on a memory of previous sensory input and motor output. According to this theory, an internal model stored in or triggered by the cerebellum controls learned movement. Imaging studies by Shadmehr and Holcomb[92] showed that the anterior cerebellum was active during consolidation of a learned internal model of a motor task. Other investigators have also demonstrated the role of the cerebellum in integrating multiple internal models for complex motor activities and transformations.[29] If the cerebellum is damaged, the learned motor programs cannot be utilized. Movement will then be guided by slow sensory feedback loops through the cerebrum, as in learning a new skill, and incoordination will result.

If the cerebellum learns or memorizes movements, are programs retained for complex movements, such as a serve in tennis, or for simple qualities of movements? Brooks[12] suggested that the lateral and intermediate cerebellum acts to sequence simple movements that make up complex actions. The cerebellum may thus learn small, simple programs, which are then triggered in the order needed to produce the complex motion. Hikosaka and colleagues[38] hypothesized that the cerebellum, particularly the anterior cerebellum and the dentate nucleus, is important in the acquisition and execution of sequential procedures that comprise complex learned motor acts. Similarly, Molinari and co-workers[75] demonstrated impairments in procedural learning of a motor sequence and suggested that the cerebellum was important in the detection and recognition of event sequences.

Thach and associates[103, 106] first showed the role of the cerebellum in adaptation during trial-and-error learning in studies examining the changes that occur with prism glasses. Lang and Bastian[59] studied the role of the cerebellum during catching. They examined the effects of learning to adapt to a change in ball weight in a catching task. In one study the subject learned to catch a light ball and then had to catch an unexpectedly heavy ball. Following adaptation, the subject again had to catch the light ball. Lang and Bastian found that those with cerebellar disease required almost 40 trials to learn to adapt to the change in ball weight compared to fewer than two trials in the normal subjects. Further, when the ball was returned to the original weight, the subjects with cerebellar disease demonstrated no negative aftereffect suggestive of adaptation. EMG recordings indicated that the cerebellar subjects could not increase anticipatory activity to counteract the increased ball weight. Land and Bastian also reversed the presentation order and found no differences in adaptation ability if the heavy ball was used first. They concluded that the cerebellum was vital to controlling anticipatory muscle activity across several joints and vital to modification of response. It is important to remember that the client with cerebellar disease will require many more practice sessions than other clients and that alternative strategies for performance may have to be taught.[59]

Although no one knows where and how learning in the cerebellum may take place, several ideas have been proposed that put heavy emphasis on the role of the inferior olivary nucleus.[2, 68] Each olivary neuron is presumed to be activated by the cerebral cortex during a demand for an elemental or simple movement. Climbing fiber pathways are modulated during active movements in a way that prevents irrelevant sensory information from reaching the cerebellar cortex and facilitating the projection of relevant information.[5] The discharge of Purkinje cells is also affected by input from the mossy fibers, which reflects the sensory context in which the elemental movement is demanded. Possibly the climbing fiber input potentiates the mossy fiber input so that mossy fiber input to the Purkinje cell may be able to evoke an elemental movement from the Purkinje cell in the absence of input from the cortex.

Further research has demonstrated that sequence is the key to understanding the cerebellum.[10, 75] The process whereby there is a row of excitation of Purkinje cells surrounded by rows of lateral inhibition has led to speculation that these "beams" respond to sequences of events in the sensory input and then produce sequences of output information. Braitenberg and colleagues[10] hypothesized that these beams were well tuned (much like FM radio stations) and were used to refine movement sequences for the adaptation necessary for the physics of multijoint movements.

The cerebellum has been shown to be active during mental imagery or mental practice. According to Ryding and colleagues,[89] mental imagery is a pure mental activity, requiring no muscle involvement and the same amount of time as the actual motor performance. The dentate nucleus and the cerebellar hemispheres are the cerebellar areas most involved during mental rehearsal. Patients who show damage in the lateral region of the cerebellar hemispheres have a reduced or absent capacity for anticipatory cues when performing a pretrained motor task and decreased ability to image a movement.[60]

There is other evidence that the role of the cerebellum is not purely motor. There is now some evidence that the cerebellum is involved in purely cognitive and emotional activities, including thinking and verbal encoding. For example, Akshoomoff and Courchesne[1] suggested that the cerebellum can affect voluntary control of a specific cognitive operation such as rapid and accurate shifts of attention. Patients with damage to the cerebellum, such as those with astrocytoma or idiopathic cerebellar atrophy, showed a deficit in shifting attention from one sensory domain to another, where no motor action was involved. The implication is that cerebropontocerebellar action for cognitive processes does not necessarily depend on the motor control system. In essence, Akshoomoff and Courchesne believe that possibly the neocerebellum "helps us to effortlessly shift from one domain of thought to another."[1, p. 737]

No one is certain whether the cerebellum functions in all three of these capacities or predominantly in just one. If the cerebellum does perform all three of the described functions, different lesions may disturb one function more than another. Recognition of these theories and the consequences of their disruption may help a therapist more carefully examine a client and plan a therapeutic program. For example, if the cerebellum no longer functions as a comparator, movement will obviously be dysmetric. This individual will need time-consuming practice, but in selected activities that will be most useful for him or her and not in all movements. Even though the cerebellum may not automatically correct movement errors, the client may consciously be able to correct movement with practice or the remaining central nervous system (CNS) may be able to assume a role of automatic correction.

If the cerebellar function of a reflex compensator is lost, the client may display abnormal muscle tone, inappropriate postural adjustment, and loss of associated limb movements, as well as being dysmetric. The therapist may need to evoke reflexes during an activity that would assist the postural stability and progression of movement. The presumption, again, is that the client can consciously learn to control the activity or that another part of the nervous system can begin to make the reflex adjustment automatically.

The concept of learning by the cerebellum is especially important for therapists to consider. If clients have lost "learned motor programs" controlled by the cerebellum, they will obviously be dysmetric. Therapy for any neurologically involved client is offered with the hope that a long-term modification of motor behavior will take place. However, if the cerebellum is the primary area where adaptive movement can be "learned," the client may never receive much benefit from therapy. Currently, no studies quantify the ability of clients with cerebellar lesions to learn new motor skills or relearn lost skills with training. Obviously, such work would be a valuable guide to therapists in providing activities that can achieve better motor performance. Therapists, however, need to recognize that even though the best therapeutic program possible is offered, the motor learning capabilities of some clients with a cerebellar lesion may be very limited and gains will be achieved slowly at best.

IMPAIRMENTS IN CEREBELLAR DISEASE

Balance and Equilibrium

As its anatomical connections may indicate, the cerebellum is a vital structure in the maintenance of the upright posture. Lesions of the cerebellum that include the vestibulocerebellum or the fastigial nucleus result in postural sway and delayed equilibrium reactions. Use of vision is not effective in preventing loss of balance. Additionally, the person with cerebellar disease is unable to modulate long-loop postural reflexes appropriately.[9] The ability of patients with cerebellar disease to increase or decrease the size of the long-loop reflex to environmental demands is lost. (See Chapters 21 and 22 for discussions of the long-loop reflex in relationship to balance and the basal ganglia, respectively.) The person with cerebellar dysfunction does not modify the reflex, even with repeated presentations of the appropriate stimulus.

Oddly enough, patients with late cerebellar atrophy almost never fall, even though they have severe disturbances in stance and gait.[23] The absence of falling appears to be due to intact intersegmental movements between the head, trunk, and legs. In fact, the person with cerebellar disease of the vestibular portion of the cerebellum has good control of the limbs when supine or fully supported.

Control of Muscle Tone

The spinocerebellum has been linked to the problem of decreased tone or hypotonicity. This is due to the decrease in excitation from the cerebellar deep nuclei to regions of the brain that excite alpha and gamma motor neurons.[64, 65, 86, 88] The muscle itself feels less firm to palpation and when the therapist examines passive range of motion, the limb will appear heavy. In fact, if the limb is suddenly dropped, the extremity will fall rapidly without correction. The limb will move through a greater arc of motion than does a normal limb when the limb is shaken. Hypotonicity is also demonstrated by asking the client to hold the arm out against gravity. One will observe either a slow fall or a postural tremor. The person with a cerebellar lesion can correct this by attention; however, think about how much effort you would have to spend if you had to concentrate all the time on objects you were holding, such as this book. In the lower extremities, the decrease in underlying muscle activity is seen in a wide, flat footprint.

Deep tendon reflexes are typically normal but there is often a pendular movement of the limb after the initial muscle contraction response. This pendular reflex was first described by Holmes in an EMG experiment of the knee jerk.[41] The normal EMG response to quadriceps stretch is a recording of two peaks of tension (Fig. 24–3A). The initial peak is evoked by the tendon tap and is responsible for the brisk twitch of knee extension. Descent of the leg causes another stretch reflex of the quadriceps femoris muscle. The descent of the leg is actually

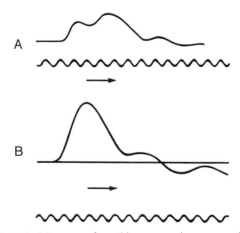

FIGURE 24–3. Myogram of quadriceps muscle on normal knee-jerk response *(A)*, and that evoked from a person with cerebellar lesion *(B)*. Time indicated below each trace by vibrations of tuning fork at 25 Hz. Note absence of second peak of tension in response of person with cerebellar disease. (From Holmes G: The Croonian lectures on the clinical symptoms of cerebellar diseases and their interpretation. Lancet 1:1181, 1922.)

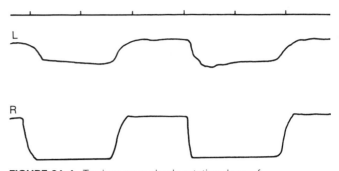

FIGURE 24–4. Tracings on a slowly rotating drum of simultaneous depression of the right (R) and left (L) arms against springs of equal tension, from a man with a lesion of the left side of the cerebellum. The tracings show delay in starting and slowness in effecting the movements, reduced and irregular exertion of power, and slowness in relaxation on the affected side. Time in seconds. (From Holmes G: The cerebellum of man. Brain 62:10, 1939.)

slowed by this second contractile response. A client with a cerebellar lesion, on the other hand, displays only the early peak (see Fig. 24–3B). The second response, which would brake the return of the limb, is not present, and the limb falls heavily. Thus, during a knee jerk, the leg behaves as a pendulum that falls by its own weight and oscillates momentarily because of momentum.

The problem here is a resultant incoordination of limb movement. The client has decreased ability to contract muscles and stabilize a limb. The client may demonstrate good distal control if the limb has external support, as in sliding the arm along a table, but is unable to reach in space. This lack of muscle control is more apparent in multijoint movements when each segment of the limb must control for the inertial forces of the other segments.[102]

Dysmetria

Dysmetria is defined as a deficit in reaching a target—usually a past pointing. It results from the deficit in accurately defining the direction, extent, force, and timing of the limb movement, one role of cerebellar function. A classic test for this is to ask the patient to touch the examiner's finger and then their own nose. Holmes[43] first described these deficits. He illustrated a slow onset in development of muscle tension, a reduced intensity, and a slow release compared to normal movement (Fig. 24–4). Other aspects of the inability to regulate force of movements are seen in dyssynergia, also described by Holmes.[41] This is tested clinically by suddenly removing a restraining force from an isometrically contracting limb. In a normal person, the limb will not change position. In contrast, the limb of a person with a cerebellar lesion will move abruptly as if still opposing the resistance.

Later studies extended the observations of Holmes and concentrated on the sequence of muscle activity.[7, 103] A ballistic motion uses a sequence of agonist-antagonist-agonist activity, a triphasic pattern[36, 69] (Fig. 24–5). The first burst from the agonist has a consistent duration of 50 to 110 ms. The antagonist muscle burst displays a

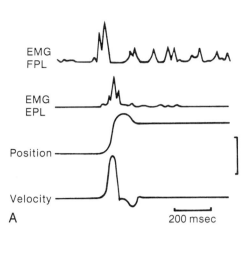

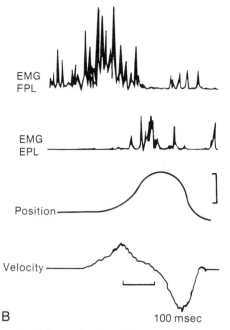

FIGURE 24–5. *A,* Fast ballistic movements in normal man. Subject flexed the distal joint of the thumb through 20 degrees. Records are, from top down, rectified electromyogram (EMG) of flexor pollicis longus (FPL), rectified EMG of extensor pollicis longus (EPL), position, and velocity. Calibration is 200 ms and 20 μV, 27 degrees or 336 degrees/sec. *B,* Fast thumb flexion from a 62-year-old man with unilateral cerebellar ataxia resulting from stroke. Records from top down are ordered as in *A.* Calibration is 100 ms and 100 μV, 25 degrees or 313 degrees/sec. Note the slower movement, inability to hold final position, and very prolonged bursts of activity in the agonist and antagonist muscle. (From Marsden CD, et al: Disorders of movement in cerebellar disease in man. *In* Rose CF (ed): Physiological Aspects of Clinical Neurology. Oxford, Blackwell Scientific, 1977.)

consistent duration of 40 to 100 ms. The duration of the second agonist muscle burst varies. The amplitude of the first agonist burst is related to the distance moved and is thought to provide the impulsive force needed to start the movement.[8] The amplitude of the antagonist muscle burst is not related to the amplitude of the movement or forces of deceleration but probably does assist in checking the movement. The amplitude of the second agonist burst varies with the accuracy of movements and might serve as a means of correction. The function of this second burst appears to be to dampen oscillations that might occur at the end of movement. This EMG pattern is a centrally programmed pattern; afferent inputs may modulate the activity but are not necessary for the activity. The studies of Berardelli and colleagues[8] showed that the cerebellum is important in the EMG bursts of voluntary movements and suggested that the cerebellum implemented the muscle force phasically.

Agonist-antagonist-agonist EMG is lost with cooling (a transient lesion) of the interposed or dentate cerebellar nuclei. Hore and Vilis[45] found that such a lesion prevented anticipatory movements in response to perturbations. They concluded that the cerebellum operates in a feedforward manner. Loss of feedforward mechanisms would mean that the animal or person could only respond with slower feedback responses. A lack of programmed deceleration was thought to be responsible for the overshoot of dysmetria and the oscillation around the end of a reaching movement. Multijoint movements were more affected than single-joint movements as control of the effects of movement of one segment on the other segments in a limb are lost. Movement of the shoulder therefore becomes separated from movement of the elbow.

Hallett and colleagues[36, 37] studied the sequence of muscle activation further. They found that when normal subjects isometrically extended their elbows against resistance and then were unexpectedly told to flex their elbows very fast, activity in the triceps muscle ceased before the onset of biceps activity. In subjects with cerebellar lesions, however, the triceps was continuously active, even during the biceps activity. This abnormal co-activation of the antagonists would lead to a delay in reversing resisted movement, or produce an overshoot.

Abnormalities are also seen in the coordination of grip in the person with a cerebellar lesion.[91] The client will use an abnormally high grip and appear to be unable to adjust the grip to environmental or task-specific demands. When resistance abruptly ends the movement, the client demonstrates a longer latency before reacting. This is another example of improper regulation of the long-loop reflexes. Serrien and Wiesendager[91] concluded that the cerebellum is therefore involved in both proactive (as demonstrated above in the EMG recordings) and reactive mechanisms of movement.

In addition to the disruptions in force and extent of movement, the cerebellum has been implicated in the initiation and timing of movement. A person with a cerebellar lesion affecting the cerebropontocerebellum or dentate nucleus displays a delay in the initiation of movement and difficulty in movements that require bursts of speed. Therefore, rapidly alternating movements are severely impaired. This is referred to as dysdiadochokinesia.

Conrad and Brooks[21] temporarily cooled the dentate nucleus in monkeys who had been trained to perform fast alternating flexion and extension of the ipsilateral elbow. Range of movement was limited by mechanical stops at the end of flexion and extension. During cooling, termination of the agonistic activity was delayed, but velocity or acceleration of motion was unaffected. For slower movements in which the spatial dimension of the movement was learned but not mechanically stopped, dentate cooling produced an overshoot or hypermetria, increased velocity, and acceleration of motion.[13] Cooling the interpositus nucleus in animals, on the other hand, leads to hypometria and decreased velocity of motion. Thus very circumscribed lesions of the cerebellum may cause different characteristics of dysmetria.[109] Specific research on human subjects is not available, but the assumption is that lesions similar to those studied in monkeys will cause similar symptoms in humans.

According to S.H. Brown and colleagues,[15] the cerebellum has a coordinative role during oculomanual tracking tasks. When there is a lesion in the cerebellum the patient takes longer to initiate purposeful limb movements on the affected side. When only the eyes are required to track a target, saccadic onset times are the same as those of normal persons. When initiation of eye and arm movements is coupled in the cerebellar patient, however, the initiation times are significantly prolonged. The cerebellum may be the center linking oculomotor and limb motor systems during a task requiring coordination of eye and limb movement.

Movement Decomposition

The person with a cerebellar lesion has difficulty performing a movement in one smooth pattern and may perform the movement in a sequence of steps. For example, if a supine client is asked to place a heel on the opposite knee, he or she may first raise the extended leg, then flex the knee, and last lower the heel to the knee. This breakdown in executing a movement as a whole is called decomposition.[42] Holmes was the first to theorize that the cerebellum functions to sequence and time simple movements into one smooth, complex act. In the absence of this function, the movement becomes separated into individual components. Much investigation on the way in which the cerebellum acts to sequence movement has occurred since Holmes's time. Cooling the dentate nucleus will produce this decomposition in monkeys.[21]

Dysdiadochokinesia

Many clients with cerebellar lesions are unable to perform rapidly alternating movements. This deficit can be demonstrated by having clients rapidly supinate and pronate their forearm or rapidly tap their hand on their knee. Compared to that of a normal person, the movement appears slow and quickly loses range and rhythm.

Holmes[39] attributed dysdiadochokinesia to an inability to stop ongoing movement rather than to a reduced velocity of motion. Use of EMG has revealed discrete, nonoverlapping bursts of antagonist muscle activity during rapid, alternating movements in normal people.[100] In people with cerebellar lesions, however, antagonist muscle activity typically overlaps, resulting in a braking action for movement such that activities like brushing one's teeth or stirring food become ineffective.

Dysdiadochokinesia is related to dysmetria in that both result from the inappropriate timing of muscle activity. The inability to stop a goal-directed movement in one direction will be displayed as hypermetria, whereas the attempt to abruptly reverse the direction of movement will reveal dysdiadochokinesia.

In monkeys trained to perform rapid, rhythmical flexion and extension of the elbow, dentate cooling increased the duration of agonist activity up to 0.1 to 0.2 second.[21] The onset of activity of the antagonist was delayed and often overlapped the activity of the agonist. No change in actual movement velocity was noted. Control of reciprocal motion by the cerebellum is also revealed by the observation that discharge of Purkinje cells in the intermediate zone of the cerebellum is related to reciprocal action of muscles. During co-contraction these same Purkinje cells become inhibited.[96] If the cerebellum is damaged, such neural discharge patterns may not occur.

Ataxia

Ataxia is one of the classic signs of cerebellar disease. It appears in the trunk, extremities, head, mouth, and tongue (speech). As may be expected, multijoint and patterns of movement are more affected than single-joint movements. Most of us have seen classic ataxia in the slurred speech and uncoordinated gait pattern of someone who is drunk.

In fact, ataxia is most often associated with disturbances of gait. Amici and co-workers[4] found ataxic gait the most frequent symptom in their clients with cerebellar tumors. Gilman and colleagues[32] likewise noted that 100 of 162 clients with cerebellar lesions displayed the phenomenon. The ataxic gait is one in which there is uneven step length, width is irregular, rhythm is absent, and the feet are often lifted too high. The individual cannot walk a straight line without lurching. The gait pattern becomes even more distorted by walking heel to toe, walking in a small circle, or walking backward. Arm swing is typically gone.

In some cases, gait may be altered without changes in limb movement, muscle tone, or equilibrium with late atrophy of the cerebellum or chronic severe alcoholism.[67, 110] In these conditions the cortex of the anterior lobe of the cerebellum is selectively involved.

The cerebellum has anatomical connections that indicate that it can play a significant role in the generation of the pattern of locomotion. The cerebellum receives inputs from the spinal cord relating to the locomotor pattern. The descending tracts, that is, rubrospinal, reticulospinal, and vestibulospinal tracts, discharge in rhythm with the swing and stance phases of gait.[82] After cerebellectomy, these rhythmical discharges disappear (Fig. 24–6). In humans the clinical problem might be observed as a total disruption of the rhythm of gait; the stance and swing phase are totally irregular in duration, and the client

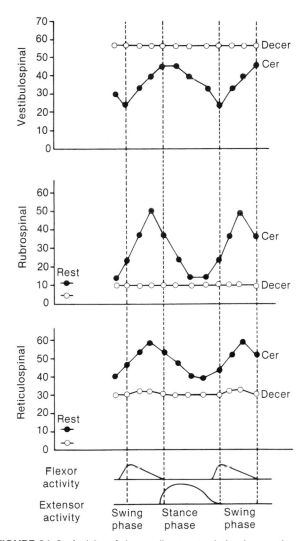

FIGURE 24–6. Activity of descending tracts during locomotion. Mean values of the discharge rate of neurons of the vestibulospinal, rubrospinal, and reticulospinal tracts are plotted as a function of the hindlimb position (ipsilateral for vestibulospinal and reticulospinal tracts; contralateral for rubrospinal tract). Curves obtained in cats with the cerebellum intact (Cer) and those who have been decerebellated (Decer) are presented. A mean value of the resting discharge rate is also presented (Rest). Flexor and extensor activity is shown schematically. (From Orlovsky GN, Shik ML: Control of locomotion: A neurophysiological analysis of the cat locomotor system. *In* Porter R [ed]: International Review of Physiology, Neurophysiology II, vol 10. Baltimore, University Park Press, 1976.)

cannot adjust for deviations in the surface on which he or she walks.

Gait disturbances can also occur due to incorrect programming of rate and force of muscle contraction, as in dysmetria. The inability to regulate posture will also decrease efficiency and smoothness of gait.

Asthenia

A lesion of the cerebellum can produce a condition of generalized weakness known as asthenia. Holmes noted that, in people with traumatic unilateral injury to the cerebellum, muscle strength on the involved side of the body may be reduced by 50% when compared with the normal limb.[39] Posture also may be poorly maintained in the client displaying asthenia. Clients complain of a sense of heaviness, excessive effort for simple tasks, and early onset of fatigue.[43] Asthenia is not as common as other symptoms accompanying cerebellar lesions. Amici and colleagues[4] noted that the symptom occurred in only 10% of their clients with cerebellar tumors. Likewise, Gilman and co-workers[32] noted it in only 2 of 162 clients with cerebellar lesions caused by a variety of problems.

The mechanism underlying asthenia is not clear. Hagbarth and associates[35] performed an experiment that offered a possible model for cerebellar asthenia. They infiltrated lidocaine about the median nerve in normal subjects, producing weakness in the hand. Lidocaine blocks conduction in thin nerve fibers, including gamma motor neurons. During voluntary contraction both alpha and gamma motor neurons to a muscle are normally co-activated. If the gamma motor neurons are blocked by lidocaine, an excitatory input to alpha motor neurons from muscle spindles will be reduced. Without the excitatory input from muscle spindles, the supraspinal drive to alpha motor neurons may have to increase to produce the voluntary movement. The normal perception of heaviness or force of effort is thought to be related to the intensity of supraspinal signals required to produce the movement.[71] Thus any increase in the supraspinal drive to produce voluntary movement will be perceived as increased effort and fatigue, which is a common complaint in asthenic clients.

A decrease in fusimotor activity is known to occur in cerebellar lesions and also has been suggested as the mechanism for hypotonicity. Hypotonicity and asthenia, however, do not necessarily accompany one another. This suggests that although the conditions may share similar features, the mechanisms for them may not be identical.

Bremer[11] theorized that asthenia is caused by a loss of cerebellar facilitation to the motor cortex, which in turn could reduce the activity of spinal motor neurons during voluntary movement. A loss of facilitation of the cortex also has been suggested as a mechanism underlying hypotonicity. If loss of facilitation of the cerebral cortex is responsible for asthenia and hypotonicity, perhaps the areas of the cortex that are affected in asthenia and hypotonicity are not identical. Future research is required to untangle the similarities and differences of these two symptoms of cerebellar dysfunction.

Tremor

People with cerebellar damage often display intention tremor, in which a hand oscillates back and forth as they try to touch their nose or the heel oscillates as they attempt to slide it down the opposite shin. The tremor has a frequency of 3 to 5 Hz and is typically enhanced during the termination of a goal-directed movement.[42]

Dentate dysfunction also influences oscillations that accompany voluntary movement. Normal movement is accompanied by very low amplitude oscillations, which are presumably the result of oscillating activity in long-loop feedback pathways. In monkeys performing a self-paced tracking task, dentate cooling causes a shift in the predominant peak of the power spectra of limb oscillation from 6 to 3 to 5 Hz. As mentioned before, intention tremor in clients with cerebellar disease also has a frequency of 3 to 5 Hz. Thus damage to the dentate nucleus could be involved in the generation of intention tremor. The slower oscillation of intention tremor might result from the time-consuming relay of sensory input to the motor cortex needed to modulate movement when the cerebellum no longer functions effectively.[3, 72, 111, 112] Thus a client with intention tremor may have trouble performing tasks requiring precision of limb placement and steadiness, such as drinking from a cup, placing a key in the door, or putting on makeup.

Another type of tremor may be seen when a person with cerebellar dysfunction is asked to maintain a posture, either to maintain position of the body as a whole or to hold an extremity against gravity. This type of tremor is referred to as postural tremor. For example, a tremor may appear in an abducted arm but will disappear if support is provided at the axilla. The frequency of this oscillation is typically about 3 Hz, and both antagonistic muscles about a joint participate.[24, 41, 95] Postural tremor is an infrequent symptom, occurring in 9% of patients (14 of 162) studied by Gilman and colleagues[32] and in 13.1% of patients studied by Amici and associates.[4]

The mechanisms for postural tremor and intention tremor may not be identical. For example, administration of levodopa will relieve postural tremor but not intention tremor.[33] Also, the two tremors are not always coincident, postural tremor being much less common than intention tremor.[4, 80] One possible mechanism for the postural tremor could be disruption of proprioceptive feedback loops. If the body shifts position, proprioceptors signal this change, and via a suprasegmental or long-loop pathway involving the cerebellum or another region in the brain, an automatic postural correction is made. When the limbs of a normal person shift because of gravity, sensory input leads to a motor output that returns the limb automatically to the desired position. The motor output occurs in time to prevent a noticeable disruption of position. An oscillation can occur in this feedback system if there is a delay in the processing of sensory input or motor output because of a lesion, a disruption in the compensatory role of the cerebellum.

Mauritz and colleagues[70] electrically stimulated the tibial nerve to excite muscle spindle afferent fibers and evoke segmental and suprasegmental stretch reflexes. They found that persons with postural tremor had delayed long-loop reflexes. Postural tremor was also produced by this stimulation technique in persons with incipient degenerative cerebellar disease. Marsden and co-workers[69] also found disruption in the long-loop reflexes in those with cerebellar disease. In their experiments, clients with cerebellar disease displayed the early stretch reflex at the same latency as normal people; however, only one (instead of two) late responses occurred with a very long latency of 80 ms.

Postural tremor may be explained by another hypothesis. Sensory feedback systems, which operate over supraspinal as well as spinal pathways, all oscillate, even in a normal person. For example, the spinal stretch reflex pathway oscillates at 8 to 12 Hz, the corticospinal pathway has an oscillation of 3 to 5 Hz, and the transcerebellar pathway has an oscillation of 4 to 6 Hz. In spite of these potentially oscillating circuits, a normal person displays no visually obvious tremor because none of the feedback pathways operate in isolation from the others. By acting together these multiple pathways effectively dampen one another's oscillation so that little oscillation is actually expressed. If one of these multiple reflex pathways is absent or delayed, however, a noticeable oscillation of the body or limbs may occur. If the transcerebellar reflex path is absent, the spinal reflex path is ineffective in dampening the low-frequency oscillation (3 to 5 Hz) induced by the corticospinal pathway.[97] Thus the body will tend to oscillate at the low frequency—that of postural tremor. This explanation is analogous to the ability of the cerebellum to adjust to the forces of movement in multiple joint segments so that smooth movement is produced.

Clients with postural tremor display the tremor only when attempting to hold a fixed position, not necessarily all the time. Any limb displays a mechanical oscillation, similar to that of a metal spring or tuning fork when perturbed. When a limb or joint changes in stiffness, as from relaxation to an attempt at stabilization against gravity, its properties of mechanical oscillation also change. The mechanical oscillations of a stabilized limb may actually reinforce the low-frequency oscillation of the limb in a client with cerebellar disease and lead to a noticeable postural tremor, but not necessarily a movement tremor.

Speech

Cerebellar lesions also disturb speech, which is a complex motor function. Grammar or word selection is not altered, but the melodic quality and the rhythm of speech are changed. The resultant disturbance is labeled *dysarthria*. Words or syllables are pronounced slowly, accents are misplaced, and pauses may be inappropriately short or long.[20] Lechtenberg and Gilman[61] noted that 19% of 162 clients with various cerebellar lesions developed dysarthria, and Amici and colleagues[4] found dysarthria in 8.5% of a large population of clients with cerebellar tumors. Clients also may display explosive speech or staccato speech.[119] The voice can become invariant in pitch and loudness, tremulous, nasal, or very soft.[14, 40, 41]

The mechanisms responsible for dysarthria are most likely similar to those producing dysmetria of the limbs. For example, inability of muscles of the larynx to initiate or stop contractions quickly or hypotonicity of the larynx could produce a slurring in the pronunciation of consonants and vowels, slow speech, prolonged pauses, or uneven stress on syllables.[14, 59] Hypotonicity of the larynx may also be responsible for the inability to increase loudness or vary the pitch of the voice.

Attempts to localize areas of speech function in the cerebellum have revealed a relatively high incidence of dysarthria in clients with damage to the left cerebellar hemisphere.[61] The left cerebellar hemisphere is influenced by the right (nondominant) cerebral hemisphere, which has among its functions perception of melodies, tone, and rhythm.[83, 93] If the left cerebellum plays a role in the melodic production of speech, input from the nondominant cerebral hemisphere seems appropriate in the context of this task.

Control of Eye Movements and Gaze

Although physical therapists are not expected to treat deviations of eye movement, they see a relatively high frequency of such problems in clients with cerebellar lesions. An awareness of the variety of problems and the underlying mechanisms should be helpful in interacting with a client who displays such phenomena. Like posture of the limbs, the resting position of the eyes is affected by cerebellar dysfunction. After an acute lesion of a cerebellar hemisphere, both eyes deviate toward the contralateral side.[27, 78]

Following cerebellar lesions, the eyes display some of the same characteristics as seen in the extremities and the speech apparatus, in this case called ocular dysmetria. The client with a cerebellar lesion is unable to move the eyes accurately to a target in the periphery. When a normal person directs gaze toward an object in the periphery, the eyes move in a rapid step called a saccade. The amplitude of the saccade must be very accurate to place the intended image on the fovea of the retina. After cerebellar damage the saccadic movement of the eyes can become too large or too small, and corrective saccades will have to be made, resulting in ocular dysmetria.[57, 85, 90] Ocular dysmetria is related to the initial position of the eyes, such that hypermetria occurs when the eyes are eccentric to the target and hypometria occurs when the eyes move from neutral to a peripheral target.

Ocular dysmetria also can occur with pursuit movements of the eyes. When a normal person follows a slowly moving object, the eyes move in a smooth, continuous fashion but stop abruptly if the object stops moving. However, if a client with cerebellar dysfunction visually pursues an object, the eyes may move only in saccades and continue to move after the object stops.[18, 19, 113] Clients are also unable to initiate conjugate eye movement and must accomplish lateral gaze by vigorous head movements.[6] Normal subjects can shift their eyes 30 degrees without accompanying head motion, but clients with cerebellar dysfunction typically move their heads within the first 30 degrees of eye movement. This is clearly seen in a degenerative disease of the cerebellum called ataxia telangiectasia.[94]

The posterior vermis, that is, the flocculus and the paraflocculus and fastigial nucleus, are involved in control of accuracy of saccades and in saccade adaptation. If either of these areas is lesioned, there is an initial hypometria in some directions and this does recover over time. However, individual saccades are less precise than before the lesion and rapid saccade adaptation is permanently lost. Without such adaptation, repetition of the same saccade results in a slow continuous reduction in the size of the eye movement. This latter decrease in saccade size is important to consistent visual function without fatigue—so that we can visually pursue objects late in the day with the same precision as early in the day.[7]

Neurons that discharge before a saccade have been located in the thalamus, cerebellum, vestibular nuclei, superior colliculus, pontine reticular formation, and mes-

encephalic aqueductal gray matter. However, the area of the brain that appears primarily responsible for the generation of the saccades is the pontine paramedian reticular formation because specific lesions at this region will produce permanent loss of saccadic eye movement.[117] Damage to this region disrupts the rapid phases of both vestibular and optokinetic nystagmus. Although the cerebellum does not initiate saccades, it does influence their accuracy. To initiate saccades, the neurons in the pontine reticular formation send a burst of activity to the motor neurons of the extraocular muscles. This burst is believed to code the difference in the visual target position and the actual eye position at the start of the saccade. Thus for this burst to move the eye to the exact location needed, the pontine reticular formation must have accurate estimates of the starting position of the eye, as well as any other short-term or long-term changes in the eye and its muscles caused by fatigue, injury, or aging. The cerebellum appears to provide this feedback to the saccadic pulse generator in the brain stem.[81]

Another common disturbance in eye movement is gaze-evoked nystagmus.[6] As the eyes move voluntarily to gaze at an object in the periphery, they move quickly in the intended direction and then drift involuntarily to neutral. The sequence is repeated as long as the effort is sustained to keep the gaze deviated toward the periphery. Clients with cerebellar atrophy may display a permanent gaze-evoked nystagmus bilaterally, whereas those with an acute unilateral lesion may display nystagmus temporarily to the ipsilateral side.[49] A rebound nystagmus often appears if gaze deviation is maintained 20 seconds or longer. The nystagmus then occurs briefly in a direction opposite to the prior gaze when the eyes are voluntarily returned to neutral.[44]

Gaze-evoked nystagmus has been explained by the loss of a holding function provided by the cerebellum. When the eyes are held steady at the end of a normal saccade, the discharge of motor neurons innervating the extraocular muscles is proportional to the position of the eyes in the head. However, the sensory systems that influence eye position transmit signals of velocity. For example, the semicircular canals detect velocity of head movement and the retina detects the velocity of the image moving across it. These signals must undergo a "mathematical" integration to code position rather than velocity. Although this process of neurointegration does not appear to occur in the cerebellum and is believed to occur in the brain stem,[16] the cerebellum is essential to the normal integration of the velocity signals. If the cerebellum is damaged, the integration undergoes a rapid decay, which is reflected in the poor maintenance of eye position. Thus the cerebellum is necessary to sustain or boost the output of the brain stem integrator of sensory signals influencing eye position.[118] The appearance of gaze-evoked nystagmus does not correlate with a specific cerebellar lesion in humans, although nystagmus occurring with downward gaze is particularly common in clients with the Arnold-Chiari malformation.[115] In addition, removal of the flocculus and paraflocculus in monkeys leads to a serious defect in the ability to sustain gaze in any direction.[118]

Cerebellar lesions also distort the vestibulo-ocular reflex movements, as well as voluntary movements of the eyes. These reflexes are crucial to maintaining an accurate visual image during head movement. The sensitivity of the vestibulo-ocular reflex can be calculated by a ratio of eye velocity to head velocity. Although the sensitivity of the reflex is not universally altered in persons with cerebellar lesions, in such problems as the Arnold-Chiari syndrome and spinocerebellar degeneration, the ratio can exceed that of normal individuals.[116, 117]

The amplitude of the vestibulo-ocular reflex will adapt to changes in internal or external conditions. For example, unilateral damage to the vestibular apparatus results in spontaneous nystagmus toward the damaged side, which typically disappears in a few weeks.[74] If one moves the head and the object simultaneously, the vestibulo-ocular reflex nearly disappears in the person without a cerebellar lesion.[116] These adaptations are lost if the cerebellum is damaged.

When a normal person watches stripes on a revolving drum moving horizontally or vertically, nystagmus develops in which the eyes snap quickly (fast phase) in the direction opposite to that of the revolving drum. The eyes then drift back slowly (slow phase) and the sequence is repeated. This phenomenon is called optokinetic nystagmus. In acute lesions of the cerebellum, the amplitude of optokinetic nystagmus is often decreased, whereas in chronic problems, the amplitude of both phases or just one of the phases of optokinetic nystagmus is often increased.[32]

Distortions of optokinetic nystagmus may be a result of disruption in the cerebellar systems, which control either smooth pursuit or saccadic movement of the eyes. For example, a client may display a loss of smooth pursuit movement and a disturbance of the slow phase of optokinetic nystagmus. Presumably, the cerebellar mechanisms responsible for these two features of eye movement are the same. Similarly, saccadic eye movement may be distorted as well as the fast phase of optokinetic nystagmus.

As might be expected, the client with a cerebellar lesion may complain of visual defects. These defects include blurred vision, diplopia, loss of perspective, and difficulty seeing when their body is in motion.[115, 116] Although these deficits are characteristic of cerebellar lesions, they also appear in lesions affecting the extraocular muscles or the vestibular system or connections between these areas.

RECOVERY FROM CEREBELLAR LESIONS

After a brain lesion there is always some level of spontaneous recovery of compensation; the level depends on the severity of the lesion and its location. For cerebrovascular accidents and head trauma, therapists do have some published guidelines for recovery patterns to which they can refer; however, such information has not been well documented for cerebellar lesions. For this reason, this chapter cannot provide a complete description of recovery patterns following cerebellar damage. Further, disruption of the cerebellum can occur in a variety of circumstances. The cerebellum can be lesioned due to a cerebrovascular accident or head trauma; it may be involved in degenera-

tive diseases such as multiple sclerosis or a variety of inherited disorders. The cerebellum is also a site of brain tumors. Lastly, the cerebellum may be damaged from toxins such as alcohol. Nonetheless, it is hoped that the information presented will provide therapists with some clarifying expectations for their clients.

Various investigators have attempted to study the recovery patterns following cerebellar damage in animal models. Poirier and colleagues[84] observed the motor behavior of monkeys for up to 1 year after various surgical lesions had been placed in the cerebellum. The most severe problems resulted from total cerebellectomy and included truncal ataxia, dysmetria of the limbs, hypotonicity, and postural tremor. These problems decreased in severity over the first 4 weeks after surgery, but improvement then reached a plateau. The animal was still severely compromised, dysmetria and postural tremor being the least obvious of the above symptoms.

Goldberger and Growdon[34] bilaterally lesioned the dentate and interpositus nucleus in monkeys. The animals displayed gross oscillations of the limbs at a frequency of two per second, hypermetria of the limb, and primitive movement locomotion during the first 2 weeks. As the animals improved over the next 50 weeks, the limbs developed a smaller and faster amplitude tremor of 6 to 8 Hz and a marked improvement in gait and accuracy of movement of the extremities. In contrast, if only one cerebellar hemisphere is damaged with no nuclear involvement in a primate, the animal displays ipsilateral dysmetria, postural tremor, and an awkward leaping gait for the first 1 to 2 weeks and becomes essentially normal over the next 2 months. If the midline structure of the cerebellum is involved, the animal's chief problem is truncal ataxia, which improves over the first 3 to 5 months but never disappears. Thus from animal work it appears that recovery is very poor from a total cerebellectomy; a bilateral lesion is more devastating than a unilateral lesion; damage to the deep cerebellar nuclei is more serious than that to the cortex; and spontaneous compensation will be complete within 6 months to a year.

Although one cannot assume that humans will respond to acute cerebellar injury exactly as primates do, the information provided by animal work does indeed provide a general framework for humans. A feature of cerebellar lesions that cannot be readily studied in animals is the effect of a degenerative disease or an expanding tumor. If a client develops a degenerative cerebellar disease or a tumor, the developing symptoms are generally milder than those produced by the same damage occurring acutely. Thus compensation appears to be concurrent with a steadily progressing lesion.

If compensation for a cerebellar lesion is possible, what other neurological structures are necessary for the compensation to take place? If the cerebellum is not totally destroyed, some available adaptation to the movement distortions may occur because of the remainder of the cerebellum. Evidence for this is the observation that compensation for a cerebellar lesion will be disrupted by a second lesion in which deficits are more serious than those that would have occurred if the second lesion had been produced alone.[4] The motor cortex is also considered to be an essential structure upon which compensation for a cerebellar lesion depends.[34]

EVALUATION AND GOALS

As for any neurologically involved client, the primary goal of therapy is to make the client as functional as possible under conditions of maximum safety, reasonable energy cost to the client, and concern for the appearance of the client. In deciding how to achieve these goals, a therapist has to determine what basic functions the client cannot achieve and the specific reasons why. Examination and evaluation of a client with a cerebellar lesion therefore should include an initial determination of basic functional capabilities such as:

Bed mobility and posture
Ability to sit up from a reclining position
Maintenance of sitting posture
Ability to stand up from a sitting position
Maintenance of a standing posture
Ambulation
Ability to dress, groom, and eat

No special tests are needed to isolate these abilities other than observing the client's attempts at each, although objective measures from disability scales are recommended for outcome measures. Description of performance can include assistance needed, level of effort involved, time to complete the activity, potential hazards to the client, and unusual accompanying movements or noticeable features unique to the client.

Once an examination of basic fundamental capabilities of clients has been completed, therapists should determine why their clients display the difficulties observed by looking carefully for the movement disorders associated with cerebellar lesions (described at the beginning of this chapter). A list of each movement disorder, a description of specific tests, and simple observations needed to determine the presence of each disturbance are presented in the following box. Both sides of the body need to be examined, even if a unilateral cerebellar lesion has been diagnosed. Although therapists are not expected to provide detailed evaluations of eye movement or speech, brief notations of obvious distortions may help clarify the total problem facing the client. If the client has multiple sites of brain involvement, the symptoms caused by cerebellar damage may be masked by spasticity or sensory loss, and tests for these features will need to be added.

The cerebellar movement disorders the client displays will help the therapist decide why any of the basic func-

---

ASSESSMENT OF MOVEMENT DISORDERS

Hypotonicity

Specific tests

1. Muscle palpation
2. Deep tendon reflexes
3. Passive shaking of limbs
4. Wet footprint
5. Hold object while conversing
6. Voluntary flexion and extension of knee or elbow supported and unsupported
7. Flex one finger only

Positive

1. Reduced firmness
2. Pendular
3. Limbs move through greater arc of motion than does normal limb
4. Print broader on involved side
5. Drops object when distracted
6. Ataxic when unsupported; controlled when supported
7. All fingers flex

Observation

1. Resting posture

1. Slack, asymmetrical

Asthenia

Specific tests

1. Maintain arm(s) in 90-degree position of flexion or abduction
2. Maximal resisted muscle contraction for major muscle groups
3. Repeat submaximal muscle contractions, such as rising on toes, pushups, squeezing tennis ball

Positive

1. Arm(s) tire quickly
2. Weaker on involved side or unable to work against resistance, which is normal for size and age
3. Tires quickly

Observation

1. Everyday activities

1. Tires easily, complains of heaviness

Continued

ASSESSMENT OF MOVEMENT DISORDERS *Continued*

Balance and Postural Control

Specific test

1. Hold limb against pull of gravity
2. Nudge client unexpectedly when sitting or standing
3. Stand on one foot or walk backward

Positive

1. Postural tremor
2. Loses balance easily
3. Loses balance easily

Observation

1. Standing posture

1. Feet apart, trunk flexed slightly, needs to hold for stability, postural tremor of legs

Dysmetria

Specific test

1. Flex arms to 90-degree position, quickly elevate overhead, and then return to 90-degree position
2. Put peg in a hole, trace circle with pencil, trace circle on floor with big toe, slide heel down shin slowly, place feet on markers when walking
3. Therapist resists client's elbow flexion and releases unexpectedly
4. Voluntarily flex and extend knee or elbow in supported and unsupported position
5. Submaximal isometric effort against force transducer
6. Electromyogram of antagonistic pair of muscles during ballistic contraction

Posture

1. Not able to resume 90-degree position without initial error
2. Intention tremor; undershoots or overshoots target
3. Arm rebounds
4. Limb ataxic whether supported or not
5. Onset and release of force of involved limb delayed
6. Duration of triphasic pattern longer than 300 ms

Gait Disturbance

Specific test

1. March to cadence
2. Walk on heels or toes
3. Walk clockwise and counterclockwise
4. Walk on uneven ground

Positive

1. Unable to follow rhythm
2. Loses balance and rhythm
3. Stumbles in one direction
4. Cannot compensate and stumbles

Observation

1. Typical gait pattern

1. Slow, stumbles easily, not rhythmical, step length and height irregular

Dysdiadochokinesia

Specific test

1. Tap hand on knee or toes on floor
2. Walk as fast as possible

Positive

1. Rapidly loses rhythm and range
2. Gait becomes very impaired only when fast

Observation

1. Activities of daily living

1. Unable to brush teeth, stir food, shake salt shaker

Movement Decomposition

Specific test

1. Supine client touches heel to opposite knee

Positive

1. Movement broken up into separate phases, does not flow

Observation

1. Typical movement

1. Activity appears as if in slow motion, mechanical like a puppet

tions cannot be performed. The therapist can then select the therapeutic activities that would best correct the movement disorder and hence improve the client's functional behavior. For example, if an individual is hypotonic, his or her resting posture while reclining, sitting, and standing will be changed. The treatment for such a client would need to include activities that enhance the tone of antigravity muscles. If asthenia exists, postural stability and ambulation will be affected. Resistive exercises to antigravity muscles during functional standing and walking may improve such a client's posture and endurance in ambulation. If a client does not display hypotonicity or asthenia but still has poor postural stability, dysmetria may be the major problem. In this situation the client needs many sessions of practice in the precise posturing of the trunk, upper extremities, or legs in an attempt to make posture an automatic function or, second best, a consciously controlled function. If a client displays gait disturbances but does not have dysmetria, hypotonicity, or asthenia, the cerebellar motor program for gait may have been selectively disturbed and attention in therapy will need to be directed only toward gait. However, if dysmetria of isolated movements in the limbs is present as well as gait abnormalities, selected coordination exercises for the extremities, as well as gait training, should be implemented. Inability to dress, feed, or groom oneself effectively may be caused by hypotonicity, dysmetria, or asthenia, but may also be specifically caused by movement discomposition or dysdiadochokinesia. The predominant distortion will need to become the focus of treatment.

TREATMENT

The program described in this section is for the client with a relatively severe but stabilized lesion of the cerebellum, as might be produced by trauma, cerebrovascular accident, or a tumor that has been surgically removed. Many parts of the program, however, could be used to help maintain function of the client with degenerative cerebellar disease or multiple sclerosis affecting the cerebellum or cerebellar pathways. The reader should be aware that success of any of the following activities has not been well documented. Thus they are to be taken only as ideas for obtaining selective goals. The reader must always remember that the client with cerebellar disorders, from whatever pathology, requires many, many repetitions of a task and task sequence for any chance of successful recovery.[107] This is true for slow movements, and even more practice is needed for execution of rapid movements. A recent study showed that the client with cerebellar degeneration demonstrated good retention of an acquired skill and improved at a faster rate in subsequent sessions than on the first day of training. Thus Topka[107] concluded that clients with cerebellar degeneration can indeed learn to perform slow movements in a near-normal manner, although they may have more difficulty learning fast movements. The authors hypothesized that the problem was a difficulty in the refinement of the movement.

It is also important that complex motor skills be presented in treatment sessions. Isaacs and colleagues[46] dem-onstrated that complex motor tasks increased the volume of parallel fiber input to the Purkinje cell. There was a concomitant increase in blood vessel supply and mitochondria to maintain this increase in volume. Klintsova and colleagues[55] trained rats on complex motor tasks following neonatal alcohol exposure and compared them with rats who had the same alcohol exposure but were allowed to run or were sedentary. The rats given "rehabilitation" showed significant improvement in tests of motor skills and this was accompanied by an increase in parallel fiber synapses in the Purkinje cells in the paramedian area. The complex motor skills used included tasks demanding balance responses and coordination of the limbs. The use of complex motor tasks during treatment can be used in cerebellar rehabilitation. Several goals toward which a therapist can work with a client having a cerebellar lesion are (1) postural stability, (2) functional transfers and gait, and (3) accuracy of limb movement during activities.

Head and Trunk Control

A client with postural instability needs to be assisted sequentially to each level of independently maintained posture. Thus a client is a candidate for sitting only when there is sufficient head and trunk control and a candidate for standing only when trunk and axial balance and posture can be maintained. If clients have inadequate head control, they can be treated in the prone position while propped on elbows with a pillow under the chest or by being placed on a wedge bolster or placed more vertical to eliminate the biomechanical disadvantage (see Chapter 4). If clients are not comfortable in the prone position, treatment can be performed with them seated with hips tucked back in a chair, feet flat on the floor, and elbows supported by a lap table or pillow. The goal is to have clients lift the head and hold it steady. This position is the same as that which a baby first learns in control of the head. It can be promoted by brushing or vibration of the neck and upper back, 3 to 5 seconds of ice to the neck extensors, stretch to the neck extensors followed by heavy resistance to extensors to maintain extension in the shortened range, and downward compression on the shoulders.[98] Theraband is a good adjunct to treatment that can be used to maintain resistance and joint approximation. To progressively promote trunk control, less support to the elbows from the pillows and bolsters should be offered. The client in the prone or semiprone position should attempt to prop on both elbows and progress to the use of just one elbow for support to promote weight shift at the shoulders (see Figs. 4–13 and 4–14 in Chapter 4 for additional information on head control treatment).

Biofeedback might be tried in an attempt to promote upright head position in the severely involved client. For example, the client could wear a helmet that provides a visual and auditory clue when the vertical position of the head is not maintained.[114]

Sitting Balance

When clients can hold their heads up and have developed some trunk control, they need to be offered progressive

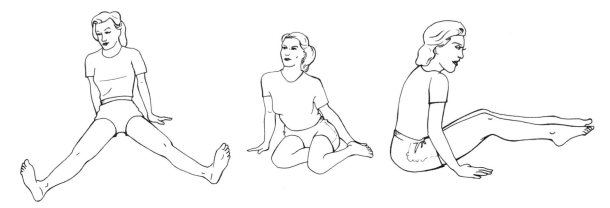

FIGURE 24–7. Alternate positions in sitting to promote control of posture and balance.

challenges in sitting balance. This can be accomplished by treating the client in a chair without arms or a back, depending on the individual's performance. If available, a safer and more versatile place to treat a client is on the edge of a mat table. To promote trunk stability, the therapist applies joint approximation at the client's hips or shoulders. To help a client sustain contraction of the trunk muscles, rhythmical stabilization for trunk rotation may be utilized. In this situation rhythmical stabilization is provided not to increase strength but to give clients the sensation of stability, which they can then attempt alone. If clients cannot sustain an isometric contraction of the trunk muscles, a pattern of slow-reversal-hold over a steadily decreasing range of trunk rotation might be attempted instead.[56] Therapists can also help clients control balance by joining hands with them and having them meet a gentle resistance through their extended arms. Push-pull activities with hands joined or with a cane or pole are also helpful in promoting co-activation needed for stability. A therapeutic ball is also a good activity as the client progresses. Gentle bouncing on the ball may also promote activity in the small trunk extensors.

Clients also need to practice weight shift in all directions while sitting. This can first be practiced with clients using both hands for support, progressing to no support from their hands. Clients also should try to sustain balance with the arms overhead and the trunk rotated because this position will be used in activities of daily living. Clients should be provided practice in maintaining different sitting positions during functional activities (Fig. 24–7). (See Chapters 11 and 16.)

Rising from Supine or Prone Position to Sitting

At the same time the client is developing control of sitting balance, work on safe and efficient ways of moving to and from the supine or prone position to sitting will be necessary. Work toward this goal also can be performed on a mat table. The procedure used will depend on the client's weight, side of involvement, and underlying muscle strength. A very heavy or weak individual may need first to roll to one side and push up from the side-lying posture or begin in sitting and eccentrically lower. The client might first lie near the edge of the table with the

knees bent and feet flat on the table. As the knees drop passively to the side, the trunk should rotate as well. If clients still have difficulty getting to side lying, their efforts can be strengthened by the therapist's providing gentle resistance in the side-lying position to flexion, adduction, external rotation of the shoulder, and trunk rotation (Fig. 24–8). As clients become stronger, the resistance can be applied when they are between the side-lying and supine positions. When clients can achieve a side-lying position alone, they can proceed to drop their legs off the edge of the table and push up with their arms to a sitting position. Ideally, clients should be taught to roll in both directions, but for practical purposes emphasis may need to be placed on one direction only. If clients have primary involvement on one side, they may find it easier to roll toward that side. However, this may create difficulty when they attempt to push up to sitting with the involved arm. Under these circumstances the therapist will have to decide the direction easier for the client.

A more natural method of rising or lowering to and from the supine position is to rely primarily on the action of the abdominal muscles. For stability, from supine a client can drop one leg off the edge of the table, placing

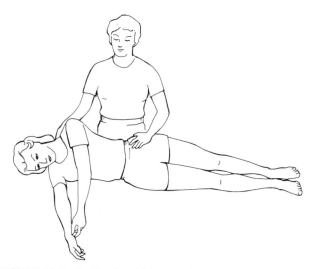

FIGURE 24–8. Position in which to apply resistance to shoulder flexion, adduction, external rotation, and trunk rotation to promote rolling from supine to side-lying.

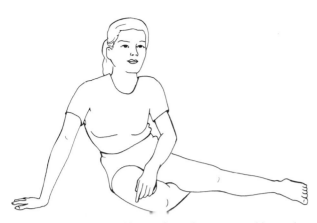

FIGURE 24–9. Client pushing up from the prone position and rotating back onto the hips to sit up.

the foot on the floor if possible. The client can then rise to a sitting position using the abdominal and iliopsoas muscles. A weak or heavy client can use this method if a side rail is provided for a pull. The difficulty with external aids for clients with dysmetria is that inaccuracy of reach may disrupt the ongoing flow of movement or actually be a hazard. If time allows, the client should practice assuming the sitting position from prone. Clients can push up on their arms and rotate their bodies backward onto their hips (Fig. 24–9). Clients also can push up on their hands and knees and drop onto a hip; however, this requires better control of balance.

Independent Transfers and Functional Activities in Sitting

If clients develop adequate sitting balance but are not considered safe candidates for ambulation, they should be taught as many independent transfers and functional activities as possible. A sliding transfer from a wheelchair to another chair or bed is the safest. A trapeze over a bed or bars in the bath may increase the level of independence if the accuracy of limb movements allows such activity. Practicing sitting during various functional activities such as dressing, grooming, or feeding again need tremendous repetition.

Preparing for Independent Standing and Ambulation

If the goal is to progress clients toward ambulation, a series of preliminary activities may be beneficial before they attempt to stand. The stability or co-activation at the hip needed for standing can be developed by working initially in the crawling or kneeling position on a mat table through impairment training. This allows the person to practice weight shifting through the hips without the harmful consequences of falling from standing. The client who is preparing to come to a standing position off the floor should be able to assume a quadruped position from sitting on the mat or assume a partial quadruped in order to sequence to kneeling and then standing. If not, the therapist can help the client achieve this position from

the prone position (Fig. 24–10). From hands and knees clients can, using the assistance of a therapist or stall bars, work their way up to a kneeling position or sit back on their heels and then straighten the trunk and legs.

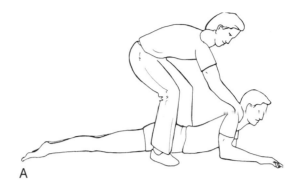

A

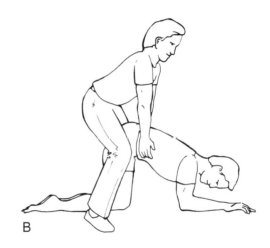

B

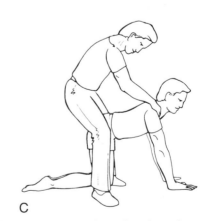

C

FIGURE 24–10. Method to assist a client from the prone to the quadruped position. *A,* While lifting the shoulders to prop client on his forearms, the therapist directs the client to lift his head. *B,* Therapist lifts the client's pelvis to bring him up on his knees. *C,* While lifting the client's shoulders to place weight on the hands, the therapist directs the client to lift his head.

If a person cannot easily practice crawling or kneeling activities because of age or other problems, postural co-activation of the hip can begin with bridging activities in the supine position. To increase lower extremity control, bridging can also be performed with the legs on a ball. This requires the client to maintain control of the hips and legs and also increases the balance demands. These activities will need to be transferred to vertical standing for task-specific carryover.

If a client has been in a wheelchair, the therapist could prepare the person's cardiovascular system for being upright by placing him or her on a tilt table. Standing activities can be started in the parallel bars to increase safety and decrease fear. Clients may not be able to assume a standing position without help. When standing up from sitting, clients need to remember to slide forward in the chair and flex their trunk considerably, placing the center of gravity over their feet. The trunk and legs should be extended only after gaining balance on the feet. This may be the most difficult step for an ataxic individual, who will either lean too far forward or extend the trunk too early and drop back into the chair. Another method a client may use to come to standing is to pull up on the stall bars from a kneeling to half-kneeling position. However, this is less practical and will be useful only if the client should end up on the floor. Whatever the method used to come to standing, it will require much repetition by the client and verbal feedback from the therapist. In addition to verbal feedback, viewing a videotape may help a client recognize and correct mistakes.

Once upright, the person should practice balancing, which can be reinforced by approximation through the hips and shoulders. Tremor may be reduced by ankle weights, a weighted belt, or the application of Theraband. Removal of distal weights may result in an increase of tremor due to the asymmetrical strength training of the agonist during movement. Rhythmical stabilization applied to rotation of the trunk may also be valuable in gaining stability. Biofeedback from a force platform may also help the person control the center of gravity. It is hoped that the client can learn to come to standing and maintain standing without pulling on the bars; however, for some people this will be impossible. Those individuals who rely on the bars will not become independent ambulators or function independently in ADL when standing, but may, with the assistance of another person, be able to get up and walk. Once standing and stable, the client needs to practice alternate lifting of the feet. These activities can be practiced in rhythm with music to promote skill. A mirror also may be valuable at this time.

Ambulation

When the person begins to walk within or outside the parallel bars, he or she may need precise verbal feedback as to step length, body rotation, accessory movements, and trunk position if the functional activity does not present itself as a whole procedural program. Sometimes, ambulation over the rungs of a ladder can be used to increase visual cues and feedback regarding foot placement. As in the initial learning of a sport, the therapist will need to isolate one problem at a time and provide practice. When the person is ready to walk outside of the parallel bars, a decision will need to be made about an ambulatory aid. Aids may be necessary but also may be an obstacle because clients will now need to control position and movement of the device as well as themselves. Although a walker is typically the most stable, it can be so only when all legs are placed down together and at a correct distance from the body. Accuracy of placement may be facilitated by weighting the legs of the device, although this again causes traction and may negatively affect the function of the arms. Also, a piece of tape placed from side to side, midway across the walker, will help keep the client from walking too far into the walker and falling backward. Crutches or canes may be used but require reciprocal movement of the arms and legs with appropriate timing and placement; this too can be very hard or impossible for some clients. The person may actually do better by using tall poles for support rather than the typical cane or crutches. Therapists can measure clients' progress in ambulation by the number of times they lose their balance in a treatment session, frequency of a specific error, the distance ambulated, or the level of assistance needed (see Chapters 14 and 28 for additional suggestions). Complementary movement approaches such as the Feldenkrais method, tai chi, or tai kwon do can, during leisure life activities, help reinforce the therapeutic outcome goals (see Chapter 33).

Activities for Temporary Reduction of Dysmetria

Clients with cerebellar lesions will be frustrated in many activities by the presence of dysmetria. A therapist attempting to modify this impairment needs to recognize that no therapeutic procedure will totally eliminate dysmetria; however, before clients practice specific functional activities, the therapist can have them perform activities that will temporarily decrease dysmetria. For example, use of proprioceptive neuromuscular facilitation (PNF) patterns of rhythmical stabilization or slow-reversal-hold for the lower extremities will allow clients to ambulate with better control.[50, 51] Similarly, functional tasks involving the arms can be preceded by PNF patterns for the arms.[77] Frenkel exercises can also be used to modify dysmetria of the lower extremities.[58] These exercises can be performed in the supine, sitting, or standing positions. Each activity is to be performed slowly with the client watching the extremity very carefully. When the client has gained reasonable control of one activity, he or she should proceed to the next.

Although Frenkel exercises are classically described for the leg (see the box on page 735), they can be modified for the arm. For example, the client can first practice flexing and extending the elbow horizontally, supported on a sliding board, then move the arm without support to place the hand on the opposite elbow, next slide the hand down and up the forearm, and, finally, place the hand in the therapist's moving hand.

Whether using Frenkel exercises or PNF patterns to improve coordination, these activities should *not* consti-

FRENKEL EXERCISES

Supine

1. Flex and extend one leg, heel sliding down a straight line on table.
2. Abduct and adduct hip smoothly with knee bent, heel on table.
3. Abduct and adduct leg with knee and hip extended, leg sliding on table.
4. Flex and extend hip and knee with heel off table.
5. Place one heel on knee of opposite leg and slide heel smoothly down shin toward ankle and back to knee.
6. Flex and extend both legs together, heels sliding on table.
7. Flex one leg while extending other leg.
8. Flex and extend one leg while abducting and adducting other leg.

Sitting

1. Place foot in therapist's hand, which will change position on each trial.
2. Raise leg and put foot on traced footprint on floor.
3. Sit steady for a few minutes.
4. Rise and sit with knees together.

Standing

1. Place foot forward and backward on a straight line.
2. Walk along a winding strip.
3. Walk between two parallel lines.
4. Walk, placing each foot in a tracing on floor.

tute the entire therapy session but should be used to prime the client to practice a subsequent functional activity. Another procedure that can reduce dysmetria of an extremity is to place weights on the extremity.[76] The weights required vary from client to client. The greater the movement error, the heavier the weight needed; however, if the weight is too heavy, dysmetria will become worse. Similarly, removal of the weight often exaggerates the dysmetria. Thus, the patient will become dependent upon this assistive device during functional activities.

The use of EMG or goniometrical biofeedback also may assist the client in receiving training in very specific acts. For example, brushing the teeth may be impossible because the toothbrush misses the mouth or hits the teeth and once inside the mouth does not effectively clean the teeth. EMG feedback from the deltoids, biceps, wrist flexors, and extensors or goniometrical position of the shoulder and elbow may be relayed to clients as they try to learn a pattern that works for them or to duplicate the pattern of signals produced by normal people when brushing their teeth.

ALCOHOLISM

Problems with Cerebellar Impairment

One metabolic problem that specifically attacks the cerebellum warrants in-depth consideration: this is the drug-induced neurological disorder that arises from overingesting alcohol. Movement disorders involve the effects of alcohol on the CNS and the effects of nutritional deficiency that are part of the alcoholic syndrome.

Alcohol, as a drug, has a direct effect on the nervous system. Alcohol ingested by a pregnant woman has a profound effect on the developing brain of the child and produces fetal alcohol syndrome. Additionally, the chronic effects of alcohol include vitamin and general nutritional deficiency. Alcohol has a high caloric value and therefore the chronic alcoholic tends to decrease food intake: the classic "drinking lunch or dinner." Thus acute intoxication, while not producing nutritional deficiency, contributes to it.

Signs and Symptoms of Acute Alcohol Intoxication

Most people are well aware of the symptoms of acute alcohol intoxication, perhaps through personal experience. Initially, alcohol produces relaxation and a loss of inhibitions. This is followed by a loss of judgment and coordination. If alcohol ingestion continues, a stuporous stage may be reached: The person "passes out" and awakens the next morning with a hangover. Drinking water and eating tend to alleviate the sick feeling, and the neurological signs are reversible at this stage. However, overly large volumes of alcohol can lead to coma and death. The symptoms of acute intoxication result from the direct effect of alcohol on the excitability of neurons, that is, inhibitory neurons become less excitable. Alcohol causes a decrease in membrane excitability. The cortex is usually affected first, and this effect descends the neuraxis. Coma is an indication of medullary involvement.

The individual with signs of acute intoxication will rarely, if ever, be seen in the clinic. The person with chronic alcohol intoxication, however, often will show neurological complications. The most prevalent problems involve cortical function, cerebellar function, and peripheral neuropathies. The cortical and cerebellar problems involve the combination of alcohol effects and nutritional deficiency; peripheral neuropathies are believed to be a result of nutritional deficiencies.[54] Because large neurons are more difficult to excite, it is possible that the large neurons of the cortex and cerebellum are more easily affected by decreases in excitability. The cerebellum and frontal lobes of the cerebral cortex are more sensitive to the deleterious effects of alcohol. The nutritional deficits further exacerbate these problems as the lack of food causes a decrease in glucose available for brain metabolism. Vitamin deficiency, especially of the B vitamins, is a further cause of the symptomatology seen.

In addition to the effects of chronic alcohol on the adult, alcohol can also be devastating to an unborn child. Because alcohol crosses the placenta, the developing brain with its high metabolic rate may be affected even in the absence of symptoms in the mother. Binge drinking by the mother can be as detrimental as chronic abuse. This has become a great enough problem with enough similarities among affected infants that fetal alcohol syndrome is a recognizable disease at birth. In addition to low birth weight and irritability, distinct facial anomalies also are associated with this disease. A long-term evaluation of these children will provide information on other neurological problems that may become more evident as the child ages. Animal research indicates that brain maldevelopment and delays in reflex and motor development are not reversible.[79] One of the areas showing a decrease in size is the frontal cortex.[79] (See Chapters 8, 9, and 10.)

Signs and Symptoms of Chronic Alcoholism

The individual suffering from chronic alcoholism can have neurological and psychological impairment. Neurological symptoms include ataxia (especially in the trunk and lower limbs), incoordination, and peripheral neuropathy. Seizures also may be a complication. The ataxia that occurs is the classic staggering, wide-based gait depicted on every television program showing an alcoholic. The person cannot perform a tandem gait (walking forward in heel-to-toe fashion on a straight line) and has difficulty maintaining an upright posture with the feet together. If weakness because of neuropathy is present, the ataxia, of course, is worsened. Vestibular deficits also are present and persist even after periods of abstinence. Abstinent alcoholics showed performance deficits on all sensory organization tests during dynamic posturography; these deficits reached statistical significance for those conditions that entailed proprioceptive conflict.[62]

The psychological problems also are probably fairly well-known. These include delirium tremens (DTs), dementia, and the Wernicke-Korsakoff syndrome. DTs are most frequently seen in any withdrawal from alcohol. This is when the alcoholic sees "pink elephants." The individual is restless, irritable, disoriented, and often hallucinates when awake; speech may be unintelligible. Temperature is elevated, and the person is dehydrated. DTs are probably caused by a type of rebound phenomenon: the depressed neuronal firing is freed from the alcohol, and neurons become overly irritable. Deep tendon reflexes are also hyperactive.

Wernicke-Korsakoff syndrome (hyphenated because the two eponymous syndromes are usually seen together) is caused by frontal lobe involvement complicated by vitamin B_1 deficiency. In Korsakoff syndrome there is a loss of memory, especially short-term and recent memory. The individual then tends to make up answers and may "remember" the physician or even the therapist as someone she or he met in a bar; a simple breakfast just completed may be described as a banquet feast. These confabulations are a classic sign of the chronic alcoholic. They are probably an attempt to function without recent memory. Wernicke syndrome includes ataxia (already described), disorientation, dementia, and ophthalmoplegia. The eye problems include nystagmus followed by lateral rectus weakness and double vision.

The peripheral neuropathies exacerbate all of these problems. The muscles are tender to touch, and there may be a burning sensation in the hands and feet, which intensifies the irritability of DTs. Muscle weakness will increase the apparent ataxia, and decreased sensation causes a further loss of proprioceptive cues the individual might otherwise use.

Pharmacological Considerations and Medical Management

The biggest factor in treatment is, of course, withdrawal from alcohol. Librium, which is synonymous with chlorpromazine and chlordiazepoxide, is used to keep the individual sedated and to reduce DTs. At the same time, the electrolyte and water balance of the body must be restored. Because alcohol usually causes dehydration, the body's fluids must be replaced, but refurnishing necessary electrolytes also requires attention. In addition, nutrition is important because the nutritional deficiencies are as harmful as the effects of alcohol itself. Large supplements of B complex vitamins should be added to the diet.

If the individual has been hospitalized fairly early, abstains from alcohol, and controls the diet, some of the symptoms of the disease can be reversed. This is especially true of the eye involvement and of much of the ataxia. Permanent memory deficits, however, often occur; the longer the alcoholism, the worse the memory. The neuropathies, if they recover, recover very slowly. Both the myelin sheath and the axon have been damaged. In long-standing alcoholism the nerve roots also become involved, lessening the chances for regeneration and recovery. The best cure therefore is prevention.

Evaluation

Before proceeding with a neurological evaluation, as one would for the person with cerebellar dysfunction, the therapist needs to assess the client's mental status (see the Mini-Mental State Examination in Chapter 26, page 798). Is there any short-term retention? Can the individual's perception of sensation be trusted as accurate? If the client cannot perform a task, is it because he or she did not understand the instructions or has forgotten them? All commands should be single commands and kept as short as possible. Because weakness and loss of sensation, especially proprioception, can produce signs similar to ataxia, it is a good idea to evaluate peripheral nerve function first. Nerve conduction tests are useful evaluation tools for the alcoholic patient. The faster myelinated nerves are the most sensitive to alcohol[30] (see Chapters 12, 20, and 28).

In assessing the degree of cerebellar involvement, static posture and movement need to be evaluated. This includes the ability to stand upright with the feet together, the width between the legs in standing or walking, and the presence or absence of equilibrium reactions. Sometimes there is a delay in equilibrium reactions that needs to be recorded. Persistent involvement of the vestibular system means that tests of vestibular function, including vestibulo-ocular reflex, optokinetic nystagmus, and balance, should be performed.

Treatment Considerations

Treatment of the alcoholic adds a few problems that may not be encountered in other cerebellar diseases. The first problem encountered is one of goal setting or prognosing, because the client may not be sufficiently mentally alert to participate in goal setting. Second, the degree of recovery is impossible to know; the therapist should strive for as much recovery as possible. Of course, the achievement of whatever goals are established depends on abstinence from alcohol.

In treatment of alcoholism, the mental status is a cru-

CASE STUDY 24–1   MRS. P

Mrs. P. sought physical therapy for a balance and coordination problem following surgery for a right acoustic neuroma. During tumor resection, branches of the superior cerebellar artery were damaged. The surgery was 6 months ago; however, Mrs. P was told that her imbalance and incoordination would get better on its own. She finally saw another physician who referred her for physical therapy. At the initial evaluation, Mrs. P walked with a cane held in the left hand. She had a wide-based gait pattern with shortened stride length and reduced speed. When she walked without her cane there was some further shortening of the stride and further reduction in speed. Additionally, she held her hands in a "medium guard" position. She was able to balance for 30 seconds with her feet together, eyes open or closed, with equal sway that was greater than expected for her age. She was unable to stand in a tandem stance nor could she balance on foam. On posturography evaluation, she had decreased ability in all conditions with the sway-referenced platform (see Chapter 21). She fell with vision occluded and the platform moving.

Mrs. P had normal tactile sensation, kinesthesia, and proprioception. Her strength was good throughout, with the right side slightly weaker than the left. Range of motion was within normal limits throughout. She demonstrated dysmetria, dysdiadochokinesia, and ataxia, right greater than left, and distal movements were more impaired than proximal movements. She had had bilateral hip replacement surgery and had lost hearing in the left ear. As a result of the acoustic neuroma resection she had lost all hearing in the right ear. She was unable to coordinate eye movements and so wore prism glasses. Her vision was now impaired enough that she could no longer drive. Her goals for treatment intervention were to improve her ability to walk without assistance, to improve her arm and hand coordination so that she could apply makeup and cook, and improve her strength so that she could remove and replace dishes in her kitchen cabinets. Before the neuroma resection she was completely independent in all activities and an excellent cook.

Treatment consisted of outpatient visits once every 2 weeks and an intensive home program of balance, strength, and coordination exercises. Her balance exercises included walking daily with and without her cane outside on uneven surfaces. The beach was highly recommended. She was also to practice balancing in a corner in a modified tandem stance, eyes open and closed, and progress to a full tandem stance. She also practiced balancing on a foam pillow with eyes open and closed. These exercises were practiced at least twice a day for 5 to 10 repetitions at a time. Initially, her home exercise program also included weight-bearing activities in the upper extremity, but these did not produce any measurable changes in function and so were discontinued. Theraband exercises for the shoulders were better for this patient and increased her ability to feel confident in lifting china plates. For coordination, she was to practice juggling, first with one ball and then with two balls. Juggling was used because it requires rapid release and catch and is a high-level skill that entails some degree of motor learning. It is also an activity in which gains can be seen easily and thus it continues to motivate the client.

During treatment sessions, Mrs. P walked on a treadmill set at her comfortable walking speed. She practiced walking without holding on, using a normal base of support, and concentrating on even steps. As she improved, she walked while turning her head, while spelling forward and backward, or while doing math problems. She walked forward and backward. There was little emphasis on sideways walking on the treadmill because of the extreme adduction that could occur. Walking while reading was begun in a treatment session and then continued at home. This was true for tandem walking with the eyes open and closed as well. While resting between weight-bearing activities Mrs. P practiced drawing straight lines with and without her glasses. Eventually, a patch had to be used for applying makeup. She also worked on upper extremity Theraband activities to increase her strength.

Mrs. P was a highly motivated client and performed her home program activities daily. Although she still relies on the cane in crowds and when she must walk long distances, Mrs. P now walks with a normal base of support and her speed and stride length have normalized. At her last visit, the therapist had to walk briskly to keep up with her as she left the clinic. She can stand on foam for 30 seconds with her eyes open and for 15 seconds with her eyes closed. Her stability score has improved in all sections of the posturography evaluation, as did the number of falls. She is able to place two dishes in the kitchen cabinet without assistance. She can juggle two balls though she has some difficulty in throwing with the right hand. Her ability to work without her glasses has not improved.

cial problem. If dementia is present, the client will not be able to use higher-level thought processes or achieve cortical control over movement. Therefore techniques that require attention or learning may have very limited success. In addition, carryover from one session to the next will be hampered because the client may have no recollection of the previous treatment or even of the therapist. The lack of attention and memory also means that, as in evaluation, all commands must be brief and simple. The treatment session should be well structured so that the client's thoughts are not allowed to wander. Sometimes it may also be advisable to adjust the length of treatment to the individual's tolerance. The addition of both physical and occupational therapy may produce a more wholistic treatment approach.

There is another consideration in the treatment of the alcoholic, and this is the effect of exercise on physical well-being in general, especially on any symptoms of asthenia. Even without neurological signs, alcoholic clients may benefit from a carefully monitored program of physical activity—carefully monitored because this client may be in a debilitated condition with generalized weakness and even respiratory problems. A study in Japan has shown that physical exercise can help the alcoholic's general rehabilitation progress.[108] As in all diseases discussed so far, the exact treatment procedures depend on the results of the evaluation. Documentation of the effects of therapy should be clear and, whenever possible, quantifiable.

This chapter has been concerned with the role of the cerebellum in movement and the effects of lesions of the cerebellum. One specific disease, alcoholism, has also been discussed.

ACKNOWLEDGMENT

The authors wish to acknowledge the contribution of Nancy L. Urbscheit to the writing of this chapter in the previous edition.

REFERENCES

1. Akshoomoff NA, Courchesne E: A new role for the cerebellum cognitive operations, Behav Neurosci 106:731, 1992.
2. Albus JS: A theory of cerebellar function. Math Biosci 10:25, 1971.
3. Allen GI, Tsukahara N: Cerebrocerebellar communications systems. Physiol Rev 54:957, 1974.
4. Amici R, et al: Cerebellar Tumors: Clinical Analysis and Physiopathologic Correlations. New York, Karger, 1976.
5. Apps R: Movement-related gating of climbing fibre input to cerebellar cortical zones. Prog Neurobiol 57:537, 1999.
6. Baloh RW, et al: Vestibulo-ocular function in patients with cerebellar atrophy. Neurology 25:160, 1975.
7. Barash S, et al: Saccadic dysmetria and adaptation after lesion of the cerebellar cortex. J Neurosci 19:10937, 1999.
8. Berardelli A, et al: Single-joint rapid arm movements in normal subjects and in patients with motor disorders. Brain 119:661, 1996.
9. Black FO, Nashner LM: Vestibulo-spinal control differs in patients with reduced versus distorted vestibular function. Acta Otolaryngol Suppl 406:110, 1984.
10. Braitenberg V, et al: The detection and generation of sequences as a key to cerebellum function: Experiments and theory. Behav Brain Sci 20:229, 1997.
11. Bremer F: Le cervelet. In Roger GH, Binet L (eds): Traite de physiologie normale et pathologique, vol 10. Paris, Masson, 1935.
12. Brooks VB: Control of intended limb movement by the lateral and intermediate cerebellum. In Asanuma H, Wilson VJ (eds): Integration in the Human Nervous System. New York, Igaku Shoin, 1979.
13. Brooks VB, et al: Effects of cooling dentate nucleus on tracking task performance in monkeys. J Neurophysiol 36:974, 1973.
14. Brown J, et al: Ataxic dysarthria. Int J Neurol 7:302, 1970.
15. Brown SH, et al: Role of the cerebellum in visuomotor coordination. Exp Brain Res 94:478, 1993.
16. Carpenter RHS: Movement of the Eyes. London, Pion, 1977.
17. Chambers WW, Sprague JM: Functional localization in the cerebellum. I. Organization in longitudinal corticonuclear zones and their contribution to the control of posture, both extrapyramidal and pyramidal. J Comp Neurol 103:105, 1955.
18. Chase RA, et al: Modification of intention tremor in man. Nature 206:485, 1965.
19. Cogan DG: Ocular dysmetria: Flutter-like oscillations of the eyes and opsoclonus. Arch Ophthalmol 51:318, 1954.
20. Cole M: Dysprosody due to posterior fossa lesions. Trans Am Neurol Assoc 96:151, 1971.
21. Conrad B, Brooks VB: Effects of dentate cooling on rapid alternating arm movements. J Neurophysiol 37:792, 1974.
22. DeLong MR, Strack PL: Relation of basal ganglia, cerebellum, and motor cortex units to ramp and ballistic limb movements. Brain Res 71:327, 1974.
23. Dichgans J, Mauritz K: Patterns and mechanisms of postural instability in patients with cerebellar lesions. Adv Neurol 39:633, 1983.
24. Dichgans J, et al: Postural sway in normals and atactic patients: Analysis of the stabilizing and destabilizing effects of vision. Agressologie 176:15, 1976.
25. Eccles JC: Long-loop reflexes from the spinal cord to the brain stem and cerebellum. Atti Accad Med Lomb 21:1, 1966.
26. Eccles JC: The dynamic loop hypothesis of movement control. In Leibovic KN (ed): Information Processing in the Nervous System. New York, Springer-Verlag, 1969.
27. Fisher CN, et al: Acute hypertensive cerebellar hemorrhage: Diagnosis and surgical treatment. J Nerv Ment Dis 140:38, 1965.
28. Fisher JD: Contributions illustrative of the functions of the cerebellum. Am J Med Sci 23:352, 1839.
29. Flanagan JR, et al: Composition and decomposition of internal models in motor learning under altered kinematic and dynamic environments. J Neurosci 19:RC34, 1999.
30. Fujimura Y, et al: Assessment of the distribution of nerve conduction velocities in alcoholics. Environ Res 61:317, 1993.
31. Gao JH, et al: Cerebellum implicated in sensory acquisition and discrimination rather than motor control. Science 272:545, 1996.
32. Gilman S, et al: Disorders of the Cerebellum. Philadelphia, FA Davis, 1981.
33. Goldberger ME, Growden JH: Tremor at rest following cerebellar lesions in monkeys: Effect of L-dopa administration. Brain Res 27:183, 1971.
34. Goldberger ME, Growdon JH: Pattern of recovery following cerebellar deep nuclear lesions in monkeys. Exp Neurol 39:307, 1973.
35. Hagbarth KE, et al: The effect of gamma fiber block on afferent muscle nerve activity during voluntary contractions. Acta Physiol Scand 79:27A, 1970.
36. Hallett M, et al: EMG analysis of stereotyped movements in man. J Neurol Neurosurg Psychiatry 38:1154, 1975.
37. Hallett M, et al: EMG analysis of patients with cerebellar deficits. J Neurol Neurosurg Psychiatry 38:1163, 1975.
38. Hikosaka O, et al: Parallel neural networks for learning sequential procedures. Trends Neurosci 22:464, 1999.
39. Holmes G: The symptoms of acute cerebellar injuries due to gunshot injuries. Brain 40:461, 1921.
40. Holmes G: The Croonian lectures on the clinical symptoms of cerebellar diseases and their interpretation. Lancet 2:59, 1922.
41. Holmes G: The Croonian lectures on the clinical symptoms of cerebellar diseases and their interpretation. Lancet 1:1177, 1922.
42. Holmes G: The Croonian lectures on the clinical symptoms of cerebellar diseases and their interpretation. Lancet 1:1231, 1922.
43. Holmes G: The cerebellum of man. Brain 62:1, 1939.
44. Hood JD, et al: Rebound nystagmus. Brain 96:507, 1973.
45. Hore J, Vilis T: Loss of set in muscle responses to limb perturbations during cerebellar dysfunction. J Neurophysiol 51:1137, 1984.

46. Isaacs KR, et al: Exercise and the brain: Angiogenesis in the adult rat cerebellum after vigorous physical activity and motor skill learning. J Cereb Blood Flow Metab 12:110, 1992.
47. Ito M: Neurophysiological aspects of the cerebellar motor control system. Int J Neurol 1:162, 1970.
48. Ito M: The Cerebellum and Neural Control. New York, Raven, 1984.
49. Jung R, Kornhuber HH: Results of electronystagmography in man: The value of optokinetic vestibular and spontaneous nystagmus for neurologic diagnosis and research. In Bender MB: The Oculomotor System. New York, Harper & Row, 1964.
50. Kabat H: Studies on neuromuscular dysfunction. XII. Rhythmic stabilization: A new and more effective technique for treatment of paralysis through a cerebellar mechanism. Permanente Found Med Bull 8:9, 1950.
51. Kabat H: Analysis and therapy of cerebellar ataxia and asynergia. Arch Neurol Psychiatry 74.375, 1955.
52. Kandel ER, Schwart JH, Jessel TM (eds): Principles of Neuroscience. New York, McGraw-Hill, 2000.
53. Kent R, Netsell R: A case study of an ataxic dysarthric: Cineradiography and spectrographic observations. J Speech Hear Disord 40:115, 1975.
54. Kissi B, Bogleiter H, eds: The Biology of Alcoholism, vol 5. New York, Plenum, 1997.
55. Klintsova AY, et al: Therapeutic motor training ameliorates cerebellar effects of postnatal binge alcohol. Neurotoxicol Teratol 22:125, 2000.
56. Knott M, Voss DE: Proprioceptive Neuro-Muscular Facilitation, 2nd ed. New York, Harper & Row, 1968.
57. Kornhuber HH: Neurologie des Kleinhirns. Zentrabl Gesemte Neurol Psychiatrie 191:13, 1968.
58. Krusen FH, et al: Handbook of Physical Medicine and Rehabilitation, 2nd ed. Philadelphia, WB Saunders, 1971.
59. Lang CE, Bastian AJ: Cerebellar subjects show impaired adaptation of anticipatory EMG during catching. J Neurophysiol 82:2108, 1999.
60. Lechtenberg R: Ataxia and other cerebellar syndromes. In Jankovic J, Eduardo T (eds): Parkinson's Disease and Movement Disorders. Baltimore, Williams & Wilkins, 1993.
61. Lechtenberg R, Gilman S: Speech disorders in cerebellar disease. Ann Neurol 3: 285, 1978.
62. Ledin T, Odkuist LM: Abstinent chronic alcoholics investigated by dynamic posteriography, ocular smooth pursuit and visual suppression. Acta Otolaryngol 111:646, 1991.
63. Llinas R: Functional Significance of the Basic Cerebellar Circuit in Motor Coordination. In Bloedel JR, Dichans J, Precht W (eds): Cerebellar Functions. Berlin, Springer, 1985, pp 170–180.
64. Luciani L: Il cervelletto: Nuovi studi di fisiologia normale e patologica. Florence, Le Monnier, 1891.
65. Luciani L: De l'influence qu'exercent les mutilations cérébelleuses sur l'excitabilité de l'écorce cérébrale et sur les réflexes spinaux. Arch Ital Biol 21:190, 1894.
66. MacKay WA, Murphy JT: Cerebellar modulation of reflex gain. Prog Neurobiol 13:361, 1979.
67. Marie P, et al: De l'atrophie cérébelleuse tardive à predominance corticale. Rev Neurol (Paris) 38:849, 1082, 1922.
68. Marr D: A theory of the cerebellar cortex. J Physiol 202:437, 1969.
69. Marsden CD, et al: Disorders of movement in cerebellar disease in man. In Rose CF (ed): Physiological Aspects of Clinical Neurology. Oxford, Blackwell Scientific, 1977.
70. Mauritz KH, et al: Delayed and enhanced long latency reflexes as the possible cause of postural tremor in late cerebellar atrophy. Brain 104:97, 1981.
71. McCloskey DI: Kinesthetic sensibility. Physiol Rev 58:763, 1978.
72. Meyer-Lohmann J, et al: Effects of dentate cooling on precentral unit activity following torque pulse injections into elbow movements. Brain Res 94:237, 1975.
73. Middleton FA, Strick PL: Basal ganglia and cerebellar loops: motor and cognitive circuits. Brain Res Rev 31:236, 2000.
74. Miles FA, Fuller JH: Adaptive plasticity in the vestibulo-ocular responses of the rhesus monkey. Brain Res 8:512, 1974.
75. Molinari M, et al: Cerebellum and procedural learning: Evidence from focal cerebellar lesions. Brain 120:1753, 1997.
76. Morgan MH: Ataxia and weights. Physiotherapy 61:332, 1975.
77. Nakamura R, Taniguchi R: Kinesiological analysis and physical

therapy of cerebellar ataxia. In Sobue I (ed): Spinocerebellar Degenerations. Baltimore, University Park Press, 1978.
78. Nashold BS, et al: Ocular reactions in man from deep cerebellar stimulation and lesions. Arch Ophthalmol 81:538, 1969.
79. Norton S, et al: Early motor development and cerebral cortical morphology in rats exposed prenatally to alcohol. Alcoholism 12:130, 1988.
80. Nyberg-Hansen R, Horn J: Functional aspects of cerebellar signs in clinical neurology. Acta Neurol Scand 48(Suppl 51):219, 1972.
81. Optican LM, Robinson DA: Cerebellar-dependent adaptive control of primate saccadic system. J Neurophysiol 44:1058, 1980.
82. Orlovsky GN, Shik ML: Control of locomotion: A neurophysiological analysis of the cat locomotor system. In Porter R (ed): International Review of Physiology. Neurophysiology II, vol 10. Baltimore, University Park Press, 1976.
83. Oscar-Barman M, et al: Dichotic ear-order effects with nonverbal stimuli. Cortex 10.270, 1074.
84. Poirier LJ, et al: Physiopathology of the cerebellum in the monkey. II. Motor disturbances associated with partial and complete destruction of cerebellar structures. J Neurol Sci 22:491, 1974.
85. Ritchie L: Effect of cerebellar lesions on saccadic eye movements. J Neurophysiol 39:1246–1256, 1976.
86. Rossi G: Sugli effetti consequenti alla stimolazione contemporanea della corteccia cerebrale e di quella cerebellare. Arch Fisiol 10:389, 1912.
87. Ruch TC: Motor systems. In Stevens SS (ed): Handbook of Experimental Psychology. New York, John Wiley & Sons, 1951.
88. Russell JSR: Experimental research into the functions of the cerebellum. Philos Trans R Soc Lond B Biol Sci 185:819, 1894.
89. Ryding E, et al: Motor imagery activates the cerebellum regionally. A SPECT rCBF study with 99mTc-HMPAO. Cogn Brain Res 1:94, 1993.
90. Selhorst JB, et al: Disorders in cerebellar ocular motor control. I. Saccadic overshoot dysmetria. Brain 99:497, 1976.
91. Serrien DJ, Wiesendager M: Grip-load force coordination in cerebellar patients. Exp Brain Res 128:76, 1999.
92. Shadmehr R, Holcomb HH: Neural correlates of motor memory consolidation. Science 277:821, 1997.
93. Shankweiler D: Effects of temporal lobe damage on perception of dichotically presented melodies. J Comp Physiol Psychol 62:115, 1966.
94. Shimizu N, et al: Eye-head co-ordination in patients with parkinsonism and cerebellar ataxia. J Neurol Neurosurg Psychiatry 44:509, 1981.
95. Silfverskjold BP: A 3 sec leg tremor in a cerebellar syndrome. Acta Neurol Scand 55:385, 1977.
96. Smith AM, Bourbonnais D: Neuronal activity in cerebellar cortex related to control of prehensile force. J Neurophysiol 45:286, 1981.
97. Stein RB, Oguztoreli MN: Reflex involvement in the generation and control of tremor and clonus. Prog Clin Neurophysiol (Basel) 5:28, 1978.
98. Stockmeyer S: An interpretation of the approach of Rood to the treatment of neuromuscular dysfunction. Am J Phys Med 46:900, 1967.
99. Strick PL: Cerebellar involvement in "volitional" muscle response to load changes. Prog Clin Neurophysiol 4:85, 1978.
100. Terzuolo TA, Viviani P: Parameters of motion and EMG activities during some simple motor tasks in normal subjects and cerebellar patients. In Cooper IS, et al (eds): The Cerebellum, Epilepsy and Behavior. New York, Plenum Press, 1973.
101. Thach WT: Correlation of neural discharge with pattern and force of muscular activity, joint position, and direction of the intended movement in motor cortex and cerebellum. J Neurophysiol 41:654, 1978.
102. Thach WT: A role of the cerebellum in learning movement coordination. Neurobiol Learn Mem 70:177, 1998.
103. Thach WT, et al: Cerebellum and the adaptive coordination of movement. Annu Rev Neurosci 15:403, 1992.
104. Thach WT: On the specific role of the cerebellum in motor learning and cognition: clues from PET activation and lesion studies in humans. Behav Brain Sci 19:411, 1996.
105. Thach WT, et al: Cerebellum and the adaptive coordination of movement. Annu Rev Neurosci 15:403, 1992.
106. Thach WT, et al: Cerebellar output: Multiple maps and modes of control in movement coordination. In Llinas R, Soto C (eds): The Cerebellum Revisited. New York, Springer-Verlag, 1992, p 283.

107. Topka H: Motor skill learning in patients with cerebellar degeneration. J Neurol Sci 158:164, 1998.
108. Tsukue I, Shohaji T: Movement therapy for alcoholic patients. J Stud Alcohol 42:144, 1981.
109. Uno M, et al: Effects of cooling the interposed nuclei in tracking-task performance in monkeys. J Neurophysiol 36:996, 1973.
110. Victor M, et al: A restricted form of cerebellar cortical degeneration occurring in alcoholic patients. Arch Neurol 1:579, 1959.
111. Vilis T, Hore J: Effects of changes in mechanical state of limb on cerebellar intention tremor. J Neurophysiol 40:1214, 1977.
112. Vilis T, et al: Dual nature of the precentral responses to limb perturbations revealed by cerebellar cooling. Brain Res 117:336, 1976.
113. Von Noorden GK, Preziosi TJ: Eye movement recordings in neurological disorders. Arch Ophthalmol 76:162, 1966.
114. Woodridge CP, Russell G: Head position training with the cerebral palsied child. An application of biofeedback techniques. Milbank Mem Fund Q 57:407, 1976.
115. Zee DS, et al: The mechanism of downbeat nystagmus. Arch Neurol 30:227, 1974.
116. Zee DS, et al: Ocular motor abnormalities in hereditary ataxia. Brain 99:207, 1976.
117. Zee DS, et al: Slow saccades in spinocerebellar degeneration. Arch Neurol 33:243, 1976.
118. Zee DS, et al: Effects of ablation of flocculus and paraflocculus on eye movements in primate. J Neurophysiol 46:878, 1981.
119. Zentay PJ: Motor disorders of the nervous system and their significance for speech. I. Cerebral and cerebellar dysarthrias. Laryngoscope 47:147, 1937.

Hemiplegia

SUSAN D. RYERSON, MA, PT

Chapter Outline

Objectives

After reading this chapter the student/therapist will:

1. Identify the various types of neurovascular disease.
2. Identify the atypical patterns of movement in clients with residual hemiplegia.
3. Identify significant primary and secondary impairments that interfere with functional movement patterns.
4. Describe a reeducation intervention strategy for improving functional limitations in clients with stroke.
5. Identify various treatment procedures and understand how they affect performance of functional movement.

OVERVIEW

The treatment of hemiplegia from vascular insult is controversial. Various treatment methods have been devised and advocated. Recent scientific theories have changed the focus of treatment from one of inhibition of abnormal tone and facilitation of normal movement to reeducation of control and weakness and functional retraining. In this chapter, pathology, impairments, and intervention strategies for clients with hemiplegia from stroke are reviewed. Although hemiplegia from neurovascular pathology is the focus of the chapter, therapists can use this information and apply it to hemiplegia in adults caused by other central nervous system (CNS) pathologies, such as tumor, trauma, multiple sclerosis, and demyelinating diseases. Normal movement is the model according to which appropriate techniques of reeducation and compensatory training are chosen to allow the person with hemiplegia to obtain the highest level of function.

Definition

Hemiplegia, a paralysis of one side of the body, is the classic sign of neurovascular disease of the brain. It is one of many manifestations of neurovascular disease, and it occurs with strokes involving the cerebral hemisphere or brain stem. A stroke, or cerebrovascular accident (CVA), results in a sudden, specific neurological deficit. It is the suddenness of this neurological deficit—occurring over seconds, minutes, hours, or a few days—that characterizes the disorder as vascular. Although hemiplegia may be the most obvious sign of a CVA and a major concern of therapists, other symptoms are equally disabling, including sensory dysfunction, aphasia or dysarthria, visual field defects, and mental and intellectual impairment. The specific combination of these neurovascular deficits enables a physician to detect both the location and the size of the defect. CVAs can be classified according to pathological type—thrombosis, embolism, or hemorrhage—or by temporal factors, such as completed, in-evolution, or transient ischemic attacks (TIAs).

Epidemiology

In the United States, stroke is the third most common cause of death, with 160,000 dying each year.[89] The National Stroke Association estimates that 730,000 new or recurrent strokes occur each year. The incidence of stroke rises rapidly with increasing age: two thirds of all strokes occur in people older than the age of 65; and after 55, the risk of stroke doubles every 10 years. With the over-50 age group growing rapidly, more people than ever are at risk. In the United States, the incidence of stroke is greater in males than in females, and it is twice as high in blacks as in whites. Cerebral infarction (thrombosis or embolism) is the most common form of stroke, accounting for 70% of all strokes. Hemorrhages account for another 20%, and 10% remain unspecified. Stroke is the largest single cause of neurological disability. Approximately 4 million Americans are dealing with the impairments and disabilities from a stroke. Of these, 31% require assistance, 20% need help walking, 16% are in long-term care facilities, and 71% are vocationally impaired after 7 years.[89]

The three most commonly recognized risk factors for cerebrovascular disease are hypertension, diabetes mellitus, and heart disease. The most important of these factors is hypertension.[20] Because high blood pressure is the greatest risk factor for stroke, human characteristics and behaviors that increase the blood pressure, including increased high serum cholesterol levels, obesity, diabetes mellitus, heavy alcohol consumption, cocaine use, and cigarette smoking, increase the risk of stroke.

Ostfeld[94] noted that mortality rates for stroke have declined, slowly at first (from 1900 to 1950) and then more quickly (from 1950 to 1970), with a sharp drop noted around 1974. Experts have speculated that the greater use of hypertensive drugs in the 1960s and 1970s started this decline, and the creation of screening and treatment referral centers for high blood pressure may account for the marked decline in the late 1970s.

Outcome

The long-term follow-up on the Framingham Heart Study revealed that long-term stroke survivors, especially those with only one episode, had a good chance for full functional recovery.[50] For those people left with severe neurological and functional deficits, studies have demonstrated that rehabilitation is effective and that it can improve functional ability.[57, 58] It has been demonstrated that age is not a factor in determining the outcome of the rehabilitation process.[3] Presently, it is thought that clients should be given an opportunity to participate in the rehabilitation process, regardless of age, unless medically contraindicated.

Prediction of ultimate functional outcome has been hampered by the inaccuracy of commonly used predictors (medical items, income level, intelligence, functional level). Computed tomography (CT), functional magnetic resonance imaging, and regional cerebral blood flow studies are used in diagnosis and, increasingly, as predictors of functional recovery following stroke. Positron emission tomography (PET) and single photon emission computed tomography (SPECT) are newer techniques that are used in research centers to define areas of dysfunctional but perhaps "salvageable" tissue.[1, 30]

Pathoneurological and Pathophysiological Aspects

Classification

The pathological processes that result from a CVA can be divided into three groups—thrombotic changes, embolic changes, and hemorrhagic changes.

Thrombotic Infarction. Atherosclerotic plaques and hypertension interact to produce cerebrovascular infarcts. These plaques form at branchings and curves of the arteries. Plaques usually form in front of the first major branching of the cerebral arteries. These lesions can be present for 30 years or more and may never become symptomatic. Intermittent blockage may proceed to permanent damage. The process by which a thrombus occludes an artery requires several hours and explains the division between stroke-in-evolution and completed stroke.[2]

TIAs are an indication of the presence of thrombotic disease and are the result of transient ischemia. Although the cause of TIAs has not been definitively established, cerebral vasospasm and transient systemic arterial hypotension are thought to be responsible factors.

Embolic Infarction. The embolus that causes the stroke may come from the heart, from an internal carotid artery thrombosis, or from an atheromatous plaque of the carotid sinus. It is usually a sign of cardiac disease. The infarction may be of pale, hemorrhagic, or mixed type. The branches of the middle cerebral artery are infarcted most commonly as a result of its direct continuation from the internal carotid artery. Collateral blood supply is not established with embolic infarctions because of the speed of obstruction formation, so there is less survival of tissue distal to the area of embolic infarct than with thrombotic infarct.[2]

Hemorrhage. The most common intracranial hemorrhages causing stroke are those due to hypertension, ruptured saccular aneurysm, and arteriovenous (AV) malformation. Massive hemorrhage frequently results from hypertensive cardiac-renal disease; bleeding into the brain tissue produces an oval or round mass that displaces midline structures. The exact mechanism of hemorrhage is not known. This mass of extravasated blood decreases in size over 6 to 8 months.

Saccular, or berry, aneurysms are thought to be the result of defects in the media and elastica that develop over years. This muscular defect plus overstretching of the internal elastic membrane from blood pressure causes the aneurysm to develop. Saccular aneurysms are found at branchings of major cerebral arteries, especially the anterior portion of the circle of Willis. Averaging 8 to 10 mm in diameter and variable in form, these aneurysms rupture at their dome. Saccular aneurysms are rare in childhood.

AV malformations are developmental abnormalities that result in a spaghetti-like mass of dilated AV fistulas varying in size from a few millimeters in diameter to huge masses located within the brain tissue. Some of these blood vessels have extremely thin, abnormally structured walls. Although the abnormality is present from birth, symptoms usually develop between the ages of 10 and 35. The hemorrhage of an AV malformation presents a pathological picture similar to that for the saccular aneurysm. The larger AV malformations frequently occur in the posterior half of the cerebral hemisphere.[2]

Clinical Findings

The focal neurological deficit resulting from a stroke, whether embolic, thrombotic, or hemorrhagic, is a reflection of the size and location of the lesion and the amount of collateral blood flow. Unilateral neurological deficits result from interruption of the carotid vascular system, and bilateral neurological deficits result from interruption of the vascular supply to the basilar system. Clinical syndromes resulting from occlusion or hemorrhage in the cerebral circulation vary from partial to complete. Signs of hemorrhage may be more variable as a result of the effect of extension to surrounding brain tissue and the possible rise in intracranial pressure. Table 25–1 summarizes the clinical symptoms and the anatomical structures involved according to specific arterial involvement.

The frequencies of the three types of cerebrovascular disease—thrombosis, embolism, and hemorrhage—vary according to whether they were taken from a clinical study or from an autopsy study, but they rank in the order presented in this section. Ischemic strokes, thrombotic or embolic, account for 80% of strokes and hemorrhagic strokes account for 20%.[101] The clinical symptoms and laboratory findings for each type are condensed in Table 25–2.

Medical Management and Pharmacological Considerations

Acute Medical Care

Thrombosis and TIAs. Although infarcted tissue cannot at present be restored, medical management of the acute stroke from thrombosis or TIA is geared toward improving the cerebral circulation as quickly as possible to prevent ischemic tissue from becoming infarcted tissue. Cells that have 80% to 100% ischemia will die in a few minutes because they cannot produce energy, specifically adenosine triphosphate. This energy failure results in an activation of calcium, which causes a chain reaction resulting in cell death.[89] Around this area of infarction is a transitional area where the blood flow is decreased 50% to 80%. Cells in the transitional area are not irreversibly damaged.[118, 127]

One of the newer drugs available for acute stroke treatment is tissue plasminogen activator (t-PA) (see Chapter 32). It is most effective if used within 90 to 180 minutes of the onset of symptoms. Recent studies indicate that 42% of patients with stroke wait 24 hours before getting care, with the average being 13 hours.[127] The importance of community-wide programs to increase awareness of symptoms and effectiveness of emergency medical responses is immense for this drug's usage. The American Heart Association and the National Stroke Association are creating community campaigns to increase awareness of the medical emergency nature of stroke symptoms.

Anticoagulant drugs are used to prevent TIAs and may stop a stroke-in-evolution. Before anticoagulant drugs are used, an accurate differential diagnosis is necessary because of the danger of excessive bleeding if hemorrhage is present. Heparin is often used in the early stage of the stroke, and warfarin (Coumadin) is commonly used in the months after the stroke. Cerebral edema, if present, is managed pharmacologically during the first few days. Antiplatelet drugs such as aspirin, dipyridamole (Persan-

tine), and sulfinpyrazone (Anturane) are used to prevent clotting by decreasing platelet "stickiness."[2]

Surgical treatment (thromboendarterectomy or grafting) is used when TIAs are the result of arterial plaques. Areas accessible to and suitable for surgery include the carotid sinus and the common carotid, innominate, and subclavian arteries. Although both surgery and anticoagulant therapy are used for TIAs, Adams and Victor[2] extensively reviewed the wide divergence of opinions. For clients who have had a stroke yet recovered quickly and well, medical care focuses on prevention. Prevention usually includes maintaining blood pressure and blood flow, monitoring hypotensive agents (if given), and avoiding oversedation, especially for sleep, to prevent cerebral ischemia.

Embolic Infarction. Management of embolic infarction is similar to that of thrombotic infarction. The primary emphasis is on prevention. Long-term anticoagulant therapy is effective in preventing embolic infarction in clients with cardiac problems such as atrial fibrillation, myocardial infarction (MI), and valve prostheses. The diagnostic use of CT is important in anticoagulant therapy to rule out hemorrhage after the infarct.

Hypertensive Hemorrhage. Medical procedures for hypertensive hemorrhage parallel those for thrombosis and embolism. Surgical removal of the clot and lowering of the systemic blood pressure to decrease hemorrhage have generally not been helpful. Again, the preventive use of antihypertensive drugs in clients with essential hypertension is the soundest medical management available.[2]

Ruptured Aneurysm. Comatose clients are not good candidates for surgery. However, if the client survives the first few days and if the state of consciousness improves, surgical intervention, whether extracranial or intracranial, is the treatment of choice. Medical treatment consists of lowering arterial blood pressures. Bed rest for 4 to 6 weeks with all forms of exertion avoided is prescribed. Antiseizure medication may be used. Often a systemic antifibrinolysin is given to impede lysis of the clot at the site of rupture. Vasospasm, resulting in severe motor dysfunction, is present with the use of drugs such as reserpine (Serpasil) and kanamycin (Kantrex). (See Chapter 32.)

Regardless of the cause of the stroke, comatose stroke clients are managed by (1) treatment of shock; (2) maintenance of clear airway and oxygen flow; (3) measurement of arterial blood gases, blood analysis, CT, and spinal tap; (4) control of seizures; and (5) gastric tube feeding (if coma is prolonged). Hypertensive hemorrhage is one of the most common vascular causes of coma.[62]

Medical Management of Associated Problems

Spasticity. Spasticity and its treatment constitute a major medical problem after stroke because clients complain about it, it may fluctuate, and it does not respond to one fixed treatment. The relationship between spasticity and movement after stroke is an area of continued

TABLE 25-1. Clinical Symptoms of Vascular Lesions

Affected Vessel	Clinical Symptoms	Structures Involved
Middle cerebral artery	Contralateral paralysis and sensory deficit	Somatic motor area
	Motor speech impairment	Broca's area (dominant hemisphere)
	"Central" aphasia, anomia, jargon speech	Parietooccipital cortex (dominant hemisphere)
	Unilateral neglect, apraxia, impaired ability to judge distance	Parietal lobe (nondominant hemisphere)
	Homonomous hemianopia	Optic radiation deep to second temporal convolution
	Loss of conjugate gaze to opposite side	Frontal controversive field
	Avoidance reaction of opposite limbs	Parietal lobe
	Pure motor hemiplegia	Upper portion of posterior limb of internal capsule
	Limb-kinetic apraxia	Premotor or parietal cortex
Anterior cerebral artery	Paralysis—lower extremity	Motor area—leg
	Paresis in opposite arm	Arm area of cortex
	Cortical sensory loss	Sensory area
	Urinary incontinence	Posteromedial aspect of superior frontal gyrus
		Medial surface of posterior frontal lobe
	Contralateral grasp reflex, sucking reflex	Uncertain
	Lack of spontaneity, motor inaction, echolalia	Uncertain
	Perseveration and amnesia	
Posterior cerebral artery		
Peripheral area	Homonymous hemianopia	Calcarine cortex or optic radiation
	Bilateral homonymous hemianopia, cortical blindness, inability to perceive objects not centrally located, occular apraxia	Bilateral occipital lobe
	Memory defect	Inferomedial portions of temporal lobe
	Topographic disorientation	Nondominant calcarine and lingual gyri
Central area	Thalamic syndrome	Posteroventral nucleus ophthalmus
	Weber syndrome	Cranial nerve III and cerebral peduncle
	Contralateral hemiplegia	Cerebral peduncle
	Paresis of vertical eye movements, sluggish pupillary response to light	Supranuclear fibers to cranial nerve III
	Contralateral ataxia or postural tremor	
Internal carotid artery	Variable signs according to degree and site of occlusion—middle cerebral, anterior cerebral, posterior cerebral territory	Uncertain
Basilar artery		
Superior cerebellar artery	Ataxia	Middle and superior cerebellar peduncle
	Dizziness, nausea, vomiting, horizontal nystagmus	Vestibular nucleus
	Horner syndrome on opposite side, decreased pain and thermal sensation	Descending sympathetic fibers
		Spinal thalamic tract
	Decreased touch, vibration, position sense of lower extremity greater than that of upper extremity	Medial lemniscus
Anterior inferior cerebellar artery	Nystagmus, vertigo, nausea, vomiting	Vestibular nerve
	Facial paralysis on same side	Cranial nerve VII
	Tinnitus	Auditory nerve, lower cochlear nucleus
	Ataxia	Middle cerebral peduncle
	Impaired facial sensation on same side	Fifth cranial nerve nucleus
	Decreased pain and thermal sensation on opposite side	Spinal thalamic tract
Complete basilar syndrome	Bilateral long tract signs with cerebellar and cranial nerve abnormalities	
	Coma	
	Quadriplegia	
	Pseudobulbar palsy	
	Cranial nerve abnormalities	
Vertebral artery	Decreased pain and temperature on opposite side	Spinal thalamic tract
	Sensory loss from a tactile and proprioceptive	Medial lemniscus
	Hemiparesis of arm and leg	Pyramidal tract
	Facial pain and numbness on same side	Decending tract and fifth cranial nucleus
	Horner syndrome, ptosis, decreased sweating	Decending sympathetic tract
	Ataxia	Spinal cerebellar tract
	Paralysis of tongue	Cranial nerve XII
	Weakness of vocal cord, decreased gag	Cranial nerves IX and X
	Hiccups	Uncertain

Adapted from Adams RD, Victor M: Principles of Neurology. New York, McGraw-Hill, 1981.

TABLE 25-2. Clinical Symptoms and Laboratory Findings for Neurovascular Disease

Disease Type	Clinical Picture	Laboratory Findings
Thrombosis	*Extremely variable* Proceeded by a prodromal episode Uneven progression Onset develops within minutes or hours or over days ("thrombus in evolution") 60% occur during sleep—awaken unaware of problem, rise, and fall to floor Usually no headache, but may occur in mild form Hypertension, diabetes, or vascular disease elsewhere in body	Cerebrospinal fluid pressure is normal. Cerebrospinal fluid is clear. EEG: limited differential diagnostic value Skull radiographs are not helpful. Arteriography is the definitive procedure; it demonstrates site of collateral flow. CT scan is helpful in chronic state when cavitation has occurred.
TIAs	Linked to atherosclerotic thrombosis Preceded or accompanied by stroke Occur by themselves Last 2–30 minutes Experience a few attacks or hundreds Normal neurological examination between attacks If transient symptoms are present on awakening, may indicate future stroke	Usually none

Embolism
Cardiac
Noncardiac
  Atherosclerosis
  Pulmonary thrombosis
  Fat, tumor, air
	Extremely variable
	Occurs extremely rapidly—seconds or minutes
	There are no warnings
	Branches of middle cerebral artery are involved most frequently; large embolus will block internal carotid artery or stem of middle cerebral artery
	If embolus is in basilar system, deep coma and total paralysis may result
	Often a manifestation of heart disease, including atrial fibrillation and myocardial infarction
	Headache
	As embolus passes through artery, client may have neurological deficits that resolve as embolus breaks and passes into small artery supplying small or silent brain area
		Generally same as for thrombosis except for following:
		  If embolism causes a large hemorrhagic infarct, cerebrospinal fluid will be bloody.
		  30% of embolic strokes produce small hemorrhagic infarct without bloody cerebrospinal fluid.

Hemorrhage Hypertensive hemorrhage	Severe headache Vomiting at onset Blood pressure >170/90; usually "essential" hypertension but can be from other types Abrupt onset, usually during day, not in sleep Gradually evolves over hours or days according to speed of bleeding No recurrence of bleeding Frequency in blacks with hypertensive hemorrhage is greater than frequency in whites Hemorrhaged blood absorbs slowly—rapid improvement of symptoms is not usual If massive hemorrhage occurs, client may survive a few hours or days secondary to brain stem compression	CT scan can detect hemorrhages larger than 1.5 cm in cerebral and cerebellar hemispheres; it is diagnostically superior to arteriography; it is especially helpful in diagnosing small hemorrhages that do not spill blood into cerebrospinal fluid; with massive hemorrhage and increased pressure, cerebrospinal fluid is grossly bloody; lumbar puncture is necessary when CT scan is not available. Radiographs occasionally show midline shift (this is not true with infarction). EEG shows no typical pattern, but high voltage and slow waves are most common with hemorrhage. Urinary changes may reflect renal disease.

Ruptured saccular aneurysm	Asymptomatic before rupture
	With rupture, blood spills under high pressure into subarachnoid space
	  Excruciating headache with loss of consciousness
	  Headache without loss of consciousness
	  Sudden loss of consciousness
	Decerebrate rigidity with coma
	If severe—persistent deep coma with respiratory arrest, circulatory collapse leading to death; death can occur within 5 minutes
	If mild—consciousness regained within hours then confusion, amnesia, headache, stiff neck, drowsiness
	Hemiplegia, paresis, homonymous hemianopia, or aphasia usually absent
		CT scan detects localized blood in hydrocephalus if present.
		Cerebrospinal fluid is extremely bloody.
		Radiographs are usually negative.
		Carotid and vertebral arteriography is performed only when diagnosis is certain.

Adapted from Adams RD, Victor M: Principles of Neurology. New York, McGraw-Hill, 1981.

interest for researchers. Recent studies have refuted the earlier belief that spasticity was inversely related to voluntary movement.[69, 110] Although therapists are more hesitant to treat spasticity now, physicians continue to treat it aggressively. Various pharmacological, surgical, and physical means are used to decrease spasticity. The pharmacological and surgical means are examined here, and therapy management is discussed later.

Two types of drugs are used to counter the effects of spasticity: centrally acting and peripherally acting. Centrally acting drugs, such as diazepam, have been used to depress the lateral reticular formation and thus its facilitatory action on the gamma motor neurons. This form of drug is used widely to treat spasticity, even though the greatest disadvantage of centrally acting drugs is that they depress the entire CNS. Drowsiness and anxiety are common side effects.

Peripherally acting drugs are used to block a specific link in the gamma group. Procaine blocks selectively inhibit the small gamma motor fibers, resulting in a relaxation of intrafusal fibers. The effect of procaine blocks is transient. Intramuscular neurolysis with the injection of 5% to 7% phenol has been used to destroy the small intramuscular mixed nerve branches.[37] Phenol blocks relieve hypertonicity and improve function, especially when followed by an intensive course of therapy.[98] They can provide relief from 2 to 12 months, and their effects have been documented to last as long as 3 years.[37, 98] Disadvantages of phenol use include its toxicity to tissue and the complications of pain that occasionally result.

Botulinum toxin A (Botox) is also used to decrease the effects of hypertonicity on functional movement in hemiplegia.[122] Local injection of the toxin into spastic muscles produces selective weakness by interfering with the uptake of acetylcholine by the motor end plate. The effect of the toxin is temporary, depends on the amount injected, and is associated with minimal side effects. Repeat injections are recommended no sooner than 12 to 14 weeks to avoid antibody formation to the toxin. Researchers report positive functional results when Botox injections are followed by intensive muscle reeducation and appropriate splinting.[33, 122]

Dantrolene sodium is used to interrupt the excitation-contraction mechanism of skeletal muscles. Trials have shown that it has reduced spasticity in 60% to 80% of clients while improving function in 40% of these clients. The side effects—drowsiness, weakness, and fatigue—can be decreased through titration of dosage. Serious side effects, including hepatotoxicity, precipitation of seizures, and lymphocytic lymphoma, have been reported when the drug has been used in high dosages over a long time.[37]

Baclofen, in pill form, is used as a skeletal muscle relaxant to decrease spasticity. It can now be delivered intrathecally into the spinal cord using a pump that is surgically inserted into the body. It relieves spasticity with a small amount of medication (10 mg/20 mL, 10 mg/5 mL). Intrathecal baclofen has had dramatic results in cases of severe spasticity, because it acts directly on the affected muscles instead of circulating in the blood. It is used for extremity spasticity that interferes with the ability to assume functional positions in patients with severe stroke, multiple sclerosis, head injury, and cerebral palsy.[95]

The surgical treatment of spasticity through tenotomy or neurectomy is considered when all other treatments fail, and it is used to correct deformity, especially of a hand or foot. A peripheral nerve block is often used as a diagnostic tool to evaluate the effect of surgical treatment. If anatomical or functional gains are made through a temporary nerve block, consideration is given to surgical release. The surgical treatment of spasticity does not necessarily result in increased movement control and, with the increased understanding of the causes of spasticity, does not seem appropriate in stroke.

Seizures. The highest risk for seizure after a stroke is immediately afterward; 57% of seizures occur in the first week and 88% occur within the first year.[11] Seizures after thrombotic and embolic stroke are usually of early onset, whereas seizures after hemorrhagic stroke are of late onset. The management of seizures after stroke is usually with antiseizure medication. Commonly used drugs include phenytoin (Dilantin), carbamazepine (Tegretol), gabapentin (Neurontin), and divalproex (Depakote).[130] Side effects that interfere with movement therapy include drowsiness, ataxia, distractibility, and poor memory.

Respiratory Involvement. Fatigue is a major problem for the person with hemiplegia. This fatigability, which interferes with everyday life processes and active rehabilitation, is attributed to respiratory insufficiency resulting from paralysis of one side of the thorax. Haas and colleagues[52] studied respiratory function in hemiplegia and found decreased lung volume and mechanical performance of the thorax to be significant factors, in addition to abnormal pulmonary diffusing capacity. Clients with hemiplegia consume 50% more oxygen while walking slowly (regardless of the presence or absence of orthotic devices) than that used by subjects without hemiplegia.[52] The decreased respiratory output and the increased oxygen demand that result from atypical movement patterns are responsible for early fatigue in persons with hemiplegia. Treatment objectives and techniques must reflect the understanding of this respiratory problem. The therapist should not overlook the use of standard respiratory functions as an objective measure of the efficacy of treatment techniques.

Trauma. If the hemiplegic client has severe trunk weakness with significant spinal asymmetries, and relies exclusively on the nonparetic extremities for function, poor balance and falls are possible. Persons with stroke fall to the affected side when protective mechanisms are inadequate or absent. Common fracture sites are the humerus, wrist, and hip.[83]

Therapy intervention for a hip fracture with a hemiplegia is complicated by increased difficulty sustaining a symmetrical trunk posture over the fractured hip, decreased strength in the leg, pain, and spasticity. In addition to the loss of balance and protective mechanisms, the development of osteoporosis from disuse is a limiting factor for functional recovery after a fracture.[100]

Thrombophlebitis. Thrombophlebitis may occur in the early stages of rehabilitation. Vascular changes are often premorbid. Deep vein thrombosis is caused by altered blood flow, damage to the vessel wall, and changes in blood coagulation times. The vascular changes are aggravated by the inactivity and dependent postures of the weak extremities. Deep vein thrombosis is many times more common in the weak leg.[22]

Reflex Sympathetic Dystrophy. Medical treatment of reflex sympathetic dystrophy includes the use of chemical sympathetic blocks and oral or intramuscular corticosteroids. The use of blocks and corticosteroids often stops the burning pain. The length of time of the relief varies from client to client. Adverse reactions from block and corticosteroids occur about 20% of the time.[25, 70] (See Chapters 12 and 29.)

Pain. The pharmacological management of pain (usually shoulder pain) includes the local injection of corticosteroids. (For additional information regarding pain and its management see Chapter 29.)

Sequential Stages of Recovery from Acute to Long-Term Care

Evolution of Recovery Process

The evolution of the recovery process from onset to the return to community life can be divided into three stages—acute, active (rehabilitation), and adaptation to personal environment.

The acute state involves the stroke-in-evolution, the completed stroke, or the TIA and the decision whether to hospitalize.

The stroke-in-evolution develops gradually with distinct demarcation of the damaged area over 6 to 24 hours. Thrombosis, the most common cause for stroke, results first in ischemia and finally in infarction. Its gradual onset has led researchers to believe that a "cure" may be found for this type of stroke. If ischemic tissue can be treated and saved before infarction occurs, the neurological damage may be reversible. Small hemorrhages also may become a stroke-in-evolution by effusing blood along nerve pathways and by attracting fluid.[80] A completed stroke has a sudden onset and produces distinct, nonprogressive symptoms and damage within minutes or hours. In contrast, the TIA has a brief duration of neurological deficit and spontaneous resolution with no residual signs. TIAs vary in number and duration.

The need for hospitalization is decided by the physician. The trend to hospitalize is more common today than years ago.[128] However, a mild stroke or TIA may produce minimal physical-mental symptoms, and the person may not even seek medical help. Cost-containment measures in hospitals and managed care have led to decreased lengths of stay and the development of critical pathway plans to deliver services more efficiently. Critical pathways are plans that describe the duration and extent of services after a stroke. These plans are created for therapy intervention services on a "best guess" basis because there are no studies that link impairment intervention with functional outcome.

The inpatient length of stay for acute stroke is currently 2 to 4 days. After the inpatient stay, the client follows one of four pathways: he or she returns home with or without home care services, goes to a rehabilitation hospital for a 2- to 4-week stay, goes to a subacute facility to become strong enough for the rehabilitation regimen, or goes to a long-term care facility for rehabilitation and/or maintenance care.

Once the stroke is completed the clinical symptoms begin to decrease in severity. A person with a stroke caused by an embolic episode may have symptoms that reverse completely in a few days; more frequently, however, improvement takes place very slowly with a marked deficit. The fatality rate is high within the first day but decreases substantially in the following months of recovery.[128] Evidence from efficacy studies of rehabilitation programs that aim at improving functional performance is limited. Studies by Bamford and colleagues indicate that early rehabilitation intervention reduces disability and improves compensatory strategies.[6]

The Framingham Heart Study has revealed that long-term stroke survivors have a good chance of returning to independent living. The greatest deficit in those persons with hemiplegia who have recovered basic motor skills and who have returned home is in the psychosocial and environmental areas.[50]

Recovery of Motor Function

Recovery of motor function after a stroke was thought historically to be complete after 3 to 6 months of onset. Research has shown that functional recovery from a stroke can continue for months or years.[5]

The initial functional gains after the stroke are attributed to reduction of cerebral edema, absorption of damaged tissue, and improved local vascular flow. However, these factors do not play a role in long-term functional recovery. The brain damage that results from a stroke is thought to be circumvented rather than "repaired" during the process of functional recovery. The CNS reacts to injury with a variety of potentially reparative morphological processes. Two mechanisms underlying functional recovery after stroke are collateral sprouting and the unmasking of neuropathways: regeneration and reorganization.[5] Research continues to provide important insights into the fundamental capabilities of the brain to respond to damage. Methods of intervention that use the environment and help the client learn lead to long-term improved recovery.

The CNS has some predictable traits in response to injury. Twitchell, in his classic study, first documented the initial loss of voluntary function.[23] Although paralysis with flaccidity initially exists, there is seldom, if ever, total paralysis. He reported both an increase in deep tendon reflexes after 48 hours and the emergence of synergistic patterns of movement.[23] The synergistic movement patterns of the upper extremity and lower extremity have been described in detail by many.[14, 24, 63] Verbal description of a visual phenomenon often leads to differences in written and spoken communication, yet the visual array or behavioral patterns may be exactly the same.[10] Synergistic patterns may not be the same as movement combinations necessary for function. Although it is stated that the leg recovers more quickly or better than the arm, a leg that is bound by an extensor synergy and that is as "rigid as a pillar" during gait has not recovered more quickly and has no better function than an arm that is flexed and held across the chest and that can only grasp in a gross pattern with no ability to release.

Although studies are investigating the exact nature of the relationship between voluntary movement and spasticity, clinical evidence demonstrates that as voluntary function increases, the dependence on synergistic movement decreases.[110] With the knowledge that the CNS is capable of reacting to injury with a variety of morphological processes, we should no longer view the effect of a stroke as a fixed event. Because the brain immediately institutes neuromechanisms that reconstitute typical functions, therapy interventions should emphasize use of movement patterns on the affected side to maximize return and to help the client achieve the highest level of function.

Predictors of Recovery

Research in motor recovery shows that, although motor recovery may continue after 6 months, functional status usually remains constant and that 86% of the variance in 6-month recovery is predictable at 1 month.[119]

Although 58% of patients regain independence in activities of daily living (ADL) and 82% learn to walk, 30% to 60% of patients have no arm function.[53] Initial return of movement in the first 2 weeks is one indicator of the possibility of full arm recovery. But failure to recover grip strength before 24 days is correlated with no recovery of arm function at 3 months.[53]

One problem inherent in prognostic research is the lack of a movement-based classification system. The clinical "predictors" in regression models are assumed to be static, whereas, in fact, they may change over time. Another problem is that there may be a lack in accuracy because of differences in researchers' objectives.[66]

As clinicians we can help minimize the problems in research methodology by precisely formulating functional goals, stating movement components and significant impairments that interfere with functional performance, and following a model when making clinical decisions to postulate cause and effect during intervention.

Classification of Atypical Movement Patterns

Although the *Guide to Physical Therapist Practice* groups patients with neurological dysfunction according to pa-

thology, therapy intervention rarely is directed by the diagnosis of stroke and resultant hemiplegia.[67] The World Health Organization (WHO) and Nagi models give us another option: classification by impairments.[87, 134] These models have given therapists an organized structure for evaluation and treatment. Both models share the impairment category, but they use different terms to title "dysfunction in task performance" and "the societal implication" of this dysfunction (Table 25–3). This semantic difference should be noted because both models are currently used by therapists. The WHO has recently modified its designations from ones with negative connotations (ICIDH-1)—*disability* and *handicap*—to more positive language (ICIDH-2)—*activities* as the nature and extent of functioning and *participation* as the measure of involvement in life situations. In this chapter the designations of the Nagi model are used.

Impairment-related classification systems for stroke are just beginning to be researched.[115] Currently, atypical movement patterns in stroke are classified according to type of lesion (embolism, thrombosis, TIA) or side of weakness. The disease and disability classification models have made it easier for therapists to identify and define the focus of their intervention for the neurological patient. These models help us organize our interventions into two categories: (1) interventions that aim at improving relevant impairments that contribute to functional limitations/disability and (2) interventions that focus on the functional limitation/disability itself. The treatment interventions in this chapter are directed at the impairment category.

Although the main focus of this chapter is the evaluation and treatment of impairments that result in loss of movement control, a stroke may result in damage to other systems that affect the client's ability to perform functional skills. There may be deficiencies in sensory processing (vision, somesthetic sensation, and vestibular systems) and disorders of cognitive integration (arousal and attention, awareness of disability, memory, problem-solving, and learning), which all have a large impact on functional retraining. Depression and, most important, problems of language and communication also contribute to the client's ability to participate in a therapy program.

Impairments Contributing to Functional Limitation and Disability

Clients with hemiplegia from stroke have movement problems—impairments—that lead to functional limita-

T A B L E 2 5 – 3. Comparison of World Health Organization (WHO) and Nagi Disability Models

Model	Disease	Loss or Abnormality	Limitation of Activity	Societal Consequence
Nagi	Pathology	Impairment Primary Secondary Composite	Functional limitation	Disability
WHO ICIDH-1	Pathology	Impairment Primary Secondary	Disability	Handicap
WHO ICIDH-2	Pathology	Impairment Primary Secondary	Activities	Participation

tions and disability. These movement problems manifest themselves as loss of movement in the trunk and extremities, atypical patterns of movement, compensatory strategies, and involuntary nonpurposeful movements of the affected side. These impairments interfere with normal functional movement and lead to loss of independence in daily life.

Impairments, as defined by the Nagi model, are the signs, symptoms, and physical findings that relate to a specific disease pathology. Schenkman and Butler were the first to apply this model of impairments to neurological physical therapy practice. Ryerson and Levit, using a similar format, specifically defined the impairment categories as primary, secondary, and composite[108, 111] (see the accompanying box).

Primary Impairments. Primary impairments are physical findings that are associated with the specific brain lesion. The primary impairments of stroke that relate to functional recovery of movement include changes in strength, changes in muscle tone, muscle activation or control changes (sequencing, firing, initiation), and changes in sensation. Cognitive/perceptual, emotional, and speech and language changes are also primary impair-

ments that have an effect on function but are less of a focus of this chapter.

Secondary Impairments. Secondary impairments involve systems of the body other than the neurological system. They occur as a consequence of the stroke and/ or because of other medical and environmental influences, such as a fall, pneumonia, or phlebitis. As they develop, they influence each other and the primary impairments. Secondary impairments influence the client's level of disability by contributing additional physical problems. There are four major categories of secondary impairments: orthopedic changes in alignment and mobility, changes in muscle and soft tissue length, pain, and edema.

Composite Impairments. Composite impairments are the combined effects of the primary and secondary impairments, motor recovery, effects of treatment, and behavioral factors. Movement deficits are the missing pieces of movement control that the client needs to move normally. Atypical movements are movements that deviate from normal coordinated movement. Undesirable compensations are alternative severely one-sided strategies used to perform a functional activity because of loss of normal movement patterns.

IMPAIRMENTS THAT INTERFERE WITH FUNCTIONAL MOVEMENT

Primary Impairments

- Changes in muscle strength
  - Paralysis or weakness
- Changes in muscle tone
  - Hypotonicity
  - Hypertonicity—spasticity
- Changes in muscle activation
  - Inappropriate initiation
  - Difficulty sequencing
  - Inappropriate timing of firing
  - Altered force production
- Changes in sensation
  - Awareness
  - Interpretation

Secondary Impairments

- Changes in alignment and mobility
- Changes in muscle and soft tissue length
- Pain
- Edema

Composite Impairments

- Movement deficits
- Atypical movements
- Undesirable compensations

Modified from Ryerson S, Levit K: Functional Movement Reeducation: A Contemporary Model for Stroke Rehabilitation. New York, Churchill Livingstone, 1997.

Patterns of Recovery

In the 1970s, "neurophysiological" theories and approaches changed therapy treatment for adults with CNS lesions. The founders of these approaches described positions and patterns of trunk and extremity movement.[14, 24, 63] These patterns were described in terms of spastic synergies, reflexive patterns, and position. Extremity movements were described as patterns of flexor or extensor synergies, arm and leg patterns were changeable according to the influence of tonic reflexes, and trunk position was always short on the affected side with scapula and pelvic retraction. The intervention techniques followed the descriptions and understanding of the movement problems. As knowledge from orthopedics, manual therapy, and motor control grew, therapists looked more closely at movement patterns and body position in clients with hemiplegia and expanded the categories. As early as 1982, new descriptions emerged that combined synergistic patterns and biomechanical influences on the musculoskeletal systems.[103] Today, descriptions of position and patterns of movement follow the impairment categories. The composite impairment category used in this chapter has three generalized movement patterns that creates one model of classification: (1) *movement deficits*, (2) *atypical movements*, and (3) *undesirable compensatory patterns.*[108]

Movement deficits result from severe weakness or paralysis with either gradual, balanced return or no significant return. Functional movement patterns and levels of independence are based on the distribution and amount of return: trunk control greater than extremity control, extremity control greater than trunk control, distal extremity return greater than proximal extremity return or vice versa, and arm control greater than leg control or vice versa. These clients do not have problems with spasticity but, when weakness is severe, have long-term problems with the secondary impairments of muscle shortening and loss of joint range.

Acutely, the arm hangs by the side, the humerus is internally rotated, the elbow is extended, and the forearm is pronated. Inferior shoulder subluxation is common. The trunk is weak, the ribs flare, and a convex lateral curve is seen on the affected side. (Appearances of lateral trunk flexion with the concavity on the affected side exist with compensatory upper and lower trunk movements.) In standing, the client has problems recruiting strength on the affected leg. The pelvis lists downward, and the hip and knee flex. The hip and knee flexion combined with a tendency to place more weight on the stronger leg places the ankle in plantarflexion, and no weight is borne on the heel. As the client learns to walk, either the knee flexes because of weakness or the patient compensates and "locks" the knee in extension.

Over time, the heavy arm pulls the upper body into flexion, creating an appearance of a low shoulder. To stand and walk, a compensatory shift of the upper body onto a cane helps the client balance. This overshifting of the upper body also makes it easier for these clients to initiate stepping with the use of pelvic elevation (Figs. 25–1 and 25–2).

Atypical movement patterns are found in clients with unbalanced muscle return and deficits in muscle activation. These clients have difficulty organizing and sequencing muscle return, quieting muscles after active firing, and grading strength of contractions. Clients with unbalanced return can be further divided into two subcategories: (1) those with greater weakness, that is, unbalanced return, with secondary problems of muscle shortening and poor alignment, and (2) those with greater return, with more problems of hypertonicity in the arm and leg.

These clients move and function with patterns that were formerly described as "spastic" or "synergistic." They have either anterior or superior shoulder subluxations, which determine the possibilities for fractionated movement in the arm. Common leg movement patterns used for walking include *swing*—proximal initiation patterns of pelvic hiking or rotation toward the affected side, hip flexion with internal rotation and knee extension, or pelvic posterior tilting with hip abduction and knee flexion—and *stance*—toe strike or foot flat, loss of hip extension, and loss of ability to use the leg to initiate forward progression.

Regardless of the proximal trunk and extremity patterns, the ankle/foot and wrist/hand patterns are predictable based on amount of distal return and the effects of proximal alignment. With weakness, the ankle plantarflexes and the wrist flexes. The foot/hand rotate on the ankle/wrist according to the pattern of and amount of return of proximal movements. Finger and toe patterns (curling/fisting or clawing) follow biomechanical rules of compensation or correlation (Fig. 25–3).

Undesirable compensatory patterns are patterns of function that arise from either of the two previously described movement categories. Undesirable compensatory patterns are one sided; they rely on movements of the uninvolved arm and leg and do not use bilateral movements in the trunk. Because the patterns are one sided, balance is often precarious and external aids are required for support. These patterns create "learned nonuse" of the affected arm and leg, foster asymmetrical postural patterns, and lead to strong patterns of spasticity. Patients who come into therapy with strongly established undesirable compensatory patterns do not respond quickly to any type of intervention. Although therapists may be tempted to train a one-sided pattern in early rehabilitation to quickly meet a stated goal, the long-term effects of "learned nonuse of one side of the body" include increased severity of secondary impairments and poor balance with increased chance of falls (Fig. 25–4).

Although the main movement problems of stroke occur because of weakness and tonal problems of hypertonicity or flaccidity, other movement disturbances, such as ataxia, do occur. In clients with ataxia, the main movement problem is one of wide swings of tone and muscle activation disturbances. In these clients, there is trunk instability, excessive extremity movement, and overshooting of distal targets. Voluntary extremity movements are usually present but uncoordinated (see Chapter 24).

EVALUATION PROCEDURES

Evaluation is a process of collecting information to establish a baseline level of performance to plan interventions and to document progress. This section reviews medical evaluations, standardized evaluations of functional performance (disability scales), evaluation of motor function and balance, and evaluation of secondary impairments that interfere with motor performance.

Medical Evaluation

After or during the evolution of a stroke, a thorough medical examination is conducted. All systems are surveyed, with emphasis placed on the level of consciousness; mental, affective, and emotional states; communication; cranial nerves; perceptual ability; sensation; and motor function.

Levels of Consciousness

Scales of varying types are used to measure the client's level of consciousness, to assess the initial severity of brain damage, and to prognosticate recovery curves. The Glasgow Coma Scale, devised by Teasdale and Jennett in collaboration with Plum,[125] has been used for nontraumatic comas caused by stroke, head injury, and cardiac disease. This scale records motor responses to pain, verbal responses to auditory and visual clues, and eye opening. It assigns numerical values according to graded scales. Plum and Caronna[99] and Levy and associates[75] have also established criteria for correlating clinical signs of coma with prognosis.

The standard descriptions of level of consciousness—normal, semistupor, stupor, deep stupor, semicoma, coma, deep coma—are categorized by objective medical data but often leave a gap in the understanding of how the client functions in life.[125] This gap was closed by the creation of a scale, "Levels of Cognitive Functioning," devised at Rancho Los Amigos Hospital. This behavioral

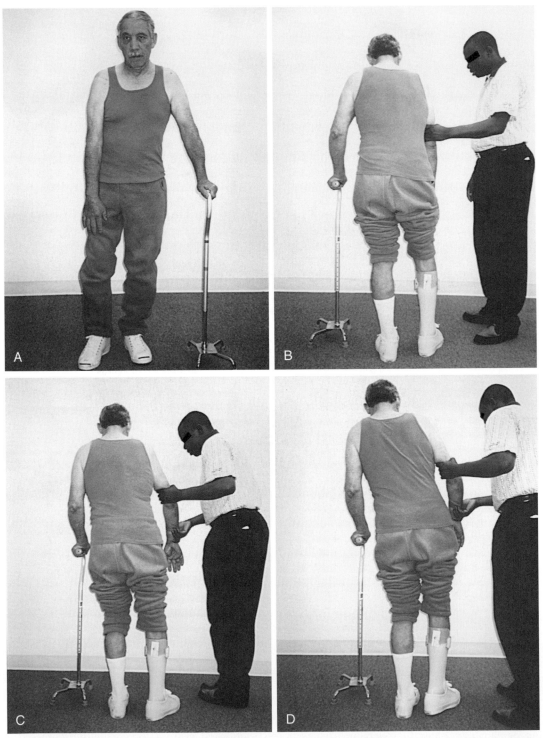

FIGURE 25–1. *A*, Client with right hemiplegia. Movement deficit: paralysis; client was unable to move arm or leg in standing or sitting. *B*, Client uses cane and tries to shift to right as he gets ready to step forward with left leg. Note how the heavy weight of the right arm pulls the upper body into forward flexion and rotation left. *C*, Client prepares to step forward with right leg. Note that his attendant has corrected upper body position. *D*, Client leans heavily onto cane (upper body translates laterally to the left), to lessen weight on the right leg. He will accomplish the "step" by rotating his upper body to left, a compensation for the loss of leg control in standing.

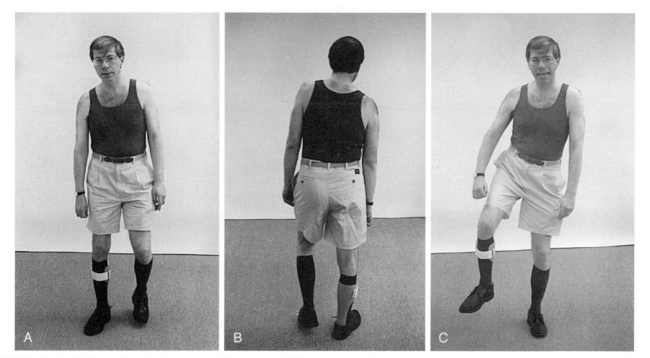

FIGURE 25–2. *A,* Client with right hemiplegia. Movement deficit: weakness; client is able to walk with a brace and does not need a cane. *B,* During stance, his upper body moves laterally to the right and his right femur internally rotates as his knee hyperextends. *C,* He has enough trunk control to stand and balance and sufficient leg control to lift the leg with knee flexion.

rating scale is not a test of cognitive skill but an observational rating of the client's ability to process information[79] (see Chapter 14).

Mental, Emotional, and Affective States

The history portion of the neurological evaluation leads to an assessment of the mental, emotional, and affective state. The client's ability to describe the illness gives information on memory, orientation to time and place,

the ability to express ideas, and judgment. If the examiner suspects a particular problem, a more thorough review is undertaken of the higher cortical function: serial subtraction, repetition of digits, and recall of objects or names. Clients with right hemiplegia may be cautious and disorganized in solving a given task, and clients with left hemiplegia tend to be fast and impulsive and seemingly unaware of the deficits present. These different response patterns stem from hemispheric involvement and prior hemispheric specialization.

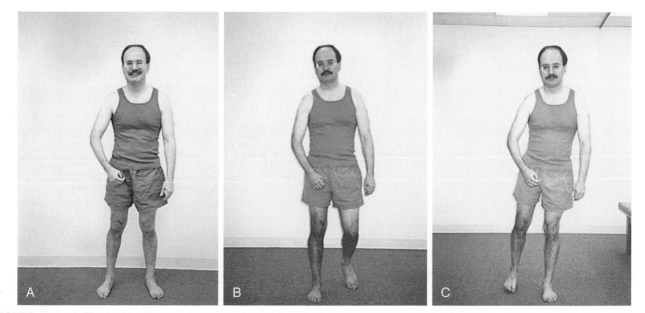

FIGURE 25–3. *A,* Client with right hemiplegia. Movement deficit: loss of control of firing patterns, timing, and sequencing. *B* and *C,* Client walking.

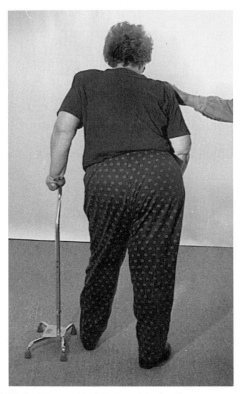

FIGURE 25–4. Client with right hemiplegia. Severe compensatory patterns. She walks with a quad cane and standby assistance. Pelvis rotates to right, upper body rotates to left, hip flexes, and knee hyperextends. There is strong lateral translation of upper body to left (to the stable cane).

Loss of emotional control often exists after a stroke. Crying is a common problem. Although excessive, inappropriate, or uncontrollable crying is usually a result of brain damage and a sign of emotional lability, crying can also be an expression of sadness as a result of depression. This difference is distinguishable by the ease with which the crying can be stopped. Other signs of emotional lability in persons with hemiplegia from stroke include inappropriate laughter or anger.

Communication

A general evaluation of communication disorders is noted while taking the history. Cerebral disorder resulting from infarct or hemorrhage can produce a loss of production or comprehension of the spoken word, the written word, or both. The therapist should be familiar with all types of communication disorders and with alternate modes of communication to establish a good client relationship.

Cranial Nerves and Reflexes

Thorough cranial nerve evaluation is necessary in hemiplegia because a deficit of a particular cranial nerve helps to determine the exact size and location of the infarct or hemorrhage. In hemiplegia, it is imperative to check for visual field deficits, pupil signs, ocular movements, facial sensation and weakness, labyrinthine and auditory function, and laryngeal and pharyngeal function.

Standard areas of reflex testing include the triceps,

biceps, supinator, quadriceps, and gastrocnemius muscles. According to Adams,[2] there are four plantar reflex responses: (1) avoidance—quick, (2) spinal flexion—slow, (3) Babinski—toe grasp, and (4) positive support.

Perception

Perceptual deficits in clients with hemiplegia are complex and are intimately linked to the sensorimotor deficit. Sensory integration theory has begun to establish norms and objective data for testing and documenting perceptual deficits in children. Presently, norms and testing procedures for adults have not been standardized, but perceptual deficits have been identified in clients with hemiplegia. Common perceptual deficits found in left and right brain damage are listed in the box on page 755.

Perceptual retraining without standardized norms for the deficit is at best difficult. The soundest course presently available appears to be one that relates perceptual and motor learning rather than retraining perception in isolation (see Chapters 4 and 11).

Sensation

Traditional sensory testing is used to assess sensory deficits in the adult with hemiplegia: light touch, deep pressure, kinesthesia, proprioception, pain, temperature, graphesthesia, two-point discrimination, appreciation of texture and size, and vibration. A comparison of the differences in the two sides of the body and qualitative as well as quantitative measurements are important features of sensory testing. Sensory testing is difficult because it relies on the client's interpretation of the sensation and on the client's general awareness and suggestibility, as well as on the client's ability to communicate a response to each test item.

The presence and quality of sensory loss must be considered during the process of reeducating motor control. Although Sherrington established the principle of interdependence of sensation and movement, current researchers have refined the concept and hypothesize that sensation modifies ongoing movement by providing feedforward, feedback, and corollary discharge. They have provided evidence that sensation is not an absolute prerequisite for movement.[123]

Evaluation of motor function includes both standardized evaluation of functional performance and evaluation of movement control. Manual muscle testing, while used by physicians to provide a general level of strength, is not widely used by therapists to measure strength in individuals with CNS dysfunction because of the insensitivity of the test to loss of trunk/limb-linked control. New measures of manual muscle testing for stroke are now beginning to be investigated.

Standardized Evaluations

Functional Performance

During the initial interview, the therapist and the client together form a list of limitations and relate them to the

PERCEPTUAL DEFICITS IN CENTRAL NERVOUS SYSTEM DYSFUNCTION

Left Hemiparesis: Right Hemisphere—General Spatial-global Deficits

Visual-perceptual deficits
  Hand-eye coordination
  Figure-ground discrimination
  Spatial relationships
  Position in space
  Form constancy
Behavioral and intellectual deficits
  Poor judgment, unrealistic behavior
  Denial of disability
  Inability to abstract
  Rigidity of thought
  Disturbances in body image and body scheme
  Impairment of ability to self-correct
  Difficulty retaining information
  Distortion of time concepts
  Tendency to see the whole and not individual steps
  Affect lability
  Feelings of persecution
  Irritability, confusion
  Distraction by verbalization
  Short attention span
  Appearance of lethargy
  Fluctuation in performance
  Disturbances in relative size and distance of objects

Right Hemiparesis: Left Hemisphere—General Language and Temporal Ordering Deficits

Apraxia
  Motor
  Ideational
Behavioral and intellectual deficits
  Difficulty initiating tasks
  Sequencing deficits
  Processing delays
  Directionality deficits
  Low frustration levels
  Verbal and manual perseveration
  Rapid performance of movement or activity
  Compulsive behavior
  Extreme distractability

client's goals and needs. The client can state his or her perceived functional limitations, or the therapist can ask the client to perform tasks. Commonly used standardized tests/scales for functional limitations/disability are listed here, and additional information is found in Chapter 3.

Scales

The *Barthel Index* is one of the oldest measures of disability.[78] It has excellent validity and reliability and is pro-foundly simple, but does not discriminate at higher levels of activity.

The *Motor Assessment Scale* (MAS) comes from the intervention theory of Carr and Shepherd.[28] Its reliability is high, it is simple to administer, and it only takes 15 minutes to perform. Although it mainly evaluates mobility skills, there is an arm and hand function section. The tests of arm function include movement patterns without tasks, and the hand function section uses object manipulation.

The *Function Independence Measure* (FIM) is commonly used in rehabilitation centers, takes 45 minutes to perform, and measures ADL, mobility, cognition, and communication.[47, 60] It has good-to-excellent reliability.

The *Rivermead Mobility Index* measures mobility only, takes 5 minutes to perform, and has been tested for reliability and validity.[31]

The *Assessment of Motor and Process Skills* (AMPS) is a standardized test that measures task performance abilities and efficiency during instrumental activities of daily living (IADL). This disability scale is used in occupational therapy evaluations.[40]

Tests of Motor Function and Balance

The *Fugl-Meyer test* is weighted with items measuring arm movement more than leg movement, factors in reflexes and sensation, has good validity and reliability, but requires approximately 45 minutes to perform.[43] The movement patterns tested follow the Brunnstrom method of intervention.

The *Berg Balance Assessment* is easy to administer, takes 5 minutes, and has norms specific to clients with stroke.[8, 9]

Functional Reach provides a measure of balance in standing. It measures control only during anterior (forward reach) weight shifts. Reliability is high, and the test is fast and easy to perform.[36]

Gait

The evaluation of gait patterns includes the assessment of the temporal characteristics of each gait cycle, the description of gait deviations, and, ideally, the assignment of a numerical score representing the efficiency of ambulation. The *Functional Ambulation Profile* (FAP) is a system that attempts to relate the temporal aspects of gait to neuromuscular and cardiovascular functioning and converts this relationship to a single numerical score.[90, 91]

The temporal characteristics of gait—step time, cycle time, step length, and stride length—can be measured with a piece of chalk and a stopwatch or with more sophisticated equipment such as a gait analyzer. These parameters provide an objective measurement of performance and a baseline from which the efficacy of treatment procedures and client progress can be assessed.

Gait deviations in persons with hemiplegia have been described according to their biomechanical and kinesiological abnormalities and in terms of the loss of centrally programmed motor control mechanisms.[65, 97]

Perry[97] described common problems of the hemiplegic person's gait as loss of controlled movement into plantarflexion at heel strike, loss of ankle movement from heel strike to mid stance (resulting in loss of trunk balance and forward momentum for push off), and loss of the normal combination of movement patterns at the end of stance (hip extension, knee flexion, and ankle extension) and at the end of swing (hip flexion with knee extension and ankle flexion).

Knutsson and Richards[65] classified the motor control problems of the hemiplegic gait into three descriptive types. Type I is characterized by inappropriate activation of the calf muscles early in the gait cycle with corresponding low muscular activity in anterior compartment muscles. In the type I activation pattern, the calf musculature is activated before the center of gravity passes over the base of support. This thrusts the tibia backward instead of propelling the body forward in a pushoff as normally occurs. The client with hemiplegia compensates for the backward thrust of the tibia by anteriorly tilting the pelvis and/or flexing forward at the hip. Type II consists of an absence of or severe decrease in electromyographic activity in two or more muscle groups of the involved lower extremity. This pattern of markedly decreased muscular activity results in the adoption of compensatory mechanisms to gain stability. Type III activation patterns consist of abnormal coactivation of several limb muscles with normal or increased muscular activity levels in the muscle groups of the involved side. This type of pattern results in a disruption of the sequential flow of motor activity.

Evaluation of Movement Control

After the standardized testing, the therapist continues on to a subjective evaluation of movement components, to gather information to answer the question "why" it is difficult to perform specific movements or tasks.

Clients with stroke have difficulty moving the trunk, arm, and leg on the affected side because of the presence of primary and secondary impairments. Objective standardized measures for the primary impairments are few; and standard muscle testing has been questioned for CNS deficits because of the numerous degrees of freedom available and the discrepancy in functional strength based on increasing degrees of difficulty of controlling linked trunk and extremity patterns as the body moves from function in supine, to function in sitting, to function in standing.

Active Movement/Strength

When assessing active movement patterns in the trunk and extremities, the therapist measures both strength and control. Paralysis, weakness, and imbalanced return are determinates of strength. Initiation pattern, sequencing, and control of firing patterns are indicators of control. Weakness and paralysis after stroke have been largely ignored because of a lingering focus on spasticity. Recent studies have shown that muscle weakness is, in fact, present and interferes with the ability to generate enough force to allow functional performance.[17, 19, 21] Motor weakness is present in 75% to 80% of clients after a stroke. There appears to be no difference in clients with left- or right-sided hemiplegia in terms of frequency or severity of weakness.[85] Although this recent research has moved

weakness back up to the top of the impairment list, there is much more to learn about reliable testing and appropriate intervention for weakness in CNS dysfunction.

The assessment of active movement in hemiplegia is commonly documented by therapists through the use of the synergistic stages as outlined by Brunnstrom[24] or by a modified version of Bobath's long evaluation form, which gradually builds series of selective/fractionated movement in the arm, trunk, and leg, in increasing levels of antigravity control.[12]

When assessing weakness and control of active movement patterns the therapist should analyze and identify the client's patterns of posture and movement in the trunk and extremities by position (supine, side lying, sitting, and standing) and in linked combinations. Active movement control is evaluated in individual muscles, movement components, and movement sequences.[108] Verbal directions or demonstrations may be necessary to help the client understand what is desired. In this phase of the evaluation, the therapist should not physically assist the client's movement but should be prepared to prevent loss of balance.

While evaluating force production or weakness in all these categories, the therapist gathers information about sequencing movements in increasingly complex patterns, timing of muscle firing, and speed of movement. Muscle activation deficits in these categories may explain why some clients with good recovery of movement control and strength do not regain spontaneous functional use of their extremities.[108]

Assisted Movement

After the evaluation of active movement, therapists use their hands while retesting the movements to gain additional information about the relationships between impairments. Whereas the use of handling must be judicious, handling is used during an assessment to:

1. Correct alignment to gather additional information about strength, control, and orthopedic impairments (Fig. 25–5)
2. Limit degrees of freedom of one of the joints to assess relationships between intralimb segments
3. Assist the movement of a weak muscle
4. Block/stabilize a joint to assess the performance of a weaker muscle group or to limit the degrees of freedom of an intralimb segment[108] (Fig. 25–6).

EXAMPLE
Step 1. *Assessment of forward reach in sitting by client with left hemiplegia.* Active movement patterns on left: client initiates movement proximally; shoulder flexes to 60 degrees, with internal humeral rotation; abducted, downwardly rotated scapula elevates during the movement; elbow flexes, forearm supinates to 10 degrees; wrist remains in flexion and radial deviation. Client leans trunk forward to assist with task but cannot reach arm forward to place it on table.

Step 2. *Clinical judgment/hypothesis 1*: weakness of scapula and humeral external rotators prevents antigravity use of elbow extensors during forward reach. Supination of forearm comes from strong proximal initiation and use of elbow flexors to lift arm. *Clinical judgment/hypothesis 2*: forearm/wrist/hand posi-

FIGURE 25–5. *A,* Client with right hemiplegia trying to perform an upper body–initiated lateral weight shift to the left. Note the spine is straight and the right hip is off the surface. *B,* Therapist uses her hands to correct and stabilize the lower trunk as the client initiates the upper body lateral movement to the left. The therapist gains information about trunk and hip control and secondary impairments of trunk muscle tightness. Note the spine is beginning to curve as the client uses eccentric activity of the right lateral musculature to control the movement. Active stretching to the right quadratus lumborum/latissimus occurs if tight muscles are present.

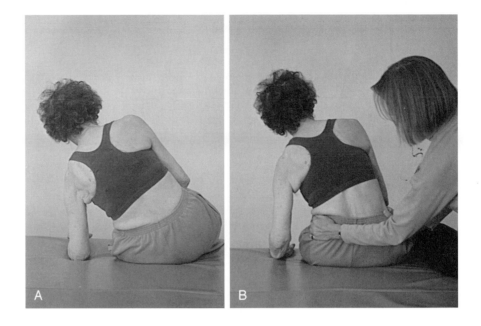

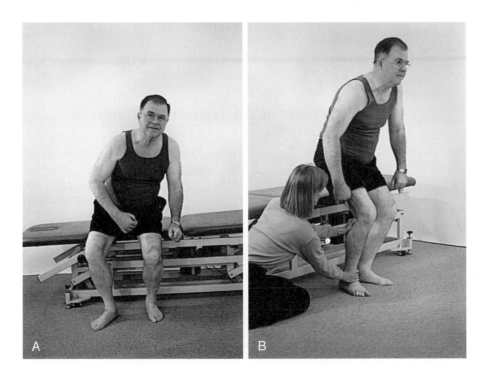

FIGURE 25–6. *A,* Client with right hemiplegia moving from sitting to standing. Note the tendency to use the left leg more than the right, the left rotation of the upper body, and the position of the right arm. *B,* Therapist uses her hands to stabilize the lower leg and to assist lower leg movements as the client initiates sit to stand. Note the change in upper body position and the decrease in arm posturing.

tion prevents distal initiation and biases shoulder in internal rotation, thus blocking use of elbow extensors.

Step 3. *Test of hypothesis 1*: therapist uses his or her hands to externally rotate humerus to neutral and asks client to reach again. *Result*: client activates elbow extension halfway through range with shoulder forward flexion and places wrist/hand on table. *Clinical intervention implication*: increased control of humeral external rotation and increased control of accompanying scapula pattern are important intervention goals to regain forward reach of arm. Retrain trunk/scapula/humeral movement patterns with emphasis on shoulder external rotation and scapular upward rotation. Assess secondary impairments of pectoral and rotator cuff tightness (rotator cuff is shortened if scapula is in an abducted position).

If result is unchanged, test hypothesis 2: therapist supports wrist and hand with wrist splint or with his or her hand and asks client to reach again. *Result*: client activates elbow extension and places the wrist/hand on the table. *Clinical intervention implication*: prevention/blocking of wrist flexion limits the degrees of freedom, changes the internal rotation moment on the distal portion of the lever arm, and allows use of existing elbow extensors. Use lightweight wrist splint during independent practice or use object to assist/preset distal segment during practice.

Tone

The evaluation of postural mechanisms must always include an assessment of tone. Over the years, leading physiologists have split into two camps over the definition of tone. During the beginning of the century, tone was thought of as postural reflexes. In the 1950s the concept of tone was thought of as a state of light excitation or a state of preparedness.[48] Granit, later, encouraged us to think of the relatedness of both these views. He believed that the same spinal organization is mobilized by the basal ganglia to produce both manifestations of tone, a state of preparedness and the postural reflexes.[49]

It is heartening to hear such discussions occurring among physiologists, because therapists are also questioned about their notations of and changes in tone, and they often have no objectively derived standard clinical system for measurement. The debate over tone continues, but clients with CNS dysfunction clinically display changes of muscle tone that result in longer rehabilitation stays and problematic secondary impairments.[39]

The response of a spastic muscle to stretch differs during passive and active movements, leading some to question the usefulness of the classic numerical test of spasticity, the *Ashworth scale*. The Ashworth scale rates the severity of tone from 1 to 5.[4]

The first noticeable change in tone is the change from the premorbid state. Clients in the acute phase of hemiplegia exhibit, for varying periods of time, a lower than normal tonal state. Clients with paralysis of the extremities exhibit low tone or hypotonicity. The extremities feel like "dead weight" as the therapist moves them. As return slowly begins, the extremities feel heavy, but some "following" of passive movement patterns is detected.

As the client becomes more active, he or she uses all available movement patterns. Ryerson and Levit have described three specific situations, which in reality have overlap, wherein tone increases (see page 766 for a detailed discussion). This increased tone, hypertonicity, or

spasticity occurs in the arm and leg if the client's trunk control is less than the demand of the task, if altered joint alignment increases the tension of the muscle, or if the voluntary movement pattern of the extremity is unbalanced and disorganized.[73, 108]

One clinical description of increased extremity tone put forth by Bobath in the 1970s is still somewhat useful today: severe hypertonicity makes coordinated movements impossible; moderate hypertonicity allows movements that are characterized by great effort, slow velocity, and abnormal coordination; slight hypertonicity allows gross movement patterns to occur with smooth coordination, but combined, selective movement patterns are uncoordinated or impossible.[13]

Equilibrium and Protective Reactions

Equilibrium reactions help us to maintain or regain our balance by keeping the center of gravity within the base of support. Equilibrium reactions are often referred to as the body's first line of defense against falling. They occur when the body has a chance of winning the battle against gravity. If equilibrium reactions cannot preserve balance, the second line of defense emerges: protective reactions. One of the best known protective responses in the arm is the "parachute reaction." Protective responses in the leg in standing include hopping and stepping.

When assessing equilibrium or balance reactions in clients with hemiplegia, the therapist remembers the distinction between equilibrium reactions and protective reactions. Equilibrium reactions should be assessed while slowly moving either the limb or trunk away from the base of support. The amount of control in the trunk and supporting limb, the size of the base of support, and the available range of motion as well as the evaluator's handling skills affect the response (see Chapter 21).

Descriptive Analysis of Functional Activities

When evaluating functional activities, the therapist assesses three phases of the movement pattern. The first phase is the *initiation* of the act, which includes the body segment initiating the movement, the direction of movement, and the establishment of antigravity control. *Transition*, the second phase, represents the point in the functional activity at which there is a switch in the muscle groups that provide antigravity control. The third phase is the *completion* of the activity, involving a final weight shift and the ability to maintain postural control.[108]

If assistive devices are used, the following questions should be asked: Is the device always used? If not, when is it used? How is the device used? Could the device be used another way that would foster trunk symmetry and allow activity of the affected extremities?

Evaluation of Secondary Impairments
Loss of Joint Range and Muscle Shortening

In hemiplegia, loss of joint range is caused by muscle shortening from poor alignment due to weakness and/or muscle activation problems. Loss of alignment occurs early in recovery, whereas muscle shortening and loss of range occur over time. When measuring joint range of motion and muscle shortening, the therapist must remember to consider the functional consequences of two-joint (multijoint) muscle tightness.

EXAMPLE

In sitting (knee bent), client has ankle joint dorsiflexion range from 0 to 10 degrees; but in standing (knee and hip straight), ankle joint dorsiflexion range is −20 degrees. This functional loss of ankle range causes significant problems for standing and walking. Loss of ankle joint range in standing may be the result of gastrocsoleus, tensor fasciae latae, and/or hamstring muscle tightness (Fig. 25–7).

Range of motion measurements should be documented in terms of functional position. Extremity muscles that cross multiple joints are the most common groups to shorten and limit joint range in hemiplegia. Muscle shifting (changes in the resting position of muscle bellies and tendons) occurs with prolonged changes in alignment and loss of joint range.

EXAMPLE

Long-standing wrist flexion may cause the ulnar wrist extensor to slip volarly and function as a wrist flexor. Similarly, a position of knee flexion with ankle plantarflexion and talar varus may lead to lateral shifting of the anterior tibial muscle belly. As the muscle shifts laterally, the tension increases distally and foot supination becomes more pronounced.

Pain

Two commonly used standardized pain measurement scales are the *Visual Analogue Pain Rating Scale* and the *McGill Pain Questionnaire*.[55, 82] These scales focus primarily on the intensity of pain but provide an objective measure of intervention effectiveness. For an in-depth discussion of the topic of pain management, see Chapter 29.

The presence of pain in hemiplegia is devastating for

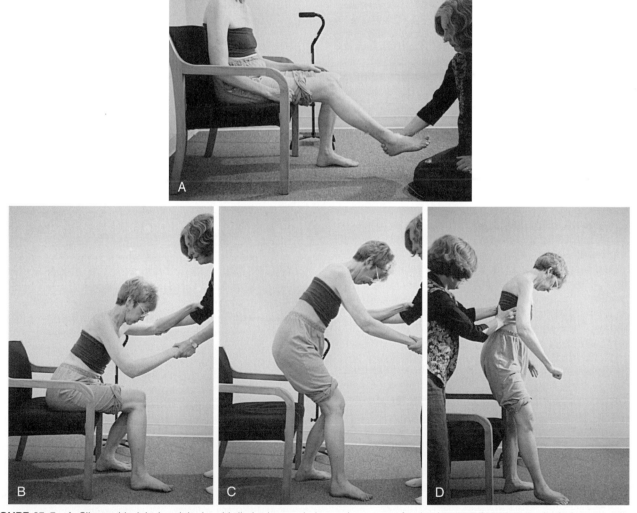

FIGURE 25–7. *A,* Client with right hemiplegia with limited range in hamstring, tensor fasciae latae, and gastrocnemius/soleus muscles. *B,* Client has sufficient range at ankle to keep foot on the floor in sitting and as she initiates the rise to standing. *C,* As she stands and reaches the limit of range of these two muscle groups, her body compensates. The pelvis rotates right, and the tight medial hamstring adducts and internally rotates the femur and pulls the knee into extension as its medial insertion becomes more anterior to the joint. *D,* As the knee extends more, the calcaneus moves into equinus and varus. The foot supinates as a result of calcaneal varus and external tibial rotation from the tight tensor fasciae latae.

QUESTIONS FOR SUBJECTIVE EVALUATION OF PAIN

- ■ Location: Where is the pain? Pinpoint the location.
- ■ Type: What does it feel like?
  - Pins and needles
  - Sharp and stabbing
  - Aching
  - Dull
  - Pulling
- ■ Occurrence: When does the pain occur?
  - At rest
  - During movement
    - Range of motion exercises
    - Weight-bearing exercises
    - A specific part of the movement

---

the client and makes movement reeducation difficult. Shoulder pain is the most frequent pain complaint after stroke.[16, 101] Pain must be evaluated specifically and should not be allowed to occur during intervention; the "no pain, no gain" message that is sometimes used in sports or orthopedic intervention should not be used in neurorehabilitation. Pain is an indicator that joint alignment or movements are incorrect. Refer to the box above for general questions.

Motor Evaluation Forms

The foregoing information, once gathered, can be placed on an evaluation form in many ways. Every medical institution seems to have its own evaluation form and its own system of recording data. Active movement at the shoulder joint may be described in one institution in terms of percentages of synergistic stages, at another institution by a narrative of degrees and planes of movement, and at still another by functional outcomes of shoulder movement. At one hospital the documentation of pain may be descriptive, and at another it may be numerical. It is important to keep in mind the substance of the evaluative material, not the form in which it is described. A detailed motor evaluation form is necessary for the establishment of realistic goals and for subsequent treatment planning, but the specific form depends both on the needs of the specific clinical setting and on the clinician's choice.

Recognizing Needs

The information obtained from the total evaluation provides the basis for answers to the following questions:

- What movements and functions are possible?
- What movements and functions are not possible?
- How do the movement impairments and secondary impairments relate to functional performance?

By understanding the impairments and their relation-

ship to functional limitations, the therapist can answer the following question: What significant movement components are missing? The answer to this question becomes the objective for treatment. How the possible is accomplished and why the impossible exists provide logical suggestions for selection of intervention techniques.

Therapy intervention occurs at either the level of disability (functional impairment) or at the level of movement-related primary and secondary impairments. The process of establishing goals and selecting activities for intervention begins with clinical decision making or problem solving.

CLINICAL DECISION MAKING/ PROBLEM SOLVING

Problem solving is a process of gathering and analyzing evaluation information from task and movement analysis, organizing and reflecting on this information to develop hypotheses for causal relationships between significant impairments and functional performance, and establishing and prioritizing goals for therapeutic intervention. The problem-solving process is also used to hypothesize how the movement problems of the trunk, arm, and leg are interrelated and how these problems relate to the ability to perform tasks. Movement control deficits, secondary impairments, and compensatory or atypical movement patterns should be identified for the trunk, arm, and leg in relation to each significant functional limitation.

Analyzing Evaluation Material

The relationship between functional performance and primary and secondary impairments in stroke has not been researched. Therefore, this relationship, which is the basis for therapy intervention, must be derived from clinical experience and judgment. Clinical intuition guides the evaluation process—what should be evaluated and how. As a result of the evaluation, the therapist has a list of functional skills that are difficult or impossible for the client to perform and a list of primary and secondary impairments that relate to the attempted performance of that task. The therapist analyzes this information with the goal of identifying common impairments in categories of tasks: Which primary impairments are major impediments in each task analyzed? Are there secondary impairments that interfere with the clients ability to perform specific critical movement components? What is the level of trunk-extremity control during task performance in each functional position evaluated? While analyzing the evaluation material the therapist pays attention to all significant factors that limit performance of tasks including cognitive, perceptual, and emotional problems.

EXAMPLE
An acute stroke patient, with left hemiplegia, cannot perform morning daily care activities at the sink while sitting in a wheelchair, cannot transfer from bed to chair, and cannot rise to stand. Common primary impairments include paralysis or weakness of the trunk and left arm and leg, inability to initiate arm movements, movements of the leg in supine against gravity but no ability to move the leg against gravity when sitting,

and loss of proprioception, or the ability to distinguish touch. Secondary impairments that begin to appear by the end of the acute stay include excessive lateral trunk flexion with the convexity of the spinal curve on the left; inferior shoulder subluxation; loss of ankle joint dorsiflexion range; tightness in pectoralis, wrist flexors, and gastrocnemius; and edema in the hand and foot.

In the rehabilitation phase of care, the primary impairments of weakness and loss of control begin to improve. Hypertonicity or spasticity may be added to the primary impairment list at this time because of the increased activity level of the client. As the client performs tasks that exceed his level of trunk strength and control, tone in the arm and leg will increase as a strategy for maintaining balance or reinforcing trunk control. Secondary impairments of shoulder pain increase, along with increasing numbers and degrees of muscle tightness and continued loss of trunk-extremity alignment.

Developing Hypotheses for Significant Impairments

The process of motor performance evaluation results in a list of multiple impairments. However, not all of these impairments directly relate to each functional limitation of the client. The therapist, using clinical judgment, hypothesizes a causal relationship between frequently occurring limitations and functional performance. These impairments, called *significant impairments*, are the ones that must be changed for measurable changes in movement and function to occur.[108] The other impairments are not forgotten but are reevaluated later as improvement begins and new functional goals are chosen. The significant impairments are often used as the focus of short- and long-term impairment goals. Because functional movement depends on the linkage of trunk and extremity movements, the therapist develops hypotheses between impairments in the extremities and specific levels of trunk control to set goals that result in improved functional performance. If weakness and control deficits of the trunk, arm, and leg are treated separately, the client may see improvement in the impairments but not see a change in function (Table 25–4). (See Chapters 3 and 4 for further discussion.)

Goal Setting

Once the therapist reviews the impairment list and selects significant impairments that interfere with functional performance, the therapist and the client together choose a practical functional goal or a category of functional goals.

● T A B L E 2 5 – 4. Movement Control Model of Postural Control

Postural tone and stability
Trunk control
  Level I: Basic movement components
    Upper body– and lower body–initiated movement
      Anterior
      Posterior
      Lateral
  Level II: Coordinated trunk and extremity patterns
  Level III: Power production
Equilibrium and protection

Functional Goals

Functional goals are based on the needs and desires of the client and on the functional impairments that have been identified by the therapist during the initial assessment. Functional goals should represent a significant change in the patient's level of independence, be practical, and reflect improvement in a specific functional limitation. They state the desired function and the expected level of performance.[108]

EXAMPLE
Client will stand independently and safely while performing self-care activities at the bathroom sink.

Long-Term Goals

A long-term goal should reflect a major improvement in a primary or secondary impairment or an increase in level of performance of an existing skill. The accomplishment of a long-term goal brings the client closer to the functional goal. The time it takes to accomplish a long-term goal varies tremendously depending on the frequency of treatment and the length of time after stroke. The therapist may set many short-term goals to achieve one long-term goal. Long-term goals may be stated in functional terms, but they usually reflect a change in a primary impairment: an increase in strength, movement control, or balance.[108]

EXAMPLES
1. Client will perform upper body–initiated movement in standing while supporting hips against a kitchen counter.
2. Client will stand against a wall and initiate upper-body lateral and rotational movements independently.

Short-Term Goals

A realistic short-term goal should be achievable quickly and should be based on the result of the patient's response to handling during the evaluation of movement. Short-term goals should directly relate to the accomplishment of the long-term goal. There are multiple short-term goals that relate to one long-term goal. Short-term goals are compiled from the list of relevant secondary impairments or desired increases of strength or movement control. These goals are measurable but do not in and of themselves result in a functional change.[108]

EXAMPLE
Client will lengthen tight hamstring and gastrocnemius muscles in standing to allow the foot to remain flat on the floor during assisted upper-body movements in standing.

When stated in terms of movement control rather than functional performance, these goals include the reestablishment of generalized movement patterns that link movement patterns of the trunk and extremities. (See the box at the top of page 762.)

Choosing Intervention Techniques

Once the problem-solving process of goal setting is finished, therapists can select specific intervention techniques and activities. Therapists have many techniques to

COMPONENT GOALS IN FUNCTIONAL TRAINING

Component goal (power): Restore strength in trunk and extremity patterns (individual muscles, components, sequences)

Component goal (structure): Minimize/eliminate secondary impairments

Component goal (control): Reeducate patterns of control (sequencing/timing)

choose from to meet their goals. Most clients with stroke will not fully regain normal movement patterns regardless of the type of intervention they receive.

Controversy exists as to the means of increasing functional mobility and performance in clients with stroke. One school of thought teaches compensatory patterns or hopes for some use of the affected side through task-specific practice without direct intervention for the neurological impairments. The other prevalent practice pattern is to increase functional movement patterns on the affected side by increasing control and strength of movement sequences of the trunk and limb through specific levels of reeducation[26, 34, 35, 108]

A combination of these two practices may be useful: impairment-based intervention strategies to reeducate movement and training strategies to foster desirable compensations—a functional reeducation strategy. This type of intervention includes strengthening trunk/extremity-linked patterns of movement, minimizing or eliminating secondary impairments that interfere with regaining control, teaching appropriate compensations, and training the client to practice functional movement patterns in context of daily tasks[81, 108] (see the box below).

For reeducation to be effective, therapists must allow the patient to initiate the active trunk/extremity pattern, must move from assisted practice to independent practice with the assistance of appropriately selected objects or verbal cues, and teach the patient appropriately staged

REEDUCATION STRATEGY FOR INTERVENTION

■ Reeducating basic trunk movement components
■ Linking trunk/extremity patterns
   • Weight bearing
   • Movements in space
■ Preventing, minimizing, eliminating secondary impairments
■ Teaching appropriate compensations
■ Teaching independent practice routines

practice patterns. Recent studies, based on the "learned nonuse" phenomenon described by Taub, have shown that when patients are encouraged to use the affected arm, rather than receiving pessimistic messages about its potential, movement and functional use, even if limited, are possible.[124, 132]

Regardless of intervention type utilized, task-performance practice or a reeducation strategy, there comes a time in the recovery process when therapists help the client select practical compensatory strategies. Compensatory strategies are taught when the client needs to function independently and cannot yet use the affected arm because of insufficient recovery or the severity of damage. To be appropriate, the strategy should incorporate the use of the involved extremities and utilize appropriate trunk movement patterns to maximize the use of future return of movement. Undesirable compensations are patterns that are so asymmetrical that they fail to incorporate available movements of the affected trunk and extremities (Fig. 25–8).

Although current literature generally applauds function-based techniques, therapists in clinical setting use hands-on approaches to increase muscle strength and control and to decrease impairments that block the emergence of new functional patterns.[108] As research in movement science and recovery of movement increases, therapists must critically analyze research findings and compare them to their own clinical experience and intuition.

COMMON IMPAIRMENTS AND INTERVENTION SUGGESTIONS

Weakness and Loss of Control

Diminished muscle strength, either paralysis or weakness, is an important category of impairment in hemiplegia. A paralyzed muscle is unable to contract to produce enough force for movement. A weak muscle contracts insufficiently for joint or body segment movement or to allow functional performance.[17, 19, 21] In a client with a severe, acute stroke, the paralysis or weakness affects the majority of muscles and results in a loss of functional movement in the face, trunk, arm, and leg. In clients with less severe strokes, some muscle groups are weak and produce movement whereas other muscles are paralyzed and cannot be activated. Other stroke patients experience no paralysis, only weakness.[87]

Weakness from stroke differs from generalized weakness and orthopedic weakness: it involves one entire side of the body and includes the trunk and extremities. Weakness in trunk muscles can exist with patterns of hypertonicity in the arm and leg. Muscle weakness in the trunk affects postural control and the ability to perform movement sequences.[41] Weakness in the extremities interferes with functional use in either weight bearing or movement in space.[46, 108]

Model of Postural Control

Trunk control allows the body to remain upright, to adjust to weight shift, to control movements against the constant

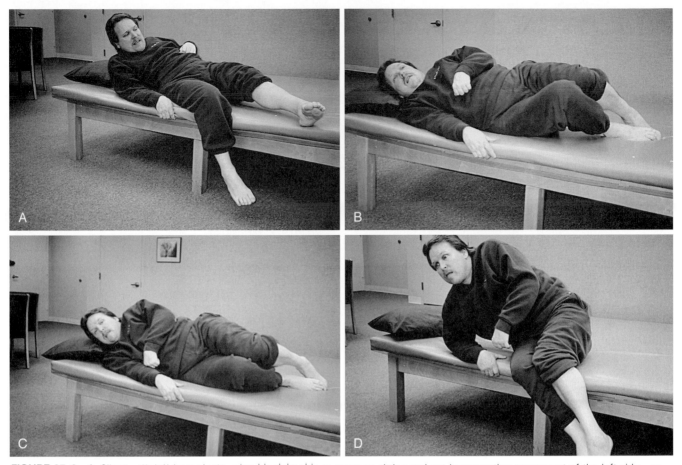

FIGURE 25–8. *A,* Client with left hemiplegia using his right side to move to sitting and not incorporating movement of the left side—an undesirable compensation. *B* to *D,* Client moving to sitting while using as much control as possible on the left side to assist the movement to sitting.

pull of gravity, and to change and control body position for balance and function. Therapy based on neurophysiological models stressed facilitation of trunk rotation to gain trunk control. Newer clinical models of postural and trunk control began appearing around 1990.[73, 84, 104] Information from motor control science has resulted in revision of therapists' thoughts on trunk control.[32, 117, 133]

In a movement component model of postural control, trunk control is part of postural control[74] (see Table 25–4). Trunk control has levels of increasing difficulty. Trunk control not only helps us remain upright but also allows weight transfer to free an arm or leg for function. For some functional movements, such as sitting, trunk control keeps the upper and lower trunk stable as we shift our weight and balance. For other tasks, such as reaching forward beyond the length of the arm, the upper trunk is stable and adjusts to the lower body–initiated anterior weight shift.[108]

Additional postural control models, based on a developmental or systems model, are well documented.[13, 54, 88, 116] Research in the field of postural control shows that the level of trunk control and trunk strength correlates with sitting balance, that extremity function correlates with trunk control, and that loss of trunk strength occurs in all planes.[15, 18, 41]

Postural Tone and Stability. Clients with hemiplegia frequently have alterations in both muscle tone and postural tone. Postural tone refers to the overall state of tension in the body musculature. Postural tone is tone that is "high" enough to keep the body from collapsing into gravity but "low" enough to allow the body to move against gravity. It is influenced by the input from the corticospinal tracts, the vestibular system, the alpha and gamma systems, and peripheral-tactile and proprioceptive receptors.[114] Normal postural tone allows a constant interplay between the various muscle groups in the body and imparts a constant readiness to move and to react to changes in the environment (internal and external). It provides us with an ability to adjust automatically and continuously to movements. These adjustments provide the proximal fixation necessary to hold a given posture against gravity while allowing voluntary and selective movements to be superimposed without conscious or excessive effort.

Trunk Control. Trunk control can be divided into levels of increasing complexity. The first level of trunk control is the ability to perform the basic movement components. Trunk strength and control at this level provides a base that allows extremity movement to be combined and used for function. Retraining strength and control of basic trunk movements in the three cardinal

TABLE 25–5. Upper Body–Initiated Weight Shift Pattern: Sitting

Weight Shift	Spinal Pattern	Muscle Activity
Anterior movement— reach down to floor	Flexes	Eccentric extensor activity
Posterior—to sit back up	Extends	Concentric extensor activity
Lateral—reach sideways to right beyond the reach of the right arm	Laterally flexes with concavity on right	Eccentric lateral activity on left
Lateral—comes back up to middle	Spine moves back to neutral	Concentric lateral activity on left

planes is a prerequisite for the coordination of trunk and extremity patterns for tasks.

Trunk movements in sitting are initiated from the upper trunk or the lower trunk according to the demand of the task. In standing, functional trunk movements are initiated from the upper trunk (if the head or arm is initiating a task) or the lower extremity. The two initiation patterns result in different spinal patterns, different types of muscular activity, and changes in the distribution of weight[108] (Tables 25–5 and 25–6). These basic movement patterns allow the body to be positioned for functional use.

EXAMPLES
While sitting, the client reaches down or sideways to the floor to pick up an object. As the arm reaches down, the upper body initiates the anterior weight shift. The lower body provides stability yet adjusts and adapts.

While sitting, the client lifts up a leg to tie a shoe. As the leg moves up, the lower body initiates a posterior weight shift. The upper body adjusts to the weight shift and to the demands of the arm and hand as they tie the shoe.

The second level of trunk control links trunk and extremity movements. This level of control allows the trunk to remain stable yet adapt to movement of the arms and legs. There are two different ways this happens: trunk movements occur as postural adjustments to extremity movement around midline, or trunk movements can precede voluntary movements to help extend the reach of the extremities. These coordinated movements can occur in supine, sitting, or standing.

EXAMPLES
1. In sitting, the lower trunk initiates a forward weight shift to extend the reach of the lifted arm. The upper body adjusts to

TABLE 25–6. Lower Body–Initiated Weight Shift Pattern: Sitting

Weight Shift	Spinal Pattern	Muscle Activity
Posterior weight shift— pelvis moves into posterior tilt	Flexion	Concentric flexor activity
Anterior weight shift— pelvis moves to neutral	Extension	Concentric extension activity to neutral

the scapula/humeral demands and yet remains relatively stable and adjusts to the forward movement of the lower body.

2. In standing, upper-trunk movements occur as postural adjustments to maintain balance and the trunk remains stable and adaptable to allow the legs to initiate the forward weight shift of walking.

The third level of trunk control allows strength and stability for power production from the arm or leg. The movement and control of the trunk are used to support power production in the extremities for propulsive activities such as stair climbing, jumping, running, throwing, hitting, and rowing.

The entire model is summarized in Table 25–4.

Extremity Weakness

Weakness in the arm and the leg results in ineffective and inefficient functional patterns in daily life. Intervention for weakness in the extremities includes reeducation of movements in space, reeducation of weight-bearing movements, and training of and appropriate initiation and sequencing of movement. Most clients with hemiplegia regain enough control in their leg to stand and walk, but those same patients may not be able to use their arm for any purpose. Today, the concept of "learned nonuse" may help therapists understand why the discrepancy between arm and leg recovery exists. Wolf and associates conclude from studies of hemiplegic patients that learned nonuse does exist in some stroke patients and suggest a program of "forced use" training.[132] Although the training model should not be transferred point by point to the clinic, these studies point out the usefulness for therapists to incorporate the use of the affected side in intervention strategies.

Distal reeducation is an important component of early reeducation that has been neglected by therapists because of a previous belief that proximal return comes before distal. Distal reeducation trains the client to be able to initiate movements from the hand or foot, instead of the common proximal initiation patterns seen during attempted reach or stepping (Fig. 25–9).

Weight bearing on either the forearm or the extended arm is used as a postural assist during transition activities such as side lying to sitting, or as a means of supporting the weight of the upper trunk in sitting or standing, and is used to stabilize objects during task performance. The activity of accepting weight through the arm is not passive but extremely active and dynamic. Forearm weight bearing in sitting or standing is used to activate trunk movements, to reestablish scapulohumeral rhythm, to maintain range of motion in the arm, or to strengthen movement sequences in the arm. It is not used to inhibit tone (Fig. 25–10). The muscles of the arm are linked with trunk weight shifts during active weight bearing.[108] Table 25–7 presents the linked trunk/arm muscle activity during active weight bearing for one functional task.

The ability to support body weight on both legs for stability and movement control is important in sitting, standing, and walking retraining. Movements of the trunk in sitting and standing occur with constant changes of muscle activity in the legs as part of the base of support, to adjust to demands of weight shifts, and to increase

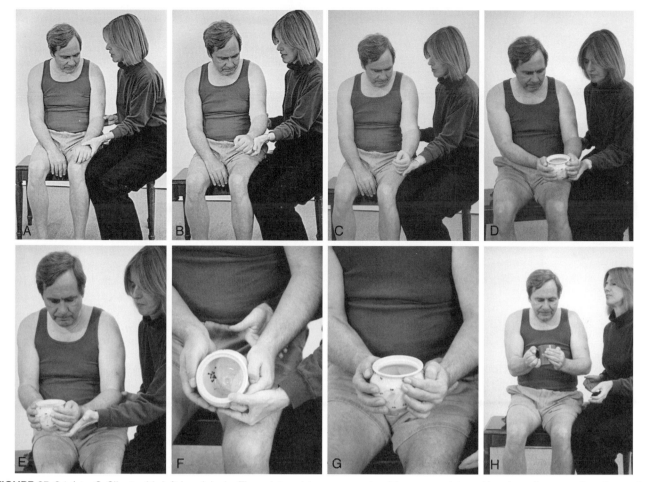

FIGURE 25–9. *A* to *C,* Client with left hemiplegia. Therapist assists movements of forearm, wrist, and hand as client practices increasing distal arm control. *D* to *F,* Therapist introduces object and assists client as he learns to control the object and the movement. *G,* Independent practice. *H,* Client uses same movements with a similar object.

activity levels of leg muscles to initiate standing weight shifts. Loss of control of weight bearing on both legs or on one leg has an immediate effect on balance. Problems of weight-bearing control of the leg may exist because of weakness; because of muscle shortening in the pelvis, hip, knee, or ankle; or because of posturing. When the leg cannot actively support body weight, undesirable asymmetrical compensations result. A significant and often overlooked prerequisite for active control of the leg in weight bearing is a stable, aligned upper body. The use of forearm or extended-arm weight bearing in standing

provides external stability to the upper body while allowing the therapist to reeducate control of bilateral or unilateral weight bearing movements in the leg.

Muscle Activation Deficits

Common muscle activation deficits include improper initiation, the inability to grade timing and force production, and the inability to sequence muscles for task performance.

Improper initiation of movement occurs when the client attempts to move the arm or leg in space and substitutes the stronger proximal muscles for weaker distal muscles.[108]

EXAMPLE
If we ask a client to lift a hemiplegic arm and reach forward for an object, he or she often initiates the movement proximally instead of distally with the hand and forearm, using the stronger elevators/abductors instead of the weaker hand and forearm muscles.

This is also seen during walking.

EXAMPLE
The client initiates swing phase of gait proximally instead of distally with the foot, using the stronger pelvic elevators or rotators instead of the weaker ankle and foot muscles.

● TABLE 25–7. Trunk/Arm-Linked Movements in Forearm Weight Bearing

Functional task: Sit at a table with both forearms supported on the table. Keepinig both arms on the table, move forward toward the table, and then move body back away from the table.

Trunk/Arm Link	Body Moves Forward	Body Moves Back
Spine	Extends	Flexes
Scapula	Adducts and depresses	Abducts and elevates
Glenohumeral joint	Less flexion	More flexion
Elbow	Flexes	Extends

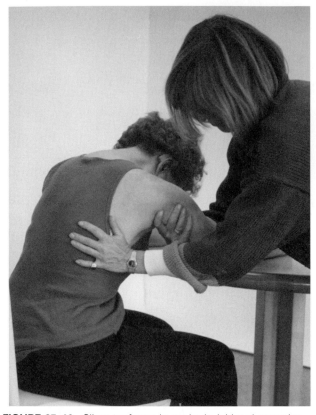

FIGURE 25–10. Client performs lower body–initiated posterior movement during forearm weight bearing at a table. The therapist uses her hands to stabilize the humerus, and as the patient moves back, the therapist's left hand slowly stretches or releases tight tissue in the rotator cuff.

Inappropriate muscle selection for the task occurs when the client substitutes a strong muscle group for a paralyzed muscle even though it is inappropriate for the function.

EXAMPLE
When the hamstrings are weak, the client may use the quadriceps to lift the leg up a step. This results in strong overshifting in the trunk and makes balance precarious.

Inappropriate sequencing includes improper initiation and excessive co-contraction. Excessive co-contraction occurs when the client activates too many muscles either at the same time or out of sequence for the task.

Excessive force production occurs when the patient activates muscles with inappropriate effort during voluntary movement. When force is excessive, the movement pattern is slow and the extremity feels stiff. Frequently, these muscles easily fatigue and the extremity slowly falls back to the starting position. Therapists often label this movement a "spastic" pattern and intervene with inhibition techniques. However, if this pattern is not from spasticity but from a muscle-activation pattern, the intervention should focus on reeducation of control, not inhibition.[108]

Hypotonicity

Hypotonic muscles offer no resistance to passive movement and are clinically associated with paralysis and weak-

ness. Clients who have experienced a severe stroke have paralysis in the trunk and extremities with low tone. As strength and control in the muscles of the trunk and extremities increase, the hypotonicity lessens. If weakness persists, they do not have problems with spasticity but have problems with the secondary impairments of poor joint alignment, muscle and soft tissue tightness, and, eventually, joint deformity or contracture.

Hypertonicity

There is considerable debate in the academic and clinical therapy community over the clinical relevance of spasticity, or hypertonicity, and the need to address it in treatment.[17, 27] Characteristics of a spastic muscle include increased velocity-dependent resistance to stretch, a clasp-knife phenomenon, and hyperactive tendon responses. Schenkman hypothesized an interesting distinction for clinical purposes: therapists can think of "hypertonicity" as tone that is higher than normal and that responds to intervention and can think of "spasticity," as researched in the laboratory, as a different type of high tone.[112] The presence or a sudden increase of its intensity is easily recognized by the therapist and the client. If hypertonicity is left untreated, the task of muscle reeducation becomes more difficult and additional secondary problems result, such as joint dysfunction, pain, and undesirable compensatory movements. In clients with hemiplegia from stroke, hypertonicity is found in the extremities, not the trunk. In severe head injury with decorticate or decerebrate posturing, trunk rigidity, a type of hypertonicity, may occur.

Clinical Hypertonicity

Although clinically the terms *spasticity* and *hypertonicity* are interchangeable, it is important to separate the types of hypertonicity that are changeable by physical and occupational therapy intervention. Therapists, although realizing that hypertonicity is not the *major* problem in hemiplegia, must understand the situations that cause it to occur. At least three different situations result in a client's increase in tone: (1) increased tone as a result of proximal instability, either insufficient trunk control for the task or instability of proximal limb musculature (e.g., hip weakness); (2) increased tension on a two-joint muscle owing to poor joint alignment and the resultant shortening and/or shifting of muscles; and (3) increased tone that is voluntarily produced during attempts at active movement, especially in the extremities.[108]

These situations are divided into three groups for ease of description, but, in reality, overlap occurs between groups. *Insufficient postural stability and control* in the trunk is the first explanation for arm and leg posturing. The extremity patterns of arm flexion or leg extension occur as an atypical balance strategy when the body is unstable.

EXAMPLE
If a client has sufficient trunk control in sitting, the arm and leg display normal resting positions. However, during the rise to stand, the arm postures in flexion. The arm postures most obviously during the transition phase of the stand when the

hips are off the surface and the center of gravity of the body is behind the feet, the new base of support.

Treatment of the increased tone, in this case, would not be directed at the arm. Rather, intervention would focus on increasing stability of the upper body during lower trunk–initiated sit-to-stand patterns and on increasing strength and control of the leg in weight bearing. As the trunk and leg gain more control, the arm hypertonicity decreases (see Fig. 25–6).

A second situation in which hypertonicity exists is when *muscle tension increases in a two-joint muscle because of changes in alignment of one of the joints.*

EXAMPLE
In sitting, tightness in the gastrocnemius muscle across the knee may not affect the ability to keep the heel on the floor. However, as the client extends the knee, the limit of tightness in the gastrocnemius is reached and the distal end of the tendon shortens and the ankle plantarflexes. When gastrocnemius tightness pulls the calcaneus into equinus, it also moves the calcaneus into varus because of the position of its insertion on the sustentaculi talus. The resultant position, ankle plantarflexion and foot supination, has been labeled a spastic foot position (see Fig. 25–7).

However, after lengthening of the gastrocnemius across the ankle and knee in standing and correction of the calcaneal position, the patient can stand and keep the foot on the floor.

EXAMPLE
In an anterior shoulder subluxation, the anterior movement of the humeral head increases tension on the biceps proximally, resulting in elbow flexion. As the tension increases, the forearm begins to supinate. As the humeral head and scapula are repositioned, the tension on the biceps is diminished. If the therapist holds this proximal correction, the elbow and forearm posturing activity stops; the forearm slowly pronates and then the elbow extends.

For the posturing to permanently stop, therapy intervention must help increase strength and control in linked trunk/scapulohumeral patterns to prevent the malalignment.

The third situation, *inappropriate voluntary muscle activation,* occurs when the client is trying to move the arm or leg. The client uses the muscles that have returning strength in the only way he or she knows how. Historically, these patterns were labeled "spastic." This label resulted in intervention strategies of inhibition. If these patterns are thought of as unbalanced or inappropriately initiated, or inappropriately sequenced, therapy intervention is more appropriately directed. The abnormally extended or flexed leg movement changes when the patient learns new activation patterns or strengthens weaker muscle sequences. Often, these are "learned" patterns and are difficult to change. Early reeducation should include training in these skills of controlling sequencing, intensity, and duration of firing.

The underlying cause of each of these situations is weakness and/or loss of control. Therefore, for changes in hypertonicity to last, treatment interventions must address the underlying causes. In each of these situations, the cause is weakness and/or loss of control of activation patterns.

In this model, generalized inhibition is inappropriate because it does not focus on the underlying cause. Intervention techniques that focus on global inhibition of extremity tone—maximal elongation, vibration, biofeedback, cold, or relaxation—rarely result in a permanent change in the tone. The temporary decrease of hypertonicity that occurs with any of these methods does not by itself directly lead to an increase in function. If used, they must be immediately followed by therapeutic exercise to create a learning environment that improves motor performance.[29, 93]

Toe Posturing

There are two patterns of toe posturing: toe clawing and toe curling. Toe clawing, metatarsal hyperextension with phalangeal flexion, is a result of loss of alignment; and toe curling, metatarsal and phalangeal flexion, is a response to instability of the trunk and leg in during standing, that is, part of a balance response.[108]

Toe curling and toe clawing interfere with comfort during standing and walking. Problems of blistering on pads of the toes and on the top of the proximal interphalangeal joint as well as toe pain occur in the intermediate and long-term stage of hemiplegia as the result of the toes rubbing on the tops of the shoes and digging into shoe soles. Relief from pressure and pain on the toepads (tips) comes with use of commercially available "hammer-toe crest pads" available from distributors (e.g., AliMed) or from medical pharmacies.

Loss of Alignment

Muscle weakness or abnormal tone in the trunk leads to atypical alignment patterns in the trunk and shoulder and pelvic girdles. This loss of alignment creates an atypical starting position for functional movement, interferes with muscle activation patterns, and limits weight transfer between extremities. Loss of alignment in the trunk in sitting and standing is analyzed and incorporated into intervention goals to reeducate functional trunk/limb-coordinated movements. The commonly described pattern of trunk shortening (lateral flexion with the concavity) on the affected side is only one of the possible alignment problems. More routinely, weakness of the trunk on one side results in a flaring of the rib cage and lateral flexion of the spine with the *convexity on the affected side.* The "appearance" of shortening on the side comes from a number of compensatory adjustments to balance or as a result of the heavy weight of a weak arm. Often therapists confuse the lower contour of the shoulder on the hemiplegic side with shortening of the trunk/concavity of the spine. The heavy weight of the weak arm pulls the upper quadrant into *excessive forward flexion.* In this position, the scapula elevates and tips forward on a flexed, rotated thoracic spine (Fig. 25–11).

Another compensatory pattern is excessive spinal flexion throughout the spine, the convexity on the weak side, and *spinal rotation toward the affected side.* Clients with this asymmetry usually shift weight onto the stronger hip. This pattern viewed from the front or rear gives the appearance of a low shoulder. This pattern of rotation to

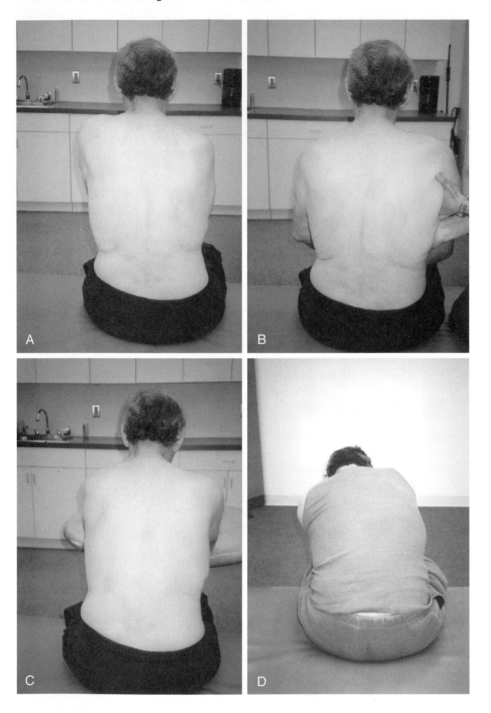

FIGURE 25–11. *A,* Client with right hemiplegia. Contour of right shoulder appears lower and longer than the left. Pelvis lists downward on right. *B,* Therapist lifts client's upper body up out of forward flexion and corrects position of glenohumeral joint. Note the contour of the right shoulder is now higher and shorter than left shoulder contour. Trunk is laterally flexed with the convexity on the right. These movement components, convexity of a lateral curve, high shoulder, and low pelvis, are compatible. *C,* Client's arms are supported symmetrically by a table. Note the convexity of the curve on the right and the low pelvis on the right. *D,* Same client moving forward and down with an upper body anterior weight shift. This position allows the therapist to evaluate the position of the trunk. Note the tendency to avoid weight on the right hip. The trunk is laterally flexed with the convexity on the right, and the right shoulder is higher than the left shoulder.

the weak side does not occur acutely but develops over time in clients who sit more than they stand or walk.

Lateral translation of the thoracic spine from the hypermobile point of T10 occurs as a means of balancing when trunk weakness results in a lateral curve, with the convexity on the affected side. This asymmetry is common in sitting when the client is encouraged to stand by pushing up with the good arm without any weight on the affected leg. It occurs in standing when quad canes or hemi-walkers are used before standing control on both legs is reeducated. The stable external cane acts as a "third stable leg," and the "long, weak" side translates laterally as the unaffected arm pushes down into the cane for stability. This pattern creates a "skin fold" on the

affected side that has been confused with shortening of the affected side (see Figs. 25–1 and 25–4).

In standing, because the need for leg stability and movement control is much greater than in sitting, trunk alignment patterns change to accommodate the demands of the leg. Often the upper body and lower body patterns are opposite one another (i.e., *counterrotational*). If the leg is in a position of ankle plantarflexion and knee extension, the hip flexes with pelvic rotation toward the affected side. The upper body then counterrotates to provide an equal and opposite balance pattern to allow the client to stand. The opposite may also exist: if the pelvis and hip rotate toward the unaffected side because of learned compensatory swing and/or stance patterns, the upper body rotates toward the affected side to provide a counterrotation for balance (see Fig. 25–4).

The atypical alignment pattern in one client may be different in sitting and standing as a result of the pattern of loss of control in the leg. In sitting, the hip is in flexion and provides support, a base, for the upper and lower trunk. Weakness in the knee and lower leg is not as critical to sitting balance and function as it is to standing functions. In standing, the hip demand is one of neutral extension to support the trunk; and complex combinations of knee, ankle, and foot movements are necessary for functional activities.

Shoulder girdle asymmetries are described in the sections on shoulder subluxation, and pelvic girdle and leg asymmetries are described in the sections on standing and walking.

Alignment problems in the distal extremity segments are related to loss of movement control and proximal alignment changes. Patterns in the distal arm and distal leg are strikingly similar. When the mid joint, elbow or knee, is extended, the proximal rotational alignment asymmetry translates down the lower segment into the hand or foot. Shoulder internal rotation translates across an extended elbow, causing the forearm to pronate and the hand to fall into carpal pronation (often confused with ulnar deviation) (Fig. 25–12A). Similarly, with knee extension, hip internal rotation asymmetries translate across the knee and cause tibial internal rotation and midfoot pronation. However, as the mid joints gain flexion activity, the proximal pattern no longer dictates distal asymmetries. The distal weight-bearing pattern or active initiation pattern causes a distal rotation that may be opposite to the proximal rotational pattern. When this occurs, the mid joint may posture with hypertonicity as a result of incompatible intralimb alignment.

EXAMPLE
As return occurs in the biceps muscle it causes the elbow to flex and the forearm to supinate. The biceps internally rotates the shoulder joint, which may already be internally rotated from shoulder subluxation. Beginning forearm supination on an internally rotated shoulder produces elbow flexor hypertonicity and a pattern that has been labeled flexion/pronation spasticity (see Fig. 25–12B).

The weakness pattern of ankle plantarflexion and calcaneal equinovarus biases return in the anterior and posterior tibialis. During movements of the leg in space with hip and knee flexion, this distal supination pattern pulls the tibia into external rotation. To place the supinated foot on the ground, the client compensates proximally by rotating the pelvis and femur, as a unit, toward the unaffected side. This incompatible tibial external rotation and femoral internal rotation result in knee hyperextension.

Muscle and tissue tightness is a common result of alignment problems. Techniques of lengthening muscle and tissue tightness must be balanced with muscle reeducation. Isolated stretching does not result in a lasting improvement in range and may decrease functional ability if not combined with activities designed to increase control. In hemiplegia, slow stretching in functional positions through active weight shifting (i.e., functional stretching) is more effective than "orthopedic" stretching because it

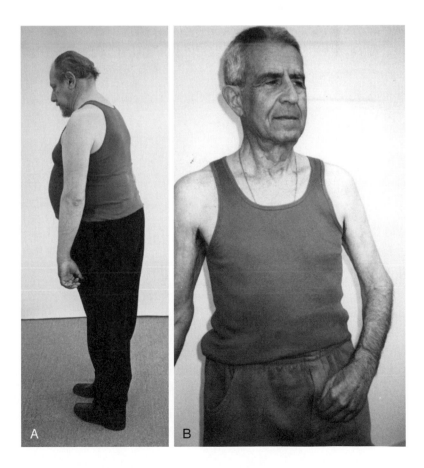

FIGURE 25–12. *A,* Client with left hemiplegia and severe weakness. The left arm and hand is in shoulder internal rotation, elbow extension, and forearm pronation. The left wrist flexes, and the hand pronates and radially deviates on the wrist. *B,* Client with left hemiplegia with atypical movements. The left arm is positioned in shoulder internal rotation and elbow flexion. As the elbow flexes, the forearm begins to supinate on the internally rotated humerus. The wrist flexes and radially deviates with finger flexion.

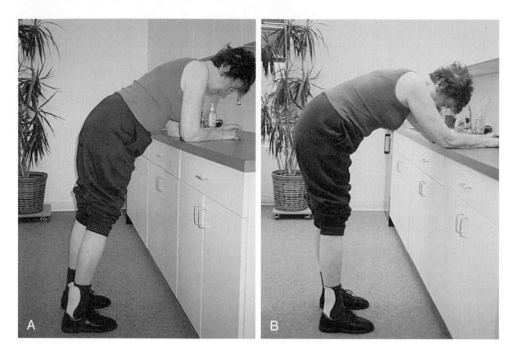

FIGURE 25–13. *A,* Client with right hemiplegia practicing home program. During standing forearm weight bearing (providing upper body stability), she initiates a lower extremity forward/backward movement. As she moves her hips and lower leg forward, she thinks of keeping her knee straight and stretching her calf. *B,* As she moves her hips backward, she may feel a stretch in the back of her thigh, on the lateral aspect of her trunk, or under her axilla.

reeducates the weakness that underlies the loss of muscle length (Fig. 25–13).

Because weakness is the underlying cause of loss of alignment and joint range, in the acute phase the *joints are hypermobile.* Over time, the tissues tighten around some joints and therapists often confuse that "feel" with joint hypomobility. Joint mobilization techniques are rarely needed because the weakness in hemiplegia renders the joints hypermobile. It is important to avoid excessive mobility in the intricate joints of the hand and foot. Tightness around a joint may indicate the need for lengthening exercises, but the joint almost never requires mobilization.

Pain

In the client with hemiplegia, arm pain can be caused by an imbalance of muscles, improper movement patterns, joint dysfunction, improper weight-bearing patterns, and muscle shortening or it may be related to diminished sensation and sensory interpretation.

Joint Pain

Joint pain is caused by poor shoulder joint mechanics during movement. Two common alignment problems are loss of scapula/humeral rhythm and insufficient humeral external rotation.[16, 102] With a shoulder subluxation, the humeral head is not seated in the fossa and passive movements of the shoulder will not occur with scapulohumeral rhythm. At 60 to 90 degrees of forward flexion, impingement of the capsule will occur and the client will report sharp pain on the superior aspect of the shoulder joint. The pain ceases when the arm is lowered. The subluxation and loss of scapulohumeral rhythm result from loss of trunk/arm movements or muscle tightness from either persistent arm posturing or weakness.

If the client reports joint pain, the therapist should lower the humerus immediately, reestablish the mobility of the scapula, reseat the humerus if necessary, and maintain appropriate humeral rotation while moving the arm up again. Trunk movements in forearm weight bearing are used to teach a self-ranging practice routine that ensures scapulohumeral rhythm.

Muscle and Tendon Pain

When a hypertonic or shortened muscle is stretched too quickly or beyond available length, a strong "pulling" type pain is often reported in the region of the muscle belly being stretched. If the amount of stretch is decreased a few degrees, the reported pain subsides.

If the inappropriate stretching is not stopped, muscle pain progresses to tendon pain. Proximal biceps tendonitis, distal biceps tendonitis radiating into the forearm, and wrist flexor tendonitis are most common. The usual cause of tendonitis is improper weight bearing, with an inactive trunk and "hanging" on the arm with forced elbow extension and shoulder internal rotation. The treatment of tendonitis is rest and modalities (i.e., heat, ultrasound or electrical stimulation) or injection of corticosteroids. When movement reeducation is restarted it is important to avoid the "exercise" that caused the pain and create a new intervention plan.

Shoulder-Hand Syndrome

The shoulder-hand syndrome begins with tenderness and swelling of the hand and diffuse aching pain from altered sensitivity in the shoulder and entire arm.[109] This pain interferes with the reeducation of movement patterns and causes a general desire on the part of the client to "protect" the arm by not moving it. Limited shoulder and wrist and finger range of motion soon occurs.

The second stage of shoulder-hand syndrome includes further loss of shoulder and hand range of motion, severe edema, and loss of skin elasticity. This is followed by the third stage, which includes demineralization of bone, severe soft tissue deformity, and joint contracture.[109]

Not every edematous hemiplegic hand leads to a shoulder-hand syndrome. Hand edema results from an upper extremity that remains dependent and that does not move for long periods of time. It is essential to teach the person with hemiplegia how to properly care for the hand and to give the responsibility for the care of the hand and arm to the client.

Levit proposes five steps for intervention of severe or chronic arm pain: (1) eliminate pain from intervention and/or the home program, (2) desensitize the arm and hand to touch, (3) eliminate hand edema, (4) introduce pain-free arm movements by reestablishing scapula mobility, and (5) beginning with guided arm movements below 60 degrees, gradually increase the variety and complexity of arm movements.[108]

Edema

Edema in the hand and foot is another common secondary impairment that develops as a consequence of loss of movement control and hospitalization factors such as intravenous infiltrates and limb positioning. Edema limits joint range and tissue mobility. The edematous fluid places the skin on stretch and acts as an interstitial "glue" that bonds the skin, fascial tissue, muscle tissue, and tendons. Hand edema is associated with the development of shoulder-hand syndrome. Foot edema is as common as hand edema, limits ankle joint dorsiflexion range, and is often ignored during intervention programs. Edema begins on the volar surface of the hand and foot, progresses dorsally, and then continues proximally across the wrist and/or ankle.

Edema interferes with the retraining of functional movement patterns by preventing the smooth glide of tissues. It must be eliminated before active reeducation begins.

Edema has defined stages. When the involved tissue feels soft and fluid, the condition responds to retrograde massage and elevation. When the tissue is gelatinous and pitting, the edematous fluid cannot be physically expressed. At this stage, it begins to adhere to underlying tissues. The edema must be softened and liquefied through trans-tissue massage. The last stage of edema is characterized by hard, lumpy tissue that does not "pit" in response to manual pressure. This stage of edema requires gentle bilateral compression to break up the hard, solid areas into regions of softness. The soft regions then act as open spaces into which fluid released by massage of hard tissue is directed. The goal is to reverse the process of hardening—from hard, to pitting, to soft and fluid. In these last two stages, when the edematous tissue no longer feels fluid, elevation, elastic gloves or bandaging, and retrograde massage are not effective. When edematous tissue is soft and fluid, active and active assistive extremity movement patterns produce muscular contractions that assist venous and lymphatic return of the fluid.[108]

Shoulder Subluxation

Shoulder subluxation occurs when any of the biomechanical factors contributing to glenohumeral joint stability are interrupted. In persons with hemiplegia, subluxation is related to a change in the angle of the glenoid fossa occurring because of muscle weakness. In the frontal plane the scapula is normally held at an angle of 40 degrees. When the slope of the glenoid fossa becomes less oblique (and more vertical), the humerus will "slide" down and out of the fossa.[7] Ryerson and Levit first described three types of subluxation in clients with hemiplegia: inferior, anterior, and superior.[107]

Inferior Subluxation

The most common type of subluxation is an inferior subluxation. It occurs in clients with severe weakness and is present in the acute stage. Weakness and the weight of a heavy arm result in downward rotation of the scapula. Downward rotation orients the glenoid fossa vertically, the unlocking mechanism of the capsule is lost, and the humerus subluxates inferiorly with internal rotation. As the humerus internally rotates, the bicipital tuberosity rolls anteriorly; this anterior prominence is often confused with an anterior subluxation.[108] As subluxation occurs, the shoulder capsule is vulnerable to stretch, especially when the humerus is dependent and resting by the side of the body. In this position, the capsule is taut superiorly, so any downward distraction of the humerus will place an immediate stretch on the upper part of the capsule. The superior portion of the capsule is reinforced by the coracohumeral ligament, which is crucial for shoulder stability. Jenson[56] has discussed the implications of rupture of this ligament as a result of forced abnormal passive motion as a cause of shoulder pain in subluxation.

Anterior Subluxation

Anterior subluxation occurs when the humeral head separates anteriorly from the glenoid fossa. Anterior shoulder subluxation occurs when the downwardly rotated scapula elevates and tilts forward on the rib cage and the humerus hyperextends with internal rotation. In an anterior subluxation, as tension increases on the proximal biceps tendon, the elbow flexes and the forearm supinates. This subluxation is found in clients with atypical patterns of return and trunk rotational asymmetries.[108]

Superior Subluxation

A superior subluxation occurs when the humeral head lodges under the coracoid process in a position of internal rotation and slight abduction. The humeral head is "locked" in this position so that every movement of the humerus is accompanied by scapula movement. The scapula position in this subluxation is one of abduction, elevation, and neutral rotation. The forearm adducts across the body as the humeral abduction and elbow flexion increase. A superior subluxation occurs in clients with inappropriate muscle firing and co-contraction.

Subluxation is not painful but results in changes in muscle length-tension relationships, muscle shortening, and permanent stretch of the joint capsule. If a subluxation exists, the therapist reduces the subluxation by correcting trunk, scapula, and humeral alignment patterns before attempting to reeducate arm movement patterns. A discussion of these subluxations, accompanying trunk movement patterns, and intervention suggestions can be found in therapy literature.[108] As the client learns to move the arm in patterns of functional coordination, subluxation and associated arm posturing decrease.

Prevention of subluxation requires (1) proper assessment of secondary alignment problems (rib cage/scapula/humeral position), (2) early reeducation of trunk/arm-linked patterns in sitting and standing, and (3) prevention of shoulder capsule stretch, including support and positioning as the client sits, stands, and practices walking.

FUNCTIONAL ACTIVITIES

Functional mobility movement analysis, intervention techniques, unilateral compensatory strategies, and suggestions for task practice are documented in therapy literature.[59, 113, 126] In this section, representative mobility skills are selected in three functional positions: supine, sitting, and standing. For each task selected, the focus is on the basic trunk and extremity control patterns used, significant impairments in addition to weakness that make it difficult for the client to perform the task, and observations from the clinic that relate to intervention and practice. Detailed description of each trunk and trunk/extremity-linked pattern is in the literature.[108]

Supine

Rolling

Basic trunk movements to be reeducated include (1) upper trunk flexion/rotation initiation, (2) lower trunk extension/rotation initiation, and (3) symmetrical lateral flexion initiation.

Trunk/Extremity-Linked Patterns. The upper-trunk flexion-rotation initiation pattern is linked with arm reach across the body. Active assistive patterns, using a bilateral arm reach, are encouraged when strength is insufficient to lift the arm against gravity or, through therapist handling, when arm muscle paralysis or weakness results in such a heavy feeling that the patient cannot control the extremity with the unaffected hand. If the therapist assists the arm, the goal of practice is for the client to initiate the active antigravity trunk pattern.

A lower trunk extension-rotation initiation pattern is coordinated with either a leg-reach pattern or a flexed-leg "push" pattern. Active assistive patterns can be implemented through therapist handling to help train the sequencing or to grade the firing patterns of the leg when it is pushing into the bed. Independent practice is performed when the control and strength in the affected leg return or both knees rotate with the pelvis and extending lower trunk. Independent practice also requires the upper body and arm to follow the movement of the lower body.

The symmetrical lateral flexion initiation pattern is known as "log rolling." In this pattern, the trunk does not rotate but is linked in a symmetrical pattern with arm and leg "reach or push" on the leading side.

Impairments That Interfere. Shoulder joint pain may occur when the client rolls onto the affected side. Pain occurs if the shoulder is trapped under the trunk as the client moves to side lying or when the humeral/scapula alignment causes the capsule to be impinged. The client should not continue to roll or lie on the painful shoulder.

In rehabilitative or outpatient care, muscle tightness in the latissimus, quadratus lumborum, biceps, and/or tensor fasciae latae may limit trunk rotation or trunk/extremity-linked movements.

Clinical Observations. Weakness in the extremities is a significant factor during rolling because the arm and the leg are used to assist the trunk initiation patterns. Rotational patterns are difficult in the acute stage because they require an integration and sequencing of flexor and extensor muscle patterns. Symmetrical rolling is an easier independent pattern to train. Active assistive strategies and strengthening need to be incorporated early in intervention. Clients have an easier time rolling to the affected side, because they use the strength of the unaffected side to initiate the roll. But they may not want to stay on that side because of shoulder pain, instability of the hip, or decreased sensation and the fear that ensues. The client may prefer rolling to the unaffected side because it is easier to rest on, but initiating the movement is difficult because of loss of control.

The family is educated to understand the nature of the loss of movement and the loss of sensation and their effects on body awareness and early bed mobility. Family members are encouraged to sit with, visit, talk to, feed, and touch the person with the hemiplegia from the client's affected side. They are instructed in simple movements, like rolling, to promote symmetry, midline control, and activation of trunk muscles. Because family members are often afraid to touch or move the client's affected side, they are educated quickly to be made a part of the intervention process.

Feeding and Swallowing

Although detailed facilitation and inhibition of oral and neck muscle movement for feeding and articulated language are a specialty of speech pathologists, the movement therapist activates trunk control to increase upper-body stability to prepare for more automatic chew and swallow.

Basic trunk patterns to be reeducated include (1) lower body anterior/posterior movement control to move toward table and back into chair and (2) upper body anterior/posterior and lateral movement control to provide control for head and arm movement.

Impairments That Interfere. Oral problems include:

- Forward head, poor lip closure, loss of saliva and food
- Facial asymmetry during function greater than at rest
- Inability to swallow
- Inability to chew
- Inability to lateralize foods
- Inability to take liquids from cup or spoon
- Muscle weakness with hypotonia

Central problems are:

- Asymmetry of trunk
- Poor postural control
- Upper body flexion with or without weight of weak arm
- Inability to feed self

Compensations include:

- Use of gravity—with head and neck extension the food flows down the throat
- Chewing on one side only
- Using the hand to place food in the mouth
- Using the hand to pull food from the cheek
- Using thicker food, which is much easier to handle than soft, liquid foods

Clinical Observations. Drooling occurs when upper-trunk extensor weakness results in excessive upper-trunk flexion. As the client tries to lift the head, it extends on the cervical spine in a forward position. As a result of the biomechanics of the forward head position, the jaw opens, automatic swallowing becomes difficult, and saliva runs out of the open mouth.

Drooling from one side of the mouth is annoying and embarrassing. The client may not be able to maintain lip closure and, in addition, may not feel the saliva running out or may not identify a need to swallow. Drooling lessens as upper-body control increases.

In the majority of cases, swallowing problems are transient in persons with hemiplegia. After the initial insult and during the flaccid period, many clients exhibit a decreased gag reflex. In acute care settings, where liquid diets are often routinely given to persons with hemiplegia, education of hospital staff to the merits of using thicker foods should be considered. Thicker, chopped food is easier to swallow than soft food. Soft food is easier to swallow than liquids. Liquids with distinct taste or texture are easier to swallow than water. Specific feeding programs are noted in Chapters 4, 8, and 9.

Sitting

Function in sitting is based on the ability to maintain the trunk in an upright position, to automatically adjust the trunk when the arms or one leg moves around midline, and to control shifting of the trunk as the arm and leg extend their reach. Control in sitting is also used to help change position, such as sitting to standing, or lying down. The reestablishment of control in sitting for function is an important early goal in rehabilitation care.

Basic trunk movements to be reeducated include:

1. Anterior, posterior, and lateral upper body–initiated movements. Upper-body movements are easier to retrain than lower-body movements because the base of support (contact of the buttocks and feet) remains on the surface.
2. Anterior and posterior lower body–initiated movements. With lower body–initiated movement, the upper body needs to be stable and yet adjust to and follow the movement of the lower body. The reeducation of upper-body control allows the therapist to begin retraining lower-body control.

3. Lateral lower body–initiated movements. These movements are the most difficult of the three movements required for sitting control because as the movement begins, the base of support narrows.
4. Rotational movements. In sitting, the easiest rotational patterns to reeducate are upper-body rotation on a stable lower body.

Trunk/Arm-Linked Patterns (Representative Examples). Postural adjustments to arm movements around midline require the trunk to be upright, to be active, and to perform small adjustments. When the hand functions in front of the body, the trunk adjusts with small posterior weight shifts and increased flexor control, while as the hand(s) move to function behind the body, the trunk adjusts with a small anterior weight shift.

The trunk moves with an arm to extend reach. If the reach is forward and down to the floor, as if to reach a shoe, the upper body initiates an anterior weight shift and the spine moves into flexion with control from eccentric contraction of the spinal extensors. If the reach is forward as if to grab an object on the far side of a table, the lower body initiates an anterior weight shift as the upper body remains stable and adjusts to the demands of the arm movement.

Trunk/Leg-Linked Patterns (Representative Examples). Small trunk adjustments occur with leg movements around midline. If the feet move back under the hips, the trunk adjusts with a small amount of anterior weight shift. When one foot is lifted up to slide into a slipper, the lower body adjusts with a small lateral weight shift. Upper-trunk stability allows lower trunk–initiated patterns when rising to stand. As the hips and knees extend to lift the buttocks off the chair, trunk adjustments accompany the changing leg pattern to provide balance.

Impairments That Interfere. Changes in alignment of the arm due to weakness and muscle shortening affect the position of the thoracic spine and rib cage. The weight of a flaccid or extremely weak arm pulls the upper trunk into forward flexion; an increase of flexor tone in the arm causes the scapula to elevate and the rib cage to rotate. Both of these alignment problems of the trunk interfere with the ability to increase strength in basic trunk movement patterns.

Shoulder subluxation results in muscle shortening (biceps, pectorals, latissimus, subscapularis), alters the line of muscle pull, and interferes with scapulohumeral rhythm. Muscle shortening contributes to loss of upper-body alignment and interferes with strengthening trunk patterns.

Loss of trunk alignment as a result of trunk weakness creates an atypical starting position for movement and limits the number and type of movement patterns that can be safely produced.

Clinical Observations. Alignment changes in the arm influence strength and control of the upper body. Therefore, intervention techniques to restore alignment and control of the arm on the upper trunk must be included in the list of short-term goals to achieve the functional goal of safe, independent task performance in sitting.

Active control of the pelvis in a neutral position is

necessary for the reeducation of lower-body lateral and rotational weight shifts. Pelvic position influences leg position. If the pelvis is held in a posterior tilt, the leg initially tends to abduct; and if it is held in an anterior tilt, the leg initially adducts.

Clients with poor hip control do not regain functional trunk patterns in sitting until they can activate and strengthen hip muscles for stability during weight shifts. Weakness of the hip joint results in a desire to shift weight to the stronger side, thus creating a spinal or pelvic asymmetry. Clients who push to the affected side in sitting need strength from the weak leg for stability as a prerequisite for midline control of the trunk.

Lower body–initiated lateral weight shift patterns are difficult to train because they require a narrowing of the base of support. Forearm weight-bearing movement patterns are used to increase the base of support to allow practice of these patterns that are needed for functional activities such as scooting, toileting, and lifting one leg off the surface. This movement is difficult to practice without upper-body stability (external or internal).

Transfers. Transfers in the half-stand, pivot pattern require upper-body control over the lower body and combined trunk/leg control patterns. The squat, pivot position is trained when leg strength and control are weak and the goal is to train the client to use the affected leg. Transfers involve interim patterns that are trained before safe standing is possible.

The client practices transfers to different objects (chair, bed, toilet) to either side. This promotes symmetry, encourages the use of the affected leg, and allows practice with varying environmental constraints. Transfers to the unaffected side have the advantage of being familiar to hospital staff because they are the "traditional" textbook way of transferring the person with hemiplegia. Nevertheless, transfers to the affected side need to be trained by therapists to allow function in either direction.

Sit to Stand. Two initiation patterns are commonly used, with or without the use of momentum, to train sit to stand. A lower body–initiated anterior weight transfer occurs with a straight spine as the shoulders move forward. Therapists should emphasize the forward weight shift component of this pattern, rather than the anterior pelvic tilt component; the requirement of sit to stand is a forward shift of the upper body and shoulders. An anterior pelvic tilt usually results in a backward movement of the shoulders. The confusion over this movement occurs because clients often sit in a position of flexion with a posterior pelvic tilt. To come to upright, they must extend the spine and move the pelvis to neutral. Although individuals with a tendency for lumbar extension may have an anterior pelvic tilt as they shift forward, the anterior pelvic tilt is not as important a component as is a forward weight shift.

An upper body–initiated anterior weight transfer during sit to stand results in spinal flexion and eccentric activity in the spinal extensors. This pattern keeps body weight over the feet, the new base of support, but does not link the extension of the legs with the lower trunk. The demand on the trunk from lift off to stand is greater than in the previous pattern because muscle contraction type must change and there is a larger requirement for strength and control as the spine moves from flexion to standing. This pattern is used in rehabilitative and extended care centers because it allows caregivers to perform safe, maximal assist transfers. Use of both legs during sitting, transfers, and sit to stand increases strength in the legs ("forced use") and promotes symmetry of the pelvis, thus enhancing control in the trunk.

During transfer and sit to stand training, techniques of directing manual pressure from the top of the knee through the tibia into the foot help the client remember to keep weight on both feet and increase the dorsiflexion moment at the ankle.

Full standing should not be attempted if loss of control in the leg results in nonuse. If the client cannot activate leg muscles in a weight-bearing position as he or she attempts to stand, the stand will be precarious with undesirable trunk compensatory patterns.

Standing

Standing Control

Control in standing is a difficult early goal to achieve because the control demands of the trunk and leg are complex. Control of basic movement patterns in standing is divided into upper body–initiated control patterns and lower extremity–initiated control patterns.[108] Upper-body control in standing includes the ability to move the upper trunk and arm in all planes with appropriate leg responses and the ability to respond and adjust to weight transfer to each leg and to provide postural stability for movements of each leg in space.

Lower-extremity control in standing has a weight-bearing component and a movement in space component. As a prerequisite for reeducation of these movements, the upper body must have enough strength and control to provide stability and postural adjustments for movements of the leg.

Basic trunk movements to be reeducated include:

1. Upper body–initiated anterior, posterior, lateral, and rotational patterns with critical corresponding adjustments in the leg (either hip, knee, or ankle strategies).
2. Control of the upper body over the lower trunk during lower extremity–initiated weight-bearing movements.
3. Linked trunk/leg patterns during movements of the leg in space. This is easiest when the leg moves around midline, and it increases in difficulty as movement in space increases in amplitude or speed.
4. Increased upper-body control to support power production of the arms for pushing, pulling, or lifting objects and increased lower-body control to support power production of the legs for jumping, running, and stair climbing.

Trunk/Arm-Linked Patterns. These patterns include:

1. Upper body–initiated flexion movements that occur with forward and downward arm-reach patterns.
2. Upper body–initiated extension that occurs when the arm reaches up or up and back.
3. Upper body–initiated lateral flexion when the arm reaches down and to one side.

4. Upper-body flexion/rotation when the arm reaches down and to one side.
5. Upper-body extension/rotation when the arm reaches up and back to one side.

Trunk/Leg-Linked Patterns in Weight Bearing. Control of the upper and lower trunk during unilateral stance on either leg is one of the most difficult patterns to retrain. Control of the trunk in unilateral stance is linked with the need for abduction control on the stance leg. In clients with hemiplegia, the complicated control demands for leg and trunk control in standing combined with the presence of weakness and control problems result in loss of alignment in multiple joints and strong compensatory patterns.

Trunk/Leg-Linked Patterns as the Leg Moves in Space. When the leg moves in space in small ranges, the movement of the upper trunk is small and occurs as a postural adjustment. The movement pattern of the femur and pelvis is a linked rhythm similar to scapulohumeral rhythm. The first 30 to 45 degrees of hip flexion occur with no pelvic movements; from 45 to 90 degrees the pelvis moves with the flexing hip with a posterior tilt; and with continued hip flexion the upper trunk flexes to maintain balance. This rhythm occurs in the other planes of movement as well. As the movement of the leg increases in range, such as when turning, the demand on the trunk increases.

1. Lower-trunk flexion occurs when the leg reaches forward and up; stepping up.
2. Lower-trunk extension occurs when the leg reaches back.
3. Lower-trunk lateral flexion occurs when the leg lifts up and out to the same side.

Impairments That Interfere. In standing, loss of alignment in the upper body on the hemiplegic side creates compensatory patterns that interfere with functional standing movements and balance. Loss of upper-body stability produces one of three common patterns: (1) forward flexion of the upper trunk, (2) upper-body rotation toward the affected side, or (3) upper-body rotation away from the affected side.

Loss of ankle joint dorsiflexion range blocks the ability of the body to use ankle strategies for leg responses to upper body–initiated movements or for leg movements and function. Loss of ankle joint dorsiflexion range is one cause of knee hyperextension in standing. Ankle range is lost within a few days after stroke and needs to be prevented to train early standing functions.

Loss of knee control during standing is the result of weakness of the trunk, pelvis, hip, ankle, or both. Loss of knee control from weakness is influenced by the position and movement control of the hip and ankle joints. Initially, the knee flexes as more weight is shifted to the unaffected side, and the pelvis lists downward. If the pelvic position is not corrected (leveled) and the client is encouraged to straighten the knee, the pelvis rotates toward the affected side to provide "length" for the knee movement. This pelvic rotation is accompanied by hip flexion as the client tries to straighten the "weak" knee. After standing and walking are practiced, the client may learn to "lock" the knee in hyperextension with unbalanced quadriceps firing as a means of gaining stability (Fig. 25–14).

The cause of early arm flexor hypertonicity and leg extensor hypertonicity in standing is insufficient trunk control. Over time, leg extensor hypertonicity results from all three previously stated situations: insufficient trunk control, altered intralimb alignment, and unbalanced

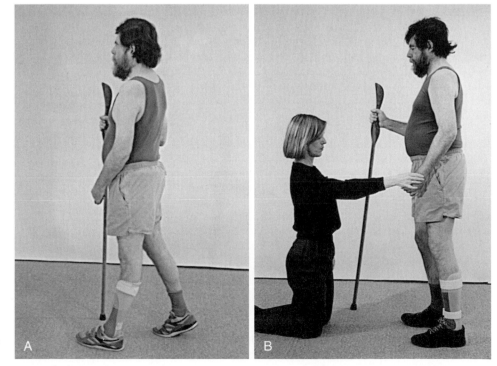

FIGURE 25–14. *A,* Client with left hemiplegia with knee hyperextension wearing a lightweight prefabricated posterior leaf-spring brace that does not control his knee hyperextension. *B,* A solid ankle brace with foot control that decreases knee hyperextension by providing distal stability.

"learned" firing. If the therapist uses handling to change one of the three situations, the previously extended knee begins to "wobble," a sign of the underlying loss of control.

Clinical Observations. In the acute phase, therapists can help the client practice standing with the hips and shoulders back against a wall to provide support for the trunk and pelvis while allowing a safe situation to practice active self-initiated leg weight-bearing movements. The client can slide down the wall, activating eccentric control in the legs, and then slide back up, activating concentric control. By using the wall to assist the stand, the therapist frees his or her hands to help correct leg alignment problems and lets the client practice the initiation of movement early, independently, and safely.

The client can practice controlled lateral weight transfer with appropriate trunk activity in this position. Whereas one study concluded that there is no relationship between lateral weight shift and walking, therapists should not conclude that unilateral weight acceptance is inappropriate functional training.[129] During intervention and independent practice many patients move laterally incorrectly by overshifting or without the prerequisite of upper-body control. The main focus of weight shift training for walking in hemiplegia should be an anterior weight shift.

Upper-extremity forearm or extended-arm weight bearing provides upper trunk stability for lower extremity–initiated practice. This practice pattern also allows a means of self-ranging for the ankle, knee, hip, and pelvis. This position is used not to inhibit tone in the extremities but to activate and strengthen the trunk and legs in linked patterns.

Walking

Independent, functional, and safe walking is difficult to retrain in the early phases of intervention because it requires refined degrees of trunk and extremity control. It requires an advanced level of trunk control, linked trunk/leg movements, and enough strength and control in the leg to support body weight, to move the multiple joints of the leg in complex patterns, and to control speed, momentum, and balance. Walking patterns in clients with stroke are characterized by slow speed, uneven step and stride lengths, impaired balance with resulting arm and leg posturing, and reliance on adaptive equipment.

In the present health care environment with the emphasis on limited therapy visits, therapists are confronted with major intervention dilemmas: Should they force the client to walk without minimal prerequisites? Should they allow undesirable compensations even though they predict future secondary problems? Should they use the benefits of the large health care systems to divide responsibility for continued gait training between therapy (inpatient, rehabilitation, home care, outpatient) divisions?

Prerequisites for functional, safe walking include:

- Upper-body control to adjust to leg movements in unilateral stance and during movements of the leg in space
- Lower-trunk control to prevent atypical pelvic alignment patterns during movements of the leg in space

- Strength and control of the leg to initiate weight shifts
- Strength and control in the leg to move in space

Because gait is the most extensively studied, analyzed, and discussed in terms of intervention, this section describes the prerequisites for walking training and common impairments that interfere with walking.[64, 120, 131] Common impairments that interfere with walking are separated into three divisions of the walking cycle: (1) forward progression, (2) single/double-limb support, and (3) swing.[96, 106]

Impairments that interfere with functional walking are summarized in Table 25–8.

Clinical Observations. If weakness in the foot and ankle creates difficulty clearing the foot during stepping, the body recruits a proximal initiation pattern: hip hiking, circumduction, or posterior pelvic tilting. If allowed to persist, this atypical initiation pattern results in a walking pattern that is difficult or impossible to change. This points to a need to consider minimal ankle/foot support during early walking as a means of creating appropriate distal initiation patterns and limiting the need for proximal compensation (Fig. 25–15). (See Chapter 31 for additional suggestions.)

After the identification of significant impairments for swing phase and stance phase, specific intervention techniques are chosen.

EXAMPLE
After the description set forth by Knuttsen,[65] in a type I motor control problem with premature activation of the calf muscles, intervention may stress lower extremity–initiated forward weight shift. Control of the ankle with appropriate knee activity allows the center of gravity to advance ahead of the foot before the activation of calf muscles pulls the lower leg backward. With a type II disturbance, training to improve control and power of the leg in standing or during sit to stand under varied conditions may be indicated. In a type III problem, intervention is directed at achieving stability control of the upper trunk during lower extremity–initiated patterns.

EQUIPMENT

Equipment for persons with CNS dysfunction can be thought of as supports or as "extra" help to allow better alignment or stabilization so that the client can move and function more independently. Too much support or equipment prevents participation in an activity and hinders the development of new movement control. Equipment should never be a substitute for treatment and should not be given without practice during treatment. One-handed equipment that is used as a substitute for trunk control is less successful than equipment that is used to compensate for loss of extremity function. Therapists should perform ongoing assessment of the appropriateness of the equipment in relation to gains made in therapy.

EXAMPLE
A "reacher" compensates for loss of trunk/limb-linked control to allow the arm to extend its reach, whereas an electric can opener designed for one-handed use substitutes for the ability to use both hands.

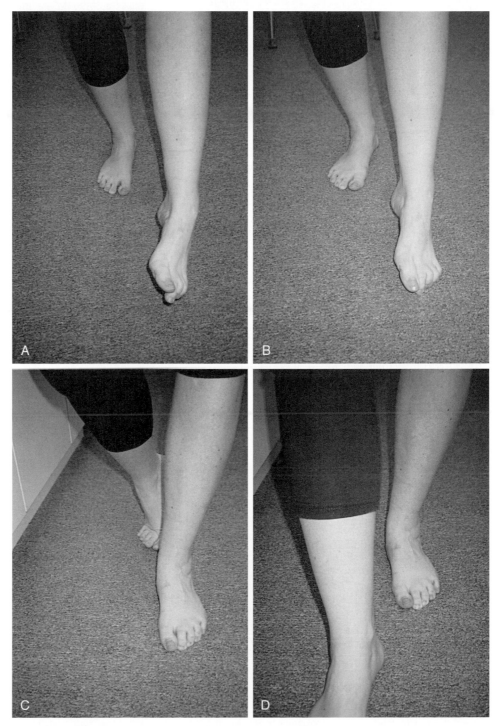

FIGURE 25–15. *A* and *B*, Client with left hemiplegia. Supination of the foot during swing and during foot contact with ankle joint plantarflexion and calcaneal varus. *C* and *D*, Compensatory pronation of the midfoot to allow the foot to contact the ground during stance.

T A B L E 2 5 – 8. Summary of Significant Functional Impairments

Forward Progression—Heel Strike to Midstance

Poor trunk control
    Loss of alignment of the upper trunk over lower trunk
    Loss of control of upper trunk as leg initiates weight shift forward
Lack of proper initiation pattern and direction
    Excessive forward trunk flexion
    Excessive lateral weight shift
Insufficient ankle joint dorsiflexion range
    Muscle tightness
    Loss of control
    Edema
Inappropriate foot contact
    Weakness of foot and ankle muscles
    Muscle tightness
    Foot posturing

Single/Double Limb Support

Insufficient trunk control to maintain position over one leg
    Asymmetries during unilateral stance
    Loss of control of upper trunk over lower trunk
Poor lower extremity control
    Hip instability
    Loss of knee control in unilateral stance
    Loss of ankle joint dorsiflexion range
    Toe clawing or curling
Loss of ability to transfer weight through foot
Inability to maintain leg on floor behind body
    Muscle tightness
    Weakness or inappropriate activation of leg muscles

Swing—Early and Late

Atypical leg muscle firing patterns
Lack of proper initiation
    Loss of ankle and foot dorsiflexion
    Inability to control trunk and lower extremity initiation pattern
    Initiation pattern
Inability of the body to continue to move forward as leg swings
Foot posturing

Bedside Equipment

In acute and rehabilitation settings, pillows, blankets, or towels are used to position the client in bed. With the client in the supine position, the head pillow can be angled so that it slips under the shoulder and scapula to prevent loss of alignment. The therapist uses a pillow to support the humerus and makes sure the shoulder joint is not hyperextended. Hyperextension of the shoulder in supine results in elbow flexion by increasing biceps tension proximally. A soft towel roll or pillow under the greater trochanter and/or knee maintains alignment of the leg in the first few days after a stroke. Once the client begins to move to both sides in bed, the use of pillows for support is not necessary.

Wheelchairs

Wheelchairs must have a solid surface to sit on and, when possible, a supportive backrest. The soft, leather seats of transport chairs act as a sling and allow the pelvis to posteriorly tilt and the spine to flex. This reinforces the preferred position of the body with paralysis or severe weakness. Solid seats and backs allow the pelvis, trunk, and extremities to be more normally aligned. Wheelchairs

specifically for clients with hemiplegia who are not expected to walk have lower seat heights and one-armed drive (two hand rims on one wheel). These adaptations make it easier for clients to propel the chair with the unaffected hand and foot.

Support for the hemiplegic arm when sitting in a wheelchair reduces the effect of the downward pull of gravity on the weak or paralyzed arm. Lapboards support both arms and provide symmetry for the upper body. In some settings, they are considered a form of restraint and cannot be used. Half-lapboards or arm troughs are used to support the arm if the client has enough perceptual awareness to be able to limit trunk movements. The use of a pillow in the lap is another option for bilateral support of the arms. If an arm support is used, the client should be taught trunk movements in relation to the support and how to protect the arm and hand while on the support.

Slings

Slings are used to support the glenohumeral joint to prevent capsular stretch, to temporarily maintain alignment that is gained in treatment, and to take some of the weight of the paralyzed arm off the upper trunk as the client begins to learn to stand and walk. They cannot reverse an existing subluxation once the capsule is stretched. Because subluxation is not inherently painful, a sling should not be used to prevent pain. However, use of a sling can help break the cycle of pain from shoulder-hand syndrome.

Various reviews and comparisons of slings are available.[86, 121] In the studies, shoulder joint position was examined without consideration of trunk or scapula position. There is no sling available that corrects a subluxation because no existing sling provides scapula upward rotation control. Slings only "hold" a correct scapulohumeral position that has been restored in treatment.

The ideal shoulder sling helps maintain the normal angular alignment of the glenoid fossa, decreases the tendency of the humerus to internally rotate, takes some of the weight of the arm off the upper trunk, and allows the upper extremity freedom of movement. Therapists should not prescribe slings that cradle the arm in front of the body, prevent any movement, and, in effect, teach learned nonuse. The orthopedic-type *envelope arm sling* was used in the 1950s and 1960s. In the 1970s, influenced by Bobath, sling usage was thought to be undesirable.[13] As more information about tone and movement became available, new slings were designed to allow the arm to be supported while movement was reeducated. Slings have different suspensions, provide different means of control for the arm, give differing "messages" to the arm and trunk, and have individual uses. Table 25–9, adapted from the work of Levit,[72] lists available slings and their characteristics.

Clients who come into therapy with a sling, but do not require one, are weaned from a supportive sling into a less-controlling one. Clients state that the *clavicle support* provides support during household tasks that require upper-body flexion, such as bedmaking or vacuuming. Cli-

TABLE 25-9. **Available Slings and Their Characteristics**

Basic Type	Supplier	Suspension	Message	Common Use
Clavicle support	DePuy (clavicle fracture sling with 1-inch soft foam axilla pad)	Figure-of-8	"Spine extend, scapula adduct"	Acute care
		Support under axilla		A minimal support To wean out of other supports
Humeral cuff	Rolyan Hemi Arm Sling	Figure-of-8 Velcro cuff support to humeral shaft	"Arm up"	Rehabilitative care
Unilateral shoulder orthosis	Bauerfeind Rolyan	Across body Elastic or spandex cuff support to humeral shaft	"Lift humerus up"	Rehabilitative care
Shoulder-saddle sling	Sammons	Saddle sits on top of shoulder	Maximal support of arm	To prevent "banging" of flaccid arm in active patients or during sports activities
		Strap across body		To provide support for the painful arm
		Forearm cuff—adjustable straps allow changes in elbow position		

ents who complain of "aching" in the arm at the end of the day like to use a support for a few hours a day.

If the arm dangles or bangs against the body during active periods, the *shoulder saddle sling* can be adjusted to protect the arm from bruising. This sling is also helpful to clients with severe shoulder-hand pain because it allows full support of the arm and can be adjusted by the client to allow the elbow to extend as the pain subsides. The *humeral cuff slings* are the least practical from a functional standpoint because they do not affect the scapula or trunk but are frequently used in acute and rehabilitation care.

Canes

Canes are given to clients with hemiplegia to provide "extra" balance, not as a means to support body weight. Canes should be used after upper-body control and lower extremity–initiated movements are practiced.

If quad canes or hemi-walkers are used before trunk and leg activity is minimally established, they encourage lateral translation of the spine or rotation of the spine and ribs. When clients shift off the weak leg onto this stable cane, the cane acts functionally as a third leg. This one-sided compensation encourages learned nonuse of the affected leg.

Single canes provide a balance assist. Often clients use their cane while walking outdoors or in crowded situations but not inside their homes. Reliance on a cane for walking eliminates the possibility of carrying objects and makes it difficult to perform one-handed tasks such as opening a door. Wrist loops allow the client to use the unaffected hand without losing the cane.

Orthotics

Ankle-foot orthoses (AFOs) are used to allow foot clearance during walking, to ensure heel strike, to provide distal stability for early standing and walking in clients with severe weakness, to provide lateral lower-leg stability in clients who need an assist to lateral hip weakness, and to control knee hyperextension caused by loss of ankle dorsiflexion control. Different design types provide different functions. Solid ankle bracing with plastic beyond the malleoli limits distal freedom but allows clients with severe weakness to practice gaining control of trunk and hip movements.

The use of polypropylene bracing to control foot posturing in adults began in the 1970s with information from pediatrics and podiatry. Foot control in a brace stops supination of the foot in swing and compensatory pronation of the foot in stance. This control is achieved through neutral rearfoot positioning and long medial and lateral foot counters. Techniques of Aquaplast fabrication have created new possibilities for inexpensive, immediate, remoldable bracing for the foot and ankle.[105]

Custom-made ankle foot orthoses provide the best fit and control, but an excellent prefabricated polypropylene brace is available through DobiSymplex, an orthotics company. Their orthoses have long medial and lateral foot edges for control of foot posturing, come in multiple models and sizes, and can be ordered with regular or long foot plates (DobiSymplex, a division of Seattle Limb System).

Clients should be encouraged to spend time standing or walking short distances without the brace, so that dependence is not established. Clients like to be able to walk to the bathroom at night without a brace. Orthopedic ankle and foot supports provide alternatives to plastic bracing. The Malleoloc ankle support controls rearfoot equinus and varus while allowing ankle and forefoot movement (Bauerfeind/AliMed). Clients with moderate supination posturing report a reassuring feeling of security with this support while walking short distances and during sports use. This support, a substitute for the Aircast and Ace support, is a good choice for sports activities such as golfing, bicycling, jumping, and running.

Functions and limitations of commonly used braces are found in Table 25–10.

Movable Surfaces

Movable surfaces such as gymnastic balls of varying sizes, large rolls, and castered adjustable stools are used as assistive devices to help clients increase trunk/extremity strength and control. To encourage trunk/leg activity, the client sits on the ball and moves it in small ranges to the limits of perceived balance. This is an activity that increases trunk and leg control but does not lead directly to improvements in standing or walking. Gymnastic balls provide symmetrical support to the rib cage when used in the hands and knees position and are used to stretch specific tight tissues. Routines of lifting the ball with either the arms or legs strengthen extremity movements in space.

When spasticity was considered the major impairment in hemiplegia, therapists often placed clients prone over balls to "inhibit" tone. This is an inappropriate technique considering advances in understanding of movement control and recovery.

Hand Splints

The practice of splinting the hemiplegic hand is controversial. Historically, the hand in clients with hemiplegia was splinted in a "resting" position. After the introduction of neurophysiological approaches, splinting became "inhibitory" in design.[38, 77, 92] Now, with the understanding

that spasticity is not the major problem, splinting the wrist and hand has undergone another change. A new splint designed in 1982 by Levit,[71] as a neutral functional splint, promotes functional retraining and hand use while minimizing secondary impairments. This splint, designed to hold the wrist and hand in a position of orthopedic neutral, decreases hypertonicity that occurs either from poor alignment or unbalanced muscle return. The splint promotes support of the wrist and hand to avoid the secondary impairments of muscle tightness, muscle shifting, and overstretching of weak wrist and finger muscles.

Therapists custom make the splints with the goals of supporting the wrist in neutral, preventing radial or ulnar deviation with long, high sides, and maintaining the palmar arches. The fingers are not incorporated into the splint but are left free to allow movement reeducation and practice.

The increased tone in finger flexors, previously labeled "spasticity," comes in part from incomplete return or weakness of finger muscle activity on a poorly aligned wrist. A position of wrist flexion results in a drop of the proximal row of carpals and a flattening of the palmar arches. If the wrist is supported in neutral and the arches are preserved, returning muscle activity is reeducated in functional patterns. Finger support in a splint should be used only when there is a serious deformity with a need to serially, systematically, and slowly lengthen tight tissues.

This functional type of splint is worn mainly during the day when arm posturing is greater and when support of critical joints allows beginning hand use. Hand posturing is less of a problem when the patient lies down because

---

T A B L E 2 5 – 1 0.   Ankle-Foot Orthoses (AFOs) Used in Clients with Hemiplegia from Stroke

Orthotic Design	Function	Limitations	Patient Types (Categories)
Solid ankle with foot control	Heel strike Distal stability Lateral hip stability Assists forward progression Assists knee control Stops foot posturing	No ankle mobility No toe break	Severe weakness in trunk and leg Need for distal stability
Modified solid ankle with foot control	Heel strike More distal mobility—less ankle control Stops foot posturing	Less knee control Less message of forward progression No control of knee	Increasing leg strength Increasing trunk/leg control
Posterior leaf spring	Toe clearance	No control of foot posturing	Good return of control in trunk and leg Need for minimal dorsiflexion assist
Articulated ankle	Free dorsiflexion Heel strike if plantar stop used	Limited control of foot posturing Bulky at ankle	Normal ankle range—if range is limited, the movement of brace is translated into foot Functional needs; climb hills, stairs, move to and from ground
Supramalleolar foot orthoses in Aquaplast	Foot control Assist heel strike Used for weaning from AFOs Used for weaning from AFOs Sports	No knee control Short shelf life of material	Increasing leg control Desire to begin increasing activity level
Foot orthoses	Balance small asymmetries of foot	No control of foot posturing No ankle or knee control	Persistent but minimal rearfoot/forefoot asymmetries
Klenzak metal, double-upright	Toe clearance Reminder of forward progression	No foot control Control of ankle and foot through shoe	Used before creation of polypropylene to provide heel strike and stop foot supination

See Chapter 32 for additional suggestions.

of decreased demands on the trunk and legs. Clients are instructed not to wear the splint at night.

Design Considerations. If joint range is limited, the therapist makes the splint to support available range. The splint can be revised as range increases. Alignment is corrected in three steps: (1) keeping the wrist in flexion, the lateral deviation is corrected by aligning the third metacarpal with the middle of the radius; (2) the carpal position is corrected (usually gently lifted up from a low position under the radius); and (3) the hand is moved to wrist neutral (see *Functional Movement Reeducation*[108] for a step-by-step analysis). The warmed, soft splinting plastic captures this corrected position as it cools. The length of palmar support is decided by the therapist after assessment of degree and distribution of muscle return and muscle tightness patterns. The thumb is supported at its base in a neutral position, not one of abduction. As beginning grip returns, the thumb hole is widened to allow function.

A variety of neutral functional splints have been designed. The neutral wrist/thumb hole splinting design is hard to keep on the hand of patients with severe weakness. They sometimes find ulnar or radial trough splints or wide opponens splints easier to keep on.

As wrist extension control against gravity emerges, the therapist can fabricate a wide opponens splint to maintain the palmar arches as the client begins practicing finger movements. The wide opponens splint supports the base of the hand and assists in maintaining carpal alignment. Patients can switch between the two splints as needed.

Clients with severe hand pain prefer a neutral wrist splint with a resting area for the thumb. This splint is fabricated with little or no correction initially but with gentle support for the wrist and palmar arches. As the pain decreases, this splint is modified to become the original neutral functional splint.

Although the move away from "inhibitory" splints and from night splinting to day-time functional splinting breaks many of the "rules" from the past, it is more compatible with concepts from research and clinical experts.

Recommended resources for practical solutions to one-handed functioning and devices that assist in independence are listed in Appendix 25–B at the end of this chapter.

PSYCHOSOCIAL ASPECTS AND ADJUSTMENTS

The suddenness of a stroke and the dramatic change in motor, sensory, visual, and perceptual performance and feedback may leave the person with hemiplegia confused, disoriented, angry, stressed, frustrated, and fearful. When a stroke occurs, time is not allowed for gradual adjustment to the resulting disability.

Psychosocial adjustments may be more detrimental than is any functional disability to long-term stroke survivors.[51] Decreased interest in social activity inside and outside the home and decreased interest in hobbies attributable to psychosocial disability hamper the hemiplegic person's return to a normal social life.[68] Feelings

of rejection and embarrassment may interfere with the hemiplegic person's interaction with people outside the home environment. Individuals with long-standing hemiplegia often become clinically depressed with symptoms of loss of sleep and appetite, self-blame, and a hopeless outlook. Suicide can result. The usual psychosocial adjustments to disability are compounded in persons with hemiplegia resulting from stroke by the issues associated with aging.

Family members and spouses may have difficulty assessing the capabilities of the hemiplegic person and may be overprotective. Overprotection among spouses may be a sign of affection and support or a sign of guilt.[61] Long-standing marriages do not tend to dissolve when one member experiences a stroke. However, previous marriage problems and personality traits may become exaggerated as a result of the presence of increased and changing demands and stresses that occur when the person returns home.

A comparison of occupational status of long-term stroke survivors in the United States and in Sweden reveals that 40% of the Swedes returned to a form of employment (including part-time work) but none of the United States group returned to work.[42] The scarcity of part-time work and a shorter treatment period dictated by third-party payers in the United States may account for this discrepancy.

Age is a general predictor for return to employment, and younger people are more attractive to employers. Barriers to return to work for the person with hemiplegia include speech, perceptual, and cognitive deficits along with a need for psychosocial support. Architectural barriers also can create severe problems for hemiplegic clients with regard to both work and recreational activities. Stroke clubs, usually organized through hospitals, the National Stroke Association, or the American Heart Association, provide educational, social, and recreational support for the hemiplegic person and his or her spouse.

The impact of psychosocial disability and the need for its long-term treatment is great. Programs need to be established and continued for years to allow clients and their families to deal with the many problems that result from the stroke.

Sexuality

The majority of persons with hemiplegia experience a decline in sexuality through a decrease in frequency of sexual intercourse without a change in the level of prestroke sexual desire.[44] On return home, the person with hemiplegia faces uncertainty about sexual skills and the risk of failure. Sexual dysfunction that results from a stroke depends on the amount of cerebral damage and includes a decreased ability to achieve erection and ejaculation in men and decreased lubrication in women.[45] The sensory, motor, visual, and emotional disturbances of hemiplegia may cause awkwardness, but these disturbances can be overcome through the education of the spouse in alternate positioning and ways to provide appropriate sensory experiences. The normal factors of aging also interfere with the sexual performance of persons with hemiplegia. A person's prestroke sexual activity is a good indicator of poststroke sexual activity. The closeness between partners achieved through satisfactory sexual relationship can add to the quality of life after stroke (see Chapter 7).

SUMMARY

This chapter reviews the neuropathology of stroke, the evaluation of impairments that interfere with functional movement patterns, and intervention planning. Both evaluation of outcomes and evaluation of movement components are described. The chapter highlights significant impairments and provides clinical observations on critical areas of intervention. A detailed process of clinical problem solving helps the therapist organize and prioritize impairments to plan intervention programs that retrain movement components and train desirable compensatory patterns to help the client gain the highest level of functional performance and independence in daily life.

CASE STUDY

A client with left hemiplegia presented 4 days after stroke on admission to a rehabilitation center. The classification of movement disorder was one of composite movement category/severe movement deficits.

Functional Limitation No. 1: Client is unable to perform morning self-care at bedside or sitting in wheelchair in front of a sink

Why? Client cannot perform anterior/posterior or lateral trunk movements in sitting without loss of balance and falling to left. Client cannot feel left arm, and it hangs by side.

Evaluation

Primary Impairments

Weakness in trunk
Weakness in left arm
Inability to initiate trunk movements
Weakness in left leg
Decreased sense of touch left arm, trunk, and leg

Secondary Impairments

Loss of trunk alignment in sitting (upper trunk flexion)
Left shoulder subluxation
Muscle tightness–pectorals, latissimus, wrist flexors
Loss of alignment of lower trunk and pelvis—left pelvis lists downward
Loss of 10 degrees of left ankle joint dorsiflexor range

Functional Limitation No. 2: Client is unable to transfer from bed to chair independently.

Why? Client cannot perform lower-body anterior weight shifts (stable upper body) to initiate transfer left. Upper body falls into flexion. Left arm hangs by side with an inferior shoulder subluxation. Left leg cannot move in sitting. Client sits up by pulling on edge of bed with right arm.

Primary Impairments

Weakness in upper trunk
Weakness in left leg and trunk/leg patterns
Inability to initiate lower-trunk patterns

Secondary Impairments

Loss of left upper-body alignment
Loss of left ankle joint dorsiflexion range
Tightness in left hamstrings and gastrocnemius

Functional Limitation No. 3: Client is unable to stand up from chair independently.

Why? Client is unable to control upper body over lower trunk during lower body–initiated transfers

Continued

CASE STUDY *Continued*

and sit to stand. Client is unable to use left leg for support and movement during the transition of sit to stand. Client is unable to keep weight (depress leg into floor) on left foot in standing.

Primary Impairments

Weakness in upper trunk
Weakness in leg and trunk/leg patterns
Inability to initiate lower-trunk patterns

Significant Impairments for Functions Evaluated

1. Loss of upper-body alignment during lower body–initiated movements, especially anterior/posterior plane
2. Shoulder subluxation contributes to loss of upper-body alignment
3. Loss of ankle joint dorsiflexion range
4. Loss of control and weakness of trunk and left arm and left leg

I. Functional Goals
   A. Transfer from chair to bed and back with contact guarding
   B. Perform morning self-care activities in wheelchair in bathroom independently
   C. Rise to standing with assistance of one person
II. Long-Term Goals
   A. Sit safely while performing tasks with right arm and leg around midline, that is, perform upper body– and lower body–initiated trunk movements in sitting independently
   B. Use left arm as a weight-bearing assist during movements of the right arm and leg in sitting and standing; that is, increase upper-body control to prepare for independent, safe, lower body–initiated movement patterns (extended-arm reach and sit to stand and standing balance)
   C. Transfer, rise to stand, and stand with minimal assistance to the upper body; that is, increase leg strength and control in trunk/leg patterns
   D. Establish a home program that the client performs independently
III. Short-Term Goals
   A. Perform basic trunk movement patterns in sitting with contact guarding
   B. Decrease trunk asymmetry; increase control in upper body to decrease shoulder subluxation
   C. Protect shoulder joint from excessive capsular stretch
   D. Be able to lift weak arm with unaffected arm, maintain sitting balance, and position arm for bathing

Secondary Impairments

Loss of left upper-body alignment
Loss of left ankle joint dorsiflexion range
Tightness in left hamstrings and gastrocnemius

   E. Increase ankle joint dorsiflexion range in standing
   F. Increase strength in leg and in trunk/leg–linked patterns during lower body–initiated transfers, during sit to stand, and in supported standing to allow assisted practice with moderate support to upper body (to maintain symmetry)
IV. Treatment Techniques
   A. Assisted trunk movements in sitting with assistance to correct alignment of upper body on lower body
   B. Independent practice of trunk movements (home program)
   C. Independent practice of trunk movements during forearm weight bearing in sitting (home program)
      1. Practice basic trunk movements
      2. Maintain arm range of motion; stretch tight muscles
   D. Independent practice of trunk/arm–linked movements
      1. In weight bearing—see earlier
      2. In space—modified cane exercises in patterns practiced in A.
   E. Standing, lower extremity–initiated movements with assistance to upper body
   F. Assisted practice of leg movements in space in sitting
   G. Standing lower extremity–initiated movements to increase length of tight gastrocnemius and hamstring muscles
      1. Forearm weight bearing in standing
      2. Standing against a wall
   H. Support arm on pillow in wheelchair, use shoulder-saddle support during transfers, sit to stand, and standing

REFERENCES

1. Adams HP, et al: Guidelines for the management of patients with acute ischemic stroke, Stroke Council American Heart Association. Circulation 90:1588, 1994.
2. Adams RD, Victor M: Principles of Neurology. New York, McGraw-Hill, 1981.
3. Adler MK, et al: Stroke rehabilitation: Is age a determinant? J Am Geriatr Soc 28:499, 1980.
4. Ashworth B: Carisoprodol in multiple sclerosis. Practitioner 192:540, 1964.
5. Bach-y-Rita P: Recovery of Functions: Theoretical Considerations for Brain Injury Rehabilitation. Baltimore, University Park Press, 1980.
6. Bamford J, et al: A prospective study of acute cerebrovascular disease in the community: The Oxfordshire Community Stroke Project 1981–1986. J Neurol Neurosurg Psychiatry 53:16, 1990.
7. Basmajian JV: Muscles Alive: Their Functions Revealed by Electromyography. Baltimore, Williams & Wilkins, 1978.
8. Berg KD, Maki BE, et al: Clinical and laboratory measures of postural balance in the elderly population. Arch Phys Med Rehabil 73:1073, 1992.
9. Berg KD, Wook-Dauphinee S, Williams J: The balance scale: Reliability assessment with elderly residents and patients with an acute stroke. Scand J Rehabil Med 27:27, 1995.
10. Bizzi E, Polit A: Characteristics of motor programs underlying movement in monkeys. J Neurophysiol 42:183, 1979.
11. Black SE, Norris JW, Hachinski VC: Post stroke seizures. Stroke 14:134, 1983.
12. Bobath B: Evaluation and Treatment. London, William Heinemann Medical Books, 1970.
13. Bobath B: Adult Hemiplegia: Evaluation and Treatment, 2nd ed. London, William Heinemann Medical Books, 1978.
14. Bobath B: Adult Hemiplegia: Evaluation and Treatment, 3rd ed. London, William Heinemann Medical Books, 1990.
15. Bohannon RW: Recovery and correlates of trunk muscle strength after stroke. Int J Rehabil Res 8:162, 1995.
16. Bohannon RW, et al: Shoulder pain in hemiplegia: A statistical relationship with five variables. Arch Phys Med Rehabil 67:514, 1986.
17. Bohannon RW, et al: Relationship between static muscle strength deficits and spasticity in stroke patients with hemiparesis. Phys Ther 67:1068, 1987.
18. Bohannon RW, Cassidy D, Walsh S: Trunk muscle strength is impaired multidirectionally after stroke. Clin Rehabil 9:47, 1995.
19. Bohannon RW, Smith MB: Assessment of strength deficits in eight paretic upper extremity muscle groups of stroke patients with hemiplegia. Phys Ther 67:552, 1987.
20. Bonita R: Epidemiology of stroke. Lancet 339:342, 1992.
21. Bourbonnais D, Vanden Noven S: Weakness in patients with hemiparesis. Am J Occup Ther 43:313, 1989.
22. Brandstater ME, Roth EJ, Siebens HC: Venous thromboembolism in stroke: Literature review and implication for clinical practice. Arch Phys Med Rehab 73(Suppl):379, 1992.
23. Brooks VB: Motor programs revisited. In Talbott RE, Humphrey DR (eds): Posture and Movement. New York, Raven Press. 1979.
24. Brunnstrom S: Movement Therapy in Hemiplegia. New York, Harper & Row, 1970.
25. Cailliet R: The Shoulder in Hemiplegia. Philadelphia, FA Davis, 1980.
26. Carr JH, Shepherd RB: A Motor Relearning Programme for Stroke, 2nd ed. Rockville, MD, Aspen Publishers, 1982.
27. Carr JH, Shepherd RB, Ada L: Spasticity: Research findings and implications for intervention. Physiotherapy 81:421, 1995.
28. Carr JH, Shepherd RB, Nordholm L, Lynne D: Investigation of a new motor assessment scale for stroke patients. Phys Ther 65:175, 1985.
29. Chan WY: Some techniques for the relief of spasticity and their physiological basis. Physiother Can 38:85, 1986.
30. Cinnamon J, et al: CT and MRI diagnosis of cerebrovascular disease: Going beyond the pixels. Semin CT MRI 16:212, 1995.
31. Collen FM, Wade DT, Robb GF, Bradshaw C: The Rivermead Mobility Index: A further development of the Rivermead Motor Assessment. Int Disabil Stud 13:50, 1991.
32. Cordo PJ, Nashner LM: Properties of postural adjustments associated with rapid arm movements. J Neurophysiol 47:287, 1982.
33. Das TK, Park D: Effect of treatment with botulinum toxin on spasticity. Postgrad Med J 65:208, 1989.
34. Davies PM: Steps to Follow: A Guide to the Treatment of Adult Hemiplegia. New York, Springer-Verlag, 1985.
35. Davies PM: Right in the Middle: Selective Trunk Activity in the Treatment of Adult Hemiplegia. New York, Springer-Verlag, 1990.
36. Duncan P, et al: Functional reach: A new clinical measure of balance. J Gerontol 45:192, 1990.
37. Easton JKM, et al: Intramuscular neurolysis for spasticity in children. Arch Phys Med Rehabil 50:155, 1979.
38. Farber S: Adaptive equipment. In Farber S (ed): Neurorehabilitation: A Multisensory Approach. Philadelpia, WB Saunders, 1981.
39. Feldman RD, Young RR, Koella WP (eds): Spasticity. Disordered Motor Control. Chicago, Year Book, 1980.
40. Fisher AG: Assessment of Motor and Process Skills. Fort Collins, CO, Three Star Press, 1995.
41. Fisher B: Effect of trunk control and alignment on limb function. J Head Trauma Rehabil 2:72, 1987.
42. Fugl-Meyer AR: Post-stroke hemiplegia—occupational status. Scand J Rehabil Med 7(Suppl):167, 1980.
43. Fugl-Meyer AR, Jaasko L, et al: The post-stroke hemiplegic patient: A method for evaluation of physical performance. Scand J Rehabil Med 7:13, 1975.
44. Fugl-Meyer AR, Jaasko L: Post-stroke hemiplegia and sexual intercourse. Scand J Rehabil Med 7(Suppl):158, 1980.
45. Garden FH, Smith BS: Sexual function after cerebrovascular accident. Curr Concepts Rehabil Med 5:2, 1990.
46. Gillian G: Upper extremity function and management. In Gillian G, Burkhardt A, et al (eds): Stroke Rehabilitation. St. Louis, CV Mosby, 1998.
47. Granger CV, Hamilton BB: The Uniform Data System for medical rehabilitation report of first admissions for 1990. Am J Phys Med Rehab 71:108, 1992.
48. Granit R: Comments. In Granit R (ed): Progress in Brain Research. Netherlands, North Holland Biomedical Press, 1979.
49. Granit R: Interpretation of supraspinal effects on the gamma system. In Granit R (ed): Progress in Brain Research. Netherlands, North Holland Biomedical Press, 1979.
50. Gresham GE, et al: Epidemiologic profile of long-term stroke disability: The Framingham study. Arch Phys Med Rehabil 60:487, 1979.
51. Gresham GE, et al: ADL status in stroke: Relative merits of three standard indexes. Arch Phys Med Rehabil 61:355, 1980.
52. Haas AL, et al: Respiratory function in hemiplegic patients. Arch Phys Med Rehabil 48:174, 1967.
53. Heller A, Wade DT, et al: Arm function after stroke: Measurement and recovery over the first three months. J Neurol Neurosurg Psychiatry 50:714, 1989.
54. Horak FB: Clinical measurement of postural control in adults. Phys Ther 67:1881, 1987.
55. Huskisson EC, Jones J, Scott PJ: Application of visual analogue scales to the measurement of functional capacity. Rheumatol Rehabil 15:185–187, 1976.
56. Jenson M: The hemiplegic shoulder. Scand J Rehabil Med 7(Suppl):113, 1980.
57. Jongbloed L: Prediction of function after stroke: A critical review. Stroke 17:765, 1986.
58. Kaira L, Dale P, Crome P: Improving stroke rehabilitation: A controlled study. Stroke 24:1462, 1994.
59. Kane LA, Buckley KA: Functional mobility. In Gillen G, Burkhardt A (eds): Stroke Rehabilitation. St. Louis, CV Mosby, 1998.
60. Keith RA, Granger CV, et al: The functional independence measure: A new tool for rehabilitation. In Eisenberg MG, Grzesiak RC (eds): Advances in Clinical Rehabilitation, vol 1. New York, Springer-Verlag, 1987.
61. Kinsella GJ, Duffy FD: Attitudes towards disability expressed by spouses of stroke patients. Scand J Rehabil Med 12:73, 1980.
62. Kistler JP, Ropper AH, Martin JB: Cerebrovascular disease. In Isselbacker KJ, et al (eds): Harrison's Principles of Internal Medicine. New York, McGraw-Hill, 1994.
63. Knott M, Voss DE: Proprioceptive neuromuscular facilitation. New York, Harper & Row, 1976.
64. Knutsson E: Gait control in hemiparesis. Scand J Rehabil Med 13:101, 1981.
65. Knutsson E, Richards C: Different types of disturbed motor control in gait of hemiparetic patients. Brain 102:405, 1979.

66. Kwakkel G, Kollen BJ, Wagenaar RC: Therapy impact on functional recovery in stroke rehabilitation. Physiotherapy 85:377, 1999.
67. Guide To Physical Therapist Practice. Phys Ther 77:1163, 1997.
68. Labi ML, et al: Psychosocial disability in physically restored long-term stroke survivors. Arch Phys Med Rehabil 61:561, 1980.
69. Landau WM: Spasticity: The fable of a neurological demon and the emperor's new therapy. Arch Neurol 31:217, 1974.
70. Lankford LL: Reflex sympathetic dystrophy. In Hunter JM, et al (eds): Rehabilitation of the Hand, 3rd ed. St. Louis, CV Mosby, 1990.
71. Levit K: Treating the hemiplegic hand. Lecture notes, Arizona State OT Conference, Phoenix, 1992.
72. Levit K: History of shoulder slings. Lecture notes, Advanced NDTA Upper Extremity Course, Alexandria, VA, 1992.
73. Levit K: Shoulder dysfunction. Presented at the 3rd Annual Magee Stroke Conference, Philadelphia, 1992.
74. Levit K: Trunk control during functional performance. Presented at the American Occupational Therapy Association Annual Conference, Baltimore, 1997.
75. Levy DE, et al: Prognosis in nontraumatic coma. Ann Intern Med 94:293, 1981.
76. Lowland C, et al: Agents and antagonist activity during voluntary upper-limb movement in patients with stroke. Phys Ther 72:624, 1992.
77. MacKinnon F, et al: The MacKinnon splint: A functional hand splint. Can J Occup Ther 42:157, 1975.
78. Mahoney F, Barthel DW: Functional evaluation: The Barthel Index. MD State Med J 14:61, 1965.
79. Malkmus D: Levels of cognitive functioning. Los Angeles, Ranchos Los Amigos Hospital, Inc., 1977.
80. Marshall J: The Management of Cerebrovascular Disease, 3rd ed. Oxford, Blackwell Scientific Publications, 1976.
81. Mathiowetz V, Bass Haugen J: Motor behavior research: Implications for therapeutic approaches to central nervous system dysfunction. Am J Occup Ther 48:733, 1994.
82. Melzack R: The McGill Pain Questionnaire: Major properties and scoring methods. Pain 1:277, 1975.
83. Mion LC, et al: Falls in the rehabilitation setting: Incidence and characteristics. Rehab Nurs 14:17, 1989.
84. Mohr JD: Management of the trunk in adult hemiplegia. Topics in Neurology. American Physical Therapy Association, 1990.
85. Mohr JP, et al: Hemiparesis profiles in acute stroke. Ann Neurol 12:156, 1984.
86. Moodie NB, Brisbin J, Morgan AM: Subluxation of the glenohumeral joint in hemiplegia: Evaluation of supportive devices. Physiother Can 38:151, 1986.
87. Nagi SZ: Some conceptual issues in disability and rehabilitation. In Sussman MB (ed): Sociology and Rehabilitation. Washington, DC, American Sociological Association, 1985.
88. Nashner LM: Adaptation of human movement to altered environments. Trends Neurosci 5:358, 1982.
89. National Stroke Association: Information Bulletin. Denver, CO, NSA Publications, 1999.
90. Nelson AJ: Functional ambulation profile. Phys Ther 54:1059, 1974.
91. Nelson AJ: Personal communication, November 1981.
92. Neuhaus B, et al: A survey of rationales for and against hand splinting in hemiplegia. Am J Occup Ther 35:83, 1981.
93. Odeen I: Reduction of muscular hypertonus by long-term muscle stretch. Scand J Rehabil Med 13:93, 1981.
94. Ostfeld A: A review of stroke epidemiology. Epidemiol Rev 2:136, 1980.
95. Penn RD, Savoy SM, Corcos D, et al: Intrathecal baclofen for severe spasticity. N Engl J Med 320:1517, 1989.
96. Perry J: The mechanics of walking. Phys Ther 47:778, 1967.
97. Perry J: Clinical gait analyzer. Bull Prosthet Res, Fall 1974, p 188.
98. Petrillo CR, et al: Phenol block of the tibial nerve in the hemiplegic patient. Orthopedics 3:871, 1980.
99. Plum F, Caronna JJ: Can one predict outcome of medical coma? In Outcome of Severe Damage to the Central Nervous System, Ciba Foundation Symposium 34. Amsterdam, Ciba Foundation, 1975.
100. Poplinger AR, Pillar T: Hip fracture in stroke patients: Epidemiology and rehabilitation. Acta Orthop Scand 56:226, 1985.
101. Roth EJ, Harvey RL: Rehabilitation of stroke syndromes. In Brad-

dom RL (ed): Physical Medicine and Rehabilitation. Philadelphia, WB Saunders, 1996.
102. Roy CW, Sands MR, Hill LD: Shoulder pain in acutely admitted hemiplegics. Clin Rehabil 8:334, 1994.
103. Ryerson S: Development of Abnormal Patterns in Adult Hemiplegia. Lecture, Barbro Salek Memorial Symposium, Newark, NJ, 1984.
104. Ryerson S: Postural control: From movement to function. Presented at the NDTA Annual Conference, San Diego, 1989.
105. Ryerson S: Neurological and biomechanical considerations in lower extremity bracing in adults with CNS dysfunction. Presented at the APTA Annual Conference, Denver, 1992.
106. Ryerson S: The foot in hemiplegia. In Hunt GC, McPoil TG (eds): The Foot and the Ankle in Physical Therapy, 2nd ed. New York, Churchill Livingstone, 1995.
107. Ryerson S, Levit K: Glenohumeral joint subluxations in CNS dysfunction. NDTA Newsletter, November 1988.
108. Ryerson S, Levit K: Functional Movement Reeducation: A Contemporary Model for Stroke Rehabilitation. New York, Churchill Livingstone, 1997.
109. Ryerson S, Levit K: The shoulder in hemiplegia. In Donatelli R (ed): The Shoulder in Physical Therapy, 3rd ed. New York, Churchill Livingstone, 1997.
110. Sahrmann S, Norton BJ: The relationship of voluntary movement to spasticity in the upper motor neuron syndrome. Ann Neurol 2:460, 1977.
111. Schenkman M, Butler RB: A model for multisystem evaluation, interpretation and treatment of individuals with neurologic dysfunction. Phys Ther 69:538, 1989.
112. Schenkman M: Lecture notes: Recent developments in motor control and their relevance to intervention techniques in adults with CNS dysfunction, NDTA Certification Course in Adult Hemiplegia, Alexandria, VA, 1990.
113. Schenkman M, et al: Whole-body movements during rising to stand from sitting. Phys Ther 70:638, 1990.
114. Scholtz J: NDTA Adult Hemiplegia Course Manual. Hartford, CT, NDTA, 1982.
115. Sheets PK, Sahrmann SA, Norton BJ: Diagnosis for physical therapy for patients with neuromuscular conditions. Neurol Rep 23:158, 1999.
116. Shumway-Cook A, Woollacott M: The growth of stability: Postural control from a developmental perspective. J Motor Behav 17:1985.
117. Shumway-Cook A, Woollacott M: Motor Control: Theory and Practical Applications. Baltimore, Williams & Wilkins, 1995.
118. Simmoons ML, et al: Individual risk assessment for intracranial hemorrhage during thrombolytic therapy. Lancet 342:1523, 1993.
119. Skillbeck CE, Wade DT, Hewer RL, Wood VA: Recovery after stroke. J Neurol Neurosurg Psychiatry 46:5, 1983.
120. Smidt G: Rudiments of gait. In Smidt GL (ed): Gait in Rehabilitation. New York, Churchill Livingstone, 1990.
121. Smith RO, Okamoto G: Checklist for the prescription of slings for the hemiplegia patient. Am J Occup Ther 35:91, 1981.
122. Snow B, et al: Treatment of spasticity with botulinum toxin: A double-blind study. Ann Neurol 28:512, 1990.
123. Taub E: Motor behavior following deafferenation in the motorically mature and developing monkey. In Rerman RM, et al (eds): Advances in Behavioral Biology. New York, Plenum, 1976.
124. Taub E, et al: Technique to improve chronic motor deficit after stroke. Arch Phys Med Rehabil 74:347, 1993.
125. Teasdale G, Jennett B: Assessment of coma and impaired consciousness: A practical scale. Lancet 2:81, 1974.
126. VanSant A: Life span development in functional tasks. Phys Ther 70:788, 1990.
127. Wardlaw JM, Warlow CP: Thrombolysis in acute ischemic stroke: Does it work? Stroke 23:1826, 1992.
128. Weinfeld D (ed): The national survey of stroke. Stroke 12(Suppl 1):2, 1981.
129. Weinstein CJ, et al: Balance training in hemiparetics. Arch Phys Med Rehabil 70:755, 1989.
130. Wiebe-Velasquez S, Blume WT: Seizures. Phys Med Rehab State Art Rev 7:73, 1993.
131. Winter D: Biomechanical and Motor Control Factors in Gait. Toronto, Waterloo Press, 1989.
132. Wolf SL, et al: Forced use of hemiplegic upper extremities to reverse the effect of learned nonuse among chronic stroke and head injured patients. Exp Neurol 104:125, 1989.

133. Woollacott MH, Bonnet M, Yabe K: Preparatory process for anticipatory postural adjustments: Modulation of leg muscles reflex pathways during preparation for arm movements in standing man. Exp
Brain Res 55:263, 1984.

134. World Health Organization: International classification of impairments disabilities, and handicaps: A manual of classification relating the consequences of disease. Geneva, World Health Organization, 1980.

Audiovisual and Literary Resources

FILMS AND VIDEOTAPES

Inner World of Aphasia—35-minute film
    American Journal of Nursing Film Library
    267 W. 25th Street
    New York, NY 10001

Candidate for Stroke—35-minute film
    American Heart Association

I Had a Stroke—35-minute film
    Filmmakers Library, Inc.
    290 West End Avenue
    New York, NY 10023

Living with Stroke
    Rehabilitation Research and Training Center
    The George Washington University
    2300 I Street, NW, Suite 714
    Washington, DC 20037

Evaluation of the Hemiplegic Patient (Sensory/Motor)
    Audio-Visual Department
    School of Allied Health
    University of Maryland
    32 Greene Street
    Baltimore, MD 21201

BOOKS
Children

First One Foot, Then the Other, by Tomie de Paola. This book explores the feelings and fears of children about a relative who has had a stroke.

Adult

How to Conquer the World with One Hand . . . and an Attitude, by Paul E. Berger. Merrifield, VA, Positive Power Publisher, 1999.

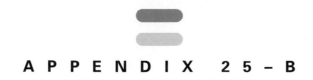

APPENDIX 2 5 – B

Resources for One-Handed Adaptations

One-Handed in a Two-Handed World
Tommye K. Mayer
Prince-Gallison Press
P.O. Box 23
Boston, MA 02113

Adaptive Resources: A Guide to Products and Services
National Stroke Association
8480 East Orchard Road
Englewood, CO 80111

A P P E N D I X   2 5 – C

Product Manufacturers

DobiSymplex—Sea Fab
9561 Satellite Blvd.
Orlando, FL 32837

AliMed
P.O. Box 9135
Dedham, MA 32703

DePuy Orthotech
700 Orthopedic Drive
Warsaw, IN 46581-0988

Smith and Nephew, Rolyan
One Quality Drive
Germantown, WI 53022-8205

Sammons Preston
P.O. Box 5071
Bolingbrook, IL 60440

Brain Function, Aging, and Dementia

OSA JACKSON, PhD, PT

Key Words

- aging
- Alzheimer's disease
- caregiver training and support
- dementia
- function
- physical therapy assessment and treatment
- problem solving
- rehabilitation
- therapeutic environment

Objectives

After reading this chapter the student/therapist will:

1. Define the basic terminology and discuss the prevalence of cognitive disturbances seen in older persons.

2. Describe normative changes in brain function with normal aging and their relevance to diagnosis of delirium and dementias.

3. Discuss how symptoms are altered with normal aging (i.e., specifically related to Arndt-Schultz principle, law of initial values, habitual biorhythms for an individual).

4. Describe normal sensory changes with aging and how they alter a person's overall ability to adapt to stress.

5. Describe how, and for what type of patient, to use the Mini-Mental State Examination as a part of the physical therapy assessment.

6. Describe common sensory changes with dementia and implications for adapting physical therapy evaluation and treatment.

7. Discuss common changes in learning styles with aging and implications for adapting physical therapy intervention so as to enhance patients' ability to perform at their highest functional level.

8. Describe how the environmental design and ergonomics can enhance patient performance in activities of daily living and instrumental activities of daily living.

9. Describe strategy to evaluate patient's emotional capacity to participate in a learning task and its clinical relevance to physical therapy.

10. Describe criteria for delirium and reversible dementia and sample strategies for modifying physical therapy evaluation and treatment procedures.

11. Discuss symptomatology and disease progression in irreversible dementia.

12. Discuss the therapist's role on the treatment team in educating key caregiver(s) and support personnel and sample training strategies.

13. Discuss treatment skills that are helpful in working with persons who have irreversible dementia.

14. Describe research activities and new findings that affect physical evaluation and treatment of the patient with dementia or delirium.

PARADIGM FOR AGING, HEALTH, YOUR BRAIN, AND YOU

Life is learning. This means that whatever goes on with us while we are alive is linked to our learning experiences and the decisions that are made by each of us based on those experiences. The brain and human nervous system have at least 3×10^{10} parts. "This is large enough for its balanced functions to obey the law of large systems. The health of such a system can be measured by the shock (stimuli) it can take without compromising the continuation of its processes."[32] Adaptability and health can be measured by the amount of stimuli or shock people can tolerate without their usual way of life being compromised. Aging is a process that requires ongoing adaptation to and compensation for the alterations that are imposed on us from the world around us and the internal physiological changes that occur with the passage of time, related to fitness, emotional state, fatigue, and the rest-activity cycle. If a person's health is altered by illness or trauma, then that person goes through an adaptive process. If too many changes happen too quickly, the brain is not able to create a functional adaptive response and the individual must alter or simplify his or her life processes or face negative mental or physiological reactions. Stress, depression, and cognitive disturbances are examples of extreme changes that occur when adaptability is wanting.

Human beings progress to adulthood through the millions of perceptions and decisions that are recorded and responded to through the developmental years. We as human beings are not born with our brain and our nervous system having the skills of an adult. As a baby our brain begins to learn during interactions with our environment. It is the kinesthetic and sensory connections that provide the data about our internal and external environments. Through this interactive learning process each human being (with a nondifferentiated nervous system) discovers new differentiations and thus new strategies for relating to the world. Differentiation for human beings does not happen uniformly. As people age, the result of this lack of uniformity is that some adults prefer to relate to the world visually, others aurally, and still others, tactilely or kinesthetically.

The adult phase of brain and central nervous system development will, for most people, involve a gradual narrowing of the focus in the development of new skills, as well as increased repetition of certain activities. The tendency is to have activity narrow more and more to the activities in which we excel or with which we feel comfortable. Intuitive or practical people continue to pursue self-knowledge and explore ways to maximize their talents. By accident or through mentoring, these people discover that lifelong learning is the gift of life itself. Ongoing and ever-increasing self-awareness allows for enhanced adaptability at any age. What if rehabilitation after illness or trauma invited a guided examination of self-awareness and habitual strategies as the basis for inventing new functional adaptive strategies? In this chapter the paradigm for aging, health, and lifelong learning presumes that:

1. The brain and central nervous system are accepted as the master system and the controller of the other human systems (e.g., digestive, cardiovascular).
2. There is a capacity for ongoing learning (self-awareness), self-regulation, and adaptability.
3. The whole (the human being) is greater than the sum of its parts.
4. Language invents our reality and our experience of life.
5. Enjoying and pacing new learning become important skills for lifelong well-being.
6. The mind and body are not separate.
7. Personal variations in learning style, preferences for relating, and so on can be utilized to maximize adaptation throughout life.
8. The activation of the limbic system for fight or flight is normal and when the crisis (real or imagined) is over, the ability to release the limbic activation and find the resting state becomes an important skill in adulthood.
9. Creation of environments that encourage safe explorations of new ideas and ways of self-expression can generate lifelong human growth and development.

The intention of clinical intervention is to provide a process for functional problem solving, therapy, or training to:

1. Create a sense of being safe, heard, understood, respected, and nurtured by the people and the environment where the patient resides (temporarily or permanently).
2. Develop functional skills to enhance the quality of life, as defined by each patient.
3. Support opportunities for self-expression and sharing that leave the individual touched, moved, and inspired.
4. Maximize the functional abilities for daily living.
5. Create a sense of community and belonging that is comfortable for each person.

FRAMEWORK FOR CLINICAL PROBLEM SOLVING

The therapist can teach, solve problems, and adapt movement and activities related to special self-care and recreation needs that are the result of impairments caused by cognitive deficits. The clinician can help the patient with cognitive deficits who may need to learn or relearn basic functional skills. In addition, therapy can be adapted to compensate for the cognitive impairments of each patient. The therapist working with patients with cognitive impairments needs to have had adequate advanced training in assessment of communication skills and neurological functioning as well as gerontology, so that he or she can work with maximal efficiency and also enjoy clinical interactions with each patient.

In 37 BC the Roman poet Virgil wrote: "Age carries all things, even the mind, away."[24] Nearly 400 years ago, Shakespeare described the last stage of human life as ". . . second childishness and mere oblivion, sans teeth, sans eyes, sans taste, sans everything."[95] This pessimistic view of the fate of the elderly persists among health care workers today[110] despite the fact that significant cognitive deficits affect only between 6.1% and 12.3% of the elderly in the United States.[37]

The clinician should not assume that an older person has impaired cognitive functioning. Perhaps the most crucial concept for clinical problem solving is that the clinician must not accept at face value what she or he sees. When a patient is observed to have altered brain function, it is necessary to describe the extent and type of the distortion of intellectual capacity and to determine the cause(s) to enable provision of appropriate and effective treatment and care.

When age or illness or medications create a temporary or permanent change in cognitive abilities, all functional training requires alteration to meet the unique cognitive abilities of the patient at the moment. Here is an example:

The therapist walked slowly into the room and greeted the patient by touching her softly on the cheek with the back of her hand. The patient looked up and smiled. The therapist smiled back and stroked the patient softly on the top of her head. The patient smiled again. The therapist kneeled down so that she was eye to eye with the lady sitting in the wheelchair. She took the patient's hand in her own hand and with her other hand slowly stroked the back of the patient's hand. The patient smiled again. The physical therapy session had begun. For this patient words were actually confusing so they were avoided.

Communication for every patient is a unique process, and for persons with cognitive disturbance, including Alzheimer's disease, the physical therapist has a unique role. Physical therapy provides the assessment, treatment, and training for others who interact with the patient on what cues (tactile, pace, proximity, eye contact, timing, visual tracking, position, temperature, etc.) can provide the desired functional participation and maximize the quality of life. All the traditional physical therapy treatment must be funneled through the fog of confusion so that the treatment does not cause emotional distress. There is the rule, "above all do no harm." The confused or disoriented patient requires ongoing assessment and problem solving

to maximize functional participation in daily life. The goal of all contact with the patient by all persons, especially physical and occupational therapists, is to eliminate fear and create a sense of peace, safety, and belonging. The favorite meditation or prayer of one patient was, "I have the power to choose and I choose love." When this was repeated slowly with the patient, from 10 to 30 times while holding her hand (authentically enjoying her company), she would allow anyone to leave her room while continuing to chant and eventually falling asleep. The goal of creating contentment and peace of mind was achieved.

Definition of Terms

There are three major categories of intellectual impairment: (1) mental retardation, (2) delirium, and (3) dementia. A definition of terms is necessary to ensure that all personnel use the same framework for clinical problem solving.

1. *Mental retardation.* A person with mental retardation (also called developmental disability) has had some degree of intellectual impairment all her or his life. A person with mental retardation also can develop delirium or dementia. Delirium or dementia differs from mental retardation in that there has been a change from the baseline level of functioning for that person.
2. *Delirium.* A person with delirium usually shows a change both in intellectual function and in level of consciousness.[68] The patient may be perplexed, disoriented, fearful, or forgetful, or all of these. The patient is often less alert than normal and may be sleepy or obtunded; however, many patients with delirium are hyperalert and may be extremely agitated and suspicious. Delirium frequently occurs in the presence of a concurrent dementia. Early identification of the symptoms and formal medical assessment and treatment are critical to ensure the return of a normal level of alertness and of intellectual function and to prevent the development of secondary functional impairments and possible dementia.[69]
3. *Dementia.* Dementia is an impairment in some or all aspects of intellectual functioning in a person who is fully alert. Some diseases that can cause dementia are treatable, and if treated early and aggressively, the patient's deterioration of intellectual function may be either reversed or prevented from worsening. Dementia usually involves cognitive impairment affecting memory and orientation and at least one of the following:

    Abstract thinking. This is a common loss and involves inability to relate to anything other than tangible reality. In dementia or Alzheimer's disease, this skill is predictably missing in most cases.
    Judgment and problem solving. This capacity decreases in early stage 1 of Alzheimer's disease and is missing by the completion of stage 1.
    Language. Language use for communication becomes altered in stage 2 of Alzheimer's disease

and by stage 3 very little verbal or no verbal communication is possible.

Personality. All the decisions that you ever made, whether you remember that you made them or not, constitute your personality. We human beings live through these decisions, they become filters for all future life experiences, and we believe that they are the truth. As caregivers and therapists, it is critical for us to be aware of how the world is perceived by the patient. It is important that the staff respect patients and their beliefs and work to minimize confrontation and agitation. We may not always like the personality of patients or their beliefs, prejudices, and biases, but the question of therapy still needs to be addressed.

Alzheimer's disease. Alzheimer's disease is not synonymous with dementia but rather one of the many causes of dementia. The term should be used only as a diagnosis when a complete clinical evaluation has been performed, a diagnosis of dementia has been made, and all other possible causes of the dementia have been ruled out. It is not possible to definitely ascertain whether a patient has this disease until an autopsy or brain biopsy has been performed. Although multiple putative causes of the disease have been proposed, the etiology and pathogenesis are unknown. Currently there is no curative treatment for Alzheimer's disease. Some drugs are available that appear to slow the process of cognitive deterioration in some patients, and patients and their families can be helped through rehabilitation to cope better with the vicissitudes of the disease (see Chapters 6 and 32).

Depression can mimic dementia.

Epidemiology

It is estimated that today more than 1 million Americans with a dementia live in nursing homes. An additional 1.5 to 2.5 million people with severe dementia are estimated to live at home, although they require continual care. An estimated 5 million persons live at home who suffer from mild or moderate dementia and who require partial care and supervision.[80, 114] It is expected that disorders causing cognitive deficits will continue to be a growing public health problem for at least the next 50 years. The projected statistics, assuming there are no cures or effective means of preventing the common causes of dementia, are that by the year 2040 there will be five times as many cases of dementia (7.4 million Americans) as today. This increase is partially the result of the increased life expectancy of Americans.[48] (The most rapid population growth in this country is in the oldest age group, and thus the increase in the prevalence of severe dementia. The prevalence of dementia rises from approximately 3% at ages 65 to 74 years, to 18.7% at ages 75 to 84 years, to 47% over age 85 years.[30]) The increasing number of persons over age 85 years will be paralleled by an increase in the incidence of dementia.

More than 70 conditions are known to cause dementia.[56] Secondary behavioral problems in the patient with dementia can be interpreted as a response to somatic, psychological, or existential stress.[106, 109] Because memory impairments, impairments of abstract thinking or judgment, or global cognitive impairments in an elderly person may be a symptom of acute physical illness,[1] the patient's physical, emotional, social, and cognitive status and physical and affective environment need to be evaluated systematically.

Gradual or sudden changes in intellectual capacity or memory function are not a normal part of the aging process. Any change, whether it develops slowly over time or happens suddenly, should be diagnosed and, where possible, the underlying cause(s) of the delirium or dementia should be treated. Even if the cause of the dementia is untreatable, it is always possible to teach the patient and significant others strategies to make the patient's activities of daily living (ADL), instrumental activities of daily living (IADL), and the effects of the cognitive deficits easier to manage.

Physical and occupational therapists are important in the comprehensive evaluation, treatment, and ongoing care of the patient with delirium or dementia. It is critical that all treatment planning occur as a part of a team effort, in which the patient, the family or significant others, the physician, nurses, social worker, physical therapist, and occupational therapist collaborate so that a consistent treatment plan and orientation are followed.

PHYSIOLOGY OF AGING: RELEVANCE FOR SYMPTOMATOLOGY AND DIAGNOSIS OF DELIRIUM AND DEMENTIAS

The Normal Brain

The brain of a normal person at age 80 years shows several significant anatomical, physiological, and neurochemical changes when compared with the brain of a younger person. It has been noted that there is a decrease in brain weight with advancing age. For example, the mean brain weight for women age 21 to 40 years is 1,260 g, whereas for women over age 80, it is 1,061 g.[85] Brody and Vijayashankar[17] have noted that although the brain loses thousands of cells daily, the areas of the brain involved in language, memory, and cognition are relatively spared of significant loss of neurons. In experimental settings, these changes are manifested by:

- Disturbance in ability to register, retain, and recall certain recent experiences
- Slowed rate of learning new material
- Slowed motor performance on tasks that require speed
- Difficulties with fine motor coordination and balance[23, 113, 115]

However, a normal, motivated elderly person who is not experiencing emotional stress will not only show few negative changes in intellectual capacity, but may actually demonstrate increase in intellectual functioning over time.[50, 67, 91, 94, 95]

Because many of the variables that need to be considered as part of the clinical evaluation of the rehabilitation potential of the person with dementia are affected by both aging and disease, it is important for therapists working with the aged patient to be aware of these variables. The therapist will explore ways to compensate for these changes, and the patient will have a greater possibility of achieving his or her potential for self-care and a meaningful existence.

A slowing of the natural pace of movement is commonly noted in people over age 80. This slowdown is manifested in the brain as a slowing of resting electroencephalogram (EEG) rhythms. At age 60, the mean frequency of the occipital rhythm is 10.3 Hz; at age 80, the mean frequency is 8.7 Hz. The average change in EEG frequency is about 1 cps per decade during these years.[118] The speed of nerve conduction in the elderly can be 10% to 15% slower than in younger persons.[11] *Because of these physiological changes, if the process and structure of evaluation and care of the healthy older person emphasize speed of execution or timed activities, the aged will appear less capable than they really are.* The therapist may need more time when working with persons over the age of 70 than is generally required with the younger adult.

The function of a normal brain requires a delicate synchronization of a large number of variables. To make normal intellectual function possible, the brain must have the following:

- No genetic defects
- A constant supply of nutrients, neurotransmitters, and other neurochemicals
- An unfailing supply of oxygen (implying appropriate blood count, collateral circulation, normal respiratory exchange, and adequate cardiac output)
- Normal blood biochemistry, especially fluid and electrolytes
- Normal hepatic and renal function
- Freedom from noxious stimuli such as trauma, infection, or toxins (including medications)
- Optimal levels of sensory stimulation and of emotional balance
- Optimal levels of intellectual stimulation

The brain is the most physiologically active organ in the body. The brain represents only 2% of the total body weight, and yet it consumes up to 20% of the oxygen and 65% of the glucose available in the circulation in the entire body.[24] The minimum cardiovascular output required to deliver this is 0.75 L/min, which is equal to 20% of the total circulation. Because of the high level of nutrient utilization by the brain, it is one of the organs of the body most likely to be affected by any acute change in homeostasis. The homeostasis of the elderly brain is more vulnerable to disruption because of the normal age-related changes already discussed, as well as the increased permeability of the blood-brain barrier and increased sensitivity of neurons to the effects of outside agents such as drugs.

Arndt-Schultz Principle

The Arndt-Schultz principle summarizes the differences between the younger and the aged brain's ability to respond to stimuli.[66]

1. The elderly require a higher level or a longer period of stimulation before the threshold for initial physiological response is reached.
2. The physiological response in the aged is rarely as large, as visible, or as consistent as noted in younger age groups.
3. The only similarity between the response of the young and the elderly to stimuli is that once the threshold is reached, the more stimuli that are provided, the greater the response.
4. On average, the range of safe therapeutic stimulation is narrower for the elderly than for the young.

The implication of the Arndt-Schultz principle for clinical problem solving is that the level of a stimulus (e.g., heat, cold, sound, light, or emotional input) needs to be adjusted to compensate for the altered physiology of the aging patient. It is possible that a level of stimulus that is therapeutic for the young may not be for the older patient because it does not reach the threshold for generating a physiological response or it goes beyond the safe therapeutic range for the older adult and becomes harmful. Therefore, when an elderly patient does not respond to treatment or presents with an unusual physical response, the clinician must ascertain whether the strength of the stimulus is too strong or too weak, and if modification of the stimulus is necessary because of factors associated with the aging process or the patient's cognitive deficits.

Law of Initial Values

The law of initial values is both a physiological and a psychological principle that states that, with a given intensity of stimulation, the degree of change produced tends to be greater when the initial value of that variable is low. In other words, the higher the initial level of functioning, the smaller the change that can be produced.[119-121] The law of initial values, when defined and applied to younger persons, presumes that homeostasis is a stable and consistent process. When the law is used to describe physiological and psychological responses in older persons, it cannot be presumed that homeostasis for any variable is predictable or consistent from one person to the next or within a 24-hour day for the same individual. In the young, it is possible to define the average times of peak activity for most physiological processes as well as for intellectual capacity. In the clinical assessment of the aged, it is necessary to define the peak times of day for awareness and intellectual capacity for each individual. For example, some patients are best able to participate in learning a new skill in the early morning and some only in the late afternoon.

Biorhythms

The body has a biological clock that controls all physiological functions in a precise temporal course, whether it be daily (e.g., secretion of some hormones), monthly (e.g., menstruation), or during a certain period of the life cycle (e.g., ability to become pregnant). Before evaluating a geriatric patient who presents with dementia or disturbance of intellectual functioning, it is helpful to examine the patient's premorbid biorhythm. The patient assessment must allow for and examine the current and past variability of individual biorhythms. It is essential to acknowledge and clearly document these biorhythms, and then maintain and reinforce their stability as much as possible. For example, if a woman has worked for 40 years as a night nurse, being primarily active from 11 AM to 7 PM, she will most likely be alert and best able to participate in a rehabilitation program during those hours. In most cases, it is possible to let the patient choose the best time for treatment. For those patients whose dementia is too severe to make this determination, the staff, by monitoring the patient's behavior, can choose a time for treatment when the client is most alert. For the elderly, and particularly for those who have dementia, the time of assessment and treatment must be documented and taken into account to maximize the client's rehabilitation potential.[53]

Sensory Changes with Aging

Aging can also be defined in terms of adaptation. Aging is the progressive and usually irreversible diminution, with the passage of time, of the ability of an organism or one of its parts to perform efficiently or to adapt to changes in its environment. The consequence of the process is manifested as decreased capacity for function and for withstanding stresses.[35] As the rehabilitation evaluation identifies functional problems, it is necessary to examine the possibility that sensory losses or disturbances (e.g., vision, hearing, touch, taste, smell, proprioception, temperature, and kinesthesia) are contributing to the functional impairments.[66] A partial or total loss of one or more of the normative sensory inputs can result in disturbance of an individual's mental status.

The more sudden the loss of a sensory function, the more difficult the adaptation to the sensory disability. This is especially true for elderly persons. Normally, adaptation to a sensory loss in one function is accomplished through an increased sensitivity of the other senses. For example, a young blind patient can adapt by using hearing and kinesthesia and usually learns to function well in spite of the loss of visual input. The older the patient is when blinded, however, the more difficulty she or he will have in making this adaptive crossover to other senses. At some time in any person's life, adaptive crossover from one sense to another becomes exceedingly difficult, if not impossible, and psychopathological or behavioral changes may occur if a sensory impairment develops.[58] This situation becomes more likely if the disruption of neurosensory input occurs in several senses and abruptly.

The poliomyelitis epidemics of the early 1950s demonstrated the relationship between sensory input and abnormal behavior. Patients with poliomyelitis who were placed in tank-type respirators developed intermittent disruptions in mental state, including hallucinations, delusions, and dreamlike experiences while awake.[35] The patients were deprived of normative input to the senses (kinesthesia and proprioception) and had severely restricted vision and hearing because of the nature of the construction of, and the noise that emanated from, the respirator. Called the sensory deprivation psychosis by Solomon,[107] this clin-

ical situation may include cognitive changes in addition to psychotic symptoms.

Sensory changes associated with normal aging can lead to the same degree of loss or distortion of significant sensory input as described earlier.[34, 63] A bilateral loss of vision may lead to agitation and disorientation. Elderly people with hearing impairments often have grave difficulty relating to the world. It is common for elderly persons who become deaf to experience some episodes of paranoid behavior.[58] The problems for hearing-impaired elderly persons are often exacerbated by health care professionals who do not know how to place a hearing aid in a patient's ear, replace a battery, adjust the volume on the aid, remove excess cerumen from the aid, or recognize a malfunctioning aid. Finally, sensory impairments may become exacerbated by surgical or medical interventions.

Certain medications, as well as some diseases, also can distort kinesthesia or retard the activity and movement of the patient. Movement is significant in the maintenance of an efficient nervous system. Anything that denies a person the ability to perform physical movement (e.g., drugs, restraints, or architectural designs not adapted to the aged) hastens and increases the difficulty of adapting to functional limitations. Movement is necessary for accurate sensation.[31, 34] Psychophysicists have demonstrated that if movement of the eyes does not occur properly, vision becomes ineffective. The same is true to a lesser degree for hearing. If movement does not occur in the course of the hearing process, hearing can become distorted and misrepresented at the central level.

Cognitive Changes in Normal Aging

As noted previously, it is a myth that cognitive decline is a necessary part of aging. This belief has been debunked by research on crystallized and fluid intelligence.[43] Crystallized intelligence involves the ability to perceive relations, to engage in formal reasoning, and to understand one's intellectual and cultural heritage. Crystallized intelligence can be affected by the environment and the attitude of the individual.[22] It is therefore possible, with self-directed learning and education, that crystallized intelligence can increase as long as a person is alive. The measurement of crystallized intelligence is usually in the form of culture-specific items such as number facility, verbal comprehension, and general information.

Fluid intelligence is not closely associated with acculturation. It is generally considered to be independent of instruction or environment and depends more on the genetic endowment of the individual.[82] The items used to test fluid intelligence include memory span, inductive reasoning, and figural relations, all of which are presumed to be unresponsive to training. Because fluid intelligence involves those intellectual functions that are most affected by changes in neurophysiological status, they have been generally assumed to decline with age. This is not true, as shown in several studies, one of which noted that during middle age, scores on tests for fluid intelligence are similar to scores in midadolescence.[59, 93]

Botwinick[13] described the classic pattern of changes in intelligence with aging. In the adult portion of the life span, verbal abilities decline very little, if at all, whereas psychomotor abilities decline earlier and to a greater extent. The period between ages 55 and 70 is a transition time and some decreases in performance are noted on many cognitive tests. A substantial decline on laboratory tests of cognitive function is generally limited to those over 75 years of age.[48] In these latter years, however, the decline in fluid intelligence is offset by the growth in crystallized intelligence for most people, unless dementia is present. Thus although changes may be demonstrated in the laboratory, they are not significant in the "real world," and the elderly are as capable as the young of participating in rehabilitation training. For elderly people to benefit maximally, however, they must control the pace of training, as the tasks that are the most difficult for the aged are those that are fast-paced, unusual, and complex.[59] All physical therapy treatment with older patients needs to be structured to encourage the patient to self-pace. Interventions should be predictable, and progress by adding one new concept at a time.

Another type of cognitive change differs from the types of changes that occur in normal aging and those that occur in patients with dementia. This type of cognitive change, the "terminal drop," involves a decline in IQ scores in persons within the year before their death. This change in intellectual function is thought to result from some predeath changes in brain physiology. It is likely that research studies that show drastic decreases in intellectual function with advanced age have a large percentage of subjects who were near death as a part of the sample.[12] If the data from these subjects are deleted, the findings are similar to those in studies on normal elderly persons.

Stress and Intellectual Capacity

Hans Selye[94] defined *stress* as the nonspecific response of the body to any demand made on it. All human beings require a certain amount of stress to live and function effectively. When a stressor (stimulus) is applied, the body predictably goes through the three stages of response called the "general adaptation syndrome." The first response is a general alarm reaction, a "fight-or-flight" response that mobilizes all senses in an effort to make a judgment about the response that is needed. The next stage involves judgment and the selective adaptation to the stressor. A decision is made as to which body action is needed, and all other body activities return to homeostasis. If the stimulus continues and goes beyond the therapeutic level, then the body system or part will gradually experience physiological exhaustion. A person in physiological exhaustion is likely to manifest abnormal responses to any new stimulus. Paradoxical reactions can result in unusual physiological or psychological responses to stimuli (e.g., an erythematous response when an ice pack is applied or a patient becoming more agitated after receiving a sedative).

When a person is under perceived stress (real or imagined), there is a predictable set of cognitive changes that can occur. These cognitive functional changes can include preoccupation; forgetfulness; disorientation; confusion; low tolerance to ambiguity; errors in judgment in relation to work, distance, grammar, or mathematics; misidentification of people; inability to concentrate, to solve problems, or to plan; inattention to details or instructions;

reduced creativity, fantasy, and perceptual field; decreased initiative; decreased interest in usual activities, the future, or people; and irritability, impatience, anger, withdrawal, suspicion, depression, and crying. It is critical to differentiate whether the patient you are working with is having a stress reaction or truly experiencing dementia.

With aging, the body undergoes physiological changes, noted later, that make the older person less physiologically efficient in her or his response to stressors. The general alarm reaction is poorly mobilized and takes longer to become activated (Arndt-Schultz principle). The stage of resistance should yield a series of responses that allows the body to economize in its response to stress. In persons of all ages who are receiving too many different stimuli, and in the elderly experiencing normal levels of stimuli, the body becomes less efficient at turning off the general alarm response and replacing it with more appropriate and limited responses. When a person is overwhelmed by these types of stress, the individual may demonstrate mild global or specific cognitive impairments, especially mild short-term memory loss.

At this time, the historical clinical data become the only means of establishing a diagnosis because there are currently no tests to distinguish acute dementia from emotional exhaustion. In cases of domestic violence that have been kept secret over the years, this can be a difficult problem. A clinical example can highlight this:

A 90-year-old man had beaten his wife a few times early in their marriage and then they had come to an agreement and their marriage had continued with only verbal abuse and no physical abuse. As he approached 85 years of age, however, he again began to get violent and would shove her during arguments. At one point she fell, broke her hip, and ended up in a nursing home for 8 weeks. Another time he was bringing her to therapy and on the way he became angry and let go of the wheelchair, and it ran into a wall. The wife chose to do nothing and say nothing. The only sign that was present was that she always cried in physical therapy when she started to relax. The client eventually confided to the physical therapist and was referred to a crisis counselor to problem-solve how to proceed. She saw the counselor weekly for over 4 years. Another incident happened in which the wife was hurt and protective services were called. The patient refused to press charges and returned to the home, stopped all counseling, withdrew in "embarrassment," and within several weeks became confused. The husband placed her in a nursing home and she was given the diagnosis of dementia and placed on haloperidol (Haldol). There were no other therapeutic services offered. It is critical to get patients access to one-on-one counseling and family therapy when it is needed.

The assessment of an elderly person, with or without dementia, must include a determination of the type, number, and severity of the patient's current stressors. It is important to realize that positive life events (e.g., marriage or the birth of a grandchild) are also stressful life events. Using scores that rate stressful life events, it is possible to identify those patients who are at greatest risk of physiological and emotional exhaustion.[49] Elderly patients, with their numerous psychosocial problems and chronic and acute illnesses, are likely candidates for physiological and emotional exhaustion and the development of psychopathology. Thus the environment and process of rehabilitation care need to be modified to counteract the effect of stress on the intellectual capacity of the older patient. *Any action that modifies stress so that a deterioration of intellectual function is stopped or reversed is an efficient and cost-effective part of the total rehabilitation effort.*

STRATEGIES FOR ASSESSING, PREVENTING, AND MINIMIZING DISTORTIONS IN INFORMATION PROCESSING

Each person acts on the available data at a specific moment. This stimulus-response cycle has four major steps, and at each step, there is a possibility for distortion or error. When a person is presented with a stimulus, all data (physiological, psychological, sociological, and environmental) are collected, and then integrated with data from past experience. Based on the results, a response is elicited, which is then followed by the behavioral concomitant of this response.

At the very outset of the process of patient assessment, it is necessary to examine the amount of verbal and written stimuli processed by the patient in relation to the amount used as a part of the testing process. Using an overview of the patient's cognitive capacity, it is possible for the rehabilitation staff to modify the process of evaluation to maximize the patient's performance. A basic assessment of the patient's fluid and crystallized intelligence at a given moment (to allow a comparison of cognitive capacity at other times in the 24-hour cycle) provides the clinician with a specific description of what aspects of intellectual function appear to be impaired and pinpoints those aspects of intellectual functioning that are still intact. Based on this approach, it is possible to proceed with the rehabilitation evaluation in a language and at a pace that is comfortable for the patient.

The Mini-Mental State Examination

The Mini-Mental State Examination (MMSE) was developed as a result of a study noting that 80% of cognitive disorders among elderly people were not detected by the general practitioner.[39, 110] Most professionals on the rehabilitation team (physicians, nurses,[20, 46] physical therapists[52] and social workers[18]) are likely to have had only minimal specialty training in gerontology and the unique symptoms and needs of the very old.

The MMSE provides a screening test for identifying unrecognized cognitive disorders in the elderly.[36, 37, 117] The MMSE (Fig. 26–1) assesses only cognition and does not examine other aspects of the traditional mental status examination such as mood, delusions, or hallucinations. The test can identify if the patient is oriented; remembers (short-term); and can read, write, calculate, and see the relationship of one object or figure to another. The examination is used to screen for cognitive dysfunctions, much as a measurement of blood pressure or blood sugar is used to screen for significant medical disorders. The MMSE also may be used in a serial fashion to quantify changes in a patient's cognitive status over time. This examination can be used as a springboard for planning how to carry out the traditional rehabilitation evaluation on a patient who has some intellectual dysfunction.[15, 71]

The MMSE has been standardized for elderly persons living in the community. The scores on this test correlate significantly with the Weschsler Adult Intelligence Scale and the Weschsler Memory Test. The MMSE is reported to have a test-retest reliability for both normal and psychiatric samples of 0.89 or greater. It has been found that when a cut-off score of 24 is used for the detection of dementia, the MMSE had a sensitivity of 87.6% and a specificity of 81.6%.[36] Several studies have noted that interviews with informants are highly consistent with elderly persons' scores on the MMSE.[51]

The examination takes only a few minutes to administer, is scored immediately, and can be administered by any member of the rehabilitation team. The entire examination grades cognitive performance on a scale from 0 to 30. A score of 24 or less usually indicates some degree of cognitive dysfunction, but some patients with dementia may score above 24, and some with depression or delirium may score significantly below 24. A low score on this examination can mean that the patient is probably suffering from dementia, delirium, mental retardation, amnestic syndrome, or aphasia. A low score on the MMSE can indicate the areas of specific cognitive impairment and gives the rehabilitation team data about how to best communicate with the patient.

A shortened version of the MMSE has been developed (using only 12 of the 20 original variables). Although the original study suggested that the shortened version of the MMSE is equally as effective as the full MMSE in identifying elderly patients with cognitive deficits, more recent studies have questioned these findings.

Sensory Changes with Dementia

Patients with dementia may have specific problems that inhibit the integration of sensory input. Aphasias and disruption of association pathways may inhibit the patient's ability to integrate accurately perceived sensory information in a meaningful way. Bassi and colleagues[10] and Fozard[38] have demonstrated that patients with Alzheimer's disease, multi-infarct dementia, and alcoholic dementia may demonstrate disturbances in visual acuity, depth perception, color differentiation, and differentiation of figure from ground when compared with normal age-matched controls and normal younger subjects.

When a patient has a distortion in cognitive capacity, all neurosensory stimuli must be reviewed. An assessment of specific sensory systems is also necessary. The challenge in rehabilitation is to design a process and environment of care so that there is compensation and modification that maximizes the ability of the elderly patient with sensory deficits to adapt to most life situations. The example of visual deficits is a case in point. One out of every two blind persons in the United States is over 65.[124] Techniques of environmental adaptation and special measures to organize care to help elderly blind people have allowed many of them to live independently in the community.[44] However, many elderly people with visual impairments are not blind. Some of the structural changes that result in mild to moderate deficits of vision include yellowing; uneven growth, striation, and thickening of the lens; increasing weakness of the muscles controlling the eye; alteration in the perception of color (especially fine

MINI-MENTAL STATE EXAMINATION

Maximum score	Score	
5	( )	ORIENTATION
		What is the (year) (season) (date) (day) (month)?
5	( )	Where are we: (state) (county) (town) (hospital) (floor)?
3	( )	REGISTRATION

Name 3 objects: 1 second to say each. Then ask the client all 3 after you have said them.
Give 1 point for each correct answer. Then repeat them until the client learns all 3. Count trials and record.

TRIALS

| 5 | ( ) | *Attention and calculation* |

Serial 7's. 1 point for each correct. Stop after 5 answers. Alternatively spell "world" backwards.

| 3 | ( ) | *Recall* |

Ask for 3 objects repeated above. Give 1 point for each correct.

| 9 | ( ) | *Language* |

Name a pencil and watch. (2 points)

Repeat the following "No ifs, ands, or buts." (1 point)

Follow a *3-stage command:* "Take a paper in your right hand, fold it in half, and put it on the floor." (3 points)

Read and obey the following: "Close your eyes." (1 point)

Write a sentence. (1 point)

Copy design. (1 point)

| 30 | ( ) | TOTAL SCORE |

Assess level of consciousness along a continuum.

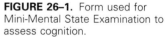

Alert   Drowsy   Stupor   Coma

FIGURE 26–1. Form used for Mini-Mental State Examination to assess cognition.

distinctions in tone and brightness); and slower adaptation to light.[38] Modifications of the environment can include good, nonglare lighting, dark and clear large-print, low-vision aids (e.g., magnifying glass), verbal orientation and escort by persons accompanying patients in a new environment, consistent furniture placement, explanation when changes occur, clear hallways, a systematic storage system for clothes and toilet articles, and the use of contrasting colors to identify doors, windows, baseboards, and corners.[20, 21, 38, 41, 42]

Older Adult Learning Styles and Communication

Learning occurs throughout life.[59] In rehabilitation the client learns new skills or relearns old adaptive skills. As with intelligence, the learning process does not change abruptly when an individual reaches old age, but differ-

ences in performance have been reported. One challenge for rehabilitation therapy is to find ways to improve the efficiency of learning by the older person.

Botwinick[13] has noted that learning and performance are not the same. Poor performance on a learning task may mean that insufficient learning has occurred or that the performance does not accurately reflect the extent of learning achieved.[82] The key variables that affect a person's ability to participate in a learning task can include intelligence, learning skills acquired over the years, and flexibility of learning style. Noncognitive factors also can have a strong bearing on an individual's performance. The noncognitive factors include visual and auditory acuity, health status, motivation to learn, level of anxiety, the speed at which stimuli and learning are paced, and the meaningfulness of the items or tasks to be learned. Therefore a rehabilitation assessment must include a review of the common alterations in learning styles seen among the elderly. This is particularly important before discharging a patient from a rehabilitation program. The rationale is that a lack of progress may not reflect the patient's lack of capacity for rehabilitation, but rather may reflect a dissonance between the patient's learning style and skills and the presentation of materials in the treatment program (i.e., verbal input has not been adapted to match the patient's level or pace of comprehension).

Interference

Interference can make the learning process less efficient in two major ways.[27] First, interference can result from a conflict between one's present knowledge and the new knowledge to be learned. Second, if two learning tasks are undertaken at the same time, they can interfere with each other. The elderly have special difficulties if they must concentrate on intake, attention, and retrieval processes at the same time.[27] Therefore the process and therapeutic environment of rehabilitation for the elderly patient must not be disturbed by background noise, other stimuli in the environment, or personal anxiety. When learning a new task, the elderly patient may require a quiet room with no other stimuli than those offered by the therapist. The need to rid the environment of distractions is particularly important when working with an elderly patient with dementia, as this patient will have greater difficulty filtering out irrelevant sensory inputs when compared with elderly patients without dementia.

Pacing

The pacing of therapeutic intervention is a significant variable in helping an elderly person learn. Elderly persons (with or without dementia) perform best if they are given as much time as they need, when learning is self-paced.[13] The major drawback of a fast pace (as perceived by the patient) is that the elderly person generally chooses not to participate rather than risk making a mistake. Nonresponse in the treatment environment is often interpreted as apathy, poor motivation, or "confusion."[6] Nonresponse is reduced when extra time to complete a rehabilitation task is offered. Following the individual assessment, group work (where concepts can be presented, reviewed, and examined at leisure) also can be used to reduce the psychological pressure of faster-paced learning. The details of therapy must be planned carefully, including how questions are asked (this involves asking clear and precise questions in nonmedical language), and, most important, setting aside enough treatment time so the patient can respond at a leisurely pace.

Organization

If data are organized in the brain as part of the learning process, the retrieval of these data becomes easier. Older persons are less likely than members of other age groups to spontaneously organize data to facilitate learning and later retrieval (memory) of that learning.[7] Elderly people who are highly verbal show fewer weaknesses in the ability to organize stimuli. Elderly persons with poor verbal skills show significant improvement when strategies for organization of data are provided by others (e.g., the therapist). Arenberg and Robertson-Tchabo[7] noted that older learners have difficulty following content because they cannot anticipate what will be taught and do not see the whole that is being presented.

Thus it is helpful to organize therapy by beginning with an overview in outline form of the entire lesson to be learned. This presents the patient with a conceptual map of the upcoming experience. The use of purposeful organizing also can help to bridge the gap between what the older person knows and the new information or task to be learned. The use of neurolinguistic programming is especially effective with elderly patients or with patients with cognitive deficits because it builds consciously—through language, kinesthesia, and visual input—a picture of a new concept from a known and familiar frame of reference.[8]

Inefficient learning, and at times an inability to learn, occurs in the older adult if material is presented in one way and the older person is expected to apply it some other way. Instructions need to be provided in the format in which they are to be used. If possible, one piece of new data should be presented at a time. A conscious transition needs to be made by the therapist from the patient's current frame of reference to the understanding of the new data, and the pace needs to be set by the patient.

There are several other strategies for maximizing the efficiency of older adult learners based on awareness of normal age-related changes. Some of the more frequently used techniques are summarized in the box on page 800.

Communication

Therapists can begin by inquiring into what the reality of the patient looks like. As people interacting with the patient, our first goal is to be able to communicate with words, gestures, positioning, and so on so that our stimuli bring out functional responses in the patient. It is true that all people have an ongoing internal dialogue. As a healthy adult, the therapist chooses to notice his or her own monologue, hear the content, and then pursue the goals and commitments that enhance interaction with the patient.

The interaction with the patient needs to be grounded in the present moment. The power for action lies in the present moment. The patient will bring his or her authentic self to the conversation or the interaction. The patient will be sensitive to our entire communication, what we say and what we withhold. The patient with cognitive problems may not understand the content but many still have the ability to sense and respond to our affective state at the moment. As we begin our communication, it is important to be clear of all previous concerns and bring no extra or extraneous emotions into the interaction. As caregivers/therapists we bring with us into the conversation the power of our intention to create a therapeutic interaction and the choice to stay on task. Patients bring whatever they bring. The patient has minimum capacity to adapt.

As therapists/caregivers it is critical that we be self-

TECHNIQUES FOR MAXIMIZING THE EFFICIENCY OF OLDER ADULT LEARNERS

1. Use mediators—the association of word, story, mnemonics, or visual inputs to help the person remember.
2. Choose learning activities that are meaningful for the client.
3. Use concrete examples to make learning easier.
4. Provide a supportive learning environment to prevent stress that can interfere with efficient learning.
5. Use supportive or neutral feedback and avoid feedback that is presented in a challenging tone.
6. Reward all responses, but reward correct responses more than incorrect responses. This can encourage elderly persons to decrease the number of errors by omission, which are often interpreted as apathy or lack of cooperation.
7. Use combinations of auditory and visual input to facilitate the learning process. This is only effective if the data presented are similar because variation between the two kinds of messages can result in interference and a decrease in the efficiency of learning.
8. Active learning is known to be more effective. A patient who moves the involved body part while getting verbal and visual input is likely to be more efficient in mastering the new skill.
9. Design the learning situation so that successful completion of the task is likely. Older people are more likely to focus on errors, which increases anxiety and lowers the self-concept. Worst of all, with all the energy focused on the error, there is a strong chance of repeating the error.

aware. What is our favorite strategy for communication? What is our favorite sentence structure? All of our habits need to be set aside because the patient needs to be the focus of our attention. This is a choice that is made if effective communication is to occur with a person with cognitive deficits. If we choose to speak as we do to a person who has no cognitive deficits, we will not have consistent results and will often agitate and upset the patient. What if we approach the patient as if he or she were a person from another culture that has its unique customs, norms, and ways of communication? The interaction becomes an inquiry where the measure of success is that the patient and the therapist are able to create the functional outcomes that are needed (e.g., the patient taking a bath and enjoying it).

Now the question becomes, What is the specific verbal category where the patient appears to be most comfort-able and feels safe? Every patient is different and it may depend on the time of day, or on whether the patient is tired or feeling threatened. It is common that a person may respond best to one particular style of communication and be predictably upset or agitated by another style. One patient may also want to joke around and be playful and this is a cue to staff that this is a workable style of communication. Another patient smiles whenever the tone of the conversation is soft, nurturing, and tender, and if staff are willing, then this is where ease of relating can occur. Other patients relate best to rules and need predictable structures and boundaries. They love to know what is coming next. Still another category is people who can relate and communicate when there is definite admiration and respect built into the conversation or when we can agree not to like something. Each patient with cognitive problems needs to have caregivers develop a chart of what works to create a sense of relatedness and ease in communication. The challenge for caregivers is that there can be ongoing change in the patient's abilities and it is still helpful for new caregivers to have some guidelines for communication when they are introduced to the patient. *It is critical that someone who is familiar and enjoys the patient introduce new staff to the patient.*

For persons with cognitive disturbances, familiarity and rituals are keys to ease of adaptability. The basis for rituals is a well-organized documentation that all caregivers have access to and contribute to on an ongoing basis. This information needs to be filtered and organized so that each shift can see what is working for the patient today. Even a nonverbal patient can relate effectively to bathing if there is a ritual to the way dressing and undressing is done (e.g., the socks always come off first). Mace and Rabins[71] spelled out the details of the importance of caregivers being aware of the power of familiarity and rituals. Mintzer and colleagues[78] reinforced the same idea in their research on the effectiveness of alternative care environments for agitated dementia patients. Hall[47] described the importance of an individualized care plan for every cognitively impaired patient. Specifically, Hall noted that it is important to be sure that the plan includes data describing the patients' culture; their habits and preferences; their remaining functional activities; regions of the brain affected; and histopathology.[47] Another detail that will require staff or caregiver attention, evaluation, and adaptation in daily care is *ideational apraxia*. LeClerc and Wells described this as "a condition in which an individual is unable to plan movement related to an object because he or she has lost the perception of the object's purpose."[62] This is especially important in relation to feeding, dressing, and bathing. The authors described a tool that can help caregivers assess the ideational apraxia and problem-solving compensations to prevent unnecessary agitation or disability, and take actions to preserve existing abilities. Savelkoul and associates[92] emphasized the importance of effective communication between staff and patients and the importance of routines for patient care to maximize functional behaviors for institutionalized elderly living in residential homes. Another key point noted was that staff corrected and tested residents too often, which can create agitation and upset. It was noted that this appeared to be related to lack of training and information on the part of the staff about the dementia and cognitive status of patients as well as to lack of support from other staff.

As a patient goes through gradual deterioration of cognitive status, as is common in Alzheimer's disease, it is critical that staff, family, and caregivers be trained in nonverbal and positional and emotional communication techniques. Many patients come to a place in their life with dementia where words are a source of confusion. It is then time to use other strategies to communicate. Sign language is initially a possible tool until the associative functions begin to disappear. Accurate assessment needs to create adaptations in communication. It may be necessary to use hand-guided communication. This is where the patient is led through a task or parts of a task in order to get his or her cooperation. At this stage of communication, ease and trust are the most important goals. It may take 5 minutes of tenderly holding a patient's hand before the patient is ready to walk to the dining room or bathroom. This requires much patience on the part of staff. Positional communication can be used, as well as simply touch. As patients begin to feel safe with our state of being, they will relax and choose to participate. At times patients will have unique needs such as only wanting to be cared for by a female caregiver or a male caregiver. It is critical to honor patient needs because the cognitively impaired may not be able to learn or adapt to the demands of the other person due to previous trauma (assault or incest, real or imagined).

As a way to summarize our considerations about communication with a person with cognitive impairment, it may be useful to examine our own intentions from moment to moment. What is my goal in this interaction? Who am I being at this moment? The task may be important and the doing of it may be critical. For the patient with cognitive disturbance, it is vital that we provide life-enhancing stimuli based on the patient's perceptions. If in our zeal to "do," we accidentally scare, intimidate, or bully the patient, then there will be damage that may not be able to be undone. The cognitively impaired patient presents a unique challenge if a threat has been created because it is often very hard to reassure and educate them to the fact that this was accidental. It is not uncommon that the patient will just need us to leave the room and may then be afraid of us for some time. The saving grace for many patients is that their short-term memory is poor so they may not remember the incident tomorrow. The problem with the agitation is that if there are other cognitively impaired clients in the area, they may also get upset.

The solution to the crisis moment, when there has been a breakdown in communication, is to effectively redirect communication and the focus of the present moment. An example of this would be that the staff member purposely bump into a chair and knock it over. Or the staff member could drop a cup of water or a book, start to sing, whistle loudly, or clap hands. At that moment a distraction is created. If the distraction works, then the patient is off the old thought and open to a new focus. It is at that moment that staff need to be intentional. The new focus needs to offer comfort or nurturing or a predictable sense of well-being (e.g., food, a picture of one of their favorite things to look at, holding a favorite item, touching a favorite comfort object, hugging).

The research findings and techniques discussed previously describe many of the aspects of the Feldenkrais approach to learning.[31, 32] The Feldenkrais method has been applied to the needs of elderly persons with good results. The principle that learning needs to be pleasurable is especially applicable to elderly clients (with and without dementia) because they are not as likely to be as motivated as young persons. Despite changes in learning style, the older person (with or without dementia) can be helped to learn more efficiently through well-planned instruction. The use of techniques to increase learning efficiency in the elderly has been demonstrated to decrease the stress that at times may result in emotional or cognitive overload and abnormal cognitive reactions.[31, 32]

ENVIRONMENTAL CONSIDERATIONS

Hypothermia

The temperature of the living environment must be carefully controlled because aged clients may not perceive that the environment is cold, as they may not experience shivering. Accidental hypothermia can develop in an older person even at temperatures of 60° F (15.5° C) to 65° F (18.3° C). Accidental hypothermia is a drop in the core body temperature to below 95° F (35° C). Patients at risk for hypothermia are presented in the accompanying box.

The symptoms of hypothermia may include a bloated face, pale and waxy or pinkish skin color, trembling on one side of the body without shivering, irregular and slowed heartbeat, slurred speech, shallow and very slow breathing, low blood pressure, drowsiness, and symptoms of delirium. The two principles of treatment of hypothermia are that the person will stay chilled unless rewarmed slowly and that he or she should be evaluated by a physician, regardless of the apparent severity of the hypothermia.[16, 82]

PATIENTS AT HIGH RISK FOR HYPOTHERMIA

- Persons over the age of 65
- Persons showing no signs of shivering or pale skin in response to cold
- Persons taking medications containing a phenothiazine (to treat psychosis or nausea)
- Persons with disorders of the hormone system, especially hypothyroidism
- Persons with head injuries, strokes, Alzheimer's disease or other dementias, Parkinson's disease, or other neurological conditions
- Persons with severe arthritis
- Persons with arteriosclerotic peripheral vascular disease, chronic ulceration, or amputation

If a person continues to be at risk for hypothermia, specific measures can be taken to prevent subsequent distortions of cognitive status. First, the room temperature should be set to at least 70° F (21° C). Second, the person should wear adequate clothing; this may include long underwear and an undershirt. Adequate nutrition also may be a factor in preventing hypothermia.

Patients and their caregivers may attempt to save money by lowering room temperatures and thus inadvertently cause accidental hypothermia. It is also common to find institutions with central air conditioning. To prevent accidental hypothermia, special accommodations for the elderly, such as a special wing of the building or individual temperature controls in the rooms, are required.[124]

Transplantation Shock

It is known that some elderly persons seem to function well in a familiar environment, but they become severely disoriented and unable to perform their ADL if taken out of their own homes. As a general rule, these persons suffer from very mild symptoms of dementia, which are not readily apparent when they remain in a structured, familiar, stable environment and maintain a consistent daily routine. When faced with the need to adapt to a new environment and being bombarded with multiple unfamiliar sensory stimuli, however, the diseased brain is unable to make sense out of this large volume of new stimuli. If a patient was oriented before admission to an institution and then becomes disoriented, it is not unusual for the patient's cognitive functioning to return to its baseline level of functioning upon return to the familiar environment. Therefore, all moves by a patient from one hospital room to another or from one institution to another, and all changes in a treatment regimen, need to be carefully planned. If a change is anticipated, the patient should be involved in the decision making. If the change is a permanent move, the patient should have a chance for one or two trial visits before the actual move. The patient should be informed of all changes well in advance and this information needs to be given repeatedly to the patient with dementia. The precautions mentioned can help the patient relocate without creating transplantation shock and related cognitive changes.

EMOTIONAL CAPACITY TO PARTICIPATE IN A LEARNING TASK

Many elderly persons who come for physical therapy are in a state of emotional "overload," as evidenced by disorientation, depression, anger, or a withdrawn and apparently uncooperative attitude. A person who is at or near the point of emotional overload needs to be evaluated as to his or her ability to be involved in learning tasks that require active participation. If the patient is in emotional overload, forms of therapeutic intervention that allow the patient temporarily to be a passive recipient of therapeutic intervention can be used. Various types of therapeutic interventions, including massage, connective tissue massage, heat, breathing exercises, relaxation exer-

cises, and Feldenkrais Functional Integration, can promote a relaxation response, lower the anxiety level, reinforce self-pacing of activity, and thereby prepare the patient to participate in more physically active types of therapeutic exercise.[31] If asked directly, most patients will state whether they feel able to actively participate.

If for any reason the patient is not able or willing to state her or his feelings, it is still possible to evaluate the patient's ability to participate. If it is possible to get a patient's cooperation, the following movements can be attempted and then evaluated. (These should be used only if active diseases involving the eyes are not present and there is no pain in doing the movements.)

1. Close eyes.
2. Close eyes and keep them closed for 30 seconds; then for 1 minute.
3. Close eyes; move only the eyes to the right and left slowly (slow movements with control is the goal).
4. Close eyes; move eyes in diagonals, right and up, then left and down; then left and up, right and down.

If a patient is unable to perform these movements, feels they require too much effort, or feels they are uncomfortable, a high level of tension is usually present. When the patient is very tense, it is necessary to begin treatment using passive therapeutic procedures. If a person can comfortably execute the movements, he or she (i.e., the central nervous system and the body) is able to receive and integrate new data and act with ease. When physical therapy requires active participation by the patient, it is important to verify psychomotor readiness to participate by using the above simple set of actions.

Distortions in intellectual and emotional capacity to receive input, integrate input, and then act on the input affect a person's ability to participate in a learning task. This section has described the most common sources of distortion in information processing that are external to the patient and therefore under the direct control of the rehabilitation team. It is possible for the rehabilitation team to make the choice to acknowledge the common age-related changes and common sources of stress response in the elderly and then to design a process and environment of care that maximizes the elderly patient's potential.

DELIRIUM AND REVERSIBLE DEMENTIA: EVALUATION AND TREATMENT

The following discussion focuses on the patient's internal environment (physiological, psychological, spiritual, and pathological) and presumes that all unnecessary external environmental stressors have been removed. Delirium and dementia have been defined earlier in this chapter. A delirium usually becomes manifested suddenly, or over a period of hours or days. Occasionally, a delirium may be chronic, but this is relatively infrequent. A dementia, whether reversible or irreversible, usually has a much longer time of onset, although an acute onset can occur.

The establishment of the diagnosis of the underlying cause of the dementia or delirium is the key to effective care. Although the diagnostic process is primarily medical, the therapist can obtain information, as part of a team evaluation, that will help establish the underlying diagnosis. Historical information needs to be obtained regarding:

- The amount of time that has elapsed since the onset of symptoms
- The progression or lack of progression of symptoms
- Associated functional impairments; associated medical signs and symptoms
- Use of prescription, over-the-counter, and illegal drugs; alcohol, caffeine, and nicotine
- Exposure to occupational or avocational toxins

Even in a patient with cognitive disturbances, this information can frequently be obtained and be corroborated by obtaining a history from significant others.

The causes of delirium and reversible dementias are many. In the elderly person, however, certain causes are more common than others (see the accompanying box). Alcohol and drugs (prescribed, over-the-counter, illegal, and home remedies) are prime offenders (see Chapter 32). The delirium may be the result of intoxication, side effects, or withdrawal syndromes.[107, 111] Indeed, one set of clinical symptoms that differentiates elderly addicts from younger addicts is the presence of cognitive deficits.[108] Benzodiazepines are among the most commonly prescribed offenders, as even a low dose (2 mg) may cause demonstrable cognitive changes.[91] Other common drugs that cause delirium or reversible dementia are alcohol, oral narcotics, psychotropic medications, steroids, antineoplastic drugs, digoxin, anesthetic agents, antiparkinsonian drugs, and antihistamines. However, all drugs have the potential to cause significant cognitive problems in the elderly.[64] These symptoms often resolve with discon-

---

COMMON CAUSES OF DELIRIUM AND REVERSIBLE DEMENTIA

Alcohol/drug abuse/dependence
Intoxication
Toxicity
Side effects
Withdrawal

Cardiovascular/pulmonary
Congestive heart failure
Cardiac arrhythmia
Hypertensive crisis
Hypoxia
Chronic obstructive pulmonary disease

Metabolic/endocrine
Electrolyte disturbance (especially hyponatremia)
Hypercalcemia
Dehydration
Overhydration
Renal failure
Hypoglycemia
Diabetic ketoacidosis
Hypothyroidism
Hyperthyroidism
Malnutrition
Vitamin B_{12}/folate deficiency
Hepatic failure
Wernicke-Korsakoff syndrome
Cushing's syndrome

Infection
Urinary tract infection
Pneumonia/acute bronchitis
Tuberculosis
Other acute infections

Neurological
Stroke
Head trauma
Mass lesion (e.g., tumor, hematoma)
Seizure

Pharmacological
Benzodiazepines
Barbiturates and other sedative-hypnotics
Antidepressants
Neuroleptics
Antihistamines
Anticholinergics
Cardiac glycosides
Steroids
Antineoplastic drugs
Narcotics
Antiarrhythmics
Antihypertensives

Miscellaneous
Sensory deprivation
Sensory overstimulation
Acute or chronic pain
Constipation/fecal impaction
Urinary retention

tinuation of the offending agent or treatment of the withdrawal syndrome. According to Chaprone, for some patients, a medication holiday of longer than 24 hours may be needed before a positive change in cognition can be noted.[53]

At times, the symptoms may be correlated clearly with the pharmacokinetic profiles of the medications taken by the client. The dose or frequency of administration of medications can be a contributing factor to a delirious state.[96] Each member of the rehabilitation team needs to document the patient's ability to participate in learning tasks and the time of the assessment, because timing of medication administration can affect functional performance. The rehabilitation team needs the input of a clinical pharmacologist who can help the team focus on concepts such as biological half-life, clearance, bioavailability of drugs, and the time course of drug concentration in plasma as a function of dose and frequency.

Several medical diseases are quite likely to cause symptoms of delirium or reversible dementia, which will also reverse with treatment of the underlying disease. Urinary tract infections, more common in women, are the cause of delirium in 23% of patients.[73] Fecal impaction is another common cause of acute cognitive change in elderly persons. Others are distended bladder caused by prostatic enlargement or drug-induced urinary retention, dehydration, malnutrition, cardiovascular disorders,[16] metabolic disturbances (particularly undiagnosed diabetes mellitus),[24] endocrine diseases, renal diseases, hematological diseases, pneumonia or bronchitis,[16] and vitamin B_{12} deficiency.

Transient (and usually mild) cognitive deficits may be the result of a cerebrovascular accident. The cognitive deficits after a cerebrovascular accident are often reversible, although they may last for several months after the stroke. The rehabilitation team needs to evaluate and regularly reevaluate the patient's cognitive capacity and build a program of care around current abilities. A program of therapeutic intervention that allows the older person to work in a self-paced program for 1 to 3 months can yield good therapeutic results and also prevent unnecessary secondary deconditioning until part or all of the patient's cognitive capacity returns.[89]

Depression is commonly misdiagnosed as dementia in the elderly.[16, 98, 99] For many years, it was thought that depression was a form of "pseudodementia" or false dementia.[65] Depression can result in mild and subtle cognitive changes affecting immediate recall, attention, and the ability to perform basic ADL. Some reports noted that as many as 31% of those thought to have dementia have depression instead.[74] However, recent research has clarified the close relationship between structural changes in the elderly brain and the onset of depression,[45, 60] thus bringing the concept of pseudodementia, or depression as a reversible dementia, into disrepute. Depression is a treatable disorder, and many patients with cognitive impairments show some improvement in their cognitive functioning if the depression is treated; however, the underlying cognitive problem does not resolve with treatment of the depression.[100, 105, 115]

Because the presence of depression can affect the process of rehabilitation through cognitive deficits or its effects on motivation, it is important for this disorder to be diagnosed early and accurately. The Geriatric Depression Scale, a 30-item yes/no questionnaire, screens for this disorder.[126] Although there is no arbitrary cutoff score that signifies depression, most individuals with a score of 15 or higher suffer from this disorder. The higher the score, the more likely that the patient not only suffers from depression but that the severity of the depression is greater.

Poststroke depression can produce a reversible decline in cognitive performance.[43] Poststroke depression is more likely to occur in patients with left hemisphere lesions, and is more likely to occur as the site of the lesion moves toward the frontal pole.[82] The relationship between site of lesion and depression also has been noted on neuropsychological testing.[12]

The treatment of major depression generally involves pharmacotherapy, psychotherapy, and environmental manipulation, which can require support from the entire rehabilitation team.[103, 116] In the treatment of a patient with depression, therapeutic techniques can promote a relaxation response and a decrease in anxiety level (massage, heat, or Feldenkrais Functional Integration) and can help bring the patient to the point where it is possible to begin aerobic training, which is known to have a beneficial effect. All aerobic training for the elderly should begin with a stress test, modified as necessary to determine the patient's exercise target heart rate. The modification most commonly required is use of the upper extremities to achieve the training effect, because lower extremity function may be limited, or use of major ADL involving the upper extremities as the stress test/training program.

The causes of delirium and reversible dementia are usually treatable, and if diagnosis and care are provided in a timely fashion, it is likely that the patient can regain full command of his or her cognitive processes. When this does not happen, it is likely that the patient had a mild irreversible dementia that had remained hidden until the onset of an acute problem that uncovered the poor cognitive functioning. The length of time in an institution (hospital or nursing home) needs to be kept as short as possible to avoid learned dependency and learned helplessness,[101, 104] which makes a return to both full cognitive functioning and independent living difficult.[99]

Therapy for elderly persons who are experiencing delirium or reversible dementia consists of treating the underlying causes of the cognitive changes. A close working relationship among all members of the rehabilitation team, including a geriatric psychiatric consultant, is necessary. Even before the cause of the disorder is elucidated, the patient should receive the same emotional and physical support as any patient with an irreversible dementia. The therapist must adapt all activities to the extent and types of cognitive losses that are present. The patient needs to feel secure, live in an environment that has as few changes as possible, and have a consistent and stable schedule for activities.

IRREVERSIBLE DEMENTIA

The course of an irreversible dementia is unique for each patient. The variation in clinical course will occur based on the cause of the underlying disease and superimposed biological and psychosocial factors, including, but not limited to, medications, concurrent illness (including delirium), the nature of the social support system, and the patient's premorbid personality structure. The causes of irreversible dementia are summarized in the box below.

Regardless of the cause of the dementia, the clinical course of these disorders has several commonalities.[81] Most of these diseases are progressive. Symptoms may be subtle early in the course of the illness, and the onset of disease is usually noted by the person with the disorder, family members, friends, or colleagues at work, rather than by a physician. The signs of impairment of mental ability are commonly memory loss, poor judgment, or incompetence at work. The patient can often succeed at hiding his or her symptoms for a while. The social consequences of the cognitive impairment usually bring the patient to the attention of health care professionals. In addition, the patient with dementia can manifest a variety of psychiatric symptoms, including mood distur-

bance, agitation, violent behavior, socially inappropriate behavior, delusions, hallucinations, catastrophic reactions, and perseveration.[70, 71] The pattern of onset and the types of psychiatric symptoms are often directly related to the underlying pathological condition.

When a physician is finally consulted, the diagnostic process can begin. When a complete diagnostic evaluation, including history, physical examination, neurological examination, neuropsychological testing, and laboratory testing (see the box below), is performed, an accurate diagnosis can be made in about 90% of patients,[56] although experienced geriatric psychiatrists can make an accurate diagnosis in more than 95% of patients.

Once the diagnostic process is completed, treatment can be started. Medications can assist in reversing underlying causes in only a small percentage of cases; patients in whom drug therapy is successful usually have had a potentially reversible dementia that has gone untreated and now have permanent sequelae of the disorder. Medications may only be able to slow down the process of an irreversible disorder (e.g., tacrine for Alzheimer's disease) or prevent further deterioration (e.g., aspirin for multi-infarct dementia). Psychotropic drugs may reverse depression or the behavioral symptoms associated with dementia.[74, 97, 102] Medical management also involves the prevention and treatment of comorbid medical conditions.

Medical management of irreversible dementias focuses on maximizing the patient's remaining functions and roles, rehabilitation of some lost functions, and family education and support.[71] Training caregivers to adapt to the patient (e.g., getting the patient out of bed, bathing), simplifying the individual's living space, and referring relatives to family support services are some of the issues to be addressed.[123] The treatment of irreversible dementias is a

---

COMMON CAUSES OF IRREVERSIBLE DEMENTIA

Degenerative

Alzheimer's disease

Parkinson's disease

Huntington's disease

Pick's disease

Fahr's disease

Multiple sclerosis

Infectious

Neurosyphilis (general paresis)

Tuberculosis

AIDS

Creutzfeldt-Jakob disease

Vascular

Multi-infarct dementia

Stroke

Binswanger dementia

Anoxia

Arteriovenous malformation

Other

Normal-pressure hydrocephalus

Mixed dementia

Alcoholic dementia

Toxins

Head trauma

Mass lesions

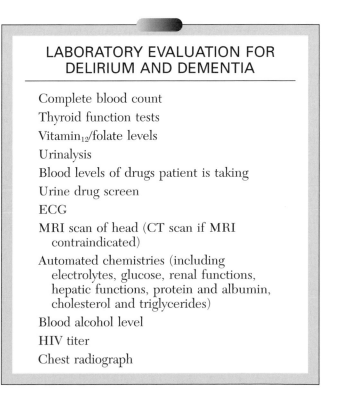

LABORATORY EVALUATION FOR DELIRIUM AND DEMENTIA

Complete blood count

Thyroid function tests

$Vitamin_{12}$/folate levels

Urinalysis

Blood levels of drugs patient is taking

Urine drug screen

ECG

MRI scan of head (CT scan if MRI contraindicated)

Automated chemistries (including electrolytes, glucose, renal functions, hepatic functions, protein and albumin, cholesterol and triglycerides)

Blood alcohol level

HIV titer

Chest radiograph

long-term process. Recent studies have found that the average duration of illness from first onset of symptoms to death was 8.1 years for Alzheimer's disease, 6.7 years for multi-infarct dementia,[9] and 5.6 years for Pick disease.[54] Medical and nursing care can extend the life expectancy of patients with dementia for up to 20 years or more.

In 1907, Alois Alzheimer[3] described the case and the neuropathology of a 54-year-old woman who developed morbid jealousy, which was followed by loss of memory, inability to read and understand, and death 4½ years after onset of the illness. Since then, it has been noted that 50% of patients with dementia suffer from Alzheimer's disease.[2] In making the diagnosis of Alzheimer's disease, all other causes of cognitive dysfunction must be ruled out. The disease can occur at any age, but the onset of the disease is almost always after age 65. The prevalence of the disease gradually increases to a rate of 20% in persons over the age of 85.[57, 76]

Alzheimer's disease can be clinically staged. The use of staging enables the family and health care team to plan ahead for the individual's needs. Staging helps the family prepare longitudinally for the process of interacting with the patient. It makes it possible for the treatment team to plan for appropriate levels of services as the individual's abilities decline. Finally, it allows the health care team to quantify change in functional and cognitive abilities over time, which helps in assessing the efficacy of the patient's treatment plan. The use of staging requires an accurate description of the patient's behavior (without the use of jargon), as well as an assessment of the patient's mental state.

Traditionally, the symptoms of Alzheimer's disease have been thought to progress in three stages. Stage 1 lasts from 2 to 4 years and involves loss of functional skills or orientation, memory loss, and lack of spontaneity. The patient is often aware of the losses and is, in many cases, able to cover up the cognitive losses by talking around the issues. During this stage the patient and family may need to deal with the issue of giving up a job, hobbies, or other types of meaningful activity because of the patient's inability to carry them out safely and independently. The patient begins to lose the ability to handle money and a personal budget, to drive a car safely, and to tell time.

The family or meaningful others may have to come to terms with the question of whether the patient can live alone. Depression is common during this stage of the disorder.[102]

In stage 2, there is progressive memory loss and the presence of a variety of neurological symptoms. Aphasias, apraxias, wandering, repetitive movements and stereotypical behavior, increased or decreased appetite, constant movement, and a peculiar wide-based gait can manifest. Psychotic symptoms (especially paranoid delusions and hallucinations), agitation, violent behaviors, and uncontrollable screaming are common symptoms during this stage of the disorder.

In stage 3, the patient develops vegetative symptoms. The patient may become mute, stop eating, and become incontinent of bowel and bladder. Muscle twitches or jerks, spasms of the diaphragm, and an inability to walk generally occur. The patient may develop seizures, and emotional responsiveness, if present, is at a very primitive level. Eventually, the patient dies from the disease.

The MMSE also may be used as a staging tool. Scores of 26 or more are generally associated with minimal, if any, dementia; and scores of 21 to 25 with mild, of 15 to 20 with moderate, of 10 to 14 with severe, and of 9 or less with profound dementia. The severity of most other symptoms correlates well with the MMSE score.

Reisberg and co-workers[86, 87] have developed a scale that defines seven stages, many with substages, of Alzheimer's disease. This scale is probably the most accurate staging system for Alzheimer's disease. In addition, the staging used by this scale closely correlates with the progression of different sets of symptoms through the course of the disease.

The Barthel Index

The Barthel Index (Table 26–1) is another profile scale. The scale rates 10 self-care, continence, and mobility criteria.[72] The specific rating guidelines used in scoring are presented in Appendix 26–A. The advantage of the Barthel Index is its simplicity and usefulness in evaluating patients before, during, and after treatment. It is functionally oriented and may be best used accompanied by a clinical evaluation.[12]

● **TABLE 26–1. Barthel Index***

	With Help	Independent
1. Feeding (if food needs to be cut = help)	5	10
2. Moving from wheelchair to bed and return (including sitting up in bed)	5–10	15
3. Personal toilet (wash face, comb hair, shave, clean teeth)	0†	5
4. Getting on and off toilet (handling clothes, wipe, flush)	5	10
5. Bathing self	0†	5
6. Walking on level surface (or if unable to walk, propel wheelchair)	10	15
7. Ascending and descending stairs	5	10
8. Dressing (includes tying shoes, fastening fasteners)	5	10
9. Controlling bowels	5	10
10. Controlling bladder	5	10

*A patient scoring 100 is continent, feeds, dresses, gets up and out of bed and chairs, bathes himself or herself, walks at least a block, and can ascend and descend stairs. This does not mean that he or she is able to live alone. The patient may not be able to cook, keep house, and meet the public, but is able to get along without attendant care.

†A score of 0 is given in the activity when the patient cannot meet the criteria as defined (see Appendix 26–A).

Modified from Mahoney FI, Barthel DW: Functional evaluation: The Barthel Index. Md State Med J 14:61, 1965.

STRATEGIES FOR TREATMENT AND CARE

Because changes in cognitive function and behavior usually happen to a person who has a circle of friends and family for support, the rehabilitation team needs to include the caregivers and the patient as much as possible in treatment planning. A very large majority of elderly people with decreased cognitive abilities live with family or friends and not in institutions. The goal of rehabilitation is to ensure that the patient remains safe, independent, and able to perform ADL and IADL for as long as is reasonable. The planning to reach these goals is best done within the context of the patient's social support system.

The rehabilitation process begins while the diagnostic workup is still in progress. At this stage of treatment, the rehabilitation plan includes basic training for the patient in performing and adapting the ADL. It also includes *caregiver training and support* for significant others, so that they can make needed environmental modifications to ensure the safety of the patient with dementia.

Once the diagnosis is established, treatment planning for long-term care at home or in an institution must be carefully made. No matter where the patient will be living, involvement of the caregivers and significant others is crucial. It is necessary to ascertain the emotional and physical resources of the patient and family or significant others who will be the caretakers. A review of the caretakers' willingness to perform basic tasks or make visits, their willingness to be taught the necessary skills, and the realistic need for respites must be determined.[61] Family training and orientation manuals that deal with all the details of caring for a person with dementia are available.[71, 75] The same detailed orientation is needed for institutional staff who care for elderly patients with dementia. It is possible, by the structure and process of care, to help patients to be maximally active in their self-care and to prevent unnecessary anxiety and catastrophic reactions.

Family, significant others, and caregivers go through their own coping and adaptive process as the patient experiences gradual or sudden cognitive disturbances. These people have a history with the patient and have expectations about what the relationship and what communication should be. As cognitive disturbance occurs, they experience a series of losses because the patient is now no longer able to respond and interact as he or she has in the past. With progressive cognitive decline, family and friends experience ongoing losses because the patient is continually changing and less able to relate. For many patients with cognitive disturbances, at the final stage all communication disappears and the family is left with only nonverbal or no communication. Staff who work with a patient over a period of time also face their own personal reactions of loss, unfulfilled expectations, and a continual need to reassess how to relate effectively to the patient. The entire burden of creating a positive relationship falls on the people who are interacting with the patient. The family and caregivers themselves need training and ongoing support in learning how to nurture and maintain an ongoing relationship with the patient. This requires that caregivers and family members be aware that they are in a healing process as they relate to the loss of the relationship that previously existed. Epstein[29] provides a workable description of the stages of healing that occur when major trauma or loss occurs. Epstein defines *healing* as "putting right our wrong relation to our body, to other people and . . . to our own complicated minds, with their emotions and instincts at war with one another and not properly understood and accepted by what we call 'I' or 'me.' The process is one of reorganization, reintegration of things which have come apart."[29] When a patient experiences cognitive changes, the first stage of response by those who care for or love this person is "suffering." There is chaos and this is a traumatic time. For example, the patient suddenly cannot understand simple directions on how to operate the new electric cart and insists on getting the old one back. The family is upset and arguments ensue. The family and patient together eventually get a medical workup and they are told that "Mom has some type of degenerative cognitive problem." They all experience a profound sense that "something is wrong." The response to helplessness for most human beings is to resist. The lesson of this stage is acceptance. When acceptance is present, then it is possible to have detachment from the emotions. With acceptance present, it is possible to begin to adapt and compensate for losses. In the example noted, this would mean that the family would return the new electric cart and have the old (familiar) model refurbished. The family would get training from the therapist in exactly what skills of interaction Mom does not have so that they can work to avoid creating situations where she feels "stupid and helpless." When a cognitive loss is truly present, training in skills only creates frustration in the patient which may lead to anger and rage. The staff and family need to be trained to understand the exact nature of the losses and provide appropriate compensations in their oral communication and how they relate to the patient.

Stage 2 was alluded to as a part of stage 1. We, the family, and caregivers search for second opinions, see other types of physicians, and try alternative treatments to gain power over our helplessness. The polarities and rhythms of this process are what this stage is about. All persons involved, even the patient, eventually begin to note that the emotions of the interactions may actually be making things worse. We move closer to accepting that there is no magic available. We all look with interest at the proposition: What can I do to make *this* life—*this* person—cope more effectively and have a reasonable quality of life (regardless of my opinion about what cognitive loss means to me personally)? The lesson at this stage is another level of acceptance.

The third stage invites an examination of the ways in which we are "stuck in a perspective." When overwhelming stimuli occur, it is common to resort to our favorite strategy from childhood. For some people the favorite strategy is to withdraw, for others it may be to eat to create a distraction, and for others it may be anger. The emotional and mental options we each create to adapt to a difficult situation are as varied as the human race is varied. We as humans dwell in the desire to know why or how to fix it. The lesson of this stage is, again, another level of acceptance and insight about how we ourselves contribute to the problem by our reactions to the moment. Stage 4 begins the process of "reclaiming your power." This is the stage where people realize that the "script" (their internal dialogue) from the last three stages is not workable or even desirable. The anger is recognized and it brings an awareness that this reaction is not helping. There is recognition that resisting is also not working because the condition of the patient is not affected in a positive way by the emotional reaction on the part of the caregiver(s). The truth of the matter is that the first four stages of healing often cause family and caregivers to be part of the problem and not part of the solution. The problem is how to support the patient to heal and adapt to the cognitive changes, whether they be temporary or permanent. Family and caregivers need to bring their healing process to their own support system separate from the patient. When caregivers attempt to share their frustration, suffering, sadness, or anger with the patient, the patient is usually upset because he or she cannot comprehend what the details of the issue really are. The patient only knows that people are upset. This will cause the patient to be further upset and agitated. It is critical to recognize the stages of healing in staff and family and create services or referral to support groups so the patient can interact with people who are able to adapt to his or her needs and not cause further upset.

Stage 5 is called "merging with the illusion" and it represents the first step in being able to "relate to the facts in a powerful way" rather than resisting or trying to manipulate the data. It is the step where family and caregivers begin to integrate the facts into their view of the world. The adult son may say, "I hate the fact that my mom cannot live alone—it makes me feel so . . . helpless or frustrated or angry or upset or inadequate." Many health care providers get very upset when cognitive losses occur in their loved ones. It is as if the cognitive loss is a failure that they take personally and this reaction is seen in many people.

Stage 6 begins with active steps to prepare for the resolution of the emotions connected with the process. Many people describe this stage as the time when they really admit that their dad or mom is never going to be able to give them advice again, or baby-sit or travel alone. The healing comes in allowing people to notice the emotions that come with accepting these big changes in our reality.

Stage 7 brings the actual physical or emotional discharge. The process can be expressed as laughter, crying, fever, the urge to be physically active, sneezing, coughing, and so on. Resolution is marked by a deep sense of peace and inner strength. The person will have gone through the six stages and the release of emotions or movement results in a deep shift away from resistance. Family and caregivers need to create these healing experiences separate from or away from the patient with cognitive losses. When we are with the patient with cognitive losses, it is critical that we create for the patient a world that works, and is safe and respectful of his or her unique abilities. In the majority of cases, the profound emotional and physical release that comes with resolution will only tend to upset the patient.

At stage 8 we are emptied and the board has been wiped clean. In the space of nothingness, there is an opportunity for new possibilities for relating to the patient. The relationship is not to be based on the past but on moment-to-moment information that comes from the patient. It is a time when we can enjoy being with the patient and we begin to feel gratitude. Family and caregivers begin to look for ways to make things work easier.

Stage 9 is a time when the caregivers and family relate to the energy of the universe and begin to see the connections to all of life around them. At this stage we begin to see that we are also a part of the great flow of time and energy and that there is an opportunity for joy now. The process of illness and dying become the focus of awe and a reason to connect with other people and appreciate other people because they are a part of the whole process of our lives.

Stage 10 is the time when we connect with the creative force of the universe. The spiritual process is brought to the issue at hand. There is a sense of great wisdom and a sense of oneness with all creation. When working from this state of being, the caregiver has the unique capacity to speak or act so that it brings out the best in others. In health care, there are caregivers who have the special gift of allowing themselves to step into the mental world of the other person and thereby create communication that will be heard and that can be acted on even by those with very limited mental capacities. The most interesting thing is that the patients can often tell if a caregiver is in this unique state because they will come and sit next to the patient or want to hold hands. This state of ease and connection can be learned. A worldwide organization called Landmark Education ([415] 981-8850) provides programs and courses that examine how people listen, what bias they bring to the communication process, and specific speech strategies to bring out the best in others.

Epstein's stage 11 is when people live day to day without being attached to the situation. Epstein notes that in this stage, "we communicate with ourselves and others through our wounds instead of from them." As healing progresses we become part of the solution in the care of the patient with cognitive losses. We know we can make a positive difference and we take action to create what needs to be done. We are able to sort out the facts of a situation from our first impression, which is often loaded with judgments and wishful thinking. As we relate to the verifiable facts, we speak to the issues at hand with power and create positive outcomes where "win-win" becomes the norm.

In the last stage, we bring our unique individuality to the service of the community. We become aware that the limits to what we can bring to the community are connected to the limits to our sense of wholeness. This insight sends us back to the earlier stages of healing to create further self-awareness and healing on other issues. Inservice training can offer a basic introduction to strategies for lifelong learning, healing, and self-awareness. What works for me? What is the easiest way to learn new skills? What strategies enhance adaptability? This type of learning is nonlinear. It is the model a scientist uses to conduct an inquiry.

Nonlinear learning begins with the posing of a question. Then data and information are collected, and additional questions are generated that are related to the first question. At some point, there is an "aha!" or an insight. A new relationship is suddenly made possible that was not possible before. Nonlinear learning is not about small gradual steps but occurs as learning balance occurs when we ride a bicycle—one minute we cannot balance and then there is the breakthrough and now we know how to balance. Nonlinear training offers precise strategies that can enhance communication with someone who has cognitive deficits. Nonlinear learning is built on scientific communication that operates based on the verifiable facts. Nonlinear learning invites each person to examine all strategies for communication to be sure that problems are not occurring as a result of misinterpretation of the facts. The fact is that communication can occur without verbal language and fear does not need to be present. When cognitive deficits exist for a patient, the art and science of human interaction needs to be precise so that we are not talking in words that are not understandable to the patient. The important fact to note is what prejudgments we bring to our interaction with the patient. Are we in a stage of awe, sharing joy in the moment, or are we suffering because this person is "difficult?" The care and therapy provided to a person with cognitive disturbances needs to be created based on the facts of the moment and carried out in a state of gratitude, vulnerability, and nurturing for the staff and the patient.

A personal note: This chapter was written for my grandmother. She had depression and related cognitive disturbances following World War II. She gradually got worse and worse in her ability to remember new information, but she could hold my hand and show me how to feed the ducks. We were great friends. I helped her to remember to turn off the stove, and I remembered where she put her glasses. She could make sandwiches, and I could always find her comb. We were empowering each other. Over 15 years she gradually grew more and more helpless in the adult skills of life. Even then she could give great hugs and loved to sit and drink tea with me. I remember her as a very frail woman. I watched the nurse's aide tuck her in, kiss her on the cheek, and hold her hand while they said prayers. The aide hummed a familiar song as she left the room. It was like those familiar songs that come from our childhood, and they wrap us in a sense of warmth and love and safety—we declare that all is well with the world and we go to sleep and dream of peaceful things. It is important that all persons with cognitive losses have access to caregivers who are trained in precise strategies for communication with people like my grandmother. It is possible to live a gracious and secure existence even when cognition is diminished if the caregivers are committed to adapting the environment and its demands to match the capacity of the patient. The challenge for health care is designing training programs that truly prepare families and caregivers to be effective, empowering communicators. A nurse's aide or physical therapist or family member needs training to create the experience I have described for a person with cognitive deficits.

As a part of the rehabilitation program, caregiver training for this group of patients needs to emphasize reassurance, hands-on interventions, and communication to allow treatment to proceed at a pace perceived as reasonable by the patient.[53] In the early and middle stages of all dementias, physical therapy intervention usually can prolong the ability to move with ease in ADL and IADL and maintain the ability to participate in some social activities. This is extremely important for caregivers, as deficits in patients' abilities to perform ADL and IADL[125] often relate to their inability to physically perform these activities under supervision. The ability to walk is lost late in most dementias,[26, 40, 55] but gait and coordination disturbances are common and can benefit from physical therapy. Therapy intervention to assist the patient and train the caregivers involves facilitation of ease of movement and motor planning and developing or refining environmental and cognitive cues to assist in carrying out complex tasks. Ultimately, caregivers will need training in how to move, lift, and otherwise assist the patient.

Cognitive impairment is a key limiting factor in the performance of ADL and IADL, as well as a limiting factor for participating in rehabilitation. Accurate assessment and training by the therapist helps the caregiver provide only the help that is absolutely needed, with patients continuing to perform for themselves as many ADL as possible. For example, when brushing the teeth, the patient needs to be able to remember the command to brush, to recognize the toothbrush, and to perform a complex but repetitive motor action. The patient may only need the help of someone placing the toothbrush in his or her hand and slowly guiding it to the mouth to be able to safely brush the teeth.

The accurate assessment of IADL and ADL is more reliable than medical diagnosis for predicting the amount of assistance and interaction a person will need in a nursing home[72] (see Table 26–1 and Appendix 26–A). The first goal of rehabilitation for patients with dementia is to create a supportive emotional and physical environment. In other words, the environment must work actively to compensate for the patient's cognitive and functional losses as they occur. The ultimate goal is to help patients feel they are capable, so that they will continue to try to do those things for themselves that they can do safely, whether they remain in their home or live in an institution. It is equally important to orient and train significant others so that they feel comfortable allowing the patient to participate safely in activities and basic self-care tasks modified to their cognitive level.

The Alzheimer's Association ([800] 272-3900) is a resource for professionals and caregivers of people with dementia. The goals of the association are:

- To support research related to the diagnosis, therapy, cause, and cure of Alzheimer's disease and related disorders
- To aid in organizing family support groups; to educate and assist affected families
- To sponsor educational programs for professional and laypersons on the topic of Alzheimer's disease

- To advise government agencies of the needs of the affected families and to promote federal, state, and private support of research
- To offer help in any manner to patients and their caregivers to promote the well-being of all involved. Through the efforts of the Alzheimer's Association, it is hoped that humane care can be provided to the patient with dementia and related disorders throughout the course of the illness. Other support groups have been tried in communities where spouses have worked to develop ongoing respite care.[14]

As a member of the rehabilitation team, the physical or occupational therapist needs to conduct an inventory of services as a part of the annual review of the quality of care that is provided for patients with dementia. A survey of persons caring for patients with dementia listed the following services in their perceived order of importance[81, 83]:

1. A paid companion who can come to the home a few hours each week to give caregivers a rest (respite)
2. Assistance in locating people or organizations that provide patient care
3. Assistance in applying for government programs, such as Medicaid, disability insurance, and income support programs
4. A paid companion who can come to the home for overnight care so caregivers can go away for one or more days (respite)
5. Personal home care for the person with dementia to help with activities such as bathing, dressing, or feeding in the home
6. Support groups composed of others who are caring for persons with dementia and other cognitive deficits
7. Special nursing home care programs only for persons with dementia
8. Short-term respite care in nursing homes or hospitals to take care of persons with dementia and other cognitive deficits while the caregiver is away
9. Adult day care providing supervision and activities away from the home
10. Visiting nurse services for care at home

In-home care, information about the availability of services and government programs, and various forms of respite care were also ranked high in the survey. Overall, caregivers (family and friends) of the patient are often able and willing to provide care for the patient throughout the illness if appropriate professional consultation can help them cope with problematic situations and if adequate respite time is provided to the caregiver(s).

Not mentioned in this study was the need for psychological support for caregivers. The stress on caregivers is extreme, and symptoms of anxiety and depression are common. Because of the relative lack of counseling services for caregivers, however, the use of (and probable abuse of and dependence on) psychotropic medications by caregivers is high.[25, 77] As these medications may impair the cognitive functioning of caregivers, the risk of harm to the patient with dementia is also high.

DEMENTIA AND DELIRIUM—NEW FRONTIERS

Most current research in delirium and dementia is focused on Alzheimer's disease. Research is under way to explore possible causes of dementias, including work that examines the roles of neurotransmitters, structural brain changes, nutrition, viruses, drugs, immunological deficits, and the role of heredity in the etiology of Alzheimer's disease. Studies to increase the diagnostic accuracy of different dementias, including a distinction between cortical and subcortical dementias, or the use of DSM-III-R criteria,[5, 83] DSM-IV criteria,[4] or neuropsychological criteria, are also under way. Newer models of dementia, including that caused by stage II or III human immunodeficiency virus infection,[79] are also being studied.

The most exciting area of research is pharmacology[113] (see Chapters 6 and 32). The advent of tacrine, a drug that slows down the progression of Alzheimer's disease in some patients, has produced an explosion of research on drugs to try to stabilize or reverse the symptoms of this disease. Although no cures are available, some drugs, such as physostigmine, ondansetron, and nerve growth factor, have shown some promise. These studies have spawned a search for new drugs not only to treat Alzheimer's disease but to treat the symptoms of other dementias.

SUMMARY

In working with the patient with dementia or delirium, the therapist can do much to make the quality of life better for the patient and caregivers.[71] A thorough listing of the details needed to develop an environment and process of care for elderly persons with cognitive deficits can be found in other texts.[70, 71, 75]

Specific examples of modifications of physical and occupational therapy assessment and treatment may include working in collaboration with other members of the rehabilitation team and developing a consultative relationship with key caregivers (professional and nonprofessional, and all shifts of institutional staff) to encourage problem solving and patient participation in self-care. Another important modification includes the evaluation of each patient's communication abilities before the therapy assessment to adapt assessment in such a way as to promote patient participation.

Modifications of treatment include the use of neurological rehabilitation techniques (e.g., the Feldenkrais method, neurodevelopmental therapy, or Brunnstrom techniques). The rationale is to decrease the presence of abnormal muscle tone and to increase the ease of movement, to increase ease of breathing (to enhance endurance and minimize the related sense of anxiety) if the rib cage is carried with massive muscle tightness, and to increase patient coordination. The therapist needs to modify the process of neurological facilitation to enhance the patient's sense of safety and motivation for self-care within the security of a supervised environment. Tasks may need to be simplified so that the patient can perform them and the caregiver is trained to perform only those tasks that the patient cannot perform.

Each month the therapist, treatment team, patient, and caregiver need to identify safe physical activities that the patient can be encouraged to perform for recreation, relaxation, and overall fitness. The goal is to enhance the performance of simple ADL and IADL tasks (e.g., washing socks, setting the table) and this can enhance patient self-esteem. In addition, the physical therapist, along with other members of the rehabilitation team and caregivers, needs to monitor the patient for new signs and symptoms of a concurrent delirium or reversible dementia so that treatment can be initiated early and further deterioration prevented.

The Hospital Patients Bill of Rights and the Nursing Home Patients Bill of Rights define the minimum quality of care required for any patient. The concepts presented in the two bills apply to the care of patients with cognitive deficits, no matter what the setting. The provision of considerate and respectful care for the patient with de-

mentia or other cognitive deficits is possible and necessary. Well-planned and gentle care prevents unnecessary distortions in cognitive function brought on by feelings of fear or being rushed, and thereby maximizes all remaining cognitive function. To use his or her remaining emotional and cognitive resources, the patient with cognitive deficits needs to live in an environment and experience a process of care that is modified to meet the special needs created by delirium or dementia.

Physical and occupational therapy are key resources for the creation of a therapeutic environment and for the effective and timely assessment and treatment of the patient with cognitive deficits. The goal of therapy is to create a process of care where the patient feels safe and the caregivers are given training and support in problem solving so as to guide the patient to participate in self-care and recreation as long as it is safe and functionally possible.

CASE STUDIES

CASE 26–1   THE COMPLEXITY OF AGING

The patient was a 78-year-old woman who had the following deficits on the Mini-Mental State Examination: was not aware of where she lived, date or year, had poor short-term memory and could not spell the word "world" backward, could not copy the two overlapping pentagons. The patient was generally happy and enjoyed having someone sit with her. The patient fractured her femur and because of the location of the fracture site, a surgical procedure was performed to allow total weight-bearing. The surgeon and the psychiatrist decided that partial weight-bearing would not be a concept that the patient could understand. The physical therapist and assistant worked together with the family and caregivers in the nursing home to develop a plan of care. At the initial care conference, the big question was whether the patient should receive physical therapy. The family was fearful that the patient would fall again if she were taught how to walk. The focus of the conference was to educate the family and other staff as to the importance of physical therapy so the patient could learn how to participate in and eventually perform transfers from wheelchair to toilet as well as to bed. The decision was made to begin physical therapy, with the initial goal being to achieve all functional ADL transfers with standby physical assistance.

The patient was not interested in walking and was fearful of falling. The key change in physical therapy intervention was in the style of communication that was used to teach basic bed mobility and the components of transfer skills. Using trial and error, it was found that the patient responded best to a smile, verbal encouragement, hand signals, and gentle manual pressure to indicate the

desired task to be performed. If the task was broken down and components were identified, the patient became frustrated and refused to participate. If the patient was invited by manual cues and verbal reassurance to stand up and sit on the bed, the patient would hesitate for up to 1 minute and then she would attempt to perform the task. It became obvious that the patient needed at least 30 to 60 seconds of waiting time between verbal requests given by staff and when she was ready to act on the request. It was also discovered that if additional time were given, the patient appeared to get frustrated and would refuse to cooperate. A sign was placed over her bed with instructions for communication: smile, reassure, use your hands to guide her to perform the desired action, and wait 60 seconds; let her feel there is plenty of time.

A sliding board was introduced in therapy, and the patient enjoyed the idea. The board allowed transfers for all ADL to involve no lifting for the staff. The patient would lean her head on the shoulder of the staff member while sitting and then she would assist in sliding across on the board. All transfers for ADL using the sliding board were possible within five visits of physical therapy. A bed was located that was 17 inches high to facilitate bed-to-wheelchair transfers. The bed could be raised to assist the nursing aide in cleaning activities. The decision was made to leave the bed at 17 inches unless the nursing staff needed to perform special in-bed procedures with the patient. The wheelchair foot rests were modified so that they formed a solid flat surface to allow the patient to rest in a natural position. The patient was only 5'2" tall and the standard wheelchair only allowed her to comfortably put both feet on

Continued

CASE 26–1   THE COMPLEXITY OF AGING *Continued*

one foot pedal and sit with her weight mostly on one buttock. A smaller wheelchair and the adapted footrest gave the patient an equal pressure on both sitting bones, and the patient began to sit at rest in a natural upright posture. The other goal of physical therapy was to teach the patient wheelchair mobility using her hands to push the chair. Once the patient was given gloves for her hands (she did not like germs), she was willing to try to push the wheelchair. The patient was instructed in the physical therapy department during two visits. The patient was next seen by the therapist on the unit to allow the nurse's aide to be a part of the physical therapy instruction. The rationale was that the nurse's aide would need to help reinforce the skills and encourage practice of wheelchair mobility skills as a part of daily activities. During the last visits the physical therapist watched daytime, afternoon, and evening staff practice with the patient and problem-solve new situations that arose. It is critical to train all caregivers on three shifts to ensure consistency of verbal and manual cuing for the patient.

Before discharge to restorative nursing, the patient's current level of functional abilities was documented using an ADL chart that specified time of day when tasks were easiest, task(s), equipment needs, special positioning, clothing and other assistive devices, verbal cuing, and other communication requirements for each critical task that had been mastered in physical therapy. The cataloging of functional skills reminded the nurse's aide of the ingredients involved in order for the patient to

successfully perform ADL. The other advantage of the detailed discharge summary to the nursing staff is that new staff could use the document and, as needed, contact physical therapy for clarifications if the patient suddenly were not able to perform the tasks (a signal of possible medical or psychosocial problems).

Key points:

1. Common goals were identified and agreed on between all team members and the patient's significant others.
2. Education was provided as needed to allow for consistency of verbal and manual cuing to the patient.
3. Physical therapy treatment began in a quiet, undisturbed area where the patient could concentrate. As mastery of a skill was achieved, the skill was practiced with supervision and instruction of other staff was provided as needed.
4. Equipment and furniture were adjusted to help the patient perform tasks with minimal assistance.
5. Discharge from therapy involved providing nursing staff with a detailed description of functional abilities and the conditions required to help maximize patient participation, sense of safety, and control (as had already been reviewed with all aides working with patient).
6. The physical therapist was designated as a resource person for nursing staff for simplifying functional tasks in patient care, problem solving, communication, and movement-related issues.

CASE 26–2   A CLIENT IN THE EARLY STAGE OF ALZHEIMER'S DISEASE

The patient was a 64-year-old man who until 1 month ago was working. He was forced to retire because he would forget the natural sequences of the work tasks. For example his partner would see him direct someone to wait for him in the waiting room and then he would forget the person was in the waiting room. On the Mini-Mental State Examination, he had difficulty with date and year and would try to redirect the question in an apparent attempt to cover up for loss of short-term memory. He could or would not spell the word "world" backward, and he poorly copied the overlapping hexagons (looked more like squares). He was a runner but now he apparently could not remember how to get home, and he would pretend to be hurt and get someone to drive him home. The man reported feeling restless.

The patient, his wife, and two sons were seen by the team at a psychiatric clinic. The wife was very upset and the family was asking for help. The

role of therapy at this early stage of Alzheimer's disease involved:

1. a. Functional assessment of basic ADL/IADL and home assessment:
   b. Orientation of spouse/significant caregivers as to the functional changes that may occur in the near future and how to compensate for current functional losses (e.g., patient had difficulty dressing in the morning and would get frustrated).
2. Orientation to the role of physical therapy in hands-on treatment related to techniques to help the patient relax. After initial evaluation, it was decided to teach caregivers massage techniques identified by the therapist as soothing and relaxing for the patient. *Note:* The emphasis in the hands-on intervention is to create slow, predictable, and nurturing contact that is perceived by the patient as soothing and relaxing.

Continued

CASE 26–2   A CLIENT IN THE EARLY STAGE OF ALZHEIMER'S DISEASE *Continued*

3. Orientation of caregivers to the use of manual contact and hand signals to communicate and reinforce the intention. Kinesthetic contact and the ability to follow kinesthetic cues can help the patient with ADL tasks at home. At this time the kinesthetic cuing may not be critical for the patient, but the caregivers need to get in the habit of cuing the patients as a compensatory tool for future cognitive losses.

4. Orientation of caregivers to the benefits of a ritualized schedule of daily events for the patient and assistance in developing the daily schedule. The predictability of the ritual will help the patient feel safe and in control. The ritualizing is especially helpful to address the frustrations with dressing in the morning.

5. Written information about local support groups, day treatment centers, and the availability of the rehabilitation team, including therapy for problem solving.

6. Participation in evaluation of patient/family need for placement in a day treatment center or use of a home health aide. Supervision was needed for cooking (would leave burners on), working in the woodshop (would leave power tools running), and in self-care to ensure his safety. It was decided to use supervision in the home with family members sharing the load. The idea of going to a new place was not positively received by the patient. *Note:* The patient may function better in the environment where he or she has lived for a long time owing to the familiarity with the details of the surroundings.

7. The therapist participated in development of the home care plan and provided for home visits to accomplish tasks described in numbers 1 to 6.

The next contact that the family made with therapy was 1 month later to address the patient's inability to settle down and be able to go to sleep at night. A home visit was made to evaluate the bedtime ritual, the relaxation strategies being used, and communication with the physician about current medications taken. It became obvious that the patient disliked bathing and undressing for bed. After discussion with caregivers the patient was allowed to go to bed in his clothes without bathing and undressing (bathing and undressing would be carried out in the morning when he was less tired). Relaxation massage was modified to involve the face, neck, hands, and feet, and the caregivers were instructed and practiced during two visits under the supervision of the therapist. A satisfactory bedtime ritual was developed and home health care was workable for the patient and the caregivers.

The next request for therapy consultation came 4 months later when the wife and the daughter-in-law (who had been taking turns being the primary caregiver) both felt the need to hire and train an attendant/companion for the patient for 8 hours a day. At this time the patient preferred to be in the home, walk in the yard, or take long walks in the local park. The therapist, in cooperation with other team members, trained the patient and aide in how to sequence for ease in ADL tasks; use of kinesthetic cuing; how to problem-solve ADL, bathing and dressing, using a slow pace and ritualized format; and sequencing the tasks and relaxation techniques to help the patient settle down and go to sleep. Foot massage was the only technique that the patient now allowed and appeared to enjoy. After three physical therapy visits over a 2-week period, the attendant was able to carry out home health care effectively for the patient.

The last request for help occurred when the family was concerned because the patient was trying to run away. The therapist made a home visit and found that the patient sat most of the day. The Mini-Mental State Examination showed that he could not give his own first or last name and had no short-term memory. Based on the evaluation, it was proposed that the family/attendant go with the patient for a walk when the patient showed an interest in leaving the house. This strategy worked for a few months but then the patient began to sit down on the sidewalk when he was tired. Another visit was made after a wheelchair was ordered to train the caregivers in use of the wheelchair and to orient the patient to the desired procedures and to reassure the patient. After this visit the patient showed gradually less interest in leaving the home over the next few months until he eventually stayed in the house constantly. At this time the patient also became incontinent of bowel and bladder. The patient refused to use the toilet and the decision was made to seek nursing home placement.

Key points:

1. Physical therapy is a part of the caregiving team for the patient and family of the patient with Alzheimer's disease.

2. Evaluation of functional skills, communication related to functional skills, and home modifications to enhance patient participation in self-care can be continued as long as the caregivers request support and problem solving.

3. Problem solving with caregivers and educating caregivers are the primary roles once the therapist has identified the intervention of choice to solve the key functional problems.

4. All therapy intervention needs to be coordinated with actions of other members of the caregiving team.

REFERENCES

1. Agate J: The Practice of Geriatrics, 2nd ed. London, Heinemann, 1970.
2. Allison RS: The Senile Brain. London. Edward Arnold, 1962.
3. Alzheimer A: Über eine eigenartige Erkrankung der Hirnrinde Allgemeine Psychiatrie Psychisch Gerichtl Med 64:146–148, 1907.
4. American Psychiatric Association: Delirium, dementia, amnestic and other cognitive disorders. In DSM-IV Draft Criteria. Washington, DC, American Psychiatric Association, 1993.
5. American Psychiatric Association: Organic mental syndromes and disorders. In Diagnostic and Statistical Manual of Mental Disorders, ed 3, revised. Washington, DC, American Psychiatric Association, 1987.
6. Arenberg D: Concept problem solving in young and old adults. J Gerontol 23:279–282, 1968.
7. Arenberg D, Robertson-Tchabo EA: Learning and aging. In Birren JE, Schaie KW (eds): Handbook of the Psychology of Aging. New York, Van Nostrand Reinhold, 1977.
8. Bandler R, Grinder J: Frogs into Princes. Cupertino, CA, Real People Press, 1979.
9. Barclay LL, et al: Survival in Alzheimer's disease and vascular dementias. Neurology 35:834–840, 1985.
10. Bassi CJ, et al: Vision in patients with Alzheimer's disease. Optom Vis Sci 70:809–813, 1993.
11. Birren JE: Handbook of Aging and the Individual. Chicago, University of Chicago Press, 1973.
12. Bolla-Wilson K, et al: Lateralization of dementia of depression in stroke patients. Am J Psychol 146:627–634, 1989.
13. Botwinick J: Aging and Behavior—A Comprehensive Integration of Research Findings. New York, Springer-Verlag, 1978.
14. Brache CI: The aging client and their family network. In Jackson O (ed): Physical Therapy of the Geriatric Patient. New York, Churchill Livingstone, 1983.
15. Braekhus A, et al: The Mini-Mental State Examination: Identifying the most efficient variables for detecting cognitive impairment in the elderly. J Am Geriatr Soc 40:1139–1145, 1992.
16. Brocklehurst JC: Textbook of Geriatric Medicine and Gerontology, 2nd ed. New York, Churchill Livingstone, 1985.
17. Brody H, Vijayashankar N: Anatomical changes in the nervous system. In Finch CE, Hayflick L (ed): Handbook of the Biology of Aging. New York, Van Nostrand Reinhold, 1977.
18. Busse EW, Pfeiffer E (eds): Mental Illness in Later Life. Washington, DC, American Psychiatric Association, 1973.
19. Calhoun RO, Gounard BR: Meaningfulness, presentation rate, list length and age in elderly adults paired association learning. J Educ Gerontol 4:49–56, 1979.
20. Campbell ME: Study of the attitudes of nursing personnel toward the geriatric patient. Nurs Res 20:141–151, 1971.
21. Carroll K (ed): Human Development in Aging—Compensation for Sensory Loss. Minneapolis, Ebenezer Center for Aging and Human Development, 1978.
22. Cattell RB: Theory of fluid and crystallized intelligence—a clinical experiment. J Educ Psychol 54:1–22, 1963.
23. Cerella J: Aging and information-processing rate. In Birren JE, Schaie KW (ed): Handbook of the Psychology of Aging, 3rd ed. San Diego, Academic Press, 1990.
24. Charatan FB: Management of Confusion in the Elderly. New York, Roerig, 1979.
25. Clipp EC, George LK: Psychotropic drug use among caregivers of patients with dementia. J Am Geriatr Soc 38:227–235, 1990.
26. Coons D, et al: Final report of project on Alzheimer's disease: Subjective experience of families. Ann Arbor, MI. Institute of Gerontology, 1983.
27. Craik IM: Age differences in human memory. In Birren JE, Schaie KW (ed): Handbook of the Psychology of Aging, New York, Van Nostrand Reinhold, 1977.
28. Elias MF, Elias PK: Motivation and activity. In Birren JE, Schaie KW (eds): Handbook of the Psychology of Aging. New York, Van Nostrand Reinhold, 1977.
29. Epstein DM: The Twelve Stages of Healing. San Rafael, CA, Amber-Allen, 1994.
30. Evans DA, et al: Prevalence of Alzheimer's disease in a community population of older persons: Higher than previously reported. JAMA 262:2551–2556, 1989.
31. Feldenkrais M: Awareness Through Movement. New York, Harper & Row, 1972.
32. Feldenkrais M: On Health. OR Feldenkrais Guild, 1979.
33. Feldenkrais M: The Elder Citizen. Berkeley, CA, Feldenkrais Resources, 1989. (Pamphlet and audio-cassette tapes.)
34. Fields WS (ed): Neurological and Sensory Disorders in the Elderly. New York, Stratton Intercontinental, 1975.
35. Foley JM: Sensation and behavior. In Fields WS (ed): Neurological and Sensory Disorders in the Elderly. New York, Stratton Intercontinental, 1975.
36. Folstein MF, et al: Mini-Mental State—a practical method for grading the cognitive state of patients for the clinician. J Psychiatr Res 12:189–198, 1975.
37. Folstein MF, et al: The meaning of cognitive impairment in the elderly. J Am Geriatr Soc 33:228–235, 1985.
38. Fozard JL: Vision and hearing in aging. In Birren JE, Schaie KW (ed): Handbook of the Psychology of Aging, 3rd ed. San Diego, Academic Press, 1990.
39. Galesko D, et al: The MMSE in the early diagnosis of disease. Arch Neurol 47:49–52, 1990.
40. George LK: The Dynamics of Caregiver Burden. Washington, DC, Association of Retired Person–Andrus Foundation, 1984.
41. Gobetz GE: Learning Mobility in Blind Children and the Geriatric Blind. Cleveland, Cleveland Society for the Blind, 1967.
42. Gobetz GE, et al: Home Teaching of the Geriatric Blind. Cleveland, Cleveland Society for the Blind, 1969.
43. Grant I, Adams K (ed): Neuropsychological Assessment of Neuropsychic Disorders. New York, Oxford University Press, 1986.
44. Gross AM: Preventing institutionalization of elderly blind. Vis Impairment Blindness 2:49–53, 1979.
45. Grossberg GT, et al: Diagnosis of depression in demented patients. In Morely JE, et al (eds): Memory Functioning and Aging-Related Disorders. New York, Springer-Verlag, 1992.
46. Gunter LM: Student attitudes toward geriatric nursing. Nurs Outlook 19:466–469, 1971.
47. Hall GR: When traditional care falls short: Caring for people with atypical presentations of cortical dementia. Gerontol Nurs 25:22–32, 54–55, 1999.
48. Hertzog C, Schaie KW: Stability and change in adult intelligence: Simultaneous analysis of longitudinal means and covariance structures. Psychol Aging 3:122–130, 1988.
49. Holmes TH, Rahe RH: The social readjustment rating scale. J Psychosom Res 11:213–218, 1967.
50. Hultsch DF, Dixon RA: Learning and memory in aging. In Birren JE, Schaie KW (eds): Handbook of the Psychology of Aging, 3rd ed. San Diego, Academic Press, 1990.
51. Jackson JE, Ramsdell JW: Use of the MMSE to screen for dementia in elderly outpatients. J Am Geriatr Soc 36:662, 1988.
52. Jackson O: Physical Therapy and the Geriatrics Patient—A Descriptive Study of Cross-Cultural Trends in Denmark and the United States, thesis. Ann Arbor, University of Michigan, 1979.
53. Jackson O: Physical Therapy and the Geriatric Patient. New York, Churchill Livingstone, 1987.
54. Jung R, Solomon K: Psychiatric manifestations of Pick's disease. Int Psychogeriatr 5:187–202, 1993.
55. Katzman R: Clinical presentation of the course of Alzheimer's disease: The atypical patient. In Rose CF (ed): Modern Approaches to the Dementias, pt 2. Basel, Switzerland, Karger, 1985.
56. Katzman R: Alzheimer's disease. N Engl J Med 314:964–973, 1986.
57. Kay DWK, et al: Old age mental disorders in Newcastle-Upon-Tyne: A study of prevalence. Br J Psychol 110:146–158, 1964.
58. Kay DWK, et al: The differentiation of paranoid from affective psychoses by patient's premorbid characteristics. Br J Psychiatry 129:207–215, 1976.
59. Knox AB: Adult Development and Learning. San Francisco, Jossey-Bass, 1977.
60. Krishnan KRR: Neuroanatomic substrates of depression in the elderly. J Geriatr Psychiatry Neurol 6:39–58, 1993.
61. Lang R, Jackson O: Model Demonstration of a Comprehensive Care System for Older People. Project Grant No. 90-A-1618, Washington, DC, Administration of Aging, 1980.
62. LeClerc CM, Wells DL: Use of a content methodology process to enhance feeding abilities threatened by ideational apraxia in people with Alzheimer's-type dementia. Geriatr Nurs 19:261–268, 1998.

63. Leighton DA: Special senses—aging of the eye. *In* Brocklehurst JC (ed): Textbook of Geriatric Medicine and Gerontology. New York, Churchill Livingstone, 1985.

64. Levinson AJ (ed): Neuropsychiatric Side Effects of Drugs in the Elderly. New York, Raven Press, 1979.

65. Libow LS: Pseudo-senility: Acute and reversible organic brain syndromes. J Am Geriatr Soc 21:112–120, 1973.

66. Licht S: Therapeutic Heat and Cold. New Haven, CT, Elizabeth Licht, 1960.

67. Light LA: Interactions between memory and language in old age. *In* Birren JE, Schaie KW(ed): Handbook of the Psychology of Aging, 3rd ed. San Diego, Academic Press, 1990.

68. Lipowski ZJ: Delirium (acute confusional states). JAMA 258:1789–1792, 1987.

69. Lipowski ZJ: Delirium in the elderly. N Engl J Med 320:578–582, 1989.

70. Mace NL (ed): Dementia Care: Patient, Family, and Community. Baltimore, Johns Hopkins University Press, 1990.

71. Mace NL, Rabins PV: The 36 Hour Day—A Family Guide to Caring for Persons with Alzheimer's Disease, Related Dementing Diseases and Memory Loss in Later Life. Baltimore, Johns Hopkins University Press, 1981.

72. Mahoney FI, Barthel DW: Functional evaluation: The Barthel Index. Md State Med J 14:63, 1965.

73. Manepalli J, Grossberg GT: Recognition and treatment of depression. *In* Szwabo PA, Grossberg GT (eds): Problem Behaviors in Long-Term Care: Recognition, Diagnosis, and Treatment. New York, Springer-Verlag, 1993.

74. May BJ: An Integrated Problem Solving Curriculum for Physical Therapists. Washington, DC, American Physical Therapy Association, 1976.

75. McDowell FH (ed): Managing the Person with Intellectual Loss (Dementia or Alzheimer's Disease) at Home. White Plains, NY, Burke Rehabilitation Center, 1980.

76. McKahann G, et al: Clinical diagnosis of Alzheimer's disease. Neurology 34:939–944, 1984.

77. Meyers BS, Cahenzli CT: Psychotropics in the extended care facility. *In* Szwabo PA, Grossberg GT (eds): Problem Behaviors in Long-Term Care: Recognition, Diagnosis, and Treatment. New York, Springer-Verlag, 1993.

78. Mintzer JE, et al: Effectiveness of a continuum of care using brief and partial hospitalization for agitated dementia patients. Psychiatr Serv 48:1435–1439, 1997.

79. Morgan MK, et al: AIDS-related dementia: A case report of rapid cognitive decline. Psychology 44:1024–1028, 1988.

80. Nissen T, et al: Dementia evaluated by means of the Mini-Mental State Examination—clinical neurological patient material. Tidsskr Nor Laegeforen 109:1158–1162, 1989.

81. Office of Technology Assessment, U.S. Congress, Congressional Summary: Losing a million minds: Confronting the Tragedy of Alzheimer's disease and other dementias. OTA-BA-324. Washington, DC, Superintendent of Documents, US Government Printing Office, 1990.

82. Peterson D, Orgren RA: Older adult learning. *In* Jackson O (ed): Physical Therapy of the Geriatric Patient. New York, Churchill Livingstone, 1983.

83. Rabins PV, et al: Emotional adaptation over time in care-givers for chronically ill elderly people. Age Aging 19:185–190, 1990.

84. Rebok GW, Folstein MF: Dementia. Neuropsychiatry 5:265–276, 1993.

85. Reichel W (ed): Clinical Aspects of Aging. Baltimore, Williams & Wilkins, 1978.

86. Reisberg B: Clinical presentation, diagnosis, and symptomatology of age-associated cognitive decline and Alzheimer's disease. *In* Reisberg B (ed): Alzheimer's Disease: The Standard Reference. New York, Free Press, 1983.

87. Reisberg B, et al: The Global Deterioration Scale (GDS): An instrument for the assessment of primary degenerative dementia (PDD). Am J Psychiatry 139:1136–1139, 1982.

88. Robinson RG, et al: Mood disorders in stroke patients. Brain 107:81–93, 1984.

89. Rodstein M: Characteristics of nonfatal myocardial infarction in the aged. Arch Intern Med 98:84–90, 1956.

90. Ross E: Effect of challenging and supportive instructions in verbal learning in older persons. J Educ Psychol 58:261–266, 1968.

91. Salzman C, et al: Cognitive improvement following benzodiazepine discontinuation in elderly nursing home residents. Int J Geriatr Psychiatry 7:89–93, 1992.

92. Savelkoul M et al: Behavior and behavioral determinants in the management of demented people in residential homes. Patient Educ Counseling 34:33–42, 1998.

93. Schaie KW: Intellectual development in adulthood. *In* Birren JE, Schaie KW (eds): Handbook of the Psychology of Aging, 3rd ed. San Diego, Academic Press, 1990.

94. Selye H: Stress without Distress. New York, JB Lippincott, 1974.

95. Shakespeare: As You Like It, 3,1.

96. Simonton DK: Creativity and wisdom in aging. *In* Birren JE, Schaie KW (eds): Handbook of the Psychology of Aging, 3rd ed. San Diego, Academic Press, 1990.

97. Sky AJ, Grossberg GT: Aggressive behaviors and chemical restraints. *In* Szwabo PA, Grossberg GT (eds). Problem Behaviors in Long-Term Care: Recognition, Diagnosis, and Treatment. New York, Springer-Verlag, 1993.

98. Solomon K: The depressed patient: Social antecedents of psychopathologic changes in the elderly. J Am Geriatr Soc 29:297–301, 1981.

99. Solomon K: The elderly patient. *In* Spittel JA Jr (ed): Clinical Medicine, vol 12. Hagerstown, MD, Harper & Row, 1981.

100. Solomon K: The older man. *In* Solomon K, Levy NB (eds): Men in Transition: Theory and Therapy. New York, Plenum, 1982.

101. Solomon K: Social antecedents of learned helplessness in the health care setting. Gerontologist 22:282–287, 1982.

102. Solomon K: The subjective experience of the Alzheimer's patient. Geriatr Consult 1:22–24, 1982.

103. Solomon K: Psychosocial dysfunction in the aged: Assessment and intervention. *In* Jackson OL (ed): Physical Therapy of the Geriatric Patient, 2nd ed. New York, Churchill Livingstone, 1989.

104. Solomon K: Learned helplessness in the elderly: Theoretic and clinical implications. Occup Ther Ment Health 10:31–51, 1990.

105. Solomon K: Mental health and the elderly. *In* Monk A (ed): Handbook of Gerontological Services, 2nd ed. New York, Columbia University Press, 1990.

106. Solomon K: Behavioral and psychotherapeutic interventions in the nursing home. *In* Szwabo PA, Grossberg GT (eds): Problem Behaviors in Long-Term Care: Recognition, Diagnosis, and Treatment. New York, Springer-Verlag, 1993.

107. Solomon K, Shackson JB: Substance use disorders in nursing home patients. *In* Reichman WE, Katz PR (eds): Psychiatric Care in the Nursing Home. New York, Oxford University Press, in press.

108. Solomon K, Stark S: Comparison of older and younger alcoholics and prescription drug abusers: History and clinical presentation. Clin Gerontol 12:41–56, 1993.

109. Solomon K, Szwabo P: Psychotherapy for patients with dementia. *In* Morley JE, et al (eds): Memory functioning and aging related disorders. New York, Springer Publishing, 1992.

110. Solomon K, Vickers R: Attitudes of health workers toward old people. J Am Geriatr Soc 27:186–191, 1979.

111. Solomon K, et al: Alcoholism and prescription drug abuse in the elderly: St. Louis University Grand Rounds. J Am Geriatr Soc 41:57–69, 1993.

112. Solomon P: Sensory Deprivation. Cambridge, MA, Harvard University Press, 1961.

113. Spirduso WW, MacRae PG: Motor performance and aging. *In* Birren JE, Schaie KW (eds): Handbook of the Psychology of Aging, 3rd ed. San Diego, Academic Press, 1990.

114. Statistical abstract of the United States, 110th ed. Washington, DC, US Bureau of the Census, 1990.

115. Stern RG, Davis KL: Treatment approaches in Alzheimer's disease: Past, present, and future. *In* Weiner MF (ed): The Dementias: Diagnosis and Management. Washington, DC, American Psychiatric Press, 1991.

116. Sunderland T, et al: A new scale for the assessment of depressed mood in demented patients. Am J Psychiatry 145:955–959, 1988.

117. Vander Camman TJM, et al: Value of the Mini-Mental State Examination and informants' data for the detection of dementia in geriatric outpatients. Psychol Rep 71:1003–1009, 1992.

118. Wang HS: Special diagnostic procedures—the evaluation of brain impairment. *In* Busse EW, Pfeiffer E (eds): Mental Illness in Later Life. Washington, DC, American Psychiatric Association, 1973.

119. Wilder J: Basimetric approach (law of initial value) to biological rhythms. Ann N Y Acad Sci 98:1211–1220, 1968.
120. Wilder J: Basimetric approach to psychiatry. *In* Arieti S (ed): American Handbook of Psychiatry. New York, Basic Books, 1966.
121. Wilder J: Stimulus and response: The law of initial value. Bristol, UK, John Wright & Sons, 1967.
122. No reference cited.
123. Winograd CH, Jarvik LF: Physician management of the demented patient. J Am Geriatr Soc 34:295–308, 1986.
124. Worden H: Aging and blindness. New Outlook Blind 70:433–437, 1976.
125. Yankelovich, Shelley, and White, Inc: Caregivers of patients with dementia. Washington, DC, Office of Technology Assessment, 1986.
126. Yesavage JA, et al: The Geriatric Depression Rating Scale: Comparison with other self-report and psychiatric rating scales. *In* Crook T, et al (eds): Assessment in Geriatric Psychopharmacology. New Canaan, CT, Mark Powley Associates, 1983.

Rating Guidelines for Barthel Index*

1. Feeding

    10 = Independent. The patient can feed himself or herself a meal when someone puts the food within reach. Patient must put on an assistive device if this is needed to cut up the food alone. The patient must accomplish this in a reasonable time.

    5 = Some help is necessary (with cutting up food, etc., as listed above).

2. Moving from wheelchair to bed and return

    15 = Independent in all phases of this activity. Patient can safely approach the bed in the wheelchair, lock brakes, lift footrests, move safely to bed, lie down, come to a sitting position in the wheelchair, if necessary, to transfer back into it safely, and return to the wheelchair.

    10 = Either some minimal help is needed in some step of this activity or the patient needs to be reminded or supervised for safety of one or more parts of this activity.

    5 = Patient can come to a sitting position without the help of a second person but needs to be lifted out of bed, or if he or she transfers only with a great deal of help.

3. Doing personal toilet

    5 = Patient can wash hands and face, comb hair, clean teeth, and shave. He may use any kind of razor but must put in blade or plug in razor without help as well as get it from drawer or cabinet. Female patients must put on own makeup.

4. Getting on and off toilet

    10 = Patient is able to get on and off toilet, fasten and unfasten clothes, prevent soiling of clothes, and use toilet paper without help. If it is necessary to use a bedpan instead of a toilet, patient must be able to place it on a chair, empty it, and clean it.

    5 = Patient needs help because of imbalance or in handling clothes or in using toilet paper.

5. Bathing self

    5 = Patient may use a bathtub or a shower, or take a complete sponge bath. Patient must be able to do all the steps involved in whichever method is employed without another person being present.

6. Walking on a level surface

    15 = Patient can walk at least 50 yards without help or supervision. Patient may wear braces or prostheses and use crutches, canes, or a walkerette but not a rolling walker. Patient must be able to lock and unlock braces, if used, assume the standing position and sit down, get the necessary mechanical aids into position for use, and dispose of them when sitting. (Putting on and taking off braces is scored under dressing.)

    10 = Patient needs help or supervision in any of the above but can walk at least 50 yards with a little help.

6a. Propelling a wheelchair

    5 = If a patient cannot ambulate but can propel a wheelchair independently. Must be able to go around corners, turn around, maneuver the chair to a table, bed, toilet, etc. Must be able to push a chair at least 50 yards. Do not score this item if the patient gets score for walking.

7. Ascending and descending stairs

    10 = Patient is able to go up and down a flight of stairs safely without help or supervision. Patient may and should use handrails, canes, or crutches when needed. Must be able to carry canes or crutches when ascending or descending stairs.

    5 = Patient needs help with or supervision of any one of the above items.

8. Dressing and undressing

    10 = Patient is able to put on and remove and fasten all clothing, as well as tie shoelaces (unless it is necessary to use adaptations for this). The activity includes putting on and removing and fastening corset or braces when these are prescribed.

    5 = Patient needs help in putting on and removing or fastening any clothing. Patient must do at least half the work himself. Patient must accomplish this in a reasonable time. Women need not be scored on use of a brassiere or girdle unless these are prescribed garments.

9. Continence of bowels

    10 = Patient is able to control bowels and have no accidents. Can use a suppository or take an enema when necessary.

    5 = Patient needs help in using a suppository or taking an enema or has occasional accidents.

10. Controlling bladder

    10 = Patient is able to control his or her bladder day and night. Patients who wear an external device and leg bag must put them on independently, clean and empty bag, and stay dry day and night.

    5 = Patient has occasional accidents or cannot wait for the bedpan or get to the toilet in time or needs help with an external device.

---

*A score of 0 is given in the activity when the patient cannot meet the criteria as defined.

Modified from Mahoney FI, Barthel DW: Functional evaluation: The Barthel Index. Md State Med J 14:63, 1965.

SECTION III

Neurological Disorders and Applications Issues

Disorders of Vision and Visual-Perceptual Dysfunction

LAURIE E. CHAIKIN, MS, OTR, OD

Key Words

- anatomy of the eye

- eye diseases

- functional visual skills

- refractive error

- strabismus

- treatment

- visual perceptual dysfunction

- visual screening

Objectives

After reading this chapter the student/therapist will:

1. Understand visual anatomy and physiology as they pertain to visual function.

2. Understand the functional visual skills and how visual dysfunction may affect functional performance.

3. Understand the symptoms of visual dysfunction.

4. Develop ability to take a visual case history using behaviors and clinical observations.

5. Understand the difference between phoria and strabismus.

6. Understand the difference between visual field loss and unilateral neglect.

7. Be familiar with various pediatric and age-related disease conditions that may affect vision.

8. Learn nonoptical, and be familiar with optical, adaptations for patients with low vision.

9. Understand basic tools for vision screening.

10. Understand when to refer and document.

Vision is an integral part of development of perception. Some aspects of vision such as pupillary function are innate, but many other aspects are stimulated to develop by experience and interaction with the environment. Visual acuity itself has been demonstrated to rely on the presence of a clear image focused on the retina. If this does not occur, a "lazy eye," or amblyopia, will result. Depth perception develops as a result of precise eye alignment and will not occur unless eye alignment is corrected within the first 7 years of life. Research has demonstrated that, in fact, most visual skills such as acuity, binocular coordination, accommodation, ocular motilities, and depth perception are largely intact by age 6 months to 1 year.[56] Visual skill development parallels postural reflex integration and provides a foundation for perception.

Early in infancy visual input is associated with olfactory, tactile, vestibular, and proprioceptive sensations. The infant is driven to touch, taste, smell, and manipulate what he or she sees. Primitive postural reflexes such as the asymmetrical tonic neck reflex help to provide visual regard and attention.

At some point the young child is able to look at an object and determine both the texture and the shape without having to touch or taste it. In adults, vision has moved to the top of the sensory hierarchy, providing full multisensory associations from sight alone. Even the visualized image of eating an apple can re-create the smell, sound of crunching, taste, and feel of the experience.

Early visual impairment and later acquired impairment can affect the quality of the image presented to the brain and thus affect the learning process. In addition, damage to association centers involved with spatial perception, figure-ground, and directionality can interfere with learning and performance. It is important, therefore, to isolate the primary visual processes of seeing from the secondary or associational processes of perceiving in the evaluation of perceptual disorders. The identification of a vision problem becomes part of the differential diagnosis of a perceptual deficit. Visual screening must be done before perceptual evaluation so that visual problems do not bias or contaminate the perceptual testing. It is just as important to eliminate vision as a contributing factor to a perceptual problem as it is to find a possible vision problem.

ANATOMY OF THE EYE

An operational analogy of the eye as a camera may be useful up to a point in understanding the physical function of the structures. Once the image hits the retina and image enhancement begins, however, metaphors change to match our ever-changing comprehension of brain function.

Eye Chamber and Lens

Structures and function are discussed from anterior to posterior (Fig. 27–1). The first structure that light hits after it is reflected from an image is the cornea. Corneal tissue is completely transparent. Light is refracted, or bent, to the greatest degree by the cornea, because the light rays must pass through different media, which change in density, as in going from air to water.[42] One can observe the refraction of light by observing how a stick when placed into water appears bent where it enters the water (Fig. 27–2).

Damage to the cornea from abrasions, burns, or congenital or disease-related processes can alter the spherical shape of the cornea and disturb the quality of the image that falls on the retina. In keratoconus, the cornea slowly becomes steeper and more cone-shaped, distorting the image and causing reduced vision.[41]

Iris

Behind the cornea is the iris, or colored portion, which consists of fibers that control the opening of the pupil, the dark circular opening in the center of the eye. The constriction and dilation of the pupil controls the amount of light entering the eye in a similar fashion to the way the F stop on a camera changes the size of the aperture

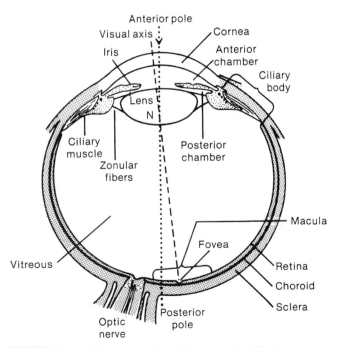

FIGURE 27–1. Horizontal section of the eye. (Modified from Wolff E: Anatomy of the Eye and Orbit, 7th ed. London, HK Lewis & Co, 1976.)

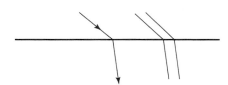

FIGURE 27–2. Refraction: bending of light at air/water interface.

to control the amount of light and depth of field.[22] Under bright light conditions the opening constricts, and under dim light conditions it dilates, allowing light in to stimulate the photoreceptor cells of the retina. This constriction and dilation are under autonomic nervous system (ANS) control with both sympathetic and parasympathetic components.[50] Under conditions of sympathetic stimulation (fight or flight) the pupils dilate, perhaps giving rise to the expression "eyes wide with fear." Under parasympathetic stimulation the pupils constrict. The effect of drugs that stimulate the ANS can be observed.[6] For example, someone who has taken heroin will have pinpoint pupils.

EXERCISE 27–1: OBSERVATION OF PUPILLARY CONSTRICTION AND DILATION

Observe pupilary dilation and constriction on a willing subject (or on yourself in a mirror) by flashing a penlight at his or her pupil. Observe the decreased size of the pupil. Remove the light and watch the pupil dilate.

Lens

Behind the iris is the lens. The lens is involved in focusing, or accommodation. It is a biconvex, circular, semi-rigid, crystalline structure that fine tunes the image on the retina. In a camera, the lens is represented by the external optical lens system. The ability to change the focus on the camera is achieved by turning the lens to change the distance of the lens from the film, which effectively increases or decreases the power of the lens, allowing near or distance objects to be seen more clearly. The same effect, a change in the power of the lens, is achieved in the eye by the action of tiny cilliary muscles, which act on suspensory ligaments, thereby changing the thickness and curvature of the lens. A thicker lens with a greater curvature produces higher power and the ability to see clearly at near. A thinner lens and flatter curvature produces less optical power, which is what is needed to allow distant objects to be clear (Fig. 27–3). The process of lens thickening and thinning is accommodation.[22, 50]

Ideally, the lens will bring an image into perfect focus

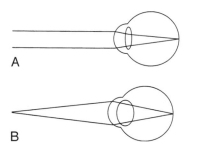

FIGURE 27–3. Accommodation. *A,* Looking far away. *B,* Looking up close.

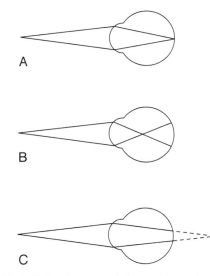

FIGURE 27–4. Refractive error. *A,* Image focused on retina; no refractive error. *B,* A near-sighted or myopic eye. *C,* A far-sighted or hyperopic eye.

so that it lands right on the fovea, the area of central vision. If the focused image falls in front of the retina, however, then a blurred circle will fall on the fovea (Fig. 27–4). In this case the lens is too thick, having too high an optical power. This can be one cause of myopia (near-sightedness). One simple remedy is to place a negative (concave) lens externally in front of the eye in glasses (or contact lenses) to reduce the power of the internal lens and allow the image to fall directly on the fovea. A similar type of problem can occur in hyperopia (farsightedness), in which the image falls in back of the retina. In presbyopia (old eyes), the flexibility of the lens fibers decreases and the lens becomes more rigid.[55] Accommodation gets weaker until the image can no longer be focused on the retina. When this occurs, a plus (positive) lens may be worn externally to aid in reading.[22]

The lens also can be affected by cataracts, in which the general clarity of vision is impaired from a loss of transparency of the crystalline lens. Incoming light tends to scatter inside the eye, causing glare problems. When vision is impaired to such a degree that it affects function, it may be removed surgically and replaced with a silicone implant placed just posterior to the iris.

Vitreous Chamber

The space behind the lens is filled with a gel-like substance and is called the vitreous chamber.[50]

Retina

The retina at the back of the eye is the photosensitive layer, like the film in a camera, receiving the pattern of light reflected from objects. The topography of the retina (Fig. 27–5) includes the optic disc, which is where the optic nerve exits and arteries and veins emerge and exit. This is also the blind spot because there are no photoreceptor cells on the disc. The macula is temporal to the optic disc and contains the fovea, or central vision. The

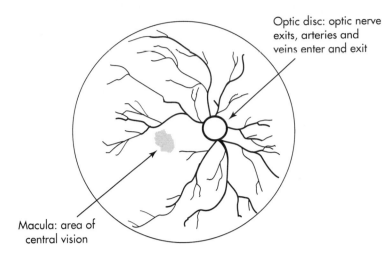

Optic disc: optic nerve exits, arteries and veins enter and exit

Macula: area of central vision

FIGURE 27–5. Retinal topography.

surrounding retina is considered peripheral vision and defines a 180-degree half-sphere.[50]

EXERCISE 27–2: BLIND SPOT

Your blind spot may be observed by doing the following: draw two dots 3 inches (7.5 cm) apart on a piece of paper. The dots can be 1/4 inch (0.5 cm). Cover your left eye and look at the dot on the left. Starting at about 16 inches (40 cm), slowly bring the paper closer. Make sure you can see the two dots—one you are looking at directly and the other peripherally. At approximately 10 inches (25 cm) the dot on the right will disappear. This is your blind spot! Why can this exercise be done only monocularly (with one eye)?

Visual Pathway

The visual pathway begins with the photoreceptor cells, which begin a three-neuron chain exiting through the optic nerve. This chain consists of the rods and cones, which synapse with bipolar cells that synapse with ganglion cells (Fig. 27–6).[30, 50]

There are two types of photoreceptor cells: rods and cones. The cone or rod shape is the dendrite of the cell. Variation in shape and slight variation in pigment give each one different sensitivities. The rod cell has greater sensitivity to dim light but less sensitivity to color, whereas the cone cell has greater sensitivity to color and high-intensity light and less to reduced light conditions. The

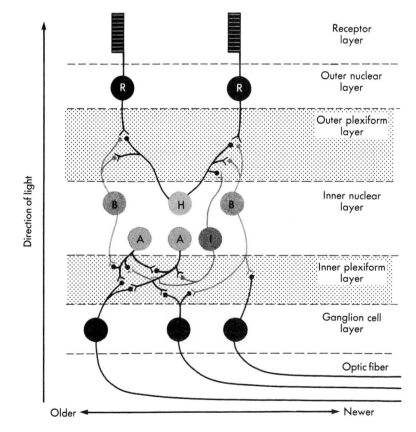

Direction of light

Receptor layer

Outer nuclear layer

Outer plexiform layer

Inner nuclear layer

Inner plexiform layer

Ganglion cell layer

Optic fiber

Older ◄————————► Newer

FIGURE 27–6. The connections among retinal neurons and the significance of prominent layers. The neurons shown are photoreceptors (R), horizontal cells (H), bipolar cells (B), interplexiform cells (I), amacrine cells (A), and ganglion cells (G). It has been suggested that ganglion cells dominated by bipolar cell inputs represent newer circuitry. The arrow indicates the direction of light as it passes through the retina to reach the photoreceptors. (From Berne RM, Levy MN [eds]: Physiology. St. Louis, CV Mosby, 1988, p 107.)

highest concentration of cone cells is in the fovea and macula, with decreasing concentration of cone cells and increasing concentration of rod cells moving concentrically away from the macula.

The phenomenon responsible for the high degree of neural representation of the foveal region and that accounts for the tremendous conscious awareness of the central view is called convergence.[50] At the periphery of the retina the degree of convergence is great; many photoreceptor cells synapse on one ganglion cell, which accounts for poor acuity but high light sensitivity. The closer to the macula, the less the degree of convergence, until, finally, at the fovea there is no convergence. This means that one photoreceptor cell synapses with one bipolar cell and one ganglion cell.

The awareness of what is seen is directly related to the amount of convergence, which reflects the extent of neural representation. The 1:1 correspondence between photoreceptor and ganglion cell at the fovea means that there is a very high degree of neural representation of the foveal image in the brain. It is even greater than the neural representation of the lips, tongue, or hands.[52] This accounts for the primary awareness of what is in the foveal field and secondary awareness of the peripheral field. Conscious awareness of the environment is whatever is in the foveal field at the moment. But continuous information about the environment is flowing over the peripheral retina, usually subconsciously. Attention quickly shifts from foveal to nonfoveal stimulation when changes in light intensity or rapid movement are registered. This type of stimulus rouses attention immediately because it could have specific survival value. For example, a person is driving down the street and picks up rapid motion off to the right. The foveas swing around immediately to identify a small red ball bouncing into the street. This information goes to the association areas, in which "small ball" is associated with "small child soon to follow." Frontal cortical centers are aroused and a decision is made to initiate motor areas to take the foot off the accelerator and onto the brake.

EXERCISE 27–3: PERIPHERAL CENTRAL AWARENESS

We have a unique ability to change our awareness by consciously shifting attention from our foveal or central awareness to our peripheral awareness. For example, as you read these words, become aware of the background surrounding the paper; notice colors, forms, and shapes; continue to expand your awareness to include your clothes, the floor, walls, and ceiling if possible. You are consciously stimulating your primitive, phylogenetically older visual system. The ability to do this has considerable therapeutic value, because a typical pattern of visual stress is associated with a foveal concentration. The ability to expand the peripheral awareness at will is a skill that can help you to relax while you drive, can improve reading skills, and can be used in visual training techniques.

The moment light hits the retina, the photographic film model must be abandoned for the image processing or computerized image enhancement model. The primary visual pathway at the retinal level is a three-neuron chain. From back to front the first neuron is the photoreceptor

cell, rods or cones. They synapse with a bipolar cell, which in turn synapses with a ganglion cell. The axon of the ganglion cell exits by means of the optic nerve. Image enhancement occurs at the two junctions between the three-nerve-cell pathway. Lateral cells at the neural junctions have an inhibitory action on the primary three-neuron pathway, and through the inhibition of an impulse the image is modulated. For example, at the first junction between photoreceptor cell and bipolar cell, there are horizontal cells. These cells enhance the contrast between light and dark by inhibiting the firing of bipolar cells at the very edge of an image. This makes the edge of the image appear darker than the central area, which increases the contrast, and thereby increases attention-getting value. After all, it is by perceiving edges that we are able to maneuver around objects. In a similar manner, amacrine cells act at the second neural junction between bipolar and ganglion cells to enhance movement detection.[31]

This image enhancement process continues throughout the visual pathway. The process has been likened to the way in which a computer enhances a distorted picture of outer space received from a satellite. The image goes through a series of processing stations in the inner workings of the computer. The computer-generated, enhanced image shown on the screen is like the end product in the brain: the perceived image.

The visual pathway continues through the brain (Fig. 27–7). The ganglion cell axons exit the eyeball by means of the optic nerve, carrying the complete retinal picture in coded electrochemical patterns. From there the patterns project to different sites within the central nervous system (Fig. 27–8). Projections to the pretectum are important in pupillary reflexes; projections to the pretectal nuclei, the accessory optic nuclei, and the superior colliculus are all involved in eye movement functions.[50] The largest bundle, called the optic tract, projects to the lateral geniculate body in the hypothalamus, where additional image enhancement and processing occurs. The next group of axons continue on to the primary visual cortex, and from there to visual association areas.

At what point does the retinal image become a perception, and with what part of the brain does one see? Current theory regarding visual perception is the result of Nobel prize–winning research by Hubel and Wiesel in the 1960s called the "receptive field theory."[39] This theory states that different neurons are feature detectors, defining objects in terms of movement, direction, orientation, color, depth, and acuity. Recent research by Hubel and Livingstone[38] was able to locate a segregation of function at the level of the lateral geniculate body. They identified two types of cells, one type being larger and faster magno cells, which are apparently phylogenetically older and color blind but which have a high contrast sensitivity and are able to detect differences in contrast of 1% to 2%. They also have low spatial resolution (low acuity). They seem to operate globally and are responsible for perception of movement, depth perception from motion, perspective, parallax, stereopsis, shading, contour, and interocular rivalry. Through linking properties (objects having common movement or depth) emerges figure-

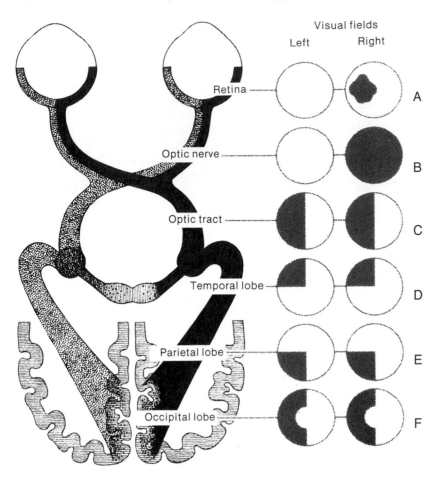

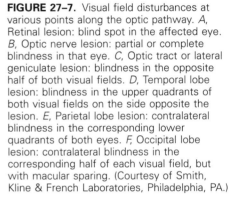

FIGURE 27-7. Visual field disturbances at various points along the optic pathway. *A*, Retinal lesion: blind spot in the affected eye. *B*, Optic nerve lesion: partial or complete blindness in that eye. *C*, Optic tract or lateral geniculate lesion: blindness in the opposite half of both visual fields. *D*, Temporal lobe lesion: blindness in the upper quadrants of both visual fields on the side opposite the lesion. *E*, Parietal lobe lesion: contralateral blindness in the corresponding lower quadrants of both eyes. *F*, Occipital lobe lesion: contralateral blindness in the corresponding half of each visual field, but with macular sparing. (Courtesy of Smith, Kline & French Laboratories, Philadelphia, PA.)

ground perception. Much of this perception occurs in the middle temporal lobe.

The other type of cells, called parvo cells, are smaller, slower, and color sensitive and have smaller receptive fields. They are less global and are primarily responsible for high-resolution form perception. Higher-level visual

association occurs in the temporal-occipital region, where learning to identify objects by their appearance occurs. It appears that these two types of cells are functionally and structurally related to the two visual systems represented in retinal topography—the foveal (central) and peripheral visual systems.

Eye Movement System

The eye movement system consists of six pairs of eye muscles: the medial recti, lateral recti, superior and inferior recti, and superior and inferior obliques (see Fig. 27–8). Together they are controlled by cranial nerves III (oculomotor), IV (trochlear), and VI (abducens). The eye movement system has both reflex and voluntary components. Reflexive movements are coordinated through vestibular interconnections at a midbrain level. The vestibular ocular reflex (VOR) functions primarily to keep the image stabilized on the retina. Through connections between pairs of eye muscles and the semicircular canals, movement is analyzed as being either external movement of an object or movement of the head or body. From this information the VOR is able to direct the appropriate head or eye movement.[50]

Two types of eye movements are the result. Smooth, coordinated eye movements are called pursuits, and rapid localizations are called saccades. Voluntary control of both these motions indicates cortical control. Pursuits are used for continuously following moving targets and are stimu-

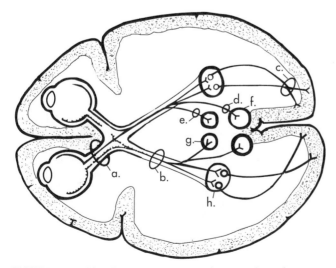

FIGURE 27–8. Visual tract system: a, optic nerve; b, optic tract; c, geniculate-occipital radiators; d, retinocolliculo radiation; e, retinopretecto tracts; f, superior colliculus (midbrain); g, pretectal area (tegmentum); h, lateral geniculate.

lated by a foveal image. Saccades are stimulated by images from the peripheral system, where a detection of motion or change in light intensity results in a rapid saccadic eye movement to bring the object into the foveal field. Either difficulties in the eye movement system or underfunctioning of the vestibular system can affect the coordinated, efficient functioning of eye movement skills.

A third type of eye movement is specifically related to eye aiming ability. This is the coordinated movement of both eyes inward toward the nose, as in crossing the eyes, or outward toward midline, as when looking away in the distance. The inward movement is called convergence, and the outward is divergence. The most important result of efficient vergence abilities is depth perception, or stereopsis. Very small errors in aiming can dramatically affect stereopsis. Problems such as double vision, wandering eyes, and strabismus are discussed in greater depth in a later section.

EXERCISE 27–4: PURSUITS, SACCADES, CONVERGENCE

Pursuits. Follow a moving target such as a pencil point as you move it across your field of gaze. Continue to move it in different directions, vertically, horizontally, diagonally, and circularly to stimulate all pairs of eye muscles. For a more challenging demonstration find a fly and follow its flight path around the room. If you lose sight of it, notice that the detection of the movement of the fly will signal your eye movement directly toward it.

Saccades. Hold two pencils about head width apart. Shift your eyes from pencil to pencil. Notice that your awareness is of the two pencils, not of the background between them. Generally, perception occurs the moment the eyes are still, rather than while moving during saccades. For a more challenging exercise, move the pencil you are not looking at, then shift quickly to it, move the other pencil while looking at the one you just moved. In other words, you will pick up the location of the other pencil peripherally and direct your eyes to the foveal region. The size and degree of blur of the peripheral image will tell the brain where the image is and how far to move the eyes. This ability again is due to the function of neural convergence, which is related to neural representation.

Convergence. Hold a pencil at arm's length along your midline. Slowly bring the pencil closer in toward you along your midline. Feel your eyes moving in (crossing). Try to bring the pencil to your nose, keeping the pencil visually single. (It is okay if you can't.) Move the pencil away now, and your eyes are diverging.

FUNCTIONAL VISUAL SKILLS

Refractive Error

Before discussing binocular coordination and the individual visual skills, it is important to describe refractive errors and how they can affect binocular coordination. Three common types of refractive errors are myopia or nearsightedness, hyperopia or farsightedness, and astigmatism.[31, 50]

The myopic eye is too long, so that the focused image falls in front of the retina. It is easily corrected with a negative or minus lens, which optically moves the image back onto the retina.

The hyperopic eye is too short, and the focused image falls behind the retina. A positive or plus lens optically moves the image onto the retina.

An eye will have astigmatism if it is not perfectly spherical. An aspherical eye will cause the image to be distorted, where part of the focused image will be in front of the retina and part in back. A person with astigmatism may see vertical lines clearly and horizontal lines as blurry, depending on the specific aspherical shape. A cylindrical type of lens is used to correct astigmatism. This lens corrects the distortion of the image so that it is placed right on the retina.

The following are examples of different refractive errors:

5.50 D.S. (diopter sphere): Myopia
+4.00 D.S.: Hyperopia
+1.50 c̄ − 1.50 × 180: Astigmatism. *Note:* × stands for the axis of the cylinder correction.

When significant refractive errors are uncorrected, they can reduce vision. Uncorrected refractive error also can interfere with binocular coordination. The symptoms are described in greater detail in the next section.

Binocular coordination is the end result of the efficient functioning of the visual skills (see the accompanying box). The individual visual skills include accommodation, eye alignment or vergence, eye movements, stereopsis (depth perception), and peripheral/central coordination. During normal activities, all the skills are inseparable.

Accommodation

Accommodation is the ability to bring near objects into clear focus automatically and without strain. Relaxation of accommodation allows distant objects to come into focus. The primary action is that of the ciliary muscles acting on the lens, and the primary system of control is the ANS with sympathetic and parasympathetic components.[50]

Accommodation is reflexly related to pupillary constriction and dilation.[22] As one focuses on a near object, the lenses thicken, allowing the near object to come into focus. At the same time the pupils constrict to increase

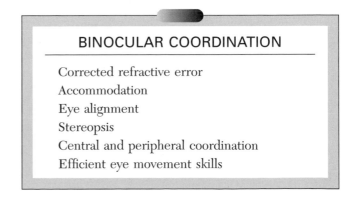

BINOCULAR COORDINATION

Corrected refractive error
Accommodation
Eye alignment
Stereopsis
Central and peripheral coordination
Efficient eye movement skills

depth of field (just as in a camera). As one looks into the distance, the lens gets flatter, relaxing accommodation, and the pupil dilates, decreasing the depth of field.

Accommodative ability is age related. A young child can focus on small objects just a few inches in front of the eyes. At about the age of 9 years, the accommodative ability slowly begins to decrease. By the mid 40s the reserve focusing power diminishes to the point that near objects begin to blur. At this stage, reading material is pushed farther away until the arms are not long enough, and then reading glasses are needed. This is called presbyopia (old eyes).

Problems in accommodation may contribute to myopia, hyperopia, and presbyopia. Symptoms include blurriness, at either near or far depending on the age and the problem.

Accommodation is important mainly for up-close activities: reading, hygiene, dressing (specifically, closing fasteners), use of tools, typing, table-top activities, and games.

EXERCISE 27–5: ACCOMMODATION

Accommodation cannot be directly observed, but it can be implied indirectly, through observation of pupillary constriction while doing an accommodative task. Cover one eye. Hold a finger in front at about 10 inches (25 cm). Focus on the finger, making sure that the fingerprint is clear. Shift focus to a distant object. Continue shifting far to near and near to far while a partner observes the pupil. He or she should be able to observe pupillary constriction/dilation as the focus is shifted.

Vergence

Vergence includes convergence and divergence. It is the ability to smoothly and automatically bring the eyes together along the midline to observe objects singly at near (convergence) or conversely to move the eyes outward for single vision of distant objects (divergence). Specific brain centers control convergence and divergence.

Vergence is reflexly associated with accommodation: convergence with accommodation, and divergence with relaxation of accommodation. The function of this reflex is to allow objects to be both single and clear, at either near or far.

Vergence has both automatic and voluntary components. Most of the time it is not necessary to think about moving the eyes inward while looking at a close object; yet if asked to cross the eyes, most people can do this at will.

Problems can occur in vergence ability when the eye movement system is out of coordination with accommodation or from damage to cranial nerve III, IV, or VI. Problems can be slight, when there is merely a tendency for the eyes to converge in or out too far, or they can be gross. Tendencies to underconverge or overconverge are called phorias and are not visible to the affected person. An individual may be asymptomatic, but problems may be elicited under conditions of increased stress or fatigue such as excessive reading or working at computer terminal or from drug side effects (licit or illicit).

Some phorias may worsen to the extent that binocularity breaks down, at which point the individual has a strabismus. There are two main types of strabismus: esotropia and exotropia. An esotropia is an inward turning of the eye, and an exotropia is a visible outward turning. A third, less common type of strabismus is hypertropia, in which one eye aims upward. Strabismus and dysfunctional phorias are discussed in greater detail in the next section.

Vergence ability is needed for singular binocular vision; thus, it is basic to all activities. At near, the patient may have difficulty finding objects; eye-hand coordination may be decreased, affecting self-care and hygiene tasks; and reading may be difficult. Distance tasks that may be affected include driving, sports, movies, communication, and, frequently, ambulation. Individuals with impaired vergence ability may also have difficulty focusing and may have decreased or no depth perception. Interpreting space can be quite difficult and confusing. If decreased vergence is a result of traumatic head injury or stroke, it may contribute to the patient's confusion, and he or she may not be able to identify or communicate the problem.

EXERCISE 27–6: VERGENCE

Hold a pencil in front of you at eye level at about 12 inches (30 cm). Look at the pencil. Look away into the distance. Looking at the pencil is convergence and looking into the distance is divergence. As you converge and diverge slowly back and forth notice any changes you may feel: changes in how relaxed you feel, how focused or spaced out you feel, feelings of dreaminess, or nothing at all. Observe a partner's eyes as they shift back and forth as well.

Pursuits and Saccades

Eye movement skills consist of pursuits and saccades. Pursuits are the smooth, coordinated movements of all eye muscles together, allowing accurate tracking of objects through space. Perception is continuous during pursuit movements. Saccades are rapid shifts of the eyes from object to object, allowing quick localization of movements observed in the periphery. The systems involved in eye movement skills are the oculomotor system with the VOR, in conjunction with coordination of the central and peripheral visual systems. The peripheral visual system is finely tuned for detecting changes in light levels and small movements.

Problems in pursuits and saccades can be the result of a dysfunctioning of any individual muscles or of the VOR. Because the VOR helps to stabilize the image on the retina and to differentiate image movement from eye movement, simple tracking can be more difficult. In addition, visual field loss, either central or peripheral, can dramatically affect localization ability. People with blind half or quarter fields can be observed to do searching eye movements rather than directly jumping to the object.

Activities affected include searching for objects, visually directed movement for fine motor tasks and gross movement and ambulation tasks, eye-hand coordination, self-care, driving, and reading.

Memory also may be affected by an eye movement dysfunction. Research by Adler-Grinberg and Stark[1] examined patterns of eye movements as subjects looked at a picture. Distinct eye movement patterns, called scan paths, became apparent. When the subject was asked to recall the picture, the same eye movement pattern was elicited as the subject recalled the picture. Perhaps a type of oculomotor motor planning is involved in recall. Applying this idea to the clinical setting, if a patient has inaccurate eye movement, inability with undershooting and overshooting, or uses 32 saccades to scan a picture rather than 10, then perhaps the stored memory is less efficiently stored and consequently the image is more difficult to reconstruct from memory. Additionally, if a patient has a type of brain damage with generalized dyspraxia, the eye movement system could quite likely be affected and might be involved in the patient's perceptual dysfunction.

SYMPTOMS OF VISUAL DYSFUNCTION

History

The identification of a visual problem begins with case history. It is important to get some idea of the client's prior visual status or any history of eye injury, surgery, or diseases. Information can be elicited by direct questioning of the client or family members or by clinical observation. Sample questions include the following:

- Are you having difficulty with seeing, or with your eyes?
- Do you wear bifocals?
- Do your glasses work as well now as before the (stroke, accident, etc.)?
- Have you noticed any blurriness? Near or far?
- Do you ever see double? See two? See overlapping or shadow images?
- Do you ever find that when you reach for an object that you knock it over or your hand misses?
- Do letters jump around on the page after reading for a while?
- Are you experiencing any eye strain or headaches? Where and when?
- Do you ever lose your place when reading?
- Are portions of a page or any objects missing?
- Do people or things suddenly appear from one side that you didn't see approaching?
- Do you have difficulty concentrating on tasks?

Clinical observations of the client while performing various activities are a valuable source of problem identification. Therapists in general are in an ideal position to observe clients in a variety of functional tasks that require near vision, far vision, spatial estimations, depth judgments, and oculomotor tasks. This situation varies considerably from the doctor's observations in the more contrived environment of the examination room. Additionally, the therapist's initial observations can be used in documenting difficulties within the therapy realm that may be amenable to visual remediation in terms that can be applied to reimbursement of therapy.

Clinical observations include the following:

- Head tilt during near tasks
- Avoidance of near tasks
- One eye appears to go in, out, up, or down
- Vision shifts from eye to eye
- Seems to look past observer
- Closes or covers one eye
- Squints
- Eyes appear red, puffy, or irritated or have a discharge (Notify nurses or doctor of these observations)
- Rubs eyes a lot
- Has difficulty maintaining eye contact
- Spaces out, drifts off, daydreams
- During activity, neglects one side of body or space
- During movement, bumps into walls or objects (either walking or in a wheelchair)
- Appears to misjudge distance
- Underreaches or overreaches for objects
- Has difficulty finding things

Near Point Blur

The first area of symptomatology is near accommodative problems. The primary symptom is near point blur. This symptom alone is not indicative of a problem in any one area, but it could indicate farsightedness (hyperopia), astigmatism, or reduced accommodative ability (insufficiency). The client may move objects or the head farther or closer, may complain of eye strain or headaches, may squint, or may even avoid near activities as much as possible. The therapist might observe excessive blinking, and the patient may complain of glasses not working well.

Distance Blur

The next problem could also indicate a number of different causes. Distance blur could indicate nearsightedness (myopia), a pathological problem (such as beginning cataracts), or accommodative spasm. Most people have some experience with accommodative spasm. After spending long periods of time either studying or reading a novel and then glancing up at the wall across the room, it may be blurry and then clear up very slowly. For some individuals, this spasm eventually becomes one component in their nearsightedness if the reading habits continue for a long time.

Clients experiencing distance blur may make forward head movements and frequently squint in an attempt to see. They may not respond or orient quickly to auditory or visual stimuli beyond a certain radius. The therapist may also note excessive blinking and a withdrawn attitude because the patient cannot see well enough to interact with the environment.

Visual hygiene can be recommended to assist in the development of good visual habits. Good lighting and posture, taking frequent breaks, and monitoring the state of clarity of an environmental cue such as a clock across the room are all beneficial.

Phoria and Strabismus

The next area of eye alignment problems can be divided into two types of problems: phoria and strabismus. A phoria can be defined as a natural positioning of the eyes in which there is a tendency to aim in front of or behind the point of focus. It may or may not be associated with symptoms. Fusion is intact to some degree, and depth perception may also be intact.

Everyone has a phoria, just as everyone has a posture. It may be within normal range, or, just as someone may have scoliosis, a high phoria may cause problems. The following phorias may cause problems:

- Esophoria: eyes are postured in front of the point of focus.
- Exophoria: the eyes are postured in back of the point of focus.

Phoria is measured in units of prism diopters, which indicate the size of the prism needed to measure the eye position in or out from the straight-ahead position.[22]

Phorias tend to produce subtle symptoms. These include having difficulty concentrating, frontal or temporal headaches, sleepiness after reading, and stinging of the eyes after reading.

A strabismus, or tropia, is a visible turn of one eye, which may be constant, intermittent, or alternating between one eye and the other. The person may have double vision, or if the strabismus is long term, the person may suppress or "turn off" the vision in the wandering eye. Suppression is a neurological function that is an adaptation to the intolerable situation of double images. It is only exhibited in long-term strabismus, because apparently the brain cannot learn to suppress past the time of peak plasticity (up to age 7 years). The developing brain must choose which eye has the visual direction, which is confirmed by motor and tactile inputs as being the "real" image. The other fovea's image is then neurologically suppressed. The peripheral vision in the suppressing eye is still normal, and the eye is not by any means blind.

The essential concept in understanding the difference between phoria and strabismus is that in strabismus fusion and depth perception are not present. Definitions of different types of strabismus are presented in the accompanying box. It is not a conclusive list; many other types and permutations are beyond the scope of this discussion. The intent here is to expose the therapist to different terms that may be used by the doctor in diagnosing the type of strabismus.

In strabismus, one eye appears to go in, out, up, or down and there is frequently an obvious inability to judge distances, especially if the strabismus is of recent onset (acquired). The client may underreach or overreach for objects, cover or close one eye, complain of double vision, or exhibit a head tilt or turn during specific activities. He or she may appear to favor one eye, have difficulty reading, appear spaced out, or avoid near activities. Additionally, especially if the patient sees double but is unable or unwilling to talk about it, he or she may be confused or disoriented.

Oculomotor Dysfunction

A client with an oculomotor dysfunction will have difficulty with activities that require smooth pursuits, tracking, and convergence and divergence. During reading tasks these patients may lose their place, skip lines, or reread

---

TYPES OF STRABISMUS

Esotropia: One eye turns in.

Exotropia: One eye turns out.

Hypertropia: One eye turns up relative to the other eye.

Intermittent: The person is strabismic at times and phoric (fusing) at times. Fatigue or stress may bring out the strabismic state.

Alternating: The person switches from using the right eye to using the left eye. The person also switches the suppressing eye. If using the right eye, the person suppresses the left, and while using the left eye, the person suppresses the right; otherwise the person would see double.

Constant strabismus: One eye is always in or out, always the same eye.

Comitant strabismus: The amount of eye turn is the same regardless of whether the person is looking up, down, right, left, or straight ahead. People who have had the condition for a long time usually have comitant strabismus. New or acquired strabismics (i.e., from stroke or head injury) usually have noncomitant strabismus, in which the amount of eye turn changes depending on which direction the eyes are looking toward.

---

lines, or they may have poor ball skills, poor eye-hand coordination, decreased balance, and clumsiness.

Visual Field Loss

Visual field loss may indicate damage at the optic chiasm, post chiasmic, in the visual radiations of the thalamus, or in the visual cortex. The resultant visual field loss is characteristic (even diagnostic) in each case. It could be bitemporal (outer half of each field), half-field (hemianopsia) with or without macular involvement, or quarter-field loss (see Fig. 27–7). Some symptoms of field loss are an inability to read or starting to read in the middle of the page, ignoring food on one half of the plate, and difficulty orienting to stimuli in a specific area of space.

Unilateral Neglect

Some clients also may have concomitant unilateral neglect. Differentiating a neglect from a hemianopia is difficult. One test to differentiate between the two involves the extinction phenomenon. Presenting first stimuli on one side followed by simultaneous presentation of stimuli on both sides and comparing the results can differentiate hemianopia from neglect if the client has neglect but not a hemianopia. Please see the discussion on inattention later in the section on visual perception.

Generally, if the patient has a field loss, it will be possible to conduct a field test and obtain fairly reliable results. The client will be able to respond more easily and tell you where the test item appears and disappears. Additionally, when doing compensation training, the client with a field loss can grasp the techniques, whereas a client with a neglect cannot without quite a bit of additional training. The client with unilateral neglect frequently has proprioceptive and tactile loss on the neglected side, and that area of space including that half of the body does not provide feedback. Therefore, if the client also has field loss, test results are unreliable and invariably inaccurate.

EYE DISEASES

Areas addressed in this section are common ocular and systemic diseases of the pediatric and geriatric populations, an introduction to low vision, and recommendations for adaptations of the treatment plan. If reduced vision (low vision) is a result of eye disease, the client may be assisted by magnification aids. Also, the therapy treatment program may need to be altered to accommodate any special visual needs of the client (lighting, working distance, inclusion of magnifiers, use of filters, contrast-enhancing devices).

Pediatric Conditions

Retinopathy of Prematurity. The incidence of retinopathy of prematurity is increasing because of the improved survival of premature infants due to improved ventilation. Immature retinal vessels are sensitive to high oxygen tension. The effect on the vessels is vasoconstriction, eventually leading to obliteration of the vessels. This creates a state of ischemia, which stimulates the growth of new blood vessels. These small, fragile vessels bleed easily, leading to fibrosis and traction on the retina. As a result of the traction, the macula gets stretched, interfering with the function of central vision.

The temporal vessels are most affected because they develop last. The degree of damage may be mild or quite severe, depending on the amount of prematurity.[55]

Retinoblastoma. Retinoblastoma is the most common malignant tumor in children.[56] The current incidence is 1 in 20,000 live births, a rate that has been increasing over the past 30 years, apparently owing to inheritance of a mutated gene.

The young child may have a strabismus due to impaired vision in the eye from the tumor. As the tumor grows the pupil may appear milky white. If not detected early, it will lead to loss of the eye; and if the tumor invades the brain, death will occur. Clearly, early detection is critical.

Mental Retardation. There is a higher number of visual problems in mentally retarded populations.[56] These individuals have a higher incidence of refractive error (myopia, hyperopia, astigmatism), strabismus, nystagmus, and optic atrophy than that in children with normal intelligence.

Cerebral Palsy. Therapists who work with children with cerebral palsy have noticed a high incidence of vision problems. Many studies confirm these observations. A study by Scheinman examining the incidence of visual problems in children with cerebral palsy and normal intelligence found the following incidences: strabismus in 69%, high phorias in 4%, accommodative dysfunction in 30%, and refractive errors in 63%.[56, 57]

Hydrocephalus. Various studies have found that the most common visual problem in children with hydrocephalus is strabismus, with an incidence of 30% to 55%. The strabismus may develop either from the hydrocephalus itself or from the shunting procedure.

Fetal Alcohol Syndrome. Children affected by fetal alcohol syndrome have several characteristic features and visual problems. Visually, they have a higher incidence of strabismus, myopia, astigmatism, and ptosis. These children frequently have some degree of mental retardation as well and are of small stature.

Age-Related Conditions

Cataracts. The most common malady affecting vision in elderly persons is cataracts. General clarity of vision is impaired from a loss of transparency of the crystalline lens of the eye.

In the senile cataract the lens slowly loses its ability to prevent oxidation from occurring, and liquefaction of the outer layers begins. The normally soluble proteins adhere together, causing light scatter.[41] Vision slowly declines as light scatter increases, until the lens must be removed.

Age-Related Macular Degeneration. Age-related macular degeneration is the leading cause of blindness in the Western world and is the most important retinal disease of the aged (affecting 28% of the 75- to 85-year-old age group).[55]

There is loss of central vision from fluid that leaks up from the deeper layers of the retina, pushing the retina up and detaching it from the nourishing layer. New vessel growth and hemorrhage and atrophy further destroy central vision.

This condition has significant implications for independent functioning. Mobility tends to be less impaired, because the peripheral visual system is still intact. All activities involving fine detail such as reading, sewing, and cooking are affected. Safety also can be affected.

Arteriosclerosis. In arteriosclerosis, vision may or may not be affected. There is a hardening of the retinal arteries, which may eventually lead to ischemia, with the areas of retina deprived of sufficient oxygen and eventually dying.

Hypertension. Hypertension is usually accompanied by arteriosclerosis. There may be retinal bleeding and edema, which can affect central vision if the macula is involved.

Diabetes. Diabetes can affect the lens. In the diabetic "sugar cataract," sorbital collects within the lens, causing an osmotic gradient of fluid into the lens, which leads to disruption of the lens matrix and loss of transparency. As the fluid increases and decreases within the lens, the patient's vision also can fluctuate, depending directly on the sugar level. This makes prescribing glasses during this time quite difficult.

The retinal effects include microvascular damage and the development of microaneurysms. Central vision may be reduced due to retinal ischemia. The ischemia leads to new vessel growth (neovascularization). These new vessels are very weak, frequently leaking and causing hemorrhage. The hemorrhage leads to fibrosis, which puts traction on the retina, pulling it off and leading to retinal detachment and blindness. Laser treatment may destroy the neovascularization, preventing retinal detachment.

Glaucoma. Glaucoma occurs in 7.2% of the 75- to 85-year-old age group.[55] It is caused by an increase in the intraocular pressure. This pressure interferes with the inflow and outflow of blood and nutrients at the optic disc. If severe enough, glaucoma can cause field loss and, eventually, complete blindness.

In one type of glaucoma called open-angle glaucoma, the outflow of aqueous humor is reduced, leading to increased intraocular pressure. There are no overt symptoms. In another type, closed-angle glaucoma, the outflow is blocked by the iris. Symptoms are a painful, red eye, which may be confused with conjunctivitis. Because corticosteroids are used to treat many conditions in the elderly for long periods of time, it is useful to be aware that side effects can include glaucoma and cataracts.

Eye Muscle Dysfunctions. Eye muscle dysfunctions causing double vision may result from several disease conditions including thyroid disease (Graves disease and others), multiple sclerosis, myasthenia gravis, and tumors. The underlying condition must be diagnosed and treated.

Visual Field Loss. Visual field loss may be either central (macular degeneration glaucoma or retinal disease) or peripheral field loss due to retinal damage or stroke at any point in the visual pathway. This is potentially the most functionally disabling form of visual impairment (see Fig. 27–7).

Implications for Functional Performance

Lighting. Lighting conditions are important and vary depending on the nature of the condition. The person with presbyopia requires more light because the aging pupil gets smaller. The smaller pupil has the advantage of increasing the depth of focus, allowing the presbyope to see clearly over a wider range, but it has the disadvantage of eliminating more light from the eye. Thus, providing a good source of direct lighting, especially on fine print, is very helpful. Direct lighting from a halogen source is helpful for some low-vision patients as well.

Glare. People who have problems with glare, such as those developing cataracts or other disease conditions, can be helped by several approaches. Incandescent lighting is preferred over fluorescent lighting. The use of a visor or wide-brimmed hat also can be helpful. For some individuals who have trouble reading because of the glare coming off the white page, a black matte piece of cardboard with a horizontal slit in it (called a typoscope) can be used to reduce the surrounding glare and enhance reading. Special antiglare lenses developed by Corning are available by prescription through the eye doctor. An antireflective coating may also help.

Low-Vision Aids. Many types of low-vision optical and nonoptical aids are available, usually by prescription by a low-vision specialist. Clients who have experienced damage to their central vision as in age-related macular degeneration or diabetic maculopathy, and who still have some reduced central vision, may be able to use various types of magnification aids. One type is a stand magnifier, which leaves the hands free for other activities. It also is useful for patients who have a tremor. Hand magnifiers are another type of aid. Some are equipped with their own internal illumination.

A telescope system can be attached to the patient's glasses frames, allowing distance viewing. High magnification also can be incorporated into special reading glasses. Some patients may need a closed-circuit TV, which allows large and variable magnification without the distortion caused by optical magnifiers.

Nonoptical aids include large print materials, available at many libraries, typoscopes, mentioned earlier, and reading stands. Talking books are available for those for whom reading is an important hobby. New developments include text-to-speech synthesizers, large-print computers, and image intensifiers.

For clients with field losses, specially designed prism or mirror systems may be used. These frequently require a bit of training to get used to and are not useful for everyone. Compensation training also can be helpful. Use of margin markers or reading slits, and holding the book sideways so that the print is vertical are other helpful techniques.

A videocamera mounted to spectacles by which the visual information was transduced to electrodes implanted in visual cortical centers allowed a low-vision patient to see the large E (20/400) and detect large contours. This is an exciting area for further research and may hold significant potential for the blind.[68]

VISUAL SCREENING

Primary visual dysfunction must be differentiated from a visual-perceptual disorder so that appropriate treatment can be addressed for each problem. Gianutsos and others[29] found that over half of the individuals in their study admitted for general head injury rehabilitation who were eligible for cognitive services had visual sensory impairments sufficient to warrant further evaluation. Visual screening can identify the need for referral for a complete eye examination. The results of the examination become part of the differential diagnosis regarding a perceptual dysfunction. See the box on page 833 for key elements in vision screening.

This section describes vision screening tools and adaptations for various populations. The following principles should be kept in mind:

- *Acuities*: Acuities should always be tested first because decreased acuities will bias other tests except for ocular motilities and the peripheral field test.
- *Positioning*: The body and head should be in good alignment or straightened with positioning devices, with the head in midline.
- *Glasses*: If the client normally wears glasses, for either distance or near, the patient should be wearing glasses for tests for which spectacle correction is required. When in doubt, try it both ways, record the best response, and note if glasses were worn.

Observations During Testing

The client's response during the test can provide important qualitative information about his or her visual system, including postural changes (head forward or back, body forward or back, head tilts or rotation [turning to either side]), squinting, closing one eye, excessive blinking, rubbing, signs of strain or fatigue, and holding the breath. Clients should be encouraged to relax, breathe normally, and not squint.

Distance Acuities

Equipment. Needed to measure distance acuity are a distance acuity chart, an occluder, a 20-ft measure, and the patient's corrective lenses if worn for distance.°

Setup. A distance chart is taped on a well-lighted wall at the patient's eye level, and 20 ft is measured off.

Procedure. One of the patient's eyes is covered and the patient is asked to read the smallest letters that he or she can see. Exposing one letter or line at a time can help if tracking or attention is a problem. The examiner should encourage the patient to guess and instruct the patient not to squint. The number of letters that were missed on the smallest line that the patient is able to see is noted. The procedure is repeated by covering the patient's other eye, and then both eyes are tested unoccluded.

°Bernell/uso, 4016 N. Home Street, Mishiwaka, IN 46545; (800)-348-2225. Complete Visual Screening Kit: Laurie E. Chaikin, OD, OTR, 20881 Redwood Road, Castro Valley, CA 94546; (510)-538-3937.

Record. The smallest line the patient was able to read is recorded. If the client missed any letters on that line then the number of letters missed is subtracted. For example, if the client read four letters correctly on the 20/30 line but missed the other two, then it is recorded as $20/30 - 2$. The scores for the client's right eye, left eye, and both eyes together are recorded.

If the patient is unable to see the top line at 20 ft, the patient is asked to move forward until he or she is able to identify the top letters. Then the distance/letter size (top line) is recorded. For example, if the patient had to move up to 4 ft to see the top line, then 4/100 is recorded. To calculate 20-ft equivalence, an equation is used where x equals the size of the letter (e.g., $4/100 = 20/x$); thus, $4x = 2000$ and $2000 \div 4 = 500$. The client's vision is 20/500 (see the box below).

For clients whose attention is very poor, the testing distance may need to be as close as 2 ft. Other testing stimuli can be used for children, such as the Broken Wheel Test° or the Lighthouse cards.° Acuity in very low functioning clients or infants can be evaluated by using preferential looking methods. Targets are usually high-contrast grating patterns of decreasing size. One such type is the Teller cards.†

Implications. A patient who fails this test may require glasses or a change in his or her current prescription.

Near Acuities

Equipment. A near point test card, an occluder, and the client's corrective lenses if normally worn for near are needed.

Procedure. The procedure is the same as for distance

°Bernell/uso, 4016 N. Home Street, Mishiwaka, IN 46545; (800)-348-2225.

†Vistech Consultants, 4162 Little York Road, Dayton, OH 45414-2566.

acuity. The standard test distance is usually 16 inches (40 cm).

Record. The smallest line read is recorded.

Interpretation/Referral. 20/20 is considered normal, 20/40 is required for reading newspaper size print, and 20/100 is needed for large print. Referral to an optometrist or ophthalmologist should be made if vision is 20/40 or worse or if a difference of 2 lines exists between the two eyes. Neurological damage can affect the accommodative system. Sometimes it corrects itself spontaneously, but not always.

Visual retraining of the focusing system may be appropriate, depending on the patient's age. This can be determined by an optometrist familiar with vision therapy.

Pursuits

Equipment. Any target that holds the patient's attention can be used, such as a pencil or small toy.

Setup. The patient is seated facing the screener.

Procedure. One pencil is held 16 to 20 inches in front of the client, and the client is asked to look directly at one part, such as the eraser, and to keep the head still, holding it if necessary. The pencil is moved around in the pattern shown in Figure 27–9, which is designed to incorporate all directions of gaze. The examiner should observe for smooth following, noticing and recording jerks and jumps, where they occur, or if the eyes stop at a certain point. If one or both eyes stop tracking, the client is encouraged to look at the pencil. If the patient is unable to do this, then the movement pattern is repeated with each eye separately and where the movement stops is recorded. Clients who have had a cerebrovascular accident (CVA) or head injury should be tested first monocularly (each eye separately).

Record. Results are rated as follows:

Poor = Difficulty following target with any accuracy,

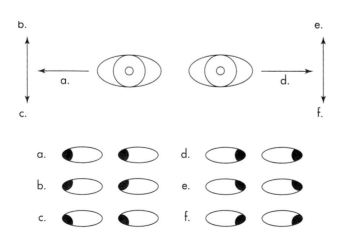

Then move from e→f, b→f, f→b, c→e to observe diagonal and midline pursuit patterns.

FIGURE 27–9. Pursuit patterns.

very jerky or jumpy, nystagmoid movements, incomplete range of motion (ROM)

Fair = Generally able to follow target, but goes off target occasionally (one to two times), with slight jerkiness

Good = Eye movements smooth with no jerkiness

If one eye stops tracking at a certain point, or if the client reports double vision (diplopia) in certain directions, the examiner should record which eye or in which direction the problem is noticed (e.g., the right eye does not pass midline when moving from left to right, or diplopia is reported on upward right gaze). This specific information can be helpful to the ophthalmologist or optometrist.

Saccades

Equipment. Tracking pencils can be used, although a few saccadic tests are available. One is the King Devick Saccadic Test; the other is the Developmental Eye Movement Test.° These both require form perception (number reading) and may be difficult, depending on the client's cognitive level.

Setup. The patient is seated facing the screener.

Procedure. A pencil is held in each hand about 17 to 20 inches from the client, and the client is told that he or she is going to be asked to look at one pencil while the other pencil is moved but he or she is not to look at it until told to look at it. The client is to move the eyes only, keeping the head still. While the client looks at the first pencil, the other pencil is moved as the screener says "shift" or "look at this pencil." The screener then moves the other pencil, says "shift," then moves the pencil, says "shift," then moves the pencil, etc., until a pattern of movement can be discerned.

This call-shift call-shift is repeated about 10 times, moving into different fields of gaze. The screener continues until the client is seen to respond. The screener observes for overshooting or undershooting the target, for the ability to isolate the eyes from the head (hold head still), for controlled eye movement, and for ability to wait until the verbal command to look. It is important to observe for the client's ability to shift to all fields of gaze. A lower level of testing would be to ask the client to move the eyes from one target to the other as quickly as possible.

Record. Results are rated as follows:

Poor = Inability to control eyes with verbal command, consistent undershooting or overshooting, inability to isolate eyes from head

Fair = Client able to maintain eyes on target with verbal command 50% of the time, with slight undershooting or overshooting, and able to isolate eyes from head with verbal reminders

Good = Client able to follow verbal commands 90%

°Bernell/uso, 4016 N. Home Street, Mishiwaka, IN 46545; (800)-348-2225. Complete Vision Screening Kit: Laurie E. Chaikin, OD, OTR, 20881 Redwood Road, Castro Valley, CA 94546; (510)-538-3937.

of the time, with no undershooting or overshooting, and complete eye from head isolation

Near Point of Convergence (NPC)

Procedure. A pencil is introduced about 20 inches away from the client's midline. The client is asked if the pencil looks single. If it is not, it is moved farther away. The client is told that the pencil will be moved toward him or her and that it will be getting blurry but to keep watching it as far in as he or she can. When the pencil appears single, it is moved toward the nose at a moderately slow rate (but not too slow). The screener should watch the client's eyes. As long as the client's eyes are tracking the pencil, the pencil is kept moving in toward the nose. At the point where one eye moves out, both eyes move out, or the eyes simply stop tracking, the distance of the pencil to the nose is measured. If the client is wearing bifocals, it is important to make sure the patient is looking through the reading segment.

Record. The break point is the distance at which the eyes were observed to stop tracking the pencil in. If the client was able to track the pencil all the way to the nose, then record this fact.

Interpretation/Referral. A score of poor or fair on saccades or pursuits suggests the need for training. NPC with a break point of 5 inches or more is suggestive of convergence problems, and recommendations for referral should be made.

Implications. Difficulties with smooth pursuit, accurate saccades, or convergence can all present tracking difficulties for the patient. These difficulties can cause loss of place in reading, rereading of words or lines, skipping lines, and lower comprehension and concentration. Inaccurate eye movements also may affect visual memory.

An eye movement problem may be the result of direct damage to the eye muscles themselves (Fig. 27–10), or the nerves controlling them, as in the case of a head injury. Damage to the vestibular center also may involve visual components. Neurons from cranial nerves III, IV, and VI synapse in the vestibular nuclei. Reflex control of eye movements occurs through the VOR and the optokinetic system.

Cover Tests

Purpose. There are two cover tests. The cover/uncover test is used to determine whether a strabismus is present. The alternate cover test determines what type of phoria is present. The magnitude of the phoria generally determines the extent of the client's symptoms.

Equipment. An occluder and a tracking pencil or a small, distinct target are needed.

Setup. The client is seated facing the screener, who is also seated.

Procedure. A pencil is held approximately 16 inches in front of the client, and the client is asked to look directly at the target and to keep it in focus.

Near Cover Tests

Cover/Uncover. *The movement of the uncovered eye is observed.* The client's right eye is covered, and the left eye is observed for movement in, out, upward, or downward. This is repeated a few times, while allowing the eyes to be uncovered for about 2 seconds between trials. Then the left eye is covered to observe for movement in the right eye.

Alternate Cover Test. *Eye movement is observed as the eye is uncovered.* An occluder is held over the right eye for a few seconds while the client looks at a near target. The occluder is moved from the right eye to the left eye while the right eye is observed for movement in, out, up, or down. After a few seconds, the occluder is moved back to the right eye, observing the left eye for movement. This is repeated back and forth several times until the screener is sure of what is seen.

Far Cover Tests

The preceding procedure is repeated with the patient looking at a distant target.

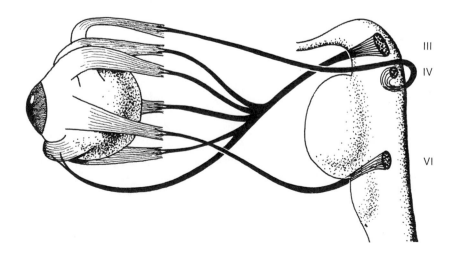

FIGURE 27–10. Cranial nerves III, IV, and VI. Oculomotor, trochlear, and abducens nerves and their innervation of the extraocular muscles. (Courtesy of Smith, Kline & French Laboratories, Philadelphia, PA.)

Interpretation/Referral. Any visible eye movement seen during the cover/uncover test with good maintenance of fixation on the target indicates a strabismus. If there is no previous history of strabismus, referral is indicated. A large eye movement seen with the alternate cover test, along with the presence of symptoms such as eye strain, headaches, or apparent difficulty in making spatial judgments, also indicates referral. In the clinic the therapist may notice that the client has difficulty finding objects in a drawer, or that the client appears cross-eyed or seems to be looking past the target. He or she may have difficulty with spatial judgments in reaching for objects or in mobility, especially with stairs or curbs.

A visible eye movement may be part of a post-CVA client's premorbid pattern. This should be determined by asking the client or the family before making a referral. Or it may be the result of neurological damage to cranial nerve III, IV, or VI from CVA, head injury, or cerebral palsy. Eye muscles are striated muscles, under voluntary control. Like other striated muscles that can be affected by neurological damage, they may recover spontaneously, they may not recover at all, or they may benefit from visual retraining. Many learning-disabled children with vestibular dysfunction have poor binocular skills. An ophthalmologist or optometrist specially trained in visual remediation can determine a patient's potential for vision therapy. Some published research has demonstrated the success of vision therapy for post-CVA patients.[16]

Stereopsis (Depth Perception)

Equipment. Any test that uses either Polaroid or red/green filters can test for stereopsis ability. Examples are the Titmus Stereo Fly, Rheindeer, and Butterfly.°

Procedure. The client is asked to point to or say which test object appears closer. If the client is able to grasp for the object in space, some stereo ability is present.

Record. The client's response should be immediate. Long delays could indicate borderline ability.

Interpretation/Referral. If the client fails this test, a referral to an ophthalmologist or optometrist is recommended. The patient must have best corrected acuities for this test; otherwise, the results are invalid.

Implications. A deficit in depth perception can interfere with all activities involving spatial judgments, in particular fine motor and eye-hand type activities in which judgments of relative depth are required (e.g., threading a needle, placing toothpaste on a toothbrush, hammering). Although ambulation itself may not be affected, ambulation involving curbs or stairs will be affected.

Vision therapy training can be helpful for clients with problems in binocular coordination. Proper diagnosis and therapy prescription are essential.

Visual Field Screening

Equipment. An occluder or eyepatch is required, and black dowels with white pins on the ends or just a wiggling finger can be used as a peripheral target.

Setup. The client is seated facing the examiner.

Procedure. The client holds the occluder over the left eye. The examiner explains that he or she is going to wiggle a finger out to the side and that the patient is to say "now" when he or she first detects the movement of the wiggling finger. The client should look at the screener's nose the entire time and ignore any arm movement. The test is begun with the examiner's hand slightly behind the client about 16 inches away from the client's head. The hand is brought forward slowly while wiggling a finger. Different sections of the visual field are randomly tested in 45-degree intervals around the visual field. The left eye is then tested after occluding the client's right eye. Alternatively, if a dowel is used, it is slowly brought in from the side until the client reports seeing the small pin at the end of the dowel.

These confrontation fields tests are considered a gross test as compared with a visual field perimeter test. Many clients cannot do the perimeter test because it requires a higher cognitive level. Confrontation fields will reveal a hemianopia and a quadrantanopia (quarter-field cut). For lower-functioning clients the examiner can observe their eye movements in the direction of the target once they have seen it to get a general idea of peripheral function.

Record. The portion of field missing for each eye is noted.

Interpretation/Referral. If any hemianopia or quadrantanopia is noted, the patient is referred to an optometrist or ophthalmologist.

Implications. A visual deficit has significant implication for the safe performance of many functional activities, including driving and mobility. Visually guided movement through space becomes impaired, as are efficient eye movements; and if central field loss is present, reading and any near activity are affected. The reader is referred to the discussion on assessment of unilateral inattention for differentiation between neglect and hemianopia.

REFERRAL CONSIDERATIONS

The final outcome of the visual screening is referral to a doctor. It is important not to make diagnostic statements but rather to indicate whether the client passed or failed the vision screening. By law, only optometrists or ophthalmologists can diagnose visual conditions.

It is not always clear-cut when to refer a client or to whom. Many doctors do not test all areas of visual function. Generally, behavioral or developmental optometrists have a functionally oriented philosophy quite similar to occupational therapy models of functional performance.°

Recommended referral guidelines are shown in the following box.

°Bernell/uso, 4016 N. Home Street, Mishiwaka, IN 46545; (800)-348-2225. Complete Visual Screening Kit: Laurie E. Chaikin, OD, OTR, 20881 Redwood Road, Castro Valley, CA 94546; (510)-538-3937.

°College of Optometrists for Vision Development has a list of behavioral doctors: P.O. Box 285, Chula Vista, CA 91912, or Optometric Extension Program, 2912 South Daimler Street, Santa Ana, CA 92705-5811.

REFERRAL GUIDELINES

1. Failure of either the distance or near acuity tests (with glasses on). This could indicate either an uncorrected refractive error, a disease process, or a neurological problem.
2. Failure of the oculomotility section only does not indicate referral because treatment of oculomotor dysfunction is currently within the scope of practice for rehabilitation.
   EXCEPTION: Failure of the pursuit test due to a reduced ocular range of motion in any direction of gaze, which indicates cranial nerve involvement.
3. Failure on the cover/uncover test indicates a strabismus and is an indication for referral unless there is a history of an eye turn.
4. A large eye movement seen on the alternate cover test, along with apparent difficulties in stereopsis, such as spatial judgments, or symptoms, such as headaches, eyestrain, or difficulty with comprehension, constitutes an indication for referral.
5. Failure of the stereopsis test alone is an indication for referral if there is no history of an eye turn, and if there is movement on either cover test.
6. Quarter field loss and half field loss (hemianopia) should be referred.

Visual Intervention

Early intervention is recommended when possible to identify ways in which a vision problem may be interfering with other therapies.[2, 16, 17, 28] Some treatments may be applied early on as well. For example, if the client has an eye muscle paresis, ROM exercises to the involved muscle can prevent the development of a contracture of the unopposed muscle.

In cases in which the client experiences double vision, a patching regimen can be instituted. One regimen is to alternate patching the eyes daily, allowing some time to experience diplopia, so that the eyes may attempt to make a fusion response. The stimulus to fusion is double vision. If one eye is always patched, spontaneous recovery may be slowed. Another patching regimen is binasal taping, and another is to use partially opaque materials to allow peripheral vision in the occluded eye. The patching regimen should be prescribed by an optometrist or ophthalmologist.

In some cases of double vision, a temporary plastic (Fresnel) prism can be applied to the client's glasses to reduce or eliminate the diplopia. This may significantly enhance the client's functioning in other therapies, particularly when spatial judgments are being made (e.g., in fine motor tasks or ambulation).

Documentation

Vision problems should be documented in functional performance terms—that is, how the vision problem affects activities of daily living. Improvement can then be monitored according to function. This will also help in reimbursement. For example, a client with an eye muscle dysfunction will have difficulty with spatial judgments such as placing toothpaste on a toothbrush, spearing objects, reaching for a cup handle, doing pegboard tasks, and using vision for balance.

THERAPEUTIC CONSIDERATIONS

Once a referral has been made, the client has been seen, and the examination report has been received, what else can be done? How the dysfunction affects therapy can be considered and some visual training can be initiated.

Accommodative Dysfunction

If the client has an accommodative dysfunction, the treatment may be the prescription of glasses for reading or table-top tasks or possibly near/far focusing exercises,[4] depending on the age of the client. "Flipper bars" are special lenses that exercise the focusing system.[4]

If the client needs glasses for near, but cannot get them for some reason, the therapist can try moving the task farther away and increasing the lighting on the task.

Eye Alignment Dysfunction

If the client has a problem in the eye alignment system, several factors should be considered. If the client is able to fuse some of the time, but loses fusion, seeing double when stressed or tired, then the most difficult tasks should be attempted when the client is least fatigued. Otherwise, if the client has constant double vision, or the client is seeing double at the time the therapist is working with him or her, patching may be prescribed by the doctor. This will reduce the client's confusion and increase attention to the task. For clients with an acquired double vision, however, it is important to provide time without a patch so that the eyes will attempt to regain fusion. Wearing the patch constantly will discourage any attempts by the brain to overcome the double vision.

Certain postures may facilitate fusion for some clients. The doctor will be able to determine which head position may be best. Frequently, many clients will automatically move around to the best position. At other times, however, head position will be used to avoid using one eye. Head and body position, therefore, are important aspects to consider.

Many convergence problems are amenable to vision therapy,[24, 25, 43] but some are not.[14] Whether a particular problem can be helped by vision therapy can be determined by an eye doctor, who can prescribe specific exercises.

Oculomotor Dysfunction

If the client has a vestibular dysfunction, tracking activities should be combined as much as possible with vestibular stimulation. Vision therapy has been demonstrated to improve reading performance and comprehension.[44, 61]

While doing any sort of tracking activity, the client is encouraged to maintain peripheral awareness. This technique will help the client keep his or her place. The oculomotor system is guided by the peripheral location of an object.

Hemianopia

For clients with hemianopia, compensation training is frequently required to allow the client to resume activities such as reading. Compensation techniques include use of margin markers and reading with a card with a slit in it (typoscope) to isolate one line or a couple of lines at a time. Holding reading material vertically also can help.

SUMMARY OF DISORDERS OF VISION

Table 27–1 summarizes primary visual deficits. Once a therapist or other specialist has eliminated the possibility of primary visual deficits, the clinician must assess whether the identified problem is due to central associative processing that is causing visual-perceptual dysfunction.

VISUAL-PERCEPTUAL DYSFUNCTION

This discussion of visual-perceptual disorders is divided into a number of categories: unilateral spatial inattention; cortical blindness, defective color perception, and visual agnosia; visual-spatial disorders; visual-constructive disorders; and visual analysis and synthesis disorders. Cortical blindness is a disorder of primary visual input; however, because variations of it may influence perceptual interpretation, it is discussed here. All other disorders listed involve direct problems with the interpretation of visual stimuli. Although each of these terms represents symptoms recognized by many authors, the reader is reminded that there are no clear boundaries between one deficit and another or one system and another. Apraxia and body image disorders are not discussed under separate categories because they are not considered "visual"-perceptual disorders per se even though their presence may influence and complicate an already dysfunctional visual-perceptual system.

Problems of Unilateral Spatial Inattention

Identification of Clinical Problems

General Category. In its purest form, unilateral spatial inattention is defined as a condition in which an individual with normal sensory and motor systems fails to orient toward, respond to, or report stimuli on the side contralateral to the cerebral lesion. Although this condition is not often seen in its pure form, inattention has been documented in persons who demonstrate no accompanying visual field defect (homonymous hemianopia) or limb sensory or motor loss.[18] In most cases, however, unilateral spatial inattention is not seen alone but is associated with (although not caused by) accompanying sensory and motor defects such as homonymous hemianopia and decreased tactile, proprioceptive, and stereognostic perception along with paresis or paralysis of the upper limb.

It is easy to become confused by the numerous terms used in the literature, for example, unilateral spatial agnosia, unilateral visual neglect, "fixed" hemianopia, hemi-inattention, or hemi-imperception. All terms describe the same deficit. *Unilateral spatial inattention* is used in this chapter because (1) in severe cases the syndrome most likely involves tactile and auditory as well as visual unawareness (i.e., a total spatial unawareness) and (2) the syndrome results in an involuntary lack of attention to stimuli contralateral to the lesion, whereas the term *neglect* implies a voluntary choice not to respond.

Unilateral spatial inattention occurs most frequently in individuals with a diagnosis of CVA, traumatic brain injury, or tumor. Most authors agree that unilateral spatial inattention occurs more often with right hemisphere than with left hemisphere lesions.[13, 21, 32, 35, 59] This frequency supports theories that the right hemisphere is dominant for visual-spatial organization. It is clear, however, that inattention may be present in individuals with left hemisphere lesions. The clinician should remember that even though the chances are statistically less, the client with right hemiplegia may exhibit inattention to right stimuli.

Unilateral spatial inattention has been associated with lesions in both cortical and subcortical structures. It is most commonly seen in inferior parietal lobe lesions[35] but has also been observed in lesions in the dorsolateral frontal lobe and in the cingulate gyrus,[34] and with thalamic[66] and putaminal hemorrhage.[36] Finally, lesions in the brain stem reticular formation have induced inattention in cats[54] and monkeys.[66]

Although a number of theories have been postulated regarding the mechanism underlying unilateral spatial inattention, no mechanism has been validly documented in human subjects. The one fact that is clear from all theoretical postulates is that inattention is a hemispheric deficit. LeDoux and Smylie[46] demonstrated this point effectively in an interesting case study of a right-sided lesion. During full visual exposure (bilateral hemispheric) of visual-perceptual slides, the affected individual made visual-spatial errors in left space. However, when the same slides were directed only to the right visual field (left hemisphere), performance improved substantially. It is as if the deficient hemisphere fails to receive or orient toward incoming information while the intact receiving hemisphere remains oblivious and goes about its own business. Treatment for inattention is problematic mainly because the mechanisms underlying unilateral spatial inattention are not clearly understood.

Theories on mechanisms underlying unilateral spatial

T A B L E   2 7 – 1. Primary Visual Deficits Associated with Central Lesions, Functional Symptoms, Management, and Treatment

Visual Deficit	Functional Deficit	Management	Treatment
Decreased visual acuity (distance or near)	Decreased acuity for distance or near tasks (reading)	Provide best lens correction for distance and near	May not be correctable
Inconsistent accommodations	Inconsistent blurred near vision	Ensure appropriate lenses are worn for appropriate activities	Accommodation training may be appropriate
		Determine if bifocal is usable; if not, provide separate lenses for distance and near	
		Enlarge target, control density, use contrast, task lighting	
Cortical blindness	Marked decrease in visual acuity	Evaluated by vision specialist to determine areas and quality of residual vision	Use headlamp to improve visual localization (i.e., functional use of residual vision)
	Severe blurring uncorrectable by lenses	Present targets of appropriate size/contrast in best area of visual field	
Visual field deficits include:	Blindness or decreased sensitivity in affected area of visual field	Be aware of normal field position in all meridians of gaze	Scanning training to facilitate compensation
Homonymous hemianopsias		Ask patient to outline working area before beginning task	Training in use of prism
Quadrantanopsias			
Scotomas		Partial press-on Fresnel prism to facilitate compensation	
Visual field constrictions			
Pupillary reactions	Slow or absent pupillary responses	Sunglasses to control excess brightness	
Loss of vertical gaze (external ophthalmoplegia)	Inability to move eyes up or down	Raise target or working area to foveal level	Prism glasses to allow objects below to be seen as directly in front
		Teach patient head movement to compensate	
Conjugate gaze deviation	Inability/difficulty moving eyes from fixed gaze position		
Lack of convergence	Diplopia or blurred vision for near tasks		Convergence exercises prescribed by vision specialist
	Decreased depth perception for near tasks		
Oculomotor nerve lesion (strabismus)	Intermittent or consistent diplopia in some or all meridians of gaze	Fresnel prism to fuse image in select cases	Oculomotor and binocular exercises with prism use prescribed by vision specialist
	Loss of depth perception	Occlude deviant eye	
Pathological (motor) nystagmus	Movement/blur of image during reading/near activities/decreased activities	Enlarge print/target to decrease blur	Rigid gas-permeable contact lens prescribed by vision specialist
		Contact lens provides feedback, reduces movement, and increases activity	
Poor fixations, saccades, or pursuits	Erratic scanning	Decrease density of material	Oculomotor exercises prescribed by vision specialist
	Unsteady fixation	Isolate targets during evaluation and treatment	Sensory integration activities
			Scanning traning
			Use of kinesthetic and tactile systems to lead visual system (eye movements)

©Copyright by Mary Jane Bouska, OTR/L, 1988.
Modified by Laurie E. Chaikin, OD, OTR.

inattention have attempted to explain it as an integrative associative defect as opposed to simply a problem of decreased sensory input. Theories include a unilateral attentional hypothesis, suggesting that inattention results from a disruption in the orienting response; that is, the corticolimbic hemisphere is underaroused during bilateral input and therefore stimuli presented to that hemisphere are neglected.[34, 35] Another theory is the oculomotor imbalance hypothesis, which suggests that individuals with inattention have a visual-spatial disorder worsened by oculomotor imbalance. The hypothesis suggests that the lesion disconnects the frontal eye fields in the damaged hemisphere from their sensory afferent nerves, resulting in an oculomotor imbalance deviating the gaze toward the lesion. This imbalance can be compensated for only momentarily by a voluntary effort to gaze toward the opposite hemispace (i.e., neglected space).[15]

Unilateral Spatial Inattention with Homonymous Hemianopia. Inattention occurs more commonly with visual field defects and is generally worse when the macula is not spared. Individuals with pure hemianopias are aware of their visual loss and spontaneously learn to compensate by moving their eyes (foveae) toward their lost visual field to expand their visual space and thereby gather information right and left of midline. On visual examination other individuals may demonstrate no visual field defect on unilateral stimulation; however, during bilateral stimulation, they extinguish the target contralateral to their lesion. Other persons may perceive both targets simultaneously, yet when engaged in activity, they may not respond to visual stimuli in one half of visual space contralateral to their lesion. These individuals are unaware of their inattention. Careful observation of their activity reveals a paucity of eye movements into the neglected space. The fovea does not appear to be directed to gather information in this space.

Unilateral Visual, Auditory, and Tactile Inattention. Inattention has been described as a multimodal sensory associative disorder involving not only visual but also tactile and auditory unawareness. Clinicians are well aware of the client with left inattention who continues to direct the head and eyes toward the right throughout an entire conversation even though the therapist is standing on the client's left side. When one conceptualizes unilateral spatial inattention as a dynamic decrease or loss of sensory information within one half of the sensory-perceptual sphere (irrespective of hypothetical mechanism), the peculiar behaviors exhibited by these clients are more easily understood.

Unilateral Spatial Inattention and Body Image. Body image is often disturbed in individuals with inattention. The defect in these persons is unusual because it affects only that half of the body that is contralateral to the lesion, for example, the left side of the body in right-sided lesions. There appears to be a lack of spatial orientation and attention for one half of intrapersonal space. Those with severe inattention fail to recognize that their affected extremities are their own and function as though they are absent. They may fail to dress one half of their body or attempt to navigate through a door oblivious to the fact that the affected arm may be caught on the doorknob or door frame. In severe cases, individuals may deny their hemiparesis, or they may deny that the extremity belongs to them. This phenomenon is called anosognosia.

Behavioral Manifestations of Unilateral Spatial Inattention. Persons with inattention orient all their activities toward their "attended" space. The head, eyes, and trunk are rotated toward the side of the lesion during much of the time, including during gait. Careful observation of eye movements (scanning saccades) during activities indicates that all or almost all scanning occurs on only one side of the midline within the attended space; the individual never spontaneously brings the eyes or head past midline into contralateral "unattended" space. Oculomotor examination always shows full extraocular movements and no apraxia for eye movements.

Inattention, like all other perceptual disorders, may be viewed on a scale from mild to severe. Mild cases of inattention may go unrecognized unless behavior is carefully observed. Scanning is symmetrical except during tasks requiring increasingly complex perceptual and cognitive demands. Leicester and coworkers[47] believe that inattention occurs mainly when the individual has a general perceptual problem with the material, that is, some

other problem with processing the task. This performance difficulty or stress brings on the additional inattention behavior; for example, neglect for matching auditory letter samples is more common in those with aphasia than in those with right hemisphere involvement without aphasia.

Independence in activities of daily living is often impossible because of inattention to both the intrapersonal and extrapersonal environment. The individual may eat only half of the food on the plate, dress only half the body, shave or apply makeup to only half the face, brush teeth in only half the mouth, read only half the page, fill out only one half a form, miss kitchen utensils, carpentry tools, or items in the store if they are located in the unattended space, collide with obstacles or miss doorways on the unattended side, and, when walking or driving a wheelchair, veer toward the attended space rather than navigating in a straight line.

Assessment

Because most tests used to measure cognitive, language, perceptual, and motor skills require symmetrical visual, auditory, and tactile awareness, it is most important to rule out inattention early in the evaluation process of any client with a central lesion. The two most common methods used to distinguish inattention from primary sensory deficits are double simultaneous stimulation testing and assessment of optokinetic nystagmus (OKN) reflexes. Double simultaneous stimuli should be applied in three modalities: auditory, tactile, and visual. Initially, stimuli should be presented to the abnormal side. If primary sensation is impaired (e.g., a visual field loss), this evaluation cannot proceed because double simultaneous stimulation testing is invalid in that modality. If responsiveness is normal, however, bilateral simultaneous stimuli should be applied. Unilateral stimuli should be interspersed with bilateral stimuli to ensure valid responses. Lack of awareness (extinction) of stimuli contralateral to the lesion during bilateral stimulation should be noted. Clients with extinction in only one sensory system often do not demonstrate inattention behaviors; however, those with extinction in more than one modality (e.g., tactile and visual) often demonstrate these behaviors. If critical diagnosis of inattention is necessary, the client may be referred for OKN testing.

One of the best evaluation tools is a keen sense of observation. The position of the client's head, eyes, and trunk should be observed at rest and during activity. Persistent deviation toward the lesion may indicate unilateral inattention. The individual should be asked to track a visual target from space ipsilateral to the lesion into contralateral space and maintain fixation there for 5 seconds. The therapist may ask the client to quickly fixate on visual targets both right and left of midline on command. Problems with searching for targets in contralateral space should be noted. Some erratic oculomotor searching is normal when making saccades into a hemianoptic field because saccades are centrally preprogrammed by peripheral input. Very slow searching or failure to search should be considered indicative of inattention.

Asymmetries in performance should be noted during

spatial tasks. Specific spatial tasks have been designed to detect inattention, including:

- Cancellation tasks. The client may be given a sheet of paper with horizontal lines of numbers or letters and asked to cross out all the 8s or As.
- Crossing-out tasks. In this test, standardized by Albert,[9] the client is asked to cross out diagonal lines drawn at random on an unlined sheet of paper.
- Line-bisection tasks. The client is asked to bisect a 4-inch to 8-inch line on a piece of paper placed at his or her midline.
- Drawing and copying tasks. The client may be asked to draw or copy a house, clock, or flower or to fill in the numbers of a clock drawn by the examiner. For copying tasks, it is important that the copy be placed in the client's attended space.

Clients with inattention demonstrate one or more of the following behaviors: failure to cancel figures or cross out lines in the unattended space; bisecting the line unequally, placing their mark toward the side of the midline ipsilateral to their lesion; placing their drawing toward the edge of the paper ipsilateral to their lesion rather than in the middle of the page; drawing only the right or left half of the house, flower, or clock; crowding all the numbers of the clock into the right or left half of the clock; or completing numbers on only one half of the clock (Fig. 27–11). When interpreting performance, the examiner is looking specifically for asymmetries in performance. Clients with inattention often have other visual-perceptual deficits that result in faulty performance on these tasks; however, these deficits are always symmetrical, that is, evident in any space to which the individual attends.

Asymmetries in performance should be carefully observed during functional activities such as eating, filling out a form, reading, dressing, and maneuvering through the environment. The therapist may note unawareness of doorways and hallways in the unattended space; turns may be made only toward one direction. As a result, these clients lose their way in the hospital or even in the therapy clinic. This behavior should be distinguished from a topographical perceptual deficit in which the individual

cannot integrate or remember spatial concepts well enough to find his or her way without getting lost. The Behavioral Inattention Test has recently been published as a standardized measure of functional inattention.[67]

Finally, various studies have shown that inattention may occur during testing that requires visual processing and therefore may invalidate test results.[12, 13, 26] Unresponsiveness to figures on one side of the page during visual, perceptual, cognitive, or language assessments may be subtle but must be documented to rule out the influence of inattention on raw score; that is, if the patient did not see the entire test display in an item, that test item is invalid. Responses to figures on the right half and left half of the test page should be counted. If the frequency of answers is noticeably less on one half of the page than would normally be expected, one may suspect that inattention may have occurred during testing. This may be used as additional evidence of inattention; but more important, this factor should be accounted for when computing the test score. Only those test items in which the correct answer was located in the attended space should be scored; that is, only those items in which the correct answer was right of midline in a client with left inattention should be scored.

Interventions

As previously stated, the mechanisms underlying unilateral spatial inattention have not been clearly elucidated. This has made development of treatment rationales difficult. A number of studies, however, have investigated the remediation of unilateral spatial inattention. They have attempted to (1) define effective remediation techniques and (2) measure changes in trained tasks as well as generalization to untrained tasks—that is, determine whether inattention training in one task carries over to other unrelated tasks such as activities of daily living. Treatment techniques used in all of these studies resulted in less inattention in trained tasks.[21, 45, 62] An overview of these studies suggests that training may decrease inattention, although extent of change and generalization to other tasks may vary widely. Discrepancies in these results may be related to neurological variables in the various client samples, severity of inattention, sample size, or tasks measured. A discussion of general principles of remediation follows.

Effort should be made to increase the client's cognitive awareness of the inattention. The individual should be made keenly aware of what a peripheral visual field loss is and how it is affecting his or her view of the world. The person with normal visual fields but with visual extinction should be treated the same as the individual with an actual visual field loss because the visual experience is similar. Pictures of the visual field deficit may be drawn for illustration. Actual performance examples in the environment should be pointed out to the client to demonstrate the biased field of view.

Visual scanning should be emphasized. Initially, the client should be made aware of how eye and eye-head movements may be used to compensate for the deficit. The individual should be trained to make progressively larger and quicker pursuits and saccades and longer fixa-

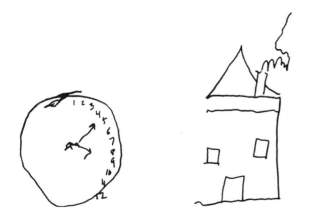

FIGURE 27–11. Drawings of a clock and house by a client with a right hemisphere parietal lobe tumor. Note the left unilateral spatial inattention in the drawings.

	0	①	2	4	5	6	7	8	9	10	
1.	① 2 3 5 4 9 7 8 0 6 3 2 10 ① 2 3 5 4 9 7										1
2.	3 4 9 6 7 10 8 ① 2 5 0 6 4 9 6 7 10 8 2 8										2
3.	8 0 6 2 ① 3 5 4 7 9 10 ① 8 0 6 2 ① 3 5 7										3
4.	5 7 3 9 6 ① 2 8 4 10 0 3 5 5 7 3 6 ① 2 5										4
5.	6 5 ① 4 2 3 8 10 9 7 9 0 6 5 ① 4 2 3 8 9										5
6.	4 8 10 0 7 6 9 1 3 2 5 6 3 4 8 10 0 7 6 9										6
7.	9 6 5 3 8 4 2 0 10 1 7 2 4 9 6 5 3 8 2 4										7

FIGURE 27–12. Underlining during visual discrimination tasks helps control eye movements (scanning).

tions into the unattended space. Training may be accomplished with interesting targets held by the therapist, for example, targets secured to the tips of pencils, such as changeable letters, colored lights, or bright small objects. Pursuit or tracking movements of the target leading the eye from attended into unattended space should be stressed first, followed by saccades into the unattended space. Initially, the client may be allowed to move the head during scanning exercises; however, eye movements without head movements should be the major goal. Individuals with inattention often move their head into the unattended space while their eye remains fixed on a target in their attended space (i.e., the visual field remains the same). The client should be taught to independently carry out a daily right-left scanning program with targets appropriately positioned by the therapist. Eventually, these targets can be moved farther into the unattended space.

Increased awareness and scanning abilities should be incorporated in increasingly complex visual-perceptual and visual-motor tasks. Because inattention often increases as task complexity increases, the therapist must select and structure tasks carefully. Examples of simple yet specific scanning tasks might include surveying a room repetitively, rolling toward and touching objects right and left of midline, assembling objects from pieces strewn on a table or the floor, completing an obstacle course, or selecting letters from a page of large print.

Scanning should be stressed during functional activities, for example, dressing, shaving, or moving through the environment. The client may be taught to constantly monitor the influence of inattention on functional performance, for example: "When something doesn't make sense, look into the unattended space and it usually will."

Diller[20] has designed a number of specific training techniques to decrease inattention during reading and paper and pencil tasks. With a little creativity, these techniques may be applied to other activities. For example, when the client is reading, a visual marker is placed on the extreme edge of the page in unattended space. The individual is instructed not to begin reading until he or she sees the visual marker. The marker is used to "anchor" the client's vision. As inattention decreases, the anchor is faded. Each line may also be numbered and the numbers used to anchor scanning horizontally and vertically. To control impulsiveness, which often accompanies inattention, clients are taught to slow down or pace their performance by incorporating techniques such as reciting the words aloud. Underlining and looping letters/words can also be used as a method to slow down impulsive scanning (Fig. 27–12). Finally, density of stimuli is reduced; decreased density appears to decrease inattention in these tasks.

To stimulate tactile awareness in clients with tactile extinction, Anderson and Choy[3] suggest stimulating the affected arm as the individual watches. A rough cloth, vibrator, or the therapist's or client's hand may be used. Eventually, this activity may be done before activities that require spontaneous symmetrical scanning, such as dressing and walking through an obstacle course.

During the early phases of treatment, when inattention is still moderate to severe, the client should be approached from the attended space during treatment for inattention or other deficits such as apraxia, balance, or speech. This ensures that the individual comprehends and views all demonstrations and treatment instructions. Subsequently, as orientation and scanning improve, activities should be moved progressively into the unattended space and the therapist should be positioned in the unattended space during treatment. In the final stages of treatment the client should be able to symmetrically scan regardless of the therapist's position (i.e., the therapist should vary position).

To enhance the integration of scanning behavior during functional tasks such as gait and dressing, the client should be reminded of scanning principles and carried through a series of scanning exercises before initiation of the activity. If inattention reappears during the activity, the therapist should stop and assist the client in becoming reoriented before resuming the activity. Inattention results in confusion, and confusion increases inattention. As will be pointed out repeatedly in the following pages, the therapist must control the perceptual environment continuously so that the client is able to sequence bits of information together meaningfully to learn or relearn.

Problems of Cortical Blindness, Color Imperception, and Visual Agnosia

Identification of Clinical Problems

Cortical Blindness. Cortical blindness is considered a primary sensory disorder as opposed to a secondary associative disorder. It is discussed here, however, because of the many variations of this lesion that may result in problems with interpretation of visual stimuli. Cortical blindness, also known as central blindness, is a total or almost total loss of vision resulting from bilateral cerebral destruction of the visual projection cortex (area 17). Similar destruction limited to one hemisphere results in a heminopia.[18] The lesion may be ischemic, neoplastic, degenerative, or traumatic. The client may perceive the defect as a "blurring" of vision or as a marked decrease in visual acuity, or may be unaware of the complete nature of the disability and even deny it, blaming the problem on eye glasses that are too weak or a room that is too dark.

Color Imperception. Color perception may be impaired in the client with brain damage. This symptom is usually associated with right hemisphere or bilateral lesions.[58] This deficit is different from color agnosia, in which there is a problem with naming colors correctly. Clients with defective color perception may see colors as "muddy" or "impure" in hue, or the color of a small target may fade into the background, decreasing the ability to differentiate it from the background.[49, 59] Total loss of color monochromatism is rare but can occur.

Visual Agnosia. A lesion circumscribed to the visual associative areas (areas 18 and 19) results in a number of unique visual disorders that are categorized as some form of visual agnosia. Lesions are usually bilateral with combined parietooccipital, occipitotemporal, and callosal lesions. Visual agnosia is defined as a failure to recognize visual stimuli (e.g., objects, faces, letters) even though visual-sensory processing, language, and general intellectual functions are preserved at sufficiently high levels.[57] It also has been described as perception without meaning; perception apparently occurs, but the percept seems "disconnected" from previously associated meaning. In this pure form, visual agnosia is a relatively rare syndrome, and there is controversy as to whether it is simply an extension of primary visual sensory deficits (variations of cortical blindness) or whether it should be considered as a separate neuropsychological entity.

Three types of agnosia have been recognized: visual, tactile, and auditory. Agnosia is most often modality specific; that is, the individual who cannot recognize the object visually will usually give an immediate and accurate response when touching or hearing the object in use. In visual agnosia, then, poor recognition is limited to the visual sphere.

Visual agnosia is divided into a number of types: visual object agnosia, simultanagnosia, facial agnosia, and color agnosia. These deficits may be seen in isolation or in various combinations, depending on size and location of lesion.

Visual Object Agnosia. During evaluation for the presence of visual object agnosia, the individual is presented with a number of common objects (e.g., key, comb, brush) and asked to name them. The evaluator may assume that the object is recognized if the client (1) names, describes, or demonstrates the use of the object or (2) selects it from among a group of objects as it is named by the examiner. If the person recognizes (describes or demonstrates) but is unable to name the object, failure is most likely a result of an anomia rather than an agnosic defect. Individuals with real visual agnosia have no concept of what the object is.[57]

Simultanagnosia. Along the same vein are visual disorders that constrict or "narrow" the visual field during active perceptual analysis (i.e., when perceptions are tested separately, the visual field is within normal limits). Simultanagnosia is a disorder in which the person actually perceives only one element of an object or picture at a time and is unable to absorb the whole. As the individual concentrates on the visual environment, there is an extreme reduction of visual span. The problem is functionally similar to tubular vision. The narrowing of the functional perceptual field decreases the ability to simultaneously deal with two or more stimuli. It appears as if the person has bilateral visual inattention with macular sparing although perimetric testing reveals full visual fields. A typical example is the individual whose visual attention is focused on the tip of a cigarette held between his or her lips and fails to perceive a match flame offered several inches away.[33]

Facial Agnosia. Another special type of agnosia that has been documented is failure to recognize familiar faces. The disorder is also known as prosopagnosia. The individual is able to recognize a face as a face but is unable to connect the face and differences in faces with people he or she knows. This person is unable to recognize family members, friends, and hospital staff by face. One must be careful not to confuse this with generalized dementia. There may be categorical recognition problems of items involving special visual experience, for example, recognition of cars, types of trees, or emblems. Facial agnosia is usually seen in combination with a number of other deficits, including spatial disorientation, defective color perception, loss of topographical memory, constructional apraxia, and a left upper quadrant visual field loss. These other symptoms are most likely not causative but rather a result of the similar neurological location of these functions.[8]

Color Agnosia. Finally, the individual may have difficulty recognizing names of colors, that is, an inability to name colors that are shown or to point to the color named by the examiner. This defect is considered agnosic (as opposed to a defect in color perception) because the client is able to recognize all colors in the *Ishihara Color Plates*[40] and is also able to sort colors by hue. The determining factor here appears to be a problem with visual-verbal association. Color agnosia is most common in clients with left hemisphere lesions and is often accompanied by the syndrome of alexia without agraphia.[57]

Assessment

Cortical blindness and variations of it should be thoroughly assessed by the vision specialist. Assessment for agnosia must be preceded by a thorough assessment for visual acuity problems, visual field deficits, and unilateral visual inattention, because these primary visual sensory and scanning deficits are often mistaken for agnosic performance. Next, basic color perception should be measured using the *Ishihara Color Plates*[40] and color-sorting or color-matching tasks. Individuals with defective color perception will have difficulty with some visual-perceptual tasks because contextual cues related to color and shading are unavailable to them. Agnosia is a valid diagnosis only if (1) the aforementioned primary visual skills are intact and (2) language skills are intact (i.e., there should be no word-finding difficulty in spontaneous speech).

Although there are no standardized tests for agnosia, commonly used assessment methods have been included. The presence of simultanagnosia is determined by keen observation of performance that indicates perception limited to single elements within objects, for example, describing only the wheel of a bicycle or, within the environment, describing only one part of a room or an activity.

Object agnosia is tested by placing common real objects (e.g., comb, key, penny, spoon) in front of the client and asking him or her to name or point to the item chosen by the examiner. In pointing and naming tasks, the therapist must be sure that the client is fixating on the appropriate target. This response is considered normal if the object is named correctly or described or its functional use demonstrated. Abnormal responses will be confabulatory or perseverative, with the individual often giving the name of a previous or similar object. Responses may also be completely bizarre and unrelated. The examiner may also present objects at an unusual angle. Abnormal responses will show lack of recognition and/or rotation of the head or body to try to view the object in the "straight on" position. The diagnosis of visual object agnosia is further confirmed if the individual can identify the object by touch or by hearing it in use. Both should be done with vision occluded.

Color agnosia is evaluated by having the client name a color and point to colors named by the examiner. Facial agnosia is evaluated by presenting the individual with photographs of famous world figures, actors, politicians, and family members.[59]

Interventions

There are no reliable studies regarding treatment of cortical blindness, color imperception, or visual agnosia. Treatment principles presented here are based on the experience of Bouska and Biddle[12] and Bouska and Kwatny.[13] If cortical blindness or simultanagnosia is suspected, the therapist must first attempt to increase the client's knowledge of foveal versus peripheral vision, that is, where the client is fixating. A small headlamp attached to the client's forehead may be used under conditions of subdued lighting. This should not be used in a completely darkened room because the client needs to use normal spatial cues from the environment. The movement of the projected light in the environment and kinesthetic input from the neck receptors augment knowledge of where the eye is fixed. To carry out this task, the client must learn to position the eyes in midline of the head. The individual is asked to move the light (i.e., head and eyes) to locate and discriminate fairly large, bright stimuli placed on a plain background (e.g., yellow block on a brown table). As acuity and localization skills improve, stimuli and background should be made smaller and more complex (e.g., paper clip on a printed background or letters printed at different locations on a large page). The client should be encouraged to accurately point to and/or manipulate targets once located with the light or to keep the light on a target as he or she slowly moves the target with one hand. In this mode, the kinesthetic input from the limb can augment visual localization abilities.[45] In patients with color imperception, treatment should initially involve materials/tasks with sharp color contrasts with minimal detail and should progress to less contrast (more hues) with more detail.

If the assessment has revealed a narrowing of the perceptual field, treatment should be aimed at progressively increasing the perception of large, bright, peripheral targets. For example, the client may be asked to fixate on a centrally placed target while another bright target is brought in slowly from or uncovered in the periphery.[5, 69] The individual is encouraged to maintain fixation on the central target while remaining alert for the presence of another target somewhere in the periphery. As the client improves, targets should be smaller, multiple, and exposed for briefer periods. Peripheral targets should always have bright surfaces that reflect light since the peripheral receptors in the retina are mainly rods (light as opposed to color receptors).

The treatment of clients with object agnosia should progress according to the abilities that return first in spontaneous recovery from agnosia. Common real objects should be used before line drawings in treatment. Presentations should be given "straight on" rather than at an angle or rotated. The client should be asked to point to objects named by the examiner before being asked to name them. Manipulation of the object with simultaneous visual input should be attempted. This may help recognition, or it may simply confuse the client; each case is unique. In general, tactile input with or without simultaneous visual input should be encouraged as a compensation method even though it may not be helpful during treatment sessions.

Color and facial agnosia may be approached by simply drilling the individual with regard to two or three names of colors or names of faces of people important to him or her. The client may be helped to pick out or memorize cues for associating names with faces.[59]

Problems of Visual-Spatial Disorders

Identification of Clinical Problems

Individuals with brain lesions, particularly in the right posterior parietal and occipital areas, may have difficulties with tasks that require a normal concept of space.[18] Disorders of this nature have been termed visual-spatial disorders, spatial disorientation, visual-spatial agnosia, spatial relations syndrome, and numerous other names. Visual-spatial abilities are complexly interwoven within the performance of many perceptual and cognitive activities such as dressing, building a design, reading, calculating, walking through an aisle, and playing tennis. An attempt is made here, however, to discuss spatial disorders in their purest form—that is, basic disorders—before dealing with visual-constructive disorders and disorders of analysis and synthesis. Constructional tasks require spatial planning, a type of planning that involves the building up and breaking down of objects in two and three dimensions. Constructional apraxia is viewed as a particular type of spatial-perceptual disorder and, therefore, is discussed separately under visual-constructive disorders and disorders of analysis and synthesis. Similarly, although perceptual skills such as figure-ground, form constancy, complex visual discrimination, and figure closure involve spatial concepts, tasks involving these skills often require the intellectual operations of synthesis and deduction. They, too, are discussed in the section dealing with analysis and synthesis.

All visual-spatial disabilities involve some problem with the apprehension of the spatial relationships between or within objects. Benton[7] has categorized them as the following disabilities:

1. *Inability to localize objects in space, to estimate their size, and to judge their distance from the observer.* The client may be unable to accurately touch an object in space or indicate the position of the object (e.g., above, below, in front of, or behind). Relative localization may be impaired so that the individual may be unable to tell which object is closest to him or her. There may be difficulty determining which of two objects is larger or which line is longer. Holmes[37] reported cases of gross disorder in spatial orientation revealed through walking; affected individuals, even after seeing objects correctly, ran into them. In another example, a man, intending to go toward his bed, would invariably set out in the wrong direction. Difficulty in estimating distances may also extend to judgments of distances of perceived sounds and lead to overly slow and cautious gait or fear of venturing into public areas.

2. *Impaired memory for the location of objects or places.* An example is not being able to recall the position of a target previously viewed or the arrangement of furniture in a room. Individuals with this difficulty often lose things because they have no spatial memory to rely on for recall.

3. *Inability to trace a path or follow a route from one place to another.* Persons without this ability, known as topographical orientation, have difficulty understanding and remembering relationships of places to one another so that they may have difficulty finding their way in space, as in locating the therapy clinic in a hospital or locating the housewares department in a store previously familiar to them. Normally functioning individuals often experience mild signs of topographical disorientation. Everyone is familiar with the disoriented feeling of not knowing how to get out of a large department store or losing a sense of direction in a familiar city. Many of the topographical errors made

by clients result from unilateral spatial inattention. For example, someone with left inattention may make only right turns. Topographical disorientation, however, may be seen in a person with no signs of unilateral inattention. This individual will demonstrate route-finding difficulties at certain points and apparently randomly choose a direction.

4. *Problems with reading and counting.* These high-level tasks require directional control of eye movements and organized scanning abilities. Eye movements (saccades) during reading bring a new region of the text on the fovea, the part of the retina where visual acuity is the greatest and clear detail can be obtained from the stimulus. During reading, the line of print that falls on the retina may be divided into three regions: the foveal region, the parafoveal region, and the peripheral region. The foveal region subtends about 1 to 2 degrees of visual angle around the reader's fixation point, the parafoveal region subtends about 10 degrees of visual angle around the reader's fixation point, and the peripheral region includes everything on the page beyond the parafoveal region. Parafoveal and peripheral vision contribute spatial information that is used to guide the reader's eye.[53] Visual-spatial disorders appear to interfere to varying degrees with the spatial schema of a page of type or numbers and the dynamic organizational scanning that must take place to gather information appropriately. Clients with unilateral spatial inattention will miss words or numbers located on one half of the page. Other spatial problems unrelated to unilateral inattention include skipping individual words within a line or part of a line, skipping lines, repeating lines, "blocking" or the inability to change direction of fixation, particularly at the end of a line, and generally losing the place on the total page. Performance usually deteriorates progressively as the individual continues to read. Eventually, such persons cannot make sense of what they read or, if counting, they complain of being lost or confused. This type of reading or counting disorder has nothing to do with recognition or interpretation of letters or numbers or their spatial configuration; rather, it represents a problem with dynamic sequential visual-spatial exploration during cognitive processing.

Other visual-spatial problems may include loss of depth perception, problems with body schema, and defective judgment of line orientation. There may also be difficulties with discrimination of right and left. Although unilateral spatial inattention is considered a visual-spatial disorder by many, it has been discussed separately in this chapter to increase clarity. Problems with judging line orientation (slant) and/or unilateral spatial inattention often interfere with a client's spatial ability to tell time when using a standard watch or clock. Perception of the vertical may also be considered a visual-spatial skill. Verticality perception is the interpretation of internal and external cues to maintain body balance. This maintenance is a complex neuromuscular process involving visual, proprioceptive, and vestibular systems. Clients with right lesions, particularly in the parietooccipital region, have more difficulty perceiving verticality than those with left lesions. This may affect posture and ambulation.[19]

Assessment

The client should be asked to accurately touch a number of targets in all parts of the visual field while fixating on a central point. Mislocalization should be noted as well as that part of the visual field in which it occurred. Mislocalization within the central field is infrequent; however, defective localization of stimuli on one or both extramacular fields is more frequently seen.[18] The client should be asked to determine which of a number of small cube blocks (placed perpendicularly in front of him or her) is closest, which is farthest, and which is in the middle. Differences in binocular (stereoscopic) and monocular viewing should be measured in this and other tasks. Impairment in both of these types of depth perception and subsequent inaccuracy in judging distances have been described in individuals with brain injury.[7]

With regard to memory for the location of objects or places, clients should be asked to describe the position of objects in their room from memory. They may also be asked to duplicate from memory the position of two or more targets (on a table or piece of paper) that have been presented for a 5-second period. As the number of targets increases, individuals with short-term memory for spatial localization will begin to make errors in spatial placement. Visual memory per se should be ruled out as a conflicting variable.

Topographical sense is assessed by asking clients to describe a floor plan of the arrangement of rooms in their house or to describe familiar geographical constellations, such as routes, arrangement of streets, or public buildings. After therapy these persons may also be asked to find their way back to their room after being shown the route several times. Failure suggests a topographical orientation problem. Finally, such a client may be asked to locate states or cities on a large map of the United States. In all of these procedures, the examiner must be sure to separate unilateral spatial inattention errors from topographical errors.

The influence of spatial dysfunction on reading and counting written material may be measured simply by asking the client to read a page of regular newsprint. The examiner should observe performance carefully and document type and frequency of errors. If errors occur, eye movements should be observed to gather additional information. Pages of scanning material (letters or numbers) often give additional information on spatial planning during reading. These are pages of print in which the size and density of the print are controlled. Scanning behavior may be demonstrated by asking the client to circle specific letters. Switching direction in the middle of a line, skipping letters or lines, perseveration, or any other abnormal performance behavior should be noted. Benton's Judgment of Line Orientation Test[9] may be used to document problems with directional orientation of lines. If there is no indication of apraxia, the client may simply be given a ruler and asked to match it to the directional orientation of the examiner's ruler.

Interventions

Treatment for visual-spatial deficits should follow basic developmental considerations progressing from simple to more complex tasks. As with children, if the evaluation suggests disorders in body scheme, tactile or vestibular input, or right-left discrimination, these should be dealt with first.

Clients who do not know where they are in space need to internalize a spatial understanding before they can make judgments regarding the space around them. In gross motor spatial training, clients can be asked to roll and reach toward various targets. In supine, prone, sitting, and standing, with vision occluded, clients should try to localize tactile stimuli (various body locations touched by the therapist) and auditory stimuli (e.g., snapping fingers or ringing a bell) presented above, below, behind, in front of, and right and left of their bodies. The individual should state where the stimulus is and then point, roll, crawl, or walk toward it; this verbal, kinesthetic, and vestibular input augments spatial learning. In the occupational therapy kitchen the client, once oriented to the room, may be asked to retrieve one type of object (e.g., cup) from "the top cupboard above your head," from "the bottom cupboard below your waist," from "the table behind you," or from "the drawer on your right or left." These clients may also place objects in various positions within a room. They should then stand in the middle of the room, close their eyes, and from memory visualize, verbalize, and point to where the objects are in relation to themselves. Having localized them, the clients should then walk through the space and retrieve the objects in sequence. Functional carryover should always be emphasized, such as having individuals remember through visualization where they put their glasses in the living room before they begin searching. Visualization is defined as the internal "seeing" of something that is not present at that moment: a vision without a visual input or internal visual imagery.[23] Visualization (spatial and other) is part of all perceptual tasks and may be used effectively as a treatment strategy. As previously discussed, a small feedback light placed in the middle of the client's forehead can help teach spatial localization through eye-hand movements.

More complex spatial skills may be taught by asking clients to "partition" space and then localize within it. An excellent activity is one in which clients use a yardstick to divide a blackboard into four or more equal parts and then number each section.

Objects may be presented to clients, who must select the largest, the farthest away, or the one placed at an angle; they may be asked to place various objects in certain relationships to each other. As shape, size, and angle begin to "make sense" to these individuals, form boards, simple puzzles, and parquetry blocks may be added to training.

Topographical abilities should improve as clients begin to better conceptualize space; however, they may be trained directly. The therapist may help such clients organize a basic floor plan of their hospital room and the furniture within it while looking at the room. They may then be asked to do this from memory. Activities can progress to drawing plans or larger areas with a number of rooms. These clients should first "navigate" tactually through the area with their finger. Eventually, they should walk or wheel through the route themselves, visualizing and repeating the route until spatial concepts are learned. Imaginary routes also may be taken through maps of cities, states, or countries.

Organized visual-spatial exploration (eye movements) during reading or other scanning and cancellation tasks may be taught. Number and letter scanning sheets may be used for such training. Initially, size of numbers and spaces between numbers should be large; this places less stress on visual acuity while training scanning. Before beginning, clients should orient themselves to the page spatially by numbering the right and left edges of each line. These numbers are used as additional spatial localization cues if needed during the scanning task.[20] Clients should then be asked to circle a specific number (or numbers) whenever it occurs. To control erratic or impulsive eye movements, they should be instructed to use a pencil to underline each line and then loop the selected letter as it comes into view (see Fig. 27–12). They may also be asked to read each letter. Underlining allows the kinesthetic and tactile receptors of the arm to control eye movements; verbalization allows the language and auditory systems to influence eye movements. Visual-spatial exploration exercises should progress to large-print magazines, books, or newspapers. The *New York Times* and *Reader's Digest* are both available in large print. In all training activities it is most important that, before the activity begins, clients fully comprehend the total space in which they will work. It is equally important that they reorient themselves at any point where errors occur. Those who lose their place during reading will eventually lose it again if the therapist simply points to where they should be. Chances are better that they will not lose their place again if they reorient themselves to the page spatially when an error occurs.

Problems of Visual-Constructive Disorders

Identification of Clinical Problems

Clients with lesions in either the right or left hemisphere may have problems when trying to "construct." Lesions in the parietal, temporal, occipital, and frontal lobes have been documented in individuals with visual-constructive disorders.[18, 48] The normal ability to construct, also known as visual-constructive ability and constructional praxis, involves any type of performance in which parts are put together to form a single entity. Examples include assembling blocks to form a design, assembling a puzzle, making a dress, setting a table, and simply drawing four lines to form a square (graphic skills). The skill implies a high level of dynamic, organized, visual-perceptual processing in which the spatial relations are perceived and sequenced well enough among and within the component parts to direct higher-level processing to sequence the perceptual-motor actions so that eventually parts are synthesized into a desired whole. Visual-constructive ability may be compromised if any part of this process is disturbed.

Typical tasks used to measure this ability include building in a vertical direction, building in a horizontal direction, three-dimensional block construction from a model or a picture of a model, and copying line drawings such as house, flower, and geometric designs.[8]

Clients with visual-constructive deficits, especially those with right lesions, often also have visual-spatial deficits. These individuals may rotate the position of a part erroneously, place it in the wrong position, space it too far from another part, be oblivious to perspective or a third dimension, or simply be unable to complete more than two or three steps before becoming entirely confused. This is usually evidence of breakdown because of faulty or inadequate spatial information.

Other clients, usually those with left lesions, have an "executional" or apraxic problem; they seem to have difficulty initiating and conducting the planned sequence of movements necessary to construct the whole. The problem seems to be in planning, arranging, building, or drawing rather than in spatial concepts. This deficit in its purest form is known as constructional apraxia. Constructional apraxia lies clinically outside the category of most other varieties of apraxia and is considered a special kind of "perceptual" apraxia. It occurs frequently in aphasic individuals; therefore, the underlying mechanisms of aphasia and constructional apraxia may be related.[60]

Assessment

Constructional abilities are generally measured through tasks that require (1) copying line drawings such as a house, clock face, flower, or geometric designs (drawing may also be done without copy); (2) copying two-dimensional matchstick designs; (3) building block designs from copy or model; or (4) assembling puzzles. (Table 27–2 lists common tests.) The more complex the picture or design to be copied, the more complex the constructional tasks. The following are examples of drawing and block construction deficits:

1. Clients may crowd the drawing or design on one side of the page or in one corner of the page or available space on the working surface, usually a result of the influence of unilateral spatial inattention.
2. Lines in drawings may be wavy or broken, too long or short.
3. One line may not meet another accurately, or lines may transect each other; in block designs, parts may not be neatly placed but rather may have small gaps.
4. There may be "overdrawing" of angles or parts of the figure because of graphic perseveration (scribble),

TABLE 27–2. Common Tests Used to Assess Visuoconstructive Skills

Test	Standardization
Drawing pictures or shapes with or without copy	Not standardized
Reproducing matchstick designs	Not standardized
Assembling puzzles	Not standardized
The Bender Visual Motor Gestalt Test	Standardized for children only
Kohs' Blocks Test	Standardized for adults
WAIS Block Design Test	Standardized for adults
Benton's Three-Dimensional Constructional Praxis Test	Standardized for adults

spatial indecision, or problems with executive planning.

5. Clients may superimpose their copy on the model or superimpose one of their drawings on top of another. In block design construction, they may become confused between the model and their reproduction and use part of the model to complete their design. This has been termed the "closing-in" phenomenon, a failure to distinguish between model and reproduction.[18]

6. Parts of the drawing or design may be reversed. Horizontal reversals are more common than vertical reversals.

A note might be appropriate here regarding dressing apraxia. This problem occurs most frequently with right hemisphere damage. It is considered a "perceptual" apraxia rather than a motor apraxia because the inability to dress is believed to result from body scheme, spatial, and visual-constructive deficits rather than difficulty in motor execution. Persons with dressing apraxia cannot correctly orient their clothes to their body. They often put clothes on backward or inside out. Failure to dress one side of the body is also often noted and is directly related to unilateral spatial inattention.

Interventions

It must be remembered that both visual-constructive and visual analysis synthesis skills are often used almost simultaneously during task performance. Thus, treatment should not separate the two skills but rather should be a precise interrelationship of activities that require finer and finer levels of each facility. For example, arranging an office filing system is both an analytical/synthetical and a visual-constructive task. The individual must first analyze overall needs and translate them into an imagined visual-spatial plan (preliminary synthesis of the whole) that will help organization. Then the organizer begins to use his or her hands to categorize (segment visual space). This building is a visual-constructive task. Intermittently during building, new ideas of the whole surface, and visual-constructive tasks change in response to a "better idea" (final synthesis of the whole). Task performance, except for tasks that are rote, usually follows similar perceptual processes. Treatment therefore must be integral. Visual-constructive skills, however, may be emphasized more than visual analysis and synthesis skills or vice versa.

As previously mentioned, visual-constructive disorders are thought to result from different underlying problems in different individuals (e.g., visual-spatial disorders in persons with right hemisphere lesions and executive, planning, or synthetic disorders in those with left hemisphere lesions). There are few reliable studies on treatment strategies for visual-constructive disorders. One possible treatment strategy is known as *saturational cuing*.[10] This method involves presenting controlled verbal instruction on task analysis and sequence and presenting cues on spatial boundaries (cuing is also response related).

If there are problems with planning and sequencing of steps necessary to accomplish a visual-constructive task, the therapist should begin with simple tasks that require only three to four steps, such as positioning one place setting at a table. The client should discuss the plan and sequence of steps before initiating the activity, while looking at the parts to be used, such as silverware, plate, and glass. These steps may even be written down for additional input. The client should be helped to reorient the plan at any point during task breakdown. Eventually, tasks should increase in complexity (e.g., setting a table for five), and the client should be encouraged to function more independently. Another technique often used by clinicians is known as *backward chaining*. This involves presenting a partially completed task and asking the client to complete the final steps, for example, placing the knife and glass on a partially completed place setting. The perceptual cues of the task already begun appear to stimulate constructional abilities. As the client progresses, he or she should complete more steps.

Intervention for problems with spatial planning during visual-constructive tasks should begin with simple spatial exercises discussed previously. If problems still exist, the individual may be asked to draw around shapes (blocks) one by one. These shapes should first have been placed in a simple two-dimensional design. The client is then asked to rebuild the design with the shapes alone. Therapy should progress from horizontal to vertical to oblique designs, from two-dimensional to three-dimensional designs, and from tasks with common objects to tasks involving abstract designs. For example, spatial problems with drawing, such as placing windows in a house or numbers on a clock face, are usually a result of underlying spatial disorder. The client should use a ruler or protractor to segment the space and plan placement before drawing. Dot-to-dot tasks may be designed that actually lead and sequence the drawing into a spatial whole. Simple puzzles also may be used to increase visual-spatial abilities during visual-constructive tasks. Finally, if task breakdown results from impulsive visual or motor behavior, these symptoms should be dealt with before further visual-constructive treatment continues.

Examples of visual-constructive tasks that may be designed for therapeutic use are:

- Setting a table for one to five people
- Wrapping a gift
- Assembling a piece of woodwork, a toy, a tool, a motor
- Changing a tire on a car
- Organizing a shelf in a library or a kitchen
- Organizing a filing system or cabinet
- Putting pieces of a sewing pattern together
- Addressing an envelope
- Rearranging furniture according to a preset plan
- Assembling a craft according to a preset plan
- Drawing from memory or copy
- Copying two-dimensional block designs
- Copying three-dimensional designs with oblique components

The key to effective visual-constructive learning, however, is not the task itself but rather how carefully the therapist organizes it and monitors performance. Clients with visual-constructive disorders are often visually or motorically impulsive; they often move or draw parts before analysis has taken place. Once a part is placed inappropriately, it begins to confuse the whole visual-perceptual process. This confusion increases anxiety and contributes to further breakdown in analysis and synthesis. Treatment should be directed at the underlying causes of task breakdown if these can be determined.

Problems of Visual Analysis and Synthesis Disorders

Identification of Clinical Problems

This separate discussion of visual analysis and synthesis is arbitrary. There is never any clear demarcation between the processes of visual-spatial orientation, visual-construction, and visual analysis and synthesis. Analysis of likes and differences, relationships of parts to one another, and reasoning and deduction occur simultaneously with more basic spatial and constructive percepts. The final visual concept of a task (e.g., what a place setting on a table should look like) is necessary before the task is begun. Similarly, synthesis of one part of a task may be necessary before synthesis of the entire task can occur. For example, the person who is setting a table for four people must be able to conceptualize one place setting before conceptualizing the table with four place settings. Those points during perceptual processing when there is a colligation or blending of discrete impressions into a single perception are known as synthesis. This final stage of coordination and interpretation of sensory data is thought to be deficient in many individuals with perceptual problems. Deficits may be present with either left or right hemisphere damage but are more common and more severe with right lesions.[51, 65]

Visual-perceptual skills considered to be analytical and synthetic in nature include making fine visual discriminations, particularly in complex configurations; separating figure from background in complex configurations (figure-ground); achieving recognition on the basis of incomplete information (figure closure); and synthesizing disparate elements into a meaningful entity, as, for example, conceptualizing parts of a task into a whole.[8]

Assessment

Many tests have been designed to measure the capacity for analysis and synthesis. Test items include complex figures in which small parts of a figure differ from another figure. The client is asked to select the one that is different. Studies have shown that basic discrimination of single attributes of a stimulus such as length, contour, or brightness is intact in many clients.[11, 63, 64] The problem appears when these individuals are asked to discriminate between more complex configurations with subtle differences. Tests also measure figure-ground ability; the client must select the embedded figure from the background. Functional examples of this problem are the inability of a client to find his or her glasses if they are lying on a figured background, to find a white shirt on a white bedspread, and to find his wheelchair locks. Figure closure is measured by asking the client to complete an incomplete figure, such as part of the outline of a common shape. Finally, synthesis of parts into a whole, also known as visual organization, is measured by asking the

TABLE 27–3. Common Tests Used to Assess Visual Analysis and Synthesis

Test	Use
Hooper Visual Organization Test	Standardized for adults
Motor-Free Visual Perception Test	Standardized for adults
Raven's Progressive Matrices	Standardized for adults
The Embedded Figure Test	Standardized for adults
Southern California Figure-Ground Test	Standardized for children only

client to conceptualize and organize the whole picture by, for example, looking at separate segments of the picture (e.g., cup or key) that have been divided and placed in unusual positions. This type of synthesis is necessary for high-level constructional tasks. Table 27–3 outlines examples of tests used to evaluate visual analysis and synthesis.

Interventions

Intervention for deficits in visual analysis and synthesis should follow developmental considerations described in the children's section. Visual discrimination tasks should begin with simple figures and obvious differences in complex figures. Color, size, texture, lighting, and verbal direction may help the client "cue in" on subtle differences among objects or figures. The therapist should determine the threshold at which the client is capable of discriminating differences and vary the dimension, contrast, and functional activity at this level. For example, if the individual cannot select a can of vegetables from a kitchen shelf stocked with cans of similar size, the therapist may simply change the task to fit that person's level of visual discrimination by removing some of the cans (decreasing the density of the display), replacing some of the cans with boxes of food (increasing the spatial contrast), moving the can to be selected forward or to one edge of the display (decreasing figure-ground difficulty), removing the label from the can (increasing the light and color contrast), or giving cues regarding what to search for (verbal direction). This example is described not as a method of compensation but rather as an approach to be used therapeutically in slowly building the client's visual discrimination abilities. Eventually, high-level visual discrimination skills should be incorporated within tasks requiring three or more steps, such as selecting a can of vegetables, opening the can (which involves selecting the can opener from the utensil drawer), and emptying the vegetables into a specific bowl (which involves selecting the bowl from among other bowls). Visual discrimination and figure-ground skills may appear normal until the client is required to do multiple-step activities, is given time constraints, or becomes anxious or confused. Table-top games that require high levels of visual discrimination along with cognitive strategies may be therapeutic and motivating. Examples include Monopoly and card games such as solitaire. Matching and sorting tasks also may be helpful in enhancing visual discrimination. Examples include matching picture cards and sorting laundry, tools, silverware, or files.

Drawings of figures with subtle differences also may

be used for therapy. The client should be encouraged to point to, verbalize, or outline the subtle differences in two or more pictures; this enhances visual attention to detail. If the individual cannot select the discrepant detail(s) among three or more figures, the problem most likely results from an inability to select one feature and compare it with elements in the other figures. This is a fairly high-level skill that requires selective attention and analysis with internal visualization while the individual is still viewing the complete figures. This type of client should practice feature detection and then begin systematic comparisons of similarities and differences between two figures, eventually progressing to three or more figures. The therapist may number or outline similar areas of each figure to help the client (1) direct attention to similar areas of all figures and (2) sequence comparisons appropriately. The client should verbalize, draw, or write details concerning similarities and differences in individual aspects of the figures. This enhances visual analysis and also informs the therapist about how the individual is selecting and comparing features. Eventually, speed should be stressed, the highest level being presentation of tachistoscopic designs.

Visual organization may be emphasized by presenting the client with activities that have multiple parts that must be sequenced together into a whole. Activities involving this type of synthesis are discussed in the preceding section on treatment of visual-constructive disorders. Figure closure may be emphasized by presenting parts of figures or objects (e.g., half a plate covered by a towel) and asking the client for identification. Figure-closure task difficulty may be increased by placing many objects on a table, some of which partially occlude others. Identification of objects in such a task requires figure closure simultaneous with figure-ground abilities.

Visual analysis and synthesis deficits reflect a disruption in cognitive function with specific regard to visual-perceptual features. The affected client may function normally when analytical tasks require another system, for example, language. In others with generalized brain damage (e.g., traumatic head injury and senile dementia), general cognitive analysis and synthesis may be at fault rather than visual analysis. Because most cognitive performance requires visual processing, however, increased ability to analyze and synthesize visual-perceptual material often generalizes to an increase in cognitive function.

PERCEPTUAL RETRAINING WITH COMPUTERS

During the past 15 years, numerous computer programs have been developed for rehabilitation of brain damage symptoms including cognition (e.g., attention, sequencing, or memory) and perception. Because the computer is so highly visual, it becomes an obvious tool for treatment of visual-perceptual dysfunction. Treatment with computers has been coined "computer-assisted therapy." No large treatment studies have yet defined the outcome significance of computer-assisted therapy versus conventional treatment programs. However, reports indicate that computer-assisted therapy is very motivating for patients with poor attention and motivation. Advantages of computer-assisted therapy include control/flexibility of perceptual variables during treatment (e.g., number, size, speed), immediate feedback of performance, and automatic control for learning (i.e., items are repeated if incorrect to facilitate learning). Visual-perceptual training with computers, if used, should be viewed as one part of a patient's treatment program. One should always remember that the computer, monitor, and keyboard are just that: they do not require the many perceptual, vestibular, and motor responses typical of daily performance (e.g., scanning requirements may be bilateral, but they are not global and associated with head movement). A patient's total program may include computer-assisted therapy as an additional tool; however, it should never be substituted for more significant training within the multidimensional environment. Some computer programs for visual-perceptual training are listed in the following box.

SUMMARY OF VISUAL-PERCEPTUAL DYSFUNCTION

Careful organized evaluation should delineate deficits well enough to result in a visual-perceptual function profile for each client, including both primary and associative visual skills. Clients rarely come with isolated visual-per-

---

COMPUTER PROGRAMS FOR VISUAL-PERCEPTUAL TRAINING

Visual Perceptual Diagnostic Testing and
   Training Programs
H. Greenberg and C. Chamoff
Educational Electronic Techniques, Ltd.
1886 Wantagh Avenue
Wantagh, NY 11793

Captain's Log Cognitive Training System
J. Sandford and R. Browne
Computability Corporation
101 Route 46 East
Pine Brook, NJ 07058

Psychological Software Services Programs
Odie Bracey
Psychological Software Services
P.O. Box 29205
Indianapolis, IN 46229

Life Science Associates Programs
R. Gianutsos
Life Science Associates
1 Fenemore Road
Bayport, NY 11705 (Diagnosis and Training)

Cognitive Rehabilitation Series
Hartley Courseware
2023 Aspen Glade
Kingwood, TX 77339

ceptual deficits; more often they exhibit a combination of visual-perceptual deficits usually interrelated with motor, language, and cognitive dysfunctions. For example, a visual-perceptual function profile may reveal a strabismus, left unilateral visual inattention, visual-spatial deficits, visual-constructive deficits, and problems with visual analysis and synthesis, all affecting daily function. Treatment should be organized to progressively build skills emphasizing one component more than another. The goal of treatment is eventual generalization of improvements in individual skills to spontaneous high-level function.

The presentation of information in this chapter is an attempt to use isolated and mechanistic terms to define a system that is extremely subtle, integrated, and complex. The reader is reminded that much of the normal and abnormal perceptual system has not been well defined. Preliminary studies cited throughout this chapter, however, suggest that disorders may be responsive to management and treatment. Research is needed to standardize evaluation procedures well enough to further define deficits and to investigate the effectiveness of various treatment approaches with various client populations.

REFERENCES

1. Adler-Grinberg D, Stark L: Eye movements, scanpaths and dyslexia. Am J Optom Phys Optics 55:557–570, 1978.
2. Aksionoff E, Falk N: Optometric therapy for the left brain injured patient. J Am Optom Assoc 63:564–588, 1992.
3. Anderson E, Choy E: Parietal lobe syndromes in hemiplegia: A program for treatment. Am J Occup Ther 24:13, 1970.
4. Andrezejewska W, Baranowska G: Accommodative disorders after head injury and cerebral contusion. Klin Oczna (Poland) 30:431, 1969.
5. Balliet R, et al: Rehabilitation of visual function in occipital lobe infarctions. Paper presented at the American Congress of Rehabilitation Medicine and the 43rd Annual Assembly of the American Academy of Physical Medicine and Rehabilitation, San Diego, November 1981.
6. Bartlett J, Jaanus S: Clinical Ocular Pharmacology, 2nd ed. London, Butterworths, 1989.
7. Benton A: Disorders of visual perception, disorders of higher nervous activity. In Vinken PJ, Bruyn GW (ed): Handbook of Clinical Neurology, vol 3. Amsterdam, North-Holland Publishing, 1975.
8. Benton A: Visuospatial and visuoconstructive disorders. In Heilman K, Valenstein E (ed): Clinical Neuropsychology. New York, Oxford University Press, 1979.
9. Benton A, et al: Judgment of Line Orientation Test, Forms H and V. Department of Neurology, University Hospitals. Iowa City, University of Iowa Press, 1975.
10. Ben-Yishay Y, et al: Ability to profit from cues as a function of initial competence in normal and brain-injured adults: A replication of previous findings. J Abnorm Psychol 76:378, 1970.
11. Bisiach E, et al: Hemispheric functional asymmetry in visual discrimination between invariate stimuli: An analysis of sensitivity and response criterion. Neuropsychologia 14:335, 1976.
12. Bouska MJ, Biddle E: The influence of unilateral visual neglect on diagnostic testing. Paper presented at the American Speech, Language and Hearing Association Annual Conference, Atlanta, November 1979.
13. Bouska MJ, Kwatny E: Manual for application of the Motor-Free Visual Perception Test to the adult population. Temple University Rehabilitation Research and Training Center No. 8, Philadelphia, 1980.
14. Carroll R, Seaber J: Acute loss of fusional convergence facility following head trauma. Am Orthop J 24:57–59, 1974.
15. Chedru F, et al: Visual searching in normal and brain-damaged subjects: Contribution to the study of unilateral inattention. Cortex 9:94, 1973.
16. Cohen A: Optometric management of binocular dysfunction secondary to head trauma: Case reports. J Am Optom Assoc 63:569–575, 1992.
17. Cohen A, Rein L: The effect of head trauma on the visual system: The doctor of optometry as a member of the rehabilitation team. J Am Optom Assoc 63:530–536, 1992.
18. Critchley M: The Parietal Lobes. New York, Hafner Publishing Co, 1966.
19. DeCencio DV, et al: Verticality perception and ambulation in hemiplegia. Arch Phys Med Rehabil 51:105, 1970.
20. Diller L: The development of a perceptual remediation program in hemiplegia. In Ince L (ed): Behavioral Psychology in Rehabilitation Medicine. Baltimore, Williams & Wilkins, 1980.
21. Diller L, et al: Studies in Cognition and Rehabilitation in Hemiplegia. Rehabilitation Monograph No. 50. New York, New York University Press, 1974.
22. Fannin T, Grosvenor T: Clinical Optics. Boston, Butterworths, 1987.
23. Forrest EB: Visualization and visual imagery: An overview. J Am Optom Assoc 51:1005, 1980.
24. Gallaway M, Schieman M: The efficacy of vision therapy for convergence excess. J Am Optom Assoc 68:81–86, 1997.
25. Garriot RS, Heyman CL, Rouse MW: Role of optometric vision therapy for surgically treated strabismus patients. Optom Vis Sci 74(4):179–184, 1997.
26. Gianotti G, Tiacci C: The relationship between disorders of visual perception and unilateral spatial neglect. Neuropsychologia 9:451, 1971.
27. No reference cited.
28. Gianutsos R, Ramsey G: Enabling survivors of brain injury to receive optometric services. J Vis Rehabil 2:37–58, 1988.
29. Gianutsos R, Ramsey G, Perlin R: Rehabilitative optometric services for survivors of acquired brain injury. Arch Phys Med Rehabil 69:573–578, 1988.
30. Glaser J: Neuro-ophthalmology. Philadelphia, JB Lippincott, 1990.
31. Gregory RL: Eye and Brain, 2nd ed. New York, World University Library, McGraw-Hill Book Co, 1972.
32. Hacean T: Aphasic, apraxic and agnosic syndromes in right and left hemisphere lesions; disorders of speech perception and symbolic behavior. In Vinken PJ, Bruyn GW (eds): Handbook of Clinical Neurology, vol 4. Amsterdam, North-Holland Publishing Co, 1969.
33. Hacean T, de Ajuriaguera J: Balint's syndrome (psychic paralysis of visual fixation) and its minor forms. Brain 77:373, 1954.
34. Heilman K: Neglect and related disorders. In Heilman K, Valenstein E (eds): Clinical Neuropsychology. New York, Oxford University Press, 1979.
35. Heilman K, Valenstein E: Mechanisms underlying hemispatial neglect. Ann Neurol 5:166, 1979.
36. Hein DB, et al: Hypertensive putomental hemorrhage. Ann Neurol 1:152, 1977.
37. Holmes G: Disturbances of visual orientation. Br J Ophthalmol 2:449, 1918.
38. Hubel DH, Livingstone MS: Color and contrast sensitivity in the lateral geniculate body and primary visual cortex of the macaque monkey. J Neurosci 10:2223–2237, 1990.
39. Hubel DH, Wiesel TN: Receptive fields and functional architecture of monkey striate cortex. J Physiol 195:215–243, 1968.
40. Ishihara Color Plates, Tokyo, Kanehara & Co, Ltd, 1977. Available from Berneil Corp, P.O. Box 4637, South Bend, IN 46634-4637.
41. Kanski JJ: Clinical Ophthalmology: A Systematic Approach, 2nd ed. London, Butterworth-Heinemann, 1989.
42. Keating M: Geometric, Physical and Visual Optics. Boston, Butterworths, 1988.
43. Krohel GB, Kristen RW, Simon JW, Barrows NA: Post-traumatic convergence insufficiency. Am J Ophthalmol 18:101–102, 104, 1986.
44. Kulp MT, Schmidt PP: Effect of oculomotor and other skills on reading performance, a literature review. Optom Vis Sci 73:283–292, 1996.
45. Kwatny E, Bouska MJ: Visual system disorders and functional correlates: Final report. Temple University Rehabilitation Research and Training Center No 8, Philadelphia, 1980.
46. LeDoux JE, Smylie C: Left hemisphere visual processes in a case of right hemisphere symptomatology: Implications for theories of cerebral lateralization. Arch Neurol 37:157, 1980.
47. Leicester J, et al: Some determinants of visual neglect. J Neurol Neurosurg Psychiatry 32:580, 1969.
48. Luria AR: Higher Cortical Functions in Man, 2nd ed. New York, Basic Books, 1980.

49. Meadows JC: Disturbed perception of colors associated with localized cerebral lesions. Brain 97:615, 1974.
50. Moses R, Hart W: Adler's Physiology of the Eye, Clinical Application. St. Louis, CV Mosby, 1987.
51. Newcombe F, Russell WR: Dissociated visual perceptual and spatial deficits in focal lesions of the right hemisphere. J Neurol Neurosurg Psychiatry 32:73, 1969.
52. Nilsson L: Behold Man. Boston, Little, Brown, 1973.
53. Rayner K: Eye movements in reading and information processing. Psychol Bull 85:618, 1978.
54. Reeves AG, Hagman WS: Behavioral and EEG asymmetry following unilateral lesions of the forebrain and midbrain of cats. Electroencephalog Clin Neurophysiol 30:83, 1971.
55. Rosenbloom A, Morgan M (eds): Vision and Aging, General and Clinical Perspectives. New York, Professional Press Books, Fairchild Publications, 1986.
56. Rosenbloom A, Morgan M: Principles and Practice of Pediatric Optometry. San Francisco, JB Lippincott, 1990.
57. Rubens A: Agnosia. In Heilman K, Valenstein E (eds): Clinical Neuropsychology. New York, Oxford University Press, 1979.
58. Scotti G, Spinnler H: Colour imperception in unilateral hemisphere–damaged patients. J Neurol Neurosurg Psychiatry 33:22, 1970.
59. Seiv E, Freishat B: Perceptual Dysfunction in the Adult Stroke Patient: A Manual for Evaluation and Treatment. Thorofare, NJ, Charles B Slack, 1976.
60. Semenza C, et al: Analytic and global strategies in copying designs by unilaterally brain-damaged patients. Cortex 14:404, 1978.
61. Solan HA, Feldman J, Tujak L: Developing visual and reading efficiency in older adults. Optom Vis Sci 72:139–145, 1995.
62. Stanton K, et al: Teaching compensation for left neglect through a language-oriented program. Paper presented at the American Speech, Language and Hearing Association Annual Conference, Atlanta, November 1979.
63. Taylor AM, Warrington E: Visual discrimination in patients with localized brain lesions. Cortex 9:82, 1973.
64. Teuber HL, Weinstein S: Ability to discover features after cerebral lesions. Arch Neurol Psychiatry 76:369, 1956.
65. Warrington E, James M: An experimental investigation of facial recognition in patients with unilateral lesions. Cortex 3:317, 1967.
66. Watson RT, Heilman RM: Thalamic neglect. Neurology 29:690, 1979.
67. Wilson B, Cockburn J, Halligan P: Behavioral Inattention Test. Hants, England, Thames Valley Test Co, 1988.
68. www.artificialvision.com
69. Zihl J: Blindsight: Improvement of visually-guided eye movements by systematic practice in patients with cerebral blindness. Neuropsychologia 43:71, 1980.

ADDITIONAL READINGS

Arnadottir G: Neurobehavioral Assessment in Adult CNS Dysfunction. St. Louis, CV Mosby, 1989.
Humphreys G, Riddoch MJ: To See but Not to See: A Case Study of Visual Agnosia. Hillsdale, NJ, Laurence Erlbaum, 1987.
Scheiman M: Understanding and Managing Vision Defecits, A Guide for the Occupational Therapist. Thorofare, NJ, Slack Incorporated, 1997
Vision Therapist: Hot Topics. Santa Ana, CA, Optometric Extension Program, 1993.
Vision Therapist: Working with the Brain Injured. Santa Ana, CA, Optometric Extension Program, 1993.
Zolton B (ed): Visual system dysfunction, Head Trauma Rehabil 4(2) (entire issue), June 1989.

APPENDIX 27-A

Helpful Websites

Annotated References List: www.vision-therapy.com/books.html

College of Optometrists in Vision Development: www.covd.org

Computerized home vision therapy system: www.homevisiontherapy.com

Neuro Optometric Rehabilitation Association (NORA): www.noravc.com

Optometric Extension Program Foundation: www.oep.org

Parents Active for Vision Education (PAVE): www.pave-eye.com/~vision

Position Statement on Optometric Vision Therapy (includes excellent reference list): www.aoanet.org/ia-op-vis-ther.html.

Vision Therapy Information and Referrals: www.visionhelp.com

Electrodiagnosis and Electrotherapeutic Interventions

CHARLENE NELSON, MA, PT • JON D. HACKE, MA, PT, ATC • KAREN L. MCCULLOCH, MS, PT, NCS

Chapter Outline

Key Words

- biofeedback
- clinical electromyography
- electrical muscle stimulation (EMS)
- electrical stimulation therapy (EMS)
- electrodiagnosis
- electromyographic biofeedback (EMGBF)
- evoked potential tests
- functional electrical stimulation (FES)
- nerve conduction tests
- neuromuscular electrical stimulation (NMES)

Objectives

After reading this chapter the student/therapist will:

1. Identify electrodiagnostic tests used in neurological clients.
2. Describe general procedures for electrodiagnostic tests.
3. Recognize basic normal and abnormal findings of electrodiagnostic tests.
4. Discuss indications for electrodiagnostic tests in neurological clients.
5. Recognize the implications of findings of electrodiagnostic tests in planning and modifying intervention programs.
6. Appreciate the value of electrodiagnostic tests as part of overall client evaluation and management.
7. Understand the basic mechanisms of neuromuscular electrical stimulation (NMES), electrical muscle stimulation (EMS), and electromyographic biofeedback (EMGBF).
8. Describe appropriate stimulus parameters for use of NMES, EMS, and EMGBF.
9. Discuss types of equipment available for NMES, EMS, and EMGBF.
10. Describe the potential benefits of NMES, EMS, and EMGBF.
11. List indications and contraindications for use of NMES, EMS, and EMGBF.
12. Provide examples of use of these modalities for a variety of neurological problems.

13. Describe considerations for use of these modalities with neurological clients.

14. Describe decision-making processes for evaluation of intervention efficacy; suggest modifications in NMES, EMS, or EMGBF program based on results.

15. Demonstrate awareness of feedback principles that relate to use of EMGBF.

16. Summarize research findings examining the efficacy of NMES, EMS, and EMGBF.

INTRODUCTION

The goal of this chapter is to enhance the therapist's ability to recognize indications for the more commonly used electrodiagnostic tests and to integrate knowledge of these test indications and findings into the overall management of clients with neuropathological dysfunction. To help the therapist attain this goal, the first section presents a basic description of the electrophysiological tests and the neuroanatomical structures, as well as the functions involved in each test. Normal and abnormal test findings are discussed. The major emphasis is on explaining how knowledge of these tests can assist the therapist in client evaluation. The second section provides a basic introduction to the physiology, indications, contraindications, equipment, and applications of neuromuscular electrical stimulation (NMES), electrical muscle stimulation (EMS), and electromyographic biofeedback (EMGBF). The information integrates electrotherapeutic interventions into program planning for common neurological impairments and their subsequent functional limitations and disabilities. A review of the literature examining efficacy is also included to assist the therapist in making choices about the use of these tools in the clinic.

ELECTRODIAGNOSIS

Rather than thinking of electrophysiological tests as a distinct and exclusive entity used by others for diagnostic evaluation, the therapist is encouraged to view these tests as part of differential diagnosis and as useful adjuncts that can guide decisions in logical planning and modification of programs for intervention or referral. In addition, having an informed perspective on the application of electrophysiological tests should benefit the therapist's interaction and communication with other members of the medical and health management community.

Most of the electrophysiological tests described here require application of an external electrical stimulus to a nerve or muscle, and observation and assessment of the muscle or nerve response. Exceptions are the clinical electromyogram (EMG) and the single-fiber electromyogram (SFEMG), which involve monitoring and recording the electrical activity produced by the muscle tissue, either while at rest or during muscle contraction.

Electrical tests commonly used at this time are motor and sensory nerve conduction tests, including F wave and H reflex response measurements, repetitive stimulation, somatosensory evoked potential (SSEP) tests, and EMG. Another electrical test, which has been used in the past but is now rarely applied specifically, is the test for reaction of degeneration (RD).

Electrodiagnostic tests are performed by physical therapists and other medical practitioners who have education, training, and experience in these procedures. Several references at the end of the chapter should be useful to therapists who have less experience with these procedures.

Before implementing electrodiagnostic tests, review of the client's history, a relevant systems review, and a clarifying physical examination are invaluable. The clarifying examination should be directed toward those factors that will guide the examiner in selecting the appropriate electrical tests and the sequence of test procedures. The client's neurological signs, muscle strength and tone, sensation, range of motion (ROM), and cognition are among the data important to the examiner in planning and administering electrical tests.

Reaction of Degeneration and Strength Duration Tests

Recall a fundamental physiological feature of nerve and muscle electrophysiological response: an electrical stimulus applied to a motor nerve can result in muscle contraction only if the stimulus amplitude (strength or intensity) and duration meet minimal criteria.[45, 59, 63, 80, 128] The lowest amplitude of electrical stimulus required to produce a response in nerve or muscle when using a pulse of long duration (over 100 ms) is the *rheobase* or threshold. The shortest pulse duration that can elicit a response when using a stimulus amplitude twice the rheobase value is the *chronaxy*. Because the chronaxy of normal peripheral motor nerves is generally less than 0.5 ms, a stimulator with a pulse duration of 0.5 ms or less can produce an effective muscle contraction. Chronaxy of a denervated muscle is considerably longer than that of a muscle with normal innervation; therefore, a stimulator with a pulse duration longer than the muscle chronaxy is necessary to produce a contraction in a peripherally denervated muscle.[59] Knowledge of these minimal criteria for rheobase and chronaxy is basic to understanding the rationale of electrophysiological testing and also is basic to effective application of electrical stimulation for treatment of peripheral nervous system (PNS) disorders.

Although the test for RD is infrequently used as a specific test, many therapists indirectly use a modified form of the RD test when they apply a neuromuscular electrical stimulator (NMES) to facilitate contraction of weak or paralyzed muscles. The standard small, portable NMES units produce a relatively short-duration electrical impulse (pulse), generally less than 0.5 ms in duration, and are discussed later in this chapter.

If a muscle contraction does not occur when using an NMES on a client with a weak or paralyzed muscle, the therapist must establish whether the technique of application should be modified or if the muscle has a compromised peripheral innervation. This use of the NMES is similar to the first part of the traditional RD test. Before development of nerve conduction testing and EMG, the part of the grossly qualitative RD test just described would be followed by a second part, that is, application of a stimulus of infinitely long duration and assessment of the response of the muscle. The problem would then likely have been further evaluated using a strength duration test, which would provide somewhat more quantitative information on the electrical excitability of the muscle, namely, the chronaxy value, and a curve describing the interrelationship of the stimulus amplitude and duration.[45, 128] Characteristics of this curve represent the status of the peripheral nerve supplying the muscle being tested. This may vary from normal innervation, to partial degeneration or regeneration, to complete denervation. The RD and strength duration tests have generally been replaced by the more objective nerve conduction and EMG tests.

Muscles that are weak or paralyzed because of involvement of the central nervous system (CNS) should contract when the NMES is applied. Therapists should recognize the reason a muscle is not responding when using an NMES and, if appropriate, refer the client for electrodiagnostic examination.

Nerve Conduction Tests

A general overview of nerve conduction tests (NCTs) is presented here to provide the reader with an understanding of their application and indications. For details of the techniques, many excellent texts are available.[56, 91, 96, 126, 130]

Motor and sensory NCTs can provide data that are helpful in establishing the presence of pathological conditions in the PNS. The tests may differentiate the anatomical level, such as a localized peripheral mononeuropathy or a plexopathy. In addition they may further localize the site of compromise, such as a median nerve compression at the wrist, a lesion of the lateral cord of the brachial plexus, or a cervical radiculopathy. Nerve conduction velocity is faster in myelinated nerve fibers and increases with increased temperature. Each of these characteristics varies independantly and supports the need for nerve conduction testing for differential diagnosis of impairments that primarily involve axonal degeneration and those that are primarily peripheral demyelination.[56, 96, 130] The severity or extent of the problem may be determined, for example, a mild, localized compressive disorder of the myelin (neuropraxia), a more severe lesion in which the nerve and its surrounding connective tissue have been completely disrupted (neurotmesis), or a demyelinating and axonal degenerating polyneuropathy.[96, 160] In the event that findings of the NCT and EMG are normal, the clinician may be able to rule out most conditions involving the PNS and look for CNS or other pathology. Knowledge of this rationale for NCT and EMG should help the therapist decide when the tests may be indicated and understand the reasoning behind reports of tests that have already been performed on their clients.

Motor Nerve Conduction

In motor nerve conduction tests (MNCTs), the peripheral nerve is stimulated at various sites, and the evoked electrical response is recorded from a distal muscle supplied by the nerve. Surface electrodes are usually used for both stimulating and recording. Electrode configuration for MNCT is shown in Figure 28–1. The response represents the electrical activity of muscle fibers under the recording electrode and is sometimes called the compound muscle action potential (CMAP). It is also called the M wave or response. Measurements are taken of latency (the time in milliseconds required for the impulse to travel from each stimulus site to the recording site), and the amplitude of the response in millivolts. The shape and duration of the response are assessed, and motor nerve conduction velocity (MNCV) is calculated for each segment of interest by dividing the distance between stimulus sites (in millimeters) by the difference in latency measured at each respective site.

Velocities, latencies, and the shape and amplitude of the responses are studied and compared with established normal values and often with values taken from tests of the uninvolved extremity. In infants and children, nerve conduction is slower than in adults and reaches adult values by age 4 years.[130] Nerve conduction time gradually slows after age 60 years[96, 130] but generally remains within the outer limits of normal.

Sensory Nerve Conduction

Sensory nerve conduction can be measured from many superficial sensory nerves, such as the superficial radial and sural nerves. It also can be measured from mixed motor and sensory nerves by placing either the stimulating or the recording electrode over a sensory branch of a nerve and recording the sensory nerve (afferent) action potentials (SNAPs) (Fig. 28–2). Response latencies and amplitudes are measured, and sensory nerve conduction velocities (SNCVs) are calculated for each segment by dividing the distance between two adjacent stimulus and recording sites, or two stimulus sites, by the latency (conduction time) between these same sites. Sensory nerve responses are considerably smaller than motor responses; therefore their amplitudes are measured in microvolts.

F Wave Latency

The F wave latency is a measure of the time required for action potentials of alpha motor neurons elicited by stimulating a nerve in the periphery to be transmitted centrally to the motor neuron cell body, and then return

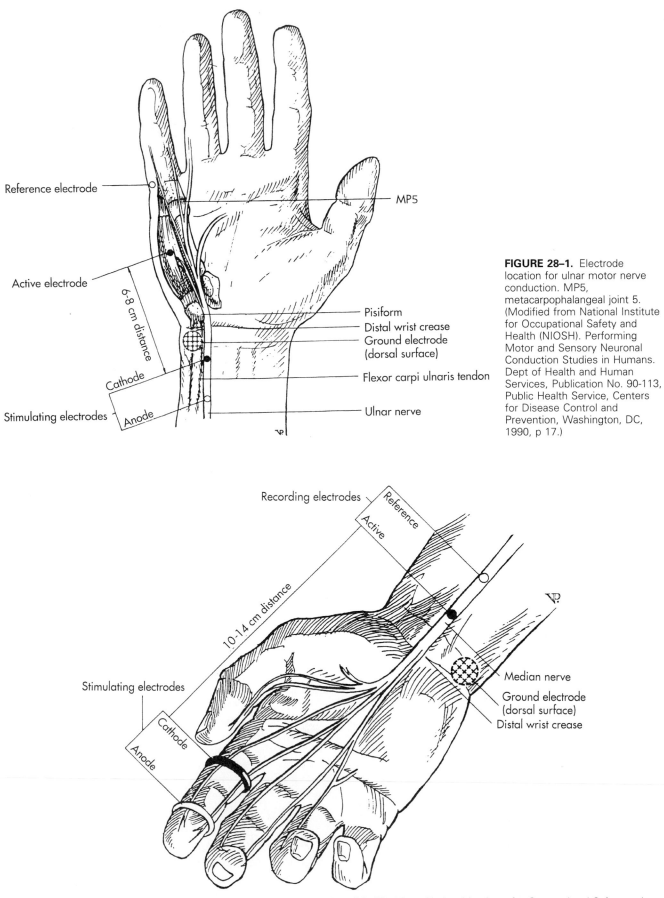

Reference electrode

MP5

Active electrode

6-8 cm distance

Pisiform
Distal wrist crease
Ground electrode
(dorsal surface)

Cathode

Flexor carpi ulnaris tendon

Stimulating electrodes — Anode

Ulnar nerve

FIGURE 28–1. Electrode location for ulnar motor nerve conduction. MP5, metacarpophalangeal joint 5. (Modified from National Institute for Occupational Safety and Health (NIOSH). Performing Motor and Sensory Neuronal Conduction Studies in Humans. Dept of Health and Human Services, Publication No. 90-113, Public Health Service, Centers for Disease Control and Prevention, Washington, DC, 1990, p 17.)

Recording electrodes — Reference
Active

10-14 cm distance

Stimulating electrodes

Cathode

Anode

Median nerve
Ground electrode
(dorsal surface)
Distal wrist crease

FIGURE 28–2. Electrode location for median sensory nerve conduction. (Modified from National Institute for Occupational Safety and Health [NIOSH]. Performing Motor and Sensory Neuronal Conduction Studies in Humans. Dept of Health and Human Services, Publication No. 90–113, Public Health Service, Centers for Disease Control and Prevention, Washington, DC, 1990, p 13.)

as a recurrent discharge along the same neuron, to activate the muscle from which the recording occurs.[96, 128, 130, 161] No synapse is involved, and therefore the F wave is not a reflex response but rather only a measure of motor neuron conduction. Specific conditions of electropotential must exist at the somadendritic cell membrane to reactivate the efferent axon; therefore the occurrence of the F wave response is inconsistent and variable in latency and waveform.[161]

Although F wave latency is useful in evaluating conduction in conditions usually involving the proximal portions of the peripheral motor neurons (e.g., Guillain-Barré syndrome and thoracic outlet syndrome), its value is considered questionable by some authors because of its variability. Normal values of F wave latency are 22 to 34 ms in the upper extremity (stimulating at the wrist), 40 to 58 ms in the lower extremity (stimulating at the ankle), and 12 ms central latency[196] in the upper extremity, with a bilateral difference in latency of no greater than 1 ms.

H Reflex Response

The H reflex response latency is a measure of the time for action potentials elicited by stimulating a nerve in the periphery to be propagated centrally over the Ia afferent neurons to the spinal cord, to be transmitted across the synapse to an alpha motor neuron, and then to travel distally over this neuron to activate the muscle. The response therefore measures conduction in both the afferent and efferent neurons.[96, 130] It also is referred to as a "late" response.

The H wave is readily identified, because it is constant in latency and waveform, and it occurs with a stimulus usually below the threshold level required to elicit the M wave response. This monosynaptic reflex response is found most easily by stimulating the tibial nerve at the popliteal area and recording from the soleus muscle. Braddom and Johnson[29] reported a mean latency of 29.8 ms (±2.74 ms) for the tibial nerve in normal adults, and a bilateral difference of no greater than 1.2 ms. The H wave latency is a valuable measure of conduction over the S1 nerve root in differentiating suspected proximal plexopathy and radiculopathy from a herniated disk or foraminal impingement. Sabbahi and Khalil[153] have reported a technique for recording the H wave from the flexor carpi radialis muscle when stimulating the median nerve. In normal humans over the age of 1 year, the H wave is usually seen only in the tibial and median nerves. It can be elicited from several nerves in infants and in conditions of CNS dysfunction in adults.

Repetitive Stimulation Tests

A variation of motor nerve conduction testing, the repetitive stimulation (RS) test is used in evaluating transmission at the neuromuscular junction. RS tests are helpful in the differential diagnosis of disorders such as bronchogenic carcinoma and myasthenia gravis. One protocol uses a series of supramaximal electrical stimuli applied to a peripheral nerve at a distal site (e.g., median or ulnar nerve at the wrist) at a rate of three to five per second for five to seven responses, and assesses changes in amplitude of the muscle response. Precise technical requirements are specified to prevent movement artifacts and other testing errors. Detailed descriptions of the RS test can be found in other texts.[96, 131] Under normal conditions, the amplitude does not change more than 10% from that of the initial response in a series of 10 stimuli, recorded before and after resistive exercise. An amplitude decrease in the fifth or sixth response of more than 10% is considered abnormal and is compatible with a physiological defect at the postsynaptic receptor site of the neuromuscular junction, as in myasthenia gravis.

In another RS protocol, stimuli are applied to a nerve, first at a slow rate and then at a faster rate, usually 10 to 20 per second for up to 10 seconds. Normally, the amplitude can decrease up to 40% from the initial amplitude. In some defects at the presynaptic site, the response may be lower than normal, with a slow stimulation rate, but show a significant amplitude increase at the higher rate. Amplitude increases greater than 100% over the initial response are consistent with presynaptic neuromuscular junction defects such as seen in small cell bronchogenic carcinoma (Pancoast tumor) and in botulism. In 1957 Eaton and Lambert[57] reported this phenomenon as a myasthenic syndrome.

Gilchrist and Sanders[67] reported another protocol referred to as a double-step RS test, which measures amplitude before and after a temporarily induced ischemia of the extremity. They found the double-step RS test to be slightly more sensitive than the routine RS test, but only 60% as sensitive as the SFEMG technique. The SFEMG test is described later in this chapter. The RS test is a good alternative test for neuromuscular transmission when the SFEMG is not available, but the examiner must meticulously adhere to technical details when conducting the test.

Clinical Evoked Potentials

Electrical potentials elicited by stimulation of nerves or sense organs in the periphery can be recorded from various sites as the impulses are transmitted centrally along the neuronal pathway and from the representative area on the brain.[38, 39, 76, 96] SSEP procedures are particularly useful in assessing the integrity of afferent pathways in the CNS. They are helpful in differentiating among lesions in areas such as the plexus, spinal cord, brain stem, thalamus, and cerebral cortex. Evoked potential tests have the advantage of providing objective data about the integrity of both peripheral and central neuronal pathways, including transmission across axodendritic synapses.

The SSEP is valuable in assessing damage and continuity of spinal cord tracts in early spinal cord injury (SCI). For example, if an electrical stimulus is applied at the popliteal area over the tibial nerve, responses can be recorded with surface electrodes placed over the spine at the L3 and C7 spinal segments and from the lumbar representation of the contralateral sensory cortical area. Conduction time and other parameters of the response waveforms can be measured from the recordings.

This simplified example of an SSEP illustrates how conduction over both motor and sensory peripheral nerves and afferent pathways to the cerebrum can be studied. The median nerve is usually tested to evaluate the integrity of peripheral and central pathways and their synaptic connections as the impulses travel from the upper extremity to the contralateral cortical area.

In visual evoked potential (VEP) procedures, visual stimuli, such as variable light flashes of changing patterns, are applied to one or both eyes under highly controlled conditions. The response is recorded from the scalp over the representative area of the cerebral cortex.[39, 76, 96] The term *pattern reversal evoked potentials* (PREPs), a more descriptive term for these procedures, is recommended by the American Electroencephalographic Society.[38] These tests and other VEP procedures are useful in assessing pathology of retinal photoreceptors, the optic nerve, the chiasm, and postchiasmal pathways. Abnormal conduction findings have been reported when using VEP studies in central demyelinating disorders such as multiple sclerosis and optic neuritis.

Auditory evoked potential tests are used to evaluate neurological function of the cochlear division of the auditory nerve (eighth cranial nerve), central auditory pathways and synapses in the brain stem, and the receptor areas on the cerebral cortex.[38, 39, 76, 96] Brain stem auditory evoked potentials are frequently referred to as BAEPs. A series of high-intensity clicks is applied to auditory receptors in the ears through headphones, and several components of the response waveforms are recorded using surface electrodes over the representative cortical areas. The BAEP is an effective test procedure for localizing and evaluating acoustic neuromas and other space-occupying lesions in the brain stem. This test is also used for assessment of brain damage and to determine the integrity of CNS pathways in patients who are comatose as a result of traumatic head injury. Robinson and Rudge[150] recommend caution when using BAEP tests for this purpose because other factors, such as defective receptor organs, can cause abnormalities in BAEPs.

The evoked potential tests described in this chapter all require application of appropriate external stimuli, which are rapidly repeated many times; the response is electronically averaged to sort out the desired signal from interference signals. The conduction times (latencies), waveform shape and amplitude, and sometimes conduction velocities are measured and compared with normal values. Absence of a response, increased latencies, decreased amplitudes, and slowing of conduction velocities are all abnormal findings. Normal values and details describing techniques for the evoked potential tests are described elsewhere.[38, 39, 76, 96]

Therapists with special interest and training administer evoked potential tests for neurological applications—more frequently the SSEP. Because of the highly specialized techniques necessary to administer the VEP for ophthalmological applications and the BAEP for hearing dysfunction, these procedures are usually performed by persons who specialize in these procedures.

Clinical Electromyography

An understanding of the basis of findings reported in EMG studies should assist neurological therapists in planning and modifying therapeutic management programs of their clients. EMG is particularly useful in showing electrical changes that occur in skeletal muscle when there is pathology in lower motor neurons or in muscle itself. Certain patterns of motor unit recruitment activity also are associated with CNS disorders. Details of contraindications and special precautions are described by Currier and colleagues.[46]

A small-diameter, sterile recording needle electrode is inserted in several representative muscles, and the electrical activity produced by the muscle is studied during relaxation or rest, slight contraction, and strong contraction. Characteristics of the muscle action potentials seen in these three conditions and the pattern of recruitment monitored during progressively stronger contractions are assessed by the examiner to determine whether they are normal or whether the electrical changes observed are consistent with those found in neuropathic, myelopathic, or myopathic conditions. EMG findings are not pathognomonic; therefore they must be carefully studied within the context of other laboratory and clinical findings. During acute stages of trauma or insult to the neurological systems, EMG is not usually indicated. As the client's condition stabilizes and as recovery begins, EMG may be valuable both for evaluation and for planning the therapeutic program. EMG can be useful, particularly with sequential follow-up testing, in determinations of progress and prognosis. Many excellent resources are available for readers interested in details of the equipment and procedures for EMG.[2, 46, 56, 91, 96]

Explanation of the technique and clear communication of instructions to the client, along with patience on the part of the examiner, can allay the client's anxiety and minimize discomfort. Although client cooperation during EMG testing is important, some aspects of the muscle electrical activity can be studied in the client who is unable to move or who has only involuntary or reflex activity. For example a client recovering from a head injury and with residual hemiplegia has abnormal extensor responses in the upper extremity and weak flexor responses in the lower extremity, except for flaccid ankle and foot responses. An EMG (and NCTs) of the leg and foot muscles may detect abnormal resting potentials, for example, fibrillation and positive sharp waves, and no motor unit potentials in muscles normally innervated by the deep peroneal nerve, but normal potentials in the tibial nerve distribution. These findings would guide the physician and therapist in looking for a possible peripheral nerve lesion concomitant with the CNS dysfunction. The treatment program in this situation would differ from that for a client without peripheral nerve pathology.

Motor unit potentials (MUPs) appear only during contraction of muscle fibers activated voluntarily or involuntarily, and in both isotonic and isometric contractions. In normal conditions, motor units are seen with voluntary movement; however, reflex activation of muscle also produces MUPs having certain normal characteristics. In CNS disorders with symptoms of spasticity, hypertonic or spastic muscles produce recordable MUPs only when they are actively shortening or contracting. MUPs are not seen in spastic muscles in a shortened but noncontractile condition. Characteristics of EMG potentials seen in normal and pathological conditions are shown in Table 28–1.

TABLE 28–1. Characteristics of Normal and Abnormal EMG Potentials

Neuro-muscular Status	At Rest		Minimum Contraction Motor Unit Potentials			Strong Contraction	
	Insertion Activity	Spontaneous Activity	Amplitude	Duration	Waveform	Recruitment Pattern	Amplitude
Normal	Brief discharges	None	100–3,000 μV	3–15 ms; average = 7 ms	Biphasic and triphasic	Full or complete interference (>75%)	Concentric: 2,000–5,000 μV
		End plate potentials			10% polyphasic potentials		Monopolar: 2,000–8,000 μV
Abnormal	Absent response	Fibrillation	Absent	<5 ms	Polyphasic potentials >10%–15%	Decreased (<75%)	<2,000 μV
	Increased or prolonged	Positive sharp waves Fasciculation	Low or >5,000 μV	>15 ms	Myotonic potentials	Discrete potentials Single unit	Concentric: >5,000 μV Monopolar: >8,000 μV
	Decreased	Complex repetitive discharges Myotonic potentials on percussion				Early recruitment	

Modified from Currier DP, et al: Guidelines for clinical electromyography. J Clin Electrophysiol 5:2–19, 1993.

As electrical tests are being conducted, the findings are continuously studied and are used by the examiner as a guide in continuing with or modifying the plan for the examination. Data from EMG and nerve conduction studies are analyzed by the examiner to determine the extent and anatomical distribution of abnormal electrical responses. The examiner then interprets the findings to establish whether they fit the characteristics usually found in pathological groupings of abnormal patterns. As stated earlier, the results of electrodiagnostic tests must be correlated with the clinical findings.

Summary of Clinical Electromyographic and Nerve Conduction Studies

Reviewing a summary of the more characteristic EMG and nerve conduction changes associated with selected groupings of neurological disorders may help the therapist understand reports of these studies and recognize changes that may be seen in sequential tests during the course of the disorders. The reader is cautioned that the following is a simplified grouping of electrical changes and that actual electrodiagnostic studies show considerably more detail and frequent variations of these findings.[2, 46, 56, 91, 96]

Electrical testing in CNS disorders typically shows normal motor and sensory nerve conduction. In the EMG, spontaneous activity is seen infrequently, and individual motor units seen on muscle contraction usually have normal parameters. The recruitment pattern may show a slower than normal MUP discharge frequency, with an incomplete and irregular interference pattern. In the presence of tremor and other involuntary movements, bursts of MUPs occur, consistent with the muscle contrac-

tion pattern. The tests are important in differential diagnosis between a CNS and a PNS problem, but often they are not used when clinical examinations demonstrate the problem to be definitely in the CNS.

In myelopathies, which include upper and lower motor neuron disorders (e.g., amyotrophic lateral sclerosis [ALS], poliomyelitis, cervical spondylitis, and syringomyelia), motor and sensory nerve conduction are usually normal, although there may be slight slowing.[96] The characteristic EMG changes, which usually appear in the more chronic stages of the disorders, are increased amplitude and duration of motor units because of the variable impulse conduction time in sprouting axon terminals. An increased number of polyphasic potentials with increased duration is usually found. Spontaneous activity is often seen, and on strong contraction, a reduced number of rapidly firing large MUPs are recruited, resulting in a single-unit or partial interference pattern.

Peripheral neuropathies show a variety of electrical changes, depending on the type and location of the pathology. In proximal pathologies (e.g., radiculopathies), motor and sensory nerve conduction generally remain normal, except for F waves and H reflex responses in specific spinal cord segments. If motor nerve roots are compromised, spontaenous activity and increased polyphasic potentials appear, and reduced recruitment of MUPs results in an incomplete interference pattern. In more chronic stages MUP amplitude and duration can be increased. As the lesion improves, spontaneous activity decreases and the recruitment pattern becomes more normal. If only sensory roots are injured, no EMG changes occur.

Lesions of peripheral nerves, which range from a focal mononeuropathy to plexopathy, frequently show abnormalities in motor and sensory nerve conduction, depending on which components of the nerve are involved. In the EMG, spontaneous activity, particularly fibrillation and positive sharp waves, is very common; if the lesion is complete, no MUPs are found. The presence of even a few MUPs suggests a more optimistic prognosis. Often the location of the lesion can be identified by the distribution of the electrical changes. With regenerating axons, low-amplitude polyphasic MUPs gradually appear. In the chronic stage, the amplitude and duration of MUPs are often increased. Spontaneous activity decreases with reinnervation, but it may persist for several years.

In generalized, systemic peripheral polyradiculoneuropathies of the primarily demyelinating type, such as Guillain-Barré syndrome (see Chapters 12 and 13), motor and sensory nerve conduction and F waves become markedly slow. The EMG changes usually do not occur, except for a reduced recruitment pattern consistent with weak muscle contraction. With primarily axonal polyneuropathies, such as uremic neuropathy, isoniazid and cisplatin toxicity, and lead poisoning, motor and sensory nerve conduction is mildly slowed or may remain normal. The duration and amplitude of the response, however, decrease. During advanced stages, many polyneuropathies develop both demyelinating and axonal pathology (e.g., diabetic neuropathy). On EMG, spontaneous activity is commonly seen. These electrical changes generally become more severe with worsening of the pathology, but they also improve if the pathology is reversed.

With myopathic disorders, motor and sensory nerve conduction are generally normal unless neural tissue is also affected. In advanced stages, however, severely atrophied muscles can produce decreased amplitude and distorted nerve conduction responses. The characteristic findings on EMG are short-duration, low-amplitude potentials. Some spontaneous potentials, particularly fibrillations and positive sharp waves, may be found but are much more frequent in the inflammatory myopathies such as polymyositis. Spontaneous activity also is seen in some neuromuscular transmission disorders (e.g., botulism). Specific myotonic potentials appear in certain myopathic disorders (e.g., myotonia congenita). The recruitment pattern shows many low-amplitude MUPs, appearing in a full pattern, with little voluntary effort. This type of recruitment pattern is referred to as early recruitment.

Single-Fiber Electromyography

Electrical activity can be recorded from two or more muscle fibers innervated by the same motor unit using a specially designed single-fiber needle electrode. SFEMG is, at this time, the most sensitive test for evaluating neuromuscular transmission defects such as myasthenia gravis and myasthenic syndrome. It also is used to evaluate peripheral neuropathies, motor neuron diseases, and myopathies.[96, 166]

During a carefully controlled minimal voluntary contraction, a 25-μm-diameter needle is inserted into the muscle, and several potentials from muscle fibers within the recording area are stored. Equipment with a trigger and delay line is necessary to "time-lock" the tracings of the potentials. The slightly different conduction time or interpulse interval (IPI) required for impulses to be transmitted from a single motor neuron to each of its terminal end plates, cross the neuromuscular junction, and activate the muscle fiber is called *jitter*. This time difference is collected from several tracings and is converted into a mean consecutive time difference (MCD), which normally ranges from 5 to 55 μs. Values shorter or longer than this range are considered abnormal. The impulses from some axons to their muscle fibers may fail to be transmitted. This is referred to as blocking. Another capability of SFEMG is the measure of fiber density, that is, the average number of muscle fibers within the needle recording area. Fiber density is increased in reinnervation and also with certain myopathies because of axonal collateralization or splitting.[40]

Macro-Electromyography

A variation of SFEMG utilizes a macroelectrode to record the majority of muscle fibers of a single motor unit as they are triggered by an initial potential, which is then time-locked with all the other muscle fiber potentials recorded from a different part of the same or a nearby needle.[96, 165, 168, 198] Two recording channels are used. Maximum amplitude of the potentials from several muscles has been reported by Stålberg.[165] The findings are analyzed, along with findings of jitter, fiber density, and conventional EMG, to evaluate the status and prognosis of various neurological and neuromuscular disorders, such as motor neuron disease, peripheral nerve lesions, and myopathies.

Automatic Analysis

Instruments with computer-assisted analysis are now available for studying EMG signals in greater detail than in earlier years.[40, 96, 167, 168] Parameters of the waveform, including amplitude, duration, frequency spectrum, number of turns, or phase polarity reversals and *area*—which is the integral or total voltage of a waveform—can be automatically analyzed. The data are then compared electronically with predetermined patterns of electrical changes, which correlate with categories of neuromuscular disorders such as myelopathies and neuropathies. Instruments with this capability are not in routine use in most clinics at this time, but rapidly changing technology will probably make this detailed automatic analysis more available in the near future.

ELECTRICAL STIMULATION AND ELECTROMYOGRAPHIC BIOFEEDBACK INTERVENTIONS

Equipment

Among the tools available for facilitation of muscle control are neuromuscular electrical stimulation, electrical muscle stimulation, and electromyographic biofeedback. Although the mechanisms of action are different for these modalities, they may be used in conjunction with each other to meet goals of improving or modulating muscle activation, with the intent of improving function.

Although this section deals with general details of interventions, there are many other references available for the reader interested in more detail concerning specific intervention protocols.[8, 10, 51, 53, 66, 129, 133, 149] For excellent discussions of neuromuscular electrical stimulation for clients with neurological impairment, the reader is referred to DeVahl,[53] Gardner and Baker,[65] and Packman-Braun.[133] EMGBF devices and protocols are addressed later in the chapter.

Typically, electrical stimulators may be either small, portable battery-operated units or larger wall- or line-powered clinical models. Portable units are particularly convenient for use by the client who requires stimulation over multiple intervention sessions or over a greater length of time, for example, home treatment. Clinical models usually have a greater choice of parameters and quite often are able to store customized programs for individual patients, but advancements in technology are minimizing the differences between devices. The major difference that must be considered when choosing a suitable device is its ability to produce the desired level and timing of muscle contractions. There is some evidence to suggest that battery-powered devices do not produce the high contractile forces needed for strengthening that is achieved by most clinical wall-powered units. This may have an effect on the rate of improvement of force production from the target muscle.[52] In many functional situations, however, strength may not be the most important factor. Attention must be paid to timing, endurance, and learning during the activity. This situation likely does not require high levels of stimulation.

Neuromuscular Electrical Stimulation

Parameters

WAVEFORM

The waveform of the stimulus of most NMES units is usually either a symmetrical or an asymmetrical biphasic pulse. The two phases of each pulse continually alternate or reverse in direction between positive and negative polarity. With the asymmetrical biphasic pulse, the cathode (negative) and anode (positive) electrodes can be identified; therefore the therapist can selectively apply the negative electrode over the target muscle, producing a more effective contraction. Because the polarity of the symmetrical biphasic waveform is continually reversing in direction and the two phases in each pulse are equal in amplitude, both electrodes alternately become active electrodes, and one is not more effective than the other.[1, 59, 124] Some stimulators use a monophasic waveform, which can be set as either a negative or a positive pulse at the active electrode. Using the negative polarity at the active electrode (over the target muscle) produces a muscle contraction with less current amplitude (intensity) than when using the positive polarity. While an ideal waveform for NMES has not been agreed upon, some studies have shown the symmetrical biphasic waveform to be more comfortable than either the asymmetrical biphasic or the monophasic waveform.[7, 8, 112] The symmetrical biphasic

pulse, when compared with others, is also considered to be the waveform of choice due to the low total pulse charge.[92]

DURATION

Stimulators with a phase duration of 1 to 300 μs (0.3 ms) can be used to activate muscles with intact innervation. A set duration of 300 μs has been reported as preferred, compared with shorter durations.[27, 71] Shorter-duration waveforms require a greater current amplitude to produce a muscle contraction and will likely be more comfortable, but they may not possess the charge needed for good contraction levels. Longer-phase durations may be used but are less comfortable.

FREQUENCY

The stimulus frequency should be set at a rate sufficient to produce a smooth, sustained (tetanic) muscle contraction. While this varies with different muscles, a frequency of 30 to 50 Hz (pulses per second [PPS]) is usually effective, although slower frequencies may be used if a satisfactory contraction is obtained.[59] Higher stimulus frequencies can cause fatigue, so the frequency should be set no faster than that which produces a smooth contraction.

Currently, commercial stimulators produce pulses with consistent interpulse intervals producing what may be called "constant frequency trains." Recently, studies examining "variable frequency pulse trains" and their effects on muscle force production and fatigue have been reported. It appears that there will be some advantage to the use of this type of stimulation parameter for enhancing muscle force and reducing the effects of fatigue.[21, 105, 117, 152]

AMPLITUDE

Amplitude or intensity of the stimulus is gradually increased until the desired level of activation is obtained in the muscle(s) being stimulated. This level depends on the goal for the program. The client should be encouraged to participate actively by contracting the muscle(s) and synchronizing his or her effort with the timing of the external stimulus. With very weak muscles, a lower level of training is used, and it may be necessary to use gravity-eliminated positions to assist movement through as much of the available range as possible. With stronger muscles, higher current amplitudes are used, with a goal of activating the muscle to the strongest level of force indicated for the exercise program. In all situations, muscle fatigue should be avoided or minimized by using the lowest amplitude necessary to produce a satisfactory contraction.[20, 22] The therapist must keep in mind that the NMES is being used to supplement, not substitute for, exercise.

MODULATIONS

In addition to the parameters of the basic individual stimulus pulses (i.e., waveform, phase and pulse duration, pulse frequency, and amplitude), several modulations are necessary to enhance the effectiveness of the NMES program. The stimulus is applied in a repetitive "train" of pulses, which can be periodically interrupted or turned on and off in rhythmical "bursts" or cycles, ramped, and delivered with preset duty cycles.

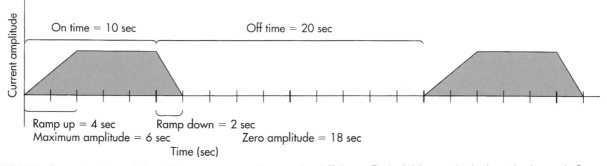

FIGURE 28–3. Example of the relationship between ramp times and on/off times. Each division on the horizontal axis equals 2 seconds. Note that the ramp-up time is considered part of the on time, while the ramp-down time is considered part of the off time. (From DeVahl J: Neuromuscular electrical stimulation (NMES) in rehabilitation. *In* Gersh MR [ed]: Electrotherapy in Rehabilitation. Philadelphia, FA Davis, 1992.)

On Time and Off Time. Neuromuscular electrical stimulation for facilitation of muscle contraction should be used to supplement exercise, and goals for stimulation should be consistent with the goals of the exercise program. To simulate isotonic or isometric muscle contractions, as in voluntary movement for exercise, the stimulator must have the capability of setting bursts or cycles of on and off times; thus the period of muscle contraction is followed by a period of relaxation[53, 59] (Fig. 28–3). In most cases, a shorter on time than off time is desirable to avoid fatigue, for example, a 5-second effective on time, and 25-second off time in a cycle, which would produce an on-off ratio of 1:5.[132] If the goal is to reduce edema by providing a muscle pumping action, a ratio of 1:1 or 1:2 may be preferred.

Packman-Braun[132] investigated ratios of stimulation to rest time with NMES for wrist extension in a group of hemiplegic patients. Results supported the on-off time of 1:5 (stimulus time–rest time) as being the most beneficial in training programs of 20 to 30 minutes because of the deleterious effects of fatigue with lower ratios (1:1, 1:2, 1:3, 1:4). The question remains whether ratios with a greater proportion of rest time might prove more beneficial.

Ramping. Ramping is another modulation that can be set by the therapist. Ramp-up is the time it takes each train of pulses to sequentially increase amplitude or intensity from zero (no current flow) to maximum. Ramp-off is the time period set at the end of the train of maximum intensity pulses to sequentially decrease from maximum to zero amplitude (see Fig. 28–3). Thus ramp time can be adjusted so that the stimulation more nearly resembles a pattern of gradually contracting and relaxing muscles. For clients with hypertonicity or spasticity and a goal of facilitation and strengthening of the antagonist muscle, a longer ramp-up time may avoid or minimize activation of the stretch reflex in the hyperactive agonist muscle. Shorter ramp times may be effective when the goal is to increase ROM or decrease edema.

Duty Cycle. The term *duty cycle* is sometimes confused with the on-off time ratio. Duty cycle is the percentage of time a series or train of pulses is on, out of the total on and off time in a cycle.[8, 59] As an example, if the train of pulses is on 10 seconds and off 30 seconds, the total cycle time is 40 seconds. The duty cycle would be 25%, that is, 10 seconds of the total 40-second cycle. The actual on time and off time of the pulses in a cycle is a more informative description than using either the duty cycle or the on-off ratio.

Mechanisms

Muscle recruitment patterns triggered by electrical stimulation therapy differ from those observed in normal muscle activation. In a voluntary muscle contraction, motor units fire asynchronously, with a larger proportion of type I, fatigue-resistant muscle fibers of the smaller motor units being recruited first. The order of muscle fiber firing occurs as a result of motor neuron size and the anatomy of synaptic connections.[19] Conversely, an electrically stimulated muscle contraction elicits initial responses from larger motor units, which contain a greater number of fatigable, type II muscle fibers.[22] A study of healthy subjects demonstrated recruitment of these higher-threshold motor units at relatively low NMES training levels. This phenomenon is not possible with voluntary exercise, as much greater exercise intensity is required for activation of these larger motor units.[22] This provides support for observed increases in strength with low NMES training intensities, as muscle fibers usually only accessible by high-intensity training participate in muscle activation and improve torque production.[175] Firing order in this scenario is a result of neuronal axon size, proximity of the electrical stimulus, and the intensity of the stimulation.[69]

Synchronous recruitment of muscle fibers is obtained with electrical stimulation, a situation that does not occur with volitional activation. Careful attention to the intensity of stimulation, stimulus frequency, and timing of rest periods is required to minimize fatigue.[22] Because the character of the neuronal excitation for a muscle contraction is different with electrical stimulation than with the physiological response of voluntary muscle activation, stimulation should be discontinued when the client can adequately activate the muscle, so that volitional strengthening can occur.

Higher stimulus frequencies cause fatigue sooner than

lower frequencies. In some instances, the frequency of stimulation may be dictated by the goal of NMES, for instance, sufficient stimulation intensity to move a limb through the desired ROM. In general, stimulation intensity should be set at the lowest level possible to get the desired response to minimize fatigue.[22]

Numerous potential benefits are identified for NMES. Among them are improvement in ROM, edema reduction, treatment of disuse atrophy, and improvement of muscle recruitment for muscle reeducation.[53]

Muscle Reeducation

After an insult or injury affecting the CNS, problems with motor control are frequently manifest. One of the common goals of therapy is to facilitate movement in the areas where control is lacking. If active movement is not present, NMES allows movement to occur via stimulation, which may be followed by resumption of active movement, possibly triggered by the proprioceptive and sensory experience that accompanies the stimulation. When active movement is present but is weak or not well controlled, the therapist may choose to use NMES to supplement and "strengthen" the muscular contraction already present. In the presence of hypertonicity, the muscles serving as antagonists to the spastic muscle may be targeted for NMES, not only to strengthen the antagonist but to inhibit the spastic muscle by reciprocal inhibition.[53, 133]

Functional Electrical Stimulation

The term *functional electrical stimulation* (FES) has been used casually to describe various applications of NMES. However, FES is defined by the Electrotherapy Standards Committee of the Section on Clinical Electrophysiology as the use of NMES (on innervated muscles) for orthotic substitution.[59] Baker and colleagues[5] use the term to describe external control of innervated, paretic, or paralytic muscles "to achieve functional and purposeful movements." While NMES generally is considered to have therapeutic applications, such as increasing ROM, facilitation of muscle activation, and muscle strengthening, the key to application of FES is to enhance or facilitate functional control. It is used with clients with spinal cord injury (SCI), traumatic brain injury, (TBI), cerebrovascular accident (CVA), and other CNS dysfunction who have intact peripheral innervation.

An example of FES application, the electrical stimulation of the peroneal nerve to enhance ankle dorsiflexion during gait in patients with hemiplegia, was reported by Liberson in 1961.[106] Numerous other uses of FES have been described since then, ranging from isolated motor control activities, such as decreasing shoulder subluxation and reduction of scoliosis, to the highly technical computerized gait and bicycling capabilities, sometimes referred to as CFES.[3, 60, 74, 94, 145, 146, 162] The trigger, which activates muscle contraction in synchrony with the functional activity, can be initiated manually by the client, set within the stimulator to automatically trigger on and off cycles, or programmed into a complex computer system for bicycling or gait.

Stimulation is generally applied in short-duration pulses with a frequency sufficient to provide smooth, tetanizing muscle contractions, for example, 25 pps, and adjusted to cycle on and off, with adequate ramp functions, as indicated by the speed and time needed to synchronize the stimulation with the functional activity. The length of the intervention depends on the purpose and may vary from a few contractions during the functional activity, building to multiple 30-minute sessions working up to several hours, repeated daily or three to five times per week. An obvious goal and benefit of FES is to facilitate or substitute for specified functional activities. With the more complex computerized systems (e.g., REGYS I/ERGYS I, Therapeutic Alliances Inc., 333 N. Broad St., Fairborn, OH 45324) used with clients with complete spinal cord lesions, electrically activated functional movements are the mechanism to achieve physiological and psychological benefits, although in some situations, assisted function also is an important goal.[61, 85, 86, 136, 137, 139, 145, 162, 177] Hooker and co-workers[85] evaluated physiological effects of using an ERGYS I leg-cycle ergometer on seven persons with paraplegia and seven with quadriplegia. Subjects were stimulated for 30 minutes with low-power output levels to avoid fatigue. Compared with resting levels, significant increases were found in cardiac output, heart rate, stroke volume, respiratory exchange rate, pulmonary ventilation, and other physiological phenomena. The authors concluded that no inappropriate or unsafe physiological responses occurred in their subjects.

Computerized FES for cycle ergometry and ambulation also has been shown to increase muscle mass, electrically induce muscle strength and endurance,[138, 140, 146] increase circulation, increase aerobic capacity, decrease edema, and have a beneficial effect on self-image.[84, 140, 162] Mutton and colleagues[123] also reported significant improvements in aerobic capacity and submaximal physiological parameters in complete SCI patients (n = 11) who performed a "hybrid" exercise of leg plus arm training immediately following FES and lower extremity cycling. Results were compared with a protocol of FES and lower extremity cycling alone. The improvements were measured with clients exercising just two times per week, in sessions ranging from approximately 17 to 20 weeks. The twice-weekly exercise regimen enhancement of cardiorespiratory fitness is supported by at least one other study.[87] Baldi and associates[9] looked at prevention of muscle mass loss in 26 subjects with acute SCI. Subjects performing FES with cycle ergometry had lean body mass loss prevented at both 3- and 6-month intervals after program initiation. The findings were significant when compared with individuals performing FES with isometrics and controls. Significant hypertrophy occurred in the cycle group after 6 months of continued training. Detraining following cessation of an exercise may be less of an issue than earlier thought. Gurney and colleagues[75] reported partial maintenance of both central distribution adaptations and peripheral muscle adaptations in six individuals with SCI, 8 weeks following completion of a 12-week computerized FES lower extremity cycling and arm ergometry program.

The demonstrated benefits of FES clearly indicate that it is a valuable tool for supplementing functional activities. The practicality and cost of applications of the more complex computerized systems clearly need further study and technological development.

Electrical Muscle Stimulation

Mechanisms

For clients with PNS dysfunction (e.g., peripheral nerve injuries or peripheral neuropathy), EMS may be helpful in preserving the contractility and extensibility of denervated muscle tissue and in retarding muscle atrophy.[16, 58, 170] There is no doubt that literature highlights controversy over the benefits of EMS for peripheral neuropathies and continues to bewilder and lure therapists, physicians, and other researchers to deliberate on and study its efficacy.[45, 164] Many studies on animals[101, 142, 180] and a few on humans[26, 151, 178] demonstrate that electrical stimulation enhances circulation and decreases venous stasis, thereby improving nutrition; reduces (not prevents) muscle atrophy; and assists in maintaining ROM and the contractile properties of muscle. The goal, then, is to keep muscle tissue healthier and viable until reinnervation is established. Electrical stimulation does not hasten regeneration of injured nerve tissue.

Opposing this goal are studies reporting that EMS may have the detrimental effect of retarding reinnervation at the terminal end plate and neuromuscular junction.[107, 141] In addition, the time and cost of treatment are major factors, because reinnervation at the rate of 1.5 to 2.0 mm/day dictates a recovery period of months or even 1 to 2 years. Others argue that the studies are flawed and that stimulation is not detrimental to terminal nerve growth if stimulus parameters are wisely selected and the amplitude is applied at a level that does not fatigue the regenerating nerve or stress the healing tissue.[164] The following discussion should help the reader in making the decision on whether to use EMS for clients with denervated muscles.

Parameters

A number of electrical stimulators with pulses of sufficiently long duration to evoke contractions in denervated muscle are available. Pulse duration, usually monophasic, must be equal to or longer than chronaxy of the denervated muscle. Tests of chronaxy are rarely performed, but, historically, tests have shown that pulse durations of 20 to 100 ms are required to produce responses in denervated muscle.[44, 80] The shortest effective duration is preferred, because a lower amplitude is required to elicit a response, making the stimulation more comfortable and less fatiguing to the muscle. Therefore stimulators with adjustable pulse durations are preferred, but few are available.

Pulse frequencies of 10 to 30 pps, applied in bouts of 5 to 20 stimulations to each involved muscle, should be followed by a rest time longer than the stimulation time (on-off time ratio of no less than 1:5). The bouts of stimulation are then repeated two to three times in each session.[45, 101, 178] Treatment sessions are more effective if repeated two to three times a day and if initiated early in the course of the impairment.

Some reports advocate use of a stimulus amplitude strong enough to cause a maximal contraction through the available ROM.[164] Because of possible detrimental effects to the regenerating terminal axons and neuromuscular junction, however, strong submaximal muscle contractions may be a better choice. A stimulus amplitude high enough to produce at least a visible contraction is necessary.

If the prognosis for nerve regeneration is good, or at least fair, and the blood supply is viable, EMS may be useful in maintaining optimal conditions of blood flow, nutrition, and muscle tissue contractility, so that if or when regeneration occurs, return of motor activation and function may be facilitated. If the EMS does not elicit an effective muscle contraction, stimulation should be discontinued after a 2- to 3-week trial period. If effective contractions can be elicited, the stimulation program should be continued 2 to 6 weeks past the time predicted for complete reinnervation, as evidenced by visible active muscle contraction. Frequent visits to a physical therapy department for exercise and EMS over the long reinnervation periods are not practical in terms of time or cost. Small, portable, and inexpensive EMS units that can deliver pulses of sufficiently long duration are available for home use. Supplementing a carefully planned therapeutic exercise home program with electrical stimulation should be seriously considered (Fig. 28–4A,B).

Electromyographic Biofeedback

Mechanisms

EMGBF has several well-documented applications, including alteration of physiological responses such as heart rate, temperature, and muscle tension.[10] These applications may prove beneficial for clients with neurological dysfunction, if relaxation is required for pain reduction, for instance. The focus of this review is primarily the use of EMGBF for improvement of active movement, which may include hypertonicity reduction, in addition to muscle reeducation. Current technology provides for a variety of EMGBF units, from very basic single-channel portable models to clinical units with multiple channels and multiple options for provision of feedback (audio or visual, or both).

EMGBF may be utilized to assist a client in attaining greater levels of muscle activation in paretic muscle, decrease levels of muscle activation in spastic muscle, or attain a balance between agonist and antagonist muscle pairs.[191] For the majority of practicing clinicians, EMG levels are monitored through the use of surface electrodes. Monitoring of activation of deep muscles therefore may not be feasible, but attention to size and specific electrode placement is critical to ensure feedback that will be most useful to the client. Smaller electrodes will allow more specific placement, although higher impedance also will be encountered; therefore skin must be carefully prepared to take this into account.[11] Because the EMG information recorded represents the sum of action potentials from motor units between the electrodes, larger interelectrode distance will increase the area of muscle recorded. This may be desirable for large muscle groups or when minimal activity is present in muscle groups. Smaller interelectrode distances are preferable if

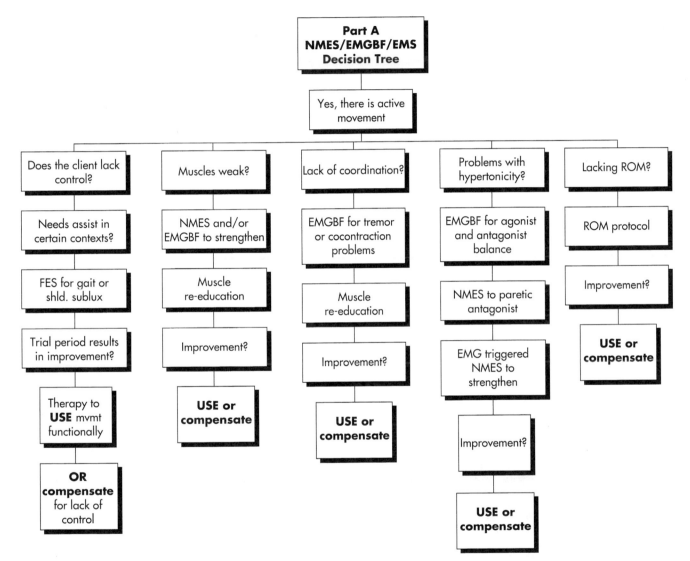

FIGURE 28–4. *A,* Decision tree for clients that exhibit active movement in the targeted treatment area. NMES, neuromuscular electrical stimulation; EMGBF, electromyographic biofeedback; EMS, electrical muscular stimulation; ROM, range of movement; FES, functional electrical stimulation.

Illustration continued on following page

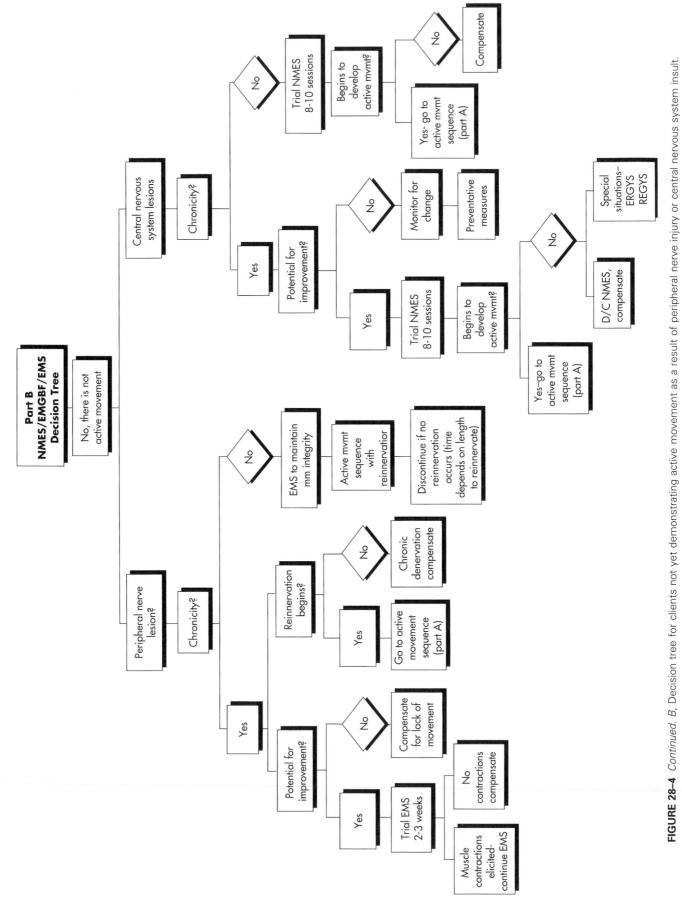

FIGURE 28-4 *Continued. B,* Decision tree for clients not yet demonstrating active movement as a result of peripheral nerve injury or central nervous system insult.

there is a risk of interference from "crosstalk" or "volume conduction" from muscles or motor units not part of the target group. Basmajian and Blumenstein[11] provide an excellent review of electrode placements for the face, trunk, and upper and lower limbs.

Reduction of Hypertonicity

DeBacher[50] has described a progression of intervention with EMGBF designed to reduce spasticity. The program utilizes three stages of intervention: (1) relaxation of spastic muscles at rest even in the presence of distraction, mental effort, or use of muscles not targeted for EMGBF training; (2) inhibition of muscle activity during passive static and dynamic stretch of the spastic muscle, beginning with static stretch at the extremes of motion, then progressing to passive movement speed at a speed of 15 degrees per second, and gradually increasing movement speed at increments of 15 degrees per second up to 90 degrees per second; and (3) isometric contractions of the antagonist to the spastic muscle, with relaxation of the spastic muscle, progressing to prompt muscle contraction and relaxation of the spastic muscle, and grading of muscle contractions with movement for various force output requirements. Application of a similar training approach with a group of four young adults with cerebral palsy demonstrated improvement in the resting levels of involuntary muscle activity, as well as reduction in resting and active tonic reflex activity.[127] Consistent functional improvements were not observed, however, as a result of these altered EMG levels.

Investigation of agonist and antagonist upper extremity muscle activity in a population of stroke patients points to the importance of focusing attention on the weak agonist as opposed to relaxation of the antagonist.[70] EMG levels of targeted muscle groups were monitored in healthy control subjects during the performance of six upper extremity movements in order to describe the appropriate agonists and antagonists for each movement. Patients unable to perform movements demonstrated reduced levels of agonist activity as opposed to increased levels of antagonist muscle activation. Our assumptions about abnormal co-contraction preventing movement from occurring[23] may require further investigation.

The presence of hypertonicity and spasticity following neurological insult or injury may be problematic for some clients, as these problems may exist in conjunction with lack of active control. Assumptions about the functional importance of spasticity per se seem to be changing as studies demonstrate reduction of spasticity without improvement of motor control. Persistence of control problems may be related to lack of force production, deficits in speed of muscle activation, and lack of reciprocal interaction of muscle groups.[103] Nevertheless, EMGBF can be useful in helping a client decrease abnormal muscle activation. Several questions remain: (1) Will the ability to relax a muscle at rest effect a change in muscle activation patterns with movement? and (2) Will alteration in EMG patterns result in functional improvement for the client?

Muscle Reeducation

Therapists may opt to use biofeedback to provide information about the quality of the muscle contraction di-

rectly to the client. The client can then attempt to alter the contraction in accordance with guidelines provided by the therapist, whether the focus be to facilitate stronger contraction, decrease apparent hyperactivity, or modulate a balance of muscle activity during a functional task.

One such application of EMGBF is concurrent assessment of muscle activity (CAMA),[194] where the therapist utilizes biofeedback as an adjunct in evaluation of client response to therapeutic exercise. In this procedure, the therapist must decide which muscle group(s) are desired for activation, and adjust client position or therapist intervention accordingly to achieve the desired muscle responses.[194] CAMA may allow judgment of efficacy of exercise intervention based on actual EMG responses rather than presumptions about what one expects to occur with a particular technique or activity.

Several authors suggest the use of biofeedback signals from homologous extremity muscles as a model for how the hemiplegic client needs to alter muscle activity in a particular function.[185, 192] Described as a "motor copy" representation by Wolf and colleagues,[192] this procedure was compared to a more traditional targeted training procedure in a group of 20 clients with stroke and 6 clients with head injury. Although improvements in functional activity level, ROM, and EMG activity were observed for both motor copy and targeted training groups, many of the improvements in the motor copy group appeared on follow-up evaluations (after a series of 10 treatments), whereas improvements in the targeted training group were observed only during the treatment process. Wissel and co-workers[185] used a similar training procedure with monitoring of the uninvolved limb as a model for the hemiparetic upper or lower extremity in the functional tasks of grasping and drinking from a glass and ambulation. Most patients demonstrated improvements in maximum integrated surface EMG, upper extremity movement, multiple stage ratings of walking and drinking from a glass; but the subject group size (n = 11) was too small to draw conclusions statistically. More recent studies support the practice of patterning or copying EMG activity from other muscles as a potentially useful tool for individuals with C4–7 SCI.[147, 174] Questions of efficacy naturally arise when considering intervention options. Is the intervention chosen likely to produce a quicker or more profound response than conventionally accepted therapies? This topic was addressed in a meta-analysis that compared EMGBF with conventional physical therapy for upper extremity function in individuals following stroke.[115] After assessing published research articles from 1976 through 1992, only six met the indicated criteria for inclusion. From the results of those articles, the authors concluded that neither approach was superior to the other. Even though the study sample was small, the authors were able to recommend that cost, ease of utilization of equipment, and patient preference be considered prior to choosing an approach.

Integrating Neuromuscular Electrical Stimulation and Electromyographic Biofeedback

An alternative application that has merit is the use of EMG-triggered NMES, where NMES is initiated once the client achieves a predetermined level of EMG activity in the targeted muscle. The threshold of EMG for the onset of NMES can be manipulated by the therapist to engage increasing levels of client active control. The success of this application is emphasized for patients with hemiplegia in increasing levels of EMG activity (improvements in 90% of chronic patients with stroke selected for eight treatment sessions) and subsequent improvement in ROM in the involved arm and leg.[62] Threshold levels of EMG activity could gradually be increased as the client gains the ability to activate muscles independently with eventual discontinuance of the NMES as strength and active control allows. Francisco and colleagues[64] obtained significant gains in upper extremity aspects of both the Functional Independence Measure (FIM) and Fugl-Meyer Motor Assessment when measured against controls. These results followed two daily 30-minute interventions for the duration of the rehabilitation.[64]

A variation of this application is NMES triggered by positional feedback, such that NMES is initiated once the patient actively moves through a portion of the available ROM at a joint.[28] The therapist may set the threshold angle in accordance with the patient's goals and abilities. This methodology was effective in improving wrist motion in patients following stroke, although it was not as effective in altering control of the knee in a similar patient group.[184]

Although discussions of EMGBF, EMS, FES, and NMES are often presented separately, the use of these modalities can be intertwined to achieve desired muscle control. Processes of clinical decision making are represented in Figure 28–4 A and B, beginning with a determination of whether the movement control problem is a result of a CNS or peripheral nerve lesion. NMES or FES may be initiated in the absence of active control (although lower levels of muscle activation may be discovered and facilitated with EMGBF). Once return of active control begins, EMGBF may be utilized to refine the control. One should not assume that an increase in muscle EMG will automatically translate to an improvement in functional use of that muscle in daily activities. Consequently, NMES and EMGBF need to be integrated into daily functional activities, so that appropriate muscle activity is elicited and used in its appropriate functional context.

Feedback Considerations

Mulder and Hulstyn[120] provide a review of the features of feedback related to motor control and motor learning theories, with discussion of the characteristics of normal feedback (see Chapter 33 for additional information). Feedback (in most instances provided verbally by the therapist) may be motivational, but it may be relatively subjective and dependent on the skill of the therapist to attend to the client, observe accurately what occurs, and provide information to the client in a timely manner. Feedback in this form generally is provided with some delay after the activity. EMGBF has the benefit of being provided simultaneously with the client's movement, consisting of accurate and objective information about muscle activity (given careful electrode application and equipment in good working order), and not requiring the same level of therapist skill as verbal feedback provision. EMGBF therefore may be beneficial for clients with deficient sensory feedback systems. The frequency of feedback provision, however, may require close scrutiny by the therapist, as demonstrated by the following studies.

Experiments examining feedback frequency in the learning of motor tasks support the use of less than 100% relative frequency for the subject to learn the task. In other words, feedback provided on every trial may improve performance but degrades learning in healthy subjects.[158] The application of this concept to the use of EMGBF was investigated by Bate and Matyas,[14] who used EMGBF with two groups of stroke patients attempting a pursuit tracking task. Comparisons were made of performance in a pretest, training test, and post-test phase. The biofeedback provided information about the contractions of the spastic antagonist (elbow flexors) for the movement task for the experimental group. The control group performed the task without the benefit of biofeedback. Posttesting revealed that the use of continuous feedback had a negative transfer effect on learning of the movement task, suggesting that the experimental learners became dependent on the external feedback in performance of the task. It is imperative, therefore, that the clinician structure the use of external feedback carefully so the client begins to develop a sense of muscle activation or relaxation, which is present without the EMGBF apparatus. Biofeedback may be used with the screen turned away from the client (or the audio signal turned off) so the client can transfer the learning without feedback, and the clinician can evaluate client performance and judge actual client learning of the muscle activation patterns.

Applications

The application of the common principles of EMGBF and NMES to different patient populations emphasizes the role of the therapist in tailoring intervention to meet specific client needs. Many investigators have evaluated the use of NMES and EMGBF in subjects with stroke. FES has been used extensively with clients with SCI. Other populations that demonstrate neuromuscular impairment or dysfunction have not been as thoroughly studied, as the heterogeneity of these groups may create difficulty in research design. Perhaps patients with cerebral palsy, brain injury, and Guillain-Barré syndrome gain or regain active control in therapy through conventional means; therefore therapists do not consider use of NMES or EMGBF. Nevertheless, there are documented applications of these modalities with a variety of patient populations. These results are reviewed.

Stroke

Wolf and Binder-Macleod[190] examined client characteristics that are critical to success with biofeedback retraining for upper and lower extremity control following stroke (see also Chapter 25). In a group of 52 clients with stroke, no significant relationships between outcome and age, sex, number of EMGBF treatments, or side of hemiparesis were found. Lower extremity treatment was associated with a greater probability of success, and this success did not seem related to chronicity of stroke sequelae. In contrast, success of upper extremity treatment did appear to be related to length of time since onset of stroke, and poorer outcomes were noted if clients had received physical therapy to the involved arm for more than 1 year before EMGBF training. Improvements in elbow and shoulder function were obtained in this group of patients, but obtaining improvement in functional use of the hand was limited. Aphasia did emerge as a slight limitation to achieving improvement, but proprioception deficits were more significant in restricting functional gains. The role of client motivation in success with EMGBF training was emphasized. On follow-up over 12 months, the improvements made in the initial intervention were maintained in the 34 clients evaluated, with one exception, where deterioration in motor function was attributed to possible organic cause (transient ischemic attacks).[193]

A number of researchers have published papers discussing the muscle recruitment problems observed following CVA.[70, 77, 78, 154] Knowledge of these problems is a prerequisite for determination of the appropriate application of EMGBF or NMES. It appears that delayed recruitment of agonist and antagonist is a relatively consistent finding. Some studies demonstrate delayed termination of muscle activity once initiated[154] and the presence of co-contraction of agonist and antagonist muscle groups.[77, 78] Other investigators have discovered a lack of co-contraction[70] and problems with maintenance of agonist muscle contractions.[77] The possibility of these conflicting presentations underscores the benefit of use of EMGBF so that the actual muscle activation patterns can be observed in a given client, and treatment can progress.

Four studies were included in a 1996 meta-analysis of electrical stimulation and recovery of strength in individuals following stroke.[68] Duration of therapy following the stroke ranged from 1.5 to 29.2 months. Interventions included stimulation applied to the neuromuscular system of the involved hemiparetic extremity. Comparisons were made to changes in muscle strength without stimulation. The authors reported a statistically significant effect ($P<.05$) between the two conditions and concluded that the results supported use of electrical stimulation for strength improvement following stroke.

UPPER EXTREMITY MANAGEMENT

EMGBF. EMGBF has been studied extensively, but success of treatment is mixed, with difficulty in interpretation complicated by focus on measures that are not directly related to function in a number of studies. A reduction in co-contraction has been observed,[143] as well as improvement in several neuromuscular variables[90, 189, 190]; however, a lack of significant improvement in functional skill was noted. Given the challenge of improving upper extremity functional ability following stroke, Wolf and Binder-Macleod suggested consideration of several key factors in predicting which clients may benefit from EMGBF: ". . . those patients who achieve the most substantial improvement in manipulative abilities initially possess voluntary finger extension; comparatively greater active ROM about the shoulder, elbow, and wrist; and comparatively less hyperactivity in muscles usually considered as major contributors to the typical flexor synergy."[189] Attention to the chronicity of motor dysfunction also

appears critical in anticipating success with EMGBF, as clients 2 to 3 months after stroke demonstrated stronger functional gains following intervention with biofeedback compared with clients 4 to 5 months after stroke.[13]

NMES. Common upper extremity applications of NMES for the stroke patient include reduction of shoulder subluxation (FES) and facilitation of elbow, wrist, and finger extension. Electrode placements for shoulder movements are detailed by Baker and Parker,[5] including shoulder extension, flexion, and abduction, and scapular muscle stimulation.

FES was utilized with 63 stroke patients (mean of 46 days post onset for the control group, and 49 days post onset for the experimental group) to evaluate the effects of this treatment on shoulder subluxation as measured by radiography.[5] The treatment protocol included stimulation of the posterior deltoid and supraspinatus muscles to reduce shoulder subluxation, with gradual increases from three half-hour sessions to one 6- to 7-hour cycle per day with a 1:3 on-off ratio. The FES was used for 6 weeks. Radiographs at the end of the intervention period showed improvements in the study group from 14.8 to 8.6 mm, with a 1 to 2 mm loss of reduction when evaluated 3 months later. The control group began with a mean subluxation of 13.3 mm, and the same amount of subluxation was noted after the 6-week intervention time. Three months after the study, the control group demonstrated no change in subluxation. No direct relationship between pain and amount of subluxation was noted. It may be argued that the chronicity of stroke sequelae of this patient population played a role in the success of the FES in altering shoulder subluxation and that this intervention may prove more beneficial if used in the initial stages to prevent subluxation, rather than attempting to reduce it once it has occurred.

Faghri and colleagues[61] implemented FES as a preventive measure in a group of acute patients. An experimental and control group each received conventional physical therapy, but the experimental group also received FES to reduce shoulder subluxation, gradually increasing up to 6 hours per day and continuing for 6 weeks. Comparisons of arm function, arm muscle tone, posterior deltoid EMG activity, upper arm girth, shoulder ROM (to test for pain), and shoulder subluxation (by radiography of both shoulders) were performed at the beginning of the intervention, at the completion of the 6-week program, and 6 weeks after completion of the program. The experimental group exhibited significantly greater range without pain than the control group and significantly less subluxation (6 mm initially, decreasing to 2.46 mm after treatment, and then increasing slightly to 3.46 mm 6 weeks later, as compared to values of 4 mm, 9.85 mm, and 9.35 mm for the control group). Both groups demonstrated functional improvement with higher values (although not significantly different) for the experimental group. Chantraine and colleagues,[37] in a controlled study over 24 months, followed 120 individuals after hemiplegia onset. Subjects in the stimulation group received 5 weeks of FES in addition to the Bobath rehabilitation protocol that all subjects experienced. Variables of ROM, pain, and radiographic measurements of subluxation were assessed at the time of stroke, between the second and fourth weeks following onset, as well as after 6, 12, and 24 months. The FES group showed significant ($P<.01$) improvements in pain relief and arm ROM as well as reduction of subluxation ($P<.05$).

FES for shoulder subluxation reduction appears beneficial for prevention of pain and subluxation, especially if utilized during the early stages of recovery. The functional benefits of this intervention are not clear, even in studies with relatively extensive (6 weeks, with 6 to 7 hours of stimulation each day) intervention. Careful cost-benefit analysis is recommended when considering this modality for shoulder subluxation reduction.

FES has also been investigated as an upper extremity orthosis following hemiplegia, utilizing movement of the uninvolved shoulder to trigger stimulation of elbow extension and hand opening.[13] After extensive training periods, patients were able to demonstrate functional use of the involved hand for basic reach and grasp. Systems with more than two channels of stimulation have proved difficult for patients to use.[179]

Extensor forearm FES was utilized in a controlled study of 46 individuals with acute stroke.[36] The 28 subjects who completed the FES protocol were compared with the control group, which received placebo stimulation over the same area of the forearm. Sessions were daily for 1 hour with a total of 15 applications. Variables assessed, in a blinded format, at pre- and post-intervention as well as 4 and 12 weeks following intervention, were the upper extremity components of the Fugl-Meyer Motor Assessment and the self-care component of the FIM. Fugl-Meyer scores were significantly improved ($P<.05$ to .06) at all stages except pre-intervention. FIM scores showed no difference at any stage of assessment. While it was felt the sample size was too small to detect changes in self-care, there was ample evidence that the FES did enhance motor recovery of the forearm after acute stroke.

Three-month interventions with EMG-triggered NMES, low-intensity NMES, proprioceptive neuromuscular facilitation (PNF) exercise, or no treatment (control group) were compared in a group of chronic stroke patients.[102] Evaluations performed before treatment, at completion of treatment, and at 3- and 9-month intervals after treatment demonstrated improvements in those patients receiving therapy. Fugl-Meyer scores improved 18% for the PNF group, 25% for the patients receiving low-intensity NMES, and 42% for the group treated with EMG-triggered NMES. The control group scores did not change.[102] These findings lend support to use of NMES and EMGBF and NMES as an adjunct to physical therapy.

LOWER EXTREMITY MANAGEMENT

EMGBF. Several studies evaluating EMGBF for retraining lower extremity control following stroke have focused on improvement of tibialis anterior control and reduction of gastrocnemius muscle activity. Results support increases in strength and ROM in ankle dorsiflexion[12, 31, 155] with carryover into ambulation[12] and maintenance of this improvement on follow-up evaluation.[12, 31]

Wolf and Binder-Macleod[190] examined a number of variables at the hip, knee, and ankle in a controlled group study of the effects of EMGBF. Subjects were assigned to one of four groups: (1) treatment of the lower extremity only with EMGBF, (2) EMGBF treatment of the upper extremity only, (3) general relaxation training, and (4) no treatment. No significant changes were observed between experimental and control groups for EMG levels and ROM at the hip, but improvements were noted in knee and ankle active motion for the experimental group. Although subjects in the experimental group increased in gait speed, these changes were not significantly different from the comparison groups.

Utilization of EMGBF with the intent of improving ambulation may require use of feedback during the task of ambulation instead of during static activity as demonstrated in this study. Positional biofeedback about ankle position and traditional EMGBF were compared in a group of hemiplegic patients.[110] A computerized system provided audiovisual feedback during ambulation for both groups. Pretreatment and post-treatment measures of ankle motion, gait, and perceived exertion were conducted for the two treatment groups and a control group. The group receiving positional biofeedback during ambulation increased their walking speeds relative to the other groups, with improvements maintained at follow-up intervals of up to 3 months. The consideration of integrating feedback into functional tasks bears further investigation.

NMES. Peroneal nerve stimulation has been documented as an assistance for patients with hemiplegia to improve ambulation.[106, 114, 173, 181] Chronic stimulation via implanted electrodes has proved effective in improving gait patterns, but not without significant drawbacks, including difficulty eliciting balanced dorsiflexion, infection with nerve damage in a few cases, and problems with equipment maintenance.[181, 182] In a few patients studied over a 10-year period, the need for stimulation eventually was eliminated, as patients regained the ability to dorsiflex independently.[182] Technology may provide smaller, more sophisticated versions of these devices so that such treatments may be more realistic in the future.

Shorter-term use of peroneal nerve stimulation as an adjunct to traditional physical therapy may be considered. In a controlled study examining the use of 20 minutes of peroneal nerve stimulation six times per week for 4 weeks, the stimulated group demonstrated dorsiflexion recovery three times greater than the control group, as measured by an average of 10 maximal dorsiflexion contractions. These improvements were observed regardless of site of lesion, age, or time since lesion.[114] This type of stimulation is more easily applied than the chronic stimulation described earlier, and may prove more effective. Two studies utilizing a surface peroneal nerve stimulator on individuals with chronic hemiplegia and various other neurological conditions were reported by Burridge and colleagues.[32, 33] Each study showed improvement in gait parameters and a decreased physiological cost when the stimulator was used. One study utilized a control group for comparison. There was no carryover effect from use of the stimulator.

A series of studies from researchers in Ljubljana suggest the use of multichannel electrical stimulation as an intervention to expedite recovery of ambulation in hemiplegia following CVA or brain injury.[24, 25, 108, 179, 188] Through the use of stimulation (as an adjunct to traditional therapy) in daily sessions in a group of 10 patients over a 2-

to 3-week period, a 61.6% increase in gait velocity, 46.3% increase in stride length, and significant decreases in mean stride time were observed during the use of FES. The significantly positive effects of multichannel stimulation were reinforced and the factors of standing and weight shift,[109] as well as gait restoration in nonambulatory chronic hemiplegia,[82] were also improved in two separate studies involving 11 subjects each. Carryover of these effects to ambulation without the stimulation was observed to varying degrees.[24] A comparison of patients treated with this form of stimulation with patients treated by conventional rehabilitation demonstrated faster and greater recovery rates for variables of step length and gait velocity in the stimulated group vs. the control group. At follow-up evaluation 8.4 months after the conclusion of therapy, however, the differences between groups had faded.[108]

Cozean and colleagues[43] utilized NMES for ankle dorsiflexion triggered by heel switch contact during gait and biofeedback to improve active recruitment of ankle dorsiflexors or relaxation of ankle plantarflexors in a study of 36 hemiplegic patients. Patients were divided into four groups: (1) control, (2) NMES, (3) EMGBF, and (4) combined EMGBF and NMES. Those patients assigned to the combined therapy group demonstrated significantly improved knee and ankle range parameters more rapidly than the NMES, EMGBF, or control groups. This result was better maintained in the combined therapy group at follow-up 1 month later. Although all groups improved in gait cycle times, the combined therapy group improved to a greater degree. The authors speculated that the reason for this success may be the benefit at the muscular level achieved by NMES and the focus on retraining central control through the use of EMGBF, which interact synergistically to allow the patient to use the hemiplegic limb more effectively.[43] Granat and co-workers[72] also studied peroneal muscle stimulation effects on multiple gait parameters and the Barthel Index in individuals following stroke onset. Length of time following stroke was 3 to 36 months with an average of 7 months. Individuals were evaluated before and after a 4-week control period and following an intervention period of the same length. Following intervention, the 19 subjects showed significant control of eversion on multiple surfaces and symmetry on a linoleum surface. The Barthel Index score also improved significantly following intervention. There was, however, no improvement in parameters when the subjects were not using the stimulator. This indicates that carryover did not occur with this intervention, the most likely reason being too short an intervention period, especially for this length of time after stroke onset.

UPPER AND LOWER EXTREMITY MANAGEMENT

A few studies have addressed upper and lower extremity retraining procedures simultaneously.[62, 79, 88, 189, 191] The use of actual EMGBF, simulated EMGBF, and no EMGBF was compared in a group of patients with stroke undergoing conventional physical therapy.[88] The simulated EMGBF was generated by the examiner contracting a muscle simultaneous to each patient attempt, so the feedback was positive, but not the actual patient EMG. After a 2-week treatment period, EMG responses from the deltoid and anterior tibial muscles and average ROM measures were compared. The two groups receiving feedback of some form in addition to physical therapy demonstrated significant improvements over the control group. Because the simulated feedback was provided by a therapist by observation of patient effort, it was not completely unrelated to the EMG activity of the limb. The specificity of the feedback did not appear to be critical, raising questions about the mechanism by which improvement occurs with this intervention.

Fields[62] used a technique of EMG-triggered EMS with a group of 69 outpatients with stroke, targeting wrist extension and ankle dorsiflexion initially, but progressing to other movements over the course of several months of four to five 45-minute treatment sessions per week. As previously described, the intervention allowed for setting gradually increased EMG threshold levels, which subjects had to meet before the onset of NMES to assist targeted muscle contraction. Peak unassisted voluntary EMG levels were used as quantitative indications of progress, despite difficulty normalizing these values. Measurable functional progress (improved active ROM and ambulation) was noted in greater than 90% of the patients treated in this study, with those patients unsuitable for this intervention being identified after the first several trials. This form of stimulation is commercially available (Electronic Medical Instruments, Bellevue, WA) and may offer an alternative to traditional NMES or EMGBF.

EFFICACY

Several reviews are available regarding the use of EMGBF with patients following stroke.[54, 62, 157, 186, 188] Well-designed studies with experimental and control groups support the efficacy of EMGBF in improving muscle activation and functional control of the upper and lower extremity, as demonstrated through a meta-analysis,[157] although only eight studies met the strict inclusion criteria for this analysis. Wolf[186] provided support for the use of biofeedback in retraining control of the upper and lower extremity following stroke, yet raised numerous questions for future investigation. Areas of possible study include correlation of feedback intervention with functional outcomes, carefully designed treatment protocols with control groups addressing acute and chronic stroke patients, clarification of site and extent of the lesion as factors in the efficacy of EMGBF, and continued consideration of the factors of age, duration of previous intervention, and sensory and communicative skills in examination of treatment effects.[186, 188]

Much of the literature evaluating the use of EMGBF and NMES involves patients with CVA. Although these studies have many significant results to share, interpretation of these findings with relation to what is recommended for clinical intervention is not as clear-cut. Improvements in generation of EMG activity and active movement appear well documented; the functional implications of these gains are not as well established. Clearly, in the current practice environment much of the focus is on function, so that these techniques to improve muscle activation patterns must be put to functional use in the context of therapy. The therapist must consider the relevant factors that may predict success and critically evaluate outcome during trial use of these modalities. Cost-benefit analyses must accompany any intervention using technology, with the goal of regaining necessary movement as quickly as possible and eliminating the use of equipment when practical. These processes may be illustrated through the use of a case example (see Case 3).

Spinal Cord Injury

NMES has a variety of applications for clients who have sustained SCI (see Chapter 16). Muscle strengthening may occur for muscles innervated by segments just above a complete SCI, or a variety of strengthening applications may be appropriate in the case of incomplete SCI. EMGBF may be used to identify muscle activity in very weak musculature, as a tool to judge improvement in muscle activation, and as a method of facilitating increased strength.[187] Applications of EMGBF for individuals with SCI also include facilitation of unassisted ventilation in high-level quadriplegia[116] and use of biofeedback for muscle reeducation with incomplete SCI in the acute stages when immobilization may be required.[125]

The use of NMES, EMGBF, and other physical therapy was examined in a group of clients with incomplete cervical SCIs over a total treatment period of 16 weeks. Clients were randomly assigned to one of four groups, receiving either physical exercise, NMES, or EMGBF administered in 8-week blocks. Group 1 received EMGBF followed by physical exercise, group 2 received EMGBF followed by NMES, group 3 received NMES followed by physical exercise, and group 4 received 16 weeks of physical exercise only. Measures of muscle strength, self-care ratings, mobility scores, and voluntary EMG were conducted at baseline, treatment midpoint, and conclusion of the interventions. All groups demonstrated improvement across the treatment period on all measures except for voluntary EMG; however, there were no significant differences among the four groups.[97] At least one other study compared conventional intervention, EMGBF, electrical stimulation, and combined stimulation with biofeedback over 6 weeks in individuals with tetraplegia. An examiner, blinded to the intervention protocol, evaluated 45 subjects in the four treatment groups. All groups improved in the parameters evaluated, and no significant difference between groups was noted.[99] These results again emphasize the need to carefully consider cost as well as time and effort for setup and equipment operation in intervention planning.

UPPER EXTREMITY MANAGEMENT

The use of electrically stimulated hand orthotic systems for patients with C6 and higher-level SCI have been refined to allow greater functional independence for a select group of patients.[94, 136, 137, 144, 156, 159, 174] Because hand function does not occur in a cyclical pattern, the onset and termination of stimulation must be controlled by the patient in some manner, with a myoelectric[136] or contact closing switch. Multichannel stimulation is then applied with intramuscular electrodes for the flexors and extensors of the fingers and thumb, with computer-configured interplay between the different muscles to achieve a functional grasp. A chest-mounted position transducer (operated by shoulder elevation or depression and protraction or retraction) allows the user to initiate stimulation and

"lock" the stimulation to maintain a grasp, as well as "unlock" it for release. A toggle switch mounted on the chest allows a choice between electrically stimulated lateral or palmar grasp patterns.[94, 137] Other investigators have utilized contralateral shoulder slings,[163] as well as elbow accelerometers[73] to trigger the needed stimulation. Multiple authors have described successful implantation and utilization, with a few drawbacks, of upper extremity FES prosthesis.[49, 81, 95, 119] Use of this type of system may allow patients with SCI at the C5 level to operate at the same or even higher level of independence as those with C6 quadriplegia with tenodesis, gaining the ability to perform more activities of daily living (ADL) without an attendant. Patients with SCI at the C6 level may be able to manipulate a greater variety of objects without special adaptations.

LOWER EXTREMITY MANAGEMENT

Standing. In an excellent review of the utilization of FES for the purpose of standing patients with SCI, Gardner and Baker[65] described the easiest approach to stimulating the quadriceps femoris in conjunction with upper extremity support to allow paraplegic clients to stand. More complex systems may incorporate stimulation of the gluteus maximus, gluteus medius, hamstring, adductor magnus, gastrocnemius, and soleus muscles for longer duration and better-quality standing performance. Multichannel surface[18] and implantable systems have been and continue to be developed for assistance in sit-stand and transfer activities.[48, 176] Surgical procedures, client selection, and technology are also factors cited in successful interventions. Despite these efforts, the duration of standing with electrically stimulated systems ranges from a few minutes to several hours. The client with SCI may be able to utilize this technology to perform functional activities that require standing. The use of these systems depends on the functions unavailable to a client without use of the technology, and the ease with which a system can be used and maintained. Peripheral to, but no less important, are the reactions of joints to these interventions. Two studies have reported positive benefits to the structure and functions of lower extremity joints of adolescents with SCI, after participating in FES programs.[17, 148]

Cycling. The use of systems to electrically stimulate reciprocal lower limb motions has increased for stationary cycling. The benefits of these interventions for the client with SCI may relate to prevention of cardiovascular disease in the wheelchair-dependent client. Physiological changes noted with electrically stimulated cycling include improvement of peripheral muscular and cardiovascular fitness, as demonstrated by increased power output following training with leg cycle ergometry.[60, 85, 86, 138, 140] Combining FES and lower extremity cycling with upper extremity ergometry induced a higher level of cardiovascular fitness than lower extremity ergometry alone.[123] Exercise session frequency as little as two times per week induced positive changes in cardiovascular fitness.[87, 123] When testing of paraplegic and quadriplegic clients is conducted with arm crank ergometry following a training program with electrically stimulated leg cycle ergometry, clients do not demonstrate differences in pretest and post-test measures of hemodynamic and pulmonary responses. These findings may relate to the specificity of the leg exercise training or the presence of a peripheral rather than a central circulatory response to the training procedure.[86] As noted earlier, many cardiovascular factors can be improved and retained for at least 8 weeks following a program of FES ergometry.[75]

An additional possible benefit of use of lower extremity NMES with the SCI client is the improvement of circulation, as occurred in conjunction with cycling training in a case report.[177] Through the use of an initial program to strengthen the quadriceps femoris, stimulation can be applied with resistance added to the limb in gradual increments, until the client is able to tolerate the training protocol for electrically stimulated cycling (the REGYS system; see above). Further research is required to validate the potential effects of decreased edema, increased blood flow, and concomitant improved wound healing as a result of electrically stimulated cycling.

Ambulation. As technology continues to progress, the use of electrically stimulated systems for ambulation[47, 98, 139] may become more practical and useful for the patient with SCI. Acceptance and use of the systems by clients outside the clinic is mixed but has been shown to have positive effects on characteristics of ambulation.[118, 183] Improvements in functional applications and use will also take place as our ability to select appropriate candidates improves.[4, 100] Benefits of these systems may include increased muscle bulk, a reduced risk of pressure sores and osteoporosis, and psychological benefit. Generally, it is expected that improvements in functional ability produce positive psychological factors. Addressing psychological factors specifically, Bradley,[30] in a study measuring the effects of participation in an FES program on the affect of 37 individuals with SCI, demonstrated that positive affect was not altered significantly. There were, however, significant changes in negative affect, with particular items of hostility and depression evident in those individuals in the treatment group who had unrealistic expectations. The author noted that these individuals need to be identified and monitored through the course of rehabilitation. Other drawbacks relate to the expense of the equipment and personnel and the lack of long-term efficacy studies. The speed with which a client with a complete SCI is able to walk with electrically stimulated systems remains relatively slow (2 to 54 m/min) compared with normal rates of 78 to 90 m/min (1.3 to 1.5 m/sec).[121, 122] Many of the published reports do not provide information on the maximal distance clients are able to walk with these systems, but reported distances range from 100 to 400 m.

The use of electrically stimulated reciprocal thigh movements in conjunction with a reciprocating gait orthosis (RGO) appears to be helpful in reducing the energy expenditure to ambulate (as compared with other orthotic interventions such as long leg braces or the RGO alone).[83] However, in another study, comparison of energy expenditure between ambulation with the RGO alone and the RGO with stimulation of the thigh muscles produced no significant improvement in the measured parameters after 5 minutes of walking.[171] Independent home use of the RGO with and without electrical stimulation also appears to be low, although measurement of utilization met with

some difficulty.[172] Stallard and Major,[169] in a comparison of different reciprocal ambulation systems, reported significant energy cost reductions with increased stiffness in the lateral or abduction component of the device. Yang and colleagues[197] measured improvements in walking speed and step length, and a reduced energy cost occurred with improvements in the hip flexion-extension ratio. With only potential energy savings and low rate of utilization at home, the use of such a system at the current time is primarily for exercise as opposed to functional ambulation. Improvements in device design and support may assist with further reductions in energy consumption and increased use.

Some clients may perceive the technology of electrically stimulated standing, cycling, or walking as moving them toward a cure for their paralysis. With a complete injury, however, the stimulation occurs passively, without expectation that voluntary control will return.[30] In cases of incomplete injury, electrically stimulated ambulation may assist the client in using and bolstering active control, so that movement without the stimulation is more feasible. In considering use of electrically stimulated cycling or ambulation, discussion of the goals of treatment and the costs of the procedure must be discussed openly with the client to allow an educated choice to be made about the use of this expensive technology.

Brain Injury

NMES may be a useful tool with clients having sustained brain injury, with potential benefits of managing contractures by increasing ROM, facilitation of active control, and reduction of spasticity by strengthening the antagonist to a spastic muscle.[6] In cases where an understanding of the purpose and principles of NMES is not feasible for the client, the comfort of the stimulation may be critical in ensuring its continued use. Comfort may be enhanced with increasing the ramp on-time and selection of waveforms that allow stimulation at lower amplitudes yet obtain the desired muscle contraction.[198] Use of NMES with a client in Rancho level IV and below is not appropriate, as the client may not be able to understand the purpose or meaning of the stimulus, and thereby perceive the stimulus as noxious.[198] The therapist may find greater success with use of NMES in functional activities if stimulation can be triggered by a heel switch or hand switch so that the stimulation coincides appropriately with the goal of therapy.

EMGBF applications for clients with brain injury can be similar to those used with stroke, given similar motor presentations.[104] Therapists must consider residual cognitive deficits following brain injury in determining the appropriateness of EMGBF. (See also Chapter 13.)

Guillain-Barré Syndrome

EMGBF in clients with Guillain-Barré syndrome demonstrated improvements in muscle strength in upper and lower extremities,[41, 89] although inconsistent improvement in functional use of the upper extremities was noted.[89] Treatment regimens consisted of EMGBF for 10 trials per muscle, conducted in 45-minute treatment sessions twice a week, in one case for 78 weeks and in the other case for 46 weeks.[89] (See also Chapter 13.)

Pediatric Applications

Interest in the application of NMES interventions for neurological diagnoses in children appears to be growing. In 1997, the Section on Pediatrics of the American Physical Therapy Association published a special issue of its journal, addressing this subject (vol. 9, no. 3). Research articles and case studies address general physiology, cerebral palsy, and SCI. These articles and their citations show the positive impact electrical stimulation can have on these populations. The issue is recommended for anyone considering use of electrical devices with children or adolescents.

Special considerations for this population need to be made when addressing the use of electricity. While contraindications and precautions are the same as for adults, acceptance and tolerance of these devices are not. Fear and apprehension of electricity, for both child and parent, must be addressed. The clinician must take extra care in explanation and demonstration, perhaps on themselves and possibly the parent, before placing the device on the child. Allowing the child as much control as possible in device operation may assist with acceptance. Of course the attention span of the child must also be addressed.

CEREBRAL PALSY

The use of NMES with children with cerebral palsy has been addressed to some degree, with several case study reports.[34, 35, 55] Carmick[34, 35] described a variety of applications with children at 1.6, 6.7, and 10 years of age, integrating NMES into a treatment regimen that focused on a "task-oriented model of motor learning." Improvements were noted in upper and lower extremity movement and functional use across a variety of tasks appropriate to the age and movement dysfunction each child demonstrated.

Advancements in technology allow for use of EMGBF in increasing contexts, such as the computer-assisted feedback (CAF) system, which can be used to provide feedback about muscle activity during ambulation.[42] Pilot data examining use of this system to provide feedback about the level of triceps surae activity during gait of children with cerebral palsy suggest potential improvements in gait symmetry, velocity, and appropriate muscle activation patterns as a result of this intervention. Use of this modality as an adjunct to physical therapy may prove beneficial.

SPINA BIFIDA

Five subjects with spina bifida (aged 5 to 21 years) were treated with daily NMES over an 8-week period to strengthen the quadriceps femoris muscles. Increases in maximum quadriceps torque production were observed in two of the five subjects in the treated limb. Improvements in functional activity speeds were noted for all of the subjects. Lack of improvement in torque production by three subjects was speculated to be related to lack of adherence to the exercise regimen and the heterogeneity of the subject sample.[93] Further investigation of this modality with spina bifida is indicated.

Threshold or Therapeutic Electrical Stimulation

In 1988, a different application of electrical stimulation was introduced: threshold or therapeutic electrical stimulation. Expected improvements include increases in muscle mass as well as functional improvements in the treated areas. The original article[134] described its use on children with cerebral palsy, but use has expanded to include spina bifida, brachial plexus injuries, and SCI among others. The technique utilizes long-term sensory level stimulation on the target muscle(s) during night and daytime protocols. The suspected mechanisms include increased nighttime blood flow and trophic hormonal secretion.[134] Beck[15] described the protocols and parameters in a case study. Currently, other information and publications can be found at a website devoted to this application: www.maya-tek.com

Contraindications and Precautions

Any electrical stimulation application is contraindicated for clients who have epilepsy or demand-type cardiac pacemakers. In addition, there are contraindications to applications over the transthoracic area or the uterus in pregnancy, as well as in the area of cancer and the carotid sinus. Other factors require precaution, but are not strict contraindications, such as sensory deficits, skin problems (sensitivity to stimulation, electrodes, gel; edema; open wounds), tolerance of stimulation intensity sufficient to elicit muscle contraction, client's capability to participate in the training process, and financial considerations.[44, 53, 66, 129]

Matthews and colleagues[111] reported changes in blood pressure and heart rate suggestive of autonomic dysreflexia when electrical stimulation was applied in seven subjects with SCI above the T6 level. FES to the quadriceps produced the noted changes as stimulation intensity was increased. The mechanism for this reaction is unclear. It would be wise for clinicians to monitor vital signs in clients with SCI (and possibly all clients), at least during the initial application of electrical stimulation.

Use of stimulation modalities by clients outside of clinical therapy sessions requires a degree of cooperation and motivation to take care of the stimulation unit, use it as instructed, and observe precautions. Long-term use of NMES (e.g., FES) may not be feasible for clients who do not have the financial resources (insurance or otherwise) to rent or purchase a unit or do not have reasonable access to support for equipment maintenance.

EMGBF does not require as many precautions because the procedure only monitors muscle activity. Utilization of this form of feedback by the client requires a basic level of attention and cognitive skill to understand the meaning of, as well as act on, the feedback to effect a change in muscle performance. Client motivation and interest in use of this modality are also required, as the client must be able to develop sensitivity to the degree of muscle activation independently, so that feedback is no longer required. EMGBF may be used in some instances that do not require the cognitive skills of the client to utilize this information, for example, as an evaluative tool for the therapist to gather information about muscle activation patterns in order to plan intervention strategies.[194]

SUMMARY

The concepts, descriptions, and applications of electrodiagnosis presented in this chapter are intended to enrich the therapist's comprehension of these studies as applied to clients with neurological conditions. Integration of the results of these tests in differential diagnosis and in subsequent planning of intervention is invaluable.

Clearly, there are numerous possibilities for the use of NMES and EMGBF with clients of all ages who have sustained neurological insult or injury. There is preliminary support for improvement of movement control in some applications, although the paucity of well-controlled group research in populations other than stroke and adult SCI underscores the need for further investigation to support the efficacy of these modalities. As the therapy environment changes in response to time and funding constraints, therapists must carefully evaluate the benefits of a variety of available tools to assist their clients in regaining motor control and functional ability. An additional benefit of FES or EMGBF is the ability of the client to work autonomously (i.e., at home) after becoming familiar with the treatment regimen, with the therapist periodically updating a home program. This protocol allows therapy time to be used for direct intervention. NMES and EMGBF may efficiently assist in attaining improvement in control, and may also be used in the context of functional activities, but these tools alone will not effect functional changes. Trial use of EMGBF or NMES for 2 to 4 weeks (daily to three times a week) with careful outcome assessment may assist the therapist in judging treatment efficacy for each client.

CASE STUDIES

CASE 28-1   C8–T1 RADICULOPATHY

Subjective Examination. A 48-year-old man was involved in a rear end motor vehicle collision 6 months ago. He sustained a cervical strain/whiplash injury along with a contusion of the right medial elbow with no fracture. He had a brief bout (about 1 month) of headaches and cervical pain, which have resolved. For the past 3 months he has complained of weakness of his right hand, numbness, and pain and tingling in the medial three digits, resulting in difficulty with grasp and fine motor control and with typical ADL.

Objective Examination. *Posture:* Forward head; rounded shoulders, right greater than left.

ROM: Cervical flexion full, extension 50% with sharp central pain at end range, left rotation full, right rotation and left side-bending each decreased 25% with pain at upper trapezius, right side-bending full, but pain produced at C7–T1 and right scalenes on end range. Gross upper extremity ROM is without restrictions.

Strength (manual muscle test): Cervical and upper extremity isometric break tests are all 5/5 without pain.

Neurological: Reflexes C5–6 biceps and C7 triceps present and equal bilaterally, C7–8 wrist extension depressed on right; Sensory—light touch and sharp dull intact and equal bilaterally; diminished over medial forearm and medial three digits of right hand.

Special tests: Palpation. Tender to moderate palpation at right medial elbow, upper trapezius, scalenes, and C7–T1 facet areas. Thoracic outlet tests: Adson test, costoclavicular, and hyperabduction are negative. Tinel sign—ulnar nerve negative at wrist and elbow. Cervical axial compression in right side-bending, rotation, and extension is positive for pain locally at right C7–T1. Upper limb tension testing is positive to the right side.

Impression. Normal conduction in all nerves tested with exception of slow F wave latencies of right ulnar nerve. EMG abnormalities seen in muscles of right upper extremity innervated by C8–T1 spinal cord segment and right lower cervical paraspinals. No EMG abnormalities are seen in left upper extremity or left cervical paraspinals (see page 877).

Evaluation. Electrical test findings are consistent with a C8–T1 cervical radiculopathy on the right. Electrical changes do not indicate a peripheral plexopathy or a localized peripheral nerve lesion.

Prognosis. Guarded; improvement expected over 1 to 2 months with intervention, depending on response to intervention and results of further imaging.

Intervention. No electrical stimulation intervention is needed for functional or strengthening activities. Possible use of transcutaneous electrical nerve stimulation for pain control or high-volt pulsed current in the cervical and medial elbow area for inflammation or healing could be considered. Other interventions would include postural exercise, stretching, and mobilization techniques. Their effects on the symptoms would determine these activities and their progression.

Continued

CASE 28–1 C8–T1 RADICULOPATHY *Continued*

Electrophysiological Examination

Nerve Conduction	Distal Latency (ms)			Amplitude			Velocity (m/s)			F wave (ms)		
	Rt	Lt	Norm	Rt	Lt	Norm	Rt	Lt	Norm	Rt	Lt	Norm
Ulnar motor (above elbow–wrist)	2.8	2.6	<4.0	6	11	>5 mV				34	29	<32
							59	55	>45			
Ulnar sensory (digiti V–wrist)	2.8	3.1	<3.6	10	10	>6 μV	50	45	>38			
Median motor (elbow–wrist)	3.0		<4.2	15		>5 mV				30	30	>32
							50		>45			
Median sensory	3.2		<3.6	18		>10 μV	43		>38			

Electromyography	Spontaneous Activity	Motor Units	Recruitment
R abductor digiti minimi	Fibrillations, positive sharp waves	Increased polyphasic potentials	Reduced
R 1st dorsal interosseus	Fibrillations, positive sharp waves	Increased polyphasic potentials	Reduced
R flexor carpi ulnaris	Fibrillations, positive sharp waves	Increased polyphasic potentials	Reduced
R abductor pollicis brevis	Fibrillations, positive sharp waves	Increased polyphasic potentials	Reduced
R extensor carpi ulnaris	Fibrillations, positive sharp waves	Increased polyphasic potentials	Reduced
R flexor pollicis longus	Fibrillations, positive sharp waves	Increased polyphasic potentials	Reduced
R flexor carpi radialis	None	Normal	Slightly reduced
R extensor carpi radialis	None	Normal	Normal
R biceps	None	Normal	Normal
R cervical paraspinalis	Fibrillations, positive sharp waves in low cervical spine	Increased polyphasic potentials	Normal
L flexor carpi ulnaris	None	Normal	Normal
L abductor digiti minimi	None	Normal	Normal

CASE 28–2 PERIPHERAL NEUROPATHY

J.R. is a 36-year-old woman with an 8-year history of renal disease. She has been receiving dialysis for 14 months. Over the past 4 or 5 months she has developed increasing weakness and decreased feeling in both lower extremities. She reports she has been falling recently.

Examination. Bilateral lower extremity examination shows depressed deep tendon reflexes in quadriceps, hamstrings, dorsiflexors, and plantarflexors. Sensation of vibration and light touch is markedly decreased in a stocking pattern in legs beginning just below the knees. ROM is within functional limits. Muscle strength is 3+ in knee flexors and extensors, 1 to 2+ in muscles about the ankles. Toe muscle strength is 0 on the right and 1+ on the left. Sensation, range, and strength of upper extremities are WFL and without symptoms. The client walks with a wide-based, shuffling gait with little or no push-off bilaterally.

Impression. NCT shows increased motor and sensory latencies and slow velocities of both lower extremities with normal conduction in the upper extremities. EMG shows abnormalities of fibrillations, positive sharp waves, and increased polyphasic potentials in distal leg muscles bilaterally.

Evaluation. The pattern of clinical findings is suggestive of a peripheral polyneuropathy. Results of nerve conduction and EMG studies are consistent with incomplete axonal degeneration and confirm the clinical findings. EMG of upper extremities is normal. Review of medical management by the referring practitioner would be a key factor in treatment decisions for this client. Some of the pathological changes seen in peripheral neuropathies may be reversible or at least reduced with good compliance and clinical management.

Prognosis. Depending on stabilization of renal function, functional improvement would be expected in gait status, strength, and sensation in the short term after beginning intervention. The long-term prognosis is unknown, depending on stabilization of disease process.

Intervention. Ankle-foot orthoses (AFOs) for both lower extremities would enhance gait and also serve a protective function. The client's instructions should emphasize compliance with the medical plan and integumentary protective measures along with the exercise intervention.

Electrophysiological Examination

Nerve Conduction	Distal Latency (ms)			Amplitude			Velocity (m/s)			F Wave (ms)		
	Rt	Lt	Norm	Rt	Lt	Norm	Rt	Lt	Norm	Rt	Lt	Norm
Peroneal motor	No response	8.4	<5.5		1.2	>2 mV		27	>40	No response		>57
Tibial motor	7.8	7.2	<6	1.8	2.0	>2 mV	32	37	>40	68	66	<57
Sural	No response	5.9	<4.2	No response	3.0	>5 µV		24	>34			
Ulnar motor		3.1	<4.0		6.2	>5 mV		55	>45		26	<32
Median motor	3.5		<4.2	6.5		>5 mV	52		>45	27		<32
Ulnar sensory		2.7	<3.6		16	>6 µV		52	>38			
Median sensory	3		<3.6	19		>10 µV	47		>38			

Electromyography Rt and Lt	Spontaneous Activity	Motor Units	Recruitment
Tibialis anterior	3+ fibrillations and positive sharp waves	↑ Polyphasic potentials ↑ Duration	Markedly ↓
Peroneus longus	3+ fibrillations and positive sharp waves	↑ Duration	Markedly ↓
Gastrocnemius	3+ fibrillations and positive sharp waves	↑ Duration	Markedly ↓
Quadriceps	None	Normal	Normal
Hamstrings	None	Normal	Normal

EMGBF/NMES options for Case 28–2

Client problem	Goals	Modality parameters	Measures to determine efficacy	Considerations
Lack of ankle dorsiflexion.	Improve activation of intact motor units of the anterior tibialis to maximize dorsiflexion at heel-off and eccentric control at heel-strike for distances approximating those at home.	FES b.i.d. or t.i.d. for 10- to 15-minute sessions; sessions should be fatigue-controlled. Due to extreme weakness begin 10:50-second on-off time with slow on-off ramping; advance to more aggressive 10:30 to 10:20 ratios if improvement is seen. Surface EMGBF could be a first choice for volitional enhancement of intact motor units with fatigability the signal for end of session; involve the peroneals depending on need to balance eversion with dorsiflexion.	Monitor each session for ability to dorsiflex foot against gravity; depending on disease progression or regression may or may not advance to use of a heelswitch for gait control without AFO. Trial use 2 to 4 weeks, stopping if no improvement in status.	(1) Multiple daily sessions require rental of portable EMG or FES unit; cost of unit rental and supplies requires dual channel units for bilateral activity. (2) A high level client and family compliance is needed for success, requiring increased time to teach use of device; time may be recovered by use of units at home rather than during sessions. (3) Frequent use requires close monitoring of skin integrity secondary to reactions from stimulation or electrodes. (4) Electrode location for stimulation requires placement over area of compromised sensation; stimulation may require higher levels of intensity than usual; determine general levels of stimulation over nearest intact sensory area. (5) Partial denervation may produce areas of no reaction to FES; it may be necessary to increase pulse duration, decrease frequency to 20 to 25 pps, and increase intensity to higher levels. (6) Intense levels of contraction in a denervated muscle may be detrimental to reinnervation process if present.
Lack of ankle plantarflexion.	Increase control of gastroc/soleus for increased postural control as well as propulsion for short standing/gait time and distance.	EMGBF for enhanced activity during standing/stance especially for soleus, utilize increasing thresholds during activity as improvements in contractility are noted, 2- to 5-minute sessions involving body sway/perturbations to activate postural control, FES parameters as with dorsiflexion.	Monitor standing balance for time and control, strength/endurance by level and number of contractions of plantarflexors.	Same as with dorsiflexion.
Weakness of quadriceps/hamstrings.	Maximize strength/endurance of musculature for improved ambulation for distances approximating home.	Use of FES or EMG is potentially unnecessary due to strength level present; standard therapeutic exercise should be sufficient if situation stabilizes.	Standard muscle testing, monitor gait parameters.	Decrease of strength/endurance may require further electrodiagnostic testing and consideration of electrotherapeutic programs.

CASE 28–3   LEFT MIDDLE CEREBRAL ARTERY CVA

A 68-year-old woman is referred 3 weeks status post left middle cerebral artery CVA with residual right hemiparesis affecting the upper extremity to a greater degree than the lower extremity.

Examination. The client's left extremities appear well controlled with at least functional strength. She exhibits a two-finger breadth right shoulder subluxation, with pain at the extremes of shoulder flexion (150 degrees), abduction (135 degrees), and external rotation (30 degrees), and hypertonicity in a stereotypical flexor pattern affecting the shoulder horizontal adductors and internal rotators and elbow, wrist, and finger flexors. She is beginning to develop upper extremity movement with the ability to shrug her shoulder, abduct, and flex through partial range (with elbow flexed), full-range elbow flexion, partial-range elbow extension against gravity, and no wrist or finger extension. Right lower extremity ROM is within normal limits, although control is limited at the ankle (dorsiflexion only with hip and knee flexion, no eversion actively) and knee control is decreased (reduced eccentric quadriceps control, difficulty isolating knee flexion with hip extension). Ambulation is accomplished with the use of a quad cane and an articulating AFO on the right for limited distances with standby assistance. The complete absence of right wrist and finger extension raises the question of secondary radial nerve pathology. Nerve conduction and EMG studies are indicated to help differentiate this problem. This client lives at home with her husband, who is very supportive of her rehabilitation. Both of them are retired, but they have an active calendar of participation in volunteer and leisure activities. Insurance coverage is good.

Impression. Nerve conduction values are approaching the outer limits of normal but are within normal limits for the considered client's age. EMG shows no electrical evidence for peripheral denervation. A few single normal motor units were seen in wrist and finger extensors.

Evaluation. The nerve conduction values are not unusual for clients over 65 years of age. The normal nerve conduction is compatible with a CNS disorder. On EMG, spontaneous activity is rarely seen with upper motor neuron lesions, and if motor units are found, they generally have normal characteristics. Therefore, the EMG findings are also consistent with a CNS rather than a PNS disorder.

The fact that radial nerve degeneration has been ruled out and the encouraging presence of some single motor unit potentials on EMG are important objective findings that should guide the therapist in management of this client.

Prognosis. Independent or isolated motor function is promising for continued improvement in the condition of the client. The fact that there appears to be no peripheral nerve involvement and motor units were found in the wrist and finger extensors would support return of function as expected with this type of CVA. Lower extremity impairments are expected to be minimized as the return of motor control progresses. Quad cane use should continue until isolated hip and knee action improves. A need for AFO is expected for an indefinite time period.

Intervention. Interventions including utilization of EMG or NMES would assist in accelerating improvement in functional control.

Electrophysiologic Examination

Nerve Conduction	Distal Latency (ms)			Amplitude			Velocity (m/s)		
	Rt	Lt	Norm	Rt	Lt	Norm	Rt	Lt	Norm
Radial motor	3.4	3.3	<3.5	3.5	3.2	>2.5 mV	47	47	>45
Radial sensory	3.2	3.3	<3.5	8.0	8.0	>10 μV	44	42	>40
Ulnar motor	3.7	3.8	<4.0	5.5	5.2	>5 mV	49	48	>45
Ulnar sensory	3.4	3.4	<3.6	7.0	7.5	>6 μV	40	41	>38

Electromyography	Spontaneous Activity	Motor Units	Recruitment
R extensor digitorum	None	↓ Amplitude, normal duration and phase	Single units
R extensor carpi radialis	None	↓ Amplitude, normal duration and phase	Single units
R extensor pollicis brevis	None	↓ Amplitude, normal duration and phase	Single units
R extensor indicis	None	↓ Amplitude, normal duration and phase	Single units
R triceps	None	Normal	Moderately reduced, irregular pattern

EMGBF/NMES options for Case 28–3

Client problem	Goals	Modality parameters	Measures to determine efficacy	Considerations
Shoulder subluxation.	Decrease subluxation to 1 finger width, with pain manageable within patient's daily routine.	Portable FES for home use, begin with 10:30 second on/off ratio for 15-minute periods t.i.d., amplitude to generate mm contraction without shoulder elevation. Increase on time and treatment time as tolerated so that reduction is maintained majority of day.	Trial use x 1 month. Measure amount of palpable subluxation, pain-free ROM; if improvement is not observed, discontinue FES, with instruction to maintain shoulder flexibility, consider lapboard or arm tray when sitting, support when standing.	(1) Requires rental of portable FES unit; patient/family compliance is needed for success in home program. (2) Cost of rental of FES and supplies. (3) Frequent use for reduction of subluxation requires close monitoring of skin for possible reactions to stimulation, gel, or electrodes. (4) Integrate scapular movement and stabilization exercises into program.
Lack of active ankle dorsiflexion.	Increase active control of ankle dorsiflexion with knee extended, allowing heel-strike without AFO for short-distance ambulation.	FES, b.i.d. for 15-minute duration; 10:20 second on-off ratio with slow ramping on-off; as active movement improves, consider EMGBF to further focus attention on balanced dorsiflexion (with eversion). Use of heelswitch requires decreased ramp time to minimum patient can tolerate. Switch should activate at heel-off to control dorsiflexion through the swing phase.	Monitor each session for increased active dorsiflexion in sitting, standing, and ambulation. Integrate use of heelswitch during ambulation without AFO. Trial use over 2 to 3 weeks. Discontinue if not seeing increase in voluntary control-compensate with AFO.	(1) If client rents unit for shoulder subluxation, may also use stimulator at home instead of requiring time during therapy session. (2) Similar cost, convenience issues as above. (3) Additional education necessary if stimulator settings are to be switched for dorsiflexion and shoulder subluxation interventions.
Lack of full active wrist and finger extension.	Control of active wrist and finger extension to allow release in gross grasp.	NMES and/or EMGBF b.i.d. for 10-minute sessions initially, with gradual increase in duration up to 20 minutes if fatigue does not alter the quality of the contractions. Other parameters as described for ankle dorsiflexion.	Active movement in finger extensors with wrist in neutral position. Functional ability to release grasp of objects of varying shapes and sizes. Trial period of 2 to 3 weeks; discontinue if voluntary motion is not changing significantly.	May utilize portable stimulator as described for ankle or shoulder interventions, with similar considerations.
Muscle imbalance, lack of right upper extremity functional movement.	Decrease hypertonicity in flexor muscle groups; increase extensor control for gross arm movements (i.e., positioning).	EMGBF to decrease flexor muscle activity (resting and with passive movement) and increase extensor activity. May utilize methodology described by DeBacher.[50]	Speed and control with reciprocal elbow motions, especially with extension. Use of this motion for functional activity (positioning the arm, reaching activity, etc.).	Focus on increased extensor control may prove more effective than simply decreasing flexor hyperactivity.

CASE 28–4   CEREBRAL PALSY

Examination. A 9-year-old boy was referred with upper extremity impairment secondary to a diagnosis of cerebral palsy. He has received physical therapy intervention for several years that brought him, currently, to a high level of activity with the exception of utilization of the forearm and hand. He has had no improvement in use of the wrist and hand for some time. As there was no improvement, his primary therapist discharged him to a home program. The client is involved in increasing levels of athletic activity, and he and his parents would like to explore the use of electrical stimulation as an avenue for improved use of the extremity. His goal is to use the hand in activities such as basketball.

Objective. Independent function of the wrist, hand, and finger musculature; however, it is poorly coordinated. Grasp activities allow for closure of the fingers, but without the needed wrist co-contraction and positioning. When the wrist was placed in the proper position he was able to maintain the needed wrist extension with a measured grip strength of 20 lb, 50% of the opposite side. The wrist flexors are the primary movers, which leaves the hand and wrist in a flexed position the majority of the time. Increased intensity of requested action increases the pattern of wrist flexion.

Impression. Function at 3-month follow-up shows continuation of independent function of muscles. Challenge of grip and grasp of the wrist and hand automatically brought the limb into the proper position.

Evaluation. At initial examination the client's ability to utilize the upper extremity in functional tasks was poor to nil as evidenced by the need for the therapist to position the part for proper use. The lower levels of individual muscle force and grip corroborated this. Follow-up visit showed improvements in strength and functional ability, but there was no change in girth.

Prognosis. Initial: The client is an intelligent, active, and motivated individual. He is able to understand and comprehend the use of the device. He is also able to control his impulse to play with the device. The prognosis is unknown, as there has been no recent improvement with other therapy interventions. It is also unknown if he or his family are motivated enough to stay with the long-term requirements of the intervention. It is expected that a consistent intervention should produce change within 2 to 3 months.

Follow-up. Continued improvement of functional ability and strength is expected. The client and family have shown themselves to be diligent in application of the intervention, missing only a few of the requested daily sessions. Maximum level of improvement is unknown as is carryover after cessation of the intervention. It is expected that the program will continue for at least 6 months total. If improvement continues, the recommendation is for purchase of the unit, with continued utilization over the next 1 to 2 years.

Intervention (Daily). *Daytime exercise:* Two-channel, neuromuscular stimulator with a symmetrical biphasic waveform. Channel 1 electrodes are placed on the motor points of the wrist extensors; channel 2 electrodes are placed to contract the finger flexors without activating wrist flexion. Electrode size was adjusted to achieve the desired results from the musculature. Timers were set so that channel 1 activated for wrist extension, followed approximately 2 to 3 seconds later by channel 2. Both channels shut off at the same time. The on-off ratio was at 10:30 seconds. The rate was 35 pps. The level of stimulation was at the maximum contraction tolerated. The client was asked to contract the muscles along with the stimulator and squeeze a small ball. Total time was 30 minutes for the exercise.

Nighttime. As an adjunct, a nighttime program was added. The electrode setup was the same as the day program. Timers were adjusted to on-off of 15:15 seconds and intensity was at the light sensory level only. The rate remained at 35 pps. There was no contraction of the muscle. The client wore the unit throughout the night.

● Measurements

Manual Muscle Test	Initial	3-month Follow-up
Elbow flexion/extension	4+/4+	5−/5−
Wrist flexion/extension	3+/3+	4/4
Thumb/finger	3+ all	3+ all
Girth (3 in. distal to lateral epicondyle)	6¾ in.	6¾ in.
Grip (dynamometer position 2)	20 lbs	26 lbs

ACKNOWLEDGMENT

The authors wish to acknowledge the contribution of Karen L. McCulloch to the writing of this chapter in the previous edition.

REFERENCES

1. Alon G: Principles of electrical stimulation. *In* Nelson RM, Currier DP (eds): Clinical Electrotherapy, 3rd ed. Stamford, CT, Appleton & Lange, 1991.
2. Aminoff MJ: Electrodiagnosis in Clinical Neurology, 4th ed. New York, Churchill Livingstone, 1999.
3. Axelgaard J, Brown JC: Lateral electrical surface stimulation for the treatment of progressive idiopathic scoliosis. Spine 8:242–260, 1983.
4. Bajd T, et al: Use of functional electrical stimulation in the lower extremities of incomplete spinal cord injured patients, Artif Organs 23:403–409, 1999.
5. Baker LL, Parker K: Neuromuscular electrical stimulation of the muscles surrounding the shoulder. Phys Ther 66:1930–1937, 1986.
6. Baker LL, et al: D: Neuromuscular electrical stimulation for the head-injured patient. Phys Ther 63:1967–1974, 1983.
7. Baker LL, et al: Effects of waveform on comfort during neuromuscular electrical stimulation. Clin Orthop 233:75–85, 1988.
8. Baker LL, et al: Neuromuscular Electrical Stimulation: A Practical Guide, 2nd ed. Downey, CA, Los Amigos Research and Education Institute, 1993.
9. Baldi JC, et al: Muscle atrophy is prevented in patients with acute spinal cord injury using functional electrical stimulation. Spinal Cord 36:463–469, 1998.
10. Basmajian JV: Biofeedback Principles and Practice for Clinicians, 3rd ed. Baltimore, Williams & Wilkins, 1989.
11. Basmajian JV, Blumenstein R: Electrode placement in electromyographic biofeedback. *In* Basmajian JV (ed): Biofeedback Principles and Practice for Clinicians, 3rd ed. Baltimore, Williams & Wilkins, 1989.
12. Basmajian JV, et al: Biofeedback treatment of foot-drop after stroke compared with standard rehabilitation technique: Effects on voluntary control and strength. Arch Phys Med Rehabil 56:231–236, 1975.
13. Basmajian JV, et al: EMG feedback treatment of upper limb in hemiplegic stroke patients: A pilot study. Arch Phys Med Rehabil 63:613–616, 1982.
14. Bate PJ, Matyas TA: Negative transfer of training following brief practice of elbow tracking movements with electromyographic feedback from spastic antagonists. Arch Phys Med Rehabil 73:1050–1058, 1992.
15. Beck S: Use of sensory level electrical stimulation in the physical therapy management of a child with cerebral palsy. Pediatr Phys Ther 9:137–138, 1997.
16. Bergmans J, Senden R: Electrical stimulation of denervated muscle. *In* Gorio A, et al (eds): Posttraumatic Peripheral Nerve Regeneration: Experimental Basis and Clinical Implications. New York, Raven Press, 1981.
17. Betz R, et al: Effects of functional electrical stimulation on the joints of adolescents with spinal cord injury. Paraplegia 34:127–136, 1996.
18. Bijak M, et al: Personal computer supported eight channel surface stimulator for paraplegic walking: First results. Artif Organs 23:424–427, 1999.
19. Binder MD, Mendell LM: The Segmental Motor System. London, Oxford University Press, 1990.
20. Binder-Macleod SA, McDermond LR: Changes in the force-frequency relationship in the human quadriceps muscle following electrically and voluntarily induced fatigue. Phys Ther 72:95–104, 1992.
21. Binder-Macleod SA, Russ DW: Effects of activation frequency and force on low-frequency fatigue in human skeletal muscle. J Appl Physiol 86:1337–1346, 1999.
22. Binder-Macleod SA, Snyder-Mackler L: Muscle fatigue: Clinical implications for fatigue assessment and neuromuscular electrical stimulation. Phys Ther 73:902–910, 1993.
23. Bobath B: Adult Hemiplegia: Evaluation and Treatment, 3rd ed. Oxford, Heinemann, 1990.
24. Bogataj U, et al: Restoration of gait during two to three weeks of therapy with multichannel electrical stimulation. Phys Ther 69:319–327, 1989.
25. Bogataj U, et al: The rehabilitation of gait in patients with hemiplegia: A comparison between conventional therapy and multichannel functional electrical stimulation therapy. Phys Ther 75:490–502, 1995.
26. Bowden REM, Gutmann E: Denervation and re-innervation of human voluntary muscle. Brain 67:273–309, 1944.
27. Bowman BR, Baker LL: Effects of waveform parameters on comfort during transcutaneous neuromuscular electrical stimulation. Ann Biomed Eng 13:59–74, 1985.
28. Bowman BR, et al: Positional feedback and electrical stimulation: An automated treatment for the hemiplegic wrist. Arch Phys Med Rehabil 60:497–502, 1979.
29. Braddom RL, Johnson EW: Standardization of H reflex and diagnostic use in S1 radiculopathy. Arch Phys Med Rehabil 55:161–166, 1974.
30. Bradley MB: The effect of participating in a functional electrical stimulation program on affect in people with spinal cord injuries. Arch Phys Med Rehabil 75:676–679, 1994.
31. Burnside IG, et al: Electromyographic feedback in the remobilization of stroke patients: A controlled trial. Arch Phys Med Rehabil 63:217–222, 1982.
32. Burridge J, et al: Experience of clinical use of the Odstock dropped foot stimulator. Artif Organs 21:254–60, 1997.
33. Burridge J, et al: The effects of common peroneal stimulation on the effort and speed of walking: A randomized controlled trial with chronic hemiplegic patients, Clin Rehabil 11:201–210, 1997.
34. Carmick J: Clinical use of neuromuscular electrical stimulation for children with cerebral palsy, pt 1: Lower extremity. Phys Ther 73:505–513, 1993.
35. Carmick J: Clinical use of neuromuscular electrical stimulation for children with cerebral palsy, pt 2: Upper extremity. Phys Ther 73:514–527, 1993.
36. Chae J, et al: Neuromuscular stimulation for upper extremity motor and functional recovery in acute hemiplegia. Stroke 29:975–979, 1998.
37. Chantraine A, et al: Shoulder pain and dysfunction in hemiplegia: Effects of functional electrical stimulation. Arch Phys Med Rehabil 80:328–331, 1999.
38. Chatrian GE: American Electroencephalographic Society: Guidelines for clinical evoked potential studies. J Clin Neurophysiol 1:3–53, 1984.
39. Chiappa KH: Evoked Potentials in Clinical Medicine, 3rd ed. Philadelphia, JB Lippincott–Raven, 1997.
40. Chu-Andrews J, Johnson RJ: Electrodiagnosis: An Anatomical and Clinical Approach. Philadelphia, JB Lippincott, 1986.
41. Cohen BA, et al: Electromyographic biofeedback as a physical therapeutic adjunct in Guillain-Barré syndrome, Arch Phys Med Rehabil 58:582–584, 1977.
42. Colborne GR, et al: S: Feedback of triceps surae EMG in gait of children with cerebral palsy: A controlled study, Arch Phys Med Rehabil 75:40–45, 1994.
43. Cozean CD, et al: Biofeedback and functional electrical stimulation in stroke rehabilitation. Arch Phys Med Rehabil 69:401–405, 1988.
44. Cummings J: Electrical stimulation of healthy muscle and tissue repair. *In* Nelson RM, Currier DP (eds): Clinical Electrotherapy, 2nd ed 2. Norwalk, CT, Appleton & Lange, 1991.
45. Cummings JP: Electrical stimulation of denervated muscle. *In* Gersh MR (ed): Electrotherapy in Rehabilitation. Philadelphia, FA Davis, 1992.
46. Currier DP, et al: Guidelines for clinical electromyography. J Clin Electrophysiol 5:2–19, 1993.
47. Cybulski GR, et al: Lower extremity functional neuromuscular stimulation in cases of spinal cord injury. Neurosurgery 15:132–146, 1984.
48. Davis R, et al: Initial results of the nucleus FES-22–implanted system for limb movement in paraplegia. Stereotact Funct Neurosurg 6:192–197, 1994.
49. Davis SE, et al: Self-reported use of an implanted FES hand system by adolescents with tetraplegia. J Spinal Cord Med 21:220–226, 1998.
50. DeBacher G: Biofeedback in spasticity control. *In* Basmajian JV

(ed): Biofeedback Principles and Practice for Clinicians, 3rd ed. Baltimore, Williams & Wilkins, 1989.

51. Delitto A, Robinson AJ: Electrical stimulation of muscle: Techniques and applications. In Snyder-Mackler L, Robinson AJ (eds): Clinical Electrophysiology: Electrotherapy and Electrophysiologic Testing. Baltimore, Williams & Wilkins, 1989.

52. Delitto A, et al: Electrical stimulation of muscle. In Robinson AJ, Snyder Mackler L (eds): Clinical Electrophysiology, Electrotherapy and Electrophysiological Testing, 2nd ed. Baltimore, Williams & Wilkins, 1995.

53. DeVahl J: Neuromuscular electrical stimulation (NMES) in rehabilitation. In Gersh MR (ed): Electrotherapy in Rehabilitation. Philadelphia, FA Davis, 1992.

54. DeWeerdt W, Harrison MA: The efficacy of electromyographic feedback for stroke patients: A critical review of the main literature. Physiotherapy 72:108–118, 1986.

55. Dubowitz L, et al: Improvement of muscle performance by chronic electric stimulation in children with cerebral palsy. Lancet 1(8585):587–588, 1988.

56. Dumitru D: Electrodiagnostic Medicine. Philadelphia, Hanley & Belfus, 1995, p.177.

57. Eaton LM, Lambert EH: Electromyography and electrical stimulation of nerves in diseases of motor unit. Observations on myasthenic syndrome associated with malignant tumors. JAMA 163:1117–1124, 1957.

58. Eichron KF, et al: Maintenance, training, and functional use of denervated muscle. J Biomed Eng 6:205–211, 1984.

59. Electrotherapy Standards Committee of the Section on Clinical Electrophysiology: Electrotherapeutic Terminology in Physical Therapy. Alexandria, VA, American Physical Therapy Association, 1990.

60. Faghri PD, et al: Functional electrical stimulation leg cycle ergometer exercise: Training effects on cardiorespiratory responses of spinal cord injured subjects at rest and during submaximal exercise. Arch Phys Med Rehabil 73:1085–1093, 1992.

61. Faghri PD, et al: The effects of functional electrical stimulation on shoulder subluxation, arm function recovery, and shoulder pain in hemiplegic stroke patients. Arch Phys Med Rehabil 75:73–79, 1994.

62. Fields RW: Electromyographically triggered electric muscle stimulation for chronic hemiplegia. Arch Phys Med Rehabil 68:407–414, 1987.

63. Fischer, E: Physiology of skeletal muscle. In Licht S (ed): Electrodiagnosis and Electromyography, 3rd ed. New Haven, CT, Elizabeth Licht, 1971, p 80.

64. Francisco G, et al: Electromyogram-triggered neuromuscular stimulation for improving arm function of acute stroke survivors: A randomized pilot study. Arch Phys Med Rehabil 79:570–575, 1998.

65. Gardner ER, Baker LL: Functional electrical stimulation of paralytic muscle. In Currier DP, Nelson RM (eds): Dynamics of Human Biologic Tissues. Philadelphia, FA Davis, 1992.

66. Gersh MR (ed): Electrotherapy in Rehabilitation. Philadelphia, FA Davis, 1992.

67. Gilchrist JM, Sanders DB: Double-step repetitive stimulation in myasthenia gravis. Muscle Nerve 10:233–237, 1987.

68. Glanz M, et al: Functional electrostimulation in poststroke rehabilitation: A meta-analysis of the randomized controlled trials. Arch Phys Med Rehabil 77:549–553, 1996.

69. Gorman PH, Mortimer JT: The effect of stimulus parameters on the recruitment characteristics of direct nerve stimulation. IEEE Trans Biomed Eng 30:407–414, 1983.

70. Gowland C, et al: Agonist and antagonist activity during voluntary upper-limb movement in patients with stroke. Phys Ther 72:624–633, 1992.

71. Gracanin F, Trnkoczy A: Optimal stimulus parameters for minimum pain in the chronic stimulation of innervated muscle. Arch Phys Med Rehabil 56:243–249, 1975.

72. Granat MH, et al: Peroneal stimulator, evaluation for the correction of spastic foot drop in hemiplegia. Arch Phys Med Rehabil 77:19–24, 1996.

73. Grill JH, Peckham PH: Functional neuromuscular stimulation for combined control of elbow extension and hand grasp in C5 and C6 quadraplegics. IEEE Trans Rehabil Eng 6:190–199, 1998.

74. Grimby G, and others: Changes in histochemical profile of muscle after long-term electrical stimulation in patients with idiopathic scoliosis. Scand J Rehabil Med 17:191–196, 1985.

75. Gurney AB, et al: Detraining from total body exercise ergometry in individuals with spinal cord injury. Spinal Cord 36:782–789, 1998.

76. Halliday AM (ed): Evoked Potentials in Clinical Testing, 2nd ed. Edinburgh and New York, Churchill Livingstone, 1992.

77. Hammond MC, et al: Recruitment and termination of electromyographic activity in the hemiparetic forearm. Arch Phys Med Rehabil 69:106–110, 1988.

78. Hammond MC, et al: Co-contraction in the hemiparetic forearm: Quantitative EMG evaluation. Arch Phys Med Rehabil 69:348–351, 1988.

79. Handa Y, et al: Application of functional electrical stimulation to the paralyzed extremities. Neuro MedChir 38:784–788, 1988.

80. Harris R: Chronaxy. In Licht S (ed): Electrodiagnosis and Electromyography, 3rd ed. New Haven, CT, Elizabeth Licht, 1971.

81. Hart RL, et al: A comparison between control methods for implanted FES hand grasp. IEEE Trans Rehabil Eng 6:208–218, 1998.

82. Hesse S, et al: Restoration of gait by combined treadmill training and multi-channel electrical stimulation in non-ambulatory hemiparetic patients, Scand J Rehabil Med 27:199–204, 1995.

83. Hirokawa S, others: Energy consumption in paraplegic ambulation using the reciprocating gait orthosis and electric stimulation of the thigh muscles. Arch Phys Med Rehabil 71:687–694, 1990.

84. Hirokawa S, et al: Energy expenditure and fatiguability in paraplegic ambulation using reciprocating gait orthosis and electrical stimulation, Disabil Rehabil 18:115–122, 1996.

85. Hooker SP, et al: Physiologic responses to prolonged electrically stimulated leg-cycle exercise in the spinal cord injured. Arch Phys Med Rehabil 71:863–869, 1990.

86. Hooker SP, et al: Physiologic effects of electrical stimulation leg cycle exercise training in spinal cord injured persons. Arch Phys Med Rehabil 73:470–478, 1992.

87. Hooker SP, et al: Peak and submaximal physiologic responses following electrical stimulation leg cycle ergometer training. J Rehabil Res Dev 32:361–366, 1995.

88. Hurd WW, et al: Comparison of actual and simulated EMG biofeedback in the treatment of hemiplegic patients. Am J Phys Med 59:73–82, 1980.

89. Ince LP, Leon MS: Biofeedback treatment of upper extremity dysfunction in Guillain-Barré syndrome. Arch Phys Med Rehabil 67:30–33, 1986.

90. Inglis J, et al: Electromyographic biofeedback and physical therapy of the hemiplegic upper limb. Arch Phys Med Rehabil 65:755–759, 1984.

91. Johnson EW, Pease WS: Practical Electromyography, 3rd ed. Baltimore, Williams & Wilkins, 1997.

92. Kantor G, et al: The effects of selected stimulus waveforms on pulse and phase characteristics at sensory and motor thresholds. Phys Ther 74:951–962, 1994.

93. Karmel-Ross K, et al: The effect of electrical stimulation on quadriceps femoris muscle torque in children with spina bifida. Phys Ther 72:723–730, 1992.

94. Keith MW, et al: Functional neuromuscular stimulation neuroprostheses for the tetraplegic hand. Clin Orthop 223:25–33, 1988.

95. Kilgore KL, et al: An implanted upper-extremity neuroprosthesis. Follow-up of five patients. J Bone Joint Surg Am 79:533–541, 1997.

96. Kimura J: Electrodiagnosis in Diseases of Nerve and Muscle: Principles and Practice, 2nd ed. Philadelphia, FA Davis, 1989.

97. Klose KJ, et al: Rehabilitation therapy for patients with long-term spinal cord injuries. Arch Phys Med Rehabil 71:659–662, 1990.

98. Kobetic R, et al: Muscle selection and walking performance of multichannel FES systems for ambulation in paraplegia. IEEE Trans Rehabil Eng 5:23–29, 1997.

99. Kohlmeyer KM, et al: Electrical stimulation and biofeedback effect on recovery of tenodesis grasp: A controlled study. Arch Phys Med Rehabil 77:702–706, 1996.

100. Konishi N, et al: Electrophysiologic evaluation of denervated muscles in incomplete paraplegia using macro-electromyography. Arch Phys Med Rehabil 79:1062–1068; 1998.

101. Kosmon AJ, et al: The influence of duration and frequency in electrical stimulation of muscles. Arch Phys Med 29:559–562, 1948.

102. Kraft GH, et al: Techniques to improve function of the arm and hand in chronic hemiplegia. Arch Phys Med Rehabil 73:220–227, 1992.

103. Landau WM, Hunt CC: Dorsal rhizotomy, a treatment of unproven efficacy. J Child Neurol 5:174–178, 1990.

104. Lazarus JC: Associated movement in hemiplegia: The effects of force exerted, limb usage and inhibitory training. Arch Phys Med Rehabil 73:1044–1049, 1992.

105. Lee SC, et al: Effects of length on the catchlike property of human quadriceps femoris muscle. Phys Ther 79:738–748, 1999.

106. Liberson WT, et al: Functional electrotherapy: Stimulation of the peroneal nerve synchronized with the swing phase of the gait of hemiplegic patients. Arch Phys Med Rehabil 42:101–105, 1961.

107. Lomo R, Slater CR: Control of acetylcholine sensitivity and synapse formation by muscle activity. J Physiol 275:391–402, 1978.

108. Malezic M, et al: Therapeutic effects of multisite electric stimulation of gait in motor-disabled patients. Arch Phys Med Rehabil 68:553–560, 1987.

109. Malezic M, et al: Restoration of standing, weight shift and gait by multi-channel electrical stimulation in hemiparetic patients. Int J Rehabil Res 17:169–179, 1994.

110. Mandel AR, et al: Electromyographic versus rhythmic positional biofeedback in computerized gait retraining with stroke patients. Arch Phys Med Rehabil 71:649–654, 1990.

111. Matthews JM, et al: The effects of surface anesthesia on the autonomic dysreflexia response during functional electrical stimulation. Spinal Cord 35:647–651, 1997.

112. McNeal DR, Baker LL: Effects of joint angle, electrodes and waveform on electrical stimulation of the quadriceps and hamstrings. Ann Biomed Eng 16:229, 1988.

113. Merletti R, et al: Electrophysiological orthosis for the upper extremity in hemiplegia: Feasibility study. Arch Phys Med Rehabil 56:507–513, 1975.

114. Merletti R, et al: A control study of muscle force recovery in hemiparetic patients during treatment with functional electric stimulation. Scand J Rehabil Med 10:147–154, 1978.

115. Moreland J, Thompson MA: Efficacy of electromyographic biofeedback compared with conventional physical therapy for upper-extremity function in patients following stroke: A research overview and meta-analysis. Phys Ther 74:534–543, 1994.

116. Morrison SA: Biofeedback to facilitate unassisted ventilation in individuals with high-level quadriplegia: A case report. Phys Ther 68:1378–1380, 1988.

117. Mourelas N, Granat MH: Evaluation of patterned stimulation for use in surface functional electrical stimulation systems. Med Eng Phys 20:319–324, 1998.

118. Moynahan M, et al: Home use of a functional electrical stimulation system for standing and mobility in adolescents with spinal cord injury. Arch Phys Med Rehabil 77:105–113, 1996.

119. Mulcahey MJ, et al: Implanted functional electrical stimulation hand system in adolescents with spinal injuries: An evaluation. Arch Phys Med Rehabil 78:597–607, 1997.

120. Mulder T, Hulstyn W: Sensory feedback therapy and theoretical knowledge of motor control and learning. Am J Phys Med 63:226–243, 1984.

121. Murray MP: Gait as a total pattern of movement. Am J Phys Med 46:290–329, 1967.

122. Murray MP, et al: Walking patterns of normal women. Arch Phys Med Rehabil 51:637–650, 1970.

123. Mutton DL, et al: Physiologic responses during functional electrical stimulation leg cycling and hybrid exercise in spinal cord injured subjects. Arch Phys Med Rehabil 78:712–718, 1997.

124. Myklebust BM, Kloth L: Electrodiagnostic and electrotherapeutic instrumentation: Characteristics of recording and stimulation systems and the principles of safety. In Gersh MR (ed): Electrotherapy in Rehabilitation. Philadelphia, FA Davis, 1992.

125. Nacht MB, et al: Use of electromyographic feedback during the acute phase of spinal cord injury: A case report. Phys Ther 62:290–294, 1982.

126. National Institute for Occupational Safety and Health, Division of Safety Research: Performing Motor and Sensory Neuronal Conduction Studies in Adult Humans (No. 90–113). Washington, DC, US Department of Health and Human Services, Public Health Service, Centers for Disease Control and Prevention, 1990.

127. Neilson PD, McCaughey J: Self-regulation of spasm and spasticity in cerebral palsy. J Neurol Neurosurg Psychiatry 45:320–330, 1982.

128. Nelson C: Electrical evaluation of nerve and muscle. In Gersh MR (ed): Electrotherapy in Rehabilitation. Philadelphia, FA Davis, 1992.

129. Nelson RM, Hayes RW, Currier DP (eds): Clinical Electrotherapy, 3rd ed. Stamford, CT, Appleton & Lange, 1999.

130. Oh SJ: Clinical Electromyography: Nerve Conduction Studies, 2nd ed. Baltimore, Williams & Wilkins, 1993.

131. Ozdemir C, Young RR: The results to be expected from electrical testing in the diagnosis of myasthenia gravis. Ann N Y Acad Sci 274:203–235, 1976.

132. Packman-Braun R: Relationship between functional electrical stimulation duty cycle and fatigue in wrist extensor muscles of patients with hemiparesis. Phys Ther 68:51–56, 1988.

133. Packman-Braun R: Electrotherapeutic applications for the neurologically impaired patient. In Gersh MR (ed): Electrotherapy in Rehabilitation. Philadelphia, FA Davis, 1992.

134. Pape KE: Therapeutic electrical stimulation (TES) for the treatment of disuse muscle atrophy in cerebral palsy, Pediatr Phys Ther 9:110–112, 1997.

135. Pape KE, et al: Threshold electrical stimulation in the rehabilitation of children with cerebral palsy. Pediatr Res 23:656A, 1988.

136. Peckham PH, et al: Restoration of key grip and release in the C6 tetraplegic patient through functional electrical stimulation. J Hand Surg [Am] 5:462–469, 1980.

137. Peckham PH, et al: Restoration of functional control by electrical stimulation in the upper extremity of the quadriplegic patient. J Bone Joint Surg Am 70:144–148, 1988.

138. Petrofsky JS, et al: Bicycle ergometer for paralyzed muscles. J Clin Eng 9:13–19, 1984.

139. Petrofsky JS, et al: Computer synchronized walking: An application of an orthosis and functional electrical stimulation. J Neurol Orthop Med Surg 6:219–230, 1985.

140. Phillips WT, et al: Effect of spinal cord injury on the heart and cardiovascular fitness. Curr Probl Cardiol 23:641–716, 1998.

141. Pinelli P, et al: In tibialis anterior reinnervation by collateral branching with or without electrotherapy. In Proceedings of the Fourth Congress of the International Society of Electrophysiology and Kinesiology Boston, 1979, pp 106–107.

142. Pockett S, Gavin RM: Acceleration of peripheral nerve regeneration after crush injury in rat. Neurosci Lett 59:221–224, 1985.

143. Prevo AJH, et al: Effect of EMG feedback on paretic muscles and abnormal co-contraction in the hemiplegic arm, compared with conventional therapy. Scand J Rehabil Med 14:121–131, 1982.

144. Prochazka A, et al: The bionic glove: An electrical stimulator garment that provides controlled grasp and hand opening in quadriplegia. Arch Phys Med Rehabil 78:608–614, 1997.

145. Ragnarsson KT: Physiologic effects of functional electrical stimulation-introduced exercises in spinal cord-injured individuals. Clin Orthop 233:53–63, 1988.

146. Ragnarsson KT, et al: Clinical evaluation of computerized electrical stimulation after spinal cord injury: A multicenter pilot study. Arch Phys Med Rehabil 69:672–677, 1988.

147. Rakos M, et al: Electromyogram-controlled functional electrical stimulation for the treatment of the paralyzed upper extremity. Artif Organs 23:466–469, 1999.

148. Rizzo M, et al: Magnetic resonance imaging data in the evaluation of effects of functional electrical stimulation on knee joints of adolescents with spinal cord injury. J Spinal Cord Med 21:124–130, 1998.

149. Robinson AJ, Snyder Mackler L (ed): Clinical Electrophysiology, Electrotherapy and Electrophysiological Testing, 2nd ed 2. Baltimore, Williams & Wilkins, 1995.

150. Robinson K, Rudge P: Centrally generated auditory potentials. In Halliday AM (ed): Evoked Potentials in Clinical Testing. London, Churchill Livingstone, 1982.

151. Rosselle N, et al: Electromyographic evaluation of therapeutic methods in complete peripheral paralysis. Electromyogr Clin Neurophysiol 17:179–186, 1977.

152. Russ DW, Binder-Macleod SA: Variable-frequency trains offset low frequency fatigue in human skeletal muscle. Muscle Nerve 22:874–882, 1999.

153. Sabbahi MA, Khalil M: Segmental H-reflex studies in upper and lower limbs of healthy subjects. Arch Phys Med Rehabil 71:216–222, 1990.

154. Sahrman SA, Norton BJ: Relationship of voluntary movement to spasticity in upper motor neuron syndrome. Ann Neurol 2:460–465, 1977.

155. Santee JL, et al: Incentives to enhance the effects of electromyo-

graphic feedback training in stroke patients. Biofeedback Self Regul 5:51–56, 1980.

156. Saxena S, et al: An EMG-controlled grasping system for tetraplegics. J Rehabil Res Dev 32:17–24, 1995.

157. Schleenbaker RE, Mainous AG: Electromyographic biofeedback for neuromuscular reeducation in the hemiplegic stroke patient: A meta-analysis. Arch Phys Med Rehabil 74:1301–1304, 1993.

158. Schmidt RA: Feedback and knowledge of results. In Schmidt RA (ed): Motor Control and Learning, 2nd ed. Champaign, IL, Human Kinetics, 1988.

159. Scott TR, et al: Tri-state myoelectric control of bilateral upper extremity neuroprostheses for tetraplegic individuals. IEEE Trans Rehabil Eng 4:251–263, 1996.

160. Seddon HJ: Three types of nerve injury. Brain 66:237–288, 1943.

161. Shiller HH, Stålberg E: F responses studied with single fibre EMG in normal subjects and spastic patients. J Neurol Neurosurg Psychiatry 41:45–53, 1978.

162. Sipski ML, et al: Functional electrical stimulation bicycle ergometry: Patient perceptions. Am J Phys Med Rehabil 68:147–149, 1989.

163. Smith BT, et al: Development of an upper extremity FES system for individuals with C4 tetraplegia. IEEE Trans Rehabil Eng 4:264–270, 1996.

164. Spielholz NI: Electrical stimulation of denervated muscle. In Nelson RM, Hayes KW, Currier DP (eds): Clinical Electrotherapy, 3rd ed. Stamford, CT, Appleton & Lange, 1999.

165. Stålberg E: AAEE minimonograph #20, macro EMG. Muscle Nerve 6:619–630, 1983.

166. Stålberg E, Trontelj J: Single Fibre Electromyography. Old Woking, Surry, UK, Miraville Press, 1979.

167. Stålberg E, and others: Automatic analysis of the EMG interference pattern. Electroencephalogr Clin Neurophysiol 56:672–681, 1983.

168. Stålberg E, et al: Multi-MUP EMG analysis—a two year experience in daily clinical work. Electroencephalogr Clin Neurophysiol 97:145–154, 1995.

169. Stallard J, Major RE: The influence of orthosis stiffness on paraplegic ambulation and its implications for functional electrical stimulation (FES) walking systems. Prosthet Orthot Int 19:108–114, 1995.

170. Sunderland S: Nerves and Nerve Injuries, 2nd ed Edinburgh, Churchill Livingstone, 1978.

171. Sykes L, et al: Energy expenditure of walking for adult patients with spinal cord lesions using the reciprocating gait orthosis and functional electrical stimulation. Spinal Cord 34:659–665, 1996.

172. Sykes L, et al: Objective measurement of use of the reciprocating gait orthosis (RGO) and the electrically augmented RGO in adult patients with spinal lesions. Prosthet Orth Int 20:182–190, 1996.

173. Takebe K, et al: Peroneal nerve stimulator in rehabilitation of hemiplegic patients. Arch Phys Med Rehabil 56:237–240, 1975.

174. Thorsen R, et al: Functional control of the hand in tetraplegics based on residual EMG activity. Artif Organs 23:470–473, 1999.

175. Trimble MH, Enoka RM: Mechanisms underlying the training effects associated with neuromuscular electrical stimulation. Phys Ther 71:273–282, 1991.

176. Triolo RJ, et al: Implanted functional neuromuscular stimulation systems for individuals with cervical spinal cord injuries: Clinical case reports. Arch Phys Med Rehabil 77:1119–1128, 1996.

177. Twist DJ: Acrocyanosis in a spinal cord injured patient: Effects of computer-controlled neuromuscular electrical stimulation: A case report. Phys Ther 70:45–49, 1990.

178. Valencic V, et al: Improved motor response due to chronic electrical stimulation of denervated tibialis anterior muscle in humans. Muscle Nerve 9:612–617, 1986.

179. Vodovnik L and others: Recent applications of functional electrical stimulation to stroke patients in Ljubljana. Clin Orthop 131:64–69, 1978.

180. Wakim KG, Krusen FH: The influence of electrical stimulation on the work output and endurance of denervated muscle. Arch Phys Med Rehabil 36:370–376, 1955.

181. Waters RL, et al: J: Experimental correction of footdrop by electric stimulation of the peroneal nerve. J Bone Joint Surg Am 57:1047–1054, 1975.

182. Waters RL, et al: Functional electric stimulation of the peroneal nerve for hemiplegia: Long term clinical follow-up. J Bone Joint Surg Am 67:792–793, 1985.

183. Wieler M, et al: Multicenter evaluation of electrical stimulation systems for walking. Arch Phys Med Rehabil 80:495–500, 1999.

184. Winchester P, et al: Effects of feedback stimulation training and cyclical electrical stimulation on knee extension in hemiparetic patients. Phys Ther 7:1096–1103, 1983.

185. Wissel J, et al: Treating chronic hemiparesis with modified biofeedback. Arch Phys Med Rehabil 70:612–617, 1989.

186. Wolf SL, Electromyographic biofeedback applications to stroke patients: A critical review. Phys Ther 63:1448–1459, 1983.

187. Wolf SL: Electromyographic feedback for spinal cord injured patients: A realistic perspective. In Basmajian JV (ed): Biofeedback Principles and Practice for Clinicians, 3rd ed. Baltimore, Williams & Wilkins, 1989.

188. Wolf SL: Use of biofeedback in the treatment of stroke patients. Stroke 21(Suppl 2I):II-22–II-23, 1990.

189. Wolf SL, Binder-Macleod SA: Electromyographic biofeedback applications to the hemiplegic patient: Changes in upper extremity neuromuscular and functional status. Phys Ther 63:1393–1403, 1983.

190. Wolf SL, Binder-Macleod SA: Electromyographic biofeedback applications to the hemiplegic patient: Changes in lower extremity neuromuscular and functional status. Phys Ther 63:1404–1413, 1983.

191. Wolf SL, Binder-Macleod SA: Neurophysiological factors in electromyographic feedback for neuromotor disturbances. In Basmajian JV (ed): Biofeedback Principles and Practice for Clinicians, 3rd eds. Baltimore, Williams & Wilkins, 1989.

192. Wolf SL, et al: EMG biofeedback in stroke: Effect of patient characteristics. Arch Phys Med Rehabil 60:96–102, 1979.

193. Wolf SL, et al: JL: EMG biofeedback in stroke: A 1-year follow-up on the effect of patient characteristics. Arch Phys Med Rehabil 61:351–354, 1980.

194. Wolf SL, et al: Concurrent assessment of muscle activity (CAMA): A procedural approach to assess treatment goals. Phys Ther 66:218–224, 1986.

195. Wolf SL, et al: Comparison of motor copy and targeted biofeedback training techniques for restitution of upper extremity function among patients with neurologic disorders. Phys Ther 69:719–735, 1989.

196. Wu Y, et al: Axillary central latency: Simple electrodiagnostic technique for proximal neuropathy. Arch Phys Med Rehabil 64:117–120, 1983.

197. Yang L, et al: Further development of hybrid functional electrical stimulation orthoses. Spinal Cord 34:611–614, 1996.

198. Zablotny C: Using neuromuscular electrical stimulation to facilitate limb control in the head-injured patient. J Head Trauma Rehabil 2:28–33, 1987.

Pain Management

LINDA MIRABELLI-SUSENS, MS, PT

Key Words

- ANS pain: complex regional pain syndrome

- acute pain; chronic pain

- behavioral manipulations: exercise; operant conditioning; hypnosis; biofeedback

- CNS pain: thalamic pain

- cognitive strategies: relaxation exercises; body scanning; humor

- cryotherapy

- iontophoresis

- joint mobilization

- massage

- myofascial release

- nociceptor

- pain intensity measurements: visual analog scale (VAS); simple descriptive pain scale (SDPS); pain estimate; faces pain scale

- pain localization tools: pain drawing

- pain modulation: gate control theory; neurotransmitters; neuromodulators

- pain pathway

- pain quality measurements: McGill Pain Questionnaire (MPQ); pediatric verbal descriptor scale; caregiver checklists

Objectives

After reading this chapter the student/therapist will:

1. Describe the pain pathways.

2. Describe how pain is modulated within the nervous system.

3. Identify the causes of acute and chronic pain.

4. List the signs and symptoms of CNS, ANS, and peripheral pain and give an example of each.

5. Perform a comprehensive pain evaluation, including taking a pain history, measuring pain intensity, measuring pain character, and examining the client.

6. Design a comprehensive pain management program that addresses the objective and subjective aspects of the pain experience.

– point stimulation

– TENS

– therapeutic touch

– thermotherapy: superficial heat;
   short-wave diathermy; microwave
   diathermy; ultrasound;
   phonophoresis

Chronic pain has a profound impact on all aspects of an individual's life. It influences relationships with family members, friends, coworkers, and health care providers. It affects the ability to fulfill responsibilities, work, and participate in social activities. Perhaps more than any other factors in an individual's life, the presence of chronic pain and the response to it determine the overall quality of an individual's life.

Chronic pain is prevalent. The American Pain Society reports that 45% of all Americans seek medical care for chronic pain at some point in their lives,[2] and chronic back pain is the second most common reason people seek medical attention.[29] Yet, studies of physicians, nurses, and therapists who treat individuals with chronic pain show that most do not have even a basic understanding of the concepts of pain management.[12, 13, 86] The result is inadequate or inappropriate care.[48, 86, 125]

This chapter deals with the complex issue of chronic pain management. In the first section a brief overview of the anatomy and physiology of pain is presented. In the second section, pain evaluation is explained. In the third section a number of treatment interventions are suggested. Finally, case studies are presented to guide clinicians through the problem-solving process when designing pain management programs.

DEFINING PAIN

Pain is a sensation with more than one dimension. To the individual, pain is both an objective and a subjective experience. The objective dimension is the physiological tissue damage causing the pain. The subjective dimensions include[89]:

- A *perceptual component:* the client's awareness of the location, quality, intensity, and duration of the pain stimulus.
- An *affective component:* the psychological factors surrounding the client's pain experience, including the client's personality and emotional state.
- A *cognitive component:* what the client knows and believes about the pain resulting from his or her cultural background and past pain experiences (both personal pain experiences and those of others).
- A *behavioral component:* how the client expresses the pain to others through communication and behavior.

All of these components taken together constitute the client's pain experience. Thus, all of these components must be addressed for a successful pain management program. When the subjective components of the pain experience are ignored, it is entirely possible to correct the client's underlying tissue damage without curing his or her pain.

In addition, recognizing that pain is more than simply an injury helps to explain some of the inconsistencies observed in patients with chronic pain: Why is a client's pain report out of proportion to the magnitude and duration of the injury? Why is pain intolerable to one person and merely uncomfortable to another? And why is pain tolerable in one instance but overwhelming to the same individual when experienced at a different time?

The answers lie in the interconnectedness of the nervous system and the fact that pain transmission involves several higher centers. To select the most appropriate intervention, it is important for clinicians to have at least a general idea of the pain pathways. Therefore, a brief overview of pain anatomy and physiology is in order.

PAIN ANATOMY

Pain arises from the stimulation of specialized peripheral nerve endings called nociceptors. Nociceptors found in interstitial tissues become excited with extreme mechanical, thermal, and chemical stimulation,[37] whereas nociceptors found in vessel walls become excited with these stimuli plus marked constriction and dilation of the vessels.[111]

Nociceptive input travels on A-delta and C fibers into the dorsal horn of the spinal cord, where the gray matter is laminated. The first-order A-delta and C fibers synapse with second-order neurons in lamina I, II (the substantia gelatinosa [SG]), and V. The second-order neurons do one of three things. A small number synapse with motor neurons causing reflex movements (e.g., withdrawing the hand from a hot object). Others synapse with autonomic fibers causing responses such as changes in heart rate and blood pressure and localized vasodilation, piloerection, and sweating. The majority, however, travel a multisynaptic route to the higher centers by means of the ascending tracts.[37, 55]

Nociceptive input ascends in the contralateral spinothalamic tract. This tract is divided into two parts. The neospinothalamic tract (also known as the lateral spinothalamic tract) is somatotopically organized and carries information about the location and character of the stimulation. The paleospinothalamic tract (also known as the anterior spinothalamic tract) is involved with the affective responses to pain. Both tracts project to the thalamus, although the neospinothalamic tract takes a direct route whereas the paleospinothalamic tract synapses several more times before reaching the thalamus.[37, 55]

The thalamus relays information to several higher centers.[111] Each projection serves a specific purpose. Projections from the thalamus to the postcentral gyrus are responsible for pain perception. It is from this projection that pain can be localized and characterized. Projections from the thalamus to the frontal lobes and limbic system are concerned with pain interpretation. It is from all these projections that an individual perceives pain as hurting. Projections from the thalamus, as well as from the limbic system and sensory cortical areas, to the temporal lobes are responsible for pain memory; and projections from the thalamus to the hypothalamus are responsible for the autonomic response to pain.

PAIN MODULATION

Nociceptive transmission is modulated at several points along the neural pathway by both ascending and descending systems.

The Gate Control Theory. The SG contains an ascending gating mechanism to block nociceptive impulses from leaving the dorsal horn of the spinal cord. The first-order neurons for both nociceptive and nonnociceptive information synapse with second-order neurons in the SG. The second-order neurons for both types of information project to specialized neurons named T (transmission) cells in lamina V. For pain transmission to occur, T cells must be stimulated while the SG is inhibited. The input from A-delta and C fibers stimulates the T cells and inhibits the SG (Fig. 29–1). Therefore, A-delta and C fiber input opens the gate, allowing pain transmission to the higher centers. On the other hand, when the SG and the T cells are both stimulated the T cells are inhib-

ited and the gate is closed to pain transmission. The input from nonnociceptive A-beta fibers carrying information from pressoreceptors and mechanoreceptors stimulates both the T cells and the SG. Therefore, A-beta fiber input closes the gate, blocking pain transmission.[88]

The gate control theory is thought to be the underlying mechanism for the effectiveness of the physical modalities in relieving pain.

Descending Pain Modulation System. There are at least two descending pain modulation systems. One involves the action of chemical messengers called neurotransmitters, including serotonin, dopamine, norepinephrine, and substance P. High concentrations of brain serotonin[108] and L-dopa (a precursor of dopamine)[114] have been found to inhibit nociception, whereas norepinephrine appears to enhance nociception.[90, 91, 113, 116] Substance P is thought to be the neurotransmitter for neurons transmitting chronic pain.[87]

The second descending modulating system is mediated by neuromodulators, chemicals capable of directly affecting pain transmission. The neuromodulators include enkephalin and beta-endorphin, which are referred to as endogenous opiates because they have morphine-like actions and are found in areas of the central nervous system (CNS) that correspond to opiate binding sites.[78] Endogenous opiates are believed to modulate pain by inhibiting the release of substance P. They have been shown to have a profound effect on nociception and mood.[56, 93, 122] Their levels in the brain and spinal cord rise in response to emotional stress, causing an increase in the pain threshold and providing a possible reason that acute stress decreases acute pain.[107, 123]

Although serotonin is not classified as an endogenous

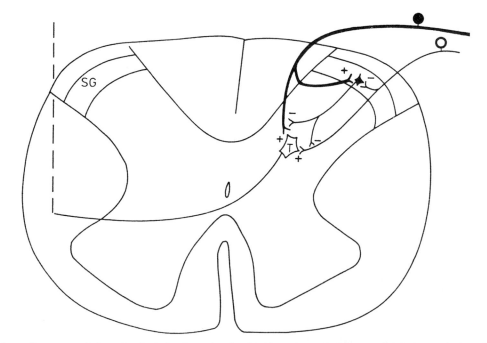

FIGURE 29–1. Schematic representation of spinal structures involved in the gate control theory of pain transmission. Afferent input by means of both large- and small-diameter fibers is theorized to influence the transmission cell (T) directly and through small internuncial neurons located within the substantia gelatinosa (SG). (From Nolan MF: Anatomic and physiologic organization of neural structures involved in pain transmission, modulation, and perception. In Echternach JL [ed]: Pain. New York, Churchill Livingstone, 1987.)

opiate, it exerts a profound effect on analgesia and enhances analgesic drug potency. High concentrations of serotonin lead to decreased pain by inhibiting transmission of nociceptive information within the dorsal horn,[4, 77] whereas low concentrations result in depression, sleep disturbances, and increased pain.[104]

The success of several therapeutic modalities, including noxious counterirritation (e.g., brief intense transcutaneous electrical nerve stimulation [TENS] or acupressure) and diversion (including hypnosis) is attributed to raising the level of endogenous opiates in the body.[123]

CATEGORIZING PAIN

Pain is grouped into several categories: acute, chronic, and referred and central, autonomic, and peripheral.

Acute pain is a warning. It alerts the individual that tissues are exposed to damaging or potentially damaging noxious stimuli. Acute pain is localized, in proportion to the intensity of the stimuli, and lasts only as long as the stimuli or the tissue damage exists.[128] Although acute pain is associated with anxiety and increased autonomic activity (increased muscle tone, heart rate, and blood pressure),[82] it is usually relieved by interventions directed at correcting the injury. The pain experience is usually limited to the individual.[124]

Chronic pain is a disease. It is defined as pain that continues after the stimulus is removed or the tissue damage heals. Physiologically, chronic pain is believed to result from hypersensitization of the pain receptors and enlargement of the receptor field in response to the localized inflammation that follows tissue damage.[45] Chronic pain is poorly localized, has an ill-defined time of onset, and is strongly associated with the subjective components outlined previously. It does not respond well to interventions directed solely at correcting the injury. The effects of the pain experience extend beyond the individual and affect the family, the workplace, and the social sphere of the individual.[124]

Referred pain is felt at a point other than its origin. Pain can be referred from an internal organ, a joint, a trigger point, or a peripheral nerve to a remote musculoskeletal structure. Referred pain usually follows a specific pattern. For example, cardiac pain is frequently referred to the left arm or jaw and the referral pattern for trigger points is exact enough to be used as a diagnostic tool. Referred pain is the result of a convergence of the primary afferent neurons from deep structures and muscles to secondary neurons that also have a cutaneous receptive field.[23]

Although it is now recognized that all neuropathic pain results in abnormal activity within the CNS,[15] pain arising from injury or disease of the CNS is referred to as *central pain.* Central pain is diagnosed by its defining neurological signs and symptoms; it is verified with neuroimaging tests that identify a CNS lesion and rule out other causes. Central pain can be caused by vascular insult; traumatic, neoplastic, and demyelinating diseases; and surgery (including vascular compromise during surgery).

The onset of central pain is variable. Central pain can occur immediately after the injury or come on much later. Pain originating from a cerebrovascular incident and spinal cord injury usually begins weeks or months after the insult, whereas pain originating from tumors may take years to begin.[15]

Individuals with central pain report burning, aching, pricking, squeezing, or cutting pain after cutaneous stimulation, movement, heat, cold, or vibration. In some cases the pain begins spontaneously.[35] Pain intensity varies, but it does seem to be associated to some degree with the location of the lesion.[15] Allodynia (pain arising from usually nonpainful stimuli) is common, and one of the characteristic features of central pain is that the clinical symptoms persist long after the stimulus is removed.

Central pain is topographical. The site of the lesion determines the location of the symptoms. The pain may involve half the body, an entire extremity, or a small portion of one extremity.[15] It is frequently migratory. Thalamic pain is the classic example of central pain.

Central pain is very difficult to treat. Surgery is not helpful for most individuals with central pain, and medications have not been effective in permanently relieving the symptoms.[37] Therefore, the treatment of clients with central pain stresses coping strategies and disability prevention.

Under normal conditions, there is a fine balance between the parasympathetic and sympathetic branches of the autonomic nervous system (ANS). Parasympathetic activity maintains homeostasis, whereas sympathetic activity functions to make "fight or flight" changes in response to stress. Stimulation of the autonomic efferent fibers is not normally painful. However, the balance between afferent input and the descending sympathetic nervous system is disrupted when there is injury, resulting in exaggerated and prolonged sympathetic activity, allodynia, and hyperalgesia (increased response to normally painful stimuli)—hence, *autonomic pain.*

Allodynia is a product of the phenomenon of central sensitization.[119] After injury, new axons sprout from the sympathetic efferent neurons. These fire spontaneously and, because they synapse on the cell bodies of the primary afferent neurons, cause them to fire as well. In addition, the dorsal horn neurons themselves become more excitable. They show an enlargement in their receptive field and also become more sensitive to mechanical, thermal, and chemical stimulation. The result is an increase in the neuronal barrage into the CNS and the perception of pain with usually nonpainful stimuli.

Complex regional pain syndrome (CRPS) is an example of pain that arises from abnormal activity within the ANS.[14] CRPS has been classified into two distinct types[84]: CRPS type I (formerly reflex sympathetic dystrophy) follows mild trauma without nerve injury and CRPS type II (formerly causalgia) follows trauma with nerve injury. CRPS type I generally begins within the month after the injury, whereas CRPS type II can occur any time after the injury.[8]

The main features of CRPS type I are constant burning pain that fluctuates in intensity and increases with movement, constant stimulation, or stress. There are also allodynia and hyperalgia, edema, abnormal sweating, abnormal blood flow and trophic changes in the area of pain, and impaired motor function. CRPS type I is relieved by blocking the sympathetic nervous system, indicating that the pain is sympathetically maintained.[8]

CRPS type II occurs in the region of a limb innervated by an injured nerve. The nerves most commonly involved in CRPS type II are the median, sciatic, tibial, and ulnar; involvement of the radial nerve is rare. Pain is described as spontaneous, constant, and burning and is exacerbated by light touch, stress, temperature change, movement, visual and auditory stimuli, and emotional disturbances. Allodynia and hyperalgia are common and may involve the distribution of more than one peripheral nerve. As with CRPS type I, edema, abnormal sweating, abnormal blood flow, trophic changes, and impaired motor function occur. The symptoms spread proximally and can involve other areas of the body. Evidence also points to sympathetic involvement in CRPS type II.[8]

The treatment of CRPS is complex and must be carefully coordinated between the physician and the therapist. Please refer to Case 29–3 for interventions for clients with CRPS.

Peripheral pain results from noxious irritation of the nociceptors. The character of peripheral pain depends on the location and intensity of the noxious stimulation as well as on which fibers carry the information into the dorsal gray matter. As noted previously, information carried on A-delta fibers is sharp and well localized, begins rapidly, and lasts only as long as the stimulus is present, whereas information carried on C fibers is dull and diffuse, has a delayed onset, and lasts longer than the duration of the stimulus. The treatment of peripheral pain is covered in detail in Chapter 12.

EXAMINATION OF THE CLIENT WITH PAIN

The examination of a client with pain can be very challenging because the therapist must frequently weed through the individual's emotions, behaviors, and secondary gains in an attempt to identify the source of the symptoms. Many clients are not referred to therapy until they have participated in weeks, months, even years of failed interventions, and their expectations and patience are at low levels. They often approach therapy anticipating more instructions, more frustration, and more pain. Despite these obstacles, therapists must strive to complete pain evaluations that include measurable, reproducible information that identifies the source of pain, that provides direction toward treatment that is both beneficial and cost effective, and that assists in establishing attainable goals.

Pain History

Every evaluation of a client with pain should begin with a comprehensive pain history. It is important to have a standardized format to decrease chances of missing important information and to minimize having the client "lead the interview." The following alphabetic mnemonic device may prove helpful:

- *Observation:* observation of the client from the moment

of entry until (and sometimes beyond) the moment of exit from the clinic. By observing the client outside of the evaluation, the therapist is able to assess the client's movement when he or she is not aware that movement is being observed.

- *Origin/onset:* date and circumstances of the onset of pain. How did the pain start? Gradually or suddenly? Was there a precipitating injury? If so, what was the mechanism of injury? If not, can the client correlate the onset to a particular activity or posture?
- *Position:* location of the pain. Have the client demonstrate where the pain is located rather than relying on description alone. In addition to being more accurate, demonstration allows another observation of the client's ability and willingness to move. Clients can also be asked to draw their symptoms on a schematic, such as the pain drawing, which is described later.
- *Pattern:* pattern of the pain. Is the pain constant or periodic? Does it travel or radiate? Which activities and postures increase or decrease the pain? Does medication or time of day have any effect on the pain? Have there been any recent changes in the pattern? Does the client believe that the pain is improving, worsening, or remaining the same?
- *Quality:* characteristics of the pain. Does the client use adjectives indicating mechanical (pressing, bursting, stabbing), chemical (burning), neural (numb, "pins and needles"), or vascular (throbbing) origin? Two tools for describing pain character are described later.
- *Quantity:* intensity of the pain. How has the pain intensity changed since the onset? Several methods that allow for monitoring change in pain intensity are presented later.
- *Radiation:* characteristics of pain radiation. Does the pain radiate? What causes the pain to radiate? Can the radiation be reversed? How?
- *Signs/symptoms:* functional and psychological components of the pain. Has the pain resulted in any functional limitations? Has it caused any changes in the client's lifestyle, including employment and recreational activities? Does the client's personality contribute to the pain, or has the pain caused changes in the client's emotional stability? Does the client benefit from the pain? How? It may be necessary to interview the client's significant others for an accurate picture.
- *Treatment:* previous/current treatment and its effectiveness including medications and home remedies. It is also important to determine the client's attitude and expectations concerning therapy in addition to obtaining a treatment history.
- *Visceral symptoms:* physical symptoms of visceral origin that can accompany and be responsible for the pain (see the box on page 892). Visceral causes for pain require referral to the client's physician for further investigation before the initiation of treatment by a therapist.

Pain Measurement

Research has shown that pain memory does not provide an accurate measure of pain intensity.[74] Therefore, pain measurement tools are designed to provide information about the intensity, location, and character of a client's

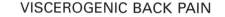

VISCEROGENIC BACK PAIN

- General signs and symptoms:
  - Pain does not increase with spinal stresses/strains
  - Pain is not relieved with rest
  - Visceral symptoms accompany back pain

- Gastrointestinal tract signs and symptoms:
  - Pain is accompanied by altered bowel habits
  - Pain is related to eating
  - Peptic pain is relieved with vomiting

- Kidney signs and symptoms:
  - Increased pain with diuresis indicates hydronephrosis

- Pelvic signs and symptoms:
  - Low back pain associated with vaginal bleeding or discharge

- Prostate signs and symptoms:
  - Low back discomfort associated with micturition

- Lung signs and symptoms:
  - Posterior thoracic pain associated with respiration in chronic obstructive pulmonary disease

- Vascular signs and symptoms:
  - Deep, boring, pulsating low back pain associated with a palpable abdominal aortic aneurysm
  - Back pain with/without calf pain after walking and relieved with standing still; possibly impaired lower extremity pulses and trophic skin changes associated with occlusive disease of the internal iliac artery or its branches

From Makofsky H, Willis GC: Non-mechanical and pathological causes of low back pain. Phys Ther Forum, May 15, 1989, p 12.

symptoms *at the time of the evaluation*. This information can then be merged with the pain history and the physical findings to identify the cause of pain. A number of pain measurement tools are available. The applications and limitations of several are discussed below.

Measuring Pain Intensity

Pain intensity rating tools are scales that have the client rate the current level of pain by marking a continuum or assigning a numerical value to the pain intensity (Fig. 29–2).

Each of the first three tools described here has been found to be reliable over time when used to measure pain that is present at the time of the rating. In general,

however, clients who are depressed or anxious tend to report higher levels of pain and clients who are not depressed or anxious tend to report lower levels of pain on all three of these scales.[65]

Visual Analog Scale (VAS). The client rates the pain on a continuum that begins with "no pain" and ends with "maximum pain tolerable." This tool provides an infinite number of points between the extremes, making it sensitive to small changes in pain intensity. However, it has not been found reliable for individuals who have impaired abstract thinking skills[11] and may be unable to translate their pain intensity into a corresponding point on a line.

Simple Descriptive Pain Scale (SDPS). The client rates the pain on a continuum that is subdivided using descriptors that gradually increase in intensity. Sample descriptors are "no pain," "mild pain," "moderate pain," "severe pain," and "maximum pain tolerable." This tool is more useful than the VAS for clients with impaired abstract thinking because it is easier for them to identify with the pain descriptors than with the line found in the VAS. However, clients have been found to favor the points corresponding to each descriptor rather than the points between, resulting in a less sensitive tool than the VAS.[54]

Pain Estimate. The client assigns a numerical rating to the pain, staying within defined limits (most commonly between 0 and 100, where 0 represents no pain and 100 represents maximum pain tolerable). Because it provides a numerical range of scores, this tool is valuable for statistical analysis purposes. However, whereas some clients find assigning a numerical rating to their pain intensity easy, clients with impaired abstract thinking may have difficulty similar to that encountered with the VAS.

Faces Pain Scale. The client selects one of seven schematic faces representing gradually increasing pain intensities. The scale begins with a face representing no pain and ends with a face representing the most pain possible. This tool is designed for use with young children who do not have the ability to use any of the three previous tools. The Faces Pain Scale has been found to be valid across cultural lines[110] and to have a strong correlation with other pain measures.[11] It is simple to use, does not require verbal skills, and requires very little instruction. It has been used successfully with children as young as 3 years as well as with individuals who are limited in verbal expression.

Localizing Pain Symptoms

Pain Drawings. The client is asked to draw his or her symptoms on a schematic of the human body using a provided list of symbols (Fig. 29–3). The result is a diagram describing the nature and location of the client's pain that can be compared with the client's verbal report. In addition to providing a database, the pain drawing has been found to be useful in identifying individuals who have a heavy psychological or emotional component to their pain, making it also helpful in identifying clients who would benefit from further psychological evaluation.[95]

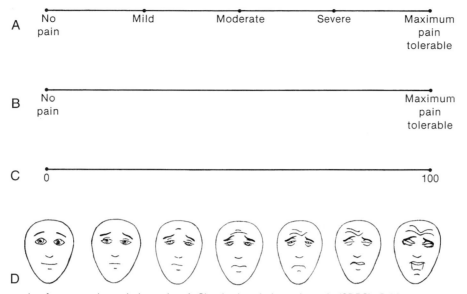

FIGURE 29–2. Rating scales for measuring pain intensity. *A*, Simple descriptive pain scale (SDPS). *B*, Visual analog scale (VAS). *C*, Pain estimate. *D*, Faces pain scale. (*D*, Reprinted from Bieri D, et al: The faces pain scale for the self-assessment of the severity of pain experienced by children: Development, initial validation, and preliminary investigation for the ratio scale properties. Pain 41:139–150, 1990, with permission from Elsevier Science.)

Describing Pain Quality

McGill Pain Questionnaire (MPQ). One of the most popular scales to rate pain quality is the McGill Pain Questionnaire, which includes 20 categories of descriptive words covering the sensory (numbers 1–10), affective (numbers 11–15), and evaluative (number 16) properties of pain (Fig. 29–4). Sensory properties are measured using temporal, thermal, spatial, and pressure descriptors. Affective properties are measured using fear, tension, and autonomic descriptors. And evaluative properties are measured using pain experience descriptors.[80] Each word has a numerical value based on its position within its category.

The client is instructed to "select the word in each category that best describes the pain you have now. If there is no word in the category that describes the pain, skip the category. If there is more than one word that describes the pain, select the word that best describes the pain."

The MPQ can provide several types of information[80]:

- A pain-rating index based on the sum of the values of all the words selected
- A pain-rating index based on the sum of the values of all the words in a given category
- The total number of words chosen

The MPQ has been studied extensively and found valid for adults with acute and chronic pain as well as for those with a variety of specific pathological states.[19, 66, 96] It provides clues into the specific cause of pain because it describes the client's symptoms.

However, the MPQ does pose some disadvantages. It is time consuming, requiring more time to complete than any of the previously described rating scales. Thus, it is not appropriate for quick estimates of pain after treatment. Clients, especially children, are frequently unfamiliar with some of the descriptors and ask the evaluator to assist by defining words. However, reliability and validity of this test are based on examiner objectivity and care must be taken to avoid the introduction of evaluator bias by helping the client to select appropriate descriptors.[80] This issue can be dealt with by telling the client, "If you do not recognize a word, it probably does not apply to you."

Pediatric Verbal Descriptor Scale. Because a child's description of pain is limited by a smaller vocabulary, Wilkie and associates[121] have developed a verbal descriptor scale specifically for use with children (Table 29–1). Their list includes 56 words commonly used by children aged 8 to 17 to describe their pain experience. The word list is divided into the four categories found in the MPQ.

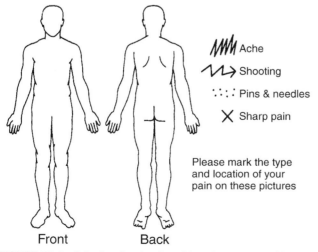

Ache

Shooting

Pins & needles

Sharp pain

Please mark the type and location of your pain on these pictures

Front   Back

FIGURE 29–3. Pain drawing for describing the nature and location of a client's pain symptoms. (From Cameron MH [ed]: Physical Agents in Rehabilitation. Philadelphia, WB Saunders, 1999.)

What Does Your Pain Feel Like?

Some of the words below describe your present pain. Circle ONLY those words that best describe it. Leave out any category that is not suitable. Use only a single word in each appropriate category—the one that applies best.

1	2	3	4
Flickering	Jumping	Pricking	Sharp
Quivering	Flashing	Boring	Cutting
Pulsing	Shooting	Drilling	Lacerating
Throbbing		Stabbing	
Beating		Lancinating	
Pounding			

5	6	7	8
Pinching	Tugging	Hot	Tingling
Pressing	Pulling	Burning	Itchy
Gnawing	Wrenching	Scalding	Smarting
Cramping		Searing	Stinging
Crushing			

9	10	11	12
Dull	Tender	Tiring	Sickening
Sore	Taut	Exhausting	Suffocating
Hurting	Rasping		
Aching	Splitting		
Heavy			

13	14	15	16
Fearful	Punishing	Wretched	Annoying
Frightful	Grueling	Blinding	Troublesome
Terrifying	Cruel		Miserable
	Vicious		Intense
	Killing		Unbearable

17	18	19	20
Spreading	Tight	Cool	Nagging
Radiating	Numb	Cold	Nauseating
Penetrating	Drawing	Freezing	Agonizing
Piercing	Squeezing		Dreadful
	Tearing		Torturing

FIGURE 29–4. The McGill Pain Questionnaire used to rate pain quality. (Reprinted from Melzak R: The McGill pain questionnaire: Major properties and scoring methods. Pain 1:277, 1975, with permission from Elsevier Science.)

TABLE 29–1. Pediatric Verbal Descriptor Scale

Dimension	Word	Dimension	Word	Dimension	Word	Dimension	Word
A	Annoying	S	Biting	S	Itching	A	Crying
	Bad		Cutting		Like a scratch		Frightening
	Horrible		Like a pin		Like a sting		Screaming
	Miserable		Like a sharp knife		Scratching		Terrifying
	Terrible		Pinlike		Stinging		
	Uncomfortable		Sharp			A	Dizzy
			Stabbing	S	Shocking		Sickening
E	Aching				Shooting		Suffocating
	Hurting	S	Blistering		Splitting		
	Like an ache		Burning			E	Never goes away
	Like a hurt		Hot	S	Numb		Uncontrollable
	Sore				Stiff		
		S	Cramping		Swollen		
S	Beating		Crushing		Tight		
	Hitting		Like a pinch				
	Pounding		Pinching	A	Awful		
	Punching		Pressure		Deadly		
	Throbbing				Dying		
					Killing		

S = sensory; A = affective; E = evaluative.

Reprinted from Wilkie DJ, et al: Measuring pain quality: Validity and reliability of children's and adolescents' pain language. Pain 41:151–159, 1990, with permission from Elsevier Science.

The evaluators' research has shown the list to be useful for children with a variety of diagnoses because it is relatively free of gender, ethnic, and developmental bias.

Caregiver Checklist. Clients who are unable to communicate verbally because of neurological disabilities may be unable to use any of the just described pain measurement scales. However, because of pain associated with their medical conditions, extensive and repeated surgery, and behavioral oddities that might limit pain expression, these individuals are at high risk for having their pain go unrecognized. McGrath and colleagues[79] have attempted to develop and categorize a checklist of demonstrated pain behaviors identified by caregivers of severely handicapped individuals. Although their list did not pass validity criteria, the researchers propose clinicians develop a client-specific checklist that could be used to gauge changes in the client's pain from the information gained during the caregiver interview portion of the evaluation of nonverbal handicapped clients.

In addition to qualifying and quantifying the client's pain, pain measurement tools have an additional value. They can be used to identify inconsistencies between a client's pain report and the clinician's objective findings. For example, a client with normal objective findings would not be expected to give a high pain report or draw symptoms over the entire pain drawing. Conversely, a client with a multitude of objective findings within the severe range would be expected to provide a high pain rating. In addition, as objective symptoms subside, it is expected that the client will report a similar decline on the rating scales. Inconsistencies between the client's pain descriptions and the therapist's findings should serve to alert the clinician that the client might require cognitive or affective intervention in addition to physical treatment.

EVALUATION OF THE CLIENT

The clinical assessment should begin the moment the client enters the door. Clients frequently change posture and affect when they are being formally evaluated, and it is important to gain an accurate view of pain behavior during spontaneous activities to assess the validity of their complaints. The formal assessment should include the following:

- Observation of gait and movement patterns, including the use of assistive devices.
- Notation of body type and anomalies.
- Assessment of sitting and standing posture, including both the normal posture and that assumed because of the pain. (Observe the client during activities, if possible, to differentiate movement patterns altered by intent versus automatic adjustments.)
- Inspection of the skin for pliability, trophic changes, scar tissue, and other abnormalities.
- Palpation of the soft tissue structures to identify changes in temperature, swelling, tenderness, and areas of discomfort.
- Palpation of the anatomical structures to determine end feel, the sensation felt at the end of the available movement.[30]

  – Bone-to-bone: hard—normal, for example, at the end range of elbow extension.
  – Spasm: muscular resistance—abnormal
  – Capsular feel: rubbery—normal at the extreme of full range of motion (ROM); abnormal when encountered before the end of ROM
  – Springy block: rebound—abnormal
  – Tissue approximation: soft tissue—normal at the extremes of full passive flexion
  – Empty feel: no physiological resistance, but client resists movement because of pain.
- Measurement of ROM: active ROM is performed to assess the client's willingness to move and to identify any limitations or painful areas; passive ROM testing is used to further refine the observations.[30]
  – When active and passive movements are painful and restricted in the same direction and the pain appears at the limit of motion, the problem is arthrogenic.
  – When active and passive movements are painful or restricted in opposite directions, the problem is muscular.
  – When there is relative restriction of passive movement in the capsular pattern, the problem is arthritic.
  – When there is no restriction of passive movement but the client cannot perform the movement actively, the muscle is not functioning, either from intrinsic problems within the muscle or interruption in the neural pathway (central or peripheral).
- Measurement of muscle strength[30]
  – When the movement is strong and painful, there is a minor lesion in the muscle or tendon.
  – When the movement is weak and increases the pain, there is a major lesion that needs to be identified with further testing.
  – When the movement is weak but does not increase the pain, there is the possibility of either complete rupture of the muscle or tendon or a neurological disorder.
  – When all resisted movements are painful, the pain may be organic or the patient may be emotionally hypersensitive.
  – When movement is strong and painless, the test is normal.
- Assessment of bilateral neurological function
  – Reflexes: peripheral lesions tend to diminish deep tendon reflexes (DTRs). CNS lesions tend to intensify DTRs, and testing frequently elicits a clonic reaction.[63] Note any asymmetries in response.
  – Sensation: test light touch, sharp (noxious) touch, and vibration. Pressure on a nerve usually affects conduction on the large, myelinated fibers first. Therefore, vibration is the first sensation to be diminished. Where there is decreased perception of touch and noxious stimuli, the lesion is more severe.[63] Note any asymmetries in response.
  – Allodynia and hyperalgesia: delineate areas of allodynia and hyperagesia to touch, hot, and cold. Exact descriptions of these areas, along with areas of decreased perception of vibration, will provide information concerning A-beta versus C fiber involvement in the production of pain.[120]
  – Coordination.
  – Stretch and pressure tests to nerve trunks.

It is not always possible to complete a pain evaluation in one session. Clients may not be able to tolerate all of the required activities at one time, or there may be enough inconsistencies for the therapist to want a second appointment to refocus on specific tests. However, with the limitations on number of visits common with managed care, the therapist may feel pressured to identify a cause for the client's pain in the initial visit. This is not necessary. It is far better to take more than one visit and be accurate than to take only one visit and develop a treatment plan that is not appropriate for the client's needs.

TREATMENT OF THE CLIENT WITH PAIN

There are three broad avenues of intervention for pain management: physical interventions, cognitive strategies, and behavioral manipulations.[36] Each avenue addresses a different aspect of the pain experience, and each requires a different level of participation from the client.

Physical interventions are directed at the client's body with the goal of healing the tissue injury. Examples include medication, surgery, and the therapy modalities. Physical interventions are of use most frequently with acute pain or recurrent pain due to reinjury. Physical interventions are often passive and, for the most part, soothing. When used long term, they promote dependence on the clinician. Therefore, it is best to use them as a short-term adjunct in the overall treatment program.

Cognitive strategies are directed at the client's thoughts with the goal of changing the client's pain paradigms. Cognitive strategies include body scanning and reinterpretation of self-statements. Cognitive strategies are self-initiated and performed independently; therefore, they encourage personal responsibility and independence.

Behavioral manipulations involve a behavioral change on the part of the client to bring about the desired response. They include exercise, biofeedback, hypnosis, relaxation exercises, and operant conditioning. There is usually a brief learning period until the client becomes proficient with these techniques; however, once learned, behavioral manipulations can be initiated and performed independently. Behavioral manipulations also encourage personal responsibility and independence.

A brief review of the benefits, indications, contraindications, and precautions for many of the interventions provided by therapists should provide an overview of the complexity of pain management. The purpose of this section is to provide guidance in the selection of one treatment option over another so that intervention will be based on sound physiological principles. Readers who wish to explore an intervention in greater depth are directed to the references listed at the end of this chapter.

Physical Interventions

Thermotherapy

The physiological effects of heat depend on the method of application, the depth of penetration, and the rate and magnitude of temperature change. Cellular metabolic rate increases with rising temperature until the tissues reach 113° F (43°C), after which there is a gradual slowing of metabolic activity until cell death results from denaturation of the protein within the tissue.[85] Speed of skeletal muscle contraction increases until the optimal temperature for metabolic processes is reached. Then speed, too, gradually decreases.[38] Muscle strength declines immediately after heat application. Strength restoration and then a temporary strength gain beginning about 30 minutes later follow this decline.[25]

Blood flow increases, both in the treatment area and systemically. Although a number of physiological mechanisms appear to be responsible for vasodilation,[28, 40] the results of local and systemic vasodilation are the same. If the area remains below core temperature, increased blood flow results in a transfer of heat from the core. If the area becomes warmer than the core, heat is carried centrally. Capillary permeability, capillary hydrostatic pressure, and capillary filtration rate all increase. There is an escape of protein into the interstitial space, leading to edema. Anastomoses that connect arterioles to venules open and blood is shunted past the capillaries. Because venules are longer than capillaries, blood remains in the area longer, allowing greater time for heat transfer to the tissues.

Muscle spasm decreases as a result of decreased activity in gamma motor efferents, decreased excitability of muscle spindles, and increased activity of Golgi tendon organs.[71, 98] This will decrease peripheral pain.

Ischemic pain is relieved by the influx of oxygen-rich blood into the dilated vessels, and muscle tension pain is decreased by interruption of the pain/spasm cycle. In addition, the pain threshold, itself, rises through gating at the spinal cord level.[7, 72]

Because of these effects, several precautions are required when using superficial heat as a modality. Heat should be used with caution in very young and elderly individuals because of their inability to thermoregulate adequately. Superficial heat should be used with caution in individuals with impaired circulation, diminished sensation, and open wounds because of the potential for tissue injury. Superficial heat should be used with caution in individuals with inadequate cardiac or respiratory reserves because of the increased cardiac demands associated with vasodilation. Superficial heat should also be used with caution directly over areas where topical creams and ointments containing counterirritants have recently been applied because the vessels under the counterirritants may not be able to dilate further in response to the heat application.[22]

The application of superficial heat is contraindicated during acute thrombophlebitis because of the increased risk of emboli. It is also contraindicated over a malignancy because the increased blood flow could nourish the tumor and increase the chance of metastases. Superficial heat should not be used where there is hemorrhage or recent trauma.[105]

Superficial heat can be applied by conduction, convection, or radiation. Conductive heating involves the exchange of heat down a temperature gradient by two objects that are in contact. The depth of penetration with conductive heating is usually 1 cm or less.[38] Moist heat packs and paraffin are examples of therapeutic conductive heating. Convective heating involves heat transfer through the flow of hot fluid. Therapeutic convective heating takes place during hydrotherapy and fluidotherapy. Molecules with a temperature greater than absolute zero are in an excited state and emit energy, thus creating radiant heat. Objects that are warmed by the energy are heated by radiation. Therapeutic radiant heat is applied with infrared or ultraviolet light.

Clients can be taught how and when to apply superficial heat independently. Once they demonstrate independence, responsibility for the application of superficial heat should be transferred to the client or his or her caregiver.

The deeper tissues can be heated using conversion, the alteration of one form of energy into another. Heating by conversion is applied with shortwave diathermy, microtherm, and ultrasound.

During shortwave diathermy, the client is placed into an oscillating magnetic field. The systemic ions create friction as they attempt to line up with the continuously reversing current, resulting in an increase in tissue temperature deep within the body. Diathermy using capacitive plates is more effective for heating superficial structures, whereas diathermy using inductive coils is more effective for heating deeper structures.[115] Shortwave diathermy is indicated for diffuse heating of the tissues.

Microwave is diathermy delivered at a higher frequency than shortwave diathermy, allowing the electromagnetic radiation to be focused. Microwave diathermy is far more exact than shortwave diathermy and is indicated where heating of specific deep structures is desired.

In addition to the general precautions outlined for the application of heat, there are several contraindications for the use of shortwave and microwave diathermy. Both are also contraindicated for clients with metal implants because of the potential for the implant to become hot and burn the surrounding tissues. Both are also contraindicated for clients with cardiac pacemakers because of the pacemaker's metal components and because the electromagnetic radiation may interfere with the pacemaker's operation. They should not be used for clients with cancer and for clients who are pregnant and should not be used over the eyes, the reproductive organs, or growing epiphyses. Therapists should avoid prolonged exposure to shortwave diathermy and microwave diathermy because some research has demonstrated a possible negative effect on pregnancy outcome and fetal development.[61]

Ultrasound

Ultrasound is another modality that heats deep tissues by conversion. As its name implies, ultrasound consists of sound waves delivered at a frequency too high to be perceived by human hearing. Ultrasound waves are longitudinal, with alternating areas of compression and rarefaction, which move along the line of propogation. Because of this, the waves are repeatedly refracted as they encounter tissues of differing acoustical resistance while traveling through the skin toward the bone. As the waves change direction at each interface, energy is transferred to the tissues (Fig. 29–5). This also includes the interface between the sound head and the client's skin. Because ultrasound does not travel through air, it is important to

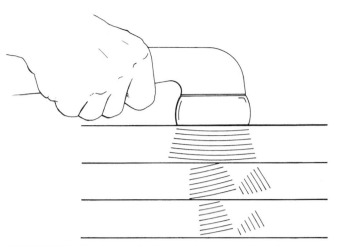

FIGURE 29–5. The longitudinal wave of ultrasound is refracted at tissue interfaces where it encounters tissues of differing acoustical resistance. When the wave changes direction, energy is transferred to the tissues, resulting in the production of heat.

utilize an appropriate transmission agent to minimize energy loss to the environment. A study evaluating various transmission agents found that creams and gels made specifically for ultrasound transmission deliver more energy to the tissues than creams and oils not made for this purpose.[97] Ultrasound can also be applied subaqueously but, because much of the energy is lost to the water, adjustments need to be made in the dosage to ensure a therapeutic level reaches the tissues.

Ultrasound can be delivered in two modes: continuous and pulsed. Ultrasound delivered in the continuous mode is responsible for the temperature increase in the deep tissues. Tissues with high collagen content (tendon, ligament, fascia, and joint capsule) are heated more efficiently than tissues with low collagen content (fat, muscle). The extent of the temperature increase is related to the dosage of ultrasound delivered. As the dosage of ultrasound is increased by increasing the treatment duration or intensity, more energy is available to the tissues and the heating effect increases.[90] However, the higher the frequency of ultrasound delivered, the more superficial the effect. Ultrasound delivered at 1 MHz heats tissues at depths to 5 cm, whereas ultrasound delivered at 3 MHz heats tissues in the upper 2 cm.[32]

The thermal effects of ultrasound can be used to increase tissue extensibility, increase cellular metabolic processes, increase circulation, decrease pain and muscle spasm, and change nerve conduction velocity. The number of impulses traveling along the nerve decreases at low dosages but begins to rise slowly beginning at 1.9 W/cm² Sounding of C fibers yields pain relief distal to the point of application, whereas sounding of large-diameter A fibers brings relief of spasm by changing gamma fiber activity, making the muscle fibers less sensitive to stretch.[34] Because it is impossible to treat C or A fibers selectively, ultrasound provides both pain relief and relief from muscle spasm, making it effective in the treatment of peripheral neuropathies, neuroma, herpes zoster, and muscle spasm associated with musculoskeletal pathology, including sprains, strains, and contusions.[103]

In addition to thermal effects, ultrasound has nonthermal effects that come from the mechanical effects of the ultrasound wave on the tissues. Ultrasound causes cavitation, the development and growth of gas-filled bubbles, in the tissues. Ultrasound also causes tissue fluid to move or stream. The movement of fluid around the gas bubbles formed by cavitation is called microstreaming, and the movement of fluid within the ultrasound delivery area is called acoustic streaming. The nonthermal effects of ultrasound include accelerating metabolic processes, enzyme activity, and the rate of ion exchange, as well as increasing cell membrane permeability and the rate and volume of diffusion across cell membranes. These effects are thought to explain the role of ultrasound in enhancing the healing of soft tissue and bone.[33, 49, 94] The nonthermal effects of ultrasound can be achieved without raising tissue temperature by applying ultrasound in the pulsed mode.

Phonophoresis

Because of these nonthermal effects, ultrasound can be rendered even more effective as a pain reliever during phonophoresis, the use of ultrasound to deliver pain-relieving chemicals to the tissues. Chemicals are delivered to the cells by the ultrasound wave, where they are broken down into ions and taken up into the cells (Fig. 29–6).

The following pain-relieving chemicals can be administered with phonophoresis:

- 5% Lidocaine ointment (Xylocaine) for acute conditions where immediate pain relief is the primary goal
- 10% Hydrocortisone cream or ointment, where pain is the result of inflammation[64]
- 10% Salicylate cream or ointment (from Iodex with methyl salicylate [Lee Pharmaceutical Co., S El Monte, CA 91733] or Gordogeic Creme [Gordon Labs, Upper Darby, PA 19082]) where a combined analgesic antiinflammatory agent is needed

After phonophoresis, measurable quantities of these molecules have been found at tissue depths of up to 2 inches.[44] The contraindication to use of any chemical

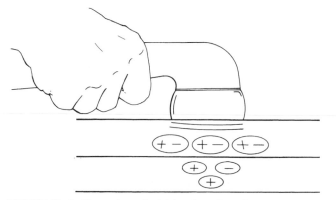

FIGURE 29–6. Phonophoresis. Molecules of a substance are driven into the tissues by the ultrasound wavefront. They are not free for use by the body until they are broken down into chemical ions.

during phonophoresis is having an allergy to that chemical. Clients should be questioned about any adverse reactions to dental local anesthesia (lidocaine) or aspirin.

Phonophoresis should not be performed subaqueously. The dissipation of the wavefront by the intervening water reduces the driving forces, and the water-soluble ointments are diluted beyond functional levels. For the same reason phonophoresis cannot be administered within solutions. It is advised that a coupling agent be applied over the chemical before the application of ultrasound to preserve the ultrasound energy and because many of the ointments used in phonophoresis are too viscous for favorable transmission when used alone.[60] The chemicals used in phonophoresis are drugs and should not be used for phonophoresis if the client has an allergy to the drug or is taking the drug systemically.[22]

Cryotherapy

The physiological effects of cold make it superior to heat for acute pain from inflammatory conditions, for the period immediately after tissue trauma, and for treating muscle spasm and abnormal tone. Peripheral nerve conduction velocity in both large myelinated and small unmyelinated fibers decreases 2.4 m/per degree C of cooling. As a result, pain perception and muscle contractility diminish.[109] Peripheral receptors become less excitable.[109] Muscle spindle responsiveness to stretch decreases; as a result, muscle spasm diminishes.[34]

Local blood flow initially decreases, local edema decreases, the inflammatory response decreases, and hemorrhage is minimized. However, cold application for longer than 15 minutes results in increased local blood flow. Known as the "hunting response," this protective mechanism brings core temperature blood to the surface and prevents tissue injury resulting from prolonged cooling.[38] Cellular metabolic activities slow. The oxygen requirements of the cell decrease.[109]

As with heat, several precautions must be taken when using cold as a therapeutic modality. Cryotherapy is contraindicated in individuals with Raynaud's phenomenon or cold allergy. Cryotherapy should not be used in individuals with rheumatic disease who, with the application of cold, have increased joint pain and stiffness. Cryotherapy should be used with caution in very young, frail, or elderly individuals and those with peripheral vascular disease, circulatory pathological processes, or sensory loss.[105]

Cryotherapy is applied in three ways. Convective cooling involves movement of air over the skin (fanning) and is rarely used therapeutically. Evaporative cooling results when a substance applied to the skin uses thermal energy to evaporate, thereby lowering surface temperature. Most commonly, this substance is a vapocoolant spray. Conductive cooling uses local application of cold, either by ice packs, ice massage, or immersion. Cooling is accomplished as heat from the higher temperature object is transferred to the colder object down a temperature gradient. Conductive cooling is the most commonly used form of therapeutic cold application.

Because muscles, tendons, and joints respond differently, the best method of cold application depends on which tissues are causing the pain.[21] Acute injuries are best treated with cryotherapy along with rest, compression, and elevation (RICE). Muscle spasm is decreased with cold packs and stretching. Trigger points, irritable foci within muscles, are best treated with vapocoolant spray, deep friction massage, and stretching. Tendinitis responds well to ice massage and exercise. Cold packs are often the only source of pain relief in acute disk pathology. The inflamed joints of rheumatoid arthritis frequently respond to cold packs or ice massage with decreased inflammation, increased function, and long-lasting pain relief.[58, 105]

Clients and caregivers can be taught how and when to perform cryotherapy independently. Once they demonstrate their proficiency, responsibility for the use of cryotherapy should be transferred to the client or the client's caregiver.

Transcutaneous Electrical Nerve Stimulation

Transcutaneous electrical nerve stimulation (TENS) is the use of electricity to control the perception of pain. The exact mechanism by which TENS modulates pain still is not completely clear. It appears that, at a high rate, TENS selectively stimulates the low-threshold, large-diameter A-beta fibers, resulting in presynaptic inhibition within the dorsal horns,[18] either directly through the gating mechanism or indirectly through stimulation of the tonic descending pain-inhibiting pathways.[17] Research has shown that the neurons in the brain stem fire in synchrony with the TENS stimulation frequency,[126] and although the significance of this is not known at this time, it does indicate that the action of high-rate TENS is not limited to the dorsal columns. TENS delivered at a low rate is thought to facilitate elevation of the level of endogenous opiates in the CNS.[106]

Stimulation frequencies between 1 and 250 pulses per second (pps) decrease pain. Frequencies between 50 and 100 pps have proven most effective for sensory level (high rate) TENS, and frequencies between 2 and 3 pps are most effective for motor level (low-rate) TENS.[77] Stimulation at exactly 2 pps causes an increase in the pain threshold.[51] As the frequency is decreased, more time is needed before the onset of relief but the effects are more longlasting.[99] Pulse width duration determines which nerves are stimulated. Sensory nerves are stimulated at widths between 20 and 100 msec and motor nerves between 100 and 600 msec.[102]

There are a variety of modes of TENS delivery. Each mode relieves pain through a specific physiological mechanism and is, therefore, most beneficial for a specific type of pain.

When TENS impulses are generated at a high rate (greater than or equal to 50 pps) with a relatively short duration, the stimulation is referred to as sensory level or conventional or high-rate TENS. Sensory level TENS produces mild to moderate paresthesia without muscle contraction throughout the treatment area. Sensory level TENS is thought to control pain through the gating mechanism in the spinal cord. The onset of relief is fast (seconds to 15 minutes)[77] because the gate is closed at the onset of stimulation. The duration of relief after stimulation stops is short lived (at best up to a few hours).

Sensory level TENS has been found to be beneficial for acute pain syndromes and for some deep, aching chronic pain syndromes.

When the impulses are generated at a low rate (less than or equal to 20 pps) and have a relatively long duration (100 to 600 μs), the stimulation is referred to as motor level or acupuncture-like or low-rate TENS. Motor level TENS produces strong muscle contractions in the treatment area with or without the perception of paresthesia. Motor level TENS is associated with deployment of endogenous opiates within the CNS. The onset of relief is delayed 20 to 30 minutes, presumably the time it takes to deploy the opiates. Relief frequently lasts hours or days after treatment. Because motor nerves are not stimulated in isolation, sensory fibers are also excited, causing the gating mechanism to come into play.[102] Motor level TENS has been found to be beneficial for chronic pain syndromes and where sensory level TENS has not been successful.

Stimulation using a high rate and long-duration impulses is called brief-intense TENS. Brief-intense TENS decreases the conduction velocity of A-delta and C fibers, producing a peripheral blockade to transmission.[77] Brief-intense TENS is useful in the clinical setting for short-term anesthesia during wound débridement, suture removal, friction massage, joint mobilization, or other painful procedures.

Modulating TENS parameters is one way to avoid the negative aspects of each of the treatment modes. Rate modulation is most commonly utilized to avoid neural accommodation during sensory level TENS. By setting the initial pulse rate so that, even with the programmed decrement, it will remain within the treatment range, there will be continuous variation in the stimulus and neural accommodation will be avoided.

Width modulation is most commonly utilized with motor level TENS. By setting the initial pulse duration so that, even with the programmed decrement, the impulses are able to recruit the desired motor units, there will be a continuous variation in perceived strength of the muscle contraction, rendering motor level TENS more tolerable.

Stimulation in which the impulses are generated in pulse trains is called burst TENS. Burst TENS is another form of TENS modulation. The stimulator generates low-rate carrier impulses, each of which contains a series of high-rate pulses. Because burst TENS is a combination of high-rate and low-rate TENS, it provides the benefits of each. The low-rate carrier impulse stimulates endorphin release, and the high-rate pulse trains provide an overlay of paresthesia. The advantage to burst TENS is that muscle contractions occur at a lower, more comfortable amplitude, and accommodation does not occur. Burst TENS is beneficial whenever motor level TENS cannot be tolerated and sensory level TENS is ineffective because of neural accommodation.[78]

TENS, like all electrical stimulation, is contraindicated for clients with pacemakers, in the low back and pelvic regions of pregnant women, and over areas with thrombus. TENS should be used with caution for clients who have decreased sensation in the area being stimulated and for clients who have difficulty with understanding or expression. TENS electrodes should not be placed over areas of skin irritation, the eyes, or the carotid sinuses. It should also not be used in the immediate area of an operating diathermy unit.

TENS appears to be of greatest benefit for acute conditions with focal pain, chronic pain syndromes, postoperative incision pain, and during delivery. It has been found least effective with psychogenic pain[75] and pain of central origin.[81] For additional information on TENS, see Chapter 28.

Clients and caregivers can be taught how and when to apply TENS independently. Once they demonstrate independence, responsibility for the use of TENS can transferred to the client or to the caregiver.

Iontophoresis

Iontophoresis is a process in which chemical ions are driven through the skin by a small electrical current. Ionizable compounds are placed on the skin under an electrode which, when polarized by a direct (galvanic) current, repels the ion of like charge into the tissues. Once subcutaneous, the ions are free to combine with the physiological ions, resulting in a physiological effect dependent on the characteristics of the ion (Fig. 29–7). Ions that are known to be effective analgesics are:[60]

- 5% Lidocaine ointment (Xylocaine) administered under the positive electrode for an immediate, although short-lived, decrease in pain. Iontophoresis with lidocaine is recommended before ROM, stretching, and joint mobilization and when immediate relief of acute pain (as in bursitis) is the object of treatment.
- 1% to 10% Hydrocortisone administered under the positive electrode for relief of inflammatory pain in conditions such as arthritis, bursitis, or entrapment syndromes. Iontophoresis with hydrocortisone has a delayed onset but a prolonged effect, and it frequently eliminates the underlying cause of pain.
- 2% Magnesium (from Epsom salts) administered under the positive electrode for relief of pain from muscle spasm or localized ischemia. High levels of extracellular magnesium inhibit muscle contraction, including the smooth muscle found in the walls of the vessels, leading to localized vasodilation.
- Iodine (from Iodex ointment [Lee Pharmaceutical Company, S. El Monte, CA 91733]) administered under the negative pole for relief of pain caused by adhesions or scar tissue. Iodine "softens" fibrotic, sclerotic tissue, thereby increasing tissue pliability.
- Salicylate (from Iodex with methyl salicylate [Lee Pharmaceutical Company] or Gordogesic Creme [Gordon Labs, Upper Darby, PA 19082]) administered under the negative pole for relief of pain from inflammation. Salicylate is effective for arthritic joint inflammation, myalgia, and entrapment syndromes.
- 2% Acetic acid administered under the negative pole to dissolve calcium deposits.
- 2% Lithium chloride or lithium carbonate administered under the positive pole to dissolve gouty tophi. In both acetic acid and lithium iontophoresis, the insoluble radicals in the deposits are replaced by soluble chemical radicals so the deposits can be broken down through natural processes.

The contraindication to the use of any ion is an allergy to that ion. Because most clients will not have had iontophoresis previously, it is important to inquire about experiences that might indicate an allergy. For example, intolerance to shellfish may be the result of an allergy to iodine, and a poor reaction to dental local anesthesia may indicate a problem with lidocaine.

Massage

Massage has been recognized as a remedy for pain for at least 3000 years. Evidence of its beneficial effects first appeared in ancient Chinese literature, and then in the writings of the Hindus, Persians, Egyptians, and Greeks. Hippocrates advocated massage for sprains and dislocations as well as for constipation.[69]

Massage decreases pain through both direct and indirect means. Massage movements increase circulation through mechanical compression of the tissues, resulting in reflex relaxation of muscle tissue and direct relief from ischemic pain. Massage also indirectly stimulates A-delta and A-beta fibers, causing activation of the gating mechanism and the descending pain modulating system.[124]

Massage movements are classified by pressure and the part of the hand that is used.[127] Stroking involves running the entire hand over large portions of the body. Stroking causes muscle relaxation and elimination of muscle spasm or improved circulation depending on the depth and force of the strokes. Compression is applied with intermittent pressure using lifting, rolling, or pressing movements meant to stretch shortened tissues, loosen adhesions, and assist with circulation. Friction massage is performed by using the fingertips to perform circulatory cross-fiber movements that break up adhesions. Percussion is performed to stimulate circulation. Hacking involves using the ulnar border of the hand or the fingers to perform a series of brisk, rapid, alternating contacts with the skin. Clapping is done with the palms flat, whereas cupping is done with the palm formed into a concave surface.

Massage is useful in any condition where pain relief will follow the reduction of swelling or the mobilization of the tissues. These include arthritis, bursitis, neuritis, fibrositis, low-back pain, hemiplegia, paraplegia, quadriplegia, and joint sprains, strains, and contusions. Massage is contraindicated over infected areas, diseased skin, and thrombophlebitic regions.

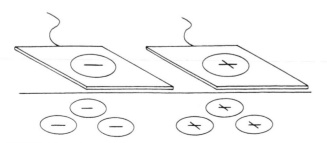

FIGURE 29–7. Iontophoresis. Chemical ions are driven into the tissues by a small electrical current. Once subcutaneous, they are immediately free to take part in chemical reactions within the body.

Clients or caregivers can be taught how and when to perform massage. Once they demonstrate independence in the appropriate technique, responsibility for the performance of massage should be given to the client or caregiver. Health care dollars should not be used if massage is the primary intervention.

Myofascial Release

Fascia is connective tissue that plays a supportive role within the body. It forms an uninterrupted framework around the viscera, stabilizes articulations, provides a constantly fluctuating biochemical equilibrium to assist in the maintenance of homeostasis in the surrounding tissues, and, in conjunction with muscle activity, assists in the movement of blood and lymph. Fascia contains sensory nerves and tension bands of varying thickness.[53]

Ideally, the fascial system is in constant three-dimensional motion: right to left, side to side, and front to back.[53] Under abnormal physical and chemical conditions, such as faulty muscle activity, alteration in the position or relationship of the bones, altered vertebral mechanics, or unnatural postures, the fascial connective tissue can thicken and shorten, creating hypomobile areas with increased tension[117] that can, because the fascia represents one continuous system, affect movement in remote areas of the body by restricting motion of that fascia. Because the fascia contains sensory nerves, areas of increased tension, sudden tension, or traction are painful.[53]

Myofascial release (MFR) techniques are used to release the built-in imbalances and restrictions within the fascia and to reintegrate the fascial mechanism. The therapist palpates the various tissue layers, beginning with the most superficial and working systematically toward the deepest, looking for movement restrictions and asymmetry. Areas of altered structure and function are then "normalized" through the systematic application of pressure and stretching applied in specific directions to bring about decreased myofascial tension, myofascial lengthening, and myofascial softening,[117] thereby restoring pain-free motion in normal patterns of movement. MFR is useful in treating musculoskeletal injuries, chronic pain, headaches, and adhesions/adherent scars.[3]

MFR is contraindicated over areas with infection, diseased skin, thromboembolus, cellulitis, osteomyelitis, and open wounds. In addition, it should not be used with clients who have osteoporosis, advanced degenerative changes, acute circulatory conditions, acute joint pathology, advanced diabetes, obstructive edema, or hypersensitive skin.[3] (See Chapter 33 for more in-depth information regarding MFR.)

Joint Mobilization

There are two forms of movement available to each joint: physiological movement and accessory movement. Physiological movement is the gross ROM (defined as flexion, extension, and rotation). Accessory movement is the fine motion that occurs between the surfaces of the opposing bones (defined as distraction, slide, glide, and tilt). Physiological movement can be performed by the individual's muscles; accessory movement requires the application of external force.

Normal accessory movement is necessary for normal physiological movement. When the collagen fibers of the joint capsule become thickened or bound down, accessory movements become restricted, preventing full ROM. Because the joint capsule is richly innervated, pain is produced when the soft tissue structures are stretched in an attempt to produce full gross movement.[100]

Joint mobilization consists of passive oscillations that allow the collagen fibers to rearrange and loosen, thereby restoring normal accessory movements.[100] In addition, the rhythmical repetition of the motions provides pain relief through the spinal gating mechanism.[83]

The oscillations involved in joint mobilization are graded as follows.[76]:

Grade I: small-amplitude movements performed at the beginning of the available ROM

Grade II: larger-amplitude movements performed farther into the available ROM

Grade III: large-amplitude movements performed at the end of the available ROM

Grade IV: small-amplitude movements performed at the end of the available ROM

Grade V: high-velocity thrust (manipulation) performed at the end of the available ROM

Grades I and II oscillations are performed to maintain joint mobility and for pain relief, making them the choice for subacute conditions where pain and potential loss of motion are the primary considerations. Grades III and IV oscillations are performed to increase joint mobility and are indicated for chronic conditions where regaining lost motion is the goal. Grade V thrusts are performed to regain full joint mobility.[100]

Joint mobilization is contraindicated with rheumatoid arthritis, bone disease, advanced osteoporosis, and pregnancy (pelvic mobilization), as well as in the presence of malignancy, vascular disease, or infection in the area to be mobilized.[74]

Joint mobilization is covered in Chapter 11 of the third edition of Gould's *Orthopaedic and Sports Physical Therapy* as well as in several excellent texts addressing musculoskeletal disorders.

Therapeutic Touch

Eastern philosophy views human life as one of the many energy forces that coexist and interact with each other within the universe. Ancient Sanskrit writings equate health and illness with energy called "prana." According to the writings, health represents an overabundance of prana and illness represents a deficit. One person can heal another by activating their personal prana and transferring it to another at will. Healing through energy exchange is also recorded in the hieroglyphics, cuneiform writings, and pictographs of the earliest literate cultures.[67]

Western philosophy has been slow to accept the view of humanity as interconnected with the universe, preferring, instead, to view us as a distinct entity. However, the treatment technique of therapeutic touch (along with the supporting research) has done much to change the view of Western clinicians.

Basic to therapeutic touch is the concept that the healthy human body has an excess of energy, which can be shared with another for the purpose of healing. The healer serves as a conduit, directing personal and environmental energy to a client who then internalizes and directs the energy to restore balance and perform self-healing.[68]

During therapeutic touch the healer contacts the client's energy field by slowly scanning the client's body with his or her own hands. It is not necessary to touch the client to perceive areas of accumulated tension. When tension is encountered, the healer slowly moves his or her hands over the area to redirect the accumulated energy.

Therapeutic touch results first in an energy transfer from the healer to the client, then in a repatterning of the client's energy state.[62] Clients report a subjective sense of heat in the diseased/painful area followed by an overall sense of well-being and relaxation.

Kreiger,[67] who first described and taught therapeutic touch, conducted research on clients receiving the treatment. She compared the posttreatment hemoglobin values in clients receiving therapeutic touch with clients who had been scanned by individuals who let their minds wander. The results were startling. In three different studies clients receiving therapeutic touch showed higher mean hemoglobin values after treatment than did clients who received placebo treatments. In other studies involving plant growth, plants watered with water treated with therapeutic touch grew larger and faster than plants watered with untreated water. Kreiger's research has shown that the technique is effective even if the client does not believe in therapeutic touch, as long as the healer has faith in the technique and is intent on helping the patient heal.

Therapeutic touch has been effective in treating painful conditions resulting from anxiety and tension. Ninety percent of individuals treated with therapeutic touch experienced tension headache relief, and 70% had continued relief for more than 4 hours; only 37% of the placebo group expressed sustained relief.[62]

Although therapeutic touch as well as other approaches are being more widely accepted, the therapist must continue to be diligent in using outcome studies to substantiate the use of any complementary therapy. (See Chapter 33 for additional information.)

Point Stimulation

The ancient Chinese were the first to become aware of acupuncture points, which are areas of the skin that become sensitive with internal disease states. Over time they mapped out imaginary lines connecting the points with each other. They believed that energy and nutrients flowed to all parts of the body along these "meridians" and that, when there is disease, the energy flow is interrupted. The most effective sites for treatment, they reasoned, are the acupuncture points.[112]

It is interesting to note that acupuncture points frequently correspond in location to trigger points, which are tight, elevated bands of tissue that are extremely sensitive when palpated and have a characteristic pattern of radiation to remote regions of the body. Trigger points appear to be areas of "focal irritability" that are myofascial in origin and are usually the site of small aggregations of nerve fibers that produce continuous afferent input when stimulated.

Needling of acupuncture points stimulates the release of endorphins,[112] most probably through the central modulating pathway that originates in the periaqueductal gray matter.[111] Acupressure (i.e., finger pressure applied to acupuncture or trigger points) is thought to decrease their sensitivity through the same mechanism. The therapist applies deep pressure in a circular motion to each point for 1 to 5 minutes, until the sensitivity subsides. Pressure must be applied directly to each point for the treatment to be effective. Acupressure can be accompanied by the use of a vapocoolant spray to provide additional sensory stimulation.

Sensitive points also can be stimulated using electricity. A point locator is used to identify points along the appropriate meridians that are sensitive to stimulation or more conductive to electricity. Each is then stimulated at the client's level of pain tolerance for 30 to 45 seconds. The points farthest from the site of pain are treated first.

Points that are most sensitive to stimulation are beneficial sites for TENS electrode placement. When point stimulation alone does not provide sufficient pain relief, TENS can be used between sessions for continuous stimulation for more prolonged relief. (See Chapter 33 for additional information on electrical acupuncture.)

Cognitive Strategies

The extent to which an individual perceives and expresses pain is a result of his or her emotional state, expectations, personality, and cognitive view. Each individual feels and responds to pain differently. Melzak and Wall[83] identified three nonphysical components to pain that interact and determine how an individual will respond to pain:

(1) the individual's sensory/discriminative interpretation of the pain,
(2) the individual's motivation and attitudes relating to the pain, and
(3) the individual's cognitive/evaluative thoughts and beliefs concerning the pain experience.

Cognitive strategies are part of a wholistic approach to health that looks at the total person and the interaction between the three components of body, mind, and spirit. Cognitive strategies recognize that the mind is not separate from the body, accept that there is a mental component to pain, and utilize the inner resources of the mind to influence the pain experience.

Cognitive strategies work in two ways. First, they activate the descending cortical modulating systems and, second, they teach the individual to control, rather than be controlled by, the pain. Used in conjunction with other modalities necessary for physical relief, these approaches can play a significant role in long-term pain management and should not be overlooked when seeking a viable pain management alternative.

Relaxation Exercises

People who are in pain experience stress. Chronic stress can trigger increased pain. Both pain and stress cause an increase in sympathetic nervous system (SNS) activity, including increased muscle tension. Relaxation exercises can bring about muscle relaxation and a generalized parasympathetic response.[57] Benson[6] has named this effect the relaxation response and reports that it is accompanied by an increase in alpha brain waves.

Relaxation reduces ischemic pain by normalizing blood flow to the muscles by making way for more oxygen to be delivered to the tissues. In addition, relaxation reduces muscle tension, resulting in an interruption in the pain spasm cycle.[24]

Relaxation exercises all have two elements in common: a single focus and a passive attitude toward intruding thoughts and distractions. The end product of relaxation is a lowered arousal of the SNS and a lessening of the symptoms caused by or worsened by stress.[16]

Deep relaxation can be achieved through progressive relaxation and attention-diversion exercises. Progressive relaxation involves alternately tensing and relaxing the muscles until, eventually, the entire body is relaxed. This activity teaches the individual how to recognize and relieve muscle tension within the body.

Attention diversion is an active process in which the individual directs his or her attention to nonnoxious events or stimuli in the immediate environment to achieve distraction from the pain. Attention diversion is defined as passive or active. Passive attention diversion includes meditation and involves concentrating on a visual or auditory stimulus rather than the painful sensation, whereas active attention diversion involves active participation in a task (e.g., serial subtraction).

Meditation involves quieting the mind and focusing the attention on a thought, word, phrase, object, or movement. The individual becomes more alert to the constant stream of conversation taking place within the mind. Meditation calms the body through the relaxation response and keeps the attention focused in the present moment. Individuals in Eastern cultures have traditionally focused on a mantra, a word with spiritual meaning; however, there are no rules for where to focus the attention. The word or object should bring the individual a sense of peace and allow the attention to be pleasantly directed toward the immediate moment.

Imagery is another form of attention diversion. During imagery the individual uses his or her imagination to produce images with pain weakening potential. This can take two forms. In one, the individual imagines experiences that are inconsistent with the pain (e.g., imagining rolling in snow to alleviate burning pain). In the other, the individual imagines experiences that modify specific features of the pain experience (e.g., imagining that the pain is the result of a sports injury or that the sensation is "numbness" rather than pain).

Attention diversion works by activating the relaxation response and by diverting the individual's attention from the pain. However, attention diversion has also been found to activate the higher brain centers and may have an inhibitory effect on pain through the spinal gating mechanisms.[36, 83] Lauterbacher and colleagues[70] found that individuals who utilized attention diversion for pain management reported decreased intensity and unpleasantness of their pain.

Clients can be taught to perform relaxation exercises independently and should be encouraged to perform them regularly because the benefits of these exercises are gained through regular practice.

Body Scanning

Clients with chronic pain frequently become one with their suffering; they do not view themselves as individuals with pain, but, rather, as painful individuals. Body scanning is a technique that endeavors to separate the individual from the pain.[59]

During body scanning the client is taught to achieve a meditative state, then focus attention on each body area, one area at a time. The client is instructed to breathe into and out from each area, relaxing more deeply with each exhalation. When the area is completely relaxed, the client "lets go" of the region and dwells in the stillness for a few breaths before continuing. Painful areas are scanned in an identical manner as nonpainful areas. The client notes, but does not judge, changes in sensation, thoughts, and emotions during scanning of each area.

Individuals who practice this technique report new levels of insight and understanding concerning their pain experience. They separate the pain experience into three parts[59]:

1. An awareness of the pain sensation and their thoughts and feelings about it.
2. An awareness of a separation between the pain sensation and their thoughts and feelings about it.
3. An awareness of a separation between themselves and their pain because they are able to objectively examine the sensation and their thoughts and feelings about it.

Once clients accept that they are not their pain or their reaction to the pain, they can determine how much influence and control pain will have in their lives.

Studies of chronic pain patients at the Stress Reduction Clinic at the University of Massachusetts Medical Center revealed that 72% of patients who used body scanning along with traditional medical interventions experienced at least a 33% reduction on their McGill-Melzak Pain Rating Index.[59] In addition, at the end of an 8-week training period, the individuals perceived their bodies in a more positive light, experienced an increase in positive mood states, and reported major improvements in anxiety, depression, hostility, and the tendency to be overly occupied with their bodily sensations.

Humor

Ever since Cousins reported in his book *Anatomy of an Illness* that he used humor to manage pain and enhance sleep during his illness, the role of humor in healing has been well studied.[27] Humor has been found beneficial for both acute and chronic pain management.[17, 73]

Laughter increases blood oxygen content by increasing ventilation. It helps to exercise the heart muscle by speeding up the heart rate and enhancing arterial and venous circulation, resulting in more oxygen and nutrients being delivered to the tissues.[42] Laughter decreases serum cortisol levels (cortisol levels increase with stress and are thought to have a negative effect on the immune response)[9, 10] and increases the concentration of circulating antibodies.[42] As little as 10 minutes of belly laughter a day has been found to decrease the erythrocyte sedimentation rate and provide 2 hours of pain-free sleep.[27] Finally, laughter releases energy and emotional tension and is followed by generalized muscle relaxation.[41, 42]

Therapeutic humor can be used to provide distraction from pain and as a coping mechanism to decrease the anxiety and tension associated with chronic pain. The muscle relaxing effect can be used to interrupt the pain-spasm cycle.

Therapeutic humor should not be used with individuals who do poorly with humor. This includes individuals who despise or misunderstand humor, individuals who find joy threatening or guilt inducing, and narcoleptic individuals who become cataleptic with laughter.[26]

Very few clients will benefit from all of these cognitive strategies, and it may take some trial and error to find the appropriate congitive strategy for an individual client. Some clients will have no difficulty learning and practicing cognitive strategies, whereas others will not be able to perform any of these techniques independently. It may be beneficial to provide the client with an individualized relaxation tape or to have the client repeat coping affirmations over and over throughout the day. The success of cognitive strategies is dependent on applying the appropriate strategy to the appropriate client and fine-tuning the strategy so that it matches the client's needs.

In conclusion, it is important to reemphasize that all individuals with chronic pain have some degree of emotional and/or congitive involvement in their pain experience. Many clients will live with pain regardless of any treatment they receive. Therefore, it is imperative for health care practitioners to address the emotional and cognitive components of each client's pain to allow him or her to function at the highest level and as comfortably as possible and to find joy in each day.

Behavioral Manipulations

Exercise

Deconditioning is a major source of disability with chronic pain. Pain causes an intolerance for activity, which in turn leads to physiological and pathological changes in the organ systems. Exercise improves overall functional performance by improving range of motion, muscle strength, neuromuscular control, coordination, and aerobic capacity.

All three types of exercise are beneficial for pain management. ROM and stretching exercises restore normal joint mobility and correct muscle tightness. The joints are held in normal alignment and are subjected to normal stresses during movement. ROM and stretching exercises are indicated where there is decreased mobility.

Strengthening exercises increase muscle strength and cardiovascular endurance. When performed with high intensity for a short duration, strengthening exercises result in increased muscle mass, improved neuromuscular con-

trol, and improved coordination. When performed at low intensity for a long duration, they increase aerobic capacity of the muscles.

Aerobic exercises improve cardiovascular fitness. More oxygen is supplied to the tissues because there is an increase in the number and size of capillaries and a decrease in the diffusion distance between the capillaries and the muscles. The tissues use oxygen more efficiently, and the individual has a higher energy level.

All exercise has an analgesic effect through the gating mechanism by stimulation of the A-delta neurons and a pain-modulating effect through activation of the descending systems.

It is important to include exercise in all pain management programs. Clients should be taught the appropriate exercises beginning with the first treatment session and encouraged to perform the exercises consistently when not at therapy.

Operant Conditioning

Coping strategies are learned. Individuals with chronic pain express their pain with behaviors that provide them with consistent positive rewards. For example, wincing might result in attention from a family member or limping might allow the individual to avoid performing a particular task. Over time, the individual with pain becomes conditioned to perform certain behaviors for the behavior's rewards rather than as a reaction to the pain. Similarly, individuals with chronic pain also can condition their nervous systems through learning. If an individual expects to experience pain as the result of a particular level of activity, the individual will always experience pain at that level of activity.

Operant conditioning addresses the learned (or conditioned) aspects of pain.[39] Operant conditioning involves unlearning or separating the behavior and the response from the pain experience. If the goal of treatment is to lessen social reinforcement of the client's pain behaviors (and thus extinguish those behaviors), the client and the family or other involved individuals are shown how their behaviors and responses provide social reinforcement for the client's reaction to pain. The involved individuals are provided with specific new responses to the client's behavior. Family members might be instructed to ignore wincing, groaning, or the verbal report of pain. They might be told not to perform activities that are the client's responsibility just because the client reports pain. In time, the client will become conditioned to the new response, and pain in those situations will diminish.

If the goal of treatment is to increase the client's pain-free activity level, operant conditioning can be utilized to condition the nervous system to a higher level of activity before responding with pain. If the client's usual pattern is to remain active until the onset of pain (negative reinforcement for activity) and then rest (positive reinforcement for pain), the client is instructed to remain active to just below the pain threshold and then rest (positive reinforcement for activity). In this way the nervous system unlearns the connection between activity and pain, and the client's activity level increases.

Hypnosis

Hypnosis is a state in which the body and conscious mind are deeply relaxed while the subconscious mind remains alert, focused, and open to suggestion.[16] This has been demonstrated physiologically by electroencephalography, which shows an increase in the number of theta waves, which are associated with enhanced attention.[20] When a hypnotized individual is given a suggestion that is in alignment with his or her existing belief system, it is accepted by the subconscious mind as reality. The suggestion is not filtered through the conscious mind, which is critical and judgmental. Hypnosis allows the individual to bypass his or her critical beliefs.[43] For example, if the individual believes that a certain activity will cause pain (critical belief), that activity is sure to cause pain. If, however, during hypnosis, the individual accepts the suggestion that the activity does not cause pain, it will no longer cause pain.

When hypnosis is used for pain management, a client is first assisted to achieve complete relaxation, then given suggestions that reinterpret the pain experience. For example, a client might be guided to reframe the pain into a messenger and then be encouraged to listen to its message to gain understanding of the meaning behind the pain. Or a client might be guided to view the pain as an indication to stop a particular activity to avoid being injured. Or a client might be instructed to feel less pain. Finally, where harmless activities have become painful through learning, the client can be guided to disconnect the activity from his or her pain.

Biofeedback

Biofeedback is a training process in which the client becomes aware of and learns to selectively change physiological processes with the aid of an external monitor. A monitoring instrument is placed on the appropriate area of the body. The machine provides an initial readout. The client is instructed how to change the monitored process, and as change occurs the machine "feeds back" that information. By mentally changing a biological function, the client learns to gain control over it. In time, the client learns to control the process without needing an assist from the instrument.

Muscle tension, pulse rate, blood pressure, skin temperature, and electromyography (EMG) and electroencephalography (EEG) readings are some of the physiological processes that can be consciously modified with biofeedback.[57]

Biofeedback is proving to be an effective pain management tool for headaches, muscle spasms, and other physical dysfunction that lead to or increase chronic pain (see Chapters 28 and 33).

GENERAL TREATMENT GUIDELINES

As noted earlier, chronic pain management using the medical model has not been found effective. Treatment limited to correcting pathology promotes dependence on the therapist, as well as making full resolution of symptoms the measure of success.

The disablement model addresses the functional losses associated with impairments. Therapeutic interventions are not focused on pathology, but they are directed at improving the individual's function and preventing or improving disability. This does not mean that the impairment is ignored, however. Most times, addressing the individual's functional losses involves treating the impairments that caused them.

For example, clients with chronic pain frequently become sedentary, leading to the impairments of limited ROM, muscle weakness, and deconditioning. These factors can then, of themselves, cause pain, creating a cycle that spirals upward until the individual becomes disabled. During therapy, interventions are directed at the impairments with the goal of restoring function. Therapeutic interventions are selected based on their ability to improve functional outcome. Impairments that do not affect function do not become the focus of therapy; therapeutic interventions that do not address functional deficits are not utilized.

The development of an appropriate treatment plan may seem overwhelming when confronted with a client who has chronic pain that has not responded to previous interventions or who has a chronic condition that has pain as one of its characteristics. The key is to identify the client's functional deficits and then develop a treatment plan that addresses the causes of those deficits. In some cases this may mean not treating the pain itself but, rather, its causative factors.

For example, if the client has chronic pain because of joint hypomobility, the treatment plan includes interventions to increase joint mobility. Conversely, if the client's pain is due to joint hypermobility, the treatment plan includes interventions to increase support around the hypermobile joints. Merely addressing the joint pain by applying modalities will do little to resolve the pain because it does nothing to correct the precipitating cause.

When a client has pain because of a chronic disease and the treatment plan will include instruction in pain-relieving interventions, it is important for the therapist to understand the specific causes of the pain to select the appropriate intervention. For example, pain from rheumatoid arthritis most commonly is the result of either joint inflammation or biomechanical stress on unstable joints. A client would be instructed in pain-relieving modalities for the former and instructed to wear splints to support the joints for the latter. One intervention would not be appropriate for both causes.

CASE STUDIES

The following case studies demonstrate a problem-solving approach to the treatment of clients with chronic pain.

CASE 29–1 ● FIBROMYALGIA

K.E. is a 35-year-old computer programmer with a diagnosis of fibromyalgia. She reports a 6-month history of generalized muscular pain and fatigue that increase when she performs repetitive motions or holds a position for a prolonged period of time. K.E. is currently unable to work because she is no longer able to perform data entry without increased neck and shoulder pain. She states she awakens from pain and leg cramps several times during the night. She awakens each morning with a headache and low back pain; she does not get much relief from pain medication. K.E. states she has not been out with friends in several months. She states she is "nervous, unable to concentrate, and depressed." She has been evaluated by several physicians. All medical tests are negative.

K.E.'s objective examination reveals pain with digital palpation to distinct points in the muscles of her neck and shoulder girdles, over both lateral epicondyles and greater trochanters, in her gluteal muscles, and just above the medial joint lines of the knees. Pain is referred from the tender points distally. K.E. sits and stands with a forward head and elevated protracted shoulders, and her cervical ROM is restricted slightly at end range because of her posture and muscle guarding. Muscle strength is 4/5 throughout. All other musculoskeletal and neurological tests are normal.

K.E. presents with the impairments of pain, poor posture, decreased cervical and shoulder ROM, and decreased endurance, resulting in the disabilities of interrupted sleep, decreased tolerance for activity, and the inability to work at her profession.

The long-term goals of treatment for K.E. are independence with self-management of pain, normalization of posture, restoration of normal sleep, independence with a home exercise program, and return to work and appropriate social activities. The short-term goals include decreasing K.E.'s pain, proper sleep positioning, correcting her postural abnormalities, improving her limited endurance, and assessing/correcting the ergonomics of her workstation. K.E. also needs intervention to address the emotional and cognitive aspects of her condition.

The lowered pain threshold and magnified pain perception seen with fibromyalgia results from a complex combination of muscle tissue microtrauma, neuroendocrine abnormalities, and changes in the levels of CNS neurotransmitters. The muscles of individuals with fibromyalgia show abnormal energy metabolism, poor tissue oxygenation, and localized hypoxia. Their blood shows decreased levels of the inhibitory neurotransmitter serotonin and increased levels of the facilitory neurotransmitter substance P. This combination, which is unique to fibromyalgia, is thought to cause changes in the dorsal horn neurons and, eventually, in the areas of the brain responsible for the sensory-discriminative and affective-motivational aspects of pain.[119]

Fibromyalgia pain has been shown to respond favorably to interventions that work through the gating mechanism. These include sensory level TENS, light massage, muscle warming, and gentle stretching. K.E. can be taught to apply localized heat or to take a warm bath before gentle stretching of her tight muscles. She should be cautioned to stretch slowly to the point of resistance and to hold the stretch for 60 seconds to allow the Golgi tendon organs time to signal the muscle fibers to relax. Quick stretching to the point of pain will cause increased tightness and pain through the pain-spasm cycle. It is important for K.E. to understand that these measures address the pain of fibromyalgia but do not have any long-term effect on the course of her condition.

Individuals with fibromyalgia, and most individuals with chronic pain, experience a variety of emotions, including depression, anger, fear, withdrawal, and anxiety.[5] These individuals have been helped with hypnosis, biofeedback, and cognitive restructing.[5, 119] In addition to giving them a sense of control over their pain, these interventions are known to bring about an increase in the individual's level of endogenous opiates, thereby activating one of the descending pain modulation systems. K.E. can be taught to perform these techniques independently.

K.E. should be asked to demonstrate her sleeping posture. Because the muscles of individuals with fibromyalgia do not relax easily, K.E. should be shown how to use pillows to support her neck and back so that they are encouraged to relax while she sleeps. This will help to decrease the frequency of morning headaches and back pain and help her to sleep through the night. She might also benefit from a warm bath before going to bed.

K.E.'s therapist can use gentle MFR to help correct the biomechanical imbalances causing her poor posture. K.E. can then be taught to selectively stretch the shortened muscles of her neck and shoulder girdles using the technique already described and to selectively strengthen their weakened antagonists using light resistance. To counter deconditioning, K.E. should be placed on a nonimpact aerobic program (walking, pool exercises, or stationary bicycle) with a goal of 30 minutes three to four times a week at 70% max heart rate (220 minus her age). If she is unable to tolerate 30 minutes of exercise at one time, she can be started

Continued

CASE 29–1 FIBROMYALGIA *Continued*

at 3 to 5 minutes twice or three times daily and gradually progressed to three sessions of 10 minutes, then two sessions of 15 minutes, and finally one session of 30 minutes. K.E. may require a significant amount of coaxing and education to motivate her to participate in exercise; many individuals with fibromyalgia do not wish to move because movement initially increases their pain.

Before she returns to work, K.E. should be assisted with the ergonomics of her workstation. Research[101] has shown that individuals who work at computers need to vary their positions throughout the day even if their sitting posture is appropriate. Further research[1, 47, 92] has shown that correct mouse placement is important to minimize stress to the arms and shoulders.

CASE 29–2 PHANTOM LIMB PAIN

A.R. is a 60-year-old carpenter who underwent below-knee amputation of his right leg 4 weeks ago after a motor vehicle accident. He now reports a constant burning, piercing, throbbing sensation in the distal portion of his missing limb. He states that immediately after the amputation he was aware of an itching or tickling in the missing portion of the leg, but the sensation gradually changed to pain. He notes that the leg feels as if it is shortening, as if the missing foot is moving closer and closer to his hip. A.R. has been fitted with a shrinker but does not wear it because of fear of increasing the pain. He does not believe he will be able to wear a prosthesis and is concerned because his employer will be unable to find work for him if he is wheelchair bound.

A.R.'s objective examination reveals a healing surgical incision and a poorly shaped stump. Right lower-extremily hip and knee strength are 3/5 and 2+/5, respectively. Sensation for light touch is diminished in the area of the incision. All other musculoskeletal and neurological tests are normal. A.R. ambulates short distances using a walker but relies on a wheelchair for locomotion outside his home.

A.R. presents with the impairments of a below-knee amputation, phantom limb pain, and decreased strength in the right lower extremity, resulting in the disabilities of inability to prepare his leg for a prosthesis, inability to ambulate, and inability to work in his profession.

The long-term goals of treatment for A.R. are independent use of a prosthesis and return to work with modified job tasks. The short-term goals include resolution of his phantom limb pain, preparation of his stump for a prosthesis, at least 4/5 right hip and knee strength, and, when appropriate, gait and balance training with the prosthesis.

There are two theories of the cause for phantom limb pain. At one time it was thought that phantom limb pain occurred as the result of the formation of a terminal neuroma at the site of the amputation[35]; however, this theory did not explain phantom phenomena in individuals with congenital amputations or individuals with complete spinal cord injuries who also experience painful and nonpainful sensations in their missing or anesthetic limbs. This led researchers to look at the role of the CNS in phantom phenomena, and the latest theories suggest the previously described changes in the dorsal horn neurons[31] and changes in the spinal cord caused by the sudden loss of afferent impulses after amputation.[50]

These theories are supported by the effectiveness of interventions that stimulate the large nerve fibers and provide inhibitory input through the gating mechanism. Phantom limb pain is relieved by stroking, vibration, TENS, ultrasound, heat applications, and the use of a prosthesis. A.R. can be taught a progressive desensitization program. He should be encouraged to wear the shrinker both to prepare his stump for a prosthesis and to decrease pain. Because phantom limb pain is adversely affected by emotional stress, exposure to cold, and local irritants, he should be taught to avoid these factors as much as possible.

A.R.'s adjustment to a changed body image, a changed lifestyle, and the use of a prosthesis can be aided with any of the cognitive strategies described previously. He might also benefit from referral to an amputee support group.

It is important for A.R. to be aware of his abilities and limitations so that he remains safe when he returns to work. If appropriate, the therapist should accompany A.R. to his job and perform a job task analysis, making suggestions for necessary modifications. If this is not possible, the therapist could discuss needed modifications with A.R. based on his descriptions of his job tasks.

CASE 29–3 COMPLEX REGIONAL PAIN SYNDROME

P.S. is a 45-year-old right-handed secretary who sustained a Colles fracture of the right wrist 6 months ago. The wrist was placed in a cast for 6 weeks, during which time P.S. avoided using the extremity. Two weeks after the cast was removed, P.S. developed pain, swelling, and stiffness in the wrist and hand. She returned to her physician who diagnosed CRPS type I. She has received four sympathetic nerve blockades. The first provided 4 weeks of pain relief. The second and third provided 2 weeks of relief each. She has just received her fourth injection along with a referral for therapy.

P.S. is wearing a sling. She presents with 30-degree flexion contractures of her right fingers, along with swelling and stiffness of the wrist and hand. Her right wrist, elbow, and shoulder show limited motion as well. P.S. describes constant burning pain that becomes worse with any stimulation, even air blowing over the skin. She rates her pain as 4/10 since the block, but she states the pain had slowly been escalating toward 10/10 before the injection. Her hand and wrist are cool, and the skin appears mottled and shiny. P.S. states she is not using her arm and needs assistance at home for activities of daily living and homemaking chores.

P.S. presents with the impairments of pain, swelling, stiffness, and decreased ROM of the right wrist and hand resulting in the disabilities of decreased ability to use the right upper extremity for functional activities including activities of daily living, job tasks, and homemaking activities. In addition, because she is not using the extremity and carries the arm in a sling, P.S. is at risk for developing shoulder-hand syndrome.

The long-term goal of treatment for P.S. is restoration of pain-free use of her right upper extremity. The short-term goals include quieting the SNS, decreasing P.S.'s pain and edema, and restoring normal ROM of the shoulder, elbow, wrist, and hand.

Successful treatment of CRPS involves a coordinated effort by the physician and the therapist. The treatment of choice is interruption of sympathetic activity with nerve blocks and therapy.[52]

Interventions included in a pain management program for CRPS should be chosen for their ability to quiet the SNS as well as accomplish the desired outcome. For example, thermotherapy is more beneficial than cryotherapy because of its ability to decrease pain without stimulating a sympathetic response.[52]

A successful rehabilitation program for CRPS cannot be limited to therapy visits. Clients need to be instructed in interventions that they then perform three, four, or even five times daily. Therefore, the therapist needs to become a guide with the responsibility for performing the pain management program given over to the client or caregiver.

Pain reduction is the first priority. This can be accomplished through the gating mechanism or through the deployment of endogenous opiates. Thermotherapy and TENS have both been found effective for pain management with CRPS. If P.S. cannot tolerate electrode placement on the right arm, the electrodes can be placed on the opposite arm or along the spinal roots of the involved segments.[60, 77] P.S. can be instructed in any of the superficial heating modalities. Stroking massage along the paravertebral muscles beginning in the cervical region and continuing to the coccyx has also been found effective in quieting the SNS.

Before P.S. can regain mobility of her wrist and fingers, the edema must be resolved. This can be accomplished with elevation, massage, and compression. P.S. can wear a compression glove or, if she is able to tolerate it, receive intermittent compression to the arm. She should be instructed to keep the arm above heart level as much as possible.

P.S. should be advised to discontinue use of the sling and begin frequent weight bearing through her arm. Immobility increases the symptoms of CRPS. Movement of the extremity is important to increase proprioception and circulation, both of which have an inhibitory effect on the SNS.[52] Therefore, P.S. should be encouraged to begin using her hand as much as possible throughout the day. If she is reluctant to use the arm, the therapist can design a functional activity program that allows her to use the arm during simple activities, which can be progressed as her symptoms improve.

There are two forms of exercise that are beneficial with CRPS. The first is active ROM, which should be performed frequently throughout the day within the pain-free range to regain motion, increase circulation, and provide nonnociceptive input. The second is stress loading,[118] which involves active compression and traction activities without joint motion. For example, P.S. can use a coarse bristled brush to scrub a piece of plywood and apply as much pressure as possible without causing pain (compression activity). Or she can carry a briefcase or purse in her affected hand (traction activity). Compression and traction both provide increased proprioceptive input.

P.S. should also begin performing desensitization activities, which can be modified as she is able to tolerate more stimulation to her extremity. P.S. may benefit from biofeedback to gain control over the circulation in her arm and from relaxation activities to stimulate the relaxation response and enhance parasympathetic function.

Once P.S. becomes independent in the performance of her program, therapy can be decreased to once or twice weekly to monitor and modify her pain management regimen.

REFERENCES

1. Albin T: To tell the truth. Phys Ther Products, May-June:68–71, 1999.
2. American Pain Society: The Facts on Intractable Pain. Skokie, IL, American Pain Society, 1994.
3. Barnes J: MFR: A Comprehensive Evaluatory and Treatment Approach. MFR Seminars, Paoli, PA, 1990.
4. Basbaum AI, Fields HL: Endogenous pain control systems: Brainstem spinal pathways and endorphin circuitry. Annu Rev Neurosci 7:309–338, 1984.
5. Bennett R: Principles of treating fibromyalgia. http://www.myalgia.com/overview.htm.
6. Benson H: The Relaxation Response. New York, Avon Books, 1975.
7. Benson TB, Copp EP: The effects of therapeutic forms of heat and ice on the pain threshold of the normal shoulder. Rheumatol Rehabil 13:101–104, 1974.
8. Berger JN, Katz RL: Sympathetically maintained pain. In Ashburn MA (ed): The Management of Pain. New York, Churchill Livingstone, 1998.
9. Berk LS: Modulation of human natural cells by catecholamines. Clin Res 2(1):115, 1984.
10. Berk L, Tau S: Neuroendocrine influences of mirthful laughter. Am J Med Sci 298:390–396, 1989.
11. Bieri D, et al: The faces pain scale for the self-assessment of the severity of pain experienced by children: Development, initial validation, and preliminary investigation for ratio scale properties. Pain 41:139–150, 1990.
12. Bonica JJ: Importance of the problem. In Aronoff GM (ed): Evaluation and Treatment of Chronic Pain. Baltimore, Urban & Schwarzenberg, 1985.
13. Bonica JJ: Cancer pain: A major national health problem. Ca Nurs 1:313, 1978.
14. Bonica JJ: Causalgia and other reflex sympathetic dystrophies. In Bonica JJ, et al (eds): The Management of Pain, 2nd ed. London, Lea & Febiger, 1990.
15. Borsook D, et al: Central pain syndromes. In Ashburn MA (ed): The Management of Pain. New York, Churchill Livingstone, 1998.
16. Borysenko J: Minding the Body, Mending the Mind. Reading, MA, Addison-Wesley Publishing Co, 1987.
17. Bottoroff J, et al: Comforting: Exploring the work of cancer nursing. J Advanced Nurs 22:1077–1084, 1995.
18. Bromage RR: Nerve physiology and control of pain. Orthop Clin North Am 4:897, 1976.
19. Byrne M, et al: Cross-validation of the factor structure of the McGill pain questionnaire. Pain 13:193, 1982.
20. Callahan J: The healing power of hypnosis. http://www.infinityinst.com/articles.nartica.html.
21. Cameron MH: Thermal agents: Physical principles, cool and superficial heat. In Cameron MH (ed): Physical Agents in Rehabilitation. Philadelphia, WB Saunders, 1999.
22. Cameron MH: Ultrasound. In Cameron MH (ed): Physical Agents in Rehabilitation. Philadelphia, WB Saunders, 1999.
23. Cervero F: Persistent Pain. New York, Grune & Stratton, 1983.
24. Chapman SL, Shealy CN: Relaxation techniques to control pain. In Brena SF (ed): Chronic Pain: America's Hidden Epidemic. New York, Atheneum Publishers, 1978.
25. Chastain PB: The effect of deep heat on isometric strength. Phys Ther 58:543–546, 1978.
26. Cohen M: Caring for ourselves can be funny business. Hol Nurs Prac 4(4)1–11, 1990.
27. Cousins N: Anatomy of an Illness. New York, Bantam Books, 1979.
28. Crockford GW, et al: Thermal vasomotor response in human skin mediated by local mechanisms. J Physiol 161:10–15, 1962.
29. Cypress BK: Characteristics of physicians' visits for back symptoms, a national perspective. Am J Public Health 73:389, 1983.
30. Cyriax J: Textbook of Orthopaedic Medicine, 8th ed. London, Bailliere Tindall, 1984.
31. Davis RW: Phantom limb sensation, phantom pain, and stump pain. Arch Phys Med Rehab 74:79–91, 1993.
32. Draper DO, et al: Rate of temperature increase in human muscle during 1 MHz and 3 MHz continuous ultrasound. J Orthop Sport 22(A):142–150, 1995.
33. Dyson M, Suckling J: Stimulation of tissue repair by ultrasound: Survey of the mechanisms involved. Physiotherapy 63:105–108, 1978.
34. Eldred E, et al: The effect of cooling on mammalian muscle spindles. Exp Neurol 2:144, 1960.
35. Evans JH: Neurology and neurological aspects of pain. In Swerdlow M (ed): Relief of Intractable Pain: Monographs in Anesthesiology, vol 1. New York, Excerpta Medica, 1974.
36. Fernandez E: A classification system of cognitive coping strategies for pain. Pain 26:141–151, 1986.
37. Fine PG, Ashburn MA: Functional neuroanatomy and nociception. In Ashburn MA (ed): The Management of Pain. New York, Churchill Livingstone, 1998.
38. Fischer E, Solomon S: Physiological responses to heat and cold. In Licht S (ed): Therapeutic Heat and Cold. Baltimore, Waverly Press, 1972.
39. Fordyce WE: Behavioral Methods for Chronic Pain & Illness. St Louis, CV Mosby, 1976.
40. Fox JJ, Hilton SM: Bradykinin formation in human skin as a factor in heat vasodilation. J Physiol 142:219, 1958.
41. Freud S: Jokes & Their Relation to the Unconscious. Vienna, Deuticke, 1905.
42. Fry WF: The physiological effects of humor, mirth, and laughter. JAMA 267:1857–1858, 1992.
43. Gannon C: 21st Century Medicine and Hypnosis. http://www.infinityinst.com/articles/med&hyp.html.
44. Griffin JE: Physiological effects of ultrasonic energy as it is used clinically. Phys Ther 46:18, 1966.
45. Grubb BD: Peripheral and central mechanisms of pain. Br J Anesth 81:8–11, 1998.
46. Halfers R, et al: Determinants of pain assessments by nurses. Int J Nurs Stud 27:43, 1990.
47. Harvey R, Peper E: Surface electromyography and mouse use position. Ergonomics 40:781–789, 1997.
48. Hauck SL: Pain: Problem for the person with cancer. Ca Nurs 9:66, 1986.
49. Heckman JD, et al: Acceleration of tibial fracture healing by noninvasive, low intensity pulsed ultrasound. J Bone Joint Surg Am 76:26–34, 1994.
50. Hill A: Phantom limb pain: A review of the literature on attributes and potential mechanisms. J Pain Symptom Management 17(2):125–142, 1999.
51. Holmgren E: Increase in pain threshold as a function of conditioning electrical stimulation. Am J Clin Med 3:133, 1975.
52. Hooshmand H: Chronic Pain: Reflex Sympathetic Dystrophy, Prevention and Management. Boca Raton, CRC Press, 1993.
53. Hubbard RP: Mechanical behavior of connective tissue. Handout material from seminar entitled Myofascial Release Concepts, Palpatory and Treatment Skills. East Lansing, MI, September, 1986.
54. Huskisson EC: Measurement of pain. Lancet 2:1127–1131, 1974.
55. Ignelzi RJ, Atkinson JH: Pain and its modulation: I. Afferent mechanisms. Neurosurgery 6:577–583, 1980.
56. Ignelzi RJ, Atkinson JH: Pain and its modulation: II. Efferent mechanisms. Neurosurgery 6:584–590, 1980.
57. Isele FW: Biofeedback and hypnosis in the management of pain. NY State J Med 82:38, 1982.
58. Jacob J: Inflammation revisited: Inflammatory pain and mode of action of analgesics. Agents Actions 2, 1981.
59. Kabat-Zinn J: Full Catastrophic Living. New York, Delacorte Press, 1990.
60. Kahn J: Principles and Practice of Electrotherapy, 3rd ed. New York, Churchill Livingstone, 1992.
61. Kallen B, et al: Delivery outcomes among physiotherapists in Sweden: Is non-ionizing radiation a fetal hazard? Arch Environ Health 37:81–84, 1982.
62. Keller E, Bzdek V: Therapeutic touch and headache, Nurs Res 35:101–105, 1986.
63. Kessler R, Hertling D: Management of Common Musculoskeletal Disorders. Philadelphia, Harper & Row, 1983.
64. Kleinkort JA, Wood AF: Phonophoresis with 1% versus 10% hydrocortisone. Phys Ther 55:1320–1324, 1975.
65. Kremer E, et al: Measurement of pain: Patient preference does not confound pain measurement. Pain 10:241, 1981.
66. Kremer E, et al: Pain measurement: The affective dimensional measure of the McGill pain questionnaire with a cancer pain population. Pain 12:153, 1982.

67. Kreiger D: Therapeutic touch: The imprimatur of nursing. Am J Nurs 75:784–787, 1975.
68. Krieger D, et al: Therapeutic touch: Searching for evidence of physiological change. Am J Nurs 79:660–662, 1979.
69. Krusen F, et al: Handbook of Physical Medicine and Rehabilitation. Philadelphia, WB Saunders, 1971.
70. Lautenbacher S, et al: Attentional control of pain perception: The role of hypochondriasis. J Psychosm Res 44:251–259, 1998.
71. Lehmann JF, DeLaterer BJ: Therapeutic heat. In Lehmann JF (ed): Therapeutic Heat and Cold, 4th ed. Baltimore, Williams & Wilkins, 1990.
72. Lehmann JF, et al: Pain threshold measurements after therapeutic application of ultrasound, microwave and infrared. Arch Phys Med Rehabil 39:560–565, 1958.
73. Leise CM: The correlation between humor and the chronic pain of arthritis. J Hol Nurs 11:82–85, 1993.
74. Linton SJ, Melin L: The accuracy of remembering chronic pain. Pain 13:281, 1982.
75. Long D: The Comparative Efficacy of Drugs vs. Electrical Modulation in the Management of Chronic Pain: Current Concepts in the Management of Chronic Pain. Miami, Symposia Specialists, 1977.
76. Maitland G: Peripheral Manipulation. Ontario, Butterworth & Scarborough, 1976.
77. Mannheimer JS, Lampe GN: Clinical Transcutaneous Electrical Nerve Stimulation. Philadelphia, FA Davis, 1984.
78. Mayer DJM, Price DD: Central nervous system mechanisms of analgesia. Pain 2:379–404, 1976.
79. McGrath PJ, et al: Behaviours caregivers use to determine pain in non-verbal cognitively impaired individuals. Dev Med Child Neurol 40:340–343, 1998.
80. Melzak R: The McGill pain questionnaire: Major properties and scoring methods. Pain 1:277, 1975.
81. Melzak R: Prolonged relief of pain by brief, intense transcutaneous somatic stimulation. Pain 1:357, 1975.
82. Melzak R, Dennis SG: Neurophysiological foundations of pain. In Sternbach RA (ed): The Psychology of Pain. New York, Raven Press, 1978.
83. Melzak R, Wall P: Pain mechanisms: A new theory. Science 150:971, 1969.
84. Mersky H, Bogduk N: Classification of Chronic Pain Syndromes and Definitions of Pain Terms, 2nd ed. Seattle, IASP Press, 1994.
85. Miller MW, Ziskin MC: Biological consequences of hyperthermia. Ultrasound Med Biol 15:707–722, 1989.
86. Myers JS: Cancer pain: Assessment of nurses' knowledge and attitudes. Oncol Nurs Forum 12:62, 1985.
87. Nicolls ML: Transmission of chronic nociception by spinal neurons expressing the substance P receptors. Science 286:1558–1561, 1999.
88. Nolan MF: Anatomic and physiologic organization of the neural structures involved in pain transmission, modulation and perception. In Echternach JL (ed): Pain. New York, Churchill Livingstone, 1987.
89. Nolan MF: Pain: The experience and its expression. Clini Management 10:22, 1990.
90. Nyborg WN, Ziskin MC: Biological effects of ultrasound. Clin Diagn Ultrasound 16:24, 1985.
91. Paalzow G, Paalzow L: Morphine-induced inhibition of different pain responses in relation to the regional turnover of rat brain noradrenaline and dopamine. Psychopharmacologia 45:9–20, 1975.
92. Paul R, Nair C: Ergonomic evaluation of keyboard and mouse tray designs. In Proceedings of the Human Factors Society, 40th annual meeting, Santa Monica, CA, 1996.
93. Piercey MF, Folkers K: Sensory and motor functions of spinal cord substance P. Science 214:1361, 1981.
94. Pilla AA, et al: Non-invasive low-intensity ultrasound accelerates bone healing in the rabbit. J Orthop Trauma 4:246–253, 1990.
95. Ransford AO, et al: The pain drawing as an aid to the psychologic evaluation of patients with low back pain. Spine 1:127–133, 1976.
96. Reading A: A comparison of the McGill pain questionnaire in chronic and acute pain. Pain 13:185, 1982.
97. Reid DS, Cummings GE: Factors in selecting the dosage of ultrasound with particular reference to the use of various coupling agents. Physiotherapy 25:5, 1973.
98. Rennie GA, Michlovitz SL: Biophysical principles of heating and superficial heating agents. In Michlovitz SL: Thermal Agents in Rehabilitation. Philadelphia, FA Davis, 1996.
99. Richard RL: Causalgia: A centennial review. Arch Neurol 16:339, 1967.
100. Saunders HD: Evaluation, Treatment, and Prevention of Musculoskeletal Disorders. Eden Prairie, MN, Author, 1985.
101. Sauter SL, et al: Work posture, work station design, and musculoskeletal discomfort in a VDT data entry desk. Hum Factors 33:151–167, 1991.
102. Selkowitz DM: Electrical currents. In Cameron MH (ed): Physical Agents in Rehabilitation. Philadelphia, WB Saunders, 1999.
103. Shealy C: Transcutaneous electroanalgesia. Surg Forum 23:419, 1973.
104. Shealy C, et al: Effects of transcranial neurostimulation upon mood and serotonin production: A preliminary report. Pain 1:13, 1979.
105. Sherman M: Which treatment to recommend? hot or cold. Am Pharmacol 20:46, 1980.
106. Sjolund B, Eriksson M: Electro-acupuncture and endogenous morphines. Lancet 2:1085, 1976.
107. Snyder SH: Opiate receptors and internal opiates. Sci Am 240:44–56, 1977.
108. Sternbach RA, et al: Effects of altering brain serotonin on human chronic pain. In Bonica JJ (ed): Advances in Pain Research and Therapy, vol 1. New York, Raven Press, 1976.
109. Stillwell GK: Therapeutic heat and cold. In Krusen FH, et al: Handbook of Physical Medicine and Rehabilitation. Philadelphia, WB Saunders, 1971.
110. Stuppy DJ: The faces pain scale: Reliability and validity with mature adults. Appl Nurs Res 11:84–89, 1998.
111. Swerdlow M: The Therapy of Pain. Philadelphia, JB Lippincott, 1981.
112. Tappan FM: Healing Massage Techniques: Holistic, Classic and Emergency Methods. Norwalk, CT, Appleton & Lange, 1988.
113. Torebjork E, et al: Noradrenalin-evoked pain in neuralgia. Pain 63:11–20, 1995.
114. VanderWende C, Spoerlein MT: Role of dopaminergic receptors in morphine analgesia and tolerance. Res Commun Chem Pathol Pharm 5:35–43, 1973.
115. Verrier M, et al: A comparison of tissue temperature following two shortwave diathermy techniques. Physiother Canada 29(1):21–25, 1977.
116. Wallin BG, et al: Preliminary observations on the pathophysiology of hyperalgia in the causalgic pain syndrome. In Zotterman Y (ed): Sensory Functions of the Skin in Primates. Oxford, Pergamon Press, 1976.
117. Ward RC: The myofascial release concepts. Handout material from course entitled Myofascial Release Concepts, Palpatory and Treatment Skills, Lansing, MI, September 1986.
118. Watson HK, and Carlson L: Treatment of reflex sympathetic dystrophy of the hand with active stress loading program. Am J Hand Surg 12(5 pt 1):779–785, 1987.
119. Weigent DA, et al: Current concepts in the pathophysiology of abnormal pain perception. Am J Med Sci 315:405–413, 1998.
120. Weinstein SM: Physical examination. In Ashburn MA (ed): The Management of Pain. New York, Churchill Livingstone, 1998.
121. Wilkie DJ, et al: Measuring pain quality: Validity and reliability of children's and adolescents' pain language. Pain 41:151–159, 1990.
122. Willer JC, et al: Stress induced analgesia in humans: Endogenous opioids and naloxone reversible depression of pain reflexes. Science 212:689–691, 1981.
123. Willer JC, et al: Psychophysical and electrophysiological approaches to the pain-relieving effects of heterotrophic nociceptive stimuli. Brain Res 107:1095–1112, 1984.
124. Wittink H, Michel TH: Chronic Pain Management for Physical Therapists, Boston, Butterworth-Heinemann, 1990.
125. Wolff MS, et al: Chronic pain assessment of orthopedic physical therapist's knowledge and attitudes. Phys Ther 71:207, 1991.
126. Wolf S: Perspectives on central nervous system responsiveness to transcutaneous electrical nerve stimulation. Phys Ther 58:1443, 1978.
127. Wood E: Beard's Massage. Philadelphia, WB Saunders, 1974.
128. Woolf C: Generation of acute pain: Central mechanisms. Br Med Bull 43:523–533, 1991.

The Pelvic Floor Treatment of Incontinence and Other Urinary Dysfunctions in Men and Women

BEATE CARRIÈRE, PT, CIFK

Key Words

- evaluation of clients with
  incontinence

- functional physical therapy
  exercises

- recoordination of the functions of
  the abdominal compartment

- clinical problem solving for pelvic
  floor dysfunction

Objectives

After reading this chapter the student/therapist will:

1. Be familiar with causes leading to incontinence.

2. Understand the neurophysiology involved in pelvic floor dysfunctions.

3. Be aware of the different layers of the pelvic floor and their functional connection.

4. Be able to correct faulty breathing patterns.

5. Understand why diaphragmatic breathing has to be recoordinated with pelvic floor activity.

6. Apply motor learning principles when instructing exercises.

7. Be able to select from various treatment approaches to improve pelvic floor function.

INTRODUCTION: OVERVIEW OF THE CLINICAL PROBLEM

History of Pelvic Floor Exercises

A different focus on how to view the pelvic floor and the problem of incontinence has to evolve from new knowledge about neurophysiology and motor learning. Kegel[34-36] must be considered the great American pioneer who recognized in the late 1940s the importance of exercises to help women who suffered from urinary incontinence (UI). Dr. Kegel, a Los Angeles physician, found that many women did not have any awareness of the function of the pelvic floor and that they were not always successful with the exercise he prescribed: drawing in the perineum. He therefore developed a pneumatic apparatus, the perineometer, which measured each muscle contraction, visible to the patient. He instructed his patients to perform the exercise for 20 minutes three times daily, or a total of 300 contractions, and suggested weekly visits for instruction.[34, 35] Kegel also recognized that there was evidence of bladder weakness in some women before childbearing, and he emphasized the importance of training the pubococcygeus muscle to achieve continence.[35, 36] Even though his approach to exercises demonstrates visual feedback combined with declarative learning,[33, 72, 73, 74] which must have been considered visionary at that time, the treatment has not changed much since. Given the complexity of the role of the pelvic floor muscles, procedural learning, sensory awareness, and functional retraining are now part of the treatment.

Prevalence of Incontinence

The prevalence of incontinence in men and women is high and very costly. Fantl and colleagues[26] reported in 1996 that 10% to 35% or 13 million adult Americans suffer from UI. It is estimated that more than half of the 1.5 million nursing home residents in the United States are incontinent and that the most common reason for placing a family member in a home is incontinence.[26, 54] Women over 60 years old have twice the prevalence of incontinence of men of that age.[26] The majority of patients with incontinence are parous women and older persons.[54] Britton and associates[9] conducted a study of urinary symptoms in 578 men over 60 years of age. Thirty percent of the men reported increased daytime frequencies and 27% reported urgencies and a variety of other urinary symptoms. Incontinence can also be found in the younger population. Nygaard and co-workers[50] investigated UI in nulliparous elite athletes and found that gymnastics and sports that include jumping, high-impact landings, and running appear to score higher in the prevalence of UI than swimming or playing golf. Since exercises and activities during field traning of soldiers can be very strenuous, it is not surprising that one third of 450 female soldiers experienced UI.[63] Baumann and Tauber[5] reported that 17% of boys between the age of 5 and 14 years are incontinent. Obesity can contribute to incontinence and make the treatment more difficult.[22] Cigarette smoking augments incontinence for three reasons: (1) it has been shown to interfere with collagen synthesis, (2) it is likely that neuromuscular and anatomical changes occur from smoking, and (3) it causes coughing.[10]

Individuals with neurological diseases often suffer from urinary problems. The Agency for Health Care Policy and Research[53] reported that it is most prevalent in persons with spinal cord injuries (SCIs) and people with multiple sclerosis (MS). Eighty percent of SCI patients experience urinary tract infections (UTIs) and 70% to 90% of individuals diagnosed with MS develop bladder dysfunction. Patients affected by spina bifida also can have various neurogenic urinary tract dysfunctions. Depending on the severity of the dysfunction, they may become socially dry with conservative therapy.[42] Individuals with Parkinson disease, cerebrovascular disease, or traumatic brain injury can also suffer from voiding dysfunction. Walters and Karram[78] provide a list of neurological diseases that are known to cause urinary problems, some of which are described later.

Cost of Incontinence

The cost of urinary incontinence escalated from 8.2 billion in 1984, to 16.4 billion in 1993, to 26.3 billion, or $3,565 per individual with UI, in 1995. According to Wagner and Hu,[75] this increase can be attributed to three major changes in the last 10 years:

1. Introduction of more continence-related products to the market
2. Change in the age composition of the U.S. population
3. Change in prevalence of UI

The authors stated that the cost for people younger than 65 years old was not included in the study and that the true cost may be much higher because UI is underreported.

Definition of Incontinence

Urinary incontinence is defined as involuntary loss of urine that is sufficient to be a problem.[26] Incontinence can have one or more causes and in over 90% of the cases it can be improved or cured.[54] Treatment should be only instituted after a careful thorough history and physical examination.[54] In non-neurological patients the most common forms of incontinence are stress, urge, and mixed incontinence. Weak pelvic floor muscles usually cause stress incontinence; urge incontinence is due to detrusor instability, an involuntary contraction of the muscle of the bladder before it is full. It is associated with a sudden urge to void. The urge can be so irresistible that it can result in loss of urine before the individual reaches the bathroom. The combination of both forms of incontinence is referred to as mixed incontinence.

ETIOLOGY

The causes of stress and urge incontinence in non-neurological clients are as follows: (Fig. 30–1):

1. Functional causes include not being able to undress in a timely fashion and being unable to reach a bathroom.

Overview of bladder dysfunctions		
Bladder dysfunction	**Non-neurological**	**Stress:** *Weakness* of the pelvic floor muscles. Reasons: Injury from childbirth; decreased function because improper use when coughing, lifting, breathing; straining with constipation or fecal impaction, estrogen deficiency, genetic make-up (possible collagen deficiency)	
		Urge: *Detrusor instability* Sudden urge to go to the bathroom, with or without loss of urine. Possible reasons: infection, prolapse of vagina, cystocele, weakness of the pelvic floor	
	Neurological	**Retention:** *Inadequate emptying* of the bladder; can be associated with pressure/pain in the lower abdomen	**Overflow:** *Overdistention* of the bladder; it empties by constant dribbling of urine when the capacity is exceeded
		1. Lesions in higher cortical areas and suprapontine: *Possible causes:* MS, stroke, Parkinson's disease, traumatic brain injury (TBI), tumors, dementia, alcoholism, Alzheimer's disease, Huntington's disease	**Possible symptoms:** Retention, inability to control the micturation reflex resulting in detrusor hyperreflexia
		2. Lesions in the upper motor neuron (spinal cord): *Possible causes:* Spinal cord injury (SCI), MS, tumors, back injuries and prolapse of a disk, stenosis of the spinal canal, inflammatory and vascular diseases (e.g., transverse myelitis), infections (e.g., syphilis–tabes dorsalis), diabetes mellitus, cauda equina syndrome, herpes zoster	**Possible symptoms:** Detrusor sphincter dyssynergy with danger of urethrovesical reflux
		3. Lesions in the lower motor neuron, peripheral nervous system, and in the autonomic nervous system: *Possible causes:* Injuries to the spinal cord, radiculitis (e.g., herpes zoster), tabes dorsalis, radiation, radical abdominal/perineal surgeries, diabetes mellitus, autonomous neuropathy, Guillain-Barré syndrome	**Possible symptoms:** Areflexia of the detrusor muscle, decreased sensation, incontinence, void by straining. Autonomic nervous system symptoms can include diffuse pain
	Other causes	**4. Psychogenic:** Non-neurogenic neurogenic bladder (Hinman syndrome), hysteria, schizophrenia, depression **5. Endocrine:** e.g., diabetes, hypothyroidism **6. Hormonal deficiencies**: e.g., lack of estrogen **7. Inflammatory**: e.g., cystitis, vulvovaginitis, and prostatitis **8. Obstructive**: e.g., tumor, prolapse **9. Pharmacological**: e.g., some over-the-counter medications, medication for treatment of hypertension, depression	**Possible symptoms:** Retention, frequency, urgency, and stress incontinence

FIGURE 30–1. Overview of reasons for incontinence of non-neurological and other causes.

2. Weakening of the pelvic floor structures can result from childbirth, hysterectomy, prolapse (rectocele, cystocele, vaginal prolapse), straining with constipation, and poor biomechanics when lifting. UTIs can also irritate the bladder.

3. Inadequate fluid intake (either too much or too little), as well as drinking fluids which may be stimulants to the bladder, can cause urge incontinence or frequent trips to the bathroom. Smoking, obesity, and postmenopausal estrogen deficiency contribute to the problem.[10, 22, 26, 77, 78]

4. Over-the-counter medications with anticholinergic agents can cause retention, overflow, and frequency; antipsychotic medications can cause sedation, rigidity, and immobility; and diuretics can worsen impaired continence. Medication for treatment of hypertension can also contribute to incontinence.[26, 54, 77, 78]

5. Retention in non-neurological clients can occur in men with prostate problems[4, 9] and in men or women secondary to inability to relax the pelvic floor muscles when in a hurry and squeezing rather than relaxing the muscles, or as a result of stressful situations and poor habits.

6. An overdistended bladder can cause overflow incontinence. It can present as constant or intermittent dribbling, sometimes combined with urge or symptoms of stress incontinence. Patients often have high residuals and feel that their bladder does not empty properly.

Additional causes of bladder dysfunctions are as follows:

1. Lesions in the higher cortical areas and suprapontine lesions can be found in MS, strokes, Parkinson's disease, traumatic brain injury, tumors, and dementia. These diseases can cause retention, and inability to control the micturition reflex, resulting in detrusor hyperreflexia with coordinated urethral relaxation.[15, 77, 78]

2. Lesions in the upper motor neurons affect the spinal cord. Common problems resulting in urinary dysfunction are SCI, MS, cauda equina syndrome, tumors, inflammatory diseases such as transverse myelitis, infectious diseases such as syphilis (tabes dorsalis), injuries to the spinal column, prolapse of a disk, or stenosis of the spinal canal. Typical bladder problems are detrusor hyperreflexia without coordinated urethral relaxation (detrusor-sphincter dyssynergy.)[15, 77, 78]

3. Lesions to the peripheral or lower motor neurons such as injuries from childbirth, traumatic injuries, radiculitis (e.g., from herpes zoster), or tabes dorsalis can cause retention and detrusor areflexia. The inability to feel when the bladder is full can lead to an overflow bladder with symptoms of dribbling and incomplete or strained voiding. Patients may need to learn clean intermittent catheterization.[15, 26, 49, 54, 77]

4. Lesions stemming from injuries to the autonomic nervous system can be caused by surgery in the pelvic area, such as hysterectomy, rectum resection, and radical prostatectomy; injury; or inflammations. Autonomic lesions can contribute to diffuse pain,[80] swelling, and altered sensory awareness. Urinary problems can cause the feeling of having cold feet.[24, 62]

5. Psychogenic causes of urinary dysfunction include schizophrenia and depression. Patients can suffer from incontinence, hesitation, retention, and pain. A non-neurogenic neurogenic bladder is called Hinman syndrome.[78]

6. Endocrine causes are hypothyroidism and diabetes, which may lead to a flaccid or areflexic bladder, and require clean intermittent self-catheterization.[49, 78] Diabetes can also increase the frequency of urination.

ANATOMY AND PHYSIOLOGY OF THE PELVIC FLOOR

The pelvic floor consists of all the muscles which close the pelvic cavity. It is part of the abdominal compartment which can be defined by the pulmonary diaphragm cranially, the pelvic and urogenital diaphragms caudally, the muscles of the abdominal wall ventrally, and the muscles of the back dorsally. This compartment houses the internal organs and the viscera.[54, 67, 71, 78] There are essentially three layers of the pelvic floor: (1) the endopelvic fascia, (2) the pelvic diaphragm, and (3) the perineal membrane.

The Endopelvic Fascia

The endopelvic fascia suspends and supports the organs within the pelvis. It is a mesh of connective tissue composed of collagen, elastin, blood and lymph vessels, and nerves. A thick fibrous part of the endopelvic fascia, the pubocervical fascia, attaches to the cervix in a slinglike fashion and assists in supporting the urethra and the bladder. Laterally it connects to the fascia white line, the tendinous arch of the levator ani muscle. Injuries to this important fascial support can contribute to weakness of the pelvic floor, prolapse, and leakage with increased abdominal pressure.[54, 71, 77]

The Pelvic Diaphragm

The pelvic diaphragm (Fig. 30–2) consists mostly of the paired levator ani muscle. The levator ani is shaped like a hammock and has several parts. In the sagittal plane the muscle originates at the pubic bone and attaches to the coccyx, hence the name pubococcygeus muscle. The medial part of the pubococcygeus loops around the rectum and therefore is named the puborectalis muscle; other fibers form a sling around the vagina or prostate (pubovaginalis and levator prostate muscles). Each side of the muscle meets in the midline with the other half and attaches to the perineal and anococcygeal bodies.

The posterior part of the levator ani has two paired sections. The coccygeus (or ischiococcygeus) muscle covers the sacrospinous ligament. The muscle arises at the spine of the ischium and extends to the lowest part of the sacrum and the coccyx. The iliococcygeus lies between the coccygeus and the puborectalis and passes in a diagonal direction between the coccyx to the spine of the ischium and the tendinous arch of the levator ani. This fibrous band of the arcus tendineus is suspended between the pubic bone and ischial spin.[18, 54, 71, 77, 78] The levator ani is a skeletal muscle with a high resting tone; it consists of approximately 70% slow twitch fibers and 30% fast twitch fibers.[11, 43, 71, 76, 77] Wall[77] and Bump[11] and their co-workers consider the high resting tone critical for pelvic support and for keeping the hiatus of the levator closed. Since the levator ani muscle is under voluntary control, it can be actively contracted and provide closure during increase of abdominal pressure, for example, when coughing or sneezing.[43, 48, 76, 77] According to Retzky and Rogers,[54] the innervation of the levator ani muscles is under dual control: on their pelvic surface by motor efferents of the sacral nerve from S2–4, and on the perineal surface by the pudendal nerve.

The Perineal Membrane

The perineal membrane, or urogenital diaphragm, is the outer layer of the pelvic floor. It is a thick fibrous and muscular layer of triangular shape immediately below the levator ani. In women the perineal membrane attaches the edges of the vagina to the ischiopubic ramus; in men it forms an uninterrupted sheet of tissue. The fibers of the deep and superficial transverse perineal muscles run primarily in a frontal plane, the ischiocavernosus muscle in a diagonal direction, and the bulbocavernosus muscle in a sagittal plane. The external sphincter muscle of the anus is part of the perineal membrane and is connected to the transverse perineal and bulbocavernosus muscle by the perineal body, which contains fibrous tissue. The dorsal attachment of the perineal membrane is achieved through the anococcygeal raphe, which connects the external anal sphincter to the coccyx.[43, 77]

The muscles of the perineal membrane contain both smooth and striated muscles. The muscles become tight when the levator ani tone remains relaxed.[77] The anterior portion of the perineal membrane is closely connected to the urethral musculature. According to Wall and co-workers,[77] the perineal membrane does not contribute substantially to pelvic support; it is mostly the levator ani which is much greater in strength and bulk and can exert upward traction when contracting to maintain outlet support. The ischiocavernosus, bulbocavernosus, and superficial transverse perineal muscles function mainly in sexual responsiveness, serving to enhance and maintain penile erection in males and maintaining erection of the clitoris in females.[71, 77] Trigger points in these muscles can cause a degree of impotence and pain with intercourse.[74] According to Claes and colleagues,[17] strengthening exercises of the muscles of the perineal membrane can significantly improve impotence. In women, the perineal membrane is often torn or injured during childbirth and if not properly repaired, can cause sexual dysfunction and low self-esteem.

The complicated innervation of the pelvic area, including the perineal area, has been well described by Wesselmann and associates.[80] The pudendal nerve, diverges from the sacral plexus, intermingles with the autonomic nerves, and then branches into several directions, innervating the external anal sphincter, and the anterior perineal muscles.

The Mucosal Coaptation of the Urethra

In addition to the three pelvic floor layers described above, an important contributor to continence is the mu-cosal coaptation, which is the arteriovenous complex between the epithelial lining and the smooth muscle coat of the female urethra. It is sensitive to estrogen, and with deficiency of this hormone, the resting pressure of the urethra can decrease and cause leakage.[54] Wall and colleagues[77] compared it to an "inflatable cushion," helping to fill the urethral wall and sealing the 3- to 4-cm-long urethra in women. Estrogen, often prescribed and applied to the vaginal area, therefore can help some menopausal women to increase the resting tone of the urethra and improve closure. The male urethra is not estrogen-dependent. Its mucosal coaptation is highly vascular and probably influenced by testosterone. In addition, the prostrate gland and the length of the male urethra may contribute to a sealing effect.

The Internal Sphincter of the Urethra

The internal sphincter muscle at the junction of bladder and urethra (urethrovesial junction) is an involuntary smooth muscle, which is under autonomic control in both males and females. Its shape is circular and formed by the trigone, a smooth muscle in the bladder, as well as by two U-shaped loops of muscles, which derive from the bladder muscle. In females the urethra rests on a hammock of connective tissue (pubocervical fascia) and is held in a position that prevents descent into the vagina. The external sphincter muscle is able to close the middle portion of the female urethra.[54]

Incontinence usually happens when several factors come together. For example, males frequently leak after a radical prostatectomy because the smooth internal sphincter urethra may be damaged by the surgery and the pelvic floor muscles have to learn to substitute and provide closure of the urethra. In healthy individuals the external sphincter and levator ani muscles serve as a backup system for continence. However, weakness of these structures leads to decreased bladder neck and urethral support and can lead to incontinence, especially with activities that increase the abdominal pressure.

THE VOIDING MECHANISM OF THE BLADDER

Many of the neurophysiological connections involved in functioning of the bladder and the surrounding muscles are not fully understood. A complicated coordination of many systems is involved in a properly functioning bladder and other pelvic organs. It is impossible to elaborate in this chapter on all the neural interactions, which take place at all levels. Wesselmann and co-workers[80] and Burnett and Wesselmann,[13] provide comprehensive information about the neurobiology of the pelvis.

Sympathetic Innervation (Fig. 30-3A)

The sympathetic innervation to the bladder, rectum, and sexual organs originates at the thoracolumbar segment of the spinal cord (T10 to L1–2), as well as from the hypogastric plexus (the sympathetic hypogastric nerve), which descends from the aortic plexus (Fig. 30–3A). The hypo-

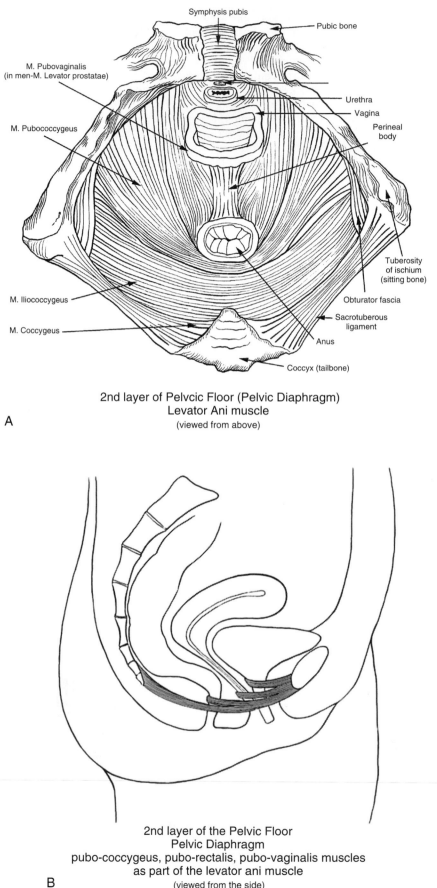

Symphysis pubis

Pubic bone

M. Pubovaginalis
(in men-M. Levator prostatae)

Urethra

Vagina

Perineal
body

M. Pubococcygeus

Tuberosity
of ischium
(sitting bone)

M. Iliococcygeus

Obturator fascia

M. Coccygeus

Sacrotuberous
ligament

Anus

Coccyx (tailbone)

2nd layer of Pelvcic Floor (Pelvic Diaphragm)
Levator Ani muscle
(viewed from above)

A

2nd layer of the Pelvic Floor
Pelvic Diaphragm
pubo-coccygeus, pubo-rectalis, pubo-vaginalis muscles
as part of the levator ani muscle
(viewed from the side)

B

FIGURE 30–2. Anatomy of the pelvic floor.
A, Pelvic diaphragm viewed from above.
B, Pelvic diaphragm viewed from the side.

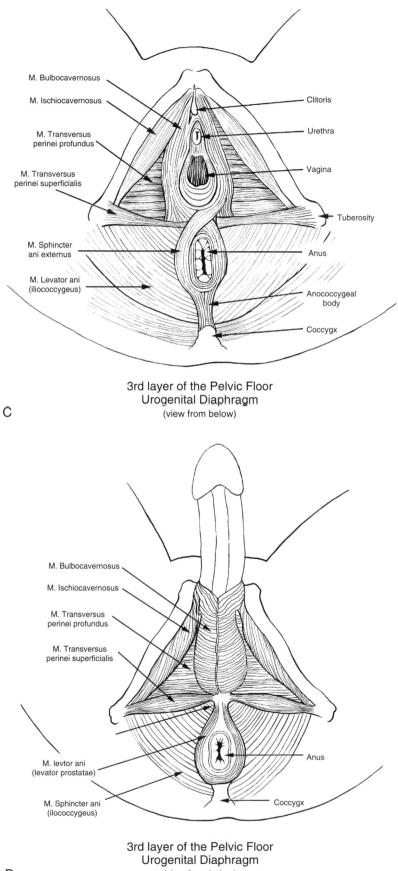

3rd layer of the Pelvic Floor
Urogenital Diaphragm
(view from below)

C

3rd layer of the Pelvic Floor
Urogenital Diaphragm
(view from below)

D

FIGURE 30–2 *Continued. C,* Urogenital diaphragm (perineal membrane) viewed from below. *D,* Urogenital diaphragm (perineal membrane) viewed from below.

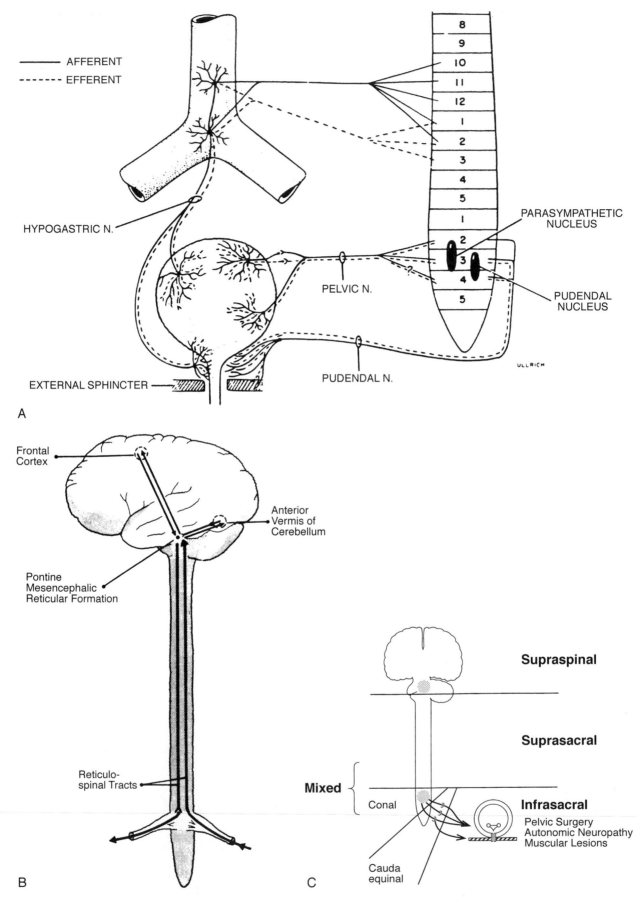

FIGURE 30–3 *A–C.* Neurophysiology of the pelvic floor. (*A* from Blaivas JG: Management of bladder dysfunction in multiple sclerosis. Neurology 30[2]:12–18, 1980; *B* from Bradley WE, Brantley SF: Physiology of the urinary bladder. *In* Campbell's Urology, 4th ed. Philadelphia, WB Saunders, 1978, p 106; *C* from Braddom RL: Physical Medicine Rehabilitation, 2nd ed. Philadelphia, WB Saunders, 2000.)

gastric nerve feeds into the inferior hypogastric (pelvic) plexus, which is the major neuronal integrative center for multiple pelvic organs.[1, 13, 80] Both the sympathetic and parasympathetic divisions of the autonomic nervous system innervate the pelvic viscera, which are also innervated by the somatic and sensory nervous systems. The sympathetic innervation inhibits the bladder and stimulates the muscles of the trigone and the internal sphincter muscles of the bladder, as well as the muscles of the rectum.

Parasympathetic Innervation

The parasympathetic innervation exits the spinal canal at the level of S2–4. The nerves join the splanchnic nerve before entering the inferior hypogastric plexus (see Fig. 30–3A). The parasympathetic fibers stimulate the bladder and other pelvic organs, including the sexual organs.[1, 5, 31, 80] The parasympathetic fibers ending in the bladder are especially sensitive to overstretching, infection, or fibrosis.[78] This explains the urge of wanting to urinate frequently under such conditions.

Somatic Innervation

The somatic innervation of the pelvic floor comes from the sacral plexus of S2–4 (see Fig. 30–3A). The pudendal nerve leaves the spinal cord at S2–4 and branches to innervate the striated muscles of the levator ani, the external sphincter muscles of both the urethra and rectum, as well as the muscles of the perineal membrane. The sacral plexus provides both efferent and afferent innervation; some of the fibers of the pudendal nerve intermingle with the autonomic pelvic nerves.[31, 78, 80] The somatic nerves can modulate the autonomic system. The complexity of the innervation of the pelvis and the influence of neurotransmitters in the bladder wall, as well as the control of higher, central nervous system regulation (see Fig. 30–3B and C), can be appreciated when observing the filling and emptying phases of the bladder. Owing to its topographical position the pudendal nerve is very susceptible to nerve injury from stretching or compression during childbirth, especially during delivery of large babies.[54]

Sensory Innervation

The sensory innervation comes primarily from proprioceptive nerve endings in the bladder and urethra. It is an afferent neuronal visceral system, which probably enters the spinal cord via the sacral and lumber segments. These afferent nerve tracts may regulate pain, the absence of pain, and the feeling of having a full bladder.[31, 78]

Filling Phase

The bladder is a smooth involuntary muscle with voluntary control. It stores the urine until it is emptied voluntarily. The normal bladder is a low-pressure system, which accepts urine without a concomitant rise of internal pressure.[54, 77] This is produced by sympathetic stimulation of the β-adrenergic receptors in the bladder wall. The

sympathetic nervous system inhibits the parasympathetic activity at the same time as sympathetic stimulation of the α adrenergic receptors in the internal sphincter muscle cause constriction and a rise in urethral pressure.[54, 77] During the filling phase the bladder is inactive until it holds approximately 350 to 500 mL of urine, even though a first sensation of filling may occur with 150 to 250 ml of urine in the bladder.[31] When the bladder is full the receptors send a signal to the cortical centers of the brain and as a result a voluntary micturition reflex is initiated to empty the bladder (see Fig. 30–3B).[31, 54, 77]

Involuntary contractions of the detrusor during the filling phase cause frequency and urgency. In neurological patients this is called hyperreflexia; if idiopathic, it is considered bladder instability.[77, 78] Individuals with a hypersensitive bladder have to empty their bladders frequently, which results in a functionally small bladder. When the sensation of the bladder is decreased, the bladder will overfill and urine can back up into the kidneys causing dysfunction. Symptoms of overflow from the overstretched bladder frequently cause dribbling.

Emptying Phase

Micturition, or voiding, depends on the coordinated activity of the urethra and the detrusor muscle. It is known that the pelvic floor (levator ani and external sphincter muscles) has to relax when the detrusor muscle contracts. This occurs with activation of the parasympathetic cholinergic receptors in the bladder muscle. An afferent stimulus from the pelvic nerve (see Fig. 30–3A) reaches the pontine micturition center via the spinal cord. Efferent tracts inhibit the activity of the pudendal nerve, which results in relaxation of the external sphincter and levator ani. At the same time sympathetic activity at the bladder neck is inhibited and postganglionic parasympathetic neurotransmitters are stimulated. This results in detrusor contraction.[5, 31, 54, 78]

From the pontine micturition center, signals are also sent to the cerebral cortex which allows voluntary control. An individual therefore can override the signal to empty the bladder and wait to empty it later, or can empty the bladder when there is no signal that it is full. Suprapontine control of bladder function is due to the modulating control of the brain stem, hypothalamus, and the cerebral cortex.[31]

There are many reflexes involved in urine storage and voiding at various levels. The sacral reflex, for example, can be elicited by light stroking at the lateral aspect of the anus and it should result in a symmetrical contraction of the anal sphincter ("anal wink"). Absence of the anal wink can be an indication of a neurological problem at S2–4 resulting in weakness or paralysis of the pudendal nerve.[54] The micturition reflex, on the other hand, depends on an intact pontine micturition center in the brain stem.[31]

PHARMACOLOGICAL TREATMENT OF PELVIC FLOOR DYSFUNCTION

The great number of receptors in the bladder wall, as well as the ability to influence skeletal muscles with muscle relaxants, is the basis for pharmacological treatment of the symptoms found in patients with incontinence. Other treatments of urinary dysfunction address the hormonal deficiency. Estrogen, for example, is prescribed for many postmenopausal women with symptoms of leakage and feeling of dryness in the vaginal area.[15, 54, 77, 78]

Individuals with enuresis (bed-wetting) or urge incontinence frequently receive oxybutinin (Ditropan) as the drug of choice. Another prescribed drug is imipramine, an antidepressant. Patients with instability of the detrusor often receive anticholinergic agents or antispasmodic medications.

α-Adrenergic agents such as phenylpropanolamine or ephedrine increase striated muscle tone and therefore are used with stress incontinence. α-Adrenergic antagonists, such as drugs for treatment of hypertension, can worsen incontinence. Caffeine, alcohol, and diuretics can increase urinary frequency, urgency, and stress incontinence.[2, 26, 54, 78] Antipsychotic agents are also α-adrenergic antagonists, they reduce urethral pressure and can be used for treatment of urinary retention.[54] The problem with pharmaceutical treatment is the side effects, some which may affect the pelvic floor adversely, such as constipation. Other clients describe severe dryness in their mouth and have to constantly drink or suck on a candy. There are many other side effects described by the people taking these drugs, ranging from dizziness to blurred vision and somnolence. The motivation to achieve a functioning pelvic floor, therefore, is very high. Physical therapy may be the main contributor to reaching that goal.

EVALUATION AND INTERVENTION

Medical Evaluation

Before a referral to physical therapy, a physician, preferably a urologist, or gynecologist, should evaluate a patient with any urinary dysfunction. The patient's history will lead the physician to select appropriate diagnostic tests, including a urodynamic test, which helps to explore the extent of the lesion, rule out causes that require other treatments, and determine if physical therapy may help.[15, 54, 77, 78] Adams and Frahm[2] provide an excellent overview to physical therapists of the causes as well as the evaluation and treatment possibilities. Part of the evaluation process should be a bladder diary or voiding log over several days, so that a clear picture emerges about fluid input-and output, as well as when frequencies and incontinence episodes occur and to what extent. If the physician has not done this evaluation it should be included in the physical therapy evaluation. Physicians should also include a muscle strength test of the levator ani,[2, 43, 77] when seeing a client with symptoms of UI to determine how much the muscle weakness contributes to the problem. Frequently, therapists working with clients referred to them because of incontinence assess the muscles themselves. A common test for evaluation of the extent of leakage in patients with stress incontinence is the pad test,[2, 45, 77, 78] which can be performed by physicians or therapists.

Conceptual Framework for Treatment

Therapy begins with an evaluation. This is necessary to determine which structures and systems are involved, and what kind of impairment or disability[3, 32, 73] can be identified. The information gathered leads to the prognosis and selection of the intervention and, hopefully, the most efficacious treatment.

Therapists working with female clients suffering from incontinence have to ask about childbirth and related trauma or surgery, prolapses, and surgery such as hysterectomy or slingsuspension. Different questions need to be asked when a male patient is evaluated, because the reason for his pelvic floor dysfunction may be very different.

Evaluation of Female Clients with Incontinence

An example of an evaluation process which might be used for female clients with incontinence is shown in Figure 30–4.

Question 1: This information gives the therapist a general idea of why the client was sent and how long the problem exists.

Question 2: The therapist learns from this information whether there may have been damage to the muscles or nerves supplying the pelvic floor, as well as whether the surgery coincided with worsening, improvement, or the onset. Since surgery produces scars, the possibility of scars being part of the problem has to be considered.

Thought Process. If the heaviest childs weighed 9 lb at birth, pudendal nerve damage could be contributing to the pelvic floor problem. (The question of diabetes is important in the medical history, because diabetic mothers are known to sometimes have big babies.) The scars have to be evaluated, especially if the client complains of pain or constipation. With a hysterectomy, the bladder is not "stabilized" by the vagina, which normally leans against the bladder.

Question 3: Scars especially in the pelvic and abdominal region can cause pain, which can radiate into the hips or pelvic region. It can also contribute to constipation.

Thought Process. Any surgery can cause scar tissue or muscle weakness in the area surrounding the pelvic floor. Observation and palpation of the abdominal cavity may be necessary. If the surgery was recent, vigorous exercises have to be avoided, and a review of body mechanics and lifting may be indicated.

Question 4: Diabetes and heart conditions can lead to increase fluid input and output. Diabetes also often causes a decreased sensory awareness of the bladder. Cancer can cause bony involvement, swelling, pain, and so on. Back pain can be caused by injuries to the back or injuries to the pelvic area, including the viscera. Pulmonary conditions may cause frequent coughing.

Thought Process. Urine output can be increased in a patient with diabetes. A patient with frequent bladder infection may not drink enough water. The type of drink may stimulate the bladder, while the influence of medications on the medical condition may affect the muscle tone of the pelvic floor. Exercises need to be altered in clients with back pain or metastasis. Emphasis on tightening the

---

EVALUATION FORM

1. Medical Diagnosis: Onset:

2. Childbirth information: **3. General Surgical History:**
How many gestations?   births?   *Abdominal surgeries (please circle): hernia,*
weight of heaviest child?   *appendix, gallbladder, kidney, laparoscopy,*
Cesarean, Y/N   episiotomy   *hemorrhoids, other?*
Vaginal/abdominal surgeries:
bladder suspension   hysterectomy
other?

4. Medical History: **5. Medications:**
Diabetes: Y/N   heart problems Y/N
hypertension Y/N cancer Y/N
kidney/bladder infections Y/N
back pain Y/N neck pain Y/N asthma Y/N
bronchitis Y/N
other (e.g., neurological conditions)

                                                       7. Urination pattern:
                                                       How often do you have to urinate?
6. Current Symptoms: *day   night*
Do you have (please circle if yes) any leakage: *How often do you leak?*
with coughing, sneezing, straining?   *daily   times a week   infrequent*
While running and going up- or downstairs?   *Do you use one of the following during*
When resting? Are any other activities   *the day (d) or night (n)?*
causing leakage?   *(Please circle and indicate how many):*
Do you have: hesitancy, urgencies, do you push   *liners d n   pads d n*
or strain?   *adult protection d n*
(Please circle when applicable)
Does your problem cause you to have
sexual dysfunction?
Do you have any pain? If yes, please describe: **9. Bowel habits:**
                                                        Regular Y/N incontinent of bowel Y/N
                                                        gas Y/N constipation Y/N Do you use
8. Daily Fluid Intake (cups, glasses):   *stool softenersY/N fiber rich-dietY/N*
How much do you drink?
* water   coffee   tea   soda*
* alcohol   citrus*
* other:*   **11. Psychosocial history:**
                                                        Current/previous employment: does it
10. History of treatment: *involve lifting?*
Have you ever been treated for this condition   *Hobbies, sports:*
before? Y/N   Did you do Kegel exercises? Y/N
Other treatments? Y/N
Please describe:

12. Treatment goal of client:

13. Objective:
(Evaluate posture, ability to do diaphragmatic breathing, pelvic tilt, ability to "feel" the activity of pelvic
floor muscles; evaluate muscle tone and strength of the pelvic floor muscles and of the surrounding
muscle if indicated; evaluate scar tissue when applicable; check for contraindications.)

14. Evaluation/Goal: **15. Intervention:**

FIGURE 30–4. Evaluation form.

pelvic floor before coughing needs to be addressed first in clients with pulmonary conditions.

Question 5: It is important to remember that antihypertensives, diuretics, antidepressants, cough medicines, and so on can affect continence.

Thought Process. Is the client aware of what drugs may affect the incontinence problem?

Question 6: Information from this section gives information about the extent of the problem of the pelvic

floor dysfunction and which other areas may need to be addressed.

Thought Process. Which impairment needs to be addressed first and does the medical diagnosis match the symptoms? Are there physical or emotional reasons for sexual dysfunction and pain?

Question 7: The pattern has to be seen in light of the history and daily fluid intake. The information of the voiding diary should match the urinary pattern. Normal urination is six times per day at a volume of about 250 ml (9 oz) with an average maximum of 500 ml. It is normal for many adults to get up once a night; elderly people may need to get up twice each night to urinate.[78]

Question 8: It is normal for women to drink and void between 1500 and 2500 ml (50 to 80 oz) a day. Except for water, all mentioned drinks are bladder irritants and can cause urgency or frequency.

Thought Process. A client who drinks below-average amounts of fluid may create frequency because the bladder is no longer used to store normal volumes. A person who drinks sodas or alcohol before going to bed needs to evaluate if a change of drinking habits affects the incontinence or urgency.

Question 9: There are many reasons for being constipated; it can be related to difficulty going to the bathroom at work, being always in a hurry, or not relaxing the pelvic floor because of improper leg support.[79] Eating hastily and constipating foods can contribute as well. Gastrointestinal problems, especially when combined with chronic pelvic pain or low back pain, can be the result of sexual abuse.[58]

Thought Process. Eating habits may have to be reviewed, as well as behavior during defecation. Straining during defecation secondary to constipation weakens the pelvic floor muscles and does not help clients who have prolapse. The abdomen needs to be evaluated and possibly treated. Is there any reason to suspect sexual abuse? Does the client appear to have low self-esteem? Are there signs of fear or nervousness during the evaluation, or a cluster of symptoms which could indicate sexual abuse?

Question 10: It is very important for a therapist to find out if the patient has been treated for this condition before, and if the treatment was successful or not.

Thought Process. In order to motivate a patient it is important not to begin a treatment with exercises or modalities which have been used unsuccessfully in the past. The selection and explanation of the treatment intended is critical to success.

Question 11: Information about employment gives the therapist input about how the work may contribute to the problem. How much does the posture affect the pelvic floor dysfunction? How can exercises be integrated with activities at work? Hobbies and sports can be important motivational factors, but it is also important to review how the exercises or hobbies are done.

Thought Process. If poor postural alignment is part of the problem, stretching and strengthening exercises may have to be practiced to achieve a neutral posture. A client who can train the pelvic floor while doing his or her favorite exercises will be highly motivated. If the exercises can be incorporated while doing, for example, lifting at work, the training effect will be greater.

Question 12: Ideally client and therapist goals should match.

Thought Process. If there is a great discrepancy, more explanations may be required or other questions need to be addressed in the objective evaluation. Try to set a goal with the client, which is achievable within a reasonable time frame. Then set new goals. Initially, the goals can be fewer episodes of wetness, sleeping through the night, having to wear a reduced number of pads, going less frequently to the bathroom, and so on.

Question 14: Summarize the findings, and also consider the general cognitive status of the client and her or his mood. The therapist's goal should reflect the prognosis and the extent of the impairment or disability.

Thought Process. A client who is cognitively impaired may require a different treatment approach. Individuals with good body awareness usually learn exercises and correct breathing patterns much faster and may require fewer treatments before seeing changes.

Question 15: There are many treatment possibilities to chose from. Often various concepts lead to the same goal. The selection also depends greatly on the therapist's experience and preference for a certain type of treatment.

Case Studies

Before presenting another case study, the conventional treatment approach to incontinence will be discussed

---

CASE 30–1   FEMALE WITH INCONTINENCE

A 56-year-old woman was sent to therapy for biofeedback training and proper instruction in Kegel exercises. This very alert librarian had a long history of mixed incontinence. Its onset was about 19 years ago, but improved for 3 to 4 years after a hysterectomy and bladder suspension surgery in 1989. The client had two vaginal deliveries, one episiotomy, and her heaviest child was 8½ lb. The client had urges more than once an hour, and used one or two pads a day; wetting occurred one to three times a week. The client drank one cup of coffee in the morning and about two sodas. Her diet was regular, but she suffered from constipation and took stool softeners.

The client liked to do brisk walking but had problems pursuing her hobby because of the leakage. The client had received instructions for Kegel exercises elsewhere but they did not help her. There was a history of chronic back and sciatic pain. The objective evaluation revealed a good sitting and standing posture. As the client exhibited a sensory awareness of the pelvic floor muscles, a strength test at that time was deferred. Her general strength appeared to be good and the muscle tone of the abdomen was within functional limits.

Impairment. The client had a poor awareness of a pelvic tilt motion and was a chest breather. There was dyscoordination of breathing with activity of the abdominal and back muscles, and the pelvic floor muscles.

Disability. The client was unable to exercise without leakage and was required to wear one or two pads during the day. The assessment: a very alert, motivated client.

Goals. Ability to cough and sneeze without leakage, not to have to wear pads during the day, and to resume walking. Ability to do home exercises independently. She received a total of 8 to 10 treatments within 3 months.

Intervention. Breathing exercises, coordination of diaphragmatic breathing with pelvic floor contraction, instruction in Swiss ball exercises for strengthening the pelvic floor muscles in all planes and during bouncing[67]; colon massage[29] and treatment of scar tissue[44] if indicated; biofeedback or electrical stimulation or both if no improvement with previous exercises after three to five treatments.

The client returned 6 days after the initial visit and reported decreased leakage with laughing. She received a colon massage and gentle scar

tissue massage as well as more challenging exercises using the Swiss ball and TheraBand. Instruction of proper lifting with contraction of the pelvic floor was part of the treatment. A return visit was scheduled 3 weeks later for an additional treatment for the abdomen and exercises. The patient reported feeling better, with improvement of the back pain, which she had had for 2 years. The abdomen had felt much looser after the treatment and leakage with coughing and sneezing was further reduced. The plan was to review the exercises in 4 to 6 weeks. The patient called 3 months later to report that she did not need further treatments. She was able to hold urine for 2 to 3 hours without wearing pads. There were no more wetting episodes and for safety she only wore pads when doing brisk walking for 45 minutes. Only occasionally did the client get up at night to urinate.

---

briefly and then the Tanzberger concept will be described in more detail.

Conventional Treatment Options for Stress, Urge, and Mixed Incontinence

Most therapists treating patients with incontinence are familiar with the following treatment options for urinary stress and urge incontinence, which are often used in combination with Kegel exercises:

1. Kegel exercises
2. Biofeedback
3. Electrical stimulation
4. Vaginal cones

A brief description of the Kegel exercises was given in the introduction to this chapter. Kegel exercises have provided only limited success. Henalla and colleagues[27] found that 65% to 69% of patients in two hospitals became dry or significantly improved with exercises only. Wall and Davidson[76] stated that exercise programs have a place in prevention of treatment of genuine stress UI. Miller and associates[48] demonstrated how tightening the pelvic floor muscles before a cough significantly diminished leakage from the bladder. Bø and co-workers,[7, 8] found that intensive exercises taught by physical therapists over a long period provided better results, which was in agreement with a Danish study by Tilbæks.[70] Meaglia and colleagues[47] stated that the motivation, close supervision, and encouragement are important for a successful treatment. Holley and co-workers[28] found that a great number of patients dropped their exercises because of lack of motivation. Bump and associates[11] found that brief verbal instructions in Kegel pelvic floor muscle exercises were not sufficient. Byl and colleagues[14] investigated the effect of repetitive movements (3 to 400 trials per day) in skeletal muscle in primates compared to variable repetitive movements and found that the repetitive movements caused interference with motor control. Variable trials preserved motor control. The question must be

asked: Is it beneficial to do pelvic Kegel exercises 300 times a day? The question is appropriate because these exercises train the muscle in isolation and not as part of a functional activity. Is it possible that individuals feel that Kegel exercises do not help and therefore discontinue them? Similarly, a therapist would not ask a client

---

CASE 30–2   MALE WITH INCONTINENCE

Obviously, adjustments are required in taking the history when evaluating a man with pelvic floor problems. The evaluation in Figure 30–5 serves as an example. The client's answers are written in script typeface. A summary of the result of the intervention (Fig. 30–6) illustrates the success that can be achieved with clients with incontinence. By the first return visit 4 weeks after the initial evaluation, the client was able to hold urine for longer periods and only needed to get up once during the night. The client also reported being able to attend water aerobics classes without loss of urine. He was exercising for approximately 20 to 30 minutes each day. The exercises, based on the Tanzberger concept,[65, 67] were reviewed with the client and new exercises added. The client purchased a Swiss ball and a return visit was scheduled approximately 3 weeks later. Before the next scheduled visit the client called, reporting that he was doing fine, no longer suffered from leakage, and did not need to wear adult protection at night; he resumed all other activities without problems. He was able to exercise at home independently and did not require further treatment. His next attempt was to maintain his condition without the bladder medication tolteridine (Detrol).

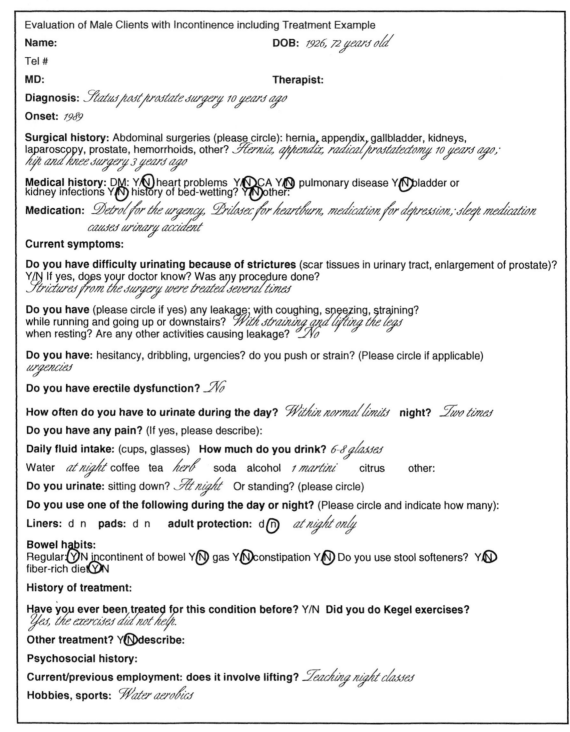

Evaluation of Male Clients with Incontinence including Treatment Example

Name: **DOB:** *1926, 72 years old*

Tel #

MD: **Therapist:**

Diagnosis: *Status post prostate surgery 10 years ago*

Onset: *1989*

Surgical history: Abdominal surgeries (please circle): hernia, appendix, gallbladder, kidneys, laparoscopy, prostate, hemorrhoids, other? *Hernia, appendix, radical prostatectomy 10 years ago; hip and knee surgery 3 years ago*

Medical history: DM: Y/Ⓝ heart problems Y/ⓃCA Y/Ⓝ pulmonary disease Y/Ⓝbladder or kidney infections Y/Ⓝ history of bed-wetting? Y/Ⓝother:

Medication: *Detrol for the urgency, Prilosec for heartburn, medication for depression; sleep medication causes urinary accident*

Current symptoms:

Do you have difficulty urinating because of strictures (scar tissues in urinary tract, enlargement of prostate)? Y/N If yes, does your doctor know? Was any procedure done? *Strictures from the surgery were treated several times*

Do you have (please circle if yes) any leakage; with coughing, sneezing, straining? while running and going up or downstairs? *With straining and lifting the legs* when resting? Are any other activities causing leakage? *No*

Do you have: hesitancy, dribbling, urgencies? do you push or strain? (Please circle if applicable) *urgencies*

Do you have erectile dysfunction? *No*

How often do you have to urinate during the day? *Within normal limits*   night? *Two times*

Do you have any pain? (If yes, please describe):

Daily fluid intake: (cups, glasses) **How much do you drink?** *6-8 glasses*

Water *at night* coffee tea *herb* soda alcohol *1 martini* citrus   other:

Do you urinate: sitting down? *At night* Or standing? (please circle)

Do you use one of the following during the day or night? (Please circle and indicate how many):

Liners: d n **pads:** d n   **adult protection:** dⓃ *at night only*

Bowel habits:
RegularⓎN incontinent of bowel YⓃ gas YⓃconstipation YⓃ Do you use stool softeners? Y/Ⓝ fiber-rich dietⓎN

History of treatment:

Have you ever been treated for this condition before? Y/N **Did you do Kegel exercises?** *Yes, the exercises did not help.*

Other treatment? Y/Ⓝdescribe:

Psychosocial history:

Current/previous employment: does it involve lifting? *Teaching night classes*

Hobbies, sports: *Water aerobics*

FIGURE 30–5. Evaluation of male clients with incontinence, including treatment example.

to do isometric exercises of a skeletal muscle 300 times a day and continue 80 times a day for the rest of his or her life once improvement became noticeable. Thus it does not seem any more appropriate if done with the pelvic floor muscles.

In a recent study by Salamey and Nof,[56] approximately 72% of the questioned therapists stated that they felt prepared to instruct patients in pelvic floor (Kegel) exercises. Only 18% of therapists were prepared to discuss UI with their patients, and the majority were not prepared to do electrical stimulation or biofeedback or other conservative treatments. Kegel exercises are what the majority of therapists learn in the United States as treatment for incontinence. Biofeedback and electrical stimulation, as well as vaginal cones, are recognized treatments for incontinence. They are used either in combination with exercises or alone.° The effect of electrical stimulation alone on stress and urge incontinence has been conflicting.[6, 41]

°References 2, 6, 12, 20, 21, 30, 41, 46, 51, 52, 57.

POSTEVALUATION PROCESS

What is your treatment goal? *To be able to lift legs and do water aerobics without leaking, not to have to wear "Healthdry" at night.*

Objective: (evaluate posture, ability to do diaphragmatic breathing, pelvic tilt, ability to "feel" the activity of pelvic floor muscles; evaluate muscle tone and strength of the pelvic floor or surrounding muscles when applicable; evaluate scar-tissue when applicable)

Patient with a good posture and good mobility of the pelvis. Because the patient became aware of his pelvic floor during the evaluation, muscle testing of the pelvic floor was deferred. The patient was also a chest-breather and was instructed in diaphragmatic breathing.

Impairment: *poor awareness of the pelvic floor muscles, dyscoordination of diaphragmatic breathing with the pelvic floor while lifting legs, coughing, etc.*

Disability: *unable to lift legs or do water aerobics without leakage of urine. Leakage at night, urgencies at night*

Assessment: *very motivated client who stated during the evaluation that he now understood the function of the pelvic floor.*

Intervention: *teaching of diaphragmatic breathing and coordination of breathing with the muscles of the entire abdominal compartment.*

Goal: *having to get up at night no more than once. No Healthdry at night; ability to lift legs, do water aerobics without leakage of urine.*

Plan: *teaching correct breathing and functional exercises based on the Tanzberger concept[66] to restore pelvic floor function in 6-8 treatments over 3 months or until patient feels independent with the home exercise program.*

SIGNATURE: _____ **Date:** _____

FIGURE 30–6. Postevaluation process.

Bø[6] recommended its use only when a person is not able to contract the pelvic floor muscles. She proposed continuing with the exercises when the individual can contract the pelvic floor muscles. A recent study by Bø[7] found pelvic floor exercises superior to electrical stimulation, vaginal cones, and no treatment. The Tanzberger concept, the most common form of exercises for continency, taught in Germany[81] is not taught in the United States.

THE TANZBERGER EXERCISE CONCEPT

The German physical therapist Tanzberger,[65–69] developed exercises, derived from Klein-Vogelbach,[39, 40] using the Swiss ball for treatment of incontinence.[16, 38] The goal of the exercises is to integrate the function of the entire abdominal compartment as a procedural program. If the client is to use the pelvic floor muscles correctly, restoration of diaphragmatic breathing is vital, as is coordination with all muscles of the abdominal compartment. The following elements are part of the Tanzberger concept.

Client Education

A client needs to know where the pelvic floor muscles are and what their function is. The therapist has to provide a clear picture of these muscles so that the client can visualize them and understand their function.

Restoration of Proper Diaphragmatic Breathing

Every breath changes abdominal pressure. Forced exhalation increases the pressure; so does coughing and sneezing. Leaning forward or backward also changes abdominal pressure. Clients should learn to coordinate the contraction of the pelvic floor with changes of pressure. In addition, these activities cannot be done without the cooperation of the abdominal and back muscles. Exercises designed to restore pelvic floor function, therefore, have to include coordination of all muscles involved. A great number of individuals with incontinence are chest breathers, possibly owing to a poor habit of as constantly pulling the stomach in to appear more slender. Restoration of diaphragmatic breathing, therefore, is the first priority for clients with incontinence.

It may also be argued that better breathing can help to provide more oxygen to the pelvic region. Knowing how to control breathing may help a client to relax when nervous or anxious (Fig. 30–7A and B).

Sensory Awareness of the Pelvic Floor

The pelvic floor muscles have the shape of a hammock. Their resting tone is high[43, 77] and learning to relax the

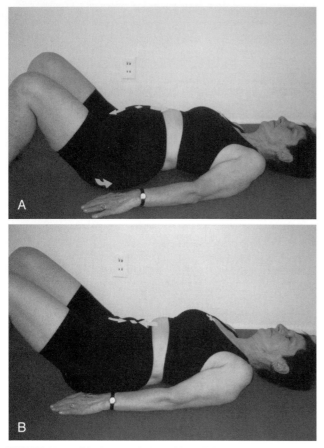

FIGURE 30–7. Diaphragmatic breathing. *A,* Inhalation. *B,* Exhalation.

pelvic floor is needed during urination and defecation, as well as during delivery and sexual activity. Thus sensory awareness is an important aspect of retraining the pelvic floor muscles. For all individuals, activities such as coughing, sneezing, lifting, and sexual activity require contraction and relaxation of pelvic floor muscles. The ability to relax and contract these muscles is a problem for clients with incontinence. In order for individuals to regain this control and sensitivity within the pelvic floor, certain treatment protocols need to be established.

First a client can feel landmarks such as the coccyx, the pubic bones, and ischium. Sitting on a firm surface, the client can first contract the gluteal muscles, then relax them, and try to feel the contraction of the anal sphincter and the muscles around the vagina by imagining holding a small object with those muscles.

In the side-lying position, the client can place a hand over the gluteal muscles while touching the anal sphincter with a fingertip (Fig. 30–8). The client can now try to pucker the anal sphincter, similar to puckering the mouth, which is at the other end of the digestive tract. The contraction can be faint but is correct if the gluteal muscles remain relaxed. Tightening of the levator ani can be palpated at the perineum, between anus and vagina, or at the side of the tip of the coccyx. Clients learn that contraction of these muscles has to precede any contraction of the surrounding pelvic floor muscles, such as the gluteal, adductor, and abdominal and back muscles.

In the same position the client can also feel how a cough moves the pelvic floor muscles in a caudal direction. During proper breathing there is a gentle, rhythmical downward movement during inhalation. The client then tries to tighten the pelvic floor muscles prior to coughing and feels less caudal movement of the pelvic floor muscles.

Coordination of Breathing with Pelvic Floor Muscle Activity

The client learns to contract the pelvic floor muscles while exhaling and to relax those muscles while inhaling. This can be done in different positions, such as supine, side lying, on all fours, sitting, or standing. When coughing, sneezing, lifting, and changing positions, as from supine to side lying, the pelvic floor contraction has to precede the activity (Fig. 30–9A and B). By contracting the pelvic floor before saying an explosive word such as a forceful "kick," then relaxing the pelvic floor by saying slowly "aaaaand," before tightening once more before saying "kick" again, the sequence of contraction and relaxation is learned.

Strengthening Exercises

Strengthening exercises of the pelvic floor muscles have to include fast twitch muscle fiber training with quick fast twitch muscle contraction, which can be done by bouncing on the ball as demonstrated by the 12-year-old boy (Fig. 30–10A and B).

Slow twitch muscle fiber training requires holding the contraction at the end for 5 to 10 seconds. This is demonstrated in Figure 30–11, where the client tightens the pelvic floor, gives herself resistance in a diagonal direction, and holds the contraction of the pelvic floor muscles for 5 to 10 seconds. The right ischial tuberosity initiates the movement toward the left knee, which should not move in space, as indicated by the X. The chest also is a "fixed" point marked by an X. All movement comes from the pelvis.

Because the pelvic floor muscle fibers run in a sagittal and frontal plane, as well as in a diagonal direction,

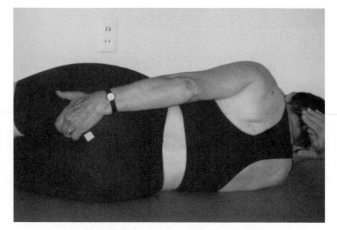

FIGURE 30–8. Feeling the pelvic floor.

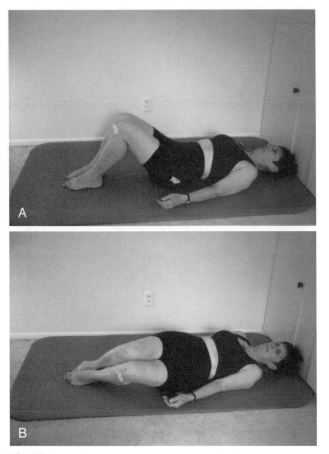

FIGURE 30–9. Turning from lying on the back *(A)* while tightening the pelvic floor, to the side *(B)*.

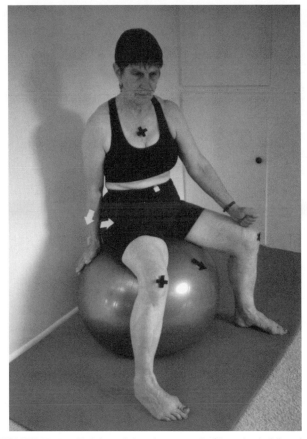

FIGURE 30–11. Training of the slow muscle fibers by holding the contraction for 5 to 10 seconds at the end.

movements in different directions should be included to maximize the benefit of strengthening exercises. The Swiss ball allows for movements in all directions as a functional activity. When two persons sit back to back on a ball (Fig. 30–12), one person can pull the ischium in the direction of the knees, which do not move, while the other person tries to slow down the movement. This requires eccentric activity of the pelvic floor muscles.

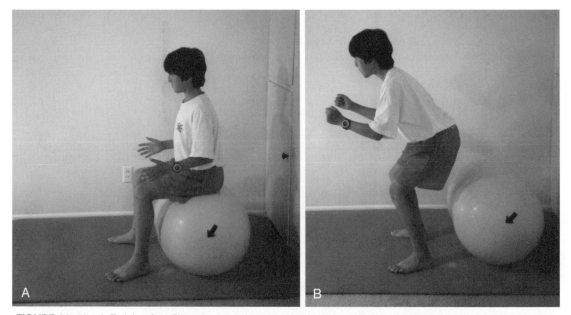

FIGURE 30–10. *A,* Training fast fibers by bouncing on a double ball. *B,* Tightening the pelvic floor while lifting up.

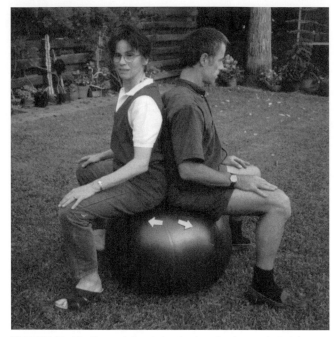

FIGURE 30–12. Two adults sitting back to back on a ball doing eccentric and concentric pelvic floor contractions.

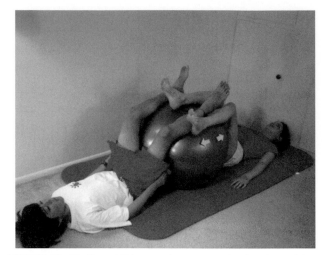

FIGURE 30–13. Two children work on strengthening the pelvic floor during exhalation.

Isometric muscle activity occurs when both pull at the same time with the same force. In Figure 30–13 two 12-year-old children tighten their pelvic floor muscles during exhalation while pulling the ball with the feet. There are many exercises with or without the ball, which can be adapted using the Tanzberger concept. Muscle strengthening is not done in isolation but is trained during functional movement activities.

Programming of Functional Activities

Pelvic floor muscle activities have to be tied into a function, such as getting up from a chair and tightening the pelvic floor muscles during exhalation (Fig. 30–14A and B). The exercises have to be repeated many times in different combinations until they become automatic. The process of acquiring these skills is part of procedural learning.[64, 72, 73] The client must be empowered to make changes in lifestyle activity and be motivated to achieve the changes. Only then will the client be willing to exercise for months until the task becomes automatic.[64, 73, 74] In order to improve motor control of a task, the exercises selected have to be meaningful and varied, as well as challenging. Mental practice, visualization, part-to-whole task practice, prepractice instructions, appropriate feedback, and guidance[23, 59, 60, 82, 83] are all part of motor learning, and are incorporated in the Tanzberger approach.

Precautions

For clients who do not feel safe on a ball, a double ball, a ball base, or a flat ball, which fits onto a chair (Figs.

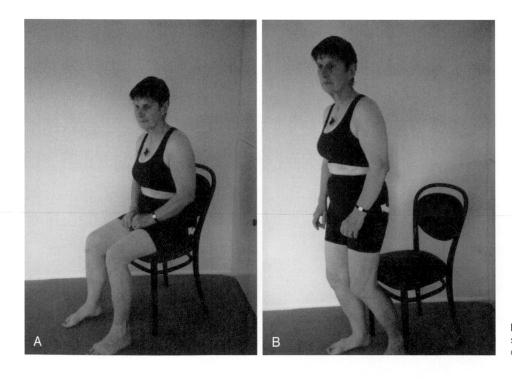

FIGURE 30–14 A and B. Sit to stand can be done with integration of pelvic floor activity.

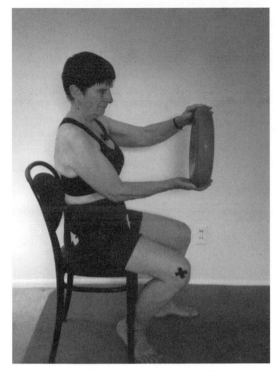

FIGURE 30–15. Flat ball (sit fit).

30–15 and 30–16), can be used. All are commercially available. Exercises also can be done between two chairs or in a corner, so that the ball cannot roll away. When learning the exercise, a belt can be used at first to hold onto a client. It is common sense not to use a ball if a severe cognitive deficit makes the activity unsafe. Any

medical condition that endangers a client on a ball makes these exercises contraindicated and requires a change of exercise and equipment.

In addition, therapists must be aware of other systems involvement, such as the autonomic system or the limbic system. The patient may be nervous or fearful, depressed, and sleep-deprived or suffer from pain in addition to the incontinence problem.[55] Some clients may have been abused, which may be manifested in multisystem involvement.[58] It is important to create an environment of trust and understanding and sensitivity toward the client's problems.

Clinical Application of the Tanzberger Concept

After a therapist has defined those aspects of pelvic floor dysfunction that require retraining, a specific exercise program can be custom-tailored to the patient.

Case Studies

In none of the four clients discussed in this chapter was biofeedback or electrical stimulation used for treatment, and most of the clients had done Kegel exercises without success. In clients who are unable to learn to feel their pelvic floor muscles, electrical stimulation or biofeedback can be helpful. Functional activities, including proper breathing, should be performed during biofeedback. Isolated contractions of the pelvic floor muscles using a device without incorporating functional activities does not seem to restore the many different functions of the pelvic floor. Therefore, the use of cones without proper pelvic floor muscle training remains questionable. All the clients mentioned in the case studies were extremely motivated, which is not uncommon in patients who suffer from pelvic dysfunctions. They are more than willing to follow their regimen. Problems arise when the client is cognitively impaired or when an illness affects motivation.

TREATMENT OPTIONS FOR ――― PELVIC FLOOR DYSFUNCTIONS
(Fig. 30–17)

Cognitively Impaired Clients

Adjustments have to be made and functional barriers decreased to help cognitively impaired clients maintain or achieve continence. Prompted voiding and timed voiding[11, 19, 25, 61] and medicine can be used when a client has cognitive problems and cannot go to the bathroom independently. In prompted voiding, clients are asked at regular intervals whether they have to go to the bathroom. In timed voiding, a client is placed on a commode or toilet at regular intervals. Many clients who are cognitively impaired probably would not be incontinent if they could reach a bathroom and if help were available to unbutton or unzip clothes, open a door, or assist in other aspects of toileting.

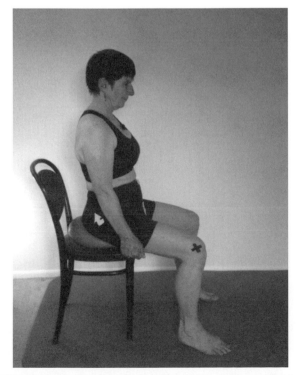

FIGURE 30–16. Exercise for the pelvic floor: sitting on a flat ball.

CASE 30–3   FEMALE WHEELCHAIR-DEPENDENT CLIENT

A 25-year-old female client, wheelchair-dependent secondary to myelomeningocele, was referred to therapy for upper extremity strengthening exercises. The diagnosis was left biceps tendonitis, left wrist strain, and lumbar discogenic pain. During treatment the young women was questioned about her bladder and bowel condition.

The patient had a history of bladder surgery as a child and placement of a suprapubic catheter and bowel reconstruction surgery were done at age 15. She reported that 50% of the time she leaked loose stool and she frequently did not make it to the bathroom in time. She was wearing up to two Depends pads per day.

The client was provided with a model of the pelvic floor muscle. Although her sensory awareness of the perineal area appeared to be reduced, she stated that she could feel a faint contraction when trying to pucker the anal sphincter. The client was a chest breather and she was instructed in abdominal breathing techniques. She then was instructed to try to coordinate the puckering with exhalation and work on relaxation of the pelvic floor, especially during defecation. She was told to place a stool in front of the toilet, so she could rest her short legs when sitting on the toilet.

The highly motivated client returned 3 weeks later: "I am very happy, I do not leak anymore and did not have to use any pads the last few weeks. I also feel my sphincter muscle now. The muscles around the suprapubic catheter seem to have a tighter fit." The client had a total of six treatments. Four treatments were devoted to her arm and trunk problems (which resolved), the last two treatments to the pelvic problem. Treatment then was discontinued as all goals had been met.

Clients with a Cerebrovascular Accident, Multiple Sclerosis, or Parkinson's Disease

The first therapeutic problem with clients who have neurological deficits is that they usually are not asked whether they have a urinary dysfunction. Not all clients with such diseases have incontinence or retention. Very often improvement can be achieved by identifying the dysfunction, explaining the anatomy and physiology to the client, and then giving him or her treatment options. Usually the coordination of diaphragmatic breathing with pelvic floor muscle activity can be integrated to varying degrees. A client with retention can learn to emphasize relaxation of the pelvic floor muscles during urination through breathing, proper seating on the toilet, and self-relaxation.

	Functional exercises and breathing	Biofeedback	Electrical stimulation	Cones	Prompted voiding	Timed voiding	Abdominal treatment. Scar-treatment	Self-catheterize
Stress incontinence	X	(x)	(x)	(x)			(x)	
Urge incontinence	X	(x)					(x)	
Mixed incontinence	X	(x)	(x)				(x)	
Anal incontinence	X	(x)	(x)				(x)	
Constipation	X	(x)	(x)				x	
Retention of urine	X					x	(x)	(x)
Overdistention of bladder	X	(x)			(x)	x	(x)	(x)
Areflexia of bladder, anus	(x)	(x)	x		(x)	x	(x)	x

FIGURE 30–17. Possible combinations of treatment options for incontinence.

CASE 30–4   CLIENT WITH VAGINAL PROLAPSE, ANAL SPHINCTER WEAKNESS, AND MIXED INCONTINENCE

This client benefited from colon treatment and gentle mobilization of the abdominal scar tissue.[29, 44, 62] The 38-year-old woman was referred to therapy because of anal sphincter weakness and incontinence of flatus for 5 to 6 years. She stated that she also had a prolapse. The client reported having incontinence when laughing and running and during sexual intercourse, which affected her self-esteem (as she explained during a later visit). She suffered from urgencies, which made her run to the bathroom every hour during the day and get up twice each night. The bladder was painful when full. There was also pain in the lower abdomen. The client suffered from constipation and had to strain during defecation. The surgical history was remarkable for difficult deliveries, one with forceps, and two others with episiotomies. The patient also had gallbladder surgery and hysterectomy approximately 15 years ago. The possibility of surgery for treatment of the prolapse and reconstruction of the vaginal area was discussed with the client and her physician. She had been instructed to perform Kegel exercises but they did not help. The client worked in an electrical assembly plant. The client's goals were to rid herself of the flatus and avoid surgery.

Objectively, there was decreased muscle tonus in the abdominal area and weakness of the abdominal and gluteal muscles. In addition, the client had dyscoordination between breathing and pelvic floor function. She developed some awareness of the pelvic muscles during the first evaluation. The impairment and the disabilities were considerable, the prognosis more guarded, but still the goal was to achieve the client's goals: to achieve anal continence, to prevent surgery, and to decrease urgencies. The client was very motivated.

The client was seen in therapy for 15 visits over 7 months, at first weekly, then every 2 weeks, and then for periodic reexaminations 3 to 4 weeks apart. Treatment began with teaching diaphragmatic breathing exercises and sensory awareness of the sphincter muscle. The client was able to distinguish between the activities of the anal sphincter and gluteal muscles and was also able to feel a faint contraction in the vaginal area. It was difficult for her at first to coordinate breathing with contraction and relaxation of the pelvic floor muscles, even when she practiced it at home. At the second visit the client received a colon massage and gentle mobilization of the abdominal scars with connective tissue massage.[29, 44, 62] Home exercises for breathing and pelvic floor contraction and relaxation were reviewed with the client. At the third visit, the client reported that the flatus problem had improved, and that the abdominal treatment helped with her constipation. New exercises were instructed using the Swiss ball in supine and sitting positions. At the fourth visit, the client said, "I have less flatus, and I am able to control the sphincter. The pelvic floor is still a problem because of the prolapse; no more back pain after the visceral treatments." The client was also instructed in how to do exercises with decreased load on the pelvic floor (supine, supine with the feet on the ball, side-lying, on all fours, etc.). The client was also instructed in how to self-massage the abdomen. At the fifth visit, the client said, "I am now taking medicine to help control the urgencies and can hold urine now for 3 hours. My husband massages my abdomen, which decreases the constipation. The bowel movements are now every 1 to 2 days instead of once a week."

The client reported only occasional pain with a full bladder, a reduction in the number of times she had to get up at night, and her ability to hold urine for 3 hours without pressure from the prolapse. The grateful client stated that her self-image had improved since she was no longer leaking urine during intercourse. According to the client's wishes, surgery was deferred. As the strength of the pelvic floor improved, the client stopped taking medication for the urgencies and was still able to hold urine for 3 hours and sleep through the night. The client continued occasional follow-up sessions to monitor her progress and to provide her with more challenging exercises.

Often functional barriers can be eliminated or help can be provided. Some clients may benefit from prompted voiding as well. With those clients who also need strengthening exercises for the pelvic floor and have difficulty sitting on a ball, a flat ball can be used in a chair, or exercises can be adapted to the client's ability without any devices.

Overdistended Bladder

It does not matter whether the cause of the overdistended bladder is neurogenic or not. In many cases the client has to learn to time herself or himself to void at regular intervals. In other cases the client may learn to do clean intermittent catheterization and carefully monitor the output of urine. The residual urine in the bladder should be low, approximately 50 ml, and if consistently higher requires further evaluation by an urologist.[78] Proper relaxation of the pelvic floor is important; men often can relax the pelvic floor better when urinating in a seated position. Abdominal breathing and coordination with pelvic floor muscle activity are very important for these clients and should be restored if there is a problem.

Areflexia

Education is always the most important part of intervention and is done at the beginning. Many clients may need to learn clean intermittent catheterization and timed intervals. In some clients, electrical stimulation or biofeedback may help to restore some function of the pelvic floor activity; exercise may improve the strength of the pelvic floor muscles once there is some return of function. Obviously, all therapeutic interventions depend on the extent of the lesion, but as described in Case 3, it is important to talk to the client and to explore treatment options. This client probably could have been spared wearing diapers for the last past 10 years. She also could have been condemned to wearing diapers for the rest of her life without intervention. All that was needed in her case was to ask about the problem and instruct her in achieving continence at two sessions.

Anal Incontinence

Inability to hold wind or leaking stool can also occur in neurogenic and non-neurogenic disorders. As with all clients with pelvic floor dysfunction, careful evaluation and education must be completed before beginning the treatment. In the presence of constipation, a careful abdominal evaluation and possible treatment of the viscera, such as colon massage,[29] may be indicated, because constipation can also be present in clients who leak stool. Electrical stimulation or biofeedback can, in some cases, be an adjunct or precede treatment of functional exercises of the abdominal compartment.

SUMMARY

Every client suffering from urinary incontinence, male or female, needs a thorough evaluation. In order to give the best possible chance for recovery, exercises have to be custom-tailored and modalities used with discretion. Electrical stimulation or biofeedback cannot replace functional exercises. Modalities may be helpful at the beginning of the treatment if the client has no sensory awareness of the pelvic floor, but should be used in combination with exercises. Treatment of the viscera should be considered in some clients to achieve full rehabilitation of the pelvic floor dysfunction.

REFERENCES

1. Acland RD, Riggs GH: The Trunk. *In* Human Anatomy, videotape 3. Baltimore, Williams & Wilkins, 1998.
2. Adams C, Frahm J: Genitourinary system. *In* Myers RS (ed): Manual of Physical Therapy Practice. Philadelphia, WB Saunders, 1995, pp 459–504.
3. American Physical Therapy Association: Guide to physical therapy practice. Phys Ther 77:1177–1284, 1997.
4. Barry MJ, Fowler FJ, O'Leary MP et al.: The American Urological Association symptom index for benign prostatic hyperplasia. J Urol 148: 1549–1557, 1992.
5. Baumann M, Tauber R: Inkontinenz beim Mann. Krankengymnastik 43:1372–1386, 1991.
6. Bø K: Effect of electrical stimulation on stress and urge urinary incontinence. Acta Obstet Gynecol Scand Suppl 168:3–11, 1998.
7. Bø K, Hagen R, Kvarstein B, et al: S: Pelvic floor muscle exercise for the treatment of female stress urinary incontinence. Neurol Urodynamics 9:489–502, 1990.
8. Bø K, Talseth T, Holme I: Single blind, randomised controlled trial of pelvic floor exercises, electrical stimulation, vaginal cones, and no treatment in management of genuine stress incontinence in women. BMJ 318:487–493, 1999.
9. Britton JP, Dowell AC, Whelan P: Prevalence of urinary symptoms in men aged over 60. Br J Urol 66:175–176, 1990.
10. Bump RC, McClish DK: Cigarette smoking and urinary incontinence in women. Am J Obstet Gynecol 167:1213–1218, 1992.
11. Bump RC, Hurt WG, Fantl A, Wyman JF: Assessment of Kegel pelvic muscle exercise performance after brief verbal instruction. Am J Obstet Gynecol 165:322–329, 1991.
12. Burgio KL, Robinson JC, Engel BT: The role of biofeedback in Kegel exercise training for stress urinary incontinence. Am J Obstet Gynecol 154:58–64, 1986.
13. Burnett AL, Wesselmann U: History of the neurobiology of the pelvis. Urology 53:1082–1089, 1999.
14. Byl NN, Merzenich MM, Cheung S, et al: A primate model for studying focal dystonia and repetitive strain injury: Effects on the primary somatosensory cortex. Phys Ther 77:269–284, 1997.
15. Cardenas DD, Mayo ME, King JC: Urinary tract and bowel management in the rehabilitation setting. *In* Braddon RL (ed): Physical Medicine Rehabilitation. Philadelphia, WB Saunders, 1996, pp 555–572.
16. Carrière B: The Swiss Ball. Berlin, Springer-Verlag, 1998.
17. Claes H, Van Kampen M, Lysens R, Baert L: Pelvic floor treatment of impotence. Eur J Phys Med Rehabil 2:42–45, 1995.
18. Clemente CD: Gray's Anatomy of the Human Body, 30th ed. Philadelphia, Lea & Febiger, 1985.
19. Colling J, Ouslander J, Hadley BJ, et al: The effect of patterned urge-response toileting (PURT) on urinary incontinence among nursing home residents. J Am Geriatr Soc 40:135–141, 1992.
20. Dumoulin C, Seaborne DE, Quirion-DeGiardi C, Sullivan SJ: Pelvic floor rehabilitation. Pt 1: Comparison of two surface electrode placements during stimulation of the pelvic floor musculature in women who are continent using bipolar interferential currents. Phys Ther 75:1067–1074, 1995.
21. Dumoulin C, Seaborne DE, Quirion-DeGiardi C, Sullivan SJ: Pelvic floor rehabilitation. Pt 2: Pelvic floor reeducation with interferential currents and exercises in the treatment of genuine stress incontinence in postpartim women—a cohort study. Phys Ther 75:1075–1081, 1995.
22. Dwyer PL, Lee ETC, Hay DM: Obesity and urinary incontinence in women. Br J Obstet Gynaecol 951:91–96, 1988.
23. Efferson L: Disorders of vision and visual perceptual dysfunction. *In* Umphred DA (ed): Neurological Rehabilitation, 3rd ed. St Louis, Mosby, 1995.
24. Enderlein K: Bindegewebsmassage—Behandlungshinweise und-voraussetzung. Physikalische Ther (6)3:71–252, 1985.
25. Engbert S, McDowell BJ, Donovan N, et al: Treatment of urinary incontinence in homebound older adults: Interface between research and practice. Ostomy Wound Manage 43:18–26, 1997
26. Fantl JA, Newman DK, Colling J, et al: Managing Acute and Chronic Urinary Incontinence, Clinical Practice Guideline, No. 2, Update. Rockville, MD, US Department of Health and Human Services, 1996.
27. Henalla SM, Kirwan P, Castleden CM, et al: The effect of pelvic floor exercises in the treatment of genuine urinary stress incontinence in women at two hospitals. Br J Obstet Gynaecol 95:602–606, 1988.
28. Holley RL, Varner E, Kerns DJ, Mestecky PJ: Long-term failure of pelvic floor musculature exercises in treatment of genuine stress incontinence. South Med J 88:547–549, 1995
29. Hüter-Becker A, Thom H: Physiotherapie, Vol 6. Massage, Kolonbehandlung. Stuttgart, Thieme Verlag, 1996, pp 162–182.
30. Jackson J, Emerson L, Johnston B, et al: Biofeedback: A noninvasive treatment for incontinence after radical prostatectomy. Urol Nurs 16:50–54, 1996.
31. Jänig W: Vegetatives Nervensystem. *In* Schmidt RF, Thews G (eds): Physiologie des Menschen, 26th ed. Berlin, Springer-Verlag, 1995, pp 340–369.
32. Jette A: Physical diasablement concept for physical therapy research and practice. Phys Ther 74:380–386, 1994.

33. Jewell MJ: Overview of the structures and function of the central nervous system. *In* Umphred DA (ed): Neurological Rehabilitation, 3rd ed. St Louis, Mosby, 1995.

34. Kegel AH: Progressive resistance exercises in the functional restoration of the perineal muscles. Am J Obstet Gynecol 8:238–248, 1948.

35. Kegel AH, Powell TO: The physiological treatment of urinary stress incontinence. J Urol 63:808–813, 1950.

36. Kegel AH: Physiologic therapy for urinary stress incontinence. JAMA, 146:915–917, 1951.

37. Kendall FP, McCreary EK, Provance PG: Muscles: Testing and Function, 4th ed. Baltimore, Williams & Wilkins, 1993, pp 69–118.

38. Klein-Vogelbach S: Ballgymnastik zur funktionellen Bewegungslehre, 3rd ed. Berlin, Springer-Verlag, 1990.

39. Klein-Vogelbach S: Functional Kinetics. Berlin, Springer-Verlag, 1990.

40. Klein-Vogelbach S: Therapeutic Exercises in Functional Kinetics. Berlin, Springer-Verlag, 1991.

41. Knight S, Laycock J, Naylor D: Evaluation of neuromuscular electrical stimulation in the treatment of genuine stress incontinence. Physiotherapy 84:61–71, 1998.

42. Knoll M, Madersbacher H: The chances of a spina bifida patient becoming continent/socially dry by conservative therapy. Paraplegia 31:22–27, 1993.

43. Laycock J, Wyndaele JJ, Dougherty M, et al: Understanding the Pelvic Floor. Dereham UK, NEEN Health Books, 1994.

44. Lörenz F: Ambulante krankengymnastische Behandlung nach Brustkrebsoperation. Krankengymnastik 50:1147–1157, 1998.

45. Lose G, Rosenkilde P, Gammelgaard J, Schroeder T: Pad-weighing test performed with standardized bladder volume. Urology 32:78–80, 1988.

46. McIntosh LJ, Frahm JD, Mallett VT, Richardson DA: Pelvic floor rehabilitation in treatment of incontinence. J Reprod Med 38:662–665, 1993.

47. Meaglia JP, Joseph AC, Chang M, Schmidt JD: Post-prostatectomy urinary incontinence: Response to behavioral training. J Urol 144:674–676, 1990.

48. Miller JM, Ashton-Miller JA, DeLancey JO: A pelvic muscle precontraction can reduce cough-related urine loss in selected women with mild SUI. Am Geriatr Soc JS 46:870–874, 1998.

49. Mostwin JL: Urinary incontinence (editorial). J Urol 153:352–353, 1995.

50. Nygaard IE, Thompson FL, Svengalis SL, Albright JP: Urinary incontinence in elite nulliparous athletes. Obstet Gynecol 84:184–187, 1994.

51. Pages IH: Komplexe Physiotherapie der weiblichen Harninkontinenz. Schweiz Physiother Verband 1:5–10, 1997.

52. Pages IH: Die Behandlung der weiblichen Harninkontinenz durch Elektrostimulation. Krankengymnastik 52:1528–1534, 1999.

53. Prevention and Management of Urinary Tract Infections in Paralyzed Persons. Summary, Evidence Report/Technology Assessment. Rockville, MD, Agency for Health Care Policy and Research, January 1999, No. 6.

54. Retzky SS, Rogers RM: Urinary incontinence in women. Clin Symp 47:3, 1995.

55. Rosenzweig BA, Hischke D, Thomas S, et al: Stress incontinence in women, psychological status before and after treatment. J Reprod Med 36:835–838, 1991.

56. Salamey J, Nof L: Physical practice pattern and perceptions related to urinary incontinence. J Womens Health, 23:8–13, 1999.

57. Sand PK, Richardson DA, Staskin DR, et al: Pelvic floor electrical stimulation in the treatment of genuine stress, incontinence: A multicenter, placebo-controlled trial. A J Obstet Gynecol 173:72–79, 1995.

58. Schachter CL, Stalker CA, Teram E: Toward sensitive practice: Issues for physical therapists working with survivors of childhood sexual abuse. Phys Ther 79:248–261, 1999.

59. Schmidt RA, Lange C: Optimizing summary knowledge of results for skill learning. Hum Mov Sci 9:325–348, 1990.

60. Schmidt RA, Young DE, Swinnen S, Shapiro DC: Summary knowledge of results for skill acquisition. J Exp Psychol 15:352–359, 1989.

61. Schnelle JF: Treatment of urinary incontinence in nursing home patients by prompted voiding. J Am Geriat Soc 38:356–360, 1990.

62. Schuh I: Bindegewebsmassage. Stuttgart, Gustav Fischer Verlag, 1986, pp 62–253.

63. Sherman RA Davis GD: Behavioral treatment of exercise-induced urinary incontinence among female soldiers. Mil Med 162:690–694, 1997.

64. Shumway-Cook A, Woollacott MH: Motor Control. Baltimore, Williams & Wilkins, 1995, pp 23–43.

65. Tanzberger R: Krankengymnastik nach der Geburt. Krankengymnastik 43:967–970, 1991.

66. Tanzberger R: Krankengymnastische Therapie bei Inkontinenz. Krankengymnastik 43:1364–1371, 1991.

67. Tanzberger R: Der weibliche Beckenboden—Krankengymnastik bei Inkontinenzbeschwerden. Krankengymnastik 46:322–324, 1994

68. Tanzberger R: Incontinence. *In* Carrière B: The Swiss Ball. Berlin, Springer-Verlag, 1998, pp 327–358.

69. Tanzberger R: Beckenboden-/Sphinktertraining bei Dysfunktionen. Krankengymnastik 7:1174–1180, 1998.

70. Tilbæks S: Effekt af bækkenbundtræning hos stress og blandet stress/urge inkontinente kvinder. Dan Fysioterapeuter 2:10–13, 1994.

71. Travell JG, Simons DG: Myofascial Pain and Dysfunction, vol 2. Baltimore, Williams & Wilkins, 1992, pp 110–131.

72. Umphred DA: Classification of treatment techniques based on primary input systems. *In* Umphred DA (ed): Neurological Rehabilitation, 3rd ed. St Louis, Mosby, 1995.

73. Umphred DA Introduction and Overview. *In* Umphred DA (ed): Neurological Rehabilitation, 3rd ed. St Louis, Mosby, 1995.

74. Umphred DA Limbic Complex. *In* Umphred DA (ed): Neurological Rehabilitation, 3rd ed. St Louis, Mosby, 1995.

75. Wagner TH, Hu TW: Economic costs of urinary incontinence in 1995. Urology 51:355–361, 1998.

76. Wall LL, Davidson TG: The role of muscular re-education by physical therapy in the treatment of genuine stress urinary incontinence. Obstet Gynecol Surv 47:322–331, 1992.

77. Wall LL, Norton PA, DeLancey JOL: Practical Urogynecology. Baltimore, Williams & Wilkins, 1993

78. Walters MD, Karram MM: Clinical Urogynecology. St Louis, Mosby, 1993.

79. Wennergren HM, Ölberg BE, Sandstedt P: The importance of leg support for relaxation of the pelvic floor muscles. Scand J Urol Nephrol 25:205–213, 1991.

80. Wesselmann U, Burnett AL, Heinberg LJ: The urogenital and rectal pain syndromes. Pain 73:269–294, 1997.

81. Wiedemann A, Zumbé J: Stand der Physiotherapie in der Harninkontinenzbehandlung—Ergebnisse einer bundesweiten Umfrage. Krankengymnastik 51:1547–1551, 1999.

82. Winstein CJ: Knowledge of results and motor learning—implications for physical therapy. Phys Ther 71:140–149, 1991.

83. Winstein CJ, Pohl PS, Lewthwaite R: Effects of physical guidance and knowledge of results on motor learning: Support for the guidance hypothesis. Res Q Exerc Sport 65:316–323, 1994.

Orthotics: Evaluation, Prognosis, and Intervention

WALTER RACETTE, BS, CPO

Key Words

- ankle-foot orthosis (AFO)
- anterior/toe lever arm
- double adjustable ankle joint
- knee-ankle-foot orthosis (KAFO)
- posterior/heel lever arm

Objectives

After reading this chapter the student/therapist will:

1. Understand the force system produced by the use of an orthosis.

2. Understand prescription rationale gained from orthotic evaluation.

3. Know the variables considered by the orthotist to optimize outcome during orthotic intervention.

OVERVIEW

The advancements of and access to medical technology have had a profound effect in the field of orthotics. The evolution of plastic technology has dramatically improved the ability to control, support, and protect all areas of the human body. Today, patients are fitted for custom-made and prefabricated orthotic devices that provide a variety of functions in both a timely and cost-effective manner. These factors have led physicians to routinely prescribe orthoses for a wide range of medical conditions, whereas in prior decades, the lack of availability and a shortage of experienced orthotists restricted patient access and narrowed the use of orthoses.[4] Today, orthoses are important treatment options in postoperative management, acute fracture management, and adjunct treatment, in addition to their more traditional uses in past decades. For many, the proliferation of prefabricated orthoses signaled a dilution of quality orthotic care, but in reality it has had just the opposite effect. The availablity of cost-effective prefabricated orthoses has not taken orthotic use out of the hands of orthotists but has put it into the minds of physicians. As with all new technological advancements, there has been incorrect application and utilization. It is not that many of these prefabricated orthoses are difficult to apply but rather that there is a need that a clear understanding of the indications, contraindications, and limitations of these devices be made known to not only orthotists but also other health care professionals.

No discussion involving the evaluation, prognosis, and intervention of orthotics would be complete without mentioning the effects of government and private regulations. Government regulations have dramatically changed the course of the orthotic profession from the beginning of the Medicare program to diagnostic-related groups (DRGs) to managed care. Medicare was the first national program to cover the cost of both orthotic and prosthetic devices, and before that point only a special few had access to "braces and limbs." DRGs put the responsibility of paying for prescribed orthoses into the hands of the local hospital. Once the specific diagnosis was made, the government would allow a specific amount for reimbursement and left the decision of how to do that with the physician or hospital. This policy change created many new innovations. Hospitals, interested in reducing the length of hospital stays, challenged physicians to change the way they treated their patients. Patients no longer are immobilized for long periods in hospital beds but are sent home sooner or discharged to a less acute setting or to skilled nursing facilities. The use of orthotic devices to expedite care has increased dramatically, and halo fixation systems, thoracic lumbar sacral orthoses (TLSOs), and fracture orthoses are but a few examples of devices that aid reduction in hospitalization. Another significant effect of the DRG decade on orthotics was the need to reduce delivery times and be as cost effective as possible. Orthoses needed to be delivered in hours, not days, and careful

937

evaluation needed to be developed in regard to use of prefabricated custom-fitted versus custom-made orthoses. Challenges to improve traditional methods of fabrication and higher utilization spawned the rapid growth of a wide range of orthoses for patient care.

Government-inspired changes in insurance coverage and managed care have created wide-ranging effects on the entire medical delivery system that are both positive and negative. The full impact on the orthotic profession has yet to be seen, but there are several areas that have changed patient care. Cost-containment pressure led to the need for small and large private orthotic facilities to reduce customary fees to enable them to continue caring for long-term patients as the rush to join health maintenance groups spread throughout the country. For many professionals, the years of creating awareness, value, and benefit for providing orthoses were now challenged by an additional layer of administrative personnal that had little or limited knowledge yet questioned cost necessity and, rarely, medical necessity. The need to learn the new rules required clinical staff to do less patient care and more administrative work at a reduced fee. Both the lack of ability to deal with all these changes and the fear of failure had a profound effect on reshaping the orthotic and prosthetic industry. In a time when the orthotist saw many new technologies emerge and patient care outcomes were exceeding those of previous decades, managed care challenged our ability to make these advancements possible for the majority of our patients and restricted access through exclusive contracts with providers. Cost/value questions are essential in quality care; unfortunately, our profession did not have the scientific data or justification ready for this health care revolution. The professional relationship between physical occupational therapy and orthotics is very important as the evolution of managed care continues. Identifying patient functional goals and a variety of predictable outcomes is critical not only for managed care but also for patient care. Orthotists must embrace the challenge of measured improvement in function from the care they provide and use it to develop a standard of care like the rest of the medical profession. It is in that spirit that I challenge the wide range of understanding of the evaluation, prognosis, and intervention of orthotics in neurological rehabilitation.

An orthosis (Fig. 31–1) is an external device that when applied to the body produces a force that biomechanically affects the body in such a way as to correct, support, or stabilize the trunk and/or extremity. The goals in patient care with orthotic use vary from permanent use, after other treatment to maintain gains, to temporary use. Many factors enter into the decisions on use and type of orthosis, but it is essential that when the need for orthotic intervention is determined that the least-complicated orthosis that fits the patient's needs be used. The rehabilitation team must build a priority list of desired outcomes and accept that there are times that all of the items on the list may not be achieved either by the orthosis or by the patient/team combination. As an example, an excessive amount of plastic ankle-foot orthoses (AFOs) have been used, both custom made and custom fitted, because they are more cosmetic and lighter than a metal and

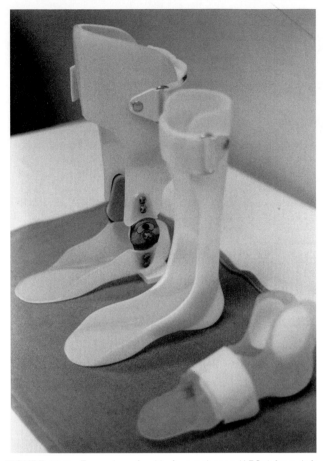

FIGURE 31–1. Examples of ankle-foot orthoses (AFOs) from *left,* ground reaction type adjustable AFO, fixed 90-degree AFO, and supramalleolar AFO.

leather type AFO. There certainly are times when all higher-priority goals can be achieved so that down the list cosmesis and light weight can be considered; however, in the case of a patient who has had a cerebrovascular accident (CVA) and who has 5 degrees of plantarflexion and a tendency to go into genu recurvatum, use of such an orthosis will not be successful. The typical pattern that follows is that the patient's knee pops back and hurts with the heel rubbing on the back of the orthosis. When the patient sits down, plantarflexion increases and the cycle continues.

Coordination between health care professionals in the development of patient treatment goals is essential during the evaluation process. Without communication, adequate care of the patient may be considered unsuccessful, owing to design criteria omission as simple as placing a loop closure on the side the patient could not reach. A sound understanding of orthotic principles, biomechanical understanding, and skilled patient management techniques must be employed in this patient population to be successful.

There are similarities in orthotic management of orthopedic and neurologically impaired patients; however, the neurological population presents additional factors that challenge prescription criteria for the rehabilitation team. Lack of proprioception, sensation (hyper- or hyposensitivity), and spasticity represent some of these special considerations, and possible problems with communication add to these patient management complications.

BASIC ORTHOTIC FUNCTIONS

Alignment of the extremities and spine is a common function in orthotic use. The orthosis can provide either temporary or permanent function. A TLSO may be prescribed for stabilizing alignment after spinal fusion in the case of a spinal cord injury. A supramalleolar orthosis is a commonly prescribed orthosis to hold the foot in proper alignment. When the goal of orthotic intervention is to correct alignment, one must evaluate if the pressure required to maintain that corrected alignment will be tolerated by the overlying soft tissue, if the malalignment being corrected is due to a muscle weakness, and if the new position will create an unstable joint. Remember that aligning one joint may result in the proximal or distal joint's being placed in malalignment. For example, the correction of a knee with genu valgum may seem easy, but in what alignment does that put the ankle joint; does the subtalar joint have the mobility to pronate?

Stability is often required when caring for the neurologically deficient patient. These patients frequently lack the muscle control and strength necessary to maintain trunk balance or to ambulate. Patients with muscular dystrophy benefit from TLSOs to help maintain trunk stability for sitting balance (Fig. 31–2) However, the decision regarding an orthosis must take into consideration maximum stability and flexibility while not restraining

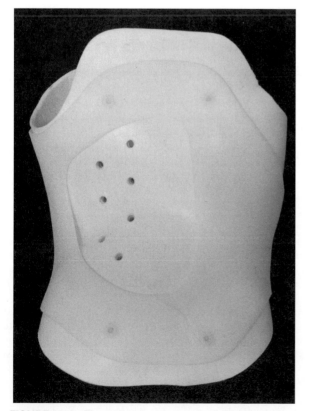

FIGURE 31–2. Thoracolumbosacral orthosis (posterior view).

breathing capability. An AFO that limits both dorsiflexion and plantarflexion can stabilize the ankle and the knee for the CVA patient.[5] Although this patient may only require medial-lateral ankle stability, controlling the anterior-posterior lever arms at the ankle can provide knee stability. The orthosis functions by producing a posterior movement acting to extend the knee, because most patients requiring this type of stability function with a foot flat gait pattern instead of a heel strike gait pattern.

Preventing deformity is a common use for an orthosis in the neurologically impaired patient. These deformities result from a lack of proprioception and/or significant muscle imbalance (e.g., spasticity) over an extended period of time. Wrist-hand orthoses (WHOs) are used to prevent flexion and ulnar deviation in the care of the CVA patient. These orthoses are static as opposed to dynamic because introduction of a dynamic force usually triggers a spastic response. In this example, preventing deformity will assist caregivers to maintain hygiene.

The patient with a closed-head injury presents a significant challenge to the rehabilitation team, and his or her orthotic care is no exception [5] The lower-extremity pattern is usually one of equinovarus with strong spasticity. Use of an orthosis to prevent or control the deformity requires maximum control, taxing skin tolerance. If not treated early and aggressively this deformity can cause major deformity of the knee—genu recurvatum and genu varum. Tone reduction and contracture prevention are vital. Maintaining long-term function in this patient population is difficult.

Contracture reduction is a goal of many orthotic uses in the patient with a neurological problem. These types of orthoses are either dynamic or static and are used in conjunction with different therapeutic modalities to reduce the contracture. Dynamic contracture-reducing orthoses employ a spring-type mechanism that uses a low force over extended time to gain range of motion (ROM). Static-type orthoses range from serial casting placed on at manual stretch, to custom-made cylinder devices designed to spread force over larger areas, to custom-fitted devices with some type of quick adjustability. Dynamic-type orthoses are usually contraindicated for the neurologically impaired patient, because even at low tension they tend to trigger spasticity; the exception occurs in the patient with a lower motor neuron impairment. To reduce contractures one must be cautiously aggressive, because the amount of force required to get results often borders on the soft tissue's ability to tolerate the pressure of the orthoses. Experience, frequent sessions, and close communication with other members of the rehabilitation team and the patient and patient's family are critical factors for success.

EVALUATION

The evaluation of the neurologically impaired patient must be comprehensive. One must not read a medical diagnosis and assume a specific clinical picture. The medical diagnosis should alert the evaluator to patterns associated with the identified impairments and should be used to confirm potential findings. Complete patient evaluations do not end with ROM evaluation, muscle testing, and assessment of proprioception, skin sensitivity or lack, and integrity of the affected limb or spine. The clinician ordering an orthotic device must assess the total picture of the client to determine what limitations initiating orthotic care may have on other important functions. Last, but not least, the evaluation must include a patient management assessment:

- What is the client/family motivation?
- How much componentry can the client tolerate/function with?
- What chance of success does the client/family have once the client leaves the clinical setting?
- How significant are the risks associated with orthotic intervention?

As stated, the total evaluation of the patient and patient's environment is important in developing the treatment plan, as is the communication between the physical/occupational therapist and the orthotist. Whether done together or, more realistically, in separate sites, the details of a treatment plan must be discussed. The neurologically impaired patient often presents a series of complex issues that include biomechanical, communication, and visualization factors, among others. Incomplete information and a lack of effort in communicating by these professionals will not lead to a comprehensive treatment plan.

When conducting an evaluation, the review of the medical diagnosis and the gathering of a history are extremely important. A complete impairment/disability diagnosis will indicate important information to the team. For example, if a client has poliomyelitis, the orthotist is aware that the client has a lower motor neuron lesion and that proprioception is intact. This person will have the benefit of skeletal balance and therefore will require durable orthotic fabrication and components. Compare this to a similar result in muscle testing and ROM for a paraplegic with an incomplete T12 level injury. Patients with this upper motor neuron lesion lack proprioception and require other stimulation to simply get a sense of standing balance. A lightweight orthosis is required because they rarely use orthoses as major means of locomotion. Gathering patient history is not only a vital part of the evaluation but also, more importantly, an opportunity to establish a productive patient management environment. Patients and family members have important information regarding the initial injury, previous medical care, reason they sought additional care, desired outcomes of new treatment, and so on. In these times of efficiency, most of this information can be gathered as either the therapist or the orthotist begins other areas of their respective professional evaluations. These are important client/family management skills. One must hear from clients/family why they came to see you and what their expectations of care are. Don't assume you know without asking, because often the expectations of the clients and families are higher than the clinicians' expectations. Communicating at a level that is understood is vital and also demonstrates to the client/family that you are a concerned professional and worthy of their trust and confidence.

Evaluation of the Spine

Each area of the spinal column has a variety of combinations of motion and function. At the lumbar level the spinal column serves as the base for the upright position. It also protects vital organs and serves as a supporting structure for the lungs. It aids the upper extremities in reaching and carrying objects, and it protects the nervous system pathway for the body and controls the upright position and motions of the head. The individual segments of the spine have relatively few complicated orthotic challenges. However, it is rare that only one segment is involved in the neuropathic patient, and it is common that two or more areas of the spine will be involved in orthotic fitting. For example, supporting the head in a functional position is a major goal of orthotic intervention, but to accomplish this the orthosis must encompass the thoracic as well as the cervical spine to distribute the forces to pressure tolerance.

When evaluating the cervical spine and head, one must, in addition to muscle testing, determine at what angulation the upright position of the head cannot be recovered. Limiting the head from nonfunctional positions (i.e., extreme extension) is an easier orthotic function than to have to fabricate an orthosis that will hold the head upright. Many neurologically impaired patients have the strength to move in a 15-to 20-degree range of flexion/extension, lateral bend, and rotation but do not have the strength to reposition the head in greater angles. Even the best soft tissue about the head does not tolerate long-term pressure from an orthosis; therefore, intermittent control/relief is critical in design. Pressure directly on the ear is not tolerated at any time.

The thoracic and lumbar areas of the spine are rarely treated separately by orthotics in the neurologically impaired patient. The major reasons for orthotic intervention in this area are to stabilize the trunk for balance, to protect surgical correction/stabilization, and to maintain respiration. The pelvis is generally used as a base to prevent distal migration of the orthosis, thus the S equals sacral in TLSO. One must closely evaluate the degree of deformity, prominence of bone structure, skin sensation, and condition of soft tissue coverage.

Many neurological patients also have other medical conditions that need to be considered in orthotic design, such as colostomy and gastrointestinal tubes. Scoliosis and kyphosis are common conditions in this patient group. The rehabilitation team must reach a balance between the advantages of correcting the spinal deformity to maintain respiratory function and the disadvantage of a tightly-fitting TLSO and the skin pressure it creates.

The evaluation of the spine and the potential need for orthotic intervention would not be complete without recognizing the effect the desired orthosis may have on the extremities, whether the patient is ambulatory or non–weight bearing. What movements of the spine are present during ambulation, and would immobilizing the spine significantly affect the patient? Will the orthosis restrict needed shoulder elevation and arm movements?

Evaluation of the Upper Extremities

The evaluation of the upper extremities requires multiple input from health care professionals, patients, family, and teachers because of the wide range of specific functions a person performs daily. Unique to this area, multiple functions generally require multiple orthotic devices. Typical functions of orthoses of the upper extremities include maintaining a functional wrist/hand position, reducing contracture or tone, transferring force available in one area to another, and supporting subluxations due to denervation in addition to various assistive orthoses necessary for activities of daily living. The neurologically impaired patient commonly requires several orthoses, each with different functions for use throughout the course of the day. Strength, ROM, condition of soft tissues, and sensation are all important evaluation factors. In addition, ambulatory status, bilateral or unilateral condition, status of vision, and condition of the spine and head must be factored into the indications and contraindications of formulation of the orthotic needs of the patient.

Many more critical muscle tests must be made in the upper extremity as opposed to the lower extremity because minor increases or decreases in strength dramatically change orthotic need. For example, the C5 quadriplegic has the ability to function with WHOs with enough wrist extension to use the tenodesis effect, which can produce a three-jaw chuck grip. The difference between a functioning and nonfunctioning orthosis is very minor, not only because of less muscle strength but also because of inefficiency in the tenodesis splint (e.g., friction or malalignment). A patient with unilateral involvement has far different needs than the patient with bilateral involvement. For example, in a patient who has sustained a CVA a typical orthotic intervention may be a positional WHO to prevent contracture and prevent injury and a supporting shoulder orthosis for shoulder subluxation. In this situation, the other extremity becomes dominant and there is little need to fabricate complex orthoses for use of the affected extremity. The patient with bilateral involvement presents a much different picture. Conservation for grooming, feeding, mobility, and so on must be factored into the desired expectation during evaluation.

Orthotic intervention for the neurologically impaired patient is complex because this patient typically has involvement of the trunk, head, and lower extremity. Specialized wheelchairs and seating systems are required. Evaluation is most effective when all rehabilitation team members work together to establish a treatment plan. Orthotic treatment must maximize what little muscle strength and ROM that these patients have. Orthoses that are used during the day to maximize function are replaced by positional orthoses at night to preserve gains and prevent decline. The occupational therapist provides the majority of functional and positional orthoses for the upper extremity. New materials and fabrication techniques have been developed that have significantly improved the quality and availability of upper extremity orthoses. In today's medical environment many occupational therapists work directly with orthopedic hand specialists and trauma physicians to use low temperature materials to mold custom devices specifically designed for protecting surgical reconstruction, for promoting or maintaining ROM, and/or for use as an assistive device.

Evaluation of the Lower Extremities

Evaluation of the lower extremities offers many challenges because of the role of ambulation and its value in the independence of the patient and other family members. ROM, strength, an existing deformity, proprioception, tone, and soft tissue sensation must be evaluated, and, where appropriate, weight-bearing/existing gait analysis is done.[2] Patient/family assessment as related to ability to understand and follow instructions is extremely important because the potential for injury may outweigh the benefit of orthotic intervention to transform a patient from non–weight bearing to limited ambulation. Lack of ROM at the hip and knee will significantly decrease the duration of potential ambulation or may totally inhibit ambulation. Lack of ROM at the hip and knee is more critical than lack of strength, and in the foot and ankle the need for normal ROM is more critical for efficient standing balance and ambulation.

Orthoses of the lower extremity function by providing a combination of force lever arms acting about a joint and are significantly compromised by the lack of ROM. These force lever arms substitute for the lack of strength; for example, the anterior lever arm provided by blocking dorsiflexion of the ankle provides a posteriorly directed force that provides knee stability. If the patient lacks the ability to get even to neutral, this tightness provides its own lever arm, which will result in a variety of undesirable actions (Fig. 31–3). Genu recurvatum, foot/ankle varus, shortened stride length on the nonaffected side, and the heel raising out of the shoe are common signs of this problem.[5] These issues are further complicated when lack of proprioception, spasticity, and lack of sensation are present. This is discussed further in the clinical examples presented later in the chapter. Lack of ROM at the ankle creates many symptoms in the lower extremity but is often missed during evaluation as the cause of these problems.

Genu varum and genu recurvatum are common deformities of the neurologically impaired patient, and there are a number of factors that create them. In addition to the ankle, leg-length differences, lack of quadriceps strength, and lack of proprioception can create deformities about the knee. The patient with poliomyelitis may have both a short extremity and weak knee extensors, which lead to genu recurvatum and genu valgum; but correcting the deformity without protecting against unde-

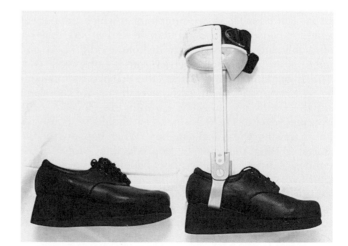

FIGURE 31–3. Modifications made in the orthosis and shoes to accommodate heel cord contracture.

sirable knee flexion would be a mistake. These patients with lower motor neuron disease have excellent proprioception, which is the reason they protect the unstable knee by hyperextending it by applying force with their upper extremity pushing posteriorly on the femur. A similar upper motor neuron–impaired patient (e.g., one with a CVA) has a similar knee presentation; however, the usual cause of this patient's deformity is a tight heel cord and/or lack of proprioception, and orthotic design is very different.

Reduced or lack of strength and ROM limitations about the hip limit effective ambulation and leave the patient much more reliant on trunk stability and upper-extremity ambulatory aids. Hip flexors are more critical than hip extensors because they serve to advance the limb in reciprocating gait, whereas lack of hip extensors are substituted by the strong hip ligaments that tighten in extension. The lack of ROM to at least neutral about the hip creates major problems for the patient even if the patient has excellent upper-extremity strength. This lack of ROM will not allow stability in standing once force is removed from the upper-extremity ambulatory aids. Hands-free standing balance is a highly desirable outcome resulting from orthotic intervention.

GOALS OF ORTHOTIC INTERVENTION

The patient evaluation and clinical experience must be used to create a plan of treatment expectation. The value of our experience is now tested to predict what outcome is likely to occur after following the treatment plan. Only a well-thought-out plan, thoroughly communicated to all participants, will be successful. All too frequently we assume that the patient and family know the goals of orthotic intervention; not listening to patient/family concerns before initiating the treatment plan is also common. These are both major patient management mistakes. Several factors play key roles in the success of orthotic intervention. To improve function without complication or patient risk, the clinician must be sure to address the client's major complaint and why he or she came to see either the therapist or orthotist. It is important to establish a baseline of function so that results of intervention are measurable. There are situations in which the patient benefit is very clear and immediate and others that require concentrated instruction, orthotic modification, and time before improved function can be observed. The process of donning and doffing the orthosis as independently as possible enhances the overall goal for the client and the family and must be carefully developed by the experienced clinician. The therapist should be conservative in setting these expectations. What happens in the clinical setting may not be reproducible easily in the home situation. Instructing the patient to stabilize the knee by using the hamstrings in the clinical setting may create risk when the patient is discharged home, whereas providing an AFO with an anterior stop at the ankle that would provide a mechanical knee-stabilizing effect may prove much safer in the long term.

Keep the orthotic interventions as simple as possible:

What is the least amount of orthotic intervention that will provide the expected goal? Although this is an obvious statement, the balance between too much and not enough can challenge the clinician's skill and experience. The use of trial orthoses can provide valuable information during the evaluation, and these devices are commercially available. Although the benefits of various types of thermomoldable plastics have been invaluable for many indications, there are times when their use adds risk and complications without improvement, compared with a traditional AFO fabricated with metal and leather attached to the patient's shoe (Table 31–1). For example, if the patient requires ankle and knee stability yet lacks sensation in the foot and ankle, the double upright metal orthosis attached to the patient's shoe presents less risk for possible skin breakdown when a rigid ankle plastic orthosis is prescribed if the family is lucky enough to find a shoe big enough to allow the patient to easily don the orthosis. Introduction of biomechanical forces to the extremities may cause unwanted movements or restrictions, and careful selection of componentry is essential to keeping the focus on the orthotic plan. For example, a patient who sustained a CVA may need more anterior lever force for knee stability, so one would plantarflex the orthotic joint (Table 31–2). However, this knee-stabilizing effect in stance phase would cause a toe drag during swing phase. A simple fix is to provide the opposite side with a ¼-inch heel and sole lift for additional clearance during the swing phase of the affected extremity.

Treatment goals must be realistic and manageable. All too often treatment plans are only in the minds of the clinicians and are never or poorly communicated to the patient/family. One should expect that the patient or the parents of the patient would always think that the benefits of this effort would be far above what you know are possible. The time to address those gaps is before treatment, not when the patient/family realize expectations regarding functional gains may not become reality. If that occurs, you have lost and so has the patient. Discussing realistic achievable goals of treatment, assessing all factors (e.g., medical, home situation, individual motivation) with the patient/family in language they understand, is critical if success of orthotic intervention is to be achieved. The goal of orthotic care for a patient with CVA is to provide safe standing balance for transfer and minimal ambulation in the home. Patients and family will realize the major benefit this will have on the home situation. However, without this identified as the goal before orthotic care, they may leave the therapeutic environment wondering why the patient cannot walk normally. This clinician error is an all too frequent patient management mistake.

A cost-effective orthosis must be provided in a timely manner. With today's vast number of orthotic devices, the orthotist must stay abreast of the wide array of choices at his or her disposal to meet the needs of the patient. The focus of cost containment is not a recent event in the orthotic profession because funding for these devices has always been challenged, and it has assisted in the development of more cost-effective alternatives, such as the prefabricated orthosis. The introduction of thermo moldable plastics into orthotics in the late 1960s and early 1970s on a custom basis replaced to a large extent the need to

TABLE 31–1. Comparison of Metal and Plastic Orthoses

Factor	Metal and Leather	Polypropylene	Lamination/Graphite	Polyethylene
Adjustability	Yes	Yes w/heat	No	Yes w/heat
Patient change shoes	No	Yes	Yes	Yes
Strength weight bearing	Yes	Yes	Yes	No
Skin at risk	Yes	Yes, close observation	No	Yes
Best spinal use	No	Yes	No	Yes
Long-term wear	Yes	Less	Yes	Least
Weight (lightest =1)	4	2	3	1
Adjustability to changing clinical picture	Yes	Limited, unless initial articulation fabricated	No	No
Short-term need	Yes	Yes	No	Yes
Requires corrective force with patient good sensation	Fair	Good	Fair	Good
Questionable patient compliance ability/ direction	Best	Questionable	No	Fair
Clinician wants ability to change angulation, ankle or knee	Best	Limited°	No	Not indicated above for weight bearing
Upper extemity fabrication—direct mold highest frequency	Limited	Yes	Limited	Yes

°Used in combination with metal joints produces best results.

TABLE 31–2. Indications for Common Orthotic Modifications/Additions

Modification/Addition	Description
SACH modification	This modification is done by cutting out a triangular wedge in the heel of the shoe and securing a softer material. The solid ankle cushion heel (SACH) modification is used to dampen the effect of the heel/posterior lever arm at heel strike. This force produces an anterior force to destabilize the knee, which may be undesirable.
Heel and sole buildup	Adding a ¼-inch heel and sole buildup to the unaffected side can create additional swing clearance needed on the affected side. This modification is indicated if additional dorsiflexion of the orthotic joint creates knee instability or if the patient lacks dorsiflexion range of motion.
Rocker-bottom heel and sole modifications	There are several different styles of rocker-bottom build up. Although the roll built into this modification may differ, the basic results are the same—to add motion and rotation of the center of gravity forward when the ankle and/or knee orthotic joint is locked.
Long tongue stirrup/extended steel shanks	A stirrup is the metal attachment to the shoe. The utilization of a long tongue (a steel extension that goes distal between the bottom of the shoe and the heel and sole) is necessary to transfer the force created by restriction of ankle motion. Without this type of fabrication, the force produced at midstance will not be controlled. The steel shank produces the same control but is not part of the stirrup and may be used alone in combination with a rocker bottom.
Medial/valgus control T-strap; lateral/varus control T-strap	These straps, leather on traditional double upright orthoses or plastic/padding modifications on plastic ankle-foot orthoses, produce a force to reduce valgus (a medial T-strap) or varus (a lateral T-strap). A medial T-strap attaches to the shoe medially, and the beltlike strap goes around the lateral upright and is tightened. The lateral T-strap is opposite.
Heel buildup	A heel buildup is used to accommodate heel cord tightness. The tibia must be at least 90 degrees to the floor for safe balance and ambulation. Common signs of the need to build up the heel are genu recurvatum and the heel slipping out of the shoe. The amount of heel buildup must be matched with the same heel and sole buildup on the opposite side.
Instep and figure-of-8 straps	This orthotic modification is used to keep the heel back in the shoe or plastic ankle-foot orthosis when a tight heel cord is present. These straps fit across the dorsum of the foot with a posterior attachment point.
Swedish knee orthosis	This prefabricated knee orthosis is an effective method to prevent genu recurvatum on a temporary basis. It is typically indicated after a cerebrovascular accident for the patient who lacks proprioception and whose knee pops back, creating pain and slack knee ligaments. It can be used temporarily as a training orthosis or permanently when persistent pain and instability are present.

mold leather and/or metal to fabricate an orthosis. This not only improved the total contact fit but also dramatically reduced the time and skill level for manufacturing. From this beginning, today's orthotist has a multitude of devices from which to choose to meet the needs of the patient, from the custom-made fit from a patient mold to the ready-made prefabricated fit. A thorough understanding of the indications and contraindications for each of these devices is essential to meet patient needs. The lack of understanding of biomechanical principles, the limitations of prefabricated orthoses, and the lack of knowledge of custom fitting can lead to failure. All orthoses produce a force field, some desirable and some not. It requires an experienced clinician to make the most appropriate choices, because all too often the failure of treatment is blamed on an orthosis when it usually is the result of an inappropriate initial selection of orthotic componentry, the lack of custom made/custom fit, or the fact that the patient was not an orthotic candidate from the beginning. Prefabricated custom-fitted orthoses are only cost effective if they produce the desired goal over a period of time. As a general rule, one should consider prefabricated custom-fitted orthoses for patients who have a normal anatomy and/or who need the orthosis for a short period of time; one should consider custom-made orthoses for extremities/spine that have deformity, an unusual size, and/or must be used indefinitely.

CLINICAL EXAMPLES

Paraplegia

Orthotic consideration for the paraplegic patient is generally considered at the T12 level in the complete lesion.[3] Complete lesions higher in the cord leave the patient without enough trunk stability to effectively utilize bilateral orthoses. Although a thoracic extension can be added to bilateral knee-ankle-foot orthoses (KAFOs) this addition greatly increases the difficulty of donning the orthosis independently, and most patients will have great difficulty getting from sitting to standing.

The orthoses for a T12 complete paraplegic are bilateral KAFOs. The patient generally uses a swing-to or swing-through gait, and successful use of orthoses requires excellent standing balance. There are three significant design requirements for these KAFOs: shallow thigh and calf bands, bail or French knee locks, and adjustable ankle joints with long tongue stirrups with strutter bars to the heads of the metatarsals (Scott-Craig design) (Fig. 31–4). The shallow bands force the center of gravity forward, inducing lordosis so the patient can rest on the Y ligaments of Bigelow. The knee locks are automatic, because the patient requires the upper extremities for standing. The bail/French joint will lock as the patient stands and bends over the rigid ankle joint, forcing the knee joints into extension. The lock then will catch on the back of a wheelchair seat or other chair and bend at the joint when the patient sits. The foot/ankle complex forms the basis for balance. A few degrees of adjustment at the double adjustable ankle joint can make the difference between safe standing balance and limited standing

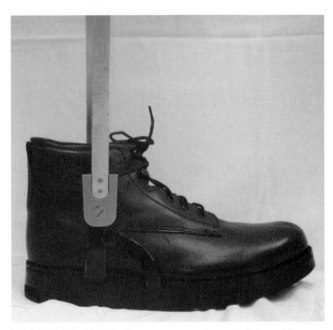

FIGURE 31–4. Modifications necessary to control the ankle setting in a client with spinal cord injury (Scott-Craig shoe/stirrup modifications).

balance. The long tongue stirrup extends at least to the heads of the metatarsals and farther if the patient is taller and heavier than normal. The use of a strutter bar from the upright of the stirrup extending to a transverse bar at the heads of the metatarsals ensures rigidity as complete as necessary. A balance between effective standing balance and ambulation is reached after training and ankle adjustment. Patients must have full ROM at the hips, knees, and ankles for use of these devices to be successful.

CASE 31–1   A.M.

A.M. is a 21-year old with incomplete T12-level paraplegia secondary to a gunshot wound. A.M. has normal upper-extremity strength and ROM. He has had surgery for spinal fusion. Trunk strength is 4/5, left hip is 3/5, knee is 2/5, right hip is 1/5, and right knee is 0/5. ROM is full at hips, knees, and ankles. A.M. can transfer independently and has the goal of household ambulation, although he is aware that it "takes a lot of work." A.M. was fitted with a right KAFO with shallow bands, drop lock knee joints, and double adjustable ankle joints locked in five degrees of dorsiflexion (Fig. 31–5). Drop locks were used instead of bail locks because of the use of a unilateral KAFO. A.M. had balance, strength, and a foot orthosis on the left side. The left lower extremity was fitted with an AFO, double upright, and double adjustable ankle joints adjusted to match the right orthosis. The distal attachment to the shoes was with long tongue stirrups and strutter bars. The patient was able to ambulate with forearm crutches.

Hemiplegia

Patients who have suffered a CVA can vary widely in their need for orthotic intervention, from a simple AFO to assist toe clearance, to an AFO to stabilize both ankle and knee, to an orthosis used temporarily for training purposes.[6] The use of a KAFO for the hemiplegic patient is rarely indicated. Even though the more affected patient does not have knee stability, he or she rarely ambulates with a heel strike that would destabilize the knee and therefore can use an AFO with an anterior limited-range ankle joint. Additionally, patients cannot don the KAFO with the use of one upper extremity. With the lack of hip flexors and knee instability on the affected side, the orthotic intervention may be to assist in transfers. As a general rule, orthotic intervention for the client with a CVA ranges from a static-toe pick-up orthosis to a double adjustable ankle joint with the ankle locked. The use of spring components is not effective, because they will initiate spasticity. The lack of ROM into dorsiflexion and even neutral causes the biggest problem for these patients. The ankle that lacks range prevents advancement of the center of gravity and produces a lever arm that induces genu recurvatum and pain, and either the heel comes out of the shoe or the ankle rolls into varus. Because these patients lack proprioception, this constant force directed posteriorly will, over the course of a few months, be significant, the patient will hurt and not ambulate, the heel cord will shorten more, and the cycle will continue. Heel cords rarely gain length long term once the patient is discharged from the rehabilitation setting,

and one must consider the family/home situation. Heel buildups on the affected side are used to bring the tibia into 90 degrees. Buildups of 1 to 1½ inches are not uncommon. Remember to balance the opposite shoe. If a patient presents on the border between different orthotic components, it is best to choose the more stable orthosis. The use of trial orthoses during evaluation is invaluable as well as helpful initially as the patient improves, requiring less or no orthosis. A three-point pressure orthosis for the knee, such as a Swedish knee cage (Fig. 31–6), is also a valuable training orthosis and, in the case of some post-CVA patients, is used daily when the degree of recurvatum exceeds the patient's ability to control the force. The stirrup, the metal attachment to the patient's shoe, must be firm and extend under the sole and heel to the heads of the metatarsals. Although this adds weight to the orthosis, it is necessary to transmit knee-stabilizing forces. Stirrups attached under the heel will only allow undesirable motion and not provide the required stability.

Paralytic Spine

There are many neuropathic diagnoses that affect the spinal column. Spinal muscle atrophy, teraplegia, myelomeningocele, and Duchennes muscular dystrophy can all require orthotic intervention. Although materials, padding/no padding, trim lines, length of time used, and optional area openings can vary with different conditions, most spinal stabilizing orthoses are TLSOs. Orthoses used for postsurgical stabilization tend to be of more rigid material to support the healing spine. The paralytic spine

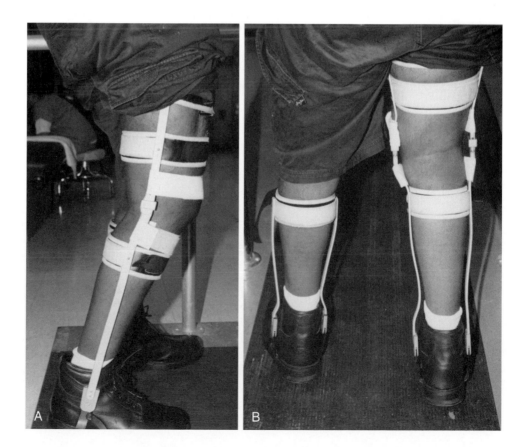

FIGURE 31–5. Patient standing wearing a right knee-ankle-foot orthosis. *A*, Lateral view; *B*, posterior view.

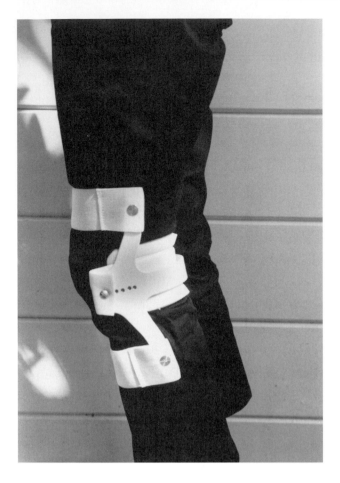

FIGURE 31–6. Prefabricated three-point pressure knee orthosis (Swedish knee cage) to control genu recurvatum.

that is not surgically stabilized can have either a flexible or a rigid curvature. An orthosis for a patient with a rigid curvature is used to avoid further deformity and differs from that used by the patient with a flexible curvature. In this case, the orthosis will be used to hold some of the correction that can be obtained. These patients are usually casted for custom orthoses, and although non–weight-bearing supine casts can greatly reduce the curve, many patients will not tolerate the pressure once in the upright sitting position. Orthotic intervention usually has one or more of the following goals: improved sitting balance, support of surgical stabilization, prevention of further spinal deformity, and use as an assistive positional device for better utilization of head and upper extremities and improved respiratory function. Most TLSOs for these patients are total circumferential designs using rigid materials (polypropylene) to less rigid materials (polyethylene) to combination padding with a rigid/semi-rigid frame to the heat-formable plastazote. Fabrication and fitting of these orthoses requires an experienced orthotist and adherence to detail. Establishing the distal and proximal trim lines of the orthosis will require a fine balancing act between providing enough length to support the spine but not break down the skin in accomplishing that goal. Several clinic visits are necessary to obtain the desired outcome.

Spastic Diplegic Cerebral Palsy

The goals of orthotic intervention in the cerebral palsy patient are to control tone, to prevent contractures, and/or as a secondary support after a surgical procedure.[1] Although it is not within the scope of this chapter to describe and discuss the current treatment protocol for cerebral palsy, orthotic intervention varies from region to region. What is clear is that careful evaluation, clinical experience, treating each patient individually, and a cohesive rehabilitation team are critical factors in successful orthotic intervention. As a general rule, the use of one orthosis to prevent contracture should be different from the orthosis for ambulation. Some of the new designs incorporate modules that can key into each other or can be used separately. This feature allows flexibility, assists in donning, especially in the spastic patient, and meets several treatment objectives. Modular articulating joints with various settings and functions to use with thermoplastic orthoses greatly increase the options that are available today. With the goals of orthotic intervention stated earlier, total contact type orthoses are generally the desired option. As with any total contact orthosis and hypersensitive or hyposensitive skin, a cautious balance between correction/holding and skin tolerance must be reached. The fitting and follow-up of these types of orthoses requires experience, knowledge, and patience. Combi-

CASE 31–2   D.M.

D.M. is a 58-year old who had a left CVA, resulting in a right hemiplegia almost 2 years ago. She is being evaluated at the request of her physician because of increased knee pain and poor standing balance. D.M. was fitted with a plastic AFO fixed at 90 degrees 14 months ago. She is wearing the orthosis, but the heel will not stay in her shoe. Evaluation shows that the patient lacks 15 degrees from getting the foot to neutral (in plantarflexion), has no active dorsiflexion or plantarflexion, and has a fair minus knee extension and flexion. She also walks with the aid of a quad cane and has 10 degrees of genu recurvatum and slight genu varum at midstance. Her goal was to walk with less pain and to be more stable. D.M. was fitted with bilateral upright, double adjustable locked ankle joints with long tongue stirrups and a 1½-inch heel buildup (Fig. 31–7). The left shoe was built up 1½ inches in the heel and sole to balance the right shoe (Fig. 31–8). A Swedish knee orthosis was also used initially to help train the patient and be a positive hyperextension control. Although the double adjustable ankle joint does give total flexibility to change the angle, a 90-degree posterior stop can also be used. Patients who lack this much ROM provide an "anatomical" anterior stop.

CASE 31–3   S.G.

S.G. is a 13-year-old with spastic cerebral palsy with involvement of all four extremities. She is nonambulatory with significant scoliosis. Her hip range of motion is from minus 25 degrees to 135 degrees of flexion. S.G. is fully dependent and lacks upper-extremity use. The goal of orthotic intervention was to prevent further deformity, maintain the thoracic and lumbar column for internal organs, and provide trunk stability for seating balance in her wheelchair. She was fitted with a custom TLSO fabricated from a cast impression (Fig. 31–9). It has 1/4-inch padding with a polypropylene outer layer, which has been modified over bony prominences for skin tolerance. S.G. wears her TLSO not only while seated in her chair but also in bed. Frequent checks of the skin were made during the first few weeks of use to establish trim lines and window type modifications.

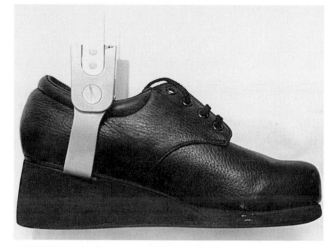

FIGURE 31–7. Shoe modification with double-adjustable ankle.

and wears it out faster than most other orthotic patients if, as in the case of a child, he or she does not outgrow it first. This should be considered in the design and fabrication.

SUMMARY

All orthoses create a force system. It is important to understand and integrate the appropriate force to achieve

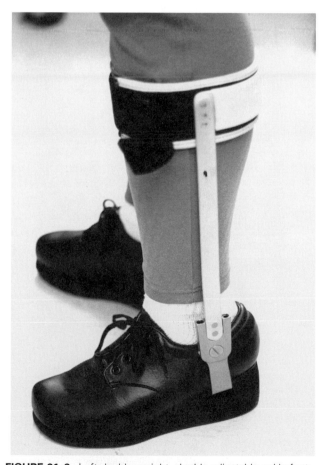

FIGURE 31–8. Left double-upright, double-adjustable ankle-foot orthosis with balancing right buildup.

nations of padding, wedging, straps, and heat relief are often necessary to enable the patient to wear the orthosis for a significant time on a daily basis. The spastic diplegic cerebral palsy patient relies heavily on his or her orthosis

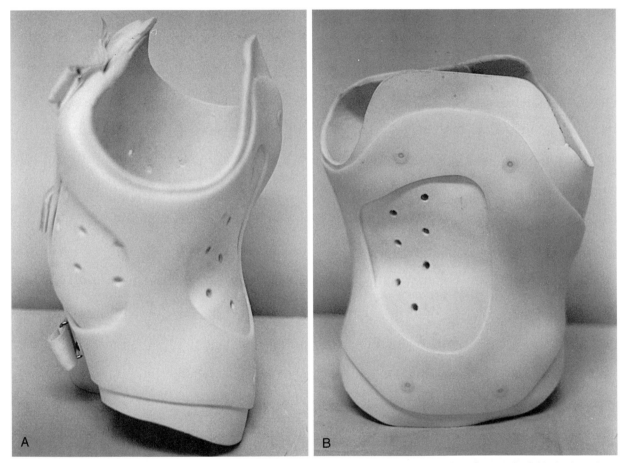

FIGURE 31–9. Thoracolumbosacral orthosis with anterior opening. *A*, Lateral view. *B*, Posterior view. Cutouts in rigid plastic to inner soft foam are for expansion and comfort.

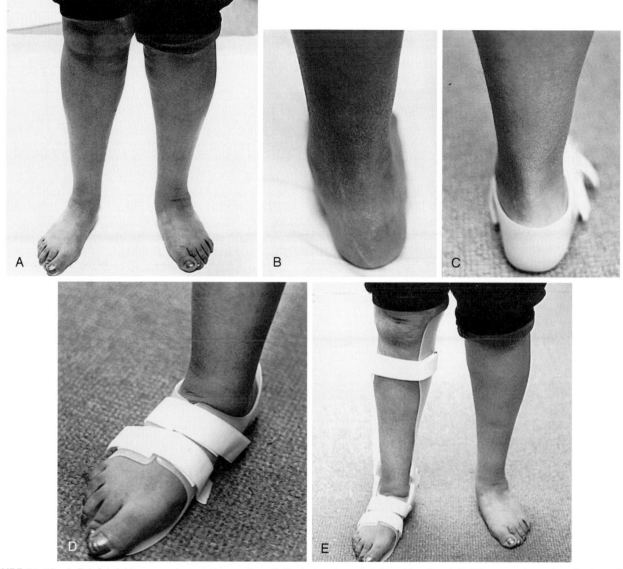

FIGURE 31–10. *A,* Painful right genu valgus and pronation. *B,* Posterior view of right ankle. *C* and *D,* Client wearing submalleolar orthosis with pronation corrected. *E,* Patient in submalleolar ankle-foot orthosis extended to knee to control genu valgus.

CASE 31–4 R.B.

R.B. is a 41-year old with spastic diplegia cerebral palsy. She has tight heel cords bilaterally, minus 5 degrees. Plantarflexion strength is fair plus, and dorsiflexion is fair bilaterally. The patient has 5 to 7 degrees of varus in the calcaneus. The left lower extremity is asymptomatic. The right side has pain in the mid femur and at the knee. She has a bilateral genu valgum deformity of 5 to 7 degrees (Fig. 31–10A). ROM at the knees is full, and strength of the quadriceps and hamstrings rate as good. Her hips are normal except for some internal rotation; leg lengths are equal, and sensation is good. Because the right lower extremity was painful at the knee and ankle (see Fig. 31–10B), the patient was fitted with an AFO that extended medially and proximally to the medial tibial condyle; ankle joints that had a posterior adjustment to limit plantarflexion; and a medial heel wedge and heel buildup of ⅜ inch. The ankle was fitted with a submalleolar orthosis that fitted inside the AFO (see Fig. 31–10C and D). The submalleolar orthosis controlled enough pronation of the ankle along with the medial heel wedging and exerted a varus force at the knee (see Fig. 31–10E). The heel buildup reduced the posteriorly directed force from midstance to toe off. The patient's symptoms were reduced, allowing her to be more active.

the desired outcome of intervention. A thorough initial evaluation and clinical knowledge of the multiple orthotic options available are vital to reach treatment goals. There has been a dramatic increase in material technology, far greater access to orthotics, and a much wider range of indications for orthotic intervention. This should challenge the rehabilitation team to establish measurable goals and then develop outcomes resulting from various orthotic treatment interventions for future patients.

REFERENCES

1. Bunch W, Dvonch V: Cerebral palsy. In Atlas of Orthotics. St. Louis, CV Mosby, 1985, pp 259–269.
2. Fish D: Characteristic gait patterns in neuromuscular pathologies. J Prosthet Orthot 9:163–167, 1997.
3. Freehafer A: Orthotics in spinal cord injuries. In: Atlas of Orthotics. St. Louis, CV Mosby, 1985, pp 287–297.
4. Otto J: Playing the numbers game: How demographics data impact orthotics and prosthetics. O and P Business News, January 2000, pp 1, 31–35.
5. Waters R, Garland D, Montgomery J: Orthotic prescription for stroke and head injury. In Atlas of Orthotics. St. Louis, CV Mosby, 1985, pp 270–286.
6. Yamamoto S, Ebina M, Miyazaki, Kubota T: Development of a new ankle-foot orthosis with dorsiflexion assist: I. Desirable characteristics of ankle-foot orthoses for hemiplegic patients. J Prosthet Orthot 9:174–179, 1997.

The Impact of Drug Therapies on Neurological Rehabilitation

TIMOTHY J. SMITH, PhD, RPh • HOWELL RUNION, PhD, PA-C

Key Words

– adverse drug reactions
– disease
– drug interactions
– drug therapy
– impairment
– pharmacist

Objectives

After reading this chapter, the student/therapist will:

1. Understand how drugs may positively or negatively affect neurological rehabilitation.

2. Given a disease state, understand how drugs may affect that disease state and the implications for neurological rehabilitation.

3. When considering one or more impairments, recognize the influence of drug therapy on these impairments and the implications for neurological rehabilitation.

4. Recognize the importance of a collaborative approach in resolving drug-related issues and neurological rehabilitation.

Drugs used for the management of a wide variety of disease states may have unintended and/or undesirable effects on a therapeutic plan for neurological rehabilitation. Although the occupational or physical therapist may not be responsible for monitoring all aspects of a client's therapeutic plan, it is important to recognize the scope of drug-related complications. A client's pharmacist, who is acutely aware of the prescribing practices of the client's physician(s), may be instrumental in resolving the drug-related impact of any medication on a therapeutic plan. The client will benefit greatly from an effective collaboration that includes the therapist and a pharmacist. Focusing on drug effects, diseases, and impairments, the discussion in this chapter addresses these interactions from two perspectives. First, a disease or pathology-driven model focuses on the pharmacological approaches used in drug therapy of major diseases that are often concurrent with

rehabilitation. Second, an impairment/disability-driven model focuses on the effects of drugs on the impairment/disability and the impact on the therapeutic plan. Although it is not possible within the scope of this chapter to define every problem associated with a class of drugs or among patients with a particular impairment, it is important to highlight common difficulties.

A DISEASE PERSPECTIVE

A number of diseases and their treatment regimens may be concurrent with neurological rehabilitation. The pharmacological interventions for these conditions and their implications from both a body system and disease/pathology model are addressed.

Parkinson's Disease

Parkinson's disease is a degenerative disorder involving a progressive loss of dopaminergic neurons in the substantia nigra. This deficit in dopaminergic function results in resting tremor and difficulty in the control of voluntary movement. Cardiovascular function, bowel motility, and cognitive function are often compromised. Although not directly associated with the motor system pathology, the functional deficits are emotionally devastating to the patient, resulting in depression and other mood disorders. The predominant pharmacological approach in the management of Parkinson's disease is the enhancement of dopaminergic function in the affected brain regions. Among the earliest successful approaches was the use of L-dopa, a precursor of dopamine in the central nervous system (CNS). The use of this agent (as with all agents to date) only enhances the dopaminergic function in remaining neurons. This approach has no effect on the progressive loss of neurons. In addition to central conversion of L-dopa to dopamine in the substantia nigra, a similar conversion occurs in the limbic system, a brain center associated with the regulation of behavior. Excessive dopaminergic influence in the limbic system has been associated with aberrant behaviors, including paranoia, delusions, hallucinations, and related psychiatric disturbances that may influence sleep and mood. These behavioral changes are obviously antagonistic to any therapeutic plan. In addition to L-dopa, a dopamine precursor, agents that inhibit the breakdown of dopamine, enhance the release of dopamine, or have dopaminergic agonist activity will have similar behavioral effects (Table 32–1). Dopaminergic agents may produce postural hypotension and syncope, by virtue of their ability to produce vasodilation, based on CNS and peripheral actions.[27, 31] If clients are unable to take their medication, there is increasing danger (with extended therapy) that movement may be impossible and the normal chest wall expansion and contraction may be compromised (see Chapter 22).

Cancer

Cancer may interfere with neurological rehabilitation in various ways. Tumors within the brain may interfere with cognitive and motor function as well as autonomic and metabolic control (see Chapter 23). Peripherally, tumors may interfere with peripheral nerve function and associated motor control or by producing pain. In addition, drugs that reduce cancer pain may interfere with cognitive and motor function.[16] Among these, morphine and related opiate derivatives are notable (Table 32–2). A significant degree of tolerance to the CNS depressant effects of these agents will develop with chronic administration. In cancer chemotherapeutic regimens, many antiemetic agents are used. These include dopaminergic antagonists (which may produce motor deficits similar to Parkinson's disease), dronabinol (a chemical component of marijuana, which can affect cognitive function), as well as high-dose corticosteroids (affecting mood). Some antitumor agents may be neurotoxic. These include a reduction in deep tendon reflex, paresthesias, and demyelination associated with vincristine (Oncovin).[38] Naturally, any change in drugs that involves a cancer treatment regimen (directly or indirectly) requires the approval of the client's oncologist.

Seizure Disorders (Epilepsy)

Epilepsy is associated with a diverse group of neurological disorders resulting in motor, psychic, and autonomic manifestations. Many of the antiseizure medications may produce drowsiness, ataxia, and vertigo (Table 32–3). Some may produce cognitive disorders in children and adults.[8, 41] Sudden discontinuation of antiseizure medications may result in status epilepticus, which may be fatal.

Stroke, Hypertension, and Related Disorders

Stroke, by virtue of the interference of blood flow and oxygenation, produces both reversible and irreversible

TABLE 32–2. Examples of Narcotic Analgesics, Morphine, and Related Agents*

morphine (Contin-MS)	hydromorphone (Dilaudid)
codeine	levorphanol (Levo-Dromoran)
fentanyl (Duragesic)	nalbuphine (Nubain)
meperidine (Demerol)	oxycodone (Roxicodone)
methadone (Dolophine)	oxymorphone (Numorphan)
buprenorphine (Buprenex)	pentazocine (Talwin)
butorphanol (Stadol)	propoxyphene (Darvon)
hydrocodone (Vicodin)	tramadol (Ultram)

*Effects on motor systems are systemic or indirect.

TABLE 32–1. Agents Facilitating Dopaminergic Activity in the Management of Parkinson's Disease*

Agents Converted to Dopamine
L-dopa (in Sinemet)

Agents That Stimulate Release of Dopamine
amantadine (Symmetrel)

Agents Reducing Breakdown of Dopamine
carbidopa (in Sinemet)
selegiline (Eldepryl)
tolcapone (Tasmar)

Agents That Are Dopaminergic Agonists
bromocriptine (Parlodel)
pergolide (Permax)
pramipexole (Mirapex)
ropinirole (Requip)

*The effects of these agents on muscle tone are complex and dose dependent. See text for an explanation.

TABLE 32–3. Anticonvulsants*

carbamazepine (Tegretol)	phenytoin (Dilantin)
clonazepam (Klonopin)	primidone (Mysoline)
ethosuximide (Zarontin)	tiagabine (Gabatril)
felbamate (Felbatol)	topiramate (Topamax)
gabapentin (Neurontin)	valproic acid (Depakene)
lamotrigine (Lamictal)	vigabatrin (Sabril)
phenobarbital (various brand names)	zonisamide (Zonagen)

*Effects on motor systems are direct and may decrease tone at higher doses. Direct effects on muscle are minimal.

TABLE 32–4. Commonly Used Antihypertensive and Cardiovascular Drugs*

Beta-Adrenergic Blocking Drugs

acebutolol (Sectral)	nadolol (Corgard)
atenolol (Tenormin)	penbutolol (Levatol)
betaxolol (Kerlone)	pindolol (Visken)
bisoprolol (Zebeta)	propranolol (Inderal)
carvedilol (Coreg)	sotalol (Betapace)
labetalol (Trandate)	timolol (Blocadren)
metoprolol (Lopressor)	

Calcium-Channel Blocking Drugs

bepridil (Vasocor)	nifedipine (Procardia)
diltiazem (Cardizem)	verapamil (Calan)

Other Antihypertensive Drugs

captopril (Capoten)	clonidine (Catapress)
enalapril (Vasotec)	doxazosin (Cardura)
lisinopril (Zestril)	prazosin (Minipress)
ramipril (Altace)	terazosin (Hytrin)

*Effects on motor systems are predominantly systemic or indirect.

neurological deficits (see Chapter 25). To reduce the damage associated with thromboembolism in such cases, tissue plasminogen activator has been recommended. However, the agent is most effective when given within an hour after the attack. Drugs with other mechanisms used to improve the prognosis of stroke are under development. However, drugs used for concurrent conditions (atherosclerosis and hypertension) before and after a stroke will be complicating factors for progressive rehabilitation outcomes. These drugs include beta-adrenergic antagonists, which reduce heart rate and correspondingly reduce exercise tolerance. Occasionally, calcium channel blockers, alpha-adrenergic blockers, and related agents may cause similar effects, including weakness, dizziness, syncope, and cognitive disorders. Changes in serum electrolytes induced by diuretics may affect the heart, the vasculature, and skeletal muscle and ultimately affect impairments such as strength of contraction.[14, 30] Table 32–4 lists many of these drugs. Many of the cholesterol synthesis inhibitors (agents used to reduce serum cholesterol) may induce muscle weakness[24, 48] (Table 32–5). The client with hypertension who discontinues these medications, resulting in uncontrolled hypertension, increases dramatically his or her risk of stroke and related disorders.

Anxiety and Depression

Agents used in the management of anxiety, whether due to acute or chronic disease, must be titrated carefully. Among these agents are the benzodiazepines, whose anxiolytic (anxiety-reducing) dosage range immediately precedes a dose that may affect motor skills and cognitive

TABLE 32–5. Hypolipidemic Drugs (HMG-CoA Reductase Inhibitors)*

atorvastatin (Lipitor)	lovastatin (Mevacor)
cerivastatin (Baycol)	pravastatin (Pravachol)
fluvastatin (Lescol)	simvastatin (Zocor)

*May rarely produce muscle damage through a direct effect on the muscle.

TABLE 32–6. Anxiolytics (Benzodiazepines)*

alprazolam (Xanax)	clorazepate (Tranxene)
lorazepam (Ativan)	diazepam (Valium)
oxazepam (Serax)	halazepam (Paxipam)
chlordiazepoxide (Librium)	prazepam (various brand names)

*Reduce muscle tone through a direct effect on motor systems at higher doses.

function (Table 32–6). In subjects of all ages, but especially the geriatric population, administration of benzodiazepines may produce paradoxical excitement, confusion, and behavioral changes.[33] Although benzodiazepines may have variable effects on learning and declarative memory, these effects may differ among the benzodiazepines, displaying considerable variation among individuals. If producing sleep alone is desired, ambien (Zolpidem) is an attractive alternative, noting that this agent does not have anxiolytic effects.[32] Although the anxiolytic agent buspirone (Buspar) is relatively free of benzodiazepine-like effects, the onset time for the desired anxiolytic effect is characteristically delayed.[36] Lack of compliance with anxiolytic agents may increase panic attacks and reduce effective interactions with a therapist.

The emergence of the serotonin-selective reuptake inhibitors (SSRIs) has revolutionized the treatment of depression. The older agents, such as the tricyclic antidepressants (TCAs) are just as effective in the management of several forms of depression; however, their adverse effect profile is somewhat different. The tricyclics often produce drowsiness and orthostatic hypotension, effects that complicate any rehabilitation regimen.[37] Although these effects may be produced by SSRIs, their incidence is much reduced. Certain TCAs, by virtue of their ability to inhibit the reuptake of norepinephrine in adrenergic nerve terminals, may be used at lower doses for neuralgias.[26] Although these low-dose regimens are usually not associated with the side effects listed earlier, some subjects may be more sensitive to these effects than others. This requires increased vigilance for the care team in determining iatrogenic versus pathological sources of somnolence and syncope. A partial list of antidepressants is presented in Table 32–7. Noncompliance with antidepressant therapy may result in lack of interest in any therapeutic regimen.

TABLE 32–7. Antidepressants: Examples of Tricyclic and Serotonin-Selective Agents*

Tricyclic Antidepressants	Serotonin-Selective Reuptake Inhibitors
amitriptyline (Elavil)	citalopram (Celexa)
clomipramine (Anafranil)	fluoxetine (Prozac)
doxepin (Adapin)	fluvoxamine (Luvox)
imipramine (Tofranil)	paroxetine (Paxil)
nortriptyline (Pamelor)	sertraline (Zoloft)
protriptyline (Vivactil)	

*These agents may produce complex direct and indirect effects on motor systems with minimal effect directly on muscle.

Patients with stroke as well as other neurological diagnoses often suffer from depression, which reduces motivation and decreases compliance with a therapeutic regimen. Although obviously linked, the degree of functional restoration after a stroke does not always correlate with resolution of depression.

Arthritis and Autoimmune Disorders

In the management of rheumatoid arthritis, the therapeutic approach may influence the progress of rehabilitation. Aggressive treatment with glucocorticoids may reduce joint pain and facilitate movement, but it may produce changes in mood and muscle wasting.[43] Although this is reversible and limited to systemic administration of high-dose corticosteroids, its impact cannot be overlooked and will certainly affect physical or occupational therapy prognosis. Prednisone and related glucocorticoids may often produce a false sense of well being that may exceed the ability of the patients to engage safely in certain exercise regimens. From the patient's perspective, this pharmacological effect is perceived as a "cure" and does not provide the motivation to continue with exercise therapy. The same problems may exist with the use of corticosteroids in other autoimmune disorders.[11]

Nonsteroidal antiinflammatory agents (Table 32–8) have long been used for the relief of pain with arthritis; however, depletion of prostaglandins in the gastric mucosa has produced bleeding that has limited their usefulness.[28] The development of newer agents that are more selective for isoforms of cyclooxygenase that are involved in joint inflammation are a major advance. An example is celecoxib. Although bleeding disorders are dramatically reduced, the incidence of ataxia with these agents may be increased.[20] Thus, clients with neurological diseases or pathological processes with problems requiring antiinflammatory medications may develop side effects that interact and confound existing motor deficits. Failure to comply with arthritis medications will likewise reduce effective movement.

Infectious Diseases

Both bacterial and viral diseases may produce neurological disorders (see Chapter 17). It is important to recognize the neurological impact of treatments and prophylactic measures. Although this may be readily apparent for drugs, vaccines have also been implicated in causing similar problems. The association of a hypotonic-hyporesponsive episode with the pertussis vaccine is such an example.[10]

In the course of treating bacterial diseases, many antibiotics/ antiinfective agents may compromise sensory, motor, and cognitive function. These functions may be compromised temporarily or permanently and may be patient specific. First, in the critically ill patient, aminoglycosides (gentamicin, tobramycin, and amikacin) and vancomycin may produce ototoxicity, such as hearing loss (reversible and irreversible) and vestibular damage (dizziness, vertigo, and ataxia). Minocycline is also associated with vestibular toxicity.[46] Extra precautions may be necessary to prevent falls during and after therapeutic exercise sessions. Fall prevention programs must be developed in these cases.

A wide variety of viral diseases interfere with neurological function. Polio is historically the most widely recognized (see Chapter 19). Acquired immunodeficiency syndrome (AIDS) may be manifest as a wide variety of neurological disorders (see Chapter 18). A recent finding is that protease inhibitors, which reduce the assembly of viral particles, may dramatically reduce and possibly reverse the neurological manifestations of AIDS.[47] Although adverse effects associated with antiviral and antibiotic agents may be intolerable, noncompliance may result in increased resistance of the virus or microorganism to retreatment.

Diabetes

The development of peripheral neuropathy (see Chapter 12) is a progressive problem in diabetics. This neuropathy compromises sensory and motor control. In addition to long-term management of diabetes from a glucohomeostatic perspective, other agents are showing promise. Treatment of diabetic neuropathy with trazodone and mexilitine[23, 50] are examples.

A more acute problem is swings in blood glucose level from inappropriate diet, exercise, insulin, and oral hypoglycemic drug administration. The balance of these factors is important, and monitoring of blood glucose level is essential. Swings in blood glucose level are often associated with changes in behavior and sensorium. This may pose a safety concern, because cognitive and motor function may be impaired as a result. An increase in exercise will decrease the blood glucose concentration, thereby reducing insulin requirements. These factors should be carefully considered in any exercise regimen for the diabetic.[21] A list of oral hypoglycemic agents is presented in Table 32–9. Lack of glucose control because of noncompliance with medications that are useful in controlling diabetes will only return the client to an accelerated course to peripheral neuropathies and related sequelae.

Pulmonary Diseases

Many clients with neurological problems have pulmonary disease as well. The treatment of pulmonary diseases presents an unusual challenge. Many drugs used for treat-

---

● **TABLE 32–8. Commonly Used Nonsteroidal Antiinflammatory Agents***

aspirin	fenoprofen (Nalfon)
diclofenac (Voltaren)	flurbiprofen (Ansaid)
etodolac (Lodine)	ibuprofen (Advil, Motrin, Nuprin)
indomethacin (Indocin)	ketoprofen (Orudis)
ketorolac (Toradol)	naproxen (Aleve, Naprosyn)
sulindac (Clinoril)	oxaprozin (Daypro)
tolmetin (Tolectin)	choline magnesium
mefenamic acid (Ponstel)	trisalicylate (Trisilate)
nambutone (Relafen)	diflunisal (Dolobid)
meloxicam (Mobic)	salsalate (Disalcid)
piroxicam (Feldene)	

*Only at higher doses will these agents affect motor systems directly. Most problems are through systemic or indirect effects.

TABLE 32–9. Oral Hypoglycemic Agents*

acetohexamide (Dymelor)	glimepiride (Amaryl)
chlorpropamide (Diabinese)	glipizide (Glucotrol)
tolazamide (Tolinase)	glyburide (Micronase)
tolbutamide (Orinase)	

*May produce direct and indirect effects upon motor systems through hypoglycemia.

ment of asthma, emphysema, and chronic obstructive lung disease are intended to have direct effects on the lung, yet systemic effects are often unavoidable. Adrenergic bronchodilators, such as albuterol, epinephrine, and metaproterenol, may increase heart rate and tremor.[40] If tremor is first manifested due to a neurological insult, then these drugs may exaggerate the motor impairment. Although ipratropium is an anticholinergic with bronchodilator properties, the associated systemic anticholinergic effects (such as urinary retention with prostatic hypertrophy) are not well tolerated in geriatric males.[39] Prednisone and related corticosteroids may dramatically reduce the degree of pulmonary hyperresponsiveness but often produce systemic effects noted previously. These are often reduced (but not necessarily eliminated) with the use of inhaled corticosteroids, such as beclomethasone, budesonide, flunisolide, and triamcinolone. The use of theophylline in asthma and obstructive pulmonary diseases can produce changes in cognitive function, including delusions and hallucinations with higher doses. General CNS stimulation, including nervousness, insomnia, and seizures, is well recognized.[2] Tremor and nausea are often produced with theophylline, even with dosage regimens commonly accepted in the clinic. Finally, the increase in diuresis by theophylline in patients with prostatic hypertrophy is certainly troublesome.[15] The metabolism of this drug is often changed by other medications, complicating therapy. These changes in drug metabolism may increase toxicity or decrease efficacy.[13] A newer class of disease-modifying agents known as the leukotriene modifiers (montelukast and zafirlukast) are being used in asthma. Although cardiovascular and neurological side effects of these drugs appear to be dramatically reduced when compared with other agents, they have been implicated in several important drug interactions.[25] Lack of compliance with these medications will decrease pulmonary gas exchange, ultimately decreasing motor performance.

Gastrointestinal Disorders

Among the wide variety of agents used in the treatment of gastrointestinal disorders, problems with agents affecting gastrointestinal motility are among the most frequently encountered. Antiemetics that are dopaminergic antagonists, such as prochlorperazine (Compazine), chlorpromazine (Thorazine), and promethazine (Phenergan), may produce extrapyramidal side effects resembling Parkinson's disease through a drug's actions in the basal ganglia.[12] Dronabinol (Marinol), a cannabinoid derivative from marijuana, is an effective antiemetic but may pro-

duce cognitive and sensory disturbances. These include drowsiness, dizziness, ataxia, disorientation, orthostatic hypotension, and euphoria.[5] The serotonin-selective antagonists dolasetron (Anzemet), granisetron (Kytril), and ondansetron (Zofran) are effective and valuable antiemetics, especially in cancer chemotherapy. The most common adverse effect is severe headache.[44] The benzodiazepine lorazepam is an effective adjunct for control of emesis. Problems associated with benzodiazepines have been discussed previously. Corticosteroids such as dexamethasone should be included among the antiemetic agents, and their adverse effects have been previously discussed.

In producing normal motility, metoclopramide (Reglan), domperidone (Motilium), and cisapride (Propulsid) are often used. The adverse effects of metoclopramide are primarily through dopaminergic antagonism. Domperidone was developed to reduce these CNS effects and has been used to treat diabetic gastroparesis with some success.[3] Cisipride, another prokinetic agent, may have a wide variety of CNS effects, including dizziness, mood disorders, vision changes, hallucinations, and amnesia, although with very low incidence in contrast to reports of arrhythmias.[19] Compliance with medications that reduce problems with the gastrointestinal system may have little direct effect on motor performance but may prove very troublesome to the client's quality of life.

AN IMPAIRMENT PERSPECTIVE

In the first section, each disease that may exist concurrently with an impairment was discussed along with potentially interfering or complicating therapeutic regimens. In this section, different forms of neurological impairments are discussed and appropriate drugs are identified that either reduce or increase the degree of impairment.

Sensory Impairment

Drugs that affect hearing, vision, and touch may influence any type of sensory, cognitive, and motor impairment. In the impairment model (Fig. 32–1), the processing of accurate sensory information is crucial to modify and adjust procedural programming during movement. A subject must be able to visually, manually, or through auditory cues (even through olfactory means) relate to or recognize the relevance of the external environment, engage the specific motor programming centers that reach consensus regarding the specific motor response, and produce the series of signals that may progress uninterrupted through spinal mechanisms and the motor endplate to a regional muscle group for an appropriate response. Any impairment or drug that affects any component within these systems, whether early or late in this sequence, will affect the motor performance. As discussed previously, certain drugs may influence hearing (as indicated earlier in the discussion on infectious diseases), or produce tinnitus (aspirin), which may be distracting and thus ultimately affect motor performance.[46] Changes in the visual field (ethambutol and anticonvulsants) are likewise important. Analgesics and topical anesthetics may dangerously affect surface heat/cold discomfort and undermine avoidance cues.

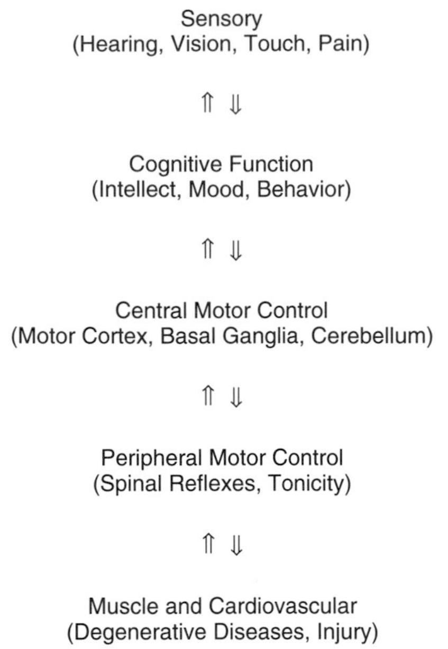

Sensory
(Hearing, Vision, Touch, Pain)

⇑ ⇓

Cognitive Function
(Intellect, Mood, Behavior)

⇑ ⇓

Central Motor Control
(Motor Cortex, Basal Ganglia, Cerebellum)

⇑ ⇓

Peripheral Motor Control
(Spinal Reflexes, Tonicity)

⇑ ⇓

Muscle and Cardiovascular
(Degenerative Diseases, Injury)

FIGURE 32–1. Neurological impairment and levels of drug modification.

However, elimination of excessive pain (peripheral and central) may enhance cognitive focus and learning. In the impairment paradigm (see Fig. 32–1), note that all steps are reversible, enabling peripheral effects of agents to modify central systems. This is especially true with regard to rehabilitation techniques and drug therapy. The reader must remember that the CNS functions with consensus of multiple interactions and thus the model could be represented by arrows extended between every system at all the levels within the CNS.

Cognitive and Central Motor Control Impairment

Disorders of mood (anxiety and depression) reduce initiative in the rehabilitation process. In this context, anxiolytics and antidepressants may have a positive impact. However, if the dose is not titrated carefully, drowsiness and anterograde amnesia will cloud effective response and learning. Both antidepressants and many of the benzodiazepines may exhibit these effects (see discussion of agents used in treatment of anxiety and depression). Behavioral disorders, especially those associated with untreated psychoses or dementia, impede cognitive function. Although antipsychotics may correct these disorders, the dopaminergic antagonism associated with these may interfere with the function of the basal ganglia and facilitation of movement. Many newer antipsychotic agents (also known as the atypical antipsychotics) have, in addition to dopaminergic activity, serotonin antagonist activity, which may reduce the extrapyramidal side effects of the earlier agents, when analyzed as movement dysfunction (Table 32–10).

Vertigo, Dizziness, Balance, and Coordination

Many agents with histamine antagonist and anticholinergic activity have been used for treatment of vertigo and

T A B L E   3 2 – 1 0. Examples of Antipsychotic Agents

Typical Antipsychotics*	Atypical Agents†
chlorpromazine (Thorazine)	clozapine (Clozaril)
thioridazine (Mellaril)	olanzapine (Zyprexa)
loxapine (Loxitane)	quetiapine (Seroquel)
molindone (Moban)	risperidone (Risperdal)
fluphenazine (Prolixin)	
haloperidol (Haldol)	
perphenazine (Trilafon)	

*May produce a parkinson-like effect through dopaminergic antagonism.
†Direct effects on motor systems least dependent on dopaminergic systems.

dizziness. Meclizine and related antihistamines are primary examples.[29] Occasionally, sinus congestion can result in impaired vestibular function and dizziness. An indirect-acting adrenergic agonist such as ephedrine or pseudoephedrine can reduce this congestion and improve this condition.[4]

Cardiovascular Impairment

In the management of hypercholesterolemia, the HMG-CoA reductase inhibitors (see Table 32–5) may produce myopathies to various degrees (see earlier). Changes in hemodynamics due to antihypertensive regimens must be monitored, because these agents can produce syncope and lower exercise tolerance (see earlier). Weakness from intermittent claudication is a challenge that can be managed in part with cilostazol.[6] Any drug that is used to decrease spasticity as a consequence of stroke and related cerebrovascular disorders may impair motor control and thus affect motor learning. A discussion of these drugs is outlined in the next section.

Spasticity and Muscle Tone

Muscle spasms may be controlled with centrally acting and peripherally acting agents, all of which produce drowsiness, dizziness, and muscle weakness to various degrees.[7] Commonly used agents are listed in Table 32–11. Pharmacological management of muscle tone, spasticity, and coordination of movement is of primary importance in neurological rehabilitation.

With regard to spasticity, several additional options are available. Tizanidine (Zanaflex) is the newest of the alpha-adrenergic agonists that are available to reduce spasticity, primarily through activation of descending noradrenergic inhibitory pathways.[49] Clonidine (Catapres) has similar actions. Intrathecal administration of baclofen (Lioresal)

T A B L E   3 2 – 1 1. Muscle Relaxants and Antispasmodics*

baclofen (Lioresal)	dantrolene (Dantrium)†
carisoprodol (Soma)	metaxalone (Skelaxin)
chlorzoxazone (Paraflex)	methocarbamol (Robaxin)
cyclobenzaprine (Flexeril)	orphenadrine (Norflex)

*Direct effects on motor systems to reduce tone.
†Direct effects on muscle to reduce tone.

produces an antispasmodic effect through enhancement of gamma-aminobutyric acid (GABA)nergic function, both central and spinal.[18] Likewise, enhancement of GABAnergic function and reduced spasticity can be realized through the antiseizure drug gabapentin.[22] Selective motor neurons can be inactivated through local injection of botulinum toxins.[35] These agents inhibit the release of acetylcholine at the neuromuscular junction. The investigational agent 4-aminopyridine has been shown to reduce spasticity in spinal cord injury.[42]

The involvement of serotonin in maintenance of muscle tone and spasticity is complex and controversial. Cyproheptadine, a relatively nonselective serotonergic antagonist, can reduce spasticity and maintain muscle tone.[34] However, serotonin-selective reuptake inhibitors used as antidepressants may occasionally increase spasticity,[45] and clozapine (Clozaril), a serotonin-selective antagonist, may produce muscle weakness.[17]

In addition to spinal cord injuries, multiple sclerosis may exhibit spasticity as a complication. Although several interferons have been used in the management of multiple sclerosis, interferon beta 1b has been shown to increase spasticity.[9]

Neuroplasticity

The effects of drugs on plasticity is highly controversial. In Alzheimer's disease a loss of plasticity may be realized through deficits in hippocampal and cortical function leading to memory loss. Many anticholinesterase agents improve memory and may provide evidence of a class of agents that may enhance neuroplasticity.[1] This rapidly evolving area of research may provide interesting avenues for treatment of other neurological disorders in addition to Alzheimer's disease.

RESEARCH AND DEVELOPMENT PROSPECTUS

It is difficult to accurately predict which areas of pharmacological research will have the most valuable impact on the management of neurological disorders and the resulting residual impairments. The reader must understand that drug development is a continuous process, although this text must have a definitive endpoint. The authors also must stress that many drugs with outstanding promise for treating neurological diseases will have adverse effects that may be less acceptable than the neurological problem (or in fact may be lethal) and may require removal from the market. In spite of these disappointments, there are many reasons for optimism.

Among the burgeoning areas of biotechnology that will have an influence on neurology will be the discovery, characterization, and application of neuronal growth factors, related growth modifiers, and cellular implants, which may have the long-term promise of restoring nerve function either partially or completely. Although these developments are unlikely to have extensive application within the next few years, over a period of decades these and related developments will take root and revolutionize

our understanding and treatment of a wide variety of neurological disorders.

The pharmacist stands as a valuable resource for the future. Pharmacists must participate in the management of drug therapies that may be related to each area discussed in this chapter. The reader should be urged to consult the pharmacist about new drug developments as well as discuss potential problems that these new drugs may have on neurological rehabilitation. This is especially true when new drugs not mentioned in the text are being administered to your client. These discussions can illuminate intended and adverse effects that may affect interventions.

SUMMARY

In the therapeutic jungle of drug therapies, the clinician must be wary of trouble that lurks ahead. This degree of vigilance can yield greater rewards for the client in terms of effective management of multiple diseases and reduced interference with rehabilitation. Resolving problems with therapies requires a team approach. When drugs are involved with management of these problems, the client's physician, pharmacist, therapist, nurse, and caregiver must be aware that drugs pose a certain degree of risk with every positive step. The team must work closely to adequately address inquiries into possible drug problems and opportunities for therapeutic success.

CASE STUDIES

The two case studies presented in this section illustrate the importance of obtaining complete medical history before initiating therapy. Unfortunately, and all too often, physical and occupational therapists are asked by the referring physician to look only at a specific problem, for example, "improve upper limb mobility" and are not given background medical history other than perhaps a one-word descriptor, such as "stroke," or a short note, "weakness in upper and lower extremities." Unless the therapist has access to a full medical history, including prescription and over-the-counter drugs, the therapy requested may be less than fully successful, as many drugs have adverse side effects that may alter cognitive function or the patient's ability to learn and redevelop impaired motor functions.

Therapists must know and understand the underlying pathophysiology of the referred patient's diagnosis to evaluate the impairment that is causing motor dysfunction. In addition, therapists need to understand how drugs affect the specific physical impairment that is altering the quality of life of day-to-day activity and in some cases hour-by-hour functioning. For example, drugs given to patients can either alter or promote their depression and can interfere with intellectual, cognitive, and pain levels, all of which can alter their abilities to fully participate in physical and occupational therapy. Often patients' cognitive abilities are modified by either their organic problem or the medical drug therapy. If a cognitive impairment is present, the therapist needs to assess how severe it is to

CASE 32–1   MULTIPLE SCLEROSIS DIAGNOSIS

C.G. is a 42-year-old white man with relapsing remitting multiple sclerosis (MS) who had an Extended Disability Status Score (EDSS) of 1 when first seen. He now has an EDSS score of 3.1. C.G. is no longer able to work. He had been a building contractor/builder and for a short period after his MS diagnosis continued working until he lost the use of his legs. He is currently confined to a wheelchair, is incontinent for both bowel and bladder, has lost the ability to stand, and is unable to dress or transfer from any seated position, for example, to toilet himself or shower independently. In addition, he is no longer able to prepare his own meals during the 8 to 10 hours per day he spends alone from his family.

Past History. C.G. had been treated unsuccessfully with two of the interferon drugs (interferon beta-1a and -1b Avonex and Betaseron) used to retard MS progression. He is now on glatiramer acetate (Copaxone), a third MS suppressive drug, and is currently stabilized. Unfortunately, he has sustained considerable damage to both his brain and spinal cord.

Although MS is a crippling disease of motor function and of cognitive functions, C.G. remains cognitively intact but suffers from slowed thinking. He also has lapses in immediate recall and occasional indiscretions of judgment that result in inappropriate conversation with outside family members. He expressed suicidal ideation and was treated effectively with paroxetine hydrochloride (Paxil) for his depression. Paxil, a serotonin reuptake inhibitory drug, was specifically chosen because of its minimal cognitive blunting effects.

All of C.G.'s identified disabilities occurred gradually, but with a sudden progression of his disease, his motor impairments progressed from poor lower extremity ambulation and postural control to involvement of his upper extremities and dependence on a wheelchair. He needed therapy initially for ambulation and more recently for wheelchair use and transfer techniques. As his MS status deteriorated, control of his upper extremities began to decline. Again therapy was ordered to teach him alternate ways to accommodate to these new losses in upper motor control and strength. He was retaught how to get dressed, use the toilet, shower, and feed himself.

Drugs used in the management of MS patients must be considered in any therapy plan, but most clinicians do not share this information with you, or only list it as a part of the patient's chart. At the initial referral of C.G. for gate therapy, he was on baclofen (Lioresal) for management of muscular spasms and associated pain. This drug, however, has the potential to increase weakness and fatigue as well as to introduce some central nervous system depression. This is important information, as C.G.'s MS was already responsible for motor weakness, but the need to reduce painful muscle spasticity outweighed the loss of muscle strength. If the therapist had not known that C.G. was taking baclofen, the PT therapy plans would have been jeopardized significantly because the therapist would have assessed C.G. as being weak simply because he had MS. The therapy plan needs to include exercises and maneuvers that compensate for the drug-induced motor weakness. C.G. was also on oxybutynin chloride (Ditropan) for bladder control, a drug that has a potential side effect of drowsiness; in C.G.'s case the Ditropan dose was minimal and was not a cognitive concern. As noted, he had been placed on paroxetine, which also can contribute to muscle weakness, but in his case this did not increase his upper extremity weakness.

Recall that C.G. was referred to therapy for functional learning, such as transferring from his wheelchair to a bed, shower stool, or toilet; dressing; and eating. Understanding the patient's environmental status, which includes his family situation, is also important in creating a therapy plan. C.G.'s therapy was through home health and incorporated a therapy plan appropriate to C.G.'s environment. C.G. is married and has two children. His wife must work to support the family. The children are not yet in high school and are gone much of the day. Thus, there is an imperative need for C.G. to manage self care while the family is away during the day. Understanding how drug therapy enhances or interferes with physical or occupational therapy interventions is the only way to optimize the interaction of both and to enhance the quality of life for C.G.

Postscript: Unfortunately with MS, the demyelinating of neurons is relentless and progressive. At this writing, C.G. has begun to lose additional upper extremity mobility following an MS exacerbation 6 months after his last OT treatments were prescribed. He has recently been taught to use assistive tools to grasp and pull items to him, for example, books, utensils, and door knobs. The assistive tools were introduced by the therapist treating C.G., thus extending CG's self-reliance and security during time alone.

CASE 32-2   PARKINSON'S PLUS SYNDROME

Background. Mrs. N is a 72-year-old married woman with Parkinson's plus syndrome, whose disease status has progressed over the past 5 years, resulting in impaired gait, periods of severe rigidity, dystonia, occasional oculomotor dysfunction, significant behavioral and cognitive changes, and some speech impairment. She is a highly educated woman who had been a speech and special education therapist-administrator. In addition to the aforementioned problems, she now has attention span difficulty, is emotionally labile, and tends to ramble on tangentially to questions posed or simply on her own. Mrs. N is still oriented to time and place, but to a large extent she is now housebound.

Mrs. N is currently wheelchair dependent and has had extensive therapy over the past 5 years to keep her mobile and to reduce muscle atrophy. She has been given hydrotherapy to facilitate both limb motion and flexibility. Her right hand and both arms are frequently immobilized for short periods of time by rigidity secondary to levodopa blood level peaks. These have been recently modulated by the addition of ropinirole (Requip, a dopamine agonist), and this drug, along with therapy to decrease upper extremity impairments, has improved her ability to carry out voluntary hand and arm movements. Mrs. N's limb movements are characteristically slow and deliberate secondary to the pathology of Parkinson's disorders. She does not have any cogwheeling of the biceps, hands, or head so frequently seen in Parkinson's patients. Her muscle mass is reduced secondary to disuse atrophy and noncompliance with home-instructed daily exercise. She continues, with poverty of motion, to feed herself but depends on her husband for assistance in dressing and transferring from her wheelchair to the toilet, bed, and shower despite the fact she could do these maneuvers on her own if she chose to do so.

She remains in a long-term stable relationship with a highly supportive husband, who is slowly being driven to exhaustion by her constant demands for attention. She scores well on mental status examinations and does not yet demonstrate marked signs of dementia but frequently has appeared slightly groggy. Mrs. N's chief complaint has been one of poor motor control and strength in both her upper and lower extremities. She is still able to stand but now requires assistance during walking. She is unable to sleep normally, finds it difficult to roll over or change position in bed, and wakes her husband to rotate her frequently throughout the night.

Her Parkinson's is less than successfully treated with standard antiparkinsonian therapy, that is, levodopa/carbidopa. With the addition of Requip, she has improved somewhat. One of the telltale characteristics of a Parkinson's plus syndrome is that patients do not respond as well to levodopa therapy as do persons with pure Parkinson's disease. Thus, the importance of adjunctive physical and occupational therapy to assist Mrs. N in maintaining mobility cannot be overstated.

Mrs. N has several other problems that affect her quality of life and her therapy. She, like many other patients with a parkinsonian syndrome, has significant joint pain for which she uses over-the-counter drugs (nonsteroidal anti-inflammatory agents) in addition to gabapentin (Neurontin, an anticonvulsant drug with neuropathic pain-relieving properties). Mrs. N has painful muscle spasms that have been moderately well managed with baclofen. She has a nocturnal sleep problem that is lessened by using zolpidem tartrate (Ambien), which helps her get 3 to 4 hours of quality sleep. However, her daytime inactivity has resulted in significant night-time sleep disturbance that even zolpidem does not always cover.

Unfortunately, Mrs. N, like so many patients with chronic problems, has sought secondary sources of pain and fractured sleep relief without informing her medical and physical/occupational therapy team until such time as she was experiencing a new set of problems, secondary to her polypharmacy, prescriptive, or over-the-counter agents. She has been reluctant in the past to disclose her use of these additional agents, several of which have clouded our assessment of her therapy. This is not an uncommon occurrence with patients who have progressively degenerative conditions.

As clinicians, we must routinely ask about patients' drugs and specifically about the use of over-the-counter drugs at each visit. For example, Mrs. N complained at one recent visit that she was having a hard time following her therapist's instructions and participating in the sessions. She was sure the therapist was "not paying proper attention to my needs." This not being the case, I asked, "So, Mrs. N, refresh my mind and save me some time from looking it up. What medicines are you now taking?" She responded, "Sinemet, as you told me to; Requip; Ambien at bedtime; Synthroid; Klonopin; and a new pill I got at the health food store for sleep." She was taking two drugs—Klonopin and the over-the-counter drug melatonin—both of which would account for the therapist's response that Mrs. N. appeared groggy and was not able to follow directions. The Klonopin she got from a psychiatrist friend of the family. She had put herself on these three sleep drugs, one long-acting and the other two short-acting, but in combination additive. In addition to this, the drug gabapentin, which was managing her neuropathic pain, and in a dose of 1200 mg per day, contributed to her level of drowsiness—a

Continued

CASE 32-2 PARKINSON'S PLUS SYNDROME *Continued*

known side effect of gabapentin. Mrs. N was already on the short-acting non–sensorium-clouding zolpidem that had been given to her for her sleep disorder. Zolpidem does not cause daytime hangover drowsiness. The key to her new daytime lethargy was found in the Klonopin and melatonin.

The offending drugs were discontinued with an explanation of why she should not add drugs. Mrs. N. subsequently returned to therapy, and her therapist found her once more able to participate in the therapy plans that had been worked out for her. Asking patients to review the drugs they are on is vital to the entire health care team and to their ultimate success.

With the recently confirmed diagnosis of Mrs. N's Parkinson's plus syndrome, all that can now be offered to her is supportive therapy, both medical and physical. She is in a class of Parkinson's patients who do not respond well to the antiparkinsonian drugs. Her medical management now depends on her participation in therapy and her resisting the temptation to add other drugs that will only cloud her senses and not improve the underlying pathology. Mrs. N and her husband have now accepted this, and she is indeed doing better.

---

adjust instructions and plan of therapy to a level at which the patient can succeed. The cognitive level, along with the primary medical diagnosis, shapes the physical and occupational therapy prognosis.

Knowledge of the drugs currently being used by the patient provides guidance in structuring therapy and may determine whether the plan of care will be effective. For example, will a patient on pain medicine have a cognitive level that permits a full understanding of what is being asked during therapy? Will drug therapy provide adequate pain management to enable physical manipulation by either the therapist or the patient in response to the commands? When is the pain medication administered, and is the time relationship to the appointment appropriate? How long does the drug work, and does it have negative effects on cognition?

These are only a few examples of the kind of questions that therapists need to ask to design and implement therapy programs that enhance the patients' abilities to recover motor functions, prevent physical regression, and perhaps even retard or stop some aspects of mental regression caused by either drug therapy or endogenous depression. Clinicians must keep in mind the potential for both positive and negative drug-induced changes and ways that these can alter or improve the overall physical and mental status of the patient.

REFERENCES

1. Allain H, Bentue-Ferrer D, Gandon JM, et al: Drugs used in Alzheimer's disease and neuroplasticity. Clin Ther 19:4–15, 1997.
2. Baker MD: Theophylline toxicity in children. J Pediatr 109:538–542, 1986.
3. Barone JA: Domperidone: A peripherally acting dopamine$_2$-receptor antagonist. Ann Pharmacother 33:429–440, 1999.
4. Baser B, Kacker SK: A simple, effective method of treating vertigo patients. Auris Nasus Larynx 17:165–171, 1990.
5. Beal JE, Olson R, Laubenstein L, et al: Dronabinol as a treatment for anorexia associated with weight loss in patients with AIDS. J Pain Symptom Manage 10:89–97, 1995.
6. Beebe HG, Dawson DL, Cutler BS, et al: A new pharmacological treatment for intermittent claudication: Results of a randomized, multicenter trial. Arch Intern Med 159:2041–2050, 1999.
7. Borenstein DG, Lacks S, Wiesel SW: Cyclobenzaprine and naproxen versus naproxen alone in the treatment of acute low back pain and muscle spasm. Clin Ther 12:125–131, 1990.
8. Bourgeois BF: Antiepileptic drugs, learning, and behavior in childhood epilepsy. Epilepsia 39:913–921, 1998.
9. Bramanti P, Sessa E, Rifici C, et al: Enhanced spasticity in primary progressive MS patients treated with interferon beta-1b. Neurology 51:1720–1723, 1998.
10. Braun MM, Terracciano G, Salive ME, et al: Report of a US Public Health Service workshop on hypotonic-hyporesponsive episode (HHE) after pertussis immunization. Pediatrics 102(5):E52, 1998.
11. Brown ES, Suppes T: Mood symptoms during corticosteroid therapy: A review. Harv Rev Psychiatry 57:239–246, 1998.
12. Caligiuri MP, Lacro JP, Jeste DV: Incidence and predictors of drug-induced parkinsonism in older psychiatric patients treated with very low doses of neuroleptics. J Clin Psychopharmacol 19:322–328, 1999.
13. Cupp MJ, Tracy TS: Cytochrome P450: New nomenclature and clinical implications. Am Fam Physician 5:107–116, 1998.
14. Daniels V, Casey A: Antihypertensives. Phys Med Rehabil Clin North Am 10:319–335, 1999.
15. Ellis EF: Theophylline toxicity. J Allergy Clin Immunol 76(2 pt 2):297–301, 1985.
16. Foley KM: Misconceptions and controversies regarding the use of opioids in cancer pain. Anticancer Drugs 6 (Suppl 3): 4–13, 1995.
17. Galletly C: Subjective muscle weakness and hypotonia during clozapine treatment. Ann Clin Psychiatry 8:189–192, 1996.
18. Gianino JM, York MM, Paice JA, Shott S: Quality of life: Effect of reduced spasticity from intrathecal baclofen. J Neurosci Nurs 30:47–54, 1998.
19. Gibson D: A review of the adverse effects of cisapride. J Ark Med Soc 95:384–386, 1999.
20. Goldenberg MM: Celecoxib, a selective cyclooxygenase-2 inhibitor for the treatment of rheumatoid arthritis and osteoarthritis. Clin Ther 21:1497–1513, 1999.
21. Gonder-Frederick LA, Clarke WL, Cox DJ: The emotional, social, and behavioral implications of insulin-induced hypoglycemia. Semin Clin Neuropsychiatry 2:57–65, 1997.
22. Gruenthal M, Mueller M, Olson WL, et al: Gabapentin for the treatment of spasticity in patients with spinal cord injury. Spinal Cord 35:686–689, 1997.
23. Jarvis B, Coukell AJ: Mexiletine: A review of its therapeutic use in painful diabetic neuropathy. Drugs 56:691–707, 1998.
24. Jeppesen U, Gaist D, Smith T, Sindrup SH: Statins and peripheral neuropathy. Eur J Clin Pharmacol 54:835–838, 1999.
25. Katial RK, Stelzle RC, Bonner MW, et al: A drug interaction between zafirlukast and theophylline. Arch Intern Med 158:1713–1715, 1998.
26. Kingery WS: A critical review of controlled clinical trials for peripheral neuropathic pain and complex regional pain syndromes. Pain 73:123–139, 1997.
27. Koller WC, Rueda MG: Mechanism of action of dopaminergic agents in Parkinson's disease. Neurology 50(6 Suppl 6):S11–S14, 1998.
28. Laszlo A, Kelly JP, Kaufman DE, et al: Clinical aspects of upper

gastrointestinal bleeding associated with the use of nonsteroidal antiinflammatory drugs. Am J Gastroenterol 93:721–725, 1998.

29. Lauter JL, Lynch O, Wood SB, Schoeffler L: Physiological and behavioral effects of an antivertigo antihistamine in adults. Percept Mot Skills 88(3 pt 1):707–732, 1999.

30. Maxwell CJ, Hogan DB, Ebly EM: Calcium-channel blockers and cognitive function in elderly people: Results from the Canadian Study of Health and Aging. Can Med Assoc J 161:501–506, 1999.

31. Mendis T, Suchowersky O, Lang A, Gauthier S: Management of Parkinson's disease: A review of current and new therapies. Can J Neurol Sci 26:89–103, 1999.

32. Mintzer MZ, Griffiths RR: Triazolam and zolpidem: Effects on human memory and attentional processes. Psychopharmacology 144:8–19, 1999.

33. Moore AR, O'Keeffe ST: Drug-induced cognitive impairment in the elderly. Drugs Aging 15:15–28, 1999.

34. Norman KE, Pepin A, Barbeau H: Effects of drugs on walking after spinal cord injury. Spinal Cord 36:699–715, 1998.

35. Palmer DT, Horn LJ, Harmon RL: Botulinum toxin treatment of lumbrical spasticity: A brief report. Am J Phys Med Rehabil 77:348–350, 1998.

36. Pecknold JC: A risk-benefit assessment of buspirone in the treatment of anxiety disorders. Drug Saf 16:118–132, 1997.

37. Pollock BG: Adverse reactions of antidepressants in elderly patients. J Clin Psychiatry 60 (Suppl 20):4–8, 1999.

38. Postma TJ, Benard BA, Huijgens PC, et al: Long-term effects of vincristine on the peripheral nervous system. J Neurooncol 15:23–27, 1993.

39. Pras E, Stienlauf S, Pinkhas J, Sidi Y: Urinary retention associated with ipratropium bromide. DICP 25:939–940, 1991.

40. Pringle TH, Riddell JG, Shanks RG: Characterization of the beta-adrenoreceptors that mediate the isoprenaline-induced changes in finger tremor and cardiovascular function in man. Eur J Clin Pharmacol 35:507–514, 1998.

41. Read CL, Stephen LJ, Stolarek IH, et al: Cognitive effects of anticonvulsant monotherapy in elderly patients: A placebo-controlled study. Seizure 7:159–162, 1998.

42. Segal JL, Pathak MS, Hernandez JP, et al: Safety and efficacy of 4-aminopyridine in humans with spinal cord injury: A long-term, controlled trial. Pharmacotherapy 19:713–723, 1999.

43. Shanahan EM, Smith MD, Ahern MJ: Pulse methylprednisolone therapy for arthritis causing muscle weakness. Ann Rheum Dis 58:521–522, 1999.

44. Shuster J: Ondansetron and headache. Nursing 29:66, 1999.

45. Stolp-Smith KA, Wainberg MC: Antidepressant exacerbation of spasticity. Arch Phys Med Rehabil 80:339–342, 1999.

46. Tange RA: Ototoxicity. Adverse Drug React Toxicol Rev 17 (2–3): 75–89, 1998.

47. Tepper VJ, Farley JJ, Rothman MI, et al: Neurodevelopmental/ neuroradiologic recovery of a child infected with HIV after treatment with combination antiretroviral therapy using the HIV-specific protease inhibitor ritonavir. Pediatrics 101(3):E7, 1998.

48. Thompson PD, Zmuda JM, Domalik LJ, et al: Lovastatin increases exercise-induced skeletal muscle injury. Metabolism 46:1206–1210, 1997.

49. Wagstaff AJ, Bryson HM: Tizanidine: A review of its pharmacology, clinical efficacy and tolerability in the management of spasticity associated with cerebral and spinal disorders. Drugs 53:435–452, 1997.

50. Wilson RC: The use of low-dose trazodone in the treatment of painful diabetic neuropathy. J Am Podiatr Med Assoc 89:468–471, 1999.

Alternative and Complementary Therapies: Beyond Traditional Approaches to Intervention in Neurological Diseases, Syndromes, and Disorders

JENNIFER M. BOTTOMLEY, PhD, PT • MARY LOU GALANTINO, PhD, PT
• DARCY A. UMPHRED, PhD, PT • CAROL M. DAVIS, EdD, PT • DONNA J. MAEBORI, MS, PT

Key Words

- alternative/complementary/transdisciplinary models
- energetic-based theories
- evidence-based practice
- integrating theories
- movement therapies

Objectives

After reading this chapter the student/therapist will:

1. Differentiate the four worldviews of health care delivery.

2. Analyze how complementary/alternative-based health care practices overlap with an allopathic medical delivery model.

3. Analyze how mind, body, and spiritual interactions have the potential to lead to health and healing.

4. Compare and contrast the various models discussed and identify similarities and differences between them and the traditions of Western medical practice.

INTRODUCTION

The use of alternative and complementary therapies in the treatment of neurological disorders is evolving into common practice as clinicians and patients/clients seek nontraditional approaches for relieving signs and symptoms of neurological diseases, syndromes, and disorders, and attempt to alter the progression of diseases of the central nervous system (CNS) through nonconventional movement and manual therapies. It is important that professionals in rehabilitation medicine understand the principles and practices of transdisciplinary, complementary, and alternative approaches to treatment beyond traditional interventions, as many of these therapeutic ap-

proaches are being proposed as options in the management of neurological problems. The clinician needs to be cautious in the application of these treatment modalities. We do not want to get drawn into alternative therapies as intervention solutions without significant evidenced-based research substantiating the use of these approaches.

This chapter presents a sampling of alternative therapeutic models and philosophies that are available for potentially assisting patients/clients with CNS problems. Although most of the techniques discussed in this chapter have been firmly established by sound research, some less evidenced-based models are also included, such as therapeutic touch and medical intuitive diagnostics. Clinicians are continually being exposed to the therapeutic potentials of these less scientifically established theories, and therefore need to be aware of their existence and potential. Creating evidence-based practice is not an all-or-none principle nor do we suggest that models that do not have a strong research base may not have efficacy. We do suggest that to adopt a model because of belief or the charisma of the founder will be and should be challenged by colleagues today and in the future. Models whose theoretical constructs are based on sound rationale or that link evidence-based practice across multiple areas, yet have not established that research base, need to be scrutinized and approached more cautiously. In time, if those models maintain their sound base, research will be developed and their efficacy established. New models will also be created in the future that link and integrate theories with practice and our professions will continue to evolve and offer quality care to the consumer.

HISTORICAL PERSPECTIVE

Donna J. Maebori, MS, PT,
Jennifer M. Bottomley, PhD, PT
Darcy A. Umphred, PhD, PT

A historical perspective of how complementary and alternative therapeutic approaches have evolved to become increasingly part of the medical and rehabilitation landscape can be helpful to obtaining a broader comprehension. The language and rationale encountered in alternative methods can seem confusing and foreign to clinicians unfamiliar with modalities outside the realm in which they were taught. With many of our patients/clients seeking alternative methods of intervention beyond the traditional Western medical model, the time has arrived for us to explore and understand the scientific basis for the apparent effectiveness of these interventions. The positive results experienced by many of our patients/clients who have received alternative interventions cannot be ignored. This is the impetus for the growing acceptance by the general public and many health care practitioners of alternative forms of therapy. Can we explain scientifically the effects of complementary and alternative interventions? And if so, how can we best integrate complementary and alternative approaches into our current approaches in neurological rehabilitation?

In their book, *The Second Medical Revolution*, Laurence Foos and Kenneth Rothenberg described levels of academic learning as being three-tiered.[4, 154] Starting at the top, the third tier is the applied studies and subjects for therapists, such as therapeutic exercise and electrotherapy. The second tier is the pure sciences upon which these subjects are founded, such as anatomy, chemistry, physiology, and biology. The first tier is the "assumption of reality" (day-to-day observations) upon which the pure sciences are based. This first tier is the basic assumptions found in "worldviews" today. Different worldviews yield different scientific bases, whether pure or applied. Alternative methods in medicine and rehabilitation are well established in "premodern" and "postmodern" worldviews. This is in contrast to the "modern worldview" customarily taught in current Western medical training.

To present these methods in overview, it would be helpful to discuss these world views, and how physical and occupational therapy may fit into the scheme.

Essentially, there are four worldviews[5]: the premodern, modern, "fracturing or splintering," and postmodern views.

The first worldview developed during prehistoric times and lasted until the sixteenth century. This is called the premodern view. In this perspective, time is cyclical rather than linear. In other words, the sun, the moon, and the star circle around the earth, the tides ebb and rise cyclically, and the seasons circle back again and again, using the same patterns each time, connecting with "deep time." Deep time is compared with profane time. Profane time is tangible, as in the time it takes rice to boil; or visible, as in the sundial; or sensible, as in the heartbeat. In deep time such perceptions are suspended, profane time stands still, and one becomes a part of time. It is in deep time that premodern man finds reality. Infused in this thinking is that life and death, the earth and the sky, are mysterious or mystical. In other words, they contain truth beyond human comprehension.

This is a hard perspective for many to grasp, yet the role of the scientist is to be a passive observer. Numbers were used to describe observed events, such as the days between the circling of the sun and the moon, the number of hours between the ebb and high tide, but "there was no widespread assumption in the western world that natural processes in general had any intrinsic relation to numbers, to mathematics."[3] In other words, in Western science, these perspectives were not tangible, visible, or sensible . . . and so, historically, science moved on.

The second worldview began with Copernicus and is known as the modern worldview. It is the one with which the majority of the Western population would be most familiar and feel at home. In this view time is linear, progressing from start to finish. "The world is a rational, predictable, clockwork universe. Every bit of it can be predicted if you know one part of it. Purpose in life is to describe, generalize, predict, and control. Human beings are fairly mechanistic, separate, discrete entities from the rest of the universe."[5]

René Descartes (1596–1650) French philosopher and mathematician, and Isaac Newton (1642–1727), were two of the most important figures ushering in the "modern era." To Descartes, the world was logical, predictable, and intrinsically expressible through mathematics. The whole was obviously equal to the sum of the parts—categorical and hierarchical. The role of the scientist became that of an active, experimental, objective observer. If the numbers didn't fit, it couldn't be real.

The modern era of the second worldview spanned the 1500s through the twentieth century. However, the near perfection of the view began to falter in the very early 1900s with important discoveries in the field of physics. Although the hold of the second worldview on Western culture is still immense, it is splintering, as can be seen within our own professions.

Worldview 3 is about this fracturing, about the realization that the categorical, orderly clockwork is not a complete or necessarily accurate picture. It is a prelude to worldview 4. A small but growing number of people see the world in worldview 3, and fewer yet in worldview 4, but the effects are starting to be felt.

Worldview 4, postmodern, is complex, integrated, and nonlinear. It is about self-organizing and self-regulating systems, looking for patterns, and knowing that a very small variation in the pattern can produce large changes. Time is a dimension, interwoven with the dimensions of space. Time and space can change, expand, or shrink, speed up and slow down. Rituals are an important means for creating order. The whole is greater than the sum of the parts, and "we know and yet don't know." Worldview 4 has a lot of similarities with worldview 1. The pure sciences that arise from this worldview include systems theory, quantum physics, cybernetics, and fractal mathematics, which in turn affect many other fields of study, such as meteorology, ecology, business and economics, medicine, theology, movement science, and computer science, to name but a few. Research parameters, technology, and interpretation differ significantly from the assumptions of worldview 2, as scientific description is no longer considered purely objective, but rather, *epistemology* (the view from which knowledge is gathered) is becoming "an integral part of every scientific theory."[1]

Today we practice within the paradigms of our professions that have in the past aligned with Western medicine. Thus, for our ease, we can first start where we are, look at the medical profession, and discuss models or strategies that parallel the worldviews.

The roots of Western medicine extend back to Hippocrates, 400 BC, who provided a wholistic picture of the state of health, writing that "Health depends upon a state of equilibrium among the various internal factors which govern the operations of the body and the mind, the equilibrium in turn is reached only when man lives in harmony with his external environment."[4, p.23] The basic assumption in this perspective is that health depended on a balance with mind-body and nature or the environment, and disease was a disturbance of this balance. Preserving the balance was the priority for the practitioner. Three means were used to ascertain the characteristics of an illness: a dialogue with the patient, observational assessment of the patient's appearance, and palpation of the soft tissues and pulses. The most important component of this approach was considered the dialogue with the patient/client. It was believed that the patient's/client's meaning of the illness, attitude, and expectation was a valuable diagnostic, as well as prognostic, factor.

The shift from a preservative approach for mind-body-environment integrity to the conventional curative thinking found in medicine today was largely initiated by Descartes. He conceptualized reality as having two separate domains, one the body or matter, the other the mind. "The body is a machine," said Descartes, "so built up and composed of nerves, muscles, veins, blood and skin, that though there were no mind in it at all, it would not cease to have the same [functions]."[4, p.32] His ideas were closely tied to newtonian physics, which conceives the universe as a harmonious and well-ordered machine. These concepts gave rise to the view that matter and nature were separate from humans, and thus one could observe without affecting what was being observed. The physician, then, could have complete objectivity when assessing the patient. The patient could be viewed as a biological organism whose function was reducible to interrelating physical parts.

The resulting medical model, known as biomedicine, was fully in place by the middle of the nineteenth century. Its characteristics may be considered as follows:

1. Disease or dysfunction is a "deviation from the norm of measurable biological parameters."[4, p.23] A patient/client is a biological organism whose dysfunction is reduced to the identified deviations. Treatments or procedures are then used to cure or at least improve the deviations, which in turn improves the biological condition.
2. Objectivity provides the basis for diagnosis or assessment and the subsequent rationale for treatment. Patients'/clients' descriptions of what they are experiencing and the clinician's observation are considered "subjective" and not given as great a value as the "objective" findings, such as laboratory or other measured tests.
3. Eventually biomedicine can address virtually all medical problems at least adequately, if not fully, through more knowledge and research.

It goes without saying that the biomedical model has produced stunning and tremendous accomplishments. Yet, its restriction to physical causes of disease, in light of diseases and dysfunctions that are more widely recognized as having multiple causes, is creating a search for other answers. More of the public and some physicians and other health professionals are turning to alternative forms of intervention and healing. As stated in *Life* magazine in September 1996, "Why have alternative therapies in this country started to migrate from the margins to the center? One reason is that as allopathic medicine, a term commonly used to describe western techniques, becomes better at what it *can* do well, its limitations become more conspicuous. Allopathy is clearly superb at dealing with trauma and bacterial infections. It is far less successful with asthma, chronic pain and auto-immune diseases."[2]

Many of the alternative practices utilized in a medical setting today clearly come from premodern worldview sources, such as acupuncture, yoga, meditation, herbal remedies, and prayer. Just how some of these therapies work to restore health is difficult to perceive from a linear worldview 2 perspective. Very frequently what happens is that alternative approaches are used to address areas of limitations in the biomedical model, in a complementary fashion. Alternative practices used this way do not supplant traditional medicine; rather, they support and enhance the options available in health care. A new worldview and medical model would not necessarily arise from this relationship, and yet the conceptual framework is no longer cohesive. Ideas from ancient sources, as well as postmodern sources, are changing the previously complete-and-adequate image of the second worldview and consequent medical model. Grappling with these issues places one in worldview 3.

Evidence of these dynamics is apparent in the professions of physical and occupational therapy. In neurorehabilitation, for example, proprioceptive neuromuscular facilitation and neurodevelopmental techniques were developed in the middle of the twentieth century, at a time when "rehabilitation" was being established as an integral part of unquestioned biomedical order. Both approaches, in their early form, worked primarily with the nervous system, and both used hierarchy and order. Patients/clients were to progress through a sequence of skills, such as the *developmental sequence*, that was invariable. The hierarchy was also found regarding the role of the therapist as the professional who could identify the pathokinesiology and "fix" it with the appropriate technique. The patient was the recipient of the treatment. With the advent of *motor control* and *motor learning* theories over the last couple of decades, these two approaches have changed as the new concepts have influenced them. The developmental sequence is now termed *learning sequence* and no longer utilizes a strict hierarchy. Its treatment approach is moving away from emphasizing the therapist's role in identification and resolution of pathological movement, and moving toward the role of the patient in his or her own capacity to problem-solve and self-monitor. Lastly, an entirely new entity of neurorehabilitation has been formed recently as a result of concepts from motor control, motor learning, and dynamical systems theory, which is known as the "task-oriented approach."

One of the tenets of dynamical systems theory, as noted in the journal of the American Physical Therapy Association (APTA) in 1990, is that "biological organisms are complex, multidimensional, cooperative systems. No one subsystem has logical priority for organizing the behavior of the system."[6, p.770] The nervous system, then, is no longer a dominant subsystem with neurological patients. Rather, it is part of a self-organizing system that has multiple subsystems such as arousal, gravity, learning style, weight, center of gravity, cardiovascular function, and so on. "No one subsystem contains the instructions for [an action] . . . The behavior of the system is instead an emergent property of the interaction of multiple subsystems."[6, p.771] (See Chapters 3 through 6.)

Added to these developments was the emergence in the 1980s of a new field of therapy intervention: vestibular habilitation—posture and balance, which is multisystem and multifunctional and inherently demands the use of motor control and motor learning, and systems theories. Systems concepts are used for both balance and the task-oriented approach, the concept being that "movement emerges from an interaction between the individual, the task, and the environment."[8] (See Chapters 14 and 21.)

Orthopedic, or manual, physical therapy appears to be firmly committed to the biomedical model, yet there is interest found in "being wholistic" and treatment and exercise approaches are continually being developed that endeavor, to various degrees, to work with movement and function in a broader and more integrated manner. (See Chapter 12.)

Thus, we find that therapists are experimenting with systems concepts, motor control, and motor learning theory, and experimenting with ancient sources of healing, such as yoga, tai chi, acupressure, and meditation, as well as refining skills in the traditional biomedical aspects of therapy. For our professions, it is awkward, confusing, and exciting all at the same time.

Worldview 2 still remains the dominant model. Two distinct observations may be made that show the prevalence of a worldview 2 approach. The first is that, for the most part, we continue to consider ourselves to be objective observers separate from our patients. The second is that we endeavor to understand ancient, modern, and postmodern therapeutic concepts and research, frequently from a linear, mechanistic, categorical worldview 2 epistemology. Yet, such a view at times does not suffice to explain what is happening. That is the dilemma of worldview 3.

Further changes will be experienced when a critical mass of the population turns fully, in all aspects of personhood, to "worldview 4," which, again, has great similarities to worldview 1. A big difference, though, is that at this time in history, we have scientific methodology for understanding our nonlinear, complex, evolving, multidimensional, multilevel, continually interacting, irreducible world. Through systems theory we can handle, with sophistication, this multitude of complex detail, by working with its "sweeping simplicity and order in overall design."[7] Throughout the twenty-first century, as the growth of worldview 4 continues to evolve on many levels and in many fields of endeavor, it is entirely possible that it and its sciences will indeed replace, and not simply complement, worldview 2. And from there, the future has yet to be conceptualized and belongs to future students willing to venture beyond what is comfortable in order to best meet the health care needs of a world society.

ALTERNATIVE MODELS AND PHILOSOPHICAL APPROACHES
Darcy A. Umphred PhD, PT

Approaches to patient management that do not fall within a traditional allopathic medical model are often considered alternative or complementary. Although many of these therapeutic approaches have not been able to show efficacy in totality as an approach to medical management, neither has Western medicine. Future research will help validate many aspects of Western medicine and areas will be discarded. Similarly, research will show the efficacy of many components of complementary approaches, although some components will need to be eliminated and new creative ideas and therapeutic techniques developed. One research problem encountered with complementary approaches is that these approaches consistently focus on the patient as a total human being with all the interactions of all bodily systems. This philosophy of the whole does not coincide with the linear, reductionistic physical research accepted by Western medicine. Until research models are developed and instrumentation becomes available that measures multiple systems at multiple levels of consciousness simultaneously, it will be difficult to prove the strengths of many aspects of alternative approaches to patient management. That does not mean the efficacy is not there. It means our research skill may not have developed to the level of measuring all the influences that are interacting simultaneously during a complementary approach intervention. Finding those research models with supporting instrumentation is and will continue to be a challenge to therapists who choose to incorporate these interventions as part of their professional management of patients with neurological disabilities.

All of the models presented in this chapter for patient management have a common thread. All approaches focus on helping the patient/client maintain or regain a quality of life that is within that person's potential. The specific philosophy or conceptual framework embraced by any one approach varies. As various approaches are introduced in the following sections, subheadings will help the reader categorize similarities of philosophies.

Movement Therapy Approaches

Feldenkrais

Donna J. Maebori, MS, PT

OVERVIEW

Moshe Feldenkrais, physicist, engineer, and judo master, developed a method of movement exploration and improvement during the 1950s through the 1980s known as the *Feldenkrais Method*. One of the central premises of the method is that people can change and all people can learn. Awareness of movement in one's body is used as a means of realizing potential for growth and learning. Another premise is that all movement is in relation to the environment. Improving movement capacities makes it possible, then, to relate more effectively to one's environment, and, interacting with that experience, one can continue to improve one's functional abilities.

The Feldenkrais Method has two components. One is *Awareness Through Movement* (ATM), which is verbally directed movement lessons. These lessons frequently last 45 minutes, but some take an hour or just 5 minutes. Physical and occupational therapists can learn lessons through classes, books, or cassette tapes, and begin to experiment with them, both for themselves and with their patients. *Functional Integration* (FI), which is one-on-one hands-on nonverbal dialogue regarding movement awareness and options, is the other component. It involves a high degree of sensitivity on the part of the person conducting this interaction. Although anyone is welcome and encouraged to take lessons and interact with the movements and ideas, to do actual Feldenkrais work in either of its components, and to state that one does so, completion of a professional training program is required. Students in these programs meet 8 weeks per year for 4 years, at the end of which one then becomes certified in the method.

With Feldenkrais, movement is the medium by which one learns, essentially, how to learn. The work is entirely kinesthetic, or sensing, moving in the design of the skeleton without stress or strain, working with the breath, playing with different movement strategies. There are no notions of predetermined correct movements. Rather, diverse influences are used, such as constraints (i.e., keep the knee balanced over the foot as you roll) that disrupt habitual patterns of movement. This confusion activates neural pathway connections in the brain, and by experimentation the learner finds new ways to move, which unlock old postural habits and create new options from which to choose actions.

The intention of Feldenkrais is not to teach how to move. Rather, the interest is in creation of conditions in which learning is easy, spontaneous, and safe. This kind of learning is not goal-oriented. Instead, it is about a process of inquiry, and the acquiring of sensitivity, awareness, and ability to teach oneself.

CLINICAL APPLICATION AND RESEARCH

As the application of the Feldenkrais Method is completely diverse, it has use in many fields, such as theater performance, education, psychology, athletics, music performance, art, and interpersonal communication, as well as rehabilitation. In rehabilitation, the Feldenkrais approach can be used in multiple settings, it being particularly effective for pediatrics, gerontology, vestibular and balance dysfunctions, chronic pain, pulmonary dysfunction, sports medicine, and neurology.

Research in nonreductionistic systems work is entirely different from research based on the traditional medical model. To realize one gain, such as increased cervical range of motion, or a more normal gait, becomes arbitrary and irrelevant. Questions arise, such as, What is the point of increased range of motion? Is it helpful, and for what? From what cultural perspective does any definition of "normal" arise? To whom is it "accurate?" Moreover, the multiplicity of emergent factors are constantly dealt with in nonreductionistic research, with outcomes, accordingly, needing to reflect multiplicity of aspects.

An example of research on Feldenkrais is found in "Responses to Ten Feldenkrais Awareness Through Movement Lessons by Four Women with Multiple Sclerosis," by Stephens and colleagues.[10] In this study, six themes emerged from a series of 10 class lessons: awareness of movement, improved flexibility, improved balance, decreased effort, reorganization of movement, and improved mental outlook. In a 1-year follow-up with the women, "the two major themes were greater ease of movement and better functional balance and a pervasive sense of improved quality of life and mental outlook."[10]

CASE 33–1   CHRISTINE

Christine, a 59-year-old white woman, came to physical therapy a few months ago with a 3-year history of multiple sclerosis. Walking with a cane, she had started falling 2 months before her first appointment. Actual falls occurred about once a month, but serious loss of balance and near falls were occurring two to three times a week. Two weeks earlier she had hit her head in one of the falls and had had dizziness since then.

My assessment of Christine began with greeting her in the waiting room. Remaining seated to shake my hand, her grip was firm and she made

Continued

CASE 33–1   CHRISTINE *Continued*

full eye contact with me. Sit-to-stand involved leaning forward markedly with the torso, and standing required effort. Her gait showed hesitancy with each step, with a tendency to lean forward through the hips, decreased stride lengths, subtalar pronation, and slightly rounded shoulders.

The initial "subjective" portion of the evaluation from a Feldenkrais perspective tends to be essentially the same as for physical and occupational therapists. In goal setting, however, my tendency is to simply ask, "What things would you like to do better or more easily?" Then I record whatever the client says. Christine's goals were to relieve the vertigo, improve her balance, be able to get up from the floor, walk stairs safely, stand with security and ease, and walk and exercise for endurance. Her ability to state goals suggested uncomplicated concrete thinking, good motivation, and aptitude for generalizing any skills learned into various aspects of her life.

Further evaluation by a Feldenkrais teacher tends to seem cursory and brief. Typically, I observe a client's posture, breathing, and organization for movement during the talking for history taking. Then the client stands and I quietly observe posture, and touch the patient very lightly and briefly to acquaint myself with the person's way of holding herself or himself, that is, muscle tone distribution, and a tendency toward initiation of movement. This takes 5 to 10 minutes. The idea is not to figure out what needs to be treated. The idea is to create an environment for learning and find what emerges through the process, which starts with the manner in which the greeting, initial interview, and initial assessments are conducted, and develops further in the course of the movement lessons through either ATM or FI.

In Christine's case, I chose to evaluate for vestibular function. The ability to track an object moving in front of her eyes resulted in visual blurring and oscillopsia. Seated, lowering and turning her head toward the right knee or the left knee, the main result was remarkable equilibrium challenge on returning to upright, as she showed considerable swaying for several seconds until regaining her balance. Ability to stand with her feet together, eyes open, lasted only 1 second with very strong jerking action at the hips (hip strategy) occurring immediately.

On her first visit, she tried a bath bench for possible use in the shower for safety and independence. Liking it very much, she purchased one for herself. She also found that a Nova-style walker afforded definite security, good speed, and actions, and she obtained one for full stride to her gait and follow-through actions, and she obtained

one for exercise purposes. Then she was taught sitting posture with underlying concepts of organizing herself around her vertical axis and keeping herself in settled coherence throughout her skeleton. She also learned to gaze on an object in front of her, for balance stability, yet keep the eye action quiet to prevent unnecessary head and neck tension.

Her next session a week later involved one ATM lesson, which was to sit and slide her hands down her legs as far as she could with ease. Christine was able to go a very small distance in a manner that included the pelvis rolling forward, then backward to return herself to upright. She played with this action with a speed and distance that gave just a mild balance challenge, and worked with variables such as smoothness of movement, breathing, going a little to the right or left, learning to keep full attention on her actions.

The next two visits were with another therapist who gave further balance activity: standing alignment, standing (feet apart) weight shifts, and standing on one leg holding on to a counter. The therapist had taken several yoga and Feldenkrais classes for therapists and taught the patient in a manner congruent with Feldenkrais. She also provided canalith repositioning,[10] which improved the vertigo and other vestibular symptoms significantly. Canalith repositioning, also known as the Epley maneuver, is a procedure in which the head is tilted in four different positions for 3 minutes each. It is suggested that during these positional changes crystals that may be loose in the semicircular canals migrate back to the otoliths for reabsorption.[10]

On her next visit with me, Christine worked with very slow, smooth actions of sitting, sliding her hands down her upper legs, then onto a chair seat in front of her until her pelvis lifted just slightly, then smoothly reversing. The action of sliding her hands forward onto the chair seat was repeated, and then she went into partially standing and pivoting toward that chair. The action was very slow, smooth, and in the range of a very mild balance challenge only, keeping the breathing easy and working with keeping settled through herself, and being able to reverse the action at any time. The lesson at her next visit had similar concepts with a lesson in side lying, and served to deepen the concept of turning smoothly around her vertical axis.

She received a second canalith repositioning from the therapist, which completely resolved her vertigo. The standing balance exercises were reviewed. At the last appointment, we worked with getting up from the floor. She found that with half-kneeling (one knee and one foot on the floor),

Continued

hands on the chair seat, using a spiral turn through the hips, and keeping her head low, she could get up with only minimal assistance.

On the last appointment, and in a telephone follow-up conversation 3 weeks later, the patient reported she had had no near or complete falls since her second therapy session, and the vertigo remained completely cleared since the second canalith reposition. She stated that keeping in mind her "centering" helps her to keep her balance. Multiple sclerosis yields "good" and "bad" days, but on her good days she is able to function more than she used to with use of the skills she has learned.

CONCLUSION

The Feldenkrais Method allows every therapist to build on the best aspects of their education and training to enhance the effectiveness of patient/client interaction. If a traditional approach is working with your patient, then don't "fix" it. However, if a patient treatment is not progressing well and the patient is not making progress, then it is time to consider a shift in paradigms for treatment. The Feldenkrais Method is a strategy for exploring new and more effective ways to help an individual achieve maximal functional outcomes in the shortest period of time.[9] The Feldenkrais Method appears to support the intentions that can be summarized as the general mission of rehabilitation: the actions of the team and of the patient's significant others are designed to promote the self-determination and the maximal functional recovery possible for each patient and help him or her develop the strategies necessary to shape their own life. The Feldenkrais Method is not a system of physical exercise such as calisthenics; these exercises are, as Feldenkrais practitioners call them, *somatopsychic explorations* that foster improvement by accessing inherent neurological competencies and facilitating new learning. The Feldenkrais Method is aimed primarily at those whose symptoms relate to inefficient movement, such as those seen in multiple sclerosis, following a stroke, or in physical deconditioning.

Tai Chi

Jennifer M. Bottomley, PhD, PT

The use of tai chi is an alternative therapeutic approach that can greatly enhance the practice of physical therapy. It is a form of exercise that recognizes the mind-body connection.[32] The movements are graceful, the tempo is slow, and the benefits are great. It can positively augment physical therapy programs aimed at improving balance and posture, coordination and integration of movement, endurance, strength, flexibility, and relaxation.[°] Tai chi exercise has cardiovascular,[22, 23, 27] neuromuscular,[19, 28, 31, 34, 35] and psychological[12, 17, 32] benefits that are clinically observed. It is a form of exercise that allows the individual to assume an active role in obtaining maximal health and focus on the prevention of disease, rather than the passive acceptance of illness as a consequence of life, aging, fate, or genetics. It is an exercise form that is particularly helpful in an elderly population because of its slow, con-

trolled, nonimpact-type movement that displaces, thereby "exercising," the center of gravity. This exercise form incorporates all of the motions that often become restricted with inactivity and aging. It improves respiratory status, stresses trunk control, expands the base of support, improves rotation of the trunk and coordination of isolated extremity motions, and helps to facilitate awareness of movement and position.[19, 28, 31, 34, 35] An additional benefit is the social interaction, as most tai chi is done in group settings.

What is tai chi? Tai chi is an ancient physical art form, originally a martial art, where the defendant actually uses the attacker's own energy against the attacker by drawing the attack, sidestepping the attacker, and throwing the opponent off balance. There are numerous forms of tai chi[25] involving as many as 108 posturings and transitions of controlled movement, each based on slightly different philosophical foundations. Family surnames came to be associated with the different styles of tai chi that have been passed on from generation to generation (e.g., Wu style, Yang style, Ch'en style, Chuan style). Each style is distinctive, but all follow classic tai chi principles.

Tai chi is a way of life that has been practiced by the Chinese for thousands of years. It is a Taoist philosophical perspective that forms the foundation of an exercise regimen developed to balance mind and body. Unlike Western civilization, which separates body from mind and allows spiritual development only in terms of religions and mystical beliefs, tai chi integrates the connections between mind, body, and spirit in a quest for the highest form of harmony in life through the combination of exercise and meditation.[21, 26, 33] The Chinese conceived the human mind to be of an unlimited dimension and focused on simplification of beliefs. They also viewed the human body as limitless in its physical capabilities. These beliefs were the keystone for the evolution of what we know as tai chi chuan today.[25]

Since ancient times, Taoist philosophy has been concerned with the question of how to reproduce and maintain the essential kind of energy required to prolong life and enhance the creativity of the individual. The answer can be found in the tai chi methods of Taoist meditation, in which a combination of movement, breathing, and mental concentration is used to purify the essential life energies, distill out its pure yang aspect, the vital energy (chi), and transmit it through the eight body-mind channels to every cell in the body. The regular practice of these methods has been shown to result in longevity, good

---

°References 12, 17, 19, 22, 23, 27, 28, 31, 34, 35.

health, vigor, mental alertness, and creativity far beyond what is experienced by most people.[18]

To obtain the full benefit from the practice of tai chi, it is essential to understand the principles underlying the methods. Hence, the aim of this section is not only to describe the methods of meditation and exercise but also to explain how they are based on the philosophy of Taoism.

The "spiritual" component of tai chi is what makes many Westerners uncomfortable with this and other Eastern practices.[21, 26, 33] However, the concentration required to accomplish the rhythmical and coordinated movement patterns and to integrate these motions with respiration in tai chi induces a level of concentration that edges on meditation.[17, 32] Movement is vital to preventing disability and maintaining health and well-being. The capability of cognitively understanding the movements is an essential element in the successful practice of the tai chi exercise form. Tai chi requires practice (preferably throughout the life cycle) and commitment.[12, 17] There would be a total lack of consistency and benefit from this exercise form if the mind-body connection were not made.

PHILOSOPHICAL BACKGROUND

Behind every tai chi movement is the philosophy of yin and yang. The yin-yang principle has been the basis of the Chinese understanding of health and sickness since ancient times. Good health requires a balance between opposing forces within the body. If one or the other is too predominant, sickness results. It is the aim of Eastern medical practices, including acupuncture, qi gong, and herbal medicine, to discover the source of the imbalance and restore the forces to their proper proportions. In the Western world, exercise concentrates on outer movements and the development of the physical body. Tai chi develops both the mind and body.[32] It embodies a philosophy that not only promotes health but can be applied to every aspect of life. Tai chi emphasizes the development of the whole person, promoting personal growth in all areas.[18]

Tai chi means "the ultimate" energy. This ultimate power is *chi*. According to the legendary theory of yin and yang, chi exercises its power by creating a balance between the positive and negative energies of nature.[25] Tai chi's philosophical basis is directed toward improving and progressing toward the unlimited and immense interrelationship between the self and all other things in existence. Tai chi is guided by the theory of opposites: the yin and the yang, the negative and the positive. This is the *original principle* of Taoist thought. According to the tai chi theory, the abilities of the human body are capable of being developed beyond their commonly conceived potential. Creativity has no boundaries, and the human mind should have no restrictions or barriers placed upon its capabilities.

The fundamental principle of Taoist philosophy, the joining together of opposites, is the basis for the practice of tai chi. The Taoist philosophy that underlies tai chi exercise and meditation is somewhat more complex in its application of the relationship between yin and yang within the body. It is not denied that a general balance is necessary to avoid illness; however, it is the aim of medita-tion to greatly increase the yang and to reduce and diminish the yin. One of the fundamental beliefs of Taoist philosophy is that the reason people become old and weak and eventually die is that they lack essential energy (chi) that sustains life.[13, 18, 25] Thus, the goal of exercise is to greatly reduce yang and to increase and enhance yin.[13, 18] The combined practice of meditation and exercise balances these opposing energies.

One reaches the ultimate level of health and physical and mental well-being through exercise and meditative means of balancing the opposing powers and their natural motions: yin, the negative (yielding) power, and yang, the positive (action) power. The theory is that the interplay and balance between opposite, yet complementary, forces of equal strength promote health. These two opposing manifestations have universal significance and apply to the phenomena of the cosmos, as well as to the operations of the human body. On the largest scale, heaven is yang, while earth is yin. Day is yang, while night is yin. Bright and clear weather is yang; dark and stormy weather is yin. On the scale of living things, the male is yang, the female yin. Spirit is yang, body yin. This opposition applies to the parts of the body and their functions as well. In the circulatory system, the arteries are yang, the veins are yin. Muscle contraction is yang, relaxation is yin. In breathing, exhalation is yang, inhalation is yin. In human activities, movement is yang, rest is yin.[14]

Hundreds of years ago, those who searched for a way to elevate the human body and spirit to their ultimate level developed the ingenious system known as tai chi exercise. It has since proved to be the most advanced system of body exercise and mind conditioning ever to be created.[14, 16, 24, 25] It makes intuitive sense from a clinical perspective to apply the idea of a natural harmony and a balancing of life forces to the integration of body and mind.

PRINCIPLES

An important insight to be attained through an understanding of Taoist philosophy concerns the way in which the practice of exercise, such as tai chi chuan, and meditation should complement one another. The relationship between them manifests as a subtle interweaving of opposite tendencies. This relationship can be seen in the famous diagram known as the tai chi t'u, the Diagram of the Supreme Ultimate (Fig. 33–1). This diagram represents rest; the black portion is called the "greater yin," and the white portion, representing movement, is called the "greater yang." Within each figure there is a smaller circle of the opposite color. The black circle within the white figure is called the "lesser yin" and the white circle within the black portion is called the "lesser yang." This inner component represents the way in which each of the opposing forces, yin and yang, contains its opposite and continuously originates from its opposite. Tai chi, essentially a form of movement, is yang—the white portion. Meditation, which involves quiet and rest, is yin—the black segment. This distinction takes into account only the external aspects of these activities. To perform tai chi exercise effectively requires inner peacefulness and quiet while executing outwardly visible movements. Conversely, the meditator uses breath and mental concentration to

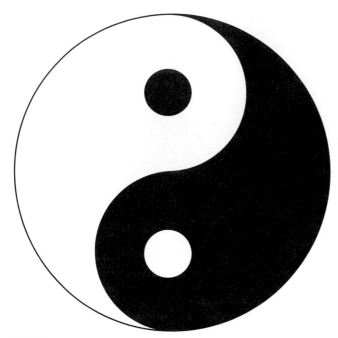

FIGURE 33–1. Yin and yang: Diagram of the Supreme Ultimate: Tai Chi T'u.

move the vital energy through the psychic channels while remaining externally at rest. Thus, the inner aspect of each of these practices is opposite to its outer aspect. In other words, just as the greater yang contains the lesser yin within it, the greater yin embraces the lesser yang. The diagram is a pictorial representation of how exercise and meditation grow out of one another as alternating practices. The movements of tai chi tend to increase the yang side of the yin-yang balance. When the yang reaches a high point of energy and vitality, it generates the need to sit quietly—meditation, which produces a more peaceful condition and increases the yin side of balance. This is cyclical. When yin reaches its peak, it generates a need to increase the yang once again. Thus, it is through the alternate practice of these two opposite methods that one obtains the beneficial effects of this form of exercise/meditation: tai chi.[13, 14, 16, 18, 24]

The traditional Chinese concept of the human body differs somewhat from the Western one. Physiological foundations are based on descriptions of chi, or vital energy. The body is hypothetically composed of eight energy (psychic) channels and has 12 meridians that run along the surface of the body. These channels and meridians form the basis of the highly sophisticated theories of acupuncture and acupressure.[18, 21, 33]

The eight channels systematically include all parts of the trunk and extremities. These energy channels are represented in Figure 33–2. The *tu mo*, or channel of control, runs along the spinal column from the coccyx through the base of the skull and over the crown of the head to the roof of the mouth. The *jen mo*, or channel of functions, goes through the center and front of the body from the genital organs to the base of the mouth. The *tai mo*, or belt channel, circles the waist from the navel to the small of the back. The *ch'ueng mo*, or thrusting channel, passes through the center of the body between

tu mo and jen mo, extending from the genitals to the base of the heart. The *yang yu wei mo* is the positive arm channel beginning at the navel, passing through the chest, and going down the posterior aspect of the arms to the middle fingers, while the *yin yu wei mo*, or negative arm channel, extends along the inner aspect of the arms from the palms, ending in the chest. Likewise, there are positive and negative channels for both lower extremities. The *yang chiao mo* is the positive channel that goes down the sides of the body and down the outer aspect of the lower extremity, ending at the soles. The negative channel is called the *yin chiao mo*, and starts in the soles and extends upward on the inside of the legs through the center of the body to a point just below the eyebrows.[14]

Twelve "psychic centers" of the human body are identified in Taoist thought.[11, 14, 25] They are represented in the *I Ching*[11] by 12 hexagrams that signify not only the 12 pathways in the body but also the 12 months of the year and the 12 times of the day. According to Taoist thought, the circulation of energy through these 12 psychic centers reflects the cyclical pattern of the universe that brings about the alternation of light and darkness as well as the changing of the seasons.[14] Figure 33–3 relates the 12 psychic centers to the 12 hexagrams that symbolize them, and indicates how the cycle reflects the times of the day and year and the center of the body that they represent.

According to Chinese astrologists, the yang movement begins with the eleventh month, which is identified with fu. This yang movement increases through the twelfth month up to the fourth month as represented by the increase in solid lines in the hexagrams. At the fifth month, the yang movement begins to decrease until it reaches the tenth month, when yin reaches complete dominance. The yin movement is the opposite of the yang.[11, 14, 18]

In addition to the psychic centers, there are 12 pathways of energy at the surface of the body called meridians. The 12 pathways take their names from the specific inner organs to which they correspond. The development of the tai chi postures and movements is related to these meridians in the human body.[14, 18, 25] The transition from one posture to the next, combined with breathing, reflects the flow of energy through these meridians.

The importance of breathing techniques has long been stressed in Chinese medicine as a means of preventing illness, prolonging youth, and achieving longevity.[15] The rationale behind this is that, besides oxygen, the air we breathe contains many other essential elements, such as iron, copper, zinc, and magnesium,[13–15, 18, 25, 30] and that the combination of exercise and breathing provides an efficient and effective method of taking these precious elements in and getting rid of wastes and poisons. It is believed that the breathing technique of abdominal or "inner" breathing facilitates the flow of energy throughout the body. Inhalation "stores" energy, whereas exhalation "releases" energy.[30]

The classic methods of tai chi combine movement with breathing. The movements are performed to assist and guide the circulation of vital energy, chi, through the eight channels and 12 meridians. The mind consciously "lifts" the energy during inward breathing from the solar plexus region, which is considered the central energy

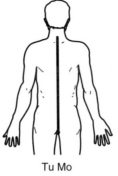
Tu Mo

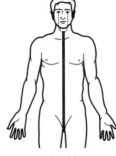
Jen Mo

Tai Mo

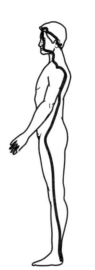
Ch'ueng Mo

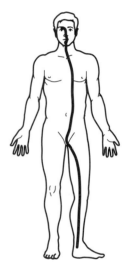
Yang Chiao Mo

Yin Chiao Mo

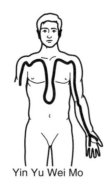
Yin Yu Wei Mo

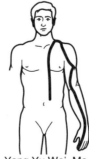
Yang Yu Wei Mo

FIGURE 33–2. The eight energy channels.

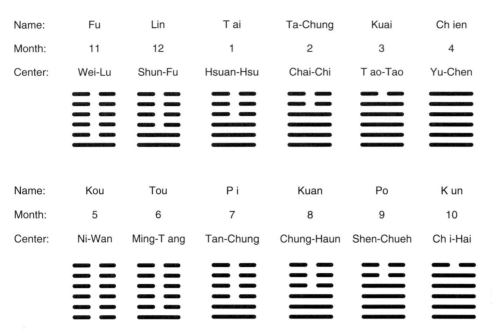

Name:	Fu	Lin	T ai	Ta-Chung	Kuai	Ch ien
Month:	11	12	1	2	3	4
Center:	Wei-Lu	Shun-Fu	Hsuan-Hsu	Chai-Chi	T ao-Tao	Yu-Chen

Name:	Kou	Tou	P i	Kuan	Po	K un
Month:	5	6	7	8	9	10
Center:	Ni-Wan	Ming-T ang	Tan-Chung	Chung-Haun	Shen-Chueh	Ch i-Hai

FIGURE 33–3. The waxing and waning of energy represented by the *I Ching* hexagrams.

source of the body.[13, 14, 25, 30] During exhalation, concentrated directing of the energy is from the solar plexus region toward the lower abdomen.[13, 14, 18, 25, 30] It is through this conscious directing of the energy that each of the eight channels is supplied with energy during the movement of tai chi. It is hypothesized that in tai chi exercise, the circulation of chi through the channels does not occur automatically as a result of the arm and leg movements combined with breathing. Rather, it is the mind's power of concentration that combines with the breathing to move the chi through the channels. The outer movements aid and guide the inner concentration. Tai chi is regarded as a method of "moving meditation."[13, 14]

Both the movements of the limbs and the way they are coordinated with the breathing cycle constitute the tai chi form of exercise. The movements are relatively simple, involving only the bending and unbending of the knees while the hands are lowered or raised. The movements are an effective way of directing the flow of energy through the channels. Several kinds of movement of the body and limbs during tai chi exercise involve movements such as shifting the weight from one leg to another, rotating the body to the right or left, taking a step, moving forward or backward, and fine hand and foot movements, all put together and coordinated in more or less complicated combinations and sequences.

PREVENTIVE QUALITIES

More than 80% of all illness has been shown to have stress-related etiologies.[20] Medical and rehabilitation practices that seek only to "fix" the physical symptoms (body) without addressing the impact of emotional well-being on disease are missing the target. Although the origins of tai chi exercise are based on ancient Eastern philosophy, it is a suitable form of exercise for tense Westerners. It has the advantage of regular exercise* combined with an emphasis on the gracefulness and slowness of pace that

Western society so conspicuously lacks. Tai chi can provide those who live in a fast-paced environment a compensating factor in their lives.

From ancient Chinese medicine, it has long been recognized that there are mental as well as physical aspects of disease.[15, 16, 20, 24, 30] Traditionally, according to Eastern philosophies, the mental state of the individual is considered to be *more* important than the physical symptoms. Recently, a new basic science of Western medical research, called psychoneuroimmunology, has emerged.[12, 17, 20, 32] This area of science is the study of the effects of emotions on the immune system. The new studies strongly indicate that virtually every illness, from a common cold to cancer and heart disease, can be influenced either positively or negatively by an individual's mental status. Today, Western health care professionals in both the physical and mental health professions are increasingly recognizing the role of the mind in the prevention and cure of illness. The health practitioner may encounter clients who do not seem to respond to traditional health care. Psychoneuroimmunology confronts these problems by employing the health traditions of other cultures and viewing the body and mind as a balanced whole.[32]

Tai chi is a specific technique for attaining peaceful mental states and therefore, by extrapolation, it may help prevent or reverse disease processes. Tai chi integrates the body and mind through breathing and movement. The open and closed movements of tai chi are coordinated with breathing. The benefits seem to be based on the fundamental combination of movements and breathing techniques in the basic tai chi exercise routines. The entry level of exercise has many similarities with medical treatments for respiratory illness (e.g., deep breathing exercises, segmental expansion exercises) and with walking exercise, the most recommended aerobic exercise for patients with coronary artery disease.[22, 23, 27]

In a study by Lai and colleagues,[23] it was determined that the elderly tai chi exercisers showed a significant improvement in Vo₂ uptake compared with an age-

---

*References 12, 17, 19, 22, 23, 27, 28, 31, 32, 34, 35.

matched control group of sedentary elders. The authors concluded that the data substantiated the practice of tai chi as a means of delaying the decline in cardiorespiratory function commonly considered "normal" for aging individuals. In addition, tai chi was shown to be a suitable aerobic exercise for older adults.[23] A subsequent study by Lai and co-workers[22] further substantiated that tai chi exercise is aerobic exercise of moderate intensity. In the past, it was believed, although never studied, that tai chi exercise forms did not have a significant cardiorespiratory component and therefore were deemed nonaerobic. It has been clearly demonstrated in these studies that, despite the slow, steady, smooth pace of tai chi exercise routines, there is a significant positive effect on the cardiorespiratory system.[22, 23, 27]

The potential value of tai chi exercise in promoting postural control, improving balance, and preventing falls has also been substantiated by several researchers.[19, 28, 31, 33, 34] Tse and Bailey[31] found that tai chi practitioners had significantly better postural control than sedentary nonpractitioners. Province and associates[28] found that treatments directed toward flexibility, balance, dynamic balance, and resistance, all components of tai chi exercise, reduced the risk of falls for elderly adults. Wolfson and colleagues[35] demonstrated that short-term exposure to "altered sensory input or destabilizing platform movement" during treatment sessions, in addition to home based tai chi exercises, elicited significant improvements in sway control and inhibited inappropriate motor responses. The outcome measure of functional balance improved more substantially in the exercise group that combined the treatment sessions with the home program of

tai chi. Wolf and co-workers[34] compared a balance training group, in which balance was stressed on a static-to-moving platform using biofeedback, with a group of tai chi exercisers. A third group served as a control for exercise intervention. This article did not provide information on the results of the effects of the two different exercise approaches on balance and frailty measures, although it provided a superb set of assessment tools for measuring balance. In a subsequent interview with Wolf, he spoke positively about the therapeutic value of exercise forms such as tai chi in delaying or possibly preventing the onset of frailty.[29] The benefits of tai chi in prevention of falls has also been supported by a study by Judge and colleagues,[19] who demonstrated improvements in single-stance postural sway in older women after tai chi exercises.

The stress reduction effects of tai chi exercise, as measured by heart rate, blood pressure, and urinary catecholamine and salivary cortisol levels, were compared with the levels in a group of brisk walkers, meditators, and quiet readers.[17] In general, it was found that the stress-reducing effect of tai chi characterized those physiological changes produced by moderate exercise. Heart rate, blood pressure, and urinary catecholamine changes for the tai chi exercise group were similar to these changes occurring in the walking group. Additionally, it was reported that the tai chi group expressed the enhancement of "vigor" and a reduction in anxiety states. In a study by Brown and associates,[12] unequivocal support is provided for the hypothesis that tai chi exercise, which incorporates a cognitive strategy as part of the training program, is more effective than exercise lacking a structured cognitive component in promoting psychological benefits.

CASE 33-2   MR. K

Mr. K is an 84-year-old white man, admitted to the nursing home from home in a markedly deconditioned state, with a diagnosis of coronary heart disease, tuberculosis, confusion, a recent history of falls, depression, and malnutrition. He was referred to physical and occupational therapy for screening and recommendations. Screening by physical therapy resulted in an initial evaluation that revealed a significantly compromised cardiopulmonary response to any activity, flexed posturing in standing with occasional loss of balance during directional changes, ambulation with moderate assistance of one requiring verbal cuing, and a fluctuating cognitive status. He was quite congested and occasionally expectorated blood, especially with exertion. He had remarkable shortness of breath at rest and significant rubor of all extremities with 1+ pulses distally. He was withdrawn, minimally verbal, and obviously quite depressed. Based on our assessment, his prognosis was deemed poor for functional recovery to his premorbid state and discharge unlikely.

Mr. K was placed on a fall prevention program

that included trunk extensor strengthening, extremity strengthening, and flexibility exercises. Deep breathing exercises were initiated and a reconditioning walking program using a 12-minute test protocol was started. Buerger-Allen exercises were initiated for his circulation and to promote postural changes and mobility. He was also referred to a nutritionist and the nursing staff was consulted regarding his skin and circulatory status. Patient's gains were marginal in both physical and occupational therapy over a 3-week period. He continued to require minimal to moderate assistance during ambulation, had a poor physiological response to activity of any sort, remained short of breath at rest, and was still withdrawn, now being virtually nonverbal and severely depressed.

Due to the restrictions placed on duration of intervention in a managed care delivery system driven by critical pathways, aggressive "skilled" intervention could no longer be justified. The insurer agreed to a 4-week trial of tai chi exercises to be done 5 days per week in a group setting. The patient was initially instructed in breathing

Continued

CASE 33–2 MR. K *Continued*

techniques and standing postures utilizing a set of tai chi movements that did not significantly displace his center of gravity. Remarkable improvements were noted in respiratory status (i.e., he was no longer short of breath at rest) and standing posture was distinctly improved by the end of the first week. It was noted that this elderly man was much more alert and responsive to his surroundings and appeared to be less depressed. The tai chi routine was expanded to encompass his increasing capabilities and weight-shifting postures were started, although one-legged stance tai chi activities were still omitted from his routine. By the end of the second week, the patient was walking to and from all activities with standby assistance and no verbal cuing. His extremity pulses had improved to 2+ with no extremity rubor. He still experienced shortness of breath on exertion, although he was no longer short of breath at rest and was not expectorating blood. He was noted to be spontaneously telling stories and joking with the staff and other residents. He reported amiably "where" his energy was going from time to time and stated that he was "eating everything on my plate."

Mr. K continued to progress in all areas of functional status. By the end of the third week he was walking to all activities independently and safely. He was alert and obviously happy. We were able

to start one-legged stance postures in his tai chi routine. He was independently taking a shower (which pleased him no end). He was fondly appreciated by his fellow residents for his sense of humor, optimism, and compassion for their concerns.

By the end of the fourth week, Mr. K, a happy man, was discharged on a home program that included tai chi exercises. Since his discharge, he has enrolled in a tai chi program at a local martial arts facility, in which he participates for 2 hours, three times a week. He comes back to the nursing home twice a week to assist as an instructor in the tai chi classes.

Perhaps Mr. K's progress sounds too good to be true, but the reality of his improvement has been observed in many of our patients who participate in the tai chi classes. Beyond the physical aspects of this exercise form, the most notable improvement appears to be in the area of "outlook." Elderly individuals participating in the tai chi classes express pure enjoyment in the slow, rhythmic movements and the group interaction. They report that they "feel stronger," "more balanced," and that they feel as if they were "dancing, not exercising." And, the insurers are overwhelmed with the functional successes that seem to be inherent in this mode of exercise. Tai chi is a low-cost, low-tech group activity.

CONCLUSIONS

The increasing body of research related to the use of tai chi as a valuable therapeutic intervention substantiates our need as professionals, in a cost-containment arena, to evaluate the merits of this exercise form.* Tai chi is viewed as an "alternative" therapy, has been observed clinically, and has been shown to enhance function in our elderly patients. Recently, the use of tai chi has been identified by the National Institutes of Health as one of a list of "alternative therapies" that will be targeted for research funding as a legitimate area for investigation. We should seize the opportunity to provide leadership in this emerging area in rehabilitative medicine. Tai chi, although it is a "nontraditional" approach to therapeutic intervention, merits further scientific analysis to quantify its apparent therapeutic validity.

Taekwondo

Clint Robinson, 8th Degree
Darcy A. Umphred, 4th Degree, PhD, PT

PHILOSOPHY

The overall philosophy of Taekwondo (TKD) can be summed up in the student oath recited by all practitioners at the beginning of each class: "I shall observe the tenets of Taekwondo: courtesy, integrity, perseverance, self-con-

trol and indomitable spirit." The tenets are to be practiced outside as well as inside the training hall in all aspects of life. All aspects of these tenets reflect CNS control and incorporate the cognitive, emotional, and motor aspects into an integrated whole. The oath continues with, "I shall respect the instructors and seniors," which refers to having respect for all people, our teachers, our parents, our peers, which reflects all individuals with whom the student may interact through a lifetime. "I shall never misuse Taekwondo." No matter what motor skill a student develops, it is not to be used to build one's ego or to injure another unnecessarily. "I will be a champion of freedom and justice." Individuals are expected to develop a sense of responsibility for those less fortunate than themselves and be an active participant in the development of mankind as a whole. "I will build a more peaceful world." Understanding that change begins with self, thus by developing and integrating the mind, body, and spirit while helping others do the same, will set an example not only in the classroom but in our society, so that others may improve themselves. The overall goal of TKD training is the development of self-sufficiency through rigorous physical and mental practice. Students are expected to strive for their own personal excellence versus comparing that skill with another's. Thus, individuals with physical challenges are always encouraged to participate. Their challenges and expectations are different, but achieving personal excellence gives them the

---

*References 12, 17, 19, 22, 23, 27, 28, 31, 32, 34, 35.

same respect and confidence that any other student would receive. Thus, TKD as a movement science empowers participants to regain a feeling of body control over the mind, the spirit, and the physical body.

PHILOSOPHY OF TRAINING

Training in TKD consists of three primary components: forms, breaking of solid objects, and sparring. The practice of tai chi focuses on the first component, but with practice a Taekwondo student would have the skill to perform both breaking and sparring.

Poomsee (a prearranged dance of defensive and offensive techniques against an imaginary opponent). The practice of poomsee increases the practitioner's memory, coordination, balance, and body awareness. All poomsee components have predetermined patterns of movement that include various stances and hand and kicking techniques, along with a proper beginning and ending point.

Kyukpa (breaking of solid objects such as boards, concrete, and bricks using a body part as a weapon). Kyukpa represents overcoming limitations and obstacles and facing fear. It requires tremendous concentration and belief in one's abilities. Additionally, it allow its practitioners to demonstrate the power they have attained, thereby increasing self-confidence. Self-confidence is the primary attribute in conflict resolution skills and leads to the understanding that there are very few situations in life in which physical confrontation is necessary.

Kyorugi (actual sparring between two people utilizing both defensive and offensive techniques one has learned through fundamental TKD practice). Kyorugi can be further broken down into two types: (1) In one-step sparring, the practitioners take turns initiating a prearranged attack while the other defends. This allows the practitioners to engage each other without risk of injury to either party. It also allows them to practice proper distancing and execution of the techniques. This develops confidence in the ability to utilize the techniques properly if the need arises. (2) In free sparring, neither opponent knows what the other is going to do. Although free sparring may appear dangerous to one untrained in TKD, it is a relatively safe activity. Free sparring requires respect for your partner and absolute controlled motions at all times. It is an exercise in which the aim is for all involved to increase their skill level. It develops the practitioner's reflexes, confidence in their abilities, and overall awareness.

Although both offensive and defensive techniques are viewed as equally important, all training is begun with blocking techniques to indicate that TKD never allows any initial offensive attack in its technique. Blocking techniques are practiced diligently so that they may function equally as offensive techniques. This way one can defeat an opponent, whether in the classroom or in real life, without either suffering or inflicting serious injuries. This builds self-confidence and replaces a perception of the "role of a victim."[41]

In TKD training, all students begin in the same place. There is no concern for one's status in life. The white belt is utilized to denote the beginning student. With all students beginning at that level, it allows another aspect of training that is critical to all students and very individualized. Training encompasses setting and achieving goals or empowering oneself to one's own quality of life. In TKD, there is a belt ranking system and the object is to progress through the various levels of proficiency, culminating in the black belt. Everyone, regardless of social status or physical skill, has the same opportunity to advance in TKD. Students who persevere and obtain a first-degree black belt learn that they have only begun their circle of growth and learning. With additional years of training, students may advance in black belt ranks that should reflect a greater understanding and acceptance of those initial tenets. The circle of growth will always lead to further integration of mind, body, and spirit and an inner peace and balance.[42] The balance of mind, body, and spirit is the core of other complementary therapy paradigms and ultimately seems to be an element linked to health and healing.

TAEKWONDO AND COMPLEMENTARY THERAPY[36–38, 40, 42–44]

Although TKD is a martial arts style whose original intent was not to heal a disease or pathology as a medical practice, the concepts and procedures learned, repetitively practiced, and transformed into life behavior, have established the foundation for health and healing in individuals who have impairments within the CNS, whether the deficits are motor, cognitive, or affective.[39, 45] Similarly, with identified disease, TKD can help maintain motor function, cognitive integrity, and emotional balance, and a feeling of self-worth in the face of a long-term and possibly progressive neurological problem.

As in all martial arts, TKD requires active participation by the student. When looking at any TKD movement pattern, certain motor control components are seen to be interacting. There are a variety of activities that generally occur during a class. First, there are warm-ups, after which the student will work on (1) his or her respective form or poomsee or hyung (dancelike patterns that may have 18 to 100 different movement sequences) depending upon the level of advancement; (2) sparring, which is either done with one partner moving with an identified pattern while the other stays in one position or with both moving and learning to respond to the movements or feints of the other; or (3) learning to focus and perform specific strikes or blows that will lead to skills in board or brick breaking or defending oneself against a life-threatening attack.

During warm-up, a student stretches and builds up power, using specific movement, balance, timing, concentration, and cardiopulmonary functions that set the stage for the remainder of the class. When doing the forms, the student will need to work on balance, postural tone, the state of the motor generator, synergistic patterns of movement, trajectory, speed, force, directionality, sequencing, reciprocal patterns, and the context within which the movement is being done. Similarly, memory of the specific pattern, movement sequences, and direction of the movements requires concentration. If other students are also practicing in class, then each individual needs to be aware of the total environment in order to respect the space of all other students.

When students are learning and practicing either one-step sparring or free sparring, they are not only working on learning combinations of movement patterns and how they interact or conflict with those of their partners, they are also learning how to control their emotional responses to threatening situations. Very little in life is worth hurting another—a basic principle of TKD. During sparring, the potential of injury is directly correlated with the control over the force and direction of movement. That control can be dramatically affected by emotion. (See Chapter 6.) Once students learn to control the emotional aspect, their skill and techniques become procedural, which allows their cognitive analytical ability to drive responses. (See Chapter 5.) The student is then ready to begin study of the mind, body, emotional, and spiritual connections that need to intertwine and become harmonious if the student is to learn the true meaning of TKD. Sparring is a controlled environment in which injury or damage to another person is never acceptable.

Board and brick breaking is the time a student can demonstrate force production as it interlocks with trajectory, speed, and position in space. If any of these perceptual or motor variables are incorrect, the student will not succeed at going through the obstacle. These skills are taught and practiced not to damage or destroy the wood or brick, but rather to learn to go beyond or through the obstacle. Once the specific body part used as a trajectory goes beyond the obstacle, it no long remains an obstacle and the student feels great satisfaction. In reality, to be successful at these tasks, the hand, elbow, or foot that is used to go through the brick or wood is only an extension of the body. Success is based on the learner's ability to tie the entire body's motor response—its rotation, its balance, its trajectory, its force, and its speed—into a motor program that will project through one or more obstacles as a knife cuts butter. If the student, emotionally, believes the obstacle will not break, it will not! The student will stop the movement before completing the task and often empower the wood or brick as a successful obstacle versus empowering himself or herself to overcome that obstacle as if it were never there. That, again, is a critical element of TKD. It is also a critical component of any client's learning of any motor program and turning the program into a functional activity and improving one's quality of life.

Those that respond best to TKD training to maintain motor function are individuals who are motivated to move, enjoy interactions with others, have cognitive integrity, and have some control over their motor system. When instructing a TKD club of individuals who had all suffered traumatic head injuries, the teacher (TKD instructor) and a therapist who had worked for over 25 years in the area of neurological rehabilitation found that using therapeutic skills through TKD movement patterns augmented the students' learning and helped them to regain motor function through guided activities without the students ever realizing there was therapeutic intervention. To those students, they were learning and advancing in a martial arts style, tested and judged according to their development of skill, and feeling accomplishment as an adult participating in an adult activity. Carryover and improvement in balance, postural integrity, reciprocal patterns of movement, and control of trajectory, force, and speed, as well as development of emotional stability and confidence, could be easily identified and evaluated using standard objective measurement tools if so desired. Expected outcomes would be improvement in those areas of motor control just mentioned. As long as the student continued training, improvement would be expected and carryover into other life activities anticipated.

Energetic Therapy Approaches

Therapeutic Touch

Eve Karpinski, BS

Therapeutic touch (TT) is a nursing intervention developed by Dolores Krieger and Dora Kunz. Karilee Shames defines *therapeutic touch* as: "a specific technique of centering intention used while the practitioner moves the hands through the recipient's energy field to assess and treat imbalance" (*Holistic Nurses Handbook*, American Holistic Nurses' Association). According to Dr. Janet Quinn at the Center for Human Caring at the University of Colorado, TT is based on a set of assumptions: people are energy fields, we are each unique patterns of energy, and we are in a universal web of energy.[55]

The intent of the practitioner is essential to the successful administration of TT, but the mechanism is grounded in the principles of physics. Several researchers have explored the properties of the skin in respect to direct current (DC) and electromagnetic energy.[48, 56] The results of these studies concluded that the human body generates subtle yet measurable alternating current (AC) and DC at all times. In physics, it is well understood that any time a current moves through a linear pathway, such as electrons through a wire, a field is produced around the structure through which energy passes. This is precisely the intent of TT, where the practitioner facilitates a change in the bioelectromagnetic field around the patient.

Connell and Meehan[46] explored the effects of TT on the experience of acute pain in postoperative patients by testing the hypothesis that there will be a greater decrease in posttest acute pain experience scores in subjects treated by TT than in subjects treated by sham TT. Keller and Bzdek[50] examined the effects of TT on tension headache pain, building on previous work by Heidt[40] and Quinn,[54] which indicated that TT reduced anxiety. Gagne and Toye[47] investigated the effects of TT in a psychiatric facility. A statistically significant reduction in reported anxiety was attained. Fedoryk studied the effects on infants in neonatal, intermediate, and intensive care units.[52] The analysis indicated that there was a significant difference between infants treated with TT and those treated with sham TT. Other studies discussed the role of TT in outcomes for wound healing. In a classic study, Krieger[51] reported a significant increase in hemoglobin values in response to TT versus routine hospital care. These studies all point to attempts to quantify the efficacy of TT.

The ability to do TT is considered a natural potential, which anyone who is basically healthy and has a pure intent to help may develop with knowledge and practice.[52] Macra[53] stated that to practice TT one needs to be in good health, to empathize with those who are suffering, to have a desire to help others without motivation for personal gain, and to possess self-discipline because TT is a highly refined skill that is developed through regular practice.

According to Nurse Healers–Professional Associates International, the purpose of TT is "a contemporary interpretation of several ancient healing practices, is an intentionally directed process of energy exchange during which the practitioner uses the hands as a focus for facilitating healing. The intervention is administered with the intent of enabling people to repattern their energy in the direction of health. Indications for use include, but are not limited to, reduction of pain and anxiety, promotion of relaxation, and facilitation of the body's natural restorative processes. In addition, Therapeutic Touch can be used alone or with other healing modalities."

In my practice as a nurse, I have found that doing TT enhances the trust relationship with the client. Many studies have found that TT can provide and promote a deep sense of relaxation, facilitate comfort, support the healing process, reduce anxiety, and reduce the need for analgesic medication.

Sessions usually do not last over 30 minutes. Clients such as neonates, children, people with psychiatric disorders, and the debilitated person are more sensitive to the process. Many nursing curricula teach the skills of TT and nursing research has been at the forefront of research in this area. Physical therapists and occupational therapists continue to perform manual contact skills with good results. The additional aspect of TT may be added to the occupational and physical therapy interventions to maximize the available options, especially with chronic conditions. Collaborative efforts in rehabilitation research may elucidate more studies of TT in the future.

ORGANIZATIONS PROVIDING INFORMATION ABOUT THERAPEUTIC TOUCH

The American Holistic Nurses' Association
PO Box 2130
Flagstaff, AZ 86003
800-278-AHNA
e-mail: *AHNA-flag@flaglink.com*
http://www.ahana.org

Nurse Healers–Professional Associates
  International
3760 South Highland Drive
Suite 429
Salt Lake City, UT 84106
801-273-3399
e-mail: *nhpa@nursecominc.com*
http://www.therapeutic-touch.org

Medical Intuitive Diagnostic

Carol Ritberger, PhD, Medical Intuitive

The practice of medicine as traditionally defined is undergoing an exciting transformation. Through modern technology and research, many ancient concepts are being validated. No longer are those involved in the health and healing modalities able to ignore the effectiveness of ancient therapeutic and diagnostic tools, nor are they able to deny the presence of the subtle energy body. The use of intuitive diagnosis is reemerging as a complementary method of identifying illness. Intuitive diagnosis works with the human energy system for the purpose of identifying imbalances and malfunctions in the physical body.[61]

The human energy system (the aura) is in actuality an extended sensory system that is an integral part of the communication network connecting the mind and the body.[63] It is electromagnetic in nature and acts as an antenna that is sensitive to both internal and external stimuli. The primary function of this energy system is to receive, interpret, transmit, and store information. It is rich in both biographical and biological information. Biographically, its electromagnetic interpretation instructs the cellular structure of the body, through an electrochemical dialogue, to store all emotional reactions of our thoughts and experiences. Biologically, it directly reflects the DNA structure and the state of all of the body's major systems. The energy body, like the physical body, has predetermined communication pathways that instruct it in how to make known the state of health or lack of it in the physical body.[62]

The pathways of the energy body include the endocrine and chakra systems. In the physical body, the master glands of the endocrine system manufacture the major hormones that control the chemical production of the body and, as a result, the biochemical dialogue in our cellular structure.[58] The locations of the seven major endocrine glands are also the locations for the seven major spiritual centers of the body. These spiritual centers are called chakras. The chakras function at the etheric and subtle levels. Consequently, the chakra and endocrine systems pair up to act as energetic pathways (transducers) from the subtle level to the physical level.[59, 60]

Persons who have developed their intuitive skills to the point that they can access the information found in the human energy system are called medical intuitives. The role of the medical intuitive is to the read the body both energetically and physically and to link all of the information together to provide a comprehensive analysis of a person's state of health and overall well-being. As a diagnostician, a medical intuitive looks at the physiological, psychological, and psychospiritual characteristics of the energy system. Through the use of intuition, a medical intuitive is able to analyze a person's energy for the purpose of:

- Identifying where energetic imbalances are occurring
- Determining the origin sites of the imbalances
- Clarifying what is triggering the imbalances, for example, emotional, psychological, or spiritual issues
- Identifying how these imbalances are affecting the physical body

- Analyzing all of the parts of the body that are being affected
- Determining what needs to be done to restore energetic and physical balance

The primary goal of this type of diagnostic process is to lead a person to self-knowledge and then to describe ways for that person to facilitate the healing process. Medical intuitives can do the following:

- They can provide a comprehensive picture of what is creating the potential for illness because they work with all aspects of a person's well-being: physical, mental, emotional, and spiritual.
- They can offer insight into the deeper struggles in a person's life that are creating blockages.
- They can reveal what needs to be done to restore balance to a person's life.
- They can help the person connect with issues that are preventing them from having the life and health they desire.

In clinical terms, the use of medical intuition as a diagnostic tool is effective when analyzing a multitude of illnesses. Since medical intuitive diagnosis is not a treatment modality, it does not require repeated visits. Some clients do choose, however, to continue to work with a medical intuitive as a means of evaluating the progress of treatment processes.

COMPLEMENTARY MEDICAL TEAMS OF THE FUTURE

As we move forward in the twenty-first century, there appears to be an open-mindedness toward the integration of complementary healing modalities. Many major teaching institutions, as well as hospitals, are currently offering a complementary medical clinic with teams including physicians and alternative practitioners (medical intuitives

---

CASE 33–3   MICHAEL

Michael, age 56 years, is an example of how a medical intuitive assesses the energy body for the purpose of diagnosis.

Energy Analysis. Michael shows overall depletion of the energy system. He suffers from physical exhaustion and shows signs of chronic fatigue. There are electrical storms in the head area. Other signs are mental disarray, chemical imbalance in the brain, and damage to and malfunction of areas in the right side of the brain. There is very little energy activity on the right side of the brain. Energy flow in both arms is erratic, more so on the left side. He has tremors in both hands, but more so in the left hand. There is red energy protrusion in the area of the brain where the brain stem originates. This energy buildup is affecting motor skills, causing energy blockages in the upper spine, primarily the second, third, fourth, and fifth cervical vertebrae. There are signs of nerve degeneration. He has severe muscle tension in the shoulder area and midback. Auric colors indicate buildup of toxins and waste in muscle structure. He has signs of depression. Reddish-brown color as seen by the medical intuitive indicates the CNS is affected. Most of his energy is focused in the upper torso area. Lower extremities show very little energy flow. He has poor circulation in the legs and feet. His weak sites are the chest, neck, and upper shoulders (fourth and fifth chakras),[59] and specifically the cerebrospinal nervous system.

Diagnosis. Michael was examined by an allopathic physician 4 months after the medical intuitive evaluation. The diagnosis was Parkinson's disease.

Psychological and Psychospiritual Causes. Michael showed extreme unwillingness to deal with change and an overwhelming need to control. He believed that if he did not have complete control of everything, his life would fall apart. He lacked belief in himself and had emotional issues pertaining to low self-esteem, a lack of drive, and lack of courage to go after what he wanted. He always felt he was not worthy of having what he had. Childhood experiences and the negative emotions he attached to them affected his self-worth. He believed that his life had no meaning or purpose. He lived with the belief that it was a mistake that he was ever born. His mother told him at a very young age that she never wanted to have him. Michael had lived his life based on the erroneous perception that he would never be loved or be worthy of getting what he desired.

There was a strong energy loss around his spiritual belief system. This was contradictory because Michael was raised in a structured and strict religious belief system that should have strengthened rather that disconnected him from his beliefs. Michael said that he felt that his God had abandoned him because he was an unwanted child.

The session revealed that Michael was afraid of change and that he never took the time to reevaluate the beliefs that were limiting him. As a result, he was not able to get in touch with his insecurities. The struggle between his emotional and spiritual issues caused him to disconnect from himself. His life focus was more on existing than on discovering his true talents.

Energetically, Parkinson's disease reflects an unwillingness to change and a lack of faith in God and life. It also represents a feeling of being alone and feeling unsafe in an uncaring world.

being one). In essence, the combination of allopathic medicine and alternative medicine can be of great value to the patient for the following reasons:

1. Each practitioner brings particular expertise, skills, and training to the diagnostic and healing process. The physician and the healing practitioner work with the patient to restore balance and health to the physical body, and the medical intuitive assists in providing a more comprehensive assessment of the root cause of the illness.
2. Each practitioner has a way of gathering the necessary information to determine the cause of illness. The physician works with the standard medical history of the person, and the medical intuitive works with the person's beliefs and biographical history.
3. The physician works to heal the body, the medical intuitive assists to determine the origin of the malfunction, and the alternative practitioner works to heal both body and spirit.
4. When each practitioner's assessment is part of the evaluation and diagnostic process, then the treatment process can be potentially accelerated because the recommended approaches will treat both cause and effect.

Thomas Edison stated, "The doctor of the future will give no medicine, but will interest his patients in the care of the human frame, in diet, and in the cause and prevention of disease."[57]

MEDICAL INTUITIVE DIAGNOSTICS AS A PROFESSION

Medical intuition as a profession is in its infancy in terms of its acceptability by allopathic medicine. There is not, at the time of this writing, a national organization with a referral listing base of medical intuitives. It was not until the late 1990s that the use of medical intuition came into awareness and the medical profession began to use these services. There are currently educational programs being developed that will teach medical intuitive diagnostics.

Physical Body Systems Approaches

CranioSacral Therapy
John Upledger, DO
Mary Lou Galantino, PhD, PT

INTRODUCTION

CranioSacral Therapy (CST) is a gentle, noninvasive, and yet very powerful and effective treatment approach that relies primarily upon hands-on evaluation and treatment. It focuses upon the normalization of bodily functions that are either part of or related to a semiclosed hydraulic physiological system, which has been named the *craniosacral system*.

STRUCTURE OF THE CRANIOSACRAL SYSTEM

The anatomy of the craniosacral system includes a watertight compartment formed by the dura mater, the cerebrospinal fluid (CSF) within this compartment, the inflow and outflow systems that regulate the quantity and pressure of the bones to which the dura mater attaches, the

joints or sutures that interconnect these bones, and other bones not anatomically connected to the dura mater. The bones of the cranium, as well as the second and third cervical vertebrae, the sacrum, and the coccyx, are also included in the structures of the craniosacral system.[73, 76]

In combination with the message sent to the patient through the intentional touch of the therapist is the corrective work that is done on a very basic physiological level by gentle hands-on manipulations applied both directly and indirectly to the craniosacral system. The semiclosed hydraulic system includes the dural sleeves, which invest the spinal nerve roots outside of the vertebral canal as far as the intervertebral foramina, and the caudal end of the dural tube, which ultimately becomes the cauda equina and blends with the coccygeal periosteum. The fluid within the semiclosed hydraulic system is CSF. The inflow and outflow of CSF are regulated by the choroid plexuses within the brain's ventricular system and arachnoid granulation bodies, respectively. CSF outflow is not rhythmically interrupted but its rate may be adjusted by intracranial membrane tension patterns, which are broadcast primarily via the falx cerebri and tentorium cerebelli to the anterior end of the straight venous sinus, where an aggregation of arachnoid granulation bodies is located. This concentration of arachnoid granulation bodies is known to affect venous backpressure, which has an effect upon the rate of reabsorption of CSF into the blood-vascular system.[65, 66, 69]

TECHNIQUE

The therapist, after mobilizing bony restrictions, focuses upon the correction of abnormal dural membrane restrictions, perceived CSF activities, and energy patterns and fluctuations as they relate to the craniosacral system. It is during this time that the patient very often moves from a phase of being corrected and having obstacles removed to a phase of self-healing, with the therapist serving as a facilitator of the process. The tenets of CST include the concept that the dura mater within the vertebral canal (dural tube) has the freedom to glide up and down within that canal for a range of 0.5 to 2.0 cm. This movement is allowed by the slackness and directionality of the dural sleeves as they depart the dural tube and attach to the intertransverse foramina of the spinal column.[73]

A basic assumption in CST, as it has evolved, is that the patient's body contains the necessary information for the discovery of the cause of any health problem. The treatment relies primarily upon hands-on evaluation and treatment. The hands-on contact is tender and supportive. It is accompanied by a sincere intention to assist the patient in any way that is possible. In short, the therapist serves primarily as a facilitator of the patient's own healing processes. The rapport that develops during the patient-therapist interaction lends itself powerfully to the positive therapeutic effect that many patients experience.

Western medicine imparts a therapeutic modality for curative measures, whereas CST fosters facilitation, wherein the client directs the treatment session. The inherent participation of the patient through CST promotes a wholistic approach to healing. Conventional medical diagnosis will usually be more closely related to what the therapist views as the result rather than the cause.

For example, the therapist would search for a cause of strabismus within the intracranial membrane system and the motor control system of the eyes, rather than considering strabismus as a diagnosed condition to be corrected by surgery. The cause of strabismus can be found as an abnormal tension pattern in the tentorium cerebelli. The therapist then searches for the cause of the abnormal tentorial tension pattern. Quite often, these tension patterns are referred from the occiput or from the low back or the pelvis. If this is the case, the CST "diagnosis" would be intracranial membranous strain of the tentorium cerebelli due to occipital or low back and pelvic dysfunctions, individually or severally, resulting in secondary motor dysfunction of the eyes (strabismus). The therapist would focus on the sacrum, the pelvis, the occiput, and then the tentorium cerebelli. Correct evaluation and treatment would be signified by a "spontaneous correction" of the strabismus.

SomatoEmotional Release is a technique that involves the bodily, and usually conscious, reexperiencing of episodes, the energies for which have been stored in the totality of body tissues. A powerful emotional content is typically connected with this technique and it has proved to be extremely effective in cases of severe posttraumatic stress disorder. It was tested through qualitative research with a group of six Vietnam veterans in 1993. It proved to be successful in all six of these patients.[73, 75–77]

OUTCOMES

Objective responses to CST are based upon the removal of obstructions to smooth and easy physiological motions of the patient's body, the absence of energy cysts, the free movement of the dural tube in the spinal/vertebral canal and the rate and quality of the craniosacral rhythm, the absence of pressing responses during the SomatoEmotional Release process, and statements from the deeper levels of consciousness via dialogue with various images encountered in the session that "all is well."[73, 75, 76]

Subjectively, clients report an increased sense of well-being, improved sleep patterns, reduced manifestation of stress, reduction or disappearance of pain, increased energy levels, and fewer episodes of transitory illness. How long it takes to achieve these results is extremely variable, and dependent upon the complexity of the layers of adaptation, the defense mechanism, and the level of spiritual evolution of the patient.

USE IN TREATMENT INTERVENTION

CST is useful as a primary treatment modality and as an adjunct to a wide variety of visceral dysfunctions. It works well to balance autonomic function, specifically reducing sympathetic nervous system tonus. It has proved beneficial in chronic headache problems, temporomandibular joint problems, whiplash sequelae, and chronic pain syndromes. We have used it as intensive treatment for persons rehabilitating from head injuries, craniotomies, spinal cord injuries, poststroke syndromes, transient ischemic attacks, seizure disorders, and a wide variety of rare brain and spinal cord dysfunction problem.[67, 68] Little positive effect has been reported in amyotrophic lateral sclerosis (ALS). However, there has been some remarkable success seen in multiple sclerosis.[74]

In children, CST has been used extensively and very effectively in a high percentage of persons with spastic cerebral palsy, seizure disorders, Down syndrome, and a wide variety of motor system disorders, including problems with the oculomotor system, learning disabilities, attention deficit disorder, speech problems, childhood allergies, and autonomic dysfunctions.[64, 70, 71]

We have used CST for people living with human immunodeficiency virus (HIV) disease who are suffering from HIV-related peripheral neuropathy and other chronic musculoskeletal and neurological problems. Pain management techniques can be employed by the therapist and also taught to family members to implement for a home program.[72] Future studies addressing the interaction of the immune system with the craniosacral system would be helpful in elucidating the neuroendocrine response to this technique.

TRAINING

The prerequisites for training in CST by the Upledger Institute, Inc, are quite simple. It is believed that any kind of therapist who has a license to see and treat patients/clients might find CST, in its more basic form, a useful adjunct to his or her practice. Therefore, a license as health care practitioner is all that is required to enroll in the Upledger Institute's CST seminar series.

There are six levels of training within the series that are required before one can enroll in the advanced-level workshops. The workshops are all 4 or 5 days in length, and are about evenly divided between academic work and hands-on supervised practice. The training program is designed to develop the sense of touch, motion, and energy perception slightly before the academic material is presented. A certification process started in 1995 is now in place.

There is a newly formed International Association of Healthcare Practitioners of which the American Cranio-Sacral Therapy Association is a subdivision. The American CranioSacral Therapy Association, a nonprofit organization, was founded by a group of therapists and concerned laypersons in 1994. Its stated objectives are to bring CST into public awareness, to enhance networking between practitioners who use CST to develop a certification program that will result in recognition of CST as a specialty for persons who are licensed as health care practitioners in other fields, and to ultimately develop CST as an independently licensed and freestanding profession.

Reimbursement by third-party carriers is done largely on a case-by-case basis. A few insurance companies have recognized CST, but there is much work to be done on this front. The Upledger Institute publishes a book listing all the practitioners who have completed training. It is available to health care professionals.

Myofascial Release (Barnes Method)
Carol M. Davis, EdD, PT

Myofascial release is a manual energetic therapy designed to treat the myofascia that surrounds every cell and tissue in the body. John Barnes, the physical therapist credited for developing this wholistic treatment technique, has pointed out that it is a mistake to think of muscle as being a tissue in and of itself. Just as we now recognize that the mind and body cannot be separated, we also realize that there is no such entity as muscle; rather, the fascial-muscle unit is the more accurate anatomical and physiological entity. As Janet Travell[83] first described it, the fascia that surrounds each muscle fiber and fibril is inextricably interconnected with the muscle, and it is impossible to treat the muscle alone. Until the fascial barriers are released, the muscle, no matter how often stretched or contracted, will tend to resume its original shape. If that shape is distorted by central or peripheral nervous system pathology, as is so often the case with our clients, or distorted from hypertonicity, if the muscle group has taken a postural position of ease from prolonged positioning or emotional protection, or if the fascia surrounding the cells of skin nearby is contorted from a surgical scar, then the muscle is not free to contract in the way it was created to function.

THE PHYSIOLOGY OF THE FASCIAL SYSTEM

In order to understand how myofascial release is administered, and why it seems to result in such positive outcomes to patients, it is necessary to understand the physiology of the fascial system. Fascia exists as a three-dimensional web surrounding all of our cells, from the top of our head to the bottom of our feet. Functional biomechanical movements depend on intact, properly distributed fasciae.[79] There are three different types of fascia, but each is composed of a web of connective tissue of similar structure. The fascia just below the dermis is known as *superficial* fascia. The fascia that surrounds and fuses with bone, muscle, nerves, blood vessels, and organs is termed *deep* fascia. The third type of fascia is the *dura*, which surrounds the brain and spinal cord. Fascia is the connective tissue that plays a largely unrecognized but vital role in holding the body together. Without fascia, the body could not remain intact and erect, supported by bones, joints, tendons, and ligaments alone. The fascia functions much like the stays of a tent, supporting the structure of the body and also facilitating metabolism and blood and lymph flow and separating organs and other structures from each other, down to the cellular level.[79]

INTERVENTION

In contrast to traditional stretching of tissue, during myofascial release practitioners and their clients experience a sensation of softening, or stretching, like pulling taffy. Once tight tissue is located by palpation or observation, the slack is taken out of the tissue under the hands, and the therapist gently leans into his or her hands and waits for the tissue to respond. Within 90 to 120 seconds, a feeling of flow results, and the therapist then simply follows that twisting and deepening flow of tissue until it stops, when he or she again waits, maintaining slight tension until the tissue begins to flow again, and the therapist can follow the fascia, as it flows or releases, to the next collagenous barrier. The collagen fibers seem to be rearranging themselves back to a position of alignment,

or self-correction. Very often an area of heat and redness under the release occur, but curiously, at times an area of erythema occurs distant from the release itself.[80]

The effect of myofascial release can be enhanced by prolonged, corrective positioning using postural wedges or therapeutic balls or both to sustain the appropriate pressure to release the fascia over time. For example, for a rotated pelvis, wedges will sustain a correcting derotation while lying supine or prone.[79] The purpose of myofascial release is to lengthen the fascia that has been abnormally constricted, thus allowing a more efficient and effective contraction of muscles, a more barrier-free blood and lymph supply to nerves and organs, and an upright posture that responds in a neutral way to the forces of gravity. Myofascial release, along with soft tissue mobilization, therapeutic exercise, and movement reeducation is an excellent wholistic therapeutic approach for musculoskeletal, neuromuscular, and integumentary disorders in function.

MYOFASCIAL RELEASE INTERVENTION

Myofascial release treatment consists of a thorough examination of the client, including an in-depth history of symptoms and a thorough musculoskeletal and neuromuscular examination, noting pain, impairments in strength, range of motion endurance, and any disorders in function. The client's posture and, specifically, the position of the pelvis are noted. In many people, the hips will appear uneven, palpation of the anterior superior iliac spines will reveal an iliac rotation, and many times there will be a leg length discrepancy associated with pelvic rotation. In the case of stroke, traumatic brain injury, or cerebral palsy, abnormal tone will have resulted in fascia frozen along with their spastic muscles as a result of disorganized nerve conduction. No matter what the cause of the fascial tightening, the treatment remains to release the connective tissue, the fascia. This is done with manual releases, soft tissue mobilization techniques, positioning on wedges, facilitating whole-body release (unwinding), cranosacral techniques, and a technique called "rebounding." The technique of rebounding, which is especially useful with CNS pathology, involves a passive rocking of tissue, exploiting the hydrophilic aspect of tissue to the maximum. As the therapist rhythmically rocks chest, legs, thorax, or arms, the tissue reverberates with the rhythm of the motion, often resulting in a spontaneous release of tense and hypertonic tissue. Patients respond very positively to this technique.

The actual techniques of myofascial release, a wholistic complementary therapy, may at first appear to be exactly like mechanical manual therapies, but soon the novice recognizes the need to quiet the mind and body, learns to wait and feel gently with an enhanced proprioceptive sense for the tissue to "move up into the hands," and then gently to follow it as it twists and turns. It is an art that is greatly enhanced by a calm and centered proprioceptive listening that is not linear or mechanical in nature, but energetic and wholistic.[81] Palpating for the cranial rhythm takes the same centered, quiet "listening with one's hands." Eventually, we learn to feel with the whole self.[82]

Models of Health Care Belief Systems

Traditional Acupuncture

Jeff Kauffman, MD, Certified Acupuncturist

INTRODUCTION

It has been very gratifying to see Western medicine, as it is practiced by allopathic physicians, come around to include many of the wholistic practices that were once considered quackery. This is happening with chiropractic, massage, and other forms of body work; nutrition and diet; and exercise practices like hatha yoga and tai chi, and so on. A research study designed by David Eisenberg of Harvard Medical School, published in the *New England Journal of Medicine* in 1993 and again in 1998,[84, 85] showed just how extensive alternative or wholistic practices are and how a very large percentage of patients are using these practices, with or without knowledge of their personal physicians. Alternative health therapeutic modes are on the rise, are being used by more and more of the general population of the United States, and are being more and more accepted by Western medical practitioners. Many medical schools now have courses teaching alternative healing practices to medical students.

The question arises as to why people are drawn to therapeutic approaches outside the medical sphere. The answer is relatively straightforward. They are not getting everything they need in health care from traditional allopathic, Western-trained medical doctors. People are looking for something that works better. More and more people are disenchanted by the lack of compassion of a large percentage of the medical profession. This involves the patient being approached by the physician as a disease rather than a person, as a gallbladder case or a case of appendicitis or chronic fatigue instead of Sherri Jackson or Marvin Jones. This involves the hurried 5- to 10-minute visits created and encouraged by health maintenance organizations (HMOs). It involves the use of pharmaceuticals over the use of any other therapeutic modality. The side effects of such medications add to the problem. Along with the decrease in or lack of compassion comes the inability of many doctors to develop rapport with their patients.

There is one other very important principle that separates allopathic medicine as it is practiced in the United States from wholistic healing, and that is the attention paid to the symptoms. Allopathic medicine traditionally treats the symptoms. In fact, the diagnosis is usually the symptom with the name changed to something that has "-itis" on it at the end as a suffix. For example, *arthritis* means inflammation of the joints, *appendicitis* means inflammation of the appendix, and *iritis* means inflammation of the iris. Tension headache or migraine headache is simply a headache. It means an ache or pain in the head. Western medicine is essentially treating the symptoms, most commonly with drugs. Even the medications are named after the symptoms—for example, anti-inflammatories, antihypertensives, antimetabolites, antacids, antiarrhythmic agents, and diuretics (to increase output of fluid through the urine).

On the other hand, wholistic healing is aimed at determining the cause of the disease (even the Western medical term *disease* means dis-ease or lack of ease). In determining the cause of disease, one looks for the underlying imbalances that all human beings have. None of us is born with a perfect body-mind that never breaks down. We all have an underlying imbalance or constitutional imbalance that is the weak or vulnerable area of our body-mind that will always be the first to show symptoms and illness when under pressure or stress.

The pressure or stress coming from the outside world, outside of our body, can be in the form of physical agents like physical trauma (accidents), which cause bruised tissues, strained or torn ligaments, or broken bones, toxic agents from the environment, like poison or chemicals in the water or foods or air, carcinogens from contaminants, or poor nutrition and poor diet, not taking in enough nutrients or taking in too much of a particular kind. There are also external causes that are related to weather, such as excessive exposure to heat or cold or humidity or dryness or wind or dampness, being struck by lightning or near-drowning. Then there are the much more common causes of illness that come from the inside. These would be in the mental or emotional spheres. Generally, it is an emotion that is in excess or deficient in the person's life, like too much fear or not enough, too much grief or not enough expression of grief, too much anger or not enough, too much joy (that's right, too much joy or inappropriate joy) or not enough, too much sympathy or not enough. Feelings and emotions that are in excess or in deficient states affect particular organs which, in turn, can cause imbalance, symptoms, and disease in a particular organ, which then manifests as a heart attack or arthritis or constipation or cancer, and so on. This occurs with our thoughts as well, where we can focus to excess on particular negative thoughts that then create imbalance, illness, and disease.

There is also the most important sphere for all human beings, which is the spirit, and there can be, and often are, imbalances in this realm that have everything to do with not recognizing one's true value, which means not acknowledging the spirit that lives inside each and every human being. When one is aware of the spiritual energy inside and focuses on it daily, then that person knows and experiences the infinite energy of spirit whose nature is bliss. Unfortunately, most human beings have lost sight of this and consequently are suffering deep inside due to a lack of recognition of self-worth or self-esteem. This, in turn, causes physical or mental disease.

There are also genetic causes of disease that are not adequately addressed. Generally, this is rather a cross that the person must bear and balancing of the body, mind, and spirit, integration, still helps that person lead an enjoyable and valuable life. Imbalances can also come from excess or deficiencies of other things like too much work or not enough, too much exercise or not enough, too much sex (or not enough?), too much food or not enough. These are usually related to underlying emotional imbalances as well. Wholistic modes of therapy address either these external causes or the internal causes, or preferably both.

Once alternative health practices are well entrenched in medical training in medical colleges, their efficacy could be proved easily over a 5-year period by simply measuring monies spent on pharmaceuticals, as well as the quantities of pharmaceuticals used before, during, and after wholistic programs are introduced. This would also include measuring and comparing outpatient visits to doctors, visits to emergency rooms, hospital admissions, need for surgery, and some kind of standard for measuring quality of life. Some of these categories have already been proved in research studies done by Herbert Benson, MD,[86] noting the effect on patients using his relaxation response (a form of meditation) on a daily basis for 3 years.

HISTORY

Acupuncture as it is practiced in the United States is a huge conglomerate of different styles of acupuncture coming from China, Japan, Korea, Thailand, Vietnam, and western Europe. The styles differ radically depending on who is doing the acupuncture, where he or she learned it, and how much of their own individuality they have instilled into their practice. Within this discussion, the similarities between practices are described followed by an in-depth analysis of the style that I use.

Acupuncture is one of the five categories that makes up Chinese medicine. The other four are herbal medicine, diet and nutrition, exercise, and massage. Acupuncture is a healing method that tunes a human being. Just as a piano tuner tunes a piano or one tunes a guitar or an auto mechanic does a tune-up on your car, it is possible to tune a human being. After this process, or intervention, is done, the body-mind functions more efficiently in a balanced, harmonious fashion. As a result, the aches and pains often are eliminated and illnesses and diseases reversed. Acupuncture can be used by itself and, even better, in combination with other wholistic and traditional Western medical methods.

METHODS

Acupuncture involves the use of very tiny needles made of stainless steel, their diameter two or three times the width of a human hair, sharpened by a diamond. These needles are put into particular points on the surface of the body. There are at least a thousand of these points all over the human body. They have a lower electrical potential compared with the surrounding skin, as is evidenced by a galvanometer. These points are also known as acupuncture points, acupressure points, trigger points, and perhaps by other names as well. These points are about 1 mm in diameter and are located pretty much in the same place for everyone, according to bony landmarks, skin landmarks, anatomical structures such as nipples, umbilicus, fingernails and toenails, eyes, ears, nose and mouth, and so on. The points can be found easily by the trained finger. There are electrical instruments that can help locate these points but their reliability has not been established. Needles are put into these acupuncture points, and after being inserted, the needles are turned either clockwise or counterclockwise one revolution. They are either taken out immediately or left in for a period of time, depending on the individual patient's imbalance and illness.

EXAMINATION AND EVALUATION

Deciding where to insert the needles is really the key and the most difficult and important part of acupuncture diagnosis. This is where styles of acupuncture come into play. There is a spectrum of acupuncture styles or methods that ranges from completely symptomatic to perfectly wholistic, just as there is in traditional Western medicine. The symptomatic methods are simply putting needles into acupuncture points at anatomical sites that are specifically related to symptoms. For example, for shoulder pain, or arthritis or bursitis, an acupuncturist using a symptomatic method would select acupuncture points that are in or around the shoulder area. Headache would be treated with needles in the head area. Constipation would be treated with needles in the belly area. Hemorrhoids would be treated with needles around the anus and coccygeal area. This method pays little attention to where the constitutional imbalance exists within each person. An opposite philosophy, which is called wholistic acupuncture, treats the underlying constitutional imbalance within the person. Described earlier, these are considered the vulnerable, or weak, links in the chain in each human being, that part that always gives out first because it is not as strong or disease-resistant as the rest of the body-mind. The type of acupuncture I use is a wholistic form. Specifically, it is called five-element acupuncture. It is based on the Law of Five Elements, which is a law of nature that comes from Chinese philosophy and is one of the basic foundations of Chinese medicine. It is sometimes known as the Five Phases and is considered the most wholistic form of acupuncture available.

THE LAW OF FIVE ELEMENTS

The Law of Five Elements states that there are five elements in nature (fire, earth, metal, water, and wood) and that these elements all relate to one another in a very particular fashion (Fig. 33–4). The diagram in Figure 33–4 shows an outer creative cycle (known as Shen) that goes in a clockwise fashion and demonstrates that fire creates earth, earth creates metal, metal creates water, water creates wood, and wood creates fire again. Also, a star-shaped control, or destructive cycle (known as K'o) shows that fire destroys or controls metal, metal does the same to wood, wood to earth, earth to water, and water to fire. These two cycles, the creative and destructive cycles, are necessary to keep balance in nature. These five elements are also found in human beings because the body is composed of elements that come from nature and return to nature when the body dies. The emotions and feelings in our personality align themselves with these same elements (Fig. 33–5).

People in Western society have not been taught to think of their bodies in elemental forms but nevertheless these elements are there. The concept of fire is present in each and every cell. The cells burn glucose to survive and this is referred to as "burning calories." It is this burning that causes our body temperature to remain at 98.6° F throughout most of our lives. It is not difficult to picture each cell of the body having a little bonfire in the center with mitochondria sitting around roasting pieces of glucose on a stick. Obviously, water is present in our bodies. Students in grammar school are taught that our bodies are 98% water with all the tears and urine and lymph and blood. Similarly, metal can be found in the body in the form of calcium in the bones and iron in the

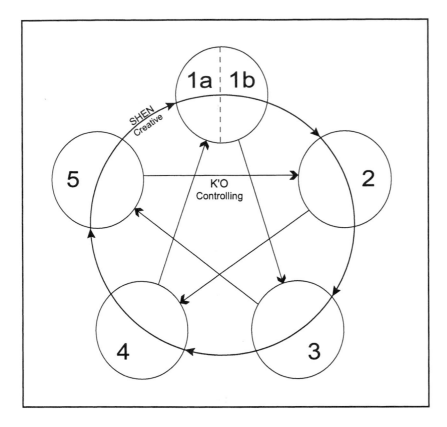

FIGURE 33–4. Law of five elements: Demonstrating the Shen (creative) and K'o (controlling) cycles.

blood, in our teeth, and so on. The concept of wood is most easily seen in the fingernails and toenails, which are similar to the bark of a tree. Also, the ligaments and tendons are much like a very strong fiber. The concept of earth is best seen in the gastrointestinal tract. Picture taking a microscopic journey down the gastrointestinal tract starting from the mouth, going down the esophagus into the stomach and the intestines; the further down you get, the more the material seems very earthlike, until it is excreted into the outside world.

Each of the elements has a particular color that emanates from the facies, a particular emotion that comes from the personality, a particular odor that comes from the body, and a particular sound that comes from the voice, as well as a particular taste, season, climate, secretion, and body part or system that it fortifies.

Every human being has a constitutional imbalance in one of these elements. The explanation for how this happens lies in spiritual law. Suffice it to say that this imbalance is well engrained some time during the first 5 years of life. Diagnosing this constitutional imbalance is both an art and a science and is done primarily by determining the color, emotion, odor, and sound belonging to each human being. The reader probably has noticed these colors, emotions, odors, and sounds previously with friends or even with strangers. Yet the realization that these are diagnostic clues that reveal a person's constitutional imbalance may not be as self-evident. The person who is always angry, no matter what, is displaying the emotion that goes with the wood element. The person who is always happy, joyful, bubbling over goes with the element of fire. The person who is always very sympa-

	1a	1b	2	3	4	5
Element	Fire		Earth	Metal	Water	Wood
Meridian	Small Intestine	Three Heater	Stomach	Colon	Bladder	Gall Bladder
Organ	Heart	Heart Protector	Spleen	Lung	Kidney	Liver
Color	Red		Yellow	White	Blue	Green
Emotion	Joy		Sympathy	Grief	Fear	Anger
Odor	Scorched		Fragrant	Rotten	Putrid	Rancid
Sound	Laughing		Singing	Weeping	Groaning	Shouting

FIGURE 33–5. Law of five elements linking fire, earth, metal, water, and wood with interlocking variables.

thetic and loves to take care of you or is always caring for children is displaying the emotion of sympathy and that goes with earth. The person who is always grieving, has tremendous loss in their life and can't seem to get over it, goes with the element of metal. And the person who is always fearful, paranoid, afraid of life fits into the water element. People have different sounds to their voice. People who laugh excessively and are always humorous go with the fire element. People who shout a lot, their voice being very powerful and strong, knocking you over, go with the wood element. People who have a singsong quality to their voice go with the earth element; groaning goes with the water element; and a weeping sound of the voice, even though the person is not crying, goes with the metal element. You have probably smelled people who have a strong body odor and wondered why they didn't bathe or use deodorant. There are five different odors and each one belongs to one of these elements. And perhaps you have seen a person who is green with envy or ash white, white as a sheet, or has pallor in the face. Each one of these colors goes with an element as described in the diagram (see Fig. 33–5).

Each element also has organs germane to it, with energetic pathways, called meridians, that are housed by that element. These pathways, or meridians, are just under the surface of the skin, throughout the body, and serve as channels for an electrical form of energy that flows in all human beings. This energy is the life force. In Chinese it is called chi. In the East Indian culture it is known as prana. This life force is always circulating round and round the body-mind along these pathways. And the acupuncturist can get in touch with this energy at certain points on these meridians, which are the acupuncture points.

INTERVENTION

Once the examination is complete and the diagnosis is made, with the elemental constitutional imbalance determined, it is simply a matter of treating the points along the meridians that are housed by that element on a week-to-week basis. Generally, this tunes the human being and everything starts to function more efficiently and more harmoniously, enhancing the person's quality of life.

There are 12 major meridians, two in each element, except for fire, which has four. Each of these meridians is named after the organ that it is connected to, which is also described in the diagram. Each meridian has from 9 to 67 points on it. Each point has a name described by the Chinese that has been translated into English. It is the names as well as the functions of the different points that allow the acupuncturist to decide which points are to be used on which day and time and treatment. Taking the history at each visit, as well as determining blockage of the chi energy flowing in the meridians, is used as well to select the points used in treatment.

As patients get better, not only do their symptoms decrease in intensity and dissolve and often totally disappear with time, their emotional and feeling state also changes for the better. People tend to become more happy and peaceful and calm, more able to handle stress. They often will say "I feel better in myself." The reason for this is that the patient is not just having his or her

symptoms treated. This form of acupuncture, the five-element style, treats the body, the mind, and the spirit and integrates these three spheres of the human being. The point names are particularly revealing. There are names connected to nature and physical objects such as "small sea," "greater mountain stream," "blazing valley," "sea of chi," and "skull breathing." There are also point names that have to do with emotions and feelings, like "palace of weariness," "gate of hope," "rushing the frontier gate," "intermediary," "little merchant," and "abdominal sorrow." And then there are the points that relate to the spiritual qualities of life, like "spirit burial ground," "heavenly ancestor," "heavenly pond," "heavenly window," "gate of destiny," "inner frontier gate," "soul door," and "spirit deficiency." When these spirit points are used, the person's spirit is buoyed up, turns back on.

Each treatment lasts 15 to 60 minutes depending on the individual practitioner. The practitioner can also include any of the following in the treatment sessions: conversation, history taking, massage, joint adjustments, instructions on diet and nutrition, psychosocial counseling, exercise recommendations, and so on. The initial visit takes longer because a history and physical examination are done and sometimes the initial treatment as well. This depends on the technique and abilities of the practitioner. Generally, the treatments are done twice a week for the first two to four visits and then once a week as the patient starts to get better. The interval continues to lengthen to every 2 to 4 weeks and, as the patient improves, the optimal interval is once every 3 months or once every season, the patient coming in for a tune-up for maintenance and prevention. Generally, a series of 10 treatments is a good way to start this type of therapy. Improvement in the patient's condition may be noticed as soon as the first treatment is done. It may take 5 or 10 treatments before it is noticed by the patient. Depending on the ability of the practitioner, improvement in the patient's condition generally occurs in 80% to 90% of patients. This, of course, is also dependent on the severity of the patient's imbalance and illness.

When acupuncture treatment is combined with psychosocial counseling, nutritional advice, exercise instruction, massage, or other forms of body work, in which the person is touched with warmth, peace, and love by another human being, great healing can take place.

BENEFITS OF INTERVENTION

Five-element acupuncture can be used for all sorts of clinical problems: physical, mental, emotional, and spiritual. Any and every type of person can and does respond. There are always exceptions to this but the general rule is one of success. This includes acute problems as well as chronic, outpatients as well as hospitalized patients. In China, all stroke victims are automatically treated with acupuncture as well as more traditional Western methods. It works on babies, toddlers, and adolescents as well as the elderly. It can be used as a primary form of therapy to which other therapies are added or it can be an adjunct to surgery, radiation, and medication, or to other wholistic therapies.

FUTURE TREATMENTS

The amount of time it takes for a person to heal depends on how long they've been ill. A rule of thumb is that for every year a person has had a particular physical or mental problem, it's going to take about a month's worth of treatment, with each session done weekly. So, if you've had arthritis for 20 years, expect 20 months of treatment.

On the other hand, if symptoms have been present for only a month or two, it is very possible that they could go away with one or two treatments unless it is some kind of serious illness, such as the sudden onset of cancer or heart disease or something that has been present for 1 or 2 years but has been subclinical. The general average is 10 treatments over a 4- to 8-week period, with a good possibility of illness being relieved partially or almost completely during that period, depending on the severity.

SUMMARY

In summary, acupuncture is a healing therapy that is both an art and a science, that comes from the Orient, specifically starting in China approximately 4,500 years ago. There are many styles of acupuncture, and the most wholistic style is known as five-element acupuncture. It truly helps to integrate the body, mind, and spirit. When combined with teaching the patient how to live a more healthy lifestyle, including diet, reducing stress, making healthy choices, thinking healthy thoughts, and including fun and relaxation, true healing can occur. Because of the chronic and degenerative nature of many illnesses in the United States, it is possible that total healing would not occur. Nevertheless, this type of therapy, along with the adjuncts mentioned earlier, should definitely help to create a more healthy human being.

Native American Healing

Richard V. Voss, DPC, MSW

Native Americans are understandably wary of the written word. Some may criticize the inclusion of this section in this chapter. This criticism is understandable, for often the written word objectifies understandings and can be manipulated outside of the relationship in which the understanding was shared. However, not to include a discussion of Native American views about medicine and health care is also a concern, because it perpetuates the invisibility of the Native American. The purpose here is to honor the continuing journey of understanding between medical science practitioners and traditional Native American medicine practitioners to see how these two medicine paths can help restore health to the people, and to bring about increased understanding—*wo 'wableza*—among peoples.

TRENDS IN CONTEMPORARY NATIVE AMERICAN HEALTH CARE

In a report to the National Institutes of Health, *Alternative Medicine: Expanding Medical Horizons*,[87] the Lakota (a Sioux people) were cited for the use of healing ceremonies by specialists who are essentially shamanic in their approach to treatment. In order to understand Native American medicine ways, one cannot rely solely on written accounts. While written ethnographical studies may provide a wealth of descriptive data, it is best to talk to authoritative sources personally. Professionals interested in learning more about traditional approaches to help and healing should contact any one of the federally recognized tribal headquarters and the tribally sponsored Native American colleges and universities for more specific information. Many colleges conduct summer courses on Lakota culture and philosophy that are open to non–Native Americans, as well as Native Americans, interested in learning their culture. This information may be found on the Internet under Tribal Colleges and federally recognized tribes.

Today, many of the old Native American healing traditions are experiencing a renaissance and are beginning to be viewed with a renewed sense of respect and credibility as an alternative and complement to more invasive or secular Western medical models of treatment.[87–90, 94, 95, 97] For example, on the Cheyenne reservation at Eagle Butte, Montana, the tribe approved alcohol treatment programs as well as delinquency prevention programs based on traditional methods and approaches to helping people with alcoholism, which is viewed as a problem with social, emotional, physical, and spiritual dimensions.[89, 90, 95, 97] These traditional methods include the *inipi*, or purification ceremony (popularly called the "sweat lodge"), the *hanblecaya*, or pipe fast (often called the "vision quest"), and the *wiwang wacipi*, or the Gazing at the Sun dance. The inclusion of these ceremonies within the treatment process has collectively been called the "Red Road approach."[89, 90, 97]

A number of medical facilities on various reservations include medicine men as consultants on a formal and informal basis,[91–93, 97] and the use of traditional ceremonies in health care settings is encouraged and respected.[93, 96] Where the ceremonial burning of sage (a common medicinal herb burned for purification) had been discouraged in the past, hospital staff report increased acceptance of this practice, and now arrange appropriate space for traditional ceremonial practices both within the health care facility and outside on hospital grounds.[93, 98] One Lakota friend commented on his recent hospitalization at an allopathic hospital. He was visited by a medicine man who placed a bundle of sage under his pillow. This made him feel better, and showed how simple cooperation among allopathic medicine, health care practices, and alternative, complementary health care practices can be.

A LAKOTACENTRIC PERSPECTIVE ON HEALTH

A traditional Native American perspective on health care and medicine begins with the spiritual reality of the human being who is part of all creation and dependent upon creation. Traditional understanding views human beings as intimately related to plants, and all other creations in the natural world that sustain life. Reality is not linear, it is circular. Everything is connected to everything else. Good and bad, sickness and health, doctor and patient are not separate processes, they are all related aspects and part of the whole. For the Lakotas and other traditional Native American peoples there is no split or dualism in reality or creation. This traditional view challenges the intervention model, and offers a prevention model as the starting place for social health and assistance. The emphasis from a Lakotacentric view is on building up the immune system and seeing the important role of the community in promoting good health care and well-being, a cultural emphasis often overlooked in conventional health care practices.

Traditional Lakota values of health and well-being emphasize the participation of the family in the healing process, including the extended family, as well as the larger kinship community, to bring about good health to the individual. The health of the individual is connected to the health of the community, so there is an important tribal dimension to this understanding. The help and healing process in not impersonal, but highly personalized and individualized around specific needs. The roles of medicine practitioners are multidimensional, and include those of healer, counselor, politician, and priest.

Another important contribution of the Native American perspective on health is that it provides a rich topology of spirit. The human creation, like all creations, is a spirit being composed of multilayered aspects of spirit. "Spirit" here is not some supernatural reality outside the human being, but an intrinsic dimension of everything that is, including the human creation (person). To speak of human beings is to speak of spiritual reality. Medical treatment or any kind of social, human, or mental health service is first and foremost a spiritual endeavor.

It is time for the diverse medical and health care disciplines to learn more about Native American ways of healing and health. The benefits of this cross-cultural collaboration affect not only Native American people but everyone in the larger culture as well who will benefit from greater access to a more wholistic health care model that recognizes the physiological and the spiritual causes of disease and sickness, as well as the efficacy of biological and spiritual remedies.

Allopathic Links to Models of Health Care Belief Systems

Electroacupuncture

Mary Lou Galantino, PhD, PT

Acupuncture, a part of traditional Chinese medicine (TCM), has been used for over 4,500 years. Mapping of 12 meridian points, which are named primarily after the visceral organs they traverse, incorporates 361 regular points. There are also "Ashi points," which are typically tender points that are used primarily for treatment of pain syndromes.[116] The acupuncturist must make a decision as to which acupuncture points to stimulate based on a specific diagnosis. The goal is to balance chi, which is considered vital energy. If there is an imbalance due to disease, the altered flow of chi can be detected and subsequently treated through needles or electrical stimulation over specific acupuncture points.

The use of acupuncture is growing in popularity in most Western countries,[113] and the effectiveness of electroacupuncture as a modality for the treatment of pain has been shown by significant decreases in visual analog scale scores.[110] The therapeutic effects of acupuncture have been the subject of several Chinese investigations for many years.[104, 108, 112] Western interest in acupuncture has generally been for the treatment of pain; with the increasing acceptance of acupuncture as an effective modality for pain relief, the scope of research on this modality has widened considerably to include other health conditions. The intensive research efforts on other therapeutic effects of acupuncture have produced encouraging results.[103, 111, 114] These results point to a reduction in pain and spasticity, improvement in motor function, better balance, and improved gait; the results therefore have a neurophysiological basis and should require a neurophysiological interpretation. Some of the possible mechanisms by which acupuncture may affect motor functions include the following:

1. A stimulation of the release of endogenous opioids.[107]
2. Changing the amplitude of end plate potential and thus facilitating events at the neuromuscular junctions. It has been suggested that peripheral factors contributing to the potentiation of a reflex (e.g., the H reflex) may affect the afferents and the neuromuscular junction.[105]
3. Stimulation of the sensory system will result in integrative actions at the spinal cord level where acupuncture may facilitate the stretch reflex arc through both the gamma and alpha motor neurons. Facilitation may depend upon the intensity and timing of the stimuli used to activate muscle afferents.[107]
4. Neuroimaging of acupuncture in patients with chronic pain reveals changes in cerebral blood flow associated with pain and acupuncture analgesia that correspond to areas of the brain involved in such phenomena.[99]

Training for acupuncture is varied throughout the United States. Because needling is considered an invasive technique, physical therapists are prohibited from using it. Therefore, an alternative to needle acupuncture is noninvasive electroacupuncture. Concerning the effects of electrical neurostimulation, there are various interpretations of the methodologies and underlying physiological mechanisms. One mechanism is neural.[110] Another study indicated that electrical stimulation applied to acupuncture points may activate neurological and endocrine functions that control pain.[100] Anderson and Lundeberg's study supported the release of beta-endorphin and oxytocin, which are important for the control of pain and the regulation of blood pressure and body temperature.[100]

My colleagues and I studied the effects of electroacupuncture on HIV-related neuropathy and found significant reduction in pain, which suggests an excitatory effect on the neuromuscular system. Such an effect may be on membrane potential (possibly through influencing ionic transport) and improvement in body fluid circulation.[106] The effect on the sympathetic system is often reported and more or less explained. The same explanation is proposed for the action of electrical stimulation on pain, with some effects on pain-mediating neurotransmitters at the level of the spinal cord and an endogenous modulation from the brain stem.[102]

Although there may be several mechanisms underlying the physiology of electroacupuncture, it would be prudent for physical therapists to consider maximizing the benefits of electrical modalities in various musculoskeletal and neurological disorders.[101] One prospective study[115] investigated the physiological effects of stimulation of ST36 and ST39 with Dynatron 200 microcurrent. Hemodynamic functions and skin temperature were monitored, with no significant differences found. However, further research is necessary to elucidate the nature of physiological effects of specific surface electrodes and various types of stimulation in order to determine efficacy of electroacupuncture treatment.

Biofeedback

Jennifer M. Bottomley, PhD, PT

The suggestion that hemiplegia, migraine and tension headaches, asthma, hypertension, cardiac arrhythmias, torticollis spasms, pain, hyperkinesis, and functional disorders of any of the body's systems may be relieved by a single form of treatment sounds more like a nineteenth-century pitch for snake oil than a true reflection of research. Yet biofeedback has been investigated extensively and has promising clinical applications in an astounding number of conditions.

The last two decades have seen an increasing convergence of body and mind therapies. These new therapies are often labeled *psychosomatic* or *psychophysical* medicine.[133] As both names imply, these approaches to healing deal with the effect of the mind on the body. With them, tremendous strides have been made in understanding mental influences on body systems ranging from the muscular to the immune system. This has led to treatment procedures that exploit this connection between mind and body. Biofeedback techniques for stress-related disorders and dysfunction and mental imaging using autogenic (a method of mind-over-body control based on a specific discipline for relaxing parts of the body by means of autosuggestion) feedback to enhance the responsiveness of the autonomic nervous system or the immune system response[138, 153] are two good examples of this process. Biofeedback is one of the earliest and most accepted ways that rehabilitation professions have employed that integrates rather than separates the mind and body.[164]

Biofeedback is a process of electronically utilizing information from the body to teach an individual to recognize what is going on inside of their own brain, nervous system, and muscles. Biofeedback refers to any technique, be it visual, auditory, or kinesthetic, that uses instrumentation to give a person immediate and continuing signals on changes in a bodily function that she or he is not usually conscious of, such as fluctuations in blood pressure, brain wave activity, or muscle tension. Theoretically, and very often in practice, information input enables the individual to learn to control the "involuntary" function.

Biofeedback acts as an output-input system whereby output is based in the motor unit and the input is via sensory pathways comprising proprioceptors, exteroceptors, and interoceptors.[164] Biofeedback provides a means of measurement of a physiological response using an electronic device. It aids the sensory side of a feedback mechanism assisting a compensated sensation, as with a cerebrovascular accident or other brain injury, in responding appropriately (i.e., motor unit training) by increasing conscious awareness of intact, but usually unfelt, sensation. Basically, biofeedback acts as a sixth sense by providing an artificial proprioception feedback. Via operant conditioning, a new association between a stimulus and a response is developed. The action the learner takes is voluntary and under their own control. The response is instrumental in producing a reward or removing a negative stimulus, and this reinforcement shapes behavior and function with successive stages.

Biofeedback transfers the responsibility for final success to the patient. Often, individuals seek medical help, hoping to place the responsibility of "curing" their problems on the clinician, while the patient takes an almost passive role in the treatment process. This is commonly known as an external locus of control. Patients should understand that they have the ability, with assistance from the appropriate medical professionals, to help themselves. Biofeedback provides a modality to accomplish this.

PRINCIPLES OF BIOFEEDBACK

The prefix *myo-* is derived from the Greek word for muscle. In combination with the Greek word *graphos*, to write, and the additional prefix, electro-, the word becomes *electromyograph* (EMG), an instrument for recording the electrical activity of the muscles. EMG biofeedback is a modality for measuring and displaying muscle activity, and is used primarily where any modification of muscular behavior is indicated. With its use, an individual can learn to become more aware of his or her own muscle activity, and thus gain more complete control of functional activity. It also provides an ideal method for rehabilitation practitioners to record a patient's day-to-day progress.

The biofeedback device imparts objective information about the degree of activity occurring in a muscle through surface electrodes, in audio, visual, or audiovisual form, in much the same way that an electrocardiogram provides information about cardiac activity or an electroencephaliogram displays brain wave activity. In an EMG biofeedback system, the electrical signal originating in the muscle under study is amplified and then translated into sound and visual readings, which correspond to increased and decreased muscle activity. EMG is the process of recording and interpreting the electrical activity of muscle. When a muscle contracts, it produces a characteristic spike (pulse) waveform that can be detected easily by placing an electrode on the skin over the muscle belly. For example, if you grasp an object tightly in your hand, the muscles in your arm will generate a specific electrical voltage, usually measured in millivolts or microvolts. As you squeeze the object tighter, the electrical voltage will increase as more motor units are recruited. As you relax your hand, the electrical voltage will decrease dramatically. EMG is, therefore, a direct physiological index of muscular activity and the state of relaxation.

The motor unit is a basic configuration of neuromuscular activity. It consists of a collection of muscle fibers controlled by a singe nerve fiber. When the nerve provides the "triggering" electrical impulse, the muscle fibers contract practically simultaneously. A motor unit may have only a few muscle fibers or thousands, and many motor units are needed to provide the mechanical force required to impart movement to the body.[164, 188] (See Chapter 28.)

Both surface and needle electrodes have been used in EMG. Although the voltage from a single muscle fiber can be monitored by the use of a fine-tipped needle electrode, surface electrodes are commonly used for biofeedback in the rehabilitation setting. The voltage picked up by the surface electrodes is actually an average of the many muscle fibers below and near the electrodes. Although muscle action potentials as picked up by the electrodes could possibly be as high as 1000 μV, values between 100 and 500 μV are more representative.[188]

The principle advantage of needle electrodes is their high sensitivity to individual motor unit potentials, usually without interference from nearby muscles.[164] Therefore, they are usually used for diagnostic purposes. However, because therapists normally use EMG biofeedback for muscle reeducation and relaxation purposes, surface electrodes have a number of advantages. For example, they eliminate the necessity of keeping all materials sterile and can be used easily at home by the patient.

EMG biofeedback has been reported as being a successful procedure for assisting the rehabilitation of patients with a wide variety of neuromuscular problems, providing muscle reeducation or muscle relaxation in conditions that may include the folllowing:

- Relaxation in spasmodic torticollis.[164]
- Migraine headache pain[119, 121, 135, 136, 143, 163, 176]
- Tension headache pain[119, 121, 135, 136, 143, 163, 176]
- Improvement of functional deficits in paraplegia and quadriplegia[144, 158]
- Improvement of postural instability, proprioception, and reduction in falls[140, 148, 158]
- Treatment of children with cerebral palsy for muscle reeducation and relaxation[161, 191]
- Cerebrovascular accident rehabilitation[141, 149, 150, 172, 177, 183, 190]
  - Footdrop and other gait problems
  - Posture and muscle tone improvement
  - Improved voluntary control of involved muscles
  - Muscle relaxation in associated reactions
  - Speech problems
- Muscular training after nerve, muscle, ligament, or tendon injury, repair, or transfers[162, 168, 184, 192]
  - Carpal tunnel syndrome
  - Rotator cuff and other shoulder pathologies
  - Lateral epicondylitis
  - Thoracic outlet syndrome
  - Patellofemoral pain
  - Achilles tendon repairs
- Early joint mobilization after surgery[162, 168, 184, 192]
  - Total joint replacements and other orthopedic surgeries
  - Reeducation of affected muscle following radical mastectomy
- Measurement of endurance with sustained activity[139, 147]
- Functional training and reduction of myoclonus following brain injury[129, 145]
- Control of urinary incontinence and other pelvic floor disorders°
- Relaxation for intractable constipation symptoms[118, 185]
- Respiratory control in asthma, emphysema, and chronic obstructive lung disease[120, 150, 160]
- Modification of hypertension[152, 187]
- Autogenic training of temperature control in diabetes,

vascular disease, and symptoms of intermittent claudication[169, 176]
- Parasympathetic control of cardiac arrhythmia[167]
- Stress management[123, 134, 146, 157, 175, 186]
- Intervention for dysphagia and other swallowing disorders[125, 182]
- Muscle reeducation following Bell palsy[173, 174]
- Pain management and reduction in chemotherapy-related symptoms in cancer patients°

CONCLUSION

As a literate civilization, we are now more than 5,000 years old. Physical needs have always kept the mind well occupied. Technologies have given us a modicum of control over our environment. Yet these technologies are costly. It is clear that medical problems can be caused or aggravated by the mental status of the individual. Western medicine has concentrated its efforts on developing extensive drugs and elaborate surgical techniques to deal with physical and mental compensations. With the evolution of managed care, the trend is now to seek less costly alternative care. This involves reaching inward and developing technologies that will allow us some insight into our inner world. It is time to balance the scales and attempt to solve some of the physical manifestations of pathologies from within.

Biofeedback has shown a remarkably positive benefit on the functional and treatment outcomes of numerous conditions.[127] Biofeedback instrumentation has been a growing part of physical therapy practice for over 20 years,[185] and physical therapists have contributed to researching its efficacy in treating various conditions. Sophisticated contemporary equipment does much more to quantify the worth of biofeedback techniques than was originally envisioned. The importance of relating quantified movement-based data to functional measures has influenced the level of appropriate reimbursement for physical therapy services utilizing biofeedback. Physical therapy, as a integral member of the medical community, needs to continue to investigate self-awareness and self-control as a probable rehabilitative tool in the treatment of a multitude of conditions.

Case Example of Integration of Various Approaches

Carol M. Davis, EdD, PT
Darcy A. Umphred, PhD, PT

The intervention with the following patient reflected awareness by the therapist of using myofascial release, CranioSacral Therapy, and Feldenkrais, as well as more traditional therapeutic interventions. The reader must remember that any one of the other approaches presented within this chapter might also have been implemented as part of this client's treatment given another therapist's experience, education, and therapeutic sensitivity, as well as the cultural biases of the client and her family. No judgment is being placed on the method or methods selected for this client or any other. What is critically important are the objective outcomes measures following the intervention.

°References 124, 137, 142, 151, 154, 155, 165, 166, 178, 180.

°References 117, 122, 126, 128, 130–132, 156, 171, 179, 181.

CASE 33–4 MRS. P.K.

Mrs. P.K., a 66-year-old woman, presented herself 2 years ago once she let her diagnosis of Parkinson's disease penetrate her consciousness. It was inconceivable to her that she might have the same illness that affected her grandmother and the same illness that the attorney general could not seem to mask in front of the public. As a seasoned lobbyist, she worked with politicians and traveled in powerful circles. Using her intellect and her considerable skill in negotiation, she successfully persuaded powerful people to see things her way for the benefit of her clients. Under no circumstances was anyone to know that she had Parkinson's disease, for she was short (5 feet tall), and weighed 105 lb, and she feared that her illness would be regarded as a weakness. Fortunately for her, her only symptom was a slight right upper extremity tremor on waking each morning, and some "stiffness," especially in flexion and extension of her right shoulder and extension of her right knee. This aspect of the case is critical. Her endless motivation to exercise was based on this fear of exposure, which she regarded, in spite of her therapist's attempts to work through this with her, as a death knell for her professional life.

Mrs. P.K. had exercised much of her life, and walked a mile on her treadmill each morning at 3.8 mph. Her husband was familiar with massage and Rolfing, and, at her request, he stretched her hips and lower extremities each day as prophylaxis against the return of a low back pain problem years earlier. Initial examination revealed the following deficits:

Active right shoulder flexion 130/170

Active right wrist flexion 45/85

Cervical rotation, right 60/80

Cervical rotation, left 45/80

Gait. Mrs. P.K. tended to walk with a narrow stance, heels close together, but with good heel strike. She was unable to ascend or descend stairs, looking straight ahead without severe slowing. She had very little head movement or thoracic rotation; her gait looked rather robotic.

Skin. There was slight edema on the right side of the face, with slight swelling of the upper right lip.

Posture. Mrs. P.K.'s pelvis was rotated down to the right, she had a slightly forward head, and although she did not have rounded shoulders per se, the fascia was drawn tight over her pectorals toward her sternum. The fascia of her legs was taut, and revealed a lack of tissue hydration.

Mrs. P.K. had no limitations in function. Her primary clinical goal was to prevent physical manifestations of the onset of the rigidity secondary to Parkinson's disease. If and when the disease itself

progressed, we reasoned that the more fluid her tissue was, and the more physically fit she was, the less the impact of a dopamine deficiency, and the more efficient her medication (selegiline) would be in controlling the progression of her symptoms. An intervention plan was developed that included a combination of traditional exercises for Parkinson's disease, complemented by myofascial release and CranioSacral Therapy, and Feldenkrais exercises to increase her awareness of her movement.

After receiving the referral from her neurologist, her treatments were scheduled for twice monthly, with home exercises. We explained how myofascial release "works" to keep the fascia loose, but how it seems to facilitate a sense of calm and peacefulness when done in conjunction with craniosacral rhythm was not known. Given the lack of basic science efficacy, she still willingly signed her informed consent. The plan of intervention integrated myofascial release techniques (along with Feldenkrais exercises) with her traditional therapeutic interventions focusing upon the impairments caused by Parkinson's disease. These exercises stressed active rotation, spinal segmental exercises, and controlled, active relaxation of the antagonists. Her prognosis was good, for she was beginning intervention in the very early stages of the disease, which would preclude secondary complications; she was fully functional and she was physically fit, if not well hydrated, and was very motivated. She was encouraged to drink more water.

Treatment began with several minutes bouncing on the Swiss ball, working on spinal segment articulation and spinal proprioception, and on lateral and backward balancing to relearn where her center of gravity was in her cone of stability. Next, with the assistance of the therapist, she moved to the bolster where she lay supine with knees flexed and worked on lower extremity extension and balance. On the mat she worked with Feldenkrais exercises and rotation of her shoulders and hips in opposite directions, with head rotation, and reviewed the pelvic exercises in her home program to help her differentiate her pelvis from her hips, and to keep her lumbosacral junction and sacroiliac joints mobile.

From there she moved to the plinth, where wedges were positioned to derotate her pelvis in the supine position. Myofascial treatment then began by gently palpating her cranial rhythm, asking her to relax, take three large breaths, and in her mind's eye, "go on vacation." This was very difficult for her, for her mind is very active, constantly thinking about work. As she relaxed, her breathing slowed, and her cranial rhythm became more pronounced. At this point the thoughts of the clinician

Continued

CASE 33–4   MRS. P.K. *Continued*

became very centered and progressed through various activities. First, there was focused intention and reflective thought that asked that energy from the clinician be used to bring about the highest good for the client. Conscious centering included taking deep breaths, and visualizing a grounding of the clinician and by seeing that energy flow went deep into the earth. Next, the clinician focused attention within the heart (heart chakra according to medical intuitives), and felt deep appreciation for the client, and for the opportunity to help her using wholistic techniques.

This exchange of healing energy was a very important moment for both client and clinician. It might be conjectured that the therapist consciously tapped into the universal healing energy that surrounds all of us at all times, and became a kind of transformer for that energy to be used to facilitate the flow of the client's own chi or healing energy that has been disrupted. No matter the verbal explanation used for this interaction, it created a strong bond of trust and respect that would continue to influence the outcome of the interventions.

The clinician continued treatment by moving into an occipital lobe release, followed by cranial releases and a sphenoid release, reasoning that this would assist the myofascia in the cranium to help ensure proper alignment of the cranial bones, and facilitate blood supply to and from the CNS. At this point in the treatment, the clinician would usually allow clinical perception or clinical intuition to guide decision making regarding the next movement. In reality, the therapist might just follow the guidance of the client's innate healing or centering aptitude. Occasionally, more time was spent on neck and upper thorax, with supine or side-lying scapular releases, and cervical spine work. Sometimes, after the wedges were removed and seeing that the symphysis pubis was in place, a leg pull or diaphragm release was done. If the clinician noticed tightness or imbalance, or if the client indicated that the "fascial voice" was speaking to her, for example, along her right rib cage as the leg pull was carried out, the clinician would follow the lead of what was happening in the body of the client disregarding any obvious symptoms that needed attention.

This concept is an important facet of myofascial release and many other complementary medical practices. Myofascial release would prescribe that, clinically, it is often shortsighted to go directly to the area of symptoms for treatment, for the problem is often caused by fascial restrictions distant from that area. Specifically, myofascial release as a type of complementary therapy seems to involve subtle or very low-intensity nonmaterial stimuli

known as "energy medicine." Although various explanations are offered for energy medicine in terms of a vital force or life energy, there is no agreed upon scientific understanding or precise meaning of these ideas in Western scientific concepts. Two proposed mechanisms for healer interventions are (1) that consciousness is causal, that is, the conscious intention of the healer through prayer or other means may physically improve the health and well-being of the patient, and (2), subtle energies may be exchanged or otherwise be involved, for instance, a condition of physical resonance between the energy fields of healer and patient, which may mediate the beneficial effects.

During the 2 years of Mrs. P.K.'s, treatment, she experienced a partial left rotator cuff tear and pain in the right fibular head area of her knee, both of which responded positively to myofascial release: cross-hands release work and soft tissue mobilization. Routinely, her right wrist was mobilized following an arm pull, and both scapulae were released in side lying following cross-hands release to the pectoral area.

On days when the pelvic area stiffness could not be relieved, 5 to 10 minutes of the myofascial release technique of rebounding was used, where her body and extremities were passively rocked back and forth. This helped the stiffness to release, after which Mrs. P.K. always remarked how much more "alive" her body felt. The treatment usually ended on the plinth with a side-lying dural tube release, helping her balance her energy gently.

Once the myofascial release and craniosacral work was completed, Mrs. P.K. might be asked to lie prone for further scapular extension exercise, or go onto all fours for "cat and camel" spinal mobility work, with wrist extension, along with partial push-ups to work on active elbow extension. From there she would go to the stairs where she practiced step-over-step maneuvers, forward and back and with "grapevine twists," working on fluidity of motion and on masking her tendency to keep her right fingers extended in a parkinsonian posture. A critical component of her intervention was working on her ability to trust herself without needing to watch her feet.

Her home program consisted of pelvic mobility exercises and opposite rotation of arms and legs with cervical rotation. Extra shoulder exercises were added for her rotator cuff injury, and passive lower extremity stretch over the side of the bed for iliotibial band release for her knee problem, along with fibular head mobilizations. She also lay supine on a 6-inch rubber ball, which she would roll segmentally up her spine to music to help with segmental mobilization. She then walked the treadmill for 1 mile.

Continued

CASE 33–4   MRS. P.K. *Continued*

The 3-month follow-up on impairment outcomes revealed the following:

Active right shoulder flexion 45/180

Active right wrist flexion 5/85

Cervical rotation, right 70/80

Cervical rotation, left 60/80

Gait. There was improved distance between heels. Stair agility was much improved, with ability to ascend and descend on most days looking straight ahead. Her braiding motion was smooth and continuous without needing to look at her feet. In Mrs. P.K.'s own words: "I feel stronger and more limber inside and outside. I feel I look better and function better."

Skin. The edema in the face was reduced and on most days is not noticeable at all.

The degenerative progression of Parkinson's disease varies with the individual, but Mrs. P.K. has been fortunate. With careful regulation of her med-

ication, her home program, and her twice-monthly therapy sessions, there has been extraordinary success in preventing any obvious signs of rigidity from becoming manifest, which was her goal and thus a primary target outcome for the clinician. No one knows how much of the relief of symptoms was due to her medication, although she was taking the medication for 3 months before she began therapy without showing the results achieved with therapeutic intervention. With this therapeutic intervention demonstrating effective outcomes, it could be argued by both clinician and client that myofascial release and CranioSacral Therapy helped keep the fascial system elongated and functioning in a self-corrective way. Similarly, integrating traditional personalized exercises with complementary interventions has enhanced the accomplishment of the client's goals for therapy and helped her to regain and maintain a higher quality of life.

The preceding case study was presented not to negate but rather to integrate traditional therapeutic interventions with complementary approaches. With limitations in health care benefits, frustration by the consumer regarding access to providers such as physical and occupational therapists, and many chronic problems remaining unanswered by allopathic medicine, many clients are looking elsewhere. When individuals no longer can look toward the Western medical system to regain or maintain health or healing, the only available options exist outside traditional Western medicine. As individual practitioners we can be part of that transition or be left behind with traditional Western medicine. It is interesting that branches of Western medicine are turning toward complementary philosophies and some medical schools are incorporating this training into student physicians' education. If physical and occupational therapy remain tethered to the portion of Western medicine that is linear, reductionistic, and focuses upon research that is univariable, not system interaction–based, then these two professions have the same potential future as traditional medicine. That future is not clear, but certainly traditional medicine is going to play a significantly reduced role in health care delivery. Our future in neurorehabilitation is up to the breadth and limitations of our leaders and to the willingness of our younger colleagues to follow or become leaders themselves. The future possibilities for both professions are enormous, not only in integrating complementary and alternative medicine into intervention of clients with chronic and degenerative illnesses, but also in acute care and in health and wellness maintenance. The answers to efficacy and functional outcome measurements will play a role in the future direction of competency-based interventions. Until the measurement tools are available to analyze the interactions of multivariables, clinicians are going to have to use objective outcomes

measures to determine whether the intervention should be stopped, continued, or altered. Selecting intervention strategies based on belief only without simultaneously measuring objective outcomes will always lead to questions regarding whether the intervention was worth the financial investment. The challenge will be to remain open and willing to discover new alternatives while keeping grounded in the ethical responsibility to establish efficacy for the practice of physical and occupational therapy.

CONCLUSION

Darcy A. Umphred, PhD, PT

Before anyone embraces any complementary approach, each clinician needs to identify which philosophy or paradigm matches his or her own belief system and emotional safety issues. Tethering an understanding of any approach to an established scientific base will allow clinicians to stretch beyond their respective comfort paradigm. When treating patients, clinicians are not recommended to jump from one theory to another or from one intervention strategy to another without analytically problem solving why those choices have been made. Therapists, during their professional education, are taught Western medicine, and the client and the variables that might influence that client are considered external to medical management (Fig. 33–6). Similarly, students are accepting that there is a transdisciplinary interaction between professional disciplines and that each profession not only uniquely affects the client but also has an interactive effect that is dependent upon other professions and their respective impact on the patient's health, wellness, and potential to attain a maximal quality of life (Fig. 33–7).

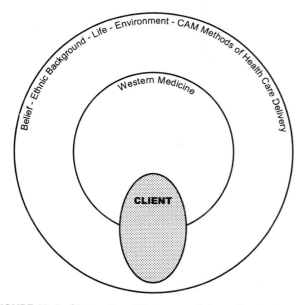

FIGURE 33–6. Client enters Western medicine owing to disease/pathology or disability/impairment.

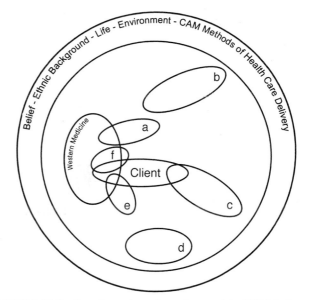

FIGURE 33–8. Complementary alternative models (CAMs) of health care delivery. a, Some CAMs interact with Western medicine: a, f, e; b, Some alternative models do not interact with Western medicine: b, c, d; c, Some alternative models meet needs of the client: c, e, f; d, Some alternative models do not meet the needs of the client: a, b, d.

When complementary and alternative approaches to health care are introduced into our model, then our colleagues need to determine which approaches interact with Western medicine and which do not (Fig. 33–8). Why one approach interacts with the patient and another does not is based upon the client's beliefs, needs, and responses to intervention. Because the professions of occupational and physical therapy have always been tethered to Western medicine, therapists need to critically analyze the interactions of those approaches that clearly overlap with our existing paradigm before we let go of the tether and venture totally into the unknown (Fig. 33–9). Those components of alternative approaches that obviously overlap with acceptable practice need to be identified and their efficacy established (Fig. 33–10). With

the establishment of those clear clinical correlations, the remaining components of identified alternative paradigms seem naturally to become part of the established delivery system. As a result, a new model for Western health care practice as identified by physical and occupational therapy is formed, which continues to allow the therapist to be

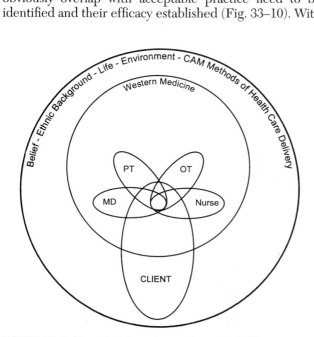

FIGURE 33–7. Transdisciplinary interactions within Western medical model.

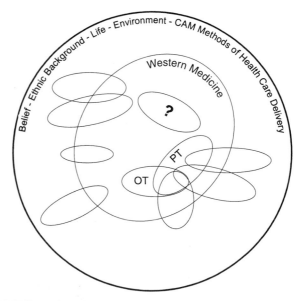

FIGURE 33–9. Complementary alternative models interacting with Western medicine. Some models interact to a large extent with Western medicine and some to a small extent. Some models interact with both Western medicine and other complementary models. The extent of complementary interactions with either physical or occupational therapy or both reflect which models fall within respective scopes of practice and thus become part of the professional's treatment tools.

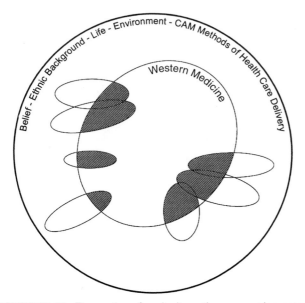

FIGURE 33–10. The portion of each alternative or complementary model that overlaps with allopathic medicine and traditional occupational and physical therapy has been the focus of this chapter. As efficacy is established for those components that interlock, therapists will more readily accept these approaches as part of their practice.

tethered while enlarging or stretching a professional comfort zone to encapsulate alternative models without feeling as if the grounded neuroscience background is jeopardized (Fig. 33–11). A clinician must always be cognizant of the fact that no matter what methods, philosophies, or interventions he or she selected to help a client reach a

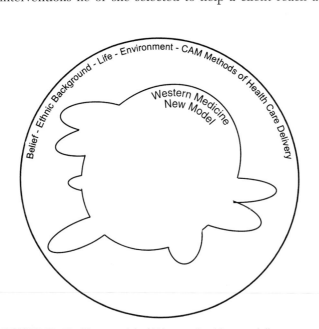

FIGURE 33–11. New model of Western health care delivery beyond complementary therapies. As the overlapping components of each alternative model are accepted as part of existing Western health care delivery practice, the barriers to the remaining aspects of these models become transparent. With barriers disappearing a new model with a different shape and different alternative becomes what will be known as traditional medicine in the future.

desired functional outcome, there is no way to eliminate the fact that other aspects of human system processing may also be active and affecting the outcome. For a century, master clinicians have been observed treating clients. Often colleagues comment that although those masters seem to use the same methods, they get very different outcomes. The question is: are those masters using other alternative interventions without those techniques ever being brought to consciousness? That is, if as a therapist I use myofascial techniques along with traditional intervention, am I also affecting craniosacral rhythm, or affecting chakras and energy fields and setting the stage for the nervous system to learn by narrowing the window and allowing it to select better options for motor responses? If so, what truly is leading to somatosensory retraining, motor learning, and neuroplasticity? It may be that master clinicians use *all* approaches but just verbalize the paradigm he or she is most comfortable with and capable of verbally explaining.

REFERENCES

Historical Perspective
1. Capra F, Steindl-Rast D: Belonging to the Universe. New York, HarperCollins, 1991, p xiii.
2. Colt GH: See me, feel me, touch me, heal me. Life, September 1996, p 36.
3. Dossey L: Time, Space, and Medicine. Boston, Shambala, 1982, p 12.
4. Foos F, Rothenberg K: The Second Medical Revolution, Boston, Shambala, 1987.
5. Jones J: Presented to the Feldenkrais Professional Training Program, Eugene, OR, June 16, 1995. Razummy D, Razummy E (eds), Berkeley, CA, Movement Studies Institute.
6. Kamm K, Thelen E, Jensen JL: A dynamical systems approach to motor development. Phys Ther 7:763–775, 1990.
7. Laszlo E: The Systems View of the World. Cresskill, NJ, Hampton Press, 1996, p 60.
8. Reynolds JP: Balance strategies: 2000 and beyond. PT Magazine June 1997, p 29.

Feldenkrais
9. Jackson-Wyatt O: Feldenkrais Method and rehabilitation: A paradigm shift incorporating a perception of learning. *In* Davis CM (ed): Complementary Therapies in Rehabilitation: Holistic Approaches for Prevention and Wellness. Thorofare, NJ, SLACK, 1997.
10. Stephens J. Cal S, Evans K, et al: Responses to ten Feldenkrais Awareness Through Movement lessons by four women with multiple sclerosis: Improved quality of life. Phys Ther Case Stud 2:62, 1999.

Suggested Readings
Feldenkrais M: Awareness Through Movement. San Francisco, Harper Collins, 1972.
Feldenkrais M: The Case of Nora. New York, Harper & Row, 1977.
Feldenkrais Guild: Questions regarding classes, Feldenkrais teachers in your location, cassette tapes of Awareness Through Movement lessons. 800-775-2118.
Shafarman S: Awareness Heals: The Feldenkrais Method for Dynamic Health. Reading, MA, Addison-Wesley, 1997.
Website: http://www.feldenkrais.com

Tai Chi
11. Blofeld J (transl and ed): I Ching: The Book of Change. New York, EP Dutton, 1965.
12. Brown DR, Wang Y, Ward A, et al: Chronic effects of exercise and exercise plus cognitive strategies. Med Sci Sports Exerc 27:765–775, 1995.
13. Da Liu: T'ai Chi Ch'uan and I Ching. New York, Harper & Row, 1987.

14. Da Liu: T'ai Chi Ch'uan and Meditation. New York, Schocken Books, 1991.
15. Fung Yu-lan: A History of Chinese Philosophy, vol 2. Princeton, NJ, Princeton University Press, 1953, pp 136–144.
16. Huai-chin Nan: Tao and Longevity. New York, Weiser, 1984, pp 8–12.
17. Jin P: Efficacy of T'ai Chi, brisk walking, meditation, and reading in reducing mental and emotional stress. J Psychosom Res 36:361–370, 1992.
18. Jou, Tsung Hwa: The Tao of T'ai Chi Chuan Way to Rejuvenation. Shapiro S(transl and ed). Warwick, NY, Tai Chi Foundation, 1988.
19. Judge JO, Lindsey C, Underwood M, Winsemius D: Balance improvements in older women: Effects of exercise training. Phys Ther 73:254–262 [discussion 263–265], 1993.
20. Kirsta A: The Book of Stress Survival: Identifying and Reducing Stress in Your Life. New York, Simon & Schuster, 1986.
21. Kronenberg F, Mallory B, Downey JA: Rehabilitation medicine and alternative therapies: New words, old practices. Arch Phys Med Rehabil 75:928–929. 1994.
22. Lai JS, Wong MK, Lan CL, et al: Cardiorespiratory responses of T'ai Chi Chuan practitioners and sedentary subjects during cycle ergometer. J Formos Med Assoc 92:894–899. 1993.
23. Lai JS, Lan C, Wong MK, Teng SH: Two-year trends in cardio-respiratory function among older T'ai Chi Chuan practitioners and sedentary subjects. J Am Geriatr Soc 43:1222–1227, 1995.
24. Legge J: The Texts of Taoism, vol. 1. New York, Dover, 1962, pp 256–257
25. Liao W: T'ai Chi Classics: New Translations of Three Essential Texts of T'ai Chi Chuan. Boston, Shambhala, 1990.
26. Lynoe N: Ethical and professional aspects of the practice of alternative medicine. Scand J Soc Med 20:217–225, 1992.
27. Ng RK: Cardiopulmonary exercise: A recently discovered secret of t'al chi. Hawaii Med J 51:216–217, 1992.
28. Province MA, Hadley EC, Hornbrook MC, et al: The effects of exercise on falls in elderly patients. A preplanned meta-analysis of the FICSIT Trials. Frailty and injuries: Cooperative studies of intervention techniques. JAMA 273:1341–1347, 1995.
29. Reynolds JP: Profiles in alternatives: East and West on the information superhighway: T'ai Chi. PT Magazine, September 1994, pp 52–53.
30. Sohn RC: Tao and T'ai Chi. Rochester, VT, Destiny Books, 1989.
31. Tse SK, Bailey DM: T'ai Chi and postural control in the well elderly. Am J Occup Ther 46:295–300, 1992.
32. Wanning T: Healing and the mind/body arts: Massage, acupuncture, yoga, t'ai chi, and Feldenkrais. AAOHN J 41:349–351, 1993.
33. Wardwell WI: Alternative medicine in the United States. Soc Sci Med 38:1061–1068, 1994.
34. Wolf SL, Kutner NG, Green RC, McNeely E: The Atlanta FICSIT study: Two exercise interventions to reduce frailty in elders. J Am Geriatr Soc 41:329–332, 1993.
35. Wolfson L, Whipple R, Judge J, et al: Training balance and strength in the elderly to improve function. J Am Geriatr Soc 41:341–343, 1993.

Taekwondo
36. Berger D: A mind/body approach. PT Magazine, September, 1994, pp 66–75.
37. Fosnaught M: The quest for wellness. PT Magazine, September 1994, pp 38–44.
38. Jackson WO: Not a hamster on a wheel: The Feldenkrais method. PT Magazine, September 1994, pp 58–65.
39. Kandel, ER, Schwartz JH, Jessel TM: Principles of Neural Science, 4th ed. New York, McGraw Hill, 2000.
40. Moyers B: Healing and the Mind. Garden City, NY, Doubleday, 1993.
41. Mueller, BM: Tae Kwon Do: A therapy adjunct. Clin Manage 11:64–66, 1991.
42. Postollec ML: Complementary movement therapies. Adv Phys Ther, August 1998, pp 8 to 10.
43. Reichley ML: What's a crane doing in PT? Adv Phys Ther, December 1993, pp 10–11.
44. Reynolds JP: Profiles in alternatives: East and West on the information superhighway. Tai Chi. PT Magazine, September 1994, pp 52–59.
45. Schmidt RA: Motor learning principles for physical therapy. In Lister MJ (ed): Contemporary Management of Motor Control Problems. Norman, OK, Foundation for Physical Therapy, 1990.

Suggested Readings
Hyams J: Zen in the Martial Arts. New York, Bantam Books, 1982.
Jampolsky G: The Tao of Healing. San Rafael, CA, New World Library, 1993.
Soho T: The Unfettered Mind. New York, Kodansha, 1986.
Soho T: The Martial Arts Explorer Manual. Nanuet, NY, Future Vision Multimedia, 1994.

Therapeutic Touch
46. Connell M, Meehan M: The effect of therapeutic touch on the experience of acute 1985 pain in post-operative patients. Dissertation Abstracts Int 46:795B, 1985 (University Microfilm No. DA8510765).
47. Gagne P, Toye RCA: The effects of therapeutic touch and relaxation therapy in reducing anxiety. Arch Psychiatr Nurs 8:184–189, 1994.
48. Gerber R: Vibrational Medicine. Santa Fe, NM, Bear, 1988.
49. Heidt P: Effect of therapeutic touch on the anxiety level of hospital patients. Nurs Res 30:57–66, 1991.
50. Keller E, Bzdek VM: Effects of therapeutic touch on tension headache pain. Nurs Res 35:101–106, 1986.
51. Krieger D: Healing by the "laying on" of hands as a facilitator of bioenergetic change: The response on in-vivo human hemoglobin. Psychoenergetic Syst 1:121–129, 1979.
52. Krieger, D: Therapeutic Touch: How to Use Your Hands to Help or to Heal. New York, Simon & Schuster, 1990.
53. Macrae J: Therapeutic Touch: A Practical Guide, 2nd ed. New York, Knopf, 1994.
54. Quinn JF: An Investigation of the Effects of Therapeutic Touch on Anxiety of Open Nursing Research. Grant No. R23 NU 01067, 1984.
55. Quinn JL: Therapeutic Touch Healing Through Human Energy Fields, videocassettes. New York, National League for Nursing, 1996.
56. Tiller WA: Explanation of electrodermal diagnostic and treatment instruments; pt 1. Electrical behavior of human skin. J Holistic Med 4:105–127, 1982.

Suggested Readings
Ayers LL: The Effect of Therapeutic Touch on the Relief of Pain as Reported by Cancer Patients Receiving Narcotic Agents, thesis. Richmond, VA, Virginia Commonwealth University, School of Nursing, 1983.
Blumberg, K: Therapeutic touch, promoting function, videocassette. University of Maryland at Baltimore, 1995.
Cotanch PH, Harrison M, Roberts J:. The use of therapeutic touch in the management of pain. In Adaptation to Chronic Illness. Philadelphia, WB Saunders, 1987.
Gehlhaart C: Therapeutic touch as adjuvant therapy for cancer pain management. Cancer Pain Update 35(summer):5–6, 1995.
Heidt P: Effect of therapeutic touch on anxiety level of hospitalized patients. Nurs Res 30:32–37, 1981.
Krieger D: Accepting Your Power to Heal. Santa Fe, NM, Bear, 1993.
Leller E, Bzdek B: Effects of therapeutic touch on tension headache pain. Nurs Res 35:101–105, 1986.
Meehan TC: Therapeutic touch—postoperative pain: A Rogerian research study. Nurs Sci Q 6:69–79, 1993.
Orlock C: The healing power of touch. Arthritis Today 8:34–37, 1994.
Wirth D: Effect of non-contact therapeutic touch on the healing rate of full thickness dermal wounds. Subtle Energy 1:1–24, 1992.

Medical Intuitive Diagnostics
57. Ackerman JM: The Biophysics of the VAS in Energy Fields of Medicine. Kalamazoo, MI, John A Fetzer Foundation, 1989, p 124.
58. Bailey AA: Esoteric Healing, vol 4. A Treatise on the Seven Rays. New York, Lucis, 1977.
59. Leadbetter CW: The Chakras. Wheaton, IL, Theosophical Publishing House, 1969.
60. Powell AE: The Etheric Double. London, Theosophical Publishing House, 1960.
61. Ritberger C: Your Personality, Your Health. Carlsbad, CA, Hay House, 1998.

62. Tiller W: Energy Fields in Medicine. Kalamazoo, MI, John A. Fetzer Foundation, 1989, p 257.
63. Tiller W: Science and Human Transformation. Walnut Creek, CA, Pavior, 1997.

CranioSacral Therapy
64. Gilmore NJ: Right brain, left brain asymmetry. ACLD Newsbriefs, July/August 1982.
65. Retzlaff EW, Roppel RM, Becker-Mitchell FL, Upledger JE: Craniosacral mechanisms. J Am Osteopath Assoc 76:288–289, 1976.
66. Retzlaff EW, Mitchell FL, Upledger JE, Biggert T: Nerve fibers and endings in cranial sutures. Research Report. J Am Osteopath Assoc 77:474–475, 1978.
67. Retzlaff EW, Upledger JE: Cranial suture pain. J Am Osteopath Assoc
68. Retzlaff EW, Vredevoogd J, Upledger JE: A proposed mechanism for drugless pain control. J Am Osteopath Assoc 1997.
69. Roppel RM, Upledger JE: Bioelectric phenomena in relation to neural function. J Am Osteopath Assoc 1976.
70. Upledger JE: Cranial therapy proves successful with some ADD children. Assoc for Retarded Citizens Advocates 1980.
71. Upledger JE: Craniosacral function in brain dysfunction. Osteopath Ann 11:318–324, 1983.
72. Upledger JE: Thermographic view of autism. Osteopath Ann 118:356–359, 1983.
73. Upledger JE: CranioSacral Therapy II. Seattle, Eastland Press, 1987.
74. Upledger JE: The therapeutic value of the craniosacral system. Massage Ther 1988.
75. Upledger JE: SomatoEmotional Release and Beyond. Palm Beach Gardens, FL, UI Publishing, 1990.
76. Upledger JE, Vredevoogd J: Therapy. Chicago, Eastland Press, 1983.
77. The Vietnam veteran's interview videotapes. Palm Beach Gardens, FL, Upledger Institute, 1993.

Myofascial Release (Barnes Method)
78. Barnes JF: Myofascial Release/The Search for Excellence. Paoli, PA, Rehabilitation Services, 1990.
79. Barnes JF: Myofascial release—The missing link in traditional treatment. In Davis C (ed): Complementary Therapies in Rehabilitation—Holistic Approaches for Preventions and Wellness. Thorofare, NJ, SLACK, 1997.
80. Hall D: The aging of connective tissue. Gerontology 13:77–89, 1968.
81. Rubik B: Energy medicine and the unifying concept of information. Altern Ther Health Med. 1:34–39, 1995.
82. Rubik B, Pavek R, Greene E, et al: Manual healing. In Swyers J, et al [11 member editorial board] (eds): Expanding Medical Horizons: Report to the NIH on Alternative Medicine. Washington, DC, US Government Printing Office, 1996.
83. Travell J: Myofascial Pain and Dysfunction. Baltimore, Williams & Wilkins, 1983.

Traditional Acupunture
84. Eisenberg D, et al:. Unconventional medicine in the United States. N Engl J Med 328:246–252, 1993.
85. Eisenberg D, et al: Trends in alternative medicine use in the United States: 1990–1997. JAMA, 28:1569–1575, 1998.
86. Benson H: Timeless Healing: The Power and Biology of Belief. Schriber, 1996.

Suggested Readings
Alavi A, LaRiccia PJ, Sadek AH, et al: Neuroimaging of acupuncture in patients with chronic pain. J Altern Complement Med 3(Suppl):47–53, 1997.
Ernst E, White AR: Acupuncture for back pain: A meta-analysis of randomized controlled trials. Arch Intern Med. 158:2235–2241, 1998.
Melzak R, Stillwell DM, Fox EJ: Trigger points and acupuncture points for pain: Correlations and implications. Pain 3:3–23, 1987.
NIH Consensus Development Panel on Acupuncture. JAMA 280:1518–1524, 1998.
Pomeranz B: Scientific basis of acupuncture. In Stux G, Pomeranz B (eds): Acupuncture: Textbook and Atlas. Berlin, Springer-Verlag, 1987.
Pomeranz B: Acupuncture research related to pain, drug addiction and
nerve regeneration. In: Pomeranz B, Stux G(eds): Scientific Basis of Acupuncture. Berlin, Springer-Verlag, 1989.

Native American Healing
87. Alternative Medicine: Expanding Medical Horizons. A Report to the National Institutes of Health on Alternative Medical Systems and Practices in the United States. Washington, DC, US Government Printing Office, 1992.
88. Babor TF: Alcohol treatment in American Indian populations: An indigenous treatment modality compared with traditional approaches. Ann N Y Acad Sci. 472:168–178, 1986.
89. Chante P: The Red Road to Sobriety, videotape. San Francisco, Kiraru Productions, 1995.
90. Chante P: The Red Road to Sobriety Video Talking Circle, videotape. San Francisco, Kiraru Productions, 1995.
91. Clifford M: Personal communication, June 10, 1997. Member of Pine Ridge Sioux Tribe, Rapid City, SD.
92. Douville V: Personal communication, June 12, 1997. Member of Rosebud Sioux Tribe, Sinte Gleska University, Mission, SD.
93. Erikson J: Personal communication, 1997. Intake Social Worker, Indian Health Services Hospital, Rosebud, SD.
94. Hall R: Distribution of the sweat lodge in alcohol treatment programs. Anthropology 26:134–135, 1985.
95. Red Dog L: Personal communication, June 24, 1997. Member of Cheyenne River Sioux Tribe, On the Tree, SD.
96. Richards M: Personal communication, June 16, 1997. Social Worker and Discharge Planner, Rapid City Regional Hospital, Rapid City, SD.
97. Thin Elk G: Appendix: Wounded Warriors: A Time for Healing. In The Red Road Approach. St. Paul, MN, Little Turtle Publications, 1995, pp 319–320.
98. DuBray W, Sanders A: Interactions between American Indian ethnicity and health cae. J Health Soc Policy 10:67–84, 1999.

Suggested Readings
Braswell M, Wong E, Wong HD: Perceptions of rehabilitation counselors regarding Native American healing practices. J Rehabil 60:33–43, 1994.
Means R, Wolf MJ: Where White Men Fear to Tread: The Autobiography of Russell Means. New York, St Martin's Press, 1995.

Electroacupuncture
99. Alavi A. LaRiccia PJ, Sadek AH, et al: Neuroimaging of acupuncture in patients with chronic pain. J Altern Complement Med 3:S47–S53, 1997.
100. Anderson S, Lundeberg T: Acupuncture—from empiricism to science: Functional background to acupuncture effects in pain and disease. Med Hypotheses 45:271–281, 1995.
101. Balogun JA, Biasci S, Han L: The effcts of acupuncture, electroneedling, and tanscutaneous electrical stimulation therapies on peripheral haemodynamic functioning. Disabil Rehabil 20:41–48, 1998.
102. Camels P: A scientific perspective on developing acupuncture as a complementary medicine. Disabil Rehabil. 21:1291–130, 1999.
103. Chen A: Effective acupuncture therapy for stroke and cerebrovascular diseases, pt 1. Am J of Acupunct 21:105–122, 1993.
104. Chen CH, Chou P, Hu HH, Tsuei J: Further analysis of a pilot study for planning an extensive clinical trial in traditional medicine–with an example of acupuncture treatment for stroke. Am J Chin Med 22:127–136, 1991.
105. Eke-Okoro ST: The H-reflex studied in the presence of alcohol, aspirin, caffeine, force and fatigue. Electromyogr Clin Neurophysiol 22:579–589, 1982.
106. Galantino ML, Eke-Okoro ST, Findley TW, Condoluci D: Use of noninvasive electroacupuncture for the treatment of HIV-related peripheral neuropathy: A pilot study. J Altern Complement Med 5:135–142, 1999.
107. Hans JS, Terenius L: Neurochemical basis of acupuncture analgesia. Annu Rev Pharmacol Toxicol 22:193–220, 1982.
108. Hu HH, Chung C, Liu et al: A randomized controlled trial on the treatment for acute partial ischemic stroke with acupuncture. Neuroepidemiology 12: 106–113, 1993.
109. Jankowska E, Perfilieva EU, Ridell JS: How effective is integration of information from muscle afferents in spinal pathways? Neuroreport 7:2337–2340, 1996.
110. Kumar A, Tandon OP, Bhattacharya A, et al: Somatosensory

evoked potential changes following electroacupuncture therapy in chronic pain patients. Anaesthesia 50:411–414, 1995.

111. Naeser MA, Alexander MP, Stiassy-Elder D, et al: Laser acupuncture in the treatment of paralysis in stroke patients: A CT scan lesion site study. Am J Acupunct 23:13–28, 1995.

112. Raoqi K: Treatment of apoplectic hemiplegia with scalp needling, using withdrawing-replenishing method plus physical exercise; A clinical observation. Int J Clin Acupunct 3:175–178, 1992.

113. Senior K: Acupuncture: Can it take pain away? Mol Med Today 2:150–153, 1996.

114. Shoukang L: Acupuncture therapy for apoplectic hemiplegia. Int J Acupunct 2:333–335, 1992.

115. Shrode LH: Treatment of facial muscles affected by Bell's palsy with high voltage electrical muscle stimulation. J Manipulative Physiol Ther 16:347–352, 1993.

116. Xinnong C (ed): Chinese Acupuncture and Moxibustion. Beijing, Foreign Languages Press, 1987, pp 439–441.

Biofeedback

117. Ahles TA: Psychological approaches to the management of cancer-related pain. Semin Oncol Nurs 1:141–146, 1985.

118. Anismus and biofeedback, editorial. Lancet 339:217–218, 1992.

119. Arena JG, Bruno GM, Hannah SL, Meador KJ: A comparison of frontal electromyographic biofeedback training, trapezius electromyographic biofeedback, and progressive muscle relaxation therapy in the treatment of tension headache. Headache 35:411–419, 1995.

120. Blanc-Gras N, Esteve F, Benchetrit G, Gallego J: Performance and learning during voluntary control of breath patterns. Biol Psychol 37:147–159, 1994.

121. Blanchard EB: Psychological treatment of benign headache disorders. J Consult Clin Psychol 60:537–551, 1992.

122. Blum RH: Hypothesis: A new basis for sentry-behavioral pretreatments to ameliorate radiation therapy-induced nausea and vomiting [review]. Cancer Treat Rev 15:211–227, 1988.

123. Blumenstein B, Breslav I, Bar Eli M, et al: Regulation of mental states and biofeedback techniques: Effects on breathing pattern. Biofeedback Self Regul 20: 169–183, 1995.

124. Brubaker L, Kotarinos R: Kegel or cut? Variations on his theme [review]. J Reprod Med 38:672–678, 1993.

125. Bryant M: Biofeedback in the treatment of a selected dysphagic patient. Dysphagia 6:140–144, 1991.

126. Burish TG, Jenkins RA: Effectiveness of biofeedback and relaxation training in reducing the side effects of cancer chemotherapy. Health Psychol 11:17–23, 1992.

127. Cassetta RA: Biofeedback can improve patient outcomes. Am Nurse 25:25–27, 1993.

128. Contanch PH: Relaxation techniques as an independent nursing intervention for oncology patients [review]. Cancer Nurs 10(Suppl 1):58–64, 1987.

129. Duckett S, Kramer T: Managing myoclonus secondary to anoxic encephalopathy through EMG biofeedback. Brain Inj 8:185–188, 1994.

130. Ferrell BR, Ferrell BA: Easing the pain. Geriatr Nurs 11:175–178, 1990.

131. Filshie J: The non-drug treatment of neuralgic and neuropathic pain of malignancy [review]. Cancer Surv 7:161–193, 1988.

132. Foley KM: The treatment of pain in the patient with cancer [review]. CA Cancer J Clin 36:194–215, 1986.

133. Ford CW: Where Healing Waters Meet. Tarrytown, NY, Station Hill Press, 1989.

134. Freedman RR, Keegan D, Rodriguez J, Galloway MP: Plasma catecholamine levels during temperature biofeedback training in normal subjects. Biofeedback Self Regul 18:107–114, 1993.

135. Grazzi L, Bussone G: Effect of biofeedback treatment on sympathetic function in common migraine and tension-type headache. Cephalalgia 13:197–200, 1993.

136. Grazzi L. Bussone G: Italian experience of electromyographic-biofeedback treatment of episodic common migraine: Preliminary results. Headache 33:439–441, 1993.

137. Glazer HI, Rodke G, Sencionis C, et al: Treatment of vulvar vestibulitis syndrome with electromyographic biofeedback of pelvic floor musculature. J Reprod Med 40:283–290, 1995.

138. Gruber BL, Hersh SP, Hall NR, et al: Immunological responses of breast cancer patients to behavioral interventions. Biofeedback Self Regul 18:1–22, 1993.

139. Hatfield BD, Spalding TW, Mahon AD, et al: The effect of psychological strategies upon cardiorespiratory and muscular activity during treadmill running. Med Sci Sports Exerc 24:218–225, 1992.

140. Hawken MB, Jantti P, Waterston JA: The effect of sway feedback and loss of sensory cues in older women with a history of falls. In Woollacott MH, Horak F (eds): Posture and Gait-Control Mechanisms, vol 2. Eugene, OR, University of Oregon Books, 1992, pp 263–266.

141. Howard S. Varley R: Using electropalatography to treat severe apraxia of speech. Eur Disord Commun. 30:246–255, 1995.

142. Jones KR: Ambulatory bio-feedback for stress incontinence exercise regimes: A novel development of the perineometer. J Adv Nurs 19:509–512, 1994.

143. King TI: The use of electomyographic biofeedback in treating patients with tension headaches. Am J Occup Ther 46:839–842, 1992.

144. Klose KJ, Needham BM, Schmidt D, et al: An assessment of the contribution of electromyographic biofeedback as an adjunct in the physical training of spinal cord injured persons. Arch Phys Med Rehabil 74:453–456, 1993.

145. Kwolek A. Pop T: Use of biological vicarious biofeedback in the rehabilitation of patients with brain damage (in Polish). Neurol Neurochir Pol 1(Suppl):321–327, 1992.

146. Lehrer PM, Carr P, Sargunaraj D, Woolfolk RL: Stress management techniques: Are they all equivalent, or do they have specific effects? Biofeedback Self Regul 19:353–401, 1994.

147. Leisman G, Zenhausern R, Ferentz A, et al: Electromyographic effects of fatigue and task repetition on the validity of estimates of strong and weak muscles in applied kinesiological muscle-testing procedures. Percept Mot Skills 80(3 pt 1):963–977, 1995.

148. Leonhardt C: Posture biofeedback for improved sitting (in German). Fortschr Med 110:33–34, 1992.

140. Leplow B, Schluter V, Ferstl R. A new procedure for assessment of proprioception. Percept Mot Skills 74:91–98, 1992.

150. Mass R, Dahme B, Richter R: Clinical evaluation of respiratory resistance biofeedback training. Biofeedback Self Regul 18:211–223, 1993.

151. McCandless S, Mason G: Physical therapy as an effective change agent in the treatment of patients with urinary incontinence [review]. J Miss State Med Assoc 36:271–274, 1995.

152. McGrady A: Effects of group relaxation training and thermal biofeedback on blood pressure and related physiological and psychological variables in essential hypertension. Biofeedback Self Regul 19:51–66, 1994.

153. McGrady A, Conran P, Dickey D, et al: The effects of biofeedback-assisted relaxation on cell-mediated immunity, cortisol, and white blood cell count in healthy adult subjects. J Behav Med 15:343–354, 1952.

154. McIntosh LJ, Frahm JD, Mallett VT, Richardson DA: Pelvic floor rehabilitation in the treatment of incontinence. J Reprod Med 38:662–666, 1993.

155. Milam DF, Franke JJ: Prevention and treatment of incontinence after radical prostatectomy [review]. Semin Urol Oncol 13:224–237, 1995.

156. Moher D, Arthur AZ, Pater JL: Anticipatory nausea and/or vomiting [review]. Cancer Treat Rev 11:257–264, 1984.

157. Montgomery GT: Slowed respiration training. Biofeedback Self Regul 19:211–225, 1994.

158. Moore S, Woollacott MH: The use of biofeedback devices to improve postural stability. Phys Ther Pract 2:1–19, 1993.

159. Moreland J, Thomson MA: Efficacy of electromyographic biofeedback compared with conventional physical therapy for upper-extremity function in patients following stroke: A research overview and meta-analysis. Phys Ther 74:534–547, 1994.

160. Nahmias J, Tansey M, Karetzky MS: Asthmatic extrathoracic upper airway obstruction: Laryngeal dyskinesis. N J Med 91:616–620, 1994.

161. Nashner LM, Shumway-Cook A, Marin O: Stance posture control in select groups of children with cerebral palsy—Deficits in sensory organization and muscular coordination. Exp Brain Res 49:393–409, 1983.

162. Palmerund G, Kadefors R, Sporrong H, et al: Voluntary redistribution of muscle activity in human shoulder muscles. Ergonomics 38:806–815, 1995.

163. Penzien DB, Holroyd KA: Psychosocial interventions in the man-

agement of recurrent headache disorders: Description of treatment techniques. Behav Med 20:64–73, 1994

164. Peper E (ed): Mind/Body Integration: Essential Readings in Biofeedback New York, Plenum, 1979.

165. Phillips HC, Fenster HN, Samson D: An effective treatment for functional urinary incoordination. J Behav Med 15:45–63, 1992.

166. Rayome RG, Johnson V, Gray M: Stress urinary incontinence after radical prostatectomy, J Wound Ostomy Continence Nurs 21:264–269, 1994.

167. Reyes del Paso GA, Godoy J, Vila J: Self-regulation of respiratory sinus arrhythmia. Biofeedback Self Regul 17:261–275, 1992.

168. Reynolds C: Electromyographic biofeedback evaluation of a computer keyboard operator with cumulative trauma disorder. J Hand Ther 7:25–27, 1994.

169. Rice BI, Schindler JV: Effect of thermal biofeedback-assisted relaxation training on blood circulation in the lower extremities of a population with diabetes. Diabetes Care 15:853–858, 1992.

170. Saunders JT, Cox DJ, Teastes CD, Pohl SL: Thermal biofeedback in the treatment of intermittent claudication in diabetes: A case study. Biofeedback Self Regul 19:337–345, 1994.

171. Schafer DW: The management of pain in the cancer patient. Compr Ther 10:41–45, 1984.

172. Schleenbaker RE, Mainous AG III: Electromyographic biofeedback for neuromuscular re-education in the hemiplegic stroke patient: A meta-analysis. Arch Phys Med Rehabil. 74:1301–1304, 1993.

173. Segal B, Hunter T, Danys I, et al: Minimizing synkinesis during rehabilitation of the paralyzed face: Preliminary assessment of a new small-movement therapy. J Otolaryngol 24:149–153, 1995.

174. Segal B, Zompa I, Danys I, et al: Symmetry and synkinesis during rehabilitation of unilateral facial paralysis. J Otolaryngol 24:143–148, 1995.

175. Shahidi S, Salmon P: Contingent and non-contingent biofeedback training for Type A and B healthy adults: Can Type A's relax by competing? J Psychosom Res. 36:477–483, 1992.

176. Sheffied MM: Psychosocial interventions in the management of recurrent headache disorders: Policy considerations for implementation. Behav Med 20:73–77, 1994.

177. Shumway-Cook A, Anson D, Haller S: Postural sway biofeedback—Its effect on reestablishing stance stability in hemiplegic patients. Arch Phys Med Rehabil 69:395–400, 1988.

178. Smith DA, Newman DK: Basic elements of biofeedback therapy for pelvic muscle rehabilitation. Urol Nurs 14:130–135. 1994.

179. Steggles S, Fehr R, Aucoin P, Stan HJ: Relaxation, biofeedback training and cancer: An annotated bibliography, 1960–1985. Hospice J 3:1–10, 1987.

180. Stein M, Discippio W, Davia M, Taub H: Biofeedback for the treatment of stress and urge incontinence. J Urol 153(3 pt 1):641–643, 1995.

181. Stoudemire A, Cotanch P, Laszlo J: Recent advances in the pharmacologic and behavioral management of chemotherapy-induced emesis [review]. Arch Intern Med 144:1029–1033, 1984.

182. Sukthankar SM, Reddy NP, Canilang EP, et al: Design and development of probable biofeedback systems for use in oral dysphagia rehabilitation. Med Eng Phys 16:430–435, 1994.

183. Sunderland A, Tinson DJ, Bradley EL, et al: Enhanced physical therapy improved recovery of arm function after stroke. A randomized controlled trial. J Neurol Neurosurg Psychiatry 55:530–535, 1992.

184. Thomas RE, Vaidya SC, Herrick RT, Congleton JJ: The effects of biofeedback on carpal tunnel syndrome. Ergonomics 36:353–361, 1993.

185. Turnbull GK, Ritvo PG: Anal sphincter biofeedback relaxation treatment for women with intractable constipation symptoms. Dis Colon Rectum 35:530–536, 1993.

186. Van Zak DB: Biofeedback treatments for premenstrual affective syndromes. Int J Psychosom 41:53–60, 1994.

187. Vasilevskii NN, Sidorov YA, Kiselev IM: Biofeedback control of systemic arterial pressure. Neurosci Behav Physiol 22:219–223, 1992.

188. Wirth DP, Barrett MJ: Complementary healing therapies. Int J Psychosom 41:61–67, 1994.

189. Wolf SL: The relationship of technology assessment and utilization. Electromyographic feedback instrumentation as a model. Int J Technol Assess Health Care 8:102–108, 1992.

190. Wolf SL, Binder-MacLeod SA: Electromyographic biofeedback applications to the hemiplegic patient. Phys Ther 63:1404–1413, 1983.

191. Woolridge CP, Russell G: Head position training with the cerebral palsied child.—An application of biofeedback techniques. Arch Phys Med Rehabil 57:407–414, 1976.

192. Young MS: Electromyographic biofeedback use in the treatment of voluntary posterior dislocation of the shoulder: A case study. J Orthop Sports Phys Ther 20:171–175, 1994.

CHAPTER 1

1. Contrast the medical and wholistic models of health care delivery.

2. Identify approaches that you take to care for your client that you or a therapist did not use 5 years ago.

3. Do those approaches fall into the definition of wholistic care? Cite evidence that they are making a difference in the outcome of your process.

4. Analyze the DEP method of documentation and identify its strengths and weaknesses.

5. Describe what evidence-based practice means and why it is relevant to the evolution of the health care community.

6. What is the difference between a diagnosis by a physician and those made by physical and occupational therapists?

7. Why does a therapist need to understand his or her preferential learning style and how that will affect the client's performance?

8. Identify the three basic central nervous system components within a client profile. Discuss how this type of information could aid the therapist in understanding the total client.

CHAPTER 2

1. Using the information collected during the history and physical examination (including tests and measures), the therapist in Differential Diagnosis Phase 1 may:
   a. Diagnose the patient as having Parkinson's disease.
   b. Communicate with a physician to report concerns about a patient's health status.
   c. Determine whether the patient is suffering from delirium or depression.
   d. Diagnose the patient as having a specific impairment and resulting disability.

2. Using the information collected during the history and physical examination (including tests and measures), the therapist in Differential Diagnosis Phase 2 may:
   a. Diagnose the patient as having Parkinson's disease.
   b. Communicate with a physician to report concerns about a patient's health status.
   c. Determine whether the patient is suffering from delirium or depression.
   d. Diagnose the patient as having a specific impairment and resulting disability.

3. Which of the following items carries the greatest weight as a risk factor for the presence of occult disease?
   a. A previous personal history of having the disease
   b. Age of the patient
   c. A second cousin having a positive history for the disease
   d. A sedentary lifestyle

4. Screening the integumentary system should take place for which of the following scenarios?

   a. The patient complains of paresthesia of both hands.
   b. The patient reports a history of falling down.
   c. This system is screened in all patients.
   d. This system is screened only if the patient has not been examined by a physician.

5. The pulmonary system should be screened if the patient complains of pain in
   a. The facial area.
   b. The thoracolumbar junction.
   c. The groin area.
   d. Multiple peripheral joints.

CHAPTER 3

1. Differentiate between the term *impairment* and the term *disability*.

2. Determine whether the following items are impairments (I) or disabilities (D).
   _____ Decreased muscle strength in the hip and knee
   _____ Absent touch and proprioceptive sensations from the foot to the knee
   _____ Decreased range of motion in the right shoulder
   _____ Hypertonicity within the extensor muscle groups in the lower extremities
   _____ Fascial tightness in the low back region
   _____ Volitional or reflexive synergies
   _____ Inability to transfer from bed to wheelchair without assistance
   _____ Inability to ambulate independently

3. Discuss some considerations when choosing the most appropriate functional test for a patient or client.

4. Name the factors to consider in choosing the appropriate examination tool.

5. Discuss how a clinical decision-making matrix may be utilized to link impairments and disabilities to interventions.

CHAPTER 4

1. Discuss two variables that relate to motor learning that are controlled by systems other than motor and two that are motor-specific.

2. What is the most important variable for neuroplasticity?
   a. The intact somatosensory lobe
   b. An attended, goal-directed activity
   c. The client's willingness to be a passive participant
   d. Third-party payers' willingness to accept experimental treatment

3. Describe the differences among somatosensory retraining, functional retraining, and augmented intervention strategies.

4. What are coincident-based connections, and why are they relevant for somatosensory retraining?

5. Cortical neuronal plasticity in children is represented by
   a. Top to bottom level of control.
   b. Progressive, multiple-staged skill learning.
   c. The rate of conduction of sensory input.
   d. Automatic progressive stages of development.

6. Functional training is
   a. The best way to intervene with clients who have CNS deficits.
   b. An intervention that focuses on correction of impairments.
   c. An intervention that utilizes repetitive practice of functional tasks.
   d. Training that does not worry about what the client cannot do.

7. Critical pathways
   a. Are the most direct way to get a patient to an outcome.
   b. Are established to direct the practitioner and will lead to maximal independence for the patient.
   c. Work well with all clients for whom pathways have been established.
   d. Work best for predictable diseases, diagnoses, and surgical procedures.

8. When analyzing augmented input, a sensory classification schema helps the learner differentiate types of extrinsic feedback. Pick one sensory system and two interventions and discuss how they will optimally facilitate or inhibit learning.

9. Why is it important for a clinician to understand the autonomic nervous system?

10. If a client lacks the ability to hold up his or her head, why might you start treatment in a vertical position? Why might vertical kneeling be more effective than vertical sitting?

CHAPTER 5

1. Why are there many models for motor control?

2. Differentiate between sensation and perception?

3. Why should therapists use an evaluative model to assess parameters such as timing, force production, and sequencing rather than spasticity, rigidity, and the like.

4. Why are the concepts of degrees of freedom and synergies important?

5. Differentiate loss of balance due to volitional sway, unexpected perturbation, and interaction with the environment.

6. Can all balance reactions be classified as an ankle strategy or a hip strategy?

7. When assessing clients for motor control problems, what parameters need to be considered?

CHAPTER 6

1. What are the four basic functions of the limbic system?

2. Discuss why the limbic system might be considered a second motor system.

3. Why is the F²ARV continuum considered to be the same continuum that triggers abusive behavior?

4. Why would understanding the general adaptation syndrome be important for therapists who work with patients who have CNS deficits?

5. Anger can be identified with specific motor responses. A clinician would not expect to see
   a. A client having an easier time coming out of standing.
   b. A client having a difficult time returning to sitting from standing.
   c. A client having difficulty reaching into the closet.
   d. A client having difficulty holding up his or her head.

6. Describe your interpretation of intuition.

7. How might spirituality or the belief that one will get better affect the outcome of interventions?

CHAPTER 7

1. Describe the difference between impairment and disability.

2. Is adaptation and adjustment a flexible and flowing process?

3. Describe five elements of the grief process that deal with age, cognition, and developmental level.

4. Describe five aspects of sensuality and sexuality, and explain how they could affect treatment.

5. Describe five ways that you would integrate the family of the client and the client's styles of coping into therapeutic treatment.

6. Describe how the elements of problem solving, loss, cognitive functioning, coping, sensuality, and significant others' coping and learning styles can be worked into the treatment process to encourage adaptation.

CHAPTER 8

1. Discuss the neuropathological and clinical differences between a brain injury occurring during the late second or early third trimester of pregnancy (i.e., 24 to 32 weeks' gestational age) and an injury occurring at term. Include the following:
   a. Common or likely mechanisms of brain injury
   b. Location of brain damage
   c. Type of brain damage (e.g., hemorrhage, infarction, ischemia)
   d. Evidence of brain injury seen by imaging (ultrasound, CT scan, or MRI)
   e. Clinical consequences

2. Describe characteristic differences between the neuromotor function of full term infants and preterm infants (at age corrected for prematurity) during the first year of life.

3. You are a therapist working in a high-risk infant follow-up clinic. You are assessing a 4-month-old infant (corrected age if born prematurely). You observe that when the baby is in prone position, that is, on her tummy, she has difficulty raising her head and pushing up onto her elbows. Provide **three** possible hypothetical reasons for this delay. For **each** hypothesis describe:
   a. The presumed reason for the delay. Include a likely medical/environmental history for the child.
   b. What you would do during your evaluation process to confirm or disprove this hypothesis as a probable explanation for the motor delay. In other words, what findings

from the child's history or from your examination would confirm or contradict this hypothesis.

   c. What intervention or course of action you would recommend.

4. You are a physical therapist working in a high-risk infant follow-up clinic. You are assessing a full term 4-month-old infant whose mother used cocaine, alcohol, and tobacco during the pregnancy. The baby's mother had no prenatal care until the sixth month of pregnancy, at which time she entered a residential drug treatment program. She is currently living independently with ongoing surveillance by child protective services. The mother says that she thinks her baby is developing appropriately, except that sometimes he is "shaky or jittery." Her primary concern is that she has heard that "crack babies have lots of problems," and she asks you, "What will be his long-term outcome?" In your assessment you observe that the baby's gross motor milestones are appropriate for his age but he shows some tremulousness in his arms and he is immature in his reaching and fine motor skills. Answer the following:

   a. What type of intervention would you recommend for this baby (e.g., home program, individual therapy, comprehensive developmental program)?

   b. What specific activities would you suggest that his mother either do or not do?

   c. How would you respond to this mother's questions regarding developmental expectations for her baby:
     (1) Short term (i.e., next 6 to 8 months)?
     (2) Long term (preschool, school age)?

   d. Outline an appropriate follow-up program for this child over the next 6 years. Include discussion of the concerns and potential "red flags" that should be addressed on follow-up.

5. Identify the structural and physiological factors that predispose preterm infants to cardiopulmonary instability and musculoskeletal risk during examination and intervention by the neonatal therapist. Describe experience and precepted training components for preparing the neonatal therapist to avoid inadvertent risk or harm to neonates who have been unstable physiologically.

6. Why is the NICU an inappropriate practice environment for student therapists, therapist assistants, therapy aides, and therapists with general practice backgrounds?

7. What theoretical frameworks and models guide neonatal therapy practice?

8. Describe a typical caseload of newborn infants referred for neonatal therapy services. What examination and intervention options are available? What postural, movement, and functional impairments of infants would the neonatal therapist be likely to analyze and incorporate into care plans with the neonatal nurse?

9. How does the neonatal therapist support parents and families in the NICU? What unique stresses are parents experiencing in the NICU that may reduce their effectiveness and energy in participating in developmental or other physical therapy activities?

CHAPTER 9

1. Why is early intervention important with children who have received the diagnosis of cerebral palsy?

2. Discuss the parameters of the diagnosis of cerebral palsy.

3. Discuss the differences among hypotonicity, athetosis,

ataxia, and spasticity as they relate to the diagnosis of cerebral palsy.

4. Discuss the role of the therapist in both direct and indirect intervention.

5. Discuss when special equipment should be recommended and when it should not.

CHAPTER 10

1. Genetic disorders can be subdivided into four major categories. Which of the following are major categories: (1) chromosome disorders, (2) single gene disorders, (3) autosomal dominant disorders, and (4) mitochondrial disorders.

2. Cystic fibrosis is a sex-linked inherited disorder.
   True   False

3. The genetic defect in trisomy 21, Down syndrome, includes partial deletion of chromosome 21.
   True   False

4. Identify the three modes of inheritance for single gene disorders.

5. Describe the intended purpose of each of the following assessments used in program planning for children with genetic disorders: (1) Peabody Developmental Motor Scales (PDMS), (2) Movement Assessment of Infants (MAI), and (3) School Function Assessment (SFA).

6. Discuss the role of the therapist in providing family-centered goals or objectives.

7. Identify three medical treatments that may used for children with genetic disorders to ameliorate the effects of the disorder.

8. What is a pedigree?

CHAPTER 11

1. When evaluating the individual with learning disabilities, what are the five dimensions of disablement that may affect performance?

2. Identify several reasons why it is more difficult to recognize nonverbal learning disabilities than verbal impairments in children.

3. Considering the diversity of clinical profiles in individuals with learning disabilities, what might you identify as the cause or causes of the difficulties? How can we develop greater knowledge in this area?

4. What are some of the possible ramifications to the belief that children with motor coordination deficits will outgrow their motor problems?

5. To compile a complete picture of motor functioning in the child with learning disabilities and coordination disorders, what areas should be assessed?

6. Discuss the important factors to consider when determining whether a child receives intervention and what model of intervention is chosen.

7. How can the therapist provide the best intervention for a child with learning disabilities and motor deficits?

CHAPTER 12

1. Describe the changes that occur at the mechanical interface with intraneural and extraneural movements.

2. Describe the changes in length and tension that occur in a nerve with intraneural and extraneural movements.

3. Describe the theoretical basis for the development of a "double crush" injury.

4. Describe the theoretical basis for the development of neurovascular entrapment.

5. Describe the adaptive responses to pathological pain.

6. Describe how to assess for the presence of neural irritability and sensitivity.

CHAPTER 13

ALS

1. Massive loss of anterior horn cells of the spinal cord and the motor cranial nerve nuclei in the lower brain stem results in _____ and _____ (amyotrophic). Demyelination and gliosis of the corticospinal tracts and corticobulbar tracts caused by degeneration of the Betz cells in the motor cortex result in _____ (lateral sclerosis).

2. The etiology of ALS is unknown; however, numerous theories have been proposed. Increased lead and aluminum levels, viral influences, and abnormalities in concentration in calcium and magnesium levels have been suggested, and more recently, _____.

3. Although the atrophy and weakness component of ALS is most obvious, 80% or more of patients show early clinical evidence of _____.

4. The pattern of ALS onset is highly varied, with several patterns identified by primary area of onset. The most typical patterns of presentation are (give 3): _____.

5. Despite the pattern of onset, the eventual course of the illness is similar in most patients with _____. Death is usually related to _____.

6. When determining therapeutic goals and treatment, one must consider the _____.

7. What are the appropriate goals for therapeutic interventions at the end of phase I (Independent), during phase II (Partially Independent), and during phase III (Dependent)?

8. When planning an exercise program for a patient with ALS, you must consider two important factors: _____ and _____.

9. Disuse atrophy contributes to the patient's level of functional loss and disability because _____.

10. Kilmer and Aitkens defined seven exercise prescription recommendations for patients with ALS. List at least six.

11. Review Figure 13–3: Exercise window for normal and damaged muscles. If you exercised a person with ALS in the "plateau range" for a person with normal muscles, your patient would be exercising in the _____ range for someone with an impaired muscle.

12. Your patient is a 54-year-old computer analyst working at home. He is walking about the house but uses a wheelchair outside the home. He is independent in eating but needs assistance with hygiene and dressing. He is in stage II: Partially Independent. Plan a treatment program for him. Before his illness, he was an active golfer and gardener.

13. Although it is important for a caregiver to give a patient the opportunity to talk about dying and to feel comfortable with the topic, each patient's personal style in talking about death _____.

14. Therapists must also consider caregiver issues. As a physical or occupational therapist, what factors should you consider?

Guillain-Barré Syndrome

15. GBS in both children and adults is characterized by a rapidly evolving, relatively symmetrical _____.

16. Motor impairment may vary from mild weakness of distal lower extremity musculature to _____.

17. ANS symptoms are noted in about 50% of patients. Typical ANS symptoms are (identify 5).

18. Your patient is recovering from GBS and had total paralysis of swallowing and oral-motor functions. Basic treatment goals are the prevention of choking and aspiration and the stimulation of effective swallowing and eating. You are a rural-based therapist. Briefly describe your treatment interventions.

19. Your patient has been totally paralyzed for 14 days. On day 3 the physician orders "stretching exercises." You talk with the physician and recommend splinting. What does the research show about splinting versus stretching?

20. Soryal and others hypothesized a number of possible mechanisms for the limitations in range of motion found in patients with GBS. Identify at least three.

21. In patients with GBS, use of heat before range of motion exercises might be contraindicated. Why?

22. The most important concept to remember in designing an exercise program for a patient with GBS is _____.

23. The major goal of therapeutic management of a patient with GBS is _____.

24. The rule in developing an exercise program for patients with GBS is _____.

25. The safe exercise range differs for normal and impaired muscle, with the therapeutic window being _____ for muscles undergoing reinnervation.

26. Bensmen recommended that once the patient has stabilized, active exercise may begin as follows: _____.

27. The major warning about exercise for a patient with GBS is _____.

28. The diagnostic criteria for GBS are _____.

Muscular Dystrophy

29. The abnormal gene for DMD has been detected on the X chromosome at band Xp21 encodes for _____, a 427-kD cytoskeleton protein in the membrane.

30. Because it has an X-linked, recessive pattern, the disease affects _____ almost exclusively.

31. Laboratory studies show serum _____ is elevated more than 100 times what is normal in early stages of the disease. Muscle biopsies show _____.

32. The most common cause of death in persons with DMD is _____; death occurs most commonly between the ages of _____ and _____.

33. Although the relationship between lower IQ and DMD was initially thought to be related to limited life experience caused by the disease, recent studies have shown that dystrophin _____.

34. The earliest obvious manifestations of DMD may be _____.

35. The typical progression of weakness is (also note which muscles and functions are usually spared) _____.

36. A typical child with DMD will continue walking until about age _____, at which time use of a wheelchair becomes imperative. A rapid decrease in strength may occur after _____.

37. A distinctive feature of DMD is the _____ in which the child gets up from the floor by _____.

38. Muscle imbalance occurs in typical patterns secondary to weakness and contractures. Describe the patterns.

39. The typical changes in gait pattern over time are identified in Figure 13–7. Many factors influence how long a child will be able to ambulate. Contributing factors are _____.

40. Although no cure for DMD looms in the immediate future, researchers have most recently _____.

41. With increasing weakness of the respiratory musculature and the development of scoliosis, physical therapy interventions, such as _____ and _____, are invaluable in preventing early death from respiratory failure.

42. Scoliosis tends to occur in two basic patterns. Describe them.

43. Orthopedists responsible for spinal fixation surgery to stabilize the development of a scoliosis suggest that a forced vital capacity (FVC) be _____ % of normal before surgery can be performed.

44. Orthopedists must attend to how the spine is positioned with fixation. If the curve cannot be completely corrected, the curves should be balanced to create a _____ pelvis.

45. Typical therapy goals for the child with DMD are _____.

46. Preliminary evidence suggests that respiratory endurance can be improved in children with DMD. Although respiratory exercise cannot reverse the process of respiratory failure, attention to pulmonary hygiene and breathing exercise can _____.

47. The development of contractures can decrease the length of time a child with DMD can ambulate. What measures can a therapist take to prevent or minimize contractures?

48. In general, research suggests that exercise consisting of brief periods of low- or high-intensity activity can improve strength for patients with _____. However, exercise programs have no effect on strength of muscles already _____.

49. A safe indicator of extent and intensity of exercise is that the patient should _____.

50. When contractures at the hip, knee, and ankle show evidence of interfering with the child's ability to stabilize each joint during stance, most children are referred for surgery to restore functional joint motion. Surgeries typically include subcutaneous releases of the Achilles tendons and hamstring muscles and fasciotomies of the iliotibial bands. Surgeons recommend that surgery be followed by intensive physical therapy. Describe a postsurgical physical therapy program for an 11-year-old boy.

51. For the child with DMD and his or her family, transition times are often accompanied by _____.

52. In all three conditions—ALS, GBS, and DMD—the therapist is challenged to design a therapy program that will provide the patient with the impetus to become or remain as active as possible without _____.

53. In some patients with ALS and DMD, intermittent positive pressure ventilation (IPPV) by nasal mask has been effective in controlling oxygen desaturation at night. Nighttime mechanical ventilatory support seems to provide relief for symptoms such as _____.

54. In patients with ALS and DMD, external ventilation support is used initially at night, then intermittently throughout the day until respiratory support is required at all times. What factors must be considered when making a decision to use HMV?

CHAPTER 14

1. List three prognostic indicators for a good outcome after coma.

2. What is the average age and sex of the brain-injured individual?

3. What is the most common cause of brain injury?

4. What is meant by *diffuse axonal shearing*?

5. List two ways that vegetative state is different from coma.

6. Discuss the types of amnesia seen after TBI.

7. Explain how a client who fails memory tests such as the Mini-Mental State Examination might demonstrate memory formation.

8. Explain the consequences of low blood pressure in the client with increased intracranial pressure.

9. List three medications that assist with normalizing increased intracranial pressure, and discuss the mechanisms by which they work.

10. List three problems that result in poorer outcome from brain injury.

11. Discuss the factors that result in a better life satisfaction score post discharge for brain-injured clients.

12. Discuss Beinstein's theory of movement.

13. By what method does the brain handle the many degrees of freedom available at joints?

14. Why is hand control different from other movements?

15. Describe and discuss similarities between anticipatory and adaptive responses.

16. Describe and discuss support for interventions by the therapist to make permanent changes in motor behavior.

17. Discuss the Rancho Los Amigos Hospital scale of cognitive function.

18. Explain the "executive functions."

19. Discuss the appropriate types of feedback for clients who are functioning at higher levels and those for clients who are functioning at lower levels.

20. Discuss how you would determine a subtask component of a task. Give an example.

21. Explain on a neurophysiological level how skills are acquired.

22. Match the following examinations with the function that they test:

WAIS _____   a. Declarative memory
GOAT _____   b. ADL
Naming tests _____   c. Upper extremity function
FIM _____   d. Aphasia
FAM _____   e. Lower extremity function
Nine hole peg test _____   f. Cognitive function
Frenchy arm test _____

23. Discuss how the same disability with the same therapeutic intervention may or may not have the same outcome.

24. How is treatment different for two clients with the same impairment, one of whom is unable to make changes in the impairment whereas the second one is?

25. Discuss the pros and cons of treating "spasticity."

26. Discuss how sensory losses may affect gait or hand function.

27. Describe what movement might look like in a client who is lacking synergistic organization for function.

28. How might a client be encouraged to develop adaptability in his or her responses? Give examples.

29. Why is strength important in clients with neurological deficits?

30. Discuss intervention strategies for a client who cannot sit up secondary to poor postural control and poor head control. List examinations that you might use for this client.

CHAPTER 15

1. Why are children with spina bifida prone to fractures? What can be done to aid in prevention of fractures in these children?

2. What is the cause of reflexive movements in the lower extremities in a child with spina bifida? What is the importance of recognizing reflexive movements?

3. What is the major physical therapy goal for stage II: after surgery, during hospitalization?

4. What is necessary for the development of sitting balance, and why is sitting balance so important for the child in the infant-to-toddler stage (stage III)?

5. When should a standing device be introduced to the child with spina bifida?

6. Except for the child with a very low level lesion, children must master what skills in standing before ambulation?

7. During what stages is skin injury more of a problem? Why?

8. What are some reasons why an adolescent might stop walking?

9. What factors are involved in the lack of progress in the area of sexual function and reproductive issues for the child with MM?

10. What do we know about the sexual abilities of the female with spina bifida?

CHAPTER 16

1. Matching the following clinical syndromes with their characteristics:
   a. Brown-Séquard syndrome
   b. Cauda equina syndrome
   c. Central cord syndrome
   d. Posterior cord syndrome
   e. Anterior spinal artery syndrome
   _____ Results from compression by tumor or infarction of the posterior spinal artery
   _____ Causes bleeding into the central gray matter of the spinal cord; results in more impairment of function in the upper extremities than in the lower
   _____ Motor function and pain and temperature sensation lost bilaterally below the lesion; prognosis poor for return of bowel and bladder function, ambulation, and hand function
   _____ Results in flaccid paralysis with no spinal reflex activity present
   _____ Characterized by ipsilateral loss of motor function and position sense and contralateral loss of pain sensation several levels below the lesion; good prognosis for recovery

2. Discuss which pharmacological agent lessens secondary injuries to surrounding tissues.

3. List some factors that are included in goal setting as they may limit functional outcomes.

4. Identify the basic goals for seating the patient with SCI.

5. List at least five basic seating concepts of proper postural alignment for the patient with SCI.

6. What is the most reasonable explanation for why a person with a complete spinal cord injury at the T12–L1 level would choose to discard lower extremity orthoses?

7. The most common and potentially life-threatening secondary complication associated with SCI is_____.

8. Serial casting contraindications include:
   a. Skin compromise/edema
   b. Heterotropic ossification
   c. Fluctuating tone
   d. Inconsistent monitoring systems
   e. a and b
   f. All of the above

9. To ensure an effective bowel program, the following should be considered:
   a. The bowel program can be done any time of day.
   b. Follow a diet high in fiber.
   c. Drink a cold drink 30 minutes before beginning the program.
   d. Perform the program in an upright position as opposed to lying in bed.
   e. b and d.

CHAPTER 17

1. What is the most common category of organisms causing meningitis? encephalitis? Can other categories of organisms be responsible for these diagnoses?

2. Explain the mechanism underlying the development of increased intracranial pressure in bacterial meningitis.

3. What is nuchal rigidity? Describe the clinical tests to determine the presence of nuchal rigidity.

4. Describe the syndrome of symptoms that are typically present in viral encephalitis.

5. Explain the following statement: Procedural learning can occur even though declarative learning processes are damaged.

6. Explain the purposes of conducting peripheral sensory tests.

7. Discuss the process of assessing an individual's ability to learn movement tasks.

8. What is the rationale for incorporating activities requiring reversal of movements into the intervention sequence?

9. Generate an example of how the therapist could construct the intervention program to incorporate problem solving by the patient.

CHAPTER 18

1. In 1993, the Centers for Disease Control and Prevention revised its definition of AIDS. What three clinical conditions were added to the list of AIDS-defining diseases?

2. What is the difference between cell-mediated and humoral immunity?

3. What are the psychoneuroimmunological changes that can occur with exercise?

4. What does the combination of the diagnostic tests Viral Load and CD4 count provide for clinical management?

5. What constitutes the wasting syndrome?

6. All systems of the body are affected by HIV. From a cardiopulmonary perspective, we have recently witnessed the complications of lipodystrophy. What are the clinical signs and symptoms of this side effect?

7. What treatments have been effective for HIV-related peripheral neuropathy?

8. There are many neuropsychiatric findings in HIV. What is most common?

CHAPTER 19

1. The primary impairments associated with postpolio syndrome are:

2. What are the primary musculoskeletal goals for intervention?

3. Identify an intervention procedure and discuss what precautions regarding overuse and fatigue of muscles would be counterproductive with an individual who has postpolio syndrome.

4. Discuss adaptive equipment that should be considered in clients with PPS.

5. Discuss the psychosocial considerations of clients with PPS and the ways their learned behaviors regarding exercise may hinder their potential quality of life.

CHAPTER 20

1. What is the target of the immune system attack in MS?

2. What are the most common symptoms of MS?

3. Describe the four possible courses of MS.

4. What is the MSQLI? Describe its component sections.

5. List strategies for managing tremor in MS.

6. Describe strategies to address cognitive deficits found in MS.

7. List several work accommodations that might be helpful for employment retention for MS patients.

CHAPTER 21

1. What is the relationship among the center of gravity (COG), the base of support (BOS), and the limits of stability (LOS) in standing?
   a. Which balance tests challenge voluntary COG control?
   b. Which of these—COG, BOS, LOS—can be manipulated to make balance exercises more difficult?
   c. How does the relationship among COG, BOS, and LOS change during locomotion?

2. List the four main components of the dynamic equilibrium model.
   a. Choose three common neurological diagnoses, and use the model to describe common impairments that might affect postural control in each one.
   b. How does this model reflect the interaction among the individual, the task, and the environment?
   c. List two tests associated with each main component that might be part of a comprehensive balance evaluation.

3. What are the two primary reflexes subserving postural control?
   a. What stimulus triggers each reflex?
   b. What symptoms accompany deficits in each of these two reflex pathways?
   c. Which balance tests determine whether these reflex pathways are intact?

4. What are the six sensory conditions in the Sensory Organization Test (SOT) and its clinical counterpart, the Clinical Test for Sensory Interaction on Balance (CTSIB)?
   a. In which conditions would a client who is *visually dependent* for balance have the most difficulty?
   b. Your client does very well in conditions 1 through 4 but falls on every trial of conditions 5 and 6. What problem do you suspect?
   c. Your client does fine in the eyes-closed conditions but not in the conditions with eyes open in a sway-referenced visual surround (or dome). Which processes may be deficient?

5. Draw the vestibular receptor (end organ) and the pathways connecting it to the central nervous system.
   a. Differentiate the function of the otoliths versus the semicircular canals.
   b. What complaints are most common with otolith lesions and which with semicircular canal lesions?
   c. Would a client with complete bilateral vestibular loss

complain more of dizziness or gaze stabilization problems? Why?

6. What is "BPV"?
   a. Which semicircular canal is most often implicated in BPV?
   b. What is the definitive test for BPV?
   c. Describe the most effective intervention for BPV.

7. What are automatic postural responses?
   a. List the four commonly identified strategies.
   b. Describe one "high-tech" and one "low-tech" balance test to identify automatic postural response deficits.
   c. How would you help your client progress from voluntary performance of these strategies to their automatic use?

8. What possible interventions could you use to address the following problems:
   a. A client who has difficulty maintaining balance when rising from or descending to a chair?
   b. A client who holds the head and trunk rigid while walking, and turns "en bloc"?
   c. A client who can go up and down a curb quickly and easily with a handrail but is fearful of doing so without the manual contact?

CHAPTER 22

1. Relate the electrophysiological studies of the basal ganglia to the function(s) of the basal ganglia in motor control.

2. Relate these functions to the symptoms seen in basal ganglia disease.

3. Relate these functions to treatment ideas for the person with Parkinson's disease; with dystonia.

4. Why is it important that the therapist be familiar with the possible surgeries for those with basal ganglia disease and intervene early after surgery?

5. Why are breathing exercises crucial in intervention for basal ganglia disease, especially Parkinson's disease?

6. Why is there such emphasis on Parkinson's disease in this chapter?

7. Discuss the role of assistive devices for those with basal ganglia disease.

8. Name the other professionals who would be involved in a comprehensive program for the person with basal ganglia disease.

CHAPTER 23

1. Contrast the treatment plan, inclusive of goal setting, for a 44-year-old woman with a meningioma and a 52-year-old man with a recurrent frontal glioblastoma.

2. Describe some physical, cognitive, and emotional factors that might preclude completion of a planned therapy session. Recommend modifications that will accommodate these factors.

3. What are some signs and symptoms that may indicate a decline in the client's status? Discuss the possible causes for these changes and outline appropriate referral recommendations.

4. Using the principles of the motor learning theory, describe a skill to be learned and specific intervention techniques to facilitate learning.

5. How can a clinician provide psychosocial support to a client with a brain tumor? What kind of relationship is necessary and how can this be established?

CHAPTER 24

1. Relate the anatomical and physiological studies of the cerebellum to the function(s) of the cerebellum in motor control.

2. Relate these functions to the symptoms seen in cerebellar disease.

3. Relate these functions to treatment ideas for the person with cerebellar disease.

4. Explain the cause of hypotonia in a patient with cerebellar disease.

5. Define asthenia and distinguish it from hypotonicity and from the fatigue seen in patients with Parkinson's disease or multiple sclerosis.

6. Describe the examination for the disruption in the direction, extent, force, and timing of movement characteristic of cerebellar disease.

CHAPTER 25

1. Name three clinical features for each of the three types of neurovascular disease: thrombosis, embolus, and hemorrhage.

2. Describe the mechanism and effects of botulinum toxin injections on spastic muscles.

3. As an acute care therapist you are caring for a 60-year-old man who had a stroke resulting in a left hemiplegia. You have treated him for 5 days and are writing a note supporting your belief that he is a candidate for inpatient rehabilitation. State what is important to include in this note: recovery of motor function, predictors of recovery, severity of primary impairments, presence or absence of secondary impairments.

4. List four categories of primary impairments and four categories of secondary impairments for clients with a hemiplegia from stroke.

5. In the past decade therapists have shifted their philosophical understanding of intervention strategies for stroke from a neurophysiological basis to a motor control and learning basis. This has led to a change in language when describing movement problems; low tone/high tone, spastic/flaccid are no longer sufficient or desirable. Using the definitions from the impairment schema, describe two or three possible patterns of atypical movement in clients with hemiplegia.

6. Describe three situations in which "tone" increases (spasticity/hypertonicity) in the arm or leg. Describe the focus of therapeutic intervention for each situation.

7. Loss of control and/or weakness in the trunk often results in atypical alignment of the spine, ribcage, and pelvis. Describe three common trunk alignment patterns for clients with hemiplegia. Refer to one of these patterns with a photograph (figure) from the chapter.

8. Working in an outpatient setting, you have a client with right hemiplegia, with complaints of shoulder pain during range-of-motion exercises, an inferior subluxation, and the ability to move the shoulder, elbow, and wrist through 1/3

range in sitting. The client wears a Rolyan Hemi Arm sling. Describe your thought process as you solve the following problem: the type of shoulder pain, the relationship of an inferior subluxation to pain and to a range-of-motion home exercise program, and the advisability of sling usage at this point in the intervention process.

9. You are the therapy representative for an outpatient brace clinic. Describe your choice of foot orthosis and your rationale for the following clients:
   a. Client with a left hemiplegia and severe trunk and leg weakness; cannot stand independently, cannot move the leg against gravity in standing or in sitting. Goal: ambulation with assistive device and contact guarding.
   b. Client with a right hemiplegia with severe foot posturing during swing and stance. Client has a prefabricated posterior leaf spring brace and walks with a quad cane. During swing, the right foot supinates out of the brace; foot contact is on the outside border of the foot. During stance, the right knee hyperextends and the foot pronates onto the medial aspect of the plastic brace. This pronation has caused a reddened sore over the navicular. Goal: independent ambulation with a straight cane, decreased foot posturing to allow reddened area on foot to heal.
   c. Client with a left hemiplegia ambulates independently and uses a straight cane and an articulated ankle orthosis. Her goal is to walk without her cane and to begin to learn how to jog and practice hitting tennis balls against a backboard.

10. You are planning an intervention program for a client with a right hemiplegia who cannot stand independently. Describe the primary and secondary impairments that may interfere with the function, the critical trunk movement patterns, the prerequisite for lower extremity control, and two specific intervention techniques (feel free to create your own using principles from the chapter).

11. You are a participant in a panel discussion entitled "Current physical therapy trends in stroke rehabilitation." Your role is to discuss the strengths of interventions that focus on improvement of impairments. Outline three points that highlight these strengths. For each point, use an example of a common impairment following stroke that interferes with a functional skill.

CHAPTER 26

1. Differentiate the behavioral manifestations of delirium and dementia, and discuss how these two cognitive conditions might affect treatment outcomes.

2. Why might an awareness of a client's biorhythms affect therapeutic outcomes?

3. Describe how, and for what type of patient, to use the Mini-Mental State Examination as a part of the therapeutic assessment.

4. Discuss the cognitive and noncognitive changes in learning style that might occur as an individual ages and how these will affect the design of therapeutic interventions.

5. How do environmental considerations such as temperature, familiarity with the environment, and emotional issues regarding feeling in control or safe affect the elderly population?

6. Depression in any client can have an adverse effect on outcomes of intervention. Discuss variables related to

seniors that lead to depression or precipitate that emotional response.

7. Why might a diagnosis of functional skills or ADL by a physical or an occupational therapist be a better indicator of therapeutic outcomes than a medical diagnosis?

CHAPTER 27

1. What is the part of the eye that controls accommodation?

2. Where does image processing occur: the retina, the lateral geniculate body, the visual cortex, or all of the above?

3. What three cranial nerves control eye movements?

4. Name three activities that could be affected by an accomodation problem.

5. Name three activities that can be affected by a vergence eye problem.

6. What is the difference between a phoria and a strabismus?

7. Name the one test that should always be done first in the visual screening.

8. What is the proper testing distance for near visual acuities?

9. During near point of convergence testing, what is the "break point" and what distance is suggestive of problems?

10. What type of information does the alternate cover test give the tester?

11. Does the cover/uncover test allow fusion to occur between trials?

12. Is the confrontation fields test done monocularly or binocularly and why?

CHAPTER 28

1. Nerve conduction velocity is known to be slower than normal or at the lower limit of normal before age 5 and after 60 years of age. What are the electrophysiological reasons for these slower values?

2. A somatosensory-evoked potential test (SSEP) of the tibial nerve is administered to a client who is in a coma. No response is obtained when recording from the contralateral cerebral cortex. What are possible sites of impairment, and what additional electrophysiological tests may be helpful in differentiating the problem?

3. Nerve conduction tests and an EMG of a client with unexplained weakness of both lower extremities that has progressively increased over a 2-month period show normal motor and sensory conduction and no EMG abnormalities except for a slightly irregular recruitment pattern. Which of the following is consistent with the electrophysiological test findings in this client (more than one answer may be correct)?
   a. Malingering
   b. Bilateral peripheral neuropathy
   c. Myopathy
   d. Central nervous system impairment
   e. Lower motor neuron impairment

4. Which electrophysiological tests are more likely to show abnormalities in a demyelinating polyradiculoneuropathy, such as Guillain-Barré syndrome, and what is the explanation for the answer?

5. Which factors are responsible for increasing fatigability in muscle that is stimulated electrically?

a. Frequency, order of motor unit recruitment, on/off ratio
b. Frequency, ramping, duration of pulse/phase
c. Duration of pulse, on/off ratio, ramping
d. Order of motor unit recruitment, wave form, amplitude

6. Discuss the benefits that individuals with SCI may derive when exercising involved musculature utilizing electrical stimulation in concert with exercise devices (i.e., stationary bicycles).

7. EMGBF has been utilized to reduce spasticity/hypertonicity in individuals with neurological insult. Describe the three stages of intervention with this modality, as detailed by DeBacher in reference 50.

8. Application of electrical stimulation has been problematic in pediatric populations. Describe the factors that may create these problems.

CHAPTER 29

1. Describe the components of the pain experience.

2. Briefly outline the pain pathways.

3. How is pain transmission modulated?

4. Differentiate among acute, chronic, peripheral, central, and autonomic pain.

5. List and describe the appropriate use of eight pain measurement tools.

6. Describe the three avenues of intervention for pain management, and state when each is appropriate.

7. Describe the role of physical interventions in pain management.

8. Describe the role of cognitive interventions in pain management.

9. Describe the role of behavioral manipulations in pain management.

CHAPTER 30

1. Which are the most common forms of urinary incontinence in non-neurological patients?

2. Name at least three anatomical or physiological factors that contribute to continence.

3. When performing evaluations of a client with urinary incontinence, define the steps that need to be taken.

4. Explain how the Tanzberger concept contributes to motor learning and achieving functional control of the pelvic floor muscles.

5. What could be the reason to begin the pelvic floor treatment with electrical stimulation?

6. What treatment possibilities for urinary incontinence are commonly used for cognitively impaired clients?

CHAPTER 31

1. What is a prefabricated orthosis? Describe the advantages and disadvantages in selections.

2. Describe how an ankle-foot orthosis can stabilize a knee that lacks knee extensors. What components are necessary?

3. What considerations must be given to the patient with a neuropathic foot when utilizing an AFO?

4. What are the major goals of orthotic intervention in the neuropathic spine?

5. What level of cervical lesion must be intact for use of a wrist-driven tenodesis orthosis? What are the critical factors for success?

6. You are evaluating a complete T12 paraplegic for orthotic consideration. What are the critical elements in patient evaluation for the patient to utilize bilateral KAFOs?

7. You have evaluated a patient who has minus 10 degrees of dorsiflexion (in 10 degrees of plantar flexion.) What problem does this represent for the patient, and what type of orthotic modifications can be made to minimize this lack of range of motion?

8. What is the importance of discussing the patient's major complaint and expectations?

CHAPTER 32

1. An 85-year-old woman is undergoing rehabilitation after a hip replacement. Her caregiver notices that the patient often complains of dizziness and is noticably unsteady after taking her medications. Which of the following most likely contributes to her problem?
a. Oxazepam
b. Diclofenac
c. Amantadine
d. Simvastatin

2. MJ, a 75-year-old man with Parkinson's disease, is effectively maintained on levodopa/carbidopa (Sinemet). On diagnosis of cancer, MJ receives chemotherapy and requires medications to control nausea and vomiting. Which of the following would most likely interfere with MJ's therapy for Parkinson's disease?
a. Lorazepam
b. Chlorpromazine
c. Dexamethasone
d. Dronabinol

CHAPTER 33

1. How might the movement-based therapies be grounded in motor learning theories? How can tai chi, tae kwon do and Feldenkrais be incorporated into therapeutic exercise?

2. What is the Law of Five Elements? How might it relate to the aspects of Native American perspectives?

3. Describe the nature of homeostasis as it relates to present rehabilitation treatments and how balance is attained in the realms of Chinese acupuncture and Native American healing.

4. How is myofascial release and craniosacral therapy similar from a manual therapy approach?

5. State the similar aspects of biofeedback and therapeutic touch in terms of the law of physics.

6. Describe the role of a medical intuitive. How might it relate to the novice versus master PT/OT clinician?

7. What movement modalities foster enhanced balance? Which one addresses all of the four practice patterns?

8. How might you incorporate complementary therapies into your daily life?

Answers

CHAPTER 1

1. Refer to the section Changing World Health Care, subsection In-Depth Analysis of the Wholistic Model (pp. 5–6), with sections throughout this chapter describing allopathic medical practice.

2. Refer to the section on intervention (p. 13) as well as to the sections on diagnosis (p. 10) and prognosis (p. 11). Additional answers can be found in every chapter of this book.

3. Refer to the section on wholistic model (p. 8) and documentation (p. 11).

4. Refer to the section on documentation with focus data, evaluation, and performance measurement (p. 12).

5. Refer to the section on efficacy with specific emphasis on efficacy-based practice and its relevance to third-party payers, the consumer, and the professional bases of both occupational and physical therapy (pp. 9–10).

6. Diagnosis by a physician is based on disease and pathology, whereas that of PTs and OTs is based on impairments and disabilities. Refer to Phase 2: differential diagnosis within a therapist's scope of practice (pp. 10–11).

7. Refer to the section on concept of the learning environment (pp. 15–20).

8. Refer to the subsection on the client profile (pp. 24–27).

CHAPTER 2

1. b

2. d

3. a

4. c

5. b

CHAPTER 3

1. Impairment is the loss or abnormality of physiological, psychological, or anatomical structure or function. Disability is restriction of the ability to perform a physical action, an activity, or a task in an efficient, typically expected, and competent manner.

2. Answers:
   - __I__ decreased muscle strength in the hip and knee
   - __I__ absent touch and proprioceptive sensations from the foot to the knee
   - __I__ decreased range of motion in the right shoulder
   - __I__ hypertonicity within the extensor muscle groups in the lower extremities
   - __I__ fascial tightness in the low back region
   - __I__ volitional or reflexive synergies
   - __D__ inability to transfer from bed to wheelchair without assistance
   - __D__ inability to ambulate independently

3. Refer to the section "The Diagnostic Process."

4. The ability to choose the appropriate examination tool(s) for a particular client depends on several factors:

a. The client's current functional status (ambulatory vs. nonambulatory).

b. The client's current cognitive status (intact vs. confused/disoriented).

c. The clinical setting in which the person is being evaluated for treatment (acute hospital vs. rehab vs. outpatient vs. skilled care vs. home care).

d. The client's primary complaints (pain vs. weakness vs. impaired balance).

e. The client's goals and realistic expectation for recovery.

5. Following the identification of the disabilities or functional limitations, and the impairments that may be causing them, the clinician may decide among three possible intervention scenarios: (1) the correction of impairments, which may lead to the correction of disabilities; (2) the correction of the disability itself through the enhancement of existing strengths; or (3) compensation for noncorrectable limitations through alterations in the external environment. Refer to Figure 3–2 and the discussion beginning on page 47.

CHAPTER 4

1. Refer to the section on motor learning concepts beginning on page 57. Variables controlled from outside the motor system begin on page 59, and those directly affected by the motor system begin on page 60.

2. b

3. Refer to sections on somatosensory retraining (pp. 121–122); functional retraining (pp. 73–74); and augmented intervention strategies (pp. 77–80).

4. Refer to section 3 under Neuroplasticity: Principles of Neural Adaptation (pp. 65–71).

5. b

6. c

7. d

8. Refer to the section on augmented therapeutic intervention classification (pp. 77–105).

9. Refer to the section on autonomic nervous system within augmented therapeutic intervention classification (pp. 97–98) as well as Chapter 6.

10. Refer to the last section on clinical problems; lack of head control and the neurophysiological relationships within the motor system (pp. 113–116).

CHAPTER 5

The answers contain phrases that are important considerations.

1. Investigators have different interests and training; theories and models are abstract representations of movement; every model has limitations and strengths; all theories have hypotheses that need to be tested; theories and models change as new knowledge is discovered.

2. Sensation and perception are processed at different levels; use of receptors to encode sensations; use of memory to process sensations for perception; sensation is not influenced by learning, but perception is influenced by learning.

3. Spasticity is a clinical syndrome that has many degrees of severity; timing, force production, and sequencing may be influenced by current neurorehabilitation procedures; spasticity is a naturally occurring process that cannot be resolved through neurorehabilitation.

4. Efficiency of the neural system in terms of metabolic requirements and preferred movement patterns generated by the individual; reduces a high-dimensional system to a low-dimensional system; limits the number of movement patterns that can be used; speed of the neural system to select and generate a movement.

5. Volitional sway occurs during everyday activities when the COG moves toward the limits of the COG. Anticipatory balance responses occur. Unexpected perturbation occurs when the COG is unexpectedly moved toward or outside the BOS. Compensatory balance responses occur. Interaction with the environment. The COG is constantly moved in the BOS or outside the BOS during performance of everyday activities. Both anticipatory and compensatory activities occur.

6. No. These strategies were defined for the lower extremity and trunk during a laboratory condition. The individual was unexpectedly perturbed in a linear direction (forward or backward). Balance responses include the interaction of all body parts with one another and with the environment to maintain the head in an upright position (face vertical, mouth horizontal). Balance responses occur during all routine activities of daily living.

7. Parameters of movement such as force, timing, sequencing; age, cognition, and current and previous activity level; preferred movement patterns; status of the physiological systems; neurological condition and prediction for recovery or functional level.

CHAPTER 6

1. Motivation/declarative memory, olfaction/smell, visceral/autonomic nervous system, and emotion.

2. Refer to subsystem entitled The Limbic System MOVEs US.

3. Fear or frustration leads to anger. Anger not controlled or modified can lead to internal chaos, which can lead to violence in some people. Refer to the subsection entitled "F²ARV Continuum."

4. Clients with CNS deficits have a much more fragile CNS and are often much more autonomically unstable than are individuals with other pathologies/diseases or impairments/disabilities. For that reason, this client population is more susceptible to developing a GAS syndrome, and is a client who progresses down the continuum at risk for a dangerous outcome.

5. A client will have difficulty overcoming the postural extension elicited by the anger.

6. Discussed on pages 174–175 beginning with paragraph 3.

7. Refer to the section on the limbic connections to the "Mind, Body, Spirit" paradigm, page 173 to paragraph 2 on page 174.

CHAPTER 7

1. With regard to adjustment, impairment relates to the ability to cope, and disability relates to the inability to enjoy life (p. 179).

2. Yes, we are in a constant process of adjusting to life. If we are rigid or inflexible, we will become maladjusted (pp. 182–186).

3. Kerr's five stages of adjustment can all be influenced by age, cognition, and developmental level (pp. 180–186).

4. The therapist should help the client to learn to enjoy the body, develop a sense of ownership of the body, and accept the body, thus encouraging the client to feel positively toward the body and the self. The therapist may also communicate to the client that "normal" sex roles and sexuality may be accomplished in the future with adaptation (pp. 186–189).

5. The family can be incorporated into therapy using crisis management, giving them a sense of control, use of role playing, stimulating problem solving, education about the disability and adjustment, and use of support groups (p. 190).

6. The therapist can stimulate family problem solving and educate the family regarding loss, cognition, coping, and learning styles to encourage a sense of control and empowerment (p. 190).

CHAPTER 8

1. See the section Neuropathology of Movement Disorders (pp. 207–210).

2. See the section Difference Between Preterm and Term Infants Neuromotor Function (pp. 242–243).

3. See the section Clinical Decision Making Pathway, Decision Step #2, choice #2 on p. 246.

4. See the sections Parent Support/Parent Teaching (p. 231) and In Utero Exposure to Drugs and Other Substances (pp. 243–244).

5. See the sections Indication for Referral, especially Biological Risk (pp. 211–212), and Educational Requirements for Therapists (p. 211).

6. See the section Educational Requirements for Therapists (p. 211).

7. See the section Theoretical Framework (pp. 204–207).

8. See the sections on Clinical Management: Neonatal Periods, introduction (pp. 210–211), Examination (pp. 212–217), and treatment planning and strategies (pp. 231–232).

9. See the section Parent Support (pp. 231–232).

CHAPTER 9

1. Refer to the section definitions, parameters, anticipated changes (pp. 259–262, especially paragraph 5 on p. 260).

2. Include a discussion of the various sensorimotor impairments, the family structure and involvement, and the psychosocial components. These can be found throughout the chapter.

3. Refer to the section Diagnostic Categorization of the Characteristics of Cerebral Palsy (pp. 263–265).

4. Refer to the sections on the roles of the therapist in direct and indirect intervention (pp. 270–272).

5. Refer to criteria for equipment recommendations (pp. 277–278) as well as Chapter 31.

CHAPTER 10

1. 1, 2, and 4. Autosomal dominant disorders are a subdivision of single gene disorders.

2. False. Cystic fibrosis is an autosomal recessive disorder.

3. False. The pathophysiology of trisomy 21 includes the presence of an additional chromosome, #21, which is the basis for the term *trisomy.*

4. Autosomal dominant, autosomal recessive, and sex-linked inherited recessive.

5. PDMS—a discriminating measure used to assess the motor development level in the gross motor and fine motor domains for children age birth to 7 years. A normative score and scaled score can be obtained.
   MAI—a predictive measure used to assess muscle tone, reflex development, automatic reactions, and volitional movement in infants in the first year of life.
   SFA—evaluative measure used to assess student performance in the school environment. The test includes items to assess the student's participation in school activities, supports needed for participation, and the student's activity performance at school.

6. Goal and objective setting should be collaborative with those of the family, determining their vision and the therapist acting as a consultant and resource to assist the family in achieving their vision.

7. Refer to the chapter section on medical management (pp. 303–304).

8. A pedigree is a family tree that is constructed by the genetics counselor or geneticist to determine the familial history of a genetic disorder.

CHAPTER 11

1. See under model of Disablement (pp. 310–311).

2. In subgroups: section on learning disabilities overview, p. 315.

3. In perspectives on the causes of LD, pp. 311–313.

4. Some information in Causes of DCD (pp. 319–320), Descriptions of Children with DCD (pp. 320–322), and Lifespan Disabilities (pp. 336–338).

5. Qualitative assessment of motor deficits (pp. 323–324).

6. Linking assessment to intervention (p. 328), intervention of the child with LD and DCD (pp. 328–330), and Service Delivery Models (pp. 317–318).

7. Assessment of and Intervention for the Child with Learning Disabilities (pp. 316–317), linking assessment to intervention (p. 328), and Intervention for the Child with Learning Disabilities (pp. 328–330, 336, 338).

CHAPTER 12

1. Discussed in Mobility of the Peripheral Nervous System (pp. 352–353).

2. Discussed in Mobility of the Peripheral Nervous System (pp. 352–353).

3. Discussed on page 353, column 2, paragraph 2.

4. Discussed on page 353, column 2, paragraph 3, to page 354.

5. Discussed in Adaptive Responses to Pain (p. 354).

6. Discussed in Clinical Examination and Treatment (p. 354).

CHAPTER 13

ALS

1. Muscle atrophy and weakness; upper motor neuron symptoms

2. Deficiency of nerve growth factor, an excess of extracellular glutamate in the central nervous system, and an autoimmune process.

3. Pyramidal tract dysfunction (i.e., hyperreflexia in the presence of weakness and atrophy, spasticity, and Babinsky and Hoffman reflexes.

4. Lower extremity onset is slightly more common than upper extremity onset, which is more common than bulbar onset.

5. An unremitting spread of weakness to other muscle groups, leading to total paralysis of spinal musculature and muscles innervated by the cranial nerves; respiratory failure

6. Rate of the patient's disease progression, the extent and areas of involvement, and the stage of illness.

7. See box on exercise and rehabilitation programs for rehabilitation patients with ALS according to stage of disease.

8. Disuse atrophy and overwork damage.

9. Disuse weakness lowers muscle force production and reduces muscle endurance. Disuse atrophy in combination with pathological weakness and spasticity of specific muscle groups contributes to poorly coordinated, less efficient movements that require more energy expenditure.

10. Answers:
    a. To improve compliance, consider both a formal exercise program and enjoyable physical activities.
    b. Include activities with opportunities for social development and personal accomplishment.
    c. Strengthening programs should emphasize concentric rather than eccentric muscle contractions.
    d. High-resistance strengthening programs probably have no benefit over moderate-resistance programs.
    e. Muscles with less than antigravity strength have little capacity to improve: the program should focus on stronger muscles.
    f. Periodically monitor muscle strength to assess for possible overwork weakness, particularly in unsupervised programs.
    g. Activity modifications should include periods of physical activity with rest.

11. Damaged

12. See section on therapeutic interventions.

13. Must be respected

14. See section on caregiver issues (p. 382).

Guillain-Barré Syndrome

15. Ascending weakness or flaccid paralysis

16. Total paralysis of the peripheral, axial, facial, and extraocular musculature.

17. Low cardiac output, cardiac dysrhythmias, and marked

fluctuations in blood pressure, peripheral pooling of blood, poor venous return, ileus and urinary retention.

18. See section on GBS: Respiratory and dysphagia function (pp. 389–390).

19. Research has shown that mild continuous stretching maintained for at least 20 minutes is more beneficial than stronger, brief stretching exercises. Therefore, use of splints for prolonged positioning is superior for maintaining functional range than short bursts of intermittent, manually applied passive stretching.

20. (1) Therapists and nurses may have been reluctant to make patients who complained of marked pain during passive movement perform range of motion exercises fully; (2) the contractures may have been secondary to pain or damage caused by inappropriate excessive passive movement of hypotonic and sensory impaired joints and muscles; (3) the paralysis may have resulted in lymphatic stasis with accumulation of tissue fluid in tissue spaces and nutritional disturbances; and (4) vasomotor disturbances resulting from autonomic neuropathy may have led to adhesions and fibrosis.

21. Heat should not be used on a patient with a sensory deficit, particularly an inability to distinguish differences in temperature. Heating muscle and tendon tissue before sustained stretching, however, was a mainstay in prevention of contractures caused by muscle spasms secondary to poliomyelitis, and it may have a place in treatment of muscle spasm and contractions in GBS provided there is no sensory impairment.

22. That exercise will not hasten or improve nerve regeneration, nor will it influence the reinnervation rate during the rehabilitation process.

23. To maintain the patient's musculoskeletal system in an optimal "ready" state, to prevent overwork, and to pace the recovery process to obtain maximal function as reinnervation occurs.

24. That muscle fatigue must be avoided and rest periods must be frequent.

25. Smaller

26. Answers:
    a. Short periods of nonfatiguing exercise appropriate to the patient's strength.
    b. An increase in activity or exercise level only if the patient improves or if there is no deterioration after 1 week.
    c. A return to bed rest if a decrease in function or strength occurs.
    d. A program of exercise directed at strengthening for function rather than strength itself.
    e. A limit of fatiguing exercise for 1 year, with a gradual return to sport activities and more strenuous exercise.

27. When neural recovery begins, the initiation of active exercise must be implemented with a clear understanding that excessive exercise during early reinnervation, when there are only a few functioning motor units, can lead to further damage rather than the expected exercise-induced hypertrophy of muscle.

28. See box on page 387.

Muscular Dystrophy

29. Dystrophin

30. Males

31. Creatine kinase; degeneration with gradual loss of fiber, variation in fiber size, with a proliferation of connective and adipose tissue.

32. Pure respiratory failure or respiratory failure secondary to infection; 18 and 25

33. Is also found in brain tissue. This suggests a possible relationship between the gene defect, which may cause decrease in dystrophin in brain tissue, and impaired IQ.

34. The delay of early developmental milestones, particularly crawling and walking.

35. Symmetrical from proximal to distal, with marked weakness of the pelvic and shoulder girdle musculature preceding weakness of the trunk and extremity muscles. Muscles innervated by cranial nerves (except the sternocleidomastoids) are not involved, and bowel and bladder function is usually spared.

36. 12; prolonged periods of immobilization secondary to illness, injury, or surgery.

37. Gowers' maneuver; using the arms to crawl up his or her own legs

38. See section Progression of Lower-Extremity Weakness (p. 399).

39. See section Progression of Gait Pattern Changes (p. 399).

40. Attempted to implant the normal precursor muscle cells or myoblasts directly into dystrophic mice and, in several cases, into children with DMD to precipitate the proliferation of normal donor muscle cells into the host muscles of dystrophic subjects, but results have not led to significant improvement to date.[162] Most recently, researchers have been working on recombinant adenovirus vector-mediated dystrophin gene transfer to Duchenne dystrophy patients.

41. Postural drainage and breathing exercises

42. The early onset form (approximately 23%), which becomes evident before the child becomes wheelchair dependent, and the late onset form, which develops, on average, 4 years after wheelchair dependency.

43. At least 35

44. Horizontal

45. (1) Prevent contractures that can lead to further disability and pain, (2) maintain maximal strength/prevent disuse atrophy, (3) facilitate maximal functional abilities using appropriate adaptive equipment, (4) maintain maximal respiratory muscle strength and movement of secretions, and (5) foster realistic child and family expectations within the context of the environment.

46. Help the child cope more effectively with respiratory infections and the discomfort accompanying respiratory compromise.

47. See section on prevention of contractures (pp. 404–405).

48. Minimal to moderate weakness; severely weakened

49. Recover from exercise fatigue after a night's rest.

50. See section on maintenance of ambulation (pp. 406–408).

51. Depression, withdrawal, and anxiety.

52. Causing possible muscle damage from excessive exercise demands or overwork.

53. Insomnia, progressive drowsiness, morning headaches, dyspnea, and anxiety.

54. Many significant treatment and ethical decisions must be made by the patient, family, and care providers when submitting to prolonged HMV: caregiver issues, financial issues, home versus hospital-based care, and psychosocial issues for both patient and caregiver.

CHAPTER 14

1. a. Glasgow coma score of 8 or better
    b. Reactive pupillary response
    c. Duration of coma of less than a week
    d. Intact brain stem function
    e. Spontanous eye movements

2. Male, 15 to 24 years old.

3. Motor vehicle accidents.

4. The axons from cortical neurons to lower centers are injured, resulting in spotty and variable patterns of neurological loss.

5. There may be spontaneous motor activity; patients may track with their eyes.

6. Retrograde and post-traumatic. Retrograde is an inability to remember events that occurred immediately before the accident. The period may vary. Post-traumatic amnesia is the time after injury until normal memory is restored and is generally related to severity of the injury. Anterograde amnesia is an inability to form new memories after the brain injury.

7. The client might show procedural memory in which he can repeat physical or cognitive functions to which he was previously exposed. Because this is an unconscious type of automatic learning, the client cannot verbalize this learning.

8. The increased pressure means that for blood to flow to the brain, it must equal or exceed the intracranial pressure in order to bring oxygen. When the ICP is higher than the blood pressure, brain injury can extend and continue.

9. Vasopressor drugs such as phenylephrine keep blood pressure high for good cerebral profusion; barbiturates lower ICP; glucocorticoids may or may not be effective in controlling edema.

10. Mild to moderate lesion on CT; cerebral edema; frontal lesion on late MRI or focal frontotemporal atrophy; low score on the Glasgow Coma Scale; post-traumatic amnesia; extended time in stupor or coma.

11. Family is happy with outcome; employment; married; good memory; bowel independence; not blaming oneself for the injury.

12. See motor control section: synergistic organization (p. 423).

13. Through synergies.

14. Hand control has a large cortically controlled function.

15. They both help modify motor responses to environment demands. Anticipatory responses occur before a movement and are feedforward, and adaptive responses occur after an experience and are feedback. They are both dependent on sensory information.

16. Experiments showing peripherally driven changes in CNS organization and function such as those of Wiesel, Byl, and Devor are the most efficacious. See Intervention Efficacy (pp. 424–425).

17. The scale includes both cognitive and behavioral components of function. It is used for brain-injured clients and looks at behavior and appropriateness of behavior, especially agitation.

18. These are higher level cognitive functions usually thought to be frontal cortex functions. There are 4: choosing a goal, developing a plan, executing a plan, evaluating the execution of the plan.

19. Random, summary feedback for more advanced clients; more frequent and specific feedback for lower level clients.

20. Can use changes in direction or speed of movement to identify subtasks.

21. Neurons are networked or connected together and work as a motor program so that new behaviors are formulated based on practice, feedback, environment, and other factors.

22. Match as follows:
WAIS a, f
GOAT a,
Naming test b, d
FIM b, e
FAM a, b, f
Nine hole peg test c, f
Frenchy arm test c

23. Factors such as family support, motivation, cognitive function, available equipment, and societal beliefs all affect whether a person will have a handicap.

24. The first client will need training of aides and family members, equipment to substitute for impairment losses, and changes in the environment to accommodate his or her problems. The second client will need treatment to improve physical function with direct treatment.

25. See Tone (p. 429), Strength (p. 434), and Tone (pp. 435–436).

26. Client not be able to accommodate to different surfaces, angles, or moving inclines with loss of vision, somatosensory functions, or vestibular loss in gait. May not be able to shape hand appropriately, grasp with appropriate strength, or prevent slipping or dropping of objects in the hand.

27. Sequence, timing, and the selection of muscles used in a movement can be disorganized, resulting in co-contraction, ataxia, and slowed and ineffective movements, which use more energy.

28. Changing the environment in which he or she works.

29. Atrophy occurs with prolonged bedrest, muscle fibers change functions in spasticity, and the ability to move and control both movement and posture are dependent on a certain level of strength or recruitment of muscle fibers.

30. See the box on page 426 and Figure 14–2 for ideas on examination areas and review of interventions within this chapter. See also Chapter 4 and Figures 4–13 and 4–14.

CHAPTER 15

1. Because the paralyzed limbs of the child with spina bifida have increased amounts of unmineralized osteoid tissue, they are prone to fractures, especially after periods of immobilization. Early mobilization and weight-bearing can aid in decreasing osteoporosis.

2. When a spinal cord is damaged, segments distal to the injury may respond to stimuli in a reflexive manner. This reflexive movement results from preservation of the spinal reflex arc and is known as "distal sparing." Because distal sparing causes reflexive, nonvolitional movements in response to muscle stretch, it is important to distinguish this movement from voluntary muscle functioning for the results of an MMT to be valid.

3. Teaching the family ROM and positioning to enhance development. Attaining good head and trunk control and eliciting head-righting reactions through weight shifting in the prone-on-elbows and sitting positions are major goals.

4. The development of adequate strength and control for head and trunk righting reactions and equilibrium and protective extension reactions will ultimately lead to improved sitting balance. The attainment of hands-free sitting with good balance allows the child to play easily in sitting. Hands-free sitting ability also appears to be a determinant of children who will become functional ambulators.

5. When the child attempts to pull to standing or would be expected to do so (10–12 months of age), a standing device should be introduced. Even if the child cannot assume a vertical position unaided, he or she should experience vertical at a developmentally appropriate time.

6. First the child must learn to weight shift in standing; the child combines weight shift with forward rotation of the non–weight-bearing side.

7. During stage III, the child begins to use some form of prone progression. During this phase of high mobility, anesthetic skin must be checked frequently for injury, and extra protection through the use of heavier clothing may be necessary (stage III paragraph 5). Also if the child becomes wheelchair dependent during stage V, skin care will become a priority for the constant sitter.

8. The energy cost of walking becomes too high. The child wants to keep up with peers. As the child grows bigger and heavier, the child's limited physical abilities cannot keep up. Strength does not increase in the same proportion as body weight.

9. Severity of mental handicap, poor manual dexterity, lack of education, overprotective parents, and difficulty of health care personnel in addressing sexuality issues with patients who are physically disabled and their families.

10. Generally the sexual capacity is near normal; that is, she has potential for a normal orgasmic response, is fertile, and can bear children. The pregnancy may be considered high risk depending on existing orthopedic deformities.

CHAPTER 16

1. __D__ results from compression by tumor or infarction of the posterior spinal artery
   __C__ causes bleeding into the central gray matter of the spinal cord; results in more impairment of function in the upper extremities than the lower
   __E__ motor function and pain and temperature sensation lost bilaterally below the lesion; prognosis poor for return of bowel and bladder function, ambulation, and hand function
   __B__ results in flaccid paralysis with no spinal reflex activity present
   __A__ characterized by ipsilateral loss of motor function

and position sense and contralateral loss of pain sensation several levels below the lesion; good prognosis for recovery

2. Methylprednisolone. High doses of methylprednisolone enhance the flow of blood to the injured spinal cord, preventing the decline in white matter, extracellular calcium levels, and evoked potentials. This acts to prevent progressive post-traumatic ischemia.

3. Age, body type, medical problems, cognitive ability, psychosocial, spasticity, endurance, strength, ROM, funding sources, and motivation.

4. Page 524.

5. Page 524.

6. Page 521, column 1, paragraph 6.

7. Respiratory; see pages 499–502.

8. f

9. e

CHAPTER 17

1. The infecting agents may be bacterial, fungal, viral, protozoan, or parasitic. The most common agents producing meningitis are bacterial; the most common agents producing encephalitis are viral. However, bacterial encephalitis and viral meningitis also are disease entities.

2. The circulation of CSF spreads the infecting organism through the ventricular system and the subarachnoid spaces. The pia mater and arachnoidea mater become acutely inflamed, and as part of the inflammatory response, a purulent exudate forms in the subarachnoid space. The exudate may undergo organization, resulting in an obstruction of the foramen of Monro, the aqueduct of Sylvius, or the exit foramen of the fourth ventricle. The supracortical subarachnoid spaces proximal to the arachnoid villi may be obliterated, resulting in a noncommunicating or obstructive hydrocephalus as a result of the accumulation of CSF. As the CSF accumulates, the intracranial pressure rises. The increased intracranial pressure produces venous obstruction, precipitating a further increase in the intracranial pressure.

3. Nuchal rigidity is indicative of an irritative lesion of the subarachnoid space. Cervical flexion is painful because it stretches the inflamed meninges, nerve roots, and spinal cord. The pain triggers a reflex spasm of the neck extensors to splint the area against further cervical flexion; however, cervical rotation and extension movements remain relatively free. See page 533 for the Kernig test.

4. Viral encephalitis presents a syndrome of elevated temperature, headache, nuchal rigidity, vomiting, and general malaise (symptoms of aseptic or viral meningitis), with the addition of evidence of more extensive cerebral damage such as coma, cranial nerve palsy, hemiplegia, involuntary movements, or ataxia.

5. Deficits in cognition may be evident as problems in the area of explicit (declarative) or implicit (procedural) learning. Explicit learning is used in the acquisition of knowledge that is consciously recalled. This is information

that can be verbalized in declarative sentences, such as the sequential listing of the steps in a movement sequence. Implicit or procedural learning is used in the process of acquiring movement sequences that are performed automatically without conscious attention to the performance. Procedural learning occurs through repetitions of the movement task. Because explicit and implicit learning utilize different neuroanatomical circuits, implicit learning can occur in individuals with deficits in the components underlying explicit learning (awareness, attention, higher order cognitive processes).

6. In addition to determining the integrity of the peripheral sensory pathways and recognition of the input, it is important to assess the individual's ability to process more complex presentations of cutaneous input. Difficulties in the cortical level processing of cutaneous stimuli are identified through tests of sharp-dull discrimination, stereognosis, tactile localization, texture recognition, two-point discrimination, and bilateral simultaneous stimulation.

7. The therapist should intertwine an appraisal of the individual's ability to learn motor tasks (or elements of the task). The therapist attempts to determine whether the client can maintain a change in the ability to perform a movement throughout a therapy session and into the next session. The client's ability to capture and integrate changes into the movement repertoire is fundamental to the success of the intervention program. The program can focus on the learning of movement sequences and the generalization of these sequences to movements within other contexts. Individuals with lowered levels of consciousness (typically Rancho Los Amigos stages 1–3) will be unable to learn or will have difficulty learning and generalizing new motor skills. Therapy sessions may be more successful if the focus remains on the performance of motor tasks that were previously "overlearned" and automatic. Although the therapist may be able to guide the individual manually in coming to sitting on the edge of the bed, until the individual demonstrates a higher level of processing, it may be unrealistic to expect that the person will consistently reposition the legs without cueing before attempting the movement sequence.

8. Incorporating reversal of movement patterns within the intervention program prepares the client to deal with situations that mandate unexpected adjustments in the movement sequence.

9. As the therapist works with the client on an intervention program, situations arise that require problem solving to determine a way to accomplish a task. If the task is to accomplish an independent transfer from a wheelchair into a bathtub, decisions must be made concerning the sequence of movements. Therapists can approach this situation in two ways. They can instruct clients step-by-step in what to do, or they can involve clients to the extent possible in the process of deciding what to do. If the therapist instructs the client step-by-step, the client may master the task but may not be able to perform it under different conditions. If the therapist involves the client in the decision-making process, the client may be learning not only how to accomplish the specific task, but also how to accomplish the task under varied conditions. The intervention process should lead to the ability to respond to the demands of a situation, and involvement of clients in the problem-solving process helps prepare them for independence. The therapist must structure the client's role in decision making to the level of the client's ability to participate so that the experience is not frustrating.

Although the client's participation may initially increase the time required to complete a task, it promotes skills that may lead more quickly to independence of function.

CHAPTER 18

1. Pulmonary tuberculosis, recurrent pneumonia, and invasive cervical cancer.

2. Acquired immunity is divided into humoral and cell-mediated responses. Humoral depends on the production of antibodies. Cell-mediated response is required to destroy infected cell-surface pathogens.

3. Immunological changes include improvement in CD4 cells; psychological alterations include decreased depression and fatigue.

4. Viral Load (VL) is a measurement of HIV viral RNA and is the standard component for the management of HIV-infected patients. Clients with a higher VL progress more rapidly, both immunologically in terms of CD4 cell count decline and clinically in terms of AIDS-defining illnesses.

5. Involuntary loss of more than 10% of baseline body weight and chronic diarrhea or unexplained weakness and fever.

6. Adverse changes in lipids, glucose, and insulin have been reported. Hyperlipidemia is also a finding with lipodystrophy. The physical changes are fatty distributions in the following areas: abdominal girth, dorsocervical fat pad, benign symmetrical lipomatosis, and breast hypertrophy.

7. Electroacupuncture with microcurrent or TENS, balance, and gait retraining.

8. Endogenous depression.

CHAPTER 19

1. a. Pain
   b. Fatigue
   c. Neuromuscular weakness
   d. Sleep disorder
   e. Cold intolerance
   f. Joint dysfunction

2. See box on page 581.

3. See pages 582–583.

4. Correction of posture and gate, orthotics (pp. 585–587).

5. Psychosocial considerations (pp. 589–590).

CHAPTER 20

1. Myelin.

2. Fatigue, weakness, paresthesia, unsteady gait, double vision, tremor, and bowel/bladder dysfunction.

3. (1) Relapsing-remitting MS (characterized by clearly defined relapses, episodes of acute worsening, followed by recovery and disease stability); (2) primary progressive MS (characterized by continuous worsening, steady progression, not interrupted by distinct relapses); (3) secondary progressive (characterized by relapsing remitting disease followed by progression with or without occasional relapse, minor remission, or plateau); (4) progressive relapsing (characterized by progressive disease from the

onset with clear, acute relapse that may or may not resolve. Periods between relapses are characterized by continued progression).

4. The Multiple Sclerosis Quality of Life Inventory, an assessment tool specific to MS. It includes health status (SF-36), fatigue (Modified Fatigue Impact Scale—MFIS), pain (Most Pain Effects Scale—PACE), sexual function (Sexual Satisfaction Scale—SSS), bladder function (Bladder Control Scale—BLCS), bowel function (Bowel Control Scale—BWCS), visual impairment (Impact of Visual Impairment Scale—IVIS), cognitive deficits (Perceived Deficits Questionnaire—PDQ), mental health status (Mental Health Inventory—MHI), and social support (Modified Social Support Survey—MSSS).

5. Functional activities, strengthening of fixation musculature, weighted cuffs, biofeedback, and drug therapies.

6. Compensatory strategies: use of memory book, electronic organizer (e.g., Palm Pilot), timers and alarms, Post-it note reminders.

7. Part-time/flexible time schedule, work at home option, memory aides, adapted computer keyboard, voice-operated software, office relocation (closer to bathroom and elevator), hands-free telephone, air conditioning.

CHAPTER 21

1. Pages 618–619.
   a. Pages 625–629.
   b. Pages 629–632.
   c. Pages 654–655.

2. Page 619.
   a. Pages 620–623.
   b. Pages 620–623.
   c. Pages 625–642.

3. Pages 623–624.
   a. Page 629, column 2, paragraphs 3 and 4.
   b. Page 629, column 2, paragraphs 3 and 4.
   c. (1) Tests of nystagmus (pp. 632–633).
      (2) Tests of semicircular canals (pp. 634–635).
      (3) Tests of visual and vestibular interaction (p. 635).

4. Pages 629–632.

5. Figure 21–2 (p. 621) and Table 21–1 (p. 617).
   a. Pages 620–621.
   b. Page 620, column 2, paragraphs 2 and 3.
   c. Page 632, column 2; pages 634–635.

6. a. See posterior canal, page 635.
   b. Pages 634–635.
   c. See canalith repositioning (pp. 650–652).

7. Pages 624–625.
   a. Pages 624–625.
   b. Pages 625–629, 655.
   c. Pages 653–655.

8. a. Page 653.
   b. Page 654.
   c. Pages 654–655.

CHAPTER 22

1. The basal ganglia are not directly connected to the spinal cord or to the motor neurons. Rather, they appear to be involved in enabling movement to occur easily and to be timed correctly. They are more involved in complex, sequential movements than in simple, single-joint movements. There is also a decrease in the ability to eliminate all but the desired motor activity. Further specifics can be found on pages 664–665.

2. In diseases we see problems of initiation and execution of movement at the right speed and for the right circumstance or for the present environment. There are difficulties in organization of sequential activities and/or performing more than one activity at a time. These symptoms are termed bradykinesia and akinesia and are also related to dyskinesia, chorea, or dystonia. The reader may find the precise symptoms in the discussion of each of the diseases listed.

3. For the person with Parkinson's disease, it is important that the treatment intervention include a lot of practice, more so than for the person without Parkinson's disease. In addition, the person must practice responding to a variety of environmental conditions and stimuli with differing sequences and speeds of movement. Details are listed on page 676, column 2, paragraph 4, to page 678 for early stages of the disease when this type of treatment is most effective.
   For the person with dystonia, the treatment is similar to that listed above but must also include some sensory re-training. The client must attend to sensory stimuli and be forced to make the appropriate, properly graded response. More specifics for this client are listed on page 690, column 1, paragraph 5, to column 2.

4. If surgery creates a lesion and increases the possibility of plastic changes, then the therapist's interventions may make a difference in the success of surgery. See page 674, column 1, paragraph 6.

5. The muscles of respiration are striated muscle and subject to changes in tone; almost all of the diseases of the basal ganglia end in rigidity. There is then a decrease in chest expansion and, with disease progression, there is decreased mobility and increased incidence of pneumonia, the leading cause of death.

6. Parkinson's disease affects approximately one third of all individuals older than 85 (see pages 669–670). As the population ages, this means that a large number of individuals referred for therapy will have Parkinson's disease.

7. These devices require the ability to move the device as well as the feet. This is difficult for those with PD and those in the later stages of HD or full body dystonias. The therapist must pay attention to the environment of the client as well as to his or her cognitive ability. For specifics for PD, see page 680, column 2, paragraph 2.

8. In addition to a physical therapist, occupational therapist, speech therapist, and neurologist, there should also be a dietitian, social worker, and psychologist and/or psychiatrist on the team. Usually, a nurse practitioner is also involved.

CHAPTER 23

1. See sections on glioblastoma (p. 698), meningioma (p. 699), goal setting (p. 707), and intervention (pp. 708–709).

2. See sections on side effects and considerations (pp. 707–708).

3. See section on rehabilitation: overview (P. 706).

4. See section on intervention, page 709, column 1, paragraph 2.

5. See sections on side effects and considerations (p. 707) and psychosocial care (pp. 713–714).

CHAPTER 24

1. The cerebellum is not directly connected to the spinal cord or to the motor neurons. It does appear to be involved in several aspects of movement based on the anatomic connections of the cerebellum, which include the vestibular system, the sensory information carried from the proprioceptors and rapidly adapting tactile receptors, and the initiation of movement and motor learning.

2. In diseases we see problems of balance, postural control, initiation and execution of movement, and disruption in the ability to learn a new skill. These symptoms are more apparent with movement of several joints than in single joint movement. They are also more apparent in fast movements than in slower movements. These difficulties are termed dysmetria, dyssynergia, dysdiadochokinesia, postural tremor, and intention tremor. See pages 721–726.

3. For cerebellar disease, it is important that the treatment intervention include a lot of practice, more so than for the person without cerebellar disease. In addition, the person must practice responding to a variety of environmental conditions and stimuli with differing sequences and speeds of movement. Intervention for the person with cerebellar disease may need to include compensatory strategies if the ability to relearn movements or adaptations has been lost. Details are listed on page 728.

4. See Control of Muscle Tone (p. 722), the box on pages 729–730, and Treatment (p. 731). The hypotonia may make movement even more difficult and poorly controlled. Resistance exercises may decrease these symptoms.

5. See pages 731 to 734 and Chapters 20 and 22.

6. See pages 729–731, particularly the box on pages 729–730.

CHAPTER 25

1. See Table 25–1 (p. 745).

2. See page 747, column 1, paragraph 4.

3. See Sequential Stages of Recovery (pp. 748–749).

4. See box on page 750.

5. See Patterns of Recovery (pp. 750–751).

6. See Clinical Hypertonicity (pp. 766–767).

7. See Loss of Alignment (pp. 767–768) and Figs. 25–1, 25–4, 25–11, 25–12.

8. See Pain (p. 770), Subluxation (pp. 771–772), Slings (pp. 778–779), Table 25–9.

9. See Orthotics (p. 779) and Table 25–10 (p. 780).
   a. See Orthotics (p. 779) and Table 25–10 (p. 780).
   b. See Orthotics (p. 779) and Table 25–10 (p. 780).
   c. See Orthotics (p. 779) and Table 25–10 (p. 780).

10. See Standing (pp. 774–776).

11. See entire chapter.

CHAPTER 26

1. Refer to the subsections on delirium and dementia (pp. 802–804) and the potential outcomes of the specific medical diagnoses if a client has impairments and is simultaneously receiving therapy (pp. 807–810).

2. If an elderly client with dementia has a time during the day when he or she is more coherent and alert, there are greater chances that learning will take place during those times.

3. Refer to the subsection entitled The Mini-Mental State Examination on page 797.

4. Refer to the section Older Adult Learning Styles and Communication on pages 798–799.

5. Refer to the section Environmental Considerations on pages 801–802.

6. Refer to the section Delirium and Reversible Dementia: Evaluation and Treatment, page 804, column 1, paragraphs 5 and 6, through column 2, paragraph 2.

7. Cognitive impairments are key limiting factors in the performance of ADL and IADL, as well as a limiting factor for participating in the learning environment. Medical diagnoses are pathology- or disease-related and are not necessarily reflective of functional skills. For additional information, refer to the section Strategies for Treatment and Care (pp. 807–810).

CHAPTER 27

1. Answer in section on Lens (p. 823).

2. Answer in section on Visual Pathway (pp. 824–826).

3. Answer in section on Eye Movement System (pp. 826–827).

4. Answer in section on Functional Visual Skills: Accommodation (pp. 827–828).

5. Answer in section on Vergence (p. 828).

6. Answer in section on Phoria and Strabismus (pp. 829–830).

7. Acuities.

8. Sixteen inches.

9. Answer in section on near point of convergence (p. 835).

10. Answer in section on vision screening (Cover Tests) (p. 835).

11. Answer in Cover Tests (p. 835).

12. Monocularly. See section on Visual Field Screening (p. 836).

CHAPTER 28

1. Myelination of peripheral nerve fibers contributes to the velocity of nerve conduction. Myelination occurs during the early developmental period and reaches maturation between 4 and 5 years of age. Slowing of conduction velocity may occur after 60 years of age because of changes in myelination and decreased temperature in peripheral tissue.

2. Abnormal or absent responses in the SSEP may result from impairment in afferent neuronal pathways between the stimulus and the recording sites, as well as from direct damage of tissue at the recording site. Sensory nerve conduction tests, including the H-reflex test, may be helpful in differentiating between peripheral and central nervous system impairment.

3. a and d

4. Nerve conduction tests, including F wave tests. These

tests would be helpful because conduction velocity slows with demyelination, and the F wave test measures conduction in the more proximal portion of nerves, which is the area in which impairment is more severe in radiculopathies.

5. a

6. Exercise performed on these devices will stimulate the body systems to respond as they would in most individuals. Even after withdrawal of the exercise, parameters of fitness may be evident up to 8 weeks following cessation of the program.

7. Page 869.

8. Page 876.

CHAPTER 29

1. Answer is found in Defining Pain (p. 890).

2. Answer is found in Pain Anatomy (pp. 890–891).

3. Answer is found in Pain Modulation (pp. 891–892).

4. Answer is found in Categorizing Pain (pp. 892–893).

5. Answer is found in Pain Measurement (pp. 893–894).

6. Answer is found in Treatment of the Client with Pain (p. 898, paragraph 1).

7. Answer is found in Physical Interventions (pp. 898–904).

8. Answer is found in Cognitive Strategies (pp. 904–906).

9. Answer is found in Behavioral Manipulations (pp. 906–907).

CHAPTER 30

1. See Etiology (pp. 914–916) and Figure 30–1.

2. See pages 916–917.

3. See pages 922–927.

4. See pages 927–931.

5. See Case Studies on page 931.

6. See Cognitively Impaired Clients (p. 931).

CHAPTER 31

1. A prefabricated orthosis is one that has been manufactured into different predetermined sizes. Prefabricated orthoses are manufactured from the same materials utilized in custom-made orthoses: thermoplastics, cloth, metal, leather, and elastic. The advantages of prefabrication are that they reduce delivery time, are less costly, and are readily available. The disadvantages generally involve poor selection criteria. Prefabricated orthoses work well if they are utilized for the proper indication and if the person fitting the orthosis has the knowledge and skill to custom fit the device. As a general rule, prefabricated orthoses should be utilized for temporary need on patients who have normal vascular and neurological function and no significant deformity.

2. An ankle-foot orthosis can produce a force system that will not allow forward motion of the tibia at midstance to toe off. This is accomplished by locking the dorsiflexion of the ankle. The components necessary are ones that are adjustable, metal, or plastic anterior stop. In the case of a metal joint, a long tongue stirrup must be used. If a rigid plastic orthosis is utilized, it must extend to the heads of the metatarsals and be thick enough to provide a posterior force to stabilize the tibia against forward motion during stance phase.

3. Many patients with neuropathic deficits have some type of hyper- or hyposensation. The neuropathic foot requires special attention when considering introducing a force system with some type of orthosis. One must consider a well-fitted shoe, possible plastazote foot inserts, and careful daily inspection. Total contact plastic orthoses are indicated only in cases when holding the alignment is highly desirable, as the risk of skin breakdown is high.

4. The goals of orthotic intervention in the paralytic spine are to maintain trunk balance, to improve or maintain respiratory function, and to provide a base for best function of the upper extremities and head balance. This is achieved by a TLSO that balance rigidity to maintain spinal alignment, open abdominal/pectoral area for respiration, and well-fitted distal and proximal trim lines so as not to restrict sitting balance or upper extremity function.

5. Cervical level 5 must be intact, as the patient must have the long wrist extensors to operate a wrist-driven tenodesis orthosis. This motion produced the three-jaw chuck, thumb, index and middle finger prehension. The major factor in patient acceptance of this orthosis depends on whether the patient can produce the force to grasp different objects. The proper alignment of the orthosis is critical. Excess radial deviation further detracts from the efficiency of the orthosis. Successful use also depends on early intervention.

6. Full range of motion at the hips, knee, and ankles allows the widest base of support for balance. Compromised range requires modifications to the orthoses, which will reduce the patient's ability to balance without the aid of the upper extremities. Patients who have minimal spasticity are more successful. The patient's desire, along with understanding and accepting realistic expectations, plays a critical role.

7. The patient's lack of range of motion creates a posteriorly directed force to the ankle and the knee. Without making modifications to an orthosis or a shoe, other problems will be short stride on the nonaffected side, varus ankle, and a heel that comes out of the heel of the shoe. Shoe modifications can be made to minimize this lack of range. Building up the heel to match the degree of lack of neutral and providing a rocker-bottom sole allows the patient's center of gravity to advance. A buildup to balance the overall length must be made on the nonaffected side. An instep strap or figure 8 strap will also help keep the heel in the place in the shoe for patients with spasticity but will not take the place of the heel buildup.

8. A critical portion of the evaluation must be to address why the patient is seeking medical help and what he or she expects to accomplish from your care. Although observation may show you the major reason the patient is in your office, giving the patient the opportunity to explain why and what is expected expect is vital. Many times, patients and their families have unrealistic goals that are nearly impossible to achieve, and it is better to address these during the initial evaluation to reach more realistic expectations. Identifying the major complaint, explaining the course of intervention related to the complaint, and describing what the intervention will achieve are values of your clinical experience and a key in gaining the confidence of the patient and family.

CHAPTER 32

1. a. Oxazepam is a benzodiazepine that may cause sedation and dizziness. See Table 32–6 and Chapter 32, page 953 for discussion.

2. b. Although this antipsychotic agent has been used successfully to reduce nausea and vomiting in many situations, it antagonizes dopaminergic pathways in the basal ganglia, reducing the effectiveness of levodopa/carbidopa. See Tables 32–1 and 32–10 and Chapter 32, pages 952 and 956.

CHAPTER 33

1. Refer to Chapter 4 on Motor Learning Theories and examples of movement therapy within this chapter (pp. 966, 968, 974). Refer to the section on example of movement therapies and Chapter 4 on functional and somatosensory retraining for link between movement therapies and therapeutic exercise.

2. Law of Five Elements is located in the Acupuncture section on page 983. Refer to the section on a Lakotacentric perspective on health (p. 986).

3. Refer to both sections on examples of health care belief systems (pp. 987, 988) and Chapter 4 and 6 regarding mind, body, and spiritual interactions with health, wellness, and healing.

4. Refer to Examples of Physical Body Systems Approaches (pp. 979–981) and Chapters 4 and 12 (sections on interventions).

5. Refer to the sections on Biofeedback (p. 988) and Therapeutic Touch (p. 976), with emphasis on biomechanical and learning.

6. Refer to the section on Medical Intuitive Diagnostic (p. 977) and Chapter 6 on master clinicianship and intuition.

7. Refer to the section on Movement Therapy Approaches (pp. 966–976) and both the Practice Guides for Physical Therapy and Occupational Therapy.

8. Refer to the concluding section (pp. 992–994), which looks at models for practice. The learners first have to identify their own learning styles, their preferences for treatment intervention options, and to what extent they feel they can stretch their learned paradigms and alternative models.

APPENDIX B

Standardized Evaluation Tools Discussed in the Text and Screening Tools

CHAPTER 2

Discussion of screening tools for medical screening at a systems level

CHAPTER 3

Entire chapter focuses on differentiating assessment of impairments from disabilities as examination tools in relation to clinical decision making.

Summary of functional versus impairment versus health status/quality of life examintion tools: Appendix 3–A

CHAPTER 4

Discussion of assessment of somatosensory function

CHAPTER 8

Dubowitz and Dubowitz: Clinical assessment of gestational age in the newborn infant
Ballard: Newborn maturing rating
Prechtle: Neurological examination of full-term infants
Brazelton: Neonatal Behavioral Assessment Scale (NBAS)
Dubowitz and Dubowitz: Neurological assessment of the preterm and full-term newborn infant
Als: Assessment of preterm infant behavior (APID)
Als and others: Neonatal individualized developmental care and assessment program
Neonatal Oral-Motor Assessment Scale (NOMAS)
Nursing Child Assessment Feeding (NCAF)
Bayley Scales of Infant Development (BSID-II)
Chandlers: Movement Assessment of Infants (MAI)
Chandlers: Movement Assessment of Infants Screening Test (CMAI-ST)
Alberta Infant Motor Scale (AIMS)
Peabody Developmental Motor Scales (PDMS)

CHAPTER 10

Bayley Scales of Infant Development
Motor assessment of the developing scales (AIMS)
Gesell and Amatruda developmental and neurological examination
Bruininks-Oseretsky test of motor proficiency
Hawaii early learning profile (HELP)
Pediatric Evaluation of Disability Inventory (PEDI)
School function assessment (SFA)

CHAPTER 11

Wechsler Intelligence Scale for Children (WISC)
Refer to Appendix 11–A: summary of standardized motor tests
Bruininks-Oseretsky test of motor proficiency
Movement Assessment Battery for Children (MOVEMENT-ABC)

Peabody Developmental Motor Scales
Quick neurological screening test
Miller assessment for preschoolers
First STEP (Screening Test for Evaluating Preschoolers)
Test of motor proficiency of Gubbay
The sensory integration and praxis tests
Bender Gestalt Test for Young Children
Development test of visual-motor integration (VMI), 3rd revision
Test of visual motor skills (TVMS-R)
Evaluation of children's handwriting (ETCH)
Purdue Pegboard Test

CHAPTER 13

Amyotrophic lateral sclerosis severity scale (box, pp. 366–368)
Daily activity log
Manual muscle testing
Range of motion
Energy expenditure index

CHAPTER 14

Functional Independence Measure (FIM)
Functional Assessment Measure (FAM)
Disability Rating Scale
Motor Assessment Scale (MAS)
Glasgow Coma Scale (box, p. 421)
Glasgow Outcome Scale (box, p. 423)
Rancho Los Amigos Scale of Cognitive Function (box, p. 427)

CHAPTER 15

Manual Muscle Test (MMT)
Sensory testing
Alberta Infant Motor Scale (AIMS)
Milani-Comparetti Motor Development Screening Test: Revised
Peabody Developmental Motor Scales (PDMS)
Pediatric Evaluation of Disability Inventory (PEDI)
Bayley Scales of Infant Development, 2nd edition (BSID-II)
Motor-free visual perceptual skills (MVPT-R)
Test of visual perception (TVPS)

CHAPTER 16

Functional outcomes for complete lesions (Table 16–2)
Sensory assessment
Motor assessment (MMT)
Modified Ashworth Scale
Functional assessment form (ADL)
Functional independence measure (FIM) (Fig. 16–10)
ASIA neurological examination (Fig. 16–11 and 16–12)

CHAPTER 20

Functional Independence Measure (FIM)
Barthel Index

Kutzke Disability Status Scale
References to a variety of functional measurements (reference 12 or www.cmsc.org).
Multiple Sclerosis Quality of Life Index (reference 12)

CHAPTER 21

Romberg Test
One-legged-stance tests (OLST)
Nudge/push tests
Postural stress test
Functional reach test
Limits of stability test
Sensory organization test (SOT)
Clinical test for sensory interaction on balance (CTSIB)
Hallpike-Dix maneuver
Vestibular Ocular Reflex Test (VOR)
Fukuda stepping test
Timed up and go
Tinetti performance oriented assessment of balance and gait
Fugl-Meyer sensorimotor assessment of balance performance
Dizziness Handicap Inventory (DHI) (Table 21–6)

CHAPTER 22

Hoehn and Yahr Scale (Fig. 22–6)
Unified Parkinson's Disease Rating Scale (UPDRS)

CHAPTER 23

Integrated functional assessment of cancer patients: O'Toole
Karnofsky Performance Scale (Table 23–1)

CHAPTER 24

Examination tools related to specific cerebellar impairments listed in box on pages 729–730.

CHAPTER 25

Glasgow Coma Scale
Barthel Index
Motor Assessment Scale (MAS)
Functional Independence Measure (FIM)
Rivermead Mobility Index
Fugl-Meyer Test
Berg balance assessment
Functional reach
Functional ambulation profile (FAP)

Ashworth Scale
Visual Analogue Pain Rating Scale

CHAPTER 26

Mini-Mental State Examination (MMSE)
Barthel Index and rating guidelines (Table 26–1 and Appendix 26–A)

CHAPTER 27

Visual screening tests for
 Distance acuity
 Near acuity
 Visual pursuit
 Saccades
 Near point of convergence
 Near cover test
 Far cover test
 Depth perception
 Visual field screening

CHAPTER 28

Reaction to degeneration (RD) test
Strength duration test
Nerve conduction test (NCT)
 Motor nerve conduction (MNCT)
 Sensory nerve action potential (SNAPs)
 Sensory nerve conduction velocities (SNCVs)
Evoked potentials
 Visual (VEP)
 Auditory (AEP)
 Pattern reversal (PREPS)
 Brainstem auditory (BAEPs)
 Sensory stimulation (SSEP)
 Motor unit potentials (MUPs)
Neuromuscular electrical stimulation (NMES)

CHAPTER 29

Pain rating scale (Fig. 29–1)
Simple descriptive pain scale (SDPS) reference 54
McGill Pain Questionnaire (MPQ) (Fig. 29–4)
Pediatric Verbal Descriptor Scale (Table 29–1)

CHAPTER 30

Evaluation form for female incontinency (Fig. 30–4)
Evaluation form for male incontinency (Fig. 30–5)

GLOSSARY

abulia A loss or deficiency of will power.

ACTH (adrenocorticotropic hormone) A hormone released by the adenohypophysis, which stimulates the adrenal cortex to secrete its entire spectrum of hormones. Thought to be immunosuppressive and antiinflammatory in treating multiple sclerosis.

acute That period of time immediately following spinal cord injury when the management of all primary injuries and the prevention of further complications are the emphasis of care.

acute pain Pain that arises from stimulation of the nociceptors and functions as a warning system of impending or actual tissue injury.

adaptive response An appropriate response to an environmental demand. Adaptive responses require good sensory integration; they also allow the sensory integrative process to progress.

adjustment The ongoing process of responding to the world with a positive adaptive response that allows the person and significant others to grow and mature in regard to all aspects of life.

agraphia Loss of ability to write.

alcoholism A disease characterized by chronic, heavy consumption of alcohol, which may lead to peripheral nerve disease, cerebellar degeneration, and other systemic and psychiatric symptoms that impair health and function.

alexia Word blindness: inability to recognize or comprehend written or printed words.

Alzheimer's disease A term used as a diagnosis when, based on the symptoms of confusion and impaired intellectual functioning, all other possible causes have been eliminated. It is not possible to ascertain whether a client has this disease until an autopsy or brain biopsy has been done. At present, there is no known cause or treatment for Alzheimer's disease, but clients and families can be helped to cope better with the presenting losses of intellectual functioning.

amblyopia Dimness of vision not caused by refractive error or organic disease of the eye.

Amigo A scooter-like, battery-operated vehicle.

amniocentesis A procedure in which a needle is passed through the mother's abdomen into the amniotic sac of the fetus. Amniotic fluid is withdrawn and analyzed to detect a variety of abnormalities.

amygdala A nuclear mass within the anterior portion of the temporal lobe involved with limbic function, especially arousal, motivation, and declarative learning.

angiography The visualization of blood vessels by injection of a nontoxic radiopaque material.

ankle-foot orthosis (AFO) An external device which controls the foot and ankle complex, and can be utilized to generate forces about the knee.

ANS (autonomic nervous system) pain Pain arising from injuries within the sympathetic or parasympathetic nervous systems.

anterograde amnesia The inability to establish new memories.

anticholinergic Blocking the passage of impulses at cholinergic postsynaptic receptor sites; also an agent that so acts.

anticipatory responses The use of information about the environment and from past experience to plan and program intended actions for the immediate future.

anxiolytic An agent that reduces anxiety.

aphasia An impairment caused by brain damage, which interferes with the ability to process language symbols. It is disproportionate to impairment of other intellectual functions and is not caused by dementia, sensory loss, or motor dysfunction.

apraxia of speech An articulatory disorder resulting from the inability to program the position of speech muscles and the sequence of muscle movements in order to volitionally produce speech. The disorder results from an impairment arising from brain damage.

Arnold-Chiari malformation A deformity in which the medulla and pons are reduced in size, and the cerebellum herniates into the spinal canal.

aspiration The act of inhaling fluids or substances into the lungs or the removal of fluids and gases from a cavity by suction.

asthenia Chronic lack of strength and energy.

ataxia Loss of muscular coordination.

ataxia-telangiectasia An inherited disorder characterized by progressive ataxia, oculocutaneous dilation of terminal arteries and capillaries, sinopulmonary disease, and abnormal eye movements.

athetosis From the Greek origin of the word: "without posture"; a dyskinetic condition that includes inadequate timing, force, accuracy, and coordination of movement in the limbs and trunk.

augmented intervention The use of therapeutic intervention strategies, such as the therapist's hands, to augment or enhance the patient's ability to perform or participate in a functional activity or therapeutic procedure.

autism A disorder that in childhood is characterized by withdrawal behavior, reduced socialization, perseveration, bizarre behavior, lack of purposeful verbal communication, and echolalia.

autogenic movement patterns (AMPs) Movements of body segments (e.g., head, limbs, trunk) that are the result of spontaneous activity of motor neurons; in contrast to reflexive or volitional (voluntary) movements.

autoimmunity Disease in which the body produces a disordered immunological response against its own tissue. Antibodies against normal parts of the body are produced to an extent that causes tissue injury.

automatic postural responses Functionally organized, long-loop responses that produce muscle activation to bring the body's center of gravity into a state of equilibrium. Examples: ankle strategy, hip strategy.

automatic speech   Words or phrases spoken without voluntary control, such as curse words, expletives, and greetings.

autonomic dysfunction   An uncompensated reaction from either the parasympathetic or sympathetic division of the autonomic system following disease, injury, or chemical imbalances; more often observed within the sympathetic system as a reaction to a noxious stimulus that exhibits itself as a visceral response, such as sweating or increased heart rate.

axonotmesis   Interruption of the axon with subsequent wallerian degeneration; connective tissue of the nerve, including the Schwann cell basement membrane, remains intact.

babbling   A stage in speech development characterized by the production of strings of speech sounds in vocal play.

balance   The ability to control the center of gravity over the base of support in a given sensory environment.

ballistic movement   High-velocity movement, such as a tennis serve or boxer's punch, requiring reciprocal organization of agonistic and antagonistic synergies.

basal ganglia   A collection of nuclei at the base of the cerebral cortex. It includes the caudate nucleus, putamen, globus pallidus, and functionally includes the substantia nigra and subthalamic nucleus.

base of support   The surfaces of the body that experience pressure as a result of body weight and gravity, and the projected area between them.

Betaseron (interferon beta-1b)   A drug distributed by Berlex Labs (Richmond, CA) licensed by the U.S. Food and Drug Administration in 1993 for the treatment of relapsing/remitting multiple sclerosis (MS). The drug is based on interferon beta, which is a protein formed by the body when cells are exposed to viruses. The drug has an immunomodulatory effect and in clinical trials reduced disease activity in relapsing/remitting MS.

biasing motor generators   Modulatory influence through synaptic excitation and inhibition over the resting state of the motor generators.

biofeedback   A cognitive treatment technique in which the client becomes aware of and learns to selectively change physiological processes with the aid of an external monitor.

bite reflex   This pathological reflex is a swift biting action produced by stimulation of the oral cavity. The bite may be difficult to release in some cases when an object such as a spoon or tongue depressor has been introduced into the mouth.

body scanning   A cognitive treatment technique in which clients are taught to view their pain objectively in order to separate themselves from their pain.

bonding   The process of creating a connection that results in trust and respect between two or more individuals.

brain abscess   A localized collection of pus in a cavity formed by the disintegration of brain tissue.

caregiver training and support   (1) Organizing educational experiences to assist caregivers to be better able to assist or perform needed tasks for patients; (2) organizing experiences (group or individual) to assist caregivers to cope with the challenges of performing as a caregiver. The support can be in the form of physical assistance or psychosocial activities.

causalgia   ANS pain characterized by intense burning and hyperesthesia throughout the distribution of an incompletely damaged peripheral nerve.

center of gravity   An imaginary point in space about which the sum of the forces and moments equals zero (equilibrium).

cerebellar atrophy (spinocerebellar degeneration)   A general term for several familial disorders in which the cerebellum deteriorates.

cerebral evoked potentials (EPs)   Study of potentials evoked from the cortex, including *visually evoked potentials* (VEPs) stimulated by light, *auditory evoked potentials* (AEPs) stimulated by sound, and *somatosensory evoked potentials* (SEPs) stimulated by electrical stimulation of the peripheral sensory nerves.

cerebral palsy   A diagnostic term applied principally to a history of anoxia for a variety of reasons shortly before, during, or after the birth process, up to 2 years of age. The same conditions or experiences are often labeled with alternate diagnostic terms that vary with the geographical area and the clinic policy.

chewing reflex   Pathological signs elicited in brain-damaged adults when the mouth is stimulated and repetitive chewing motions ensue.

childhood aphasia   A disturbance of the capacity to process language resulting from brain dysfunction in childhood.

chorea   Involuntary movements of the face and extremities that are of short duration, spasmodic, irregular; frequently involve a component of rotation.

chronic pain   Pain that occurs without a clear stimulus to the nociceptors, in response to innocuous stimulation or in a prolonged exaggerated fashion to noxious stimulation.

climbing fibers   One of two fiber types carrying input to cerebellar cortex; terminates in 1:1 relationship on a Purkinje cell.

clinical electromyography   An electrophysiological evaluation encompassing the observation, recording, analysis, and interpretation of bioelectric muscle and nerve potentials detected by means of needle electrodes inserted into the muscles for the purpose of evaluating the integrity of the neuromuscular system.

clinical problem solving   A method of analyzing specific questions that are difficult or perplexing, whose solution will be founded on actual observation and treatment of a patient as distinguished from data or facts obtained by experimentation or pathology.

closure   Visualization of the whole figure when only a portion is visible.

CNS pain   Pain arising from central nervous system lesions.

cognition   The mind processes that allow the individual to perceive and be aware of the self, objects, and others in a person's internal or external environment.

cognitive-behavioral methods   Treatment methods

that deal with the sensory/discriminative, motivational/affective, and cognitive/evaluative aspects of pain.

cold application The use of cooling modalities to accomplish a therapeutic goal.

coma A complete paralysis of cerebral function, a state of unresponsiveness. Clients do not obey commands, speak, or open their eyes.

communication A reciprocal act of social interaction and sending/receiving information through conventional symbol systems (e.g., language) and affective messages (e.g., smiling). Customary rules of communication are established within individual social cultures.

complete lesion A lesion in which there is absence of sensory and motor function in the lowest spinal segment.

complex spatial relations Relationship of one figure or part of a figure to another.

computed axial tomography (CT or CAT scan) An x-ray technique designed to show detailed images of structures on separate planes of tissue. When combined, these images can often detail multiple sclerosis lesions and other neurological deficits.

concentric contraction Controlled shortening of the muscle.

conceptual disorders A disturbance in thought processes, in cognitive activities, or in the ability to formulate concepts.

configuration Overall shape or enclosure of a figure.

constancy The invariant quality of distinctive features in spite of valuation in location, rotation, size, or color.

contrecoup injury Injury to the brain produced distant to the part sustaining the blow.

coping Behaviors used to respond to positive or negative stressors in a person's environment in an effort to overcome or deal with them.

copolymer 1 (Copaxone, glatiramer) A drug under study by TEVA Pharmaceuticals (Kulpsville, PA), which in clinical trials is reported to reduce the frequency of exacerbations in early exacerbating/remitting MS.

cor pulmonale Heart disease due to pulmonary hypertension secondary to lung disease with right ventricular hypertrophy.

cortisone, prednisone Synthetic adrenal glucocorticoids, used in multiple sclerosis to reduce edema and other aspects of inflammation. They are immunosuppressive and have also been shown to be useful in improving nerve conduction in demyelinated fibers.

coup injury Injury to the brain at the site of the impact.

cryosurgery Technique of exposing tissues to extreme cold to produce well-demarcated areas of cell destruction. The cold is usually produced by use of a probe containing liquid nitrogen; in rare cases, used to destroy thalamic tissue in persons with MS to control severe tremor and other involuntary movements.

declarative memory The mental registration, retention, and recall of past experiences, sensations, ideas, knowledge, and thoughts. This memory has a high cognitive basis to it. The original data must relay through the amygdala or hippocampal nuclear structures before long-term storage is possible.

decorticate rigidity A term derived from animal transections, sometimes used to describe abnormal posturing in humans, that is characterized by exaggerated flexor responses in the upper extremities and exaggerated extensor responses in the lower extremities. In reporting, it is preferable to describe the posture observed.

decubitus ulcer An ulcer resulting from pressure to an area of the body, usually from a bed or chair; the heels, sacrum, ischia, and trochanters are most prone to the development of these ulcers.

deep vein thrombosis The existence of a blood clot within a deep vein.

Deiter nucleus One of the vestibular nuclei, also known as the lateral vestibular nuclei; located in the brain stem.

delayed language Failure of language to develop at the expected age because of any number of causes such as hearing loss, emotional disturbance, or brain injury.

delirium A delirious person shows both a change in intellectual function *and* in the level of consciousness. The client is less alert than normal and may be confused, disoriented, forgetful, and/or sleepy. Other commonly used terms to describe this condition are acute brain syndrome and reversible brain syndrome. If the underlying medical or emotional problem(s) is treated in a timely fashion, the level of alertness and intellectual function will return to normal.

dementia An impairment in some or all aspects of intellectual functioning in a person who is clearly awake. Other terms used to describe this condition are organic brain syndrome, senility, senile dementia, hardening of the arteries, and shrinking of the brain. Some diseases that can cause dementia are treatable. In these diseases the distortion of intellectual capacity is reversed when treatment is given and/or the intellectual functioning is prevented from becoming worse.

demyelination The process of breakdown or destruction of the myelin sheath surrounding the axons of nerve tissue.

dentate nucleus One of the deep cerebellar nuclei; found lateral to the emboliform nucleus, within the cerebellar hemisphere; receives fibers from the lateral zone of the cerebellar cortex; fibers leave nucleus via brachium conjunctivum; is considered part of the neocerebellum.

developmental dyspraxia A disorder of sensory integration characterized by an impairment in the ability to plan skilled nonhabitual movement.

developmental handling Moving a child through part or all of the developmental sequence to enhance the expression of normal movement patterns (i.e., righting and equilibrium reactions).

diagnosis by a physical or occupational therapist The conclusions drawn following a thorough examination that clearly identify the functional limitations of the individual and the system and subsystem impairments that are causing those limitations. These profession-specific conclusions are measurable and lay the foundation for prognosis and selection of treatment interventions and are based on disablement/enablement or human performance-based models

dioptric power Unit of measurement of the refractive power of an optic lens.

diplopia Double vision.

direct intervention Hands-on therapy to enhance the possibility of new motor learning when movement and postural control is inadequate.

disability Any restriction or lack of ability to perform an activity in a normal manner or within the normal range. Examples: requires a cane to walk, requires assistance to transfer, etc.

disablement model An evaluation and treatment model based on the specific impairment, functional loss, and quality of life attainable, not on the medical diagnosis of the injury or disease process.

distal sparing The spinal cord below the congenital lesion remains intact. The reflex arc through the spinal cord therefore remains but is unmodified by supraspinal influences. This results in spastic movements distal to the level of the lesion.

drug disposition Refers to the absorption, distribution, metabolism, and excretion of a drug.

ductions Movements of one eye from the primary position into the secondary or tertiary positions of gaze.

dynamic equilibrium Ability of clients to adjust to displacements of their center of gravity by appropriately changing their base of support.

dysarthria A disorder of articulation resulting from impairment of the central or peripheral nervous system in the control of the muscles of speech—errors in articulation of speech sounds.

dysdiadochokinesia Inability to perform rapidly alternating motion.

dysesthesias Sensation is impaired, but not absent. Often used when referring to "pins and needles" sensation.

dyskinesia A defect in voluntary movements.

dysmetria An inability to position the limbs accurately with respect to another object.

dysphagia A disorder of swallowing.

dystonia An abnormal involuntary sustained movement or posture involving the contraction of a group of muscles.

dystrophin Protein that is missing or defective in Duchenne muscular dystrophy which is localized to the sarcolemma of the muscle cell membrane. Its absence results in abnormal cell permeability, which may lead to cell destruction.

eccentric contraction Controlled lengthening of a muscle.

echolalia Automatic reiteration of words or phrases that have been heard.

ecology Study of the environmental relations of organisms.

ego-dystonic Destructive to self-enhancement.

ego-syntonic Supportive of self-enhancement.

electrical stimulation Study of muscle response to electrical currents including reaction of degeneration (RD), rheobase and chronaxy, strength-duration (SD), and galvanic-tetanus ratio tests.

electroencephalography (EEG) Study of the electrical activity of the brain.

electroglottography Process of measuring changes in electrical potential across membrane of the glottal tissue.

electromyographic biofeedback (EMGBF) Use of electronic instrumentation to elevate normally subconscious electromyographic potentials to a conscious level through auditory or visual signals, so that muscle contractions may be facilitated, inhibited, or coordinated for neuromuscular activity.

electroneuromyography (ENMG) The electrical activity of the muscles and their associated motor and sensory nerves.

electronystagmography Study of eye movements to evaluate vestibular function.

electrophoresis The movement of charged particles through the medium in which they are dispersed as a result of changes in electric potential; useful in analysis of protein mixtures because protein particles move with different velocities.

electroretinography Study of the potentials produced by the light-sensitive tissues of the retina.

emboliform nucleus One of the deep cerebellar nuclei in humans; receives input from intermediate zone of the cerebellum; involved in control of posture and voluntary movement.

emotional behavior Motor behavior activated by chemical reactions induced by emotional responses. The motor patterns activated by specific emotions elicit specific pattern generators.

empowerment The process by which power or authority over all aspects of self is reassumed by the client.

encephalitis Inflammation of the brain tissue.

encephalomeningitis Inflammation of the meninges and the brain substance.

end-feel Sensation experienced by therapist at the end of a patient's passive range of motion. May be springy or an abrupt halt, bone-to-bone, capsular, or tissue approximation.

endogenous opiates Naturally occurring substances that produce opiate-like effects, including analgesia.

endoscopy Examination of organs accessible to observation through an endoscope (small tube with light camera), which is inserted through the mouth.

epicritic Pertaining to the somatic sensations of fine discriminative touch, vibration, two-point discrimination, stereognosis, and conscious and unconscious proprioception.

ergotropic Combinations of cortical alpha rhythm, sympathetic nervous system activity, and somatic muscle activation; activity or work state.

evoked potentials The electrical manifestation of the brain's reception of and response to an external stimulus; a way of measuring efficiency in the CNS.

exacerbating-remitting An unpredictable disease course characterized by episodes of symptom appearance or worsening followed by partial or complete recovery.

experimental autoimmune encephalomyelitis (EAE) An induced, laboratory model of multiple sclerosis characterized by inflammation and demyelination.

exteroceptive Receptors activated primarily by stimuli from the external environment.

extrafusal muscle Striated muscle tissue found outside the muscle spindle.

extrinsic ophthalmoplegia Paralysis of the extrinsic ocular muscles.

eye disease Any systemic or local disease that affects visual function; may cause a reduction in visual acuity (being able to see clearly with central vision), or some type of visual field defect.

F²ARV continuum This continuum begins with fear or frustration and proceeds to anger, range, and violence in that order. This is a highly volatile emotional reaction and escalates as the emotions mount.

family involvement The interactions of significant others in a person's life that relate to an individual's development and coping.

family priorities Importance of services and intervention goals based on family values and preferences.

fast pain The sensation first perceived after injury; it is localized, easily qualified, and lasts as long as the duration of the stimulus.

fastigial nucleus One of the deep cerebellar nuclei; receives input from the medial zone of the cerebellum; involved in the control of equilibrium and posture.

fine motor coordination Motor behaviors involving manipulative, discrete finger movements, and eye-hand coordination; require corticospinal tract innervation for intentional fine motor control.

flaccidity The absence of voluntary, postural, and reflex movements resulting in muscle laxity and lack of resistance to passive stretch; this condition results from destruction of all or practically all peripheral motor fibers supplying a muscle.

forced use The term used for an intervention strategy that requires the patient to use an extremity while participating in a functional activity. It may require either restraining the opposite extremity or require bilateral use of two extremities.

functional electrical stimulation (FES) Use of electrical stimulation of the peripheral nervous system to activate muscle contractions to assist in functional activities, such as walking or upper extremity function.

functional skills Ability to accomplish necessary daily activities.

functional training The intervention strategy that uses a functional activity as the treatment itself and assumes that the functional movement strategy necessary for that activity is available to the patient to practice.

functional visual skills These include eye aiming, eye alignment or eye posture, oculomotilities, and depth perception.

gag reflex Also known as the pharyngeal reflex, this involuntary contraction of the pharynx and elevation of the soft palate is elicited in most normal individuals by touching the pharyngeal wall or back of the tongue.

gate control theory The pain modulation theory developed by Melzak and Wall, who proposed that presynaptic inhibition in the dorsal gray matter of the spinal cord results in blocking of pain impulses from the periphery.

gaze-evoked nystagmus Abnormal oscillation of the eyes when attempting to fixate gaze on an object.

gestalt Form, space, concept; the configuration of separate units into a pattern that itself seems to function as a unit or a whole.

gliosis An excess of astroglia in damaged areas of the central nervous system.

globose nucleus One of the four deep cerebellar nuclei in humans; receives input from intermediate zone of the cerebellar cortex; involved in control of posture and voluntary movement.

goal-oriented movements These used to be called voluntary movements in contrast to reflexive movements. These are movements that are organized around behavioral goals, environmental context, and task specificity.

gross motor coordination Motor behaviors concerned with posture and movement, ranging from early developing behavioral patterns to finely tuned, highly complex functional activities. Based on axial/trunk movement patterns versus distal control and requires the regulation over the ventral/medial and lateral descending motor tract systems.

habilitate To supply with the means to develop maximum independence that has never been obtained.

handling In this context refers to physical contact with the client's body to guide directly the movement and postural adaptation to a more normal pattern; usually refers to functional movement patterns used in daily care.

heat application The use of heating modalities to accomplish a therapeutic goal.

higher cortical processing Refers to the functions of the many association areas of the cerebral cortex. This includes memory, learning, and associating multiple information from a variety of sensory and motor sources. Outcomes of this processing include something as relatively simple as stereognosis or complex as mathematical processing, abstract thinking, or art. Simply stated, higher cortical processing results in gnosis (knowing).

hip-knee-ankle-foot orthosis (HKAFO) Essentially a device to control all lower extremity segments.

hippocampus A nuclear complex forming the medial margin of the cortical mantle of the cerebral hemisphere. It forms part of the limbic system and projects by way of the fornix to the septum, anterior nucleus of the thalamus, and the mamillary body.

holistic The spiritual dimension of a health care model.

homeostasis The maintenance of a steady state, in particular, the maintenance of the internal (physiological milieu) and the maintenance of safety or viability in the external environment.

homonymous hemianopsia Loss of the same side of the field of vision in both eyes.

humoral Pertaining to any fluid or semifluid of the body.

Huntington disease An inherited disease with degeneration of the basal ganglia and cerebral cortex; characterized by choreiform movements and loss of cognitive functions.

hyperbaric oxygen Oxygen under greater pressure than at normal atmospheric pressure (usually at 1 1/2 to 3 times absolute atmospheric pressure). Thought to be immunosuppressive in treating multiple sclerosis.

hypermetria Distortion of target-directed voluntary movement, in which the limb moves beyond the target.

hypesthesias Abnormally decreased sensitivity to stimulation.

hypnosis A cognitive treatment technique that involves changing pain perception while the client is deeply relaxed.

hypometria Distortion of target-directed voluntary movement, in which the limb falls short of reaching the target.

hypotonicity Reduced resistance to passive stretch; displayed as inability to hold resting posture against gravity; limp, "floppy" extremities during passive movement.

immunoglobulin Any one of several proteins that are capable of acting as antibodies. May be found in plasma, urine, and cerebrospinal fluid. IgG is an immunoglobulin.

impairment Any loss or abnormality of psychological, physiological, or anatomical structure or function. Examples: loss of joint mobility, weakness, sensory loss.

impairment training An intervention strategy that assumes that with specific system or subsystem training, the individual will regain control over a specific or multiple functional activities.

imprinting casting The application of casting material to subject the body part to consistent input for a specified period of time. This allows the central nervous system to "learn" the warranted response.

incomplete lesion A lesion in which partial preservation of sensory and/or motor function is found below the neurological level and includes the lowest sacral segment.

indirect intervention Instruction of parents and other caregivers to modify their daily care of the child or individual to open new possibilities for motor learning and preventing expression of abnormal movement patterns.

inferior olivary nucleus A large nucleus in the anterolateral medulla; origin of climbing fibers to the cerebellum.

inpatient services Services delivered to the patient during hospitalization.

input systems or modalities The ways specific information enters into the nervous system to inform the brain about the external world.

intention tremor An abnormal tremor of 4 to 6 Hz that occurs during voluntary, goal-directed movement.

interferon A protein formed when cells are exposed to viruses and other stimuli. Noninfected cells exposed to interferon are protected against viral infection. Thought to be of use in treating multiple sclerosis.

intermediate region of the cerebellum cortex A longitudinal zone of the cerebellar cortex; located on either side of the median zone; involved in the control of posture and voluntary movement; projects to globose and emboliform nucleus in humans and the interpositus nucleus in lower animals.

internal ophthalmoplegia Paralysis of the intrinsic muscles of the eye—those of the iris and ciliary body.

interoceptive receptors Receptors activated by stimuli from within visceral tissues and blood vessels.

interpositus nucleus One of the deep cerebellar nuclei in lower animals (globose and emboliform in humans); receives input from intermediate region of the cerebellar cortex; involved in the control of posture and voluntary movement.

intrafusal muscle Striated muscle tissue found within the muscle spindle.

iontophoresis The use of electricity to drive chemical ions into the body for therapeutic purposes.

isometric contraction Muscle tension without shortening.

isotonic contraction Contraction associated with shortening or lengthening of the muscle tissue; can be either concentric or eccentric.

jaw jerk Closure of the mouth caused by striking the lower jaw while it hangs passively open. This reflex is rare in normal individuals.

joint mobilization Graded passive oscillations at a joint for the purpose of increasing range of motion.

kinesiological electromyography Study of the muscle activity produced on motion.

knowledge of results Augmented information provided about success or errors in achieving environmental goals.

kyphosis The exaggeration or angulation of the normal posterior curve of the spine.

language A code for representing feelings and ideas about the world through a conventional system of signals (such as sign language) or symbols (such as spoken or written words). Language includes understanding and producing the conventional symbols and the rules for combining and using symbols.

language disorder A complete or partial disruption in the ability to understand and produce the conventional symbols or words that constitute one's native language, not directly attributable to sensory loss (e.g., blindness, hearing loss) or motor impairments.

laser A device that produces a coherent, monochromatic beam of light that can be used therapeutically for pain management, as well as for surgical procedures.

lateralization The tendency for certain processes to be more highly developed on one side of the brain than on the other. In most people, the right hemisphere develops the processes of spatial and musical thoughts, and the left hemisphere develops the areas for verbal and logical processes.

lateral region of the cerebellar cortex A longitudinal zone of the cerebellar cortex; located lateral to intermediate zone; comprises bulk of cerebral hemispheres; involved in the control of skilled voluntary movement; receives projection from motor cortex and has output to dentate nucleus.

learning disability A disorder in one or more of the basic physiological processes involved in understanding or using spoken or written language. This may be manifested in disorders of listening, thinking, talking, reading, writing, spelling, or doing arithmetic. They include conditions that have been referred to as, for example, perceptual handicaps, brain injury, minimal brain dysfunction, dyslexia, and developmental aphasia. They do not include learning problems that are primarily caused by visual, hearing, or motor handicaps, mental retardation or emotional disturbance, or environmental disadvantage.

learning environment   All the conditions (internal and external), circumstances, and influences surrounding and affecting the learning of the client.

learning theory   The theoretical basis used to describe changes in behavior or performance, whether declarative, procedural, or some combination of both.

leptomeningitis   Inflammation of the arachnoid and pia mater layers of the meninges. The same condition may be referred to as meningitis.

ligation   Application of a ligature (a ligature being any material used for tying a vessel or to constrict a part).

limbic system   A group of brain structures that include amygdala, hippocampus, dentate gyrus, cingulate gyrus, and their interconnections with hypothalamus, septal areas and brain stem.

limits of stability (LOS)   The boundary or range that is the farthest distance in any direction a person can lean away from vertical (midline) without changing the original base of support (stepping, reaching, etc.) or falling.

lipofuscin   Any of a class of fatty pigments formed by the solution of a pigment in fat.

long-loop stretch reflex   Stretch reflex mediated through centers above the spinal system.

loss and grief   The process of dealing with the removal of function or roles in a person's life.

magnetic resonance imaging (MRI)   A scanning technique using magnetic fields and radio frequencies to produce a precise image of the body tissue; used for diagnosis and monitoring of disease.

massage   Manipulation of the soft tissues of the body for the purpose of affecting the nervous, muscular, respiratory, and circulatory systems.

McGill pain questionnaire   A pain character measurement tool in which clients are asked to select words that describe their pain from a series of word categories.

medial zone of cerebellar cortex   The longitudinal zone of the cerebellar cortex, which includes the vermis and the flocculonodular lobe; involved in control of equilibrium and posture; projects to fastigial and vestibular nuclei.

meningitis   Acute inflammation of the meninges covering the brain and spinal cord.

metencephalon   The cephalic part of the rhombencephalon, giving rise to the cerebellum and pons.

minimal brain dysfunction   A mild or minimal neurological abnormality that causes learning difficulties in the child with average intelligence.

model of human occupation   A model that addresses the motivation for occupation, the patterning of occupational behavior into routines and lifestyles, the nature of skilled performance, and the influence of environment on occupational behavior.

modulation   A variation in levels of excitation and inhibition over sensory and motor neural pools.

morphogenesis   The morphological transformation including growth, alterations of germinal layers, and differentiation of cells and tissues during development.

mossy fibers   One of two fiber types carrying information to the cerebellar cortex.

motor control   The ability of the central nervous system to regulate and/or direct the musculoskeletal system in purposeful acts.

motor control theory   Theoretical basis for understanding how the motor system is controlled within the human body.

motor coordination   Functions that are traditionally defined as motoric. Includes gross motor, fine motor, and motor planning functions.

motor dysfunction, motor deficit, motor disorder, motor disturbance   Generic terms for any type of disorder found in learning-disabled children that has a motor component.

motor lag   A prolonged latent period between the reception of a stimulus and the initiation of the motor response.

motor learning   The acquisition of skilled movement based on previous experience and functional outcomes.

motor learning stages   The process through which a learner acquires, refines, and retains a new motor skill, in which performance of the skill occurs with diminishing errors and greater efficiency and flexibility.

motor learning theory   Theoretical basis for understanding how the central nervous system *learns to* control, modify, and regulate the motor system in order to respond and react to the internal and external environment within which that body functions.

motor planning (praxis)   The ability to plan and execute skilled nonhabitual tasks.

motor skill   The ability to execute coordinated motor actions with proficiency.

movement decomposition   Distortion of voluntary movement in which the movement occurs in a distinct sequence of isolated steps, rather than in a normal, smooth, flowing pattern.

movement speed   The time elapsed between the initiation of a movement and its completion.

multiple sclerosis   A chronic disease of the white matter of the central nervous system characterized by inflammation, demyelination, and the development of hardened plaques. The symptoms and signs are numerous; the course is erratic; its etiology appears to be autoimmune.

myelencephalon   The lower part of the embryonic hindbrain from which the medulla oblongata develops.

myelin   A fatlike substance forming the principal component of the sheath of nerve fibers in the CNS.

myelin basic protein (MBP)   A protein component of myelin which has been the subject of considerable study in MS research. An injection of MBP can induce a demyelinating condition reminiscent of MS in animals called experimental allergic encephalomyelitis (EAE).

myelination   The process of forming the "white" lipid covering of nerve cell axons; myelin increases the conduction velocity (speed) of the neuronal impulse; forms the white matter of the brain and spinal cord (as opposed to the gray matter).

myelography   Radiographical inspection of the spinal cord by use of a radiopaque medium injected into the intrathecal space.

myasthenia gravis   A disorder of neuromuscular function, thought to be due to the presence of antibodies to acetylcholine receptors at the neuromuscular junction.

Clinically, there is fatigue and exhaustion of the muscular system with a tendency to fluctuate in severity and without sensory disturbance or atrophy.

myofascial release Manipulation of the soft tissues of the body for the purpose of interrupting built-in imbalances and restrictions within the fascia and reintegrating the fascial mechanism.

natural environments All integrated community settings.

neocerebellum Those parts of the cerebellum that receive input via the corticopontocerebellar pathway.

neologism A new, meaningless word, often spoken by fluent aphasic clients.

nerve conduction tests Measurement of the electrical conductivity of motor and sensory nerves by application of an external electrical stimulus to the nerve and evaluation of parameters such as nerve conduction time, velocity, amplitude, and shape of the resulting response, as recorded from another site on the nerve or from a muscle supplied by the nerve.

neurapraxia Interruption of nerve conduction without loss of continuity of the axon.

neurography Study of the action potentials of nerves.

neuromechanism A neurological system whose component parts work together to produce central nervous system function.

neuronal sprouting The process of regrowing a neuronal process, e.g., axon, in an injured neuron attempting to reestablish innervation with a target structure.

neuropathy Any disease or dysfunction of the nerves.

neuroplasticity Anatomical and electrophysiological changes in the central nervous system in response to demands from the internal and external environment.

neurotmesis Damage to the axon and the endoneurial tube with the nerve remaining macroscopically intact, or complete transection of the nerve. Regeneration is less successful than in axonotmesis.

neurotransmitter A specific chemical agent that is released from presynaptic cells and travels across the synapse to stimulate or inhibit postsynaptic cells, thereby facilitating or inhibiting neural transmission.

neurotrophic Nutrition and maintenance of tissues as regulated by nervous influence.

nociceptor A peripheral nerve ending that appreciates and transmits painful or injurious stimuli.

nosocomial Hospital-acquired.

nuchal rigidity Reflex spasm of the neck extensor muscles resulting in resistance to cervical flexion.

nystagmus A series of automatic, back-and-forth eye movements. Different conditions produce this reflex. A common way of producing them is by an abrupt stop following a series of rotations of the body. The duration and regularity of postrotary nystagmus are some of the indicators of vestibular system efficiency.

occupational based performance Involves performance that requires the individual to have competence.

occupational therapy The therapeutic use of purposeful and meaningful goal-directed activities (occupations), which engage the individual's body and mind in meaningful, organized, and self-directed actions that maximize independence, prevent or minimize disability, and maintain health.

ocular dysmetria Inability to fix gaze on an object or follow a moving object with accuracy.

oligoclonal banding A process by which cerebrospinal fluid IgG is distributed, following electrophoresis, in discrete bands. Approximately 90% of clients with multiple sclerosis show oligoclonal banding.

oligodendroglia Myelin-producing cells in the CNS.

operant conditioning A cognitive treatment technique in which a voluntary, nonautomatic behavior is paired with a new stimulus through reinforcement or punishment.

ophthalmoplegia Paralysis of ocular muscles.

opisthotonus Position of extreme hyperextension of the vertebral column caused by a tetanic spasm of the extensor musculature.

optokinetic nystagmus Nystagmus induced by watching stripes on a drum revolving around one's face.

oral myelin (Myloral) An oral bovine myelin therapy for MS currently under study by Autoimmune, Inc. (Lexington, MA), which is based on the theory of "oral tolerance" to reduce immune activity against myelin. Oral tolerance refers to the ability of the immune system associated with the digestive tract to protect against immunoreactions to foreign proteins that are ingested.

orthostatic hypotension A dramatic fall in blood pressure when a patient assumes an upright position, usually caused by a disturbance of vasomotor control decreasing the blood supply returning to the heart.

orthosis An external device utilized to apply forces to a body part to limit movement, increase the velocity or power of a movement, stop movement, or hold the body part in a particular position. Previously called brace or splint.

outpatient Services provided to the patient following discharge from inpatient hospitalization, or services provided to a patient referred to the therapist directly from the physician.

pachymeningitis Acute inflammation of the dura mater.

pain character measurement Any of the tools used to define the character of a client's pain.

pain estimate A pain intensity measurement in which clients rate pain on a scale of 0 to 100.

pain intensity measurement Any of the scales used to quantify pain intensity.

pain modulation Variation in the intensity and appreciation of pain secondary to CNS and ANS effects on the nociceptors and along the pain pathways, as well as secondary to external factors such as distraction and suggestion.

pain pathway The route along which nerve impulses arising from painful stimuli are transmitted from the nociceptor to the brain, including transmission within the brain itself.

papilledema Edema of the optic disk.

parallel talk A form of speech used during play therapy with children in which the clinician verbalizes actions such as what is happening or what the child is doing without requiring answers from the child. For instance,

"I'm making a cake. Mine is good. You're making a cake, too." The clinician often repeats utterances of the child correctly and parallels the child's activities.

paranodal myelin intussusception   The ultrastructural change that occurs at Ranvier node because of acute focal compression of a nerve, resulting in a neuropraxic lesion.

paraplegia   The impairment or loss of motor and/or sensory function in the thoracic, lumbar, or sacral (but not cervical) segments of the spinal cord, secondary to damage of neural elements within the spinal canal.

paraxial   Lying near the axis of the body.

paresthesia   An abnormal spontaneous sensation such as burning, pricking, tickling, or tingling.

Parkinson disease; parkinsonism   A degenerative disease of the substantia nigra; cause is unknown for idiopathic parkinsonism; disease is characterized by slow movements, rigidity, a resting tremor, and postural instability.

patterned responses   The programs either preprogrammed or created by the motor system to succeed at the presented task in the most efficient and integrated response possible at that moment in time.

pendular knee jerk   Upon elicitation of the deep tendon reflex of the knee; the lower leg oscillates briefly like a pendulum after the jerk, instead of returning immediately to resting position.

perceptual-motor   The interaction of the various channels of perception with motor activity, including visual, auditory, tactual, and kinesthetic channels.

perceptual-motor match   The process of comparing and collating the input data received through the motor system and through perception.

peripheral pain   Pain arising from injury to a peripheral structure.

phantom limb pain   The sensation that an amputated part is still present, often associated with painful paresthesia.

phenol block   An injection of phenol (hydroxybenzene) into individual nerves; used as a topical anesthetic and produces a selective block of these nerves; sometimes used to control severe spasticity in specific muscle groups.

phonophoresis   The use of ultrasound waves to drive chemical molecules into the tissues for therapeutic purposes.

physical therapy   A profession with an established theoretical base and widespread clinical application in the preservation, development, and restoration of optimal physical function. Interventions focus upon movement function and dysfunction, which encompass treating musculoskeletal, cardiopulmonary, integumentary, and neuromuscular problems that affect the individual during life activities such as work, leisure time, or daily living skills.

physiological flexion   The excessive amount of flexor tone that is *normally* present at birth because of the existing level of CNS maturation and fetal positioning in utero.

plaque   A multiple sclerosis lesion characterized by loss of myelin and hardening of tissue.

plasmapheresis   A process by which whole blood is removed from the client, plasma is discarded and replaced by normal plasma or human albumin, and reconstituted blood is then returned to the client. In treating multiple sclerosis this process is believed to rid the blood of antibodies or substances that are damaging to myelin or that impair nerve conduction.

plasticity   The ability to change (refer to neuroplasticity when discussing nervous system plasticity).

pneumoencephalogram   Radiographical examination of ventricles and subarachnoid spaces of the brain following withdrawal of cerebrospinal fluid and injection of air or gas via lumbar puncture.

point stimulation   The stimulation of sensitive areas of skin using electricity, pressure, laser, or ice for the purpose of relieving pain.

polyradiculopathy   Inflammation of multiple nerve roots.

polysomnography   Monitoring of physiological activity during sleep.

position in space   Direction in which figures point, relationship of one body part to another, or the entire body's relationship to objects or others in space.

posttraumatic amnesia   The time elapsed between a brain injury and the point at which the functions concerned with memory are determined to have been restored.

postural background movements   The subtle, spontaneous body adjustments that make overt movements of the hands easier, for example, reaching for a distant object. These postural adjustments depend on good vestibular and proprioceptive integration.

postural tremor   A pathological tremor of 3 to 5 Hz that appears in a limb or the trunk when either is working against the pull of gravity.

posture   In the strictest sense, the position of the body or body part in relation to space and/or to other body parts. Functionally, the anticipation of and response to displacement of the body's center of mass.

pragmatics   The study of language as it is used in context.

problem solving   The process of logically or intuitively overcoming barriers in an individual's environment.

procedural memory   The specific motor programs learned and retained to run motor programs or combinations of programs in order to perform functional activities

proprioceptive   Receptors that respond to stimuli originating primarily from muscle spindles, Golgi tendon organs, and joints.

protopathic   Pertaining to the somatic sensations of fast, localized pain; slow, poorly localized pain; and temperature.

Pro-Ven   A processed mixture of cobra, krait, and water moccasin venoms developed by Florida physicians to treat multiple sclerosis. The FDA has banned the sale of Pro-Ven until it is tested for safety and effectiveness.

pulmonary embolism   An obstruction of the pulmonary artery or one of its branches usually caused by an embolus from a lower extremity thrombosis.

Purkinje cells   Large neurons found in the cerebellar cortex that provide the only output from the cerebellar cortex after the cortex processes sensory and motor signals from the rest of the nervous system.

quadriplegia Term used to describe paralysis in all four extremities; often used when describing the movement dysfunction in individuals following cervical neck spinal cord injury.

reaction of degeneration The condition in which a short-duration electrical stimulus (usually less than 1 ms) applied to a motor nerve results in a sluggish or absent muscle response, rather than the normally brisk contraction. The reaction may be partial or complete, depending on the extent of neuropathology. This electrophysiological reaction can be used as a screening assessment of peripheral nerve integrity.

rebound phenomenon Inability to stop a resisted muscle contraction, such that movement of the limb occurs when the resistance is unexpectedly withdrawn from the limb.

red nucleus Large, vascular nucleus found in mesencephalon, involved in transmission of cerebellar communications to the motor cortex and thalamus.

reflux Backflow of urine from bladder to ureters.

refractive error Nearsightedness (myopia), farsightedness (hyperopia), astigmatism, or presbyopia. All conditions are improved with corrective lenses.

rehabilitation The restoration of a disabled individual to maximum independence commensurate with his or her limitations.

relaxation techniques A cognitive treatment technique that addresses muscle tension accompanying pain.

response speed The time elapsed between presentation of a stimulus and the client's initiation of movement.

retardation A retarded person has had some degree of mental impairment all his or her life. A retarded person can also develop a delirium or dementia. A delirium or dementia differs from retardation in that there has been a change from what was normal for that person.

retrograde amnesia The inability to recall events that have occurred during the period immediately preceding a brain injury.

reverberating loops or circuits A process by which closed chains of neurons when excited by a single impulse will continue to discharge impulses from collateral neurons back onto the original neuronal pool. The end result may produce a higher level of excitation than the original input itself.

rhizotomy A neurosurgical intervention at the level of the cauda equina, or lower level of the spine, to interrupt abnormal sensory feedback that appears to maintain hypertonus. The procedure was developed in 1908 and has been modified by a series of neurosurgeons, with the objective of reducing hypertonus associated with CNS dysfunction to allow the expression of functional postural control.

rigidity Resistance to passive range of motion that is not velocity-dependent and affects the muscles on both sides of the joint.

rooting reflex This normal reflex in infants up to 4 months of age consists of head turning in the direction of the stimulus when the cheek is stroked gently.

saccadic eye movement An extremely fast movement of the eyes, allowing the eyes to accurately fix on a still object in the visual field.

saccadic fixations A rapid change of fixation from one point in a visual field to another.

scanning speech An abnormal pattern of speech characterized by regularly recurring pauses.

scoliosis Lateral curvature of the spine; this usually consists of two curves, the original abnormal curve and a compensatory curve in the opposite direction.

sensorimotor therapy Therapy planned to enhance the integration of motor learning and the emergence of voluntary motor behaviors concerned with posture and movement.

sensory conflict Situations in which sensory signals that are *expected* to match ("agree") do NOT match, either between systems (vision, somatosensory or vestibular) or within a system (two proprioceptive inputs such as the joint and the muscle).

sensory deprivation An enforced absence of the usual repertoire of sensory stimuli. The continued decrease or absence of adequate, normal stimuli can produce severe cognitive, motor, and emotional changes, including hallucinations, anxiety, depression, neglect of an extremity or body part, and inadequate motor response to the environment.

sensory environment The conditions that exist in the real world around us which affect balance, i.e., darkness, visual movement, compliant surfaces, etc.

sensory integration The organization of sensory input for use, a perception of the body or environment, an adaptive response, a learning process, or the development of some neural function.

sensory integrative dysfunction A disorder or irregularity in brain function that makes sensory integration difficult. Many, but not all, learning disorders stem from sensory integrative dysfunctions.

sensory integrative therapy Therapy involving sensory stimulation and adaptive responses to it according to a child's neurological needs. Treatment usually involves full body movements that provide vestibular, proprioceptive, and tactile stimulation. It usually does not include desk activities, speech training, reading lessons, or training in specific perceptual or motor skills. The goal is to improve the brain's ability to process and organize sensations.

sensuality Responding to sensory input in a positive manner, resulting in the person deriving bodily or sensory pleasure.

septicemia Systemic disease associated with the presence and persistence of pathogenic microorganisms or toxins in the blood.

serial speech Overlearned speech involving a series of words such as counting and reciting the days of the week.

sexuality The behaviors that relate psychological, cultural, emotional, and physical responses to the need to reproduce.

slow pain The second sensation perceived after injury; it is poorly localized and outlasts the duration of the stimulus.

smooth pursuit movement of the eyes When the

eyes are following a slowly moving object, they move together at a steady velocity, not in saccades.

soft neurological signs Mild or slight neurological abnormalities that are difficult to detect.

somatosensory retraining An intervention strategy used to retrain the somatosensory association areas in order to remap the sensory component of functional activities; used most often following repetitive strain injuries which result in distal focal dystonia.

spastic diplegia An increase in postural tonus that is distributed primarily in the lower extremities and the pelvic area.

spastic quadriplegia An increase in postural tonus that is distributed throughout all four extremities. These findings are often coexistent with relatively lower tone in the trunk and severe difficulty in controlling posture.

spasticity A motor disorder characterized by a velocity-dependent increase in tonic stretch reflexes with exaggerated tendon jerks, resulting from hyperexcitability of the stretch reflex. Spasticity is one component of the upper motor neuron syndrome.

speech The meaningful production and sequencing of sounds by the speech sensorimotor system (e.g., lips, tongue, etc.) for the transmission of spoken language.

speech pathology Speech/language pathology, speech therapy, or communicative disorders: terms used to specifically identify the professional scope of practice that focuses upon communication as a receptive, interactive, and expressive function of humans. This profession deals with the cognitive, emotional, and motor impairments that deal with human language and communication.

spinal cord injury An insult to the spinal cord that results in neurological deficits.

spirituality That aspect of human thought and communication that focuses upon belief that man has more than a physical body and that aspect does or may join a universal energy that has a higher power source than any one individual. This may or may not have a direct connection with formal religion.

spirometry (pneumatometry) The measurement of air inspired and expired.

static equilibrium Ability of an individual to adjust to displacements of his or her center of gravity while maintaining a constant base of support.

stereognosis The ability to recognize the sizes, shapes, and weights of familiar objects without the use of vision.

stereopsis Quality of visual fusion.

strabismus Oculomotor misalignment of one eye.

sudomotor Denoting the nerves that stimulate the sweat glands.

synaptogenesis The process of forming synaptic connections between nerve cells, or between nerve cells and muscle fibers; the basis of neuronal communication.

synergy Fixed set of muscles contracting with a present sequence and time of contraction.

systems interactions The ways the various CNS systems affect or interact with one another to provide a more integrative and functional nervous system.

systems model A conceptual representation which incorporates a set of major functional divisions or systems within the CNS which interlock and interrelate to create the functional whole. Although each division may be considered a whole in and of itself with multiple subsystems interlocking to form its entire division, each major component or division influences and is influenced by all others and thus the totality of the CNS is based on the summation of the interactions, not individual function.

systems model/approach An interactive framework for understanding movement and postural control which includes (1) environmental stimuli, (2) sensory reception, perception, and organization, and (3) motor planning, execution, and modification.

systems theory A theory describing movements emerging as a result of an interaction among many peripheral and central nervous system components with influence changing depending on the task.

tactile defensiveness A sensory integrative dysfunction characterized by tactile sensations that cause excessive emotional reactions, hyperactivity, or other behavior problems.

telereceptive The exteroceptors of hearing, sight, and smell that are sensitive to distant stimuli.

tenotomy Surgical section of a tendon used in some cases to treat severe spasticity and contractures.

TENS *T*ranscutaneous *e*lectrical *n*erve *s*timulation; the use of electricity for pain management.

tetraplegia Impairment or loss of motor and/or sensory function in the cervical segments of the spinal cord due to damage of neural elements within the spinal canal.

thalamic pain CNS pain caused by injury to the thalamus and characterized by contralateral and sometimes migratory pain brought on by peripheral stimulation.

therapeutic environment Organizing all aspects of the environment in a systematic way so that they enhance a patient's ability to perform desired tasks and activities (mental, emotional, functional).

therapeutic touch The exchange of energy from one person to another for the purpose of healing.

thermotherapy The use of heat or cold for therapeutic purposes.

thrombophlebitis Inflammation of a vein associated with thrombus. formation.

thyrotropin-releasing hormone A hormone from the hypothalamus which stimulates the anterior lobe of the pituitary gland to release thyrotropin.

tongue-thrust swallow An immature form of swallowing in which the tongue is projected forward instead of retracted during swallowing.

topognosis The ability to localize tactile stimuli.

total lymphoid irradiation (TLI) Radiation therapy targeted to the body's lymph nodes; in the treatment of multiple sclerosis, the goal is to suppress immune system functioning (reduce the number of lymphocytes in the blood).

transcutaneous nerve stimulation (TNS) A procedure in which electrodes are placed on the surface of the skin over specific nerves and electrical stimulation is carried out. Stimulation of the CNS in this manner is thought to improve CNS function, reduce spasticity, and control pain.

traumatic head injury An insult to the brain caused by an external physical force that may produce a diminished or altered state of consciousness resulting in impairment of cognitive abilities, emotional control, or functioning.

treatment Application of or involvement in activities/stimulation to effect improvement in abilities for self-directed activities, self-care, or maintenance of the home.

trophotropic Combination of parasympathetic nervous system activity, somatic muscle relaxation, and cortical beta rhythm synchronization; resting or sleep state.

truncal ataxia Uncoordinated movement of the trunk.

ultrasound A therapeutic modality using sound waves.

universal cuff An adaptive device worn on the hand to hold items such as utensils, shaver, or pencil, allowing an individual with weak grasp to participate in self-care activities.

verbal rating scale A pain intensity measurement in which clients rate pain on a continuum that is subdivided from left to right into gradually increasing pain intensities.

vergence Movement of the eyes in the opposite direction.

vermis Forms the unpaired medial region of the cerebellum.

version Movement of the eyes in the same direction.

vestibular-bilateral disorder A sensory integrative dysfunction characterized by short-duration nystagmus, poor integration of the two sides of the body and brain, and difficulty in learning to read or compute. The disorder is caused by underreactive vestibular responses.

vestibuloocular reflex A normal reflex in which eye position compensates for movement of the head, induced by excitation of vestibular apparatus.

visual analog scale A pain intensity measurement in which clients rate pain on a continuum that is without subdivisions.

visual analytical problem solving The ability to look at a complex array of visual stimuli, identify the critical attributes, and then use appropriate strategies to solve simple to complex problems.

visual-motor coordination The ability to coordinate vision with the movements of the body or parts of the body.

visual-motor function The ability to draw or copy forms or to perform constructive tasks.

visual-perceptual dysfunction May include deficits in any of the areas of visual perception: figure-ground, form constancy, or size discrimination; distinct from deficits in functional visual skills and tested separately.

vision screening Can include distance and near visual acuities, oculomotilities, eye alignment or posture, depth perception, and visual fields.

volitional postural movements Movement patterns under volitional control that relate specifically to controlling the center of gravity, as in skating, ballet, gymnastics, etc.

wallerian degeneration The physical and biochemical changes that occur in a nerve because of the loss of axonal continuity following trauma.

wholistic A model or approach to health care that takes into account all internal and external influences during the process. It incorporates the mind, the body, and the spirit as a total or whole.

zero-to-three infant stimulation groups Groups that provide therapeutic services for children from birth to 3 years of age, since this age group is not yet eligible for public school placement.

Index

Note: Page numbers in *italics* refer to figures; those followed by t refer to tables.

A fibers, 81t
Abdominal binders, with spinal cord injury, 502, *502*
Abnormal responses, in cerebral palsy, evaluation of, 266–268, *267*
Abscess(es), of brain, 532
Abstract thinking, in dementia, 792
Accommodation, visual, 827–828
  assessment of, 431
  disorders of, 837
  dysfunction of, 839t
Acetic acid, for pain, 902
Acetylcholine (ACh), basal ganglia and, 668, 660, *669*
  memory and, 170–171
Acid-base imbalances, with traumatic brain injury, 417
Acoustic neuromas, 699
Acquired immunodeficiency syndrome (AIDS), 553, 554. See also *Human immunodeficiency virus (HIV) infection.*
Action potentials, sensory nerve, 857, *858*
Active response, in adaptive process, 181
Activities of daily living (ADLs). See also specific disorders and activities.
  in multiple sclerosis, 613
  team interaction on, 607t
  in spinal cord injury, 502–503, 504t–505t, 505–509
Activities of daily living scales, 54–55
Activity level, assessment of, motor control and, 143–144
Activity logs, in amyotrophic lateral sclerosis, 371, *372*
Acupuncture, electroacupuncture and, 987–988
  traditional, 982–986
    examination and evaluation in, 983
    historical background of, 983
    intervention using, 985
    Law of Five Elements and, 983–985, *984*
    methods in, 983
    treatment duration with, 985–986
Adaptation, psychosocial. See *Psychosocial adaptation/adjustment.*
  self-reinforcing, in adaptive process, 181–182
Adaptive equipment, for Guillain-Barré syndrome, 394
  for spinal cord injury, assessment for, 485
Adaptive training, for motor function, following traumatic brain injury, 425
A-delta fibers, 890, 891
Adenomas, pituitary, 699
Adjustment, psychosocial. See *Psychosocial adaptation/adjustment.*
Adjustment stage, of adjustment, 181

ADLs. See *Activities of daily living (ADLs).*
Adolescents, adaptation to losses, 185–186
  spina bifida in, management of, 470–473
  with learning disabilities, 336, 337–338
Adults, brain-injured, therapeutic interventions for, 194
  older. See *Aging; Elderly people.*
  sexuality in, 188–189
  with learning disabilities, 336, 337
Aerobic capacity, spinal cord injury and, assessment of, 484–485
Affective state, evaluation of, in hemiplegia, 753–754
Afferent pathways, of basal ganglia, *663*, 663–664
Age correction, for premature infants, 234
Aging. See also *Elderly people.*
  case study of, 811–812
  cognitive function and, 792–793
  eye diseases associated with, 831–832
  of brain, 791. See also *Dementia.*
    Arndt-Schultz principle and, 794
    biorhythms and, 794–795
    cognitive changes and, in normal aging, 795–796
      stress and, 796–797
    law of initial values and, 794
    sensory changes associated with, 795
Agnosia, visual, 843, 844
AIDs (acquired immunodeficiency syndrome), 553, 554. See also *Human immunodeficiency virus (HIV) infection.*
AIDS Health Assessment Questionnaire, 563t
AIDS Specific Functional Assessment, 563t
Akinesia, in Parkinson's disease, 670–671
Alberta Infant Motor Scale, 237, 238–239, 461
Alcohol intoxication, acute, signs and symptoms of, 735–736
Alcoholism, 735–737
  cerebellar impairment in, 735
  evaluation of, 736
  limbic lesions in, influence on therapeutic environment, 164, *164*
  medical management of, 736
  signs and symptoms of, 735–736
  treatment of, 736–737
Alignment, of eyes, disorders of, 837
  problems with, in hemiplegia, intervention for, 767–770, *768–770*
Allergy(ies), to latex, with spina bifida, 454
  vestibular disorders and, 618
Allodynia, 892
Allopathic approaches, 987–989
  biofeedback as, 988–989
  electroacupuncture as, 987–988
Alpha motor neurons, influences over, 82

ALS. See *Amyotrophic lateral sclerosis (ALS).*
Alternative and complementary therapy(ies), 962–994
  acupuncture as, 982–986
  allopathic, 987–989
    biofeedback as, 988–989
    electroacupuncture as, 987–988
  energetic therapy approaches to, 976–979
    medical intuitive diagnosis as, 977–979
    therapeutic touch as, 976–977
  historical background of, 963–965
  integration of, case example of, 989–992
  integration with Western medicine, 992–994, *993, 994*
  movement therapy approaches to, 966–976
    Feldenkrais Method as, 966–968
    Taekwondo as, 974–976
    tai chi as, 968–974
  Native American healing as, 986–987
  physical body systems approaches to, 979–981
    CranioSacral Therapy as, 979–980
    myofascial release as, 980–981
Alzheimer's Association, 809–810
Alzheimer's disease, 793
  case study of, 812–813
  limbic lesions in, influence on therapeutic environment, 164–165
  stages of, 806
  tools for, 55
Amantadine (Symmetrel), for fatigue, in multiple sclerosis, 603
  for Parkinson's disease, 674
Ambulation, following spinal cord injury, ambulation trial criteria for, 521
  synergistic organization and, 424
  with cerebellar impairments, intervention for, 734
  preparing for, *733*, 733–734
  with Duchenne muscular dystrophy, maintenance of, 406–408, *407*
  with hemiplegia, 776, *777*, 778t
  with multiple sclerosis, 611
    team interaction on, 607t
  with postpolio syndrome, to decrease muscle workload, 584
  with spina bifida, 470, 471
  with spinal cord injury, 512
    assessment for, 485
    functional electrical stimulation for, 875
American Spinal Injury (Association), assessment and, 487, *488*, 489
Amnesia, following traumatic brain injury, 419
Amygdala, memory and, 171
Amygdaloid circuits, learning and memory and, 170
Amygdaloid complex, structure and function of, 167, *168*